AF668426

FOGSI's POSTGRADUATE GYNAECOLOGY

A TEXTBOOK

FOGSI's POSTGRADUATE GYNAECOLOGY

A TEXTBOOK

Volume 2

Editor-in-Chief

Alpesh Gandhi

MBBS DGO FICOG FRCOG Post PG (Hospital Management)
Senior Consultant, Obstetrics and Gynecology
Critical Care in Obstetrics and
High-risk Pregnancy Expert
Arihant Women's Hospital, Ahmedabad, Gujarat
President, The Federation of Obstetric and Gynaecological Societies of India (FOGSI), 2020

Editors

Parikshit Tank

MD DNB DGO DFP MNAMS FICOG FRCOG
Senior Consultant Obstetrician and Gynecologist
Ashwini Maternity and Surgical Hospital
Jupiter Hospital, Mumbai, Maharashtra, India
Honorary Professor, Assisted Reproduction
Pacific Medical College and Hospital
Udaipur, Rajasthan, India
Treasurer, The Federation of Obstetric and Gynaecological Societies of India (FOGSI), 2021-2024
Joint Secretary, FOGSI, 2012
Joint Treasurer, FOGSI, 2018-2020
Chairperson, Safe Motherhood
FOGSI, 2014-2017

Ameya Purandare

MD DNB FCPS DGO DFP MNAMS FICMCH FICOG Fellowship in Gyne Endoscopy (Germany)
Senior Consultant Obstetrician and Gynecologist
Purandare Hospital, KJ Somaiya Medical College and Hospital
Sir HN Reliance Foundation Hospital and Research Centre
Bhatia Hospital, Masina Hospital, Mumbai Police Hospital
Mumbai, Maharashtra, India
2nd Vice President Elect, The Association of Maharashtra Obstetric and Gynaecological Societies (AMOGS), 2022-2024
Joint Secretary, FOGSI, 2019
Chairperson, Food, Drugs and Medical and Surgical Equipments Committee, FOGSI, 2015-2017
Assistant Administrator, FOGSI Manyata Project

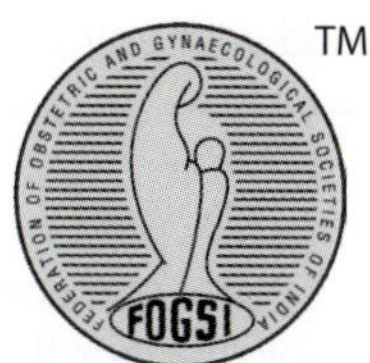

An Official Publication of
The Federation of Obstetric and Gynaecological Societies of India

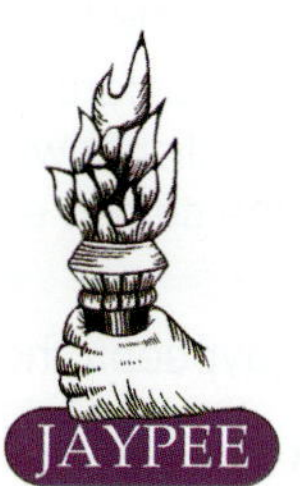

JAYPEE BROTHERS MEDICAL PUBLISHERS

The Health Sciences Publisher

New Delhi | London

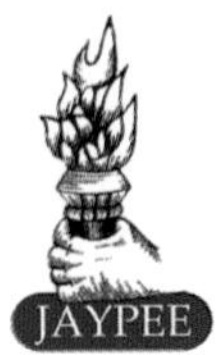

Jaypee Brothers Medical Publishers (P) Ltd

Headquarters

Jaypee Brothers Medical Publishers (P) Ltd
EMCA House, 23/23-B
Ansari Road, Daryaganj
New Delhi 110 002, India
Landline: +91-11-23272143, +91-11-23272703
+91-11-23282021, +91-11-23245672
Email: jaypee@jaypeebrothers.com

Corporate Office

Jaypee Brothers Medical Publishers (P) Ltd
4838/24, Ansari Road, Daryaganj
New Delhi 110 002, India
Phone: +91-11-43574357
Fax: +91-11-43574314
Email: jaypee@jaypeebrothers.com

Overseas Office

JP Medical Ltd
83 Victoria Street, London
SW1H 0HW (UK)
Phone: +44 20 3170 8910
Fax: +44 (0)20 3008 6180
Email: info@jpmedpub.com

Website: www.jaypeebrothers.com
Website: www.jaypeedigital.com

Inquiries for bulk sales may be solicited at: jaypee@jaypeebrothers.com

FOGSI's Postgraduate Gynaecology: A Textbook

First Edition: **2022**

ISBN: 978-93-5465-662-0

Printed at: Samrat Offset Pvt. Ltd.

Dedicated to

The students of Obstetrics and Gynecology, especially the postgraduates and their teachers

And

The girls and women of our country whom they are privileged to take care of

Section Editors

Amita Maheshwari MD
Professor and Head
Department of Gynecologic Oncology
Tata Memorial Centre, Mumbai, Maharashtra, India
President Elect, Association of Gynaecologic Oncologists of India

Anuradha Khanna MD FAMS FAICOG FUICC MANAMS FICS FUWAI
Former Professor and Head
Department of Obstetrics and Gynecology
Institute of Medical Sciences, Banaras Hindu University
Varanasi, Uttar Pradesh, India

Gokul Das MD FICOG FICMCH
Former Professor and Head
Department of Obstetrics and Gynecology
Gauhati Medical College, Guwahati
Founder Professor and Head
Department of Obstetrics and Gynecology
Tomo Riba Institute of Health and Medical Sciences
Nagarlagun, Arunachal Pradesh
Senior Consultant and Head
Department of Obstetrics and Gynecology
Health City Hospital, Guwahati, Assam, India
Vice President, FOGSI 2014

JB Sharma MD FRCOG FAMS PhD FICOG DNB
Professor, Department of Obstetrics and Gynecology
All India Institute of Medical Sciences
New Delhi, India

PK Shah MD DGO DFP FCPS
Former Professor and Unit Head
Department of Obstetrics and Gynecology
Seth GS Medical College and KEM Hospital
Mumbai, Maharashtra, India
President, FOGSI 2012

Pratima Mittal MD FICOG FICMCH PGDHHM FRCOG (Hon)
Former Professor and Head
Department of Obstetrics and Gynecology
Vardhman Mahavir Medical College and
Safdarjung Hospital
New Delhi, India

Pushpa Junghare MD
Professor and Head
Department of Obstetrics and Gynecology
Dr Panjabrao Deshmukh Memorial Medical College
Amravati, Maharashtra, India

Suyajna Joshi MD (OBG) DNB
Head
Department of Obstetrics and Gynecology
District Hospital, Ballari
Consultant
Geetha Medical Center
Ballari, Karnataka, India

Contributors

Abha Singh MS FICOG FIMCH
Director Professor and Former Head, Department of Obstetrics and Gynecology, Lady Hardinge Medical College and Smt Sucheta Kriplani Hospital
New Delhi, India

Abhishek Chandavarkar MD DNB DGO
Assistant Professor
Department of Obstetrics and Gynecology
DY Patil Medical College
Navi Mumbai, Maharashtra, India

Achla Batra MBBS DGO DNB
Professor and Unit Head
Department of Obstetrics and Gynecology
Vardhman Mahavir Medical College and Safdarjung Hospital
New Delhi, India

Ajay S Shetty MS MCh (Urology)
Consultant Andrologist and Microsurgeon
Lilavati Hospital and Research Centre
Mumbai, Maharashtra, India

Akanshi Madan MBBS MD
Consultant
Department of Obstetrics and Gynecology
Tanvir Hospital
Hyderabad, Telangana, India

Alka Kriplani FIMSA FICMCH Fellowship FRCOG MD
Consultant Gynecologist and Obstetrician
Former Professor and Head
Department of Obstetrics and Gynecology
All India Institute of Medical Sciences
New Delhi, India
Member of Menstrual Disorders Committee, FIGO

Amala Khopkar Nazareth MBBS MD
Specialist Obstetrician and Gynecologist
Prime Healthcare Group
Dubai, United Arab Emirates
Past Secretary General, Emirates Medical Association—Obstetrics and Gynecology

Ameet Patki MD DNB FCPS FICOG FRCOG (UK)
Medical Director
Fertility Associates
Mumbai, Maharashtra, India

Ameya Purandare MD DNB FCPS DGO DFP MNAMS FICMCH FICOG Fellowship in Gyne Endoscopy (Germany)
Senior Consultant Obstetrician and Gynecologist
Purandare Hospital, KJ Somaiya Medical College and Hospital, Sir HN Reliance Foundation Hospital and Research Centre Bhatia Hospital, Masina Hospital Mumbai Police Hospital, Mumbai, Maharashtra, India
2nd Vice President Elect, The Association of Maharashtra Obstetric and Gynaecological Societies (AMOGS) 2022-2024
Joint Secretary, FOGSI, 2019
Chairperson, Food, Drugs and Medical and Surgical Equipments Committee, FOGSI, 2015-2017
Assistant Administrator
FOGSI Manyata Project

Anand Kumar Jaiswal MD (Radio-diagnosis)
Associate Professor
Department of Radio-diagnosis
Pt Jawahar Lal Nehru Memorial Medical College, Raipur, Chhattisgarh, India

Anand Sharma MBBS MD (Internal Medicine)
Principal Medical Officer
Department of Internal Medicine
Government Medical College
Kota, Rajasthan, India

Anant Ramaswamy MD
Associate Professor
Department of Medical Oncology
Tata Memorial Centre
Mumbai, Maharashtra, India

Anita Singh MBBS MS DGO DNB FICOG
Chief Consultant
Jyoti Punj Hospital and Jan Chikitsa Hospital, Patna
Former Professor, Patna Medical College and Hospital, Patna, Bihar, India
Vice President FOGSI (EZ), 2020
Chairperson, Endocrinology Committee FOGSI, 2014–2016
Secretary, IFS, Bihar Chapter

Anita Soni MBBS MD (Obs & Gynec) DGO
Consultant Gynecologist
Department of Obstetrics and Gynecology
Dr LH Hiranandani Hospital
Mumbai, Maharashtra, India

Anju Singh MBBS MS
Assistant Professor
Department of Obstetrics and Gynecology
All India Institute of Medical Sciences
New Delhi, India

Anshu Baser MBBS MS (Obs & Gynec)
Consultant
Department of Obstetrics and Gynecology
Akash Hospital
Indore, Madhya Pradesh, India

Anu Agarwal MD
Director
Vansh Fertilty Centre
Varanasi, Uttar Pradesh, India

Anupam Gupta MBBS MD (Obs & Gynec)
Gynecologist and Obstetrician
Arva Medical and Gyne Centre
New Delhi, India

Anuradha Khanna MBBS MD MNAMS FICOG FUICC FICS
Professor and Former Head
Department of Obstetrics and Gynecology
Institute of Medical Sciences
Banaras Hindu University
Varanasi, Uttar Pradesh, India

Anuradha Ridhorkar MD DGO FICMCH FICOG
Consultant - Gynecologist
Ridhorkar Hospital
Nagpur, Maharashtra, India

Archana Baser MS DNB FRCOG FICOG
Director, Akash Hospital, Indore
Vice President FOGSI, 2020
Organizing Secretary, AICOG 2021 (Indore)
Managing Committee Member, ISAR 2018-20
Fellow Representative, AICC RCOG WEST Zone
Managing Committee Member, IAGE 2018-19
Managing Council Member, ICOG 2017-19
Chairperson, FOGSI Imaging Science Committee, 2015-2017
Founder Secretary, MP ISAR
Organizing Secretary, ISAR 2016

Ashok Kumar MD PhD
Managing Director
Department of Obstetrics and Gynecology
Maulana Azad Medical College
New Delhi, India

Ashwini Bhalerao Gandhi MD DGO DFP FCPS DNB FICOG
Consultant Gynecologist
PD Hinduja National Hospital and Research Center
Mumbai, Maharashtra, India

Ashwini Neelakanthi MS DNB
Assistant Professor
Vydehi Institute of Medical Sciences and Research Centre
Bengaluru, Karnataka, India

Aswathy Kumaran MS DGO DNB FNB (Reproductive Medicine)
Assistant Professor
Manipal Assisted Reproductive Centre
Department of Obstetrics and Gynecology
Kasturba Medical College
Manipal Academy of Higher Education
Manipal, Karnataka, India

Atul Ganatra MBBS DGO MD (Obs & Gynec)
Consultant
Department of Gynecology
Fortis Hospital
RJ Ganatra Nursing Home
Mumbai, Maharashtra, India

Atul Munshi MD DGO FICOG
Consulting Obstetrician and Gynecologist
Kalpana Munshi Hospital LLP
Ahmedabad, Gujarat, India

Basab Mukherjee MD FRCOG FICOG
Consultant Obstetrician and Gynecologist
Columbia Asia Hospital
Kolkata, West Bengal, India

Bharti Maheshwari MBBS MD
Obstetrician and Gynecologist
Muzaffarnagar Medical College and Hospital, Meerut, Uttar Pradesh, India

Bhawna Khera MRCOG (UK) MICOG MCCG
Consultant
Department of Obstetrics and Gynecology
Raj Chandra Hospital and Research Centre
Director
Mom Friendly Clinic and Cosmic-o-Laser Centre
Lucknow, Uttar Pradesh, India

Bhumika Kotecha Mundhe DGO DNB (Obs & Gynec) MNAMs (India)
Consultant Gynecologist, Saifee Hospital
Wockhardt Hospital, SRCC Hospital
St Elizabeth Hospital, Masina Hospital
Apollo Spectra Hospital
Managing Committee Member, Mumbai Obstetrics & Gynaecological Society

Bindiya Gupta MD MAMS FICOG
Associate Professor
Department of Obstetrics and Gynecology
University College of Medical Sciences and Guru Teg Bahadur Hospital
New Delhi, India

BL Nayak MBBS MD (Obs & Gynec)
Associate Professor
Department of Gynecologic Oncology
Acharya Harihar Postgraduate Institute of Cancer, Cuttack, Odisha, India

Chaitanya Nagori MD DGO
Director
Dr Nagori's Institute for Infertility and IVF
Co-director, Ian Donald Inter-University School of Medical Ultrasound
Ahmedabad Branch
Ahmedabad, Gujarat, India

Chandravati MS DGO DFPA FICS FICMCH FN RS FI COG
Professor Emeritus
Department of Obstetrics and Gynecology
KG Medical College, Lucknow
Proprietor Director, Krishna Medical Centre, Lucknow
Chairman/Patron, Indian College of Maternity and Child Health (ICMCH) (NARCHI)
Patron, Indian Infertility Society (UP Chapter) and Lucknow Obstetrics and Gynaecology Society

Charmila Ayyavoo MD DGO DFP FICOG
Obstetrician and Gynecologist
Parvathy Ayyavoo Fertility Centre
Director, Aditi Hospital and Parvathy Ayyavoo Fertility Centre
Tiruchirappalli, Tamil Nadu, India

Chirag Patel MBBS
Resident Doctor
Department of Obstetrics and Gynecology
Nanavati Hospital
Mumbai, Maharashtra, India

CN Purandare MD MA OBST (IRL) DGO DFP DOBST RCPI (DUBLIN) FRCOG (UK) FRCPI (Ireland) FACOG (USA) FAMS FICOG FICMCH PGD MLS (Law)
Emeritus Dean
Indian College of Obstetrics and Gynecology
Emeritus Professor of Obstetrics and Gynecology, Grant Medical College and Sir JJ Group of Hospitals
Former President, FIGO (2015-2018)

D Gayathri MBBS
Junior Resident
Ramakrishna Medical Centre LLP
Tiruchirappalli, Tamil Nadu, India

Damodar Rao MD (Obs & Gynec) MBBS
Gynecologist, Laparoscopic Surgeon (Obs and Gynec)
Infertility Specialist, Obstetrician
Rao Hospital
Coimbatore, Tamil Nadu, India

Darshana Legha MBBS MD
Assistant Professor
Department of Obstetrics and Gynecology
Mahatma Gandhi Institute of Medical Sciences, Wardha, Maharashtra, India

Deepti Gupta MBBS MS
Consultant
Department of Obstetrics and Gynecology
Fortis Hospital, Shalimar Bagh
New Delhi, India

Deepti Prasad MRCOG DGO DNB (Obs & Gynec)
Former Assistant Professor
Department of Obstetrics and Gynecology
Grant Government Medical College and Sir JJ Group of Hospitals
Mumbai, Maharashtra, India

Divya Pandey MBBS MS (Obs & Gynec)
Associate Professor
Department of Obstetrics and Gynecology
Vardhman Mahavir Medical College and Safdarjung Hospital
New Delhi, India

Dinesh Wade MBBS MS
Managing Director
Department of Obstetrics and Gynecology
Dr Shankarrao Chavan Government Medical College
Nanded, Maharashtra, India

Duru Shah MD FRCOG FCPS FICOG FICMCH DGO DFP
Scientific Director and Infertility Expert
Gynaecworld –The Center for Women's Health and Fertility
Mumbai, Maharashtra, India

Eshani Sharma MBBS DNB
Senior Research Scholar
Department of Obstetrics and Gynecology
All India Institute of Medical Sciences
New Delhi, India

Fessy Louis T DGO DNB FAGE MNAMS DPS MICOG FICOG
Senior Consultant and Associate Professor
Department of Reproductive Medicine and Surgery
Amrita Fertility Centre
Amrita Institute of Medical Sciences
Kochi, Kerala, India

Foram Vora MS (Gynec Endoscopic Surgeon)
Consultant
Fortis Hospital (FMRI)
Jyoti Maternity Hospital and Minimum Invasive Surgery Centre
Ahmedabad, Gujarat, India

Freni Shah MS (Obs & Gynec)
Consultant
Department of Obstetrics and Gynecology
Chhatrapati Shivaji Maharaj Hospital
Mumbai, Maharashtra, India

Gargee Mulye MD
Senior Registrar
Department of Radiation Oncology
Tata Memorial Hospital
Mumbai, Maharashtra, India

Gayathri V MBBS DGO DNB (Obs & Gynec)
Gynecologist
Women Wellness Clinic
Coimbatore, Tamil Nadu, India

George Paul MBBS MS
Consultant Gynecologist and Endoscopic Surgeon, Paul's Hospital
Centre for Advanced Endoscopy and Infertility
Kochi, Kerala, India

Gillian Ryan MB BCh BAO MRCPI MRCOG MD
Maternal and Fetal Medicine
Fellow, Department of Obstetrics and Gynecology
The National Maternity Hospital
Dublin, Ireland

Gokul Das MD FICOG FICMCH
Former Professor and Head
Department of Obstetrics and Gynecology
Gauhati Medical College, Guwahati
Founder Professor and Head
Department of Obstetrics and Gynecology
Tomo Riba Institute of Health and Medical Sciences
Nagarlagun, Arunachal Pradesh
Senior Consultant and Head
Department of Obstetrics and Gynecology
Health City Hospital
Guwahati, Assam, India
Vice President, FOGSI 2014

Gorakh Mandrupkar MBBS DGO FCPS FICOG PGDCR PGDMLS
Director, Mandrupkar Clinic
Islampur, Maharashtra, India

Haritha C DGO MBBS
Consultant Gynecologist
Thrissur District Cooperative Hospital
Thrissur, Kerala, India

Harmi Thakkar BSc MS (Biotechnology)
Research Assistant
Akanksha Hospital and Research Institute
Anand, Gujarat, India

Harshad Parasnis MD DNB FCPS DGO FICOG FICS
Consultant Gynecologic Oncologist
Head of Gynecologic Oncology Unit
Associate Professor, Bharati Medical College, Pune
Visiting Gynecologic Oncologist
BJGMC and Sassoon General Hospital
Pune, Maharashtra, India
Chairperson, Oncology Committee, FOGSI (2009-2011)
President, Pune Obst-Gyn Soc, 2020-2021

Hrishikesh Pai MD FRCOG (UK-HON) FCPS FICOG MSc USA
Medical Director, Bloom IVF Group
Director
Lilavati Hospital in Mumbai and Fortis Hospitals in New Delhi, Gurugram
Faridabad, Mohali and Navi Mumbai
Past President, ISAR
Past President, MOGS
Past Senior VP, FOGSI
Past President, Indian Society of Gynecological Endoscopists

Jai Bhagwan Sharma MBBS MD FRCOG FAMS
Professor
Department of Obstetrics and Gynecology
All India Institute of Medical Sciences
New Delhi, India

Jaideep Malhotra MD FICMCH FICOG FICS FMAS FIAJAGO FRCOG FRCPI
Director ART Rainbow IVF
President ISPAT
President SAFOMS
Immediate Past President, ISAR
Past President, FOGSI, ASPIRE, IMS
Regional Director South Asia Ian Donald School of USG
Professor Dubrovnik International University, Croatia
Editor-in-Chief SAFOG and SAFOMS Journal
Past Vice Chairman ICOG
Member of FIGO Committee of Reproductive Endocrinology and Infertility and FIGO Working Group on RDEH

Jayaraman Nambiar M MBBS MD
Professor
Department of Obstetrics and Gynecology
Kasturba Medical College
Manipal, Karnataka, India

Jayashree Natarajan MBBS MS (Obs & Gynec) FRM
Consultant, ESJAY Craft Fertility Center
Coimbatore, Tamil Nadu, India

Jaydeep Tank MBBS MD (Obs & Gynec) DNB
Fellow of College Of Physicians and Surgeons (FCPS)
Obstetrician and Gynecologist
Infertility and IVF Specialist
Ashwini Maternity and Surgical Hospital
Mumbai, Maharashtra, India

Jwal Banker MD DNB
Fellow in Reproductive Medicine
IVI RMA, Madrid, Spain

Jyoti Jaiswal MD (Obs & Gynec) FICOG FMAS
Professor and Unit Head
Department of Obstetrics and Gynecology
Pt Jawahar Lal Nehru Memorial Medical College
Raipur, Chhattisgarh, India

Kamini A Rao MBBS DGO DORCP DCH MCH FRCOG FNAMS PGDMLE
Medical Director
Milann Fertility Centre
Bangaluru, Karnataka, India

Kanthi Bansal MD DGO FICOG
Director, Safal Fertility Foundation
Ahmedabad, Gujarat, India

Karishma Thariani MBBS MS (Obs & Gynec) DNB (Obs & Gynec) Fellowship in Urogynecology
Urogynecologist, Gynecologist and Obstetrician
Center for Urogynecology and Pelvic Health
Vardhman Mahavir Medical College and Safdarjung Hospital, New Delhi, India

Kavita Singh FRCOG MRCOG MD MBBS
Gynecologist and Gynecological Cancer Surgeon
Consultant Gynecological Oncologist
Pan-Birmingham Gynecological Cancer Centre, Hamburg, Germany

Kavita V Kapadia MBBS DNB DGO DFP FCPS DAES
Obstetrician and Gynecologist
Ramaben Hospital
Navsari, Gujarat, India

Keshav Malhotra Master of Clinical Embryology MBBS
Lab Director–Rainbow IVF, Agra
Director- Global Rainbow Healthcare
Director of Training Rainbow IVF
Joint Treasurer, Delhi Chapter of ISAR (Indian Society of Assisted Reproduction)-(2015-2017)
National Committee Member, Quality Control and Accreditation Committee ISAR 2016 onwards
Committee Member, Quality Control and Accreditation ASPIRE 2016 onwards
Member Managing Committee, Indian Society of Assisted Reproduction 2018

Kiran Pandey MBBS MD FICOG FICMCH FIMSA MAMS
Professor and Head
Department of Obstetrics and Gynecology
Ganesh Shankar Vidyarthi Memorial Medical College
Kanpur, Uttar Pradesh, India

Krishnendu Gupta MBBS MD DGO
Professor and Unit Head
Department of Obstetrics and Gynecology
Vivekananda Institute of Medical Sciences
Kolkata, West Bengal, India

Krithika Meenakshi MS OG
Consultant
Apollo Hospitals
Chennai, Tamil Nadu, India

Kunal Doshi MBBS DGO FCPS (Mid. & Gynec)
Laparoscopic Surgeon
Department of Obstetrics and Gynecology
Ashish Women Care and Fertility Clinic
Mumbai, Maharashtra, India

Kunal Thakkar MBBS MD (Internal Medicine) DM (Endocrinology)
Endocrinologist
Sterling Ram Krishna Speciality Hospital
Gandhidham, Gujarat, India

Kurush P Paghdiwalla MD DNB
Consultant Obstetrician and Gynecologist
Breach Candy Hospital, Saifee Hospital
Masina Hospital and Parsee General Hospital
Mumbai, Maharashtra, India

Kusum Lata Singhal MBBS MS (Obs & Gynec)
Consultant
Koteshwar Hospital
Gwalior, Madhya Pradesh, India

KV Divya MD
Senior Resident
Department of Obstetrics and Gynecology
Maulana Azad Medical College and Lok Nayak Hospital, New Delhi, India

L Krishna MS
Professor and Head
Emeritus Professor
Department of Obstetrics and Gynecology
PES Institute of Medical Sciences and Research, Bengaluru, Karnataka, India

Lavanya Gurram MD
Assistant Professor
Department of Radiation Oncology
Tata Memorial Hospital
Mumbai, Maharashtra, India

Laxmi Shrikhande MBBS MD (Obs & Gynec)
Medical Director and Consultant
Shrikhande Hospital and Research Centre
Nagpur, Maharashtra, India

Lila Vyas MBBS MS
Senior Consultant
Cocoon Hospital, Jaipur
Former Professor
Department of Obstetrics and Gynecology
SMS Medical College
Jaipur, Rajashthan, India

Lucy Das MD
Professor
Department of Obstetrics and Gynecology
SCB Medical College
Cuttack, Odisha, India

Madhu Nagpal MBBS MD
Gynecologist and Obstetrician
Nayyar Superspecialty Hospital
Amritsar, Punjab, India

Madhuri Mehendale MBBS DGO DNB FCPS Diploma in Advanced Laparoscopy (Kiel)
Assistant Professor
Lokmanya Tilak Municipal Medical College
Mumbai, Maharashtra, India
Managing Council Member, MOGS

Madhva Prasad S MS DNB PGDMLS PGDCR
Associate Professor
Department of Obstetrics and Gynecology
Vydehi Institute of Medical Sciences and Research Centre
Bengaluru, Karnataka, India
National Corresponding Editor, Journal of Obstetrics and Gynaecology of India

Mala Arora FRCOG (UK) FICOG FICMCH DA (UK)
Consultant
Department of Obstetrics and Gynecology
Fortis La Femme Hospital, New Delhi
Director
Noble IVF Center
Noble Hospital
Faridabad, Haryana, India
Past Chairperson, ICOG

Mandakini Megh MD DGO FICMCH FICMU FICOG
Director and Consultant Gynecologist of Dr Megh's Gynaec-Care Clinic
Mumbai, Maharashtra, India
Chairperson, ICOG
International Vice President of Medical Women's International Association (MWIA), Central Asia

Manish Banker MD FICOG
Medical Director, Nova IVF Fertility
Ahmedabad, Gujarat, India
Past President, ISAR

Manjitkaur Mohi MD MBBS
Consultant
Department of Obstetrics and Gynecology
Fortis Hospital
Mohali, Punjab, India

Manjulata Verma MD PDCC (Fetal Medicine)
Associate Professor
Department of Obstetrics and Gynecology
King George's Medical University
Lucknow, Uttar Pradesh, India

Manu Sobti MS (Gen Surgery) MCh (Urology) DNBE (Urology) (Sp. Urology)
Urologist and Urological Surgeon
Holy Family Hospital
Medical Research Center
Mumbai, Maharashtra, India

Maya Padhi MD (Obs & Gynec)
Professor
Department of Obstetrics and Gynecology
SCB Medical College
Cuttack, Odisha, India

Meenu Handa MS DNB FICOG Fellow Reproductive Medicine (Gold medalist)
IVF Consultant
Fortis Bloom IVF Centre
FMRI, Gurugram, Haryana, India
Treasurer, Haryana ISAR

Meeta MBBS MD
Consultant
Department of Obstetrics and Gynecology
Tanvir Hospital
Hyderabad, Telangana, India

Meghana Shedge MBBS DGO
Gynecologist and Obstetrician
Thunga Hospital
Mumbai, Maharashtra, India

Minal Dhanvij MS (Obs & Gynec)
Consultant
Department of Minimally Invasive Gynecology, Akanksha Hospital
Mumbai, Maharashtra, India

Molina Patel MBBS MD (Obs & Gynec)
Gynecologist
Akanksha Hospital and Research Institute
Anand, Gujarat, India

Mrinmayi Dharmadhikari MBBS MD DNB
Clinical Fellow
Fertility Associates
Mumbai, Maharashtra, India

Mukta Jain MBBS MS (Gynecology)
Gynecologist and Obstetrician
Indore, Madhya Pradesh, India

Munjal Pandya MS
Assistant Professor
Department of Obstetrics and Gynecology
AMC MET Medical College
Sheth LG Hospital
Ahmedabad, Gujarat, India

Muralidhar V Pai MBBS MD (Obs & Gynec)
Professor and Head
Department of Obstetrics and Gynecology
Kasturba Medical College
Manipal, Karnataka, India

N Rajamaheswari MD DGO MCh (Urology)
Consultant Urogynecologist
Urogynecology Research Center
Chennai, Tamil Nadu, India

N Sanjeeva Reddy MD DGO
Professor and Head
Department of Reproductive Medicine and Surgery
Sri Ramachandra Institute of Higher Education and Research (DU)
Chennai, Tamil Nadu, India

N Shailaja MBBS MS (Obs & Gynec) DGO
Former Professor
Department of Obstetrics and Gynecology
PES Institute of Medical Sciences and Research, Kuppam, Andhra Pradesh, India

Nalini Anand MD
Professor and Head
Department of Obstetrics and Gynecology
Government Medical College
Bhavnagar, Gujarat, India

Nalini Shah MD
Professor and Head
Department of Pediatric Endocrinology
King Edward Memorial Hospital
Seth Gordhandas Sunderdas Medical College
Mumbai, Maharashtra, India

Nandan Roongta DNB DGO DFP
Consultant Gynecologist
Bloom IVF Centre, Lilavati Hospital
Mumbai, Maharashtra, India

Nandita Palshetkar MD FCPS FICOG
Director and Senior Consultant
Bloom IVF Group, New Delhi/Mohali/Vashi and Lilavati Hospital Mumbai
Trustee, DY Patil Medical College, Mumbai and Group
Past President, MOGS
Past President, FOGSI, President, AMOGS

Narendra Malhotra MD FICOG FICMCH FRCOG FICS FMAS AFIAP
Managing Director
Global Rainbow Healthcare, Agra
Prof. Dubrovnick International University
Vice President, WAPM (World Association of Prenatal Medicine)
President, ISPAT (2017-2019)

Nayana Patel MD (Obs & Gynec)
Managing Director and Medical Director
Infertility Specialist, Akanksha Hospital and Research Institute
Anand, Gujarat, India

Neerja Bhatla MBBS MD
Professor and Head of Unit
Department of Obstetrics and Gynecology
All India Institute of Medical Sciences
New Delhi, India

Neerja Sachdev MS (Obs & Gynec)
Consultant, Rainbow IVF
Agra, Uttar Pradesh, India

Neha Agarwal MBBS MD
Assistant Professor
Department of Obstetrics and Gynecology
SN Medical College
Agra, Uttar Pradesh, India

Neha Seehara MBBS MS
Assistant Professor
Department of Obstetrics and Gynecology
Government Medical College
Kota, Rajashthan, India

Neharika Malhotra MD (Obs & Gynec) FICMCH FMAS DRM (Germany) Fellowship in Reproductive Medicine Fellowship in Ultrasound
Infertility Consultant
Rainbow IVF Hospital
Agra, Uttar Pradesh, India

Nidhi Shah Gandhi DGO DNB (Obs & Gynec) IFCPC-IARC Fellowship in Colposcopy
Obstetrician ad Gynecologist
Women Care Clinic, Opera House
Mumbai, Maharashtra, India

Niket Patel MBBS MD (Obs & Gynec)
Director and Gynecologist
Akanksha Hospital and Research Institute
Anand, Gujarat, India

Nikhil Datar MBBS MD (Mid & Gynec) DGO FCPS (Mid & Gynec) DNB (Obs & Gynec)
Gynecologist, Obstetrician, Laparoscopic Surgeon
Department of Obstetrics and Gynecology
CloudNine Hospital
Mumbai, Maharashtra, India

Nikhil Parwate MBBS MD (Obs & Gynec)
Senior Consultant
Chief Colposcopist
Gynec-Onco and Robotic Surgeon
Aditya Birla Memorial Hospital
Pune, Maharashtra, India

Nikhil Shetty BBS MS (Obs & Gynec)
Associate Professor
Department of Obstetrics and Gynecology
Kasturba Medical College
Mangaluru, Karnataka, India

Niranjan Chavan MD FCPS DGO DICOG MICOG (Mum) Diploma in Endoscopy (USA)
Professor and Unit Chief
LTMMC and LTMG Hospital, Mumbai
Director
Chavan Maternity and Nursing Home
Mumbai, Maharashtra, India
Chairperson, FOGSI Oncology and Trophoblastic Tumors Committee (2012-2014)

Nirmala Sharma MBBS MS (GYNAE) MICOG
Professor and Head
Department of Obstetrics and Gynecology
Government Medical College
Kota, Rajasthan, India

Nisha Rani MBBS MD DGO
Gynecologist and Obstetrician
Nisha Rani's Clinic
New Delhi, India

Nitin Raithatha
Professor
Department of Obstetrics and Gynecology
Pramukh Swami Medical College
Bhaikaka University
Karamsad, Gujarat, India

Parikshit Tank MD DNB FCPS DGO DFP MNAMS FICOG FRCOG
Senior Consultant Obstetrician and Gynecologist
Ashwini Maternity and Surgical Hospital
Jupiter Hospital
Mumbai, Maharashtra, India
Honorary Professor
Assisted Reproduction
Pacific Medical College and Hospital
Udaipur, Rajasthan, India
Treasurer, Federation of Obstetrics and Gynaecological
Societies of India (FOGSI), 2021-2024
Joint Secretary, FOGSI, 2012
Joint Treasurer, FOGSI, 2018-2020
Chairperson, Safe Motherhood, FOGSI, 2014-2017

Parvathy T MBBS MD DNB
Assistant Professor
Department of Reproductive Medicine and Surgery
Amrita Fertility Centre
Amrita Institute of Medical Sciences
Kochi, Kerala, India

Pavika Lal MBBS MD
Assistant Professor
Department of Obstetrics and Gynecology
Ganesh Shankar Vidyarthi Memorial Medical College
Kanpur, Uttar Pradesh, India

PB Hiremath MD
Professor and Head
Department of Obstetrics and Gynecology
Sri Venkateshwaraa Medical College Hospital and Research Center
Puducherry, India

PC Mahapatra MD
Associated Professor
Department of Obstetrics and Gynecology
SCB Medical College
Cuttack, Odisha, India

PG Paul MBBS DGO
Consultant Gynecologist and Endoscopic Surgeon
Paul's Hospital, Centre for Advanced Endoscopy and Infertility
Kochi, Kerala, India

Phiroze Soonawala MBBS MS (General Surgery) FRCS (General Surgery) MCh (Urology) DNB (Urology/Genitourinary Surgery)
Urologist, General Physician
Breach Candy Hospital
Mumbai, Maharashtra, India

Poonam Varma Shivkumar MBBS MD
Professor and Head
Department of Obstetrics and Gynecology
Mahatma Gandhi Institute of Medical Sciences
Wardha, Maharashtra, India

Prabha Lal MD (Obs & Gynec)
Professor
Department of Obstetrics and Gynecology
Lady Hardinge Medical College and Smt Sucheta Kriplani Hospital
New Delhi, India

Pragnesh Shah MD FICOG
Director and Gynecological Endoscopic Surgeon, Jyoti Hospital
Ahmedabad, Gujarat, India

Prakash Trivedi MBBS DGO MD (Obs & Gynec) FCPS (Mid. & Gynec)
Gynecologist, Obstetrician, Infertility Specialist
Dr Trivedi's Total Woman Health Care Centre
Mumbai, Maharashtra, India

Pranav Mandovra MBBS MS General Surgery FMAS FCRS FACRSI
Fellow Colorectal Surgery
Zen Hospital
Mumbai, Maharashtra, India

Pratap Kumar MD DGO FICS FICOG FIMCH
Professor
Manipal Assisted Reproductive Centre (MARC)
Department of Obstetrics and Gynecology
Kasturba Medical College
Manipal Academy of Higher Education
Manipal, Karnataka, India

Prathamesh Kane MBBS
Consultant Gynecologist
TN Medical College and BYL Nair Charitable Hospital
Mumbai, Maharashtra, India

Preeti Sharma MBBS MS
Senior Consultant
Department of Obstetrics and Gynecology
Cocoon Hospital
Jaipur, Rajashthan, India
DNB Guide

Priti Kumar MD (Obs & Gynec) FICOG
Director, Sunflower Medical Centre
Lucknow, Uttar Pradesh, India
Chairperson, Safe Motherhood Committee, FOGSI (2020-22)
Vice President, Lucknow Obstetrics and Gynaecology Society

Priya Ballal K MBBS MD (Obs & Gynec)
Professor and Head
Department of Obstetrics and Gynecology
Kasturba Medical College
Mangaluru, Karnataka, India

Pushpa Junghare MD
Professor and Head
Department of Obstetrics and Gynecology
Dr Panjabrao Deshmukh Memorial Medical College
Amravati, Maharashtra, India

Radha Vembu MBBS DGO DNB PhD (Reproductive Medicine and Surgery)
Associate Professor
Department of Reproductive Medicine and Surgery
Sri Ramachandra Institute of Higher Education and Research (DU)
Chennai, Tamil Nadu, India

Ragini Agrawal MBBS MS (Obs & Gynec) Fellow Clinical Gyne Endoscopy (UK)
Clinical Director, W-Pratiksha Hospital
Gurugram, Haryana, India

Rajal Thaker MD FICOG
Professor
Department of Obstetrics and Gynecology
SCL Hospital
Smt NHL Municipal Medical College
Ahmedabad, Gujarat, India
Past President, AOGS (2018-19, 2020-21)
National Coordinator, Adolescent Committee, FOGSI

Rajashree Dayanand Katke MD (Obs & Gynec) FIGOG FMAS
Professor and Head
Department of Obstetrics and Gynecology
Grant Government Medical College and Sir JJ Group of Hospitals, Mumbai
Former Professor and Head
Department, SRTR Medical College
Beed, Maharashtra, India

Rajendra Sankpal MD DNBE FCPS DGO DFP MB Fellowship 3-D Ultrasonography (USA) Diploma Adv. Lapascopy (USA)
Gynecologist, Infertility Specialist
Obstetrician, Sage Hospital
Mumbai, Maharashtra, India

Raji Raj MBBS DGO MS
Senior Consultant - Obsterics and Gynecology
Department of Obstetrics and Gynecology, Rajagiri Hospital
Aluva, Kerala, India

Rajrani Sharma MS (Gynec)
Senior Professor and Head
Department of Obstetrics and Gynecology
Pacific Medical College and Hospital
Udaipur, Rajasthan, India

Ramprasad Dey MBBS (Cal) MD (Cal) FICOG FMAS DCH (Cal)
Professor
Department of Obstetrics and Gynecology
Chitta Ranjan Seva Sadan
Kolkata, West Bengal, India
Joint Editor, Journal of ISOPARB

Reeti Dutta Mehra MD (Obs & Gynec)
Professor
Department of Obstetrics and Gynecology
Government Medical College and Hospital
Chandigarh, India

Revathy Janakiram MD DGO MNAMS FICOG FICMCH
Former Director
Institute of Obstetrics and Gynecology and Government Hospital for Women and Children, Chennai, Tamil Nadu, India
Vice President, FOGSI 2016

Richa Deshmukh MBBS DGO
Gynecologist
Lokmanya Tilak Municipal Medical College and General Hospital
Mumbai, Maharashtra, India

Richa Jha MD DGO
Consultant
Holy Promise Hospital, Patna
Former Assistant Professor
Department of Obstetrics and Gynecology
Netaji Subhas Medical College and Hospital
Patna, Bihar, India

Rishma Dhillon Pai MD DNB DGO FCPS FICOG
Consultant
Gynecologist and IVF Expert
Lilavati and Jaslok Hospitals
Mumbai, Maharashtra, India
Past President, Indian Society of Assisted Reproduction
Past President, IAGE
Past President, FOGSI
President, MOGS

Ritu Hinduja MD MRM (UK) DRM (Germany) Fellowship in Reproductive Medicine (India, Spain, Israel) Certificate in Genetic Counseling
Senior Consultant, Reproductive Medicine
Nova IVF Fertility
Mumbai, Maharashtra, India
Member of Managing Committee, Indian Society of Assisted Reproduction

RM Saraogi MD FCPS FICOG DGO
Emeritus Professor
Seth GS Medical College
Former Honorary Consultant and Head
Dr RN Cooper Hospital
Senior Consultant
Nanavati Hospital
Director, Saraogi Group of Hospitals
Mumbai, Maharashtra, India
Trustee and Founder Member of AFG
President, Society of Vaginal Surgeons of India –Maharashtra Chapter

Rohan Krishnakumar MBBS DGO
Consultant Gynecologist-Obstetrician
JK Women Hospital
Thane, Maharashtra, India

Rohan Palshetkar MS (Obs & Gynec) FRM
Associate Professor
Department of Obstetrics and Gynecology
DY Patil School of Medicine
Mumbai, Maharashtra, India

Roy Patankar MBBS MS FRCS
Gastrointestinal Surgeon and Laparoscopic Surgeon
Department of Digestive Disease Centre
Zen Multispecialty Hospital
Joy Hospital
Mumbai, Maharashtra, India

Ruchi Shah MBBS MD (Pediatrics)
Consultant Pediatric Endocrinologist
Endo KIDS Clinic
Ahmedabad, Gujarat, India

Rujuta Fuke MD
Associate Professor
Department of Obstetrics and Gynecology
Government Medical College and Hospital
Nagpur, Maharashtra, India

Rupin Shah MS MCh (Urology)
Consultant Andrologist and Microsurgeon
Lilavati Hospital and Research Centre
Mumbai, Maharashtra, India

S Sampathkumari MD DGO FICOG
Professor
Department of Obstetrics and Gynecology
Institute of Obstetrics and Gynecology
Madras Medical College
Chennai, Tamil Nadu, India

Sabina Hasan Ali Moman MBBS DGO
Senior Registrar
Aditya Birla Memorial Hospital
Pune, Maharashtra, India

Sai Charisma MBBS
Resident
Department of Obstetrics and Gynecology
Maulana Azad Medical College and Lok Nayak Hospital
New Delhi, India

Sanghamitra Thakur MBBS MS
Assistant Gynecologist
Paul's Hospital
Centre for Advanced Endoscopy and infertility
Kochi, Kerala, India

Sanket Pisat MS (Obs & Gynec) DNB (Obs & Gynec) MBBS
Laparoscopic Surgeon
Department of Obstetrics and Gynecology
Akanksha Maternity and Surgical Hospital
Mumbai, Maharashtra, India

Saritha Shamsunder MD FRCOG
Consultant and Professor
Department of Obstetrics and Gynecology
Vardhman Mahavir Medical College and Safdarjung Hospital
New Delhi, India

Saroj Singh MBBS MS (Obs & Gynec)
Professor and Head
Department of Obstetrics and Gynecology
SN Medical College
Agra, Uttar Pradesh, India

Saumya Prasad MBBS MS (Obs & Gynec)
Assistant Professor
Atal Bihari Vajpayee Institute of Medical Sciences and Ram Manohar Lohia Hospital
New Delhi, India

Sayali Jahagirdar MD
Assistant Professor
Consultant
Department of Obstetrics and Gynecology
Dr Panjabrao Deshmukh Memorial Medical College
Amravati, Maharashtra, India

Seema Singhal MBBS DGO
Associate Professor
Department of Obstetrics and Gynecology
All India Institute of Medical Sciences
New Delhi, India

Seeru Garg MD DNB
Consultant Gynecologist and Obstetrician
Dr LH Hiranandani Hospital
Mumbai, Maharashtra, India

Shalini Rajaram MD FAMS FICOG MCh
Professor and Program Coordinator
Gynecologic Oncology
Department of Obstetrics and Gynecology
All India Institute of Medical Sciences
Rishikesh, Uttarakhand, India

Shally Gupta DGO DNB MRCOG-1 FICOG
Fellowship in Reproductive Medicine
Consultant, Rainhow IVF
Agra, Uttar Pradesh, India

Shantanu Abhyankar MD (Obs & Gynec) FICOG
Consultant
Modern Clinic, Wai
Satara, Maharashtra, India

Sheela HS MD
Professor
Department of Obstetrics and Gynecology
Vydehi Institute of Medical Sciences and Research Centre
Bengaluru, Karnataka, India

Sheela Mane MBBS MD
DNB Faculty
KC General Hospital
Consultant Gynecologist
Anugraha Nursing Home
Bengaluru, Karnataka, India

Shehla Jamal DNB (Diploma) MBBS
Associate Professor
Gynecologist and Obstetrician
Sharda Hospital
Greater Noida, Uttar Pradesh, India

Shikha Sachan MBBS EDIC MD (Anesthesia and Critical care)
Assistant Professor
Department of Obstetrics and Gynecology
Institute of Medical Sciences
Banaras Hindu University
Varanasi, Uttar Pradesh, India

Shikha Singh MBBS MS
Professor
Department of Obstetrics and Gynecology
SN Medical College
Agra, Uttar Pradesh, India

Shirish S Sheth MD FACOG (Hon) FRCOG (Ad Eundem)
Consultant Gynecologist
Breach Candy, and Saifee Hospitals
Mumbai, Maharashtra, India
President, International Federation of Gynecology and Obstetrics (FIGO) 2000-2003

Shobha Gudi MBBS MD DNB FICOG CIMP
Senior Consultant
Department of Obstetrics and Gynecology
Manipal Hospital
Bengaluru, Karnataka, India

Shobhana Mohandas MD DGO FICOG DIP. Endoscopy (Germany)
Gynecological Endoscopic Surgeon
Sun Medical Centre
Thrissur, Kerala, India

Shraddha Mevada MBBS
Assistant Professor
HBT Medical College and Cooper Hospital
Mumbai, Maharashtra, India

Shweta Shah MS DNB OBGY FMIS
Gynecologist, Laparoscopic Surgeon
Infertility Specialist, CloudNine Hospital
Mumbai, Maharashtra, India

SK Giri MD FICOG
Honorary Professor
Department of Gynecologic Oncology
Acharya Harihar Postgraduate Institute of Cancer, Cuttack, Odisha, India

Sona Dharmendra Phd
Senior Research Fellow
Department of Obstetrics and Gynecology
All India Institute of Medical Sciences
New Delhi, India

Sonal Panchal MD
Consultant Sonography Specialist
Dr Nagori's Institute for Infertility and IVF
Director, Centre of Excellence for Ian Donald School Inter-university of Medical Ultrasound, Ahmedabad, Gujarat, India

Soumil Trivedi MBBS DNB (Obs & Gynec)
Gynecologist, Laparoscopic Surgeon
Infertility Specialist
Dr Trivedi's Total Woman Health Care Centre, Mumbai, Maharashtra, India

SP Somashekhar MBBS MS (Gen Surg) MCh (Surgical Oncology) FRCS (Gen Surg)
Surgical Oncologist
Chairman and Head
Department of Surgical Oncology
Gynecological Oncology
Robotic Surgery, Manipal Hospital
Bengaluru, Karnataka, India

Subash Mallya MBBS DGO DNB MNAMS Diploma in Endoscopy (Germany)
Senior Consultant
Gynecologist, Infertility Specialist and Laparoscopic Surgeon
PVS Hospital and Baby Memorial Hospital
Calicut, Kerala, India

Subhash Ch Biswas MBBS (Cal) MD (PGI Chd.) FICOG FMAS FIMSA
Professor
Department of Obstetrics and Gynecology
IPGME and R, Kolkata, West Bengal, India
Member, Uro-Gynae Committee, FOGSI
National Corresponding Editor, JOGI (2011-13)
Member, Publication Committee, IUGA

Sucheta Kinjawadekar MBBS MD (Obs & Gynec)
Obstetrician and Gynecologist
Kamalesh Mother and Child Hospital
Navi Mumbai, Maharashtra, India

Suchita Dabhadkar MBBS MD (Obs & Gynec) FICS FAIMER Fellow
Fellow, Gynec-Oncology Unit
Associate Professor
Department of Gynecological Oncology
Bharati Medical College
Pune, Maharashtra, India

Sudeep Gupta MD
Professor
Department of Medical Oncology
Director, Advanced Centre for Treatment Research and Education in Cancer
Tata Memorial Centre
Mumbai, Maharashtra, India

Sudha Prasad MBBS MD FICMCH FICOG
Director and Professor
Department of Obstetrics and Gynecology
All India Institute of Medical Sciences
New Delhi, India

Suma Natarajan MBBS MD DGO FIC MCH FAGE
Head
Department of Obstetrics and Gynecology
Ganga Women and Child Centre
Coimbatore, Tamil Nadu, India

Sunil Shah MBBS MS FICOG
Consultant Gynecologist and IVF Specialist
Sarvamangal Hospital
Ahmedabad, Gujarat, India

Sunita Arora MD FICOG FICS
Senior Consultant
Bloom IVF Centre, Fortis la Femme Hospital
New Delhi, India

Sunita Tandulwadkar MD (Obs & Gynec)
Infertility Specialist, Gynecologist and Obstetrician
Chief IVF Consultant and Endoscopist
Ruby Hall Clinic
Solo Clinic IVF and Obstetrics and Gynecology, Pune, Maharashtra, India

Surveen Ghumman MBBS MD (Obs & Gynec)
Director and Head
IVF and Reproductive Medicine
Max Multispecialty Hospitals
New Delhi, India
Chairperson, Endocrinology Committee AOGD, Treasurer, Indian Fertility Society

Susheela Rani BS MBBS MD (Obs & Gynec)
Gynecologist
Manjushree Speciality Hospital
Bengaluru, Karnataka, India

Suvarna Khadilkar MD (Obs & Gynec) DGO FICOG Diploma Endocrinology (UK)
Consultant
Obstetrics and Gynecology
Bombay Hospital and Medical Research Centre, Mumbai, Maharashtra, India

T Ramani Devi MD DGO FICS FICOG
Consultant
Ramakrishna Medical Centre and Janani Fertility Centre
Tiruchirappalli, Tamil Nadu, India
Chairperson, Endometriosis Committee of FOGSI 2014–2016
EC Member of SAFOG Endometriosis Committee

Tanvir MBBS MS (Obs & Gynec)
Obstetrician and Gynecologist
Tanvir Hospital
Hyderabad, Telangana, India

Thiencherry Rema MBBS MSc (Ultrasound)
Consultant in Sonology
Udhagamandalam, Tamil Nadu, India

Trupti Nadkarni MBBS MD DNB DGO FCPS
Gynecologist/Obstetrician
The Bai Jerbai Wadia Hospital
Nowrosjee Wadia Maternity Hospital
Wadia Hospital
Mumbai, Maharashtra, India

Uma Jain MBBS MS
Senior Consultant
Department of Gynecology and Obstetrics
BLK-Max Superspecialty Hospital
New Delhi, India

Uma Singh MS
Professor and Head
Dean (Faculty of Medicine)
Department of Obstetrics and Gynecology
King George's Medical University
Lucknow, Uttar Pradesh, India

Umesh Mahantshetty MD DMRT DNB
Director and Professor
Department of Radiation Oncology
Homi Bhabha Cancer Hospital and Research Centre
Visakhapatnam, Andhra Pradesh, India

Unmesh Santpur MBBS MD
Consultant - Gynecologist
Maharishi Markandeshwar University
Mullana, MM University Trust, Mullana
Ambala, Haryana, India

Usha B Saraiya MD DGO FIAC FICOG FRCOG (UK)
Gynecologist and Obstetrician
Breach Candy Hospital
Mumbai, Maharashtra, India

Vaibhav V Kapadia MD (Obs & Gynec) DGO DAES (Germany)
Consultant Obstetrician and Gynecologist, Infertility Specialist
Ramaben Hospital, Navsari, Namaha Healthcare, Mumbai, Maharashtra, India

Vaishnavy MBBS MD
Consultant
Department of Urogynecology and Gynecology, Kauvery Hospital
Tiruchirappalli, Tamil Nadu, India

Vijaya Sarthi MBBS MD (Pediatrics) DM (Endocrinology)
Endocrinologist, Diabetologist
Dr Sarathi's Diabetes, Endocrine Nutrition and Wellness Centre
Bengaluru, Karnataka, India

Vijyalakshmi Pillai MBBS DGO MRCOG (London)
Head and Senior Consultant Obstetrician Gynecologist and Infertologist
Vijayalakshmi Medical Centre
Ernakulam, Kerala, India

Vishesha Yadav MD Fellowship in Reproductive Medicine
Fertility Consultant
GynaecWorld–The Center for Women's Health and Fertility
Mumbai, Maharashtra, India

VP Paily MBBS MD MRCOG FRCOG
Senior Consultant and Head
Department of Obstetrics and Gynecology
Rajagiri Hospital
Aluva, Kerala, India

Vyshnavi A Rao MBBS MS (Obs & Gynec) FRM (Fellow Reproductive Medicine)
Consultant, Reproductive Medicine
Milann Fertility Centre
Bengaluru, Karnataka, India

Yuvraj Jadeja MBBS MD (Obs & Gynec)
Gynecologist
Akanksha Hospital and Research Institute
Anand, Gujarat, India

Preface

It is with great pride that I present to you the *FOGSI's Postgraduate Gynaecology: A Textbook.*

At the beginning of the year, we declared our wish to compile a detailed textbook that will comprehensively, yet in a concise manner, cover all the topics with the latest scientific evidences that a postgraduate student requires to thoroughly understand this subject. We believe that FOGSI being such a large and responsible federation should have its significant contribution in the curriculum for undergraduate and postgraduate education in Obstetrics and Gynecology. The content of such a curriculum should be scientifically and ethically sound, and useful in our Indian scenario.

This textbook has been a labor of love. At FOGSI, we have always believed that an investment in training and guiding future clinicians will reap the best rewards. With this in mind, we have made PG students our primary focus this whole year. This includes initiatives like the PG Forum, the PG Training Program, and the UG-PG Curriculum. This textbook is the crowning glory of the PG activities. The idea behind these activities was to promote respect and brotherhood among colleagues, to provide them with training, education and research opportunities, facilitate interactions between PG teachers and students from all over the country, to provide a mentor-mentee type experience and enable better learning; in short, to help them to become well-rounded practitioners once they go out into the world. This book is a continuation of that theme.

It is a source of great pride to have our FOGSI research and guidelines on many topics highlighted in this book. It gives our future clinicians a straightforward perspective when it comes to making decisions. It also provides a sense of uniformity to have students across the country referencing the same guidelines.

This is an exhaustive compendium, divided into 2 volumes with a total of 207 chapters, encompassing every aspect of our ever-changing and evolving field. We start with the basics of obstetrics, where we discuss anatomy, communication, counseling, and good clinical practices. We then cover normal pregnancy and fetal evaluation, stressing on newer concepts like genetics and genomics, noninvasive prenatal testing, as well as covering the gold standards like antenatal assessment and laboratory evaluation. We have five separate sections dedicated to complications in early and late pregnancy, preexisting medical conditions, and their management. We then move on to labor, its mechanisms and management, as well as its complications, anesthesia and analgesia, and rounding up with postpartum issues. We have separate sections dedicated to social obstetrics, to enlighten our readers about the steps that are being taken to tackle public health issues like maternal mortality and perinatal deaths. There is also a section on critical care, to make our future obstetricians capable of managing emergency situations with confidence.

This volume is on Gynaecology. We begin with contraception and pregnancy termination, to highlight the importance of a woman's choice to motherhood. The next sections cover the basics of the reproductive cycle, including chapters on neuroendocrine development, puberty and adolescence going on to menopause. We then cover basic ultrasound and diagnostic techniques. There are three dedicated sections on the care, management and operative aspects in general gynecological conditions. We then move on to specialized topics like infertility, endoscopy, urogynecology and oncology, giving our readers a 360-degree viewpoint of every aspect of gynecology.

It was a Herculean task, which could not have been completed successfully without the wholehearted support of the editors, Dr Parikshit Tank and Dr Ameya Purandare.

A special thanks to my amazing, energetic and efficient section editors, who worked quickly and competently to follow-up on authors, validate data, and compile this manuscript into the version you see today.

The final result is this magnum opus. We sincerely hope that it proves to be of value, not just to PG students, but to clinicians and academicians all across the country and beyond.

To quote Carl Jung, "Medicines can treat diseases, but only doctors can treat patients."

We aim to create such doctors.

We look forward to your feedback.

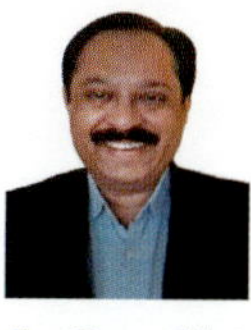

Alpesh Gandhi
President, FOGSI, 2020

FOGSI Office Bearers 2020

Acknowledgments

We thank the office bearer of FOGSI 2020. We are thankful to them for their wholehearted motivation and support throughout the year for this initiative. The entire FOGSI family has been a source of strength.

We are thankful to all the medical colleges and teachers across India for inspiring us for this useful initiative.

This book comprises 207 chapters and we had to work closely with more than 400 amazing authors for the last one and a half years. They are the experts in the subjects that they have written on. We would like to personally thank each of these brilliant authors who contributed high quality chapters for this project.

We are thankful for the immense work of editing and compilation of the chapters by our team of experienced section editors—Dr Pratima Mittal, Dr Suyajna Joshi, Dr PK Shah, Dr Pushpa Junghare, Dr Gokul Das, Dr Anuradha Khanna, Dr JB Sharma, and Dr Amita Maheshwari. It was a huge task. They worked day and night with great care and expertise to make this a high-quality textbook. We sincerely appreciate their invaluable contribution. The section editors have been helped in this work by the ablest doctors in their departments. We place on record our thanks in particular to Dr Jyotsna Suri and Dr Rekha Bharati (both Professors in the Department of Obstetrics and Gynecology, Vardhman Mahavir Medical College and Safdarjung Hospital, New Delhi, Dr Priya Ballal (Professor and Head, Department of Obstetrics and Gynecology at the KMC, Mangaluru), Dr Shweta Tahlan from Tata Memorial Hospital, Mumbai and Dr Shikha Sachan (Associate Professor, Department of Obstetrics and Gynecology, IMS, BHU, Varanasi).

We thank Jaypee Brothers Medical Publishers (P) Ltd, New Delhi, India. They are one of the most reputed and largest medical publishing houses in the world. They have been instrumental in giving us insights into the publishing process and giving much sought suggestions throughout the project.

Mr Jitendar P Vij (Group Chairman) took great personal interest and care of this project. His patience and trust was a great support. Ms Chetna Malhotra (Associate Director–Content Strategy) played the role of a seasoned and experienced facilitator. Ms Saima Rashid, Ms Kritika Dua and other team members were thorough professionals and pure perfectionists. They provided amazing support with their personal care. We sincerely appreciate their support.

TEAMWORK MAKES THE DREAM WORK.

Contents

Volume 1

PART 1: Obstetrics and Perinatology

Volume 2

PART 1: Contraception and Termination of Pregnancy

PART 3: Urogynaecology and Gynaecological Oncology

Section 13: Urogynaecology

Section 14: Gynaecological Oncology

Contraception and Termination of Pregnancy

- General
- Contraception: Spacing Methods
- Termination of Pregnancy
- Permanent Contraception
- Contraception and Pregnancy Termination for Special Groups

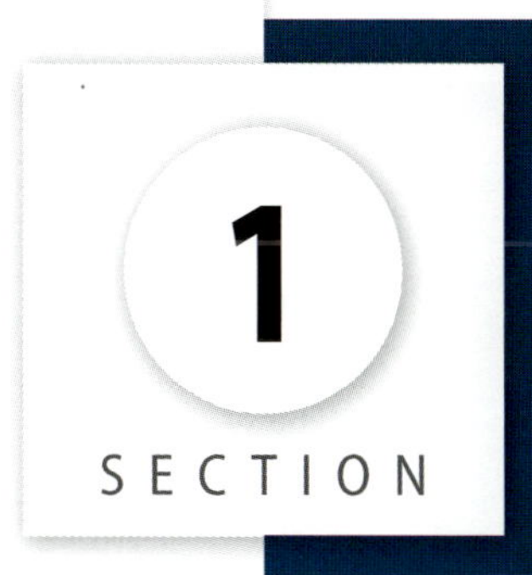

General

1.1 POPULATION DYNAMICS: THE INDIAN PERSPECTIVE

Anita Soni, Seeru Garg, Ruchi Shah

DEFINITION

Population dynamics is a portion of ecology that deals with the variation in time and space of population in size and density for one or more species.

INTRODUCTION

In population dynamics, we study short- and long-term changes in the composition, size, and age of the population along with the biological and environmental processes influencing those changes. Fundamentally, it is the study of how population changes over time.

Population dynamics overlaps with other branches of research in mathematical epidemiology (the study of infectious disease affecting population). Over the past years, population dynamics has been complemented by the evolutionary game theory, which was first developed by John Maynard Smith.

With abundant resources and favorable growing conditions, a population has the potential to increase in number from generation to generation. The population's intrinsic growth rate ("r") is considered exponential, if each generation increase is a constant percentage of the total population size. As population size approaches the carrying capacity:

- There may be increase in mortality rate and decline in the birth rate.
- The population may stabilize below the carrying capacity, known as a logistic or sigmoid (S-shape) growth curve.
- The population may overshoot the carrying capacity and then crash, resulting in repeated cycles of "boom" and "bust."
- The population may oscillate around (or below) the carrying capacity.

POPULATION TRENDS IN INDIA

Population of India is currently growing at a rate of 1.44% per year. Hence, it has been projected that India would have a total of 2 billion, i.e., 16% of world's population. As per the 2011 Census, the population was noted as 1,210 million with a percent change of 17.7%. The National Population Policy (NPP)— 2000 states that India contributes 58% to population growth on account of demographic momentum and 20% of unwanted fertility due to unmet need of contraception. As a result, a "bulge" or baby boom is moving through the age structure of population **(Fig. 1)**.

While global population has increased three times during this century from 2 to 6 billion, the population of India has increased nearly five times from 238 million to 1 billion in the same period. India's current annual increase in population of 15.5 million is large enough to neutralize efforts to conserve the resource endowment and environment.

COMPOSITION OF POPULATION

Population dynamics include birth rate (BR), death rate (DR), immigration (I), emigration (E), and age and sex composition. Birth and death rates are the most important determinants of population growth.

$$\text{Crude birth rate (CBR)} = \frac{\text{No. of live births in a area}}{\text{Mid-year population}} \times 1000$$

$$\text{Crude death rate (CDR)} = \frac{\text{No. of deaths in a area}}{\text{Mid-year population}} \times 1000$$

The *annual growth rate* for India was 1.19 in 2018. If the annual growth rate of a population is 1%, it doubles in 70 years. This law is called Malthusian model.

$$\text{Annual growth rate} = \frac{\text{Crude birth rate} - \text{Crude death rate}}{10}$$

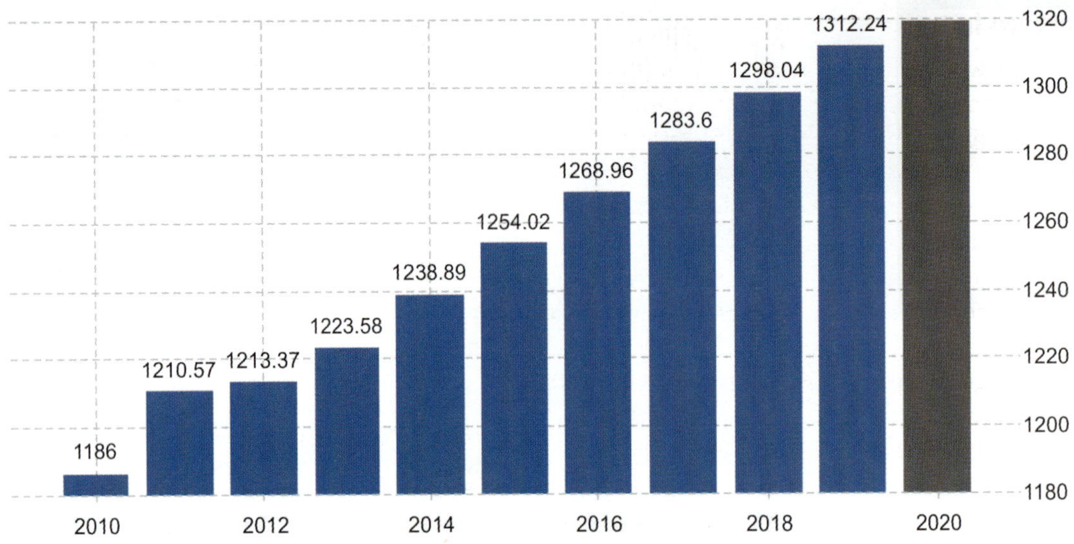

Fig. 1: Population trends in India.
Source: Tradingeconomics.com: Ministry of Statistics and Programme Implementation.

Annual growth rate:

- *<0.5%*: Slow growing population
- *0.5–1%*: Moderately growing population
- *1–1.5%*: Rapidly growing population
- *1.5–2%*: Very rapidly growing population
- *>2%*: Explosively growing population.

After the formulation of the national family welfare program, India has reduced CBR from 28.3 (1995) to 21.4 (SRS bulletin, 2013). The maximum CBR has been reported in respect of Bihar (27.7) and the minimum in respect of Kerala (14.9) (SRS Bulletin, 2013). The CDR for the country has declined from 7.1 in 2011 to 7.0 in 2012 and 2013. The maximum CDR has been reported for Odisha (8.5) and minimum for Delhi (4.2). The IMR declined from 74 per 1,000 live births (SRS bulletin, 1995) to 40 (SRS bulletin, 2013). The maximum IMR has been observed in Madhya Pradesh (56) and the minimum in Kerala (12).

DETERMINANTS OF FERTILITY IN INDIA

Education plays a very important role in population control, especially women education that affects socioeconomic and demographic indicators, which are essential for population stabilization. The Task Force of the National Commission on Population (NCP) has identified these social, economic, and demographic indicators for population stabilization in India, which are directly or indirectly affected by women education.

- Total fertility rate
- Sex ratio
- Percentage of couples using family planning methods
- Child mortality up to the age of 2 years
- Maternal mortality rate
- Percentage of women receiving skilled attention during deliveries
- Percentage of children (12–24 months) getting complete immunization
- Nutritional status of children below 6 years
- Percentage of girls marrying below 18 years of age
- Percentage of births, deaths, and marriages registered
- Literacy rate—males and females
- Enrollment of children in schools up to the age of 14 years and the rate of dropouts
- Percentage of households with safe drinking water
- Percentage of villages connected by paved roads.

There are four *fertility indicators,* which help in demographic analysis:

1. *General fertility rate (GFR)*: Total number of live births in an area among the females in reproductive age group:

$$\text{GFR} = \frac{\text{Live births}}{10} \times 1000$$

WRA = Women of reproductive age (15–49 years)

2. *Total fertility rate (TFR)*: Total number of live births a female will bear during her reproductive years, assuming: *The age-specific fertility rate (ASFR)*:

$$\text{TFR} = \frac{\text{No. of live births (ASFR)}}{\text{WRA}} \times 1000$$

Age-specific fertility rate (ASFR):

$$\text{ASFR} = \frac{\text{No. of children in a specific age group}}{\text{Total no. of female in that age group}} \times 1000$$

3. *Gross reproduction rate (GRR)*: Total number of daughters a female will bear during her reproductive years assuming the age-specific fertility pattern:

$$\text{GRR} = \frac{\text{No. of daughters (ASFR)}}{\text{WRA}} \times 1000$$

4. *Net reproduction rate (NRR)*: Total number of daughters a newborn girl child will bear during her entire life assuming the age-specific fertility and mortality pattern.

Fertility Pattern in India

The fertility levels of women in urban India are much lower in comparison to rural areas of India. The main factors behind this change are ranging between children, age of marriage, education and better healthcare, widespread acceptance of family planning measures, and socioeconomic conditions. Age-specific fertility rate (ASFR) during 1981–2011 in India has fallen for women at all ages, indicating that fertility is increasingly being controlled through adoption of family planning measures.

At the younger age group of 15–19 years, fertility decline suggests a rise in the age at marriage of girls which increased from 17 years in 1971 to 21.2 years in 2012. Moreover, earlier fertility peaked at 20–24 and 25–29 years, but now it has peaked at only 20–24 years. This shows that the average span of childbearing has declined considerably, which is due to improvement in women education level and improvement in socioeconomic condition of women.

Contraception Prevalence

Contraceptive prevalence rate is the percentage of women of age 15–49 years who are practicing any form of contraception or whose sexual partners are practicing any form of contraception. It is usually measured for women aged 15–49 years who are married or are in union. Contraceptive prevalence rate in India was reported at 53.5% in 2016, according to the World Bank collection of development indicators.

According to the data published in The Lancet, approximately 15.6 million abortions (range: 14.1–17.3 million) took place in India in 2015, giving an abortion rate of 47 (42.2–52.1) per 1,000 women of reproductive age of 15–49 years. They estimated 48.1 million pregnancies, a rate of 144.7 pregnancies per 1,000 women and a rate of 70.1 unintended pregnancies per 1,000 women. Abortions accounted for one-third of all pregnancies, while nearly half of pregnancies were unintended.

Target numbers of fertility and reproduction rates as a part of National Health Policy, 2017:

Target of NRR = 1

It gives replacement level and indicates population stabilization. To attain NRR of 1, we need TFR of 2.1 (due to unequal gender biased mortality) for which a couple protection rate desired is 60%.

SEX RATIO AND LIFE EXPECTANCY IN INDIA

Sex ratio is defined as the number of females per 1,000 males. It is one of the basic demographic characteristics of a population. The sex composition is affected by the differentials in mortality conditions of males and females, sex selective migration, and sex ratio at birth. "Female deficit syndrome" is considered adverse. A low sex ratio indicates strong male child preference and consequent gender inequalities, neglect of the girl child resulting in higher mortality at a younger age, female infanticide and feticide, higher maternal mortality, and male bias. Sex determination test, abortion services, and preconception sex services being easily available enhance this process.

Sex ratio of India has shown an increasing trend from 1991 to 2011. According to the 2011 Census, the overall sex ratio is 940 females per 1,000 males. There has been an increase in sex ratio recorded in 29 states and UTs whereas Bihar, Gujarat, and Jammu and Kashmir have shown a decline in sex ratio as compared to the 2011 Census. Kerala has the highest sex ratio of 1,084 followed by Pondicherry having 1,038. The sex ratio is lowest in Daman and Diu at 618. In 1950, the life expectancy in India (31 years) was less than half of the US (68 years). The life expectancy in India also differs by sex, which varies from state to state. In 1951, life expectancies for male and female were 38.7 and 37.1 years, respectively. However, by 2005, the life expectancy in India (64 years) was not far behind the US (77 years). The life expectancy of male and female in India reversed in recent years. In 2012, the life expectancy at birth for women was 67.7 years and for men it was 64.6 years. The overall current life expectancy for India in 2020 is 69.73 years, a 0.33% increase from 2019.

POPULATION POLICY IN INDIA

Population policies are formulated to address the unmet needs for contraception, healthcare infrastructure, and health personnel and to provide integrated service delivery for basic reproductive and child healthcare. The main objective is to achieve a stable population at a level consistent with the requirements of sustainable economic growth, social development, and environmental protection.

Five-Year Plans by the Government of India for Population Control

The central government formulated the "new national population policy" in February 2000.

The latest 12th 5-year plan (2012–2017) objectives are:

- To create 50 million new work opportunities in nonfarm sector
- To remove gender and social gap in school environment
- To enhance access to higher education
- To reduce malnutrition among children of 0–3 years
- To provide electricity to all rural areas
- To ensure 50% rural population to have accesses to safe drinking water
- To increase green cover by 1 million hectare every year
- To provide access to banking services to 90% of households.

The *Population Regulation Bill, 2019,* was a proposed bill introduced in the Rajya Sabha in July 2019 by Rakesh Sinha to control the population growth of India. According to the World Population Prospects 2019 report by the United Nations, the population of India is set to overtake that of China within a decade. The 2020 bill proposes to introduce a two-child policy per couple and aims to incentivize its adoption through various measures such as educational benefits, taxation cuts, home loans, free healthcare, and better employment opportunities. The 2019 bill proposed by Sinha talks about introducing penalties for couples not adhering to the two-child policy such as debarment from contesting in elections and ineligibility for government jobs.

The complex status of the India's population dynamics is at some point of *demographic transition*, in the process and moving to its final stage. India has already achieved the target of some demographic indicators, namely reduction of crude death rate to (7.0) and crude birth rate to (21.4) per thousand and TFR is 2.4. The cohort comprises mainly the working age group as compared with the dependent population. Hence, there can be accelerated skilled development and economic growth of India.

FURTHER READING

1. Begon M, Harper JL, Townsend CR. Ecology. Individuals, populations and communities. Oxford: Blackwell Scientific Publications; 1986.
2. Bloom DE, Canning D, Fink G. (2008). Urbanization and the wealth of nations. Science. 2008;319(5864):772-5.
3. Bloom DE. (2011). Population dynamics in India and implications for economic growth. [online] Available from: https://cdn1.sph.harvard.edu/wp-content/uploads/sites/1288/2013/10/PGDA_WP_65.pdf. [Last accessed November, 2021].
4. Census India. (2011). Decadal growth: 2011 Census of India. [online] Available from: www.censusindia.gov.in. [Last accessed November, 2021]
5. Government of India, Planning Commission. An approach to 12th five-year plan. New Delhi, India. 2011.
6. Manjul P, Rupam T. Population dynamics in India. Int J Sci Eng Res. 2016;6(1):
7. Ministry of Health and Family Welfare. (2015). Health and Family Welfare Statistics of India, 2015. [online] Available from: http://mospi.nic.in/statistical-year-book-india/2015/199. [Last accessed November, 2021]
8. Ministry of Statistics and Programme Implementation (MOSPI). Population trends in India. [online] Available from: http://mospi.nic.in. [Last accessed November, 2021].
9. Park K. Park's Textbook of Preventive and Social Medicine, 23rd edition. India: Bhanot Publishers; 2015.
10. Pritchett L. Desired fertility and impact of population policies. Popul Dev Rev. 1994;20(1):1-55.

LONG QUESTION

1. What is population policy? Describe the population policy in the Indian context and the main events or factors that have shaped it since independence.

SHORT QUESTIONS

1. What are the determinants of fertility in India?
2. What are the main fertility indicators?
3. What is contraceptive prevalence and what factors affect it?

MULTIPLE CHOICE QUESTIONS

1. If annual growth rate of a population is 1.5%, how many years will it take to double?
   a. 105 years b. 70 years
   c. 100 years d. 110 years
2. New parameter added in 2020 population regulation bill is:
   a. Unmet needs for contraception
   b. Healthcare infrastructure
   c. Health personnel
   d. Two-child policy
3. The twelfth 5-year plan includes the following objectives, except:
   a. To remove gender and social gap in school environment
   b. To enhance access to higher education
   c. To reduce malnutrition among children aged 0–3 years
   d. To ensure all rural areas to have access to safe drinking water
4. The current life expectancy for India is:
   a. 67.9 b. 64.6
   c. 69.7 d. 67.7
5. Crude birth rate is defined as:
   a. $CBR = \frac{\text{No. of live births in a area}}{\text{Mid-year population}} \times 1000$
   b. $CBR = \frac{\text{No. of live births in a area}}{\text{Total no. of births}} \times 1000$
   c. $CBR = \frac{\text{No. of total births in a area}}{\text{Mid-year population}} \times 1000$
   d. $CBR = \frac{\text{No. of live births in a area}}{\text{Mid-year population}} \times 100$
6. Sex ratio of India is:
   a. 618 b. 940
   c. 943 d. 1,048
7. All are fertility indicators, except:
   a. General fertility rate b. Total fertility rate
   c. Gross fertility rate d. Gross reproductive rate
8. Determinants of fertility in India are all, except:
   a. Total fertility rate b. Sex ratio
   c. Infant mortality rate d. Maternal mortality rate

Answers

1. a 2. d 3. d 4. c 5. a 6. b
7. c 8. c

1.2 GOVERNMENT POLICIES AND POPULATION STABILIZATION

Mandakini Megh, Bhumika Kotecha Mundhe

INTRODUCTION

This chapter considers the past, present, and future perspectives of the population stabilization and the government policies projected with regard to the same. India was the first country in the world to have launched a national program for family planning in 1952 under India's first Prime Minister Mr Jawaharlal Nehru. Over the decades, the program has undergone transformation in terms of policy and actual program implementation and currently being repositioned to not only achieve population stabilization goals but also promote reproductive health and reduce maternal, infant, and child mortality and morbidity. However, the severity of the current situation can be understood by the mere fact that India has 17% of the world's population on 2.4% of the global land. If the current trend continues, India will overtake China by 2045 and will become the most populous country of the world.[1]

A very rapid increase in the population for a long time may be termed population explosion (i.e., if the birth rate is much more than the death rate for a long time, it may lead to a population explosion).[1] The Prime Minister of India, Shri Narendra Modi, in his speech on Independence Day said that Jansankhya Visphot (Population Explosion) may affect the future of our children **(Fig. 1)**.

There are evidences of the following effects due to population explosion:[1]

- Living standards of people drop
- Rise in crime and violence
- High level of unemployment
- Thousands go hungry due to poverty and one-third of the population are below the poverty line
- *Famine*: Lack of food and cooking fuel
- Poor health
- Poor sanitation services
- Environmental degradation in terms of air, water, and soil pollution
- Deforestation and ecology modification and distribution of agriculture holdings

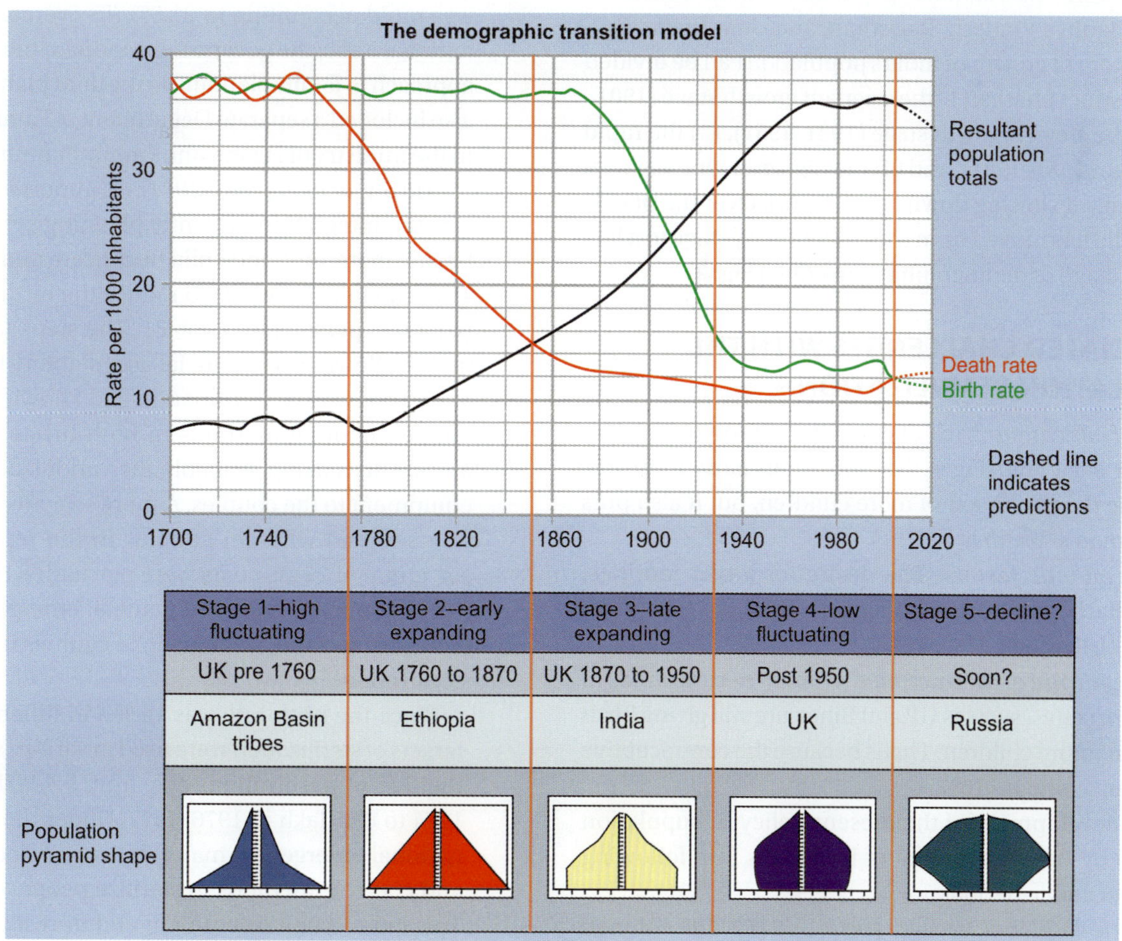

Fig. 1: Demographic transition model.
Source: http://www.coolgeography.co.uk/GCSE/AQA/Population/Demographic%20Transition/Demographic_Transition_Model.jpg

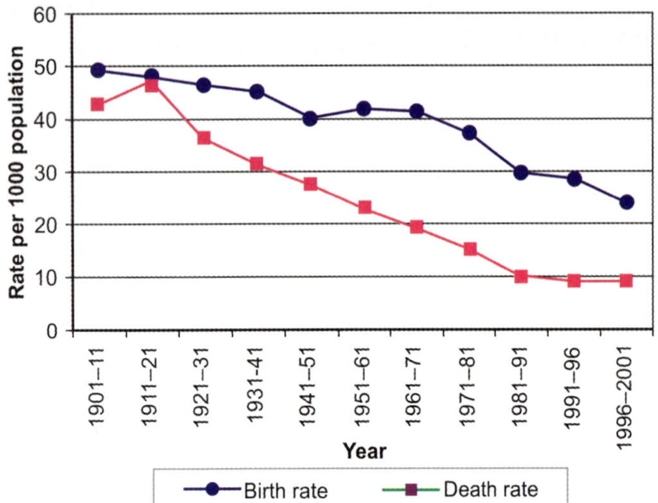

Fig. 2: Birth rate and death rate of India from 1901-2001.
Source: Registrar General of India.

- *Dissolution of family*: More divorces, separation, suicides, etc., due to unhappiness.

Bare facts[1]

- Every sixth person on the globe is an Indian and by the turn of this century, every fifth living person will be an Indian
- 49% of the increase in India's population is from four states: Bihar, Madhya Pradesh, Rajasthan, and Uttar Pradesh.

The history of growth of India's population can be divided into four distinct phases: (1) the stagnant growth stage (1901–1921), (2) the steady growth stage (1921–1951), (3) the rapid growth stage (1951–1981), and (4) the high growth stage with definite signs of slowing down (1981–2011). Over the period of time, India has moved from a high stationary stage to a late expanding stage of demographic transition **(Fig. 2)**.[2]

ASSOCIATED CHALLENGES WITH THE POPULATION STABILIZATION

- *Level of education:* Lack of education in women results in their early marriages. Not only does early marriage increase the likelihood of more children, but it also puts the woman's health at risk.
- *Socioeconomic factors:* The desire for larger families, particularly preference for a male child, also leads to higher birth rates.
- *Inadequate use of contraceptive:* Women in rural areas of northern states, such as UP and Bihar, are still giving birth to four or more children. This is because the contraceptive prevalence rate is <10%.

  The development of the present policy of population control by the government of India falls into following distinguishable periods:
- *The period of "indifference" (before 1947)*: The colonial government of Britain was largely indifferent to population growth. Though the British Government was indifferent to population control policy in India, the enlightened section of Indian public along with some politicians urged the government to develop a population control policy.

  PK Wattal was the pioneer who wrote a book on Population Problem in India in 1916. Among Indian politicians and political parties, it was supported by Jawaharlal Nehru, Mahatma Gandhi, Shubhash Chandra Bose, and Bhore Committee.
- *The period of "neutrality" (1947–1952)*: Postindependence, the early apathy of the Government to develop population policy was attributed to its preoccupation in drafting the constitution and finding India's way in international relations. Finally, 3 years after independence, the National Family Planning Program was launched in 1952.
- *The period of "experimentation" (1952–1961)*: The first 5-year plan (1951–1956) was laid with the objective of "reducing birth rate to the extent necessary to stabilize the population at a level consistent with the requirement of the national economy." One of the national sample survey reports revealed that the population of India had grown substantially, which was confirmed in 1961 census.
- *The beginning of policy of population control (1961–2000)*:
  - *Second and third 5-year plans (1956–1961 and 1961–1966)*: The population growth from 1951 to 1961 was rapid accounting to 21.5%. To overcome such a national issue, the government adopted the extension approach to family planning in the third plan. This plan also included a separate Department of Family Welfare in the Ministry of Health and Family Planning in 1966.
  - *Fourth 5-year plan (1969–1974)*: An important measure was the integration of family planning services with health, maternity, and child healthcare and nutrition. The main aim here was to reduce the birth rate to 25 per 1,000 persons by 1980–81. The steps taken were in the following areas: social acceptability for a small family, increasing information and knowledge about family planning methods in both urban and rural areas, and making available the various devices and equipment to the couples. A more selective approach was adopted wherein couples in the reproductive age group of 25–35 years were persuaded to undergo sterilization as a matter of national emergency. Also, monetary incentive was given to couples undergoing sterilization.

    Since the birth rate was varied in different states, targets of sterilization were fixed in various states. The number of sterilizations rose from 9.4 lakh in 1973–1974 to 82.6 lakh in 1976–1977. Under the banner of national emergency, many states resorted to unfair and coercive methods to sterilize people of all ages. This led to mass resentment and unrest among the people. As a result, the family planning program became very unpopular.

- *Fifth 5-year plan (1974–1979)*: The 1971 census showed a rapid growth in population by 24.6%. To control this, the fifth plan laid down the ambitious target of reducing the birth rate to 30 per 1,000 by the end of the plan (1978–79) and to 25 per 1,000 by 1983–84.

In 1977, post national emergency, the government announced the new population policy renaming the family planning program to the family welfare program. This program did have a leeway to the common man. The main features of this policy were:

- Fixing the marriage age for girls at 18 years and for boys at 21 years. This has been implemented by the Child Marriage Restraint (Amendment) Act, 1978
- Making sterilization voluntary
- Including population education as part of normal course of study
- Monetary incentive to those who go in for sterilization and tubectomy
- Private companies to be exempted in corporate taxes if they popularize birth-control measures among employees
- Use of media for spreading family planning in rural areas, etc.; this policy put an end to compulsory sterilization and laid emphasis on voluntary sterilization.

However, this slowed down the family planning program. As a result, the number of sterilizations fell from 82.6 lakh in 1976–1977 to 9 lakh in 1977–1978.

- *Sixth, seventh, and eighth 5-year plans (1980–1985, 1985–1990, and 1990–1995)*: The efforts were done to control population by determining long-term demographic aims such as net reproduction rate, crude birth rate (CBR), crude death rate, and couple protection rate.

  The government replaced the earlier Population Control Approach by the Reproductive and Child Health Approach in October 1997 with the intention to decentralize area-specific macroplanning. It led to several new schemes for improving quality and coverage of welfare services for women, children, and adolescents such as child survival, safe motherhood program, and universal immunization program (UIP), and reproductive tract infections (RTI).
- *Ninth 5-year plan (1997–2002):* During the ninth plan, the earlier approach of using NRR (Net Reproduction Rate) of 1.0 was changed to a total fertility rate (TFR) of 2.1. This level of TFR been projected to be achieved by 2026 in the plan. One of the important strategies of this plan was to undertake area-specific microplanning, i.e., at the primary health care (PHC) level.

  In 2001, the National Policy for Empowerment of Women was adopted with the ultimate objective of ensuring women their rightful place in society by empowering them as agents of socioeconomic change and development.

National Population Policy, 2000

The population of India on May 11, 2000, had risen to 100 crores from 23 crores over a period of 100 years. This meant that all efforts of population stabilization taken so far seemed to be elusive.

The National Population Policy (NPP) was announced in 2000. It had three types of objectives:

1. *The immediate objective*:
   - To address the unmet needs for contraception, healthcare infrastructure, and health personnel
   - To provide integrated service delivery for basic reproductive and child healthcare
2. *The medium-term objective*: Bring TFR to the replacement level by 2010.
3. *The long-term objective*: To achieve a stable population by 2045.

The NPP 2000 relies more on persuasive and positive measures rather than on coercive methods. It lays emphasis on both the qualitative and the quantitative aspects of population.

A major cause for worry for policy makers is that the sex ratio of children has declined for all age groups as compared to 2001. The decline is more pronounced in the younger age groups, especially below 20 years. There has been a constant decline in child sex ratio (CSR) over the last four to five censuses and there is a particularly steep decline in the report of 2011, which registered a fall from 927 girls per 1,000 boys in the age group of 0–6 years to 918 per 1,000 boys. This led to the aggressive implementation of the Preconception and Prenatal Diagnostic Techniques (PCPNDT) Act, rules and regulations by the government to improve the skewed ratios. While the sex ratio has seen a decrease, the silver lining is that there is an improvement in survival ratio and there is an upward shift for all age groups during Census 2001–2011.

The National Family Planning Program of the Ministry of Health and Family Welfare is guided by the tenets of the NPP 2000 and oversees its implementation. Under this program, the service delivery data are regularly reviewed through annual review meetings, supportive supervision visits, common review missions, etc.

As a result of the government's efforts, the successes achieved as on February, 2020 are enumerated below:[3,4]

- The TFR has declined from 2.9 in 2005 to 2.2 in 2017 (SRS)
- 25 out of 37 states/UTs have already achieved replacement level fertility of 2.1 or less
- The decadal growth rate has declined from 21.54% in 1999–2000 to 17.64% during 2001–2011
- The CBR has declined from 23.8 to 20.2 from 2005 to 2017 (SRS)
- The teenage birth rate has halved from 16% (NFHS III) to 8% (NFHS IV).

CURRENT ISSUES AND TRENDS IN POPULATION STABILIZATION

Current Issues

Population stabilization is a stage when the size of the population remains unchanged. Census data released by the Office of the Registrar General shows that at the national level, the TFR has declined from 2.5 to 2.2 during 2001–2011.[3,4] So, India has begun moving toward population stabilization showing a drop of 0.3 points in the TFR. (The TFR is the number of children born or likely to be born to a woman in her lifetime.)[3,4]

Data with the Health Ministry shows that so far, only 24 out of 35 states have achieved the TFR of 2.1 (2019) that are yet to reach the targeted TFR and 10 big states still have a higher TFR. Bihar leads at (3.4), UP (3.1), MP (2.9), Rajasthan (2.8), Jharkhand (3), Chhattisgarh (2.6), Assam and Gujarat (2.5), and Haryana and Odisha (2.3).

The proportion of married women to total number of women is at 49.9% in Census 2011 as against 47.7% in Census 2001. The corresponding figure in case of males has increased to 46% from 43.6% during the same period. For women, the average marriage age has increased from 18.3 to 19.3 years and for men from 22.6 to 23.3 years during Census 2001–2011. There are 30 million currently married women in the age group of 15–49 years.[5] The desired fertility rate is 1.8 which indicates that women in India prefer to have no more than two children.[6]

According to the NPP 2000, India should have reached a replacement-level fertility rate of 2.1 by 2010 to attain population stabilization at 145 crores by 2045. However, India expects to reach population stabilization of 2.1 TFR at 165 crores by 2040.[6]

Current Trends in Population Stabilization

NITI Aayog[7]

NITI Aayog is responsible for charting India's road map toward attaining the commitments under the Sustainable Development Goals, particularly in critical social sectors such as health and education. A 3-year action agenda and a 7-year strategy have already been prepared by the NITI Aayog and placed in the public domain.

The federal policy think tank of NITI Aayog consults subject specialists and officials to find ways of strengthening the country's population policy and family planning programs. The consultation is expected to result in recommendations that will address the regional disparities in the outcome of population stabilization programs. The NITI Aayog move comes in the wake of Prime Minister Narendra Modi flagging, in his Independence Day speech 2019, the need for controlling the explosive growth in population.

The key recommendations are likely to include helping women make informed choices about delaying pregnancy and ensuring there was a sufficient gap between childbirths, stepping up access to contraceptive choices, addressing sociocultural barriers toward contraception, increasing public spending on family planning, investing in behavior-change communication strategies, and treating population stabilization and family planning as a national priority. The NITI Aayog said that India is at a stage where birth rates are falling but population continues to grow due to the fact that >30% of the population is young and in the reproductive age group.

GOVERNMENT INITIATIVES

The government is taking several steps to sensitize people and generate awareness of the need for population control. Some of the important initiatives are as follows:[5]

- *360° media campaign*: The first phase of the campaign was launched in 2016 and the present second phase comprising TV commercials, posters and hoardings, year-long radio show, and a dedicated website on family planning was launched in 2017
- *World Population Day and fortnight* as well as *Vasectomy Fortnight* are observed every year to boost awareness.
- *Promotional activities* such as Saas Bahu Sammelans, Nayi Pehel Kits, mobile publicity vans, and advocacy meetings are undertaken to increase awareness in high-fertility Mission Parivar Vikas districts.

The government is implementing various schemes for improving access to quality family planning services, details of which are given below.

Steps being taken by the government for population control:

1. *Mission Parivar Vikas*: This was launched to increase access to contraceptive and family planning services in 146 high-fertility districts with TFR of 3 and above in seven high focus states. These districts are from the states of Uttar Pradesh, Bihar, Rajasthan, Madhya Pradesh, Chhattisgarh, Jharkhand, and Assam that itself constitute 44% of the country's population.
2. *New contraceptive choices*: New contraceptives, namely injectable contraceptive and centchroman, have been added to the existing basket of choices.
3. A new method of intrauterine contraceptive device (IUCD) insertion immediately after delivery, i.e., *postpartum IUCD (PPIUCD)*, has been introduced.
4. *Redesigned contraceptive packaging*: The packaging for condoms, oral contraceptive pills (OCPs), and emergency contraception pills (ECPs) has now been improved and redesigned so as to increase the demand for these commodities.
5. *Compensation scheme for sterilization acceptors*: Under this scheme, the Ministry of Health and Family Welfare (MoHFW) provides compensation for loss of wages to the beneficiary and also to the service provider (and team) for conducting sterilizations.

6. *Clinical Outreach Teams (COT) scheme*: The scheme has been launched in 146 Mission Parivar Vikas districts for providing family planning services through mobile teams from accredited organizations in far-flung, underserved, and geographically difficult areas.
7. Scheme for *home delivery* of contraceptives by ASHAs at the doorstep of beneficiaries.
8. Scheme for *ASHAs* to ensure spacing in births.
9. Scheme for *provision of pregnancy testing kits* in the drug kits of ASHAs for use in communities.
10. *Family planning logistic management and information system (FP-LMIS)*: This is dedicated software to ensure smooth forecasting, procurement, and distribution of family planning commodities across all the levels of health facilities.
11. *National family planning indemnity scheme (NFPIS)* under which clients are insured in the eventualities of death, complication, and failure following sterilization.
12. Ensuring *quality of care* in family planning services by establishing quality assurance committees in all states and districts.
13. Appointment of dedicated *RMNCH+A (Reproductive, Maternal, Newborn, Child and Adolescent Health) counselors* at high-case load facilities.
14. Improved demand generation activities through a 360° media campaign.

As a result of these efforts, the country is knocking on the door of replacement level fertility and is on track to achieve TFR 2.1 by 2025.

The Population Control Bill, 2019 (or Population Regulation Bill, 2019), is a proposed bill introduced in the Rajya Sabha in July 2019. The purpose of the bill is to control the population growth of India.

The 2020 bill proposes to introduce a two-child policy per couple and aims to incentivize its adoption through various measures such as educational benefits, taxation cuts, home loans, free healthcare, and better employment opportunities. Penalties for couples are not adhering to the two-child policy such as debarment from contesting in elections and ineligibility for government jobs.

Family Planning, 2020: Family planning division is working on the national and state-wise action plans so as to achieve Family Planning 2020 goals. The key commitments of Family Planning 2020 are as follows:

- Increasing financial commitment on family planning whereby India commits an allocation of 2 billion USD from 2012 to 2020
- Ensuring access to family planning services to 48 million (4.8 crore) additional women by 2020 (40% of the total Family Planning, 2020 goal)
- Sustaining the coverage of 100 million (10 crore) women currently using contraceptives
- Reducing the unmet need by an improved access to voluntary family planning services, supplies, and information.

Janasankhya Sthirata Kosh

The Jansankhya Sthirata Kosh (JSK) (National Population Stabilization Fund) has been registered in 2004–2005 as an autonomous society established under the Societies Registration Act of 1860 with Rs 100 crore grant from the government. This had an aim to promote and undertake activities aimed at achieving population stabilization at a level consistent with the needs of sustainable economic growth, social development, and environment protection by 2045.

It implemented the following schemes:

- Prerna Scheme (for delaying marriage, childbirth, and spacing)
- Santushti Scheme (Public Private Partnership for sterilization services)
- National Helpline (for information on family planning).

However, the JSK has been discontinued on 08/02/2019 vide the cabinet decision on 07/02/2018 and various schemes for population control are being supported under the National Health Mission.[8]

REFERENCES

1. Kishore J. National Health Program of India. New Delhi: Century Publication; 2012.
2. Saroha J. Demographic transition in India. IJRAR. 2017; 4(4): 193-8.
3. Ministry of Health and Family Welfare. (2020). National Population Policy. [online] Available from: https://pib.gov.in/PressReleasePage.aspx?PRID=1601839#:~:text=National%20Population%20Policy%20formulated%20in,maternal%20health%20and%20child%20survival. [Last accessed November, 2021].
4. The Pioneer. (2015). India begins population stabilization. [online] Available from: http://www.dailypioneer.com/2015/page1/india-begins-population-stabilization-html [Last accessed November, 2021].
5. Ministry of Health and Family Welfare. (2019). Population control. [online] https://pib.gov.in/PressReleseDetailm.aspx?PRID=1593004. [Last accessed November, 2021].
6. Press Information Bureau. [online] Available from: http://pib.gov.in/PressReleseDetailm.aspx?prid=133018 [Last accessed November, 2021].
7. India Today. [online] Available from: http://www.indiatoday.in/business/story/niti-aayog-to-draft-roadmap-for-population-stabilization-1629879-2019-12-19 [Last accessed November, 2021].
8. Journals of India. (2019). Jansankhya Sthirata Kosh. [online] Available from: https://journalsofindia.com/jansankhya-sthirata-kosh/. [Last accessed November, 2021].

LONG QUESTION

1. What precautions should the doctor take so that the MTP is safe medicolegally?

SHORT QUESTIONS

1. Who can perform MTP?
2. What are the pre-requisites for MTP approved center?

3. What are the indications to perform MTP.
4. Discuss: consent in MTP.
5. Judicial activism in abortion law in India: Dr Nikhil Datar Vs Union of India. Discuss

MULTIPLE CHOICE QUESTIONS

1 Inj Anti-D ______ mg should be administered in ABO incompatibility after first trimester MTP.
   a. 300 µg   b. 150 µg
   c. 50 µg   d. 200 µg
2 The permissible legal limit for MTP (under MTP Act 1971) in case of abnormal fetus is:
   a. 19 weeks   b. 24 weeks
   c. 20 weeks   d. 22 weeks
3 The amendment in 2002 in MTP Act dealt with:
   a. Increasing the permissible limit to 24 weeks
   b. Validating use of mifepristone and misoprostol
   c. Both a and b
   d. None of the above
4 The forms to be filled up in a case of MTP are:
   a. Form A + Form B   b. Form I
   c. Form I + Form C   d. All of the above
5 Medical MTP can be done uptil:
   a. 35 days   b. 49 days
   c. 63 days   d. 52 days
6 Second trimester MTP requires:
   a. Opinion of 2 RMPs
   b. Form 2
   c. Government hospital only
   d. Medical management

Answers

1. c 2. c 3. d 4. c 5. b 6. a

1.3 LEGAL ASPECTS IN MEDICAL TERMINATION OF PREGNANCY AND CONTRACEPTION

Nikhil Datar, Meghana Shedge

INTRODUCTION

Contraception and abortion are two important health rights of a woman. Social structure of male dominance, religious beliefs, and lack of health education change the outlook toward these issues. Thus, they do not remain to be pure medical issues.

In India, abortions are governed by a specific Act of the parliament, namely "Medical Termination of Pregnancy Act (MTP Act)." Contraception is not specifically covered by any law yet general principles of medical ethics, namely autonomy, justice, beneficence, and nonmaleficence, must be kept in mind by the healthcare provider.

LEGAL ASPECTS OF MEDICAL TERMINATION OF PREGNANCY

Abortion is a criminal offence according to the Indian Penal Code. This code was drafted in 1860 by the British, which is still the law of the land.

Sections 312 to 316 deal with the offences against unborn. Both a woman seeking abortion and the person helping her can be punished for this offence. Many women lost their lives while undergoing illegal abortions. In order to prevent this maternal mortality, India passed the MTP Act in 1971. It decriminalized the abortions in a limited manner. It carved out an exception to the general law, namely the Indian Penal code. Thus, abortions strictly done under the norms laid down by the MTP Act are not illegal anymore. However, if one transgresses the limits laid down by the MTP Act, a doctor can face criminal charges and may get prescribed punishment, which could be fine and/or imprisonment.[1]

The MTP Act was further amended in 2002 to introduce medical abortion by giving medications. Judicial activism by the author who filed the case, Dr Nikhil Datar Vs. Union of India, and series of cases filed in various High Courts and Supreme Court has paved way to another amendment. While this chapter is being written, the amendment to the MTP Act has been passed in both the houses of the parliament and has received the assent from the President of India. Yet the rules and regulations have not been amended and the amended law has not yet been applied. This amendment has upwardly revised the gestational age for termination to 24 weeks and above.[2]

Thus, for this article, MTP Act (1971 and 1992) and rules and regulations (1975 and 1992) have been taken into consideration.

A gynecologist must know the exact provisions of the MTP Act so as to stay clear of the potential medicolegal implications. The Act has eight sections and rules and regulations.

Section 2: Who can do MTP?

According to Section 2 of MTP Act and MTP Rules 2002, the registered medical practitioner (RMP) must be registered with state medical council and have qualification in accordance with section 2 of the Indian Medical Council Act (1956). The RMP adequate training/experience is as follows:

- Training house surgery post of 6 months in obstetrics and gynecology (OB-GYN)

- Experience of 1 year in a hospital in OB-GYN department
- RMP should have assisted 25 cases and done five cases independently in any institute which is approved as training center (for this experience, the RMP is eligible to do MTP only up to 12 weeks)
- Postgraduate degree/diploma in OB-GYN.

Section 3: In which conditions can the MTP be done?
MTP can be done:

- If there is a risk to the life of a woman
- If there is a grave injury to the physical or mental health of the mother

  The law further defines the "grave injury to mental health." It states that the below situations will be considered as grave injury:
  - Anguish caused by pregnancy alleged out of rape
  - Anguish causes by pregnancy caused due to failure of contraception by a married woman or her husband.

  While determining the risk of injury to health, "actual and reasonably foreseeable environment" should be taken into account.
- If there is a substantial risk that if the child were born, he/she shall suffer such serious mental or physical abnormalities as to be seriously handicapped.

Till what weeks of gestation can the MTP be done?
If the MTP is done to immediately to save the life of the woman, there is no upper limit on gestational age (Section 5).

For all other indications, the MTP can be done only up to 20 weeks of gestation.

Consent-taking for MTP
A written consent of the woman is mandatory. It should be taken in FORM C. The consent of the guardian is taken, if she is <18 years or lunatic. (This word is replaced by mentally ill in the amendment of 2002.)

An RMP must form his opinion in good faith while conducting the procedure.

For MTP to be done up to 12 weeks, one RMP can opine. For MTP beyond 12–20 weeks, opinion of two RMPs is required.

When MTP is done beyond 20 weeks as an "immediate necessity to save the mother's life", one RMP is enough to opine.

Section 4: Where can one do MTP?
MTP can be done only at a government hospital or hospitals approved by the government.

For medical MTP, approval of place is not required but the RMP must satisfy the criteria of qualification and experience. An RMP can provide the medical MTP only if the patients have an access to the approved center. Thus, the place must display the letter from the owner of approved place stating that the patients will be provided with the emergency services at the approved place 24 by 7.

How should nongovernmental clinics/hospitals get approval for MTP?

Approval of place is mandatory for surgical MTP.

The owner should apply in Form A to the Chief Medical Officer (CMO). The CMO inspects the place within 2 months of application and then recommends to committee, which gives an approval in form B within 2 months of inspection.

The owner has to display the certificate at a prominent place within the premises.

Section 6: The central government can make rules, which have to be passed in the parliament.

These rules are about the qualification of RMPs and the procedural aspect of approval of the place.

Section 7: States can make regulations related to MTP.

Contravention of any regulation attracts penalty of 1,000 rupees.

The regulations deal with the following:

1. There is a prescribed form in which the RMP has to register the details of cases:
   - *Form I*: The RMP/RMPs should certify his/her opinion regarding the MTP in Form I within 3 hours of such termination.
   - *Custody of forms*: The RMP has to make a sealed envelope of forms I and C and handover to the owner/head of the hospital/CMO of the state.
     - The RMP should write the serial number from the admission register and name of the RMP/RMPs. The word "Secret" should be written.
     - The owner should keep in safe custody. He/she shall make a monthly report in Form II.
     - In case MTP is done under Section 5 at a place not approved for MTP, the serial number and place shall be kept blank.
   - *Admission register:* Form III.

It is important that the register has all the 14 columns as described.
The admission register needs to be kept for 5 years from the end of the calendar year it relates to.

A fresh serial number for a new calendar year is given. The serial number will be in this format—5/2020.

It is confidential and not open for inspection except for any person under the authority of law; on application by an employed woman, the RMP can grant a certificate for the same.

The name is not to be entered in any case-sheet, operation theater register, follow-up card, or any other document or any other register. Only the serial number must be entered.

Section 8: It provides protection to the RMP from any suit related to MTP.

When MTP is done diligently and in good faith, the RMP enjoys the protection of law. Thus, if the RMP follows all the rules and regulations correctly, it can be said that the MTP is done in good faith and conscientiously. Thus, it is vital that standards laid down by the ministry are followed by the RMP while doing the MTP cases.[1]

EXAMINATION AND INVESTIGATIONS

Elaborate history should be elicited with proper examination; ultrasonography as a routine is not mandatory.

Basic blood investigation such as Hb, blood group, and urine testing to be done.

In cases of Rh incompatibility, injection Anti-D—50 µg in the first trimester and 300 µg in the second trimester should be administered.

- Another important aspect is to provide counseling before and after the MTP.
- *Medical management:* MTP can be done up to 7 weeks of gestation with mifepristone and misoprostol regimen: On day 1, mifepristone 200 mg oral tablet followed by 400 µg misoprostol oral/vaginal/sublingual on day 3. The Drug Controller of India has allowed use of combipack of mifepristone and misoprostol until 63 days of gestation. It is expected that the amendment to the rules will take into consideration this discrepancy and resolve the same.

  Also, symptomatic treatment for abdominal pain/nausea/vomiting/loose motions should be provided.
- *Treatment of failure:* If POCs are seen in cervix, digital evacuation or vacuum aspiration (VA) can be done.

  If USG suggests incomplete evacuation, additional 600 µg of misoprostol can be given.

  If no sac seen, "wait and watch" approach can be followed.

SURGICAL METHOD FOR MEDICAL TERMINATION OF PREGNANCY

- *Vacuum aspiration or dilatation and evacuation:*
  - Vacuum aspiration is preferred over the traditional dilatation and curettage. The evidence shows that there is 3–4 times higher chances of excessive bleeding, infection, and perforation as compared to D&C.
  - The need for dilatation is lesser in VA and the recovery is faster.
  - Vacuum aspiration should be done in case up to 12 weeks size for MTP/miscarriage/incomplete abortion and retained products of conceptions (RPOCs).

Priming of the cervix: Tablet misoprostol 400 µg 3–4 hours prior oral or vaginally and injection prostaglandin F2α (PGF2α) can be administered 45 minutes before.

- *Methods of second-trimester MTP*: *Surgical, medical, and miscellaneous:* Surgical method is not commonly used, but when required priming can be done by tablet misoprostol 400 µg; per vaginum 3–4 hours prior or per oral route 2–3 hours prior is preferred. Few prefer to use osmotic dilators before evacuation of uterus.

  A hysterotomy can be attempted in case of failure of medical method or if an associated gynecological procedure needs to be carried out.

  The medical method uses tablet mifepristone + misoprostol, but it is not yet approved in India.

  By the WHO regimen, misoprostol 400 µg can be given every 3 hourly for five doses.
- *Second-trimester MTP*: Mifepristone + misoprostol for second trimester is not currently recommended in India. Permitted methods are:
  1. Ethacridine lactate
  2. Dilatation and evacuation (maximum 16 weeks) and hysterotomy
  3. Adjuvant therapy which includes tablet misoprostol for priming and PGF2α/20 units of oxytocin for hastening the termination.
- *Postabortion advice*: 75% women ovulate and 6% conceive within 2–6 weeks of abortion.

  All contraceptives can be offered after first-trimester MTP including laparoscopic tubal ligation (TL).

  A laparoscopic TL cannot be done after second-trimester MTP, but abdominal TL can be done.

MTP beyond 20 Weeks: Judicial Activism

- In 2008, Dr Nikhil Datar filed his first case against the Union of India where he helped a woman with 24 weeks period of gestation with severely abnormal fetus for termination and ever since then he has helped more than 150 women to file cases for termination of pregnancy beyond 20 weeks.
- These cases paved way for the proposed amendment to the existing Act. The amendment has been formally passed in both the houses of parliament and received the assent of the President of India. It is expected that the government will notify the application of the amended Act any time in near future.

LEGAL ASPECTS IN CONTRACEPTION

As stated earlier, although there is no specific law governing the subject of contraception, the general framework of ethics and law needs to be followed. The general principles of reproductive rights include:

- The rights of men and women to be informed and to have access to safe, effective, affordable, and acceptable methods of family planning of their choice, as well as other methods of their choice for regulation of fertility, which are not against the law.
- The right of access to appropriate healthcare services that will enable women to safely go through pregnancy and childbirth and provide couples with the best chance of having a healthy infant.

Reproductive health problems can be prevented and solved by offering an array of contraceptive methods, techniques, and services. The couples should be empowered to select, change, and discontinue a method as per their needs. Proper screening, provision of contraceptive services in adherence with guidelines, management of side effects, and follow-up procedures for specific contraceptive methods are the key elements in reproductive health.

Current trends in family planning in India show a high level of knowledge among eligible couples, yet the acceptance remains low, especially for spacing methods. Female sterilization remains the most widely used family planning method in spite of efforts to popularize male sterilization.

Counseling is the cornerstone:

- A single method of family planning cannot be recommended to everyone. Family planning counseling can help a woman and/or her partner to choose which method best suits him or her.
- Counseling facilitates decision-making, promoting continuation of contraceptive, counseling about side effects, prevention of unwanted pregnancy, and also sex education.

CONCLUSION

A gynecologist plays a vital role in ensuring the reproductive health of the society. This subject is not purely medical in nature. It has ramifications into rights, ethics, and law. While treating the patients, the doctor should also stay safe and within the limits of law.

REFERENCES

1. Ministry of Health and Family Welfare. The Medical Termination of Pregnancy Act, 1971. [online] Available from: https://main.mohfw.gov.in/acts-rules-and-standards-health-sector/acts/mtp-act-1971. [Last accessed November, 2021].
2. Ministry of Health and Family Welfare. The Medical Termination of Pregnancy Amendment Act, 2002. [online] Available from: https://main.mohfw.gov.in/acts-rules-and-standards-health-sector/acts/mtp-act-amendment-2002. [Last accessed November, 2021].

LONG QUESTION

1. What precautions should the doctor take so that the MTP is safe medicolegally?

SHORT QUESTIONS

1. Who can perform MTP?
2. What are the prerequisites for an MTP-approved center?
3. What are the indications to perform MTP?
4. Discuss consent in MTP.
5. Discuss judicial activism in abortion law in India: Dr Nikhil Datar Vs Union of India.

MULTIPLE CHOICE QUESTIONS

1. Injection Anti-D ______ mg should be administered in ABO incompatibility after first trimester MTP.
   a. 300 µg b. 150 µg
   c. 50 µg d. 200 µg
2. The permissible legal limit for MTP (under MTP Act 1971) in case of an abnormal fetus is:
   a. 19 weeks b. 24 weeks
   c. 20 weeks d. 22 weeks
3. The amendment in 2002 in MTP Act dealt with:
   a. Increasing the permissible limit to 24 weeks
   b. Validating use of mifepristone and misoprostol
   c. Both a and b
   d. None of the above
4. The forms to be filled up in a case of MTP are:
   a. Form A + Form B
   b. Form I
   c. Form I + Form C
   d. All of the above
5. Medical MTP can be done until:
   a. 35 days b. 49 days
   c. 63 days d. 52 days
6. Second-trimester MTP requires:
   a. Opinion of two RMPs
   b. Form 2
   c. Government hospital only
   d. Medical management

Answers

1. c 2. c 3. d 4. c 5. b 6. a

Contraception: Spacing Methods

2.1 NATURAL AND BEHAVIORAL METHODS OF CONTRACEPTION

Vijyalakshmi Pillai

INTRODUCTION

Unintended pregnancies are estimated to be in the tune of about 42%[1] in India. Most of these unintended pregnancies are unwanted too. The practice of prevention of unintended pregnancies (birth control) is as old as human civilization. For many thousands of years, birth control was practiced based on imagination. The most practiced effective method of birth control since antiquity is *coitus interruptus*.[2] This remains to be practiced widely even today. When the man realized that sex led to pregnancy, he started practicing periodic *abstinence* as the most effective form of birth control.

Almost all couples rely on behavioral methods of contraception at least sometimes in their lifetime. As a matter of conformity, abstinence is considered the norm in adolescents. Women tend to practice abstinence at all ages. Vatsyayana's classical text from the second century CE has described various methods of birth control, including coitus interruptus.

To a large group of people with stringent religious practices, cultural taboos, and social reach and awareness, natural family planning (NFP) methods and fertility awareness methods (FAM) are probably the only acceptable methods of birth control.

Behavioral methods of contraception can be of two categories:

1. Methods that do not rely on the menstrual cycle (i.e., abstinence and coitus interruptus)
2. Methods that rely on the menstrual cycle.

Methods that rely on the menstrual cycle can be further subdivided into:

- Fertility awareness methods (FAM)
- "Natural" family planning (NFP).

Fertility awareness methods are methods that rely on a woman to monitor changes in her body during her menstrual cycle. NFP relies on the menstrual calendar to discern fertile from nonfertile days. NFP allows couples to control unplanned pregnancies irrespective of economic status and regardless of the supply chain. There is a need for better training of masses, better learning tools, and instructions in NFP to maximize the potential benefits of these methods.

HISTORY OF NATURAL METHODS OF CONTRACEPTION

In the year 1905, Theodoor Hendrik van de Velde, a Dutch gynecologist, described that woman ovulates once per menstrual cycle. In the 1930s, Kyusaku Ogino, a Japanese gynecologist, and Hermann Haus, from Austria, separately discovered that ovulation occurs about 14 days before the next menstrual period and fertilization occurs on that day. This was a breakthrough discovery that allowed the calculation of the fertile and infertile period of a woman's menstrual cycle. The Ogino-Knaus theory[3] became known as the calendar method in 1934. This was promoted by the Roman Catholic faith, which reprimands all artificial birth control methods.

In the 1930s and 1940s, enhanced perception of ovulation and associated temperature changes brought in the temperature method. In 1964, John Billings' work in understanding cyclical changes in cervical mucus led to the development of the cervical mucus method or Billings method.

By the 1990s, the symptothermal method (STM) combining all fertility indicators was developed and was found to be efficient. Various devices and smartphone applications are now available, which can monitor a woman's menstrual cycle, based on changes in temperature, urinary hormones, or saliva.

CANDIDATES FOR NATURAL FAMILY PLANNING OR FERTILITY AWARENESS METHODS

Those women who have regular menstrual cycles are fitting candidates for NFP techniques. Hence, women with polycystic ovary syndrome (PCOS) and other menstrual disturbing disorders, postpartum and postabortal women, and perimenopausal women are precluded as eligible candidates for NFP. Some medications can disrupt menstrual cycles, and women on such medications are not suitable for NFP. Concurrence of both members of the couple is mandatory for successful NFP. Users should be well counseled about emergency contraception in occasional noncompliance.

Advantages of NFP include the following:
- Acknowledgment of their fertility needs
- Dependence on their resources
- Nonreliability on distant medical services and hence practical
- Nonusage of artificial substances and their possible side effects
- Reduced resupply costs
- Intimacy with a partner due to better communication
- Coherence to religious and cultural practices.

Disadvantages of NFP include the following:
- Sexually transmitted infections are not prevented.
- Requires training from experts.
- Unrelenting to incorrect use.
- Partner concurrence and liaison are essential.
- Women with irregular cycles are inappropriate candidates.
- Diligent daily monitoring and recording are essential.

EFFICACY AND CONTINUATION RATES

The failure rate of typical users is reported as around 25%.[4] The most common reason for the actual lower effectiveness is not due to improper instructions or ignorance but conscious user noncompliance. Nevertheless, the failure rate associated with correct and compatible method users, especially using contraceptive efficacy mobile applications, is very small. Calendar method or the rhythm method has a failure rate of 9% with proper use, whereas the ovulation detection method has 3% failure, 2% for the STM, and 1% for the post-ovulation method.[5] Studies on contraceptive efficacy of certain mobile applications such as "natural cycle mobile application," which evaluated "perfect- and typical-use Pearl index," were found to be 6.9 pregnancies per 100 woman-years.[6] Widespread use of such mobile applications may come up with solutions to bridge the unfulfilled need for contraception.

NATURAL CONTRACEPTIVE OPTIONS

Abstinence

Avoiding penetrative sex prevents pregnancy 100% and prevents sexually transmitted infections as well. Many cultures insist on periods of prolonged abstinence in unmarried adults. Initiation of first sex is culturally delayed in many societies and this has a positive impact on pregnancy prevention and can have many potential benefits in health, education, and monetary.

Withdrawal or Coitus Interruptus

This is a male-controlled method and different from other contraceptive methods. It is known for several millennia. Preventing ejaculation into the vagina prevents pregnancy. This is very popular in many countries such as Romania, Turkey, Mauritius, and the Czech Republic.

Exact data regarding prevalence, acceptability, use effectiveness, and the safety of use is not clear. It offers contraceptive effectiveness like barrier methods. The best-estimated efficacy is that about 4% of couples would fail and have an unplanned pregnancy in the first year. Typical users probably would have about 19% pregnancy in the first year.[7] It is not an ideal method of contraception. It is still a choice of contraception for those who use it effectively.

Calendar Methods

In the calendar method or rhythm method, the days of the fertile period are calculated based on the past menstrual cycle length. Various versions of the calendar method exist. All of them necessitate, fixing the days for abstinence or avoiding unprotected intercourse, by calculating the probable fertile phase. The expectation is that the length of the current menstrual cycle is similar to the past cycles and thus the fertile phase is similar to previous cycles. The fertile period includes, at least, the 5 days before ovulation and the day after based on the assumption that sperm is alive 1–3 days and the egg is fertilizable up to 24 hours after ovulation. Accurate use of this method requires knowledge of at least the past six natural menstrual cycles of the practicing woman. Abstinence days are calculated by subtracting 18 from her shortest cycle number. This forms the 1st day of abstinence. The last day of abstinence happens on the day, which is calculated by subtracting 11 from the longest cycle. This is an 11–18 rule. The interval may be adjusted depending on the length of the previous cycle. Others have modified this rule as 9–19, 7–12, and 12–17. Typical use efficacy of this method is 9% in the first year of practice.[8] The calendar method is reported to be the most common of natural methods. Women with irregular and unpredictable cycles are not the ideal suiters for this method.

Standard Days Method

The standard days method (SOM)[9] is a simple fertility awareness-based method. It relies on a "standard rule" or a fixed "window" of fertility that makes it easy for women to know when they are likely to become pregnant. A mnemonic device is used to teach couples to keep track of their fertility. This can be a calendar on which women record their cycles or cycle beads (**Fig. 1**) representing the fertile and infertile days of the menstrual cycle.

Methods Based on Symptoms and Signs

Ovulation Method/Billings Method/Cervical Mucus Method

Billings method of ovulation detection is formulated based on the knowledge of changes in quantity and quality of cervical/vaginal secretions happening during an ovulatory menstrual cycle. These changes happen because of swing in estrogen and progesterone levels during a menstrual cycle. Women are taught to feel the secretions by touching with their finger or a paper against the vaginal introitus every day before urination throughout their cycle. The testing is "negative" when cervical mucous is scanty as in the initial follicular phase. As the follicular phase progresses, the vaginal mucous secretions increase slightly but remain viscous. The estrogen surge, which happens preovulatory, profusely increases the amount of these secretions and makes them clearer and elastic (creating the maximal finger-to-thumb Spinnbarkeit sign) (**Fig. 2**).

Couples are expected to practice either abstinence or use a barrier method from the time calculated when they first feel sticky mucus until 4 days after the last clear mucous secretion. Postovulation, the progestogenic influence causes mucus to thicken and become sticky again. Unprotected intercourse is allowed after 3 days of dry secretions. Women practicing the Billings method have to learn about their menstrual cycles. The best collected information is when they are practicing abstinence for about 6–9 months. They have to learn to interpret mucous patterns. The best elucidation is when they practice sex every other day. This enables her to assess her fertility without having her measurements muddled by seminal fluid or vaginal secretions. Factors that can confuse

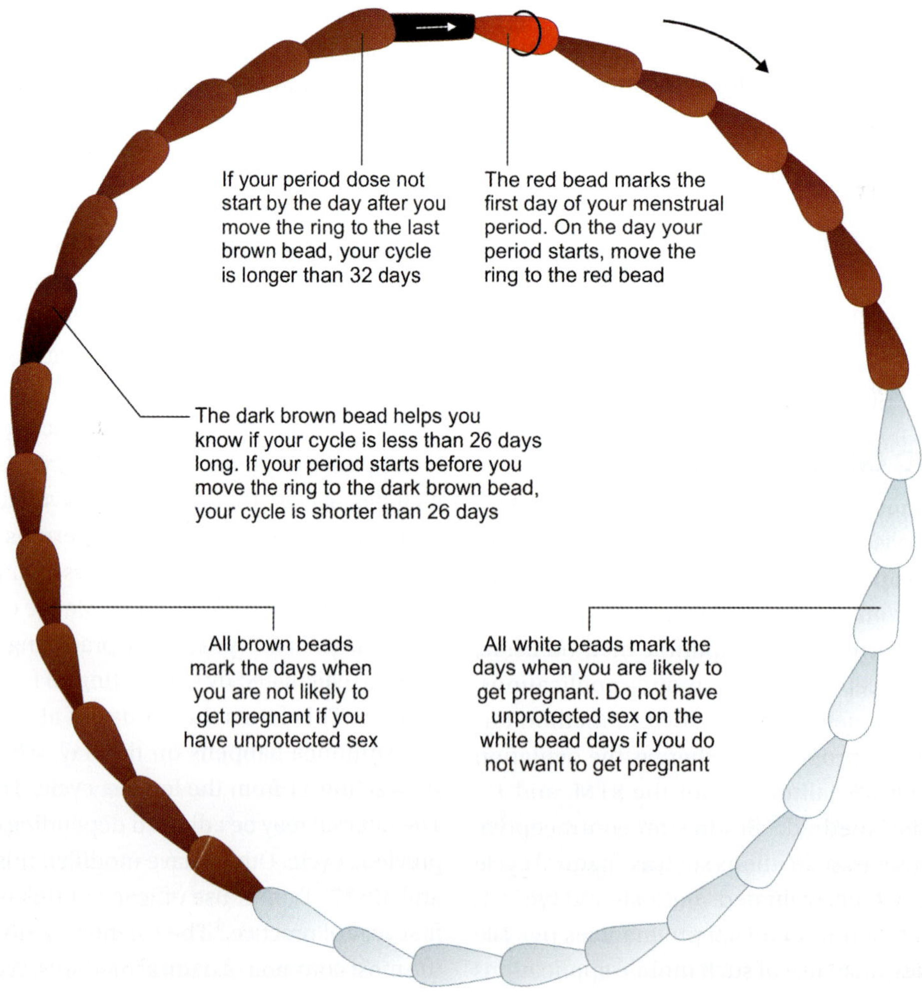

Fig. 1: CycleBeads.
Source: Institute for Reproductive Health, Georgetown University.

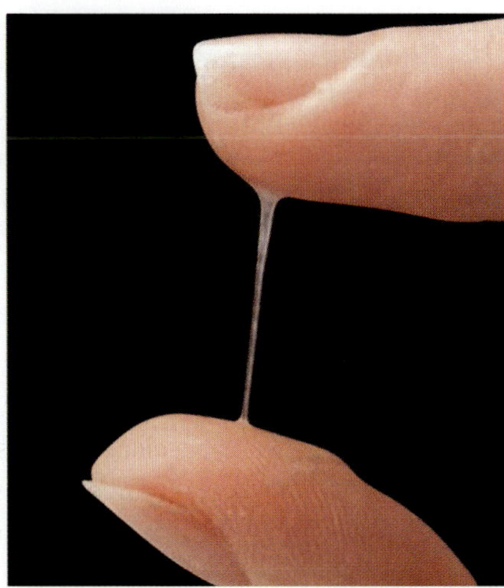

Fig. 2: Spinnbarkeit of cervical mucus.

with the interpretation of cervical mucus are vaginal infection, vaginal therapies, and douching.

The World Health Organization (WHO) data from five countries—New Zealand, India, Ireland, Philippines, and El Salvador—showed that, when best used, the first-year probability of unplanned pregnancy was 3.4%. The failure rate was 22.5% in the first year for faulty and inaccurate use.[10]

Basal Body Temperature Method

Progesterone has a thermogenic action on the hypothalamus. Body temperature increases by 0.2–0.5°C after ovulation. This rise in body temperature remains throughout the luteal phase until the end of the cycle, following a slight dip in basal body temperature (BBT). The woman practicing the BBT method should record her temperature every day, immediately after waking up before getting out of bed and starting any activity. Abstinence or protected sex is practiced from the first day of the cycle till after the third consecutive day of raised temperature. By this, unprotected sex is relegated to the postovulatory infertile time. Ovulation occurs within 48 hours of the temperature shift. The BBT method stipulates typical abstinence between 14 and 21 days, making it the most demanding among different natural methods of contraception. The effectiveness is high, if compliance from the couple is good for the schedule. The first-year probability of pregnancy is only about 2%[11] for perfect adherers. But, during typical use, the probability of pregnancy is near 20%. Failures in this method can be due to external factors, in febrile illness, if the temperature is taken at varied times each day, alcohol, emotional or physical stress, sleep disturbance, change of room temperature, change of waking time, change of climate, and recent start or discontinuation of birth control pills or antipyretic. In real life, only 80% of women have interpretable BBT patterns. The best use of BBT is as a postovulatory method or at best in combination with other methods of prediction of ovulation.

2-day Method

A relatively new easy technique using cervical secretions called the 2-day method is developed, which depends on just the presence or absence of cervical secretions to determine whether or not she is fertile each day. Each day, the practicing woman questions herself if she observed vaginal secretions that day as well as if she had observed secretions the prior day. She is considered fertile if she observes cervical secretions of any type on that day and the prior day. Practicing abstinence on such days or having protected sex helps her to achieve contraception. With proper understanding and use, this method has a first-year pregnancy rate of no more than 3% and 13.7% with typical use.[12] More than 96% of participants had no difficulty in ascertaining secretions after the third cycle. The average number of days when they had secretions was 12.1, which is akin to the "standard days method". The mean length of the period for abstinence or use of a barrier method in practicing couples is estimated to be about 10 days.

Symptothermal Technique

A combination of two of the above FAM to predict ovulation daily is the STM. It is a better method of detection of ovulation. The method typically is monitoring and charting cervical changes at ovulation such as Spinnbarkeit of mucus and cervical position (at ovulation, the cervix is softer, moist, dilates, and elevates in the vagina) and temperature changes (BBT) daily. This can also include symptoms of ovulation, such as breast tenderness, mittelschmerz, changes in libido, or light intermenstrual bleeding/spotting. The correct use of this method entails abstinence or protected sex from the first sign or symptom of ovulation up to at least 3 days after the peak day is observed. This method combines recommendations of the ovulation method to determine the beginning of a fertile period and that of the BBT method (postovulatory approach) to determine its conclusion. It helps to reduce the number of days of abstinence than when the BBT method is used alone. The cumbersome daily measurement and charting are more taxing than any of the above FAMs. The overall pregnancy rate was 1.8% after 13 cycles of use. In spite of being cumbersome, fewer couples discontinued and the discontinuation rate due to dissatisfaction was only 9.2% after 13 cycles.[13]

Ovulation Detection Monitors

Home tests and devices are available to monitor the fertile period in a cycle. Many use these in addition to traditional techniques, while others use them as a substitute. Most devices are marketed to help an infertile couple track ovulation.

Ovulation predictor kits (OPKs) are cheap and found in most drugstores. The kits work by qualitatively testing the luteinizing hormone (LH) in urine. The kits can predict LH surge which happens 12–36 hours before ovulation. They are

>90% accurate in most studies. Modern digital kits available have displays that are easier to read.

Progesterone ovulation tests: These kits are available over the counter in many drugstores. The kits are designed to test the level of progesterone metabolite in urine over several days. The metabolite pregnanediol-3-glucuronide (PDG)[14] levels typically rise 24–36 hours after ovulation. It is to determine postovulation status.

Saliva or "ferning" microscopes: These are compact microscopes, like lipstick cases, that can examine a sample of saliva. Toward ovulation, the estrogen level rises and salts in saliva increase. These salts form a fern-like pattern under the microscope while viewing through it. Hence, one looks at the saliva under a microscope to see the fern-like pattern.

Fertility monitors: They are expensive but very efficient. Most ovulation predictors can only give a fertile window of up to 2 days whereas these monitors show up to 6 or 7 days of fertile days for each cycle. These monitors work in different methods. The Clearblue Fertility Monitor predicts by measuring LH levels as well as the hormone e3G (estrone-3-glucuronide) in urine. The results are displayed on a digital screen and are simple to comprehend. The results are stored in monitor memory for easy recall. Studies presume it to be >90% accurate.

The OvaCue Fertility Monitor checks levels of electrolytes in saliva and uses computer analysis and memory. It is easy to use by just sticking a sensor in the mouth, can store data, and displays results on a screen. A vaginal sensor can confirm ovulation. The accuracy of the results is mixed.

Lady Free Biotester is a small hand-held microscope used to check for cervical mucus and the Clearplan Easy Fertility Monitor is available in the United States. It measures urinary metabolites.

A few FAMs and devices and their efficacy have been summed up in **Table 1**. The data are regarding first-year use pregnancy rates or probabilities per 100 woman-years based on a recent systematic review.[15,16]

TABLE 1: Fertility awareness methods and devices and their efficacy. The following data are regarding first-year use pregnancy rates or probabilities per 100 woman-years based on a recent systematic review.[17]

Fertility awareness methods and devices	***Efficacy—1st-year use pregnancy rates***
Standard days method	11.2–14.1
2-day method	13.7
Billings ovulation method	10.5–33.6
Marquette mucus—only method	4–18.5
Basal body temperature methods	9.0–9.8
Single-check symptothermal methods	13.2
Thyma double-check symptothermal methods	11.2–33.0
Sensiplan	1.8
Persona	25.6
Marquette monitor—only method	2–6.8
Marquette monitor and mucus method	6–7

Lactational Amenorrhea Method

The use of breastfeeding as a contraceptive method is called the lactational amenorrhea method (LAM). LAM was defined during the 1988 Bellagio Consensus Conference in Italy.[17] LAM is considered a "transitional" form of contraception. The hypothalamic-pituitary-ovarian axis is temporarily suppressed during the postpartum period. It is mostly due to lactation-induced temporary prolactin elevation. Prolactin decreases gonadotropin-releasing hormone release. The ensuing pattern of LH secretion inhibits ovarian activity. To use LAM efficiently, a woman must have amenorrhea since delivery, should be exclusively breastfeeding, and should be within 6 months of delivery. Lactational amenorrhea caused by breastfeeding in the first 6 months postpartum is an almost accurate indicator of suppression of ovulation. A fully lactating woman usually has anovulatory menstruation in the first 6 months postpartum; menstruation usually precedes ovulation. This menstruation can be utilized by women as an efficient time to adapt to other contraceptive methods to protect themselves. Mostly after 6 months of lactational amenorrhea, the first cycle is usually ovulatory. There is a possibility of a return of fertility and thereby unintended pregnancy, if she is exclusively relying on LAM beyond 6 months, especially when breastfeeding diminishes and/or more frequent supplemental feeding is initiated.

Lactational amenorrhea method is >98% effective during the first 6 months, as by many studies. LAM is a popular and efficient family planning method with high acceptance. Its efficacy is thought to be 99.5%.[18] Researches have also suggested that LAM may be reliable for perhaps up to a year after delivery.

CONCLUSION

Total sexual abstinence is the most effective method of birth control but the least observable. Poor commitment results in high rates of unplanned pregnancies. Periodic abstinence and FAMs depend on menstrual calendars. CycleBeads, BBT, the Billings method, and the symptothermal method are used to detect at-risk fertile days. Coitus interruptus has high failure rates. LAM is very effective for up to 6 months postpartum. Other practices which may not be characterized as coitus provide sexual pleasure without provoking unintended pregnancy but do not protect against STIs.

KEY MESSAGES

The oldest contraceptives, abstinence and coitus interruptus, are still practiced. Behavioral methods of contraception are of two categories—methods that do not rely on the menstrual cycle and that rely on the menstrual cycle. Methods that rely on the menstrual cycle are of two types—fertility awareness methods (FAM) and natural family planning methods (NFM). Women with regular cycles can practice NFM. These are accepted by most religions and by all cultures. They are unforgiving of incorrect use. Typical failure rate is 25%. Calendar methods, standard days method, ovulation method, basal body temperature method, 2-day method, symptothermal techniques, ovulation detection monitors, and lactational amenorrhea method are the NFMs discussed.

REFERENCES

1. Singh S, Shekhar C, Acharya R, Moore AM, Stillman M, Pradhan MR, et al. The incidence of abortion and unintended pregnancy in India, 2015. Lancet Glob Health. 2018;6(1):e111-20.
2. Carrick PJ. Medical Ethics in the Ancient World. Washington, DC: Georgetown University Press; 2001. p. 294.
3. James WH. The arithmetic of the rhythm method of contraception. BJOG. 1963;70(3):470-2.
4. Russo JA, Nelson AL. Behavioral methods of contraception. In: Shoupe D, Kjos SL, Totowa NJ (Eds). The Handbook of Contraception: A Guide for Practical Management. Totowa: Humana Press; 2006. pp. 179-94.
5. Hatcher RA. Contraceptive Technology. United States: Ardent Media; 2007. p. 941.
6. Bull J, Rowland S, Lundberg O, Berglund-Scherwitzl E, Gemzell-Danielsson K, Trussell J, et al. Typical use effectiveness of natural cycles: postmarket surveillance study investigating the impact of previous contraceptive choice on the risk of unintended pregnancy. BMJ Open. 2019;9(3):e026474.
7. Casey FE. (2020). Contraception: Practice Essentials, Overview, Periodic Abstinence. [online] Available from: https://emedicine.medscape.com/article/258507-overview. [Last accessed November, 2021].
8. Kambic RT, Lamprecht V. Calendar rhythm efficacy: a review. Database of Abstracts of Reviews of Effects (DARE): Quality-assessed Reviews. Centre for Reviews and Dissemination (UK);1996 12(2):123-8.
9. Arévalo M, Jennings V, Sinai I. Efficacy of a new method of family planning: the Standard Days Method. Contraception. 2002;65(5):333-8.
10. A prospective multicentre trial of the ovulation method of natural family planning. The effectiveness phase. Fertil Steril. 1981;36(5):591-8.
11. Bartzen PJ. Effectiveness of the temperature rhythm system of contraception. Fertil Steril. 1967;18(5):694-706.
12. Arévalo M, Jennings V, Nikula M, Sinai I. Efficacy of the new TwoDay Method of family planning. Fertil Steril. 2004;82(4):885-92.
13. Frank-Herrmann P, Heil J, Gnoth C, Toledo E, Baur S, Pyper C, et al. The effectiveness of a fertility awareness-based method to avoid pregnancy in relation to a couple's sexual behaviour during the fertile time: a prospective longitudinal study. Hum Reprod. 2007;22(5):1310-9.
14. Gifford RM, Howie F, Wilson K, Johnston N, Todisco T, Crane M, et al. Confirmation of ovulation from urinary progesterone analysis: assessment of two automated assay platforms. Sci Rep. 2018;8(1):17621.
15. Urrutia RP, Polis CB, Jensen ET, Greene ME, Kennedy E, Stanford JB. Effectiveness of fertility awareness-based methods for pregnancy prevention: a systematic review. Obstet Gynecol. 2018;132(3):591-604.
16. Urrutia RP, Polis CB. Fertility awareness-based methods for pregnancy prevention. BMJ. 2019;l4245.
17. Bellagio. (1988). Consensus Statement: Lactational Amenorrhea Method for Family Planning. [online] Available from: http://www.linkagesproject.org/LAMCD/publicationsconE.htm. [Last accessed November, 2021].
18. Van der Wijden C, Manion C. Lactational amenorrhoea method for family planning. Cochrane Database Syst Rev. 2015;(10):2015.

LONG QUESTIONS

1. NFP has yet to reach its maximum potential in spite of being the easiest available contraceptive option. Elaborate.
2. Discuss the role of AI (artificial intelligence) in fertility awareness.
3. Explain natural family planning (NFP).
4. Explain calendar method of contraception.
5. What are cycle beads and how is it used?

SHORT QUESTIONS

1. Define and classify behavioral methods of contraception.
2. Is abstinence a contraceptive choice that is universally suitable? Comment.
3. What is NFP or FAM? What are the pros and cons? Who are suitable couples for this method?
4. Enumerate FAMs based on symptoms and signs.
5. What is Billings method?
6. Write a short note on ovulation detection monitors.
7. What are the advantages and problems of the coitus interruptus method?
8. Write a short note on Standard Days Method.
9. What are the criteria to be fulfilled for Lactational Amenorrhea Method to be effective?

MULTIPLE CHOICE QUESTIONS

1. Commonest reason for high failure rates of NFP:
   a. Lack of awareness
   b. Unavailability of healthcare resources
   c. User non-compliance
   d. Inadequate studies
2. Which of the following does not affect BBT?
   a. Sleep
   b. Recent commencement of OCPs
   c. Mood
   d. BMI
3. Which of these is not a natural contraceptive option?
   a. Calendar method
   b. Standard Days method
   c. Billings method
   d. Coitus interruptus

4. Which of the following is true?
   a. There is a slight elevation in body temperature after ovulation, then remains elevated till the end of the cycle
   b. There is a slight dip in body temperature before ovulation, then rises after ovulation and remains elevated till the end of the cycle
   c. There is a slight elevation in body temperature after ovulation, then drops and remains low till the end of the cycle
   d. None of the above
5. Which of the following is not a suitable candidate for NFP?
   a. PCOS b. Women on OCPs
   c. Lactating mother d. All of the above
6 A 40-year woman, known case of breast CA on tamoxifen–preferred choice of contraception:
   a. NFP b. OCPs
   c. Barrier method d. None of the above
7. Symptothermal technique includes all, except:
   a. Cervical mucus monitoring
   b. Ovulation detection kits
   c. Mittelschmerz
   d. BBT method
8. Black beads on Cycle Beads is placed on which location?
   a. 28 & 32 b. 27 & 32
   c. 27 & 33 d. 28 & 33
9. Rise in body temperature after ovulation is due to:
   a. Progesterone b. Estrogen
   c. FSH d. LH
10. Two-day method uses:
   a. Cervical secretions b. Progesterone levels
   c. Estrogen levels d. LH levels
11. Progesterone ovulation kit tests the level of:
   a. Pregnanediol -3-glucoronide
   b. 3 alpha dihydroprogesterone
   c. Allopregnanolone
   d. 20 alpha dihydroprogesterone
12. In cervical mucus method, intercourse may be permitted after how many days of dry secretions?
   a. 6 b. 4
   c. 7 d. 3
13. Changes in quantity and quality of cervical/vaginal secretions are due to effects of swings in levels of:
   a. Progesterone
   b. Estrogen
   c. FSH and LH
   d. Estrogen and progesterone
14. The infertile beads in cycle beads are:
   a. White b. Black
   c. Brown d. Red
15. Following statements about Lactational amenorrhea method is true:
   a. A 'transitional' form of contraception
   b. The woman must remain amenorrhoeic since delivery
   c. A fully lactating woman usually has anovulatory menstruation in the first 6 months postpartum
   d. All of the above

Answer

1.	c	2.	c	3.	c	4.	b	5.	d	6.	c
7.	b	8.	b	9.	a	10.	a	11.	a	12.	b
13.	d	14.	c	15.	d						

2.2 MALE BARRIER METHODS

Rujuta Fuke

INTRODUCTION

The prevention of pregnancy is one of the most important aspects of practice of medicine. This fertility control can be achieved through various contraceptive practices.[1] This also forms the basis of management of controlling the population explosion. With the advent of science, various means of newer mechanical and chemical contraceptives are now available such as condoms, hormonal contraceptive pills, depot preparations, and intrauterine devices (IUDs).[2]

This chapter focuses on the male barrier methods of contraption such as male condoms and spermicides.

The barrier method of contraception, the most popular method worldwide, acts as a barrier to the process of fertilization preventing the union of sperms and ovum necessary for pregnancy.[3] This is the simplest, safest, cheapest, and effective method of contraception, if properly used.

Recently, the barrier method of contraception has gained much more importance as it prevents precancerous lesion and cancer of the cervix as well as acquired immunodeficiency syndrome (AIDS) and other sexually transmitted infections (STIs).[4]

The male barrier methods of contraception can broadly be divided into:

- *Male condom*: This is one of the most popular mechanical barriers and, among all of the barrier methods, the one that provides the most effective protection of the genital tract from sexually transmitted diseases (STDs).
- *Spermicidal agent*: It prevents sperm from entering the cervical canal by attacking the sperm's flagella and body,

reducing their mobility, and disrupting metabolism thereby inhibiting their nourishment. These are mainly available in the form of jellies, foam tablets, or films to be inserted in vagina just before the act of coitus.

HISTORY

Known by various names, condoms are the oldest and most widely used birth control device in the world. The mention of barrier methods of contraception dates back to 15th century when use of moistened linen was proposed as a means of protection against venereal diseases. In the 18th century, it was quite popular but only among rich and royals, as it was used to be made from the cecum of sheep and other animals.[5] With the vulcanization of rubber in 1844, condoms were made from rubber but manufacturing of rubber condoms was a laborious task and the quality of rubber used to deteriorate in a short span.[6] This drawback was overcome with the innovation of latex material in 1930s. Since then, semidry, prelubricated condoms using latex material are being manufactured with the help of automatic electronically equipped machines.[7] Lately, spermicidal condoms, which use spermicidal agent, nonoxynol-9 coated on outer and inner surfaces of condoms, are being marketed and made available in blister packages.

In 1967, the government of India established Hindustan Latex Limited to manufacture condoms to avoid the cost on imports. The growing population demanded the implementation of a public family planning program, which promoted a "Small Family, Happy Family." Oral pills and condoms were freely distributed as a part of this program. As of March 2018, condoms were the second most popular form of contraception in India after IUD insertions according to a report from the Ministry of Health and Welfare.[8]

ACCEPTABILITY AND USAGE

The barrier method is the most popular and accepted method of family planning and contraception worldwide. But the number of people using condoms as contraception is difficult to ascertain as condoms are directly available in shops and over the counter in chemist shops. In 1991, there were 45–50 million condom users throughout the world, most of them in the developed countries where 10% of married women were protected against pregnancy by the use of condoms as compared to only 3% in the developing countries.

In India, only 3–5% married women are protected against pregnancy by condoms. The use of condoms also differs in different states of India and is directly proportional to the education level. The Indian union territory of Dadra and Nagar Haveli had the highest number of condom users at around 993 users for every 10,000 unsterilized couples as of fiscal year 2020. This is a small number compared to the number of unsterilized couples in the state.

The north-eastern state of Arunachal Pradesh in India had the lowest number of condom users compared to the rest of the country, with just about 27 couples reportedly using this contraceptive method per 10,000 unsterilized couples. Overall, the data pointed to the fact that a majority of north-eastern states in the country including Manipur, Tripura, and Nagaland had low numbers of condom users but a higher share of other birth control method users.[9]

TYPES

Condoms are mostly made of fine latex rubber and are available in various sizes, shapes, colors, and textures. The condoms are available in cylindrical shapes with a circular rim at one end and closed at the other end. They are usually 15–20 cm in length, so as to fit onto an erected penis comfortably, and 3–3.5 cm in diameter. They are available in dry or semi-dry, prelubricated or nonlubricated, and with or without spermicides types. Silicon is used nowadays to produce semi-dry, prelubricated condoms. The condoms are rolled over the circular rim and packed in aluminum or plastic foils and sealed in packets of 3–12 or available in blister packets **(Figs. 1A and B)**.

Condoms are manufactured and supplied free of cost by the government of India under national family planning programs by the name "Nirodh." Some varieties such as "Nirodh Deluxe" or "Nirodh Lubricated" are supplied at the subsidized rates through chemist shops, grocery stores, and small vendor shops. Some are also available through vending machines. Prelubricated and spermicidal condoms are also manufactured in India.

Nonlatex forms of condoms are now commercially made of polyurethane, which have a longer shelf life. A new form of male condom using styrene ethylene butylene styrene (SEBS), a synthetic material such as Tactylon, is also being tried.

ADVANTAGES

- *Condoms prevent unwanted pregnancies*: Condoms are the most effective contraceptive method if used most correctly and consistently. They are also useful for old age couples, couples with less frequent sexual intercourse, during lactation, during holidays, and for people with multiple sexual partners. They are also helpful to those who cannot tolerate other methods of contraception. Their use is also recommended in teenagers and for those with premature ejaculation.
- *They protect against STIs*: In addition to preventing childbirths, condoms also give protection against STIs such as gonorrhea, syphilis, vaginal infections such as trichomoniasis, candidiasis, nongonococcal urethritis, chlamydia, herpes, and hepatitis B infections.[10]
- *They protect against infections such as HIV*: The use of condom prevents infection against HIV and thus prevents parents and their children from infection and subsequent development of acquired immunodeficiency syndrome (AIDS).[11]

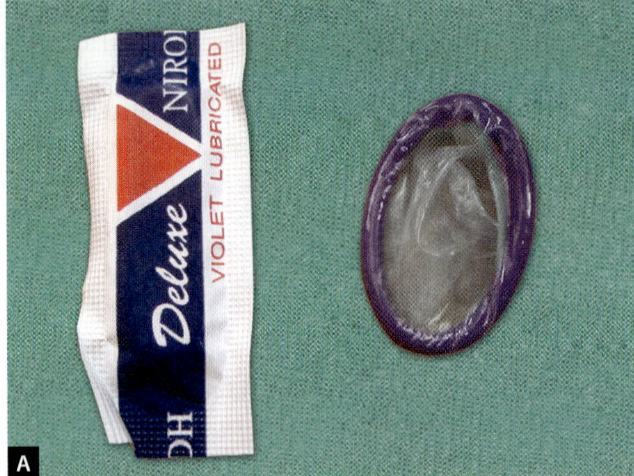

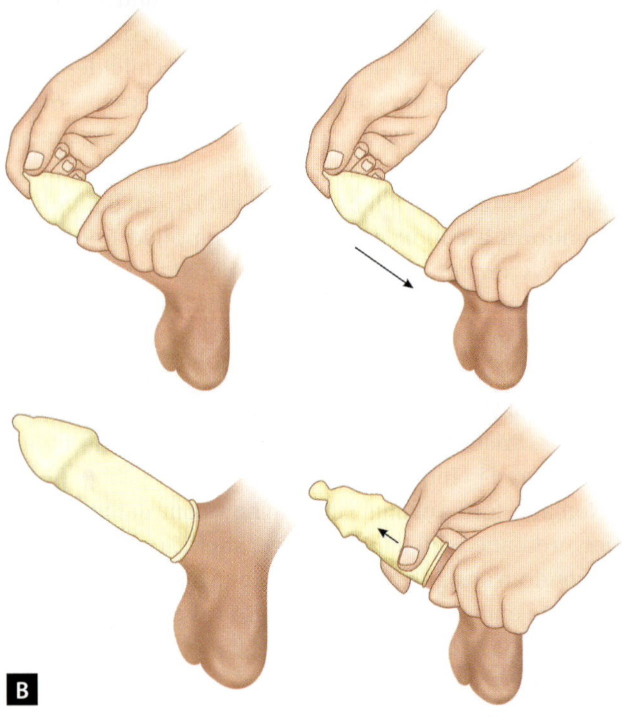

Figs. 1A and B: (A) A male condom; (B) Application of male condom.

- *Protect against carcinoma cervix*: It prevents infection against human papillomavirus, which is the etiological factor in carcinoma cervix. If used for >5 years, barriers methods reduce the chances of developing cervical intraepithelial neoplasia and thereby cervical cancer as compared to the use of oral contraceptives.[12]
- Condoms, if used during pregnancy in later months, can prevent amniotic fluid infections and neonatal sepsis.
- Condoms need no prescription and no medical advice for use and are easily available and easy to carry.
- They are the safest method devoid of any systemic or hormonal side effects.
- Used properly and consistently, barrier methods have a very less failure rate.
- They are a reversible method of contraception. Condoms are used for spacing. This method of contraception is completely temporary, reversible, and does not affect fertility.
- Compared to other methods, condoms are very cheap.
- Currently, different types of condoms are available, which can enhance the sexual pleasure with their textured surface. Others are medicated to make sex last longer and others are lubricated for smooth, hassle-free experience.
- They involve a male partner in the contraceptive choice.

DISADVANTAGES

- There are practically no disadvantages of condom use, except it can cause hypersensitivity reaction to rubber or latex in some people.
- Few couples experience decrease in sexual pleasure due to interruption in sexual act as well as decrease in sensitivity due to condom use. But this is minor and most couples adjust to the condom use with practice.
- The failure rate is higher than other contraceptives such as combined pills and intrauterine contraceptive device (IUCDs).
- Storage and disposal after use can be a problem particularly in village population.
- *Intravaginal breakage*: Nonlubricated and ultrathin condoms are more prone to breakage during intercourse. An emergency contraception has to be used in case of accidental rupture of condoms.

CONTRAINDICATIONS

- As such, there are no major contraindications to the use of condoms.
- *Allergy to latex*: It can be managed by antiallergic drugs and use of local or oral steroid preparations. In such cases of allergy, polyurethane condoms may be tried.

EFFECTIVENESS

The failure rate of condom with common use is typically 12%, but it can be as low as 3% if used correctly and consistently during each act of coitus without fail.[13] Lower failure rates (1%) are obtained with the use of spermicidal condoms or when use of condoms is combined with other contraceptive measures such as female condom, diaphragm or cervical cap and spermicidal contraceptives such as Today sponge.[14]

Common errors with condoms usage include failure to use condoms with every act of intercourse and throughout intercourse, improper lubricant use with latex condoms (e.g., oil-based lubricants), incorrect placement of the condom on the penis, and spillage due to poor withdrawal technique and using the too large or too small condoms. The dry nonlubricated variety and ultrathin condoms have more chances of breakage.

DIRECTIONS FOR USE

The condom should be unrolled on the erected penis after retracting the foreskin just before the act of coitus. Air-free space should be left at the tip by holding it upright till it is unrolled completely. This is overcome in condoms, which have teats. Prelubricated condoms are preferable. If lubrication is needed, K-Y jelly or spermicidal jellies can be used. Avoid using moisturizer or body lotions or oils. It increases the chance of rupture. A condom has to be used only once and discarded after use.

After the act of coitus, the penis has to be withdrawn from vagina carefully holding the condom without spilling its content. After use, it should be wrapped in a paper and thrown in dustbin. It should not be flushed down the toilette drain.

To increase effectiveness, it should be combined with female barrier methods such as female condom, diaphragm or cervical caps or spermicidal agents. This is known as dual method of contraception. In case of accidental rupture, emergency contraception has to be used within 72 hours.

In a November 2013 policy statement (reaffirmed 2017), the American Academy of Pediatrics (AAP) provided updated recommendations for improving the use of condoms among adolescents.[15] These include the following:

- Adolescents should be encouraged to abstain from sexual intercourse or postpone future sexual relationships.
- Pediatricians should play a role in educating adolescents and their parents about responsible sexual activity and encouraging the correct use of condoms among adolescents who are sexually active.
- Health education programs for K-12 children should provide education and counseling about sexual activity and be integrated into collaborative, community-based condom-availability programs.
- School-based condom distribution should be considered a valid means of obtaining contraception.
- Pediatricians and other clinicians should help to make condoms more available to adolescents by providing condoms directly and by encouraging better condom availability in the community.
- Pediatricians should raise awareness that the onset and frequency of sexual activity among adolescents are not increased by better access to condoms.

SPERMICIDAL AGENTS

Vaginal spermicides consist of a base combined with either nonoxynol-9 or octoxynol.[16] The actual spermicidal agent consists of a surfactant that destroys the sperm cell membrane. Bases include vaginal foams, suppositories, jellies, films, foaming tablets, and creams. These must be inserted into the vagina prior to each coital act. Nonoxynol-9 is toxic to the lactobacilli that are part of the normal vaginal flora. Adverse effects include disruption of the vaginal epithelium, possibly raising the risk of STI, and increased vaginal colonization with the bacteria *Escherichia coli*, which may predispose to bacteriuria after intercourse.

Spermicides prevent sperm from entering the cervical canal by attacking the sperm's flagella and body, reducing their mobility, and disrupting their fructolytic activity, thereby inhibiting their nourishment.

Efficacy

The perfect-use failure rate within the first year is 2%. The typical-use failure rate within the first year is 13%.[17]

Advantages

The lubrication provided by spermicides may heighten satisfaction in both partners. Another advantage is the ease of application. Either partner can purchase and apply spermicide because it is easily accessible, available over the counter, and inexpensive. Applying spermicide requires minimal patient education. It augments contraceptive efficacy of the cervical cap and diaphragm. Spermicides produce no adverse systemic effects.

Disadvantages

Spermicides may increase the risk of STI transmission. Insertion may be uncomfortable for some couples. Vaginal irritation is possible, and spermicides may cause an allergic reaction. Effectiveness of spermicides lasts less than an hour.

A traditional Indian society puts the weight of contraception and upbringing of children on the women. Hormonal contraceptives and IUDs are known to cause undesirable systemic effects. Apart from being the most widely used, safest, and effective method, male barrier methods not only protect against STDs and HIV but also ensure participation of male partner in the fertility control process. In spite of these advantages, contraception among men has declined over the years according to government sources. Education, awareness, and further improvement in quality and its easier and free distribution in India and other developing countries will go a long way to control population explosion and transmission of HIV and STDs throughout

MISCONCEPTIONS

- *Condoms can break easily.*
  Condoms do not break easily, if worn correctly.
- *Condom does not prevent pregnancy.*
  Condom is an effective method for preventing pregnancy, as it acts as a barrier for entry of sperm into vagina.
- *Condoms do not protect against STDs.*
  Using condoms correctly and consistently provides the best protection against STDs. When used correctly, condoms have a 98% rate of protecting against unwanted pregnancies and are 98–99% effective in protecting against HIV and other STDs.
- *Condoms are a man's responsibility.*
  Healthy and protected reproductive life is a combined responsibility of couples. Correct and consistent use of condom by male partner makes sex safe and free of risk of pregnancy and STDs.

REFERENCES

1. Colquitt CW, Martin TS. Contraceptive methods. J Pharm Pract. 2017;30(1):130-5.
2. Curtis KM, Tepper NK, Jamieson DJ, Marchbanks PA. Adaptation of the World Health Organization's selected practice recommendations for contraceptive use for the United States. Contraception. 2013;87(5):513-6.

3. Curtis KM, Jatlaoui TC, Tepper NK, Zapata LB, Horton LG, Jamieson DJ, et al. U.S. selected practice recommendations for contraceptive use, 2016. MMWR Recomm Rep. 2016;65(4):1-66.
4. Ministry of Health. Communication Strategy for Prevention and Control of STIs and HIV/AIDS; STD/ACP. New Delhi, India: Ministry of Health; 2004.
5. James M. "Condoms Cathedrals and Caves - Europe for Visitors". about.com. Archived from the original on February 5, 2013. Retrieved December 21, 2012.
6. Reprinted from India Rubber World (1891-01-31). "CHARLES GOODYEAR—The life and discoveries of the inventor of vulcanized India rubber". Scientific American Supplement. New York: Munn & Co. (787). Retrieved June 8, 2008.
7. "Special Topic: History of Condom Use". Population Action International. 2002. Archived from the original on July 14, 2007. Retrieved February 18, 2008.
8. Census of India. (2011). Population projections for India and states 2011–2036. Report of the technical group on population projections July, 2020. [online] Available from: https://main.mohfw.gov.in/sites/default/files/Population%20Projection%20Report%202011-2036%20-%20upload_compressed_0.pdf. [Last accessed November, 2021].
9. Statista Research Department, Oct 16, 2020.
10. Holmes KK, Levine R, Weaver M. Effectiveness of condoms in preventing sexually transmitted infections. Bull World Health Organ. 2004;82(6):454-61.
11. National AIDS Control Organisation. (2014). Condom promotion newsletter. [online] Available from: http://naco.gov.in/sites/default/files/Condom%20Promotion%20Newsletter.pdf. [Last accessed November, 2021].
12. Hariri S, Warner L. Condom use and human papillomavirus in men. J Infect Dis. 2013;208(3):367-9.
13. Sanders SA, Yarber WL, Kaufman EL, Crosby RA, Graham CA, Milhausen RR. Condom use errors and problems: a global view. Sex Health. 2012;9(1):81-95.
14. Peragallo Urrutia R, Polis CB, Jensen ET, Greene ME, Kennedy E, Stanford JB. Effectiveness of fertility awareness-based methods for pregnancy prevention: a systematic review external icon. Obstet Gynecol. 2018;132:591-604.
15. Garcia J. (2013). AAP Policy Statement: Provide Condoms to Adolescents. Medscape Medical News. [online] Available from: https://www.medscape.com/viewarticle/813290. [Last accessed November, 2021].
16. Raymond EG, Chen PL, Condon S, Luoto J, Barnhart KT, Creinin MD, et al. Acceptability of five nonoxynol-9 spermicides. Contraception. 2005;71(6):438-42.
17. Trussel J, Aiken ARA, Micks E, Guthrie KA. Efficacy, safety and personal considerations in contraceptive technology, 21st edition. New York, NY: Ayer Company Publishers, Inc.: 2018.

LONG QUESTIONS

1. What do you understand by male barrier methods? Write in detail about condom as contraceptive method.
2. What are the noncontraceptive benefits of condoms?

SHORT QUESTIONS

1. What are the recommendations of the American Academy of Pediatrics in 2013 for improving the use of condoms among adolescents?
2. Enumerate precautions to be taken while using condom as barrier method of contraception?
3. Write the various ways by which the effectiveness of condom can be increased?
4. Justify the statement—male condoms can prevent carcinoma cervix.
5. Write the different advantages of condom use.
6. What are the different types of condom available in the market?
7. What are the common misconceptions about condom use in general population?

MULTIPLE CHOICE QUESTIONS

1. Which of the following are the physical barrier methods of contraception?
   a. NuvaRing b. Oral contraceptives
   c. Male condoms d. i-Pill
2. The active chemical of spermicide coated male condom is:
   a. Nonoxynol b. Ethyl alcohol
   c. Desogestrel d. Tetracycline
3. In which year did the use of latex condom start?
   a. 1954 b. 1930
   c. 1964 d. 1945
4. Failure rate of condom with typical use is:
   a. 13% b. 18%
   c. 8% d. 3%
5. Failure rate of condom with correct and consistent use is:
   a. 12% b. 18%
   c. 8% d. 3%
6. In which year did the government of India establish Hindustan Latex Limited to manufacture condoms to avoid the cost on imports?
   a. 1967 b. 1958
   c. 1945 d. 1964
7. How many married women of India are protected against pregnancy by the use of condoms?
   a. 12% b. 18%
   c. 8% d. 3%
8. Which state of India had the highest number of condom users according to survey in year 2020?
   a. Dadra and Nagar Haveli b. Arunachal Pradesh
   c. Tripura d. Uttarakhand
9. Which state of India had the lowest number of condom users according to survey in year 2020?
   a. Dadra and Nagar Haveli b. Arunachal Pradesh
   c. Tripura d. Uttarakhand
10. Failure rate of spermicides with typical use is:
    a. 6% b. 18%
    c. 26% d. 34%
11. Failure rate of spermicides with correct and consistent use is:
    a. 6% b. 18%
    c. 26% d. 34%

Answers

1. c 2. a 3. b 4. a 5. d 6. a
7. d 8. a 9. b 10. c 11. a

2.3 FEMALE BARRIER METHODS

Shobha Gudi

INTRODUCTION

The female barrier is an important method in the basket of choices for contraception. This is a method which will give autonomy to women to exercise safe sex at all times. It is coital-dependent reversible contraception that does not interfere with fertility and is available without prescription.[1.]

FEMALE CONDOM

Female condoms account for <1% of condoms produced globally.[2] They provide a physical barrier during penetrative sex between the female and male genitalia preventing pre-ejaculatory fluid and semen from entering vagina or cervix. It thereby protects against sexually transmitted infections (STIs) as well as pregnancy.

Types

Generally, the condom has a simple structure with an outer ring or frame, which sits on introitus, anchors the condom, and is used to remove it after the act. The inner sleeve that lines the vagina and an inner ring or sponge covers the cervix. It is usually made of natural rubber latex or nitrile (a synthetic latex) or polyurethane.[3,4] It requires lubricant, but no spermicide is required.

Natural latex female condom: The World Health Organization (WHO) has approved the natural latex female condom, manufactured by Cupid Limited.[5] This is distributed in India, Brazil, Indonesia, Netherlands, South Africa, and Mozambique. The failure rate in terms of breakage, slippage, invagination (condom gets pushed into vagina and on one side, exposing the cervix to semen), and misdirection was evaluated in a trial of 300 women and was found to be similar to other forms available, e.g., FC2.[6]

- *The capsule form*: The PATH WC (Program for Appropriate Technology in Health: Woman's Condom) is made of polyurethane capsule insert, inserted into vagina (using a water-based lubricant in the pack) before coitus; it dissolves and releases the condom.[7] It clings to vaginal mucosa with hydrophilic areas on its surface. It has been approved by the WHO in 2016.[8]
- VA wow (worn of women) is made of natural rubber latex, has India Drug Control Authority approval, and is available in some parts of Europe, Asia, and Latin America. It is prelubricated and has a medical-grade sponge at one end that is used for insertion; the other end has a triangular frame to anchor it outside the vagina.[9]

FC1 was the first female condom to be marketed mainly in the western world. It was made of polyurethane and had a seam. But the most widely available one today is FC2, a soft, loose-fitting nitrile sheath with two flexible rings. One ring is in the closed end of the sheath, which helps in insertion and anchors against the cervix. The other ring is the open edge of the device; it remains outside the vagina after insertion. Silicone-based lubricant lines the inside of the condom, but additional lubrication for the inside and/or outside could be used. The condom is approximately 17 cm (6.5 inches) in length (similar to a male condom). Limited evidence available shows that FC1 and FC2 are similar in efficacy and safety, and the latter is more comfortable for couples.[10] The FC2 is approved and indicated for preventing pregnancy and transmission of HIV and other STIs and is available in approximately 100 countries.

Counseling Points

It is a safe, effective, coitus-related method, has no effect on fertility, requires no medical examination or prescription, and grants the woman autonomy to protect herself.

Correct use: To contain the pre-ejaculatory fluid and semen to protect the woman from pregnancy and STI transmission, one piece is used for one act of intercourse.

Efficacy

Studies have shown a slightly higher risk of failure (pregnancy rates) after 1 year of perfect use and typical use as 5 and 21% for female condom (regardless of the type of condom) and 2 and 13% for male condom, respectively.[11-14]

Sexually Transmitted Infections

The WHO medical eligibility criteria (MEC) clearly state that only male latex condoms are effective in prevention of HIV transmission and there is very limited data to say that female condoms are effective though trials conducted on sex workers showed significant benefit.[15,16]

Some Drawbacks

Allergy to latex or nitrile and inconsistent and incorrect use, with difficulties for insert, can make the sexual act unpleasant. It has a higher failure rate of pregnancy than male condom. Usage is limited as women find it embarrassing to buy and it is not easily available.

Comparison of Coital-dependent Methods

Female condoms in comparison with male condoms:

Advantages:

- Do not disrupt intimacy as can be placed before intercourse and are more user friendly and can be easily removed immediately after the act.[17-19]
- Made of materials such as nitrile and polyurethane, can be easily stored, are mostly nonallergic, and can be used with lubricants.

Disadvantages:
- Cost much higher and is not part of public sector methods.
- User difficulties are slippage, breakage, incorrect penetration, and invagination; all of them decrease with continued usage.[20]
- Effective against STIs but unlike the male condoms, they are not declared effective against HIV.
- Cannot be used for anal intercourse.[21]
- Cannot be reused.[22]

How does the female condom compare with the other female barrier methods?

Diaphragms, cervical caps, and sponges: Though all three devices need to be inserted prior to any vaginal sexual activity, there are some differences.
- Diaphragms are reusable devices. They always used with spermicide and should remain in vagina for 6 hours after intercourse to be effective. Only one free size is available. They are better contraceptives than female condom, (failure rate: 12% vs. 21%) but less effective in prevention of STIs.
- The cervical cap is a reusable device, needs a medical examination for size, and needs spermicide application with every use. Efficacy as contraceptive is similar but not reliable for STI prevention.
- *Comparison with spermicides and contraceptive sponge:* These methods are inexpensive and available over the counter. Efficacy as contraceptive is similar to female condoms but not reliable for STI prevention.[23]

Strategies for Promoting Effective Female Condom Use

The optimal methods of counseling to ensure correct female condom are yet to be known. The WHO advises the following steps to support the patient who wishes to use female condoms:[1]

Ensure correct understanding of use: The client should repeat the five basic steps after counseling. A plastic model of the female pelvis can be used to practice insertion and removal. A separate condom is to be used with every sexual act and should be used correctly and consistently. The basic steps of female condom use should be reviewed with the patient and her partner, if present (**Fig. 1**). A free interactive FC2 training program is available for healthcare providers online.

Review ways to discuss condom use and troubleshoot problems and encourage follow-up: Female condom use requires partner participation, and they will benefit from counseling as a couple. This conversation allows the clinician, patient, and partner to address any concerns.

Ensure supply and access to information: Local retail pharmacies and online sites should be identified for clients and they should be encouraged to keep a supply in case of breakage.
- The female condom should not be used concurrently with a male condom, as friction may cause breakage.
- It can be inserted in any position she finds comfortable and can be done up to 8 hours before intercourse. Adequate lubrication is needed for passage and to minimize noise during sex. Either water-based or oil-based lubricants can be used.
- It should be disposed off in waste containers, not in the toilet. The female condom cannot migrate into a woman's uterus or body.

Reuse: Female condoms are not recommended for reuse.[1] However, where there are cost constraints, washing, disinfecting, and reusing female condoms may be better than unprotected intercourse, although their efficacy is unknown.[24,25]

Complications or failure: The main complications are penis insertion to the side of the condom, invagination, and condom breakage. A good detail in counseling should be to instruct the client to steady the outer ring at the beginning of penetrative sexual intercourse. To avoid breakage, a new condom should be used with every act of vaginal intercourse and using adequate lubricant.

Use with lubricants and/or medications: As it is made of nitrile, a synthetic latex (rubber) female condom can be used with lubricants such as clean water, butter, and cooking oils.

Storage and expiration: Currently available female condoms are made of synthetic materials (nitrile and polyurethane) and do not have special storage requirements. The product should be used before the manufacturer's expiration date.

The Indian Council of Medical Research (ICMR) pilot study (urban and rural Indian women) on contraceptive acceptability and utilization of female condom showed it to be highly acceptable. In this study, 90% of women found it easy to store, insert, and dispose off and were comfortable to use during sex.

The failure rate at the end of 1 year was 18%.[26]

The Ministry of Health and Family Welfare (MoHFW) in India, the public sector, provides a "cafeteria approach" and only includes both male and female sterilization, intrauterine contraceptive device (IUCD), oral contraceptives, injectable contraceptives, and male condoms. For population stabilization to be achieved, it is important to expand the basket of choice and add female condoms; it would empower women to protect themselves from the risk of unintended pregnancy as well as address their infection prevention needs.

KEY MESSAGES

- Female condoms consist of an anchor (e.g., ring and frame) that sits outside the vagina, a sleeve that lines the vagina, and an inner ring or sponge that holds the device in place. They are commonly made out of nitrile (a synthetic latex), sometimes of natural rubber latex and polyurethane. The FC2 female condom is the most commonly available female condom.
- The female condom provides a physical barrier and a new one must be used correctly with every act of vaginal intercourse to be effective at preventing pregnancy and STI transmission.
- Failure rates during the first 12 months of perfect use and typical use are 5% and 21%, respectively (higher than use of the male condom: 2% and 13%).

The right way to use a female condom

Female condom dos and don't's

- **Do** use a female condom from start fo finish, every time you have vaginal sex
- **Do** read the condom package insert and check the expiration date
- **Do** make sure there are not tears or defects
- **Do** use lubricant to help prevent the condom from slipping and tearing
- **Do** store female condoms at room temperature
- **Don't** use a male condom with a female condom as this can cause tearing
- **Don't** reuse a female condom
- **Don't** flush female condoms as they may clog the toilet

How to insert and remove a female condom

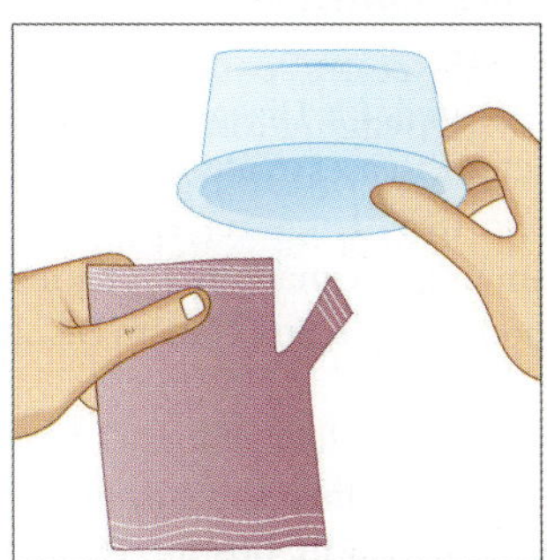

Carefully open and remove female condom from package to prevent tearing

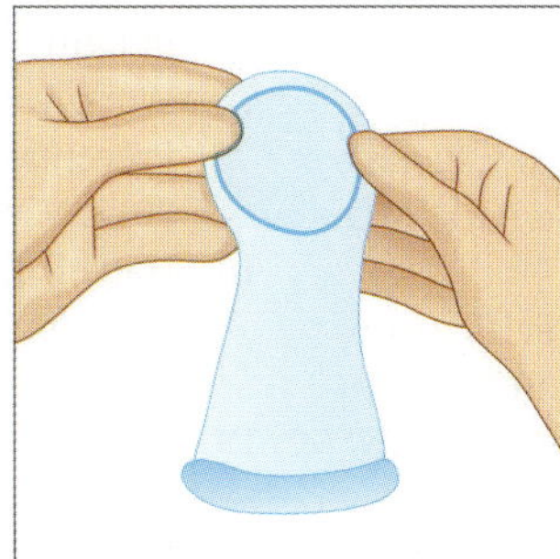

The thick, inner ring with closed end is used for placing in the vagina and holds condom in place. The thin, outer ring remains outside of body, covering vaginal opening

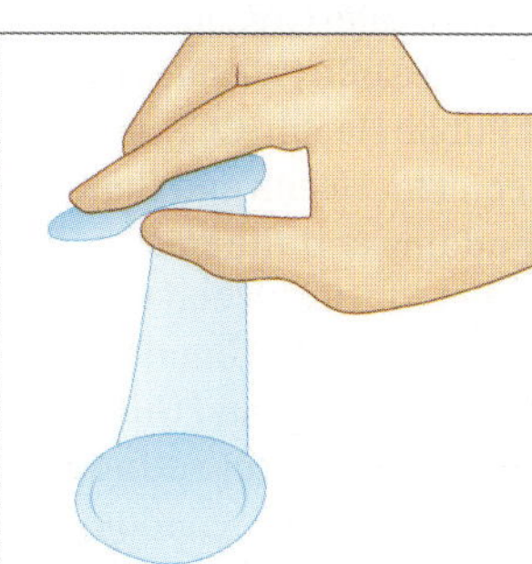

Find a comfortable position. while holding outside of condom at closed end, squeeze sides of inner ring together with your thumb and forefinger and insert into vagina. It is similar to inserting a tampon

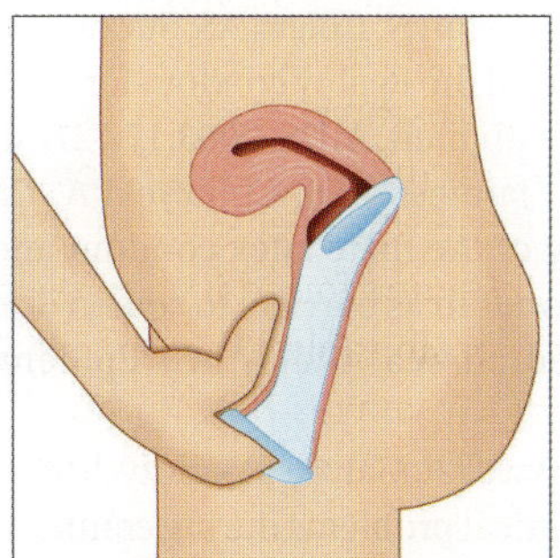

Using your finger, push inner ring as far up as it will go - near the pubic bone. The condom will expand naturally and you may not feel it

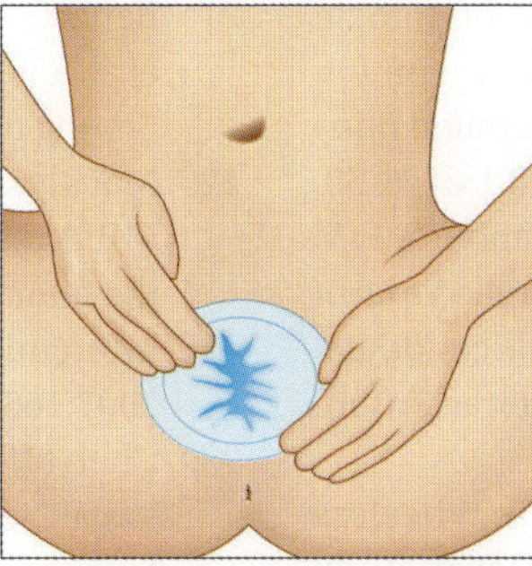

Be sure condom is not twisted The thin, outer ring should remain outside vagina

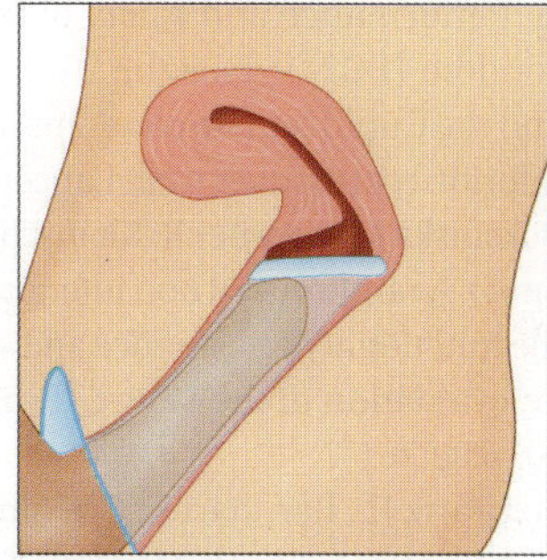

Guide partner's penis into opening of female condom. Stop intercourse if you feel penis slip between condom and walls of vagina or if outer ring is pushed into vagina

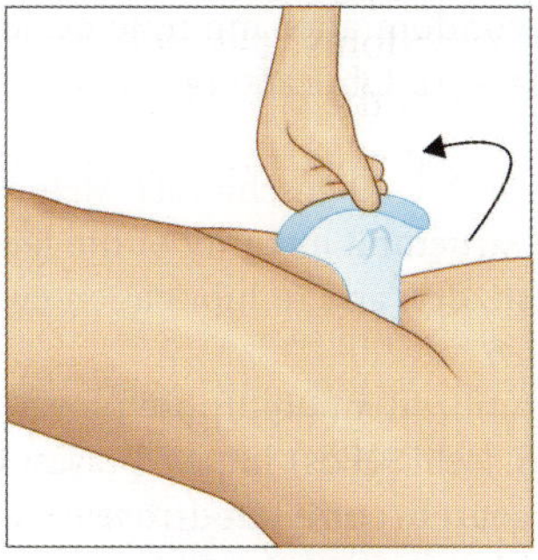

To remove, gently twist outer ring and pull female condom out of vagina

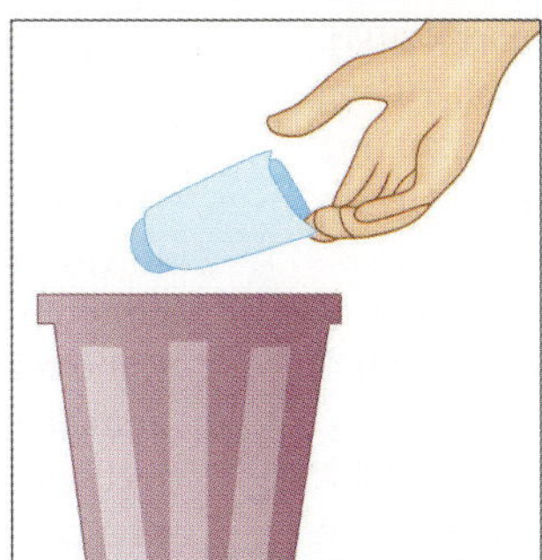

Throw away female condom is trash after using it one time Do not reuse

*Female condoms should not be used for anal sex

Fig. 1: Basic steps of female condom use.

- Female condoms are a safe, effective, reversible method of contraception. No medical examination or sizing needed prescription or special fitting. They are available over the counter and are highly useful for women at risk for STIs when the male does not use a condom.
- The only contraindication is allergy to nitrile. Other disadvantages might include problems with insertion or removal.
- It offers advantages over the male condom in being more user friendly (can be placed up to 8 hours before intercourse,

need not be removed immediately after, and can be used with either water-based or oil-based lubricants).

- The disadvantages are higher cost and cannot be used for anal intercourse. They are not intended to be reused (unlike the diaphragm or cervical cap).

REFERENCES

1. World Health Organization. Family Planning: A Global Handbook for Providers (2018 update). Baltimore and Geneva: World Health Organization Department of Reproductive Health and Research (WHO/RHR), Johns Hopkins Bloomberg School of Public Health/CCP and WHO; 2018. pp. 261-70.
2. Center for Health and Gender Equity. Saving lives now: Female condoms and the role of US foreign aid. Takoma Park, MD: Center for Health and Gender Equity; 2008.
3. WHO/UNFPA Female Condom Generic Specification, Prequalification and Guidelines for Procurement 2012.https://www.who.int/reproductivehealth/publications/family_planning/female_condom_specification.pdf
4. Beksinska M, Smit J, Mabude Z, Vijayakumar G, Joanis C. Performance of the Reality polyurethane female condom and a synthetic latex prototype: a randomized crossover trial among South African women. Contraception. 2006;73:386-93.
5. Beksinska ME, Piaggio G, Smit JA, Wu J, Zhang Y, Pienaar J, et al. Performance and safety of the second-generation female condom (FC2) versus the Woman's, the VA worn-of-women, and the Cupid female condoms: a randomised controlled non-inferiority crossover trial. Lancet Glob Health. 2013;1:e146-52.
6. Beksinska M, Greener R, Kleinschmidt I, Pillay L, Maphumulo V, Smit J. A randomized non inferiority crossover controlled trial of the functional performance and safety of new female condoms: an evaluation of the Velvet, Cupid2, and FC2. Contraception. 2015;92:261-7.
7. Schwartz JL, Barnhart K, Creinin MD, Poindexter A, Wheeless A, Kilbourne-Brook M, et al. Comparative crossover study of the PATH Woman's Condom and the FC female condom. Contraception. 2008;78:465-73.
8. http://www.asiaone.com/asia/female-condom-made-china-receives-un-and-who-approval [Last accessed September 5, 2017].
9. Zirong H, Junqing W, Coffey PS, Kilbourne-Brook M, Yufeng Z, Wang C, et al. Performance of the woman's condom among couples in Shanghai, China. Eur J Contracept Reprod Health Care. 2012;17:212-8.
10. Wang X, Xi M, Zhang L, Jia L, Wang Y, Cheng Y. Awareness of female condoms and failures reported with two different types in China. Int J Gynaecol Obstet. 2015;128:152-6.
11. Trussell J. Contraceptive efficacy. In: Hatcher RA, Trussell J, Nelson AL, Cates W, Kowal D, Policar M (eds). Contraceptive Technology, 20th edition. New York: Ardent Media; 2011.
12. Vijayakumar G, Mabude Z, Smit J, Beksinska M, Lurie M. A review of female-condom effectiveness: patterns of use and impact on protected sex acts and STI incidence. Int J STD AIDS. 2006;17:652-9.
13. French PP, Latka M, Gollub EL, Rogers C, Hoover DR, Stein ZA. Use-effectiveness of the female versus male condom in preventing sexually transmitted disease in women. Sex Transm Dis. 2003;30:433-9.
14. Fontanet AL, Saba J, Chandelying V, Bhiraleus P, Rugpao S, Chongsomchai C, et al. Protection against sexually transmitted diseases by granting sex workers in Thailand the choice of using the male or female condom: results from a randomized controlled trial. AIDS. 1998;12:1851-9.
15. Hoke TH, Feldblum PJ, Van Damme K, Nasution MD, Grey TW, Wong EL, et al. Temporal trends in sexually transmitted infection prevalence and condom use following introduction of the female condom to Madagascar sex workers. Int J STD AIDS. 2007;18:461-6.
16. Feldblum PJ, Kuyoh MA, Bwayo JJ, Omari M, Wong EL, Tweedy KG, et al. Female condom introduction and sexually transmitted infection prevalence: results of a community intervention trial in Kenya. AIDS. 2001;15:1037-44.
17. Workowski KA, Bolan GA, Centers for Disease Control and Prevention. Sexually transmitted diseases treatment guidelines, 2015. MMWR Recomm Rep. 2015;64:1.
18. Hatzell T, Feldblum PJ, Homan RK, Gmach RD. The female condom: is "just as good" good enough? Sex Transm Dis. 2003; 30:440.
19. Peterson K, Herman L, Fiske L, Marseille E, Kahn JG. Smarter programming of the female condom: increasing its impact on HIV prevention in the developing world. Boston: FSG Social Impact Advisors; 2008.
20. Beksinska M, Smit J, Greener R, Piaggio G, Joanis C. The female condom learning curve: patterns of female condom failure over 20 uses. Contraception. 2015;91:85-90.
21. Renzi C, Tabet SR, Stucky JA, Eaton N, Coletti AS, Surawicz CM, et al. Safety and acceptability of the Reality condom for anal sex among men who have sex with men. AIDS. 2003;17:727-31.
22. Macaluso M, Blackwell R, Jamieson DJ, Kulczycki A, Chen MP, Akers R, et al. Efficacy of the male latex condom and of the female polyurethane condom as barriers to semen during intercourse: a randomized clinical trial. Am J Epidemiol. 2007;166:88-96.
23. Chen MP, Macaluso M, Blackwell R, Galvao L, Kulczycki A, Diaz J, et al. Self-reported mechanical problems during condom use and semen exposure. Comparison of two randomized trials in the United States of America and Brazil. Sex Transm Dis. 2007;34:557-62.
24. Potter B, Gerofi J, Pope M, Farley T. Structural integrity of the polyurethane female condom after multiple cycles of disinfection, washing, drying and relubrication. Contraception. 2003;67:65.
25. Pettifor AE, Rees HV, Beksinska ME, Kleinschmidt I, McIntyre J. In vitro assessment of the structural integrity of the female condom after multiple wash, dry, and re-lubrication cycles. Contraception. 2000;61:271-6.
26. Female condom: an underutilized multipurpose prevention technology. In: Chandhiok N, Joshi S (Eds), https://prayaspune.org/health/index.php/research/completed-research1/2-uncategorised/209-fc-study.html

LONG QUESTIONS

1. Discuss the place of barrier methods in the expanded basket of choice of contraception and how will they help to tackle the unmet need?
2. Give an account of different types of female barriers in relation to their structure, mechanism of action, efficacy, and availability.

SHORT QUESTIONS

1. Enumerate the different types of female barrier methods.
2. Describe in brief the counseling points for optimal use of female condoms.
3. What are comparative failure rates of female barrier methods of contraception as compared to the male condom?
4. Describe the role of barrier methods of contraception in prevention of HIE.

MULTIPLE CHOICE QUESTIONS

1. Which is the most effective among female barrier methods?
   a. Female condom b. Vaginal diaphragm
   c. Cervical cap d. Vaginal sponge
2. What is the most effective protection against HIV transmission according to WHO?
   a. Female condom b. Vaginal diaphragm
   c. Cervical cap d. Male condom
3. The following is true about female condom insertion:
   a. Does not need training or instruction
   b. Examination and sizing by gynecologist mandatory before first use
   c. Efficacy better with male partner condom usage
   d. Invagination can be overcome with continued use
4. Strategies to improve female condom uptake, except:
   a. Adequate counseling session
   b. Make it accessible and available
   c. Include male partner in instructions
   d. Make it essential with male condom
5. Following are true for female barrier use, except:
   a. No lubricant needed
   b. Using spermicidal agent not necessary
   c. Should be included in basket of contraceptive choices
   d. Not suitable for anal intercourse

Answers

1. a 2. d 3. d 4. d 5. a

2.4 VAGINAL SPERMICIDES

Gorakh Mandrupkar

INTRODUCTION

Various methods for contraception are being tried. The one "easy to use" and "easily available" method is adored by couples. In barrier methods, spermicides alone or with other barrier methods are being tried since long ago. In 1885, WJ Rendell prepared a soluble cocoa-butter vaginal suppository containing quinine sulfate, which was very popular at that time.[1] Now, nonoxynol-9 is the widely used chemical. Others which are tried are benzalkonium chloride, chlorhexidine, menfegol, sodium docusate, and octoxynol-9.

DEFINITION

Spermicides are sperm-killing, chemical, contraceptive agents, which are inserted deep in vagina near cervix before sexual intercourse. Nonoxynol-9 is the widely used one.

MECHANISM OF ACTION

These agents contain nonionic surfactants, which alter the permeability of the surface membrane of sperms. This leads to osmotic changes causing breaking or slowing of sperms.[2]

AVAILABLE FORMS

These are available in various forms:

- Foaming suppositories
- Melting suppositories
- Foaming tablets
- Melting films
- Jellies
- Creams
- Cans of pressurized foam.

USE OF SPERMICIDES

Jellies, creams, and foam from cans can be used alone with a diaphragm or with condoms. Films, suppositories, foaming tablets, or foaming suppositories can be used alone or with condoms.[3]

ADVANTAGES

- Simple to use
- Over-the-counter
- Medically safe
- Inexpensive
- Provide lubrication
- Available in different forms.

DISADVANTAGES

- These give moderate protection against pregnancy (72% effective with typical use) when used alone.
- When used alone, do not offer protection against sexually transmitted diseases (STDs) though some of the old reports say so.
- Many of these cause irritation and increase the risk of STDs.
- Many of these have to be used along with other barrier contraceptives.

CONTRAINDICATIONS

- Allergy to spermicides or carrier
- Inability of proper application (knowledge gap, genital prolapse, vaginal septum)
- Personal or medical need for highly effective contraception.

INSTRUCTIONS BEFORE USE

- The package instructions must be read carefully before using any of these methods.
- When there is less time between sexual intercourse and insertion of spermicides, then cream, jelly, or foam must be used as these are immediately effective right from insertion.
- If the applicator method for cream or foam or jelly is used, first the applicator is filled, inserted high up in vagina, and spermicide is deposited near cervix and applicator is removed.
- For film or suppository, the hand must be dry. The film or suppository is taken on finger and inserted as high as possible in vagina.
- For second intercourse, spermicide should be inserted again.
- Douching is not advisable for at least 6 hours after intercourse.
- Additional supplies are essential along with back-up method.

COMMERCIAL PREPARATIONS

Lorophyn suppositories, Preceptin jelly, "Today"- Foam Tablet, Delfen vaginal foam, and C-film are available.

KEY MESSAGES

- Spermicides are sperm-killing, chemical, contraceptive agents which are inserted deep in vagina near cervix before sexual intercourse.
- Nonoxynol-9 is the widely used chemical for spermicides worldwide.
- It alters permeability of sperm membrane causing osmotic changes leading to ineffective sperms.
- These are available as foaming/melting suppositories, melting films, jellies, and creams.
- Spermicides are simple and safe to use, available over the counter, and provide lubrication.
- These are 72% effective with typical use.
- They do not offer protection against STDs.
- Many of these have to be used along with other barrier contraceptives.

REFERENCES

1. Chaudhari SK. Practice of Fertility Control: A Comprehensive Textbook. Gurugram: Elsevier Health; 2007.
2. WHO. (2018). Family planning: A global handbook for providers by WHO, 3rd edition. [online] Available from: https://www.who.int/reproductivehealth/publications/fp-global-handbook/en/. [Last accessed November, 2021]
3. University of California, UHS information. (2009). Contraception: Spermicides. [online] Available from: https://uhs.berkeley.edu/sites/default/files/Spermicides.pdf. [Last accessed November, 2021].

LONG QUESTION

1. What is the role of vaginal spermicides in the cafeteria approach to contraception? What are its pros and cons? What instructions should be provided to a couple who opts for this method?

SHORT QUESTIONS

1. What are vaginal spermicides? How do they act?
2. What are the different formulations of vaginal spermicides available?

MULTIPLE CHOICE QUESTIONS

1. Spermicides are:
   a. Sperm-killing agents b. Chemical in nature
   c. Offer contraception d. All of the above
2. Worldwide used spermicidal agent is:
   a. Nonoxynol-9 b. Chloroquine
   c. Quinine sulfate d. Orthoquinone
3. Mechanism of action of spermicidal agent is:
   a. Osmotic changes of sperm membrane
   b. Ionic blockage
   c. Reverse osmosis
   d. Receptor blockage
4. With typical use, they offer contraceptive efficacy of:
   a. 60% b. 72%
   c. 100% d. 28%
5. What is the correct sentence about spermicides?
   a. They are the best contraceptive agents when used alone
   b. When used along with barrier methods, they give better protection
   c. They are quite expensive and difficult to use
   d. None of the above

Answers

1. d 2. a 3. a 4. b 5. b

2.5 COMBINED ORAL CONTRACEPTIVE PILLS

Poonam Varma Shivkumar, Darshana Legha

INTRODUCTION

The combined oral contraceptive (COC) pills are commonly used hormonal contraceptives, which are taken orally by women. COC pills contain a combination of an estrogen (usually ethinylestradiol) and a progestogen (one of various generations). The effect of both the steroids is different and so a better protection occurs due to the different mechanism of action of both of them.

HISTORY

Oral contraceptive drug was developed long before the complex regulation of ovulation and the menstrual cycle was elucidated. The development of oral contraceptives was by a gynecologist, John Rock; a biologist, Gregory Pincus; and two feminists, Katherine McCormick and Margaret Sanger. Newer discoveries happened to reduce side effects and complications of the high doses of sex steroids. The first oral contraceptive, Enovid, was manufactured by GD Searle and supplied free for clinical trials in Puerto Rico and elsewhere. It contained 9.85 mg of the progestin norethynodrel and 150 µg of the estrogen mestranol.

Today's pills contain dramatically lower hormone doses—0.1–3.0 mg of modern progestins and 20–50 µg of estrogens. The progestins used today are much more pharmacologically specific and more focused in their drug effect. While current progestin doses are not directly comparable, the doses for both the original pill ingredients have fallen manyfold from those of the original recipe. Safety concerns were raised. The pill prompted fear of "sexual anarchy", and fear that it would encourage female promiscuity was also discussed in plenty.

In 1970–80s, empowered women began to take charge of their own health by including self-determination on issues of contraception as well as feminist interpretations and informed women demanded family planning.

This led to the development of new preparations with reduced estrogen content and progestins of different varieties, and COCs with minimum steroid dose and complications became the choice.[1]

The birth of the pill was the result of a combination of studies on the effect of sex steroids on ovulation and, paradoxically, the search for fertility enhancing and biochemical advances in the production of sex steroids and their synthetic analogs. It was observed that combining two steroid hormones controls the fertilization in a much better way and very little failure occurs.

The initial observation that the addition of estrogen reduced breakthrough bleeding was at the basis of the composition of all later pills, namely a combination of an estrogen and a progestin. Beside their proliferative effect on the endometrium, estrogens have an anti-ovulatory effect of their own. They suppress the rise of follicle-stimulating hormone (FSH) and, as a result, follicular growth. Progestins, on the other hand, add to the contraceptive effect by suppressing the ovulatory luteinizing hormone (LH) surge. They also thicken the cervical mucus, thereby hindering sperm migration into the upper genital tract, and they have an antiproliferative effect on the endometrium, making it less receptive for implantation. Both sex steroids have dose-related side effects. Progestins do not exclusively bind to the progesterone receptor but can also to a certain degree activate other steroid receptors. Estrogens promote the synthesis of several hepatic proteins and have a well-established prothrombotic effect.[2]

USES

- As a contraceptive
- As emergency contraceptive—Yuzpe method
- Noncontraceptive uses.

CLASSIFICATION

Combined oral contraceptive pills are classified based on the amount of hormones in each pill:

- Monophasic—same amount of estrogen and progesterone in each tablet
- Biphasic—amount of estrogen and progesterone in each tablet is different in two phases of menstrual cycle, constant EE—35 µg progestogens: low in first 10 days and higher in next 11 days
- Triphasic—amount of estrogen and progesterone in each tablet is different in three phases, Triquilar: –0.03 EE + 0.5 mg L-norgestrel (1–6) – 0.03 EE + 0.75 mg L-norgestrel (7–11) – 0.03 EE + 0.125 mg L-norgestrel (12–21).

Combined oral contraceptive pills have also been grouped into "generations" in the medical literature based on when they were introduced.

- First-generation COC pills are sometimes defined as those containing the progestin noretynodrel, norethisterone, norethisterone acetate, or ethynodiol acetate and sometimes defined as all COC pills containing ≥50 µg ethinylestradiol.
- Second-generation COC pills are sometimes defined as those containing the progestin norgestrel or levonorgestrel and sometimes defined as those containing the progestin norethisterone, norethisterone acetate, ethynodiol acetate, norgestrel, levonorgestrel, or norgestimate and < 50 µg ethinylestradiol.

- Third-generation COC pills are sometimes defined as those containing the progestin desogestrel or gestodene and sometimes defined as those containing desogestrel, gestodene, or norgestimate.
- Fourth-generation COC pills are sometimes defined as those containing the progestin drospirenone and sometimes defined as those containing drospirenone, dienogest, or nomegestrol acetate.[3-5]

MECHANISM OF ACTION

- *Estrogen*: This inhibits ovulation by suppressing release of gonadotropins due to negative feedback.
- *Progesterones*: The mechanism of action is by suppression of the LH surge, suppression of ovulation, development of viscous and scanty cervical mucus to deter sperm penetration, alteration of tubal motility and tubal transport, and prevention of endometrial growth and development.

VARIOUS COMBINED ORAL CONTRACEPTIVE PILLS

Combined oral contraceptives pills available in the public sector:

- *Free supply*: The available COC pill in the public sector is Mala-N. Mala-N contains levonorgestrel (0.15 mg) + ethinylestradiol (30 μg). Mala-N is supplied free of cost through government health centers and hospitals. Each strip of Mala-N contains 21 hormonal tablets and 7 nonhormonal (iron) tablets.
- *Yasmin*: Ethinylestradiol 20–35 μg, drospirenone 3 mg and ethinylestradiol increase angiotensinogen production, which acts on renin-angiotensin system (RAS) causing Na and water retention. It is reversed by drospirenone. Its advantage is that drospirenone counteracts the mineralocorticoid action of estrogen.
- *Other available combination*: Ethinylestradiol 35 μg with cyproterone acetate 2 mg. Brand names in India are Diane 35, Krimson 35, and My Pill.
- *Advantages*: Because of antiandrogenic effects, they are useful in women with hirsutism, acne, and polycystic ovary syndrome (PCOS)
- *Ultra-low-dose pills*: Combination of ethinylestradiol 15 μg and gestodene 60 μg. Clinical trials are ongoing. They are available abroad as "Minesse"[5]

ADMINISTRATION OF COMBINED ORAL CONTRACEPTIVE PILLS: HOW TO USE

- To take one pill every day for 28 days (4 weeks) in a row and then start a new pack on day 29. The last seven pills in 28-day packs of combination pills do not have hormones in them. These pills are called "reminder" or "placebo" pills—to take pill every day and start next pack on time. The reminder pills may contain iron or other supplements.
- In 21-day packs*: To t*ake one pill every day for 21 days (3 weeks) in a row. No pill to be taken for 7 days (week 4). The hormone pills will prevent pregnancy even if sex is done during the week when no pills are taken. The next pack is to be started after not taking pills for 7 days.
- In 91-day packs*: Extended pills intake*—some combination pills have 12 weeks (3 months) of hormone pills in a row, followed by up to 1 week of hormone-free reminder pills. This is to have period once every 3 months. The hormones will prevent pregnancy even if the woman will have sex during the reminder pill week.
- *Missed pills*:
  - *One pill missed*: The woman should take the missed pill as soon as she remembers and then continue taking the remaining pills. There is no need of backup contraceptive method.
  - *Two pills missed*: The woman should take two pills on the next two consecutive nights and continue with the rest of the pack as usual but should use backup contraceptive such as barriers for 1 week. She should continue with the next pack as usual.

COUNSELING POINTS

As with any other contraceptives, the GATHER and cafeteria approaches have to be followed and the women should be well explained about the contraceptive and noncontraceptive benefits, side effects, complications, efficacy, and failure rate of COCs. Also, she should be advised a thorough check-up with her gynecologist before prescribing COCs.

CLINICAL EXAMINATION AND TESTS BEFORE PRESCRIBING COMBINED ORAL CONTRACEPTIVE PILLS

Examination

- Blood pressure
- Weight (BMI) [weight (kg)/height (m)^2]
- Clinical breast examination
- Bimanual examination and cervical inspection.

Laboratory Tests (Desirable)

- Glucose
- Lipids
- Liver enzymes
- Hemoglobin
- Thrombogenic mutations
- Cervical cytology (Papanicolaou smear)
- Sexually transmitted disease (STD) screening with laboratory tests
- Human immunodeficiency virus (HIV) screening with laboratory tests.

NONCONTRACEPTIVE BENEFITS AND THERAPEUTIC USE OF THE COMBINED ORAL CONTRACEPTIVE PILL

The health benefits of COCs are numerous and outweigh the risks of their use. Definitive evidence exists regarding the protective effect of combined COCs against ovarian and endometrial cancers and, to a lesser extent, colon cancer.

The pill also reduces the incidence of benign breast disease, functional ovarian cysts, pelvic inflammatory disease requiring hospitalization, ectopic pregnancy, and iron-deficiency anemia.

Whether solely with a view to treat these symptoms or in conjunction with contraception, the pill can also be prescribed for the treatment of several gynecological disorders such as dysmenorrhea, irregular or excessive bleeding, acne, hirsutism, and endometriosis-associated pain.[6]

EFFICACY CONCERNS

There is a great gap between the theoretical efficacy (*method effectiveness*) of the pill, which approaches 100%, and the clinical efficacy (*typical use effectiveness*), which depends on patients' compliance. Several factors account for the patient-related pill failures: skipping one or more pills, starting pill intake too late in the cycle, unfamiliarity with the precautions in case of unintended cessation of pill intake, or conscious noncompliance with instructions may all be responsible. Rarely, the contraceptive efficacy is impaired by intestinal malabsorption due to vomiting or diarrhea or interactions with drugs that decrease the contraceptive estrogen and/or progestin levels.

Pearl Index is usually used to assess failure rate per 100 women in year of exposure. (Average: 0.1 – 0.5 HWY)

Usually, two Pearl Indexes are published from studies of birth control methods:

- *Actual-use Pearl Index*, which includes all pregnancies in a study and all months (or cycles) of exposure. It is as high as 3–9.
- *Perfect-use or method Pearl Index*, which includes only pregnancies that resulted from correct and consistent use of the method and only includes months or cycles in which the method was correctly and consistently used. It is as high as 0.1–0.3.

SIDE EFFECTS

Minor Side Effects

- Symptoms of nausea, vomiting, and fluid retention leading to edema
- Headache and irritability
- Depression
- Mastalgia
- Increased noninfective vaginal discharge
- Symptoms of vaginal dryness
- Cloasma, acne, and loss of libido
- Menstrual abnormalities such as hypomenorrhea, amenorrhea, or breakthrough bleeding.[7]

Major Side Effects/Complications

- Venous thromboembolic (VTE) disease is the most common vascular event affecting current COC users with VTE risk—three to six times that in nonusers. Risk is related to both the dose of estrogen and the type of progestogen, *with an approximately twofold higher risk for desogestrel/gestodene/drospirenone/cyproterone pills compared with levonorgestrel/norethisterone.*
- Blood coagulability is increased, partially by increased production of various blood coagulation factors, but more importantly, by a decreased synthesis of antithrombin III, a natural protective mechanism against intravascular coagulation. This increases thrombosis risk. Various epidemiological studies indicate a 5–10-fold increase in thromboembolism and thrombophlebitis, deep vein thrombosis, and pulmonary embolism.
- There is a correlation between contraceptive use and cerebrovascular disorders and myocardial infarction. This risk increases with age and years of pill use.
- There is a mild increase in blood pressure in long-term contraceptive use caused by increased angiotensinogen production by the liver. It is significant only for women with a history of familial hypertension, diabetes mellitus, or pre-eclampsia. Smoking increases this risk.
- Urinary tract infections are 25–50% more frequent in pill users.
- Glucose tolerance is slightly decreased.
- Findings are contradictory in their effects on cholesterol and triglyceride serum level, but the pill is contraindicated in lipid metabolism disorders as they surely alter lipids.
- There is an increased incidence in cholecystitis and cholelithiasis in pill users (70–80 additional cases/100,000 user-years). Liver diseases, intrahepatic cholestasis, occur rarely and benign liver tumors have not conclusively been proved to be caused by the pill.
- A variety of laboratory findings have been related to contraceptive use and drug interactions occur with barbiturates, rifampicin, hydantoin, and phenylbutazone.[8-10]
- Prolonged use for >5–10 years can cause cervical dysplastic changes.

RECOMMENDATIONS AS PER WHO CATEGORIES

Medical Eligibility Criteria for Contraceptive Use of COCs

Medical eligibility criteria (MEC) categories for contraceptive eligibility:

- A condition for which there is no restriction for the use of the contraceptive method

- A condition where the advantages of using the method generally outweigh the theoretical or proven risks
- A condition where the theoretical or proven risks usually outweigh the advantages of using the method
- A condition which represents an unacceptable health risk, if the contraceptive method is used

1. *Recommendations for combined hormonal contraceptive (CHC) use by age group*:
   - *<40 years*: Women from menarche through 40 years of age can use CHCs without restriction (MEC Category 1).
   - *≥40 years*: Women 40 years and older can generally use CHCs (MEC category 2).
2. *Recommendations for CHC use among breastfeeding women*:
   - <6 months postpartum (primarily breastfeeding) generally should not use CHCs (MEC Category 3).
   - *≥6 months postpartum breastfeeding*: Women ≥6 months postpartum can generally can use CHCs (MEC Category 2).
3. *Recommendations for CHC use among postpartum women*:
   - *<21 days postpartum without other risk factors for VTE*: Women who are <21 days postpartum and do not have other risk factors for VTE generally should not use CHCs (MEC Category 3).
   - *<21 days postpartum with other risk factors for VTE*: Women who are <21 days postpartum with other risk factors for VTE should not use CHCs (MEC Category 4).
   - *≥21–42 days postpartum without other risk factors for VTE*: Women who are ≥21–42 days postpartum without other risk factors for VTE can generally use CHCs (MEC Category 2).
   - *≥21–42 days postpartum with other risk factors for VTE*: Women who are ≥21–42 days postpartum with other risk factors for VTE generally should not use CHCs (MEC Category 3).
   - *42 days postpartum*: Women who are >42 days postpartum can use CHCs without restriction (MEC Category 1).
4. *Recommendations for CHC use among women with superficial venous disorders—varicose veins*:
   - Women with varicose veins can use CHCs without restriction (MEC Category 1)
   - *Very low superficial venous thrombosis (SVT)*: Women with SVT can generally use CHCs (MEC Category 2).
5. *Recommendations for CHC use among women with known dyslipidemias*:
   - Women with known dyslipidemias without other known cardiovascular risk factors can generally use CHCs (MEC Category 2).
6. *Recommendations for progestogen-only contraceptive (POC) use among breastfeeding women*:
   - *<6 weeks postpartum breastfeeding*: Women who are <6 weeks postpartum can generally use progestogen-only pills (POPs) (MEC Category 2).
   - *≥6 weeks to <6 months postpartum breastfeeding*: Women who are ≥6 weeks to <6 months postpartum can use POPs without restriction (MEC Category 1).
   - *≥6 months postpartum breastfeeding*: Women who are ≥6 months postpartum can use POPs without restriction (MEC Category 1).

CONTRAINDICATIONS

Absolute

- Heavy smokers due to significant risk for cardiovascular events and specifically deep vein thromboembolism
- Women with uncontrolled hypertension
- Uncontrolled diabetics
- Women with a history of VTE or known ischemic heart disease
- Migraines with auras
- Active or history of breast or endometrial cancer should not use OCs, as these conditions represent unacceptable health risks[9]
- 4–6 weeks prior to planned surgery
- History of chronic liver diseases such as cholestatic jaundice of pregnancy, cirrhosis of liver, porphyrias, and adenomas.

Relative

- Age > 35 years
- Previous history of jaundice
- Sickle cell disease
- Breastfeeding
- Gallbladder disease
- Unexplained headache
- Cervical intraepithelial neoplasia (CIN 1)
- Smokers
- Patients on rifampicin and antiepileptic drugs except sodium valproate
- Gross obesity.

MONITORING

Oral contraceptive pills provide patients with the option to prevent pregnancy. OCs are a choice made by the patient and her physician after adequate counseling of risks and benefits. Long-term COC use needs monitoring of blood pressure, lipid profile, liver functions, and cervical cytology every 2 years of its use.

COMBINED ORAL CONTRACEPTIVE PILLS AS EMERGENCY CONTRACEPTIVE

In this method, four pills of COCs are to be consumed, twice 12 hours apart preferably within 72 hours of intercourse.

This method has become obsolete with the availability of better methods. Still, it can be used if the pills are available with the woman.

KEY MESSAGES

Combined oral contraceptives are a very reliable method of contraception. COC is a major achievement of the last century and a boon particularly for women. It is an acceptable and feasible method of contraception. It has brought millions of women relief from the fear of unwanted pregnancy and has made it possible to avoid innumerable deaths from illegal abortion and childbirth. COCs, if used appropriately, are a very effective contraceptive and should be promoted in eligible cases.

REFERENCES

1. Baird DT, Glasier AF. Hormonal contraception. N Engl J Med. 1993;328(21):1543-9.
2. Maguire K, Westhoff C. The state of hormonal contraception today: established and emerging noncontraceptive health benefits. Am J Obstet Gynecol. 2011;205(4 Suppl):S4-8.
3. IARC Working Group. (2007). Combined Estrogen-Progestogen Contraceptives (PDF). IARC Monographs on the Evaluation of Carcinogenic Risks to Humans. [online] Available from: https://publications.iarc.fr/Book-And-Report-Series/Iarc-Monographs-On-The-Identification-Of-Carcinogenic-Hazards-To-Humans/Combined-Estrogen-Progestogen-Contraceptives-And-Combined-Estrogen-Progestogen-Menopausal-Therapy-2007. [Last accessed November, 2021].
4. Nelson AL, Cwiak C. Combined oral contraceptives. In: Hatcher RA, Trussell J, Nelson AL, Cates W Jr, Kowal D, Policar MS (Eds). Contraceptive Technology, 20th revised edition. New York: Ardent Media; 2011. pp. 253-4.
5. Committee on Gynecologic Practice. ACOG Committee Opinion Number 540: Risk of venous thromboembolism among users of drospirenone-containing oral contraceptive pills. Obstet Gynecol. 2012;120(5):1239-42.
6. American College of Obstetricians and Gynecologist. ACOG Practice Bulletin No. 110: noncontraceptive uses of hormonal contraceptives. Obstet Gynecol. 2010;115(1):206-18.
7. Shulman LP. The state of hormonal contraception today: benefits and risks of hormonal contraceptives: combined estrogen and progestin contraceptives. Am J Obstet Gynecol. 2011;205(4 Suppl):S9-13.
8. Simmons KB, Haddad LB, Nanda K, Curtis KM. Drug interactions between non-rifamycin antibiotics and hormonal contraception: a systematic review. Am J Obstet Gynecol. 2018;218(1):88-97.e14.
9. Weerasinghe M, Konradsen F, Eddleston M, Pearson M, Agampodi T, Storm F, et al. Overdose of oral contraceptive pills as a means of intentional self-poisoning amongst young women in Sri Lanka: considerations for family planning. J Fam Plann Reprod Health Care. 2017;43(2):147-50.
10. Nanda K, Stuart GS, Robinson J, Gray AL, Tepper NK, Gaffield ME. Drug interactions between hormonal contraceptives and antiretrovirals. AIDS. 2017;31(7):917-52.

LONG QUESTIONS

1. Discuss in detail about the indications, prescription, risks, and contraindications of combined oral pills.
2. Classify OCs and discuss their contraindications and side effects.

SHORT QUESTIONS

1. How are COCs used as emergency contraception?
2. Classify combined oral pills and discuss their advantages.
3. What is the mechanism of COCs in preventing fertilization?
4. How should we evaluate a woman before prescribing COCs?
5. Discuss absolute and relative contraindications of COCs.
6. What are noncontraceptive benefits of COCs?

MULTIPLE CHOICE QUESTIONS

1. A combined oral pill contains:
   a. Combination of high- and low-potency progesterone
   b. Combination of two generations of progesterone
   c. Combination of estrogen and progesterone
   d. Combination of high- and low-potency estrogens
2. Fourth-generation COCs contain:
   a. Norethisterone b. Drospirenone
   c. Desogestrel d. Levonorgestrel
3. COCs are absolutely contraindicated in:
   a. Severe nausea and vomiting
   b. Acne formation
   c. Deep venous thromboembolism
   d. Loss of libido
4. Failure rate of COCs with ideal use is:
   a. 1–2 HWY b. 5–6 HWY
   c. 0.1–0.3 HWY d. 0.9–1 HWY
5. The COC pills reduce:
   a. The incidence of benign breast disease and functional ovarian cysts
   b. Cervical dysplasia
   c. Acne formation
   d. Cholestasis

Answers

1. c 2. b 3. c 4. c 5. a

2.6 PROGESTERONE-ONLY PILLS

Nalini Anand

INTRODUCTION

Progestin-only contraceptives, as the name suggests, contain only progestins for contraceptive action, unlike combined oral contraceptive pills (COCPs), which contain both estrogen and progestin for contraceptive action. They are available as pills, implants, injectables, patches, and intrauterine device (**Figs. 1 to 4**). Progesterone-only pills (POPs) are taken without interruption unlike combined OCPs. The combined OCPs are more commonly used as oral contraceptives in comparison to the POPs. However, POPs have their own unique features, advantages, and disadvantages, which will be discussed in this segment.

TYPES OF PROGESTIN AND DOSAGE SCHEDULE

Among the various progestins that can be used as POPs, the following ones are more commonly used:

- Desogestrel 75 µg
- Levonorgestrel 30 µg
- Norethisterone 350 µg

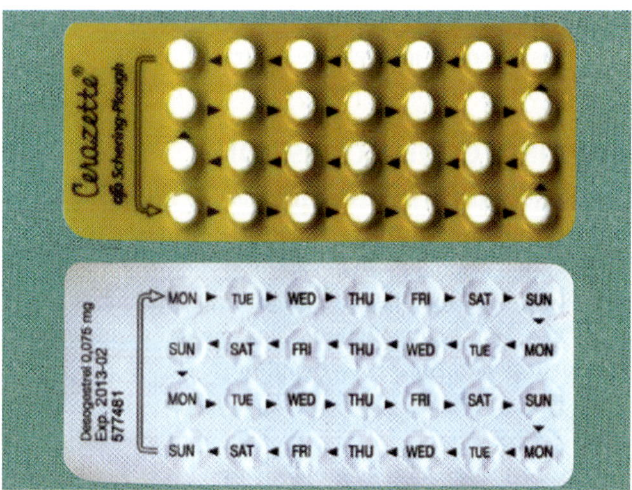

Fig. 1: Progesterone-only pill (Cerazette, desogestrel 75 µg, Merck, Sharp and Dohme Limited).

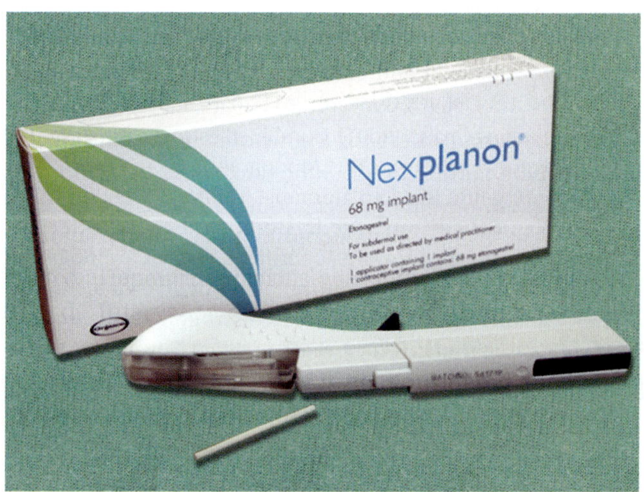

Fig. 2: Nexplanon (68 mg Etonogestrel Implant, Merck, Sharp and Dohme, BV).

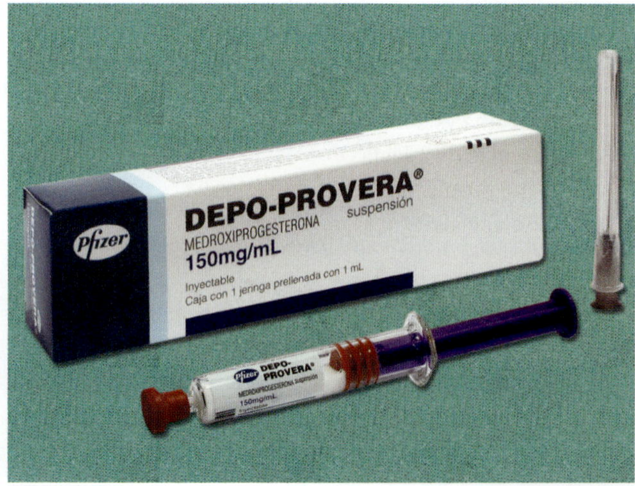

Fig. 3: Depot-medroxy-progesterone acetate (Depo-Provera, Pfizer Inc.).

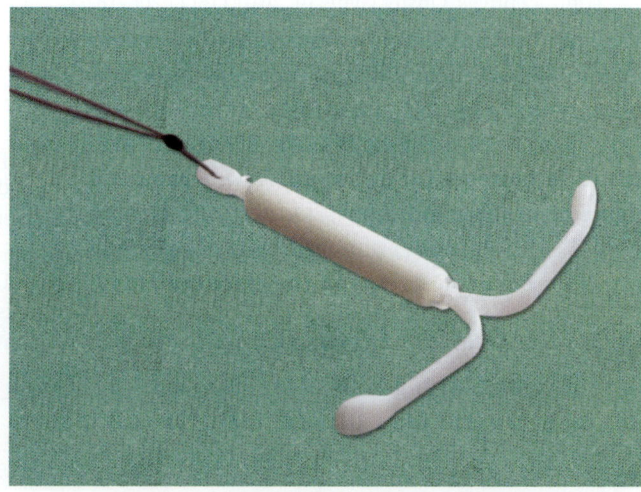

Fig. 4: Levonorgestrel intrauterine system.

- Lynestrenol 500 μg
- Norgestrel 30 μg.

In regular cycles:

- As per WHO recommendations, suggest POP to be started within first 5 days of menstrual cycle without the need of additional contraception (preferably first day).

Amenorrhea:

- Start any time after being sure that there is no pregnancy.
- Additional protection or abstinence from sex is advised for the first 48 hours.

During lactation:

- As per American CDC guidelines: Started any time after delivery
- As per WHO: Started after 6 weeks.

These pills are taken continuously without interruption. POPs are supposed to be taken daily without any break between packs and on same time every day. With a delay of >3 hours (traditional POP)/12 hours for desogestrel POP (compare this to 12 hours for combined OCP), user should immediately take the missed pills and continue the pills as per schedule. However, she should use additional contraception for next 2 days. This requirement of strict adherence to schedule can become cumbersome and make POP less suitable to many women and is one of its disadvantages.

MECHANISM OF ACTION

The primary method of action in POPs is to thicken the cervical mucus due to the high levels of progesterone. This prevents the entry of sperm and thereby fertilization of the oocyte. It also suppresses ovulation to varying degrees, in a dose-dependent manner. It inhibits ovulation in about 60% of cycles with pills containing levonorgestrel whereas POPs containing desogestrel suppresses ovulation in 97% of cycles. The increased levels of progesterone also cause thinning of the endometrium, which inhibits implantation (decidualization of endometrium). Since POPs do not completely suppress follicular development, there is endogenous secretion of estrogens which prevents negative impact on bone mineral density of the user. Ovulation may occur despite usage of POP; however, because of above-mentioned changes, fertilization and/or implantation do not occur.

FAILURE RATE

Breastfeeding women:

- Typical use: 1/HWY
- Perfect use: 0.3/HWY.

Nonbreastfeeding women:

- Typical use: 3–10/HWY
- Perfect use: 0.3/HWY.

ADVANTAGES

- *Suited ideally for:*
  - It is the oral contraception of choice in lactating women, where it neither affects the quantity nor the quality of breast milk. It is highly suitable in women who want to space their pregnancies but unwilling for postpartum intrauterine device. It is particularly useful for this indication. It can be started after 6 weeks postpartum, and unlike intrauterine devices which have high expulsion rates, POPs if used properly could provide effective contraception in the postpartum period.
  - Sickle cell anemia (best contraceptive).
  - Seizure disorder (raises seizure threshold).
- It can be used by those women, who cannot take combined OCP.
- Decreased cyclic mood changes.
- Many contraindications of COCPs like age >35 years and smoking do not apply on POPs.
- Pills are taken daily without any break, which makes it easy for the user as they do not have to worry for "off" days, as in COCPs.
- More effective than barrier methods when taken correctly.
- Rapidly reversible.
- Sex does not need to be interrupted to use contraception, making it more comfortable for a couple (*sexual freedom).*
- Can be used in many patients for whom estrogen in combined OCP is contraindicated, like those with hypertension, fibroid, diabetes, smoking, history of thromboembolism, epilepsy, etc.
- May reduce risk of endometrial cancer and pelvic inflammatory disease (PID).
- Can also be used as hormone therapy in postmenopausal women with intact uterus, thereby avoiding the risk of endometrial carcinoma.
- A POP may be preferred for safety reasons in older women with lower fertility who wish to continue oral contraception.

DISADVANTAGES

- User dependent and has to be taken at the same time each day, which can become cumbersome for some users.
- Can produce irregular menstruation (breakthrough bleeding) which can be heavy on some, abdominal cramps and amenorrhea. This can become troublesome for many of its users and is the most common reason for discontinuation of POP. However, with continued usage, most women tend to establish amenorrhea.
- Weight gain due to fluid retention is common, which may become significant for some women. A gain of >5% in the first months of usage warrants discontinuation of POP and switching to alternate contraception.

- Moderately increased risk of ovarian cysts.
- In case of failure, if pregnancy occurs—10% are ectopic.
- Small increased risk of breast cancer.
- No protection against sexually transmitted diseases such as HIV, HPV, HSV, trichomonas, and others.
- Effectiveness reduced by hepatic enzyme inducers.

SIDE EFFECTS

- Acne
- Breast tenderness and enlargement
- Altered sex drive
- Mood changes
- Headache and migraine
- Nausea and vomiting.

These side effects are most likely to occur during the first few months of POP usage and generally improve over time.

CONTRAINDICATIONS (WHO, 2008)

- *Absolute (Category 4):*
  - Breast cancer (current or past)
- *Relative (Category 3; risks outweigh advantages):*
  - Breastfeeding (<6 weeks)
  - Cardiovascular disorders
  - Current deep vein thrombosis (DVT)/pulmonary embolism (PE)
  - Current ischemic heart disease
  - Migraine with aura
  - *Liver disorders*:
    - Active viral hepatitis
    - Cirrhosis
    - Benign/malignant liver tumors
    - Drugs affecting liver enzymes (rifampicin, some anticonvulsants)
- Undiagnosed/unexplained vaginal bleeding
  - Pregnancy.

DISCUSSIONS ON PROGESTERONE-ONLY PILLS (FROM THE COCHRANE LIBRARY)

- Randomized controlled trials published to date are inadequate to compare POPs to each other or to combined oral contraceptives.
- Since POPs are commonly used during breastfeeding, when fertility is low, the impact of better efficacy of any pill would be small in this setting.
- No trial addressed the question of consistent timing of ingestion.
- *Levonorgestrel versus desogestrel*:
  - Better efficacy of desogestrel is offset by worse bleeding patterns (prolonged bleeding and absent bleeding) as compared to levonorgestrel, which leads to higher rate to discontinuation.
  - This trade-off needs to be seen in individual setting; for some women, efficacy is more important and for some regular bleeding.
  - Abnormal bleeding patterns may reflect the better suppression of ovulation with the desogestrel POP than with the levonorgestrel POP.

FURTHER READING

1. Family Planning. Chapter 2: Progestin-Only Pills. [online] Available from: https://www.fphandbook.org/chapter-2-progestin-only-pills. [Last accessed November, 2021].
2. Grimes DA, Lopez LM, O'Brien PA, Raymond EG. Progestin-only pills for contraception. Cochrane Database Syst Rev. 2013;(11):CD007541.
3. Michelle M, Deshmukh PY, Deepali K. Progesterone only pills: an effective contraceptive option for lactating women. Int J Reprod Contracept Obstet Gynecol. 2017;6(10):4399-401.
4. NHS. The progestogen-only pill. [online] Available from: https://www.nhs.uk/conditions/contraception/the-pill-progestogen-only/. [Last accessed November, 2021]
5. Trussell J. Contraceptive efficacy. In: Hatcher RA, Trussell J, Nelson AL, Cates W, Kowal D, Policar M (Eds). Contraceptive Technology, 20th revised edition. New York: Ardent Media; 2011.

LONG QUESTION

1. Discuss the advantages, disadvantages, contraindications, and side effects of POPs.

SHORT QUESTIONS

1. Why the POP should be taken every day?
2. Why it is important for a woman to take her POPs at the same time each day?
3. How effective are POPs in preventing pregnancy?
4. What are possible side effects of POPs?

MULTIPLE CHOICE QUESTIONS

1. What is a unique thing about POPs?
   a. They can be taken from the first day of menses.
   b. They are to be taken continuously without a break.
   c. They reduce milk secretion.
   d. They cause irregularities in menstruation.
2. The full form of POPs is:
   a. Progesterone-only pills b. Postoperative pills
   c. Postdelivery pills d. Postabortion pills
3. The failure rate of POPs with perfect use is:
   a. 18/HWY b. 10/HWY
   c. 0.3/HWY d. 0.03/HWY
4. POPs are contraceptive of choice for:
   a. Lactating women b. Nulliparous women
   c. Unmarried girls d. Elderly women
5. POPs are ideal for patients with:
   a. Thalassemia major b. Sickle cell anemia
   c. Cardiovascular diseases d. Nulliparity

6. Mechanism of action of POPs includes all, except:
   a. Cervical mucus thickening
   b. Ovulation inhibition
   c. Thinning of endometrium
   d. Spermicidal
7. All of the following are contraindications of POPs, except:
   a. Pregnancy b. Breast cancer
   c. Liver disorders d. Migraine
8. Following is used as POP:
   a. Levonorgestrel b. Estradiol
   c. Estriol d. Cyproterone acetate
9. This is not a disadvantage of POPs:
   a. Acne
   b. Breakthrough bleeding
   c. Increased risk of ovarian cysts
   d. Increased risk if carcinoma of breast
10. Strict adherence to time schedule for POPs is:
   a. Desirable b. Necessary
   c. Not required d. None of the above

Answers

1.	b	2.	a	3.	c	4.	a	5.	b	6.	d
7.	d	8.	a	9.	a	10.	b				

2.7 INJECTABLE CONTRACEPTIVES

Mukta Jain

INTRODUCTION

Injectable contraception is one of the convenient, safe, and reversible birth control methods of contraception. The injectable contraceptives contain synthetic hormones resembling the natural female hormones. After introduction of oral contraceptives, it was discovered that when an injectable form of a synthetic form of progesterone is administered (IM/SC) there is a slow release of hormone into the bloodstream and it provides protection from pregnancy for a long duration of time.

The injectable contraceptive is the fourth most popular family planning method worldwide, after female sterilization, intrauterine contraceptive device (IUCD), and oral contraceptive.

TYPES OF INJECTABLE CONTRACEPTION

There are two main types of injectable contraceptives:[1,2]

1. *Progestogen-only injectables* (POIs) containing only synthetic progesterone. Two types are:
   i. Depot-medroxy-progesterone acetate (DMPA)—3 monthly injection
   ii. Norethisterone enanthate (NET-EN)—2 monthly injection
2. *Combined injectable contraceptive* (CIC): Containing estrogen (usually ethinylestradiol) and progesterone—1 monthly injection
   ii. Medroxy-progesterone acetate (MPA)/estradiol cypionate (WHO and CCP, 2008).

History of DMPA

Depot-medroxy-progesterone acetate is a synthetic progesterone, developed by the Upjohn Company in 1954 for the treatment of endometriosis and habitual or threatened abortions. In early 1960s, it was noted that women receiving DMPA for premature labor subsequently had a marked delay in return of fertility. This observation led to the development of DMPA as a fertility-regulating agent. In the mid-1960s, Upjohn got a contraceptive product license for marketing DMPA as a contraceptive in many countries. Since then, DMPA has become a popular contraceptive and has been one of the most extensively researched drugs with an accumulated research experience of over 3 million women months of use with more than a thousand published scientific papers and reviews. It is now a widely used contraceptive and is approved for use in more than 130 countries.[2]

Mechanism of Action (DMPA)

- Suppresses mid-cycle peaks of luteinizing hormone (LH) and follicle-stimulating hormone (FSH) and thus inhibits ovulation.
- Thickening of cervical mucus—due to depletion of estrogen. The thick mucus prevents sperm penetration in the upper reproductive tract.
- Thinning of endometrial lining due to high progesterone and depleted estrogen making it unfavorable for implantation of fertilized ovum.

Eligibility Criteria (DMPA)

- Women of any age, including adolescents and women over 45 years old.
- Any woman, irrespective of parity, marital status, smoker, HIV infected, or at risk of sexually transmitted infection (STI)/HIV infection is eligible to receive this injection.
- Can be given in breastfeeding woman starting 6 weeks postpartum or postabortion.

Women can begin DMPA injection:

- Without a pelvic examination
- Without any blood tests or routine laboratory tests
- Without cervical cancer screening

- Without a breast examination
- Even when she is not having monthly bleeding at the time of injection, if it is certain that the woman is not pregnant.

Contraindications (DMPA)

- Breastfeeding woman <6 weeks postpartum
- Blood pressure 160/110 mm Hg
- Unexplained vaginal bleeding.

WHEN TO START INJECTABLE CONTRACEPTIVE?

- Injectable contraceptives can be started at any time of the menstrual cycle (after excluding pregnancy), preferably within the first 5 days of menstrual bleeding when no back-up method is needed. If given later in the cycle, a back-up method such as barrier (condoms) or spermicide should be used for at least the next 48 hours.
- After delivery, it can be started as early as after 6 weeks when the woman is fully or partially breastfeeding her baby. In nonlactating mothers, it can be given immediately after childbirth or any time within 6 weeks without waiting for return of menses.
- After an abortion, it can be started immediately, or in the first 7 days, or any time later after excluding pregnancy.
- Women discontinuing the use of other contraceptives can use injectable without any delay.

CLINICAL ASSESSMENT

History

- *Demographic details*:
  - Name, husband's name, address, contact number, age, marital status, occupation, religion, educational status, number of living children, and last childbirth
- *Menstrual history*:
  - Last menstrual period (LMP), length of cycles, duration, amount of flow, any dysmenorrhea, regularity of periods, any intermenstrual bleeding
- *Obstetric history*:
  - Number of pregnancies, living children, mode of delivery, date of last childbirth, and history of abortions
- Breastfeeding—full, partial or not and since when is she breastfeeding
- Contraceptive—when and which method of contraceptives used. If discontinued, then details of timing and reason
- *Medical history*:
  - Details about any medical illness
  - Drug history
  - Any allergies.

Examination

- General physical examination
- Routine abdominal examination
- Pelvic examination (not mandatory).

Investigations

- Pregnancy test
- Others if indicated.

ROUTE OF DMPA INJECTABLE CONTRACEPTIVE

Intramuscular

- Single-dose vial with disposable syringe and needle
- Prefilled syringe with needle.

Subcutaneous

- Prefilled autodisable syringe in Uniject system.

EFFECTIVENESS

- Highly effective method with effectiveness of 99.7% when used correctly
- Failure rate is 0.3% even lower than female sterilization (0.5%), IUCD (0.8%), and oral contraceptive pills (OCPs) (3%).

Factors determining effectiveness are:

- Timing of first injection
- Regularity of injections
- Injection technique
- Postinjection care.

BENEFITS

Contraceptive Benefits

- Safe and highly effective with long-term contraceptive benefits
- Easy to use and convenient (does not require daily routine or additional supplies)
- Acts for 3 months with a grace period of 4 weeks
- *Reversibility*: Completely reversible—7–10 months from the date of last injection (average 4–6 months after 3 months effectivity of last injection is over)
- A private and confidential method
- Does not interfere with sexual intercourse/pleasure
- Pelvic examination not required prior to use
- Suitable for women who are not eligible to use an estrogen-containing contraceptive
- Suitable for lactating women (after 6 weeks' postpartum), as it does not affect quantity, quality, and composition of breast milk.

Noncontraceptive Benefits[3-7]

- May decrease menstrual cramps and reduce premenstrual syndrome/tension
- Improves anemia by reducing menstrual blood loss due to menstrual changes such as amenorrhea
- Reduces the symptoms of endometriosis
- Decreases benign breast disease and ovarian cyst

- Helps to prevent uterine tumors (fibroids)
- Reduces the incidence of symptomatic pelvic inflammatory disease (PID)
- Protect against endometrial cancer and possibly ovarian cancer
- Reduces sickle-cell crises in women with sickle cell anemia
- Protects against ectopic pregnancy (since ovulation does not occur)
- Minimal drug interactions.

THERAPEUTIC USE[8-14]

DMPA to be considered for treatment in:

- Menorrhagia/dysmenorrhea
- Premenstrual syndrome
- Pain in women with endometriosis
- Hemoglobinopathies
- Seizures refractory to conventional anticonvulsant
- Menstrual hygiene problems in handicapped
- Endometrial hyperplasia
- Vasomotor symptoms in menopausal women
- Pelvic pain/dyspareunia of ovarian origin after hysterectomy
- Ovulatory pain
- Metastatic breast cancer
- Metastatic endometrial cancer.

LIMITATIONS

- No protection against STI/reproductive tract infection (RTI) and HIV infection
- Once taken, its action cannot be stopped immediately
- It causes changes in the menstrual cycle and bleeding due to its inevitable effect on a woman's body hormones
- It has to be repeated every 3 months to achieve desired contraceptive effectiveness
- Return of fertility usually takes around 7–10 months from the date of last injection
- Cannot be given in few medical conditions/diseases.

SIDE EFFECTS

- *Menstrual problems*:
  - Menstrual changes occur in almost all women using DMPA.
  - More episodes of unpredictable, irregular bleeding and spotting lasting 7 days or more during the 1st month of use.
  - The frequency and duration of these episodes decrease by increasing the duration of use.
  - After 1 year of DMPA use (four injections), 50% of women experience amenorrhea. With ongoing use, the rate of amenorrhea may increase to 75%.
- Weight gain
- Headaches
- Bloating of abdomen and breast
- Mood changes
- Reduced libido.

RETURN TO FERTILITY

The persistence of ovulation suppression after DMPA discontinuation is not related to duration of use. Return of fertility usually takes around 7–10 months from the day of last injection. It may take up to 18 months as well. Thus, counseling is an essential part before offering this as a mode of contraception. Women who wish to conceive within next 1–2 years need to choose an alternative method of contraception.[15]

FOLLOW-UP (TABLE 1)

Repeat injections are needed every 3 months.

ANTARA

It is a lipid regulatory agent called a filtrate used to treat high cholesterol and high triglyceride levels.

Antara is available in generic form.

The adult starting dose of Antara to treat primary hypercholesterolemia or mixed hyperlipidemia is 130 mg/day.

TABLE 1: Follow-up care in DMPA clients.

	Time of visit	*Action to be taken*	*Points of reinforcement*
Client	At 3 months after last injection on the scheduled date	Give DMPA injection No back-up required	Encourage to come for the next allotted date of injection Discuss if she is having any side effects and counsel accordingly
Defaulters	2 weeks earlier or up to 4 weeks later from scheduled date (within grace period)	Give DMPA injection No back-up required	Counsel her for importance of next injection Discuss if she is having any side effects and counsel accordingly
Dropouts	>4 months from the date of last injection	Rule out pregnancy If not pregnant, give DMPA injection Advise back-up method for the next 7 days (barrier method)	Ask reason for coming late If returning within 4 months is not possible, discuss other method of contraception

(DMPA: depot-medroxy-progesterone acetate)

The adult starting dose of Antara to treat hypertriglyceridemia is 43–130 mg/day based on blood lipid levels measured every 4–8 weeks.

Interaction

- Blood thinners, cyclosporine, and other cholesterol-lowering medicines.

Contraindications

- *Pregnancy:* Not to be used as possible risk to the fetus
- *Breastfeeding:* Not recommended as potential adverse events reported in 2% cases.

Side effects may include **(Table 2)**:

- Stomach pain
- Back pain
- Headache
- Runny or stuffy nose
- Infrequently cause gallstone and liver problems
- Severe such as—severe abdominal pain, tachycardia, persistent nausea, vomiting, yellowish discoloration of eyes or skin, dark urine, easy bruising, unusual bleeding, purple or red pinpoint spots under skin, chest pain, sudden cough, wheeze and rapid breathing, coughing up blood, pain/swelling/warmth/redness in one or both legs.

POSTMARKETING EXPERIENCE

Myalgia, rhabdomyolysis, pancreatitis, renal failure, muscle spasms, acute renal failure, hepatitis, cirrhosis, anemia, arthralgia, asthenia, severely depressed high-density lipoprotein (HDL) cholesterol levels, and photosensitivity reactions have occurred days and months after initiation **(Table 2)**.

TABLE 2: Adverse effects of fenofibrate versus placebo.

Adverse effect	*Fenofibrate*	*Placebo*
Body as a whole:		
Abdominal pain	4.6%	4.4%
Back pain	3.4%	2.5%
Headache	3.2%	2.7%
Digestive:		
Abnormal LFT	7.5%	1.4%
Nausea	2.3%	1.9%
Constipation	2.1%	1.4%
Metabolic and nutritional disorders:		
Increased AST	3.4%	0.5%
Increased ALT	3.0%	1.6%
Increased CPK	3.0%	1.4%
Respiratory:		
Respiratory disorder	6.2%	5.5%
Rhinitis	2.3%	1.1%

(ALT: alanine transaminase; AST: aspartate aminotransferase; CPK: creatine phosphokinase; LFT: liver function test)

SUMMARY OF KEY RECOMMENDATIONS[16]

- When administered at the recommended dosing interval, the failure rate of POI contraception is approximately 0.2% in the 1st year of use. With typical use, the failure rate is approximately 6%.
- Health professionals should be familiar with the most up-to-date UK Medical Eligibility Criteria for POI contraception.
- Amenorrhea or reduced bleeding is common in POI users and may benefit women with menstrual problems.
- Depot-medroxy-progesterone acetate use may reduce pain associated with endometriosis.
- Women should be advised about changes in bleeding patterns.
- Use of DMPA is not associated with an increased risk of ovarian or endometrial cancer and may offer some protection.
- DMPA is a contraceptive option for women with sickle cell disease and may reduce the severity of sickle crisis pain.
- Progestogen-only injectable use is associated with a small loss of bone mineral density, which is usually recovered after discontinuation.
- In women aged under 18 years, POI contraception can be used after consideration of alternative methods.
- Women using DMPA who wish to continue use should be reviewed every 2 years to assess individual situations and to discuss the benefits and potential risks.
- Women are generally advised to switch to another method at the age of 50 years. If a woman does not wish to stop using DMPA, consideration may be given to continuation, provided the benefits and risks have been assessed and the woman informed of the potential risks.
- There is possibly a weak association between the current use of DMPA and breast cancer. Any increased risk is likely to be small and reduces with time after stopping.
- A causal association between DMPA and venous thrombosis has not been demonstrated in the small number of studies that have investigated this relationship.
- From the limited evidence available, it is not possible to confirm or exclude an association between POI use and myocardial infarction or stroke.
- There is a weak association between cervical cancer and use of DMPA for 5 years or longer. Any increased risk appears to reduce with time after stopping and could be due to confounding factors.
- Health professionals should ensure that women requesting DMPA are up to date with cervical cytology screening and, if relevant, have completed the human papillomavirus (HPV) vaccination program.
- Women should be informed about the link between HPV and cervical cancer and advised about strategies that reduce the risk such as condom use, smoking cessation, regular cervical screening and, where appropriate, vaccination against HPV.

- Use of DMPA appears to be associated with weight gain, particularly in women under 18 years of age with a body mass index (BMI) ≥30 kg/m^2.
- Women who gain >5% of their baseline body weight in the first 6 months of DMPA use are likely to experience continued weight gain.
- Injection site reactions appear to be more common with use of subcutaneous (SC) DMPA than with use of intramuscular (IM) DMPA.
- While there is little evidence available to demonstrate causation, a number of possible side effects such as acne, decreased libido, mood swings, headache, hot flushes, and vaginitis have been reported with use of DMPA.
- The gluteal muscle in the buttock is the preferred site for IM DMPA administration, but it can be administered into the deltoid muscle of the upper arm. In women with deep adipose tissue in the gluteal area, standard-length needles may not reach the muscle layer and SC DMPA or deltoid administration of IM DMPA should be considered.
- SC DMPA should be injected into the abdomen or anterior thigh.
- Women should be advised to return every 13 weeks for a repeat injection of IM or SC DMPA (outside the product license for IM DMPA). An injection of DMPA can be administered up to 7 days late (up to 14 weeks after the last injection) without the need for additional contraceptive precautions (outside the product license for IM DMPA).
- If necessary, an early repeat injection of DMPA can be administered from 10 weeks and from 6 weeks for norethisterone enanthate (NET-EN) (outside product license).
- The efficacy of DMPA contraception is not reduced with concurrent use of enzyme-inducing drugs.
- No increased risk of pregnancy has been demonstrated in POI users with higher body weight, although data are limited in women with a BMI ≥ 40 kg/m^2.
- Women who discontinue their POI and who do not wish to conceive should be advised to start another contraceptive method before or at the time of their next scheduled injection even if amenorrheic.
- Women should be informed that there can be a delay of up to 1 year in the return of fertility after discontinuation of IM or SC DMPA.
- The consistent and correct use of condoms (male or female) can reduce the risk of STI transmission and should therefore be recommended as a risk-reduction strategy.
- A causal relationship between POI contraception and HIV transmission/acquisition has not been established but cannot be completely excluded.
- Women who experience unscheduled bleeding during use of a POI and who are medically eligible can be offered a combined oral contraceptive (COC) for 3 months. This can be taken in the usual cyclic manner or continuously without a hormone-free interval (outside product license). Longer-term use of the injectable and COC has not been studied and is a matter of clinical judgment.
- Women with unscheduled bleeding during use of a POI contraceptive can be offered 500 mg mefenamic acid up to three times daily for 5 days.

REFERENCES

1. WHO. (2018). Family Planning: A Global Handbook for Providers. [online] Available from: https://www.who.int/reproductivehealth/publications/fp-global-handbook/en/. [Last accessed November, 2021].
2. Family Planning Division Ministry of Health and Family Welfare, Government of India. (2016). Reference Manual for Injectable Contraceptive (DMPA). [online] Available from: https://nhm.gov.in/images/pdf/programmes/family-planing/guidelines/Reference_Manual_Injectable_Contraceptives.pdf. [Last accessed November, 2021].
3. Cullins VE. Noncontraceptive benefits and therapeutic uses of depot medroxyprogesterone acetate. J Reprod Med. 1996;41(S5):428-33.
4. Pardthaisong T, Gray R. In utero exposure to steroid contraceptives and outcome of pregnancy. Am J Epidemiol. 1991;134:795.
5. Kaunitz AM. Depot medroxyprogesterone acetate contraception and the risk of breast and gynecologic cancer. J Reprod Med. 1996;41(S5):419.
6. Lumbiganon P, Rugpao S, Prandha-Fung S. Protective effect of depot-medroxyprogesterone acetate on surgically-treated uterine leiomyomas: A multinational case-control study. Br J Obstet Gynaecol. 1995;103:909.
7. The WHO Collaborative Study of Neoplasia and Steroid Contraceptives. Depot-medroxyprogesterone acetate (DMPA) and risk of endometrial cancer. The WHO Collaborative Study of Neoplasia and Steroid Contraceptives. Int J Cancer. 1991.49:186.
8. American College of Obstetricians and Gynecologists. Uterine leiomyomata. ACOG Technical Bulletin 192. Washington, DC: ACOG; 1994.
9. Muse K. Hormonal manipulation in the treatment of premenstrual syndrome. Clin Obstet Gynecol. 1992;35:658.
10. Vercellini P, De Giorgi O, Oldahi S, Cortesi I, Panazza S, Crosignani PG.. Depot medroxyprogesterone acetate versus an oral contraceptive combined with very-low-dose danazol for long-term treatment of pelvic pain associated with endometriosis. Am J Obstet Gynecol. 1996;175:396.
11. De Ceulaer K, Hayes R, Gruber C, Serjeant GR. Medroxyprogesterone acetate andhomozygous sickle-cell disease. Lancet. 1982;2:229.
12. Mattson RH, Cramer TA, Caldwell BV, Siconolfi BC. Treatment of seizures with medroxyprogesterone acetate: Preliminary report. Neurology. 1984;34:1255-8.
13. Elkins TE, Gafford LS, Wilks CS, Muram D, Golden G. A model clinic approach to the reproductive health concerns of the mentally handicapped. Obstet Gynecol. 1986;68:185-8.
14. Fraser IS, Dennerstein GJ. Depo-Provera use in an Australian metropolitan practice. Med J Aust. 1994;160:553.
15. Schwallie PC, Assenzo JR. The effect of depot medroxyprogesterone acetate on pituitary and ovarian function, and the return of fertility following its discontinuation: a review. Contraception. 1971;10:181-202.

16. The Faculty of Sexual and Reproductive Healthcare. (2020). CEU Guidance. Progestogen – only Injectable Contraception. Faculty of Sexual & Healthcare Clinical Guidance Dec 2014 (Amended April 2019). [online] Available from: https://www.fsrh.org/standards-and-guidance/fsrh-guidelines-and-statements/method-specific/progestogen-only-injectables/. [Last accessed November, 2021].

LONG QUESTIONS

1. Elaborate the types of injectable contraceptives and their mechanism of action. Which is the most accepted form of injectable contraceptive? Discuss in detail.
2. Describe the benefits and therapeutic uses of injectable contraceptives.
3. Discuss the role of Antara as a contraceptive in detail.
4. Discuss the criteria to start a patient on injectable contraceptive. Describe in brief when to start DMPA in following conditions:
   - In regular menstrual cycle
   - Breastfeeding in postpartum women
   - After abortion
   - After taking emergency contraceptives.
5. Describe the follow-up required in case of DMPA. When can fertility return to normal after stopping it?

SHORT QUESTIONS

1. Discuss the route of administration of injectable contraceptives and its effectiveness.
2. Explain the mechanism of action of injectable contraceptives.
3. Discuss the eligibility criteria for injectable contraceptives.
4. Discuss the noncontraceptive benefits of DMPA.
5. Discuss the side effects, limitations, and contraindications of use of DMPA.

MULTIPLE CHOICE QUESTIONS

1. Progestational contraceptives primarily act by:
   a. Oviductal motility b. Uterine endometrium
   c. Altering cervix mucus d. Inhibiting ovulation
2. All are true for DMPA, except:
   a. Failure @ 0.3/100WY
   b. 150 mg/3 month delivered
   c. Weight gain
   d. Glucose intolerance occurs
3. Side effects of medroxyprogesterone acetate are all, except:
   a. Weight gain b. Irregular bleeding
   c. Amenorrhea d. Hepatitis
4. To avoid contraception, DMPA is given:
   a. Monthly b. 3 monthly
   c. 6 monthly d. Yearly
5. Which is not a contraindication for injectable contraceptive?
   a. Deep vein thrombosis b. History of breast cancer
   c. Lactating female d. Irregular menses
6. What is false about DMPA?
   a. It protects against STI
   b. It prevents endometrial cancer
   c. It may cause breast tenderness and weight gain
   d. One of the side effects is depression
7. What is the dose of NET-EN?
   a. 300 mg every 3 month b. 200 mg every 2 month
   c. 200 mg every 3 month d. 300 mg every 2 month
8. Contraceptive of choice in a couple when the female suffers from epilepsy is:
   a. Barrier b. OCP
   c. Mini-pill d. Injection DMPA
9. Least failure rates noted in:
   a. cuT b. Mirena
   c. DMPA d. OCP
10. What is the contraceptive of choice in sickle cell anemia?
    a. cuT b. Mirena
    c. DMPA d. OCP
11. Which of the following is generally increased by the use of DMPA compared with other contraceptive methods?
    a. Acne
    b. Bone fractures
    c. Hepatic neoplasms
    d. Interval to resumption of ovulation after method cessation
12. Which of the following is not considered a long-acting reversible contraceptive method?
    a. Levonorgestrel implant
    b. Copper intrauterine device
    c. DMPS
    d. All of the above are long-acting reversible contraceptive methods
13. Which of the following statements most accurately describes the injectable progestin contraceptive DMPA?
    a. When injection is given within 5 days of the onset of menses, a backup method is needed for 7 day
    b. Although irregular bleeding leads to 25% of users discontinuing within the 1st year, amenorrhea develops in 80% of users after 1 year
    c. For women desiring only a brief period of contraception, DMPA is not a good choice due to prolonged anovulation after discontinuation
    d. All of the above

Answers

1. c 2. d 3. d 4. b 5. d 6. a
7. b 8. d 9. b 10. c 11. d 12. c
13. c

2.8 NEWER ROUTES FOR CONTRACEPTIONS: IMPLANTS, RINGS AND PATCHES

Ashwini Bhalerao Gandhi, Sanket Pisat, Minal Dhanvij

INTRODUCTION

Modern contraceptive methods account for most contraceptive use worldwide. Globally in 2019, 44% women of reproductive age were using a modern method of contraception. Access to and use of family planning varies by region, and the unmet need for family planning is 10%.[1] It is estimated that if unmet need for contraception is fulfilled, then there will be 60% reduction in global maternal mortality, unintended pregnancies would drop by 70%, and unsafe abortions would decline by 74%.[2] Female sterilization is the most common contraceptive method used worldwide. In 2019, 23.7% women who were currently using contraception rely on female sterilization. Overall, 45.2% of contraceptive users rely on permanent or long-acting methods [female and male sterilization, intrauterine device (IUD), and implant], 46.1% on a short-acting method (such as male condom, the pill, injectable, and other modern methods), and 8.7% on traditional methods (withdrawal, rhythm methods, and other traditional methods).[1] Female sterilization is a permanent method, while oral contraceptives (OCs) are highly effective when used perfectly; daily adherence is a problem for many women. Many women who use OCs are therefore at unnecessary risk of unintended pregnancy and maternal morbidity. OCs offer many benefits, including immediate reversibility, cycle control, decreased pain and regular cyclic bleeding, ovulation suppression and decreased risk of endometrial and ovarian cancer. The transdermal patch and vaginal ring offer the same noncontraceptive benefits, but patch and ring users demonstrate improved compliance over OC users, as these methods do not require daily adherence. The contraceptive implant, with its progesterone-only content, avoids all estrogen-related side effects. All three methods are patient controlled and noncoitus dependent, thereby making them convenient options.

CONTRACEPTIVE IMPLANTS

The subdermal implants are available as Norplant, Jadelle (Chinese version Sino-plant II), Implanon, and Implanon NXT (Nexplanon). The Norplant "sustained-release" system consists of six capsules containing 36 mg levonorgestrel (LNG) in each capsule, Jadelle contains two rods of 75 mg LNG in each, and Implanon is single rod containing etonogestrel (ENG). All are effective up to 3 years. Implanon and Jadelle are included in WHO Model List of Essential Medicine. Norplant and Jadelle are not marketed in the United States. Implanon has been extensively marketed throughout the world with a good track record and high continuation rates.[3]

Structure

The Implanon is 4 cm in length and 2 mm in diameter (**Fig. 1**). It is composed of a solid core of ethylene-vinyl acetate (EVA)

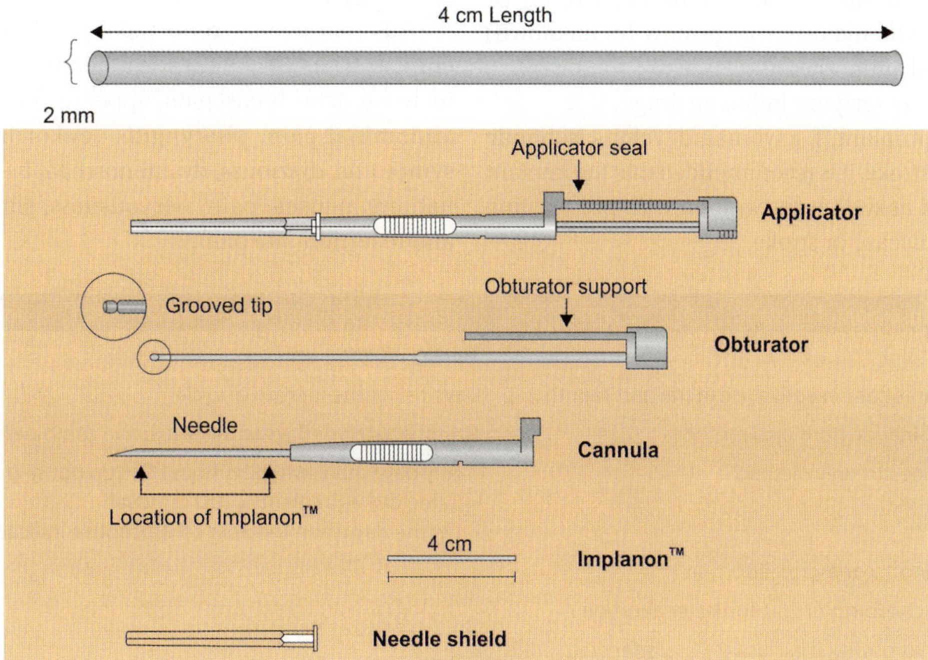

Fig. 1: Implant.

copolymer core containing 68 mg ENG imbedded within the core. Surrounding the core is a thin layer of EVA (0.06 mm thick) that controls the rate at which ENG is released. EVA has been shown to be minimally irritating on the subdermal tissue and may cause a thin fibrous capsule around the implant after insertion. The initial release rate of ENG is 60–70 µg/day, which decreases to about 35–45 µg/day at the end of the 1st year, to about 30–40 µg/day at the end of the 2nd year, and then to about 25–30 µg/day by the end of the 3rd year.[4]

Insertion

The Implant is inserted *subdermally* in the inner aspect of the upper nondominant arm in the groove between the biceps and triceps. This site was chosen because it is easily accessible. One of the many things that make the Implant unique is that it is supplied in a preloaded sterile single-use applicator which facilitates insertion. No incision or suturing is necessary for insertion and as the implant is preloaded into the applicator, the chance of contamination is minimized.

Timing of Insertion

Implants have an immediate contraceptive effect when inserted within the first 7 days of menstrual cycle, but when insertion is after 7 days, a backup method of contraception is necessary for at least 3 days[3] (**Table 1**).

Medical Eligibility

There is no age restriction making implant safe for women of any reproductive age group. There are a few medical conditions for which the risks outweigh the advantages, as defined by the WHO Medical Eligibility Criteria. These include:

- Severe hepatic disease, such as decompensated cirrhosis, hepatocellular adenoma, malignant hepatoma, or systemic lupus erythematosus with positive (or unknown) antiphospholipid antibodies
- Women taking liver enzyme-inducing drugs
- While using an implant if, a woman develops ischemic heart disease or stroke, it is recommended that the implant be discontinued as well as for women with pre-existing ischemic heart disease or stroke
- Current or past history of breast cancer, which is a contraindication to implant use, as breast cancer can be hormone sensitive
- In cases of undiagnosed vaginal bleeding, the cause should be evaluated before inserting an implant.

All reasonable efforts should be made to exclude pregnancy at the time of insertion.

Mechanism of Action

The implant works by two main mechanisms of action. First, it primarily and effectively inhibits ovulation. Contraceptive efficacy is also augmented through the thickening of cervical mucus. Since the cervix is very sensitive to changes in progestin levels, maintaining fairly consistent levels of progestin allows for a consistent effect on the cervical mucus.

Efficacy

Implants are a safe and highly effective continuous method of contraception that requires little efforts and is rapidly reversible. Each ENG and LNG implant has the same 3-year cumulative pregnancy rate of 0.4 per 100 W-Y.[5] The overall pregnancy rate reported in the National Institute for Health and Care Excellence guidelines is <0.1% over the course of 3 years (NICE Guidelines, 2014).

Side Effects

The implant use is associated with an unpredictable bleeding pattern, which includes amenorrhea and infrequent, frequent, and/or prolonged bleeding. The bleeding pattern experienced during the first 3 months is broadly predictive of future bleeding patterns for many women.[6]

Adverse events reported by >5% of subjects in the clinical trials (n = 942) were headache, vaginitis, weight increase, acne, breast pain, upper respiratory tract infection, abdominal pain, pharyngitis, leukorrhea, influenza-like symptoms, dizziness, dysmenorrhea, back pain, emotional liability, nausea, pain, nervousness, sinusitis, depression, and insertion-site pain.

TABLE 1: Timing of insertion of implant.

Scenario	*Timing of insertion*
No preceding hormonal contraceptive use in the past month	Days 1–5 of the menstrual cycle
Switching from combination hormonal methods	Anytime within 7 days of the last active combined dose
Switching from a progestin-only method	• Any day when switching from POP (do not skip any dose) • Same day as implant or IUD removal • On the day when the next contraceptive injection would be due
Within 5 days following 1st-trimester abortion	
3–4 weeks following childbirth or 2nd-trimester abortion	
After the 4th postpartum week if exclusively breastfeeding	

(IUD: intrauterine device; POP: progestogen-only pill)

Implant in Breastfeeding Women[7]

According to WHO, breastfeeding women who are <6 weeks postpartum can use LNG and ENG implants (MEC Category 2). Most studies have found no significant differences in children with regards to physical and psychomotor development. Implant placement within 48 hours of delivery does not appear to affect exclusive breastfeeding rates or alter the quantity and quality of breast milk produced, or to delay stage II lactogenesis. In fact, high continuation rates have been reported after insertion in the immediate postpartum period which is an added advantage over IUDs as the risk of expulsion is eliminated.[7]

Disadvantages

It is important to note that the Implanon is not radiopaque and therefore cannot be seen by X-ray or computed tomography (CT) scan. However, it is easily detectable by ultrasound using a high-frequency linear-array transducer or by MRI.

Serum concentrations of ENG are inversely related to body weight and decrease with time after insertion. The implant may be less effective in overweight women, especially in the presence of other factors that decrease ENG concentrations such as concomitant use of hepatic enzyme-inducing drugs. It provides no protection against the sexually transmitted infections (STIs), high up-front cost if not covered by insurance, insertion requires a doctor's visit, and device must be removed after 3 years. It may happen rarely that the implant sometimes migrates from the initial site of implantation. This can make the implant difficult for the clinician to find and remove.

Recent Advances

In 2010 (Europe) and 2011 (US), the original Implanon was replaced by second-generation Nexplanon, known as Implanon NXT, which is an evolution of older implant technology. This is radiopaque and contains 15 mg of barium sulfate at the core of the rod, which allows for its localization by two additional methods—X-ray and CT scan.

Return to Fertility

Serum concentrations of ENG were undetectable within 1 week of removal. Furthermore, there have been pregnancies reported that have occurred as early as the 1st week after implant removal. It is important, therefore, to note that if the patient is having implant removed and does not wish to become pregnant, she should be started on another contraceptive immediately after her implant is removed.[8]

Indian Council of Medical Research Data[9]

The review showed that Nexplanon has good clinical effectiveness. Studies reported Pearl index [contraception failures per 100 woman years (HWY) of exposure] of 0 or <1. Continuation rates were in a range of 6–86%, but premature discontinuation (within 3 years of insertion) was found to be between 11 and 47% at the end of 12 months of follow-up. The main reasons for discontinuation were frequent bleeding (47%) and prolonged bleeding (37%). Addition of Nexplanon to the current family planning scenario in the public health sector of India is found to be cost-effective [Indian Council of Medical Research (ICMR)].

Indian Scenario[10]

A study was conducted to determine the acceptability, efficacy, safety, and return of fertility with the implant. 200 subjects were enrolled [160 within 5 days of last menstrual period (LMP), 40 concurrent with medical termination of pregnancy (MTP)]. 74 implant removals were done (16 after tenure completion and 58 for other reasons). 16% cases discontinued the implant for polymenorrhagia, 10% for irregular bleeding, 4.5% for amenorrhea, 40% had return of ovulation within 1 month, and 95.8% conceived within 12 months. There was no failure of the implant. The study concluded that the implant is a safe, effective, and well-accepted method of contraception.

CONTRACEPTIVE PATCH

Transdermal systems represent a milestone innovation in drug delivery, offering a number of advantages over the oral route. They include multiday and more convenient dosing, especially for the sustained release of short half-life drugs (Burkman 2007). The patch is an alternative to continuous oral contraceptives (COCs) for the women who want autonomy and also provides the benefit of not taking a pill daily with similar efficacy and tolerability. Although long-acting reversible contraception (LARC) has been more popular, there is still a desire from patients to have a contraceptive method that they can control.

Structure and Usage

The ethinylestradiol (EE)/norelgestromin patch (Ortho-Evra) is an innovative, three-layer hormonal contraceptive system that provides similar efficacy to OCs, with the substantial benefit of once-weekly administration. For successful delivery of a medication through a transdermal system, the molecule must be of low molecular weight and lipophilic to permeate through the skin. Estradiol and EE are ideal molecules as therapeutic levels can be delivered easily, whereas progesterone and progestins require higher therapeutic levels.[11] The patch is applied once weekly for 3 consecutive weeks, followed by a patch-free week (**Fig. 2**).

Time of Starting

The woman should apply her first patch during the first 24 hours of her menstrual period. When switching from the pill or vaginal contraceptive ring to the patch, she should complete her current pill cycle or vaginal ring cycle and apply the first patch

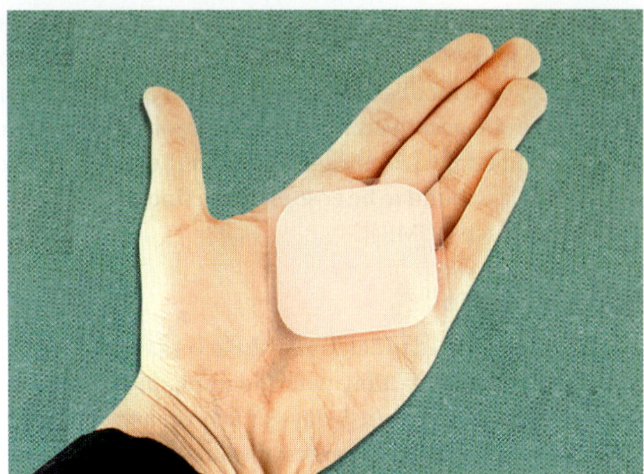

Fig. 2: Contraceptive patch.

on the day she would normally start her next pill or insert her next vaginal ring. The patch may be placed on the upper outer arm, abdomen, buttock, or back in a place where it will not be rubbed by tight clothing. Before applying the patch, the woman should make sure the skin is clean and dry. She should not use lotions, creams, oils, powders, or makeup at the patch site. It may cause the patch to fail to stick properly or to become loose.[3]

Mechanism of Action

The transdermal contraceptive EE/NGMN patch has the same mechanisms of action as combined OCs. After the patch is applied, hormones appear rapidly in the circulation, reaching a plateau after approximately 48 hours, which is maintained at this level during the 7-day wear period. On average, each EE/NGMN patch contains 750 µg EE and 6 mg norelgestromin and delivers 150 µg of norelgestromin (the primary active metabolite of norgestimate) and 20 µg of EE daily to the systemic circulation.

Efficacy

In a large epidemiological trial in the UK, patients prescribed Evra™ had an incidence of 0.34 unintended pregnancies per HWY.[12] In another European study, the transdermal contraceptive patch was shown to have a Pearl Index of 0.43 and a Pearl Index for patients who reported perfect compliance of 0.48. Thus, both indexes were comparable to those of other popular forms of hormonal contraception even if a patch change is missed for 2 days during weeks 2 and 3 of a 4-week cycle, clinical efficacy is maintained, and backup contraception is not needed.[13]

Adverse Effects

The most frequent adverse events are headache and nausea. Mild-to-moderate application site reactions and breast discomfort symptoms may occur, which generally resolve after 3 months of use. However, women with atopia and allergic skin diseases are more vulnerable to allergic reactions or local skin irritation. The patch leads to more discontinuation rates and side effects than the COC.[14] EE/NGMN patch shows no evidence of an increased risk of cerebral venous sinus thrombosis compared with LNG-containing, norgestimate-containing, and desogestrel-containing OCs. The risk of venous thromboembolism is also comparable to third-generation progestin OCs.[15-17]

Recent Advances in Contraceptive Patch

A novel transparent patch has been developed by Bayer that delivers 0.5 mg EE and 2.1 mg gestodene (GSD). GSD is a progestin contained in many COCs widely used in Europe for years. It is a favorable drug for transdermal use as it has an established efficacy and safety profile, and good skin absorption allowing for a low dose needed and small patch size.[18] The dosing of this 11 cm^2 transparent patch results in the same amount of hormone exposure as the 0.02 mg EE and 0.06 mg GSD OC.

The US Food and Drug Administration (FDA)-approved Twirla (120 µg/day LNG and 30 µg/day EE) transdermal system is a circular beige-colored 15 cm^2 matrix core with a surrounding adhesive for a total area of 26 cm^2 containing 2.3 mg EE and 2.6 mg LNG. Major differences between this and the currently marketed NGMN/EE patch are the decreased area under the curve (AUC) of estrogen and the use of LNG, which has been shown to have lower rates of venous thromboembolism (VTE) compared to other progestins.[19,20]

VAGINAL CONTRACEPTIVE RING

The vaginal contraceptive ring, Nuvaring, is a flexible and transparent ring that is used monthly. It offers continuous hormone release of estrogen (EE) plus progesterone (ENG), thereby acting as a long-acting contraceptive method.

Structure

The ring is soft, flexible, and transparent made up of EVA copolymer which contains crystals of ENG and EE. It has an outer diameter of 54 mm and a thickness of 4 mm available in one size and fits all women. It releases 120 g ENG and 15 µg EE per day (**Fig. 3**).

Usage

The ring is to be inserted after the patient had her menses. Once inserted, the ring can be kept in the vagina for 3 weeks, followed by a 1-week ring-free interval in which the patient can expect her menses. If the ring is removed and not replaced within 3 hours, it is recommended backup contraception be used until the ring has been placed for 7 days.

Vaginal administration has several advantages over other routes of administration. First, it gives a constant serum concentration because there is no risk of missing a dose.

It avoids gastrointestinal interference with absorption and avoids hepatic first-pass metabolism. The exposure to EE is half that as a standard oral contraceptive pill and the progestogen exposure (ENG) is comparable to a standard 150 µg desogestrel pill.

As described by Alexander et al., the vagina, because of its anatomy, blood supply, and innervation, is the ideal route for a drug delivery system. Details are given in **Table 2**.

Efficacy

The failure rate in the 1st year of use for the vaginal ring is estimated to be equal to that of OCs and the patch (0.3% for perfect use and 9% for typical use).[21,22] Various authors have reported a pearl index ranging from 0.25 to 1.75. The contraceptive effect of the ring also extends beyond its standard 21-day use. The efficacy persists even during extended use (at least up to 5 weeks), if the ring is accidentally removed early (3 days' use will delay ovulation) and is even effective after late insertion (up to 13 mm follicle size on ultrasound). There is a rapid return to ovulation following ring removal (mean time 19 days).[23]

Side Effects

The most common adverse reactions (≥2%) in clinical trials were vaginitis, headache (including migraine), mood changes (e.g., depression, mood swings, mood altered, depressed mood, and affect liability), device-related events (e.g., expulsion/discomfort/foreign body sensation), nausea/vomiting, vaginal discharge, increased weight, vaginal discomfort, breast pain/discomfort/tenderness, dysmenorrhea, abdominal pain, acne, and decreased libido.[24] Most of the side effects occur within the first 3 months. The most frequently reported adverse events leading to discontinuation from use are device-related events (expulsion, etc.) (2.5%), headache (1.3%), vaginal discomfort (1.0%), and nausea (1.0%). If expulsion occurs, the woman can wash the ring in warm water and reinsert it.[25]

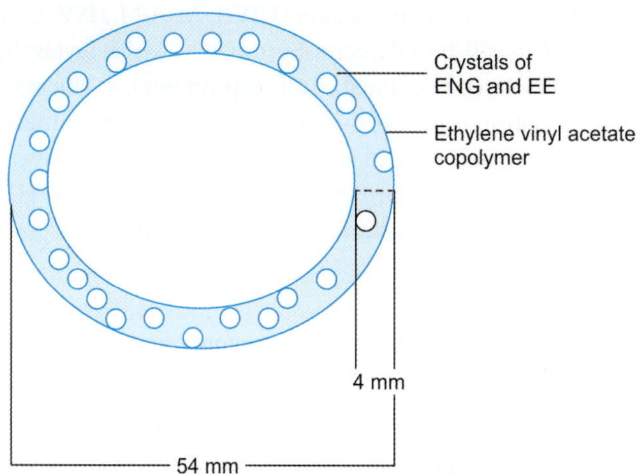

Fig. 3: Vaginal ring. (EE: ethinylestradiol; ENG: etonogestrel)

Only a few women discontinue the ring because of bleeding irregularities or vaginitis. There is a very low incidence of irregular bleeding, a predictable menstrual pattern, and a cycle control superior than OCs. The ring does not significantly contribute to weight gain any more than the pill.

Patient Acceptability

According to market research, majority of women found the ring highly acceptable and felt comfortable with the ring during intercourse. The ring tended to slightly shorten their monthly bleed and it was less painful. A significant number of women preferred it to other contraceptive methods.

Use During Lactation

Similar to combined OCs, use of the EE/ENG ring is discouraged before 6 weeks of breastfeeding is established. Between 6 weeks and 6 months, use of the ring is classified as a Category 3 according to the WHO Medical Eligibility Criteria—a condition where the risks usually outweigh the benefits. Given the lack of evidence, the decision to use the EE/ENG ring for contraception while breastfeeding should be individualized.[26]

New Developments in Vaginal Rings

- Ornibel® is bioequivalent to Nuvaring® in terms of efficacy, safety, tolerability, and acceptability. The new polymer composition provides Ornibel® with more stability and gradual hormonal release during the 1st day of use, particularly for EE.[27]

TABLE 2: Vagina is ideal route for contraceptive drug delivery.

Vaginal feature	*Benefit*
Anatomy	Nearly horizontal orientation of vagina minimizes risk of ring falling out
Vaginal rugae	Increased surface area that enhances drug absorption
Vasculature	Arteries and veins form dense plexus around the vagina; venous drainage eliminates first pass through liver
Innervation	• Lower one-fourth of vagina has a *peripheral* nerve supply, which is sensitive to pain • The nerve supply to the upper vagina is *autonomic* and is less sensitive to pain and, therefore, sensation of the ring in place is minimal
Epithelium	Stratified squamous epithelium permits easier steroid penetration to the underlying lamina propria made up of collagen and elastin which is richly vascularized

Source: Alexander N, Baker E, Kaptein M, Karck U, Miller L, Zampaglione E. Why consider vaginal drug administration? Fertil Steril. 2004;82(1):1-12.

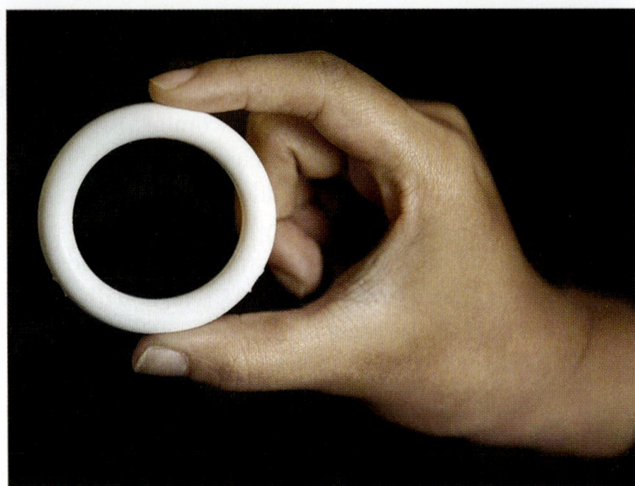

Fig. 4: Annovera ring.

- *Nestorone and EE combined hormonal vaginal ring*: Population council researchers have developed Annovera™ (segesterone acetate and EE vaginal ring), the first and only contraceptive that provides an entire year of protection against unintended pregnancy while fully under a woman's control. Annovera was approved by the US FDA in August 2018 (**Fig. 4**). Annovera is the first in a new class of contraceptives. It is a soft, reusable flexible silicone ring (2¼ inches diameter) that can be inserted and removed by a woman herself. Left in place for 21 days and removed for 7 days, it is indicated to prevent pregnancy for up to a year and does not require refrigeration, which is particularly important for distribution and use in low-resource settings.[28] Nestorone (segesterone acetate) is a potent 19-nortestosterone derivative that is not orally active but is an effective contraceptive when administered via implants, transdermal systems, and rings. NES does not bind to androgen or estrogen receptors and thus can potentially minimize some hormone-related side effects such as acne. In fact, research has shown that fewer women using transdermal NES exhibit high levels of total and low-density lipoprotein (LDL) cholesterol.[29] Since it is not orally active, it cannot affect breastfeeding babies.
- *Progesterone-releasing vaginal ring:* The progesterone-releasing vaginal ring (PVR) is a contraceptive device that was specifically designed to use among breastfeeding women in order to expand the method for this population. The device is manufactured in Chile under the trade name "Progering®". The silicone-elastomer ring has a cross-sectional diameter of 8.4 and 58 mm and contains micronized progesterone (P) that is released at an average rate of 10 mg/day over a 90-day period. For breastfeeding women, the ring is designed to use continuously for 6 months with infrequent removal approved for a maximum of 2 hours. Women who breastfeed and are of 4 or more weeks postpartum can use the PVR without restrictions (WHO MEC Category 1). Use of the PVR among women who breastfeed compares favorably to other highly effective methods of contraception and does not compromise a woman's breastfeeding performance nor adversely affect infant weight gain during the 1st year postpartum. A 1-year pregnancy rate of 1.5 per 100 women years was observed.[30]
- *Vaginal rings to prevent infection (HIV and HPV) and unintended pregnancy*: Women urgently need a self-initiated, multipurpose prevention technology (MPT) that simultaneously reduces their risk of acquiring HIV-1, HSV-2, and HPV (latter two associated with increased risk of HIV-1 acquisition) and prevents unintended pregnancy. The MZCL IVR effectively delivers the contraception and MZC combination microbicide. The MZCL IVR contains four active pharmaceutical ingredients (APIs): MIV-150 (targets HIV), zinc acetate (ZA; targets HIV and HSV-2), carrageenan (CG; targets HPV and HSV-2), and LNG (targets unintended pregnancy). The elastomeric IVR body made up of EVA-28 contains the hydrophobic small molecules of MIV-150 and LNG. The solid hydrophilic core, embedded within the IVR by compression, contains the small molecule ZA and a macromolecule CG. Hydrated ZA/CG from the core was released by diffusion via a pore on the IVR while the MIV-150/LNG diffuses from the matrix continuously for 94 days. The APIs released in vitro and in vivo were active against HIV-1, ADA-M, HSV-2, and HPV16 in cell-based assays. Serum LNG was at levels that are associated with local contraceptive effects. The result demonstrated proof-of-concept of a novel core-matrix IVR for sustained and simultaneous delivery of diverse molecules for the prevention of HIV, HSV-2, and HPV acquisition as well as unintended pregnancy.[31,32]

REFERENCES

1. United Nations Department of Economic and Social Affairs. Contraceptive Use by Method. New York: Population Division; 2019.
2. Singh S, Darroch JE, Ashford LS. Adding it up: the costs and benefits of investing in sexual and reproductive health 2014. New York: Guttmacher Institute and UNFPA; 2014.
3. Taylor H, Pal L, Seli E. Speroff's Clinical Gynecologic Endocrinology and Infertility, 9th edition. Philadelphia: Wolters Kluwer; 2020.
4. Food and Drug Administration. (2006). IMPLANON™ [package insert]. [online] Available from: https://www.accessdata.fda.gov/drugsatfda_docs/label/2006/021529lbl.pdf. [Last accessed November, 2021].
5. Bahamondes L, Brache V, Meirik O, Ali M, Habib N, Landoulsi S, et al. A 3-year multicentre randomized controlled trial of etonogestrel- and levonorgestrel-releasing contraceptive implants, with non-randomized matched copper-intrauterine device controls. Hum Reprod. 2015;30(11):2527-38.
6. Mansour D, Korver T, Marintcheva-Petrova M, Fraser IS. The effects of Implanon on menstrual bleeding patterns. Eur J Contracept Reprod Health Care. 2008;13(S1):13-28.

7. Carmo LS, Braga GC, Ferriani RA, Quintana SM, Vieira CS. Timing of etonogestrel-releasing implants and growth of breastfed infants. Obstet Gynecol. 2017;130(1):100-7.
8. Girum T, Wasie A. Return of fertility after discontinuation of contraception: a systematic review and meta-analysis. Contracept Reprod Med. 2018;3(1):9.
9. Indian Council of Medical Research. (2019). Health Technology Assessment of Long-acting Reversible Contraceptives in India". Health Technology Assessment (HTA) Resource Hub National Institute for Research in Reproductive Health. [online] Available from: https://dhr.gov.in/sites/default/files/HTA_%20LARC%20in%20India.pdf. [Last accessed November, 2021].
10. Pushpa B, Nangia S, Aggarwal S, Tewari C. Implanon: subdermal single rod contraceptive implant. J Obstet Gynaecol India. 2011;61(4):422-5.
11. Galzote RM, Rafie S, Teal R, Mody SK. Transdermal delivery of combined hormonal contraception: a review of the current literature. Int J Womens Health. 2017;9:315-21.
12. Jick SS, Hagberg KW, Kaye JA, Jick H. The risk of unintended pregnancies in users of the contraceptive patch compared to users of oral contraceptives in the UK General Practice Research Database. Contraception. 2009;80(2):142-51.
13. Grazziotin A. Safety, efficacy and patient acceptability of the combined oestrogen and progestin transdermal contraceptive patch: a review. Patient Prefer Adherence. 2008;2:357-67.
14. Lopez LM, Grimes DA, Gallo MF, Stockton LL, Schulz KF. Skin patch and vaginal ring versus combined oral contraceptives for contraception. Cochrane Database Syst Rev. 2013;2013(4):CD003552.
15. Burkman RT. Transdermal hormonal contraception: benefits and risks. Am J Obstet Gynecol. 2007;197:134e1-6.
16. Jick SS, Jick H. The contraceptive patch in relation to ischemic stroke and acute myocardial infarction. Pharmacotherapy. 2007;27:218-20.
17. Cole JA, Norman H, Doherty M, Walker AM. Venous thromboembolism, myocardial infarction, and stroke among transdermal contraceptive system users. Obstet Gynecol. 2007;109:339-46.
18. Waellnitz K, Duijkers I, Klipping C, Rautenberg T, Rohde B, Zurth C. A two-centre, open-label, randomised study of ovulation inhibition with three transdermal contraceptive patches, each containing different amounts of ethinyl estradiol and gestodene in healthy, young women. J Obstet Gynaecol. 2015;36(1):106-13.
19. Nelson AL, Kaunitz AM, Kroll R, et al. Efficacy, safety, and tolerability of a levonorgestrel/ethinyl estradiol transdermal delivery system: phase 3 clinical trial results. Contraception. 2021;103(3):137-43.
20. Kaunitz AM, Portman D, Westhoff CL, Archer DF, Mishell DR Jr, Rubin A, et al. Low-dose levonorgestrel and ethinyl estradiol patch and pill. Obstet Gynecol. 2014;123(2 Pt 1):295-303.
21. Hatcher R, Trussell J, Stewart F, Edelman AB, Aiken ARA, Marrazzo JM, et al. Contraceptive Technology, 21st edition. New York: Ardent Media, Inc.; 2018.
22. Trussell J. Contraceptive failure in the United States. Contraception. 2011;83(5):397-404.
23. Kerns J, Darney P. Vaginal ring contraception. Contraception. 2011;832011:107-15.
24. Merck and Co, Inc. Nuvaring [package insert]. Whitehouse Station, NJ. Merck and Co, Inc. 2001-2018. [online] Available from: http://www.merck.com/product/usa/pi_circulars/n/nuvaring/nuvaring. [Last accessed November, 2021]
25. Oddsson K, Leifels-Fischer B, de Melo NR, Wiel-Masson D, Benedetto C, Verhoeven CHJ, et al. Efficacy and safety of a contraceptive vaginal ring (NuvaRing) compared with a combined oral contraceptive: a 1-year randomized trial. Contraception. 2005;71176-82.
26. Brache V, Massai R, Mishell D, Moo-Young AJ, Alvarez F, Salvatierra AM, et al. Ovarian function during use of Nestorone® subdermal implants. Contraception. 2000;61:199-204.
27. Algorta J, Diaz M, de Benito R, Lefebvre M, Sicard E, Furtado M, et al. Pharmacokinetic bioequivalence, safety and acceptability of Ornibel®, a new polymer composition contraceptive vaginal ring (etonogestrel/ethinylestradiol 11.00/3.474 mg) compared with Nuvaring® (etonogestrel/ethinylestradiol 11.7/2.7 mg). Eur J Contracept Reprod Health Care. 2017;22(6):429-38.
28. Blakely KK. A new year-long combination hormonal contraceptive. Nurs Womens Health. 2019;23(2):172-6.
29. Massai R, Miranda P, Valdes P, Lavín P, Zepeda A, Casado ME, et al. Preregistration study on the safety and contraceptive efficacy of a progesterone-releasing vaginal ring in Chilean nursing women. Contraception. 1999;60:9-14.
30. Carr SL, Gaffield ME, Dragoman MV, Phillips S. Safety of the progesterone-releasing vaginal ring (PVR) among lactating women: a systematic review. Contraception. 2016;94(3):253-61.
31. Derby N. An intravaginal ring that releases three antiviral agents and a contraceptive blocks SHIV-RT infection, reduces HSV-2 shedding, and suppresses hormonal cycling in rhesus macaques. Drug Deliv Transl Res. 2017;7(6):840-58.
32. Ugaonkar SR, Wesenberg A, Wilk J, Seidor S, Mizenina O, Kizima L, et al. A novel intravaginal ring to prevent HIV-1, HSV-2, HPV, and unintended pregnancy. J Control Release. 2015;213:57-68.

LONG QUESTIONS

1. What is Implanon? Describe its mechanism of action, method and timing of insertion.
2. What is Contraceptive Patch? Write details of its efficacy, adverse effects and advantages.

SHORT QUESTIONS

1. Enumerate contraindications for Implanon.
2. Write a short note on Vaginal Ring.

MULTIPLE CHOICE QUESTIONS

1. Timing of insertion of Implanon:
   a. Anytime of the menstrual cycle
   b. Days 1 to 5 of menstrual cycle
   c. In second half of menstrual cycle
   d. None of the above
2. Which is the contraindication for insertion of implant?
   a. Hepatocellular adenoma
   b. Fibroadenoma of breast
   c. Perimenopausal age
   d. Lactation
3. Which is not a side effect of Implanon?
   a. Amenorrhea
   b. Prolonged bleeding
   c. Weight gain
   d. Heavy bleeding

4. Primary mechanism of action of implanon is:
    a. Thickening of cervical mucus
    b. Prevention of fertilization
    c. Inhibition of ovulation
    d. Prevention of ascend of sperms
5. All are disadvantages of implanon, except:
    a. It is not radiopaque
    b. Less effective in overweight women
    c. Insertion requires doctor's visit
    d. It is long acting reversible contraceptive
6. Pearl index of contraceptive patch is:
    a. 0.48
    b. 1.2
    c. 3
    d. 0.01
7. Nuvaring contains:
    a. Estrogen and progesterone
    b. Only progesterone
    c. Only estrogen
    d. None of the above
8. All are newer hormonal contraceptives, except:
    a. Implanon
    b. Vaginal ring
    c. Phexxi
    d. Contraceptive patch

Answers

1. b 2. a 3. d 4. c 5. d 6. a
7. a 8. c

2.9 INTRAUTERINE CONTRACEPTION (INCLUDING PPIUCD): COPPER DEVICES

Pushpa Junghare, Sayali Jahagirdar

"Any contraception is far safer than an unwanted pregnancy which ends up in MTP or an unwanted birth."

INTRODUCTION

Intrauterine contraceptive device (IUCD) provides very effective, safe, and long-term protection from pregnancy. It is reversible. There is prompt return of fertility upon its removal. It is cost-effective. A woman can start using IUCD at any time and at any age. It does not require daily action on the part of the user and does not depend on usage at the time of sexual activity. It does not require the woman to repeatedly go to the clinics or shops for its supply.

Intrauterine contraceptive device users in India: Only 3.1% of couples who are using contraceptives, the women are using IUCD.[1]

Intrauterine contraceptive devices available in India are:
- Copper-containing intrauterine devices (IUDs) (second generation)
- Hormone-releasing IUDs (third generation)

COPPER INTRAUTERINE CONTRACEPTIVE DEVICE

Copper wire or copper sleeves are put on the plastic frame made up of polyethylene. The various types of copper IUDs differ from each other by the amount of copper and the shape of the plastic frame **(Table 1 and Figs. 1 to 6)**.

Lippes loop, which was made of polyethylene, impregnated with barium sulfate, is no more available in India. Lippes loop was much larger than copper IUDs and had naturally more untoward side effects. Hence, the IUD was reduced in size to reduce the side effects, but copper was added to it to increase the efficacy.

Contraceptive Effectiveness

- The IUD is effective as soon as it is inserted
- It is one of the most cost-effective and long-lasting contraception methods
- It is comparable with female/male sterilization in its effectiveness and has the advantage of being reversible.

TABLE 1: Types of copper IUCDs available in India.

Frame is made of polyethylene and impregnated with barium sulfate to make it radiopaque	Copper content describes the area in mm^2 of the copper wire on the stem	Effective duration	Strings
T shaped	380	10 years	Polyethylene, white
	375	5 years	
Multiload (serrated, flexible transverse arms)	375	5 years	Monofilament nylon, blue
	250	2 years	

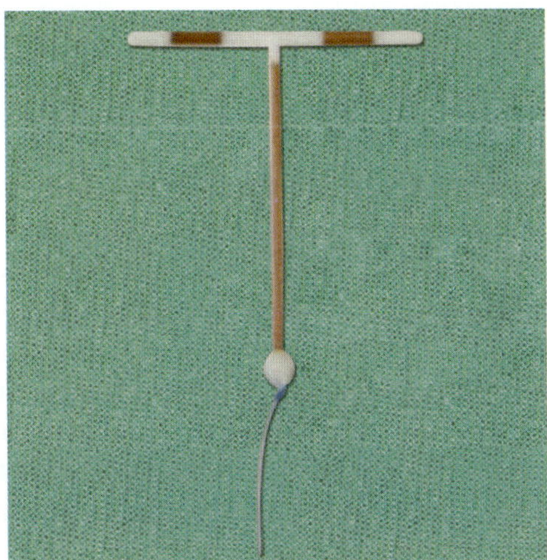

Fig. 1: Copper-T 380A.

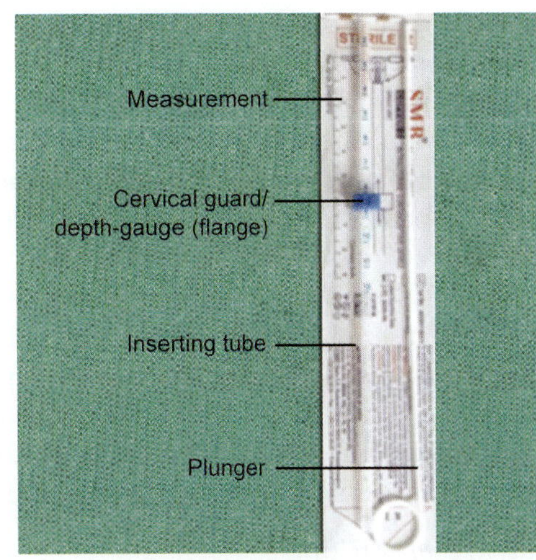

Fig. 2: Pack of copper-T Cu-T 380A.

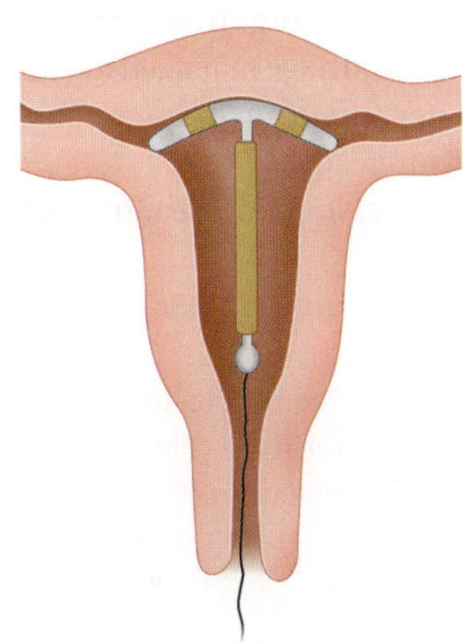

Fig. 3: Copper-T (Cu-T) 380 A in uterus.

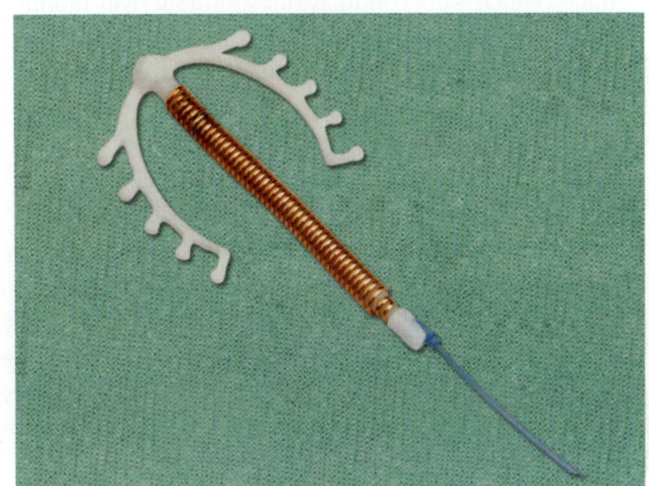

Fig. 4: Multiload 375.

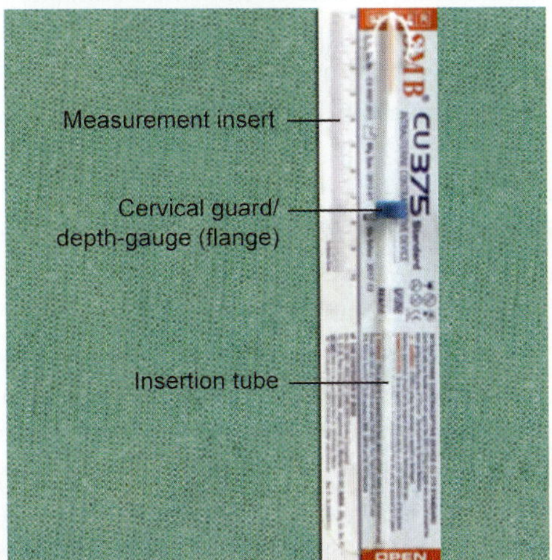

Fig. 5: Pack of Multiload 375.

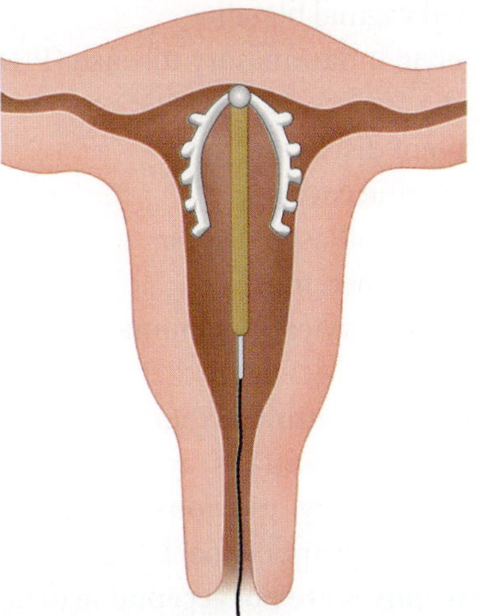

Fig. 6: Multiload 375 in uterus.

The failure rate is <1% in the 1st year of use. This means less than one pregnancy in 100 women in the 1st year of use (i.e., 6–8 women out of 1,000 users will become pregnant). The cumulative pregnancy rate for the copper T 380 A is 2.2 per 100 women year.[2]

Mechanism of Action

Mechanisms by which pregnancy is prevented are many. IUCD was initially considered to be interceptive as it was thought to prevent implantation of fertilized ovum in the uterus.

Various studies carried out suggest that the copper IUCD releases free copper and copper salt which change the intrauterine environment and the cervical mucus. This causes immobilization of sperms preventing their migration to the fallopian tube[3] and even causes decapitation of sperms making them incapable of fertilization. Actual fertilization was found to be extremely less with copper IUCD.

Copper IUD also appears to directly affect oocytes so that the ability to get fertilized is inhibited or at least reduced.[3] It prevents implantation as it stimulates foreign-body noninfective inflammatory reaction in the endometrium which releases macrophages and damages the endometrial tissue (that must be the reason to use it as an emergency contraceptive).

To summarize, copper IUCD:

- Alters the cervical mucus and affects the endometrial milieu which is not conducive for sperm survival, motility, and ascent into the fallopian tubes
- Affects the oocytes adversely making them incapable of getting fertilized
- Prevents implantation of fertilized ovum.

Medical Eligibility Criteria for Copper IUCD Use

Copper IUCD is an excellent option for majority of women. As per WHO guidelines, women are categorized into four categories. In category 1, IUCD can be used in any circumstances. In category 2, it can be generally used if the advantages of using the method outweigh the risks. In category 3, the risks outweigh the advantages; hence, it is better not used. In category 4, the use of IUCD is contraindicated.

Contraindications:

- Pregnancy
- Unexplained vaginal bleeding
- Current pelvic inflammatory disease (PID), gonorrhea, or chlamydia
- Acute purulent discharge
- Distorted uterine cavity
- Malignant trophoblastic disease
- Known pelvic tuberculosis
- Endometrial or cervical carcinoma
- Wilson's disease
- AIDS, without antiretroviral therapy for HIV.

In women with anemia, scarred uterus, fibroids not distorting uterine cavity, previous ectopic pregnancy, no children, and age <20 years, copper IUCD can be safely offered if other contraceptives are not acceptable to her.

In women having valvular heart disease or diabetes mellitus, antibiotic cover should be given whenever IUCD is inserted.

Counseling

Patient should be offered different contraceptive options and should be allowed to choose. But one has to guide the patient to use IUCD giving all its advantages, efficacy, and its duration of action. Her myths regarding IUCD should be dispelled.

Timing of IUCD Insertion

- Although it is said that IUCD can be inserted anytime during the menstrual cycle,[4] ideally it should be inserted between 8th and 14th day of cycle. Once the menses starts, one is reasonably sure that the woman is not pregnant. Insertion during menstruation increases the chances of expulsion. Postovulation/premenstrual insertion can help because of its mechanism of action of prevention of implantation, but there is a possibility that the fertilized ovum may continue to grow in the fallopian tube and result in ectopic pregnancy.
- Immediately or within 48 hours after delivery or >6 weeks postpartum.
- Immediately following first- or second-trimester spontaneous miscarriage managed medically or surgically or medical termination of pregnancy (MTP) done medically or surgically.
- During lactational amenorrhea, provided pregnancy is ruled out.
- Within 5 days of unprotected sex as an emergency contraception.

Copper IUCDs are available in sealed packs and are ethylene oxide (ETO) sterilized. The expiry date mentioned on the package is of sterilization.

Method of Insertion

Intrauterine contraceptive device should be inserted after thorough counseling and ascertaining that the women is not pregnant. Ideally, a written informed consent should be taken.

Perform per-vaginal examination to know the size and position of the uterus and to rule out vaginal infection and PID.

Clean the vulva with antiseptic solution, insert a sterile speculum to visualize the cervix, and clean the cervix and surrounding vagina with antiseptic solution.

Gently grasp the anterior lip of the cervix with a sterile vulsellum or tenaculum and apply gentle traction by holding the instrument in index finger and thumb. The remaining three fingers should be on the suprapubic region. This will straighten the cervical canal and align it with the uterine cavity.

Insert the tip of sterile uterine sound into the cervical canal up to the internal os. Direct the sound anteriorly or posteriorly depending upon the position of the uterus. Pass the sound slowly further till the resistance of the fundus is met. Remove the sound. The uterocervical length and position of the uterus are thus ascertained.

Load the copper-T (see instruction to load the copper-T at the end of this section) just prior to insertion. Multiload does not require loading.

Now, adjust the blue cervical guard over the inserter according to the UCL. The loaded copper-T is held in the right hand. The blue guard is kept horizontal so that it will be parallel to the copper-T when released in the uterine cavity. The left hand should hold the vulsellum with gentle traction to align the uterus and the cervix in a straight line.

The loaded copper-T is gently pushed through the cervical canal into the uterine cavity.

Once the cervical guard touches the external os, it means loaded copper-T is touching the fundus. The cervical guard will prevent any further advancement of the inserter with copper-T and perforation of the uterus. Now, the inserter tube is withdrawn downward, till it touches the circular thumb ring of the plunger. This will release the IUCD arms in the uterine cavity in either cornu. This is withdrawal technique to prevent/minimize uterine perforation as copper-T is not pushed but only placed in the uterine cavity. Now, the plunger is removed first. This will not cause entanglements of the strings between the plunger and the inserter. Then the inserter tube is pushed gently and carefully upward toward the fundus. This will ensure proper placement of copper-T in the uterine cavity.

In case of multiload, loading is not required. After holding the anterior lip of cervix with vulsellum, the already loaded multiload and inserter tube with the cervical guard placed in horizontal position is gently pushed through the cervical canal into the uterine cavity till the guard comes in the contact with the external os. The inserter tube is now removed.

The strings of IUCD are cut short 1–2 cm from the external os.

Loading of Copper-T

Adjust the contents of the package:

- Ensure that the vertical stem of the T is fully inside the insertion tube.
- Ensure that the other end of the insertion tube (farthest from the IUCD) is close to the sealed end of the package.

Partially open the package:

- Place the package on a clean, hard, flat surface with the clear plastic side up.
- Pull up on the clear plastic cover from the end that is farthest from the IUCD (marked open).
- Keep pulling the plastic cover until the package is open, approximately half-way to the blue length-gauge.

Place the white plunger rod in the clear insertion tube:

- Starting at the open end of the package, fold the clear plastic cover and white backing "flaps" away from each other.
- Using your free hand, grasp the white plunger rod (behind the measurement insert) by the circular thumb grip and remove it from the package.
- Place the plunger rod inside the insertion tube and gently push until the tip of the rod almost touches the bottom of the T.

Bend the "arms" of the "T" downward:

- Through the clear plastic cover, place your thumb and index finger over the tips of the horizontal arms of the T to stabilize the IUCD.
- Still holding the tips of the arms of the T, use your free hand to grasp the insertion tube and gently push it against the T. This pressure will cause the arms to begin bending downward, toward the stem of the T.
- Finish bending the arms of the T by bringing your thumb and index finger together and continuing to push against the T with the insertion tube.

Pull the insertion tube away from folded arms of the T:

- When the arms of the T are folded down enough to touch the sides of the insertion tube, pull the insertion tube out from between the arms.

Push the folded arms of the T into the insertion tube: Gently push and rotate the insertion tube back over the tips of the folded arms of the T, so that both tips are caught inside the insertion tube.

Set the blue guard to the appropriate measurement: Align the blue guard and the folded arms of the T so that they are both in a "horizontal" position.

Adverse Effects

Side effects of IUCD can be unpleasant but are not harmful to the women's health or life.[5] Usually they subside after a few months of use.

- *Abnormal uterine bleeding (AUB)*: There can be intermenstrual spotting or slight bleeding or increase in amount and/or duration of bleeding over the first few menses. This responds to nonsteroidal anti-inflammatory drugs (NSAIDs)
- Discomfort or abdominal pain during insertion and for next few days
- Menstrual cramps
- Leukorrhea.

Complications/Health Risks

- Spontaneous expulsion in 2–8% of patients which usually occurs during first menstruation; hence, patient should be followed up after her first menses after insertion.
- *Failure*: If pregnancy occurs with the IUCD in-situ, there are increased chances of spontaneous abortion, sepsis, and ectopic pregnancy. IUCD however does not affect the fetus adversely. Hence, MTP is not indicated if the patient wishes to continue her pregnancy. The IUCD should be removed only if it can be done easily.

- *Sepsis*: If asepsis is not observed while insertion, there can be pelvic infection, but per se copper IUCD does not cause infection.
- *Uterine perforation*: It can occur during insertion, especially in lactating woman whose uterus is small but soft. The perforation might be missed till the follow-up.
- *Displaced copper IUCD*: It can expel out of the uterus or descend into the cervix. It can perforate the uterus and get embedded in the myometrium or may migrate outside the uterus after perforation into the surrounding peritoneal cavity.

Follow-up

After the IUCD insertion, the patient is given few instructions. She should try to feel the strings time and again. She is told that she can have intermenstrual spotting and her first few menses can be prolonged and/or heavy. But the bleeding can be reduced with symptomatic treatment. She should come for the first follow-up immediately after her first menses. If the patient is not able to feel the strings or on examination, they are not seen then there are three possibilities:

1. The IUCD is expelled.
2. The strings might be coiled inside the cervical canal or the strings are broken and expelled out.
3. It is displaced.

In OPD, a Cytobrush can be introduced in the cervical canal and rotated. This will bring out the threads if they are coiled in the cervix.

Uterine sound can be passed in the uterine cavity to sound the device. If it is not sounded, the patient can be subjected to pelvic ultrasonography (USG) or X-ray pelvis [anteroposterior (AP) and lateral views) with uterine sound kept in the uterine cavity. The copper-T can be thus located. If it is in the uterine cavity, it will be obvious on USG. On X-ray, the copper-T image will overlap on that of the uterine sound. If displaced, it will be outside the uterus far away from the uterine sound. On USG, the uterine cavity is found to be empty and the IUCD will be seen either in the myometrial wall or somewhere else in the pelvis or abdomen. A displaced copper-T should be removed with laparoscope or laparotomy, as a copper device can erode into the bladder or small bowel. If the device is embedded in myometrium, it should be removed with copper-T removing hook or, if necessary, through hysteroscope.

The patient should periodically come for checkup or if she misses her period or fails to feel the threads. Copper-T/Multi-load 375 lasts for 5 years and copper-T 380 A for 10 years. It is advisable to reinsert new IUCD in the same sitting whenever the previous one is removed as fertility promptly returns after an IUCD removal.

Advantages of Copper IUCD

- It offers long-term, highly effective reversible contraception and fertility returns promptly on its removal.
- It is effective immediately after insertion.
- It is suitable for use by most women.
- It can be replaced as many times the woman desires contraception till she attains menopause, without any gap.
- It does not require daily attention or interruption during sexual intercourse.
- Insertion is a one-time procedure and cost-effective.
- It can be used by lactating woman.
- No side effects as with hormones or interactions with any medications.
- It can be used as an emergency contraception.

Emergency contraception: As copper IUCD also acts by affecting implantation of fertilized ovum; it can be offered as an emergency contraception, up to even 5 days of intercourse. The other benefit is that the inserted IUCD can provide ongoing contraception.[6]

POSTPARTUM INTRAUTERINE CONTRACEPTIVE DEVICE[7]

Every woman must be counseled regarding family planning options when she is admitted for delivery. She should be given the option of postpartum IUCD (PPIUCD) with respect to its advantages, limitations, effectiveness, and side effects related to the IUCD.

Contraindications should be ruled out.

Timing of PPICUD Insertion

- *Postplacental*: Insertion within 10 minutes after expulsion of placenta
- *Intracesarean*: During cesarean section after removal of placenta and before closure of uterine incision
- Within 48 hours after delivery
- *Extended postpartum*: Insertion at the end of 6 weeks after delivery.

Intrauterine contraceptive device should not be introduced after 48 hours to 6 weeks after delivery. Bacteria start colonizing over the placental site after 48 hours. Introduction of IUCD at this juncture can cause pelvic infection. At the end of 6 weeks, with involution of uterus, the placental site is completely healed.

Advantages of PPIUCD

- Convenience, saves time, and additional visit as the patient is already in the hospital.
- Patient and relatives can be motivated better, they being more receptive.
- Uterus, though soft, has thick walls and hence no chance of perforation.
- Reduced perception of initial side effects of bleeding and cramping due to the presence of normal puerperal changes.

- With lactational amenorrhea, there is no chance of having heavy menstrual bleeding.
- Lactation is not affected.

The only problem is that there is higher risk of spontaneous expulsion as the uterus is actively involuting. Moreover, special PPIUCD insertion forceps may be required for placing the IUCD properly in a very large uterine cavity as the usual instruments may fall short of length to reach the uterine fundus.

> Copper IUCD provides very effective, safe, and long-term protection from pregnancy. It is reversible with prompt return of fertility upon its removal. Failure rate is 0.8–2.2% per 100 women-year. Copper IUCD alters the cervical mucus and milieu interior of endometrial cavity and fallopian tubes. It affects the sperm migration, their quality and viability, and alters the oocytes, thereby preventing fertilization. It also brings about noninfective inflammatory reaction in the endometrium preventing implantation. Hence, it can also be used as an emergency contraceptive. Copper IUCD can be inserted immediately after delivery of placenta (PPIUCD).
>
> Patient education and dispelling the myths associated with IUCD are needed to increase the accepwvtance of this top tier, efficacious contraceptive.

REFERENCES

1. Family Planning. Available from: https://www.familyplanning2020.org/India. Report on Contraceptive use dynamics in India: a prospective cohort study of modern reversible contraceptive users, 01 March 2020. [Last accessed November, 2021].
2. Kulier R, O'Brien P, Helmerhorst FM, Usher-Patel M, d'Arcangues C. Copper containing, framed intra-uterine devices for contraception (review). Cochrane Database Syst Rev. 2008. [online] Available from: https://www.t-safe.nl/wp-content/uploads/2016/04/cochrane-review-mirena-versus-koper.pdf [Last accessed November, 2021].
3. Ortiz ME, Croxatto HB, Bardin CW. Mechanisms of action of intrauterine devices. Obstet Gynecol Surv. 1996;51(12 Suppl):S42-51.
4. Edelman D, Zipper J, Rivera M, Medel M. Timing of the IUD insertion. Contraception. 1979;19(5):449-54.
5. Kaneshiro B, Aeby T. Long-term safety, efficacy, and patient acceptability of the intrauterine copper T-380A contraceptive device. Int J Womens Health. 2010;2:211-20.
6. Planned parenthood.org. (2020). How Does the Copper IUD Work as Emergency Contraception? [online] Available from: https://www.plannedparenthood.org/learn/morning-after-pill-emergency-contraception/how-does-copper-iud-work-emergency-contraception. [Last accessed November, 2021].
7. Shahbaz FA, Tariq RO, Shahbaz F, Tahira T, Mavaid J, Zahida N. Evaluation of post placental trans caesarean/vaginal delivery intrauterine device (PPIUCD) in terms of awareness, acceptance and expulsion in services hospital, Lahore. Pak J Med Health Sci. 2016;10:338-40.

LONG QUESTIONS

1. Discuss various mechanisms of action of copper IUCD to prevent pregnancy.
2. Describe copper T 380A in details and the technique of its insertion and follow-up.

SHORT QUESTIONS

1. What are the different types of copper IUCD available in India?
2. Give a list of contraindications for copper IUCD use.
3. Enumerate the adverse effects of copper IUCD.
4. Write a note on PPIUCD.
5. Write a note on Copper T as an emergency contraceptive.

MULTIPLE CHOICE QUESTIONS

1. Failure rate of copper IUCD in 1st year of use is:
   a. 0.01 per 100 women-year
   b. 0.8 per 100 women-year
   c. 3 per 100 women-year
   d. 10 per 100 women-year
2. Absolute contraindication for copper IUCD is:
   a. Pregnancy
   b. Previous ectopic pregnancy
   c. Fibroid uterus
   d. Nulliparity
3. Mechanism of action of copper-T is:
   a. Immobilization of sperms
   b. Prevention of fertilization
   c. Prevention of implantation
   d. All of the above
4. Fertility is restored_____ after removal of Cu-T.
   a. 4 weeks b. 6 months
   c. Immediately d. 2 months
5. Copper T 380A should be inserted by:
   a. Withdrawal technique
   b. Push technique
   c. Any technique as it makes no difference
   d. Only by a gynecologist
6. Which is not a contraindication for copper-T?
   a. Wilson's disease
   b. Acute PID
   c. Breastfeeding
   d. Endometrial carcinoma
7. Missing strings of IUCD indicate:
   a. The device is expelled out
   b. The strings are broken and expelled out
   c. The device is displaced
   d. Any of the above
8. Removal of IUCD requires:
   a. Hysteroscopy
   b. X-ray screening
   c. Intrauterine instrumentation
   d. Pulling out the strings
9. The following is not a side effect of copper IUCD:
   a. Leukorrhea
   b. Heavy menstrual bleeding
   c. Dyspareunia
   d. Intermenstrual bleeding

10. PPIUCD should be inserted within:
    a. 4 weeks of delivery
    b. 2 weeks of delivery
    c. 48 hours of delivery
    d. Seconds of placental delivery
11. Copper IUCD as an emergency contraception is highly effective when inserted within___ of intercourse.
    a. 5 days
    b. 7 days
    c. 1 week
    d. 15 days

Answers

1.	b	2.	a	3.	d	4.	c	5.	a	6.	c
7.	d	8.	d	9.	c	10.	c	11.	a		

2.10 LEVONORGESTREL INTRAUTERINE SYSTEM

Priya Ballal K, Nikhil Shetty

INTRODUCTION

The search for an ideal contraceptive method has led to continuous innovations and newer contraceptives in the market. The long-acting reversible contraception (LARC) consists of copper-containing intrauterine devices (IUDs), levonorgestrel intrauterine system (LNG-IUS), and implants.[1] Due to lower pregnancy rates compared to any other reversible form of contraception and minimal ongoing effort from the patient, they have received acceptance worldwide.[1,2] LARCs have been evolving since the Lippes loop to copper-containing devices and then hormone-releasing intrauterine systems. Although initially identified for use in abnormal uterine bleeding, the LNG-IUS has found its place in current scenario with increasing use from 2.4% in 2002 to 11.6% in 2012.[3] There has been a significant reduction in unintended pregnancy rates and abortions since its widespread use. The hormonally impregnated IUDs were first introduced in 1970s with the launch of the first IUS in Finland in 1990. Addition of progestin to an IUD increases contraceptive effectiveness and reduces expulsion rates.[4] By effect of LNG on endometrium, it reduces bleeding and dysmenorrhea adding to chances of continuity and compliance.[4] By inactivating the endometrium, the LNG-IUS provides health benefits, such as prevention of anemia and endometrial protection in women on estrogen therapy.[5] Relatively low systemic serum levels compared with other hormonal methods result in fewer side effects. Among the LARCs offered to women between age groups of 14 and 45 years, majority preferred the LNG-IUS followed by implants and lastly copper-containing devices.[6]

LEVONORGESTREL: THE MOLECULE

Levonorgestrel is a 17α-ethynyl-18-methyl-19-nortestosterone derived from 19-nortestosterone with high progestational potency **(Fig. 1)**. This molecule is used in many forms of contraception such as IUS, subdermal implants, and single-agent emergency contraception.

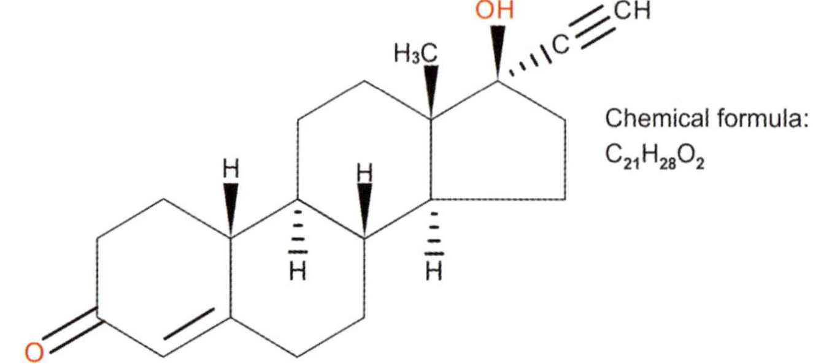

Fig. 1: Chemical composition of levonorgestrel.

The molecule may be absorbed from the gastrointestinal (GI) tract when administered orally, direct absorption into endometrium from IUDs and into the interstitium from subdermal implants. Systemic side effects are minimal and mostly due to the androgenic and weak estrogenic effects of the drug.

THE DELIVERY SYSTEM

The LNG-IUS is a T-shaped device made of polyethylene with a silastic reservoir containing LNG mixed with polydimethylsiloxane (PDMS) attached to the vertical arm. The rate-controlling PDMS covering membrane regulates the daily release rate of the hormone.[4,7] The polyethylene of the T-body is compounded with barium sulfate, which makes it visible upon X-ray examination. Two removable threads are attached to the caudal end of the T frame **(Fig. 2)**.

The total amount of LNG in the cylinder and dimensions of the device vary depending on the type of IUS **(Table 1)**. They are marketed worldwide under brand names such as Mirena, Liletta, Kyleena, Skyla, Jaydess, Fiona, Emily, and Eloira.[1,2,7]

A 52 mg of LNG-IUS initially releases at a rate of approximately 20 μg/day. This rate decreases progressively to approximately 10 μg/day after 5 years.[7] Serum levels of LNG (0.4 ng/mL) found in LNG-IUS users are much less than those observed with use of oral progestins and combine oral contraceptives. This explains the lower incidence of systemic side effects.[8]

MECHANISM OF ACTION

The contraceptive action of all IUDs is within the uterine cavity. Mechanism of action is through local foreign body reaction and inflammation on the endometrium. Progestogen added to the IUS contributes to its effectiveness by the following mechanisms.[4]

Primary mechanism of action is prevention of fertilization by causing a change in amount and viscosity of cervical mucus, thus making it impermeable to sperm (prefertilization).[3,9] Sperm capacitation, penetration, and survival are all affected by LNG contributing to contraceptive benefit.[7,8] Postfertilization action is by the direct effect of high local LNG concentrations leading to uniform suppression of endometrial proliferation, thin endometrium, and decidualization of the stroma.[5] Poor implantation is an in vitro phenomenon that could not be proven in vivo research. The very same profound changes in the endometrium are responsible for frequently observed irregular bleeding or spotting during the initial months of using the LNG-IUS, which improves with time.[7] LNG does not affect the hypothalamic-pituitary-ovarian axis and serum estradiol concentration remains unchanged.

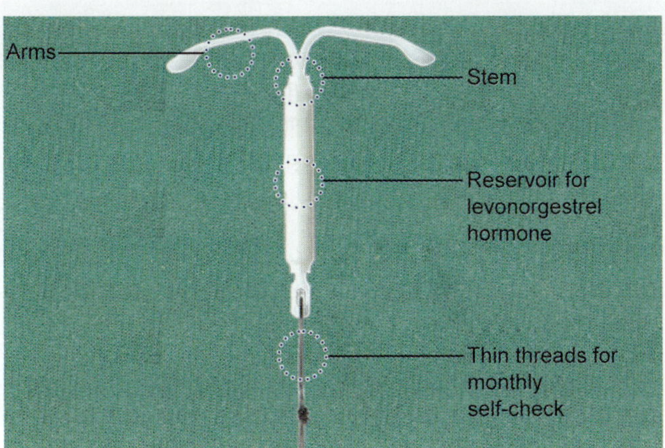

Fig. 2: Levonorgestrel intrauterine system (LNG-IUS) device (Mirena® marketed by Bayer Zydus Pharma).

Women (>75%) continue to ovulate despite being amenorrheic as ovulation is not affected.[1,7] Following removal, the normal intrauterine environment is rapidly restored ensuring reversal of contraceptive effect proven by large studies showing no delay in return of fertility regardless of duration.[7] LNG-IUS may have a role in reducing the ascent of infection through the thickened cervical mucus; however, it does not offer protection against sexually transmitted infections (STIs) and may be combined with a barrier method if required.[9] LNG-IUS is not recommended for emergency contraception unlike the CuT 380A.

CONTRACEPTIVE EFFICACY

Levonorgestrel intrauterine system, also termed the "forgettable contraception," requires almost no effort on the part of women, thus increasing compliance.[9] It is one of the most effective LARCs with a failure rate of <1 pregnancy per 100 women with LNG-IUS use over the 1st year.[2] The gross cumulative pregnancy rate at 5 years is 0.5–1.1%.[10-11] The efficacy remains the same throughout the 5-year lifespan of the IUS. Effectiveness of LNG-IUS is superior to copper-containing devices.[13]

The European Active Surveillance Study (EURAS) for IUDs found LNG-IUS superior in terms of efficacy and with low failure rate in both types of devices.[13] Serum levels of LNG with prolonged use of 52 mg LNG-IUS were detectable even beyond the licensed 5 years of use; however, since the LNG action is a local effect on the endometrium, this cannot be relied upon as proof of efficacy. Other studies have shown LNG-IUS to be effective even beyond the licensed time of use.[1]

INDICATIONS OF USE

Levonorgestrel intrauterine system is primarily used to treat heavy menstrual bleeding (HMB) with added advantage of contraception in women who desire so. It reduces menstrual blood loss both in women with HMB and in women with normal blood loss up to 90%.[8] The effect has been significantly more than those offered by nonsteroidal anti-inflammatory drugs (NSAIDs), antifibrinolytics, or oral progestins and

TABLE 1: Description of the various IUS available in the market with its dimensions, daily release rate of LNG, and approved duration of use.[7]

Device	*Brand name*	*LNG (mg)*	*LNG release rate (μg/day)*	*Dimension (mm)*	*Licensed duration of use (years)*
LNG-IUS 20	• Mirena • Fiona • Emily • Eloira	52	20	32 × 32	5
LNG 20	Liletta	52	19.5	32 × 32	4
LNG-IUS 12	Kyleena	19.5	17	28 × 28	5
LNG-IUS 8	Skyla	13.5	14	28 × 28	3

(IUS: intrauterine system; LNG: levonorgestrel)

comparable with endometrial ablation.[4] Prevention of anemia comes as an added advantage to women using LNG-IUS.[5] The use of this device has shown to be effective in primary dysmenorrhea.[1]

Levonorgestrel intrauterine system due to its strong progestational effect on endometrium and similar effect on endometrial implants has been successful in treating adenomyosis and endometriosis, especially those with complaints of dysmenorrhea.[1,8] Significant levels of LNG in peritoneal fluids explain the pain relief experienced by women with peritoneal endometriosis.[8] Efficacy of LNG-IUS is comparable to gonadotropin-releasing hormone (GnRH) analogs.[1] Treatment is effective for a longer duration of time compared to GnRH (5 years). However, hypoestrogenic side effects noted with GnRH are not seen with LNG-IUS as these do not affect serum estradiol levels.[5]

INTRAUTERINE SYSTEM INSERTION

Patient Selection

Levonorgestrel is safe to use in all age groups of patients requiring contraception. Nulliparous and nulligravida women can safely use LNG-IUS.[3] Devices with smaller dimensions are also available for use in these women.[3]

Risk factors for STIs are most important consideration in patient selection. A thorough history-taking and clinical examination is an important part of the process. Women who have multiple sexual partners, partners who have multiple sexual partners, those not in a stable sexual relationship, and alcohol and drug-dependent women are at a greater risk of pelvic infection and have to be screened during patient selection.[1]

Medical comorbidities such as diabetes, hypothyroidism, and epileptic women on anticonvulsants are not the contraindications for use of LNG-IUS.[7] Women with a previous history of ectopic pregnancy can be safely offered LNG-IUS.[7]

Contraindications to Insertion of LNG-IUS

Levonorgestrel intrauterine system contraindications are grouped in categories 3 and 4 of the WHO Medical Eligibility criteria for contraception. These categories stratify the candidates based on those in who the risks outweigh the benefit or use is absolutely contraindicated.[14] The conditions falling in such category are listed in **Tables 2 and 3.**

Prerequisites for Insertion

Intrauterine system insertion should be attempted by a trained healthcare worker. A valid consent for pelvic examination and written informed consent for insertion of IUS are mandatory.[1] A complete medical history and examination is an important prerequisite prior to LNG-IUS insertion. Relevant investigations and imaging may be used to rule out STIs and other gynecological pathologies that may contraindicate the use of IUS, especially in women with HMB. Women with STI should be offered treatment and ideally delay IUS insertion.[1,7]

TABLE 2: Indications for the use of levonorgestrel intrauterine system (LNG-IUS).

Contraceptive indications	*Other indications*
Long-acting reversible contraception	AUB due to problems with inherited, iatrogenic coagulopathy
Heavy menstrual bleeding	Adenomyosis and endometriosis causing dysmenorrhea
	Protection of the endometrium in women on postmenopausal estrogen therapy[1,2,6,7]
	Small fibroids causing AUB that do not distort uterine cavity
	To prevent endometrial hyperplasia during SERM use like tamoxifen in breast cancer patients
	Simple endometrial hyperplasia

(AUB: abnormal uterine bleeding; SERM: selective estrogen receptor modulator)

TABLE 3: Contraindications to use of an LNG-IUS, based on the WHO Medical Eligibility Criteria.[14]

Category 3—risk outweighs benefit	*Category 4—absolutely contraindicated*
Insertion 48 hours to <4 weeks postpartum	Pregnancy
Acute venous thromboembolism	Puerperal sepsis
Current/history of ischemic heart disease	Immediately postseptic abortion
SLE with unknown or positive antiphospholipid antibodies	Unexplained vaginal bleeding that has not been adequately investigated
Migraines with aura	GTN and increasing β-hCG levels
Past breast cancer	Cervical cancer
Increased risk of STI	Current breast cancer
Advanced HIV/AIDS	Endometrial cancer
Severe cirrhosis	Ovarian cancer
Hepatocellular adenoma	Uterine leiomyoma with distortion of cavity
Malignant hepatoma	Current PID or mucopurulent cervical discharge
	Distortion of the uterine cavity that is incompatible with IUD insertion
	Pelvic tuberculosis

(AIDS: acquired immunodeficiency syndrome; β-hCG: β-human chorionic gonadotropin; GTN: gestational trophoblastic neoplasia; HIV: human immunodeficiency virus; IUD: intrauterine device; LNG-IUS: levonorgestrel intrauterine system; PID: pelvic inflammatory disease; STI: sexually transmitted infection)

Routine prophylactic antibiotic use is not recommended for IUS insertion.[1,3] Prophylaxis against infective endocarditis in patients with preexistent valvular heart disease is not routinely recommended.[1,7] However, considering the risk from genitourinary infections, the decision can be made on a case-to-case basis.

Vasovagal reaction resulting in bradycardia or arrhythmias can occur during insertion following cervical stimulation which usually subsides without intervention and rarely warrants treatment with atropine.[1] The vasovagal reaction could be a serious risk in women with cardiac conditions such as Eisenmenger's physiology or single ventricle. Such high-risk cases may benefit from insertion of IUS in a hospital setting under anesthesia.

Timing of Insertion

Like all IUDs, insertion is advised within the first 7 days of cycle, preferably between days 5 and 7, when the risk of disturbing a pregnancy is minimal and also the flow of menstrual cycle has reduced. However, the LNG-IUS can be inserted any time in the menstrual cycle if it is reasonably certain that the woman is not pregnant or at risk of pregnancy.[2,3] Additional contraception may be advised in such an event. IUS may be inserted immediately after a first-trimester or second-trimester abortion. The chance of expulsion is higher when IUS is inserted following a second trimester of abortion (category 2).[3,7] Postnatal IUS insertion is ideally after 6 weeks from delivery. Insertion within 48 hours leads to higher rates of expulsion (**Table 4**).[1]

Technique of Insertion

After the patient is in position, bimanual examination to identify the position and size of uterus is done. The cervix is visualized and cleaned with antiseptic solution. Anterior lip of the cervix is held with vulsellum and gentle traction is applied. This helps in straightening the cervical canal with uterine cavity and facilitates insertion of device.[1,2] The length of the uterine cavity is measured using a uterine sound. Simultaneously, the patency of the os can be confirmed and uterine anomalies can be ruled out. The ideal length of the cavity should be 6–10 cm. A uterine cavity <6 cm has a higher chance of perforation at insertion or expulsion later.[9] If the cervix needs to be dilated, then paracervical block can be used for pain relief.[3] The device is loaded into the insertion tube; then this is passed through the cervix till the flange is 1–1.5 cm from the external os. IUS is released which takes about 15–20 seconds for the folded arms to open up, after which it is gently pushed toward the fundus for proper placement.[1,15] The ends of the threads visible are cut leaving about 3 cm length. There is no evidence from the current trials to support the use of topical lidocaine, misoprostol, or NSAIDs for improving ease of insertion or reducing pain during insertion of intrauterine system (**Fig. 3**).[1]

Interventions to Ease Insertions

Cervical ripening agents, gels-containing drugs such as nitroprusside and nitroglycerine, and oral ibuprofen have been tried with no effect.[16] Filling of bladder prior to insertion

TABLE 4: Timing of insertion in terms of various clinical scenarios and specific need for additional contraception.

Circumstance	*Timing of insertion*	*Additional contraceptive precautions required*
All circumstances	Any time in menstrual cycle if reasonably certain the woman is not pregnant or at risk of pregnancy (outside terms of product license after day 7)	Yes, required for 7 days unless inserted in the first 7 days of the menstrual cycle
Postpartum (including post-cesarean section and breastfeeding)	Within 48 hours of delivery From 4 weeks after delivery if it is reasonably certain that the woman is not pregnant or at risk of pregnancy	No Yes, required for 7 days unless inserted on day 1–7 of cycle or LAM criteria are met
Following abortion (all induced or spontaneous abortions <24 weeks' gestation)	*Postsurgical abortion IUC*: Ideally should be inserted at the end of the procedure	If an LNG-IUS is fitted after day 7 postabortion, additional precautions are required for 7 days
	Postmedical abortion IUC: Can be fitted any time after completion of the second part of the abortion (i.e., passage of products of conception confirmed by clinical assessment and/or local protocols)	
Following administration of oral EC	Should not be inserted following administration of oral EC until pregnancy can be excluded as above	Not applicable

(EC: emergency contraceptive; IUC: intrauterine contraception; LAM: lactational amenorrhea method; LNG-IUS: levonorgestrel intrauterine system)

Source: Reference 1.

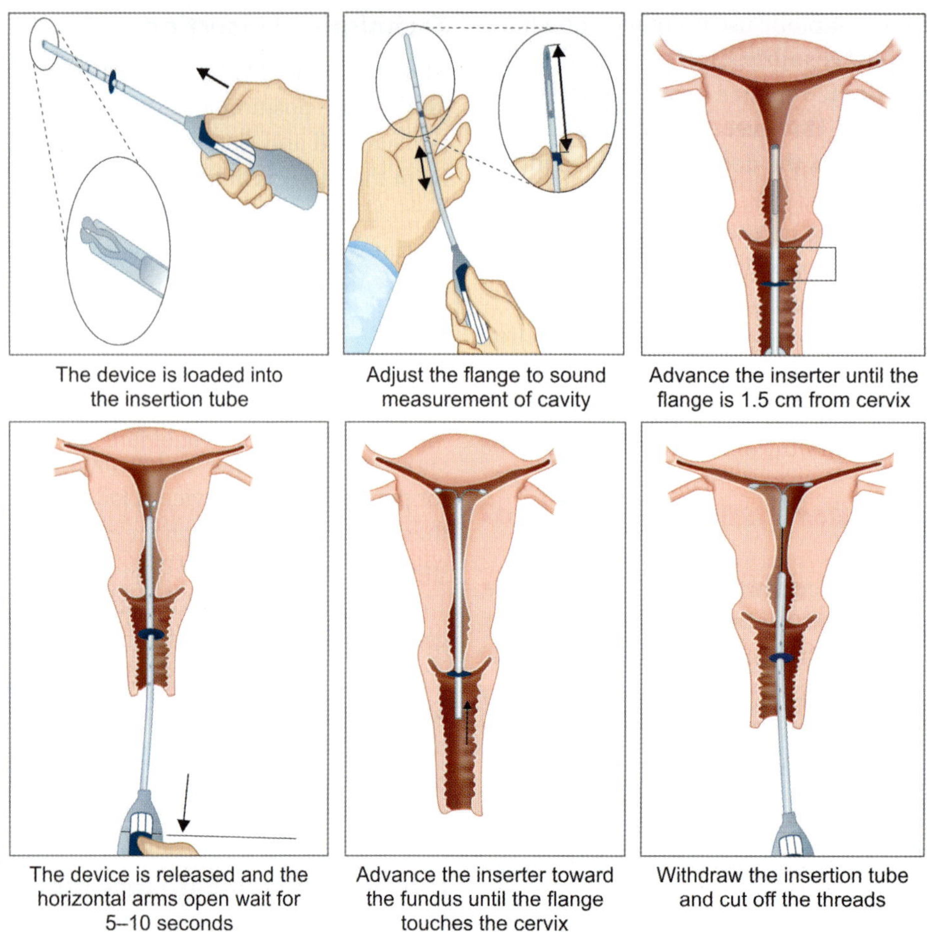

Fig. 3: Diagrammatic representation for insertion of LNG-IUS 20.15 (LNG-IUS: levonorgestrel intrauterine system)
Source: Permission for use from Bayer Zydus Pharma.

does not ease difficulty. Stabilizing the cervix with the use of vulsellum facilitates insertion by reducing flexion angle.[1,3] Use of an atraumatic instrument and slow application could reduce the pain. Routine use of paracervical block is not recommended; however, its use may be beneficial in case where dilatation of cervix is required or where difficulty is anticipated during insertion like nulliparous women or those with tightly closed cervical os.[3]

Postinsertion Counseling

Women should be instructed on how to check for the threads of IUS and counseled regarding the missing thread. Risk of device having perforated the uterus or expelled is to be clearly informed. Additional contraception is required until they seek medical advice. NSAIDs can be offered to women who experience pain after insertion.[1] Follow-up visit after the first menses or 3–6 weeks is mandatory to exclude infection, perforation, or expulsion. Complaints with regards to length of thread may be dealt with at the check-up. Date of removal or replacement could be discussed and documentation of the same confirmed. Women should be advised to report if they develop symptoms of pelvic infection, pain, abnormal bleeding, delayed menstrual period, nonpalpable threads, or palpable stem of the IUS.[1] Women are advised to wait for 6 weeks following insertion of IUS before using menstrual cup or tampons.[1]

DEVICE-RELATED COMPLICATIONS

Risk of Perforation

Perforation is a potentially serious complication that most often occurs at the time of insertion. It is uncommon, approximately 1.4 per 1,000 women, and usually occurs during involution of uterus after postpartum insertion.[9] It is important to identify perforation that occurs at the time of insertion. Confirmation by ultrasound of proper placement in cases of doubt is good clinical practice. Other than the time of insertion, perforation can occur long after insertion. Symptoms of loss of thread, lower abdominal pain, bleeding, and history of pain at the time of insertion may indicate uterine perforation and need to be evaluated. The chances for perforated IUS may cause visceral injury, lie free in the peritoneal cavity, or lie embedded in uterine musculature.[3] Confirmation by ultrasound is to be done and if required an X-ray to be performed to identify the location of the perforation of the uterus caused by LNG-IUS, followed by removal by laparoscopy or laparotomy.

Expulsion

Device partially or completely extruded through the cervical os is expulsion. It is usually associated with cramping pain, bleeding, or vaginal discharge. Expulsion is reported among 1 in 20 women, commonly in the first 1–3 months following insertion and usually during menses.[1,8] History of one expulsion increases the chance of subsequent expulsion. Chances are higher among those with postpartum or postabortal insertion, especially those wherein insertion was within 48 hours of delivery or after second-trimester abortion.[1,3] Expulsions could be asymptomatic where they just present with missing threads which could result in an unintended pregnancy. Women suspecting an expulsion should seek medical help and consider backup method of contraception. Data suggests more expulsion of copper-containing devices compared to LNG-IUS.[1]

Nonvisible Threads

The four possibilities to consider when women present with nonvisible IUS threads are thread coiled up in the cervix, expulsion, perforation, or pregnancy.[3] An important part of postinsertion counseling is identification of missing threads. They are advised to use additional contraception and seek medical help. The evaluation and management of nonvisible threads are the same as for any other IUDs.

Nonfundally Placed IUS

It is possible to find nonfundal location of the IUS when it has displaced either into the lower part of uterine body or the cervix.[3] When IUS is identified in the cervix, it should be removed as there is a risk of complete expulsion.[1] Since the LNG mechanism does not depend on location in the cavity, there may be no change in efficacy or failure rates in a downward displaced IUS. Those IUS that are nonfundal on insertion have been seen to move toward fundus within a 3-month period.[3] Hence, unless symptomatic, the IUS may be left alone.

SIDE EFFECTS (TABLE 5)

Irregular Bleeding

Symptoms of irregular bleeding are the most common cause for discontinuation of LNG-IUS after pelvic pain and cramping.[4] It usually occurs in the first 3–6 months following IUS insertion. Some women experience prolonged or irregular bleeding but tend to improve with time (>3 months).[3]

Amenorrhea or hypomenorrhea after 1 year of use is noted in 20% of users.[1] For some women, amenorrhea is worrisome enough to request removal. Postinsertion counseling could lower the incidence of such discontinuation. Oral contraceptive pills for a short duration of 2–3 months control irregular bleeding well. One should keep in mind other causes of irregular bleeding and postcoital bleeding which may need evaluation.[3] Pap smear may be done with ease by brushing aside the threads at the cervix. Similarly, a thin endometrial cannula can allow for easy sampling of the endometrium. Pelvic inflammatory disease (PID) and STIs should be ruled out. Slight increase in bleeding initially was noticed in women whose IUS was replaced after the initial 5 years of use.

The relatively low systemic blood levels result in less systemic side effects.[7] However, reports of headache, nausea, mood swings, acne, and hirsutism have been noted especially in the 1st month of use, sometimes even leading to discontinuation. The effect on libido by LNG-IUS has not been established.[1] The changes in weight gain are similar to copper-containing devices, especially in the 1st year of use. The 52-mg LNG-IUS has been found to be associated with a slight increase in the formation of benign ovarian cysts (1 in 100) that are most often asymptomatic and resolve spontaneously. There seems to be no difference among various types of LNG-IUS in terms of systemic side effects. However, irregular bleeding was found to be more frequent among the lower dose LNG-IUS.[3]

TABLE 5: Side effects of LNG-IUS.

• Changes in bleeding patterns including: – Lighter bleeding – Fewer days of bleeding – Infrequent bleeding – Amenorrhea – Prolonged bleeding – Irregular bleeding	• Acne • Headaches • Breast tenderness or pain • Nausea • Weight gain • Dizziness • Mood changes • Ovarian cysts • Pelvic pain and cramps

(LNG-IUS: levonorgestrel intrauterine system)

Risk of Ectopic Pregnancy

There is no increased risk of ectopic pregnancy in women using LNG-IUS.[1] The device can be inserted in women with a previous history of ectopic pregnancies as well.[7] Accidental exposure that occurs due to failure of LNG-IUS, however rare, should raise suspicion of ectopic pregnancy, and necessary investigations and imaging must be performed to rule out this condition.

Pregnancy

In the event of an accidental pregnancy as suggested earlier, ectopic pregnancy must be ruled out. Intrauterine pregnancy with IUS displaced into the cervix or easily accessible IUS may be removed. Women who conceive with IUS in situ have a higher chance of spontaneous abortion, septic abortion, preterm labor, and chorioamnionitis.[3] Based on limited evidence, removal of IUS early in pregnancy improves outcomes.[1,3]

Pelvic Inflammatory Disease

Pelvic inflammatory disease occurs in up to 1% of users regardless of age or IUD type.[3] Various studies have shown that LNG-IUS may have reduced incidence on PID as compared to other IUDs, possibly because of the effect of LNG on the cervical mucus.[5] PID appears to occur at insertion procedure and to the background of STIs. The chance for infection is the highest in 20 days following insertion, after which the risk remained low unless there was exposure to STIs.[3] PID when diagnosed, treatment is with appropriate antibiotic therapy without the need for removal of the IUS unless there is no clinical improvement within 72 hours.[3] Screening for STIs is not recommended as routine; however, it is important to identify those at high risk for STI.

There is some evidence that yeast binds to the IUD and forms a biofilm which protect the yeast from antifungals causing recurrent vaginal candidiasis.[1] Cytology slides of LNG-IUS users show increased presence of yeast cells, but there are no increased rates of infection. Association of bacterial vaginosis and LNG-IUS is unclear; however, women with recurrent infection are advised to choose other modalities of contraception.

Risk of Metabolic and Systemic Effects

Levonorgestrel intrauterine system has revealed no major systemic side effects attributable to low serum concentration of the molecule. Concern of affecting blood pressure, lipid metabolism, and glucose control remains theoretical. LNG-IUSs has not been shown to affect hypertension, weight gain, hyperglycemia, hyperlipidemia, or increased metabolic cardiovascular and inflammatory parameters making it safe for use in these conditions.[5] There is little or no increased risk of venous thromboembolism or myocardial infarction (MI) associated with the use of LNG-IUS.[1] Studies on bone marrow density have shown no difference between LNG-IUS and copper-containing devices.[1,3] Evidence does not support increased risk of breast cancer with LNG-IUS use; in fact, its use has been endorsed in those women with breast cancer on tamoxifen therapy to counter the estrogenic effect on endometrium.

Effect on Breast Milk

Concerns regarding negative effect of hormone-releasing IUS during breastfeeding have been at most theoretical showing no evidence in RCT results which exhibit no difference in breast milk production, newborn weight, or incidence of exclusive breastfeeding. Breast milk composition did not vary. Women considering LNG-IUS postpartum should not be discouraged on the basis of theoretical bias.

REMOVAL OF INTRAUTERINE SYSTEM

The removal/replacement of IUS recommended by Faculty of Sexual and Reproductive Healthcare (FSRH) is shown in **Flowchart 1**.

Flowchart 1: The Faculty of Sexual and Reproductive Healthcare (FSRH) recommendation for removal/replacement of IUS.

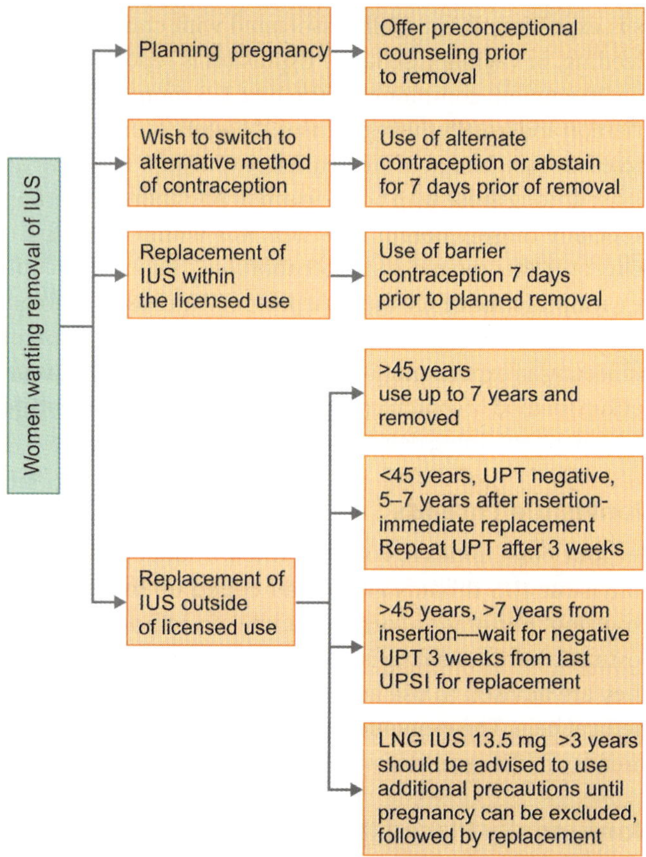

(IUS: intrauterine system; LNG: levonorgestrel; UPT: urine pregnancy test; UPSI: unprotected sexual intercourse)

ADVANTAGES OF THE LNG-IUS

- Contraceptive method with efficiency and low failure rate
- Long-acting and reversible contraceptive
- Rapid return to fertility after removal

TABLE 6: Noncontraceptive benefits.

• Treatment of heavy menstrual bleeding • Prevention of anemia • Treatment of HMB caused due to inherited disorders of coagulation • Reduction in primary dysmenorrhea and premenstrual syndrome • Treatment of dysmenorrhea secondary to endometriosis	• Reduces the need for hysterectomy for AUB • Endometrial protection during postmenopausal estrogen therapy • Prevention of endometrial hyperplasia in tamoxifen users • Reduction in endometriosis, endometrial hyperplasia, and endometrial cancer • Reduction in the symptoms and size of fibroid uterus

(AUB: abnormal uterine bleeding; HMB: heavy menstrual bleeding)

- Reduces menstrual blood loss and dysmenorrhea
- Relatively low systemic side effects when comparing with other hormonal methods
- Ease of removal compared to implants
- Noncontraceptive health benefits including treatment of heavy menstrual bleeding and potential reduction in iron deficiency anemia **(Table 6)**
- May help protect against endometrial and cervical cancer

- No further action or supplies required once the LNG-IUS is inserted—forgettable contraceptive
- Hormonal device is safe to use in perimenopausal age group.

KEY MESSAGES

- Levonorgestrel intrauterine system is currently the method of choice among long-acting reversible contraceptives.
- It has better efficacy and lesser expulsion rates compared to copper-containing IUCD.
- It may be used among all age groups, especially in those suffering from HMB.
- It has numerous noncontraceptive indication and therapeutic benefits, especially in cases of HMB, dysmenorrhea, adenomyosis, and endometriosis. It ensures immediate return to fertility on removal.
- Insertion of the device requires special training. Removal technique is easy and pain free.
- Irregular bleeding or amenorrhea is concern that has led to discontinuation of the device.
- Minor systemic side effect compared to other hormonal contraception.

FURTHER READING

1. American College of Obstetricians and Gynecologists' Committee on Gynecologic Practice; Long-Acting Reversible Contraceptive Expert Work Group. Committee opinion no 672: clinical challenges of long-acting reversible contraceptive methods. Obstet Gynecol. 2016;128(3):e69-e77.
2. French R, Van Vliet H, Cowan F, Mansour D, Morris S, Hughes D, et al. Hormonally impregnated intrauterine systems (IUSs) versus other forms of reversible contraceptives as effective methods of preventing pregnancy. Cochrane Database Syst Rev. 2004;(3):CD001776.
3. Teal SB, Turok DK, Chen BA, Kimble T, Olariu AI, Creinin MD. Five-year contraceptive efficacy and safety of a levonorgestrel 52-mg intrauterine system. Obstet Gynecol. 2019;133(1):63-70.

REFERENCES

1. Faculty of Sexual and Reproductive Healthcare. (2019). FSRH Clinical Guideline: Intrauterine Contraception (April 2015, amended September 2019). [online] Available from: https://www.fsrh.org/standards-and-guidance/documents/ceuguidanceintrauterinecontraception/. [Last accessed November, 2021].
2. World health Organisation. (2018). Family Planning - A global handbook for providers 2018 edition. [online] Available from: https://www.who.int/reproductivehealth/publications/fp-global-handbook/en/. [Last accessed November, 2021].
3. Committee on Practice Bulletins-Gynecology, Long-Acting Reversible Contraception Work Group. Practice Bulletin No. 186: Long-acting reversible contraception: implants and intrauterine devices. Obstet Gynecol. 2017;130(5):e251-69.
4. Chrisman C, Ribeiro P, Dalton VK. The levonorgestrel-releasing intrauterine system: an updated review of the contraceptive and noncontraceptive uses. Clin Obstet Gynecol. 2007;50(4):886-97.
5. Sitruk-Ware R, Inki P. The levonorgestrel intrauterine system: long-term contraception and therapeutic effects. Womens Health. 2005;1(2):171-82.
6. McNicholas C, Tessa M, Secura G, Peipert JF. The contraceptive choice project round up. Clin Obstet Gynecol. 2014;57(4):635-43.
7. Fritz MA, Speroff L. Clinical gynecologic endocrinology and infertility, 9th edition. Philadelphia: Wolters Kluwer Health/Lippincott Williams & Wilkins; 2011.
8. Kailasam C, Cahill D. Review of the safety, efficacy and patient acceptability of the levonorgestrel-releasing intrauterine system. Patient Prefer Adherence. 2008;2:293-302.
9. Costescu DJ. Levonorgestrel-releasing intrauterine systems for long-acting contraception: current perspectives, safety, and patient counseling. Int J Womens Health. 2016;8:589-98.
10. Andersson K, Odlind V, Rybo G. Levonorgestrel-releasing and copper releasing (Nova T) IUDs during five years of use: a randomized comparative trial. Contraception. 1994:49(1);56-72.
11. Sivin I, El Mahgoub S, McCarthy T, Mishell DR Jr, Shoupe D, Alvarez F, et al. Long-term contraception with the levonorgestrel 20 mcg/day (LNG 20) and the copper T 380Ag intrauterine devices: A five-year randomized study. Contraception. 1990;42(4):361-78.
12. Backman T, Rauramo I, Huhtala S, Koskenvuo M. Pregnancy during the use of levonorgestrel intrauterine system. Am J Obstet Gynecol. 2004;190:50-54.
13. Heinemann K, Reed S, Moehner S, Minh TD. Comparative contraceptive effectiveness of levonorgestrel-releasing and copper intrauterine devices: the European Active Surveillance Study for Intrauterine Devices. Contraception. 2015;91:280-3.
14. World Health Organisation. (2015). Medical eligibility criteria for contraceptive use, 5th edition. [online] Available from: https://www.who.int/publications/i/item/9789241549158. [Last accessed November, 2021].
15. Bayerhealthcare.com. (2021). Mirena full prescribing information. [online] Available from: https://labeling.bayerhealthcare.com/html/products/pi/Mirena_PI.pdf. [Last accessed November, 2021].
16. Attia AM, Ibrahim MM, Abou-Setta AM. Role of the levonorgestrel intrauterine system in effective contraception. Patient Prefer Adherence. 2013;7:777-85.

LONG QUESTION

1. Mention various types of long-acting reversible contraception. Enlist with rationale the indication for use of LNG-IUS. What are the prerequisites for LNG-IUS use and also write a short note on timing of insertion.

SHORT QUESTIONS

1. What are noncontraceptive benefits of LNG-IUS?
2. Describe the mechanism of action of LNG-IUS that leads to contraception among the users.
3. What is the complication of LNG-IUS?
4. Compare mechanism of action, side effects, and complication of LNG-IUS with copper IUD.
5. Write a short note on levonorgestrel in contraception with special emphasis on IUS systems.

MULTIPLE CHOICE QUESTIONS

1. The daily release rate of the 52 mg levonorgestrel intrauterine system (LNG-IUS) is:
   a. 5 µg b. 14 µg
   c. 20 µg d. 52 µg
2. Bleeding patterns associated with LNG-IUS use are:
   a. Amenorrhea occurs in 20% of users
   b. Bleeding patterns will remain regular throughout use
   c. Bleeding patterns are likely to be regular and heavy
   d. Irregular bleeding is usual until the last year of use
3. The primary mechanism of action of LNG-IUS is:
   a. Preventing fertilization
   b. Preventing implantation
   c. Suppressing ovulation
   d. Hostile cervical mucus changes
4. Which of the following cannot be used for emergency contraception?
   a. Copper IUD b. LNG-IUD
   c. Progesterone only pill d. Ulipristal acetate
5. Licensed duration of use for LNG-IUS 20 is:
   a. 1 year b. 3 years
   c. 5 years d. 10 years
6. With regard to LNG-IUS, which of the following sentences is false?
   a. Breastfeeding is not a contraindication to LNG-IUS use
   b. Ectopic pregnancy is one of the complications of LNG-IUS
   c. Local release of LNG results in low systemic side effects
   d. There is no role for prophylactic antibiotics during insertion
7. The most effective long-acting reversible contraception (LARC) is:
   a. LNG-IUS
   b. Copper-containing devices
   c. Implants
   d. Female sterilization
8. According to the medical eligibility criteria, the use of LNG-IUS is absolutely contraindicated in:
   a. After 6 weeks' postpartum
   b. Current breast cancer
   c. Endometrial hyperplasia
   d. Immediate postabortion
9. The following are noncontraceptive benefits of LNG-IUS:
   a. Decrease in primary dysmenorrhea
   b. Protection against endometrial hyperplasia during Tamoxifen therapy
   c. Treatment of HMB caused due to inherited thrombophilias
   d. All of the above
10. With regard to insertion of LNG-IUS, the statement that is false is:
    a. It cannot be inserted in nulliparous women
    b. Insertion is delayed in the presence of active upper genital tract infections
    c. Uterine cavity should be at least 6 cm in length
    d. Use of cervical priming agents does not improve ease of insertion

Answers

1.	c	2.	a	3.	d	4.	b	5.	c	6.	b
7.	a	8.	b	9.	d	10.	a				

2.11 EMERGENCY CONTRACEPTION

Lila Vyas, Preeti Sharma

INTRODUCTION

- Emergency contraception (EC) is a method of contraception that is used to prevent unwanted pregnancy after an act of unprotected sexual intercourse.
- Emergency contraception can be used in the following situations: unprotected intercourse, concerns about possible contraceptive failure, incorrect use of contraceptives, and sexual assault if without contraception coverage.
- Methods of emergency contraception are the copper-bearing intrauterine devices (IUDs) and the emergency contraceptive pills (ECPs).
- A copper-bearing IUD is the most effective form of emergency contraception available.
- The emergency contraceptive pill regimens recommended by WHO are ulipristal acetate, levonorgestrel, or combined oral contraceptives (COCs) consisting of estradiol plus levonorgestrel.

EMERGENCY CONTRACEPTION

Emergency contraceptives are used to prevent pregnancy after intercourse where no protective methods have been used. They should be used as early as possible within the next 120 hours.

Although EC helps to prevent pregnancy and control births, it is not a primary contraceptive method. It is used as a secondary tool to reduce the risk of unwanted pregnancy in the fertile period of menstrual cycle where either no contraceptive failure was used or contraceptive measure failed.

Drug composition of an emergency contraceptive pill (ECP) is different from abortion pills. Emergency contraceptives will not damage or terminate the pregnancy already existing.

Emergency contraception plays an important role as a spacing method of contraception for planned parenthood, but it is not a primary contraceptive.

Emergency contraceptive pills are also known as the "morning-after pill" or postcoital pill to be taken as soon as possible after unprotected sex.

INTRODUCTION OF EMERGENCY CONTRACEPTION IN INDIA

India participated in research trials of WHO Division for Reproductive Health and High-risk Pregnancy (WHO-RHR/HRP) in 1995–1997 and in 1998–2001. Research provided sound scientific foundation of efficacy and safety in Indian women. A Consortium on National Consensus for EC was held in January 2001, where the following issues were discussed for consensus:[1] (1) Dedicated method of choice for EC in India, (2) preintroduction IEC and media campaigns, (3) training of healthcare providers, (4) ideal approach for distribution to the masses, (5) client information and counseling, and (6) monitoring of the program.

The report and recommendations of the consortium were released in June 2001.[1] Subsequently, EC was approved by the Drug Controller General of India (DCGI) in September 2001, permission was granted for manufacture/import of levonorgestrel (LNG) and social marketing on prescription, and the drug was made available in the country in January 2002. There were several challenges for introducing EC in India, including the size and diversity of the country and poor awareness of both users and providers. It was made an over-the-counter (OTC) drug in 2005. At present, there are seven ECPs available in the Indian market, all of them are sold over the counter (**Table 1**).

Higher BMI reduces efficiency of oral EC but does not reduce effectiveness of copper intrauterine device (IUD).[2]

METHODS OF EMERGENCY CONTRACEPTION IN DECREASING ORDER OF EFFICIENCY[3]

- Copper IUD
- Ulipristal acetate (UPA)
- LNG
- Mifepristone
- Yuzpe method
- LNG-IUD.

*Emergency contraception is always indicated for unprotected sex and after sexual assault (**Table 2**).*[4]

WHO CAN USE EMERGENCY CONTRACEPTION?

Emergency contraceptives can be used when a woman is concerned that she might get pregnant. Emergency contraceptives can be used in all age groups. They are safe for use in all ages from adolescent girls, lactating mothers to perimenopausal women.[5] There are no absolute medical contraindications to the use of EC.[6] The criteria for use of copper IUD are same in both general use for contraception and EC.

Before giving the EC, the healthcare provider must ascertain the following:

- Duration of menstrual cycle
- Last menstrual period
- Duration since the last unprotected intercourse in hours
- Was any contraceptive method used?
- If there is any history of sexually transmitted or medical disease?

WHO CAN PRESCRIBE?

Emergency contraceptive pills can be given by doctors, nurses, pharmacist, paramedics, and other trained person and community health workers. This will help in the widespread use of emergency contraception in community.

TABLE 1: Available methods of emergency contraception.

Regimen	*Formulation*	*Timing of use after unprotected intercourse*	*Access*	*US FDA*	*Efficacy risk of pregnancy*
Selective progesterone receptor modulator	Tablet, one tablet ulipristal acetate 30 mg	Up to 5 days	Prescribing essential	Yes	1.2%
Progestin only	Tablet, one tablet levonorgestrel 1.5 mg or two tablets	Up to 3 days Up to 3 days	OTC	Yes Yes	1.2–2%
Combined progestin–estrogen pills	Tablets, 120 mg ethinylestradiol and 0.6 mg LNG Yuzpe method	Up to 5 days	Prescribing essential	No	1.2–2%
Copper IUD	CuT 380A	Up to 5 days	By clinician	No	0.1%
Mifepristone	Tablet, 10 mg/25 mg/50 mg	Up to 5 days	By clinician		0.1%

(FDA: Food and Drug Administration; IUD: intrauterine device; LNG: levonorgestrel)

TABLE 2: Indications for emergency contraceptive use.

Method of contraception	***Indication***
Hormonal methods:	
Progestin-only contraceptive pills	• More than 3 hours late from the usual time of intake of the progestogen-only pill (minipill) or delay since last pill >27 hours • Vomiting and diarrhea for >48 hours • Delay in starting new pill pack • No backup method for the first 2 days
Combined only contraceptive pills	• Three or more consecutively missed pills • Delay in starting new pill pack by >48 hours • Vomiting and diarrhea for >48 hours • No backup method for first 7 days
Patch	• Leaving the patch on for >9 days • Delay in applying new patch >48 hours • No backup method for the first 7 days
Ring	• Leaving the ring in for >35 days • Failure to reinsert ring >48 hours • No backup method for the first 7 days
Depot-medroxy-progesterone acetate injection	• More than 3 weeks late • Interval between injections >15 weeks • No backup method for the first 7 days
Barrier methods:	
Male condom	Slippage, leakage, and breakage
Female condom	Incorrect insertion, dislodgement
Diaphragm and cervical cap	Incorrect insertion, dislodgement
Spermicide	Incorrect insertion, dislodgement
Withdrawal	Incorrect or uncertain usage
Long-acting reversible methods:	
Copper IUD	• Concern for device expulsion • Device beyond duration of efficacy
LNG-IUD	• Concern for device expulsion • Device beyond duration of efficacy • No backup method in first 7 days of method
Progestin implant	• Device beyond duration of efficacy • No backup method in first 7 days of method

(IUD: intrauterine device; LNG: levonorgestrel)

All providers should have proper knowledge of EC and should be appropriately trained to counsel the patients for use of emergency contraceptives.

Need for Emergency Contraception

Annually, approximately 210 million pregnancies occur, of which 46 million (22%) end in induced abortions and 20 million in unsafe abortions.[7] Majority of these (95%) occur in developing countries, and 13% of pregnancy-related deaths are due to unsafe abortion as a consequence of unwanted pregnancy.[7] Nearly half of the pregnancies in US are unplanned.[8] Moreover, since the use of emergency contraceptives, the contribution of unsafe abortion toward maternal mortality has declined from 13 to 8%.[9]

Registered LNG-EC products **(Figs. 1A to F)** that are available over the counter without prescription are:

- E Pills
- ECee2
- i-Pill
- Pill 72
- Postinor-2
- Postpill, Pregnon
- Preventol
- Unwanted 72.

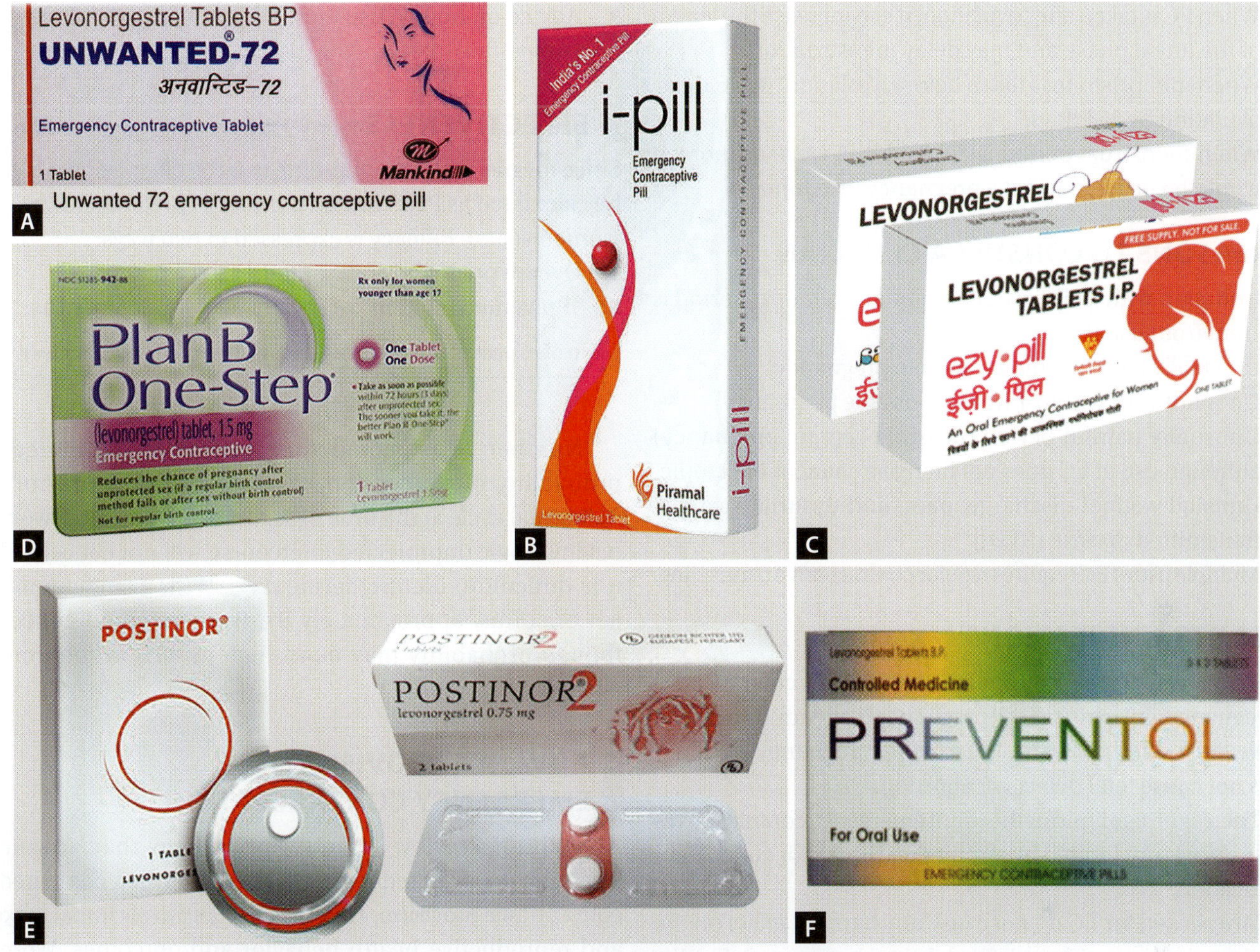

Figs. 1A to F: Registered levonorgestrel emergency contraception (LNG-EC) products that are available over the counter without prescription.

It was stated that advertisements related to EC should follow Code of Ethics and it should give information with respect to the following:

- When to take EC pills?
- How to take EC pills?
- Side effects of the EC pills.

MECHANISM OF ACTION

Mode of action of EC pills is by:

- Interrupting ovulation by preventing or delaying it
- Thickening of cervical mucus.

Prevent fertilization directly if ovulation has already happened.[10,11]

Mode of action of copper IUD is by:

- Causing a chemical change in sperm and egg before fertilization
- Interfering in transport of ovum sperm or egg, preventing implantation of fertilized egg[2]
- Interference with corpus luteum function and luteolysis.

Pregnancy will not be prevented or harmed if implantation has already occurred.[12]

Timings

Emergency contraceptives are effective if taken within 120 hours of unprotected intercourse and are most effective in the first 12 hours.

SIDE EFFECTS

- Nausea and vomiting are common with combined oral contraceptives (COC) pills but routine use of antiemetic is not recommended. Dose should be repeated if, vomiting occurs within 3 hours of taking the pill.
- Some patients may experience breast tenderness, abdominal pain dizziness, and fatigue. These side effects usually resolve within 24 hours.
- Irregular bleeding occurs in 16% of patients in the first week after use.

Change in the bleeding pattern occurs only in the cycle in which ECPs are taken; next cycle duration is not affected. It resolves on its own and no treatment is required except reassurance.

- When EC is taken before ovulation, the high doses of progestogen may induce progestogen withdrawal bleeding a few days after taking pills.

- When EC is taken after ovulation, it can increase the length of the luteal phase and may delay menstruation.
- When mifepristone is taken before ovulation, it can delay ovulation by 3–4 days.
- When menstrual period is delayed by a week or more, it would be prudent to get a pregnancy test done.

REASONS TO CONSULT A CLINICIAN

Consultation with a clinician is essential if her next period is different from usual:

- Unusually light bleeding (possible pregnancy)
- Does not start within 4 weeks (possible pregnancy)
- Unusually painful period (possible ectopic pregnancy) although use of EC does not increase chances of ectopic
- Unusual vaginal discharge, pain, and dysuria [sexually transmitted disease (STD)]
- Multiple use of EC requires regular contraceptive counseling.

CONTRAINDICATIONS

The only absolute contraindication of emergency contraceptive is pregnancy as it cannot act if pregnancy is already implanted. However, it does not harm the existing pregnancy so that it does not cause fetal defects or abortion.

There is no age limit for the use of emergency contraceptives and its use is not limited by any medical illness or concurrent medication.

Drugs used for EC do not cause any harmful effect on the existing pregnancy. There is no delay in the return to fertility after taking ECPs. Further, no clinical or laboratory tests are mandatory before administering ECPs.

MEDICAL ELIGIBILITY CRITERIA (AS PER WHO)[13]

There are no restrictions for the medical eligibility of who can use ECPs.

Some women, however, use ECPs repeatedly for any of the reasons stated above, or as their main method of contraception. In such situations, further counseling needs to be given on what other and more regular contraceptive options may be more appropriate and more effective. EC can prevent up to 95% of pregnancy only; hence, use of regular contraceptive methods must be encouraged.

Frequent and repeated use of EC can result in increased side effects, such as menstrual irregularities. Use of EC provides an opportunity to counsel and plan using an appropriate contraceptive method.

Emergency contraceptive pills were found to be less effective in obese women (whose body mass index is more than 30 kg/m^2), but they are not unsafe and can be used in obese women whenever required.

Counseling for use of ECPs should include:

- Information about other options for using regular contraception
- Advice on how to use methods correctly so that they are successful.

EFFECTIVENESS

Since the method is for one-time use, the effectiveness cannot be calculated as Pearl index (number of pregnancies per 100 women years). Efficacy is expressed in two ways:

1. Overall pregnancy rate—failure/100 women
2. "Prevented fraction" of pregnancies—calculated as:

$$\frac{\text{(No of expected pregnancies - no. of observed pregnancies)}}{\text{No. of expected pregnancies}} \times 100$$

Number of expected pregnancies is calculated by probability of conception based on the cycle day of the menstrual cycle at the time of sexual exposure. Most women having single unprotected intercourse will not conceive, but it is difficult to identify fertile days. With a single random act of coitus, approximately 8% women would conceive, though probability may be as high as 40% at the time of ovulation.[14]

ADVANCE PROVISION OF EMERGENCY CONTRACEPTION

A Cochrane review (2007)[15] has shown that advanced provision does not reduce pregnancy rate when compared to conventional provision. This does not negatively impact sexual and reproductive health behavior and outcomes. Women should have easy access to EC because it may decrease the chance of pregnancy; however, interventions tested so far have not reduced the overall pregnancy rates in the populations studied.[15]

When to Resume or Initiate a Regular Method of Contraception?

Following administration of emergency contraceptives with LNG or COC pills, the patient may resume or start any contraceptive method immediately including copper IUD.

Following use of UPA, patient may resume or start any progestogen containing method on 6th day after taking UPA. However, LNG-IUD or copper IUD can be inserted immediately.[16]

No other contraceptive protection is required if a copper IUD is used for EC.

Repeated use of EC is safe.

The use of EC may be repeated by the women who have taken it earlier.

This may be done even within the same menstrual cycle since there is no contraindication for such repeat use. Women should not be denied frequent access to ECPs whenever needed.

There is no scientific evidence for limiting the number of times women use ECPs. ECPs are safer than unintended pregnancy, especially when women do not have access to safe abortion facilities. Women can use ECPs as often as required.

EC and sexual assault: Pregnancy rates among rape victims of childbearing age are around 5% in the US;[17] about half of rape victims who become pregnant have abortions. EC is commonly used as an option for victims of sexual assault.

WHO Recommendations for Provision of Emergency Contraception

All women and girls at risk of an unintended pregnancy have a right to access EC, and these methods should be routinely included within all national family planning programs. Moreover, EC should be integrated into healthcare services for populations most at risk of exposure to unprotected sex, including postsexual assault care and services for women and girls living in shelter homes.

The WHO reaffirms its commitment to constantly reviewing emerging evidence through its continuous identification of research evidence (CIRE) system and also by regularly updating its guidance accordingly.

FUTURE OF EMERGENCY CONTRACEPTION IN INDIA

Emergency contraception can be an important tool in improving the reproductive health of women in India. It is essential to provide training modules to train providers in both the public and private sectors including chemists and pharmacists. Awareness about EC should be increased in sexually active women.

Unwanted pregnancy has a high complication rate resulting in maternal morbidity and mortality. It has both financial and social implications for the society. National guidelines for family planning should encourage the use of regular contraception. Women undergoing medical termination of pregnancy should be counseled for use of EC. No contraceptive method is 100% effective. Therefore, women may need a last-minute chance to prevent unwanted pregnancy by using EC as a backup method in the fertility period of her menstrual cycle.

REFERENCES

1. WHO-CCR in Human Reproduction. (2001). Consortium for National Consensus on Emergency Contraception in India. [online] Available from: https://www.aiims.edu/aiims/events/Gynaewebsite/ec_site/consortium.htm#:~:text=A%20Consortium%20on%20National%20Consensus,January%2011-12%2C%202001. [Last accessed November, 2021].
2. Dean G, Schwarz EB. Intrauterine devices. In: Kowal D, Hatcher RA, Nelson AL, Trussell J, Cwiak C, Cason P, Policar MS, Edelman AB, Aiken ARA, Marrazzo JM (Eds). Contraceptive Technology, 21st edition. New York: Ayer Company Publishers Inc.; 2018. p. 157.
3. Centers for Disease Control and Prevention. (2014). Effectiveness of family planning methods. [online] Available from: https://www.cdc.gov/reproductivehealth/unintendedpregnancy/pdf/family-planning-methods-2014.pdf. [Last accessed November, 2021].
4. American College of Obstetricians and Gynecologists. ACOG Committee opinion no 777: Sexual Assault. Obstet Gynecol. 2019;133:e296.
5. Upadhyaya KK; Committee on Adolescence. Emergency Contraception, Pediatrics 2019:144.
6. Turok D, Schreiber CA, Eckler K; UptoDate. (2019). Emergency contraception. [online] Available from: https://www.uptodate.com/contents/emergency-contraception. [Last accessed November, 2021].
7. Trussell J. Contraceptive failure in the United States. Contraception. 2004;70:89-96.
8. Finer LB, Zolna MR. Declines in unintended pregnancy in the United States, 2008-2011. N Engl J Med. 2016;374(9): 843-52.
9. Mittal S. Emergency contraception: Potential for women's health. Indian J Med Res. 2014;140)(Suppl S1):45-52.
10. Gemzell-Danielsson K, Berger C, Lalitkumar PG. Mechanisms of action of oral emergency contraception. Gynecol Endocrinol. 2014;30(10):685-7.
11. Gemzell-Danielsson K, Berger C, Lalitkumar PG. Emergency contraception—mechanisms of action. Contraception. 2013;87(3):300-8.
12. Food and Drug Administration. Birth Control: Medicines to Help You. Silver Spring, MD: Food and Drug Administration; 2016.
13. World Health Organization. (2018). Emergency contraception. [online] Available from: https://www.gfmer.ch/SRH-Course-2018/family-planning/pdf/Emergency-contraception-Idris-2018.pdf. [Last accessed November, 2021].
14. Wilcox AJ, Weinberg CR, Baird DD. Timing of sexual intercourse in relation to ovulation: effects on the probability of conception, survival of the pregnancy and sex of the baby. N Engl J Med. 1995;333:517-21.
15. Polis CB, Schaffer K, Blanchard K, Glasier A, Harper CC, Grimes DA. Advance provision of emergency contraception for pregnancy prevention (full review). Cochrane Database Syst Rev. 2007;(2):CD005497.
16. Hsiang D, Dunn S. Emergency contraception. CMAJ. 2016;188:E536.
17. Frost JJ, Singh S, Finer B. U.S. women's one-year contraceptive use patterns, 2004. Perspect Sex Reprod Health. 2007;39: 48-55.

LONG QUESTIONS

1. Discuss the indications for emergency contraception use in a couple who have been using some form of contraception.
2. Emergency contraception is an essential component of planned parenthood. Discuss the statement.

SHORT QUESTIONS

1. Enumerate the methods of available emergency contraception.
2. What are the implications of EC use on an unintended pregnancy?
3. Mention the general and method-specific contraindications to EC use.
4. Write a short note on the use of ulipristal in EC.

MULTIPLE CHOICE QUESTIONS

1. Which of the following statement is false?
   a. EC can be used as a primary contraceptive.
   b. EC can be used within 5 days of unprotected sex
   c. EC is safe to use in diabetic patients
   d. EC does not increase chance of ectopic
2. What is the best time to take ECP after unprotected sex?
   a. 12 hrs
   b. 48 hrs
   c. 72 hrs
   d. 120 hrs
3. Which is the most effective contraceptive?
   a. Progesterone only pill
   b. Mirena
   c. Copper IUD
   d. Oral contraceptives
4. Which of the following is true about EC pills?
   a. It has the same hormone content as most birth control pills
   b. It is effective when taken within 72 hrs after intercourse
   c. It is generally considered an abortion pill
   d. It is only available on prescription

Answers

1. a 2. a 3. c 4. b

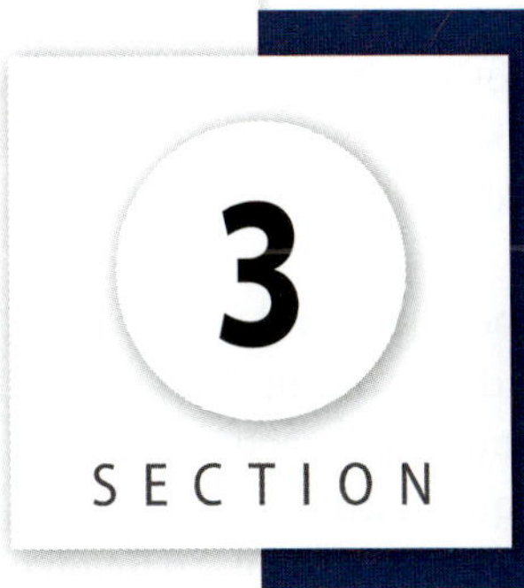

Termination of Pregnancy

3.1 TERMINATION OF PREGNANCY: COUNSELING AND EVALUATION

Chandravati, Priti Kumar, Bhawna Khera

INTRODUCTION

The provision of safe and legal pregnancy termination is a crucial aspect of women's reproductive health. In India, the Medical Termination of Pregnancy (MTP) Act 1971 legalizes abortion until 20 weeks. As providers, we must empower women with information and knowledge that help them in making informed choices about their reproductive and sexual health. In order to provide safe services, the government of India has transformed the concept of abortion care from being just a medical procedure into a woman-centered approach. The three key elements of this approach are choice, accessibility of services, and quality of services. The first element of choice includes giving woman the options to choose from the methods for the termination of pregnancy and postabortion contraception. Counseling and evaluation go hand in hand with each other in fulfilling criteria of choice. Together, both provide a firm foundation to safe termination procedures.

COUNSELING

Counseling, which is informative, empathetic, and non-judgmental, is the need of the hour. For most of women, the confirmation of an unwanted or unplanned pregnancy can be seen as a negative life event. The decision on what to do about pregnancy gives rise to different conflicts and choices to be made. These choices may have a major impact on her future personal development depending on how the choice is managed. A well-organized preprocedure counseling session fulfills this task efficiently.

Principles of good counseling session include:

- Patient and active listening
- Confidentiality
- Empathy and respect
- Appropriate unbiased information
- Open discussion and shared decision.

Role of Counseling in Pregnancy Termination

Women requesting termination should have access to counseling services. These sessions should be conducted by appropriately trained medical personnel. Wherever possible, her partner should also be involved. Most women deciding to have a termination consider many of the factors such as their relationship with their partner, the well-being of the fetus, their readiness to take on a parenting role, the needs of children they may already have, their career and financial situation, their mental and physical health, the level of support they are likely to receive from their extended family, and their moral, emotional, and religious beliefs about pregnancy, abortion, and motherhood. Three types of counseling have been appreciated in pregnancy termination settings:

1. Implication counseling where the woman wants to know about the impact of her decision of termination of pregnancy on herself, her future reproductive outcomes, and her family.
2. Support counseling where the woman or her partner needs support while going through a difficult phase.
3. Therapeutic counseling where the discussion is mainly around options available for termination, their risks and benefits, and postabortion follow-up.

Preprocedure Counseling

Preprocedure counseling is a very important component of comprehensive and safe abortion care. The steps include addressing queries and concerns about decision-making, discussing medical and surgical options available along with their implications for her, finalizing the plan with a shared decision approach, getting informed consent signed, and discussion about safe and effective postabortion contraception. Throughout the process of counseling, maintaining confidentiality, privacy, and positive relationship with the patient is imperative **(Fig. 1 and Table 1)**.

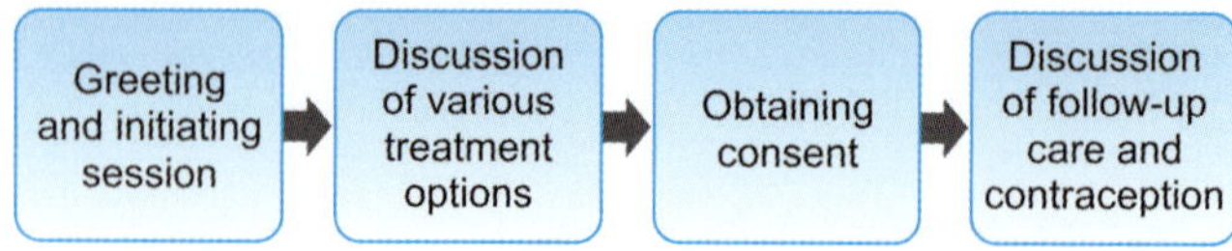

Fig. 1: Step-by-step approach for effective counseling.

TABLE 1: Communication principles.

Features	*Dos*	*Don'ts*
Interaction	Sympathetic, listens actively	• Nonsympathetic approach • Ignores answers
Language	Patient friendly and easy	Medical terminology difficult to understand
Confidentiality	Most important	Discussion with others without her consent
Information gathering	Relevant with open questions	Irrelevant with vague discussions
Decision making	Shared between clinician and patient	Clinician is taking lead and taking decision for her

Step 1: Initiating Session and Gathering Information

Whole interaction should be done very sensitively, engaging the patient and listening calmly. Building a rapport with patient and building confidence in her are of paramount importance to make communication effective. Identify why she wants pregnancy termination and what are her beliefs regarding termination. It is a very sensitive issue and she may be reluctant to discuss it. Many women undergoing abortion experience negative emotions, including guilt if their decisions are biased by family interference. Counseling is a good opportunity for her to clear all her uncertainties and take informed decision for herself. Also, it gives an opportunity to medical personnel to check if she has already tried any method for termination herself. This information is indispensable for formulating the management plan for her. Information regarding her previous contraceptive usage carries significance in discussing postabortion contraception.

Step 2: Discussion of Available Options

Once the patient has made up her mind for termination of pregnancy, now it is a responsibility of clinical personnel to discuss the range of therapeutic options available to the patient after evaluating her for gestational age. Patient-friendly language in simple words should be used throughout discussion. Avoid using medical jargon. Information should be sufficient enough to explain the benefits and risks of intended procedures and the alternative management strategies. Medical abortion may be a preferred option in cases of obese women, those with fibroids or uterine malformations, and those with cardiovascular risk factors making surgery risky. Information should be provided in a noncoercive and unbiased manner.

Diagrams, posters, flip books, booklets, and information leaflets can be used for better understanding. This step is foremost in providing a women-centric approach to abortion care. She should be allowed to ask questions and to make the decision best for her. If she requires time or wants to involve her partner or any family member, she should be given adequate opportunity to do so.

Other points of paramount importance in discussion should be care after abortion and support available at home. It should be undoubtedly explained that if termination is done safely in accordance with guidelines, this will not affect her future fertility. The immediate risk of pregnancy, if no contraceptive method is used, as fertility can return as early as 10 days after the first trimester abortion and within 4 weeks after a second trimester abortion, also needs to be highlighted.

Step 3: Obtaining Consent

The consent is said to be valid if it is fully informed, voluntary, and unbiased. The person signing consent should be able to take the required information and should be able to analyze it in her context and communicate back her decision. The process of shared understanding and decision-making between the patient and clinician must be followed diligently and firmly. The risks of the proposed procedure and the likelihood of complications should be presented in a fashion that the patient is able to understand.

The consent document should cover the nature of the procedure concerned, risks, benefits, and alternatives, along with a record of fears or concerns raised by her.

Step 4: Discussion about Safe and Effective Future Contraception

The clinician should take this valuable opportunity to discuss the various contraceptive methods suitable for her after evaluating her clinically. Benefits of methods should be explained in detail. If she is not ready to decide about the contraceptive method, she should not be denied termination, as she is likely to go to get her abortion done in an unsafe way. This information should be clearly conveyed to her. Another counseling effort can be carried out at the time of postprocedure follow-up **(Table 2)**. All contraceptive methods including long-acting contraceptive methods and sterilization can be safely prescribed immediately with first-trimester abortions. The continuation rate for postabortion insertion of intrauterine contraceptive device (IUCD) is good. Insertion of IUCD immediately after the first/second-trimester abortions is not associated with a higher risk of expulsion, infection, or bleeding.

TABLE 2: Counseling for postprocedure choice of contraception.

Contraception method	*Use after medical termination*	*Use after surgical termination*
Barrier methods	As soon as she is sexually active	As soon as she is sexually active
Cu IUCD	Inserted after day 15 of the process after ensuring complete expulsion and risk or presence of infection or any other contraindication is ruled out	Can be inserted immediately after the surgical method
Combined oral contraceptives (COCs)	Can be safely started immediately at any time after misoprostol administration	Immediately at any time after surgical evacuation
Long-term injectables: MPA (medroxyprogesterone acetate)	It can be started on day 3 with the dose of misoprostol.	Immediately after surgical procedure
Progesterone-only pills (POPs)	Can be started on day 3 with the dose of misoprostol	Immediately after surgical termination
Female sterilization	Can be done only after the first menstrual cycle	Can be performed after an abortion in the absence of any infection or severe blood loss, concurrently (both minilaparotomy and laparoscopic sterilization can be done)

(IUCD: intrauterine contraceptive device)

Counseling in Special Circumstances

- *Woman is silent or crying or anxious:* Sympathetic attitude and acknowledging her reactions to be normal are the key to rewarding session in these patients. Women's concerns usually revolve around one of two broad issues—either apprehension about her condition or anxiety about the medical care. In such circumstances, it is always good to explore first her beliefs and concerns after building confidence and then proceed with counseling.
- *Woman wants clinician to take decision for her:* Instill confidence in her. Confirm if she still has any concerns, she needs time, or she wants to discuss with her husband or family. Reassure her that you are here to provide her the best of information but she is the best judge for herself. Final decision should be taken by her.
- *Woman is illiterate:* Illiteracy does not make her incapable of taking her decisions. Use pictures, posters, flip books, etc., to make her understand the required information. Patient-friendly language can be used to deliver clear message.
- *Counseling adolescent girls:* This can be a tricky situation, needs a lot of sympathy, reassurance of confidentiality, and involvement of her family members with her consent. These young patients are more prone to emotional trauma so they need special attention. Consent from parent or guardian is required, but these girls should be included in discussions and shared decision-making.

EVALUATION OF PATIENT

The first step in providing termination of pregnancy care is to establish that the woman is indeed pregnant and, if so, to estimate the duration of the pregnancy and confirm that the pregnancy is intrauterine. The risks associated with the termination, though small when the procedure is properly performed, increase with the duration of pregnancy. Determination of the length of pregnancy is a critical factor in selecting the most appropriate abortion method, which determines the content of the information and counseling to be given to women prior to abortion. History-taking and clinical examination are the mainstay of authentic clinical examination.

Objectives of clinical evaluation are:
- Confirmation of pregnancy
- Assess period of gestation
- Exclude ectopic pregnancy
- To assess any associated risk factors pertaining to women's health
- To assess any associated medical disorders

Components of clinical assessment:
- History-taking
- Physical examination including general as well as systemic
- Abdominal examination
- Pelvic examination including speculum examination and bimanual examination
- Laboratory investigations

History

Information gathering must follow the following sequence:
- *Personal details*: Age, marital status, address, and occupation details. This information familiarizes the clinician with the patient and gives a fair idea of lifestyle of patient. Knowledge of basic information is useful in planning your counseling session well.
- *Menstrual history and date of last menstruation*: Most women begin to suspect that they are pregnant when their expected menstrual period does not occur. The woman should be asked about the 1st day of her last

menstrual period (LMP), i.e., the first day of bleeding and whether the menstruation was normal, as well as about her menstrual history, including the regularity of her cycles. Women may experience amenorrhea for reasons other than pregnancy. On the contrary, some women may experience nonmenstrual bleeding in early pregnancy, and this can be a cause of missing or misdating pregnancy. Other scenarios where women may not be sure of her dates include examples such as women who are breastfeeding may become pregnant before their first postpartum menses and women who are amenorrheic while using injectable hormonal contraception may become pregnant after missing an injection. So, a clear understanding of menstrual history goes a long way in discussing management options with her. Also, history of any self-treatment is important to prevent further complications.

- *Obstetric history:* Her parity, live births, miscarriages, details of previous pregnancy terminations (induced and spontaneous), previous cesarean section (if any), last child birth/abortion, and future fertility concerns. Information acquired plays an important role in defining her contraception counseling.
- *Sexual health and contraception history:* History of any previous or present sexually transmitted infections in herself or her partner and history of previous contraceptive usage are two most significant points in this context. This session can be utilized as an opportunity to discuss safe sex practices.
- *Medical history:* Clinical history taking should serve to identify contraindications to medical or surgical abortion methods and to identify risk factors for complications of treatment. History of bleeding disorders, hypertension, heart disease, diabetes mellitus, epilepsy, asthma, renal disease, and thyroid disease should be specifically noticed. These conditions are not contraindications to termination per se; rather they require specific considerations and precautions. Optimization of the medical disorder and follow-up with a concerned specialist is important. Anemia is a very common condition in our health scenario and if not looked upon aggressively, it might lead to many folds increasing risk of complications. Hypertension and thyroid medications should be administered on the day of surgery if surgical termination is planned.
- *Drug allergy history:* Any positive drug history should be well documented and highlighted on the case notes. Details of the severity of allergic reaction to be elicited.
- *Family support:* Risk assessment for violence or coercion is an indispensable part of history-taking. The healthcare provider must be alert to the possibility of violence or coercion, particularly in the context of unintended pregnancy.
- *Mental health:* Mental health issues such as anxiety and depression can also be manifested at these times and should be addressed appropriately by counseling or, if needed, expert advice.
- *Status of tetanus immunization:* If already done, when was the last dose given. If it was done 6 months before, it should be repeated as a part of preprocedure preparation.

Physical Examination

- *General examination:* Check pulse, blood pressure, and temperature to know about the general well-being of women. Look for pallor/icterus/cyanosis.
- *Systemic examination:* Examination of chest and cardiovascular system
- *Abdominal examination:* A thorough inspection to look for any distension generalized or localized, color of skin, surgical scar marks, or evidence of abdominal masses. Inspection should be followed by palpation to palpate any lump or mass, look for guarding and rigidity, and elicit rebound tenderness.
- *Pelvic examination:* A skilled and gentle pelvic examination is a necessary and important part of evaluation. Verbal consent should be obtained prior to all pelvic examinations. Always instruct the patient to void before examination.
- *Speculum examination:* Inspect the vaginal walls and the cervix for any ulcer, foul-smelling discharge, and bleeding. The presence of infection in the lower reproductive tract at the time of abortion is a risk factor for postsurgical sepsis. In such cases, appropriate antibiotics should be prescribed.
- *Bimanual examination:* Signs of pregnancy that are detectable during a bimanual pelvic examination as early as 6–8 weeks of gestation include softening of the cervical isthmus and softening and enlargement of the uterus. A pregnant woman's uterus that is smaller than expected could be due to:
    - A pregnancy that is less advanced than estimated from the date of the LMP
    - An ectopic pregnancy
    - A missed abortion
    - Incomplete abortion

  A uterus that is larger than expected may indicate:
    - A pregnancy that is more advanced than calculated from the date of the LMP
    - A multiple pregnancy
    - A full bladder
    - The presence of uterine fibroids or other pelvic tumors. Usually firm in consistency.
    - A molar pregnancy.

During the vaginal examination, the clinician should also assess whether the uterus is anteverted, retroverted, or otherwise positioned in a way that might affect assessment of the gestational age or complicate a surgical abortion. Tenderness on cervical movement is indicative of ectopic pregnancy while fullness or tenderness in the fornices is indicative of pelvic inflammatory disease (PID) or ectopic pregnancy.

Laboratory Testing

- Measuring hemoglobin to detect anemia is useful, particularly in cases where the clinical features of anemia are there.
- Tests for Rhesus (Rh) blood group typing should be provided to administer Rh-immunoglobulin when indicated.
- Laboratory testing for pregnancy using highly sensitive urine pregnancy test kits.
- Urine dipstick for albumin and sugar rules out chronic medical ailments.
- In case of existing infections, samples should be taken for culture for a final diagnosis of the type of infection.
- *Role of ultrasound scanning:* Ultrasound scanning is not routinely required for the provision of termination of pregnancy. A scan can help to identify an intrauterine pregnancy and exclude an ectopic one from 6 weeks of gestation. It may also help to determine gestational age, for dating a pregnancy with irregular cycles, lactation amenorrhea, clinical discrepancy or uncertainty in examination, diagnose pathologies, or nonviability of a pregnancy.

It is worth closing the counseling session by summarizing the whole discussion, reiterating the plan of management and ensuring that the woman not only understands the planned care but is also able to take a safe decision for herself and that she has been given ample opportunities to explore her concerns.

KEY MESSAGES

- Counseling and evaluation are the important tools for women-centered approach for safe and legal pregnancy termination.
- Key principles of effective counseling include active listening, confidentiality, empathy and respect, appropriate unbiased information gathering, and open discussion and shared decision.
- The ability to take a structured and focused history is the key and fundamental clinical skill and aids the clinician to establish the best option for patient.
- Thoroughly performed clinical assessment is imperative along with history to make appropriate decisions.
- No patient should be denied termination if eligible as it can have a huge negative impact on a woman's life and also can divert her to adopt illegal and unsafe methods.

REFERENCES

1. Ministry of Health and Family Welfare, Government of India. (2018). Comprehensive Abortion Care Training and Service Delivery Guidelines, 2nd edition. [online] Available from: https://nhm.gov.in/New_Updates_2018/NHM_Components/RMNCHA/MH/Guidelines/CAC_Training_and_Service_Delivery_Guideline.pdf. [Last accessed November, 2021].
2. Tank J, Maheshwari B. The Medical Termination of Pregnancy (MTP) Act, 1971: Overview and Reporting Requirements. New Delhi: Ministry of Health & Family Welfare; 2019.
3. Malhotra J, Patel MC, Goel RN, Malhotra N. (2018). FOGSI FOCUS Medico legal Issues in Obstetrics and Gynecology Practice. [online] Available from: https://www.fogsi.org/wp-content/uploads/fogsi-focus/FOGSI-FOCUS-Medicolegal-2018.pdf. [Last accessed November, 2021].
4. Royal College of Obstetrician and Gynecologist. (2002). Gynaecological Examinations: Guidelines for Specialist Practice. [online] Available from: https://elearning.rcog.org.uk/sites/default/files/Communication%20skills/rcog_gynaeexams4.pdf. [Last accessed November, 2021].
5. WHO. (2012). Safe abortion: technical and policy guidance for health systems, 2nd edition. [online] Available from: https://www.who.int/reproductivehealth/publications/unsafe_abortion/9789241548434/en/. [Last accessed November, 2021].
6. Baron C, Cameron S. Do women seeking termination of pregnancy need pre-abortion counseling? J Fam Plann Reprod Health Care. 2015;41(3):181-5.
7. United Kingdom National Health Service. Counseling Skills for Medical Termination of Pregnancy. [online] Available from: https://www.nlg.nhs.uk/content/uploads/2014/01/pub-Co-sk-MedTermPreg.pdf. [Last accessed November, 2021].
8. Ministry of Health & Family Welfare, Government of India. (2015). Ensuring access to safe abortion and addressing gender biased sex selection. [online] Available from: https://www.fogsi.org/wp-content/uploads/2015/12/mtp-guidance-handbook.pdf. [Last accessed November, 2021].
9. Faculty of Sexual and Reproductive Healthcare. (2017). New FSRH Guideline - Contraception After Pregnancy. [online] Available from: https://www.fsrh.org/documents/contraception-after-pregnancy-guideline-january-2017/#:~:text=A%20woman%27s%20chosen%20method%20of,and%20she%20is%20medically%20eligible.&text=Women%20should%20be%20advised%20that,be%20inserted%20immediately%20after%20delivery. [Last accessed November, 2021].
10. Paul M, Danielsson KG, Essén B, Allvin MK. The importance of considering the evidence in the MTP 2014 Amendment debate in India - unsubstantiated arguments should not impede improved access to safe abortion. Glob Health Action. 2015;8:10.3402/gha.v8.27512.

LONG QUESTIONS

1. Critically appraise the methods of contraception you may offer a 21-year-old woman requesting for termination of pregnancy at 11 weeks' gestation.
2. Discuss the step-by-step approach of counseling in context to a 22-year-old woman asking for termination of pregnancy at 7 weeks. She is primigravida and got married 1 year back.

SHORT QUESTIONS

1. Mrs A wishes to have a termination of pregnancy. She has read that this can be done either surgically or medically. How will you counsel her about the surgical and medical options?
2. Mrs B requests for termination of pregnancy. During the counseling session, you gathered that her date of LMP is

7 weeks back. You examined her clinically and find that uterine size is 10 weeks. How will you proceed further?

3. A newlywed couple, woman 20 years of age, is requesting for termination of pregnancy at 6 weeks' gestation. When you start taking history, you feel that she is not actively participating and not sure of her decision. What important points you will keep in mind while counseling her?

MULTIPLE CHOICE QUESTIONS

1. The key elements of women-centered approach for termination of pregnancy include:
   a. Decision making by women
   b. Addressing her concerns
   c. Accessibility of services
   d. Quality care
   e. All of the above
2. Principles of good counseling session include all, except:
   a. Patient and active listening
   b. Confidentiality
   c. Empathy and respect
   d. Appropriate biased information
   e. Open discussion and shared decision
3. What is not mandatory in preprocedure evaluation for termination of pregnancy?
   a. Information gathering
   b. General physical examination
   c. Hemoglobin estimation
   d. Blood group determination
   e. Ultrasound
4. All are the components of good communication skills, except:
   a. Sympathetic approach
   b. Easy and patient friendly language
   c. Judging her statements as right and wrong
   d. Allowing her to make her decision
   e. Gathering information in detail
5. A 17-year-old patient is requesting you termination of 7 weeks' pregnancy. How will you proceed?
   a. Refuse termination as she is <18 years
   b. Proceed with termination as she can sign her consent form
   c. Refer her to medical board
   d. Inform legal authorities and refuse her MTP
   e. Counsel her for methods available and answer her concerns but for consent, her parents or guardian signatures are needed
6. Which is not an important prerequisite for pelvic examination?
   a. Verbal consent
   b. Full bladder
   c. Adequate provision of light
   d. Privacy
   e. Warm and comfortable room
7. Objectives of clinical evaluation include all, except:
   a. Confirmation of pregnancy
   b. Assess period of gestation
   c. Exclude ectopic pregnancy
   d. To assess any associated risk factors pertaining to women's health
   e. To assess her likelihood of future conception
8. You are examining a patient who by date is 10 weeks' pregnant. But on your clinical evaluation, you find uterine size to be 6 weeks. She has a 28-day regular cycle and is sure of her dates. What could be the probable cause for this?
   a. Molar pregnancy
   b. Full bladder
   c. Missed miscarriage
   d. Fibroid
   e. Pregnancy with oligohydramnios
9. All are features of proper history-taking, except:
   a. Eye-to-eye contact
   b. Closed questions
   c. Structured pattern
   d. Welcoming postures
   e. Relevant and logical questions
10. You are counseling a woman regarding post-termination contraception counseling. She is 10 weeks' pregnant and opts for surgical option. She wants you to decide the best method for her. She does not want to get pregnant for the next 1 year. What would be your most appropriate advice for her?
    a. Best for her is Cu IUD
    b. Best for her is LNG IUD
    c. Best for her is combined hormonal pills
    d. Tell her to come after the next period
    e. Discuss the pros and cons with her of all suitable methods and encourage her to decide
11. Mrs XYZ, 40-year-old, third gravida, both previous vaginal deliveries, has come to you for termination of her 6 weeks' pregnancy. She is a known patient of hypertension and diabetes but noncompliant with medications. What would be the most appropriate next step?
    a. Tell her to take medications regularly and come after 15 days
    b. Refuse to do termination of pregnancy
    c. Refer her to a specialist concerned with her diseases and then proceed
    d. Tell her to continue pregnancy as termination is more risky for her health
    e. Call her husband or family members to discuss risk

Answers

1.	e	2.	d	3.	e	4.	c	5.	e	6.	b
7.	e	8.	c	9.	b	10.	e	11.	c		

3.2 CHOICES AND METHODS OF PROCEDURES IN PREGNANCY TERMINATION IN FIRST AND SECOND TRIMESTERS

Suma Natarajan, Gayathri V, Jayashree Natarajan

INTRODUCTION

Unsafe abortions contribute to a significant maternal mortality rate in developing countries in spite of liberalized abortion laws. Pregnancy due to contraception failure, chromosomal anomaly, medical disorders in a pregnant woman, and unintended pregnancy are the most common reasons for an abortion. 90% of them are first-trimester abortions. 80 million women worldwide go through abortion, and a significant proportion of these are unsafe.[1]

To make abortion safe and accessible to Indian woman, safe guidelines have been developed by the Federation of Obstetric and Gynaecological Societies of India (FOGSI), Indian College of Obstetricians and Gynaecologists (ICOG), and Government of India governing all aspects of termination of pregnancy.

It is essential to have thorough knowledge of the evidence-based guidelines and choice of methods available for termination of pregnancy.

PREABORTION WORKUP AND INVESTIGATIONS

Comprehensive History

- Last menstrual period (LMP) for pregnancy dating
- Obstetric history
- Medical history.

Physical Examination

- General examination
- Systemic examination
- Pelvic examination.

Investigations

- Hemoglobin
- Blood group and Rh typing
- Urine for sugar and protein
- Viral markers (HIV, HBsAg, and HCV) for surgical procedures as per institution protocols.

Role of Ultrasound: Not Mandatory

- Indicated for dating pregnancy with irregular cycles
- During lactational amenorrhea
- Clinical discrepancy or uncertainty in examination
- Exclude ectopic gestation.

Consent

Form C of the medical termination of pregnancy (MTP) regulations is to be filled for medical and surgical abortions.

Counseling

- Regarding advantages, drawbacks, risks, limitations of MTP, and contraception
- Injection anti-D prophylaxis for Rh-negative women.

Antibiotics

- Not mandatory for medical methods of abortion (MMA)
- Beneficial in nullipara, active vaginal infections, and high-risk situations[2]
- As appropriate for all surgical methods.

Analgesics

First-trimester termination: Non-narcotic analgesics.

Second-trimester termination:
- Anxiolytics, such as diazepam
- *Parenteral sedation*: Pethidine (meperidine) 50 mg
- General anesthesia, if necessary.

SPECIFIC COUNSELING FOR MEDICAL METHODS OF ABORTION (FIRST TRIMESTER)

At least two to three visits to hospital or clinic are required. Misoprostol may be given for home administration. Explain symptoms likely to be experienced, such as bleeding per vaginum (often lasts for 8–13 days), abdominal pain, nausea, vomiting, and diarrhea, which are minor side effects, and contact healthcare facility, if there is an emergency.[3] The possibility of surgical evacuation in case of failure or excessive bleeding should be counseled. Explain regarding delay of the next menstrual cycle by 1–2 weeks. Use of a contraceptive method (such as condoms) if intercourse is done during treatment and all postabortion contraceptive options should be discussed.

CHOICES OF METHODS IN TERMINATION OF PREGNANCY

- Medical
- Surgical

Medical Methods of Abortion

- Safe, effective, noninvasive, and have minimal complications
- *High rate of efficacy in early pregnancy:* 95–99%
- Does not require anesthesia or prophylactic antibiotics
- Should have access to a center where surgical methods are available in the event of complications.

Drugs for MMA

- Mifepristone
- *Mifepristone and misoprostol (PGE1)*: Most popular combination
- Methotrexate and misoprostol
- Tamoxifen and misoprostol.

Pharmacology of Drugs used in Medical Abortion

Mifepristone (RU486): Antiprogestin[4]

Pharmacodynamics: It is considered as progesterone receptor modulator (PRM):

- Acts by promoting decidual degeneration
- Release of prostaglandins
- Induces uterine contraction
- Softens the cervix.

Pharmacokinetics: Absorption: Rapidly absorbed and peak plasma concentration attained 90 minutes after ingestion. It is metabolized in liver.

Contraindications:

- History of allergy/hypersensitivity to mifepristone and misoprostol
- Confirmed or suspected ectopic pregnancy or undiagnosed adnexal mass
- Chronic adrenal failure
- Hemorrhagic disorders or concurrent anticoagulant therapy
- Inherited porphyrias.

Drug interactions:

- Ketoconazole, itraconazole, and erythromycin may inhibit metabolism of mifepristone.
- Rifampicin, dexamethasone, and some anticonvulsants may induce metabolism of mifepristone.

Misoprostol (PGE1): It is a synthetic methyl analog of prostaglandin E1.

Pharmacodynamics:

- By interacting with C receptors on myometrial cells, PGE1 decreases cyclic adenosine monophosphate (AMP) [mediated by gastrointestinal (GI) pathway], induces changes in intracellular calcium, and causes myometrial contraction.
- Results in cervical softening and uterine contractions, thus causing expulsion of uterine contents.

Pharmacokinetics: Extensively absorbed, undergoes rapid de-esterification and gets readily metabolized to free acid which is a biologically active form.

Action on uterus: The effect of misoprostol on uterine contractility has been well studied by mean time to increase tonus, which is 8, 11, 20, and 103 minutes for oral, sublingual, vaginal, and rectal administration, respectively **(Table 1)**.

Action on cervix: Misoprostol causes cervical ripening by:

- Decreasing total collagen content
- Increasing collagen solubility.

Adverse effects:

- Gastrointestinal side effects such as diarrhea, abdominal pain, nausea, flatulence, dyspepsia, and vomiting
- Shivering and hyperthermia.

Teratogenicity: Along with mifepristone causes *sirenomelia*[6] which involves complete or partial fusion of the lower limb, renal agenesis, ambiguous genitalia, imperforate anus, and blind intestinal loop. Misoprostol is associated with *Moebius syndrome* which is a type of congenital facial paralysis.

Contraindications:

- Hypersensitivity to misoprostol
- Co-administration of misoprostol + mifepristone contraindicated in suspected ectopic
- Hemorrhagic disorder or concomitant anticoagulant therapy
- Inherited porphyrias.

Medical Methods: First-trimester Protocols

Medical methods can only be administered by a gynecologist or Registered Medical Practitioner (RMP) recognized for performing MTPs (MTP Act, 1971).[7]

- *Mifepristone alone: Effectiveness*: Only 80%
- *Regime of mifepristone and misoprostol* ***(Table 2)***:

All guidelines recognize the effectiveness and safety of combining mifepristone and misoprostol for inducing abortion up to 63 days.[8-10]

In India, the following is approved for use by the Drug Controller of India:

- *Regime up to 49 days of gestation*:
  - *Day 1*: Mifepristone 200 mg orally
  - Injection anti-D prophylaxis to Rh-negative women
  - *Day 3*: Misoprostol 400 µg vaginally or orally
  - *Day 15*: Follow-up visit to assess for completion of abortion.

TABLE 1: Effectiveness of misoprostol administered by different routes.[5]

Route of administration	*Onset of action*	*Duration of action*	*Recommended route*
Sublingual	Fastest	Highest plasma levels and prolonged action	Most recommended
Buccal	Quick	Prolonged action	Recommended
Vaginal	Quick	Prolonged action	Recommended
Oral	Quick	Least duration	Least recommended

TABLE 2: Regimen for 1st trimester MTP using medical methods.

Visit	Day	Drugs used
First	One	• One 200 mg mifepristone oral • Anti-D 50 μg, if Rh negative (give 300 μg if 50 μg not available)
Second	Three	• 400 μg misoprostol (two tablets of 200 μg each) sublingual/buccal/vaginal/oral—up to 49 days[11] • Misoprostol 800 μg vaginal or sublingual or buccal—from 49 to 63 days[12] • Analgesics • Antiemetic • Offer contraception
Third	Fifteen	• Confirm and ensure completion of abortion • Offer contraception

- *Regime from 49 to 63 days of gestation*:
  - *Day 1*: Mifepristone 200 mg orally
  - Injection anti-D prophylaxis to Rh-negative women
  - *Day 3*: Misoprostol 800 μg vaginally or orally
  - *Day 15*: Follow-up visit to assess for completion of abortion.

Surgical termination is recommended if a viable pregnancy is detected at follow-up.

Very Early Medical Abortion

Very early medical abortion (VEMA) is done at gestation of <6 weeks that is too early for an intrauterine gestation to be visible in an USG.

Protocol

- Estimation of serum β-human chorionic gonadotropin (β-hCG) levels followed by mifepristone and misoprostol combination. Repeat serum β-hCG after 10 days.
- Higher than expected baseline hCG or no characteristic fall of hCG associated with medical abortion indicates a possible asymptomatic ectopic pregnancy at a very early gestational age. VEMA management may potentially detect an asymptomatic ectopic pregnancy.[13]

Medical Methods: Second Trimester

About 9–11% of all induced abortions occur in the second trimester. These abortions are responsible for two-thirds of all major complications.[14]

To avoid these, it is essential that second-trimester abortions are performed as per the criteria laid down in the MTP Act and Rules, following the appropriate method and taking all necessary precautions.

Medical methods

- Mifepristone and misoprostol regime
- Misoprostol alone regime
- Miscellaneous:
  - Hypertonic saline (20%)
  - Hyperosmolar urea (40%) injected intra-amniotically
  - Ethacridine administered extra-amniotically
  - Prostaglandin analogs administered parenterally or intra- or extra-amniotically
  - Oxytocin injected intravenously.

These methods and routes are invasive and available data regarding safety are limited.

Time to complete abortion is longer when compared to medical methods (WHO, 2012).[15]

Use of mifepristone and misoprostol for second-trimester terminations is not yet approved in India.

However, WHO and international evidences recommend VEMA as being a safe and effective method.[16]

WHO Recommended Protocol

Medical methods in second-trimester termination involve two steps:

1. Cervical priming
2. Inducing uterine contraction

- *Misoprostol (PGE1 analog)*:
  - Used for cervical priming and inducing uterine contractions
  - Less effective (75–90%)
  - Drug protocol 400 μg misoprostol, vaginal or sublingual, every 3 hours, up to five doses (WHO, 2014)
  - The mean induction–abortion interval is 11–12 hours.
- *Misoprostol + mifepristone—drug protocol (WHO, 2014)*:
  - 200 mg oral mifepristone followed 36–48 hours later by 400 μg misoprostol oral followed by 400 μg misoprostol vaginal or sublingual every 3 hours, up to five doses (including the first dose)

    Or
  - 200 mg oral mifepristone followed 36–48 hours later by 800 μg misoprostol vaginal followed by 400 μg misoprostol vaginal or sublingual every 3 hours, up to five doses (including the first dose).[17]

  During the process, the placenta should be expelled within 2 hours of fetal expulsion.

  If placenta remains, one of the following options should be used:
- Sublingual/buccal/rectal misoprostol, 400 μg
- High-dose oxytocin regimen for 2 hours, such as 20 units in 500 mL normal saline, at 50 mL/h.[18]
- *Miscellaneous*:
  - *Dinoprostone PGE2 analog:*
    - 20 mg used as vaginal suppository every 3–4 hours (maximum for 4–6 doses)
    - When used along with osmotic dilators, the mean induction to abortion interval is 17 hours
  - *Prostaglandin F2 (PGF2α)*:
    - 250 μg IM every 3 hours for a maximum of 10 doses can be used
    - Success rate—90% in 36 hours
    - Side effects—nausea, vomiting, diarrhea, and pain at injection site
    - Contraindicated in bronchial asthma

- *Oxytocin*:
  - High-dose oxytocin as a single agent can be used for second-trimester abortion.
  - Effective in 80% of cases.
  - Can be used with intravenous normal saline along with any of the medications used by intra-amniotic or extra-amniotic route in an attempt to augment the abortion process.
- *Mode of action of oxytocin*:
  - Myometrial oxytocin receptor concentration increases maximum (100–200-fold) during labor.
  - Oxytocin acts through receptor and voltage-mediated calcium channels to initiate myometrial contractions.
- *Extra-amniotic ethacridine instillation supplemented by oxytocin*:
  - Stimulates amniotic and decidual prostaglandin production
  - Commonly used method
  - When instilled extra-amniotically, it has a direct oxytocic effect on the myometrium.
  - It causes separation of membranes, which releases prostaglandins, leading to uterine contractions.
  - Ethacridine is currently not easily available.

Surgical Methods: First Trimester

Menstrual Regulation

Aspiration of the endometrial cavity can be done within 14 days of missed period in a woman with a previous normal cycle. It is done as an outpatient procedure with aseptic precautions. Sedation or paracervical block anesthesia may or may not be employed. Antibiotics are not mandatory.

Procedure ***(Fig. 1)***:

- After introducing posterior vaginal speculum, cervix is steadied with Allis forceps.
- Cervix may be gently dilated using 4- or 5-mm size dilators.
- About 5–6 mm suction cannula (Karman's) is inserted and attached to a 50 mL syringe for suction and rotated, pushed in and out with gentle strokes.
- Examine aspirated tissue by floating it in a clear plastic dish over a light source.
- Placental tissue appears fluffy and feathery when floating in normal saline.
- It helps to detect failed abortion, molar pregnancy, or ectopic pregnancy.

The procedure is contraindicated in advanced pregnancy and in the presence of local pelvic inflammation.

Vacuum Aspiration (MVA/EVA) (Figs. 2 and 3)

Various studies demonstrated vacuum aspiration as very safe and effective technique. It is successful in 98% of cases.[19]

A joint recommendation by the WHO and FIGO states that the efficacy and safety of vacuum aspiration are superior to conventional dilatation and curettage (D and C). Therefore, hospitals should abandon D and C and adopt aspiration methods.[20]

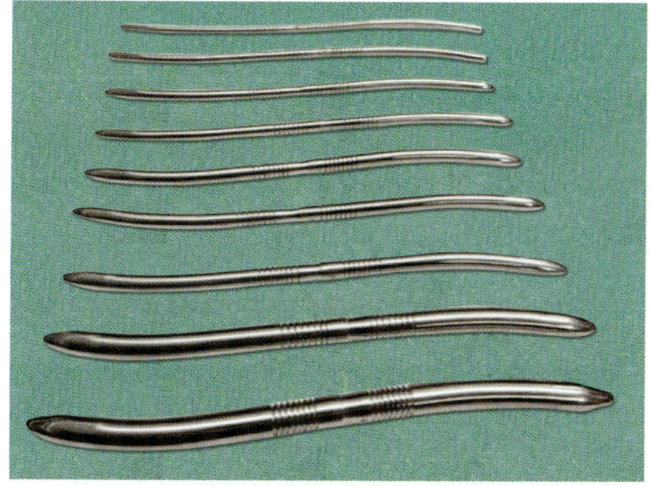

Fig. 2: Metallic hegar cervical dilators.

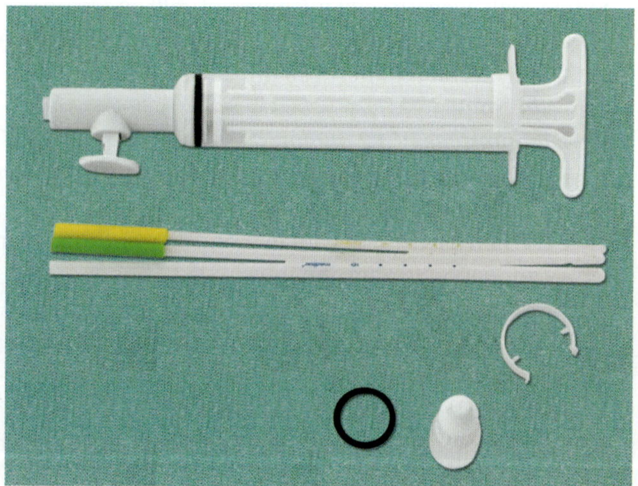

Fig. 1: Manual vaccum aspiration apparatus (MVA syringe and canulae).

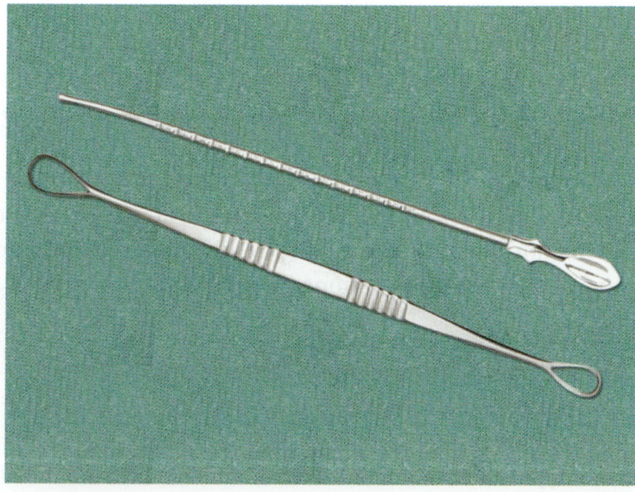

Fig. 3: Uterine sound and uterine/endometrial curette.

TABLE 3: Features of the two types of manual vacuum aspiration (MVA) equipment.

Features	*DV aspirator*	*SV aspirator*
Capacity	60 cc	50 cc
Negative pressure	26 in/660 mm Hg	26 in/660 mm Hg
Cannula size used	Up to 12 mm	Up to 6 mm

Rates of major complications are two to three times lesser than with D and C.

Vacuum aspiration can be either manual (MVA) or electrical (EVA) **(Table 3)**.

- MVA uses a handheld, portable aspirator.
- EVA employs an electricity-operated device.

Disposable, single-use cannula (Karman) or autoclavable, reusable cannula (easy grip), single or double valve, is used for MVA.

Vacuum aspiration is done up to 12 weeks with minimal cervical dilatation. It is performed as an outpatient or inpatient procedure. It is quicker (15 minutes), effective (98–100%), less traumatic, and safer than D and C.

Procedure

- Hand-operated double-valve plastic syringe is attached to a cannula.
- Cannula is inserted transcervically into the uterus and vacuum is activated.
- A negative pressure of 600 mm Hg is created.
- Aspiration of products of conception is done.

Electric Vacuum Aspiration

It is a procedure in which the products of conception are sucked out from the uterus with the help of a cannula fitted to a suction apparatus.

Preliminaries:

- Cervix dilatation—with the help of metal Hegar dilators or osmotic dilators (laminaria tents 10–12 hours before) or vaginal misoprostol 400 µg 6 hours before
- Paracervical block, sedation
- Spinal or general anesthesia.

The patient is put on the table after she empties her bladder.

Steps

- Vaginal examination is done to note the size and position of uterus and the state of cervix.
- Posterior vaginal speculum introduced and the anterior lip of the cervix is to be grasped by an Allis forceps.
- Uterine sound is to be introduced to note the length of the uterine cavity and position of the uterus.
- The cervix may have to be dilated with smaller size graduated metal dilators up to one size less than that of the suction cannula. Feeling of "snap" of the endocervix around the dilator is characteristic. Instead, laminaria tent 12 hours before (osmotic dilator) or misoprostol (PGE1) 400 µg given vaginally 3 hours prior to surgery produces effective dilatation.
- Appropriate suction cannula is fitted to suction apparatus by a thick rubber or plastic tubing. The cannula is then introduced into the uterus and the tip is to be placed in the middle of the uterine cavity.
- The pressure of the suction is raised to 400–600 mm Hg. The cannula is moved up and down and rotated within the uterine cavity (360°) with the pressure on. The suction bottle is inspected for the products of conception and blood loss. The suction is regulated by a finger placed over a hole at the base of the cannula.
- Oxytocin 5 units IM is administered or intravenous methergine 0.2 mg while aspirating.
- If ultrasound facilities are available, these can be performed under ultrasound guidance to avoid complications.
- The endpoint of suction is denoted by:
  - No more material is being sucked out
  - Gripping of the cannula by the contracting smaller sized uterus
  - Grating sensation
  - Appearance of bubbles in the cannula or in the transparent tubing.
- The vacuum should be broken before withdrawing the cannula down through the cervical canal to prevent injury to the internal os.
- It is better to curette the uterine cavity by a small flushing curette at the end of suction and the cannula is reintroduced to suck out any remnants.
- After being satisfied that the uterus is remaining firm, and there is minimal vaginal bleeding, the patient is brought down from the table after placing a sterile vulval pad.

Complications

- *Excessive hemorrhage:* May be due to incomplete evacuation or atonic uterus
- *Injury:* Cervical lacerations or uterine perforation
- Shock due to local anesthesia, excessive blood loss, or vasovagal syncope due to cervical stimulation
- *Perforation:* Injury to major blood vessels, bowel, or bladder
- *Sepsis:* Endometritis, myometritis, and pelvic peritonitis
- Hematometra
- Continuation of pregnancy (failure)—1%.

Dilatation and Evacuation (D + E)

The procedure consists of dilatation of the cervix and evacuation of products of conception from the uterine cavity with ovum forceps. With the recent advance of safe medical methods, the above procedure is rarely used.

Surgical Methods: Second Trimester

It is difficult to terminate pregnancy in second trimester **(Box 1)** with reasonable safety as in first trimester. In all

BOX 1: Complications of surgical methods of second-trimester medical termination of pregnancy.

- Cervical laceration
- Uterine perforation
- Hemorrhage
- Infection
- Incomplete abortion

Late sequelae:
- *Due to cervical lacerations:*
  - Recurrent abortions
  - Preterm labor
- *Due to infection*:
  - Infertility due to tubal block
  - Ectopic pregnancy
  - Chronic pelvic pain
- *Psychological*

Depression
Anxiety
Feeling of guilt

mid-trimester abortion, cervical preparation must be used (WHO, 1997) to make the process easy and safe. Cervical priming agents are used to reduce cervical injuries and uterine perforation.[20]

When facilities are available, the procedure can be performed under ultrasound guidance to reduce the risk of complications. Simultaneous use of oxytocin infusion is useful between 16 and 20 weeks to augment the procedure.

Surgical methods
- Dilatation and evacuation
- Hysterotomy

Dilatation and evacuation: It is a safe and effective surgical technique for abortions beyond 12–14 weeks where skilled, experienced providers are available. With the availability of medical methods, it is less commonly used in India and requires special training.

D and E is a two-step process:
1. Cervical preparation or dilatation
2. Evacuation of the uterus with a combination of suction and forceps

Cervical preparation/dilatation:
- Decreases the risk of cervical injury and uterine perforation
- Medication/devices/instruments used for cervical preparation and dilatation before evacuation of the POCs:
  - Misoprostol
  - Osmotic dilators

A. Misoprostol: 400 μg is used vaginally 3–4 hours or sublingually 2–3 hours before procedure for cervical dilatation. One additional dose of 400 μg may be given if dilatation is inadequate after 4 hours or dilators may be used.

Advantages:
- Highly effective for inducing cervical dilatation and uterine contractions
- Leads to contraction of uterus even before the actual procedure is initiated
- *Reduces:* Blood loss, possibility of perforation, and procedure time.

Disadvantage: GI side effects.

B. Osmotic dilators:
- Used to dilate the cervix before performing uterine evacuation
- These are made of hygroscopic materials, which swell up by absorbing cervical and vaginal secretions. They gradually dilate and soften the cervix and also stimulate uterine contractions. These require a minimum of 10–12 hours to be effective.

Advantage: Less incidence of cervical tears and hemorrhage since it induces gradual dilatation.

Disadvantages:
- Can lead to infection, particularly if introduced without proper aseptic care and left in the cervix for too long
- Not easily available.

Evacuation: After achieving the desired level of cervical dilatation, proceed with evacuation of uterine contents with 12–16 mm cannula and forceps. In the unlikely event that the fetus parts cannot be easily removed, administer additionally any one of the following uterotonic agents such as: 400–600 μg misoprostol orally or sublingually, injection of prostaglandin (PGF2α) 250 μg IM, injection of oxytocin 20 units in 500 mL normal saline or lactated Ringer's solution run at 50 mL/h.

INTRAUTERINE INSTILLATION OF HYPERTONIC SOLUTION

- Intra-amniotic
- Extra-amniotic

Intra-amniotic

Intra-amniotic instillation is less commonly used now. It is instilled through the abdominal route.[20]

Mode of Action

Liberation of prostaglandins takes place following necrosis of the amniotic epithelium and the decidua. This in turn excites uterine contraction and results in the expulsion of the fetus.

Procedure

Preliminary amniocentesis is done by a 15-cm 18-gauge needle. USG may be used for guiding the needle. The amount of saline to be instilled is calculated as the number of weeks of gestation multiplied by 10 mL. The amount is to be infused slowly at the rate of 10 mL/min or directly with a 20-mL syringe.

Contraindications

There is presence of cardiovascular or renal disease or severe anemia because of sodium load.

Precautions

It must be ensured that the needle is in the amniotic cavity evidenced by clear liquor coming out. If there is a bloody tap, the needle should be pushed further or the direction should be changed until clear liquor comes out. If it fails, the procedure is to be abandoned. Strict vigilance is taken during and following instillation till expulsion occurs. Routine antibiotic is given such as ampicillin 500 mg thrice daily for 3–5 days.

Success rate: 90–95% cases with an induction-abortion interval of 32 hours.

The procedure is considered to have failed when abortion does not occur within 48 hours.

Complications (Table 4)

- Minor complaints such as fever, headache, nausea, vomiting, and abdominal pain
- Cervical tear and laceration
- Retained products for which exploration has to be done
- Infection
- Hypernatremia, cardiovascular collapse—due to intravascular injection
- Pulmonary and cerebral edema
- Renal failure
- Disseminated intravascular coagulopathy
- Incidence of death rate varies from 0 to 5 per 1,000 instillations.

Instillation methods are not frequently used at present mainly because of the safe use of medical methods.[20]

Extra-amniotic

Extra-amniotic instillation using 0.1% ethacridine lactate is done. It is done transcervically through a 16 size Foley's catheter.

Mode of Action

Stripping the membranes with liberation of prostaglandins from the decidua and dilatation of the cervix by the catheter are some of the known factors for initiation of the abortion.

TABLE 4: Complications of medical methods of termination in the second trimester and their management.

Complications	*Management*
• Incomplete abortion • Retained placenta	• Dilatation and curettage
• Uterine rupture	• Surgical intervention
• Cervical laceration	• Surgical intervention
• Infection	• Antibiotics
• Hemorrhage	• Oxytocics/blood transfusion • Exclude incomplete abortion

Procedure

- The catheter is passed up the cervical canal for about 10 cm above the internal os between the membranes and myometrium; the balloon is inflated (20 mL) with saline. It is removed after 4 hours. The success rate is similar to saline instillation but is less hazardous.
- It is used in cases contraindicated for saline instillation.
- Induction abortion interval of 24–36 hours can be shortened by vaginal misoprostol.

HYSTEROTOMY

- It is not a preferred method for pregnancy termination.
- It is an operative procedure done through the abdominal route for a previable fetus from the lower part of the uterus.

It is done in the following conditions:

- Failure with the other methods
- Other associated gynecological conditions
- Placenta occupying the internal os completely.

Complications (Table 4)

Immediate

- Hemorrhage and shock
- Anesthetic complications
- Peritonitis
- Intestinal obstruction.

Remote

- Menstrual abnormalities
- Scar endometriosis (1%)
- If pregnancy occurs, chance of scar rupture
- Incisional hernia.

Postprocedure Care

After a second-trimester abortion, a woman should remain in the healthcare facility for at least 4 hours.

KEY MESSAGES

- Unsafe abortion is one of the major contributors of MMR (maternal mortality rate).
- More than 6 million in India undergo abortions.
- Guidelines have been developed by the government of India, FOGSI, and ICOG governing all aspects of termination of pregnancy.
- Choice of procedure is important and depends on the gestational age.
- First-trimester procedures are very safe compared to second trimester.
- Medical method of choice—combination of mifepristone and misoprostol is the best method with a good success rate of 95–98% **(Table 5)**.
- Antibiotic prophylaxis is only for surgical methods.
- Rh-immunoprophylaxis is for Rh-negative women.
- Preabortion procedure preparation is required.

TABLE 5: Medical versus surgical methods of termination of pregnancy—first trimester.

Parameter	*Medical methods*	*Surgical methods*
Gestation limit of the technique	Used up to 7 weeks of pregnancy	Used up to 12 weeks of pregnancy
Hospitalization	Not required	Required except for MVA
Anesthesia	Not required	Required
Time taken for procedure completion	Completed within 4–6 hours Bleeding may continue up to 8–13 days	5–15 minutes
Number of visits	Two or more Misoprostol administration	Single
Duration	Days to weeks	Single visit
Success rate	95–98%	98–100%
Bleeding	Moderate	Mild
Follow-up	Required to ensure completion	Not routinely required

(MVA: manual vacuum aspiration)

- Manual and electronic vacuum aspirations are surgical methods of choice for first-trimester abortions.
- Second-trimester abortions are technically difficult with more complications.
- Combinations of mifepristone and misoprostol again have a high success rate with second-trimester abortion also.
- Extra-amniotic instillation of ethacridine lactate is a safe and effective procedure.
- Providing clear and concise knowledge of choice and methods of abortion with its related complications leads to safe abortions.

REFERENCES

1. World Health Organization. (2018). Global abortion policies database. [online] Available from: http://srhr.org/abortion-policies/. [Last accessed November, 2021].
2. FOGSI ICOG. Good Clinical Practice Recommendation Medical Termination of Pregnancy. 2011.
3. Kulier R, Kapp N, Gulmezoglu AM, Hofmeyr GJ, Cheng L, Campana A. Medical methods for first trimester abortion. Cochrane Database Syst Rev. 2011;(11):CD002855.
4. FOGSI-MTP Committee. (2010). FOGSI FOCUS on medical abortion. [online] Available from: http://www.fogsi.org/wp-content/uploads/fogsi-focus/medical+abortion+2011.pdf.
5. Nautiyal D, Mukherjee K, Perhar I, Banerjee N. Comparative study of misoprostol in first and second trimester abortions by oral, sublingual, and vaginal routes. J Obstet Gynaecol India. 2015;65(4):246-50.
6. Bagri DR, Bagri R, Gupta RK, Mathu P, Mittal R. Mermaid syndrome (sirenomelia): With use of mifepristone and misoprostol in early first trimester with failed medical abortion and continuing pregnancy in a multipara with bad obstetric history. Scholars Journal of Applied Medical Sciences, 2016; 4(5B):1574-6.
7. American College of Obstetrics and Gynaecologists. Practice bulletin No. 143: Medical management of first-trimester abortion. Obstet Gynaecol. 2014;123:676-92.
8. Abubeker FK, Kim CR, Lavelanet A. Medical termination of pregnancy in early first trimester (≤ 63 days): a systematic review. [Evidence synthesis for a WHO guideline]. 2018 (unpublished). BMC Womens Health. 2020;20:142.
9. Schaff EA, Fielding SL, Eisinger SH, Stadalius LS, Fuller L. Low-dose mifepristone followed by vaginal misoprostol at 48 hrs for abortion up to 63 days. Contraception. 2000;61:41-6.
10. Hamoda H, Ashok PW, Flett GM, Templeton A. A randomised controlled trial of mifepristone in combination with misoprostol administered sublingually or vaginally for medical abortion up to 13 weeks of gestation. BJOG. 2005;112:1102-8.
11. Raymond EG, Shannon C, Weaver MA, Winikoff B. First-trimester medical abortion with mifepristone 200 mg and misoprostol: a systematic review. Contraception. 2013;87:26-37.
12. Abbas D, Chong E, Raymond EG. Outpatient medical abortion is safe and effective through 70 days gestation. Contraception. 2015;92:197-9.
13. Cameron S. (2018). Recent advances in improving the effectiveness and reducing the complications of abortions. [online] Available from: https://www.ncbi.nlm.nih.gov/pmc/articles/PMC6281004/. [Last accessed November, 2021].
14. Wildschut H, Both MI, Medema S, Thomee E, Wildhagen MF, Kapp N. Medical methods for mid-trimester termination of pregnancy. Cochrane Database Syst Rev. 2011;(1):CD005216.
15. World Health Organization. Safe abortion: technical and policy guidance for health systems, 2nd edition. [online] Available from: http://www.who.int/reproductivehealth/publications/unsafe_abortion/9789241548434/en/. [Last accessed November, 2021].
16. Verma ML, Singh U, Singh N, Sankhwar PL, Qureshi S. Efficacy of concurrent administration of mifepristone and misoprostol for termination of pregnancy. Hum Fertil. 2017;20(1):43-7.
17. World Health Organization. (2014). Clinical practice handbook for safe abortion. Geneva: World Health Organization; 2014 [online] Available from: http://www.who.int/reproductivehealth/publications/unsafe_abortion/clinical-practice-safe-abortion/en/. [Last accessed November, 2021].
18. Lalitkumar S, Bygdeman M, Gemzell-Danielsson K. Mid-trimester induced abortion: a review. Hum Reprod Update. 2007;13(1):37-52.
19. Ashok PW, Kidd A, Flett GM, Fitzmaurice A, Graham W, Templeton A. A randomized comparison of medical abortion and surgical vacuum aspiration at 10–13 weeks gestation. Hum Reprod. 2002;17:92-8.
20. International Planned Parenthood Federation (IPPF). First trimester abortion guidelines and protocols, surgical and medical procedures. [online] Available from: https://www.ippf.org/sites/default/files/abortion_guidelines_and_protocol_english.pdf. [Last accessed November, 2021].

LONG QUESTIONS

1. Describe the different methods of abortions in the first trimester.
2. A 26-year-old 3rd gravida with two living children comes to the clinic with 4 months amenorrhea and requests for abortion. How would you counsel her and what methods would you choose?
3. What are the complications of induced abortions?

4. Briefly describe the medical and surgical method of second-trimester abortion.
5. What are complications and contraception after MMA?

SHORT QUESTIONS

1. A 28-year-old 2nd gravida comes to the clinic with 37 days' amenorrhea and pregnancy test positive and requests for abortion. What method will you advise her? Describe.
2. Briefly describe vacuum aspiration, indications, and complications.
3. What are the surgical methods of second trimester? Discuss its complications.
4. A 40-year-old, 2nd gravida, seeks abortion for 50 days' pregnancy. What is the preabortion work-up you would do?
5. Write briefly the pharmacokinetics of different routes of misoprostol.
6. A 22-year-old woman with 18 weeks' pregnancy diagnosed to have bilateral polycystic kidneys in the fetus with severe oligohydramnios. What would be your method of termination?

MULTIPLE CHOICE QUESTIONS

1. Uterine perforation is a complication of:
   a. Vacuum aspiration
   b. Extra-amniotic ethacridine lactate
   c. Medical abortion
   d. Intra-amniotic hypertonic saline
2. Dangerous complication of intra-amniotic hypertonic saline:
   a. Pulmonary edema
   b. Disseminated intravascular coagulation
   c. Infection
   d. Both a and b
3. Mifepristone is a:
   a. Prostaglandin b. Antiprogesterone
   c. Antibiotic d. Oxytocin
4. The best method of choice for second-trimester abortion is:
   a. Medical abortion
   b. Hypertonic saline intra-amniotic
   c. Hysterotomy
   d. PGE2 analog
5. What are the preferred methods for uterine evacuation in the first trimester of pregnancy according to the World Health Organization?
   a. Medical abortion only
   b. Sharp curettage
   c. Medical abortion and vacuum aspiration
   d. Intra- or extra-amniotic instillation
6. Effectiveness of medical methods of abortion for pregnancy up to 7 weeks is:
   a. 95–99% b. 80%
   c. 82–83% d. 70–80%
7. Which of the following are contraindications to MMA?
   a. Suspected ectopic pregnancy
   b. HIV/AIDS
   c. Breastfeeding
   d. Multiple pregnancy
8. Government of India's standard MMA drug protocol (for gestation up to 49 days) is:
   a. 600 mg misoprostol followed 2 days later by 400 μg mifepristone vaginal/sublingual
   b. 200 mg mifepristone orally followed 2 days later by 400 μg misoprostol sublingual/buccal/vaginal/oral
   c. 600 mg mifepristone orally followed 2 days later by 400 μg misoprostol oral/vaginal
   d. 200 mg misoprostol orally followed 2 days later by 800 μg mifepristone vaginal/buccal
9. Which of the following is the least effective route for misoprostol administration during the MMA process?
   a. Sublingual b. Vaginal
   c. Oral d. Buccal
10. After giving misoprostol, the woman should be called for follow-up on which day?
    a. 5th b. 15th
    c. 7th d. 10th
11. What are the symptoms suggestive of complications during MMA process?
    a. Excessive bleeding, soaking more than two thick pads per hour for two consecutive hours
    b. Fever any day after the day misoprostol is used
    c. Unusual or foul-smelling vaginal discharge
    d. All of the above
12. Possible complications with MMA include:
    a. Mild cramping
    b. Uterine perforation
    c. Continuation of pregnancy
    d. Injury to cervix and uterus
13. Documentation of the MMA procedure is done in the following formats:
    a. Form C b. RMP Opinion Form
    c. Admission register d. All of the above
14. Only way to manage an incomplete abortion during the process of MMA is:
    a. Vacuum aspiration
    b. Repeat dose of misoprostol
    c. Either of the two depending on the severity of bleeding
    d. Watch and wait
15. Which contraceptive method can be started on the day of taking misoprostol?
    a. Oral pills b. Tubectomy
    c. Vasectomy d. Condoms

Answers

1.	a	2.	d	3.	b	4.	a	5.	c	6.	a
7.	a	8.	b	9.	c	10.	b	11.	c	12.	c
13.	d	14.	c	15.	d						

3.3 DIFFICULT SITUATIONS IN PREGNANCY TERMINATION

Jaydeep Tank, Kunal Doshi

INTRODUCTION

Termination of pregnancy is a human need. This is a global truth. In India, it was estimated that 15.6 million abortions (14.1–17.3 million) occurred in 2015. Overall, 12.7 million (81%) abortions were medication abortions, 2.2 million (14%) abortions were surgical, and 0.8 million (5%) abortions were done through other methods that were probably unsafe.[1] With the procedure being done so commonly, it is obvious that some situations will pose challenges and could be classified as being difficult. The difficulty could arise from a variety of reasons as depicted in **Figure 1**. The woman may have a medical condition or a pelvic pathology, the pregnancy may be at an advanced gestational age, or there could be social, legal, or difficulties with access to care. These difficulties may occur together in clinical circumstances. For example, an unmarried minor may have had a sexual assault and now presents at an advanced gestational age for termination of pregnancy. Similarly, a technically challenging situation could be a woman who has an undiagnosed pelvic pathology and a failed termination attempt with complications who does not want to continue the pregnancy. These situations present multi-level decision-making and technical challenges to accomplish the termination safely within the legal framework.

MEDICAL CONDITIONS

For women who have medical conditions, ideally, chronic care programs should include effective contraceptive advice. However, this may not always be implemented or the method may fail, leading to a need for medical termination. Medical conditions which may pose difficulties to termination of pregnancy may be classified as in **Table 1**.

Pregnancy termination is safer when it is done earlier in gestation. This is true for the general population and is especially relevant to the woman who has a medical condition, especially one which affects her general systemic status. The hemodynamic changes are the least and it is possible to perform the procedure with medical methods. This avoids the need for anesthesia and surgical intervention in a large majority of women in this condition.

The work-up of the woman who has a medical condition should be systematic. The considerations are illustrated in **Figure 2**. Specific conditions will need related preparations, precautions, and emergency drugs. These should be checked and available, especially when a surgical procedure is planned.

For termination of pregnancy in the first trimester by medications, the drug regimen is well established. The recommended combination is to use 200 mg of mifepristone orally followed by 400 µg of misoprostol (sublingually, buccally, vaginally, or orally).[2] The same combination should be used in women with medical conditions. Women with severe cardiac conditions are at risk of cardiovascular events with misoprostol administration. It would be prudent to hospitalize them or at least keep them under observation for a few hours when it is administered. Medical conditions or the drugs used to treat them in general do not have an impact on the doses of mifepristone or misoprostol as used for first-trimester pregnancy termination. There are very minimal drug interactions of other medications with either drug. Therefore, practically, there is no medical condition, which poses a difficulty from this point of view. Theoretically, mifepristone may have drug interactions with cytochrome P450 inhibitors (e.g., high doses of erythromycin, clarithromycin, ketoconazole, miconazole, ritonavir, lopinavir, saquinavir).[3]

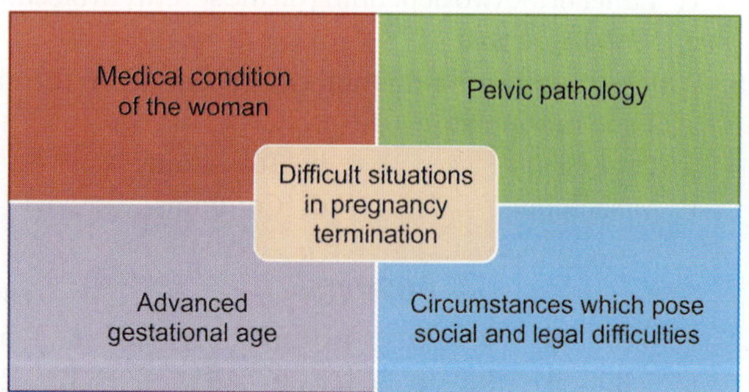

Fig. 1: Difficult situations in pregnancy termination.

TABLE 1: Medical conditions that pose difficulty for pregnancy termination.

Category of difficulty	*Examples of conditions*
General systemic compromise with a high risk of complications with anesthesia	• Severe anemia with hemoglobin <8 g/dL • Severe cardiac disease (uncontrolled hypertension, angina, valvular heart disease, and arrhythmias) • End-stage renal disease • Liver failure • Compromised neurological status or uncontrolled seizure disorders • Advanced stages of cancer • Severe respiratory disease
Medical conditions which alter surgical risk	• Conditions where there is a bleeding tendency (severe coagulopathy or thrombocytopenia) • Conditions which compromise immune function leading to a greater susceptibility to pelvic infections (AIDS, cancer on chemotherapy, and uncontrolled diabetes)

(AIDS: aquired immune deficiency syndrome)

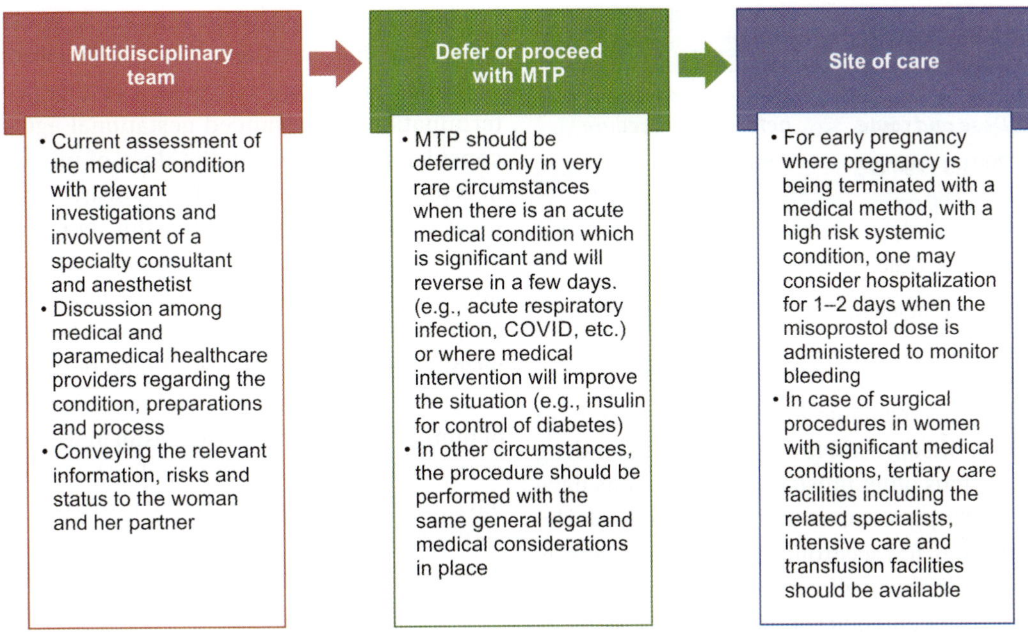

Fig. 2: Workup and preparation for medical termination of pregnancy (MTP) in women with medical conditions.

For women with medical conditions where a surgical procedure is needed for pregnancy termination, there should be due consideration for anesthesia. The procedure should be conducted in an appropriate care setting. Even if the procedure is planned under local anesthesia by paracervical block, the anesthetist should be available as standby and to monitor the woman. The least invasive and safest route of anesthesia should be considered as per the choice and preference of the anesthetist and surgeon. Regional anesthesia, though not conventionally used, may be a safer choice with severe systemic compromise and should be considered.

PELVIC PATHOLOGY

Anatomical variations in the cervical and uterine structure can result in difficulties with surgical procedures for pregnancy termination and termination at advanced gestational ages. They generally do not affect the process or outcomes of medicated abortion in the early first trimester. The pelvic pathologies that can result in difficulties are outlined in **Table 2**. These pelvic pathologies can result in excess surgical morbidity in the form of cervical injuries, uterine perforations and damage to other viscera, bleeding, creation of a false passage, incomplete evacuation, and continuing pregnancy.

Pelvic pathology may be suspected based on past history or reports and clinical examination. It should be further defined by appropriate imaging, most commonly a pelvic ultrasound. Ideally, pelvic anatomical abnormalities should be diagnosed before the surgical procedure. But this may not always be the case. On the other hand, there are certain problems which will be detected only during the surgical procedure such as difficult cervical dilatation or bleeding on dilatation.

A separate discussion is whether a particular pathology is an indication for termination of pregnancy. This is a matter which should be individualized for every clinical situation. There are no blanket rules, but usually fibroids of small-to-moderate size can largely coexist with pregnancy and do not warrant a termination of pregnancy. Cervical polyps, if symptomatic, can be removed even during pregnancy and the pregnancy can be continued. In certain circumstances such as cervical cancer, termination of pregnancy may be advised as a part of the broader treatment plan.

For first-trimester surgical procedures, many of the difficulties can be solved by planning, preparing the operation theater in anticipation of the needs, cervical priming, and the use of ultrasound guidance.

TABLE 2: Pelvic pathology that poses difficulty for termination of pregnancy.

Conditions that can be diagnosed in advance and pose technical difficulties	***Conditions that can be diagnosed in advance and to be considered for prostaglandin dose in advanced gestation***	***Conditions that are encountered on the operation table and cannot be diagnosed in advance***
Cervical polyp	Grand multiparity	Cervical stenosis causing difficult dilatation
Uterine fibroids—lower segment, cervical fibroids, fibroids that distort the uterine cavity	Previously scarred uterus—a history of cesarean section, myomectomy, hysterotomy, or uterine rupture	Bleeding with cervical dilatation
Cervical cancer, especially in advanced stages		
Mullerian anomalies		

TABLE 3: Methods for cervical priming before first-trimester pregnancy termination.

Agent	Dose and route	Timing of administration before the procedure
Misoprostol	200 µg vaginally	2 hours
	400–600 µg sublingually	2 hours
Mifepristone	200 mg orally	12–24 hours
Dinoprostone	0.5 mg vaginally	6–8 hours
Laminaria tents		12–24 hours

The various choices available for cervical priming are outlined in **Table 3**. Misoprostol is a commonly used drug for this purpose. Various other prostaglandin regimens have been described. A 200-µg misoprostol dose acts effectively, is economical, and has few gastrointestinal side effects as compared to other described regimens and agents.[4] Cervical priming allows an easier and quicker dilatation and reduces the chances of creating a false passage and bleeding.

Transabdominal ultrasound during the surgical procedure is a useful adjunct when the anatomy is altered. The passage of the dilators and cannula is by touch, but ultrasound gives guidance and prevents complications such as perforation. It allows the operator to work with a greater degree of confidence. When there is a large fibroid or a Mullerian anomaly, it is possible to miss the pregnancy entirely during a first-trimester surgical termination. Ultrasound will allow positive confirmation that the pregnancy is evacuated completely. The use of ultrasound is associated with a lower risk of complications, even in pregnancies where there is no pelvic pathology.[5]

If there is intraoperative difficulty, such as difficult dilatation, the following measures may be helpful:

- Empty the bladder.
- Remove all the instruments from the vagina and examine the woman again to assess the position of the uterus.
- Two vulsellums are applied to the anterior cervical lip to get a firm traction without tearing and slipping.
- Use a different set of dilators.
- Use a uterine sound or obturator to identify a cervicouterine path.
- Ultrasound guidance.
- Abandon the procedure without injury or complications, counsel about the events, and attempt again after a few days with cervical priming.

In some situations, there may be significant bleeding when the cervix is dilated. This could be from laceration of the cervix or perforation. The procedure can be continued and the uterus evacuated. This should be followed by sustained, firm pressure with a pack on the cervical canal for at least 10 minutes. This would usually suffice in stopping the bleeding. Further steps such as an intracervical balloon or suturing the descending cervical artery are rarely needed. If the woman is hemodynamically unstable, a greater vascular injury to the uterine vessels should be suspected. Resuscitation with fluids, investigations, blood cross-matching, and a laparotomy should be done.

Pelvic pathology can pose a challenge for pregnancy terminations at advanced gestational age. There is some consideration regarding the dose of misoprostol that can be safely used with a previously scarred uterus. However, most studies have found that the standard doses of 200–400 µg of misoprostol administered orally or vaginally at intervals of 4–6 hours are a safe regimen and do not result in greater complications in second-trimester pregnancy terminations. Adequate time should be allowed for the drug to act and polypharmacy should be avoided. The incidence of uterine rupture with misoprostol in women with previous cesarean birth is rare and found to be <1%.[6] Some authors have recommended mechanical dilatation of the cervix with a Foley's balloon with or without extraovular saline or ethacridine lactate instillation.[7] Ethacridine is no longer freely available. Mechanical priming could reduce the prostaglandin usage. With pelvic pathology, there may be a higher incidence of failed procedures and need for a hysterotomy. This requires a prior discussion with the couple and preoperative preparation. The pelvic pathology (large fibroid) may be surgically treated at the same time. This approach increases the surgical risk of time, bleeding, and related morbidity.

ADVANCED GESTATIONAL AGE

Advanced gestational age represents technical and legal issues that need to be addressed. The technical problems that can occur are:

- No response to medications
- Partial response to medications, but prolonged process beyond 48 hours
- Sepsis due to prolonged process or rupture of membranes
- Bleeding
- Uterine rupture.

The technical problems may occur more commonly when there are other pelvic pathologies associated with advanced gestational age as outlined in the previous section. The standard approach to second-trimester pregnancy termination is a combination of mifepristone and misoprostol.[8,9] The dosage regimens and schedules are mentioned earlier. Though there is no definite time point where the process has to be stopped, one should consider abandoning the medical process in the following circumstances:

- More than 48 hours of induction with prostaglandins with no appreciable cervical change. One should consider changing the type and/or route of prostaglandin administration if there is no response in the first 24 hours.
- Suspicion of complications such as sepsis, bleeding, or uterine rupture.

In such circumstances, one would resort to a hysterotomy.

In terms of legal provisions under the Medical Termination of Pregnancy (MTP) Act as it stands today, pregnancy

TABLE 4: Gestational age for pregnancy termination in India.

	MTP Act 1971	*MTP Act amendments 2021*
Up to 12 weeks	Opinion from one practitioner	Opinion from one practitioner
12–20 weeks	Opinion of two practitioners	Opinion from one practitioner
20–24 weeks	Not allowed	Opinion of two practitioner for some categories of pregnant women
After 24 weeks	Not allowed	Opinion of medical board for substantial fetal abnormalities

(MTP: medical termination of pregnancy)

termination is permitted till 20 weeks of pregnancy with the opinion of two practitioners. If the pregnancy duration is beyond 20 weeks, the woman has to approach the courts for permission. The court generally directs the case to an interdisciplinary body of medical experts from public hospitals and usually abides by its opinion. In general, the courts have looked upon these situations favorably from a humanitarian point of view and granted permission to the woman. The MTP Act has recently been amended and been passed in the Parliament in March 2021.[10] The new provisions and a comparison to the existing ones are made in **Table 4**. It should be noted that at the time of writing this chapter, these amendments are not in practice as the process framing of the standard operating procedures and related rules and regulations is awaited by various state governments.

DIFFICULT SITUATIONS FROM SOCIAL AND LEGAL ASPECTS

The MTP Act is an enabling act of law.[11] Section 8 of the MTP Act (Protection of Action Taken in Good Faith) protects the medical practitioner from suits or other legal proceedings for any damage caused or likely to be caused by anything done in good faith under the act. This last section of the MTP Act has profound implications. It protects medical practitioners, from being prosecuted under the IPC, or civil/consumer court action. However, the practitioner should be diligently functioning within the limits set by the Act, Rules, and Regulations. The MTP Act and the legal aspects about pregnancy termination have been discussed in another chapter in the book. This section looks at situations where there is a need to alter the usual process to comply with other laws, which would be relevant to a given situation.

MTP for Women Who have a History of Sexual Assault

A pregnancy resulting from sexual assault is an indication for termination of pregnancy as per the MTP Act. The woman has to be managed in a sensitive manner. The likelihood of finding evidence of the sexual assault at a time that the woman presents for an MTP is minimal. Except for gross physical injuries and bruises, there would be no obvious evidence of an assault. However, it may be prudent to collect, document, and process the samples as per the protocol for women presenting after sexual assault. It is the woman's choice whether she would be pursuing further police proceedings.

Unmarried, Separated, Divorced Woman Seeking MTP

Medical termination of pregnancy can be performed on a woman under the above circumstances under the indication of "risk of grievous injury to mental health." The provision of failure of contraception should not be used in these circumstances as it is a provision for married women as per the Act. Adequate counseling of the woman, her consent, and documentation are essential. Occasionally, the medical practitioner may face an irate, separated husband or parents of an unmarried girl seeking explanation about the procedure. These should be discussed with another party only with the consent of the woman. In all other circumstances, her confidentiality has to be maintained.

MTP for Minors or Adolescents

The Protection of Children from Sexual Offences (POCSO) Act came into effect in India in 2012.[12] As per this Act, every individual under the age of 18 years is considered as a "child" and can be prosecuted for engaging in a sexual act irrespective of her consent. The POCSO Act does not recognize consensual sexual activity below the age of 18 years. Section 19 of the Act covers Reporting of Offences and it is mandatory for any person (including medical practitioners) to report such an act. Failure to report can result in punishment and a case of child sexual abuse can be filed against the individual who intentionally omits to do so. For the situation that an adolescent approaches a medical practitioner (with or without an adult guardian) for an MTP, this would mandate the practitioner to inform the police, breaking confidentiality of the adolescent.

This Act has direct implications on criminalizing adolescent sexuality and affecting confidentiality of an adolescent. The Act adopts a protectionist approach under the assumption that a uniform age of consent would be in accordance with the UN Convention on the Rights of the Child, 1989. In effect, the Act infringes upon the right to dignity and bodily integrity, freedom of expression, right to life, and the right to privacy of adolescents engaging in consensual sexual behavior. Given these considerations, there is an urgent need for the POCSO Act to take these considerations into account and modifications are needed. A practical guide to the conflating positions and possible solutions has been published and provides important guidance for the medical practitioner.[13] As things stand today, the following should be borne in mind when faced with the situation of providing MTP for an adolescent or minor girl:

- It is mandatory for the provider to inform the police (irrespective of the wishes of the girl and/or her parents). This is applied to a married adolescent woman also. If the age is uncertain, it is prudent to report the same.
- The medical practitioner should provide a written record (medicolegal certificate) and get an acknowledgment. The National Commission for the Protection of Child Rights (NCPCR) has stated that providing a medicolegal certificate to the authorities is sufficient to comply with the reporting requirements of the POCSO Act.[14]
- The medical practitioner does not need to file an FIR and should not insist on the girl/parents to take legal action.
- The medical practitioner does not have to seek further permission or wait for police or court proceedings to perform the MTP.
- The products of conception may be considered as evidence as the sexual act that has resulted in pregnancy of the minor constitutes rape. Ideally, the products should be preserved or handed over to the police for further process. It would be considered a violation under section 201 only if a provider destroys evidence with the intent to protect the accused from legal action. Therefore, providers who dispose of the products of conception for a good faith reason (e.g., inadequate preservation facilities or following standard operating procedures) should be shielded from prosecution under Section 201.[13]

MTP and Gender Selection

Gender selection and selective abortion based on the gender of a fetus are illegal in India as per the Preconception and Prenatal Diagnostic Technique (PCPNDT) Act. This is a completely separate issue and in some forums, this has been falsely conflated with the MTP Act. The right to abortion must be differentiated from the laws against sex discrimination that are in no way in contradiction to each other. There is no conflict between the PCPNDT Act and the MTP Act. The MTP Act allows abortion, while the PCPNDT forbids prenatal sex determination to stop female feticide. By conflating the two, confusion is being created in the minds of the public against a basic right of women.[15] There has to be a rational application of both the Acts and women should not be denied abortion access under the guise of the PCPNDT Act.

CONCLUSION

There may be difficult situations in the context of various clinical situations and presentations when pregnancy termination is needed. The difficulties may be from the woman's medical condition, from technical difficulties, or from the sociolegal circumstances. An experienced operator backed with a good team, open communication, and adequate backup are needed in difficult situations. In all circumstances, the medical provider should remain within the ambit of the law and follow well-established guidelines. These practices form the cornerstone in facing difficult situations.

KEY MESSAGES

- Termination of pregnancy is a human need.
- The woman may have a medical condition or a pelvic pathology, the pregnancy may be at an advanced gestational age or there could be social, legal or difficulties with access to care.
- For women who have medical conditions, ideally, chronic care programs should include effective contraceptive advice.
- For women with medical conditions, there could be general systemic compromise with a high risk of complications with anesthesia or medical conditions which alter surgical risk.
- Specific medical conditions will need related preparations, precautions and emergency drugs.
- Medical conditions or the drugs used to treat them in general, do not have an impact on the doses of mifepristone or misoprostol as used for first trimester pregnancy termination.
- The least invasive and safest route of anesthesia should be considered as per the choice and preference of the anesthetist and surgeon.
- When terminating a pregnancy in a woman who has significant pelvic pathology, the surgical risk can be minimized by cervical priming and transabdominal ultrasound during the surgical procedure.
- There can be social and legally challenging situations in pregnancy termination. In all circumstances, the medical provider should remain within the ambit of the law and follow well-established guidelines.

FURTHER READING

1. Lawyers Collective Women's Rights Initiative (LCWRI), Government of India and UNICEF. Monitoring Guidelines for NCPCR/SCPCR for Roles and Functions of Various Stakeholders- Child Welfare Committees/ Support Persons, and Health Professionals. [online] Available from: https://ncpcr.gov.in/showfile.php?lang=1&level=1&&sublinkid=406&lid=843. [Last accessed November, 2021].
2. Prasad V. (2020). Contrived Confusions - No Contradictions Between PCPNDT and MTP Acts. [online] Available from: https://www.epw.in/journal/2015/10/web-exclusives/contrived-confusions.html. [Last accessed November, 2021].

REFERENCES

1. Singh S, Shekhar C, Acharya R, Moore AM, Stillman M, Pradhan MR, et al. The incidence of abortion and unintended pregnancy in India, 2015. Lancet Glob Health. 2018;6:e111-20.
2. Ministry of Health and Family Welfare, Government of India. (2016). Handbook on medical methods of abortion to expand access to new technologies for safe abortion. National Health Mission. [online] Available from: http://nhm.gov.in/

images/pdf/programmes/maternal-health/guidelines/MMA_Handbook.pdf. [Last accessed November, 2021].
3. Danco Laboratories, LLC. (2000). Mifeprex (mifepristone) prescribing information. [online] Available from: https://www.accessdata.fda.gov/drugsatfda_docs/label/2016/020687s020lbl.pdf. [Last accessed November, 2021].
4. Kapp N, Lohr PA, Ngo TD, Hayes JL. Cervical preparation for first trimester surgical abortion. Cochrane Database Syst Rev. 2010;(2):CD007207.
5. Acharya G, Morgan H, Paramanantham L, Fernardo R. A randomized controlled trial comparing surgical termination of pregnancy with and without continuous ultrasound guidance. Eur J Obstet Gynecol Reprod Biol. 2004;114:69-74.
6. Bahar R, Alexandroni H, Karavani G, Gilad R, Benshushan A. Safety of medical second trimester abortions for women with prior cesarean sections. Arch Gynecol Obstet. 2021;303:1217-22.
7. Li N, Wu P, Zhao J, Feng L, Qiao FY, Zeng WJ. Effectiveness and safety of double-balloon catheter versus intra-amniotic injection of ethacridine lactate for termination of second trimester pregnancy in patients with liver dysfunction. J Huazhong Univ Sci Technolog Med Sci. 2015;35:129-34.
8. Tank JD, Maheshwari B, Palshetkar N, Purandare A. (2019). Everything you need to know about abortion in India. Theme: Second Trimester Abortion. [online] Available from: https://www.fogsi.org/wp-content/uploads/committee-2020-activities/issue-2-trimester-abortions-november-2019.pdf. [Last accessed November, 2021].
9. Ministry of Health and Family Welfare, Government of India. (2021). Comprehensive Abortion Care: Training and Service Delivery Guidelines. www.nhm.gov.in. [online] Available from: https://nhm.gov.in/New_Updates_2018/NHM_Components/RMNCHA/MH/Guidelines/CAC_Training_and_Service_Delivery_Guideline.pdf. [Last accessed November, 2021].
10. Ministry of Law and Justice, Government of India. (2021). The Medical Termination of Pregnancy (Amendment) Act 2021. The Gazette of India Extraordinary. [online] Available from: https://egazette.nic.in/WriteReadData/2021/226130.pdf. [Last accessed November, 2021].
11. Ministry of Health and Family Welfare, Government of India. (1971). The Medical Termination of Pregnancy Act, 1971. Acts, Rules and Standards for the Health Sector. [online] Available from: https://main.mohfw.gov.in/acts-rules-and-standards-health-sector/acts/mtp-act-1971. [Last accessed November, 2021].
12. Ministry of Law and Justice, Government of India. (2012). The Protection of Children From Sexual Offences Act, 2012. [online] Available from: https://legislative.gov.in/sites/default/files/The%20Protection%20of%20Children%20from%20Sexual%20Offences%20Act%2C%202012_0.pdf. [Last accessed November, 2021].
13. IPAS Development Foundation. The POCSO Act and the MTP Act - Key Information for Medical Providers. (2014). [online] Available from: https://www.ipasdevelopmentfoundation.org/resourceFiles/75201803210124.pdf. [Last accessed November, 2021].

LONG QUESTIONS

1. Discuss the approach to medical termination of pregnancy in a woman with a severe cardiac disease.
2. Discuss the approach to medical termination of pregnancy in a woman with a 20-cm cervical fibroid.
3. An adult woman presents to the clinic with an ultrasound report showing a large cranial defect in the fetus at 22 weeks of pregnancy and requests for the pregnancy to be terminated. How will you proceed further?
4. Discuss the implications of the POCSO Act on the clinical situation of a 16-year-old girl who presents for a termination of pregnancy. What measures are important for the medical practitioner to bear in mind?

SHORT QUESTIONS

1. Give examples of difficult situations compounding with each other and creating a complex situation.
2. Name the contraindications to using mifepristone and misoprostol.
3. What are the drug interactions with mifepristone and misoprostol?
4. What is cervical priming? What are the agents available for cervical priming?
5. Enumerate the steps that an operator may consider when faced with difficulty in cervical dilatation at the time of a surgical termination of pregnancy.

MULTIPLE CHOICE QUESTIONS

1. What is the estimated incidence of pregnancy termination in India annually?
   a. 15 lakhs per year
   b. 15,000 per 100,000 women
   c. 15 million per year
   d. 150 million per year
2. The following is not a contraindication to using misoprostol:
   a. Angina
   b. Asthma
   c. Uncontrolled hypertension
   d. Recurrent uncontrolled seizure disorder
3. The following technical problem will be usually diagnosed only on the table during a surgical medical termination:
   a. Cervical fibroid b. Cervical polyp
   c. Cervical cancer d. Cervical stenosis
4. The following is an acceptable method of cervical priming before a surgical termination of pregnancy:
   a. 200 mg Misoprostol vaginally 24 hours before the procedure
   b. 200 μg Misoprostol sublingually 2 hours before the procedure
   c. 200 mg Mifepristone orally 2 hours before the procedure
   d. Laminaria tent inserted intracervically 2 hours before the procedure

Answers

1. c 2. b 3. d 4. b

3.4 COMPLICATIONS OF TERMINATION OF PREGNANCY

Bharti Maheshwari

INTRODUCTION

Termination of pregnancy is an integral part of the reproductive health of the woman and the essential responsibility of the clinician to conduct it successfully without complications and legally. In India, termination of pregnancy is legally allowed under certain conditions, up to 20 weeks of pregnancy under the Medical Termination of Pregnancy (MTP) Act since 1971.[1]

COMPLICATIONS

Complications of termination of pregnancy vary from minimal bleeding and pain to life-threatening complications such as hemorrhage, perforation, and sepsis, depending on the skill of provider and infrastructure available. The most important fact is that with little awareness and skilled interventions, the majority of complications are preventable.[2]

Complications of termination of pregnancy depend on:[3-5]

- Gestational age at termination
- Method of termination
- Associated risk factors
- Preprocedure work-up
- Postprocedure follow-up

Gestational Age at Termination

Usually, earlier the termination, lesser are the complications.

We have options for safe medical methods of abortion (MMA) till 9 weeks and manual vacuum aspiration till 12 weeks. Both procedures are associated with least complications; hence, all unwanted pregnancies should be terminated as early as possible with all precautions and follow-up.

Methods of Termination and Associated Complications

Termination of pregnancy can be done by medical method or surgical method according to gestational age, patient's compliance, and facility available. Medical method and manual vacuum aspiration (MVA) are safest methods and associated with least complications.

Associated Risk Factors

Advanced age, anemia, hypertension, cardiac disease, scarred uterus, coagulopathy, etc., are associated with increased risk of complications.

Preprocedure Work-up

Proper history, clinical evaluation, counseling, and planning by eligible provider at approved place with proper infection prevention practices minimize the risk of complications and the related morbidity and mortality.

Postprocedure Care

Postprocedure monitoring, early identification of complications and management, proper follow-up, and timely referral play key role in reducing morbidity and mortality after MTP.

Complications of Termination of Pregnancy[1,6-10]

Medical method of termination:
- Protocol—200 mg mifepristone followed by 400 microgram after 36 hours, till 7 weeks of gestation 800 µg misoprostol till 9 weeks of gestation
- Follow with follow-up card—at 15th day

Complications: Hemorrhage, incomplete evacuation, and continuation of pregnancy

They can be categorized according to method of abortions:

- *Medical method of abortion*:
  - Hemorrhage
  - Incomplete evacuation
  - Continuation of pregnancy
- *Surgical method of evacuation*:
  - Complication due to anesthesia
  - Hemorrhage
  - Uterine perforation
  - Fainting and syncope
  - Shock.

Complications of Medical Method

Medical methods of abortion is a method to terminate pregnancy by using combination of drugs mifepristone and misoprostol. There are proper dose protocols for particular gestational age and checklist for providing medicine and follow with proper follow-up card. If drugs are given correctly, then MMA have 95–99% success rate and only 0.1–0.2% require blood transfusion.

Proper case selection, adequate counseling, and appropriate referral are the key to the success of MMA. Also, the woman should be informed about the possible complications and where/whom to contact for emergency services.

Hemorrhage

Preabortion counseling should emphasize that bleeding is likely to be heavier than regular menses and comparable to

Flowchart 1: Algorithm for management of excessive bleeding during MMA process.

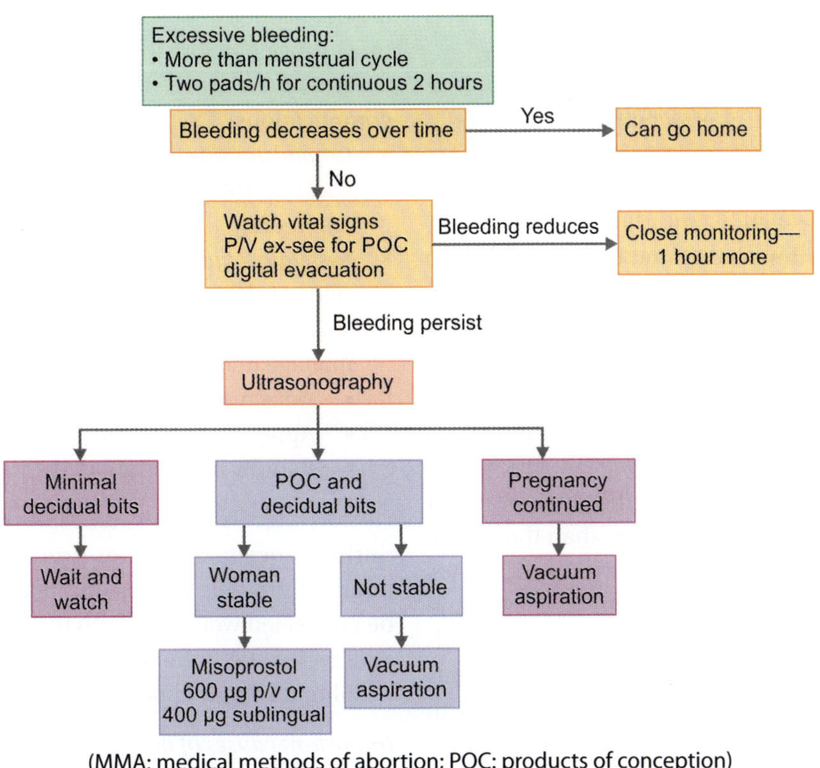

(MMA: medical methods of abortion; POC: products of conception)

that of a miscarriage. The woman should be told that soaking two pads per hour for 2 hours in a row is normal at the time of peak cramping. This is often the case during the expulsion of the products of conception (POC). However, if this persists and/or the woman is dizzy, she should consult the doctor. Vacuum aspiration may have to be done to complete the process **(Flowchart 1)**.

Incomplete abortion: Women with incomplete abortion during the process of MMA generally present with excessive/continued bleeding. On examination of vitals:

- If her condition is unstable—resuscitate and stabilize her first.
  - Stabilization should be followed by an examination and further management.
- If her condition is stable, proceed with the internal examination:
  - If POCs are felt at the os, manage with digital evacuation, followed by vacuum aspiration, if required
  - If no POCs are felt at the os, decide the line of management, based on:
    - Clinical symptoms
    - Pelvic examination
    - *Ultrasonography (USG) findings*:
      - If the USG shows incomplete expulsion of POCs, then an additional dose of misoprostol (600 µg oral or 400 µg sublingual) may be offered to the woman.

      Wait for the pregnancy to be expelled with time. The woman should be counseled to return to the clinic after 1 week to ensure that the abortion is complete.

      If bleeding continues, even after an additional dose of misoprostol (as mentioned above)—perform vacuum aspiration
      - If no gestation sac is visible on USG, but bleeding continues owing to decidua bits in the uterine cavity, manage conservatively, without any medication or intervention, as these are expelled spontaneously in most cases.

      An additional visit after 7 days will have to be planned to ensure completion of the process. If bleeding is profuse at any time during this process, VA may have to be done.
      - If USG shows continuation of the pregnancy despite use of MMA drugs, it should be terminated by vacuum aspiration.

If USG is not available, manage the woman based on her general condition, severity of bleeding, and pelvic examination findings, similar to management under table on "incomplete abortion".

- *Continuation of pregnancy*: If this is diagnosed on clinical examination, it is advisable to terminate a pregnancy surgically. If it continues after drugs for MMA have been taken, a written statement, signed by the woman, must be kept on record if surgical termination is refused making her aware of the risk of possible teratogenicity.

- *Delay or early in onset of next menses*:

Complications by surgical method of termination:
- *MVA*: Least complication indicated till 12 weeks of gestation
- *Suction evacuation in 2nd trimester*: Hemorrhage, perforation, shock, sepsis, syncope, anesthesia complications

Complications and Management of Surgical Abortion[1,11,12]

Surgical abortion can be done by suction evacuation in first trimester till 12 weeks and by dilatation and evacuation in second trimester. Manual vacuum aspiration is the golden method of termination till 12 weeks, associated with minimal resources and complications. It is successful in over 98% of cases. Incidence of cervical injury perforation, hemorrhage is two to four times lesser than curettage. The practice of D and C is to be discouraged because the rates of major complications are two to three times higher than those with vacuum aspiration. Curettage is abandoned in any trimester.

About 9–11% termination occurs in second trimester and responsible for two-thirds of major complications. Second-trimester abortions should always be done as indoor patients at tertiary center or district hospital by expert obstetrician with opinion of two registered medical practitioners. Cervix repining by misoprostol tablets or dinoprostone gel is important step to prevent cervical injury and inhibiting forceful dilatation. 200–400 µg misoprostol tablets 3–4 hours per vaginally/sublingual or 10–15 minutes orally before termination, not only soften and dilate cervix but also separate products by initiating uterine contraction and make procedure safe.

Facility for management of complications of second-trimester termination with expert should be readily available at center. Timely referral facility, if required with all life-saving resuscitative measures, should be checked before starting procedure.

Proper counseling, taking consent, and documentation are a must before starting procedure.

Nulliparous and scarred uterus:
- Proper repining of cervix is required in nulliparous cervix and in scarred uterus.
- There are chances for hysterotomy, so consent should be taken with proper counseling. Blood transfusion facility should be available.

Complications due to anesthesia: Pain relief is important part of termination procedure: Till 12 weeks, MVA can be done safely with paracervical block-local method of anesthesia. In second-trimester IV sedation, short general anesthesia (GA) may be required according to need of patient.

Local anesthesia complications: Complications and side effects are rare with the appropriate dose and when care is taken not to inject the drug into a blood vessel. However, mild side effects such as the numbness of lips and tongue, a metallic taste in the mouth, dizziness, and lightheadedness, ringing in the ears, difficulty in focusing the eyes, itching and rashes are occasionally encountered. They should be observed and must subside before the procedure is commenced.

However, one should be alert for the following complications:
- *Convulsions*: Injection diazepam 10 mg IV or phenytoin sodium 100 mg IV must be given slowly in such an emergency
- *Systemic toxic reactions are* very rare. If the woman shows signs of sleepiness, disorientation, muscle twitching and shivering, slurred speech, and respiratory depression, manage her as follows:
  - Administer oxygen
  - Apply suction to the throat to maintain patent airway
  - Rapidly infuse fluids.

Hemorrhage: It is important life-threatening complication during procedure or after procedure. Provider should be aware of possible causes and management. Patient should be counseled well. Pre-evaluation investigations are a must. Staff should be trained for resuscitative measures of patient with hemorrhagic shock.

Important causes of hemorrhage during procedure:
- Cervical injury, which may have been caused by the vulsellum or difficult dilatation
- Incomplete emptying of uterus
- Uterine atony (soft and boggy uterus)
- Perforation of uterus (instrument passed beyond the uterine wall).

Clinical features:
- Heavy, bright red vaginal bleeding with or without clots
- Tachycardia, pallor, and hypotension.

Management: In case of cervical injury: Apply pressure with a sponge and suture with chromic catgut or any other suitable absorbable suture 1-0 using a round body needle, if required.

In case of bleeding from the uterine cavity: Give tablet misoprostol 400 µg sublingual or per rectal. Bimanual uterine massage should be given.

If the bleeding continues, oxytocin infusion 10 units in 500 mL RL or NS at 40–60 drops per minute should be started.

Completion of evacuation with vacuum aspiration or ovum forceps should be carried out if POC are not completely removed. Injection methylergometrine 0.2 mg can then be given.

Uterine perforation: Experience and proper training minimize chances of perforation. Preprocedure evaluation and premedication also decrease chances of perforation. Surgeon should identify earliest and should manage in time to save life of patient.

Features of suspicion of perforation:
- Sudden loss of resistance with the instrument in utero
- Dilator or cannula penetrates further than expected

- Fat/omentum (yellow colored) or bowel seen in the cannula or at the cervix
- Difficulty in withdrawing the cannula
- Rapid pulse and falling blood pressure (signs of shock)
- Severe abdominal pain
- Abdominal rigidity and distension
- Shoulder pain
- Bowel injury during MTP **(Fig. 1)**.

Management of perforation:

- Stop the procedure as soon as possible and remove the instruments
- Keep patient in Trendelenburg position (elevate the foot end of the bed and lower the head end), if there is hypotension
- Start intravenous fluids (RL or NS)
- If the perforation is with a cannula/dilator of <8 mm, either complete the procedure immediately under USG/ laparoscopic guidance or after 48 hours, if she is stable.

If she is unstable or continues bleeding or a bigger-size cannula was in use, refer to the next higher level of care following protocols of referral.

If intestine or omentum is seen on cannula, start an intravenous infusion and antibiotics. If properly equipped with complete laparotomy facilities, perform MTP in the facility itself under USG/laparoscopic guidance or refer to a higher level facility.

During transport, a trained healthcare provider should accompany the woman: Continue oxygen, IV therapy, keep the woman warm, and keep her feet elevated.

Fainting/syncope:

Symptoms and causes: This occurs usually when the cervix is *forcefully dilated.* Severe pain is experienced and the woman faints due to a *vasovagal attack* causing marked *bradycardia.*

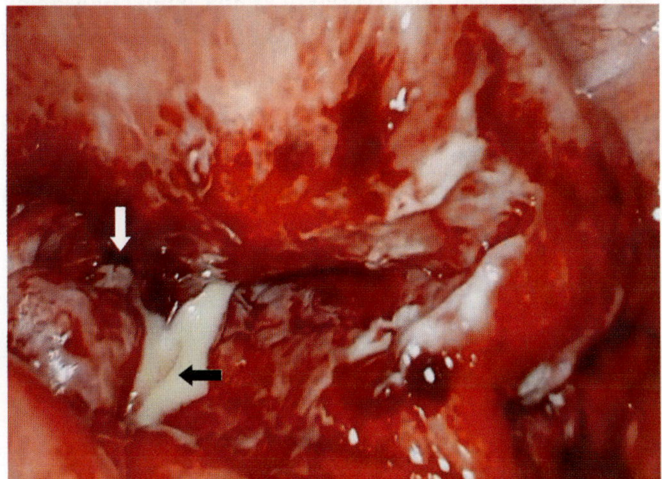

Fig. 1: Uterine (white block arrow) and bowel (black block arrow) injury being managed by laparoscopy. The pelvis is being explored one week after the injury and has pus and adhesions.
Courtesy: Dr Atul Ganatra, Mumbai.

This may last only for a few seconds to minutes, provided the pain is controlled.

Management:

- Stop the procedure immediately.
- Maintain an open airway.
- Prevent aspiration of vomitus by turning the woman's head and shoulder to one side
- Trendelenburg position (elevate the foot end of the bed and lower the head end)
- Administer injection atropine sulfate 0.6 mg IV. Repeat after 2 minutes, if response is inadequate
- If recovery is not immediate, ventilate with an Ambu bag and administer oxygen. Start intravenous fluids and monitor vital signs.

Shock (either during the procedure or later):

- Shock due to hemorrhage and sepsis may be life threatening so it should be treated at higher center. This is important cause of maternal morbidity and mortality.
- Preprocedure clinical evaluation, prophylactic antibiotic, blood transfusion facility, and infection prevention practices are important measures that should be followed.

Symptoms:

- Rapid, weak pulse (110 beats/min or more)
- Low blood pressure (diastolic <60, systolic <90)
- *Pallor*:
  - Rapid breathing (respiration 30 breaths/min or more)
  - Anxious, confused, or unconscious mental state
  - Profuse sweating or perspiration
- *Clinical evaluation*: History, physical examination, and pelvic examination
- *Investigations*: Hb, ABORh, urine, total leukocyte count (TLC), differential leukocyte count (DLC), electrolytes, urea, creatinine, and X-ray chest.

Management: Initial stabilization—follow principle of ABC (airway, breathing, circulation)

- Make sure the airway is open
- Give oxygen at 6–8 L/min (mask or nasal cannula)
- Give IV fluids (Ringer's lactate or isotonic solution) at one liter in 15–20 minutes using a large bore needle 16–18 gauge
- Keep the woman warm
- IV antibiotics
- Blood transfusion, if required

  Asses response of fluid transfusion—increase blood pressure >100 mm Hg, increase urine output >100 mL/4 h, and improving mental status.

  If stable, do specific treatment.
- Evacuate the uterus with VA for retained POC, if suspected and manage sepsis, if suspected.

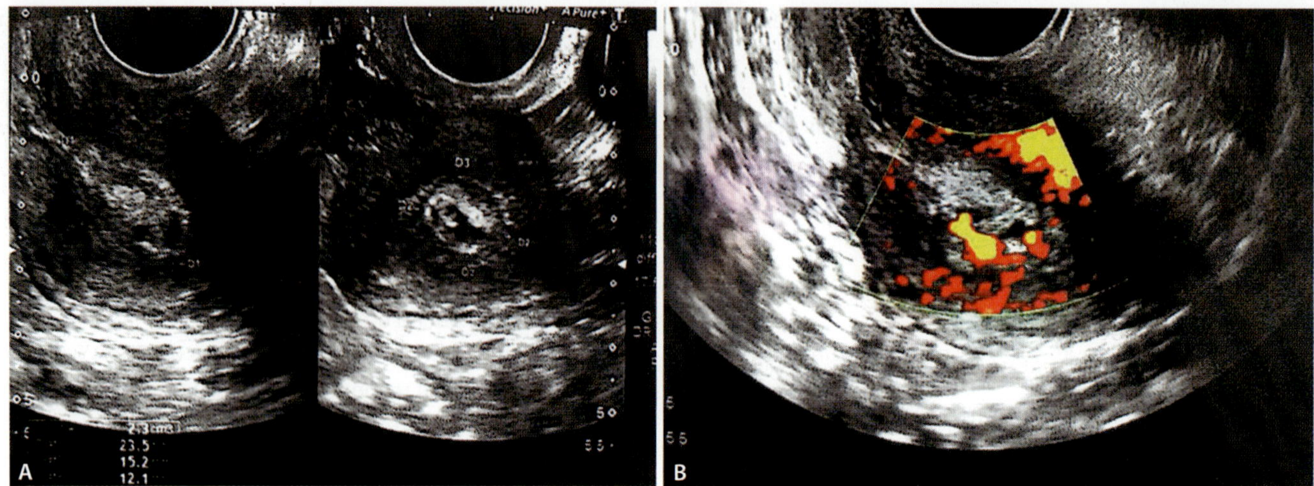

Figs. 2A and B: Retained products of conception after an incomplete termination of pregnancy on ultrasound (A) and color Doppler (B).

Delayed Complication of Surgical Methods of Abortion

1. Incomplete abortion
2. Infection/sepsis
3. Continuation of pregnancy

Incomplete Abortion

Symptoms:

- Pallor
- Excessive or prolonged bleeding per vaginam
- Fever or pain in the abdomen **(Figs. 2A and B)**.

Main cause is incomplete evacuation of all the POCs. Ideally, the bulk/quantity of the products that are removed should be assessed/confirmed. Gentle check curettage can be carried out after evacuation. The uterine walls should be felt gritty once all the products are removed. PV examination at the end of the procedure will reveal a firm uterus, with size reduced and cervix closing.

Management: Depending on the general condition of the woman and the severity of bleeding:

- Stabilize the woman first, with the measures mentioned before in the section on "Shock"
- Give tablet misoprostol 400 µg sublingual/or 600 µg orally and observe her for decrease in the vaginal bleeding
- Evacuate the uterus with VA for retained POC under antibiotic cover.

Infection/Sepsis

Symptoms:

- Chills, fever
- Foul-smelling vaginal discharge
- Abdominal pain or cramps
  - Distended abdomen
  - Rebound tenderness
  - Prolonged bleeding **(Fig. 3)**.

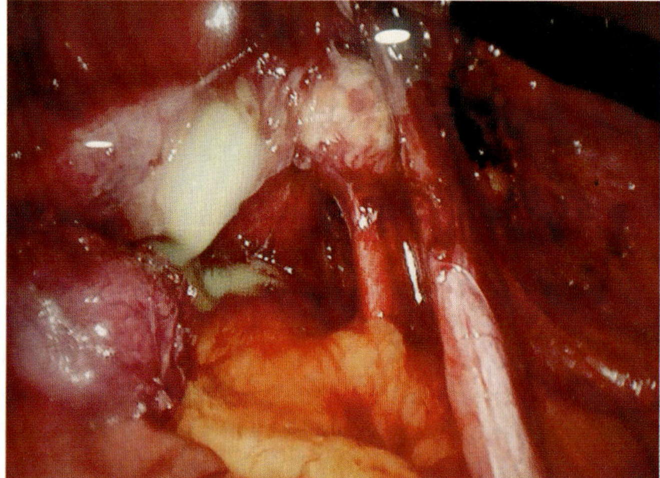

Fig. 3: Pelvic abscess after unsafe pregnancy termination managed by laparoscopic drainage and irrigation.

Clinical assessment: Detailed history, physical examination, pelvic examination, pus in cervix or vagina, tender movement of adnexa or cervix, uterine subinvolution, and foreign body in vagina.

Investigations: Abdominal X-ray in upright position, USG pelvis and abdomen, c/s of blood, urine, cervical, vaginal swab, liver function test (LFT), and kidney function test (KFT)

Main causes of sepsis:

- Retained POCs
- Asepsis not properly maintained

Management of sepsis:
Initial treatment:

- Admission
- Ensure airway is opened
- Elevate feet
- Oxygen 6–8 L/min by nasal catheter or mask
- IV fluids RL/NS with 18–20 G cannula

- Input/output chart maintained
- IV antibiotics has to be started.

On examination:

If retained products: Evacuate the uterus with VA for retained POCs. Uterine evacuation performed on an infected uterus can more easily result in perforation, so it should be done with caution.

Suspect disseminated intravascular coagulation (DIC):
- If blood does not clot
- Bleeding from venipuncture, oral mucosa, and bladder
- Coagulation profile deranged

Management: Fresh blood and component transfusion and refer to higher center.

Suspect-gas gangrene or tetanus:
- If gas in pelvic tissues on X-ray
- Painful muscle contraction
- Generalized spasm and convulsions—refer to higher center after sedation, if suspecting tetanus.

Suspect uterine perforation:
- If abdominal pain, rigidity
- Rebound tenderness
- X-ray shows—gas under diaphragm—manage accordingly.

Continuation of Pregnancy

The pregnancy may continue if pregnancy is not disturbed, may be if the cannula is not inserted in the uterine cavity and remains in the cervical canal. Another possibility is formation of false passage. Third possibility is of bicornuate uterus with the nongravid cornu being curetted.

Continuation may be prevented by confirming the presence of chorionic villi in the evacuated POC.

Women must also be counseled to report *any delay in menstruation 6 weeks* after the procedure.

This is managed by counseling and informing the woman of the condition. If she wants to get it terminated, the procedure should be repeated, if pregnancy is still within the first trimester. However, if the pregnancy has advanced to the second trimester, appropriate methods of termination should be used at an appropriate level of facility.

Remote Complications of Surgical Methods of Abortion

The following complications are rare with VA and usually the result of trauma or infection. This underlines the importance of adopting a gentle and meticulous aseptic surgical technique.

Menstrual Disturbances

Amenorrhea and hypomenorrhea may result from varying degrees of intrauterine adhesions *(Asherman's syndrome)*. Usually, it follows vigorous curettage with removal of basal layer of endometrium. Hysteroscopic adhesiolysis is now the management of choice for intrauterine adhesions.

Heavy menstrual bleeding occurs in next few cycles. Not actually a complication but can occur just like after spontaneous abortion or childbirth.

Infertility

Infertility may result from tubal factor (closure or distortion) due to postabortal infections or uterine factor due to endometrial trauma or infection and Asherman's syndrome.

Recurrent Abortion

Late (mid-trimester) abortion can occur due to cervical incompetence as a result of injury from forceful dilatation to the cervix.

Ectopic Pregnancy

Tubal distortion due to postabortal infection may increase the risk of tubal ectopic pregnancy.

Obstetric Complications

Obstetric complications may rarely occur during future pregnancies. Adherent placenta and uterine rupture may result from a previous undiagnosed perforation.

Psychosomatic Conditions

Though uncommon, depression may be reported occasionally. Psychosomatic symptoms are predisposed to by abortions carried out for medical reasons or fetal abnormality in an otherwise wanted pregnancy or when there is coercion or force by the spouse or family members. Sensitive and supportive counseling is the key to *preempting and preventing psychomotor symptoms.*

PREVENTION OF COMPLICATIONS

Role of Ultrasonography

It is not mandatory to perform an USG for all women undergoing termination of pregnancy with medical methods. USG is indicated for *the following conditions*:

- *Before the procedure*:
    - Women with a suspicion of ectopic pregnancy (symptoms such as irregular vaginal bleeding, pelvic pain, or adnexal mass or tenderness.
    - Provider's uncertainty with examination, or inability to assess the uterine size due to obesity or pelvic discomfort.
    - Women unsure of last menstrual period (LMP) or have conceived during lactational amenorrhea; have irregular cycles; and have a discrepancy between the history and the clinical findings.

- *During the procedure*: USG-guided evacuation eliminates the chances of incomplete evacuation. Also, it is useful in case of bicornuate uterus.
- *During follow-up*:
  - Clinical examination does not confirm the completion of the abortion process
  - Continued vaginal bleeding, which is more than normal menstrual periods
  - Suspicion of continuation of pregnancy.

Since it is an obstetric USG, all the protocols under the Preconception and Prenatal Diagnostic Techniques (PCPNDT) Act should be followed.

Complications of Second-trimester MTP

- Failure of induction
- Delay in induction abortion interval with chances of incomplete abortion, excessive bleeding, and sepsis.

Rh isoimmunization in case the mother is Rh negative and fetus is Rh positive.

Hence, injection anti-D should be administered to all Rh-negative mothers soon after MTP within 72 hours. After first trimester MTP 150 μg and after second-trimester MTP 300 μg is to be given.

MANAGEMENT OPTIONS AT DIFFERENT LEVELS OF FACILITIES

At primary health level [primary health center (PHC) and community health center (CHC) level]:

- Initial clinical assessment of woman coming with abortion complications
- Initiation of resuscitation/stabilization treatments including antibiotic therapy, intravenous fluid replacement, and oxytocics
- Diagnosis of the type of abortion complication
- *Investigations*: Hemoglobin, blood grouping, and cross-matching
- Preparation for definitive treatment or referral to an appropriate facility for further management and care
- Uterine evacuation.

At secondary/tertiary level hospital (district hospital and medical college):

- All services provided at the primary level
- Blood cross-matching and transfusion, USG, X-ray abdomen, and other relevant investigations
- Laparotomy and indicated surgery
- Treatment of severe complications (bowel injury, tetanus, renal failure, gas gangrene, etc.)
- Treatment of DIC.

KEY MESSAGES

- Complications such as sepsis, hemorrhage, and tissue injury are responsible for maternal morbidity and mortality related to abortion care.
- Universal stabilization measures should be provided to all cases of abortion complications and definitive management should be started immediately after establishing the diagnosis.
- Since primary-level facilities cannot treat all types of abortion complications, timely referral after stabilizing the woman helps in the definitive treatment.
- Practice safe and legal abortion with proper preprocedure workup, correct clinical protocols, implementing MTP, Protection of Children from Sexual Offence (POCSO), and PCPNDT Act with proper follow-up.

FURTHER READING

1. Ministry of Health and Family Welfare, Government of India. (2016). Handbook on Medical Methods of Abortion. [online] Available from: http://nhm.gov.in/images/pdf/programmes/maternal-health/guidelines/MMA_Handbook.pdf. [Last accessed November, 2021].
2. Ministry of Health and Family Welfare, Government of India. (2016). Post-Abortion Family Planning Technical Update. [online] Available from: http://nhm.gov.in/images/pdf/programmes/family-planing/guidelines/Post_Abortion_Family_Planning.pdf. [Last accessed November, 2021].

REFERENCES

1. Ministry of Health and Family Welfare, Government of India. (2018). Comprehensive Abortion Care, 2nd edition 2018. Ministry of Health and Family Welfare, Government of India Training and Service Delivery Guideline. [online] Available from: https://nhm.gov.in/New_Updates_2018/NHM_Components/RMNCHA/MH/Guidelines/CAC_Training_and_Service_Delivery_Guideline.pdf. [Last accessed November, 2021].
2. Hyman A, Castleman L. (2005). Woman-Centered, Comprehensive Abortion Care Reference Manual, 2nd edition. [online] Available from: https://www.researchgate.net/publication/280925082_Woman-Centered_Abortion_Care_Reference_Manual. [Last accessed November, 2021].
3. Patient Safety Network. (2019). Root Cause Analysis. [online] Available from: http://psnet.ahrq.gov/primer.aspx?primerID=10. [Last accessed November, 2021].
4. Turner KL, Huber A, Ipas. Woman-centered postabortion care: Reference manual, 2nd edition. Chapel Hill, NC: Ipas; 2013.
5. NHS Institute for Innovation and Improvement. (2008). Quality and Service Improvement Tools: Root Cause Analysis Using Five Whys. [online] Available from: http://www.institute.nhs.uk/quality_and_service_improvement_tools/quality_and_service_improvement_tools/identifying_problems_-_root_cause_analysis_using5_whys.htm. [Last accessed November, 2021].
6. Paul M, Lichtenberg ES, Borgatta L, Grimes DA, Stubblefield PG, Creinin MD. (2009). Management of unintended and abnormal pregnancy: Comprehensive abortion care. [online] Available from: http://eresources.lib.unc.edu/external_db/external_database_auth.html?A=P%7CF=N%7CID=221823%7CREL=HSL%7CSO=HSL%7CURL=http://libproxy.

lib.unc.edu/login?url=http://onlinelibrary.wiley. com/book/10.1002/9781444313031. [Last accessed November, 2021].
7. Postabortion Care Consortium. (2013). Postabortion Care (PAC) Consortium. [online] Available from: http://www.pac-consortium.org/. [Last accessed November, 2021].
8. World Health Organization (Producer). (2008). Learning from error: Patient safety workshop. Video and booklet. [online] Available from: http://www.who.int/patientsafety/education/vincristine_download/en/index. Html. [Last accessed November, 2021].
9. World Health Organization. (2014). Clinical practice handbook for safe abortion. [online] Available from: http://apps.who.int/iris/bitstream/10665/97415/1/9789241548717_eng.pdf?ua=1. [Last accessed November, 2021].
10. Ministry of Health and Family Welfare, Government of India. (2007). Infection Management and Environment Plan: Policy Framework. [online] Available from: http://toxicslink.org/docs/rulesansregulation/imeppolicyframework.pdf. [Last accessed November, 2021].
11. Ministry of Law and Justice. (1983). Medical Termination of Pregnancy Act, 1971 [online] Available from: http://www.egazette.nic.in/WriteReadData/1971/E-1383-1971-0034-61647.pdf. [Last accessed November, 2021].
12. World Health Organization. Sexual Violence. [online] Available from: http://www.who.int/violence_injury_prevention/violence/global_campaign/en/chap6.pdf. [Last accessed November, 2021].

LONG QUESTIONS

1. What are complications of termination of pregnancy in first trimester?
2. What are second-trimester termination complications, how to prevent them?
3. What is management protocols for hemorrhage after medical method of termination?
4. What is features suggestive of perforation during MTP, how you will manage?
5. Write down measures to prevent litigations with MTP procedure.

SHORT QUESTIONS

1. Describe management of failed medical method of abortion in first trimester.
2. What are the features of shock?
3. What are causes of hemorrhage after abortion?
4. Discuss complication of local anesthesia.
5. Describe management of perforation.

MULTIPLE CHOICE QUESTIONS

1. Which of the following is a drawback of suction evacuation?
   a. Cannot be used for uterus of 12-week size
   b. Needs local paracervical block anesthesia
   c. Complications such as perforation and sepsis
   d. All of the above
2. MVA can be done up to:
   a. 6 weeks b. 12 weeks
   c. 18 weeks d. 20 weeks
3. What is the most common cause of bleeding in most abortion cases?
   a. Hemorrhage due to retained products
   b. Perforation
   c. Sepsis
   d. Hematometra
4. In case of bleeding due to retained products, what is the first step in management?
   a. Curettage
   b. Uterine massage
   c. Evacuation of the uterus
   d. Laparotomy
5. In a patient following abortion, D and E was performed. How will you ensure that the procedure is complete?
   a. Grating sensation
   b. Visible bubbles
   c. No bleeding and closure of the cervix
   d. All of the above
6. In a suspected patient with uterine perforation, the treatment of choice is:
   a. Laparotomy b. Evacuation
   c. D and E d. Hysterectomy
7. Which of the following are remote gynecological complications following surgical termination of pregnancy?
   a. Menstrual disturbances
   b. Infertility
   c. Uterine synechiae
   d. All of above
8. Obstetrical complications in a patient following MTP by surgical procedures increases risk of:
   a. Preterm labor
   b. Recurrent mid-term abortion
   c. Ectopic pregnancy
   d. All of the above
9. Following are features of shock:
   a. Tachycardia b. Hypotension
   c. Decrease urine output d. All of the above
10. Suspicion of perforation is done if:
    a. Sudden loss of resistance with the instrument in utero
    b. Dilator or cannula penetrates further than expected
    c. Fat/omentum (yellow colored) or bowel seen in the cannula or at the cervix
    d. Difficulty in withdrawing the cannula
    e. All of above

Answers

1. a 2. b 3. a 4. c 5. d 6. a
7. d 8. d 9. d 10. e

3.5 COUNSELING AFTER PREGNANCY TERMINATION

Basab Mukherjee

COUNSELING

Counseling may be defined as a structured interaction in which a person voluntarily receives emotional support and guidance from a trained person in an environment that is conducive to openly sharing thoughts, feelings, and perceptions.[1]

It is the choice of the woman whether she wishes to undergo a discussion about her situation, her feelings, and decisions with the healthcare provider. If she chooses to interact, counseling provides a unique opportunity to address her physical and emotional health needs and refers her to ancillary services as and when necessary. It is understood that any woman's counseling should be guided by her needs and responses and not a predetermined checklist. Open-ended questions help in establishing a rapport and encourage her to share her concerns. It goes much beyond providing information and giving advice **(Box 1)**.

WOMEN-CENTERED COMPREHENSIVE ABORTION CARE COUNSELING

Counseling: Who, When, Where, and How?

A medical doctor may not be always necessary or available for counseling. Any staff member of the clinic who has been trained in providing comprehensive abortion care (CAC) counseling services may be employed. Midwives, nurses, and auxiliary nurses (ANMs) can be utilized effectively for pre- and postabortion counseling.

The counseling should ideally be provided before, during, and after the procedure. The preprocedure counseling will also include the consent needed to conduct the procedure.

Counseling should be done at an appropriate place where auditory and visual privacy can be maintained. Often, a separate room for counseling may not be dedicated in the clinic, but the area assigned should be both accessible and comfortable.

While counseling, the counselor needs to demonstrate empathy and there should be no time constraints for the discussion. Culturally appropriate gestures and communicating in the familiar language are important. She may or may not want to include family members in the discussion with her.

BOX 1: Tips on features of effective counseling.

- Voluntary
- Effective communication
- Respecting confidentiality
- Focusing on woman's needs
- Accepting her perception and feelings
- Supporting her decisions

Bias of Healthcare Provider toward the Client

It is often seen that consciously or unconsciously some bias creeps up in the counseling of clients by healthcare providers. These depend on preconceived ideas of the providers. Women who have repeated abortions, inconsistent users of contraception, having multiple sexual partners, or are a part of a specific race, religion or community are likely to be perceived differently from others.

To minimize these issues, value clarification exercises should be periodically conducted for healthcare professionals. This is an educational intervention that includes reflexive personal sociocultural and intercultural processes whereby one seeks to identify the value priorities that guide one's interests, choices, actions, and reactions in a variety of social contexts.[2]

Postabortion Care

Emergency Treatment of Incomplete Abortion

Surgical treatment has been the traditional method of managing incomplete abortions. Vacuum aspiration (both manual and electric) has been shown to be safer, less painful, and involves less blood loss than sharp curettage.[3] Manual vacuum aspiration (MVA) in these cases can most often be done with a paracervical block and emotional support, thus avoiding general anesthesia.

Women should also be counseled that medical management of incomplete abortion (misoprostol 400 µg sublingual or 600 µg oral single dose) in the first trimester has been found to be comparable to surgical evacuation.[4] Successful evacuation rates ranging between 89 and 99% at 1–2 weeks post-treatment have been observed without resorting to surgical intervention. This treatment can be expanded to secondary and district hospitals and addressed by mid-level clinicians with high client satisfaction rates.

Surgical evacuation is still necessary in 2–8% of women who present with persistent incomplete evacuation, infection, heavy bleeding, and an advanced gestational age.[5]

Other Aspects of Postabortion Care

Sexually transmitted infection (STI) screening and counseling for risk factors are a necessary service, which can be offered as a part of the postabortion care. Treatment for existing STIs and use of barrier contraception to prevent future STIs would be a part of the medical care. This would also be an opportunity to educate women who are at a high risk for STIs due to their lifestyle.

The psychological effects of abortion on women should not be underestimated regardless of the abortion being spontaneous or induced. Though initial distress is relieved soon after the procedure, anxiety and depression may persist in some women up to 2 years from the procedure. The healthcare worker should be made aware of signs, which may warrant referral to a mental health specialist.[5]

"If a woman comes to a hospital with an incomplete (induced) abortion, we have already failed once to help her avoid an unwanted or a mistimed pregnancy. If she leaves the facility without having any means of preventing another pregnancy in the future that may not be wanted, we have failed her twice."

Source: Cynthia Steele Verme 1994, Postabortion Care (PAC) Consortium, International Conference on Population and Development (ICPD), Cairo.

Postabortion Family Planning

Many women in the world have little to no control of the circumstances in which they become pregnant. A significant proportion of these women opt for an abortion faced with an unwanted or unintended pregnancy. In many cases, the abortion may be unsafe further risking the life of the woman.[6]

As unmet need for family planning is one of the primary causes of induced abortion, it is important that postabortion family planning is discussed and offered to women to break the cycle of repeated induced abortions. It is also necessary to understand that almost immediately after the abortion, the woman is at risk of another pregnancy unless she uses effective birth control methods.[7]

If a woman has a spontaneous miscarriage, she would still need contraception to give a preferred 6-month interval period before trying again. WHO has suggested that for an optimal future pregnancy outcome, a minimum of 6-month interval in between pregnancies is ideal. This reduces the incidence of preterm delivery, low-birth weight, premature rupture of membranes, and maternal anemia.[8]

Postabortion Family Planning in India

Consistent use of postabortion family planning is expected to minimize 90% of abortion-related maternal mortality. Since most women receiving abortion services in a facility do not return for family planning services, even if they do not want to become pregnant in the near future, immediate counseling for birth control in the facility is the best way forward. If she is unable to decide on a method or is not eligible, schedule a follow-up within 2 weeks or give her a referral appointment at a nearby family planning facility.[9]

Postabortion family planning is endorsed by the professional organizations of doctors, nurses, and midwives as a standard of practice. Governments are encouraged to provide universal access to postabortion family planning **(Box 2)**.

BOX 2: Family planning counseling messages.

- Wait for at least 6 months before trying to conceive again
- Fertility returns quickly (10–11 days after first-trimester abortions)
- She can choose from available family planning methods that can be started at once
- If a woman decides not to use immediately, she should be offered information on all available methods
- She should avoid intercourse till bleeding stops to avoid infection.
- Method-specific counseling should follow

Source: Postabortion family planning: Technical Update March 2016. Family Planning Division, Ministry of Health and Family Planning, Government of India.

INTEGRATION AND ORGANIZATION OF SERVICES

It is vital that family planning services are provided with or immediately after abortion services. The integration of both and providing voluntary contraceptive counseling at the facility has shown to rapidly increase the postabortion contraception acceptance rates.[10]

Providing postabortion contraception also is beneficial financially for the institution. It saves time and less staff may be employed in the facility. In countries such as Nigeria where safe abortion access is less, it has been calculated that the cost of tackling abortion-related complications is four times the cost of providing family planning services in the postabortion period to minimize further abortions.[11]

Institutions appreciating the importance of postabortion family planning provision should allocate space for providing the necessary services. Contraceptive supplies and necessary equipment should be made available and appropriate task sharing involving nurses and paramedical staff for counseling. Auditing the procedures and the number of women adopting a birth control method before leaving the facility would go a long way in providing quality care.

CONTRACEPTIVE CHOICES IN CLIENTS POSTABORTION

The choice of contraception in a woman would depend to some extent on her reproductive goals. Spacing methods would be appropriate if an interval of 6 months to 1 year is considered before planning pregnancy again. Long-term methods would be pertinent if longer gaps or no further childbearing is planned. Most contraceptive methods can be used in the immediate postabortion period.

Task sharing could include nurses and trained paramedical workers to provide contraception services in accordance with the state legal framework.

If a woman is starting combined oral contraceptive pills (COCPs), progestogen-only pills (POPs), centchroman, or injection depot-medroxyprogesterone acetate (DMPA) within a week of a first- or second-trimester abortion, she does not need a backup method. However, if she starts a week later, a backup method would be necessary for the first 7 days (2 days in case of POPs) **(Table 1)**.

FOLLOW-UP VISITS

Before the woman leaves the facility, it is advisable that she is advised to return for a follow-up in a couple of weeks.

TABLE 1: Time of initiation of contraceptive methods after an abortion.

	Surgical abortion	*Medical abortion*
Combined oral contraceptive pills, progestin-only pills, centchroman pills, and injection DMPA	Immediately	3rd day of protocol (on the day of misoprostol)
Condoms	Immediately	As soon as sexual activity resumes
IUCD	Immediately	Once abortion is complete (around day 15) ruling out infection
Female sterilization	Concurrently or within 7 days	After the first menstrual cycle
Vasectomy	Anytime	Anytime

(DMPA: depot-medroxy-progesterone acetate; IUCD: intrauterine contraceptive device)
Source: Postabortion Family Planning—Technical Update March 2016. Family Planning Division, Ministry of Health and Family Planning, Government of India.

This would be to assess her physical condition, rule out postabortion complications, and address any issues with the chosen method of contraception. If she did not choose the contraception earlier, this will give her another opportunity to adopt another method.

While closing a counseling session, the provider should ideally provide a summary of the discussion done. The couple needs to be asked whether they have additional queries. Some simplified reading material, written or pictorial, in the local language should be shared.

CONCLUSION

In a postabortion setting, the first priority would be to rule out an emergency and provide immediate medical care. The next step would be consent to receive counseling and the benefits of the same without any coercion. Most young women are capable of making their own decisions after being provided the necessary information. Screening for STIs and assessing the psychological response would be an important part of postabortion care. It is important to counsel women on effective and appropriate birth control and options of adopting the same before leaving the facility. Healthcare providers should try to avoid personal beliefs and bias into the counseling. Referral services should be offered whenever necessary.

KEY MESSAGES

- In a postabortion setting, the first priority would be to rule out an emergency and provide immediate medical care.
- The next step would be consent to receive counseling and the benefits of the same without any coercion.
- Most young women are capable of making their own decisions after being provided the necessary information.
- Screening for STIs and assessing the psychological response would be an important part of postabortion care.
- It is important to counsel women on effective and appropriate birth control and options of adopting the same before leaving the facility.
- Healthcare providers should try to avoid personal beliefs and bias into the counseling.
- Referral services should be offered whenever necessary.

REFERENCES

1. IPAS. (2014). Women-centered Comprehensive Abortion Care Trainer's Manual, 2nd edition. [online] Available from: https://www.ipas.org/resource/woman-centered-comprehensive-abortion-care-trainers-manual-second-edition/. [Last accessed November, 2021].
2. Kulich SJ, Chi R. Values Clarification. In: Michalos AC (Ed). Encyclopedia of Quality of Life and Well-being Research. Dordrecht: Springer; 2014.
3. United States Agency for International Development (USAID), Postabortion Care Working Group. What works: a policy and program guide to the evidence on postabortion care. Washington (DC): USAID; 2007.
4. Shochet T, Diop A, Gaye A, Nayama M, Sall AB, Bukola F, et al. Sublingual misoprostol versus standard surgical care for treatment of incomplete abortion in five sub-Saharan African countries. BMC Pregnancy Childbirth. 2012;12(1):127.
5. Huber D, Cutis C, Irani L, Pappa S, Arrington L. Postabortion care: 20 years of strong evidence on emergency treatment, family planning, and other programming components. Glob Health Sci Pract. 2016;4(3):481-94.
6. Peipert JF, Madden T, Allsworth JE, Secura GM. Preventing unintended pregnancies by providing no-cost contraception. Obstet Gynecol. 2012;120(6):1291-7.
7. Wilcox AJ, Dunson D, Baird DD. The timing of the "fertility window" in the menstrual cycle: day-specific estimates from a prospective study. BMJ. 2000;321(727):1259-62.
8. Westoff CF. Recent trends in abortion and contraception in 12 countries. DHS Analytical Studies, No. 8. Calverton, MD: ORC Macro; 2005.
9. Family Planning Division, Ministry of Health and Family Planning, Government of India. (2016). Post Abortion Family Planning - Technical Update March 2016. [online] Available from: http://nhm.gov.in/images/pdf/programmes/family-planing/guidelines/Post_Abortion_Family_Planning.pdf. [Last accessed November, 2021].
10. High Impact Practices in Family Planning (HIP). Post abortion family planning: strengthening the family planning component of post abortion care. Washington DC: USAID; 2012.
11. Lule E, Singh S, Chowdhury SA. Fertility regulation behaviors and their costs: Contraception and unintended pregnancies in Africa and Eastern Europe and Central Asia. Washington, DC: World Bank; 2007.

LONG QUESTION

1. Define counseling and discuss the key features in post-abortal counseling

SHORT QUESTIONS

1. When and which methods of contraception are to be offered after an abortion?
2. What should be the components of care during a post-abortal follow up visit?

MULTIPLE CHOICE QUESTIONS

1. All of the following are features of effective post abortal counseling, except:
   a. It should be mandatory
   b. Respecting confidentiality
   c. Focusing on woman's needs
   d. Supporting her decisions
2. Clinical scenarios which mandate a surgical evacuation are all, except:
   a. Persistent incomplete evacuation
   b. Infection
   c. Heavy bleeding
   d. Early gestational age
3. Consistent use of postabortion family planning is expected to minimize abortion-related maternal mortality by:
   a. 30% b. 50%
   c. 70% d. 90%
4. WHO has suggested that for an optimal future pregnancy outcome, a minimum interval in between pregnancies ideally should be:
   a. 2 months
   b. 6 months
   c. 12 months
   d. 18 months Respecting confidentiality
5. All of the following are complications that may be seen in pregnancies occurring too soon after an abortion, except:
   a. Preterm labor b. Maternal anemia
   c. GDM d. IUGR

Answers

1. a 2. d 3. d 4. b 5. c

3.6 ACCESS TO SAFE PREGNANCY TERMINATION

Atul Ganatra, Freni Shah

"No woman can call herself free until she chooses consciously whether she will or will not be a mother."

—**Margaret Sanger**

Access to safe abortion care at the right time is more important than ever—this is how we can keep services going through the crisis.

INTRODUCTION

Eight percent maternal death in India is due to unsafe abortions, being the third largest cause of maternal death. In absolute numbers, close to 10 women die due to unsafe abortions each day.[1] While abortion has been legal in India since 1971, available research shows that 56% of the 6.4 million abortions that take place in the country are unsafe.[2] Many severe complications that the women face are preventable through just easy access to safe abortion services. Recent census data (2011) reveals a dismal child sex ratio of 918 girls per 1,000 boys. This is down from 927 in 2001 and 945 in 1991.[3] The Medical Termination of Pregnancy Act, 1971 (the MTP Act) which was amended in 2002 legalizes abortion in India under certain conditions. The central government made the MTP Rules (amended in 2003) and the MTP Regulations, 2003 (applicable to all Union Territories). The regulations under the MTP Act prescribe forms for recording opinion of the Registered Medical Practitioner (RMP), reporting to Chief Medical Officer (CMO) and for maintaining records, etc. The state legislatures are required to make similar or appropriate regulations for the state and make them readily available to all concerned. In addition, the central government released the Comprehensive Abortion Care (CAC) Training and Service Delivery Guidelines (hereafter referred to as the National CAC Guidelines) in 2010 (updated in 2014) to strengthen access to CAC and prevent mortality and morbidity resulting from unsafe abortions. The Pre-Conception and Pre-Natal Diagnostic Techniques (Prohibition of Sex Selection) Act, 1994 (the PCPNDT Act), as amended in 2003, along with the PCPNDT Rules, 1996, as amended in 2011, 2012, and 2014, have been enacted to prevent misuse of preconception and prenatal diagnostic techniques for determining the sex of the fetus and to prevent disclosure of the sex to the pregnant woman and her relatives.

UNDERSTANDING THE MTP ACT AND ITS IMPLEMENTATION[4]

Table 1 lists out the key provisions of the MTP Act and the National CAC guidelines that must be kept in mind to ensure availability and monitoring of abortion services.

Although the abortion services were legalized in India in 1972, services for safe abortion are restricted, especially in rural areas. Use of mifepristone-misoprostol was approved for MTP in 2002 but it is mainly in primary setting only.

No matter what happens, sexual and reproductive healthcare, including access to safe abortions, will be the utmost need of a woman. There seems to be a profound impact of the crisis on people's lives which means the need

TABLE 1: Key provisions of the MTP Act and the national CAC guidelines.

Issue	*Key provisions*	*Additional information for proper implementation*
Conditions under which a pregnancy may be terminated	The MTP Act allows for termination of pregnancy on a broad range of conditions: • Continuation of the pregnancy would involve a risk to the life of the pregnant woman or it may cause grave injury to her physical or mental health • Substantial risk that the child, if born, would be seriously handicapped due to physical or mental abnormalities • Pregnancy is caused by rape (presumed to constitute grave injury to mental health) • Pregnancy is caused due to failure of contraceptive in married woman or her husband (presumed to constitute grave injury to mental health)	Sex selection is not a legal ground for terminating a pregnancy. The provider/s must ensure that the ground for termination is clearly stated in the opinion form. The opinion of the provider is adequate to certify ground/s for providing abortion service
Place where a pregnancy may be terminated	Hospital established or maintained by the government or a place approved by the government or the District Level Committee (DLC) headed by the Chief Medical Officer (CMO) or District Health Officer (DHO). As per the National CAC Guidelines, pregnancy may be terminated at government facilities up to: • 8 weeks of gestation at primary health center (PHC) • 12 weeks of gestation at Community Health Center (CHC) or 24 × 7 PHC • 20 weeks of gestation at District Hospital and above facilities. The DLC may approve a (private) place to conduct • Terminations up to 12 weeks • Terminations up to 20 weeks	The CMO shall properly examine the application for approval before making a recommendation to the DLC for approving the place
Who can terminate a pregnancy?	Medical termination of pregnancy can be legally provided only by a "registered medical practitioner" (RMP)—a medical practitioner who possesses any recognized medical qualification as defined in clause (h) of section 2 of the Indian Medical Council Act, 1956, whose name has been entered in a State Medical Register and who has one or more of the following experience or training in gynecology and obstetrics: • In the case of a medical practitioner, who was registered in a State Medical Register immediately before the commencement of the Act, with experience in the practice of gynecology and obstetrics for a period not <3 years. • In the case of a medical practitioner, who was registered in a State Medical Register after the commencement of the Act and: – Has completed 6 months of house surgency in gynecology and obstetrics Or – Has experience in any hospital for a period of not less than 1 year in the practice of obstetrics and gynecology Or – Holds a postgraduate degree or diploma in gynecology and obstetrics Or – Has assisted an RMP in the performance of 25 cases of MTP of which at least five have been performed independently, in a hospital established or maintained by the Government, or a training institute approved for this purpose by the Government	Training as detailed in 2d will enable the RMP to do only first trimester terminations (up to 12 weeks of gestation)

(CAC: comprehensive abortion care; MTP: medical termination of pregnancy)

for easy access to safe abortion is going to increase than before owing to the decision to whether continue a pregnancy which is affected by the pandemic which has caused a loss of job or other health concerns as well as increased incidences of rape and domestic violence.

The poorest and most marginalized women and girls are most affected by the coronavirus disease 2019 (*COVID-19*) crisis, making it difficult for them to access contraception and safe abortion services.

There is shortage of medications and contraceptives due to disruption in supply chain; people's ability to pay for services has been restricted due to economic insecurity; and quarantines, travel bans, and closed borders are making physical access to safe services increasingly challenging.

Of the estimated 15.6 million abortions that happen in India annually, 73% are through medical abortion (MA) drugs accessed outside of facilities, 16% in private health facilities, 6% in public health facilities, and 5% through traditional unsafe methods.[5] The nation-wide lockdown following the outbreak of COVID-19 pandemic, although necessary, leads to unintended adverse impact on access to sexual and reproductive health (SRH) services, particularly abortion access across all three points of care.

Despite abortion being designated as an "essential service", there are several barriers to access. While movement restrictions and suspension of transport facilities limited women's mobility to access facilities or chemist outlets, there has also been a shift in focus of the public health system.

Public health facilities are either converted to COVID-19 treatment centers or the facility staff is redeployed from regular duties to COVID-19 care. Moreover, closure of private health facilities due to provider unavailability and lack of protective gear and disruption in supply chain of MA drugs at both chemist outlets and facilities are other key drivers.

The Ipas Development Foundation (IDF) undertook a modeling exercise to assess the near-term impact of COVID-19 on abortion access in the first 3 months following the commencement of the lockdown (25 March 2020 to 24 June 2020). The estimation takes into consideration two key parameters—degree of restriction at the point of care and dynamic changes in the level of public restrictions over the period. We estimate that access to *1.85 million abortions (or 47% of the estimated 3.9 million abortions that would have taken place under normal circumstances) is likely to be compromised in this period due to COVID-19* ***(Fig. 1)***.

Unintended pregnancies can have serious consequences such as unsafe abortions and pregnancy-related complications, especially in lower economic countries, that may contribute to maternal morbidity and mortality.

As global SRH providers, we know the inevitable result. Restricting access to safe abortion does not prevent them but makes abortion occur at alter in pregnancy and more complex and dangerous. Each year, 25 million women resort to dangerous and unsafe methods to end an unplanned pregnancy and our teams worldwide witness and deal with the terrible consequences of this every day.

Globally, around 1.5 lakh pregnancies end in abortion every day. As the COVID pandemic continues to spread, medical services and health systems are stretched, in some places, to breaking point. The provision of safe abortion is an extremely time-sensitive, essential health service.

During this ongoing pandemic, there are effective and easily implemented solutions those can help release the pressure on the health system, free up providers, and ensure easy access to lifesaving services without affecting the quality of care.

Some solutions could be telemedicine, removal of unnecessary waiting periods, easy access of mifepristone and misoprostol, patient education initiatives, and a digital media campaign highlighting the high margin of the safety of abortion both early and late in the pregnancy and the availability of abortion in different settings to the full extent of the local law, delinking the provision of abortion to the coercive acceptance of postabortion contraception, task shifting to the extent possible in various countries.

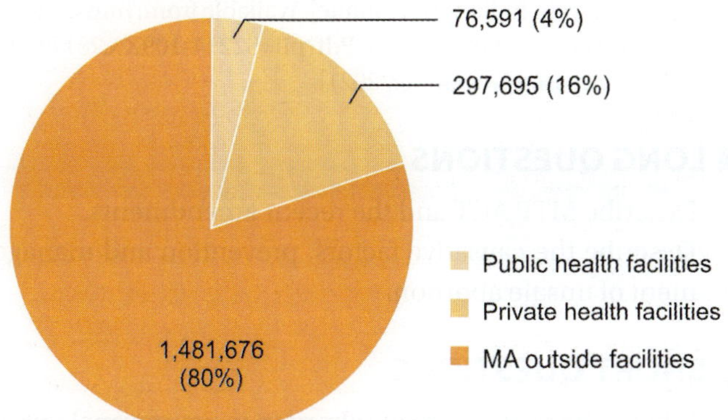

Fig. 1: Compromised abortions by points of care.

To illustrate, one answer is *telemedicine:*

- Telemedicine (SMS, WhatsApp, video call, or telephone call) is a safe and private communication method, not requiring in-person contact or visit to clinic to have an early pregnancy abortion or to screen for medical eligibility.
- It is the most convenient and vital for women living in remote area, self-isolating or who cannot leave their houses because of other responsibilities such as childcare, etc.
- There is clear evidence that for the provision of safe and effective abortion services, an in-person meeting is not essential. As per WHO recommendation, if women have access to appropriate information and to health services they need or want at any stage during MA process, it can be self-managed also.
- All prescriptions should be sent to pharmacy or clinic directly.
- Provide additional information and counseling like side effects of the drugs to be used (misoprostol may cause cramping pain, vomiting, fever, bleeding, etc.).
- Treating and managing minor side effects through telemedicine.
- Counseling on fertility awareness methods.
- Scheduling clients' individuality, maintaining adequate social distance, and/or having adequate space for clients to wait outside may be helpful in avoiding crowding in the clinic area.

The American College of Obstetricians and Gynecologists (ACOG) points out that although most abortion care is delivered as an outpatient, some cases need a hospital-based setting or access to surgical facilities. Abortion is an essential component of our healthcare system and a time-sensitive procedure. Any delay, whether days or weeks, has the potential to profoundly impact the health and well-being of women.

During the COVID-19 pandemic, access to safe abortion is compromised in public sector due to redeployment of health facilities and staffs while in private sector due to mandatory testing for COVID-19 infection and lack of resources, especially the protective gears for providers and patient care.

The findings indicate an improvement in abortion access with successive time periods. While 59% (nearly one million) of the total compromised abortions were during the first 40 days of the lockdown period, when the whole country was under the strictest conditions, the compromise is likely to reduce to 33% in the recovery period—in line with relaxations in government guidelines.

The compromise in abortion access due to COVID-19 and its management have a direct impact on the reproductive lives of women. Five possible results of compromising access to safe abortion could be the following:

1. There can be little delay, but women are able to access abortion as per their desire.
2. Women are able to access abortion; however, access might be delayed resulting in exceeding the permissible limit of 9 weeks. Thus, not as per their initial preference, but they might have to go for a facility-based surgical abortion.
3. Chances of second-trimester abortion (beyond 12 weeks) would increase.
4. Some would have to continue their unintended pregnancy.
5. Some would resort to unsafe abortions.

Access to an abortion is challenging, even at an approved facility during normal times. It becomes even more difficult if pregnancy exceeds 12 weeks. Thus, the healthcare system needs to gear up to meet the demands and needs to the women, especially during the pandemic. Our key recommendations:

Rapid mapping of facilities (public and private) to identify geographic distribution of those offering first- or second-trimester abortion.

- Assess the services provided by public and private sectors with respect to abortion, especially second-trimester abortion and strengthening the service.
- Informing about availability of services.
- Strengthening the referral linkages to enable women seeking abortion to access safe, legal services
- Streamlining the supply chain and ensuring availability of MA pills and contraceptives
- Including mechanisms to offset additional travel and out-of-pocket expenditure. Most importantly, we need continued advocacy with government and key stakeholders to prioritize the need to rapidly restore abortion services with focus on shifting needs of women.

Counseling protocol of safe abortion in the new normal after the SARS CoV2 pandemic:

- Initial counseling by phone
- Enquire for flu-like symptoms
- Discuss all the methods by video/teleconsultation
- Explain the procedure by video consultation
- Risk assessment
- Sexually transmitted infection (STI) risk assessment
- Explain side effects
- Take the mobile number of the patient
- Suggest and supply online reading material in local language
- Online consent if necessary (as suggested by local authorities)
- Consent can be sent and collected by phone
- Contact person on the day of appointment for flu-like symptoms
- Reduce contact time
- Take all precautions to avoid crowding, infection, and delay of procedures
- Ask the patient to wear a mask
- Reduce foot fall; patient has to come to clinic alone
- Maintain social distancing
- Stagger appointments
- Ask patient to wait outside if delay anticipated
- Healthcare worker (HCW) should wear personal protective equipment (PPE)
- Deep cleaning of waiting area and examination room after every patient
- Checklist and standard operating procedure (SOP) for complication.

KEY MESSAGES

- Unsafe abortion is third leading cause of maternal death in India.
- Abortion services were legalized in India in 1972.
- During the pandemic access to safe abortion will be needed more than usual.
- Approximately 1.85 million abortions were likely to be compromised due to COVID-19 pandemic.
- Continuation of access to safe abortion should be available in following ways-telemedicine, removal of unnecessary waiting periods, easy access of mifepristone and misoprostol, patient education initiatives and a digital media campaign highlighting the high margin of the safety of abortion both early and late in the pregnancy and the availability of abortion in different settings.

REFERENCES

1. Calculated estimates from RGI SRS 2001-03.
2. Duggal R, Ramachandran V. The abortion assessment project – India: key findings and recommendations. Reprod Health Matters. 2004;12:122-9.
3. Jha P, Kesler MA, Kumar R, Ram F, Ram U, Aleksandrowicz L, et al. Trends in selective abortions of girls in India: analysis of nationally representative birth histories from 1990 to 2005 and census data from 1991 to 2011. Lancet. 2011;377(9781):1921-8.
4. Ipas. Compromised abortion access due to COVID-19. [online] Available from: https://www.ipas.org/news/covid-19-restrictions-compromised-abortion-access-for-1-85-million-women-in-india/. [Last accessed November, 2021].
5. The Lancet. (2015). The incidence of abortion and unintended pregnancy in India, 2015. [online] Available from: https://www.thelancet.com/action/showPdf?pii=S2214-109X%2817%293. [Last accessed November, 2021].

LONG QUESTIONS

1. Describe MTP ACT and the recent amendments.
2. Describe the causative factors, prevention and management of unsafe abortion.

SHORT QUESTIONS

1. What is the protocol of safe abortion in new normal during COVID-19 pandemic?

2. Compromised access to safe abortion facilities may lead to which scenarios?

MULTIPLE CHOICE QUESTIONS

1. What percentage of maternal death in India is due to unsafe abortion?
   a. 10% b. 9%
   c. 8% d. 15%
2. As per recent census data, child sex ratio is:
   a. 918 females/1000 males
   b. 915 females/1000 males
   c. 907 females/ 1000 males
   d. 927 females/ 1000 males
3. Medical termination of pregnancy using mifepristone and misoprostol drugs has been legalized in India since:
   a. 2001 b. 1972
   c. 2003 d. 1971
4. Which of the following is included in the purview of MTP Act?
   a. Induced abortion
   b. Inevitable abortion
   c. Missed abortion
   d. Incomplete abortion
5. PNDT Act was renamed as PCPNDT in year:
   a. 1994 b. 2001
   c. 2003 d. 2005
6. Which of the following is not one of the reasons listed in the FORM I of the MTP ACT:
   a. Pregnancy is caused due to failure of contraceptive in married woman or her husband (presumed to constitute grave injury to mental health)
   b. Pregnancy is caused due to failure of contraceptive in woman (presumed to constitute grave injury to mental health)
   c. Pregnancy caused by rape
   d. Continuation of the pregnancy would involve a risk to the life of the pregnant woman or it may cause grave injury to her physical or mental health

7 MTP Act was passed by Parliament on:
   a. 10th August 1971 b. 10th August 1972
   c. 15th August 1971 d. 15th August 1972
8. Dose of ethacridine lactate for extra amniotic infusion for 2nd trimester abortion:
   a. 10 mL/week of gestation b. 11 mL/week of gestation
   c. 9 mL/week of gestation d. 15 mL/week of gestation
9. Which of the following are not used for cervical dilatation?
   a. Laminaria tents b. Misoprostol
   c. Metallic dilators d. Mifepristone
10. What are the maximum number of doses of misoprostol for medical abortion in misoprostol alone protocol?
   a. 3 b. 6
   c. 4 d. 5
11. Who cannot perform MTP? In the case of a medical practitioner, who was registered in a State Medical Register after the commencement of the Act and:
   a. Has completed one months of house surgency in gynecology and obstetrics
   b. Has experience in any hospital for a period of not less than one year in the practice of obstetrics and gynecology
   c. Holds a postgraduate degree or diploma in gynecology and obstetrics
   d. Has assisted an RMP in the performance of 25 cases of MTP of which at least five have been performed independently, in a hospital established or maintained by the government, or a training institute approved for this purpose by the Government
12. Access to safe abortion during pandemic can be in following ways, except:
   a. Teleconsultation
   b. Call all the patients at same time
   c. Patient education initiative
   d. Digital media campaign

Answers

1.	c	2.	a	3.	b	4.	a	5.	c	6.	b
7.	a	8.	a	9.	d	10.	d	11.	a	12.	b

Permanent Contraception

4.1 MALE STERLIZATION INCLUDING NONSCALPEL VASECTOMY: METHODS AND STRATEGIES TO IMPROVE ACCEPTANCE

Phiroze Soonawala

INTRODUCTION

Vasectomy is currently the most effective form of contraception. It was first described to sterilize dogs by Sir Ashley Cooper in 1827 and used a few years later in humans. Dr Li Shunqiang described the nonscalpel vasectomy (NSV) from China in 1974, which greatly helped to increase the acceptability of vasectomy worldwide. Approximately 5% of married couples worldwide use this method. There is a wide variation in acceptance of vasectomy, peaking in Bhutan (up to 40%), followed by New Zealand (25%), UK (20%), and the United States (up to 10%).[1] The Indian government launched the national NSV project in 1998, following which the prevalence of vasectomy in India increased from 0.7% in 1997 to about 3% in 2003. Subsequently, it has declined and current NSV acceptance in India is approximately 0.3%.[2]

SURGICAL ANATOMY (FIG. 1)

The vas deferens is a 3–5-mm thick tube, with a characteristic cord such as feel, running in the spermatic cord. It is adjacent to the vasal artery and surrounded by a thin vas sheath. The vas in its sheath and the other components of the spermatic cord (testicular artery, pampiniform venous plexus, testicular nerves, genital branch of the genitofemoral nerve, and lymphatics) are all contained in the spermatic fascia. Gentle manipulation can separate the vas from the surrounding structures, allowing easy dissection without risk to adjacent vessels and nerves.

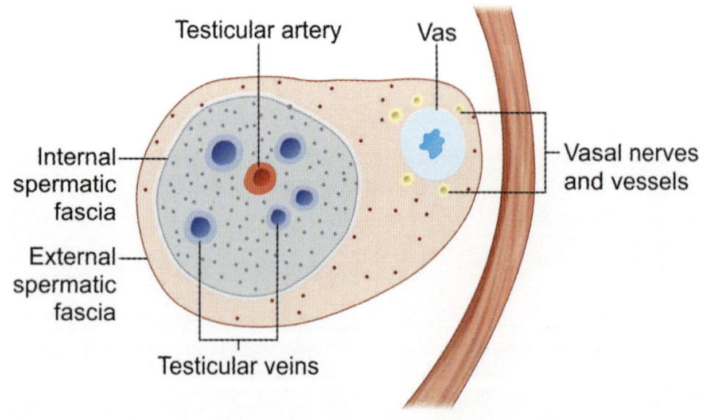

Fig. 1: Surgical anatomy.

Preoperative Evaluation

Detailed counseling should include other contraceptive options, the permanence of the procedure, the small but present risk of failure, and possible complications. It is preferable for both partners to participate in the counseling. Though not mandatory, the last child should be at least 6–12 months old and in good health. Despite success rates of 80–90% for vasectomy reversal, it should not be planning for future reversal. The procedure, including anesthesia, should be clearly explained. Since it will not be effective immediately, the need to continue contraception for at least 3 months should be emphasized.

Check history for any allergies, bleeding diatheses, and ongoing medications. A thorough physical examination of the genitalia is required. Unusually thickened cords, large scrotal hernia, or hydrocele can make the surgery difficult.

Nonscalpel Vasectomy: The Li Technique

Vasectomy is normally performed as an outpatient procedure under local anesthesia. It is best performed through a single midline puncture in the upper scrotum. However, bilateral punctures directly over each vas can be used for thickened or adherent cords, three instruments critical for the nonscalpel technique are the ringed vas forceps, fine pointed vas forceps, and fine grasping clamp **(Fig. 2)**. Vasectomy is performed in the upper scrotum where the vas is easily palpable. Infiltrate 2% plain lignocaine (without adrenaline) through a

26-g needle. A small dermal bleb is raised for local anesthesia in the midline raphe. The needle is then advanced, and 1–2 cc is injected immediately around each vas for vasal block. A total of 5 cc is usually adequate. Gentle pressure for 1 minute after infiltration minimizes cord hematomas.

With the fingers of the nondominant hand, the vas is manipulated, brought just under the midline scrotal raphe, and fixed there with the vas ring forceps. The same hand isolates the vas from the other cord structures, displacing them laterally. The scrotal skin is punctured directly over the vas with the pointed vas dissection forceps **(Fig. 3A)**, and the hole enlarged to 5–6 mm by gently spreading the jaws **(Fig. 3B)**. The vas will be visible in the depth of the skin opening. One jaw of the pointed forceps is pierced into the vas and the jaws are gently closed to grip the vas. The ring forceps is released and the vas is pulled out of the scrotum with a twisting movement of the pointed forceps **(Figs. 3C and D)**.

The vas is then separated from its sheath to ensure that only bare vas, devoid of vessels and nerves, is ligated. Usually, it is divided and both ends doubly tied with 3-0 silk **(Fig. 4A)**. Interposition of vasal fascia between the cut ends of the vas reduces failures resulting from recanalization **(Fig. 4B)**. Cautery occlusion of the lumen **(Fig. 4C)** or metal clips can also be used instead. Excision of a length of vas is not necessary and can make future reversal more difficult. Open-ended vasectomy (occluding only the abdominal end and leaving the testicular end open) can reduce postoperative testicular pain but is associated with more failures and is not advisable. Following the occlusion, the two ends of vas are carefully inspected for hemostasis and then pulled back into the scrotum. The procedure is repeated on the opposite side through the same midline puncture. After the vasectomy, the skin puncture does not require sutures and is sealed by gently crushing the edges together with a fine Allis forceps. A small Band-Aid or adhesive dressing is applied.

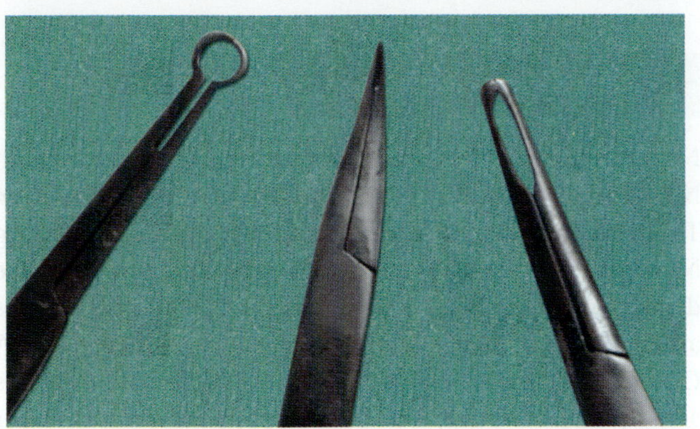

Fig. 2: Nonscalpel vasectomy instruments.

Nonscalpel Vasectomy: Modified Technique

The traditional Li technique has some drawbacks. Unlike Orientals, Indian men often have thicker and rugose scrotal skin. Fixing the vas under the skin with the ringed forceps is difficult in a thick-walled scrotum. Also, the hooking maneuver with the pointed forceps does not give a secure hold on the vas, which often slips out. This maneuver can tear or transect a thin vas. These pitfalls are overcome in the following technique.

The vas is brought to the midline of the scrotum and fixed under the skin using three fingers of the left/nondominant hand **(Fig. 5A)**. The pointed vas forceps then punctures the skin over the vas. The jaws are gently spread to create a track up to the vas with a diameter of about 5–6 mm **(Fig. 5B)**.

The ring vas holding clamp is passed through this aperture, to grip the vas and pull it to the surface **(Fig. 5C)**. This gives a very secure grip on the vas, without the risk of tearing or transection. Under direct vision, the vas fascia is separated off the vas with the pointed forceps, to bare a 1.5 cm length of vas. Vas occlusion is then completed as usual.

Postoperative Care

Though many centers do not routinely use any antibiotic prophylaxis, 3 days of postprocedure antibiotic is advised. No scrotal support is necessary but a snug-fitting undergarment helps prevent discomfort. Light activity can resume immediately but strenuous activity is restricted for 2 weeks. Sexual activity can resume after 1–2 weeks. The dressing is removed after 24–48 hours, after which the area can be left open and a full bath can resume.

A semen analysis must be done after 3 months (or 20 ejaculations) to confirm azoospermia.

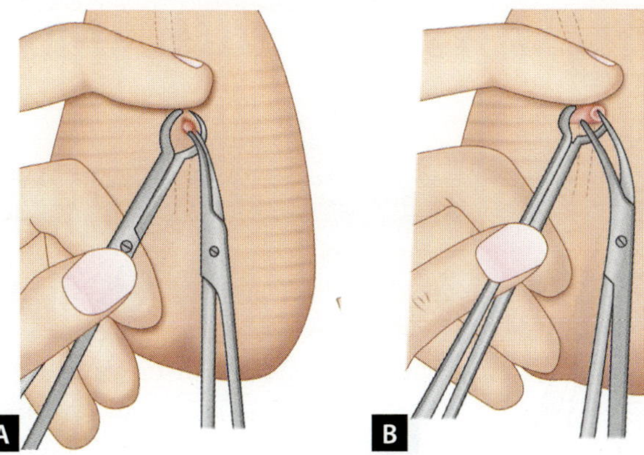

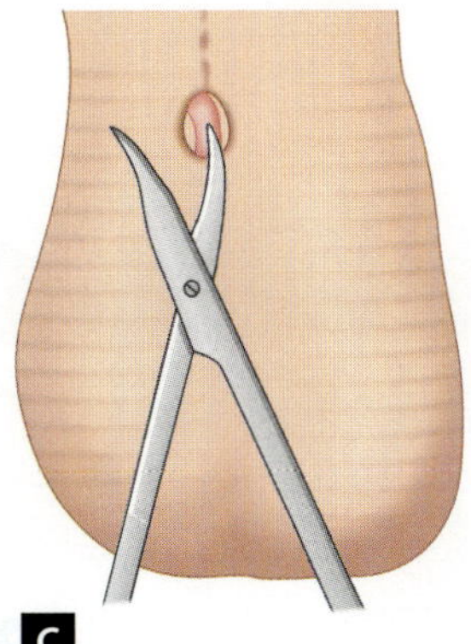

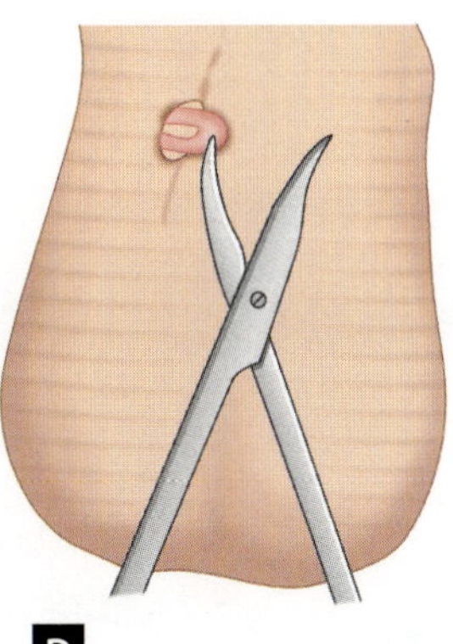

Figs. 3A to D: Vas retrieval in nonscalpel vasectomy as described by Li Shunqiang.

EFFECTIVENESS OF NONSCALPEL VASECTOMY

Vasectomy has the lowest failure rate of all the family planning methods presently available. Pregnancy rates after NSV are about 0.5%, with a range of 0–2%. The US Collaborative Review of Sterilization reports a 9.4 and 11.3 cumulative probability of failure per 1,000 cases at 1 and 5 years after vasectomy respectively.[3] Early failures are usually due to unprotected coitus before azoospermia is achieved. Late failure, seen as persistence of motile sperm in semen, is usually due to inadequate initial occlusion or early vas recanalization. The couple is advised to continue using contraception and repeat the semen every 6–8 weeks. The majority will gradually become azoospermic over time. Persistence of motile sperm beyond 6 months should warrant redoing the vasectomy.

Other late failures, indicating reappearance of motile sperm after initial confirmation of azoospermia, are rarer. These are only detected after an accidental pregnancy occurs and will need repeating the vasectomy.

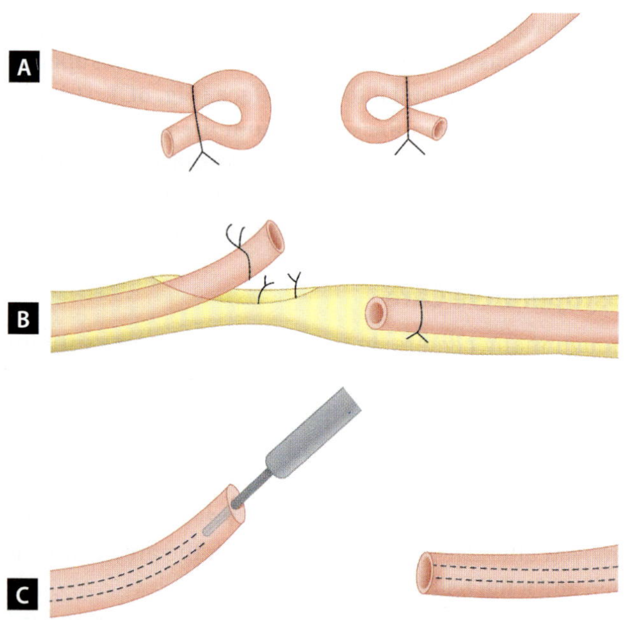

Figs. 4A to C: Common methods of vas occlusion.

EARLY COMPLICATIONS

Infection, bleeding, hematoma formation, and epididymitis are the most common and are largely dependent on operator experience. Bleeding or hematomas are seen in up to 4.6% for those performing <10 vasectomies annually and in <1.6% of those performing over 50 annually.[4] Most complications are minor.

LATE COMPLICATIONS

Chronic scrotal pain, starting weeks to sometimes years after the vasectomy, is seen in 0.4–5.1% and is the most vexing complication.[5] This results from obstructive epididymal dilatation and congestion and occasional sperm extravasation and granuloma formation. It is usually dull and resolves with time. Treatment is with scrotal support, analgesics, and antibiotics.

Antisperm antibodies are reported in 50–70% of men after vasectomy.[6] These do not require treatment but can adversely affect pregnancy rates after vasectomy reversal.

Earlier concerns of increased risk of atherosclerosis and cardiovascular disease following vasectomy have been proven to be unfounded.[7-9] Several epidemiologic studies have revealed an elevated risk of prostate cancer following vasectomy.[10] However, the majority evidence suggests no significant causative relationship between vasectomy and prostate cancer.[11,12]

Vasectomy does not have any effect on ejaculation, erectile capacity, or the male hormones.

NONSCALPEL VERSUS TRADITIONAL INCISIONAL VASECTOMY

Numerous studies now confirm that the complications with NSV are substantially lower. A large study of 1,203 cases from Thailand showed complications in 0.4% of men following NSV compared to 3.1% after incisional vasectomy.[13] Since dissection is minimal and perivasal nerves and vessels are untouched, pain and bleeding are substantially less. A Cochrane database review showed that while both methods are equally effective, the nonscalpel method has fewer complications and shorter operating times.[14] The lack of an

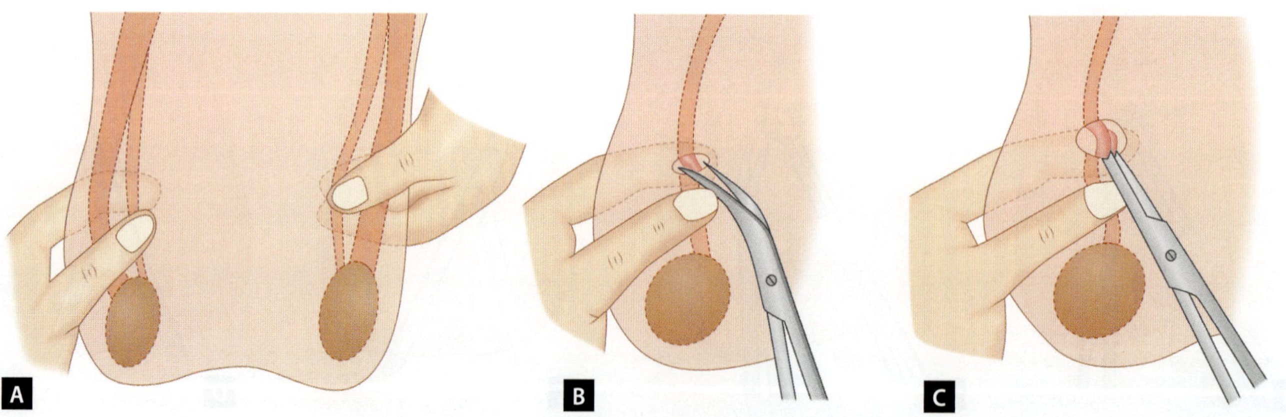

Figs. 5A to C: Nonscalpel vasectomy: Modified technique.

incision also makes it psychologically more acceptable to many men. Since no skin sutures are required, postoperative care is minimal and no dressings or suture removal is required, unlike the incisional procedure.

MALE STERILIZATION VERSUS FEMALE STERILIZATION

While tubal occlusion is far more popular than vasectomy, as a procedure, vasectomy is simpler, safer, cheaper, and probably more effective **(Table 1)**.

ALTERNATIVE METHODS OF VAS OCCLUSION

Various noninvasive methods of sealing the vas have described in an attempt to avoid surgery and make vasectomy more widely acceptable. The most common is by percutaneous injection of sclerosing agents into the vas lumen. Percutaneous insertion of a fine bipolar diathermy probe and injections of silicon-based elastomer to seal the vas lumen are also used. These are safe and associated with minimal morbidity. However, they are technically demanding as blind cannulation of the vas lumen requires considerable skill and training. Complete azoospermia is sometimes not achieved in a single attempt and they often need to be repeated. Since a variable length of vas is obstructed, there are also concerns about future reversibility. Hence, other than China, these alternatives are not commonly used in most parts of the world.

VASECTOMY REVERSAL

Less than 2% of vasectomized men will request a reversal for various reasons. Vasectomy reversal is easier and more successful than reversal following tubal ligation. Reversal is a delicate surgery, requiring training and microsurgical skill, and should be performed only by specialists.

It is usually performed under spinal or general anesthetic. The scrotum is explored and the site of vas occlusion is mobilized. The two cut ends of vas are carefully freed, preserving the vasal artery. Patency of the abdominal end of the vas is confirmed by gentle injection of 3 cc normal saline via a 24-g cannula in the vas lumen. Patency of the testicular end is checked by seeing spermatic fluid oozing from it. Microscopic examination of the fluid should reveal spermatozoa. The ends are then approximated using six to eight sutures of 9-0 or 10-0 Ethilon in a single layer, tension-free anastomosis. A double-layer anastomosis, though technically more demanding, is preferred when there is substantial disparity in the lumen of the two vas ends.

The success of reversal declines the longer it is performed after vasectomy. The Vasovasostomy Study Group reported patency rates of 97%, 88%, 79%, and 71% for reversals done <3 years, 3–8 years, 9–14 years, and beyond 15 years after vasectomy, respectively. However, pregnancy rates were only 76%, 53%, 44%, and 30% for the same periods.[15] Pregnancy rates significantly lower than patency rates have been attributed to testicular dysfunction and epididymal obstructions secondary to prolonged vas obstruction and antisperm antibodies.

TABLE 1: Vasectomy versus tubal ligation.

	Vasectomy	*Tubal ligation*
Anesthesia	Local	General
Training	Easier	More training required
Morbidity	Minimal	More (peritoneum opened)
Cost	Cheaper	More costly
Failure rate	<1–2% Most failures detectable by semen test at 3 months	1–2% Failures detected after accidental pregnancy
Reversal	Easier, more successful	More difficult, success lower

KEY MESSAGES

- Vasectomy is one of the most effective method of contraception with failures in only 1%.
- Despite this, it is underutilized, with a prevalence of <3% in India.
- It is a simple and quick procedure and can be performed under local anesthesia in any clinic setting.
- The modified NSV procedure uses the ringed vas forceps to pull the vas out of the scrotum. This is often easier to learn and perform.
- It is safe with minimal morbidity. Persistent testicular pain (in <5%) is the only common postprocedure complaint.
- Microsurgical reversal of vasectomy gives excellent results in experienced hands. However, the results decline with time after vasectomy.

REFERENCES

1. Pile JM, Barone MA. Demographics of vasectomy – USA and international. Urol Clin North Am. 2009;36:295-305.
2. International Institute for Population Sciences (IIPS), ICF. National Family Health Survey (NFHS-4), 2015-16. Mumbai: IPS; 2017.
3. Jamieson DJ, Costello C, Trussell J, Hillis SD, Marchbanks PA, Peterson HB. The risk of pregnancy after vasectomy. Obstet Gynecol. 2004;103:848-50.
4. Forste R, Tanfer K, Tedrow L. Sterilization among currently married men in the United States. Fam Plann Perspect. 1995; 27:100-7.
5. Raspa RF. Complications of vasectomy. Am Fam Physician. 1993;48(7):1264-8.
6. Ansbacher R. Sperm-agglutinating and sperm-immobilising antibodies in vasectomized men. Fertil Steril. 1971;22:629-32.
7. Walker AM, Jick H, Hunter JR, Danford A, Rothman KJ. Hospitalization rates in vasectomized men. JAMA. 1981; 245(22): 2315-7.
8. Alexander NJ, Senner JW, Hoch EJ. Evaluation of blood pressure in vasectomized and non-vasectomized men. Int J Epidemiol. 1981;10(3):217-22.

9. Goldacre MJ, Holford TR, Vessey MP. Cardiovascular disease and vasectomy: findings from two epidemiologic studies. N Engl J Med. 1983;308(14):805-8.
10. Giovannucci E, Ascherio A, Rimm EB, Colditz GA, Stampfer MJ, Willett WC. A prospective cohort study of vasectomy and prostate cancer in US men. JAMA. 1993;269(7):873-7.
11. John EM, Whittemore AS, Wu AH, Kolonel LN, Hislop TG, Howe GR, et al. Vasectomy and prostate cancer: results from a multiethnic case-control study. J Natl Canc Inst. 1995;87(9): 662-9.
12. Hayes RB. Are dietary fat and vasectomy risk factors for prostate cancer? J Natl Canc Inst. 1995;87(9):629-31.
13. Nirapathpongporn A, Huber DH, Krieger JN. No-scalpel vasectomy at the King's birthday vasectomy festival. Lancet. 1990;335(8694):894-5.
14. Cook LA, Pun A, van Vliet H, Gallo MF, Lopez LM. Scalpel versus no-scalpel incision for vasectomy. Cochrane Database Syst Rev. 2007;(2):CD004112.
15. Belker AM, Thomas AJ Jr, Fuchs EF, Konnak JW, Sharlip ID. Results of 1469 microsurgical vasectomy reversals by the Vasovasostomy Study Group. J Urol. 1991;145(3):505-11.

LONG QUESTIONS

1. What are the surgical principles of Vasectomy? What are the pros and cons of NSV over the conventional technique?
2. A man has undergone a vasectomy 2 years ago. Due to an accident, the couple have lost both their children. The couple is 34 years old. They wish to have another child. What is the approach and choices available for this couple?

SHORT QUESTIONS

1. A married couple has completed their family and approaches you for permanent contraception. Which method would you advise and why?
2. Describe in brief the technique of nonscalpel vasectomy.

MULTIPLE CHOICE QUESTIONS

1. Nonscalpel vasectomy has an overall failure rate of:
   a. <1% b. 2—4%
   c. 4–7%
2. Microsurgical reversal of a vasectomy done 10 years earlier will result in pregnancies in:
   a. 80–90% of cases
   b. 60–80% of cases
   c. 40–60% of cases
3. Which of the following is true about NSV?
   a. Libido is usually reduced after vasectomy
   b. Erectile dysfunction is common after vasectomy
   c. Ejaculation is lost after vasectomy
   d. All of the above
   e. None of the above
4. Since vasectomy has a very low failure rate, following the procedure, the couple can resume unprotected sex after:
   a. 1 week b. 1 month
   c. 3 months d. 6 months
5. The lowest failure rates are achieved with vas occlusion by:
   a. Ligation with silk
   b. Double ligation of both vas ends
   c. Diathermy of the vas lumen
   d. Ligation followed by fascial interposition between the vas ends
6. Which of the following are absolute contraindications for performing a nonscalpel vasectomy?
   a. Large hydrocele
   b. Hernia
   c. Filariasis of the cord
   d. Hypertension
   e. None of the above
   f. All of the above
7. Local anesthesia for NSV is given using:
   a. 2% lignocaine without adrenaline
   b. 2% lignocaine with adrenaline
   c. 0.5% bupivacaine without adrenaline
   d. 0.5% bupivacaine with adrenaline

Answers

1. a 2. c 3. e 4. c 5. d 6. e
7. a

4.2 FEMALE STERILIZATION: STANDARDS, SURGICAL APPROACHES, AND TECHNIQUES

Madhuri Mehendale, Shraddha Mevada

INTRODUCTION

Female sterilization is one of the most practiced and effective permanent methods of contraception. It is highly effective, safe, and has comparatively very few side effects.

According to Health Management Information System (HMIS) 2013-2014 data, in India, more than 4.1 million female sterilization procedures are done annually.[1]

ELIGIBILITY CRITERIA OF WHO CAN PERFORM FEMALE STERILIZATION[2]

- Female sterilization by the method of minilap tubectomy should be performed by an MBBS designated doctor who is trained in it.
- Laparoscopic sterilization method should be performed by a gynecologist with DGO/MD/MS qualification or a

surgeon holding an MS degree, and he/she should have been trained and certified in laparoscopic sterilization.

CLIENT ELIGIBILITY CRITERIA (TABLES 1 AND 2)

- The female must have been married.
- The age of the female clients should be below 49 years and above 22 years.
- The client should have at least one child, whose age is above 1 year.
- Females or their partners must not have undergone any sterilization procedure in the past.
- The client must be in a normal state of mind so as to understand the full implications of sterilization.
- A psychiatrist-certified document must be taken for unsound clients.

TIMING OF THE PROCEDURE

- Within 7 days of the menstrual period—interval sterilization is performed.
- 48 hours up to 7 days of delivery—postpartum sterilization
- Along with medical termination of pregnancy (MTP), female sterilization can be performed simultaneously.
- In case of spontaneous abortion, it can be performed provided the medical eligibility criteria are fulfilled.

It is advised not to do laparoscopic tubal ligation simultaneously with second-trimester abortion or in the postpartum period.

The steps for preparation for surgery are as follows: counseling, preoperative assessment, preoperative instructions, and postoperative care.

COUNSELING

Counseling is the process of helping the client make informed and voluntary decisions about fertility. Before the client signs the consent form, the following should be informed about the following:

- Among all the available methods of contraceptions, tubal ligation operation is a permanent one.
- A voluntarily informed decision should be made by the female.
- Counseling should be done in the language they understand.
- They should be informed about side effects or potential complications.
- They should be informed that it does not affect sexual pleasure or performance and does not protect against reproductive tract infection (RTI)/sexually transmitted infection (STI)/human immunodeficiency virus (HIV); reversal of surgery, if required, involves a major surgery and it is not 100% guaranteed.

CLINICAL EXAMINATION AND SCREENING OF CLIENTS

Prior to the surgery, menstrual and obstetrics history, general examination, and laboratory tests as required should be done.

INFORMED CONSENT

- Consent for sterilization should not be taken under coercion or when the client is under sedation.
- Client must sign the consent form for sterilization before the surgery.
- The consent of the spouse is not required for sterilization operation. The consent form should be in English and in local language.

SURGICAL APPROACHES TO FEMALE STERILIZATION

Two Approaches in Minilap Tubectomy (Fig. 1)

1. *Subumbilical approach* is used in the immediate postpartum period and within 7 days of childbirth (postpartum sterilization).
2. *Suprapubic approach* is used for interval minilap tubectomy.

Presurgery Checkup in Postpartum Sterilization

- Antenatal counseling and assessment for postpartum sterilization before arriving at the center for delivery are must.
- The condition of the newborn should be taken into consideration. The sterilization procedure can be postponed up to a week after delivery if the health of the newborn is not good.

TABLE 1: : WHO categories of medical eligibility criteria for contraceptive use.

Accept (A)	There is no medical reason to deny the method to a person with this condition or in this circumstance. The procedure can be performed in most clinical settings
Caution (C)	The method is normally provided in a routine setting but with extra preparation and precautions as required
Delay (D)	Provision of the method should be delayed or postponed. These conditions need to be evaluated, treated, and resolved before female sterilization can be performed. Alternatively, temporary methods of contraception should be provided
Special (S)	Certain women have conditions that make operation difficult or increase the risks. The procedure should be undertaken in a setting with an experienced surgeon and staff, equipment needed to provide general anesthesia and other back-up medical support. The capacity to decide on the most appropriate procedure and anesthesia support is also needed. Alternatively, temporary methods of contraception should be provided if referral is required or there is otherwise any delay

TABLE 2: Check list of medical eligibility criteria for female sterilization.

Caution	*Delay*	*Special*
Previous abdominal or pelvic surgery	Severe iron deficiency anemia (hemoglobin <7 g/dL)	Conditions that increase chances of heart disease or stroke, i.e., older age, smoking, high BP, or diabetes
Obesity	Current pregnancy	Blood pressure > 160/100 mm Hg
Controlled BP (140–159/90–99 mm Hg)	8–42 days postpartum	Complicated heart disease
Uncomplicated heart disease	Pregnancy with severe preeclampsia or eclampsia	Coagulation disorders
History of ischemic heart disease	Postpartum or postabortion complications (infection, hemorrhage, and trauma)	Chronic lung diseases (asthma or emphysema)
Stroke	Current DVT/PE	Endometriosis
History of cerebrovascular accident	Major surgery with prolonged immobilization	Pelvic tuberculosis
History of deep vein thrombosis or pulmonary embolism	Abdominal skin infections	Fixed uterus due to previous surgery or infection
Epilepsy	Current ischemic heart disease	Abdominal wall or umbilical hernia
Depressive disorders	Lung disease-like pneumonia	Postpartum or postabortion uterine rupture or perforation
Current breast cancer	Systemic infection	Diabetes of 20 years standing with organ damage
Uterine fibroids	Unexplained vaginal bleeding	Hyperthyroidism

(BP: blood pressure; DVT: deep vein thrombosis; PE: pulmonary embolism)

- The client should be nil by mouth for solid foods for 6 hours and liquids for 4 hours before surgery.

Positioning for surgery: Dorsal supine position.

Abdominal Preparation

The operative incision site should be cleaned with an antiseptic solution, preferably iodophor (povidone iodine) or chlorhexidine gluconate.

Alcohol preparations should not be applied to the sensitive genitalia.

Selecting Incision Site

The incision should be taken beneath the umbilicus, just below the upper border of the palpable postpartum uterus.

After late second-trimester abortion, incision for simultaneous sterilization should be just at the level of the palpable fundus of the uterus.

Abdominal Entry

Approximately a 2–3 cm transverse incision is taken. The fallopian tube is identified by its fimbriated end.

The procedure of ligation and excision of the tube is done by a modified Pomeroy technique which is the most commonly used method for minilap tubectomy.

The basic principles of the modified Pomeroy technique are as follows:

- A Babcock forceps is used to grasp and elevate a 2-cm loop of tube at its midsection (the isthmic portion), approximately 2–3 cm from the cornual portion of the tube.

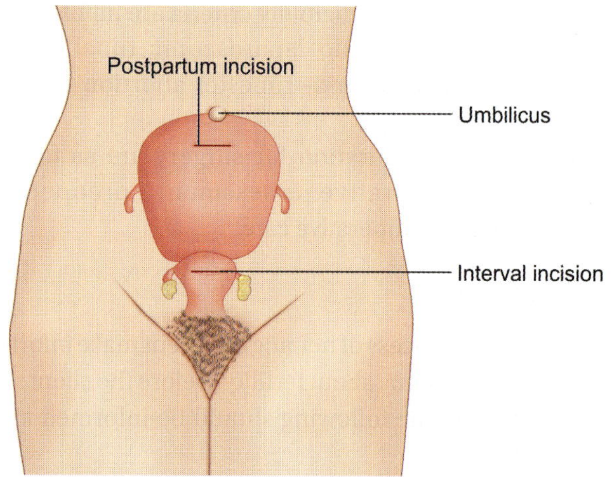

Fig. 1: Incision site landmarks in postpartum and interval abdominal tubectomy.

- A loop of the fallopian tube at an avascular area of the mesosalpinx is made.
- The next step includes placing a knot using absorbable suture, usually chromic gut, around the loop to occlude the lumen of the tube and excise a portion of the loop of the tube above the ligature to separate the two limbs of the loop so that the lumen is not connected. A similar procedure is repeated on the other side.

Suprapubic Approach in Interval Minilap Tubectomy

Incision site: The best area for the suprapubic incision is usually 2–3 cm (or 1 inch) above the border of the pubis.

Surgical Procedure: Laparoscopic Tubal Occlusion

Laparoscopic tubal occlusion is done during the "interval" phase or after first-trimester abortions.

Steps for Laparoscopic Tubal Occlusion

Preoperative steps: It has to be made sure that high-level disinfected laparoscopic instruments, fiberoptic cable, and insufflator tubing are working.

The client is given a lithotomy position. A bimanual pelvic examination is performed to assess uterine size, position, mobility, and contour of the uterus and whether there is any pelvic abnormality.

Creating Pneumoperitoneum

- The client is in a Trendelenburg position of not more than 20°.
- A small incision at the inferior umbilical margin is made.
- The shaft of the Veress needle is grasped and inserted at a 45° caudal angle to the abdominal wall. Two distinct "gives" are felt as the fascia is penetrated and the peritoneum is entered.
- Check for correct abdominal entry by placing a drop of the anesthetic on the opening of the Luer lock of the Veress needle and observing its ingress when the abdominal wall is lifted manually. Introduce carbon dioxide at the rate of 1 L/min and make sure that intra-abdominal pressure should not exceed 15 mm of mercury. The Veress needle after insufflating 1.5–2.0 L of CO_2 is removed.

LAPAROSCOPE-GUIDED TUBAL OCCLUSION

The posterior limb of the prong under is placed in the inferior aspect of the tube about 4 cm away from the cornu. Slowly, the operating slide is pushed aside to increase the forceps tongs and the occluded fallopian tube is released. Adequacy of occlusion, i.e., a 2-cm loop of tube just above the Falope ring, showing the acute angle in mesosalpinx is checked and any active bleeding, if present, is seen.

Now, place two ring adaptors in no. 2 position. In order to occlude the other tube, the same steps are repeated. The laparoscope is removed from the abdominal cavity under direct vision and the wound is sutured and cleaned followed by a small dressing.

Postoperative Care

The client should be kept under observation and may be discharged after 4 hours of procedure, when the vital clinical signs are normal and she has passed urine and can talk and walk.

During Discharge

The following postoperative instructions must be provided.

The client should:

- Take adequate rest on the same day and resume light work after 48 hours
- Make sure to avoid heavy weightlifting or putting tension on the incision for at least 1 week
- Be able to resume all activities within 1 week after surgery
- Bathe after 24 hours after the surgery
- In case of excessive pain, fever, bleeding, or pus discharge from the incision, not passing urine, flatus, and bloating of abdomen, the doctor should be notified
- If there is no period even until 2 weeks of expected date of periods then return immediately for ruling out pregnancy.

Follow-up

The first follow-up contact should be within 48 hours after the discharge.

The next follow-up visit should happen on the seventh day after surgery.

Subsequent follow-up visit should be made after 1 month.

CERTIFICATE OF FEMALE STERILIZATION

A certificate of female sterilization should be issued 1 month after the surgery or after the next menstrual period by the medical officer of the facility.

COMPLICATIONS

Female sterilization procedures are safe and very few women experience complications.

Complications occur in less than 2% of all cases, and serious complications are rare.[3] If complications are immediately and accurately diagnosed and effectively treated, the morbidity rate is low.

Complications can be classified as follows:

Intraoperative Complications

- Vasovagal attack
- Respiratory depression or cardiac arrest
- Cardiac arrest
- Convulsions to local anesthesia
- Gas embolism
- Uterine perforation
- Bleeding from the mesosalpinx
- Injury involving urinary bladder
- Injury to bowel and blood vessels.

Postoperative Complications

- Wound site sepsis
- Hematoma involving abdominal wall

- Intestinal obstruction
- Surgical site incisional hernia.

All complications, major or minor, arising during surgery or postsurgery must be reported to the district quality assurance committee.

REFERENCES

1. Manual of Female Sterilization. Family Planning Division, Ministry of Health and Family Welfare, National Heath Mission, Government of India, 2014.
2. World Health Organization. Medical eligibility criteria (MEC) and conditions for female sterilization. In Family Planning: A Global Handbook for Providers. Geneva: WHO; 2011.
3. Standards of Male and Female Sterilization Services, Ministry of Health and Family Welfare, Government of India.

LONG QUESTIONS

1. Describe the anatomy of fallopian tubes. Explain various surgical approaches of tubal ligation.
2. What are the short- and long-term complications of tubal ligation? Enumerate and explain their management and reporting?

SHORT QUESTIONS

1. Write a note on eligibility of providers for tubal ligation.
2. Enumerate case-selection criteria for tubal ligation.
3. Explain discharge and follow-up policy in operated cases of tubal ligation.

MULTIPLE CHOICE QUESTIONS

1. Which among them is an irreversible method of contraception?
   a. Levonorgestrel-releasing intrauterine system (LNG-IUD)
   b. Implanon
   c. Copper-T
   d. Laparoscopic tubal ligation
2. Fimbriectomy is also known as:
   a. Pomeroy technique
   b. Uchida's technique
   c. Kroener's technique
   d. Irving's technique
3. During Pomeroy technique of female sterilization, which portion of the tube is ligated?
   a. Isthmo-ampullary
   b. Ampullary
   c. Isthmus
   d. Corneal
4. Which of the following is not an abdominal laparoscopic technique for tubal ligation?
   a. Pomeroy
   b. Parkland
   c. Essure
   d. Irving
5. Which of the following is incorrect?
   a. Certificate of sterilization is issued 1 month after the surgery
   b. All complications should be reported to district quality assurance committee
   c. Patient should stay admitted after procedure for 24 hours
   d. Histopathology of the removed tubal part is not mandatory
6. In which of the following conditions should the tubal ligation be delayed?
   a. Hemoglobin less than 7 g%
   b. Uterine fibroids
   c. Uncomplicated heart disease
   d. BP > 140/90 mm Hg
7. In which of the following can tubal ligation be done?
   a. 35-year-old female, unmarried, one child, >5 years
   b. 20-year-old female, married, one child, >3 years
   c. 35-year-old female, married, one child, 6 months
   d. 28-Year-old female, married, one child, 2 years
8. Which of the following is not true for puerperal tubal ligation?
   a. Suprapubic incision
   b. To be done within 7 days postpartum
   c. Laparotomy
   d. None of the above
9. Laparoscopic tubal ligation can be performed by all, except:
   a. MS obstetrics and gynecology
   b. MD obstetrics and gynecology
   c. DGO
   d. Registered medical practitioner
10. Which patient needs referral to a higher center for tubal ligation?
    a. Previous abdominal surgeries
    b. Patient with obesity
    c. Known case of epilepsy
    d. BP > 160/100 mm Hg
11. Which of the following is not a prerequisite for tubal ligation?
    a. Patient should sign consent before surgery
    b. Consent of spouse is mandatory
    c. Unsound clients should be certified by psychiatrist
    d. Consent should be in English and local language

Answers

1.	d	2.	c	3.	c	4.	d	5.	c	6.	a
7.	d	8.	a	9.	d	10.	d	11.	b		

4.3 STERILIZATION FAILURE

Kiran Pandey, Pavika Lal

INTRODUCTION

Female sterilization is one of *the most common and most accepted procedures* performed worldwide mainly on healthy women at their request with the intention to occlude both fallopian tubes.[1] The most popular method of female sterilization is the *laparoscopic tubal occlusion through the application of a mechanical device* (Filshie clip, Hulka clip, or Falope ring) or electrocautery. The most common and preferred technique of sterilization which is performed during cesarean delivery and minilaparotomy is Pomeroy's method. Other related techniques (Uchida, Parkland, Kroner's Madlener, etc.) are rarely performed now a days.

Almost 5–6 million sterilization procedures are performed annually contributing to 98% of all sterilizations and roughly 62% of all contraceptive use, and majority of these (83%) have availed this service from government sector.[2]

INCIDENCE OF FAILURE RATE

Conception after sterilization is termed failure of sterilization and can occur several years after the procedure; one such case was described after an interval of 23 years.[3] According to international sources, pregnancy can occur in 1 in 200; *the estimated failure rate is 0.1–0.8% especially in the 1st year after tubal sterilization.*[2] Two large population-based studies have reported the 10-year cumulative probability of pregnancy of 18.5 per 1,000 procedures and 8 per 1,000 procedures.[4,5] The rate of failure is highest for *Hulka clip sterilization and lowest for postpartum partial salpingectomies.* Wide differences in sterilization failure rate are due to variations in the following:[6]

- *Woman's characteristics* (age and time interval from the procedure)—women younger than 28 years at the time of sterilization are at higher risk of failure for all methods as compared to women older than 34 years except for interval partial salpingectomy
- Operator experience and operating center
- Sterilization technique
- Time interval to resume the sexual activity poststerilization and its frequency
- Pre-existing gynecological pathology.

RELATIVE RISK OF STERILIZATION FAILURE BY METHOD[4]

Relative risk of sterilization failure by method is given in **Table 1**.

TABLE 1: Relative risk of sterilization failure by method.

Method	Relative risk
Postpartum partial salpingectomy	1.0
Unipolar coagulation	1.5
Silicone rubber band application (Falope ring)	2.3
Bipolar coagulation	3.2
Spring clip application (Hulka clip)	3.7

MECHANISM OF FAILURE

The mechanism of sterilization failure still remains unanswered. If the mechanism of failure is due to "tubal non-occlusion" or "wrong structure sterilization," these are considered negligent mechanisms, whereas "spontaneous tubal recanalization" or "fistula formation" mechanisms of failure are considered non-negligent. A shorter interval to failure is suggestive of negligent failure, whereas a longer time interval may be predictive of spontaneous tubal recanalization or fistula formation.

FACTORS CONTRIBUTING TO FAILURE

- *Timing of procedure*: Sterilization performed during postpartum or postabortion period is associated with higher rates of failure as compared to interval ligation.[7,8]
- *Pregnant at the time of the sterilization*: Luteal pregnancy can occur in 0.32–0.6% of sterilization cases;[9] therefore, it is very essential that interval ligation should be done between 5th and 10th day of the menstrual cycle. If performed at any other time of the menstrual cycle, effective contraception should be advised before and after the procedure and up to her next menstrual cycle to avoid luteal phase pregnancy.
- *Type of procedure*: Studies have shown no significant difference in failure rate or operative morbidity between minilaparotomy and laparoscopy approach of tubal sterilization, but the failure rate for both methods approximates to each other in recent studies.[10-12] Unipolar coagulation technique remains unpopular and has been deserted due to its association with thermal injury to bowel, whereas bipolar coagulation, although safer than unipolar, has an increased risk of ectopic pregnancy as revealed by Crest study.[4]
- *Operator dependent*: Operator error can occur due to various reasons:
    - *Failure in localizing the correct sterilization site*, i.e., placement of the device away from the midisthmic tubal site or sterilization of an adjacent structure, i.e., round ligament or peritoneum between the round ligament and tube.[13]
    - Deviation from the recommended technique for sterilization method.
    - *Failure in the systematic approach to check the sterilization method.* It is essential that the surgeon

should check the tubal fimbria and the same structure should be followed back up to the tubal isthmus to ensure proper placement of the device postprocedure.

- *Improper maintenance of laprocator.*
- *Place of surgery*: Sterilization procedure which is performed during camps have higher failure rates due to enthusiasm to perform a large number of operations as quickly as possible.

PRECAUTIONS TO DECREASE THE FAILURE RATE DURING VARIOUS PROCEDURES

- Medical record checklist to be filled properly with detailed information regarding eligibility criteria, menstrual history, obstetric history, contraceptive history, physical, local, and psychiatric information.
- General measures to decrease failure rate (laparoscopic sterilization)
    - Delineate the fallopian tubes and follow them up to the fimbrial ends.
    - Place the occlusive device 2–3 cm from the uterotubal junction.
    - Placement of the device must be adequate as per the manufacturer's instructions.
    - Gentle handling of tissues and keep tubes off the tension.
    - Deploy the devices slowly.
    - Entire tubal lumen should be occluded properly by the device.

Inadvertent transection of tube by the device may increase the risk of spontaneous regeneration of tubal lumen and thereby failure.[14]

- Specific to the procedure
    - *Falope ring* (banding procedure) (**Fig. 1**)
        - Sometimes, adhesiolysis of the tube may be required as 2 cm of fallopian tube is necessary to be pulled into the cylinder.[15]
        - Placement of the ring should be done on the applicator immediately before putting it onto the tube since *more than 5 minutes postapplication may result in permanent stretching* of the silicone.
    - *Occlusive procedure* (Filshie clip, Hulka clip)
        - *Filshie clip*: It is a hinged device composed of titanium with silicone rubber coating **(Fig. 2)**.[13]
            - Application of the clip should be perpendicular (90°) to the lumen of the tube.
            - Visualization of the bottom jaw of the Filshie clip in the area of mesosalpinx should be always ensured prior to closure of device.
        - *Hulka clip*: It is a hinged, spring-loaded plastic clip with zig-zag teeth which is designed specifically for occlusion of the isthmic portion of the tube over 48 hours **(Fig. 3)**.[16]
    - *Bipolar coagulation*: To increase the success rate[17]
        - A cutting wave form should be used at 25–35 W.

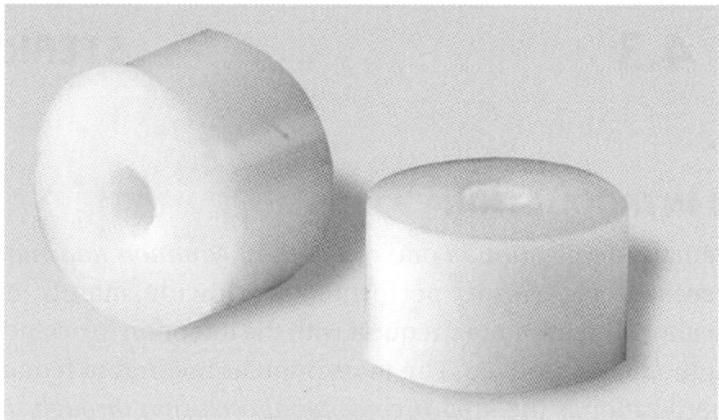

Fig. 1: Falope ring.

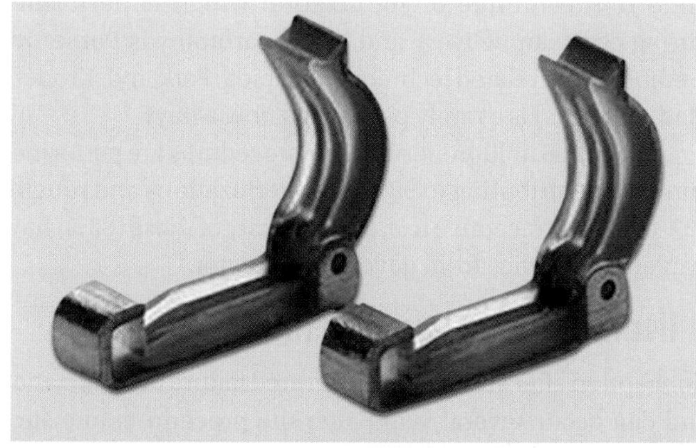

Fig. 2: Filshie clip.

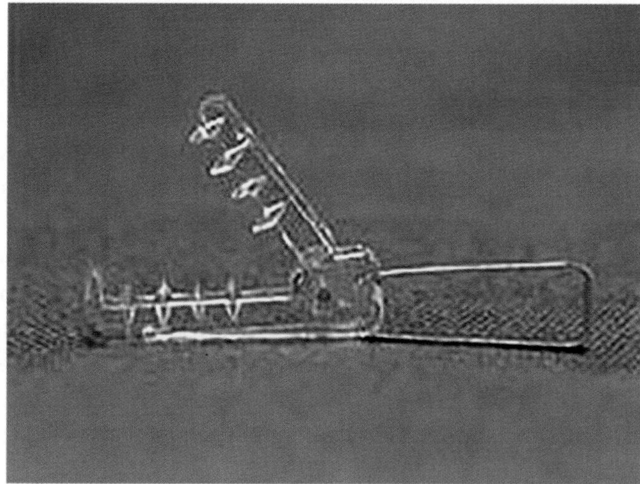

Fig. 3: Hulka clip.

        - Use a current flow meter to ensure complete electrocoagulation of 3 cm of contiguous tube with adequate energy.
    - *Pomeroy's method*: It is employed during interval or minilaparotomy procedure or postpartum which is done within 48 hours of delivery or during cesarean section (**Figs. 4A to C**).
        - Base of the loop should be tied keeping 2 cm of loop above the tie.

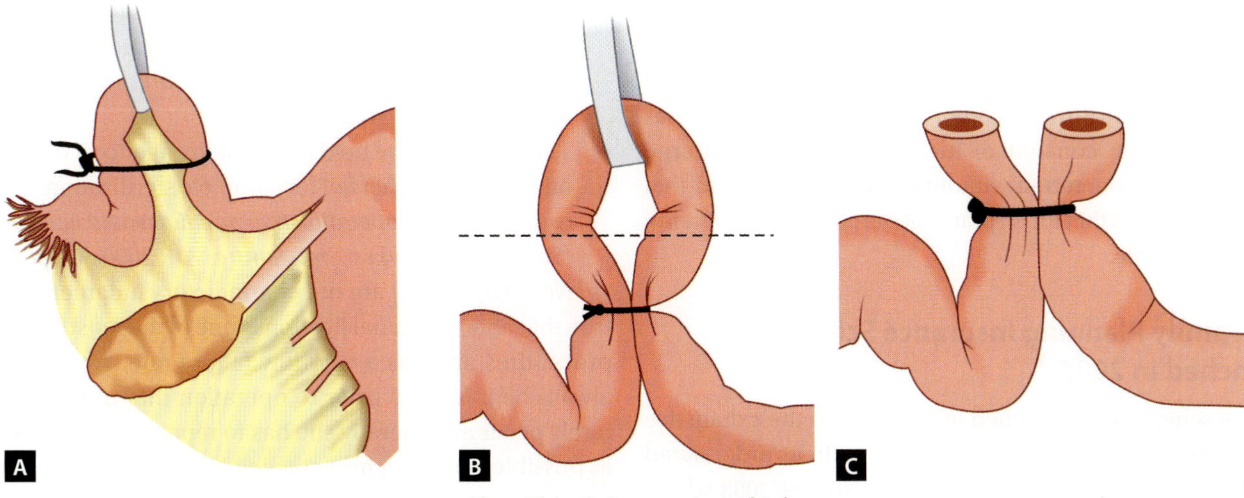

Figs. 4A to C: Pomeroy's method.

- About 1.5 cm of loop removed taking care that cut margins are not too close to tie made at the base of loop.
- Catgut stitches are used to ligate the loop as it has less chances of failure.

ADVICE ON DISCHARGE

- Patient is advised for abstinence till her next menses.
- She is also to be counseled that ligation failure can occur in 1–2% of cases, and therefore she has to report within 2 weeks to hospital if she misses her periods.
- Ligation certificate to be issued only after she has her periods and is negative for pregnancy test.

Confirm the written consent which clearly mentions about the failure rate albeit very low and advice given to the patient that whenever she misses her period in future, she should report to the hospital so that MTP can be offered in case of sterilization failure.

What to do when Sterilization Fails?[18]

Patient may present before 12 weeks when she can be offered MTP. If she comes at an advanced gestational age because of ignorance regarding failure of sterilization, the decision to continue the pregnancy or to get it aborted solely depends upon decision of the couple as well as gestational age after proper counseling. However, if after termination of pregnancy women want repeat sterilization, the following measures should be taken:

- A detailed and clear documentation to be done along with laparoscopic examination of pelvis.
- Chromopertubation of the tubes can be done if patient is not pregnant to confirm the true occlusion of the tubes.
- Once the sterilization failure occurs, repeat sterilization to be taken only after proper counseling of the couple and the mode of operation should be minilaparotomy. *The ideal procedure should be bilateral total salpingectomy* or removal of patent portion of the tube should be performed and *send for histopathological examination to identify the reason for failure.*
- Careful removal of Filshie or Hulka clips to identify the device defect.
- Operative note should be completed and noted immediately after corrective surgery.
- Government incentives (financial benefit) are not provided to patient after repeat sterilization procedure, but the procedure cost should be borne by the government.

LEGAL IMPLICATIONS

Sterilization is a permanent method of family planning and is an integral part of the National Family Planning Programme in India and facilities are provided free of charge in government sector. A breach of duty arises when an operation is not carried out in accordance with the accepted good medical practice to avoid foreseeable complications. Negligence in such operations becomes crucial and can have two major consequences:

1. Unwanted pregnancy
2. Expiry (mortality) of the patient

In either case, the patient and her family members have to undergo intense mental anguish and misery/sufferings along with financial burden to rear the child.

Moreover, the cost associated to rear a child born with serious disabilities becomes more distressing, even though the mental/physical abnormalities are not attributed to the negligence of the process of sterilization.

Guidelines by the Government of India for Sterilization[19]

- Age of the husband should not ordinarily be <25 years nor should it be over 50 years.

- Age of the wife should *not be <20 years or >45 years.*
- Motivated couple must *have one living child older than 1 year of age* at the time of operation.
- It is sufficient if the acceptor declares that he/she has obtained the consent of his/her spouse to undergo sterilization operation without undue pressure and that he/she knows that for all practical purposes, the operation is irreversible.

The Family Planning Insurance Scheme: Launched in 2005[19]

- The scheme was launched in response to the exhaustive directives issued by the Supreme Court in its order dated March 1, 2005, in Civil Writ Petition No 209/2003 where it directed the Union of India and States/UTs to ensure enforcement of the union government's guidelines for conducting sterilization procedures and norms for bringing about uniformity in sterilization procedures.
- The scheme grants a patient (or family as applicable) compensation of:
  - ₹ *1 lakh* in case of death due to sterilization while in hospital
  - ₹ *30,000* in case of death due to sterilization within 30 days of discharge from hospital
  - *A maximum of* ₹ *20,000* to cover expenses for treatment of medical complications due to the sterilization operation (within 60 days of the operation)
  - ₹ *20,000* in case of failure of sterilization (including first instance of conception after sterilization)
    - *Claim for failure can be made within 90 days of obtaining investigation reports related to the procedure.*
    - *Compensation is only entitled in patients in which the death is related to the process of sterilization and not related to pregnancy or its complications; in fact if there are any problems encountered during the procedure of termination of pregnancy, it is always advisable to abandon the process of sterilization due to the litigation involved.*

Under this scheme, all doctors (central, state, public sector as well as private sector) conducting such operations shall stand indemnified against the claims arising out of failure of sterilization.

Ascertaining Negligence

- It is an established fact that *no sterilization operation can guarantee success*, and there are always instances when conception may occur despite the surgery and in the absence of any medical negligence [State of MP v. Sundari Bai, AIR 2003 MP 284; State of Haryana v. Raj Rani 2005].
- The fact that a woman after having undergone a sterilization operation becomes pregnant and delivers a child does not imply that the surgeon is liable; *the claim can be sustained only if there is proof of negligence on the part of the surgeon [State of Punjab vs. Shivaram and others, AIR 2005 SC 3280].*
- The doctor will be held liable for negligence if the patient offered himself/herself for complete sterilization and *was assured after the operation that no child would be conceived [State of Haryana vs. Smt. Santra, AIR 2000 SC 1888].*

Note: (b) and (c) are not contradictory judgments as it is true that although tubal ligation is one of the most successful procedures and has a very low failure rate, couple should always be informed prior to operation that pregnancy can rarely occur and thereby she has to report to doctor as early as possible whenever amenorrhea occurs.

CONCLUSION

- Tubal sterilization is a safe, effective, and permanent procedure and tops among the contraceptive choices worldwide.
- The ultimate decision to undergo this procedure is totally dependent on women, which can be facilitated by the clinicians after a thorough counseling, which includes:
  - Permanence of the procedure along with its failure rate and the need to report early if menses are delayed to diagnose pregnancy in early stage and thereby reduce related morbidity.
  - Lack of protection against sexually transmitted diseases.
  - The need for continued routine gynecologic care (Pap smear, mammography, etc.).

REFERENCES

1. Varma R, Gupta JK. Predicting negligence in female sterilization failure using time interval to sterilization failure: analysis of 131 cases. Hum Reprod. 2007;22(9):2437-43.
2. Date SV, Rokade J, Mule V, Dandapannavar S. Female sterilization failure: review over a decade and its clinicopathological correlation. Int J Appl Basic Med Res. 2014;4(2):81-5.
3. Huddleston HT, Dunnihoo DR. Long-term sterilization failure: twenty-three years. J La State Med Soc. 2000;152(9):427-8.
4. Peterson HB, Xia Z, Hughes JM, Wilcox LS, Tylor LR, Trussell J. The risk of pregnancy after tubal sterilization: findings from the U.S. Collaborative Review of Sterilization. Am J Obstet Gynecol. 1996;174(4): 1161-8. (discussion 1168-70)
5. Trussell J, Guilbert E, Hedley A. Sterilization failure, sterilization reversal, and pregnancy after sterilization reversal in Quebec. Obstet Gynecol. 2003;101(4):677-84.
6. Nardin JM, Kulier R, Boulvain M. Techniques for the interruption of tubal patency for female sterilisation. Cochrane Database Syst Rev. 2003;(1):CD003034.
7. Chi IC, Siemens AJ, Champion CB, Gates D, Cilenti D. Pregnancy following minilaparotomy tubal sterilization—an update of an international data set. Contraception. 1987;35(2):171-8.
8. Hillis SD, Marchbanks PA, Tylor LR, Peterson HB. Post-sterilization regret: findings from the United States Collaborative Review of Sterilization. Obstet Gynecol. 1999;93(6):889-5.

9. Birdsall MA, Pattison NS, Wilson P. Female sterilisation: National Women's Hospital 1988–9. N Z Med J. 1994;107(990):473-5.
10. Kulier R, Boulvain M, Walker D, Candolle G, Campana A. Minilaparotomy and endoscopic techniques for tubal sterilisation. Cochrane Database Syst Rev. 2004;(3): CD001328.
11. Chi IC, Gardner SD, Laufe LE. The history of pregnancies that occur following female sterilization. Int J Gynaecol Obstet. 1979;17(3):265-7.
12. Davies GC, Letchworth AT, Diamond I. A comparison of Filshie and Hulka-Clemens clips used in sterilisation operations. J Obstet Gynaecol. 1990;10(3):251-2.
13. Filshie GM. Laparoscopic sterilization. Semin Laparosc Surg. 1999;6(2):112-117.
14. Soderstrom RM. Sterilization failures and their causes. Am J Obstet Gynecol. 1985;152(4): 395-403.
15. Sokal D, Gates D, Amatya R, Dominik R. Two randomized controlled trials comparing the tubal ring and Filshie clip for tubal sterilization. Fertil Steril. 2000;74(3):525-33.
16. Hulka JF, Omran KF, Phillips JM Jr, Lefler HT Jr, Lieberman B, Lean HT, et al. Sterilization by spring clip: a report of 1000 cases with a 6-month follow-up. Fertil Steril. 1975;26(11):1122-31.
17. Soderstrom RM, Levy BS, Engel T. Reducing bipolar sterilization failures. Obstet Gynecol. 1989;74(1):60-3.
18. Soderstrom RM. Case reports. II. Sterilization litigation. Clin Obstet Gynecol. 1988;31(1):174-8.
19. Noopur R, Sharma D. Negligence in sterilisation: the changing legal regime. Indian J Med Ethics. 2009;6(1):40-1.

LONG QUESTION

1. Discuss the approach to a woman who presents in the clinic with 12 weeks of gestation with a history of tubal ligation performed 2 years ago at the time of a cesarean done for the birth of her second child.

SHORT QUESTIONS

1. What are the common causes of failure of sterilization?
2. What is the compensation structure in case of failure of sterilization?

MULTIPLE CHOICE QUESTIONS

1. All of the following are the general measures to reduce the failure rate during female sterilization, except:
   a. Gentle handle of tissue and keep tubes at maximum tension
   b. To deploy the devices slowly and ensure that the entire tubal lumen is occluded by device
   c. Identification of fallopian tube and follow-up to fimbrial end
   d. Place the occlusive device 2–3 cm from uterotubal junction
2. Application of Filshie clip on fallopian tube should be:
   a. At 90° angle perpendicular to the lumen of the tube
   b. At 30° angle perpendicular to the lumen of the tube
   c. At obtuse angle perpendicular to the lumen of the tube
   d. At 60° angle perpendicular to the lumen of the tube
3. All of the following are the guidelines of Government of India (GOI) for sterilization, except:
   a. Age of husband should not be <35 and >55 years
   b. Age of wife should not be <20 and >45 years
   c. The motivated couple must have one living child at the time of operation
   d. It is sufficient that he/she knows that for all practical purposes that operation is irreversible
4. The family planning insurance scheme included for patient and family is:
   a. A compensation of ₹ 1 lakh in case of death due to sterilization
   b. A compensation of ₹ 3 lakh in case of death due to sterilization
   c. A compensation of ₹ 5 lakh in case of death due to sterilization
   d. A compensation of ₹ 8 lakh in case of death due to sterilization
5. All of the following measures need to be taken during the process of resterilization, except:
   a. Detailed and clear documentation
   b. Laparoscopic examination
   c. Ideal procedure to repeat sterilization is bilateral salpingectomy
   d. Removal of ring or clips is not necessary
6. The highest rate of failure of sterilization is for:
   a. Hulka clip
   b. Bipolar coagulation
   c. Unipolar coagulation
   d. Falope ring
7. All of the following are true, except:
   a. Ring should be placed as early as possible to prevent permanent stretching
   b. In Pomeroy's method, base of the loop should be tied keeping 2 cm of loop above the tie
   c. Bipolar coagulation uses a cutting wave of 45–55 W
   d. At least 2 cm of fallopian tube to be taken in cylinder to place ring
8. All of the following are true for failure of sterilization, except:
   a. Tubal nonocclusion or wrong structure sterilization
   b. Spontaneous tubal recanalization or fistula formation mechanism of failure are considered as non-negligent
   c. A larger interval to failure is suggestive of negligent failure
   d. Failure should always be documented through systematic assessment of hysterosalpingogram (HSG), fallopian tube histology, and direct visual pelvic examination
9. Unipolar coagulation has been abandoned due to:
   a. Greater association with thermal injury to bowel as compared to bipolar

b. Unipolar coagulation carries far risk of ectopic pregnancy
c. Unipolar coagulation has increased failure as compared to bipolar
d. Unipolar coagulation results in more transection than bipolar

10. All the following are factors contributing to failure of sterilization, except:
a. Timing and type of procedure
b. Failure in systematic approach for each sterilization method as well as to check the tubal fimbriae post placement of device
c. Proper maintenance of laprocator
d. Operator dependent

Answers

1.	a	2.	a	3.	a	4.	a	5.	d	6.	a
7.	c	8.	c	9.	a	10.	c				

4.4 REVERSAL OF STERILIZATION

Abha Singh, Prabha Lal

INTRODUCTION

Tubal ligation is the surgical procedure for sterilization of females where the fallopian tubes are permanently blocked/tied or removed. It is the most accepted method of permanent contraception in India. Almost 5–6 million sterilization procedures are performed annually contributing to 98% of all sterilizations and roughly 62% of all contraceptive uses. Due to male dominance in the society, male sterilization constitutes a very small percentage (6%) of the permanent method of contraception.

The most popular approach used for female sterilization in India is the laparoscopic tubal ligation. More than 85.3% of all women who have adopted this method of contraception avail this service from government facilities. Tubal sterilization is associated with an estimated failure rate of 0.1–0.8% in the first year after sterilization.

According to the Standards of Sterilization Guidelines, Ministry of Health and Family Welfare, Government of India (GOI), the site of the occlusion of the fallopian tube must be within 2–3 cm from the uterine cornu in the isthmic portion with excision of 1 cm of the tube to improve the possibility of reversal if required in the future. Use of cautery and crushing of the tube should be avoided.[1]

Conception can be achieved after reversal of sterilization by surgical tubal recanalization. However, nowadays with the advent of in vitro fertilization (IVF), patients have different choices for conception without undergoing surgical procedure.[2] The option for conception depends upon many factors such as patient age, method of sterilization, financial resources, and patient choice.

Currently in India, fertility trend is to have two or three children. There is social pressure on family to marry woman at a very young age and to complete family size also at a faster rate. On achieving desired family size, the woman and her family opt for a permanent method of contraception that is usually female sterilization.[3] Social factors, illiteracy, ignorance, and lack of women empowerment in the Indian society are other factors that contribute to the decision-making for contraception by elderly family members than the couple itself.[4,5]

REASONS FOR SEEKING REVERSAL OF TUBAL STERILIZATION

Sterilization regret among married women in India is one of the most important deciding and compelling reasons for reversal of sterilization.

By comparison, the United States Collaborative Review of Sterilization (CREST) study, a prospective cohort study of more than 11,000 women, conducted in the United States, reported an overall cumulative probability of regret of 3.9, 7.5, and 12.7% at 3, 7, and 14 years, respectively, with women under 30 years of age nearly twice as likely to experience regret. The cumulative probability of regret did not plateau over the time period but rather continued to increase substantially throughout the long period of follow-up. Furthermore, an analysis of regret among women in CREST whose husbands underwent vasectomy found that the probability of regret was similar to women who underwent tubal sterilization.[6]

Various Factors Associated with Sterilization Regret

Factors influencing sterilization regret are almost similar for both male and female sterilization.

Age

This is one of the most common reasons for women to opt for reversal of sterilization. Younger the age at time of sterilization, greater is the regret. If age at sterilization continues to decline, sterilization regret is likely to increase.

In a report of the National Health Family Survey 2005–2006, it was observed that the median age at sterilization in India declined from 27 years in 1992–1993 to 25 years in 2005–2006. Further, in 2005–2006, about 81% of women reported being sterilized before the age of 30 years. The couple should be encouraged to adopt spacing methods as long-acting reversible method of contraception (LARC) in place of permanent methods of sterilization to avert sterilization regret in future.[3] Use of LARC can also help in reducing the ligation failure rate. It has been observed over many years that sterilization failure is more common if women undergo it at a younger age.

Family Size

The current fertility norm in India is to have two or three children. The family size is completed soon after marriage. Due to high unmet needs, the couple is likely to opt for the one-time method of surgical tubal sterilization, especially in a rural setup.

Compared with women who have more children, those with fewer children at the time of sterilization are more likely to experience regret.[7]

Sex of the Child

Similarly, women who have only male children are less likely to report sterilization regret than women who have only female children.[8]

Child Loss

Women who report having experienced child loss are more likely to report sterilization regret than women without such losses. High infant mortality in underprivileged women is an important reason to undergo sterilization reversal.

In an Indian study on the reversal of sterilization in women over two decades in the year 2012, it was found that out of 220 women 25% of reversal was done for remarriage while around 80% was done for death of children.[8]

COMMON INDICATIONS FOR REVERSAL OF STERILIZATION[9]

The common indications for reversal of sterilization are listed in **Table 1**.

TABLE 1: Guidelines for reversal of sterilization.

Reversal of male sterilization	• There has been a death of the only existing child of the man from the current or any previous relationships • There has been remarriage following death of spouse, and there are no living children for both partners • Loss of unborn child when vasectomy had taken place during the pregnancy AND the couple has no living children from the current or any previous relationships
Reversal of female sterilization	• There has been a death of the only existing child of the woman from the current or any previous relationships • There has been remarriage following death of spouse, and there are no living children for both partners • Loss of the child when tubectomy had taken place after delivery AND the couple has no living children from the current or any previous relationships

SURGICAL METHODS FOR TUBAL REANASTOMOSIS

Reversal of tubal sterilization can be performed by reanastomosis of the two obstructed tubal segments. There are various methods of tubal reanastomosis which are classified according to the anatomic location of tubal damage: cornual-isthmic, isthmic-isthmic, isthmic-ampullary, ampullary-ampullary, ampullary-infundibular, neosalpingostomy tubocornual anastomosis, and tubouterine implantation.

Preoperative Workup

Patient Selection

Pregnancy rates following reversal depend upon the method of tubal ligation done. The outcome is better with the methods such as use of Hulka clip and Falope ring as there is less tubal damage compared to other methods causing destruction of a greater portion of the tube. For example, electrocoagulation, Uchida technique, and Essure sterilization cause more damage resulting in small final tubal length.

Basic Infertility Tests

Patients undergoing tubal recanalization procedures should have a basic infertility evaluation. Hysterosalpingography (HSG) and laparoscopy should be performed to assess or predict the likelihood of a successful outcome. Proximal fallopian tube segment is better assessed with HSG than laparoscopy. Laparoscopy additionally helps the surgeon to ascertain the length of the distal segments, the status of the fimbria, and presence of any peritubal adhesions altering the motility of tube.

Most patients normally conceive within 2 years after the reversal. If pregnancy does not occur within 6 months of the operation, an HSG should be done to check the patency of the anastomosis. There is evidence to show a direct relationship between the length of the repaired tube and the time required for a postoperative conception.

If tubal segments or fimbria are in a poor condition due to damage caused by sterilization surgery, the couple should be evaluated further or offered the alternative of IVF. It is important to keep the best interest of the patient in mind, and recommendations should be based on the most practical, efficacious, and cost-effective method of conception for the couple.

PRECAUTIONS TO BE EXERCISED DURING REVERSAL SURGERY FOR BETTER RESULTS

Proper Exposure of Surgical Field

The incision size and type depend upon the previous incisions and mobility of the uterus and adnexa as well as the weight of the patient. A small (5–6 cm) minilaparotomy incision can also be given to exteriorize the uterus and tubes.

Laparoscopic and robotic approach access to tubotubal anastomosis can also be used in expert hands. The technique of surgery and basic principle remain the same as in open method. However, expertise in suturing laparoscopically or robotically is required.

Microscopic Technique and use of Microsurgical Instruments

Use of microsurgical technique should be preferred for reversal of tubal sterilization, with magnification varying between 4× and 10×. A dual-headed operating microscope with variable magnification can be used for all procedures.

High magnification also helps to inspect the tubal mucosa. If normal mucosa, recognizable by the capillary vessels in the mucosal folds, has not been reached, further resection of small tubal segments should be performed until normal mucosa is found.

Magnifying glass can also be used in setups lacking facility of a dual-headed operating microscope. However, it has its inherent limitation of causing defocusing of field of surgery on head movement and restricted field of vision. Most microsurgeons agree that the use of the microscope in these procedures yields higher pregnancy rates than the use of surgical loupes.

In addition, use of microsurgical instruments such as tissue micro forceps with or without teeth, a microneedle electrode, iris scissors, fine microsurgical scissors, and micro-Babcock forceps can add to better precision to the procedure.

Heparinized Solution Irrigation

Constant irrigation is a good prophylactic measure to prevent adhesion formation as it keeps the tissue moist, thus avoiding dryness and potential trauma with future adhesion formation. It also aids in the identification of small bleeders which can be cauterized. Heparinized lactated Ringer's solution in 20–500 mL syringes with a 25-gauge needle catheter should be used. This method helps to pinpoint the bleeders so that they can be better taken care of. This also aids in the prevention of clot formation with subsequent improvement in surgical field and tissue visualization.

Achieving Good Hemostasis

The use of numerous sutures for hemostasis should be avoided; instead, the use of a bipolar coagulator is essential to minimize tissue trauma. Microbipolar cautery can be easily performed in a wet surgical field. Monopolar energy should be used for excision of peritubal adhesions.

Suture Materials and Needles

Suture materials for tubal anastomosis are 7-0 or 8-0 polydioxanone (PDS Monofilament suture, Ethicon, Inc.) or 7-0 or 8-0 vicryl (polyglactin), polyglyconate (Maxon, Davis-Geck). Absorbable sutures being less irritant can cause less tissue reaction and resulting fibrosis as compared to nonabsorbable suture does not matter how fine it may be.

PRINCIPLES OF REANASTOMOSIS IN FEMALE STERILIZATION REVERSAL

Identification of the site of occlusion should be done by subjecting the women to diagnostic laparoscopy and transcervical chromopertubation using methylene blue for proximal segment and through fimbrial end for distal end.

The site of occlusion can also be identified by inspection and also by palpation as the occluded segment is felt as an indurated segment. As the luminal diameter of the tube is not uniform, therefore, the technique may vary depending upon lumen caliber **(Fig. 1)**.

Two ends are prepared for anastomosis by excision of occluded and scarred segments with a straight scissor or a sharp microblade on either end.

Examination of cut ends of tubes under high magnification should be done to know the health status of the tube. A healthy tube is devoid of scarring and has normal muscular and vascular architecture with an intact mucosal fold.

Hemostasis should be obtained by precise electro-dessication of significant bleeders between serosa and muscularis layer. Avoid intense electrodessication to prevent devitalizing the anastomosis site.

Tubal segments are approximated in two layers. These sutures are placed in a two-layer, interrupted fashion. The first layer incorporates the muscularis and the second layer is placed through serosa 6-6, 3-3, 9-9, and 12-12 o'clock positions. Four square knots should be applied while tying, else there may be chances of slippage.

Mesosalpinx between two cut ends if long should be approximated first using a single interrupted stitch with 7-0 suture polyglactin, which brings the tubal segments in close proximity for better alignment.

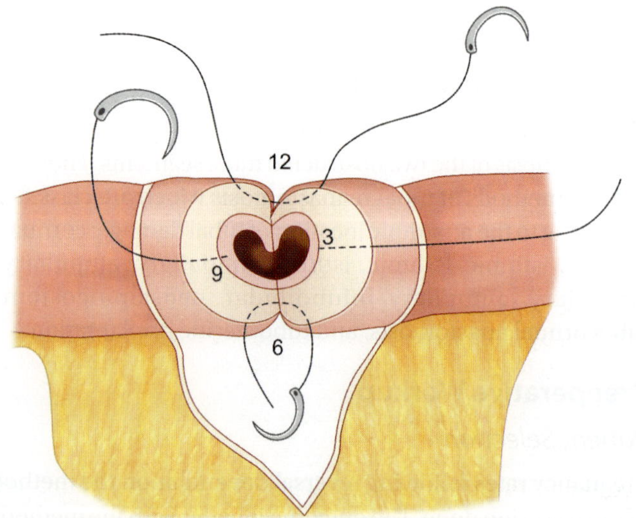

Fig. 1: Tubotubal anastomosis in two layers.

The first suture of the muscular layer should always be placed at the mesosalpingeal border at 6 o'clock position to ensure proper alignment of the two segments of the tube.

Positions of knots should be placed outside the lumen. During intraoperative time, tubal patency and water-tight anastomotic site should be demonstrated by chromopertubation after suturing the first layer.

Use of stents during suturing should be avoided as it may cause damage to cilia lining the lumen which helps in motility of fertilized ovum.

The role of hydrotubation after surgery is debatable as increased pressure in the tubal lumen may cause stitches to give way.

Steps are taken during surgery to try and minimize the formation of adhesions. Some of these include shortening surgical time, keeping the tissues moist, gentle handling of any tissues, avoid rubbing with cotton gauge, and using starch-free and latex-free gloves. For prevention of adhesions after surgery crystalloids, fluid of approximately 200 mL can be left in the peritoneal cavity for hydroflotation.

Types of Tubotubal Anastomosis

It depends upon the site of tubal sterilization or occlusive disease.

Intramural Isthmic Anastomosis

It is most commonly used for cornual disease. In post-sterilization, a short segment of tube which is frequently adherent to side of the uterus as a result of retraction of mesosalpinx may be mistaken for total absence of the proximal end. HSG and chromopertubation also can help to identify the isthmic part of the tube. In this type of anastomosis, there is no significant luminal disparity between two segments.

Isthmic–Isthmic Anastomosis

It is the simplest type of anastomosis to perform. Lumen caliber of the two cut ends are of equal size yielding best results.

Isthmic–Ampullary Anastomosis

There is considerable disparity in lumen between two segments, isthmus and ampullary parts. The basic principle of anastomosis remains the same. Disparity in lumen caliber can be overcome by enlarging the isthmic segment by making an oblique incision or 2–3 mm slit at its antimesengeal border. An alternative approach is to reduce the size of larger ampullary opening by plication of the muscularis layer surrounding the opening with interrupted sutures **(Fig. 2)**.

Ampullary–Ampullary Anastomosis

In this type of anastomosis, there is a tendency of the mucosa to prolapse through the lumen, thus causing difficulty. Excision of mucosal epithelium should not be done to avoid subsequent intratubal adhesion formation at this site. This can be replaced with irrigation fluid pressure or with the help of microforceps. Care should be taken not to include the mucosal epithelium in a suture or in knotting.

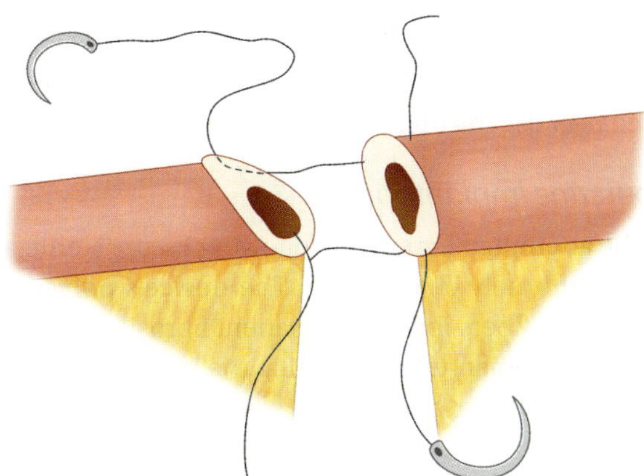

Fig. 2: Isthmic–ampullary anastomosis.

Ampullary–Infundibular

When the distal ampullary end of the tube is excised or ablated during sterilization or prior to that during removal of ectopic gestation, a circular opening is created with microscissor on the infundibular segment. A similar sized lumen is created on the ampullary end of the tube. Anastomosis is done in two layers, first layer involves muscularis and second layer consists of serosa layer.

Tubouterine Anastomosis

Tubouterine anastomosis was first described for treating women with proximal tubal occlusion unrelated to sterilization due to conditions such as chronic salpingitis, salpingitis isthmic nodosa, cornual fibroids, adhesive disease, and endometritis. Long before IVF, tubal cannulation and tubouterine anastomosis were attempted to restore tubal patency in women with proximal tubal occlusion.

Tubouterine anastomosis is classically an open procedure in which fundal hysterotomy or cornual wedge resection is performed for excision of the affected fallopian tube and reimplantation of the distal fallopian tube to the uterine cornua. Conception rates following the procedure were variable, ranging from 14 to 42% in the literature.[1,10]

When the anastomosis involves the intramural segment, four mucosal folds should be identified and free-flowing indigo carmine dye test expected. Injection of a dilute solution of vasopressin into the cornual region with a fine-gauge needle helps to reduce the oozing **(Fig. 3)**.

With the advent of a surgical microscope, tubouterine anastomosis has become a better option than tubal implantation for proximal tubal obstruction involving the entire interstitial isthmic segment.

The advantages of tubocornual anastomosis over tubal implantation are that the bleeding is less and small amount of uterine and tubal tissue is removed. Cesarean delivery is not needed because the uterine wall is not weakened.

Tubouterine Implantation

It can be attempted in reversal following Essure sterilization, which is uniquely challenging. The device's polyethylene terephthalate fibers induce permanent fibrosis along almost half of the fallopian tube, including the interstitial segment. This leaves only a short segment of the distal fallopian tube available for direct attachment to the uterus. A laparoscopic tubal reanastomosis can be performed.[11] IVF may be a better option in these cases **(Figs. 4A to C)**.

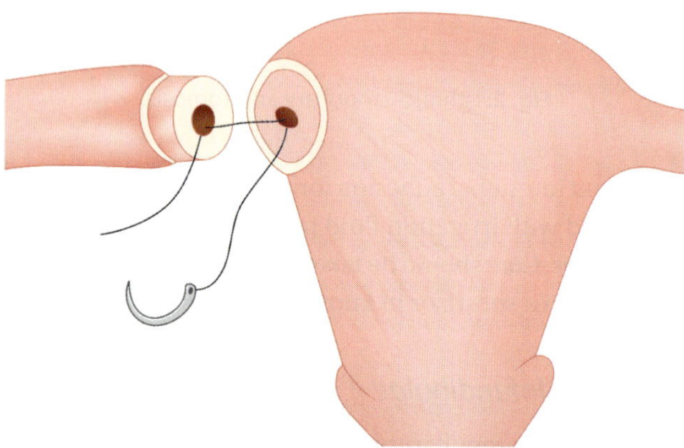

Fig. 3: Tubouterine anastomosis.[10]

Infundibular Neosalpingostomy

When the fimbrial end is damaged badly, neosalpingostomy at the ampullary portion can be done. However, the risk of ectopic pregnancy remains high.

Following reversal of sterilization, generally most patients become pregnant within 2 years after the reversal surgery. If pregnancy does not occur within 6 months of the operation, an HSG is suggested to confirm the patency of the anastomosis.

With laparoscopic tubal reanastomosis, pregnancy rate were ranging between 80 and 85%, majority of pregnancies occurred within 6 months where pregnancy rate was 67%. The results were comparable to open microsurgery but with decreased morbidity.[11]

Factors Affecting Successful Reversal of the Procedure

In India, many tubal sterilization surgeries are performed at the peripheral level and in an attempt to reduce failure, there

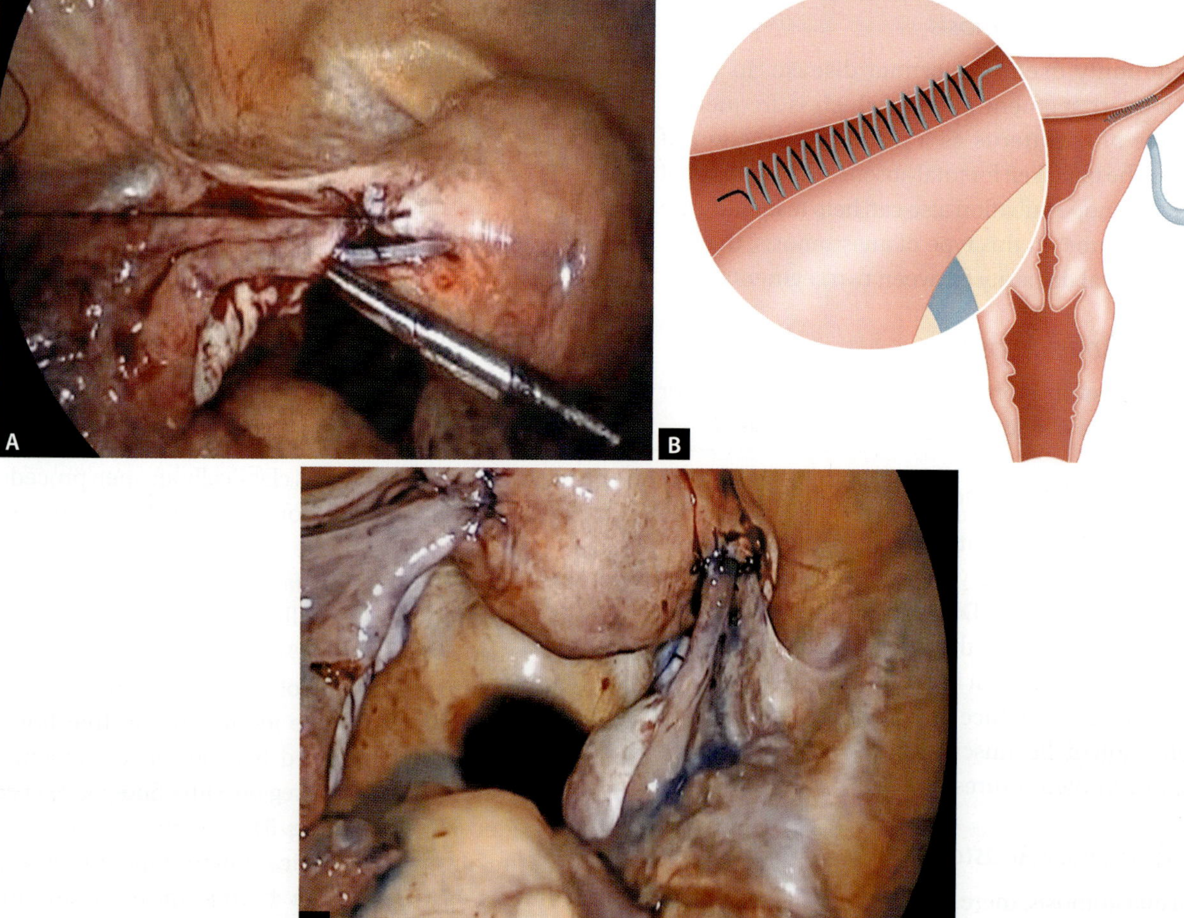

Figs. 4A to C: Tubal implantation following Essure sterilization.[11]

TABLE 2: Estimated cumulative probability of pregnancy after reversal by Falope ring and monopolar cautery by Rock.[11]

Method of sterilization	*Time after procedure in months*			
	6 months	12 months	24 months	36 months
Falope ring	28.4	48.8	69.3	87.7
Monopolar cautery	22.7	37.8	52.4	57.9

is a tendency to remove more length of the fallopian tube and doing fimbriectomy to avoid failure. Kroener sterilization (fimbriectomy) has been considered irreversible, but if at least 50% of the ampulla has been preserved, an ampullary salpingoneostomy may yield a significant live birth rate.

In a retrospective study conducted in a tertiary care center based on case records from 1995 to 2008 in India by Premlatha and Tripathi, the following important observations were made:

Isthmoampullary anastomosis was practiced in more than 30% of women, whereas the percentage of isthmoisthmic anastomosis was reducing.

The percentage of pregnancy in various sterilization types that have undergone reanastomosis was highest with isthmic–isthmic anastomosis. Up to 48% of pregnancy following reversal was associated with a tubal length of ≥6 cm at least on one side.[12]

However, another US-based study showed that reconstructed tubal length of at least 4 cm with an ampullary length of 1 cm had live birth rates of 60–80%. The tubal pregnancy rates varied with an average of 2–5%.[13]

Rock et al. estimated a cumulative probability of pregnancy after reversal of Falope ring sterilization of 28.4, 48.8, 69.3, and 87.2% at 6, 12, 24, and 36 months after the reversal surgery, respectively. On comparing this finding with 22.7, 37.8, 52.4, and 57.9% cumulative probability of pregnancy after 6, 12, 24, and 36 months after reversal of monopolar cautery sterilization, respectively, it was observed that patients in whom the final tubal length was <4 cm and who have marked luminal discrepancy tend to have lower success rates. Sterilization procedures that involve the use of clips, rings, or Pomeroy midsegment resection allow for longer, less damaged tubal segments than coagulation techniques **(Tables 2 and 3)**.[14]

To improve the efficacy, use of fibrin adhesives, tissue adhesives, and laser welding has been tried on animals. However, each procedure had severe limitations, because of foreign-body granulomatous reactions.[14,15]

Using a microsurgical anastomosis technique has a better outcome than that done without using a microscope. Careful screening with the use of preliminary laparoscopy is essential if the type of sterilization method is not known. This can be attributed to proper selection of cases and ultimately a successful outcome of the surgery.[16]

TABLE 3: Pregnancy rates for tubal reanastomosis at various anatomical sites.

Types of anastomosis	*Intrauterine pregnancy percentage*
Isthmic–isthmic	75
Cornual–isthmic	70
Isthmic–ampullary	64
Ampullary–ampullary	57

The use of magnification, minimal and gentle tissue handling, perfect hemostasis, constant irrigation, and fine nonreactive sutures all help reduce the incidence of postoperative adhesions. The role of hydropertubation, prophylactic antibiotics, and anti-inflammatory is questionable as they have not produced significant improvement in results. Use of physical barrier can sometimes help in prevention of adhesion formation. Oxidized, regenerated cellulose barriers have been proven to be an ideal physical barrier for the prevention of adhesions. Its efficacy has been evaluated during salpingolysis and fimbrioplasty to prevent the formation. Studies have shown that the physical barrier has shown twice as many tubes free of adhesions to the tubes that had microsurgery alone.[17,18]

Evaluation of Outcome of Reversal Procedure

Results of reanastomosis can be assessed by HSG and laparoscopy and ultimately by the pregnancy rate.

A study to correlate the HSG findings with laparoscopy by Letterie et al. concluded that HSG was more reliable in assessing patency with a sensitivity and specificity of 96 and 61%, respectively. However, it was associated with a high false-negative rate (60%), due to its inability to detect peritubal adhesions which can affect tubal motility during embryo transfer. Only 15% cases showed complete agreement between HSG and laparoscopy. Thus, limitations of HSG should be kept in mind while interpreting HSG in an infertile patient who has had tubal surgery. However, HSG is not routinely recommended.[19]

Complication of Surgery

Morbidity is not common, and the role of prophylactic antibiotic to improve tubal patency or pregnancy rates is not much studied. The major postoperative complications are a tubal pregnancy and reocclusion. A high index of suspicion and good precaution is to assume that there is a tubal pregnancy until an intrauterine gestation is proved otherwise.

The patient needs thorough counseling for high risk of extrauterine pregnancy with associated complications and need for early ultrasound diagnosis for location of pregnancy.

Alternative to Reversal Procedure in Irreparable Tubal Damage

The IVF technique is an alternative to irreparable tubal damage. However, the decision between IVF and tubal reversal is difficult. The choice between two methods should be based upon its costs and success rates and long-term plans. If a woman is young and wants to conceive more than once, tubal recanalization would be better. Elderly women 35 years or more who desire to conceive only once can have the better choice of IVF if facility is available. Perimenopausal women in the age group of 42–43 years would have less chances of conception by either methods. So, thorough counseling is required and informed consent should be taken.

MALE STERILIZATION REVERSAL

Because of various myths and misconceptions associated with vasectomy, most of the Indian men do not participate in contraception use may it be temporary or permanent. In a study done by the Indian Council of Medical Research (ICMR), it was observed that acceptance and prevalence of vasectomy has reduced from 74.2% in 1970 to 4.2% in 1992. Presently, its worldwide acceptance is approximately 6%. The GOI is putting all efforts to improve its acceptance. The reason for seeking reversal is almost the same as in case of female sterilization reversal.[20]

A thorough counseling and evaluation of both partners should be done before selecting a male partner for the reversal procedure. A successful outcome declines as the interval between vasectomy and reversal increases. A study done by Boorjian et al. observed a drop in pregnancy rate to 50% after 9 years of vasectomy. The failure rate can also be attributed to female factor such as with increasing age, women ≥35 years have a poor outcome despite successful reversal.[21]

Surgical Techniques

Surgical techniques, such as vasovasostomy (VV) and vasoepididymostomy (VE), can be done on the basis of vasal fluid findings during surgical exploration **(Fig. 5)**. Sperm quality categorization is done intraoperatively, which can help to decide the type of surgery to be done.[22,23]

Vasovasostomy

A small incision is made on the scrotum. The obstructed vas is visualized and palpated. The obstructed scarred site is excised. Vasal fluid from the testicular side is carefully evaluated and graded as discussed above. If sperms are present, VV is completed by joining together the two cut ends of vas deferens in two or three layers **(Fig. 6)**.

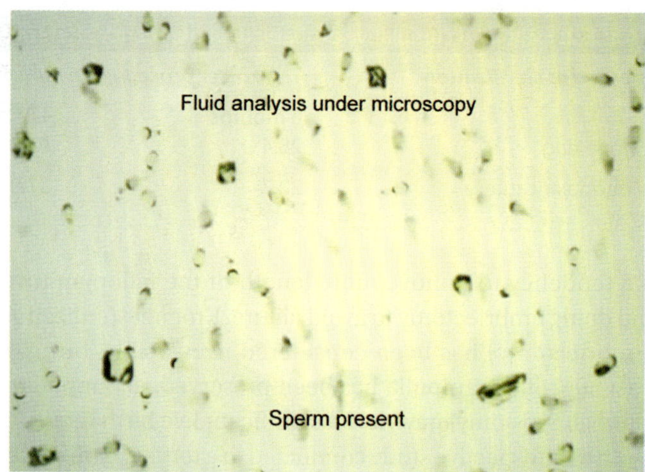

Fig. 5: Vasal fluid analysis.[24] Grade 1—mainly normal motile sperm; Grade 2—mainly normal nonmotile sperm; Grade 3—mainly sperm heads; Grade 4—only sperm heads; Grade 5—no sperm.

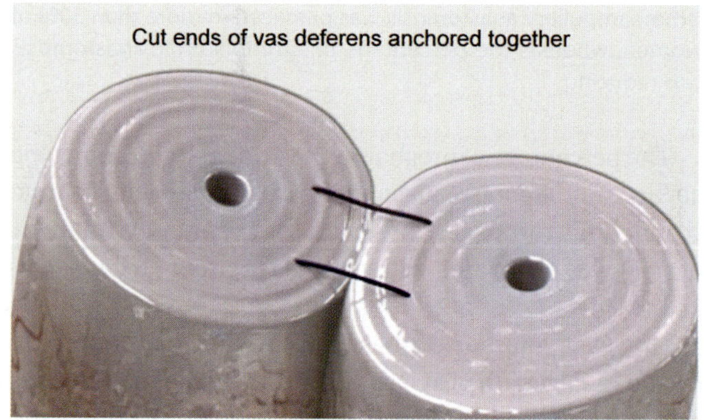

Fig. 6: Vasovasostomy.[24]

Epididymovasostomy

In the absence of sperm in vasal fluid, epididymovasostomy (EV) is the only option for reversal. Technically, EV is a difficult procedure and should be done by experienced surgeons. Here, the skin incision of VV is further enlarged so as to deliver testicles. An incision is made on epididymis. The tubes inside epididymis are incised and vas is anchored to the incision site. A small incision is made on tube and fluid is again analyzed for the presence of sperm. Anastomosis between vas and epididymis tube is made. Hematoma formation, surgical site infection, and chronic testicular pain are some of the complications which are not very common if proper instructions are followed after surgery. Imperfect technical repair, poor vas blood supply, and failure to identify epididymal obstruction can lead to failure of procedure. Repeat reversal can be attempted even if single motile sperm is present on sperm analysis done 5–6 months after surgery **(Fig. 7)**.

CONCLUSION

Laparoscopic tubal ligation is the most popular approach used in female sterilization: 85.3% Indian women have adopted this permanent method of contraception, whereas only 6% of men

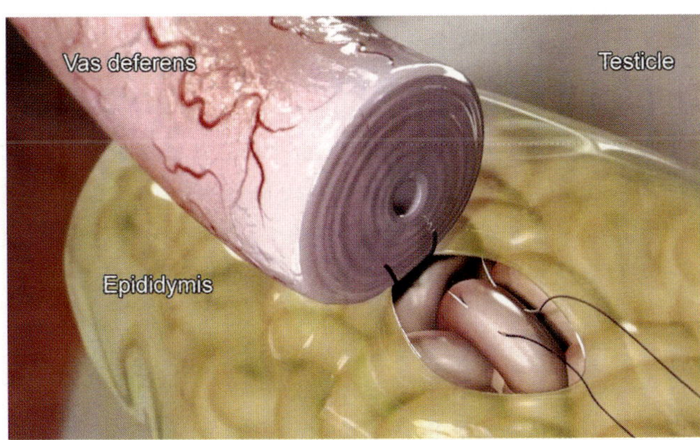

Fig. 7: Epididymovasostomy.[24]

have their contribution toward permanent contraception. In India, 25% of reversal are done for remarriage, around 80% for loss of children. High infant mortality in underprivileged women is an important reason to undergo sterilization reversal. It is pertinent to follow the guidelines of Ministry of Health and Family Welfare, GOI, to improve the possibility of reversal in case if required in future. The site of the occlusion of the fallopian tube must be within 2–3 cm from the uterine cornu in the isthmic portion and 1 cm tubal length should be excised to maintain an adequate length. Adoption of surgical techniques of ligation causing less damage, use of magnification, maintaining perfect hemostasis, constant irrigation, and use of fine delayed absorbable suture material and gentle handling of tissues can help to improve the success rate of reversal.

The success rate is better if tubotubal anastomosis is done in tubes with tubal ends of the same caliber such as isthmoisthmic anastomosis. The reversal outcome also depends upon the type of sterilization the woman had undergone. Sterilization surgeries should avoid fimbriectomy and removal of greater length of tube to avoid sterilization failure, which is detrimental to improve the success rate of reversal surgery. The chances of tubal damage are least with use of clips and Falope ring. The results of reanastomosis can be assessed by HSG and laparoscopy if women do not conceive by 6 months following sterilization.

The decision for reversal of male sterilization VV and EV depends upon the vasal sperm analysis of the testicular end of vas-deference intraoperatively. EV is a technically difficult procedure and good skill is required. Microsurgical techniques should be used to get a better outcome in both male and female reversal surgery. On failure of vasectomy, reversal frozen sperms directly collected from testicles during reversal procedure can be used for IVF.

REFERENCES

1. Standards for female and male sterilization services—Division of Research Studies and Standards, Ministry of Health and Family Welfare, GOI, 5th edition; 2006.
2. Deleon FD, Grimes EM, Peters AJ. [Online] Available from: http://.www.glown.com/section_view/heading/reversal of female sterilization/item/405.
3. International Institute for Population Sciences (IIPS) and Macro International, National Family Health Survey (NFHS-3), 2005–2006: India, Vol. 1. Mumbai: IIPS; 2007.
4. Matthews Z, Padmadas SS, Inge H, Juliet M. Does early childbearing and a sterilization-focused family planning programme in India fuel population growth? Demogr Res. 2009;20(28):693-720.
5. Krithika BK. Men say no to sterilization despite lower health risks. International Institute for Population Sciences (IIPS) and Macro International, National Family Health Survey (NFHS-3), 2005–2006: India, Vol. 1. Mumbai: IIPS; 2007.
6. Schmidt JE, Hillis SD, Marchbanks PA, Jeng G, Peterson HB. Requesting information about and obtaining reversal after tubal sterilization: findings from the U.S. Collaborative Review of Sterilization. Fertil Steril. 2000;74(5):892-8.
7. George R, Taylor PJ. A comparison of definable traits in women requesting reversal of sterilization and women satisfied with sterilization. Am J Obstet Gynecol. 1983;145:198.
8. Ramanathan M, Mishra US. Correlates of female sterilization regret in the southern states of India. J Biosoc Sci. 2000;32(4): 547-58.
9. Ipswich and East Suffolk Clinical Commissioning and Group. Partially excluded policy—PE105 reversal of female sterilization.
10. Rock JA. Reconstruction of the fallopian tube. In: Mattingly RF, Thompson JD (Eds). Te Linde's Operative Gynecology. Philadelphia: Lippincott Williams & Wilkins; 2019.
11. Smith M, Janik G. Laparoscopic tubal reanastomosis. Available at: https://www.contemporaryobgyn.net Sept4,2006.
12. Premlatha R, Tripathi MS. A study on the reversal of sterilization in women over two decades. J Obstet Gynaecol India. 2012; 62(1):62-7.
13. Gauwerky JFH, Kubli F, Fursman WG. Morphology and fertility after re-anastomosis of the rabbit fallopian tube with fibrin glue. Hum Reprod. 1988;3:327.
14. Rucker K, Baumann R, Volk M, Taubert HD. Tubal reanastomosis using a tissue adhesive. Hum Reprod. 1988;3:185.
15. Wiegerinck MA, Roukema M, Van Kessel PH, Mol BW. Hum Reprod. 2005;20:2355.
16. Gomel V. Microsurgical reversal of female sterilization: a reappraisal. Fertil Steril. 1980;33:587.
17. Hedon B, Wineman M, Winston RML: Loupes or microscope for tubal reanastomosis? An experimental study. Fertil Steril. 1980;34:264.
18. Diamond E. A comparison of gross and microsurgical techniques for repair of cornual occlusion in infertility: a retrospective study, 1968–1978. Fertil Steril. 1979;32:370-6.
19. Letterie GS, Haggety MF, Fellows DW. Sensitivity of HSG after tubal surgery. Arch Gynecol Obstet. 1992;251(4):175-80.
20. Family Planning Worldwide: 2008 Data Sheet, Population Reference Bureau; 2008.
21. Boorjian S, Lipkin M, Goldstein M. The impact of obstructive interval and sperm granuloma on outcome of vasectomy reversal. J Urol. 2004;171:304-6.

22. Belker AM, Thomas AJ Jr, Fuchs EF, Konnak JW, Sharlip ID. Results of 1,469 microsurgical vasectomy reversals by the Vasovasostomy Study Group. J Urol. 1991;145:505-11.
23. Silber SJ. Microscopic vasectomy reversal. Fertil Steril. 1977; 28:1191-202.

LONG QUESTIONS

1. Describe the various reasons for reversal of female sterilization in India.
2. What are the tubal factors responsible for outcome of reversal sterilization?
3. Explain the guidelines for female tubal sterilization.
4. What are various surgical methods of tubal reversal and which has the best outcome?
5. What precautions should be taken during surgery of reversal of sterilization?

SHORT QUESTIONS

1. What are the important selection criteria for reversal of sterilization?
2. In an irreparable damage caused to tubes following sterilization, what is an alternative method?
3. What is the alternative to retrieve sperm if vasectomy reversal fails?
4. What is the preferred method of reversal of male sterilization if sperm in vasal fluid is absent?

MULTIPLE CHOICE QUESTIONS

1. Out of the following methods of tubal occlusion which can give the best pregnancy rate following reversal of sterilization?
   a. Use of Uchida technique
   b. Use of Parkland technique
   c. Pomeroy's technique
   d. Bipolar coagulation
2. The guidelines of Ministry of Health and Family Welfare (MoHFW) for tubal sterilization is all, except:
   a. Occlusion of the fallopian tube must be within 2–3 cm from the uterine cornu.
   b. In the isthmic portion with excision of 1 cm of the tube
   c. Use of cautery for cutting the tube
   d. Avoid crushing of the tube
3. Following precautions should be exercised during reversal surgery, except:
   a. Gentle handling of tissues
   b. Use of heparinized solution for irrigation
   c. Avoid stenting of tubes
   d. Use of surgical loupe for magnification rather than double loupe microscope
4. What is the most common factor responsible for sterilization regret among Indian women?
   a. Remarriage b. Child death
   c. Small family size d. Large family size
5. HSG in preoperative evaluation is helpful mainly:
   a. For assessment of distal tubal segment
   b. For visualization of adhesions
   c. For assessment of proximal tubal segment
   d. For assessment of the entire length of the tube
6. Out of all surgical techniques done for reversal of sterilization, which has the best outcome?
   a. Tubouterine implantation
   b. Isthmo-ampullary anastomosis
   c. Isthmic–isthmic anastomosis
   d. Isthmic–ampullary anastomosis
7. For laparoscopic tubal reversal, all are true, except
   a. It should be considered experimental unless recommended by fertility surgeons
   b. Pregnancy rate is compromised during learning curve
   c. There is advantage of short hospital stay but outcome is variable
   d. Pregnancy rate is only good at skilled hands
8. Among principles of tubotubal anastomosis, all are true, except:
   a. Preparation of cut ends
   b. Use of microscopic technique
   c. Reconstruction of tubal lumen
   d. Three-layer closure
9. The following statement is not appropriate for reanastomosis outcome:
   a. Microsurgical technique gives best results
   b. Magnifying loupe use gives better result than double loupe microscope
   c. Tubal length ≥6 cm gives better result than 4 cm final tubal length
   d. Endoscopic approach is only good in skilled hands
10. For isthmic–ampullary reanastomosis, all are true, except:
    a. There is significant luminal disparity
    b. Fish-mouth opening is created at mesangial border
    c. Anastomosis is done in two layers
    d. Isthmic cut is given anteriorly at antimesenteric border
11. Regarding difficulty in ampullary–ampullary reanastomosis, all are true, except:
    a. The muscularis layer is thick
    b. Mucosal fold tends to prolapse
    c. Place more sutures than usual to approximate the ends
    d. The muscularis layer is thin
12. During intraoperative time, tubal patency and water-tight anastomotic site should be demonstrated by:
    a. Chromopertubation
    b. Hydrotubation
    c. Digital palpation
    d. Air insufflation

13. In the event of significant discrepancy between the segments and when the stumps are not free, anastomosis is brought about by:
    a. Enlarging the proximal lumen
    b. Enlarging the distal lumen
    c. Enlarge both proximal and distal lumen
    d. Suturing without enlarging lumen
14. Where the fimbrial end is damaged badly, neosalpingostomy is done at:
    a. Ampullary portion
    b. Isthmic portion
    c. Cornual portion
    d. Infundibular portion
15. The best option for male sterilization reversal if sperm is absent in vasal fluid is:
    a. Epididymovasostomy
    b. Vasovasostomy
    c. Vasoepididymostomy
    d. Use of cryopreserved sperm

Answers

1.	b	2.	c	3.	d	4.	b	5.	c	6.	c
7.	c	8.	c	9.	d	10.	b	11.	b	12.	a
13.	a	14.	a	15.	a						

Contraception and Pregnancy Termination for Special Groups

5.1 CONTRACEPTION IN ADOLESCENTS

Sucheta Kinjawadekar, Unmesh Santpur

INTRODUCTION

Adolescence is a period of physical, psychological, and social maturing from childhood to adulthood. The term adolescent "refers to individuals between the ages of 10 to 19 years."

Now the question arises as to:

Why adolescents need contraceptive methods?

Adolescents makeup about 16% of the world population; out of these, approximately 86% live in developing countries. Half of the adolescent girls in the developing countries are sexually active by the time they are 19 years, about 40% are married, and around 20% have children.[1]

About 23 million adolescent girls are at the risk of unintended pregnancy due to lack of contraception. Approximately 21% of unintended adolescent pregnancies in Asia and 50% of unintended pregnancies in Latin America and Africa end in unsafe abortion.[2]

Unmarried teenagers tend to have unpredictable lifestyles that revolve around such issues as asserting their independence and gaining acceptance among their peers. Many adolescents have difficulty adjusting to this stage in their life, especially in coping with their sexuality. Although sexual activity may be infrequent, relationships are often temporary and multiple sexual partners are possible; hence, their contraceptive needs require special consideration.

In our society, marriage of adolescents is still widespread. These adolescents face many of the same issues as teenagers of the same age who are unmarried. In addition, they are usually under pressure from their families and society to bear children soon after marriage, a practice which increases the risk of maternal and neonatal morbidity and mortality **(Fig. 1)**.[3]

CONTRACEPTIVE BEHAVIOR AND PSYCHE OF ADOLESCENT

The most notable feature of contraceptive behavior in adolescence is its inconsistency. The first coital episode is usually a spontaneous event with both partners disavowing

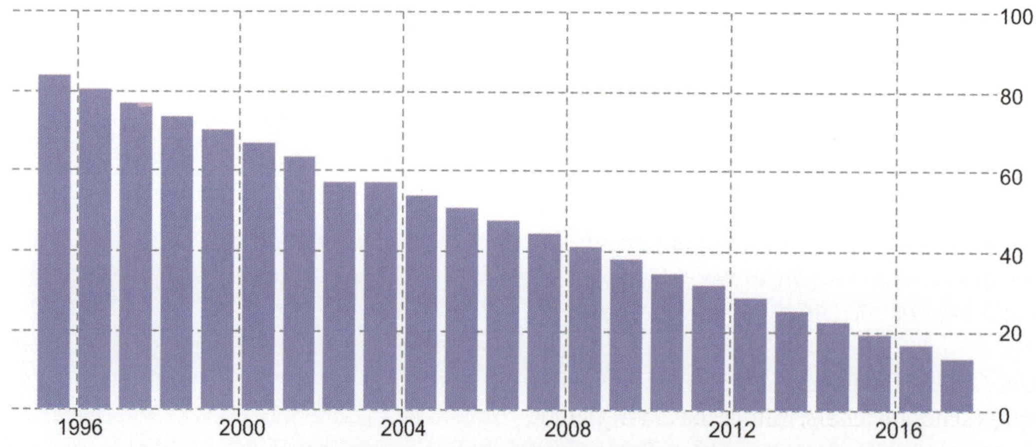

Fig. 1: The extent of adolescent fertility in India.
Source: Trading Economics. [online] Available from: https://tradingeconomics.com/india/adolescent-fertility-rate-births-per-1-000-women-ages-15-19-wb-data.html. [Last accessed November, 2021].

any conscious responsibility or advance intent. A very few adolescents engage in prior discussions or give serious thoughts to their personal contraceptive needs. Even when services are available, major factor in nonseeking them is ignorance and major degree of misinformation. Much of what young people learn is from unreliable sources—peers, hearsay, and school sex education programs which are short of ideal. Many believe that they are too young to become pregnant but have inadequate knowledge of ovulation and fertilization. Apart from inadequate knowledge, another major factor of such inconsistent behavior is complex behavior pattern typical of this age.[1]

From unmarried to married adolescent's perspective, using contraception is acknowledgment of sexual activity, having to plan ahead when not committed to coital behavior, taking initiative in a relationship in which idealized feminine role is one of passivity, thereby devaluation by partner.

Risk of discovery of contraceptive supplies with adolescents may reveal sexual behavior to parents.

Adolescent cognitive immaturity makes them think that possibility of pregnancy is less; there is defensive denial. The same immaturity makes them difficult to perceive future consequences of their present act (of indulging in unprotected sex).

These psychological and social barriers are reduced by dealing openly and honestly with adolescent sexuality, providing correct information, sex education, and promotion of decision-making skills, and this will enable teenagers to make a more rational choice with regard to their sexual activity.[1]

EXTENT OF ADOLESCENT FERTILITY IN INDIA

It is defined as number of births per 1,000 women in the 15–19 age group. The extent of adolescent fertility in India is depicted in **Figure 1**.

In a country like ours where traditional and societal norms are very rigid, education on sexuality and reproductive health for adolescents has not been widespread as seen in western countries. Providing sex education to adolescents in an appropriate and timely fashion is an opportunity by which we can reduce the abortion rate and sexually transmitted infections (STIs) and their negative consequences.[4]

This sexual and reproductive education should be commenced and should be tailored to suit the adolescent who have not begun sexual activity. They should emphasize on creating awareness and preventing unwanted pregnancy and HIV, and adolescents should know where to access such services.

Health workers should involve important members of the community such as schoolteachers, influential elderly ladies and men, local pharmacists, and youth leaders. These "gate keepers" should be sensitized to contraceptive needs of the adolescents.[4]

Emerging data suggest mobile phones and social media are promising means of increasing contraceptive use among adolescents.

Although parents and adults would prefer unmarried adolescents not to be sexually active until they are able to appreciate the risk fully, often adolescents do not wait. Married or unmarried adolescents face several potential problems in relation to their reproductive health.[5]

They are as follows:
- High risk of contracting STIs [including hepatitis B virus (HBV) and human immunodeficiency virus (HIV)/ acquired immunodeficiency syndrome (AIDS)] through unprotected sexual intercourse
- Unwanted pregnancy resulting in unsafe abortion
- Early childbearing (<19 years) results in high risk of complications for both mother and child due to the mother's physical immaturity with respect to labor and birth
- Especially for females, early childbearing leads to reduced opportunities for further education and employment that in turn affect their social and cultural development.

Therefore, it is very important that all adolescents have access to good counseling and effective family planning, regardless of their marital status.

COUNSELING THE TEENAGER

An important step in counseling adolescents is developing a rapport with them and to speak in a language they understand. The environment should be supportive and nonjudgmental ensuring confidentiality. The counselor/healthcare personnel should be trained in sexuality counseling skills, they should be able to understand the needs, concerns, and problems of adolescents. They should not be biased about sexual behavior, morality, etc.[4] The counselor should be able to explain the bodily changes and the normal and abnormal feelings and actions. Both the males and females should be counseled for responsible sexual behavior. The male adolescents are to be counseled to share the responsibility of contraception and the prevention of sexually transmitted diseases (STDs) with their female partners.

Adolescents who are subjected to sexual abuse and coercion require special support and care, and emergency contraception (EC) should be provided in such circumstances. Healthcare providers have to be sensitive and should be aware of how to access the health and social services that these adolescents need.[4]

CHOICE OF CONTRACEPTION

While helping the adolescents choose a method to use, the healthcare provider must give them knowledge about different methods explaining the merits and demerits and help them make well-informed voluntary choice of the method. The eligibility and legal issues should be considered. Adolescents and clinician misperceptions are important barriers to effective adolescent contraception. Both adolescents and clinicians have certain misapprehensions about the following issues:

- Effectiveness of contraception
- Contraindications for the use
- Preinitiation evaluation of the adolescents
- Adverse effects of various methods of contraception.

Adolescent Concerns

- *Weight gain:* Many adolescents are concerned that hormonal contraceptives cause weight gain. However, a causal relationship has not been established.
- *Effect on height:* Adolescents may be concerned that hormonal contraception may cause premature closure of the growth plates, reducing their ultimate adult height. However, by the time of menarche, most female adolescents have already undergone their growth spurt and achieved approximately ≥95% of their adult height.
- *Birth defects and infertility:* Adolescents may be concerned that hormonal contraception may cause birth defects or infertility. However, evidence to support these associations is lacking.

Choosing the Correct Contraceptive Method

Various methods of contraception are suitable for adolescents. Effective contraception for adolescents, married, or unmarried is especially important because of more serious consequences of unwanted pregnancies.[6,7] An important consideration is better protection against possible STIs. It should be remembered that adolescents may require a very highly effective form of contraception to prevent pregnancy and at the same time protection from STI.

Important factors that affect the choice of contraceptives:

- Availability
- Risk of STD taken care
- Information about uses and side effects
- Any medical conditions contraindicating the use
- Efficacy of the method.

DIFFERENT CONTRACEPTIVE METHODS

Different contraceptive measures that are available are:

Combined Oral Contraceptive (COC) Pills

Newer COC pills with respect to lower dose of ethinylestradiol (EE; 20 μg) and newer progesterone levonorgestrel (second generation) and desogestrel, drospirenone, and cyproterone (third generation) are devoid of annoying side effects and hence well accepted by motivated users.

Prerequisites

Although careful medical history and personal and family history to assess cardiovascular risk factors are a must, pelvic examination/pap smear can be deferred to a later date. In young woman, COC can be prescribed safely in World Health Organization (WHO) category A or B.

Instructions

Initiation of COC pill: It should be started on day 1 or day 2 of bleeding and she should take one pill preferably at a fixed time. (Put a reminder on mobile of the girl or her partner!) Everyday irrespective of coital activity. This point is required to be driven in users' mind as many girls/couples think that pills can be skipped if the husband is away for a day or two!

Address Issue of Missed Pill

If one forgets a pill and it is less than 24 hours from the last pill, then both the missed pill and the due pill should be taken at the same time. If more than 24 hours, then continue with the pill but has to use additional precautions.

Stop Signs

Stop signs are headache, chest pain, abdominal pain, and calf pain.

Beneficial Side Effects

Combined oral contraceptives give cycles that are pain free, premenstrual syndrome free, and anemia free as they result in "normal" blood loss. Cycles are precise and regular.

Remarks Regarding Adolescents

- COCs should be used only if the adolescent has started menstruating.
- It requires strong client motivation. Forgetfulness and irregular use increase method failure.
- Conditions requiring precautions are rare in adolescents.
- No protection against STIs (e.g., HBV, HIV/AIDS).
- Therefore, unmarried adolescents may need to use condoms as well.
- Additional benefits include regulated and reduced menstrual bleeding and reduced menstrual cramps and acne.
- Counsel regarding regular use and protocol for missed dose.

Vaginal Ring

The vaginal ring (NuvaRing) has also been used. It releases 15 μg of ethinyl estradiol and 120 μg of etonogestrel daily. NuvaRing is a round device which is flexible and measures 54 mm in diameter and 4 mm cross-sectionally. It protects against pregnancy by the release of estrogen and progestins. It is a silicon ring; once inserted in vagina, it is to be kept for 3 weeks and removed for 1 week to induce menstruation which is followed by insertion of a new ring. The patient should be instructed by demonstration by pelvic model.

Adverse effects are the same as COCs such as breast tenderness, headache, nausea, and breakthrough bleeding with additional vaginal discharge.[8]

Transdermal Contraceptive Patch

The combined hormone contraceptive patch contains 0.6 mg norelgestromin and 0.75 mg ethinyl estradiol and measures approximately 1.75 × 1.75 inch. This patch has to be placed on the abdomen, upper outer arm, or buttocks. One patch can be used for 3 weeks and then 1 week off the patch.[8]

Injectable Contraceptives

Since 1986, depot-medroxy-progesterone acetate (DMPA) is approved by the Drug Controller of India and the Indian Council of Medical Research (ICMR) and is available for use.

It acts at various levels. It reduces gonadotropin-releasing hormone (GnRH) surge and causes thinning of endometrium and also thickening of cervical mucus.

Initiation

DMPA is to be given within 7 days of menstruation or within a week of abortion or within 6 weeks of term delivery. No physical examination or investigations are needed. Injections are to be repeated every 3 months (±1 week).

Disadvantage

Return of fertility is not immediate, especially in a long-term user, and this should be told beforehand. However, this does not make this method of contraception contraindicated in a nulliparous patient.

Health Benefits

- Continued use of DMPA reduces anemia (due to oligomenorrhea or amenorrhea)
- Help preventing pelvic inflammatory disease (PID; probably thickening of cervical mucus prevents STI-causing organisms to ascend through cervix)
- Injectable contraceptives (DMPA) reduce frequency of seizures in women with epilepsy. This can be contraception of choice in women with some medical conditions such as immune thrombocytopenic purpura (ITP), chronic liver disorders, and deep vein thrombosis (DVT) where estrogen-containing formulations are contraindicated.

Remarks Regarding Adolescents

DMPA is recommended for adolescents who want intermediate or long-term effective contraception, especially if they had trouble with compliance while using another method.

They should be well counseled about the possibilities of weight gain, skin disorders, and irregular bleeding/spotting which can be bothersome.

Lack of need for supplies and nonvisibility make this method attractive to adolescents.

Some studies suggest that use of Depo-Provera in adolescents (<16) within 2 years of menarche may pose a risk of osteoporosis. Calcium supplementation and adequate exercise are advisable.

Progestin Implants Long-acting Reversible Contraception (LARC)

- A single-rod implant containing etonogestrel (active metabolite of desogestrel) also contains barium sulfate to make it visible on radiography.
- The implant is highly effective with a failure rate of less than 1%.
- It can be kept in place for 3 years.
- It is inserted into the inside of the nondominant upper arm, 6–8 cm above the elbow.
- Implants are ideal for adolescents who prefer a method that does not require scheduled adherence and who desire a long-term protection. It is a good option for delaying second pregnancy in adolescent mothers.[8]

Intrauterine Contraceptive Device

Intrauterine contraceptive device (IUCD) can be used with precaution in nulliparous and young adolescent girls. It is an excellent method of contraception for married parous women who want to space her next pregnancy.

Initiation

Intrauterine device can be inserted in postmenstrual, postabortal, and postpartum periods. Nulliparity and past history of ectopic pregnancy are no longer contraindications of IUD insertion. Minor problems should be handled by caregiver, thereby reducing emotional distress of the client and increasing compliance. Difficult insertion can be tackled by using oral, vaginal, or sublingual misoprost, thus making the cervix soft and insertion painless.

Adverse Effects

Pain and mild cramping are expected during the procedure and may last for days after insertion. These can be managed by antispasmodic/nonsteroidal anti-inflammatory drugs (NSAIDs). Slight vaginal discharge and light spotting may occur. The woman should be reassured regarding its short-term nature. If these symptoms are troublesome, IUD may be removed.

Remarks Regarding Adolescents

It can be an adequate option for parous adolescents with low risk of STIs who require long-term protection against pregnancy. It is not recommended for adolescents with multiple sex partners.[8]

Barrier Contraceptives

Among the various barrier contraceptives available are condoms (male and female), cervical cap, diaphragm, sponge, spermicidal, etc. Latex male condoms are easily available all over. They are available in lubricated, textured, colored, and flavored forms suitable for adolescents indulging in alternative sexual practice.

How to Use It

Each couple/client should be aware of all the facts mentioned below and the caregiver should not assume that client possesses proper information.

- A new condom to be used during each act.
- No oil-based lubricants to be used that may cause condom breakdown.
- Pinch and hold small receptacle at the tip and then unroll condom over the erected penis.
- After ejaculation, condom should be grasped at the base to avoid inadvertent spillage.
- Used condom should be wrapped in wastepaper before trashed (not to flush in commode).

Advantages

- Condoms' usage imparts the male partner as the responsibility of contraception
- Easy accessibility and availability
- Gives protection from STI and HIV
- Used-alone condom has failure rate of 2–20%.

EMERGENCY CONTRACEPTION

Emergency contraception, the use of nonabortifacient, hormonal medications within 72–120 hours after unprotected/ underprotected coitus for the prevention of unintended pregnancy, is an important part of the contraception counseling in adolescents.

Emergency contraception has an important place in family planning services for adolescents because young people may have difficulties in obtaining contraceptive supplies and are often likely to have unplanned and unprotected sexual intercourse. EC can be used as a back-up in case of condom breakage or improper use of the withdrawal method. It is important to publicize the availability of EC together with thorough counseling.

Indications of EC are as follows:

- Contraceptive accidents include:
  - Failed coitus interrupts
  - Condom rupture
  - Complete/partial expulsion of IUD
  - Midcycle removal of IUD
  - Missed COC
- Adolescents who are subjected to sexual abuse and coercion
- Failure to plan ahead
- Sexual assault
- Recent use of live vaccine.

Emergency contraception: EC methods that are effective and safe for use in teenagers include the following:

- Tab levonorgestrel 1.5 mg single dose or 0.75 mg two tablets to be taken within 5 days or preferably within 72 hours of contact. This drug is available over the counter.
- Tab ulipristal acetate 30 mg is another newer alternative. It, however, requires prescription.
- The original Yuzpe method consists of two 50-µg ethinyl estradiol/norgestrel pills taken as soon as possible within the 72-hour time frame, followed by two additional pills taken 12 hours later. 30- or 35 µg ethinyl estradiol pills combined with norgestrel or levonorgestrel may be used, but four must be ingested at each dose, for a total of eight pills.
- RU 486–600 mg single dose is most effective.
- IUCD insertion as EC within 5 days of act is also effective.

One should take the opportunity of providing EC as disseminating knowledge of contraceptive choices to the couple—whether they are married or unmarried. Counseling should be in a supportive and nonjudgmental way, explaining proper use of EC and discussing effectiveness and side effects. This may be the first contact point for reproductive health personnel and need for ongoing contraception can be discussed. The possibility of failure of EC should be disclosed to the couple and advised to report if any delay in menses occur by 1 week. Abdominal pain, heavy bleeding, and logorrhea in the next menstrual cycle is observed.[9,10]

Instructions for Use of Emergency Contraception

- Dose of EC to be repeated if vomiting occurs within 1 hour.
- It can be used at any time of the cycle.
- EC do not prevent STD.
- It will not protect rest of the cycle.
- Certain antiepileptic drugs reduce the effectiveness of contraceptives such as the pill or contraceptive implants that contain hormones. Medicines and Healthcare products Regulatory Agency (MHRA) advise that women taking these medications may need to take a double dose of the emergency contraceptive.[11.]
- EC is for emergency use only and cannot be an alternative to regular contraception.

SPECIAL CONDITIONS[8]

Adolescents with Disabilities

These adolescent patients have similar levels of sexual behavior and are also similarly exposed to STIs and may require counseling and support for healthy sexual development.

Adolescents who have severe physical disabilities or cognitive impairment will require hormonal contraceptives for menstrual control and hygiene. Suppression of menses can be achieved with COCs, transdermal patches, DMPA, and levonorgestrel IUDs.

Adolescents with Obesity

Obesity either with or without polycystic ovary syndrome is usually anovulatory, and these patients have oligomenorrhea. These adolescents are mainly concerned about the additional weight gain by the use of hormonal contraceptives. Use of drugs containing ethinyl estradiol and cyproterone acetate can serve the purpose of polycystic ovarian disease (PCOD) treatment as well as contraception.

Adolescents with Human Immunodeficiency Virus

Majority of adolescents with HIV acquire the infection through either unprotected sex or intravenous drug abuse. These adolescents also have similar contraceptive and sexual health needs like uninfected adolescents. But due to the risk of transmission to partners and drug interactions with antiretroviral therapy (ART), adolescents with HIV are a challenge for contraceptive prescription.

The Center for Disease Control and Prevention (CDC) and WHO have provided guidelines on prescription of different contraceptives for patients with HIV infection who are on ART.

These patients should be advised to use condoms as they decrease the risk of HIV transmission.

Adolescent Recipient with Solid Organ Transplantation

These patients who have solid organ transplantation and are on immunosuppressant medications, do not show a decrease in fertility. Patients who have established normal organ function and are stable can use hormonal contraceptives if there is no contraindication to estrogen.

Combined oral contraceptives should not be prescribed to patients with liver dysfunction or coronary artery disease.

Nonhormonal methods can be used temporarily after assessing drug toxicities.

Factors Contributing to Successful Family Planning Programs for Adolescents

- Dissemination of knowledge about the availability of services
- Convenient location of services, without risk of public disclosure on entering or leaving the premises
- Guaranteed confidentiality and protection of privacy throughout
- Afternoon clinic hours at times when adolescents are not required at school or expected home
- Brief admission procedure, with a minimum of "red tape"
- Appointment for services within 1 week of initial contact
- Services free or at nominal cost
- Positive staff attitude, with close attention to reducing embarrassment and enabling adolescents to acknowledge that contraception is both necessary and permissible if they have decided to be sexually active
- Personalized, friendly counseling
- Choice of method based on the adolescent's own preferences and patterns of sexual behavior, in addition to medical considerations
- Instruction of a backup method in case of discontinuation of primary method
- Frequent follow-up visits.[12]

MEDICAL TERMINATION OF PREGNANCY IN ADOLESCENTS

Sexual relationship among adolescents and young adults is a fact that should be understood and managed effectively. 16% of the total pregnancies in India are teenage pregnancies. 9% of total maternal deaths are due to teenage pregnancies, and abortions account for a significant number of these deaths.

Abortion in adolescence is associated with physical or psychological risk to the patient. Physical risks include cervical lacerations, hemorrhage, infections such as PID and endometritis, long-term risks of infertility, ectopic pregnancy, etc. Psychological risks include loss of self-confidence, sleep and sexual disturbances, reduced motivation, guilt and suicidal tendencies, and substance abuse.

Most of these pregnancies may be due to consensual relationships, and some may be due to rape or pressure/coercion by employers and family members.

How to Prevent Pregnancies and Abortions

Adolescents should be encouraged to have abstinence, and the women should have social support and empowerment to say no to any form of sexual abuse. The social setup should be such that sensitive issues, such as abortion, should be dealt with proper interventions and policy-level changes to reduce delays.

Adolescents should be properly educated and counseled. Adolescent clinics should be set up, and these should be patient friendly and help in removing the taboo of abortion and providing proper contraceptive measures.

MTP Act

In India, abortion has been legalized by the MTP Act since 1971. This was enacted in 1972. This act provides MTP for different social and medical reasons, but in case of minors who are below 18 years, written consent of the guardian is required.

Factors Contributing to Unsafe Abortions

- Delay in seeking abortion leading to complications
- Delay in reaching the healthcare providers

- *Social stigma:* Adolescents usually tend to go unskilled and untrained providers, especially in case of unmarried pregnancies
- Lack of knowledge
- Lack of privacy and confidentiality.

METHODS OF TERMINATION

Methods of termination of pregnancy are usually conforming to the gestational age at which the adolescent approaches the healthcare worker.

Usually, the early first-trimester pregnancies (42–50 days amenorrhea) can be terminated by medicinal methods.

Surgical techniques including suction evacuation [manual vacuum aspiration (MVA)] can also be used, but it has been observed that adolescents approach the healthcare worker or hospital in the second trimester when termination is more difficult and prostaglandins or other techniques have to be used.

REFERENCES

1. World Health Organization. Family Planning Evidence Brief: Reducing Early and Unintended Pregnancies among Adolescents. Geneva: World Health Organization; 2017.
2. Darroch JE, Woog V, Bankole A, Ashford LS, Points K. Costs and Benefits of Meeting the Contraceptive Needs of Adolescents. New York, NY: Guttmacher Institute; 2016 May.
3. Jain D, Tronic B. Conflicting abortion laws in India: unintended barriers to safe abortion for adolescent girls. Indian J Med Ethics. 2019;4(4)310-7.
4. Vikaspedia. Available from: https://vikaspedia.in/health/women-health/adolescent-health-1/management-of-adolescenthealth/contraception-for-adolescents (Last accessed June 2, 2020).
5. Chandra-Mouli V, McCarraher DR, Phillips SJ, Williamson NE, Hainsworth G. Contraception for adolescents in low and middle income countries: needs, barriers, and access. Reprod Health. 2014;11. Available from: http://www.reproductive-health-journal.com/content/11/1/1.
6. World Health Organization. WHO Guidelines on Preventing Early Pregnancy and Poor Reproductive Health Outcomes among Adolescents in Developing Countries. Geneva: World Health Organization; 2011.
7. Bellizzi S, Pichierri G, Menchini L, Barry J, Sotgiu G, Bassat Q. The impact of underuse of modern methods of contraception among adolescents with unintended pregnancies in 12 low-and middle-income countries. J Global Health. 2019;9(2):020429.
8. Ott M, Sucato G. Technical report: contraception for adolescents. Pediatrics. 2014;134(4):e1257-81.
9. Yuzpe AA, Lancee WJ. Ethinylestradiol and dl-norgestrel as a postcoital contraceptive. Fertil Steri. 1977;28(9):932-6.
10. Piaggio G, Von Hertzen H, Grimes DA, Van Look PF. Timing of emergency contraception with levonorgestrel or the Yuzpe regimen. Lancet. 1999;353(9154):721.
11. MHRA. Levonorgestrel-containing emergency hormonal contraception: advice on interactions with hepatic enzyme inducers and contraceptive efficacy. Available from: https://www.gov.uk/drug-safety-update/levonorgestrel-containing-emergency-hormonal-contraception-advice-oninteractions-with-hepatic-enzyme-inducers-and-contraceptive-efficacy. [Last accessed May 2, 2009.
12. American College of Obstetricians and Gynecologists. Women's Health Care Physicians. Health care for adolescents. American College of Obstetricians and Gynecologists 2003.

LONG QUESTION

1. What are the various methods of contraception that can be used in adolescent age group?

SHORT QUESTIONS

1. What are the noncontraceptive uses of oral contraceptive pills in adolescents?
2. Discuss the emergency contraception provision in adolescent friendly facilities.
3. Mention the pros and cons of DMPA in adolescents.

MULTIPLE CHOICE QUESTIONS

1. All of the following mechanisms of action of oral contraceptives pill are true, except:
   a. Inhibition of ovulation
   b. Prevention of fertilization
   c. Interference with implantation of fertilized ovum
   d. Interference with placental functioning
2. Contraindications to COC pills are:
   a. Heart disease b. Uterine malformation
   c. Menorrhagia d. Liver failure
   e. Epilepsy
3. Emergency contraception prevents pregnancy by all of the following mechanisms, except:
   a. Delaying and inhibiting ovulation
   b. Inhibiting fertilization
   c. Preventing implantation of the fertilized egg
   d. Interrupting and early pregnancy
4. Emergency contraception is required in:
   a. Partner not willing to use any contraceptives
   b. In emergency where sexual intercourse is done in camps in emergency floods
   c. Contraception failure
   d. Unprotected sex
5. All of the following agents may be used for postcoital contraception, except:
   a. Danazol b. Cu-T
   c. RU-486 d. High-dose estrogen
6. Emergency contraceptives are effective if administered within the following period after unprotected intercourse:
   a. 24 hours b. 48 hours
   c. 72 hours d. 120 hours
7. Side effects of DMPA are all, except
   a. Weight gain b. Irregular bleeding
   c. Amenorrhea d. Hepatitis

8. Norplant is:
   a. Subcutaneous implant b. Nonsteroidal pill
   c. Depot tablet d. IUCD
9. Prevention of transmission of STD is done by:
   a. COC pills b. IUCD
   c. Condom d. Norplant
10. Check all that apply. Sexually active youth face the following reproductive health risks:
    a. Unintended and too early pregnancy
    b. Sexual violence and unwanted sexual activity
    c. Too much influence on peers
    d. Sexually transmitted infections, including HIV
    e. Lack of communication with parents
11. What are the main reasons that unmarried, sexually active youth report they do not use contraception? Check all below that apply:
    a. Did not have permission from their parents
    b. Did not expect to have sex
    c. Lacked information about contraception
    d. Lacked access to resources
12. Please indicate whether the following statement is true or false.
    a. As many as half of pregnancies among unmarried women in developing countries are unintended
    b. Using contraception can reduce the risk of unsafe abortion among youth
    c. More than half of the women seeking hospital care for unsafe abortion in developing countries are younger than 20 years
    d. Medical complications from abortion are not serious
13. Check all that apply. Which of the following communication skills is needed by providers working with youth?
    a. Reflective listening b. Superior knowledge
    c. Closed-ended questions d. Honesty
    e. Nonjudgmental attitude
14. Check all that apply. Why are barrier methods considered particularly appropriate for young people?
    a. Many young adults are at high risk of STIs
    b. Many young people have easier access to barrier methods than to other contraceptives
    c. They are good methods for couples in long-term relationships
    d. They can be easily initiated and discontinued
    e. All of the above
15. Please indicate whether the following statements about oral contraceptives are true or false.
    a. Oral contraceptives are very safe for young women
    b. Oral contraceptives can protect against ectopic pregnancy, benign breast disease, ovarian and endometrial cancer, and some forms of pelvic inflammatory disease
    c. Fertility returns 10 months to a year after a woman stops taking the pill
    d. Oral contraceptives are usually available only through a clinic or other trained providers
    e. Progestin-only pills are the best type of oral contraception for most young women
    f. Oral contraceptives offer protection against some STIs.
16. Which of the following methods are considered appropriate for young people? Check all that apply.
    a. Complete abstinence
    b. Oral contraceptives
    c. Condoms
    d. IUDs
    e. Sterilization

Answers

1. d 2. d 3. d 4. d 5. a 6. c
7. d 8. a 9. c 10. All 11. c, d
12. a True, b True; c False, d False 13. a, b, d, e
14. a, b, d, applies
15. a True, b True; c False, d False, e False 16. b, c

5.2 PERIMENOPAUSAL WOMEN

Nisha Rani, Shikha Sachan

INTRODUCTION

Perimenopause is the phase in the aging process in which a woman passes from the reproductive to the nonreproductive stage.[1,2] During these perimenopausal years, menstrual cycles tend to become irregular, but although there is a decline in natural fertility, contraception is still necessary if unplanned pregnancies are to be avoided. The importance of contraception for the older woman is emphasized by figures from the USA, which show that the highest percentages of unplanned pregnancies have been in adolescents and in women older than 35 years.[3]

Worldwide, elderly population is increasing with women forming the majority. Those approaching the menopause often have contraceptive requirements which differ from those of younger women, but the provision of effective contraception remains equally important. Pregnancies in the late reproductive years are associated with a higher maternal as well as perinatal mortality and a greater incidence of fetal malformation. Medical disorders such as diabetes mellitus and essential hypertension are more common, and these conditions increase the risk to both the mother and fetus. If pregnancy termination is chosen, this can expose the couple to psychological trauma and carries with its significant medical risk. Various gynecological pathologies such as uterine fibroids are also more frequently encountered in perimenopausal women, and anovulatory cycles during the perimenopause may cause dysfunctional uterine bleeding or predispose to endometrial hyperplasia and carcinoma.

This chapter describes some of the theoretical advantages and disadvantages of various methods of contraception for perimenopausal women. What should be borne in mind, however, is that one of the greatest problems faced by many of the developing countries is the provision of realistic access to family planning services.[4] The age-specific fertility rates (ASFR) throw light on the fertility pattern and success of family planning plans. It is defined as number of live birth in a year to 1,000 women in any specified age group.

The goals of an effective service should be to offer a wide variety of contraceptive methods from easily accessible centers staffed by educated personnel. It is also essential that the cost of contraceptives should not be prohibitive.

HORMONAL CHANGES DURING THE PERIMENOPAUSE

During the reproductive life span, the number of ovarian primordial follicles steadily diminishes, but after approximately 40 years of age the rate at which follicles are lost starts to accelerate.[5] Despite the reduction in the number of follicles, ovulation continues in up to 98% of women over the age of 40 who have regular menstrual cycles,[6] which emphasizes the necessity for the continued use of contraception.[7,8]

TYPES OF CONTRACEPTION

Women must be advised on all available methods of contraception, including long-acting reversible contraceptives (LARCs), so they can make an informed choice. No method of contraception is contraindicated based on age alone, up to the age of 50 years. Contraceptive methods are categorized according to their risk and benefit in the presence of certain medical conditions and lifestyles. *Medical eligibility criteria* are classified as

- No restriction for use of the contraceptive methods
- Advantages outweigh the theoretical or proven risk
- Theoretical or proven risk outweigh the advantages
- Unacceptable health risk if used.

Although all forms of contraception are available to couples where the female partner is perimenopausal, certain methods may be more suitable for women in this age group on medical grounds, whereas other methods may have no medical advantage but may simply be more convenient or more acceptable. After the age of 40 years, women become less likely to use contraception, but those who do so will more frequently undergo sterilization and are less likely to use oral contraceptives than younger women.[9]

Oral Contraceptives

Oral contraception is becoming an increasingly more popular form of birth control for healthy perimenopausal women as the safety of this method has become well established, especially for women who are nonsmokers and who have no cardiovascular risk factors. Although oral contraceptives have some adverse effects, they also provide benefits apart from the contraceptive action which may have a favorable effect on the health of a perimenopausal woman.

There are a number of reasons why the use of oral contraceptives has gained popularity in recent years, particularly in older women:

- Low dose of sex steroids in combined oral contraceptive pills is now available.
- Better screening methods for complications from oral contraceptive use.
- Substantial overall decline in the number of young women suffering from myocardial infarction and stroke.[10]

Oral contraceptives are extremely effective when properly used. The failure rate of the new multiphasic and low-dose monophasic combination pills is approximately 0.1% per annum under ideal circumstances and 3.0% per annum in unselected users. The lower-dose preparations require that the tablet be taken at the same time each day, and this time restraint is even more strict for the progestogen-only pills.

Progestogen-only oral contraceptives may be considered for perimenopausal women who smoke or who have other contraindications to estrogen use or who suffer estrogen-related side effects. Cycle control is not as good as with combined oral contraceptives, and an irregular bleeding pattern is the main reason for discontinuation of treatment. This may make this form of contraception unsuitable for many perimenopausal women.[11]

Adverse effects of oral contraceptives on perimenopausal women are as follows:

- Contraceptive pills containing more than 50 mg ethinylestradiol which are associated with a higher risk of developing venous thrombosis, myocardial infarction, and stroke.[12,13] A slightly greater risk of thrombosis may also be present with 30 mg doses, but this represents only a minimal increase as it translates into one additional death per one million users per year with oral contraceptives compared with users of intrauterine contraceptive devices (IUDs).[14]
- Risk of stroke was increased in users.
- Low-dose oral contraceptives may cause an increase in blood pressure in a small proportion of users, but this appears to apply more to the monophasic than the multiphasic preparations.

- Oral contraceptives containing the newer progestogens have less effect on insulin production as reflected on glucose tolerance testing and hence have less effect on diabetes mellitus which is more likely to affect women who are perimenopausal.[15]

Beneficial effects of oral contraceptives on perimenopausal women include the following:

- Oral contraceptives provide good cycle control and reduce the volume of bleeding in perimenopausal women with dysfunctional uterine bleeding due to anovulatory cycles.
- In addition, they prevent endometrial hyperplasia and reduce the risk of endometrial carcinoma by at least 40% with more than 2 years of use.[16]
- Oral contraceptives also provide protection against ovarian carcinoma. The magnitude of the reduction in risk is less than that with endometrial carcinoma, but the effect persists for up to 15 years after discontinuation of treatment.[17,18]
- Incidence of fibroid increases at the perimenopausal age group, and for these women with uterine fibroids and menorrhagia, the use of oral contraceptives may reduce the volume of menstrual bleeding.
- Perimenopausal women may especially benefit from the protection against osteoporosis provided by oral contraceptives. Reduced concentrations of estradiol in perimenopausal women predispose to the development of osteoporosis, but bone loss may be prevented by oral contraceptive use **(Fig. 1)**.[16]

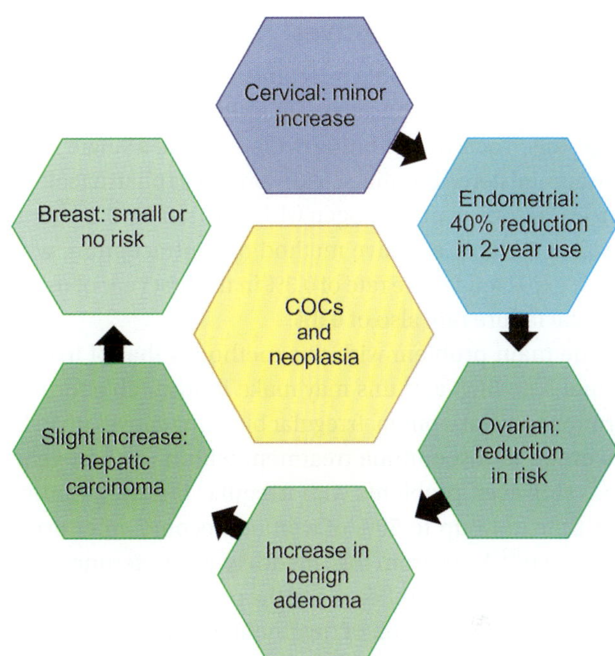

Fig. 1: Effect of oral contraceptives on different neoplasia. (COC: combined oral contraceptive).

Barrier Methods

Barrier contraception is safe to use until menopause is confirmed. Both men and women have barrier methods of contraception available to them. Condoms, diaphragms, caps, and spermicides are relatively cheap methods of contraception which do not carry any special advantages for perimenopausal compared with younger women. One of their main benefits is protection against sexually transmitted diseases, especially the human immunodeficiency virus (HIV).

Perimenopausal women are equally at risk of contracting the virus, and this factor may make condoms the safest method in many of the developing countries. Other advantages of condoms are that they are usually easy to obtain, are a reversible method of contraception, and are comparatively cheap. Condoms are 98% effective and women's barrier methods are up to 95% effective; however, the effectiveness of both methods is user dependent. Diaphragms have a relatively high failure rate, but they are more commonly used by older women with a lower rate of natural fertility.[19]

Intrauterine Contraceptive Devices

Intrauterine device is an effective and safe form of long-term contraception in women over the age of 40 years. IUDs have the advantages of being reversible and not needing frequent replacement. They are also highly effective, with the lowest expected failure rate of 0.8–2.0% during the first year of use and a typical failure rate of up to 3%. The relatively new hormonal IUD which releases 20 mg levonorgestrel (LNG) each day may be particularly useful for the perimenopausal woman. The most common indication for removal of this device is amenorrhea,[20] which is unlikely to be viewed as a disadvantage by perimenopausal women. The LNG IUD is also associated with fewer episodes of prolonged bleeding, and the constant release of progestogen protects against endometrial hyperplasia. Since they also have high efficacy and are a long-lasting form of contraception, they may be especially suitable for perimenopausal women.

Intrauterine devices can be used as both emergency and continuing contraception for a period of 5–10 years and work by interfering with fertilization and implantation. IUDs must be removed after menopause or when no longer required. IUDs have minimal systemic effects so can be safely used in women with comorbidities that are more common in perimenopausal women such as diabetes, hypertension, cardiovascular, cerebrovascular, and thrombotic diseases.

Adverse Effects

Intrauterine devices are associated with intermenstrual bleeding, spotting, and prolonged bleeding, especially within the first 3–6 months. These bleeding patterns are usually harmless and self-limiting, but counseling is necessary to prevent early discontinuation in perimenopausal women. If they persist, it is essential to exclude STIs and gynecological pathologies.

Injectable Contraceptives

The most widely available injectable contraceptive is depot-medroxy-progesterone acetate (Depo-Provera). This injectable progestogen acts by inhibiting ovulation, and a single 150 mg dose administered intramuscularly produces pharmacological concentrations of progestogen which persist for 3–4 months. It is also a highly effective method of contraception, with a lowest expected failure rate of 0.3% in the first year of use and a typical failure rate also of 0.3%.

The main problem with this method is that of irregular vaginal bleeding, and this may make it unsuitable for many perimenopausal women. Irregular bleeding causes up to 25% of women to discontinue treatment within the first year of use.[21] However, problems with irregular bleeding diminish with time, and up to 50% of women become amenorrheic after 1 year.[22] Apart from this, medroxy-progesterone acetate has relatively few side effects, and the possible delay in fertility after the discontinuation of treatment is rarely a problem for perimenopausal women.

Contraceptive Implants

The sustained-release LNG contraceptive implant (Norplant) consists of six silastic implants, each of which contains 36 mg LNG. A newer preparation consists of two rods containing a total of 70 mg LNG (Norplant-2), and these are easier to insert and to remove than the older implant. They act by inhibiting ovulation and are highly effective, with lowest expected as well as typical failure rates of 0.2% in the first year. LNG concentrations with Norplant peak at 0.4–0.5 ng/mL, but decrease to around 0.25 ng/mL after 5 years, which is the recommended duration of use.[23] Although Norplant is highly effective, skill is required to insert the implants and also to remove them if problems occur. The most common side effect leading to discontinuation of treatment is that of irregular bleeding, which means that this is another form of contraception which will be unsuitable for some perimenopausal women. Over 5 years, only 5–10% of women become amenorrhoeic and abnormal bleeding patterns develop in up to 80% of users.

The advantages for perimenopausal women are the low incidence of metabolic side effects and the long duration of action. Although Norplant is associated with a high incidence of irregular bleeding, it is not usually heavy, and for a perimenopausal woman whose only preceding problem has been menorrhagia, the use of Norplant may reduce the volume of blood loss and protect against anemia.[24]

Natural Family Planning Methods

Fertility awareness methods, also called "natural methods," include monitoring body temperature, cervical mucus, and the length of the menstrual cycle and plotting the values on a chart to predict the fertile time. Natural family planning (NFP) methods become less reliable in the perimenopause because ovulation becomes more difficult to predict as cycles become less regular and ovulation markers are difficult to interpret. Both the woman and her partner must be motivated to use this method consistently and correctly.

Withdrawal, as for example, is a natural form of contraception used by a few UK perimenopausal couples. It prevents approximately 50% of pregnancies that would have happened without using the method. With lower fertility rates in the perimenopause, withdrawal can be used as an adjunct to other methods.

Sterilization

Sterilization is the most commonly used of all methods of contraception.[25] In the USA, approximately 15% of couples choose tubal sterilization and 12% vasectomy. In the UK, over 40% of couples choose sterilization when the female partner is over 40 years of age. Sterilization involves occluding the fallopian tubes and can be done laparoscopically, via minilaparotomy, during cesarean section, or hysteroscopically. Another form of contraception must be used until tubal occlusion is confirmed after 3 months. Vasectomy has a lower failure rate after proven azoospermia. Both tubal sterilization and vasectomy are safe and effective methods of contraception and are suitable options for couples who have completed their family. Tubal sterilization has been reported to have a lowest expected failure rate of 0.2% during the first year and a typical failure rate of 0.4%.[26]

Sterilization has an advantage over contraceptive methods which must be used on a regular basis and has few unwanted effects. The main risks of the procedure involve the immediate problems of the anesthetic and the operation. Apart from the operative risks, it has been suggested that tubal sterilization may increase the chance of subsequent menstrual disturbances. The evidence is contradictory, however, as dysfunctional uterine bleeding is more common with advancing age and is especially likely to affect perimenopausal women. The balance of evidence suggests that the association between sterilization and menstrual disorders is probably coincidental,[26] and this is not thought to be a valid reason for choosing an alternative method of contraception.

Emergency Contraception

There are three methods of emergency contraception commonly available: LNG, ulipristal acetate (UPA), and copper IUD. All are safe for use during the perimenopause. LNG and UPA inhibit or delay ovulation for up to 7 days, which is beyond the natural span of sperm within the genital tract, and can both be used more than once in the same menstrual cycle.[26]

Levonorgestrel can be used up to 72 hours after unprotected sexual intercourse (UPSI) but becomes less effective as time passes. UPA remains effective up to 120 hours after UPSI. LNG works only up until the start of the preovulatory luteinizing hormone (LH) surge. Copper IUDs are the most effective form of EC and should always be offered when EC is requested. IUDs effectively prevent implantation after fertilization as soon as they are fitted. This mechanism of action should be explained because methods that act after fertilization are not acceptable to some women.

Following EC with LNG, reliable continuing contraception should be started as soon as possible—ideally straight away—along with an additional barrier method until the hormonal method becomes effective. Progesterone-containing contraceptives after UPA increases the risk of breakthrough ovulation so should not be given within 5 days of UPA. There is no evidence that failed EC results in increased fetal abnormality rates, so a request for EC should rarely be refused, even where menstrual cycles have become irregular.

TERMINATION OF PREGNANCY

Termination of unwanted pregnancy in the perimenopausal age group merits special attention due to associated comorbidities such as diabetes mellitus, hypertension, and cardiovascular morbidities. Certain gynecological conditions such as fibroid, adenomyosis, and endometrial hyperplasia also have increased incidence during this period, which should be considered while planning. The various methods of termination available are as follows:

Nonsurgical Methods

- Mifepristone in combination with misoprostol
- Mechanical dilators
- Misoprostol used alone vaginally.

Surgical Methods

- Vacuum aspiration
- Dilatation and evacuation.

Care should be taken for proper counseling and psychological support as pregnancy in the perimenopausal age group is still a taboo in many parts of India.[27] Women should also be offered contraceptive counseling at the same time. The conceptus should be sent for histopathological testing.

CONCLUSION

In the absence of accurate evidence-based advice on fertility, contraception, and hormone replacement therapy (HRT), perimenopausal women remain at risk of an unplanned pregnancy. There is no method of contraception that is contraindicated for women under the age of 50 years on the basis of age alone. HRT does not provide adequate contraception. After taking a comprehensive medical history, all women should be given information on all suitable methods of contraception so that they can make an informed choice. When giving contraceptive advice to perimenopausal women with multiple comorbidities, clinicians should carefully consider the associated risks. New research and product developments will widen the contraceptive choice for women in this age group.

There are no clearly established guidelines for when it is safe for a perimenopausal woman to discontinue contraception. Whitehead and Godfree[26] suggested that contraception should be continued for women who are 50 years or older until after 1 year of amenorrhea, and for younger women, for a period of 2 years. If a perimenopausal woman is using oral contraceptives, it may be advisable to change to another method for a few months at around 50 years of age before measuring gonadotropin concentrations to determine her menopausal status. For users of both hormonal and nonhormonal methods, the time at which it is safe to discontinue contraception provides a suitable opportunity to discuss the risks and benefits of HRT for the management of menopause **(Table 1)**.

Age itself is not a contraindication for any method of contraception or method of termination of pregnancy.

- After teenage most of the unplanned pregnancy happen in this age group.
- Increased incidence of lifestyle diseases such as diabetes and hypertension and gynecological disorders such as fibroid and endometrial hyperplasia should be given special consideration while prescribing contraception and termination.
- Levonorgestrel-releasing devices are one of the ideal choice for contraception in perimenopausal women as they have least side effects.
- Proper counseling and mental support should be provided for unwanted pregnancy termination.
- Each perimenopausal women should be individualized while prescribing.

KEY MESSAGES

- Although women's natural fertility declines after their mid-30s, effective contraception is required until menopause to prevent unintended pregnancies.
- We should be aware that the risks of fetal chromosomal abnormalities, miscarriage, pregnancy complications, and maternal morbidity and mortality increase for women aged 40 years and older.
- No contraceptive method is contraindicated on the basis of age alone. Clinicians must carefully consider comorbidities when prescribing women the most suitable contraception.
- Return of fertility can be delayed for up to 1 year after discontinuing progestogen-only injectable contraceptives; therefore, these contraceptives are not suitable for perimenopausal women considering future pregnancies.
- Contraceptive methods with a recognized postfertilization, preimplantation effect may not be acceptable to some women.
- Women should be given information about all suitable contraceptive methods to make an informed choice.
- If pregnancy termination is chosen, this can expose the couple to psychological trauma and carries with its significant medical risk.

TABLE 1: The main advantages, risks, and reliability of contraceptive methods for perimenopausal women.

Method	*Advantages*	*Disadvantages*	*Risk of failure in first year of typical nonperfect use (%)*
Combined hormonal contraception	Regular bleeding pattern Reduction in menstrual bleeding and flushes	Increased risk of thrombosis, and breast and cervical cancer Daily dosing required	9.0
Progesterone-only pills	Very few medical contraindications	Irregular bleeding Daily dosing required	9.0
Progesterone-only injectable	Long -acting method Often induces amenorrhoea	Masks menopause Bone mineral density concerns Unable to remove after injection	6.0
Progesterone-only implant	Very few contraindications Easily reversible	Irregular bleeding Requires trained operative	0.05
Copper intrauterine device	Hormone free Does not mask menopause Long-acting method	Heavy menstrual bleeding and pelvic cramps Unsuitable if woman has a distorted uterine cavity	0.8
Levonorgestrel-releasing device	Long-acting method Treatment for heavy menstrual bleeding Endometrial protection with hormone replacement therapy	Irregular bleeding Unsuitable if woman has a distorted uterine cavity	0.2

- For users of both hormonal and nonhormonal methods, the time at which it is safe to discontinue contraception provides a suitable opportunity to discuss the risks and benefits of hormone replacement therapy for the management of the menopause.

REFERENCES

1. World Health Organization. Research on the menopause. WHO Tech Rep Ser. 1981;670:8-10.
2. World Health Organization. Research on the menopause in the 1990s. WHO Tech Rep Ser. 1996;866:13.
3. Sulak PJ, Haney AF. Unwanted pregnancies: understanding contraceptive use and benefits in adolescents and older women. Am J Obstet Gynecol. 1993;168:2042-8.
4. Potts DM, Crane SF. Contraceptive delivery in the developing world. Br Med Bull. 1993;49:27-39.
5. Richardson SJ, Senikas V, Nelson JF. Follicular depletion during the menopausal transition: evidence for accelerated loss and ultimate exhaustion. J Clin Endocrinol Metab. 1987;65:1231-7.
6. Metcalf MG. The approach of menopause: a New Zealand study. N Z Med J. 1988;101:103-6.
7. Lee SJ, Lenton EA, Sexton L, Cooke ID. The effect of age on the cyclical patterns of plasma LH, FSH, oestradiol and progesterone in women with regular menstrual cycles. Hum Reprod. 1988;3:851–5.
8. Burger HG. Reproductive hormone measurements during the menopausal transition. In: Berg G, Hammar M (Eds). The Modern Management of the Menopause. Carnforth, UK: Parthenon; 1994. pp. 103-7.
9. Oddens BJ, Visser AP, Vemer HM, Everaerd WT, Lehert P. Contraceptive use and attitudes in Great Britain. Contraception. 1994;49:73-86.
10. Fortney JA. Oral contraceptives for older women. IPPF Med Bull. 1990;24:3-4.
11. Broome M, Fotherby K. Clinical experience with the progestogen-only pill. Contraception. 1990;42:489-95.
12. Mann JI, Vessey MP, Thorogood M, Doll SR. Myocardial infarction in young women with special reference to oral contraceptive practice. Br Med J. 1975;2:241-5.
13. Berel V. Mortality among oral contraceptive users. Royal College of General Practitioners' Oral Contraception Study. Lancet. 1977;ii:727-31.
14. Hirvonen E, Idanpaan-Heikkila J. Cardiovascular death among women under 40 years of age using low-estrogen oral contraceptives and intrauterine devices in Finland from 1975 to 1984. Am J Obstet Gynecol. 1990;163:281-4.
15. Becker H. Supportive European data on a new oral contraceptive containing norgestimate. Acta Obstet Gynecol Scand Suppl. 1990;152:33-9.
16. Vessey MP, Painter R. Endometrial and ovarian cancer and oral contraceptives—findings in a large cohort study. Br J Cancer. 1995;71:1340-2.
17. Cancer and Steroid Hormone Study of the CDC and NICHD. The reduction in risk of ovarian cancer associated with oral-contraceptive use. N Engl J Med. 1987;316:650-5.
18. Vessey MP, Lawless M, Yeates D. Efficacy of different contraceptive methods. Lancet. 1982;i:841-2.
19. Chi IC. The TCu-380A, (AG), MLCu375, and Nova-T IUDs and the IUD daily releasing 20 mg levonorgestrel—four pillars of IUD contraception for the nineties and beyond? Contraception. 1993;47:325-47.
20. Cromer BA, Smith RD, Blair JM, Dwyer J, Brown RT. A prospective study of adolescents who choose among levonorgestrel implant (Norplant), medroxyprogesterone acetate (Depo-Provera), or the combined oral contraceptive pill as contraception. Pediatrics. 1994;94:687-94.
21. Brache V, Alvarez-Sanchez F, Faundes A, Tejada AS, Cochon L. Ovarian endocrine function through five years of continuous treatment with Norplant subdermal contraceptive implants. Contraception. 1990;41:169-77.
22. Nilsson CG, Holma P. Menstrual blood loss with contraceptive subdermal levonorgestrel implants. Fertil Steril. 1981;35:304-6.

23. Whitehead MI, Godfree V. Hormone replacement therapy: your questions answered. Edinburgh: Churchill Livingstone; 1992. p. 215.
24. Parker-Mauldin W, Segal S. Prevalence of contraceptive use: trends and issues. Stud Fam Plann. 1988;6:335.
25. Trussell J, Hatcher RA, Cates W Jr, Stewart FH, Kost K. Contraceptive failure in the United States: an update. Stud Fam Plann. 1990;21:51-4.
26. Liskin L, Rinehart W, Blackburn R, Rutledge AH. Minilaparotomy and laparoscopy: safe, effective and widely used. Popul Rep Ser C. 1985;9:125-67.
27. Government Of India. Sample Registration System Statistical Report 2016, Office of the Registrar General and Census Commissioner India, Ministry of Home Affairs, New Delhi; 2017.

LONG QUESTIONS

1. 40 years old $G_4P_3L_3$ reports for pregnancy termination and contraception. She is a known case of hypertension since 6 years and has impaired glucose tolerance. How will you manage and counsel her?
2. What is the mechanism of action of intrauterine devices? Discuss the advantages and disadvantages of using intrauterine devices in perimenopausal age group?
3. Discuss the plausibility of prescribing oral contraceptive pills in perimenopausal age group.

SHORT QUESTIONS

1. How can a healthcare provider be reasonably certain that a woman is not pregnant?
2. What are the serious cardiovascular side effects of combined pills?
3. When to stop further contraceptive usage in a woman?
4. Write short notes on:
   a. Side effects of injectable contraceptives
   b. Pregnancy termination in a 42-year-old woman
   c. Barrier method in perimenopausal age group
   d. Pregnancy at 40 years of age.

MULTIPLE CHOICE QUESTIONS

1. Which of the following is false about stopping contraception?
   a. For women over the age of 50 years who do not use hormonal methods, contraception can be stopped after 6 months of amenorrhea
   b. Women less than 50 years contraception should be continued for 2 years
   c. For women over 50 years using progesterone-only pill, subdermal implants and IUDs should continue using for 1 year two FSH levels of >30 IU/L taken at least 6 weeks apart
   d. Women can consider stopping their method of contraception at the age of 55 years
2. Femilon has the following disadvantages, except:
   a. Reduces venous thrombosis
   b. Is cheaper than standard oral contraceptive pills (OCPs)
   c. Reduces acne and hirsutism
   d. Useful in heart disease
3. Which of the following statements about levonorgestrel-releasing intrauterine system (LNG-IUS) is incorrect?
   a. There is decreased incidence of rectovaginal endometriosis
   b. This system can be used as hormone replacement therapy
   c. It is useful in treatment of endometrial hyperplasia
   d. Irregular uterine bleeding is not a problem during initial use
4. Emergency contraceptive prevents pregnancy by all, except:
   a. Delaying ovulation
   b. Inhibiting fertilization
   c. Preventing implantation of the fertilized egg
   d. Interrupting an early pregnancy
4. The perimenopausal age group is characterized by the following:
   a. Decreasing ovarian reserves
   b. Increasing comorbidities like diabetes mellitus (DM) and HT
   c. Increased incidence of endometrial hyperplasia
   d. All of the above
5. Unplanned pregnancy is mostly seen in which age group?
   a. Adolescence b. Perimenopausal
   c. Mid thirties d. Late twenties
6. Hormonal changes characterizing perimenopausal age group are:
   a. Decrease in both LH and follicle-stimulating hormone (FSH
   b. Increase in FSH (2 to 3 times) and LH remains same
   c. No change in FSH and LH
   d. Both LH and FSH increase
7. LNG-containing intrauterine devices are not used in:
   a. Endometrial hyperplasia b. Osteoporosis
   c. Submucosal fibroids d. Irregular bleeding
8. Which of the following is not a side effect of oral contraceptive pills?
   a. Increased incidence of ovarian carcinoma
   b. Increased incidence of thrombosis
   c. Altered lipid profile
   d. Increased incidence of stroke
9. A 42-year-old $G_8P_4A_4L_4$ hypertensive and diabetic reports to the outpatient department (OPD) for pregnancy termination at 9 weeks. What contraception will be best for her after termination:
   a. OCP b. Progesterone-only pill
   c. Barrier method d. Tubal ligation

Answers

1. a 2. a 3. d 4. d 5. a 6. b
7. c 8. a 9. d

5.3 CONTRACEPTION AND PREGNANCY TERMINATION FOR WOMEN WITH MEDICAL DISORDERS

Ashok Kumar, Sai Charisma

INTRODUCTION

Ideally, all women should have a reproductive life plan and all of their pregnancies should be intended and planned.[1] In the reproductive age, many women have chronic medical conditions that are affected by pregnancy or during which the fetus is placed at an increased risk. In most of those women, ongoing medical management of their conditions is greatly improved, even compared with a decade or two ago. However, their condition is seriously exacerbated by the physiological changes of pregnancy, so their pregnancy should be planned and monitored carefully for optimal results. This requires effective and safe contraceptive use until pregnancy is desired and the medical condition is stabilized.[2] Familiarity with the appropriate options for birth control in women with medical illness is therefore an integral part of their obstetric care.

Currently available contraceptive methods are grouped into efficacy tiers by World Health Organization (WHO).[3]

Top Tier: Most Effective

- Intrauterine devices (IUDs)
- Copper IUD (Cu-IUD)
- Levonorgestrel-releasing intrauterine system (LNG-IUS): Mirena®
- Sterilization
- Female sterilization
- Male sterilization.

Second Tier: Very Effective

- Combined oral contraceptive (COC; estrogen and progestin) pill
- Progestin-only pill (POP)
- Transdermal norelgestromin/ethinyl estradiol system patch
- Etonogestrel/ethinyl estradiol vaginal ring: NuvaRing®
- Medroxyprogesterone acetate injectable suspension [depot-medroxy-progesterone acetate (DMPA)]: Depo-Provera®
- Etonogestrel (ETG) implant: Implanon®.

Third Tier: Effective

- Condom (male and female)
- Fertility awareness-based methods
- Fertility awareness-based methods overall
- Standard days method (avoiding intercourse on cycle days 9–19)
- 2o-day method (based on cervical mucus)
- Ovulation method (based on cervical mucus).

Fourth Tier: Least Effective

- Spermicides
- Sponge.

No WHO Category

- Withdrawal method
- No contraception.

Many contraceptives will also have adverse effects on some medical conditions, and there is now a considerable awareness of the complexities of some of these interactions. For this reason, the WHO has developed an excellent, simple, and pragmatic program of guidelines on a four-point scale [the WHO "Medical Eligibility Criteria" (WHO-MEC)],[4] summarizing risk of specific contraceptive methods in women with specified chronic medical conditions.

Medical eligibility criteria categories for contraceptive eligibility are as follows:

- A condition for which there is no restriction for the use of the contraceptive method
- A condition in which the advantages of using the method generally outweigh the theoretical or proven risks
- A condition in which the theoretical or proven risks usually outweigh the advantages of using the method
- A condition which represents an unacceptable health risk if the contraceptive method is used.

Table 1 lists the recommended MEC categories of some contraceptive methods.[5]

SPECIFIC MEDICAL CONDITIONS

Women with Cardiac Disease

Contraceptive Methods

Cardiac disease offers a good example of a range of related medical conditions which require specialized and individualized assessment and consideration of the risks faced by a particular woman whether she wishes to attempt a pregnancy or whether she wishes, or needs, to reliably prevent pregnancy for a period of time.[6] There is a wide range of types of congenital and acquired cardiac disease ranging from those raising only minor concern (e.g., uncomplicated valvular or congenital heart disease) to certain conditions which may be associated with substantially increased risk of maternal morbidity or mortality (e.g., pulmonary hypertension or current ischemic heart disease).[7] It needs to be recognized that pregnancy causes considerable physiological cardiovascular changes from early gestation,

TABLE 1: MEC (contraindications and cautions) with specific contraceptive methods.

Condition	*CHC*	*POP*	*DMPA*	*Implants*	*LNG-IUS*	*Cu-IUD*
Active breast cancer	4	4	4	4	4	1
Breast cancer disease free ≥5 years	3	3	3	3	3	1
Multiple cardiovascular risks	3/4*	2	3	2	2	1
Well-controlled or mild chronic hypertension	3	1	2	1	1	1
SBP ≥ 160 mm Hg or DBP ≥ 100 mm Hg	4	2	3	2	2	1
Vascular disease	4	3	3	2	2	1
Complicated heart valve disease	4	1	1	1	2	2
Acute venous thromboembolism	3/4*	3	3	3	3	1
History of venous thromboembolism	3/4*	2	2	2	2	1
Thrombophilia	4	2	2	2	2	1
Surgery with long immobilization	4	2	2	2	2	1
Major surgery without long immobilization	2	1	1	1	1	1
Diabetes >20 years or vascular disease	3/4*	2	3	2	2	1
Diabetes with end-organ failure	3/4*	2	3	2	2	1
Cirrhosis (severe, decompensated)	4	3	3	3	3	1
Liver tumors	4	3	3	3	3	1
Symptomatic gallbladder disease	3	2	2	2	2	1
Distorted uterine cavity	1	1	1	1	4	4
Enzyme inducing anticonvulsants	3	3	1	2	1	1
Lamotrigine	3	1	1	1	1	1
Current or history of ischemic heart disease	4	2/3	3	2/3	2/3	1
Stroke	4	2/3	3	2/3	2/3	1
Migraine with aura	4	2/3	2/3	2/3	2	1
Unexplained vaginal bleeding	2	2	3	3	4/2	4/2
Cervical cancer before treatment	2	1	2	2	4/2	4/2
Current PID or cervicitis	1	1	1	1	4/2	4/2
Acute viral hepatitis	4/2	1	1	1	1	1
Pelvic tuberculosis	1	1	1	1	4/3	4/3
SLE and positive or unknown APAs	4	3	3	3	3	1
SLE and severe thrombocytopenia	2	2	3	2	2	3/2
Complicated solid organ transplant	4	–	–	–	3/2	3/2

*In those methods, under start/continue columns, the first MEC number refers to whether a method may be initiated in an affected patient. For patients who initially develop the condition while using a specific method, the second number refers to risks for continuing that method.
(APA: antiphospholipid antibody; CHC: combined hormonal contraception; Cu-IUD: copper intrauterine device; DBP: diastolic blood pressure; DMPA: depot medroxyprogesterone acetate; LNG-IUS: levonorgestrel-releasing intrauterine system; PID: pelvic inflammatory disease; POP: progestin-only pill; SBP: systolic blood pressure; SLE: systemic lupus erythematosus; S/C: start/continue)

and these place substantial extra demands on the pregnant heart.[8] Hence, careful, specialized prepregnancy assessment and planning are strongly advised for the individual woman with any cardiac condition. The four categories of the New York Heart Association guidelines are still the important basis for assessment of risk for women with cardiac disease in pregnancy, modified if necessary for the local situations.[7] It is worth noting that the WHO recommends no contraindication for the use of postcoital ("emergency") contraception in women with medical problems, including cardiovascular and thromboembolic diseases. The short duration of exposure associated with single-dose hormonal therapy is unlikely to be of harm. In patients at risk for thromboembolic disease, it may be prudent, however, to favor progestin-only emergency contraceptive regimens over those that include estrogen. In cases in which women of reproductive age have significant cardiac lesions or for those who develop life-threatening cardiac complications during pregnancy, it is critical that counseling regarding effective contraception occurs. Furthermore, as most pregnancies in the general population are unplanned, women with congenital or acquired heart disease require special attention. Options for contraception include barrier methods, hormonal contraception, and sterilization. The choice of the method depends on the maternal cardiac status, associated risk factors, and consideration of the consequences of unplanned pregnancies in life-threatening situations.[9] As most barrier methods are associated with a high failure rate (up to 26%), they cannot be recommended alone as ideal contraception. However, when used in conjunction with other methods, they may confer greater confidence in conception control. The standard COC tablets are highly effective, with typical failure rates <1%. Vaginal rings and combined injectable forms of combined estrogen/progestin preparations are available in some areas but have less established use in the setting of women with heart disease. All contraceptives containing estrogen carry risks of arterial and venous thrombosis and are generally to be avoided in women with significant valvular heart disease associated with the risk of valvular or mural thrombosis or in patients with cyanotic heart disease with the potential for paradoxic embolism. Although women taking warfarin for prothrombotic heart conditions have a relative contraindication to estrogen-containing contraceptives, the efficacy of these agents may justify their use when a patient is reliably protected by anticoagulation but desiring a reversible mode of contraception. Progestin-only preparations are not contraindicated in cardiac disease as they carry minimal thrombotic risk.[10,11] The failure rates associated with progestin-only preparations are slightly higher than those for COCs and are associated with higher vaginal breakthrough bleeding rates. However, with careful use and barrier method back-up, they may provide an ideal solution for women with complex heart disease. The long-acting injectable form, depot medroxyprogesterone, provides a high degree of protection, but may be a source of bleeding and/or hematoma formation at the site of injection in women who are anticoagulated. IUDs, such as the copper device or progestin-containing intrauterine system (IUS), have very low failure rates, approaching the rates seen with sterilization procedures. Placement of these devices may theoretically predispose to bacterial endocarditis, but a similar situation applies here as to the role of infective endocarditis (IE) prophylaxis as was previously discussed for vaginal and cesarean deliveries. The WHO supports their use in women with cardiac disease. At the time of insertion, clinicians should remember that a vagal response may occur, and therefore the resulting decrease in left-sided pressures could also be undesirable in patients with intracardiac shunts. Arrhythmias at the time of IUD insertion have been reported as well.[12] Thus, in patients with shunts and those at higher risk of developing bacterial endocarditis (Eisenmenger's syndrome, uncorrected tetralogy of Fallot, patent ductus arteriosus, coarctation of the aorta, and significant mitral and aortic valve disease), IUD should be inserted with caution or placed carefully (due to the risk of uterine perforation) in the immediate postpartum period.[13] For patients who have completed their families or where the medical condition cannot be repaired and is perceived to be associated with high maternal and fetal morbidity and mortality [severe pulmonary hypertension, left ventricular dysfunction, New York Heart Association (NYHA) classes III and IV], vasectomy or tubal ligation should be offered. As tubal ligations are typically performed via a laparoscopic approach, the effect of intraperitoneal carbon dioxide insufflation and general anesthesia on cardiac output, as well as the possibility of air embolism, must be considered in patients with cyanotic lesions or pulmonary hypertension. Laparoscopic procedures usually require general anesthesia, as insufflation of the abdomen and pressure on the diaphragm are poorly tolerated by awake patients under neuraxial anesthesia. It may be a safer approach to consider a minilaparotomy as the preferred approach, under slowly titrated neuraxial anesthesia.

Termination of Pregnancy

For the patient with complex congenital heart disease in whom continuation of pregnancy presents a substantial risk of maternal morbidity or mortality, a forthright discussion of the advisability of therapeutic termination is imperative. However, the risk of termination of pregnancy increases with increasing gestational age and should be performed as soon as the decision has been made, preferably in the first trimester regardless of method; expediency in patient decisiveness is important. The therapeutic benefit of termination for patients presenting at ≥20 weeks of gestation is controversial because many of the physiological cardiopulmonary adaptations are established by this time and consequently would not necessarily be mitigated by interruption of the pregnancy.

First trimester: Surgical dilation and suction curettage represent the most common method of pregnancy termination through 12 weeks' gestation. Complication rates are low for skilled practitioners, and selection of anesthetic technique may be dictated by maternal status. The procedure should be carried out in a hospital setting where careful monitoring is accessible. Medical abortion regimens using combined antiprogesterone (mifepristone) and prostaglandin E1 (misoprostol) agents are similar in efficacy to suction curettage if administered within the first 7 weeks of pregnancy; however, because the process and subsequent hemorrhage typically occur in a relatively unpredictable manner in an unmonitored outpatient setting, this may not be an appropriate option for hemodynamically fragile patients.

Second trimester: Midtrimester medical termination can be accomplished with transvaginal misoprostol to induce labor on an inpatient basis. Disadvantages of this approach include prolonged duration (>24 hours), intrapartum discomfort, and potential requirement for uterine curettage if placental retention occurs. Surgical dilation and evacuation are more frequently performed, offering the principal advantage of effecting termination under controlled circumstances in a surgical suite. Although no studies have specifically evaluated adult patients with congenital heart disease in the general population, dilation and evacuation by experienced providers appear to have a lower complication rate than labor induction at gestational ages between 13 and 24 weeks.[14]

Women with Hypertension

Hypertension is one among the most typical complications seen in pregnancy in both developed and developing countries. The hypertension could also be further complicated by the presence of obesity, diabetes, or the metabolic syndrome, which brings a variety of additional complicating and potentially serious risks.[15] Combined hormonal methods are strongly advised against for all grades of hypertension. The WHO-MEC gives a score of 3 for most levels and a score of 4 for a woman with a systolic of >160 mm Hg or diastolic of >100 mmHg. The combined pill increases both systolic and diastolic BP by 6–8 mm Hg, and this is dose dependent. Most progestogen-only methods are given a WHO-MEC rating of 1 or 2, indicating that benefits outweigh the risks but that there are minor issues in some women which may require caution and closer monitoring. The copper IUD and LNG-IUS have a particularly favorable profile, but all patients with hypertension require regular blood pressure (BP) monitoring. Male and female sterilization are both suitable options for all these patients. Women with chronic renal disease are generally able to use all contraceptive methods, unless they have co-existing clotting disorders, cardiovascular disease of hypertension, when combined hormonal methods should be avoided. Women with a renal transplant are usually advised to wait for 1–2 years before trying to conceive, and progestogen-only methods are preferable, with the LNG-IUS and subdermal implant having an MEC classification of "1," indicating no restriction due to the transplant.[5]

Women at Risk of Thromboembolism

Some women have preexisting medical conditions, which increase their risk of experiencing venous thromboembolism (VTE).[16] The highest risks are generally experienced by those women with a familial thrombophilia, the most common in most societies being the coagulation factor V Leiden (FVL) mutation. Diabetes, obesity, and metabolic syndrome, however, also face increased risks. Women at risk of VTE should all avoid contraceptives that contain estrogen.[17] It is thought that the main culprit in increasing risk in women using combined hormonal methods is ethinyl-estradiol, but there are not yet good data to demonstrate whether there is a different level of risk in the newer combined hormonal contraceptives which are based on estradiol-17b. Although the VTE risk is significantly increased in users of combined hormonal methods, especially if they have been identified to be in a high-risk group, it is still substantially less than the risks seen in pregnancy or postpartum. The increased risk of VTE with estrogen-containing oral contraceptive pill (OCP) use is approximately fourfold; with the addition of FVL, this increases to 20–30-fold. Clinicians should discuss these absolute risks with thrombophilic women to allow them to make an enlightened and informed choice about OCP use. The lowest possible estrogen dose should be recommended as low-dose estrogen pills are associated with a lower risk of VTE. Patients with prior VTE and thrombophilia should be strongly discouraged from using estrogen-containing OCP as they will have absolute risks estimated to be 8.5% per year.[18] Progestogen-only methods, including pills, DMPA, subdermal implants and the LNG-IUS, are all recommended in the "1" or "2" categories by WHO-MEC, while a personal history of VTE or a thrombophilia carries a category "4" warning.

Choice for Termination

Surgical abortion is preferred because the onset and peak of bleeding are more predictable than during medication abortion.

Women with Autoimmune Hepatitis

Providing they have well-controlled disease, women with autoimmune hepatitis (AIH) can use any form of contraception. If hepatic impairment is present, estrogen-containing contraceptives are usually discouraged.

Women with Diabetes, Obesity, and Related Metabolic Disorders

Contraceptive Methods

These women may present with a variety of different combinations of symptoms, metabolic problems and "metabolic severity" and require careful assessment before receiving advice on the best contraceptive practices.[19] It is most important that diabetic women plan their pregnancies to enter pregnancy when metabolic features and hypertension are under the best possible control to minimize the risk for complications of pregnancy especially the first trimester.[20] All the contraceptive methods available to nondiabetic women can be used by diabetic women, paying attention to the contraindications that pertain to any woman. Natural family planning and barrier methods are safe for all but their effective use requires considerable motivation and their effectiveness in practice is less than that for IUDs and hormonal methods. For many years, IUD were avoided in diabetic women due to fear of an excessive rate of infection. However, devices containing both copper and levonorgestrel seem equally safe and effective in diabetic and nondiabetic women and they should be offered as a reasonable option.[21] As is true for all women, the doses of hormones in combined estrogen progestin oral contraceptives should be kept as low as possible. Modern low-dose combined preparations have negligible effects on glucose control and atherogenic lipid profiles in diabetic women in good metabolic control. Those women with complications of diabetes such as nephropathy, retinopathy, neuropathy, or especially long-standing diabetes and vascular disease should not be using combined hormonal methods because of risks of VTE and hypertension (MEC scores of 3 or 4). By contrast, the progestogen-only methods appear to carry very little adverse metabolic risk for the majority of women. The LNG-IUS is usually regarded as a first-choice method, because its contraceptive effectiveness is not influenced by obesity.[5] There is insufficient information regarding the use of either the contraceptive ring or the patch to recommend their use in diabetic women. These same principles apply to postpartum diabetic women.

Choices for Termination of Pregnancy

Surgical abortion for obese women may be associated with increased technical difficulty and, for second-trimester procedures, with adverse outcomes such as increased blood loss, prompt care is therefore important.[22] Ventilation difficulties with deep sedation may be more common with patients with obesity, suggesting that medication abortion may be a better option for women with obesity.

Women with Migrainous Headaches

Migraine headaches with or without aura are common in Western society, and some of these are specifically triggered at around the time of menses. Women with aura have at least a twofold increased risk of developing stroke, and this can be exacerbated by smoking and conditions such as hypertension and diabetes. Menstrually related migraines are generally triggered by fluctuations as endogenous estradiol levels. Women with a history of aura should not be given an estrogen-containing hormonal method; however, women without aura may use low-dose estrogen-containing methods provided that they do not smoke and are younger than 35 years.[23] These women should be monitored and the estrogen-containing method ceased if the headaches become worse. Women without aura do not have an increase in stroke risk. In general, there is an increasing move toward encouraging all migrainous patients to use progestogen-only methods, especially DMPA, subdermal implants, or LNG-IUS, because there is no evidence that these methods increase the stroke risk. They also have the benefit of being able to induce amenorrhea or infrequent bleeding (with only limited fluctuation of estrogen levels in those women with a "menstrual" component to their symptom).

Women with Epilepsy

The concerns with epilepsy relate to the increased risk of contraceptive failure in women taking certain anti-epileptic drugs.[24] Phenytoin, carbamazepine, primidone, and phenobarbital are all fairly potent inducers of the hepatic microsomal oxidase system which increase the metabolism of some drugs, including estrogens and progestogens. There is a pragmatic recommendation that epileptic women who wish to take a pill for their contraception should double the dose of their modern dosage pills (either combined estrogen–progestogen or progestogen-only); however, this is an uncertain advice when many factors influence the blood levels of hormones, and the enzyme inducers have different effects in different women. In general, it is probably wiser to use DMPA or a copper-bearing IUD. Copper IUD and the LNG-IUS have not been extensively studied in epileptic women, but their contraceptive effect should not be adversely affected by enzyme inducers.

Termination of Pregnancy

Women with well-controlled epilepsy may receive outpatient abortion care; those with recent onset or uncontrolled seizures may benefit from hospital-based care. The dose of mifepristone may be increased in patients who take antiepileptic drugs that augment the hepatic p450 system that metabolizes mifepristone (i.e., phenytoin, phenobarbital, carbamazepine, and oxcarbazepine).[25,26] No research data guide the choice of mifepristone dose. A mifepristone dose of up to 600 mg is approved as safe and effective for abortion care.

Women with Human Immunodeficiency Virus

Contraceptive services should be provided. Although the use of male and female condoms can prevent human immunodeficiency virus (HIV)/sexually transmitted disease (STD) transmission, they may not be highly effective in preventing pregnancies. Combination hormonal contraceptives are highly effective in preventing pregnancies. Significant drug interactions with antiretroviral agents can complicate their use among HIV-infected women. In addition, oral hormonal contraception decreases amprenavir levels and these drugs should not be coadministered. Alternative methods or back-up contraception can be used simultaneously with oral contraceptives in women receiving ART. Transdermal or intravaginal hormonal contraceptives may be other options, but their pharmacokinetics in the setting of ART have not yet been determined. Medroxyprogesterone levels appear to be unaffected by ART.[27] IUDs are safe and effective contraception for selected HIV-infected women. Studies from Kenya show equal safety of the copper T IUD among HIV-infected and uninfected women.[28] Increased HIV genital tract shedding has not been found with IUD use. The levonorgestrel-releasing IUD has an added advantage of decreased menstrual bleeding compared to the copper T IUD. Spermicides have in vitro activity against HIV but nonoxynol-9 (N-9) has been associated with increased vaginal irritation, inflammation, and decreased lactobacilli. These changes may theoretically increase HIV shedding in the genital tract.

KEY MESSAGES

- COC is contraindicated in a hypertensive, cardiac, diabetic women, liver disease, and previous thromboembolism.
- An epileptic woman who is on antiepileptics may face a higher failure rate due to drug interaction except sodium valproate.
- POP is contraindicated in liver diseases, vascular diseases, and breast cancer.
- MEC categories for contraceptive eligibility should be followed.

REFERENCES

1. CDC/ATSDR Preconception Care Work Group and the Select Panel on Preconception Care. Recommendations to improve preconception health and health care. MMWR Recomm Rep. 2006;55(RR06):1-23.
2. Cantwell R, Clutton-Brock T, Cooper G, Dawson A. Saving Mothers Lives" reviewing maternal deaths to make motherhood safer 2006-2008. The eighth report of the confidential enquiries into maternal deaths in the United Kingdom. BJOG. 2011; 118(Suppl. 1):1e203.
3. World Health Organization. Comparing Typical Effectiveness of ontraceptive Methods. Geneva: World Health Organization; 2007.
4. World Health Organization. Medical Eligibility Criteria for Contraceptive Use, 4th edition. Geneva: WHO; 2009.
5. World Health Organization. Medical eligibility criteria for contraceptive use, 5th edition. Geneva, Switzerland: WHO; 2015.
6. Siu SC, Colman JM. Heart disease and pregnancy. Heart. 2001; 85:710e5.
7. Thorne S, Nelson-Piercy C, MacGregor A, Gibbs S, Crowhurst J, Panay N, et al. Pregnancy and contraception in heart disease and pulmonary arterial hypertension. J Fam Plann Reprod Health Care. 2006;32:75e81.
8. Hunter S, Robson FC. Adaptation of the maternal heart in pregnancy. Br J Heart J. 1992;68:540e3.
9. Thorne S, MacGregor A, Nelson-Piercy C. Risks of contraception and pregnancy in heart disease. Heart. 2006;92:1520-5.
10. Vasilakis C, Jick H, del Mar Melero-Montes M. Risk of idiopathic venous thromboembolism in users of progestogens alone. Lancet. 1999; 354:1610-11.
11. World Health Organization. Cardiovascular disease and use of oral and injectable progestogen-only contraceptives and combined injectable contraceptives. Results of an international, multicenter, case-control study. World Health Organization Collaborative Study of Cardiovascular Disease and Steroid Hormone Contraception. Contraception. 1998;57:315-24.
12. Acker D, Boehm FH, Askew DE, Rothman H. Electrocardiogram changes with intrauterine contraceptive device insertion. Am J Obstet Gynecol. 1973;115:458.
13. Metcalfe J, McAnulty JH, Ueland K. Heart Disease and Pregnancy: Physiology and Management, 2nd edition. Boston, MA: Little, Brown; 1986:116.
14. Bryant AG, Grimes DA, Garrett JM, Stuart GS. Second-trimester abortion for fetal anomalies or fetal death: labor induction compared with dilation and evacuation. Obstet Gynecol. 2011;117:788-92.
15. Moodley J. Maternal deaths due to hypertensive disorders in pregnancy. Best Pract Res Clin Obstet Gynaecol. 2008;22:559-67.
16. Cohen AT, Agnelli G, Anderson FA, Arcelus JI, Bergqvist D, Brecht JB, et al. Venous thromboembolism (VTE) in Europe. The number of VTE events and associated morbidity and mortality. Thromb Haemost. 2007;98:756-64.
17. Reid RL. Oral hormonal contraception and venous thromboembolism (VTE): commentary. Contraception. 2014. in press.
18. Hoibraaten E, Qvigstad E, Arnesen H, Larsen S, Wickstrom E, Sandset PM. Increased risk of recurrent venous thromboembolism during hormone replacement therapy—results of the randomized, double-blind, placebo-controlled estrogen in venous thromboembolism trial (EVTET). Thromb Haemost. 2000;84(6):961-7.
19. Vahratian A, Barber JS, Lawrence JM, Kim C. Family planning practices among women with diabetes and overweight and obese women in the 2002 National Survey for Family Growth. Diabetes Care. 2009;32:1026-31.
20. Chuang CH, Chase GA, Bensyl DM, Weisman CS. Contraceptive use by diabetic and obese women. Womens Health Issues. 2005;15:167-73.
21. Rogovskaya S, Rivera R, Grimes DA, Chen P-L, Pierre-Louis B, Prilepskaya V, et al. Effect of a levonorgestrel intrauterine system on women with type 1 diabetes: a randomized trial. Obstet Gynecol. 2005;105:811-5.
22. Grimes DA, Shields WC. Family planning for obese women: challenges and opportunities. Contraception. 2005;72(1):1-4.
23. MacGregor EA. Menstrual migraine. A clinical review. J Fam Plann Reprod Health Care. 2007;33:36-47.
24. Gaffield ME, Culwell KR, Lee CR. The use of hormonal contraception among women taking anticonvulsant therapy. Contraception. 2011;83:16-29.
25. Davis A, Easterling T. Medical evaluation and management. In: Paul M, Lichtenberg ES, Borgatta L, Grimes DA, Stubblefield P, Creinin MD (Eds). Management of unintended and abnormal pregnancy: comprehensive abortion care.Oxford: Blackwell Publishing Ltd; 2009, pp. 78-89.
26. Sitruk-Ware, R. Mifepristone and misoprostol sequential regimen side effects, complications and safety. Contraception. 2006;74(1): 48-55.
27. Cohn SE, Watts DH, Lertora J, Park JG, Yu S. An open-label, non-randomized study of the effect of depo-medroxyprogesterone acetate on the pharmacokinetics (PK) of selected

protease inhibitors and non-nucleoside reverse transcriptase inhibitors therapies among HIV-infected women. 12th Conference on Retroviruses and Opportunistic Infections, Boston, MA, 2005.

28. Morrison CS, Sekadde-Kigondu C, Sinei SK, Weiner DH, Kwok C, Kokonya D. Is the intrauterine device appropriate contraception for HIV-1-infected women? Br J Obstet Gynaecol 2001;108:784-90.

LONG QUESTIONS

1. What is WHO Medical Eligible Criteria for contraception? What are the contraceptive choices for a postpartum woman with rheumatic heart disease?
2. How will you do contraceptive counseling for a woman with history of venous thromboembolism?

SHORT QUESTIONS

1. What is WHO Medical Eligible Criteria for contraception?
2. Discuss the drugs that interact with combined oral contraceptive pills.
3. What are the indications for medical termination of pregnancy (MTP) in women with cardiac disease?
4. What contraceptive advice will be given for women with HIV?
5. Enumerate the noncontraceptive uses of OCP.

MULTIPLE CHOICE QUESTIONS

1. Which of the following patients can safely receive combination oral contraceptive pills?
   a. 35-year-old woman with diabetes with peripheral circulatory problems
   b. 37-year-old woman who smokes cigarettes, about 1 pack (20 cigarettes) per day
   c. 25-year-old woman with persistent tension headaches
   d. 30-year-old whose blood pressure is 160/90 mm Hg
2. A 44-year-old woman who is a smoker requests sterilization as she does not want any more children. She has three children. Her partner will not consider a vasectomy. She has regular but heavy menses. She is currently using no method of contraception. What method of contraception is she medically eligible for?
   a. LNG-IUS b. CHCs
   c. Cu-T d. Both a and c
3. A 19-year-old woman who previously had a medical abortion attends a clinic requesting contraception. She is overweight and has acne but has no other medical history of note. Her mother had a deep vein thrombosis (DVT) after childbirth. Which of the following is not a suitable method for her? Choose the single best answer.
   a. Depo-Provera b. POP
   c. CHC patch d. LNG-IUS
   e. Progestogen-only implant
4. Oral contraceptive pills do not interact with:
   a. Phenobarbitone
   b. Mebendazole
   c. Ritonavir
   d. Phenytoin
5. A 25-year-old female with a single child seeks contraceptive advice. She gives history of clear mucous vaginal discharge. The cervix appears inflamed on speculum examination. Her husband is working abroad and comes home once in 2 months. Which is the best contraceptive advice?
   a. OCP
   b. Condom
   c. Intrauterine contraceptive device (IUCD)
   d. DMPA
6. A 25-year-old woman who has one child seeks contraceptive advice. She has had viral hepatitis 1 month ago. Liver enzymes are slightly elevated but coagulation profile is normal. What is the best contraceptive method for her?
   a. COCs b. Cu-T
   c. DMPA d. Progestogen implant
7. Which of the following is absolute indication for termination of pregnancy?
   a. Bronchial asthma
   b. Primary pulmonary hypertension
   c. Valvular heart disease
   d. Type 1 diabetes mellitus
8. The common familial thrombophilia that has high risk of thromboembolism is:
   a. Prothrombin defect
   b. Protein C deficiency
   c. Factor V Leiden mutation
   d. Protein S deficiency
9. A woman who has delivered her first child 6 weeks ago seeks contraceptive advice. She suffers from frequent attacks of migraine with aura. Which of the following is the best method for her?
   a. OCP
   b. Cu-T
   c. POP
   d. Progesterone implant
10. The contraceptive of choice in women with active breast disease is:
    a. CHCs b. POPs
    c. LNG-IUS d. Cu-IUD

Answers

1. c. 2. a. 3. c. 4. b. 5. b. 6. b.
7. b. 8. c. 9. b. 10. d.

5.4 CONTRACEPTION AND PREGNANCY TERMINATION IN THE POSTABORTAL PERIOD

Trupti Nadkarni

If the woman we treat for postabortion complications is there because she could not get contraception, we have failed her. If she leaves without family planning we have failed her twice. [1994, Postabortion Care (PAC) Consortium, International Conference on Population and Development (ICPD), Cairo]

INTRODUCTION

Abortion is usually the result of contraceptive method failure or of inadequacies in the family planning. After abortion, both the patient and the health personnel are highly motivated to start contraceptive use.

It is crucial to start an effective method of contraception at the time of abortion since return of fertility is rapid after first-trimester abortion. After a first-trimester abortion, the levels of estrogen and progesterone decrease to nonpregnant levels within a few days. Ovarian response to follicle-stimulating hormone (FSH) occurs within 4–9 days, while human chorionic gonadotropin (hCG) takes longer, disappearing within 38 days. Thus, the first ovulation may take place as soon as 2 weeks after first-trimester abortion and half of the women have ovulated by 3 weeks.[1] In addition, not all women return for postabortal checkup examinations, especially in our country where people are not in the habit of visiting health facilities when there is no "apparent problem."

COUNSELING FOR POSTABORTION CONTRACEPTION

Before the abortion procedure, it should be checked that the woman's physical condition and emotional situation are appropriate for counseling on contraception. The provider/counselor should respect her right to accept or refuse postabortion contraception and services are provided accordingly. The service provider/counselor should consider both the woman's clinical condition and personal situation and discuss any potential barriers to the successful adoption of contraception in a sensitive manner. The service provider/counselor should explain the characteristics, use (how it works), side effects, and effectiveness of the available methods and aid the woman in choosing a contraceptive which best suits her.

Preabortion counseling about the range of contraceptive choices is one of the cornerstones of quality of care and effectiveness in family planning services. Therefore, it is essential to review the data on the efficacy, safety, and acceptability of the postabortal use of all contraceptive measures currently available.

INTRAUTERINE DEVICES

Insertion of an intrauterine device (IUD) immediately after abortion has several potential advantages. The woman is known not to be pregnant; also the discomfort related to insertion is avoided. Any bleeding from the insertion is disguised by the expected bleeding after abortion. However, insertion of an IUD immediately after a pregnancy ends carries potential risks as well. The risk of perforation may be increased due to softening of the myometrium. Spontaneous expulsion of the device may be more common than after interval insertion since the cervical canal has been recently dilated. Another potential concern is infection if termination is not carried out under aseptic precautions. An intrauterine contraceptive device (IUCD), 380 A/Cu IUCD 375, providing contraception for 10/5 years, respectively, can be inserted as per the preference of the client. The IUCD can be inserted immediately after both first- and second-trimester abortion provided there is no evidence or potential for infection, bleeding, or other complications. The procedure of IUCD insertion after first-trimester abortion is similar to interval IUD insertion. The uterine length can be measured by the using the last cannula used. The procedure of IUCD insertion after second-trimester abortion is similar to postpartum IUD insertion and can be done using long ring forceps. The Cochrane database which reviewed the studies, which assessed the safety and efficacy of IUD insertion immediately after spontaneous or induced abortion, found IUD after abortion to be safe and practical. IUD expulsion rates appeared higher than after-interval insertion. However, IUD use was higher at 6 months with immediate than with interval insertion.[2]

ORAL CONTRACEPTIVES

Providing combined oral contraceptives (COCs) following abortion offers an opportune moment to initiate a reliable contraceptive method. COCs do not affect the recovery of the pituitary–ovarian system, even though they are introduced immediately after abortion. The combination of preceding pregnancy, abortion procedure, and immediate start of oral contraceptive (OC) containing 30 μg of ethinyl estradiol results in slight tendency toward hypercoagulability. This may be clinically insignificant, but it can be avoided by postponing OC for 7 days, without losing the contraceptive efficacy. Evidence shows that COCs can be safely initiated immediately following first-trimester abortion.[3]

Combined oral contraceptives can be started on the day of abortion or within the first 7 days. If started later than that, additional precautions need to be taken in that cycle.

Similarly, progesterone-only pills can also be started on the same day or within 5 days of the procedure.

INJECTABLE CONTRACEPTIVES

Depot-medroxy-progesterone acetate (DMPA) and Norethisterone Enanthate (NET-EN) injections can be offered to the patient after an abortion. They can be administered on the same day or within 7 days of a first- or second-trimester miscarriage. Proper counseling regarding menstrual irregularity will improve the compliance.

IMPLANTS AND LEVONORGESTREL-RELEASING INTRAUTERINE SYSTEM

The above contraceptives can be used immediately after a spontaneous or induced abortion or within 7 days. There are fewer studies evaluating the outcome of these contraceptives postabortion; information on events such as amount and duration of bleeding, spotting, pain, and other side effects is scant. One study, which evaluated the immediate postabortal contraception with the levonorgestrel-releasing intrauterine system (LNG-IUS) and implants found no clinically significant side effects in this group. The women found the levonorgestrel implants and IUDs easy and safe to use and highly effective.[4] Bleeding disturbances, including amenorrhea, were the principal features the women disliked.

STERILIZATION

As per the recommendations of the Ministry of Health and Family Welfare 2016 and the Indian College of Obstetricians and Gynaecologists-Federation of Obstetric and Gynaecological Societies of India (ICOG-FOGSI) clinical recommendations, laparoscopic tubal ligation can be carried out concurrently with first-trimester Medical Termination of Pregnancy (MTP). However, laparoscopic ligation is contraindicated after second-trimester abortion due to risk of trocar injury to the enlarged uterus. Minilaparotomy can be done after both first- and second-trimester abortion. However, the patient needs to be adequately counseled and not pushed to make a hasty decision of sterilization.

The provider must ensure that the client has signed the consent form for sterilization before surgery. The operating surgeon must ensure that the medical record and checklist are filled properly after reviewing the client's suitability for sterilization and conducting final assessment prior to surgery. It is concluded that postabortal sterilization is as safe as interval sterilization, and it is strongly recommended.

Note: In the unlikely event of failure, complications, or death attributable to sterilization operations, Family Planning Indemnity Scheme indemnifies the clients of sterilization as well as doctors performing the procedure in public health facilities and accredited private/NGO facilities. The client or her kin reports the incidence to the District Quality Assurance Committee/District FP Indemnity Subcommittee which is responsible for processing and settlement of claims and reporting these incidences to the State Quality Assurance Committees/State FP Indemnity Subcommittee for final settlement.[5]

NATURAL METHODS OF FAMILY PLANNING

These can be employed only after resumption of the normal menstrual pattern.

CONTRACEPTION AFTER MEDICAL ABORTION

Due to a rising number of medical first-trimester abortions, it is important to know how to provide the various contraceptive measures after a medical abortion. Women who have had a medical abortion can use any modern method of contraception afterward. When the woman is counseled about the abortion, the opportunity should be taken to review her contraceptive needs. Ideally, she should be provided with an effective contraceptive method immediately after the abortion.

- COC pills can be started on the day that misoprostol is administered, when expulsion usually occurs. Two prospective randomized controlled studies evaluated the effects of immediate use of COC pills versus placebo following medical abortion and found no difference in complete abortion rates, side effects, and duration of bleeding.[6,7]
- Progestogen-only methods are commonly associated with breakthrough bleeding, which may be confused with an incomplete or irregular bleeding, which may make it difficult to determine whether pregnancy has been terminated. It may therefore be preferable to start using these methods only after it has been confirmed that the pregnancy has been terminated on day 15.
- Sterilization and insertion of an IUD should be deferred until confirmation that the abortion is complete and is usually preferred after the first cycle.
- Women who choose a contraceptive method that cannot be started immediately should be encouraged to use condoms in the meantime.
- Other methods, such as caps, sponges, diaphragm, spermicidal foams, jellies, and vaginal tablets, can be used as soon as sexual intercourse is resumed, preferably when bleeding has stopped.
- Methods of natural family planning can be resumed only after the return of regular cycles.

CONTRACEPTIVE USE IN THE PRESENCE OF CLINICAL COMPLICATIONS

In the presence of complications, treatment of the condition is the first priority. Consideration of contraception can occur once the patient's medical condition is stabilized.[8]

- *Confirmed or presumptive infection related to abortion*:
  - Delay female sterilization until infection is resolved
  - Any other method can be considered immediately (Norplant, injectables, OC, condoms, vasectomy, spermicidal jelly, foams).
- *Trauma to genital tract*:
  - Delay sterilization until trauma is resolved. However, if abdominal surgery is required, sterilization can be done concurrently if no additional risk is involved.
  - Do not insert an IUD until uterine perforation or serious trauma is healed.
  - The use of female barriers and spermicides may be limited according to the extent and placement of injury.
  - Any other method can be used immediately.
- *Hemorrhage/severe anemia*:
  - Female sterilization and IUD should not be used in this situation.
  - Other methods are considered appropriate.

ADVICE FOR FOLLOW-UP VISIT

Before the woman leaves the health facility, she should be advised to:

- Come for postabortion follow-up within 1 to 2 weeks for assessment of her physical condition, ruling out continuing pregnancy, sepsis, and incomplete abortion.
- Come for a routine follow-up of IUCD/other contraception after 1 month, preferably after the next menstrual bleeding.
- Come back immediately in case she has any of these problems:
  - Persistent nausea and/or vomiting
  - Continuous and/or heavy bleeding per vagina
  - Fever
  - Pain in abdomen.

POSTABORTION FAMILY PLANNING COUNSELING MESSAGES

- She should wait for at least 6 months before trying to conceive again as it reduces the chances of low birth weight, premature birth, and maternal anemia.
- Fertility returns quickly—within 10–11 days after first-trimester abortion or miscarriage and within 4 weeks after a second-trimester abortion or miscarriage. She can choose from available family planning methods that can be started at once.
- If a woman decides not to use contraceptives at this time, providers can offer information on all available methods and from where to obtain them. Also, providers can offer condoms, OCs, or emergency contraceptive pills for women to take home and use later.
- To avoid infection, she should not have intercourse until bleeding stop—if being treated for infection or vaginal/cervical injury, she should wait until the lesion is fully healed.
- Method specific counseling should follow if she chooses any family planning method.

In conclusion, postabortal contraception is a safe, practical, and effective approach to bridge the lacunae in our family planning services. Preabortion counseling is of utmost importance in helping the woman make a choice of the contraceptive most suited and acceptable to her. Preabortion counseling combined with immediate postabortal provision of contraceptives has been shown to increase contraceptive use at 6 months postprocedure.[9]

KEY MESSAGES

- Return of fertility is rapid after first-trimester abortion; hence, it is crucial to start immediate postabortal contraception.
- IUD insertion postabortion is safe. Expulsion rates are slightly increased; however, IUD use was higher at 6 months than with interval insertion.
- COCs can be started on the day of abortion or within the first 7 days. There is slight tendency to hypercoagulability; however, this is not clinically significant.
- Injectable contraceptives, implants, and Lng-IUS can be administered on the same day or within 7 days of a first- or second-trimester miscarriage.
- Laparoscopic tubal ligation can be safely performed after first-trimester abortion but should be avoided after a second-trimester abortion.
- All methods of contraception can be safely used after a medical abortion, either on the day of misoprostol administration (oral pills, condoms, and injectable contraceptives) or after the next menstrual cycle (intrauterine device and sterilization).
- In the presence of complications, contraception must be deferred until the patient's medical condition is stabilized.

REFERENCES

1. Lahteenmaki P. Postabortal contraception. Ann Med.1993; 25(2):185-9.
2. Grimes DA, Lopez LM, Schulz KF, Stanwood NL. Immediate postabortal insertion of intrauterine devices. Cochrane Database Syst Rev. 2010;16(6):CD001777.
3. Gaffield ME, Kapp N, Ravi A. Use of combined oral contraceptives postabortion. Contraception. 2009; 80(4):355-62.
4. Ortayli N, Bulut A, Sahin T, Sivin I. Immediate postabortal contraception with the levonorgestrel intrauterine device, Norplant and traditional methods. Contraception. 2001;63(6): 309-14.
5. Post Abortion Family Planning Technical Update. Family Planning Division, Ministry of Health and Family Welfare Government of India. March 2016.
6. Martin CW, Brown AH, Baird DT. A pilot study of the effect of methotrexate or combined oral contraceptive on bleeding patterns after induction of abortion with mifepristone and a prostaglandin pessary. Contraception. 1998;58:99-103.

7. Tang OS, Xu J, Cheng L, Lee SWH, Ho PC. The effect of contraceptive pills on the measured blood loss in medical termination of pregnancy by mifepristone and misoprostol: a randomized placebo controlled trial. Hum Reprod. 2002; 17:99-102.
8. WHO. Reducing unsafe abortions: In progress No 75, 2007.
9. Ortayli N, Bulut A, Nalbant H. The effectiveness of preabortion contraception counseling. Int J Gynaecol Obstet. 2001;74(3): 281-5.

LONG QUESTION

1. Discuss in detail contraceptive use after abortion and the role of preabortion counseling.

SHORT QUESTIONS

1. Discuss the advantages and disadvantages of insertion of IUCD immediately after abortion.
2. Discuss the role of preabortion counseling in the success of postabortal contraceptive use.
3. Discuss the initiation of contraception after a medical abortion.

MULTIPLE CHOICE QUESTIONS

1. Ovulation after a first-trimester abortion can resume as early as:
   a. 2 weeks
   b. 3 weeks
   c. 4 weeks
   d. 6 weeks
2. All of the following may be the disadvantages of immediate postabortal insertion of IUCD, except:
   a. Increased rates of perforation
   b. Increased rates of failure
   c. Increased rates of expulsion
   d. Increased risk of infection
3. In case of suspected perforation during abortion, all the following methods can be safely used, except:
   a. IUCD
   b. OC pills
   c. Norplant
   d. DMPA
4. Laparoscopic tubal ligation can be performed in all cases, except:
   a. After first-trimester abortion
   b. After medical abortion
   c. After second-trimester abortion
   d. After missed abortion
5. The following hormonal contraception can be safely used after a 1st trimester abortion in a lactating patient:
   a. Combination oral contraceptive pills
   b. Progesterone-only pills
   c. DMPA
   d. Lng-IUS
6. All the following statements about postabortal contraception are true, except:
   a. IUCDs can be safely inserted on the day of abortion
   b. There is a slight increase in coagulability on immediately starting OC pills after abortion
   c. Starting OC pills immediately after abortion leads to delayed recovery of the pituitary ovarian axis
   d. All methods of contraception can be safely used following a medical abortion
7. All the following statements about postabortal contraception are true, except:
   a. Prebortion counseling with immediate postabortion provision of contraception increases contraception use at 6 months postpartum
   b. Levonorgestrel implants are safe to use after abortion
   c. All methods of contraception must be initiated on the day of abortion to be effective
   d. Laparoscopic tubal ligation after abortion is as effective as interval ligation
8. The following statements about the recovery of pituitary ovarian axis after abortion are true, except:
   a. The levels of estrogen and progesterone decrease to nonpregnant levels within a few days of the abortion
   b. Ovarian response to FSH occurs within 4–9 days
   c. HCG disappears from bloodstream in 10 days
   d. Ovulation may resume in 2–3 weeks after abortion
9. The following is true of contraception after medical abortion, except:
   a. OC pills can be initiated on the day of misoprostol administration
   b. Progesterone-only methods are better initiated on completion of abortion on day 15
   c. Sterilization is better done after first cycle
   d. Natural family planning methods can be employed in the cycle immediately after abortion

Answers

1.	a	2.	b	3.	a	4.	c	5.	a	6.	c
7.	c	8.	c	9.	d						

5.5 CONTRACEPTION IN POSTDELIVERY AND LACTATION

Kavita Singh, Deepti Gupta

Postpartum contraception is a huge area of unmet need.
Inter-pregnancy interval of >24 months can optimize maternal and neonatal outcome.
Best time to discuss is the antenatal period.
Injectable contraceptives and intrauterine devices are good long-acting reversible contraceptive options.

INTRODUCTION

A lot has been said about contraception in previous few chapters. Postdelivery and lactation comprise one subgroup which forms a large segment of women who need contraception. Worldwide:

- 9 in 10 women want to avoid pregnancy for 2 years postpartum, but 1 in 7 do not use any contraception.[1]
- More than one third of the maternal deaths can be prevented only with family planning.
- Child mortality risk highest with interpregnancy interval (IPI) <12 months.

In 2019, the number of births for India was whopping 2,41,16,002. There are numerous studies to show that short-interval pregnancies (IPI <12 months) are associated with poor maternal nutrition and adverse childhood outcomes such as low birth weight, preterm birth, neonatal death for newborn, malnutrition in newborn, infection, and increased second-year mortality for previous child.[2] Astonishingly IPI in 32% pregnancies was <12 months.[3] The National Family Health Survey (NFHS) 2015–16 has shown negative association between IPI and stunting and wasting among children. This survey also showed that irrespective of socioeconomic, demographic, and maternal care utilization, there was negative association between IPI and adverse childhood outcome.[4] IPI of 2 or more years is associated with better infant survival and reduced maternal morbidity. Clearly postdelivery/lactation contraception needs urgent attention to avoid unwanted pregnancies and increase IPI for optimal childhood outcomes.

Even though India was the first country to launch a structured family planning program as early as 1952, still female sterilization and abortion are leading means of controlling fertility in our country. Total unmet need of Family Planning is 12.9 (NFHS-IV) in our country. Sample registration system (SRS) 2017 data show that in India, spacing between two childbirths is less than the recommended period of 3 years in 50.3% of births. The NFHS-IV survey shows 53.5% use of contraceptives among married women (aged 15–49 years) and prevalence of modern method to be 47.8%[4] (**Flowchart 1, Table 1, and Fig. 1**).

AIMS OF POSTPARTUM FAMILY PLANNING

- To decide on a contraceptive method, initiate, and continue use for 24 months
- To prevent unwanted pregnancies
- To increase IPI.

Interestingly, childbirth provides an ideal and important time and circumstance to address contraceptive needs. The woman is already in the hospital setup, sure of not being

Flowchart 1: Population comprising unmet need.

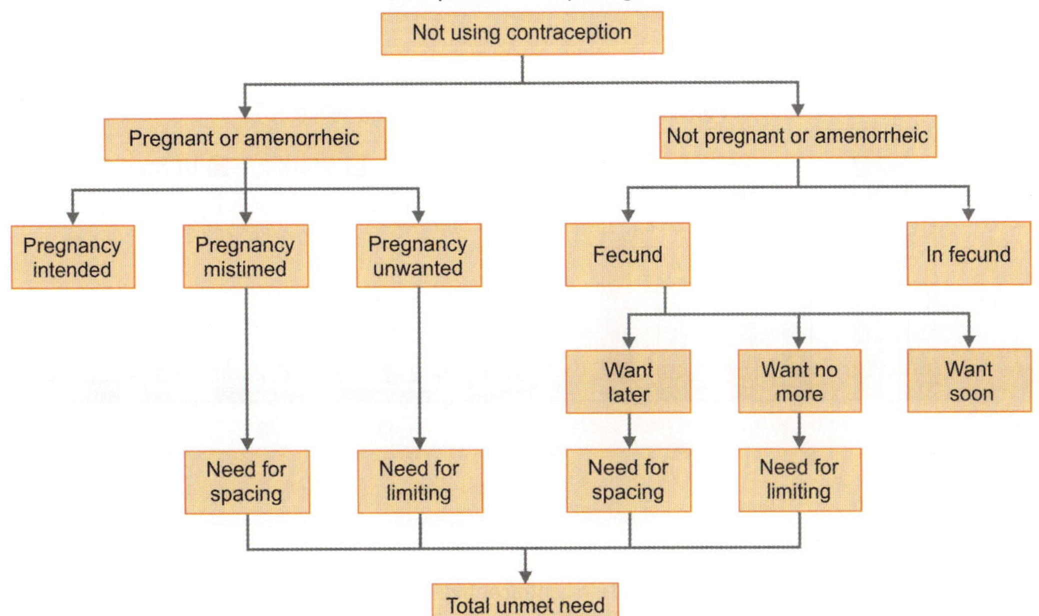

pregnant, likely motivated, and in close interaction with healthcare worker. Having undergone labor/childbirth recently, she is more receptive to contraceptive advice and birth spacing.

POSTPARTUM PHYSIOLOGY

Elevated levels of prolactin in the postpartum period are associated with ovulatory dysfunction and infertility. During pregnancy, prolactin levels rise from normal (10–25 ng/mL) starting at about 8 weeks to about 200–400 ng/mL at term.[5] There is evidence to indicate that the central action of prolactin predominates in producing lactational amenorrhea and anovulation. Till about 2–3 months postpartum, prolactin levels remain at around 40–50 ng/mL with rise of 10–20 ng/mL after each suckling. These values/patterns do not necessarily predict the duration of amenorrhea/infertility. However, on weaning, prolactin levels return to normal and ovulation may resume between 14 and 30 days. Many studies have been conducted to study correlation between breastfeeding and timing of resumption of ovulation. Only women with amenorrhea and exclusive breastfeeding including nighttime feeds have contraceptive protection of approximately 98%. All studies show that even though breastfeeding is effective in preventing ovulation, less so after 3–4 months, it is not fully effective. In addition, many women do not practice exclusive, nonsupplemental breastfeeding. One study proposed a threshold for suppression of ovulation to be around five daily feedings totaling to at least 65 minutes of suckling per day.[5] Progressively increasing supplementation and decreasing suckling time weakened the association between lactation, amenorrhea, and anovulation.

In nonlactating women, the gonadotropin levels are low to start with and return to normal by 3rd to 5th week postpartum. In a study conducted in US women, the range of first ovulation varied from 25 to 72 days in nonlactating women, with the average time being 45 ± 3.8 days.[5]

TABLE 1: Contraceptive use in India.

Contraceptive method	*Knowledge among eligible population (%)*	*Ever use (%)*	*Current use (%)*
Any method	99	55.1	48.2
For all modern methods	98.9	49.3	42.8
Combined oral pills	79 .5	8.4	2.1
IUDs	70.6	5.6	1.6
Condoms	71	7.9	3.1
Female sterilization	98 .2	34.2	34.2
Male sterilization	89.3	2	1.9
Natural methods	48.9	11 .8	5

(IUD: intrauterine device)

MECHANISM OF ACTION

Prolactin seems to act on granulosa cells inhibiting the synthesis of progesterone. It may also change the testosterone:dihydrotestosterone ratio, thus reducing aromatizable substrate. The central action predominates in inhibiting ovulation. It inhibits the pulsatile secretion of gonadotropin-releasing hormone (GnRH) by short loop positive feedback on dopamine. After weaning, prolactin levels fall and gonadotropins increase leading to ovulation within 14–30 days.

In nonbreastfeeding women, gonadotropin levels return to normal in 3rd to -5th week. Important to note here is that two third of the women ovulate before resumption of first menses so women should be clearly explained that onset of menses cannot be taken as indicator of ovulation and they

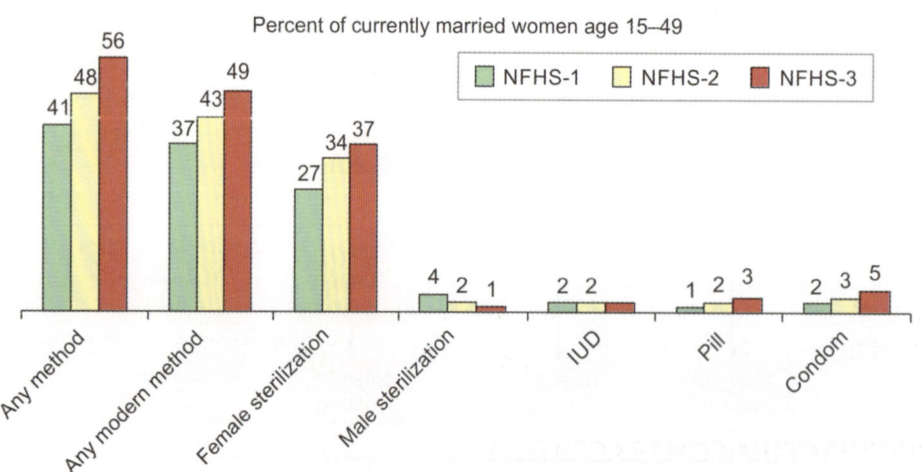

Fig. 1: Trends in contraceptive use in India.
(IUD: intrauterine device; NFHS: National Family Health Survey)

may still ovulate and conceive without menstruating after childbirth.

HYPERCOAGULABLE STATE

This is an important factor while considering contraceptive in the postdelivery period because of the persistent hypercoagulable state of pregnancy. There is an increased risk of venous thromboembolism for 2 weeks after childbirth. Therefore, estrogen-containing contraceptives are not recommended in the first 2 weeks' postpartum.

RULE OF THREES[6]

For fully breastfeeding women, contraception should begin by 3rd month of postpartum.

For supplemental or nonbreastfeeding women, it should begin by 3rd postpartum week.

POSTPARTUM CONTRACEPTION

Conventionally, the first postpartum visit was advised at 6 weeks. This was based on understanding of puerperal changes reverting to normal by 6 weeks. But many studies have shown that a lot of women are sexually active before that period. The fact that a woman may ovulate as early as 4 weeks postpartum and in the absence of menses; therefore, it seems appropriate to schedule first postpartum visit at 3 weeks. This will help initiate postpartum contraception earlier if not done already at the time of birth and help in decreasing postpartum surprises in the form of unwanted pregnancies/abortions/short-interval pregnancies.

POSTABORTION CONTRACEPTION

In cases of spontaneous/elective abortion of <12 weeks, steroid contraception may be started immediately post-abortion. But in cases of termination/abortion of >12 weeks, 3-week rule should be followed to avoid the risk of venous thromboembolism.

ROLE OF COUNSELING

Counseling for contraception should ideally begin in the antenatal period. The aim of counseling should not just be to inform about various methods, but also try to understand a woman's lifestyle involving open discussion about personal health, sexuality, impact of the chosen contraceptive on health, and lifestyle. For example, suggesting depot- medroxy-progesterone to a rural illiterate patient residing in interiors might be impractical as it will need frequent visits and administration by healthcare worker eventually leading to discontinuation.

CHOICE OF POSTPARTUM CONTRACEPTION

This needs to be based on the following factors[8] **(Fig. 2)**:

- Time since delivery
- Infant feeding choice
- Desire of temporary or permanent method.

PERIODIC ABSTINENCE/SAFE PERIOD METHOD

It is not advised as a method of contraception in immediate postpartum period until regular menses have resumed.

LACTATIONAL AMENORRHEA METHOD

This method relies on anovulatory effect of breastfeeding. It is important to note that nonsupplemental breastfeeding and amenorrhea provide maximum likelihood of contraception. Supplemental feeds, resumption of menses, or passage of >6 months increases the chances of ovulation. With correct and consistent use, the failure rate is about 0.5 per HWY for the first 6 months. But for the typical use, failure rate is 2 per HWY. This method has many advantages.

- Can be initiated immediately after birth
- Encourages best breastfeeding patterns
- No direct cost/ supplies/procedure needed
- No hormonal side effects
- Independent of coital timing.

Disadvantages: Efficacy starts decreasing after 3 months and uncertain after 6 months. Also, it does not provide any protection against sexually transmitted infections (STIs) and may even increase the risk of mother-to-child transmission in an HIV-positive mother. It may be impractical for working mothers.

Medical eligibility: The child should be <6 moths, amenorrheic, and exclusively breastfeeding including night feeds.[8]

Recommend alternative/additional contraceptive if menses have resumed, baby is more than 6 months, and not exclusively breastfeeding.

BARRIER METHODS

The advantage of barrier methods is that they do not affect lactation and are always an excellent choice for motivated couples. Uterine involution plays an important role in selecting and initiating certain barrier methods such as cervical cap and diaphragm. Lubricated condoms and spermicidal jellies are especially helpful for vaginal dryness experienced by some women in postpartum period due to low estrogen levels.

It is therefore recommended that fitting and initiation of a new device should be done after complete involution of uterus, i.e., after 6 weeks postpartum.

COMBINATION ORAL CONTRACEPTIVES

They can be offered to nonbreastfeeding women but after 2 weeks when the pregnancy-induced hypercoagulable state has near resolved. These are not the best choice for women

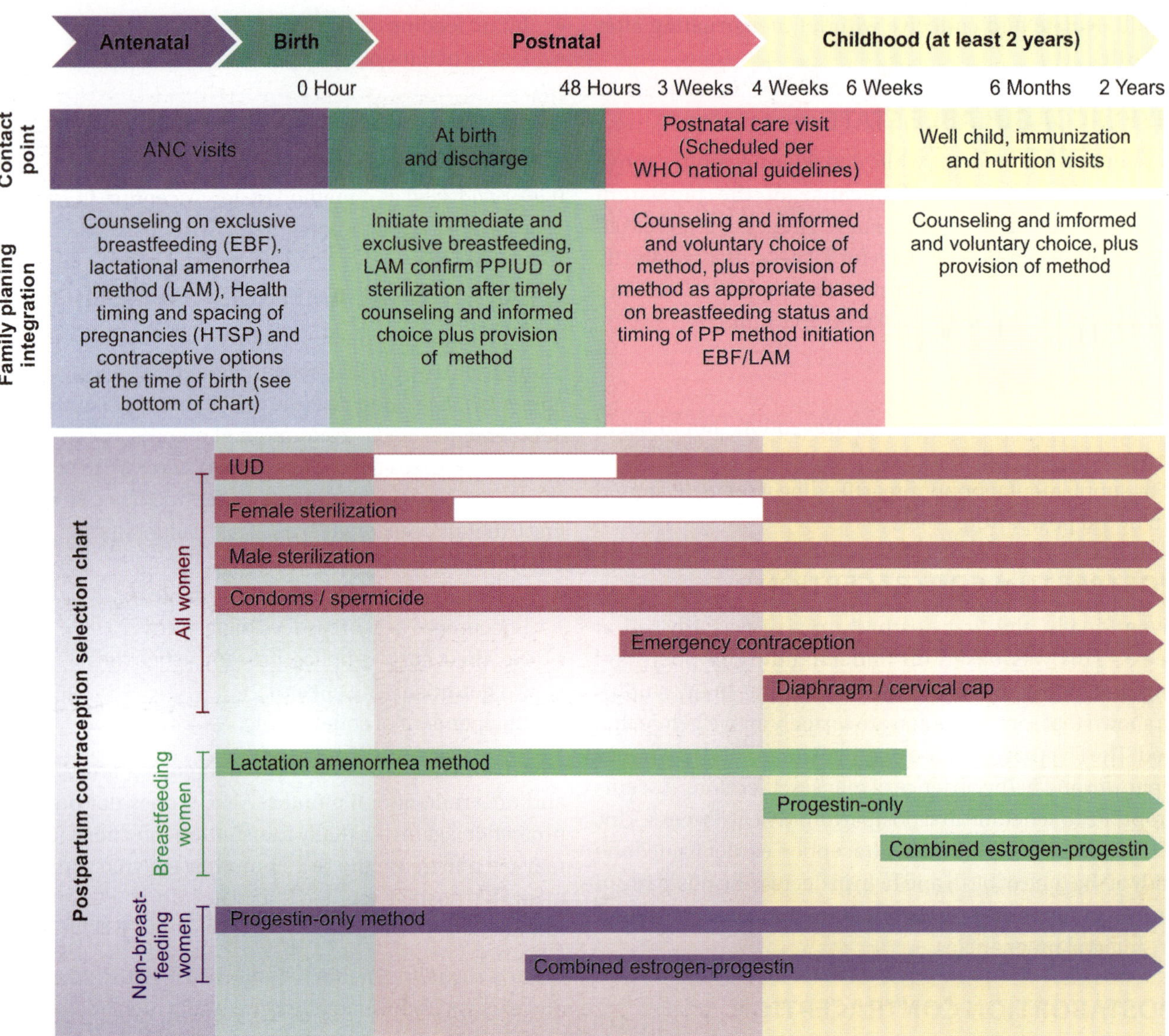

Fig. 2: Counseling and selection of postpartum contraceptive.
(EBF: exclusively breastfed; IUD: intrauterine device; LAM: lactation amenorrhea method; PPIUD: postpartum intrauterine contraceptive device)

who breastfeed because it decreases milk volume and quality. Thus, the clear recommendation is that:

- Nonbreastfeeding may initiate combined oral contraceptive (COC) from 3rd week postpartum.
- Breastfeeding may begin the same by 3rd month postpartum.

PROGESTIN-ONLY METHODS

These methods do not suppress lactation and can be used by postpartum women irrespective of the breastfeeding status.

Progestogen-only pill (POP) can be started any day up to 21 days without any additional contraceptive. An alternative method is to be used for 2 days if started beyond 21 days. The most important thing to remember with progestin-only pills is strict adherence to time. Delay of few hours also in POP tablet can cause escape ovulation and decrease cervical mucus thickening, thus decreasing efficacy.

Depot-medroxy-progesterone acetate has not shown to affect breastfeeding or infant growth and could be an excellent choice for postpartum contraception. It can be administered immediately postpartum and should always be initiated before 3rd postpartum week. An additional method is needed for 7 days if it is initiated after 21 days postpartum.

Advantages include safe, highly effective, easy to use, long-acting, and reversible; no special training/equipment needed for administration; can be discontinued without provider's help; privacy maintained; has no effect on lactation, has no dependence on sexual activity; and has certain noncontraceptive benefits too.

Disadvantages include no protection against STIs, slight delay in return of fertility, menstrual changes, and weight gain.

INTRAUTERINE DEVICES

Higher expulsion rates were a problem with older bigger plastic intrauterine devices (IUDs) when inserted before

8 weeks' postpartum. However, the newer devices can be inserted without a significant increase in expulsion rates/perforation/pregnancy rates or removal rates for bleeding or pain. It can be easily inserted immediately after normal delivery without any added risks or at the time of cesarean section. Thus, it can be inserted up to 48 hours or after 4 weeks which is also referred to as interval insertion. Few things to remember are as follows:

- It should be inserted within 15 minutes of delivery of placenta.
- Insertion should not be done in case of intrauterine infection.
- The thread should be cut flush with external os because as the uterus involutes, the thread will eventually come down in the vagina.

An intrauterine device may also be inserted immediately after a spontaneous/elective abortion as long as intrauterine infection is ruled out. Considering its low cost, easy availability, independence from coital act, only one visit for insertion/removal, and immediate return of fertility, long-acting nature IUD is the best choice for spacing method or long-acting reversible contraceptive (LARC). The myths and taboos surrounding the IUD need to be busted in order to increase acceptance. CuT 380A also known as "reversible sterilization" because of its long duration of action with immediate return of fertility **(Table 2)**.

PERMANENT METHODS

Female Sterilization

This does not protect against STIs. Surprisingly, it is the leading method of contraception in our country despite the fact that it is permanent, invasive, and requires anesthesia. The best timing for procedure is within 7 days of childbirth or after 6 weeks. The failure rate is of about 2 per 1,000.

TABLE 2: IUCD use in different countries including India.

IUCD		
Worldwide IUCD Usage		
Country	***Any method***	***IUCD***
Europe	73%	9%
North America	75%	2%
China	84%	36%
Vietnam	79%	38%
Cuba	73%	43%
Egypt	60%	38%
Jordan	56%	24%
Korea	80%	13%
India	54%	2%

(IUCD: intrauterine contraceptive device)

Male Sterilization

The failure rate is around 1 per 1,000, and this also does not protect against STIs. The failure rate is lower than female sterilization and is simpler to perform. Alternative contraceptive should be advised till confirmation of success of procedure by documenting azoospermia at 12 weeks.

Making Best Use of Opportunities for Postpartum Family Planning (Fig. 3)

In the Antenatal Clinic

- Make sure that verbal and written information about various available options is given.
- Discuss vasectomy/female sterilization if the woman is willing to limit family size.
- Allow the woman to ask questions about postpartum family planning (PPFP) at every visit.
- Document the method chosen by the woman on the antenatal card.

In Labor Ward

- Enquire if contraceptive options were discussed in the antenatal period.
- Ideally, active labor is not the right time to discuss the contraceptive choice.
- Consider IUD insertion at the time of cesarean section or postpartum insertion after due counseling and consent.

If not discussed yet, the contraceptive choice should be discussed and contraceptive administered/handed over before discharge.

Postpartum Clinic

- Do not assume on the use of contraceptive. Confirm so at every visit.
- Ensure satisfaction and compliance with chosen method at every visit.
- If not using any method yet, offer choices and start using rule of 3s.

Immunization Clinic

This opportunity can be a blessing in disguise. Women are visiting immunization clinics regularly and are sensitive to health issues of neonate. This can offer an opportunity to sensitize and reinforce postpartum contraceptive use for best childhood outcome.

What should Women Know about Postpartum Family Planning[1]

- Effectiveness and correct use of the method **(Tables 3 to 5)**
- Side effects
- Follow-up care and resupply
- Stopping the method and return of fertility
- STI prevention.

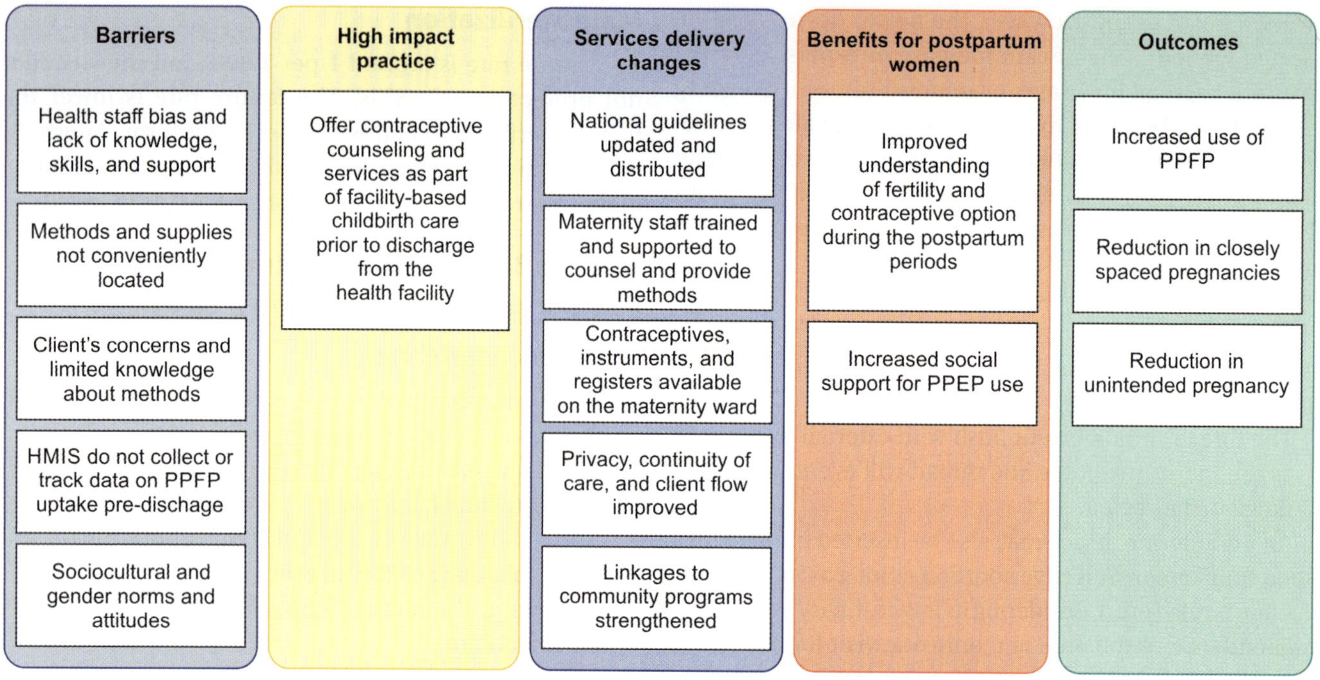

Barriers	High impact practice	Services delivery changes	Benefits for postpartum women	Outcomes
Health staff bias and lack of knowledge, skills, and support	Offer contraceptive counseling and services as part of facility-based childbirth care prior to discharge from the health facility	National guidelines updated and distributed	Improved understanding of fertility and contraceptive option during the postpartum periods	Increased use of PPFP
Methods and supplies not conveniently located		Maternity staff trained and supported to counsel and provide methods	Increased social support for PPEP use	Reduction in closely spaced pregnancies
Client's concerns and limited knowledge about methods		Contraceptives, instruments, and registers available on the maternity ward		Reduction in unintended pregnancy
HMIS do not collect or track data on PPFP uptake pre-dischage		Privacy, continuity of care, and client flow improved		
Sociocultural and gender norms and attitudes		Linkages to community programs strengthened		

Fig. 3: Optimizing and strengthening postpartum family planning services.
(HMIS: Health Management Information System; PPFP: postpartum family planning).

TABLE 3: Postpartum contraceptive methods based on effectiveness.[1]

Most effective methods	***IUD, contraceptive implants, female sterilization, male sterilization***
Effective methods	Progesterone-only injectables, progesterone-only pills, lactational amenorrhea method, combined oral contraceptives
Less effective methods	Male condoms, female condoms
Least effective methods	Withdrawal method, fertility awareness method, emergency contraception

TABLE 4: Summary of UK medical eligibility criteria for contraceptive use after childbirth.

Condition	*Cu IUD*	*LNG IUS*	*IMP*	*DMPA*	*POP*	*CHC*
Postpartum breastfeeding <6 weeks			1	2	1	4
6 weeks to 6 months			1	1	1	2
>6 months			1	1	1	1
Postpartum breastfeeding 0–3 weeks With risk factors for VTE			1	2	1	4
Without risk factors for VTE			1	2	1	3
3–6 weeks with risk factors			1	2	1	3
3–6 weeks without risk factors			1	1	1	2
6 weeks			1	1	1	1
Postpartum 0–48 hours	1	1				
48 hours to 4 weeks	3	3				
>4 weeks	1	1				
Postpartum sepsis	4	4				
History of high BP during pregnancy, now controlled	1	1	1	1	1	2
History of pregnancy related cholestasis	1	1	1	1	1	2
History of gestational diabetes now resolved	1	1	1	1	1	1

(BP: blood pressure; CHC: combined hormonal contraception; DMPA: depot-medroxy-progesterone acetate; IMP: implant; IUD: intrauterine contraceptive device; IUS: intrauterine system; POP: progestogen-only pill; VTE: venous thromboembolism)

TABLE 5: Suggested methods based on interval postdelivery.

	Unrestricted methods	*Methods not recommended or to be used with restriction*
Nonbreastfeeding <21 days postpartum	POP Progesterone-only injectables/implants Barrier methods	CHC IUD unless inserted in 48 hours Fertility awareness methods Sterilization
Nonbreastfeeding >21 days postpartum	COC POP Progesterone-only injectables/implants Barrier methods	Fertility awareness methods Sterilization IUD unless inserted in 48 hours
Breastfeeding <6 weeks postpartum	LAM POP Progesterone-only injectable/implants Barrier methods	COC IUD Fertility awareness methods Sterilization
Breastfeeding >6 weeks	LAM if amenorrheic POP Progesterone-only injectable/implants IUD Barrier methods Sterilization	COC Fertility awareness methods
Six months postpartum, except for LAM, woman may use almost any method of choice		

(CHC: combined hormonal contraception; COC: combined oral contraceptive; IUD: intrauterine contraceptive device; LAM: lactation amenorrhea method; POP: progestogen-only pill)

REFERENCES

1. RCOG. Best Practice in Postpartum Family Planning. Best Practice Paper No 1, June 2015.
2. World Health Organization and United States Agency for International Development. Programming Strategies for Postpartum Family Planning. World Health Organization; 2013.
3. Asgharpour M, Villarreal S, Schummers L, Hutcheon J, Shaw D, Norman WV. Inter-pregnancy interval and pregnancy outcomes among women with delayed childbearing: protocol for a systematic review. Syst Rev. 2017;6:75.
4. International Institute for Population Sciences (IIPS) and LCF. 2017. National Family Health Survey (NFHS-4), 2015–16: Mumbai: IIPS.
5. Speroff L, Darney DP. The postpartum period, breastfeeding and contraception. In: A Clinical Guide for Contraception. 5th edition, Chapter 10. New Delhi: Wolters Kluwer India; 2011. pp. 330-1.
6. Shulman, L, Kaunitz, A. Postpartum contraception. Glob Libr Women's Med. 2008.
7. Parihar M, Bhalerao Gandhi A. Postpartum contraceptive options: match the method to individual needs: In Contraception: Past, Present and Future, 1st edition. New Delhi: Jaypee Brothers Medical Publishers; 2006. p. 343 (Chapter 21).
8. UK Medical Eligibility Criteria for Contraceptive Use | Ukmec 2016 (Amended September 2019).

LONG QUESTIONS

1. Describe the physiology of lactation and its inhibitory role on ovulation. Discuss LAM in detail.
2. Discuss the need for postpartum contraception. Enlist how strategies can be implanted at various levels for better implementation?

SHORT QUESTIONS

1. Enumerate various postpartum contraceptives.
2. Describe how lactation suppresses ovulation.
3. Discuss the importance of postpartum contraception.
4. Discuss the evolution of family planning program of India.

MULTIPLE CHOICE QUESTIONS

1. India's first family planning program was launched in:
   a. 1966 c. 1952 b. 1977 d. 1980
2. Estimated lactation threshold for suppression of ovulation is:
   a. 10 feeds, 100 minutes per day
   b. 2 feeds, 20 minutes per day
   c. 5 feeds, 65 minutes per day
   d. 8 feeds, 80 minutes per day
3. ________ fraction of women ovulate before resumption of menses.
   a. 1/3rd c. 1/4th b. 2/3rd d. 3/4th
4. Any contraceptive containing estrogen should be avoided for ________ weeks after delivery.
   a. 1 c. 2 b. 3 d. 4
5. Correct and consistent use failure rate of LAM is:
   a. 0.5% c. 1% b. 2% d. 4%
6. IUCD can be inserted ________ after delivery.
   a. Up to 6 hours or after 6 weeks
   b. Up to 24 hours or after 6 weeks
   c. Up to 48 hours or after 4 weeks
   d. Only immediately after delivery of placenta or after 6 weeks

7. This method is also known as "reversible sterilization:"
   a. Progesterone depot
   b. Progesterone implant
   c. Intrauterine contraceptive device
   d. Combined oral contraceptive
8. Contraceptive method not to be recommended after 6 months postpartum is:
   a. Barrier method
   b. LAM
   c. COC
   d. IUCD
9. Short interval pregnancy is defined as one with an interpregnancy interval less than:
   a. 36 months
   b. 18 months
   c. 24 months
   d. 12 months
10. The average time of first ovulation after term delivery is:
   a. 25 days
   b. 75 days
   c. 45 days
   d. 95 days
11. For LAM to be effective, the following need to be fulfilled:
   a. Amenorrhea
   b. Exclusive breastfeeding
   c. Less than 6 months postpartum
   d. All of the above

Answers

1.	c	2.	c	3.	b	4.	c	5.	a	6.	c
7.	c	8.	b	9.	d	10.	c	11.	d		

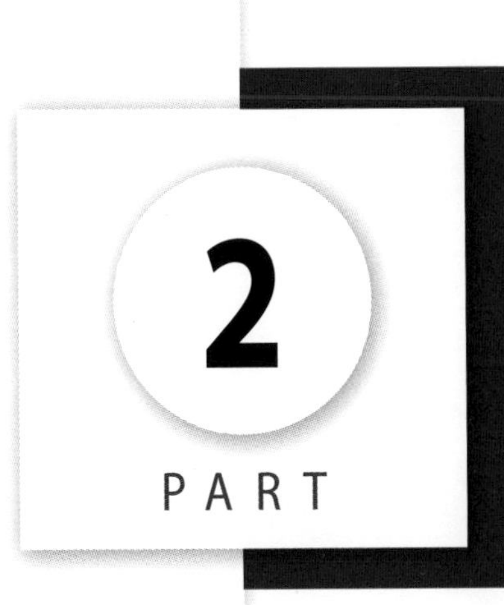

Part 2

Gynaecology

- Reproductive Physiology and Basic Sciences
- Basic Aspects of Gynaecological Care
- Puberty and Adolescence
- General Gynaecology
- Benign Gynaecological Conditions
- Endoscopy
- Reproductive Endocrinology and Infertility

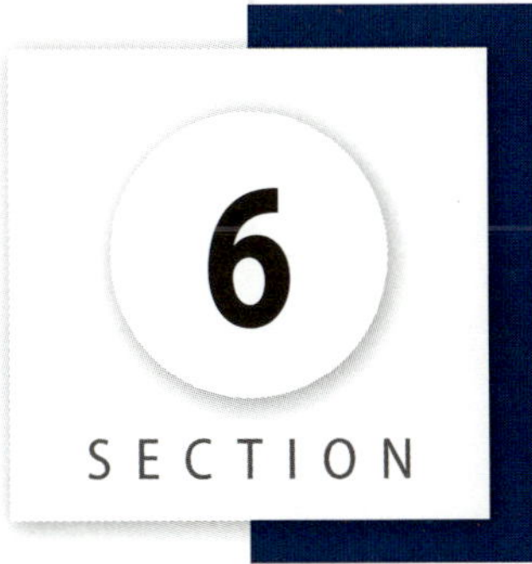

Reproductive Physiology and Basic Sciences

6.1 EMBRYONIC DEVELOPMENT AND SEXUAL DIFFERENTIATION

Madhu Nagpal, Manjitkaur Mohi

INTRODUCTION

Embryonic development and sexual differentiation are an intricate process. It is a subject related to embryology, genetics, physiology, endocrinology, molecular biology, fetomaternal medicine, and ultrasonography. During embryogenesis, a very well-coordinated growth of all fetal organ systems and placental tissues is seen. The morphological changes specifying gender differentiation are a reflection of external and internal genital organs, each being very complex at the cellular and molecular levels. All these physiological events occur under genetic and hormonal influences, observed by a sonoembryologist chronologically, forming the basis of clinical knowledge now.

Several aberrations during the development process occur and many sexual disorders are better understood now due to improved knowledge of sonoembryology, chromosomal analysis, cytogenetic studies associated with steroid hormone synthesis, and hormone receptors' functioning. Thus, some congenital anomalies, isolated genetic defects, growth of abnormal sex organs, and formation of ambiguous genitalia can be related to syndromes of genetic origin and hormonal receptor problems.

FERTILIZATION TO EMBRYO FORMATION

Human embryo development is a process in continuum that includes cell division, differentiation, cell migration, cellular rearrangement, tissue growth, organ development, system functioning, and programmed cell death (apoptosis) converting the fertilized oocyte to a zygote and then into a multicellular human being. The period from a single cell through the period of establishing various organ primordia (the first 8 weeks of human development) is known as the period of embryogenesis; thereafter, it is known as the fetal period till birth where differentiation continues as a fetus grows and gains weight.

Fertilization and First Week

A single oocyte released at the time of ovulation (oogenesis) is undergoing the second meiotic division (metaphase stage) **(Fig. 1)**. The sweeping action of tubal fimbriae moves the oocyte to the site of fertilization in the ampulla. The sperms formed by spermatogenesis in testis are stored in the epididymis; later on, they are deposited in millions in vagina in one ejaculate. As quickly as within 1 hour, several million sperms traverse through the uterus to reach fallopian tubes. Before a single spermatozoan fertilizes oocyte, sperms undergo capacitation (spermatozoan head is denuded of glycoprotein coat and seminal plasma proteins) and acrosome reaction (activation of substances such as acrosin and trypsin helping in penetrating zona pellucida).

Fertilization occurs with penetration of spermatozoon into corona radiata, zona pellucida, and oocyte cell membrane. The second meiotic division is completed when the oocyte meets the sperm. Thus, a mature oocyte and a second polar body are formed. The nucleus of a mature oocyte represents as a female pronucleus. Once the sperm enters the oocyte, the head of the sperm enlarges and gets separated from the tail to represent as the male pronucleus. During fertilization, male and female pronuclei inheriting chromosomes from both maternal and paternal origin unite in the metaphase of the first mitotic division of the zygote. This results in restoring chromosomes in diploid number and determines chromosomal sex by initiating cleavage furthering many mitotic cell divisions. After penetration of one sperm, zona pellucida becomes impenetrable to other spermatozoa **(Fig. 2)**.

As the zygote travels along the fallopian tube toward the uterine cavity, a number of smaller cells or blastomeres form by cleavage. A ball of 12 or more blastomeres, called morula, enters the uterus by the third day postfertilization. The formation of a cavity in morula converts it into a blastocyst

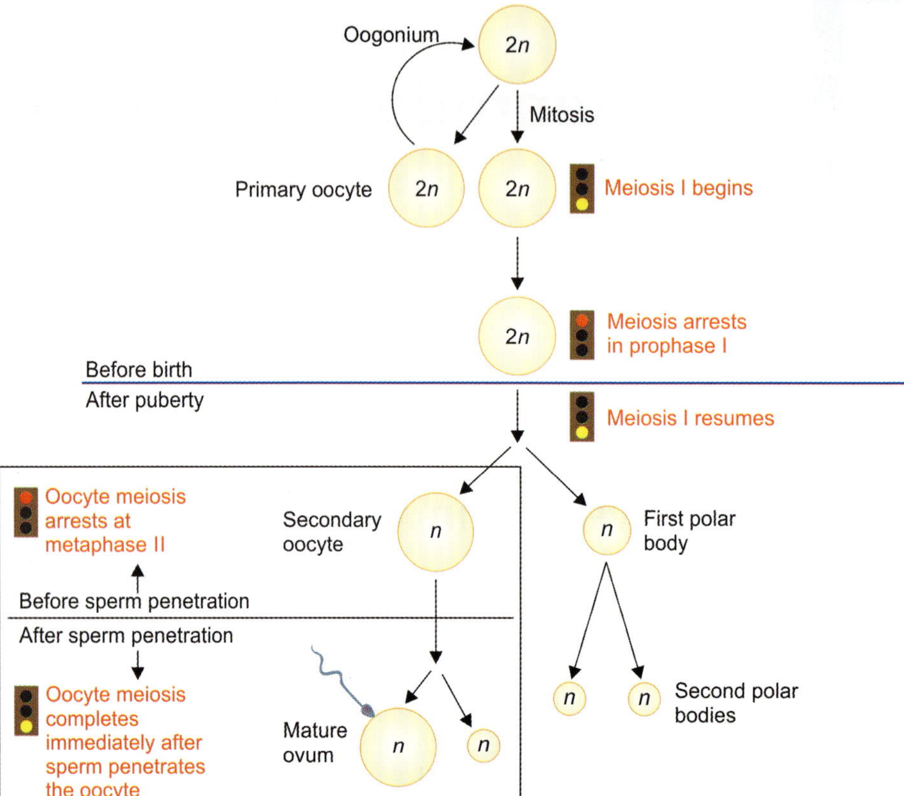

Fig. 1: Oogenesis.

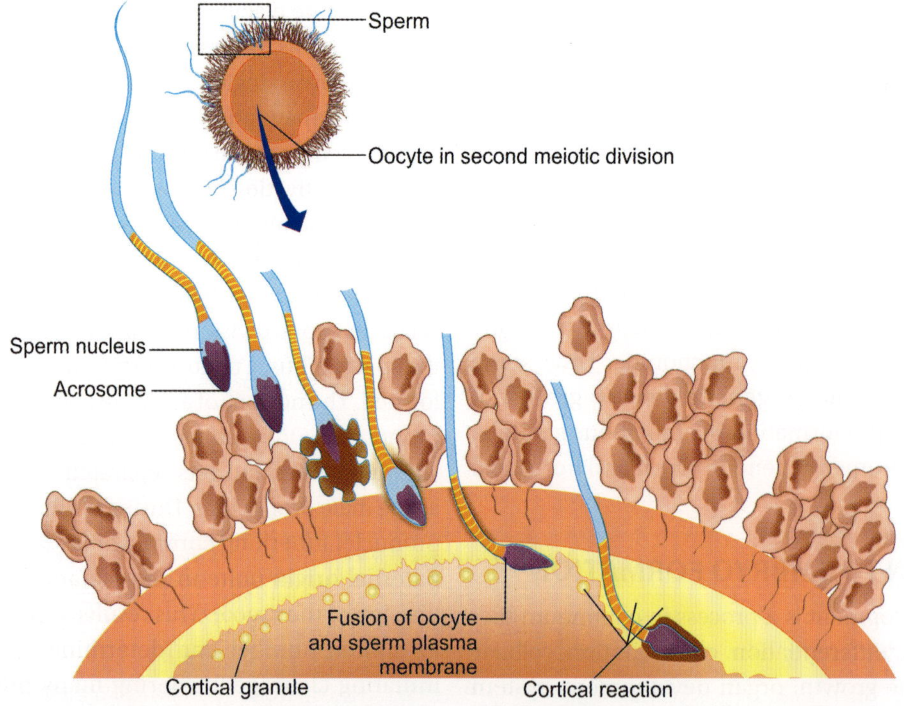

Fig. 2: Fertilization of oocyte with sperm.

with inner cell mass (embryoblast), a blastocystic cavity, and outer cell mass (trophoblast).

A definite embryo develops from embryoblast and lies at one pole of blastocyst with trophoblast surrounding it. The extraembryonic structures and embryonic part of placenta develop from trophoblast. At 4–5 days post-fertilization, zona pellucida is shed off and the trophoblast adjacent to the embryoblast or so-formed embryonic pole adheres to the endometrial layer. The trophoblast at the embryonic pole differentiates into two distinct layers, an outer

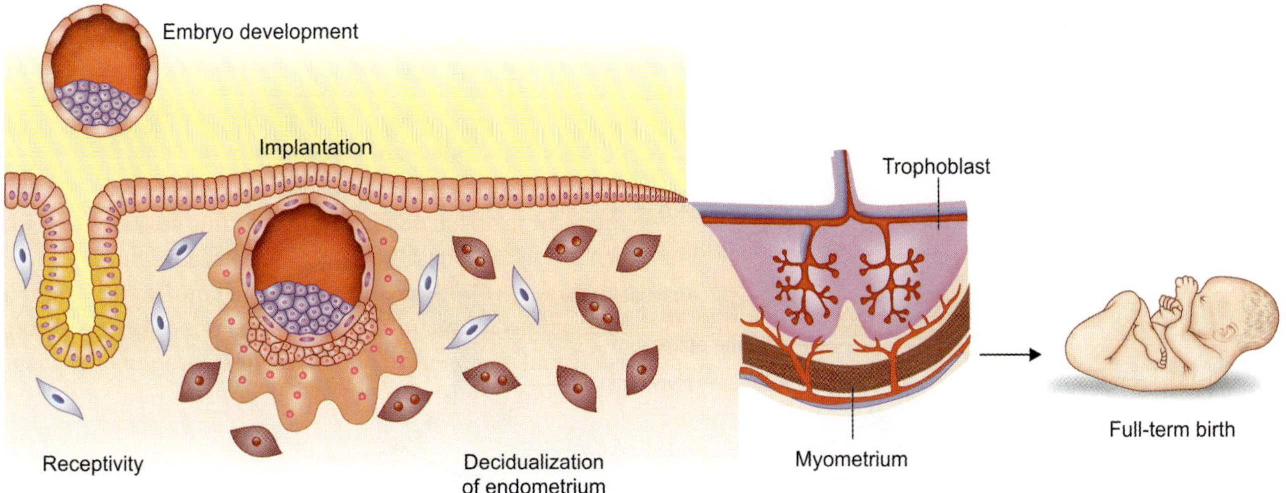

Fig. 3: Interstitial implantation in stratum spongiosum.

syncytiotrophoblast and an inner cytotrophoblast, which in an appropriately programmed window of implantation adheres to the site of invasion in a receptive endometrium bearing pinopodes. Thus, this blastocyst is ready to get implanted at the destined site of endometrium by the first week-end. The successful implantation process is an intricate graft–host reaction as a result of adaptation of tissues with a well-optimized decidual reaction and other immunological interactions called fetomaternal cross talk.

Second Week

As the second week begins, the blastocyst is embedded in the endometrial stromal tissue partially. The syncytiotrophoblast has lacunae formation by the ninth day and by the second week-end, it erodes maternal sinusoids, letting maternal blood enter this lacunar network, marking the start of a primitive uteroplacental circulation. Meanwhile, the cytotrophoblast cellular columns surrounded by syncytium penetrate called primary villi. As the second week ends, the blastocyst gets embedded in the connective tissue layer (stratum spongiosum) completely and a breach in the endometrial mucosal surface gets closed, making it an interstitial implantation **(Figs. 3 and 4)**.

At the same time, extraembryonic mesoderm develops to form a primary umbilical vesicle. The spaces start developing in this mesoderm to form extraembryonic coelom (cavity) which later on develops as chorionic cavity. Between cytotrophoblast and embryoblast, another space called amniotic cavity appears. With this, the differentiation of embryoblast into bilaminar embryonic disc as epiblast related to amniotic cavity and hypoblast related to blastocystic cavity occurs. A localized thickening of hypoblast forms a prechordal plate, which denotes the future cranial part and the mouth of embryo, thereby organizing the head region. The primary umbilical vesicle shrinks to disappear slowly while the secondary umbilical vesicle grows **(Figs. 5A to D)**.

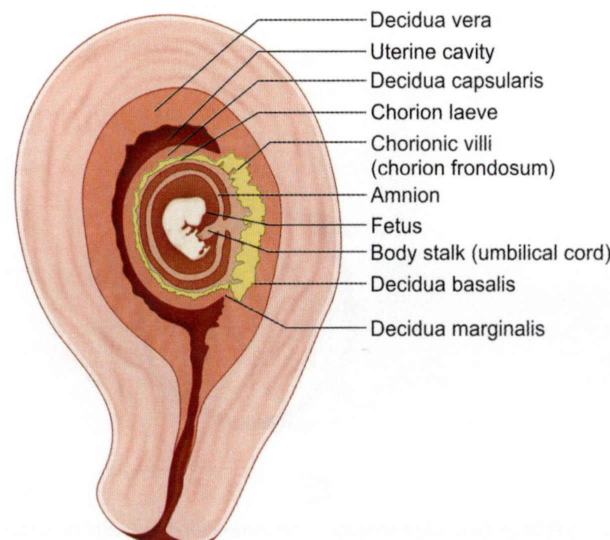

Fig. 4: In utero implantation and embryo formation.

Third Week

With acquisition of mesenchymal core, primary chorionic villi become secondary chorionic villi **(Figs. 6A and B)**.

By the end of third week, capillaries grow in secondary chorionic villi, thus changing them into tertiary chorionic villi. The cytotrophoblastic extensions unite to form stem villi anchoring chorionic sac to endometrium.

As the third week begins, a primitive streak is seen as an epiblast thickening by migration of epiblastic cells to median plane at the caudal end of the embryonic disc. Its development on the epiblast surface starts the gastrulation process changing the bilaminar embryonic disc into a trilaminar embryonic disc. From here, invagination of epiblastic cells occurs migrating mesenchymal cells ventrally, laterally, and cranially to lie between epiblast and hypoblast. When the mesenchymal cells are formed, the epiblast is known as embryonic ectoderm. Also, the embryonic endoderm now forms from the cells of epiblast that displace hypoblast. Some mesenchymal cells

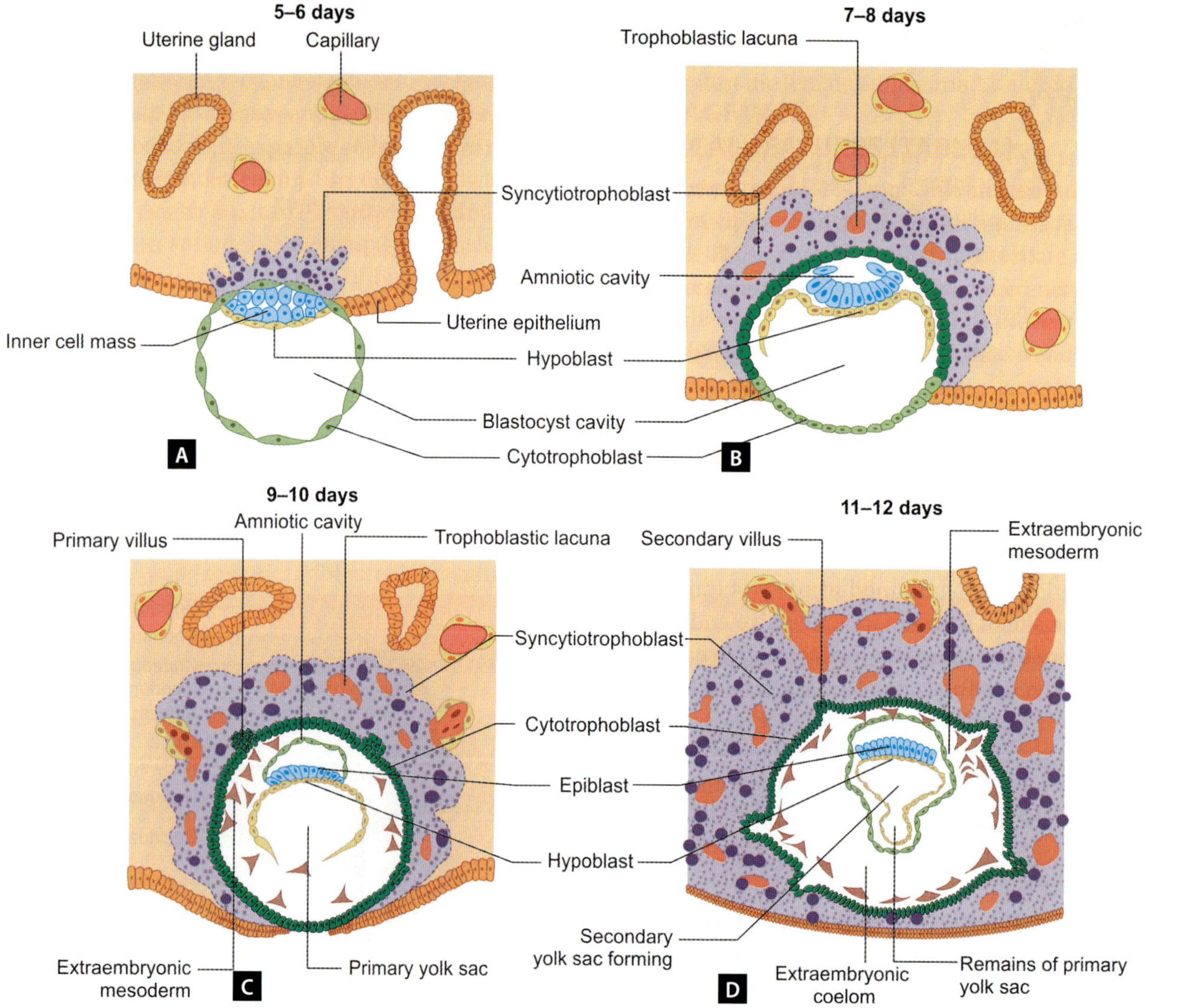

Figs. 5A to D: (A) Differentiation into inner cell mass; (B) Formation of bilaminar disc and amniotic cavity; (C) Formation of primary yolk sac and primary villus; (D) Formation of secondary yolk sac, extraembryonic mesoderm, and secondary villus.

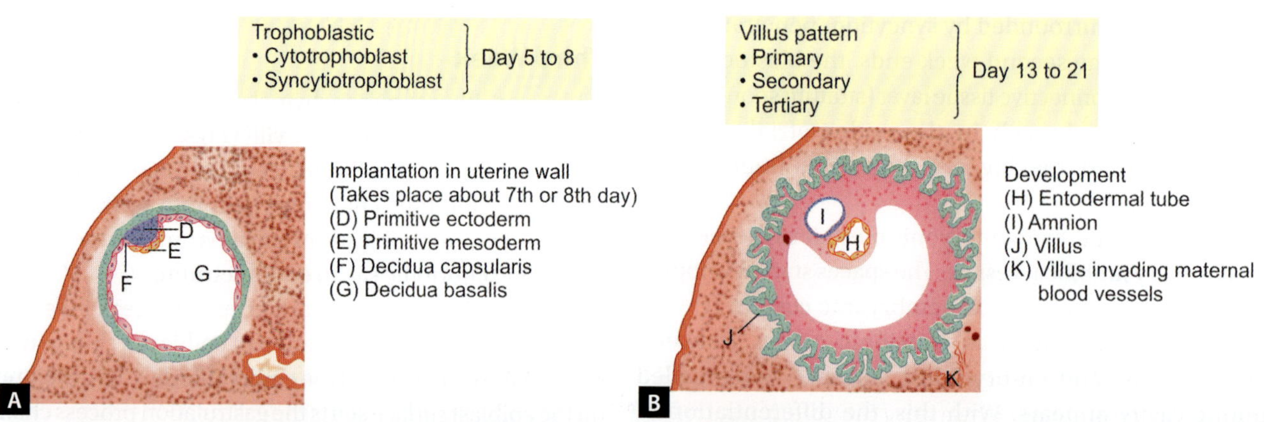

Figs. 6A and B: Genesis of placenta.

soon organize to form a third germ layer, intraembryonic (embryonic) mesoderm, occupying space between the former hypoblast and epiblast. These cells of mesoderm shift to embryonic disc edges to join extraembryonic mesoderm covering amnion and umbilical vesicle.

As the third week ends, an embryo is seen as a flat ovoid embryonic disc. The mesoderm comes between the ectoderm and the endoderm of disc all through except at the site of oropharyngeal membrane, in median plane occupied by notochord, and at the cloacal membrane.

The notochordal process develops from mesenchymal cells between embryonic ectoderm and endoderm at the start of the third week extending from a primitive node to a prechordal plate. The openings formed at the floor of the notochordal canal coalesce, leaving a notochordal plate. Finally, this plate folds in to form definitive notochord to become the primordial axis of embryo the where axial skeleton (vertebral column) develops. A thickening of embryonic ectoderm, so induced by developing notochord, is seen as a neural plate. A neural groove develops in a neural plate longitudinally to get flanked by neural folds which fuse to form a neural tube, which denotes the primordium of the central nervous system (CNS). As this fusion happens, a neural crest forms between the surface ectoderm and the neural tube by the neuroectodermal cells. Then, on either side of the notochord, the mesoderm condenses to form longitudinal paraxial mesoderm columns forming somites by the third week-end.

An isolated space as coelom (cavity) forms in embryo in lateral mesoderm and cardiogenic mesoderm. These coelomic vesicles later unite to form a single, horseshoe-shaped cavity, giving rise to various body cavities finally. First, blood vessels grow in walls of umbilical vesicle, allantois, and chorion and then in embryo soon afterward. The fetal erythrocytes come from various hematopoietic precursors. The primordial heart is represented by paired endocardial heart tubes which fuse at the end of the third week to make a tubular heart. Joining this are the vessels in embryo, umbilical vesicle, chorion, and connecting stalk to form a very primeval cardiovascular system.

In the third week, primordial germ cells appear in the endodermal lining of the wall of the umbilical vesicle and migrate to developing gonads thereafter. These cells finally form spermatogonia in males and oogonia in females.

Fourth to Eighth Week

Various tissues and organ systems originate from three germ cells and complete the initial stages of the main organ systems formation by the end of the embryonic life (10 weeks). The development of brain, heart, liver, somites, limbs, eyes, ears, and nose give an external look of the embryo. As the fourth week starts, the flat trilaminar embryonic disc becomes cylindrical C-shaped, due to infoldings in median and horizontal planes. The head, caudal eminence, and lateral folds become prominent to give a look of a constriction between the embryo and umbilical vesicle. Head-folding brings brain most cranially with the oropharyngeal membrane and heart shifting ventrally, incorporating a part of the endodermal layer to form foregut. Correspondingly, with the ventral folding of caudal eminence, a part of the endodermal germ layer forms the hindgut. The terminal part of hindgut expands to form cloaca with a folding of caudal region forming cloacal membrane and shifting allantois and connecting stalk to the ventral aspect of embryo. As the embryonic folding occurs in the horizontal plane, it incorporates a part of endoderm to form midgut and further on form primordia of ventral and lateral body walls. The midgut is connected to the umbilical vesicle by the yolk stalk (a narrow omphaloenteric duct). As the amnion expands, enveloping connecting stalk, omphaloenteric duct and allantois, an epithelial covering for umbilical cord is formed. In the fourth week, the endoderm of the umbilical vesicle forms primordial gut. Its endoderm, which is derived from epiblast, forms the epithelium of trachea, bronchi, lungs, and alimentary canal. The umbilical vesicle can be recognized early in the fifth week by ultrasound.

By the fourth week, the intraembryonic coelom converts into a horseshoe-shaped cavity in cardiogenic and lateral mesoderm. The future pericardial cavity is at a point of bend, while pleural and peritoneal cavities are from lateral extensions. During the fourth week, folding of the embryonic disc occurs and lateral parts of intraembryonic coelom come together ventrally, the caudal part of ventral mesentery disappears, and merging of right and left parts occurs to form peritoneal cavity. By the seventh week, embryonic pericardial cavity connects to the peritoneal cavity with dual pericardioperitoneal canals.

At the start of the fourth week, the neural crest cells shift to the future head and neck regions and pharyngeal arches start forming. For the first pharyngeal arches, sonic hedgehog signaling plays an important part. The first pair of arches, primordial jaws, appear as outside ridges lateral to the developing pharynx while other arches soon appear as elevations on either side. So by the end of the fourth week, four pairs of arches can be seen externally. The fifth and sixth arches are rudimentary, so they are not seen.

In the early fourth week, facial primordial appears around stomodeum (primordium of mouth) and further facial development continues under the inductive influence of developing forebrain (through sonic hedgehog morphogenic gradients), frontonasal ectodermal zone, and developing eye. The palatogenesis (regulated morphogenetic process) occurs from the end of the sixth week until the start of the ninth week involving WNT and PRICKLE1 molecular pathways. Salivary glands develop as highly branched structures from solid epithelial buds of primordial oral cavity by branching morphogenesis under the influence of notch signaling pathway, during sixth and seventh weeks. The optic groove appears around 22 days marking the onset of eye development and around 32 days an optic cup appears. A thickening of surface ectoderm, otic placode, appears in the preplacodal field at the start of the fourth week.

At 4–5 weeks, the embryonic skin has a single layer of surface ectoderm over mesoderm.

The first endocrine gland is thyroid gland, which begins to develop approximately 24 days post fertilization under effect of fibroblast growth factor signaling pathways. By the end of the fourth week, a median lingual swelling (tongue bud) is visible in the floor of primordial pharynx rostral to the foramen cecum.

During the fourth week, the lung (respiratory) bud starts forming at the caudal end of laryngotracheal diverticulum in the floor of anterior foregut (primordial pharynx) at the caudal end. It soon divides into two outpouchings called primary bronchial buds. These buds extend laterally into pericardioperitoneal canals and primordia of pleural cavities followed by development of secondary and tertiary bronchial buds. Early in the fifth week, each bronchial bud has a large connection with the trachea to form primordia of main bronchi. Other structures, such as connective tissue, cartilage, and smooth muscle, develop from splanchnic mesoderm around foregut. At the end of the fifth week, there develop in diverticulum the longitudinal tracheoesophageal folds which fuse to form tracheoesophageal septum and separate laryngotracheal diverticulum from primordial pharynx. An intricate synchronized influence of multiple signaling pathways and transcription factors results in separation of a single foregut tube into trachea and esophagus. By the seventh week, the final length of esophagus is attained. However, its recanalization occurs by the eighth week-end. During the fourth week, a slight dilation denotes the future site of primordial stomach. In early fourth week, other organs such as liver, gallbladder, and biliary duct system originate from a ventral outgrowth—hepatic diverticulum, from the distal part of foregut. In the sixth week, a ridge representing primordium of cecum and appendix as well as cecal swelling appears on the antimesenteric border of the midgut at the caudal end.

Three sets of kidneys develop in succession during embryonic growth. The first set is rudimentary called pronephroi. The second set, called mesonephroi, functions temporarily during the early fetal period. The third set, called metanephroi, forms future kidneys, the latter, as primordia of permanent kidneys, start developing in the fifth week and become functional in 4 weeks' time. During the sixth week, an amalgamation of mesenchymal cells on each side starts forming suprarenal gland cortex between the root of dorsal mesentery and developing gonad. The medulla grows from neural crest cells.

During the fifth week, on the medial side of mesonephros (primordium of a permanent kidney), a thickening of mesothelium starts which represents the beginning of gonadal development. The proliferation of this epithelium and mesenchymal tissue forms gonadal ridge and gonadal cords. Post-fertilization day 24, primordial germ cells among endodermal cells of the umbilical vesicle are first identified to have migrated along the dorsal mesentery of hindgut to gonadal ridges. During the sixth week, these germ cells constitute gonadal cords. At 6–7 weeks, Sertoli cells in fetal testes start forming testosterone—masculinizing hormone **(Figs. 7A and B)**.

The pectoral, pelvic girdles, and limb bones constitute the appendicular skeleton. During the fifth week, mesenchymal bones are seen as condensations of mesenchyme in limb buds. During the sixth week, these condensations in limbs undergo chondrification and form hyaline cartilage bone models. However, post-fertilization 8 weeks ossification of limb bones starts **(Table 1)**.

Thus, the fourth to eighth weeks of the embryonic period are the most critical period of eventful development because it constitutes the beginning of the most essential external and internal tissues and organ systems. This is called the organogenesis period. Any developmental aberration during this period can go toward major birth defects.

SONOEMBRYOLOGY: DEVELOPMENTAL MILESTONES

The advent of 2D/3D, power Doppler technology and expertise has revolutionized the study of embryological developmental events. The 3D technique is no alternative to 2D; instead, it works as a complement. The surface and transparent views

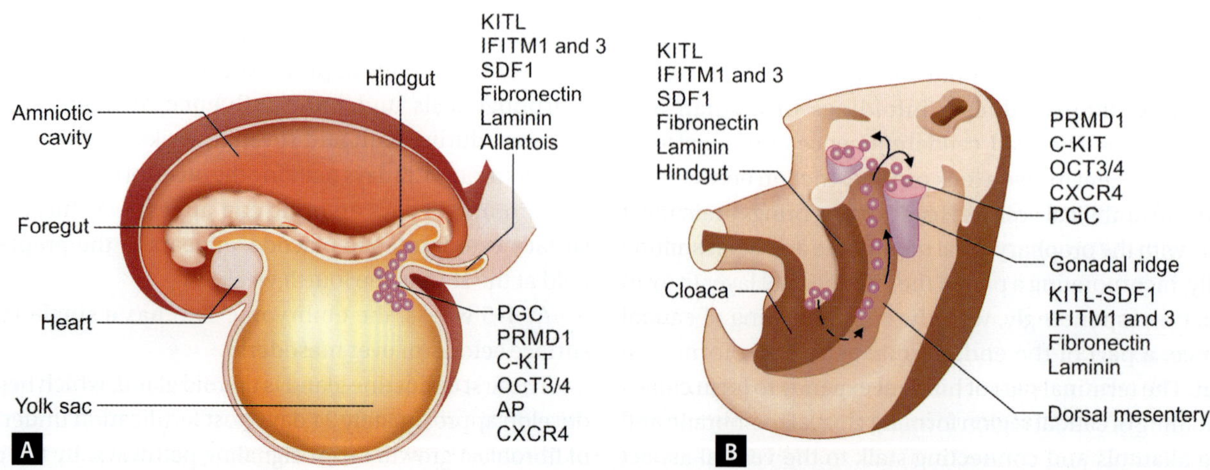

Figs. 7A and B: Embryonic development and various factors influencing growth regulating germ cell migration.

TABLE 1: Origin of various organs from germ cells.

Ectoderm	*Endoderm*	*Mesoderm*
Some part of mouths, lower part of anal canal, terminal part of male urethra, parts of female external genitalia	Epithelial lining of middle ear and eustachian tube	Kidneys and renal tubules, ureter, trigone of urinary bladder
Sensory epithelium of eye, ear, and nose (cornea, conjunctiva, external auditory meatus, outer surface of tympanic membrane)	Thyroid and parathyroid glands	Gonads, most of genital organs, fallopian tubes, uterus, upper part of vagina, testis, and its ductal system
Muscles of iris (sphincter and dilator pupillae)		Mesothelial lining of pleural pericardial, peritoneal cavity, joint cavities
Enamel of teeth		Blood and its components, lymphatics
Central and peripheral nervous systems, (pia mater and arachnoid), pituitary gland	Epithelial lining of GIT, except some parts of mouth and anal canal lined by ectoderm	Microglia, oligodendroglia, dura mater (CNS)
Skin—epidermis, appendages, hair follicles, sweat and sebaceous glands	Respiratory epithelium	Bones, cartilages, dermis of skin
Adrenal medulla and other chromaffin glands	Liver, gallbladder, pancreas	Spleen, adrenal cortex
Salivary glands	Mucosa of urinary bladder, membranous urethra, vagina	Muscles
Mucus lining of nasal cavity, paranasal sinuses	Bulbourethral, great vestibular glands	Cardiovascular system

(CNS: central nervous system; GIT: gastrointestinal tract)

can reconstruct fetal surface structures for fetal skeletal analog. The anatomical details can be visualized due to amniotic fluid. The vascular network in mother, placenta, and fetus can be observed. Lately, vascular 3D measurement as vascularization index (VI) and vascularization flow index (VFI) can be calculated. Their positive correlation can be utilized in relation to crown–rump length and chorion volume. It is useful in prenatal diagnostics by virtue of anatomical survey, structural anomaly scan for minor defects, volumetric assessment of gestational sac, yolk sac and other organs, blood flowmetry, and visualization of fetal skeleton **(Table 2)**.

SEXUAL DIFFERENTIATION

There is a potential to develop into a fetus of either sex since fertilization. The genetic sex is determined by the contribution of either 22 XX or 22 XY chromosomes to make a complete set of 46 chromosomes including two sex chromosomes in it (chromosomal sex).

In early weeks of life, the fetus has no anatomic or hormonal sex but possesses only a karyotype which distinguishes a male or a female. Since there is no sexual difference seen till the sixth week of embryonic life, destined embryos with undifferentiated gonads of XX or XY are identical. This stage is called an indifferent or bipotential stage of gonadal development. The development of testis from these primitive gonads forms the basis of sex differentiation. The absence of androgenic stimulus with 22 XX chromosomes forms ovaries and determines female sex (gonadal sex).

This complex process of embryological development and sexual differentiation is in continuum whereby an undifferentiated zygote develops into an embryo, which in due course develops into a male or a female fetus (phenotypic sex).

Male sex is due to Wolffian ducts and female sex develops from Mullerian ducts. In the initial part, all embryos are feminine unless masculinizing factors play a role and male gonads start forming. Due to many testis determining genes present on Y chromosome, undifferentiated embryonic gonads are directed to develop as testis for initiation of gender differentiation. Testosterone effects development of male sex organs and stimulates the Wolffian ducts to form spermatic ducts (ductus deferens), ejaculatory ducts, and seminal vesicles. During the third month of fetal development, Sertoli cells of testis start secreting Mullerian-inhibiting hormones causing atrophy of Mullerian duct and inhibiting the development of uterus and fallopian tubes. There is a firm concept that even if the fetus is castrated, irrespective of genetic or gonadal sex, the reproductive tract will develop according to female phenotype.

In a fetus predestined to become female, the Mullerian ducts are maintained and Wolffian ducts regress due to absent androgenic effect. The ovaries originate along Mullerian ducts and sexual differentiation to fully mature female reproductive system initiates which continues till puberty. Previously, it was thought that the mere existence of ovaries does not decide the development toward female pathway but lately some specific genes have been identified which promote ovarian development and others which regress testis development.

The gonadal attribute determined by genetic-specific domains produces hormonal differences leading to psychological and behavioral difference, whether from within or induced by social environment. Besides genetic influence, the gender identification comes from the development of specific external genitalia, internal genital organs, breast, body hair distribution, and behavioral development.

TABLE 2: Sonoembryological events marking embryonic development.

Days	*Milestones: USG parallels 2D/3D/power Doppler*
Day 0	• *Fertilization:* Endometrial thickness measurement done • Subendometrial blood flow visualized
Day 1–2	2–4-cell stage of zygote
Day 3	16-cell stage (morula), 0.1 mm diameter
Day 5	Morula enters uterine cavity, formation of blastocyst of 0.2–0.3 mm diameter
Day 6–7	• Implantation starts as zona pellucida disappears • Endometrial volume measurement—quantification better than thickness • VFI • Corpus luteum vascularization seen
Day 8	Bilaminar disc, cyto and syncitio trophoblast layers formed
Day 9–10	Blastocyst
Day 11	Implantation completed
Day 12–13	Primary villi formed, BV in extraembryonic mesoderm of yolk sac, connecting stalk, chorion
Day 14–15 4th week after menstruation	• Gestational sac seen 5 mm in size • Primary yolk sac seen as a circular well-defined echo-free area • Small amniotic cavity formed • Primitive streak replaced by secondary yolk sac • Yolk sac volume and vascularity seen • Vascular network seen—maternal, placental
Day 16 5th week	• Formation of intraembryonic mesoderm (trilaminar disc) • Fetal pole seen. CRL ~ 2.5 mm • Amniotic cavity enlarges, secondary yolk sac seen as 2–3 mm in size • CVS develops. HR 124–180 bpm by 9th week • Notochordal process appears. Deep neural groove and first somites seen • Facial primodia appears; eye and ear placodes appear • Pharyngeal arches begin to develop • Allantoic diverticulum seen • Connecting stalk distinguished, 8-mm size • Secondary villi formed, with an arteriovenous capillary network
Day 21 6th week	• CRL ~ 5 mm • Cardiac prominence distinct • Fetal heart visualized • Formation of bulky head fold • Neural groove formed, closure of neural tube occurs • Pancreatic bud, hepatic bud, primitive kidney appears • Primodia of gonads appear, adrenal glands begin to develop • Umbilical cord and vitelline duct visible • Aortic and umbilical blood flow seen • Increased VI and VFI seen. Tertiary villi formed. Fetoplacental circulation established
7th week	• CRL ~ 10 mm • Head larger than trunk, bent over cardiac prominence. • Brain vesicles seen • Trunk and neck straighten • Limb buds seen. Hand and foot plates formed, digital rays start appearing • Spine visible • Amnion seen • Early vascular anatomy of brain of skull seen, intracranial circulation seen • Discrete pulsations of interior carotid arteries detected at the base of skull • Villi seen all around the trophoblast—chorion frondosum seen separate from levae • Blood flow signals in intervillous space identified with spiral artery
8th week	• CRL ~ 10–17 mm, can be measured • Embryonic skeleton seen as cartilaginous structure • Yolk stalk formed, communication between primitive gut and yolk sac reduced • Head erects and comes over midbrain

Contd...

Contd...

Days	*Milestones: USG parallels 2D/3D/power Doppler*
	• Brain structures expand—lateral, third, and midbrain ventricles seen • Complete visualization of limbs, future hands, and feet seen at end • Shape of face begins to appear though not clear due to cranial flexion • Umbilical cord insertion on the anterior abdominal wall seen • Chorionic villi over the entire surface of gestational sac • Chorionic frondosum visualized forming placenta, chorionic levae seen • Early first-wave trophoblastic invasion in decidua seen • Fetal heart, aorta, intracranial blood flow, and umbilical artery seen • Complete fetal circulation can be seen
9th week	• CRL is ~25 mm • Head rounded separate from body, measures two-third of the body • Face well formed, external ears seen • Cerebral hemispheres develop, lateral ventricles size increases, have hyperechoic choroid plexus • Early spine as dorsal column seen • Arms with elbows and legs with knees form, hands and feet approach each other Placental margin delineated clearly
10th week	• CRL ~ 38 mm • Upper limbs develop faster than lower limbs • Fingers completely formed • Developing intestine is herniated into the proximal umbilical cord • Internal carotid arteries and intracranial vascular network are seen
11th week	• CRL ~ 45 mm • Head and neck grow • Face has nose, orbits, maxilla, and mandible • Fetal spinal vertebra, intervertebral discs, chest ribs, and long bones seen • Fetal limbs, hand, and feet grow with active movements • Midgut herniation disappears due to reposition in abdominal space • Stomach, kidneys, and urinary bladder seen—urine formed, excreted into amniotic fluid
12th week	• Fetal anatomy very clear, head and neck well formed • Brain—cerebellum visible, lateral vesicles dominate • Face broad, eyes separated • Cerebral, CVS, digestive, urinary tracts seen • Fetal sex known • Aortic branches, common iliac, renal arteries, circle of Willis, MCA pulsations seen, absent end diastolic flow seen • Placental circulation appreciable fully • Decidua capsularis adheres to decidua parietalis, space disappears

(BV: blood vessels; CRL: crown–rump length; CVS: cardiovascular system; HR: heart rate; MCA: middle cerebral artery; VI: vascular index; VFI: vascularization flow index)

The differentiation of other body parts and secondary sex characteristics is also dependent on the sexual dimorphism of skeletal structure differential in the early childhood, at puberty, and during adolescence.

Brain differentiation due to influence of sex hormones on the infant brain brings significant differences in growth potential and function with a typical adult reproductive behavior. The sex hormone receptors, such as androgen receptors and estrogen receptors, have been identified in brain. Several sex-specific genes, other than steroids, are expressed differently in male and female human brains. The differences in structural and sexual characters are appreciable by 2 years of age including those in the higher centers in brain like the size and shape of corpus callosum (larger in women), certain hypothalamic nuclei, and gonadotropin feedback response to estradiol. The male brain requires testosterone to differentiate which is released due to a gene expressed during embryonic development. Therefore, singularly absence of genes that generate male genitalia does not alone lead to a female brain, making it an intricate synchronized process again.

Testicular Differentiation: Genetic Role

The Y chromosome essentially possesses at least one gene which determines testicular formation. This gene present in the sex-determining region of the short arm of Y, identified as SRY, has been observed to stimulate the production of a protein—TDF (testis-determining factor) which then binds to DNA and induces cell differentiation in genital ridges into testis formation. The SRY alone has the potential to induce male differentiation.

The testis itself directs the sexually dimorphic fate of internal and external genitalia. So when gonadal primodes differentiate into testis, all internal and external genitalia follow a male pathway of growth, irrespective of their chromosomal inheritance. In males, thus the Wolffian ducts grow predominantly and the Mullerian ducts regress.

Testicular Differentiation: Cellular and Molecular Mechanism

The significance of Y chromosome for testicular development irrespective of the existence of X chromosome is well known. It was formerly thought that TDF on Y chromosome solely determines the male pathway till lately *SRY* gene (sex-determining region on Y) was found and established as a TDF. Now, it has been established that SRY has a weak transactivation potential; instead, it is a target gene encoding transcription factor SOX9 which is the chief regulator of testis differentiation. So the prime role of SRY lies in the pathway which stimulates the differentiation of Sertoli cells, for regulating SOX9 expression. This SOX9 is autoregulated with some feedforward-enhancing mechanisms and some opposing sets of genes which oppose ovarian differentiation.

SRY is expressed in pre-Sertoli cells, which get delaminated from the coelomic epithelium in the central part of bipotential gonad and start their differentiation. SRY is a member of DNA-binding proteins and bears high mobility group (HMG) box on the short arm of Y chromosome. Human SRY expression is present in both Sertoli cells and germ cells at fetal and adult stages **(Fig. 8)**.

The proteins SIP1/NHERF2 and KRAB-O interact with SRY in gonadal differentiation.

SRY effects are mimicked by SOX9 irrespective of SRY expression. It affects genital tract differentiation by upregulating anti-Mullerian hormone (AMH) expression—a Sertoli cell factor involved in the male pathway of the internal genitalia. SOX9 upregulates expression of FGF9 and PGD2 which maintains expression levels, accelerating male pathway in a feedforward loop.

Two other members from the SOX family (SOX8 and SOX10) triggered after SOX9 are found at low levels in the gonads and other tissues. They work in unison to autoregulate SOX9 expression.

SOX3 from the same family also induces SOX9 expression. It is ectopically present in XX gonad and works for regulation of steroid hydroxylase-nuclear receptor in hypothalamus, pituitary, gonads and adrenal glands through SFI known as Ad4BP or FT2F1- HGNC.

Other general transcription factors, such as LHX 1-EMX-2 and PAX2, under action of SFI, are found essential for intermediate mesoderm and gonadal ridge development.

DMRT1 is another member of the DM domain transcription factor family which significantly contributes to male gonad development.

Expression of steroidogenic factor 1 and Wilms tumor 1 during early human gonadal development and sex determination has also been identified.

For appropriate differentiation of fetal testis and secretion of masculinizing hormones, all the factors should be available in appropriate amounts in right cell lineage in optimum

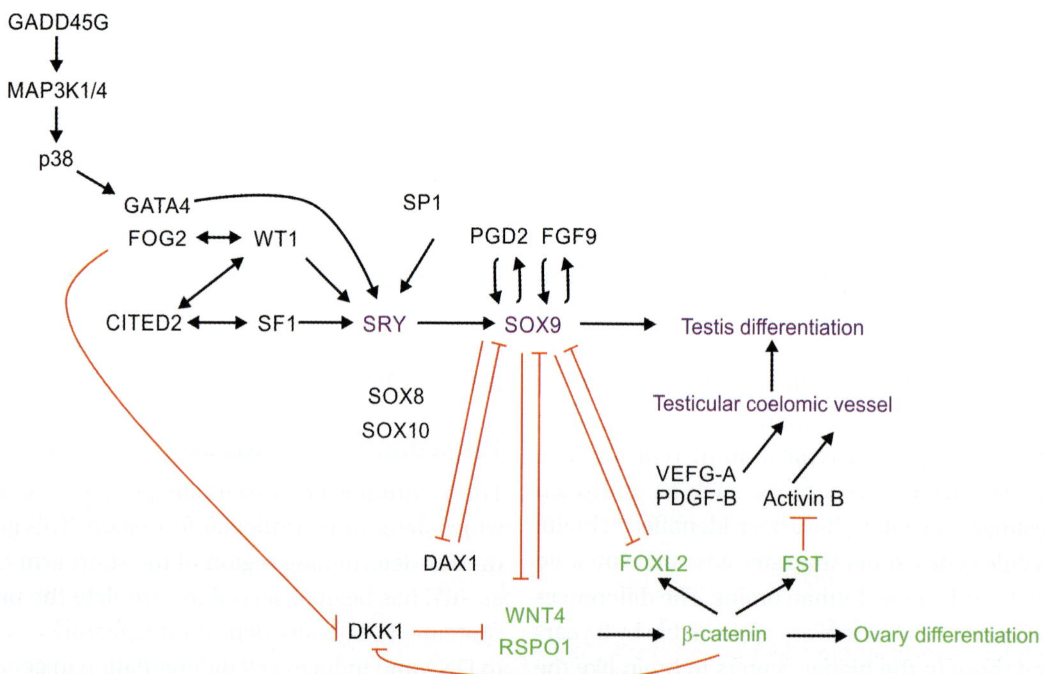

Fig. 8: Schematic representation of molecular mechanisms affecting undifferentiated gonadal ridge. Black arrows indicate a positive regulation, double arrows indicate a positive feedback loop, red lines indicate a negative regulation, and double red lines indicate a mutual antagonism.

narrow window periods which may be as small as 6 hours; for example, if activation of SOX9 is not achieved appropriately by timely SRY expression, it will lead to failed initiation of male pathway **(Figs. 9A and B)**.

Interaction of Germ Cells with Somatic Cells in Developing Testis

At 4 weeks, gonadal tissue predominantly formed of somatic cells gets inhabited by primordial germ cells originating from pluripotent cells of the proximal epiblast. They move in embryonic life through the primitive streak into the extraembryonic site at the base of allantois. Their contribution to germ cell lineage as well as extra embryonic mesoderm cells is important.

The genital system, urinary system, and adrenal cortex arise from a common location of the urogenital ridge. During the fourth week post fertilization, it segregates into urinary and adrenogonadal ridges which later on differentiate into adrenal cortex and gonads.

The gonadal ridge is indifferent and bipotential, so it can develop into an ovary or testis either. The undifferentiated genital ridge has germ cells till the fifth week-end and they proliferate by mitotic division for 1 week more, though they maintain bipotentiality. Thereafter, the primordial germ cells of extragonadal origin also get colonized in gonads.

The gonadal ridge differentiation from the intermediate mesoderm is under WT1 and SF1. The Wilms tumor gene (*WT1*) acts as a transcription factor regulating SRY expression and is later on found in Sertoli and granulosa cells. SF1 regulates steroid hydroxylases in gonads, hypothalamus, pituitary, and adrenal cortex.

The germ cells are enclosed in seminephrous cords and they differentiate into the spermatogonial lineage to enter meiosis at the onset of puberty only. This inhibition of gonocyte proliferation is by androgens, and its meiotic arrest which was originally considered to be a specific effect of male somatic cells is now realized to be protected by retinoic acid action through various factors, enzymes, and proteins simulating FGF9, CYP26B, and enzyme NANOS 2 protein repressing STRA-8 expression.

During the bipotential stage, sex differentiation of germ cells is not under the chromosomal factor alone. It is the Sertoli cells surrounding XY germ cells which differentiate into spermatogonia, while in an ovarian situation XX germ cells differentiate into oogonia much before undergoing meiosis. However, those germ cells where discordancy of karyotype with the somatic lineages exists, they fail to enter gametogenesis and apoptosis occurs later in life.

Mullerian Duct Regression

Till the end of 8 weeks, the internal reproductive tract is alike in both sexes (undifferentiated reproductive tract) with two unipotential ducts as Wolffian and Mullerian ducts. The Wolffian ducts arise lateral to somite number 8-10 in the intermediate mesoderm in a 25–30-day-old embryo. The regression of Mullerian ducts, both cranially and caudally, starts allowing male accessory organs to start developing, such as the prostatic utricle, in a 55–60-day-old embryo. The Mullerian duct regression itself is under the influence of certain factors due to deposition of periepithelial extracellular matrix. The remnant of the Mullerian duct can be seen as a fibrotic structure with condensed perimullerian mesenchyme in it.

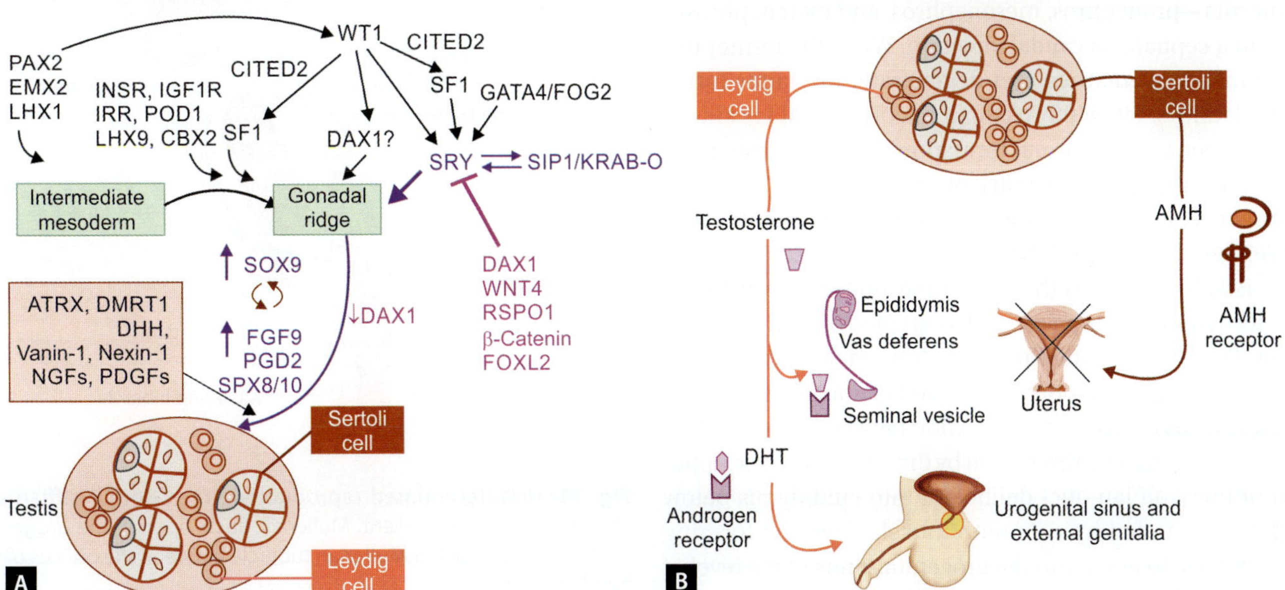

Figs. 9A and B: Male sex determination—growth factors and hormonal regulation. (A) General transcription factors, such as LHX1, EMX2, and PAX2, are necessary for intermediate mesoderm development. The gonadal ridge differentiates from the intermediate mesoderm following the action of SF1, which is regulated by LHX9 and WT1. SRY expression, activated by WT1 and GATA4, induces testis differentiation, characterized by an increase in SOX9 and a decrease in DAX1 expression. The effect of SRY overcomes the action of genes that have been proposed to repress testicular differentiation, such as *WNT4*, *RSPO*, β-catenin, and *FOXL2*; (B) Hormonal regulation of sex differentiation through AMH and testosterone.

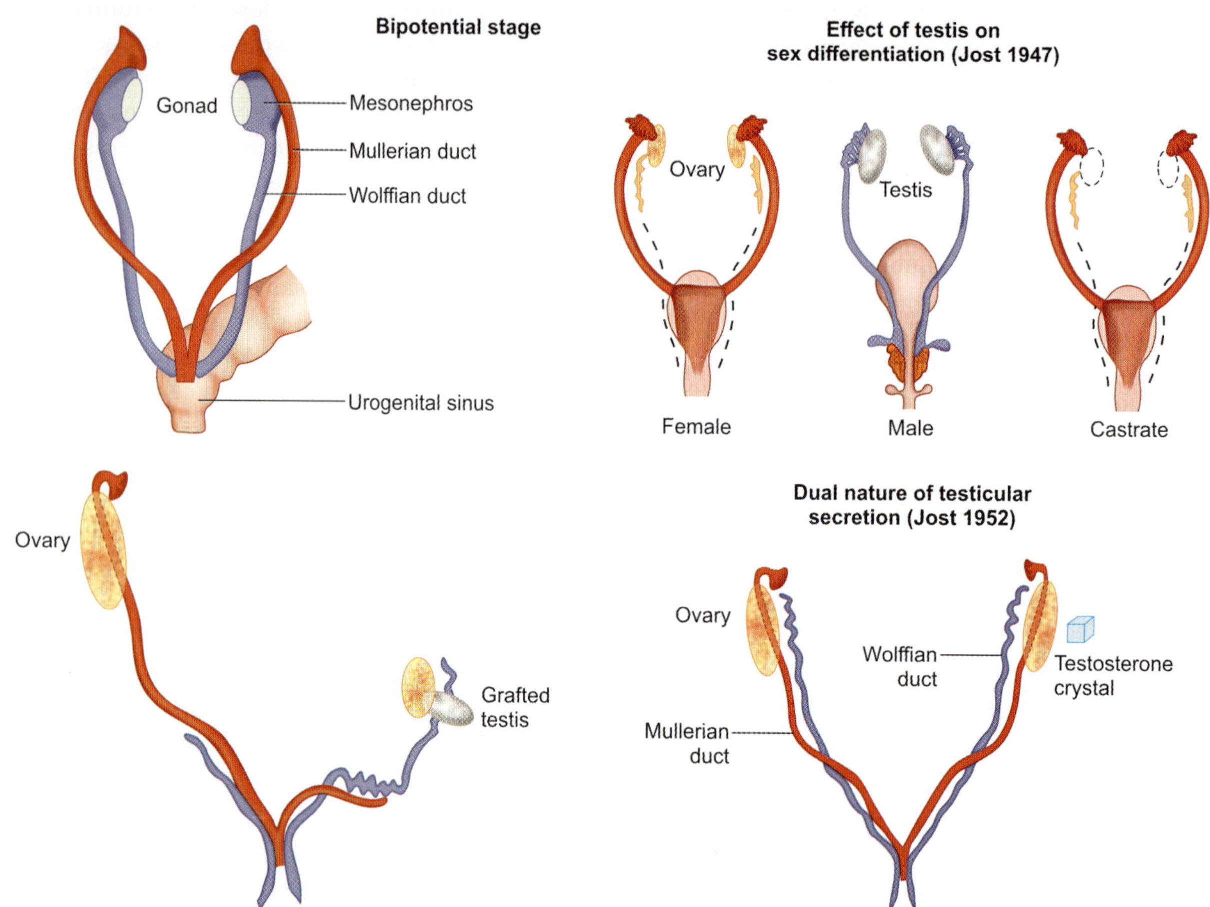

Fig. 10: Sex differentiation: Jost's pioneering experiments.

The Wolffian ducts elongate caudally and initiate the formation of nephric tubules through a mesenchymal transition process. It is from these tubules that three kidney primordia—pronephros, mesonephros, and metanephros—arise in a cephalic to caudal direction. While the former two are transient structures and degenerate, the latter forms future kidneys. Since the Wolffian duct is crucial for kidney development, its abnormal formation is usually associated with malformation of urinary or genital systems. Several factors are associated with the development and maintenance of Wolffian ducts **(Figs. 10 and 11)**.

It is subsequent to the loss of mesonephric functional activity that stabilization and differentiation of Wolffian ducts occur. The cranial tubules persist to form male efferent ducts while mesonephric nephrons and caudal tubules degenerate. The rete testis forms from connection between mesonephric tubules and gonadal primordium by the sixth week. The upper part of the Wolffian duct delineates into epididymis below to get surrounded by a smooth muscle covering forming vas deferens, to open into the urogenital sinus at the level of Mullerian tubercles between 9 and 13 weeks **(Fig. 12)**.

At 12 weeks, the terminal portion of the vas deferens dilates to form seminal vesicles. The descent of testis occurs by migration from the original pararenal position into the scrotum in many steps. Earlier, the upper pole of testis is connected by the suspensory ligament cranially to the posterior abdominal wall and a primitive gubernaculum extends from the caudal pole to the internal inguinal ring.

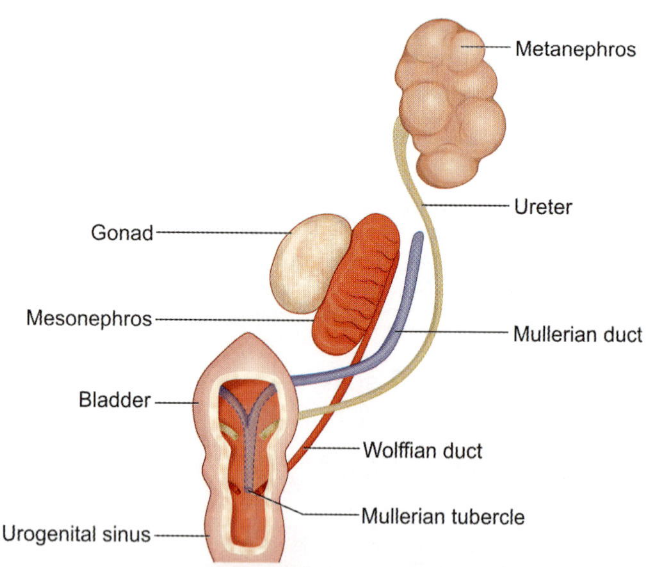

Fig. 11: Undifferentiated reproductive tract: Both Wolffian and Mullerian ducts are present. Mullerian ducts open in the urogenital sinus at the level of the Mullerian tubercle between the orifices of the Wolffian duct.

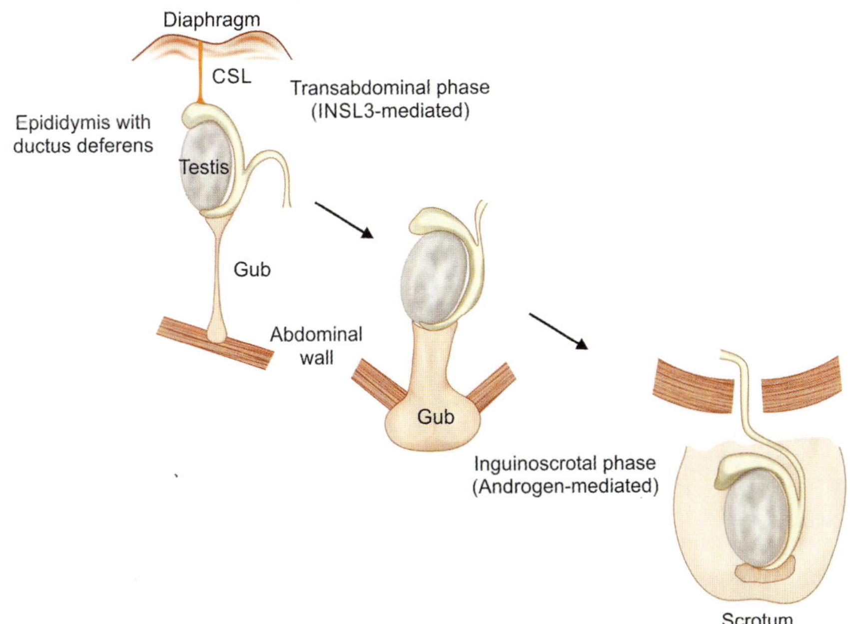

Fig. 12: Testicular descent. (Left) Initial phase: The primitive gonad located near the kidney, held by cranial suspensory ligament (CSL) and gubernaculum (Gub) testis. (Right) Transabdominal descent: Androgen-mediated dissolution of the CSL and insulin-like factor 3 (INSL3) mediated swelling of gubernaculum brings testis to the internal orifice of the inguinal canal. Inguinoscrotal migration: The testis passes through the inguinal canal into the scrotum, androgen-dependent phase.

Source: Klonisch T, Fowler PA, Hombach-Klonisch S. Molecular and genetic regulation of testis descent and external genitalia development. Dev Biol. 2004;270(1):1-18.

Ovarian Differentiation

The Mullerian ducts open in the urogenital sinus between the orifices of the Wolffian ducts at the level of the Mullerian tubercle. The Mullerian duct formation occurs in three steps **(Figs. 13A and B)**:

- *Phase I: Initiation*: The progenitor cells (PGCs) of mesonephric epithelium develop under the influence of various transcriptional factors (LHXI).
- *Phase II: Invagination:* Primordial Mullerian cells invaginate from the coelomic epithelium to reach the Wolffian duct under WNT4 fault.
- *Phase III: Elongation:* Mullerian ducts elongate, cross over Wolffian ducts ventrally, and fuse centrally near the urogenital sinus under the WNT9B signaling factor.

Ovarian Differentiation: Genetic, Cellular, and Molecular Pathways

While SRY has a predominant role in the testicular development pathway, an ovary-determining factor still remains unrecognized. The absence of SRY alone is not the only reason for gonadal ridges to form ovaries. On the contrary, complete absence of active *SRY* gene, e.g., *SRY* mutation or deletion of Y chromosome involving SRY locus, still causes some gonadal dysgenesis, insufficient ovarian differentiation, oocyte meiotic arrest, or absent follicle growth during early fetal life.

Recently, it has been concluded that several factors work in harmony for ovarian differentiation and stabilization.

The germ cells play a major role in stabilizing gonadal structure and maintaining somatic component. The germ cells effect in developing gonad in sexually dimorphic-germ cell multiplication through meiosis is of prime significance for the maintenance of the fetal ovary; otherwise, prospective follicular cells degenerate and streak gonads form. On the other side, lack of germ cells does not cause testicular developmental arrest. To conclude, in the absence of germ cells, unlike the testis which can differentiate normally, the ovarian follicles do not. If instead germ cells are lost even after the formation of follicles, these rapidly degenerate.

The initial ovarian differentiation starts with germ cell entry into meiosis under the effect of WNT4 (a protein as a paracrine factor controlling several developmental mechanisms) in unison with RSPO1 (which increases in XX gonads where SRY is absent). Both result in increasing levels of cytoplasmic β-catenin and follistatin (FST). The latter shifts to the nucleus and causes FST expression and antagonizes activin-B, which represses endothelial cell migration and coelomic vessel formation **(Fig. 14)**.

Ovarian Morphogenesis

In an XX fetus, gonads are indifferent till the 7th week histologically, but functionally estradiol production starts at the same time as testosterone in XY gonad. The PGCs proliferate by mitosis and differentiate to oogonia. The ovarian maturation starts occurring from the center to the periphery. At 10 weeks, oogonia in the deepest layer enter meiotic prophase representing the first sign of morphological ovarian differentiation. Thereafter, a single layer of follicular cells or granulosa cells is seen surrounding oogonia, which enter meiosis and become

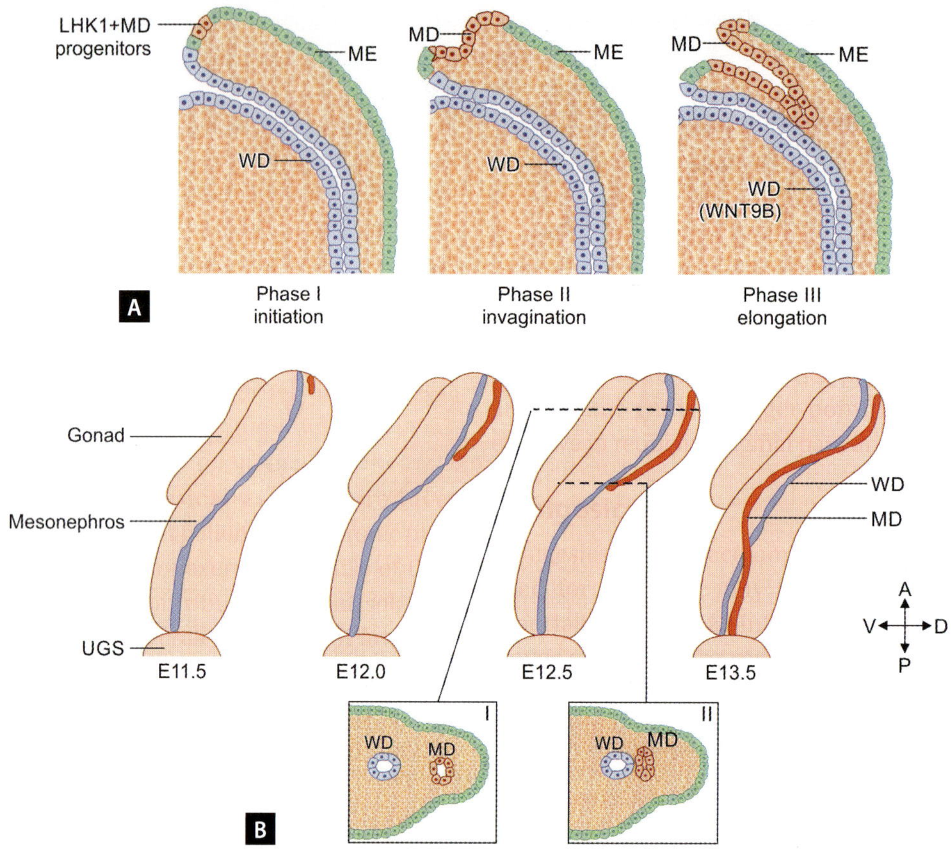

Figs. 13A and B: Müllerian duct (MD) development. (A) Phase I (initiation), Phase II (invagination), and Phase III (elongation); (B) At ~ E12.5, MD crosses over the Wolffian duct to be located medially. Elongation is complete by ~E13.5 with the MD reaching the urogenital sinus (UGS). [A = anterior (rostral); D = dorsal; P = posterior (caudal); V = ventral]

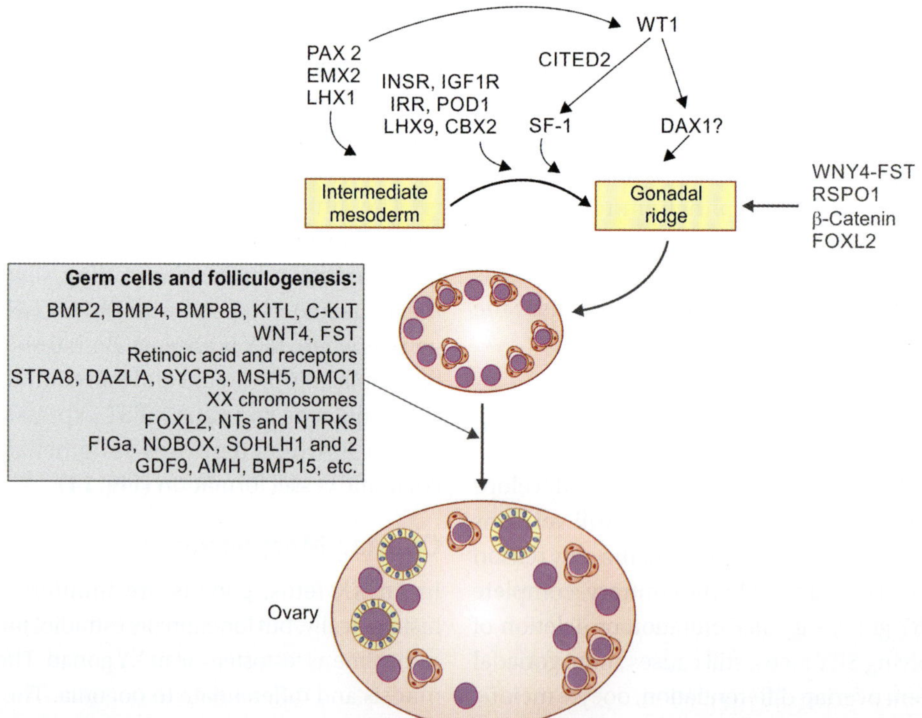

Fig. 14: Female sex determination. Like in male, general transcription factors, such as LHX1, EMX2, and PAX2, are necessary for intermediate mesoderm development. The gonadal ridge differentiates from the intermediate mesoderm following the action of SF1, LHX9, and WT1. WNT4, FST, RSPO1, and β-catenin should be expressed to antagonize testis differentiation and promote early ovarian differentiation. Germ cell development (dependent on BMP family members, KIT ligand and its receptor C-KIT, WNT4, FST, retinoic acid and its receptors, the existence of two X chromosomes as well as several factors such as DAZLA, MSH5, STRA8, and DMC1) are essential for fetal ovary stabilization.

oocytes forming primordial follicles. The meiosis in a fetal ovary is initiated by an increase in retinoic acid synthesized from retinaldehyde dehydrogenase isoform I (ALDH 1A1).

In XX gonads, only a few endothelial cells shift from the mesonephros to the gonad suggesting cortical and medullary portions being established in early gonadogenesis almost alike. The granulosa cells (like Sertoli cells) arise from three areas—ovarian surface epithelium, mesonephric cells from nearby rete ovarii, and existing mesenchymal cells of genital ridge. The theca cells (like Leydig cells) come from fibroblast-like precursors in ovarian stroma under the influence of granulosa cells. Thus, at 45 days, the absence of testicular differentiation suggests the presence of ovary. Finally, when the embryo is 14 weeks, rows of old gonad germ cells are seen in meiotic prophase. The medulla has primordial and primary follicles.

Oogenesis and Folliculogenesis: Genetic Control

The important events are germ cell migration, proliferation, meiosis, and folliculogenesis. Two X chromosomes are required for ovarian growth. With the absence of two X chromosomes, e.g., in Turner syndrome, germ cell loss and gonadal dysgenesis occur. So, all influencing factors are optimally essential for proliferation and migration of PGCs during early embryogenesis.

In female gonad, the germ cells keep undergoing mitosis. The meiosis is deferred till the end of tenth week due to suppression by polycomb repressive complex-1 (PRC-1) which in turn represses STRA-8 and other factors involved in differentiation of primordial germ cells in the early meiotic phase until retinoic acid reaches an optimum level. Retinoic acid is formed from retinaldehyde dehydrogenase in mesonephros. STRA-8 expression is induced in developing ovary by binding of retinoic acid to retinoic acid receptor (RAC) in germ cells.

A number of other genes of unknown significance are upregulated in human ovary before and during development of a primordial follicle. Similarly, several other hormonal factors are involved in ovarian folliculogenesis and follicle growth. AMH has a role in regulating the recruitment of primordial follicles in each cycle and thereafter folliculogenesis. The initial primary follicles are identified at 15–16 weeks and the first graafian follicle at 23–24 weeks. At inception, follicle number is 6–7 million at 25 weeks while only 2 million remain at term. At the end of the seventh month gestation, mitosis is halted and all germ cells remain in meiotic prophase until the adult life. Most oocytes have apoptosis and follicular atresia occurs. After 23 weeks of fetal development, AMH produced by granulosa cells from primary to antral follicles is in low quantity **(Figs. 15A and B)**.

Female Internal Genitalia Differentiation

By the end of 3 months of fetal development, it is characterized by complete regression of Wolffian ducts and only vestigial structures such as Rosenmuller organs and Gartner canals remain.

Molecular regulation of male genital duct development

- SRY is a transcription factor and the master gene for testes development; possibly acting in conjunction with the autosomal gene SOX9 a transcription regulator also inducing testes differentiation
- SOX9 binds the promoter region of the gene for antimullerian hormone/mullerian inhibiting substance (AMH, MIH) regulating this genes expression.
- At the begining SRY and/or SOX9 induce the testes to secrete FGF-9 acting as a chemotactic factor that causes tubules from the mesonephric duct to penetrate the gonadal ridge.
- Without penetration by these tubules differentiation of the testes does not continue.
- Next SRY directly or indirectly through SOX9 upregulates production of steroidogenesis factor-1 (SF-1) that stimulates differentiation of Sertoli and Leydig cells. SF1 with SOX9 increase AMH leading to regression of the paramesonephric (mullerian) ducts.
- SF1 upregulates the genes for enzymes that synthesize testosterone

A

SRY
SOX9
SF1
Other genes
Testes

Molecular regulation of female genital duct development

- WNT4 is the ovary determining gene; upregulating DAX1 which is a member of the nuclear hormone receptor family.
- DAX1 inhibits the function of SOX9.
- WNT regulates expression of other genes (TAFII105.... TATA binding protein for RNA polimerase in ovarian follicular cells) responsible for ovarian differentiation
- Mice that do not synthesize that subunit do not form ovaries
- Estrogens are involves in sexual differentiation; under their influence paramesonephric (mullerian) ducts are stimulated to form external genitalia

B

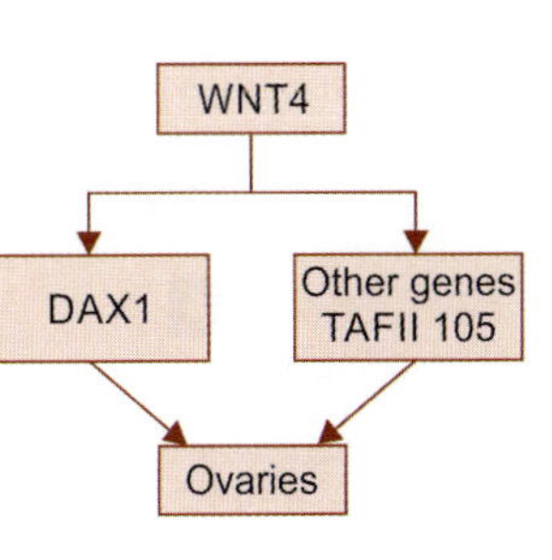

Figs. 15A and B: (A) Molecular regulation in male; (B) Molecular regulation in female.

Mullerian Duct Formation

It originates from a cleft between the gonadal and mesonephric parts of the urogenital ridge in a 10-mm embryo. It is lined by coelomic epithelium which later on forms the abdominal ostium of fallopian tubes. The solid bud of epithelial cells in the cleft caudally migrates into basal lamina and burrows in mesenchyme placed lateral to the Wolffian ducts. The Mullerian ducts persist, forming an epithelial tube from the apex to the base developing as endometrium, while the mesenchyme develops into the myometrium of uterus and fallopian tubes. The end of mesoepithelial features is marked by a decline of AMH-sensitive window of Mullerian ducts. The tube differentiates to form fimbria and ampullary folds lined by high columnar epithelium possessing ciliary and secretory activity. The uterotubal junction is seen as an abrupt widening of the uterine segment and by the presence of epithelial crypts. Earlier, the endometrium is lined with closely packed columnar cells in which other changes such as vacuolation and glandular formation happen as the gestational age advances. The distal two-third of the uterus constitutes the cervix in fetus.

Urogenital Sinus, External Genitalia: Indifferent Stages

The Mullerian tubercle demarcates the vesicourethral canal cranially and the urogenital sinus caudally. A transverse urorectal septum segregates the cloaca into the rectum dorsally and the primitive urogenital sinus in a 5-week-old embryo. The cloaca is covered with the cloacal membrane consisting of ectoderm and endoderm with no mesoderm in it **(Figs. 16 and 17)**.

In the fifth week, a pair of cloacal folds comprised of mesodermal cells is seen along the cloacal membrane forming urogenital folds along the urogenital sinus and anal folds posteriorly. These urogenital folds unite to form a genital tubercle anterior to the cloacal membrane in the midline. The cloacal membrane divided by the urorectal septum is named genital membrane anteriorly and anal membrane posteriorly. By 8 weeks, the genital membrane disappears itself.

The genital tubercle has a lateral plate of tissues comprised of ectoderm and mesoderm, seen as a medioventral projection near the ostium cranially. From the urogenital sinus, the endodermal epithelial cells invaginate into the genital tubercle to form the urethral plate in midline, forming roof of primary urethral groove extending up to phallus tip. A deep furrow called, urethral groove, is formed on the genital tubercle on the ventral surface after corpora cavernosa and glans have developed **(Fig. 18)**.

In a 6-week-old embryo, urogenital sinus opening is surrounded by paired labioscrotal swellings on either side of urogenital folds to get connected by fibrous tissue bands

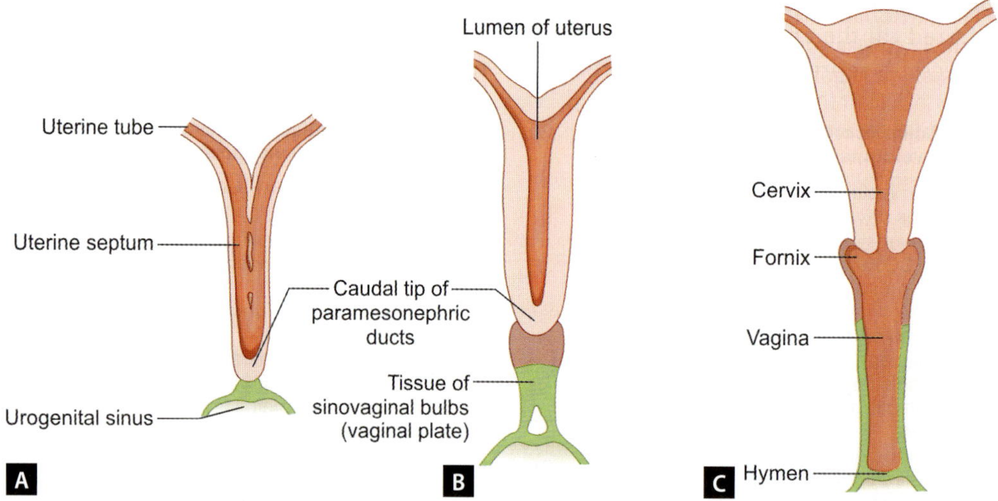

Figs. 16A to C: Development of external female genital organs.

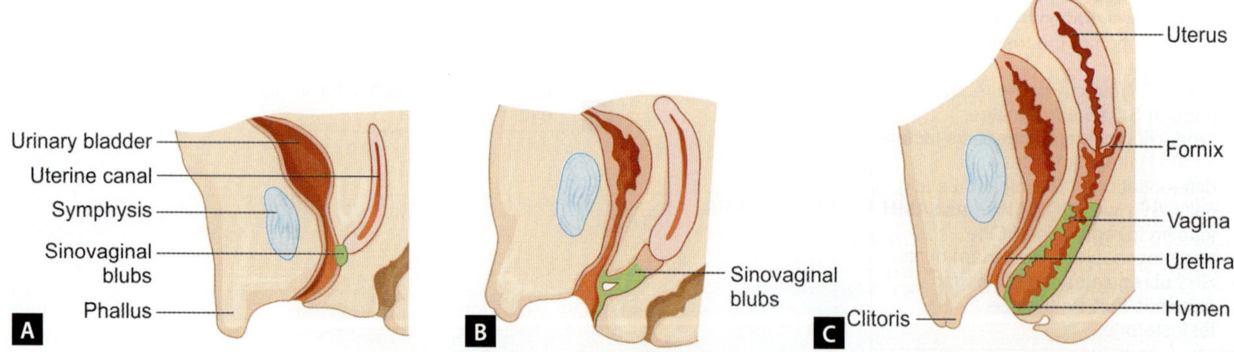

Figs. 17A to C: Development of internal female genital organs.

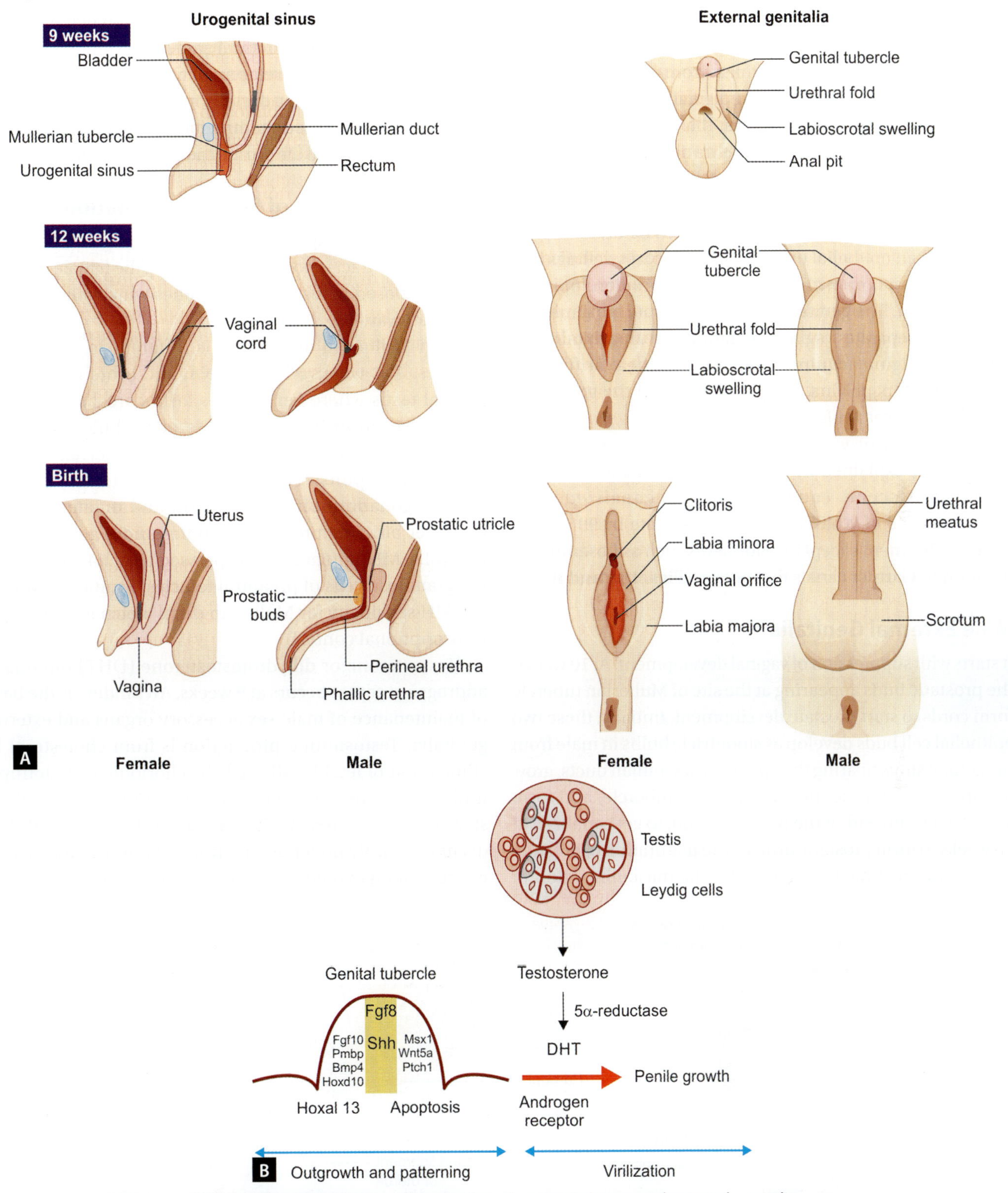

Figs. 18A and B: (A) Sex differentiation of urogenital sinus and external genitalia; (B) Growth factors regulating outgrowth and ambisexual differentiation of external genitalia.

to caudal poles of genital ridges, seen as round ligaments in females or gubernaculum testis in males.

The external genitalia do not undergo differentiation up to approximately 9 weeks.

At 12 weeks in both females and males, the vaginal primordium develops caudally from ends of the Mullerian duct and medially from urogenital sinus projections. The sinovaginal bulbs unite to form a vaginal cord or plate where desquamation of cells of the vaginal plate creates the vaginal lumen. The female character of urogenital sinus is established by the presence of a distinct vaginal orifice on the perineum and by the absence of prostatic development.

Till the end of ambisexual stage, vaginal anlage is just below bladder neck. The upper part of vagina has origin from Mullerian ducts and the lower part from sinovaginal bulbs which have origin from the fused vaginal plate, derived from the urogenital sinus. By 22 weeks, the lower end of vagina extends downward underneath urethra till vaginal rudiment to open directly on the perineum. The female external genitalia growth remains static. The anogenital distance remains same with no fusion of rims of urethral groove. The urethral plate remains as an epithelial end. The labioscrotal swellings give rise to labia majora with dorsal commissure developing at their junction. The genital folds form separate labia minora. The hymen separates vagina and diminutive urogenital sinus. When the vagina acquires a separate perineal orifice, the diminutive pars pelvina and pars phallica of the urogenital sinus become vestibule.

The atresia of vagina in Rokitansky–Kustner–Hauser syndrome is explained by failure of Wolffian and Mullerian ducts to descend caudally and get canalized. The disappearance of Wolffian ducts is complete by 90 days of fetal development except for rudiments such as Rosenmuller organs and Gartner canals that persist **(Figs. 19A and B)**.

Male External Genitalia

It starts with suppression of vaginal development. At 10 weeks, the prostatic buds appearing at the site of Mullerian tubercle form cords to start prostate development. Initially, these two epithelial cell buds develop as sinoutricle bulbs in male from urogenital sinus nearing the openings of Wolffian ducts, grow inward, fuse with the medial Mullerian tubercle, and form sinoutricle cord within the prostate gland, to get canalized at 18 weeks to form prostatic utricle. The maturation of prostate gland and prostatic utricle occurs. The masculinization of external genitalia occurs at 9 weeks by fusion of labioscrotal folds enclosing primary urethral groove. The urethra forms by 14 weeks. The penile development occurs in two stages with the male urethra forming dorsally from the urethral plate and ventrally from the fused urethral folds. The maximal phallus growth occurs in fetal life during the third trimester **(Table 3)**.

Hormonal Control of Sex Differentiation

Jost experiments explain that whatever the genetic sex, the reproductive tract is bound to grow along the female pathway unless exposed to testicular hormones which stimulate the male pathway.

Anti-Mullerian expression is different in males than females. At 8 weeks AMH, mRNA, and protein are found in fetal testis where Sertoli cells form cord-like structure destined to form future seminiferous tubules. The high amounts of these are crucial to male Mullerian ducts to lose their responsiveness. AMH expression in males is initially gonadotropin independent and in later fetal life and after birth, its production comes under gonadotropin control. AMH in females is expressed after 24 weeks from the granulosa cells of preantral follicles. So, it is the timing of AMH sensitivity for Mullerian ducts which is under tight transcriptional control.

Testosterone or dihydrotestosterone (DHT) binding to androgen receptor occurs at 9 weeks. AR binding is the basis of maintenance of male sex accessory organs and external genitalia. Testosterone production is from cholesterol by stimulation of fetal Leydig cells by chorionic gonadotropin under well-synchronized action of mainly adrenal gland steroidogenesis enzyme. It peaks at 14–17 weeks and then declines sharply under gonadotropin control so that serum concentration in both males and females is similar.

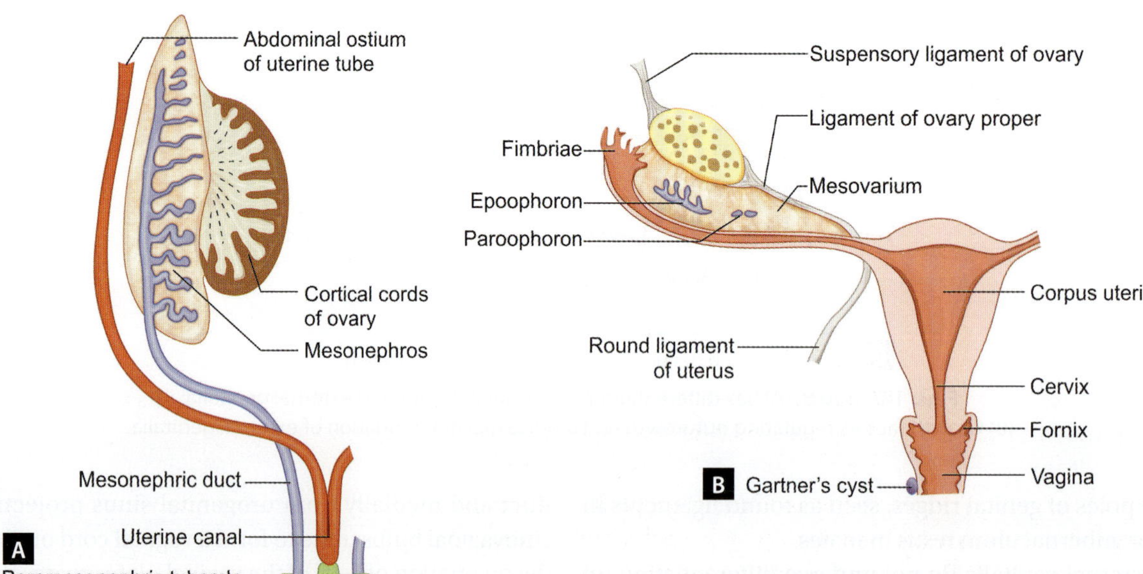

Figs. 19A and B: Remnants of the cranial and caudal excretory tubules in the mesovarium form the epoophoron and paroophoron, respectively. The mesonephric duct disappear except for a small cranial portion found in the epoophoron and a small caudal portion in the wall of uterus or vagina (Gartner's cyst).

TABLE 3: Tracking chronology of sexual development.

Age from conception	*CRL (mm)*	*Male pathway*	*Female pathway*
32 days	5	Gonadal primordia develop Growth of Wolffian ducts	
37 days	10	Primordial germ cell differentiation	Primordial germ cells near gonadal ridge Müllerian ducts' differentiation starts
42–50 days	15–20	Seminiferous cord differentiation	
55–60 days	30	Beginning of secretion of AMH Leydig cell differentiation Cranial part of Müllerian ducts regresses	
9 weeks	40	Leydig cells produce testosterone Beginning of masculinization of urogenital sinus and external genitalia	
10 weeks	45–50	Beginning of degeneration of female Wolffian ducts Male Müllerian ducts have disappeared Prostatic buds appear	Meiotic entry of oocytes in the medulla
12 weeks	55–60	Seminal vesicles develop Testis at the internal inguinal ring	Vaginal cord is formed Primordial follicles appear
14 weeks	70	Completion of male urethral organogenesis	
16 weeks	100		Primary follicles appear
20 weeks	150	Testosterone serum level is low Formation of prostatic utricle	
22 weeks	180		Vagina reaches perineum
24 weeks	200	Graafian follicles appear Beginning of penile growth	
27–30 weeks	230–265	Inguinoscrotal descent of the testis	
36 weeks	300		Secondary and tertiary follicles produce AMH

(AMH: anti-Mullerian hormone)

TABLE 4: Growth factors in urogenital development.

SOX9	Lack of ventral prostate development
WNT/β catenin	Masculinization of external genitalia
SERP1 and 2	Testicular decent
PAX8	Vaginal opening
MSX2	Disruption of vaginal epithelium and lack of caudal Wolffian regression
WT1	Wilms tumor gene 1 for early gonadal and sexual development

Estrogen, Diethylstilbestrol, and Xenoestrogens

The female sex differentiation is not directly under ovarian hormones; instead, the toxicity of diethylstilbestrol (DES) is well known during in utero exposure. An uncontrolled bisphenol (xenoestrogen) exposure can result in cryptorchidism and hypospadias. Other endocrine disrupters, such as phthalates, act as pseudoestrogens (bisphenol A), can demasculinize male gonads, and can suppress spermatogenesis by interfering in phosphodiesterase enzyme action.

TABLE 5: Proteins involved in androgen production.

Protein	*Gene*	*Chromosome*	*Purpose*
Steroidogenic acute regulatory protein	*STAR*	8p11.2	Cholesterol trafficking
P450 scc (side chain cleavage enzyme) Cytochrome P450 family 11, subfamily A, polypeptide 1	*CYP11A1*	15q24.1	Cholesterol side chain cleavage
Cytochrome b5, type A	*CYB5A*	18q22.3	Regulation of 17,20-lyase activity
Steroidogenic factor 1 (SF1)	*NR5A1*	9q33.3	Regulates many steroidogenic enzymes
5α reductase type 1	*SRD5A1*	5p15.31	Reduction of P to 17OH-P

The conclusion is that hormones as well as growth factors work in a coordinated manner during sexual differentiation and gender development **(Tables 4 to 8)**.

TABLE 6: Factors involved in early gonadal ridge development.

Gene	*Chromosome*	*Role*	*Expression*
LHX1 LIM homeobox gene1	17q12	Development of head, neural, lymphoid urogenital structures	Primitive streak, prechordal and intermediate mesoderm brain, thymus, tonsil
LHX9	1q31.3	SF1 activation in gonadal primordia	Central nervous system, fore and hindlimb, mesenchyme, urogenital system
EMX 2 homolog of spiracles homeobox gene 2	10q26.11	Induction of mesenchyme	Telencephalon, epithelial components of urogenital system
IGF1R (insulin growth factor 1 receptor)	15q26.3	Metabolic, cell proliferation	Widespread effect on brain, heart, lung, liver, small intestine, kidney, thymus, spleen, muscle, adipose tissue, cartilage
PAX2 (paired box gene 2)	10q24.31	Regulation of WT1 expression	Mesonephros, metanephros adrenals, spinal cord, hindbrain, optic, otic vesicles

TABLE 7: Factors in gonadal differentiation.

Gene	*Chromosomal localization*	*Function*	*Expression*
SRY (sex-determining region on Y chromosomes)	YP 11.31	Regulates SOX9, triggers testis differentiation	Male gonadal ridge
SP1 (specificity protein 1)	12q.13.13.	Regulation of SRY expression	Widespread effect
GATA4 (GATA binding protein 4)	8p23.1	Regulation of SRY expression	Widespread effect
SOX 9 (SRY box 9)	17q24.3	Triggers testis differentiation and regulates its genes	Testis cartilage
SOX 8 (SRY box 8)	16p13.3	Regulation of SOX9 with SF1	Gonadal tissues
SOX 10 (SRY box 10)	22q13.1	Regulation of SOX9 with SF1	Gonadal tissues
FGF9 (fibroblast growth factor 9)	13q12.11	Upregulation of SOX9 and WNT4	Gonadal tissues
VEGFA (vascular endothelial growth factor)	6p21.1	Induces vascular endothelial cell migration to gonad	Mesenchymal cells of gonadal ridge
WNT4 (wingless type MMTV integration site family, member 4)	1p36.12	Induces β-catenin and silences FGF9 and SOX9	Gonadal tissues
FST (follistatin)	5q11.2	Antagonizes activins	Widespread effect
CTNNB1 (β-catenin)	3p22.1	Upregulates WNT4, FST, FOXL2	Widespread effect
WT-1 (Wilms tumor-associated gene 1)	11p13	Urogenital ridge derivatives	Transcriptional regulation and post-transcriptional stabilization of *SRY*

TABLE 8: Null mutation effects of growth factors on genital ducts morphogenesis.

Growth factors	*Wolffian ducts*	*Mullerian ducts*	*Gonads*
β-catenin	Normal	Lack of oviduct coiling, lack of regression	Loss of germ cells in ovary, testes normal
EMX2	Early degeneration	Do not form	Absent
HOXA13	Rostral ureteral junction	Agenesis of caudal portion	Normal
Retinoic acid receptors	Agenesis of vas deferens and seminal vesicles	Agenesis of uterus and cranial vagina	Normal
IGF1	Agenesis of caudal portion	Infantile uterus	No ovulation, abnormal Leydig cells
LIM1 (LHX1)	Do not form	Do not form	Normal
PAX2	Early degeneration	Early degeneration	Normal
PAX8	Normal	Endometrium does not form	Normal
WNT4	Persists in females No regression in males	Do not form	Ovary produces testosterone

However, lately, a well-defined genetic pathway has been identified directing active ovarian function for female sex determination. Till then, the theory of testicular hormones directing male sex differentiation will remain true and the female sex differentiation remains as a default pathway.

"Homosapiens is a perfect masterpiece created by Nature"

ACKNOWLEDGMENTS

The authors acknowledge extensively helpful inputs from following articles, which have been incorporated in this manuscript for illustrations at appropriate places.

FURTHER READING

1. Allard S, Adin P, Gouédard L, di Clemente N, Josso N, Orgebin-Crist MC, et al. Molecular mechanisms of hormone-mediated Mullerian duct regression: involvement of beta-catenin. Development. 2000;127:3349-60.
2. Ashe HL, Briscoe J. The interpretation of morphogen gradients. Development. 2006;133:385.
3. Azumendi G, Kurjak A. Three dimensional sonoembryology. Donald Sch J Ultrasound Obstet Gynaecol. 2008;2(2):62-86.
4. Barnea ER, Hustin J, Jauniaux E (Eds). The First Twelve Weeks of Gestation. Berlin: Springer-Verlag; 1992.
5. Berta P, Hawkins JR, Sinclair AH, Taylor A, Griffiths BL, Goodfellow PN, et al. Genetic evidence equating SRY and the testis-determining factor. Nature. 1990;348:448-50.
6. Chemes HE, Rey RA, Nistal M, Regadera J, Musse M, Gonzalez-Peramato P, et al. Physiological androgen insensitivity of the fetal, neonatal, and early infantile testis is explained by the ontogeny of the androgen receptor expression in Sertoli cells. J Clin Endocrinol Metab. 2008;93:4408-12.
7. Fitzpatrick DR, Human embryogenesis. In Magowan BA, Owen P, Thomson A (Eds). Clinical Obstetrics and Gynaecology, 3rd edition Philadelphia: Saunders; 2014.
8. Gasser RF. Atlas of Human Embryos, Baltimore: Lippincott Williams & Wilkins; 1975.
9. George FW, Wilson JD. Conversion of androgen to estrogen by the human fetal ovary. J Clin Endocrinol Metab. 1978;47:550-5.
10. Hanley NA, Ball SG, Clement-Jones M, Hagan DM, Strachan T, Lindsay S, et al. Expression of steroidogenic factor 1 and Wilms' tumour 1 during early human gonadal development and sex determination. Mech Dev. 1999;87:175-80.
11. Hanley NA, Hagan DM, Clement-Jones M, Ball SG, Strachan T, Salas-Cortes L, et al. SRY, SOX9, and DAX1 expression patterns during human sex determination and gonadal development. Mech Dev. 2000;91:403-7.
12. Jirásek JE. An Atlas of Human Prenatal Developmental Mechanics: Anatomy and Staging. London: Taylor and Francis; 2004.
13. Jost A. Problems of fetal endocrinology: the gonadal and hypophyseal hormones. Recent Prog Horm Res. 1953;8:379-418.
14. Kim Y, Bingham N, Sekido R, Parker KL, Lovell-Badge R, Capel B. *Fibroblast* growth *f*actor receptor 2 regulates proliferation and Sertoli differentiation during male sex determination. Proc Natl Acad Sci USA. 2007;104:16558-63.
15. Klonisch T, Fowler PA, Hombach-Klonisch S. Molecular and genetic regulation of testis descent and external genitalia development. Dev Biol. 2004;270(1):1-18.
16. Moore KL, Persaud TVN, Shiota K. Color Atlas of Clinical Embryology, 2nd edition. Philadelphia: Saunders; 2000.
17. Moore KL, Persaud TVN, Torchia MG. The Developing Human Clinically Oriented Embryology, 10th edition. Philadelphia: Elsevier; 2016.
18. Mullen RD, Behringer RR. Molecular genetics of Mullerian duct formation, regression and differentiation. Sex Dev. 2014;8:281-96.
19. Racine C, Rey R, Forest MG, Louis F, Ferré A, Huhtaniemi I, et al. Receptors for anti-müllerian hormone on Leydig cells are responsible for its effects on steroidogenesis and cell differentiation. Proc Natl Acad Sci USA. 1998;95:594-9.
20. Rey R, Josso N, Chrystele R. Sexual differentiation. [online] Available from: https://www.ncbi.nlm.nih.gov [Last accessed November, 2021].
21. Saddler TW. Medical Embryology, 13th edition. Philadelphia: Wolters Kluwer Health; 2015.
22. Sekido R, Bar I, Narvaez V, Penny G, Lovell-Badge R. SOX9 is up-regulated by the transient expression of SRY specifically in Sertoli cell precursors. Dev Biol. 2004;274:271-9.
23. Sekido R, Lovell-Badge R. Genetic control of testis development. Sex Dev. 2013;7:21-32.
24. Sharpe RM. The 'oestrogen hypothesis'—where do we stand now? Int J Androl. 2003;26:2-15.
25. Shimamura R, Fraizer GC, Trapman J, Lau Y, Saunders GF. The Wilms' tumor gene WT1 can regulate genes involved in sex determination and differentiation: SRY, Mullerian-inhibiting substance, and the androgen receptor. Clin Cancer Res. 1997;3:2571-80.
26. Steptoe PC, Edwards RG. Birth after implantation of a human embryo. Lancet. 1978;2:36.
27. Suzuki T, Mizusaki H, Kawabe K, Kasahara M, Yoshioka H, Morohashi K. Concerted regulation of gonad differentiation by transcription factors and growth factors. Novartis Found Symp. 2002;244:68-77.
28. Tilmann C, Capel B. Cellular and molecular pathways regulating mammalian sex determination. Recent Prog Horm Res. 2002;57:1-18.
29. Visser JA, de Jong FH, Laven JSE, Themmen APN. Anti-Mullerian hormone: a new marker for ovarian function. Reproduction. 2006;131:1-9.
30. Yamada S, Samtani RR, Lee ES, Lockett E, Uwabe U, Shiota K, et al. Developmental atlas of the early first trimester human embryo. Dev Dyn. 2010;239:1585.

LONG QUESTIONS

1. Discuss embryological development supported by diagrams.
2. Discuss sonoembryology representing events of embryo development.
3. Discuss sexual differentiation and male pathway determining factors.
4. Discuss embryological events marking female pathway development.
5. Discuss development of male sexual pathway and factors affecting it.

SHORT QUESTIONS

1. Discuss process of fertilization and implantation.
2. Discuss neural tube formation during embryogenesis.
3. Discuss sexual differentiation of gonads in an embryo.
4. Discuss development of female genital organs.
5. Discuss factors influencing male sex pathway.

MULTIPLE CHOICE QUESTIONS

1. Second meiotic division of oocyte and release of second polar body occurs:
   a. Before sperm penetration
   b. After sperm penetration
   c. After union of male and female pronucleus
   d. At the formation of zygote
2. Urogenital ridge does not give rise to ------ in 4th week post fertilization.
   a. Genital system b. Adrenal cortex
   c. Urinary system d. Digestive system
3. Kidneys develop from which kidney primordia:
   a. Pronephros b. Mesonephros
   c. Metanephros d) Urogenital ridge
4. Neural tube closure occurs on:
   a. Day 21 b. Day 23
   c. Day 25 d. Day 27
5. What is not of significance in sexual differentiation of male pathway:
   a. Chromosomal sex b. Testes SRY gene
   c. Estrogens d. Testosterone
6. Cardiac motion in a developing embryo starts at:
   a. 4th week b. 5th week
   c. 6th week d. 7th week
7. Ectoderm arises during embryogenesis from:
   a. Epiblast
   b. Hypoblast
   c. Bilaminar disc all layers
   d. Trilaminar disc all layers
8. Somitogenesis completely occurs by:
   a. 9–10 weeks b. 7–8 weeks
   c. 5–6 weeks d. 3–4 weeks
9. Follicular cells in ovary develop in:
   a. 10 weeks b. 12 weeks
   c. 14 weeks d. 16 weeks
10. Penile growth in male sexual pathway is under effect of all factors, except:
    a. Endocrinal control
    b. Molecular growth factors control
    c. Genetic control
    d. Epigenetic control
11. Lens placode develops in:
    a. 8th week b. 6th week
    c. 5th week d. 7th week
12. Limb buds are completely formed by:
    a. 8th week b. 9th week
    c. 10th week d. 11th week
13. Circle of Willis (cerebral circulation) can be documented by 3D USG Power Doppler in:
    a. 8th week b. 7th week
    c. 10th week d. 9th week
14. Placental tertiary villus formation is complete at ~ 5 mm CRL by:
    a. 6th week b. 8th week
    c. 10th week d. 12th week
15. Early gestational sac size 5 mm is visible during:
    a. 4th week b. 5th week
    c. 6th week d. 7th week
16. Rounded bulky head and thin trunk on 3D USG can be seen during:
    a. 6th week b. 5th week
    c. 8th week d. 7th week
17. Aortic and umbilical blood flow is visible with 3D USG Power Doppler by:
    a. 6th week
    b. 8th week
    c. 10th week
    d. 12th week
18. AMH effect in male sex differentiation is independent of gonadotropin control:
    a. After birth in infancy
    b. After birth near puberty
    c. Before birth in early fetal life
    d. Before birth till late fetal life
19. SOX-9 and other members of this family result in molecular and cellular effect in:
    a. Testicular differentiation
    b. Ovarian differentiation
    c. CNS development
    d. CVS development
20. 3D USG knowledge of embryogenesis is important in Prenatal diagnostics & early embryopathy detection:
    a. True
    b. False

Answers

1.	a	2.	d	3.	c	4.	b	5.	c	6.	b
7.	a	8.	d	9.	d	10.	d	11.	c	12.	c
13.	a	14.	a	15.	b	16.	a	17.	a	18.	c
19.	a	20.	a								

6.2 NEUROENDOCRINOLOGY AND REPRODUCTIVE CYCLE

Kamini A Rao, Vyshnavi A Rao

INTRODUCTION

The regulation of reproductive function involves two major sites of action in the brain—hypothalamus and pituitary gland. Since time immemorial, the pituitary gland has been called the master gland of the body. Now, the pituitary gland is a subordinate counterpart which plays a role as part of an orchestra, along with the hypothalamus, acting through neurotransmitters transported to the pituitary via a portal vessel network. The developmental events taking place in an ovary are related to the central nervous system (CNS)-pituitary complex.

The hypothalamus along with the pituitary brings about the endocrinological changes required for ovulation executed by feedback on the anterior pituitary.

This chapter gives us a clear picture regarding the current status of reproductive endocrinology and helps the clinician in tackling gynecologic endocrinological problems encountered in clinical practice.

HYPOTHALAMIC–HYPOPHYSEAL PORTAL CIRCULATION

Hypothalamus is located at the base of the brain just above the junction of the optic nerves. The hypophyseal portal system is a system of blood vessels in the microcirculation at the base of the brain, connecting the hypothalamus with the anterior pituitary. Its main function is to quickly transport and exchange hormones between the hypothalamus arcuate nucleus and anterior pituitary gland.

The hypothalamus and the pituitary are essential for the accurate functioning of the menstrual cycle, in synchrony with the endocrine feedback by the ovary on the anterior pituitary that leads to process of ovulation. The physiology of the menstrual cycle is dependent on signaling whereby the "ovarian clock" modulates the hypothalamic–pituitary function as well as endometrial proliferation and secretion. There is thus the "ovarian cycle" and the "endometrial cycle."

The predominant hormones involved in the menstrual cycle are gonadotropin-releasing hormone (GnRH), follicle-stimulating hormone (FSH), luteinizing hormone (LH), estrogen, and progesterone. GnRH is secreted by the hypothalamus, the gonadotropins FSH and LH are secreted by the anterior pituitary gland, and estrogen and progestins are secreted at the level of the ovary. GnRH stimulates the release of FSH and LH from the anterior pituitary, which in turn stimulate release of estrogen and progestin at the level of the ovary **(Table 1 and Fig. 1)**.

Several levels of feedback to the hypothalamus exist and are known as the long, short, and ultrashort feedback loops.

TABLE 1: Pituitary-releasing factors from the hypothalamus.

Hypothalamic hormone	*Action*
Gonadotropin-releasing hormone (GnRH)	Controls the secretion of luteinizing hormone (LH) and follicle-stimulating hormone (FSH)
Corticotropin-releasing hormone (CRH)	Controls the release of adreno-corticotropin hormone (ACTH)
Growth hormone-releasing hormone (GHRH)	Regulates the release of growth hormone (GH)
Thyrotropin-releasing hormone (TRH)	Regulates the secretion of thyroid-stimulating hormone (TSH)

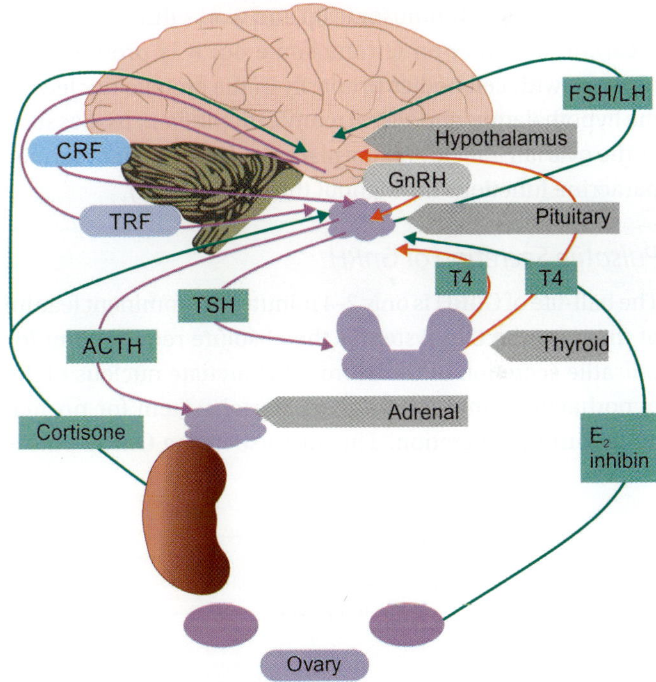

Fig. 1: The pituitary-releasing factors that control the endocrine function of the ovaries, thyroid, and the adrenal glands. Note the feedback from the target hormones (marked in blue lines).

The long feedback loop is composed of endocrine input from circulating hormones, just as feedback of androgens and estrogens onto steroid receptors is present in the hypothalamus. In short-loop feedback, pituitary hormones send feedback to the hypothalamus and serve important regulatory functions. Hypothalamic secretions may directly feed back to the hypothalamus itself in an ultrashort feedback loop.[1,2]

Pituitary

The pituitary consists of two lobes: anterior (adenohypophysis) and posterior (neurohypophysis) which are structurally different. The unique fenestrated capillaries in this region eliminate the blood-brain barrier in the median eminence and permits bidirectional feedback control. The anterior pituitary is under the influence of the hypothalamus by means of neurohormones released into this portal circulation. There also exists retrograde flow so that pituitary hormones can be delivered directly to the hypothalamus, creating the opportunity for pituitary feedback on the hypothalamus. Short vessels that originate in the posterior pituitary that in turn receives its arterial supply from the inferior hypophyseal arteries provide an additional blood supply **(Fig. 2)**.

HORMONES IN FEMALE REPRODUCTION

Gonadotropin-Releasing Hormone

Gonadotropin-releasing hormone (also called luteinizing hormone releasing hormone, or LHRH) is a vital factor for gonadotropin secretion. There is a single neurohormone (GnRH) for both FSH and LH. It is a decapeptide with the gene located on chromosome 8p and works through its own receptor, encoded on chromosome 4q. It is produced by neurons with cell bodies primarily in the arcuate nucleus of the hypothalamus and also in many extrapituitary tissues such as the ovarian follicle and the placenta. GnRH has autocrine–paracrine functions throughout the body **(Fig. 3)**.

Pulsatile Secretion of GnRH

The half-life of GnRH is only 2–4 minutes. A prominent feature of the reproductive system is the absolute requirement for pulsatile secretion of GnRH from the arcuate nucleus of the hypothalamus into the pituitary portal system for normal gonadotropin secretion. The increase in the GnRH pulses marks the onset of puberty. GnRH is unique as it regulates the secretion of two hormones—FSH and LH—and must be secreted in a pulsatile fashion within a critical range in frequency and amplitude. Knobil et al. showed that in hypothalamic-lesioned monkeys receiving GnRH, intermittent stimulation of the pituitary results in secretion of LH and FSH, whereas constant GnRH stimulation leads to suppression of gonadotropin levels.[3]

The frequency of GnRH secretion is once per 90 minutes in the early follicular phase, which increases to once per 60–70 minutes in the late follicular phase. Lower GnRH pulse frequencies favor FSH secretion and higher frequencies favor LH secretion. Pulsatile GnRH secretion is more frequent but lower in amplitude during the follicular phase. An increase in frequency and amplitude during mid-cycle favors LH surge necessary for ovulation. Slowing of pulse frequency in the late luteal phase favors FSH synthesis and allows the rise in FSH essential for the next cycle **(Fig. 4)**.

Control of GnRH Pulses

Catecholamines such as norepinephrine, dopamine, and serotonin and transmitters such as opiates and prostaglandins also appear to influence the secretion of GnRH from the hypothalamus. Norepinephrine seems to stimulate GnRH release, whereas dopamine, serotonin, endogenous opioids, and corticotroponin-releasing hormone (CRH) appear capable of inhibiting or suppressing GnRH, as witnessed by the association of stress with hypothalamic amenorrhea in some women. Biogenic catecholamines modulate GnRH pulsatile release by influencing the frequency (and perhaps the amplitude) of GnRH discharge **(Fig. 5)**.

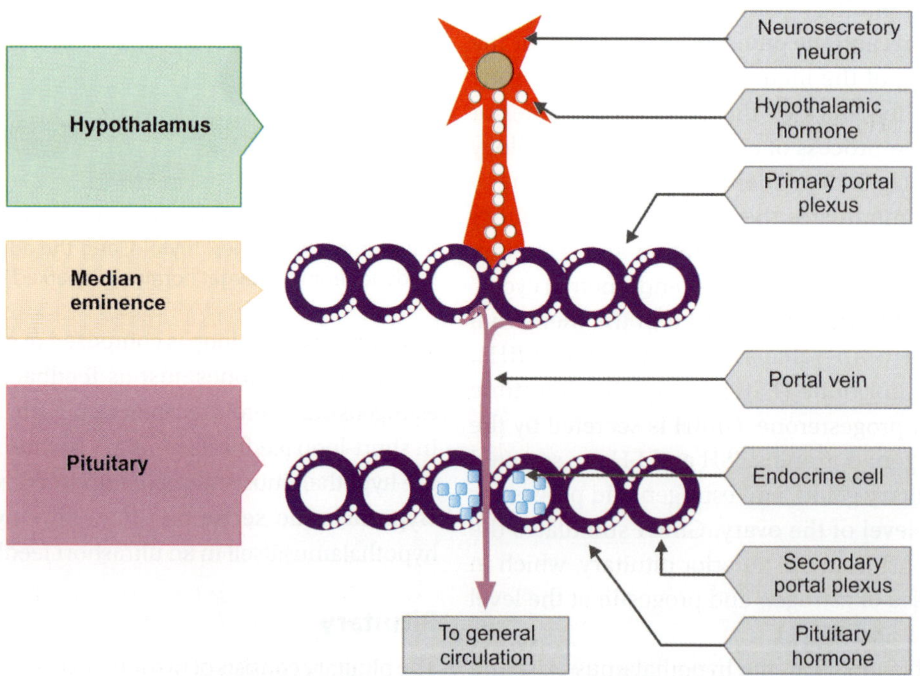

Fig. 2: Hypothalamic–pituitary axis with portal system.

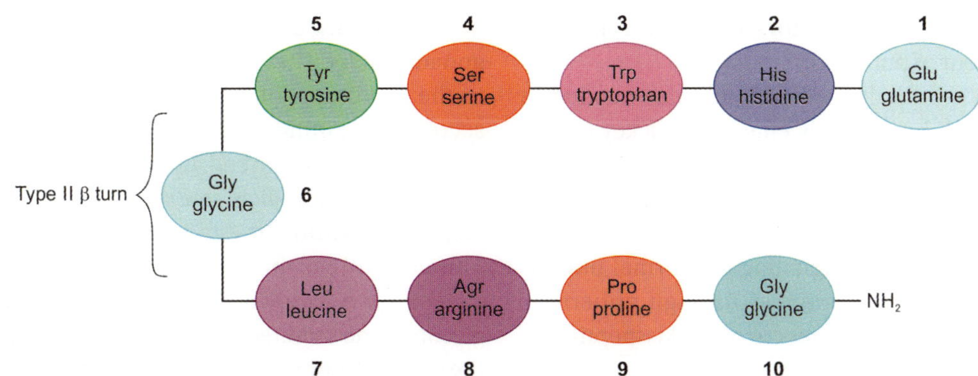

Fig. 3: Structure of a gonadotropin-releasing hormone (GnRH) molecule.

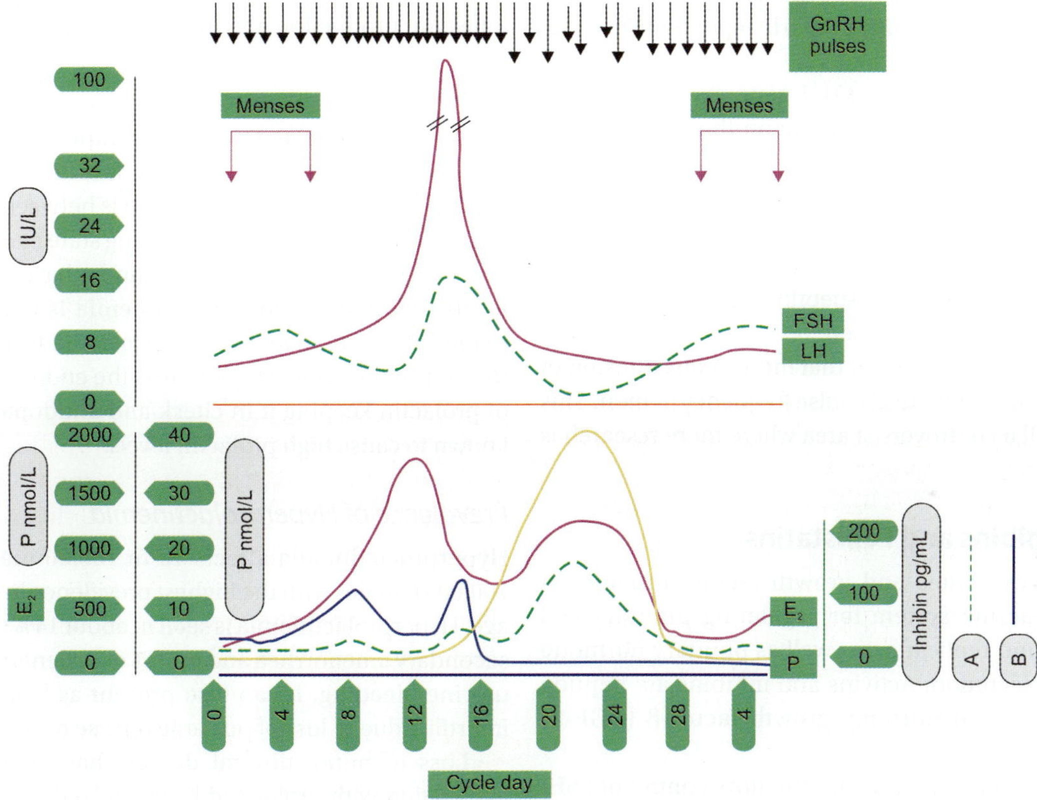

Fig. 4: GnRH pulsatility affecting gonadotropin and steroid release during menstrual cycle.

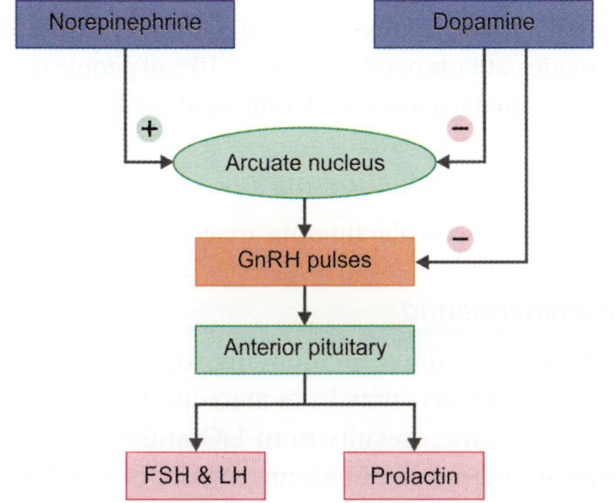

Fig. 5: Control of catecholamines and dopamine on gonadotropins. (FSH: follicle-stimulating hormone; GnRH: gonadotropin-releasing hormone; LH: luteinizing hormone)

The *dopamine* tuberoinfundibular tract arising within the medial basal hypothalamus and terminating in the median eminence provides the dopaminergic effect on the pituitary. Dopamine is directly secreted into the portal blood, thus behaving like a neurohormone. It directly suppresses GnRH activity and is transported via the portal system to directly and specifically suppress pituitary prolactin secretion.

Neuropeptide Y (NPY), a polypeptide, stimulates appetite, decreases heat production. and increases insulin and cortisol secretion. The secretion and gene expression of neuropeptide Y in the hypothalamus is regulated by gonadal steroids. It stimulates the pulsatile release of GnRH and potentiates gonadotropin response to GnRH.[4]

Kisspeptins are peptides encoded by the gene *Kiss1*, expressed in hypothalamus. The kisspeptin neurons have estrogen and progesterone receptors and are essential for normal development of puberty.[5]

Kisspeptin is a hypothalamic neuropeptide encoded by the gene *Kiss1*, which has recently emerged as a key central regulator of gonadotropin secretion. The kisspeptin neurons have estrogen and progesterone receptors and are essential for normal development of puberty.[5]

The obligatory kisspeptin signaling for normal puberty is evidenced by a failure to progress through puberty in individuals with mutations in genes encoding kisspeptin and its receptor, GPR54.[6]

Assessment of gonadotropin response to the administration of exogenous kisspeptin provides a novel investigative tool to assess GnRH neuronal function in vivo in reproductive health medicine.

Sex steroids can regulate *Kiss1* gene expression both positively and negatively, depending on the physiological environment. There are studies that showed administration of kisspeptin, as the longer kisspeptin fragment, kisspeptin-54 (Kp54), stimulates gonadotropin secretion in healthy women and in women with hypothalamic amenorrhea. However, another study suggested that kisspeptin-10 does not stimulate gonadotropin secretion in women.[7]

Various studies have shown that intravenous infusion of kisspeptin-10 can stimulate LH pulse frequency in men. This is, however, still a controversial area where more research is needed.[8]

Activins, Inhibins and Follistatins

Intrapituitary cytokines and growth factors provide an autocrine-paracrine system for regulating pituitary cell development and replication as well as pituitary hormone synthesis and secretion. Activins and inhibins are peptide members of the transforming growth factor-β (TGF-β) superfamily.

The inhibins, named for their inhibitory control of FSH, are composed of two dissimilar peptides linked by disulfide bonds. There are two forms of inhibin which are composed of one of two inhibin β subunits and a closely related α subunit to form inhibin A or inhibin B.

Inhibins are secreted by granulosa cells. FSH stimulates secretion of inhibin and inhibin suppresses FSH secretion. Inhibin blocks synthesis and secretion of FSH, prevents upregulation of GnRH receptors and in high levels may also promote degradation of gonadotropins. Inhibin B peaking in the midfollicular phase amplifies the withdrawal of FSH from other follicles allowing emergence of the dominant follicle. After appearance of LH receptors and formation of corpus luteum, it comes under control of LH and inhibin A dominates. Inhibin has little or no effect on growth hormone, adrenocorticotropic hormone (ACTH), and prolactin production.[9,10] Inhibin blocks synthesis and secretion of FSH, prevents upregulation of GnRH receptors, and in high levels may also promote degradation of gonadotropins.

Activins are derived from granulosa cells and pituitary gonadotrophs. They are composed of two subunits identical to the β subunits of inhibins A and B. They augment FSH secretion but inhibit prolactin, ACTH, and growth hormone responses.[11-13] A marked increase in activin tone helps in FSH-dependent follicle selection. Activin increases pituitary response to GnRH by enhancing GnRH receptor formation. The effects of activin are blocked by inhibin and follistatin.[13,14]

Follistatin, also called the FSH-suppressing protein, is a glycopeptide secreted by a variety of pituitary cells, including the gonadotrophs. Its main action is inhibiting FSH synthesis, secretion and the FSH response to GnRH, probably by binding to and decreasing the activity of activin.[15,16] Activin stimulates follistatin production and inhibin prevents this response.

Prolactin

Prolactin is a polypeptide of 198 amino acids secreted in a pulsatile manner from the lactotrophs of the anterior pituitary. The normal blood level of prolactin is between 25 and 30 ng/mL and usually measured in a fasting state after a well-rested night's sleep. Women are usually found to have higher prolactin levels than men. Hyperprolactinemia is diagnosed when blood values are higher than normal and tests are repeated to confirm the same. Dopamine is the endogenous inhibitor of prolactin keeping it in check and antidopaminergics are known to cause high prolactin levels.

Prevalence of Hyperprolactinemia

Hyperprolactinemia affects 10 in 100,00 males and 30 in 100,000 females with the highest prevalence in 25–35 years of age. Hyperprolactinemia is seen in about 14% of women with secondary amenorrhea and in 10% of patients with abnormal uterine bleeding. It can also present as hypogonadism or infertility due to loss of pulsatile release of GnRH.

Loss of bone mineral density has been reported in association with prolonged hyperprolactinemia, which may not revert even after normalization of serum prolactin levels. Males with even a marginal increase in prolactin present with decreased libido and features of hypogonadism, and therefore all symptomatic patients need evaluation. 10% of people may also have asymptomatic adenomas found incidentally at autopsy.

Causes of Hyperprolactinemia

The causes of hyperprolactinemia are given in **Table 2**.

Macroprolactinemia

Asymptomatic patients incidentally found to have high serum prolactin levels may have macroprolactinemia (big-big prolactin) which results from IgG antibodies binding to prolactin and is seen in about 10–25% of patients with hyperprolactinemia. The delayed renal clearance of antibody-bound prolactin causes a false elevation in prolactin levels, but it is not bioactive. It is diagnosed by doing a polyethylene

TABLE 2: Causes of hyperprolactinemia.

Physiological	*Pituitary*	*CNS disorders*	*Systemic disease*
• Pregnancy • Lactation • Stress • Nipple stimulation • Sleep • Coitus	• Prolactinomas • Hypothyroidism • Nonsecretory adenomas • Acromegaly Cushing's disease • Empty Sella turcica	• Tumors • Vascular malformations • Granulomatous • Autoimmune disease • Metastasis	• Chronic renal failure • Severe hypothyroidism • Polycystic ovarian syndrome • Chest wall trauma • Herpes zoster

glycol precipitation of the serum. If the only cause of hyperprolactinemia is confirmed to be macroprolactinemia, no further treatment is required.

Hypothyroidism

Elevated levels of thyrotropin-releasing hormone (TRH) due to hypothyroidism can cause high prolactin due to stimulatory effect on the lactotrophs. There may also be associated global pituitary enlargement which may cause hyperprolactinemia. Corrections of hypothyroidism correct hyperprolactinemia.

Tumors of Pituitary

Common tumors of the pituitary include adenomas, the most common being functional prolactinomas, and nonfunctional tumors which may cause mass effect (headache, vomiting) or visual disturbances. Stalk effect causing hyperprolactinemia occurs when compression on the pituitary causes a loss of inhibitory control of pituitary.

Drugs Causing Hyperprolactinemia

Several of commonly prescribed drugs are known to increase serum prolactin levels, and therefore patients with hyperprolactinemia must be asked about their medications' history.

The most important drugs known to cause hyperprolactinemia are the antipsychotics, antidepressants, prokinetics, H2 blockers, and antihypertensive to name a few.

Most medications such as prokinetic agents and antacids may safely be discontinued and safer alternatives found without any consequences or if required dopamine analogs may be started. However, switching to alternative drugs with less propensity to hyperprolactinemia (e.g., olanzapine, aripiprazole) is preferred compared to starting dopaminergic drugs which may worsen the psychosis in those patients with hyperprolactinemia due to antipsychotics.

Common Presentations of Hyperprolactinemia

Common presentations of hyperprolactinemia are given in **Table 3**.

TABLE 3: Common presentations of hyperprolactinemia.

Female (prolactin levels)	*Male*
• >100 µg/L—hypogonadism, galactorrhea, amenorrhea • 51–75 µg/L—oligomenorrhea • 31–50 µg/L—luteal phase defect, decreased libido, infertility • Osteopenia	Decreased libido, impotence, infertility, oligospermia, retrograde ejaculation, gynecomastia

Investigation and Management (Evidence-based Guidelines)

In patients with high suspicion of hyperprolactinemia, a fasting prolactin level is checked and if found high, the value is reconfirmed by repeating the blood test. A detailed medical history including the chance of pregnancy, history of medications, and any illness in the recent past is enquired into. Probable causes for hyperprolactinemia are looked for before imaging with contrast MRI.

Serum prolactin levels of >200 µg/L are strongly indicative of pituitary adenoma and must require imaging. Lower values can be seen due to various causes, most importantly due to medications and nonfunctioning pituitary adenomas.

Management: Management depends on the cause of the raised prolactin levels which needs to be addressed. If high blood levels of the hormone are the only concern, dopaminergic drugs are found to be highly effective. If the mass effect of the lesion is the primary concern, an initial course of medical therapy may be tried failing which surgery may be required.

Medical therapy: Dopaminergic drugs such as cabergoline or bromocriptine, are the *first-line therapy* in hyperprolactinemia and are found to be highly effective. They are known to suppress the hypogonadism and restore ovulatory functions and spermatogenesis in both females and males. Despite therapy, about 10% and 20%of patients with microprolactinomas and macroprolactinomas will continue to have high blood levels of the hormone. Cabergoline is used in bromocriptine resistance or intolerance, although bromocriptine has been used for the longest.

Surgery*:* Surgery in hyperprolactinemia is reserved for nonfunctional tumors causing visual defects or stalk effect or in those patients where medical therapy has failed or is not tolerated. Trans-sphenoidal resection is to be done with extreme caution in an experienced center. Recurrence of 20–50% has been reported.

Hyperprolactinemia and Pregnancy

A multidisciplinary approach benefits pregnant patients with hyperprolactinemia. Patients with microadenomas on medical therapy have minimal risk of tumor expansion in pregnancy. Patients with macroadenoma need to continue dopamine agonists and are evaluated every 2 months for visual field changes. Worsening of visual defects warrants prompt delivery or surgery. Most dopaminergics are found to be nonteratogenic and safe in pregnancy.

THYROID AND REPRODUCTION

The thyroid gland consists of numerous follicles made of a simple secretory epithelium around a gelatinous lumen containing thyroglobulin and thyroxine (T4).

Iodide is taken up from the blood, converted to iodine, and the resulting monoiodo- or diiodotyrosine is incorporated into the thyroglobulin. Organification occurs with the coupling of two diiodotyrosine to form T4 or one mono- and one diiodotyrosine to form triiodothyronine (T3). Both iodination and organification are done by the enzyme thyroid peroxidase (TPO). Autoantibodies to this enzyme are common and result in various pathologies of the thyroid gland.

Majority of the T4 in the circulation is bound to plasma proteins [70% to thyroid-binding globulin (TBG), 20% to transthyretin, and 10% to albumin] and changes in the protein concentration have a profound impact on the free T4 concentration.

The thyroid is one of the most important and simplest of endocrine organs. Thyroid disorders have huge reproductive implications preconceptionally, antenatally, and postnatally, even affecting the growth and well-being of the infant. Regulation of thyroid function occurs through the simple hypothalamo-pituitary-thyroid axis with T3 and T4 acting negatively on the hypothalamus and pituitary.

Correcting thyroid abnormalities are known to increase the chance of conception, although recommendations to screen for thyroid disorders are not widespread.

Functions of the Thyroid

- The thyroid controls the basal metabolic rate through T3 and T4.
- The thyroid is essential for the growth and development of the CNS, especially the brain.
- Both hypothyroidism and hyperthyroidism are known to affect reproduction.
- Patients with antithyroid antibodies are known to have adverse pregnancy outcomes despite being euthyroid.

Prevalence

Thyroid disorders are more prevalent in women than men and most of them unsurprisingly have an autoimmune etiology. The most common causes of hypothyroidism (Hashimoto's thyroiditis) and hyperthyroidism (Grave's disease) have antithyroid antibodies as the etiology.

About 2.3% of subfertile women and 1.5% of women in the general population are found to have hyperthyroidism.

About 3.1% of reproductive age women are hypothyroid with most of them having menstrual symptoms and anovulation.

Subclinical hypothyroidism, which presents with normal T4 levels (9–25 pmol/L), but raised TSH (> 4.5 µM/mL), affects 2–4% of reproductive age women.

Hypothyroidism prevents the pulsatile release of GnRH, preventing cyclical FSH and LH release subsequent anovulation. Children or adolescents with hypothyroidism present with delayed sexual development, whereas adults may manifest with menstrual irregularities such as oligomenorrhea, menorrhagia or amenorrhea, and hyperprolactinemia.

Hypothyroidism is common in infertile women and controlled ovarian stimulation causes high estradiol levels, resulting in higher binding of T4 to T4-binding globulin, temporarily making euthyroid women hypothyroid. Correcting both subclinical and overt hypothyroidism has been shown to improve implantation, pregnancy, and live birth rates and it has been therefore recommended to maintain TSH levels of <2.5 mU/L in the preconceptional period similar to the American Thyroid Association (ATA) guidelines for women in the first trimester of pregnancy.

Hyperthyroidism

Patients having hyperthyroidism typically present with palpitations, anxiety, involuntary weight loss, increased sweating, intolerance to heat. and excessive bowel movements

Women with hyperthyroidism have a higher sensitivity to GnRH causing high LH, sex hormone–binding globulin (SHBG), and total estradiol levels resulting in either *oligomenorrhea* or *hypomenorrhea*.

Most women with hyperthyroidism are *ovulatory* despite having these menstrual irregularities, and therefore treating hyperthyroidism generally does not increase the ovulation rate and does improve the quality of life in affected women. Pregnant women with thyrotoxicosis must be differentiated from those with hyperemesis gravidarum, molar pregnancies, and women having physiological changes of pregnancies.

Graves' disease, the most common cause of hyperthyroidism, occurs due to anti-TSH receptor antibodies, causing unregulated stimulation of thyroid hormone production. On examination, affected patients have a classical protuberant gaze with exophthalmos due to the paralysis of extraocular muscles with periorbital infiltration and ophthalmopathy, resting tachycardia, tremors, and proximal muscle weakness. Pregnant women affected by Graves' disease have an increased risk of fetal or neonatal thyrotoxicosis due to the transplacental transport of the antibodies.

Men with Graves' disease present with hypogonadism, with low free testosterone levels despite high SHBG and high total testosterone. Low sperm counts unresponsive to human chorionic gonadotropin (hCG) and gynecomastia may also be present.

Inflammation of the thyroid gland causes thyroiditis, with subsequent release of the stored thyroid hormone into the circulation causing thyrotoxicosis. There is an immediate hyperthyroidism, which may last up to 8 weeks followed by a transient hypothyroidism and subsequent euthyroid state in most patients. Typically, both serum thyroglobulin and erythrocyte sedimentation rate are elevated in subacute thyroiditis.

Subacute thyroiditis (de Quervain's disease) may present with the classical symptoms of neck pain, fever, and tender thyroid gland following a viral infection in the recent past.

Other causes of hyperthyroidism include toxic adenoma, where a germline mutation results in a solitary tumor autonomously producing T3 and T4 or toxic multinodular goiter.

Diagnosis of hyperthyroidism: A fasting T3, T4, and TSH is essential to make a diagnosis of hyperthyroidism in symptomatic patients.

Treatment

Thyroid and subfertility: Evidence suggests that routine screening for thyroid disorders by a TSH is beneficial. If TSH is <2.5, no further tests are needed. However, a TSH of >2.5 needs to be repeated along with antithyroid antibodies. Levothyroxine supplementation with repeat TSH measurements done 6 weeks thereafter until TSH is <2.5 is recommended. Evidence to support levothyroxine supplementation with positive antithyroid antibodies is lacking, but such patients need close monitoring of their thyroid status.

Autoimmune disorders such as antiphospholipid antibody (APLA) syndrome APLA, type I diabetes, systemic lupus erythematosus (SLE), and premature ovarian failure (POF) are common in infertile patients and the significance of antithyroid antibodies has long been debated. Common thyroid disorders such as Hashimoto's thyroid disease, postpartum thyroiditis, and Graves' disease have autoantibodies as the etiology. Most important and most common is autoimmune thyroid disease. Elevated levels of antithyroid antibodies are also seen in polycystic ovarian syndrome (PCOS) and endometriosis.

Infertile euthyroid women with antithyroid antibodies have a poorer pregnancy outcome with lower fertilization, bad embryos, and reduced pregnancy rates when compared to infertile women without autoantibodies. Higher levels of antibodies are also seen in ovarian follicular fluid with higher NK cell activity in the uterus.

Limited evidence suggests an improvement of pregnancy outcomes with the treatment of thyroid antibodies.

The most common cause of hyperthyroidism, Graves' disease, is generally treated with radioactive iodine, with no reported adverse effects in subsequent pregnancy or in offspring's health. However, women are generally advised to avoid pregnancy for at least 6 months postprocedure.

Miscarriages and Thyroid Disease

Thyroid hormone is essential for embryonic development in the first trimester of pregnancy with the transplacental migration of maternal hormone being its sole source in the fetus. Recurrent pregnancy loss has been found to be higher in women with untreated hypothyroidism and those with antithyroid antibodies.

No direct evidence of miscarriages and hyperthyroidism exist. However, a higher incidence of miscarriages is associated with antithyroid antibodies.

There is a three-fold higher incidence of miscarriage in women with antithyroid antibodies.

Hypothyroidism of Pregnancy

Higher levels of estradiol seen in pregnancy cause increased synthesis of TBG resulting in the lower fraction of the free thyroxin causing higher requirement of thyroid hormones. Patients with subclinical hypothyroidism will be unable to compensate **(Box 1)**.

Differential Control of FSH and LH Secretion

The anterior pituitary secretes the major hormone-releasing factors—FSH, LH, TSH, and ACTH—along with GH and prolactin. Both FSH and LH are glycoproteins that share identical α subunits along with TSH and placental hCG and differ only in the structure of their β subunits, which confers receptor specificity.

Although secreted from common gonadotroph, FSH and LH have markedly different functions in the control of ovarian physiology. The divergent control of FSH and LH is achieved through a combination of differential control of their synthesis and secretion by GnRH. The preferential control of FSH synthesis is by the activin/follistatin system and differential feedback by ovarian steroids and the inhibins **(Fig. 6)**.

Follicle stimulating hormone: Follicle-stimulating hormone is essential for follicular growth. It induces estrogen and progesterone secretion at the level of the ovary by activating aromatase and p450 enzymes and exerts negative feedback on GnRH secretion. FSH further induces the proliferation of granulosa cells and expression of FSH and LH receptors on granulosa cells. The rise in FSH during LH surge helps in the ovulation by stimulating plasminogen activator activity **(Box 2)**.

Luteinizing hormone: Luteinizing hormone is secreted by the anterior pituitary gland and is required for growth of

BOX 1: Effects of hyperprolactinemia on female reproductive function.

- Disrupts normal follicular development
- Inhibits aromatase enzyme
- Premature destruction of the corpus luteum

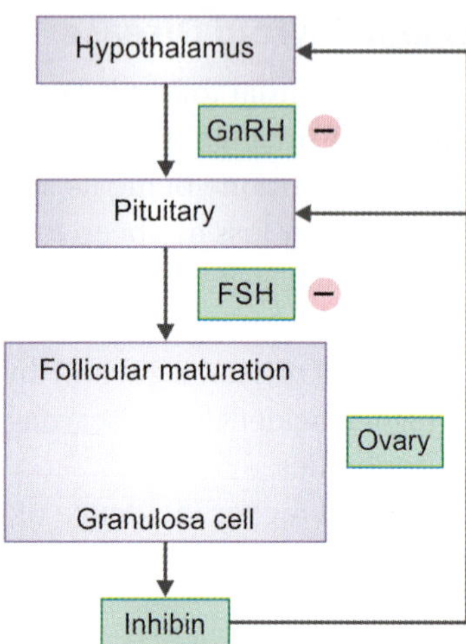

Fig. 6: Role of FSH and inhibin in the control of ovarian function. (FSH: follicle-stimulating hormone; GnRH: gonadotropin-releasing hormone)

BOX 2: Functions of FSH in menstrual cycle.

- Selection and maturation of dominant follicle
- Proliferation of granulosa cells
- Aromatization within granulosa cells
- Induction of FSH and LH receptors on granulosa cells
- *Production of autocrine–paracrine factors:* Activin and inhibin
- FSH surge helps in ovulation
- Prevents germ cells from atresia in luteal–follicular transition

(FSH: follicle-stimulating hormone; LH: luteinizing hormone)

preovulatory follicles, ovulation, and luteinization of the dominant follicle. During the follicular phase of the menstrual cycle, LH induces androgen synthesis by theca cells that is essential for robust steroidogenesis; stimulates proliferation, differentiation, and secretion of follicular thecal cells; and also increases LH receptors on granulosa cells. The preovulatory LH surge drives the oocyte into the first meiotic division and initiates luteinization of thecal and granulosa cells. The resulting corpus luteum produces high levels of progesterone and some estrogen.

The LH-dependent phase of preovulatory follicular development proceeds normally only if LH is present at concentrations within the *LH window*, which is over the threshold level and beneath the ceiling value **(Table 4)**.

TABLE 4: Impact of different concentrations of LH on the menstrual cycle.

Effects below LH threshold	*Effects within LH window*	*Effects above LH ceiling*
Absent paracrine signaling between granulosa and theca	Normal follicular growth and development	Suppression of granulosa proliferation
Inadequate androgen and estrogen synthesis	Adequate granulosa proliferation and functional maturation	Follicular premature luteinization
Compromised oocyte maturation	Normal estrogen and androgen biosynthesis	Compromised oocyte development
	Optimum oocyte maturation	

HYPOTHALAMIC–PITUITARY–OVARIAN AXIS

In the presence of a GnRH pulse, the pituitary and ovarian hormones exert mutual control over the circulating levels of one another. The complex interactions between pituitary and ovarian hormones involve forward control, positive feedback, and negative feedback mechanisms and serve to sustain a self-perpetuating monthly endocrine cycle **(Fig. 7)**.

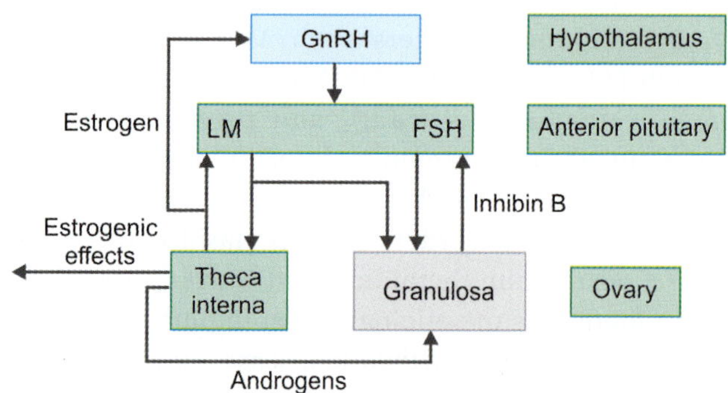

Fig. 7: Hypothalamic-pituitary-ovarian (HPO) axis.

OVARIAN FEEDBACK ON THE HYPOTHALAMUS AND PITUITARY

Estrogen

Estrogen produced at the level of the ovary is crucial for the development of the antrum and maturation of the Graafian follicle. It is predominant at the end of the follicular phase, directly preceding ovulation. Estradiol, the most potent and abundant estrogen, is primarily derived from androgens produced by thecal cells. The androgens migrate from the theca cells to the granulosa cells, where they are converted into estradiol by aromatase enzyme. The actions of estradiol include induction of FSH receptors on granulosa cells, proliferation and secretion of follicular and thecal cells, induction of LH receptors on granulosa cells, and proliferation of endometrial stromal and epithelial cells. At low circulating levels, estrogens exert negative feedback on FSH and LH secretion and at very high levels estrogens exert positive feedback on LH secretion.[17] Estrogen further induces proliferation of estrogen-converting granulosa cells and synthesis of estrogen receptors, establishing a positive feedback loop on itself. In the endometrial cycle, estrogen induces proliferation of the endometrial glands **(Fig. 8)**.

Progesterone

Progesterone is secreted at the level of the ovary, primarily by luteinized follicles. The levels increase just prior to ovulation and peak 5–7 days postovulation. It stimulates the release of proteolytic enzymes from thecal cells that ultimately prepare for ovulation. Progesterone further induces migration of blood vessels into the follicle wall and stimulates prostaglandin secretion in follicular tissues. During the luteal phase, progesterone induces swelling and increased secretion of the endometrium **(Fig. 9)**.

GnRH DYNAMICS AND PITUITARY RESPONSIVENESS

The interplay between pituitary and ovarian hormones gives rise to a stereotyped pattern of hormone levels during the menstrual cycle. The graph shows relative hormone trends in an average 28-day cycle (**Fig. 10**).

PHYSIOLOGY OF MENSTRUAL CYCLE

Following the exhaustive discussion about the neuro-endocrinological control and the hypothalamic-pituitary ovarian (HPO) axis, the understanding of the physiology of menstrual cycle becomes comprehensive. The menstrual cycle is divided into four phases based on the ovarian cycle as described here **(Fig. 8)**:

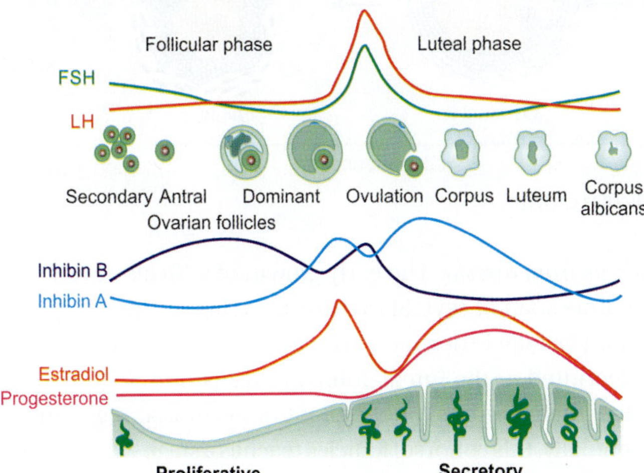

Fig. 8: Overview of hormonal and peptide variations in the menstrual cycle.

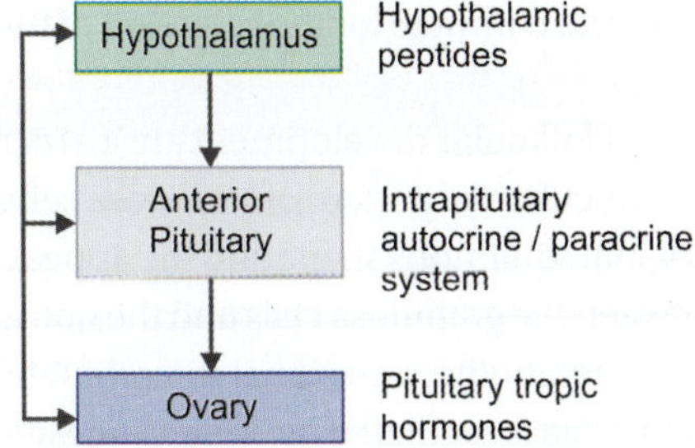

Fig. 9: Hypothalamic and ovarian control of pituitary secretions.

1. Follicular phase (further classified into early and late follicular phase)
2. Ovulatory phase
3. Luteal phase
4. Luteal-follicular transition phase.

Based on the uterine cycle, it may be divided into:

- Proliferative phase
- Secretory phase
- Menstruation.

Follicular Phase

The follicular phase of the menstrual cycle spans from the first day of menstruation until ovulation. The primary goal is to develop a viable follicle capable of undergoing ovulation. The early events of the follicular phase are initiated by a rise in FSH levels at the luteal-follicular transition attributed to a decrease in progesterone, estrogen, and inhibin levels at the end of the previous cycle and the subsequent removal of inhibition of FSH. Rise of FSH rescues a cohort of preantral follicles from apoptosis—a phenomenon called as recruitment—which requires a certain minimum concentration of FSH called FSH threshold. The time frame for which this threshold surpasses the level of FSH needs to be maintained for follicular recruitment and growth. This is called *FSH window* **(Fig. 11)**.

This requires an orderly sequence of events and a series of sequential actions of hormones and autocrine-paracrine peptides on the follicle, through a period of initial growth from a primordial follicle through the stages of the preantral, antral. and preovulatory follicle.[18,19] As folliculogenesis has already been described in another chapter, this chapter only discusses the physiological attributes of the ovarian events **(Fig. 12)**.

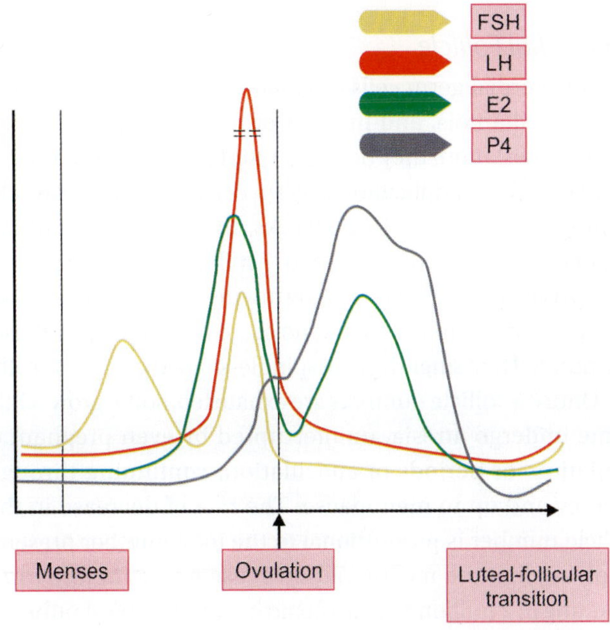

Fig. 10: Pituitary and ovarian hormonal interrelationships during the menstrual cycle.

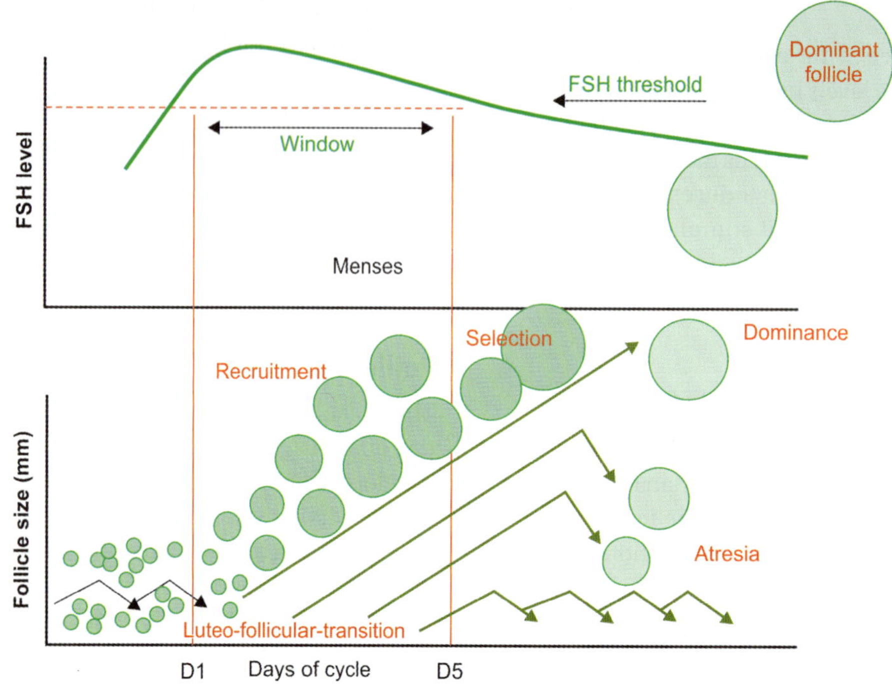

Fig. 11: Concept of FSH window and threshold.

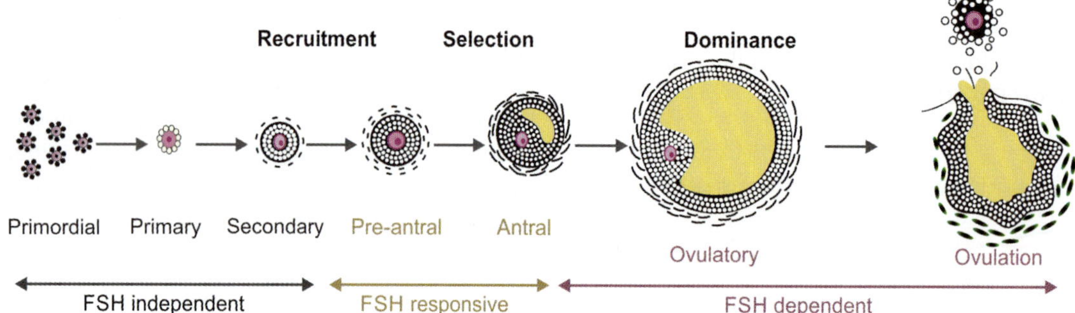

Fig. 12: Stages of follicular growth.

Primordial Follicle

The primordial germ cells originate in the endoderm of the yolk sac, allantois, and hindgut of the embryo and by 5–6 weeks of gestation, they have migrated to the genital ridge. A rapid mitotic multiplication of germ cells begins at 6–8 weeks of pregnancy, and by 16–20 weeks, the maximum number of oocytes is reached: a total of 6–7 million in both ovaries.[20] The primordial follicle is nongrowing and consists of an oocyte, arrested in the diplotene stage of meiotic prophase, surrounded by a single layer of spindle-shaped granulosa cells.

Until the follicle numbers are exhausted, some grow while some undergo atresia, uninterrupted by even pregnancy, ovulation, or periods of anovulation, continuing through infancy and up to menopause. The rate of decrease in the follicle number is proportional to the total number present, implying that the most rapid decrease occurs before birth resulting in 2 million oocytes at birth and 3,00,000 at puberty. Out of these, about 400 follicles will ovulate during a woman's reproductive years[20] **(Fig. 13)**.

Rescue from atresia: The early growth of follicles occurs over the time span of several menstrual cycles, approximately 85 days. The follicle destined to ovulate is one of a cohort which is recruited at the luteal-follicular transition.[21] Until a late stage, the growth is independent of hormonal regulation.[22] Eventually, this cohort of follicles reaches a stage where, unless recruited or rescued by FSH, it is doomed toward apoptosis, a programmed physiologic cell death.[23]

Recruitment is the process by which the cohort of follicles responding to FSH at the beginning of the cycle gets rescued from apoptosis and compete for the selection of the dominant follicle.

Early signs of follicular development are an increase in the size of the oocyte, cuboidal pattern of granulosa cells—a change from their original squamous shape and the appearance of gap junctions between the granulosa cells and the oocyte, essential for nutritional, metabolite, and signal interchange.

Follicular atresia is regulated by endocrine factors, such as FSH and LH, and by paracrine factors, including insulin-like

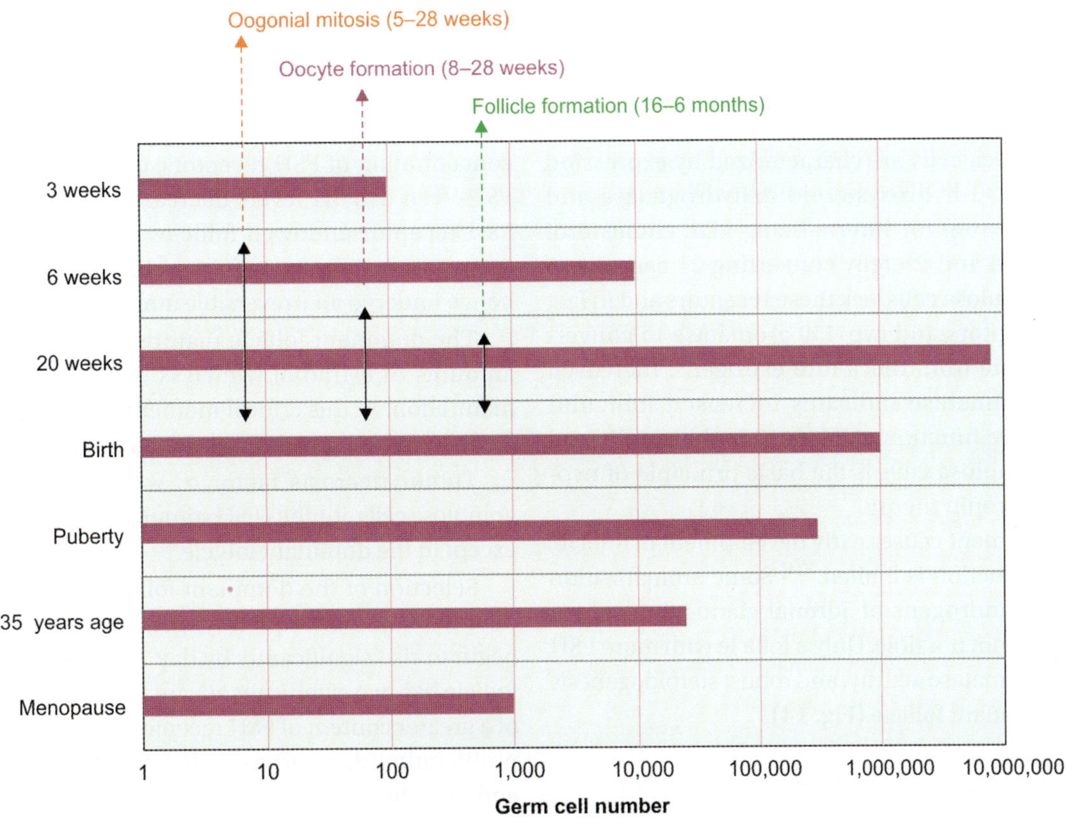

Fig. 13: Changes in germ cell numbers in relation to age.

growth factor (IGF-I), epidermal growth factor (EGF), basic fibroblast growth factor (bFGF), tumor necrosis factor α (TNFα), interleukin 6 (IL-6), and others.

Primary Follicle

With multiplication of the cuboidal granulosa cells, the primordial follicle becomes a primary follicle. The granulosa cell layer gets separated from the stromal cells by a basement membrane called the basal lamina. The stromal cells further subdivide into the theca interna and theca externa.

Preantral Follicle

With accelerated growth promoted by the gonadotropins, the granulosa cells undergo a multicellular proliferation leading to an increasing production of not only estrogen but also other steroids such as androgens and progestins. The oocyte too enlarges and is surrounded by zona pellucida, an acellular glycoprotein membrane. FSH receptors are acquired through which FSH aromatizes androgens to estrogens generating an *estrogenic* microenvironment.[24] Together, FSH and estrogen synergistically promote a rapid accumulation of FSH receptors, allowing the follicle to respond to relatively low concentrations of FSH.

Androgens have a complex role in early follicular development. In low concentrations, androgens serve as a substrate for FSH-induced aromatization to the extent of even enhancing the enzyme. But in androgen-rich environment, the limited capacity of aromatization is overwhelmed and the preantral granulosa cells instead favor the conversion of androgens to more potent 5α reduced androgens.[25] These androgens inhibit aromatase activity and FSH-induced LH receptor formation as they cannot convert to estrogen leading the follicle toward atresia.[18,19] Therefore, the fate of the preantral follicle is in delicate balance depending on the ability to convert an androgen-dominant microenvironment to an estrogen-dominated one for survival **(Box 3)**.

Antral Follicle

Follicular fluid, accumulated in the intercellular spaces of the granulosa, eventually coalesces into a cavity—the antrum. This fluid, being rich in hormones, growth factors, and cytokines, nurtures the oocyte. The granulosa cells surrounding the oocyte form the cumulus oophorus. LH is not normally present in the fluid until the mid-cycle. Antral follicles with the lowest androgen/estrogen ratios are most likely to house a healthy oocyte.[26] The synthesis of steroids is functionally compartmentalized within the follicle as the two-cell system.

Two-cell, Two-gonadotropin Concept in Follicle Selection

FSH receptors are present only on the granulosa cells. LH receptors are present only on theca cells.[27] LH optimizes the final stages of maturation. FSH-stimulated estrogen production from the granulosa cells is dependent on LH-stimulated androgen production by the theca cells. This is not fully functional till the later part of antral development. Theca cells are characterized by expression of LH receptors, 3β-hydroxysteroid dehydrogenase and cyp-P450c17 essential for internalizing LDL cholesterol into mitochondria and thereby converting 21 carbons to androgens.[28] Granulosa cells lack these receptors and in fact express FSH receptors and cyp-450 aromatase to convert androgen substrate from theca into estrogens. Increased expression of aromatase indicates increased follicular maturity. Exclusive function of P450c17 in theca cells and aromatase in granulosa cells is the basic principle of two-cell, two-gonadotropin theory.[29]

Pure FSH treatment causes early development of follicle, but estradiol production is limited.[30,31] Some aromatization occurs from the androgens of adrenal glands, but robust steroidogenesis is not possible. Only a follicle with more FSH receptors, high aromatase activity, and robust steroidogenesis is selected as dominant follicle **(Fig. 14)**.

Selection of the Dominant Follicle

The successful conversion to an estrogen dominant follicle marks the selection of a follicle destined to ovulate. This process is attributed to few of the estrogen actions, namely positive influence of estrogen on FSH within the maturing follicle and a negative feedback relationship with FSH at the hypothalamic–pituitary level serving to withdraw gonadotropin support. The dominant follicle, with its high concentration of FSH receptors, continues to acquire more FSH even as FSH levels decrease. The remaining, poorly FSH receptor-endowed follicles ultimately show reduced aromatase activity, granulosa proliferation, and function and hence undergo an irreversible atretic change.

BOX 3: Role of androgens.

- Substrate for aromatization into estrogens within granulosa cells at low levels—estrogenic microenvironment
- Enhances atresia of less mature follicles
- Systemic effect of stimulating libido periovulation

The dominant follicle matures and secretes increasing amounts of estradiol, which is essential for its complete maturation. At this critical moment, estrogen exerts positive feedback on LH, generating a dramatic preovulatory LH surge.

Tumor necrosis factor α, which is produced in the granulosa cells, inhibits FSH stimulation of estradiol secretion, except in the dominant follicle.[32]

Selection of the dominant follicle is established during days 5–7 and consequently, peripheral levels of estradiol begin to rise significantly by day 7 of cycle.[33] The dominant follicle has two significant advantages, mainly its acquisition of a greater content of FSH receptors due to rate of granulosa proliferation that surpasses the proliferation of its cohorts and also the enhancement of FS action because of its high intrafollicular estrogen concentration, a consequence of local autocrine–paracrine molecules. Thus, the dominant follicle is more sensitive to FSH, and as long as a critical duration of FSH exposure was initially present, the dominant follicle continued to develop.[34] Improved theca vascularity allowing a preferential delivery of gonadotropins to the dominant follicle also contributes.[33]

In order to respond to LH surge and become a corpus luteum, granulosa cells must acquire LH receptors.

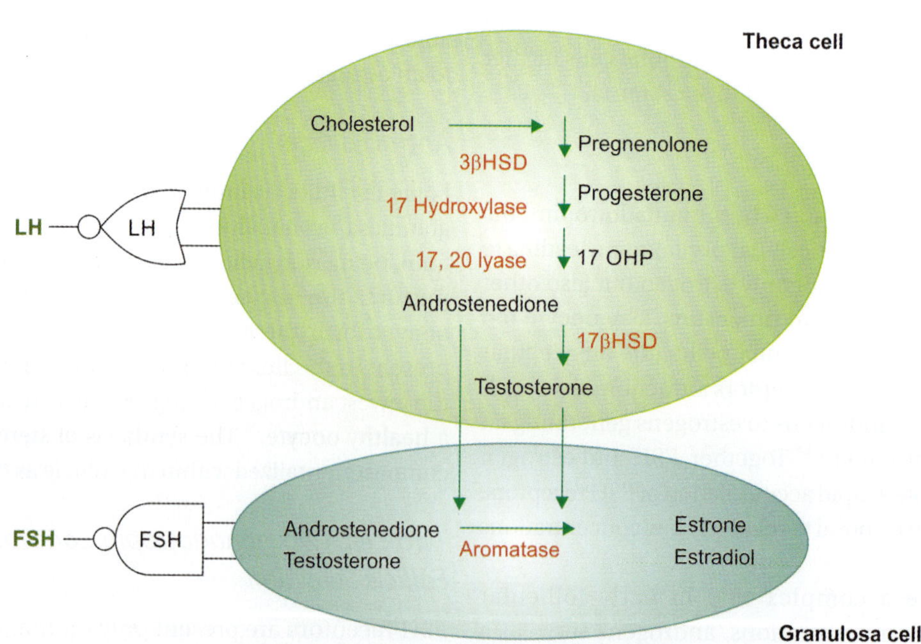

Fig. 14: Two-cell, two-gonadotropin concept.

With increasing concentration of estrogen, FSH changes its focus of action from upregulation of FSH receptors to upregulation of LH receptors.[35] Moreover, LH can induce development of its own receptors in FSH-primed granulosa cells. LH plays a critical role in final stages of follicular development, providing support for final follicular maturation.[36,37]

Feedback System

Follicle-stimulating hormone secretion is very sensitive to the negative inhibitory effects of estrogen at low levels, and at higher levels this effect of estrogen is supplemented by inhibin. In contrast, the transition from suppression to stimulation of LH release occurs as estradiol fulfils two critical events—estradiol concentration rising above 200 pg/mL and sustained for about 50 hours, usually occurring when the dominant follicle reaches 15 mm in diameter[38,39] **(Fig. 15)**.

Preovulatory Follicle

The preovulatory follicle gets a hyperemic appearance with the granulosa cells enlarging and acquiring lipid inclusions and the theca cells getting vacuolated and vascular. The oocyte too proceeds in meiosis, approaching completion of its reduction division. Approaching maturity, the preovulatory follicle produces increasing amounts of estrogen, peaking at 24–36 hours prior to ovulation.[40] The onset of LH surge occurs when peak levels of estradiol are reached. In providing the ovulatory stimulus to the selected follicle, the LH surge seals the fate of the remaining follicles, with their lower estrogen and FSH content, by further increasing the androgen superiority.

Luteinizing hormone promotes luteinization of the granulosa in the dominant follicle producing progesterone, which via its own receptors and only after adequate estrogen priming facilitates the positive feedback of estrogen on LH. If administered before the estrogen stimulus, or in doses high enough to achieve a blood level >2 ng/mL, progesterone blocks the mid-cycle LH surge. Hence, appropriate low levels of progesterone derived from the maturing follicle contribute to the precise synchronization of the mid-cycle LH and the FSH surge **(Table 5)**.

With the smaller follicles undergoing atresia, theca cells form the stromal tissue, enhancing androgen production to enhance libido and accelerate atresia.

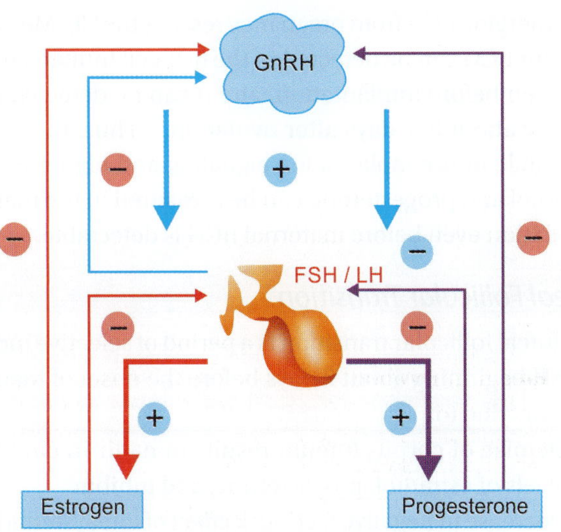

Fig. 15: Feedback mechanism.

Ovulation

Ovulation is the phase of menstrual cycle in which a mature egg is released from the ovarian follicle into the fallopian tube. In humans, ovulation occurs about midway through the menstrual cycle, after the follicular phase. The few days surrounding ovulation (from approximately days 10 to 18 of a 28-day cycle) constitute the most fertile period where the chances of pregnancy are the highest.

Ovulation occurs in the morning in springs and in the evening in autumn and winter. It occurs 55% of the time from the right ovary. Oocytes from the right ovary are said to have a higher potential for pregnancy.[41] Contralateral ovulation favors pregnancy more than ipsilateral ovulation, while ipsilateral ovulation occurs more with advancing age **(Fig. 16)**.[42]

Decline of LH Surge

Within hours after LH rise, there is a precipitous drop in plasma estrogens. This LH fall may be due to loss of the positive stimulating action of estradiol or to an increasing negative feedback of progesterone. High levels of progesterone inhibit pituitary secretion of gonadotropins by inhibiting GnRH pulses at the level of the hypothalamus. In addition, high levels of progesterone can antagonize pituitary response to GnRH by interfering with estrogen action.

The abrupt decline in LH may also reflect exhaustion of pituitary LH stores due to downregulation of GnRH receptors.[43,44]

TABLE 5: Role of midcycle surge of gonadotropins.

LH surge	*FSH surge*
Resumption of meiosis in the oocyte	Frees the oocyte from follicular attachments → Free-floating oocyte in the antral fluid
Luteinization of granulosa cells to secrete progesterone.	LH receptors on granulosa cells → adequate luteal function
Cumulus expansion	Cumulus expansion
Prostaglandin and eicosanoid synthesis → Follicular rupture	Plasminogen → Plasmin: Follicular rupture
LDL cholesterol internalization → corpus luteum steroidogenesis	

(FSH: follicle-stimulating hormone; LDL: low-density lipoproteins; LH: luteinizing hormone)

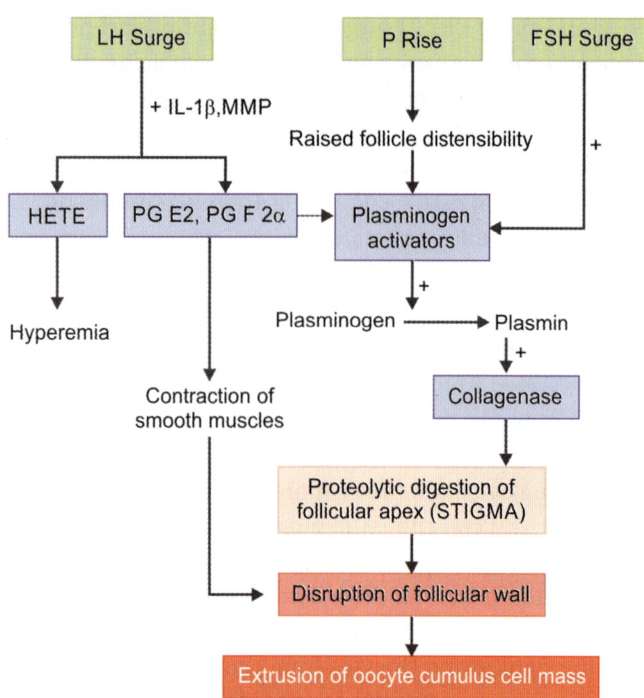

Fig. 16: Key events leading to ovulation.

Activity of a nonsteroidal ovarian substance, named gonadotropin surge-attenuating factor (GnSAF), is hypothesized to regulate the amplitude of the endogenous LH surge at midcycle, by antagonizing the sensitizing effect of estradiol on the pituitary.[45] It is produced by the granulosa cells and also has a role in prevention of premature luteinization. All these events lead to shutdown of LH surge.

Luteal Phase

Normal luteal function requires optimal preovulatory follicle development. Granulosa and theca lutein cells continue to enlarge and accumulate yellow pigment lutein. For successful steroidogenesis and supply of adequate LDL cholesterol substrate, good vascularization is required. Rapid vascularization occurs mediated by VEGF.[46] By day 8 or 9 after ovulation, a peak of vascularization is reached associated with peak levels of progesterone and estradiol in the blood. Corpus luteum has the highest blood flow per unit mass of body and spontaneous bleeding can occur specially in anticoagulated patients.

The luteal phase is defined by the luteinization of the follicles forming corpus luteum initiated by the LH surge. The major effects of the LH surge are the conversion of granulosa cells from predominantly androgen-converting cells to predominantly progesterone-synthesizing cells, the expression of new LH receptors which foster increased progesterone synthesis with some estrogen secretion. LH regulates LDL receptor binding, internalization, and processing.[47] Induction of LDL receptors in granulosa cells occurs in response to LH surge. Progesterone secretion by the corpus luteum peaks between 5 and 7 days postovulation. High progesterone levels exert negative feedback on GnRH and subsequently GnRH pulse frequency decreases leading to reduced FSH and LH secretion. The corpus luteum further loses its FSH and LH receptors. Lacking stimulation by FSH and LH, after 14 days corpus luteum undergoes atresia. With the decline of both estrogen and progesterone levels, an important negative feedback control on FSH is removed and FSH levels rise once again to initiate the next menstrual cycle.

If fertilization and subsequent implantation of the blastocyst do not occur, the corpus luteum undergoes apoptosis and becomes the corpus albicans, a white scar. Luteal apoptosis involves a loss of LH-binding receptors and is mediated by prostaglandins.

The life span of corpus luteum depends on tonic LH secretion as evident by prompt luteolysis occurring when the GnRH antagonist or agonist is continued in the cycles. Estrogen and progesterone production by corpus luteum is under control of LH. High levels of estrogen, progesterone, and inhibin A suppress new follicular growth.

The corpus luteum is not homogeneous as it is composed of luteal cells, endothelial cells, leucocytes, and fibroblasts.[48] Nonsteroidogenic cells form 70% of the cells. Endothelial cells (35%) contribute to the vasoactive compounds.[49]

Luteal cells are of two types—large cells and small cells.[50] Large cells, formed from granulosa cells, are the sites of steroidogenesis whereas small cells, formed from theca cells, contain receptors and provide a stimulus for large cells to function.[51]

Luteinizing hormone surge to menses is on an average about 14 days ranging from 11 to 17 days, with the short luteal phase occurring in about 5-6% women.[52]

The luteal phase cannot be extended for long despite continuous LH stimulation suggesting an active luteolytic mechanism. Corpus luteum rapidly declines 9–11 days after ovulation. Nitric oxide (NO), prostaglandin F2α (PGF2α), endothelin-1, TNFα, and proteolytic enzymes, such as matrix metalloproteinase (MMP), are involved in luteolysis.[53]

Emerging hCG from pregnancy rescues the CL. Messenger RNA for hCG can be detected in the 6–8-cell human embryo, i.e., even before implantation, and it can be detected in the mother about 6–7 days after ovulation.[53] Thus, the embryo is capable of preimplantation signaling and higher levels of estradiol and progesterone can be measured in the maternal circulation even before maternal hCG is detectable.

Luteal Follicular Transition

The luteal follicular transition is a period of selective increase in FSH beginning about 2 days before the onset of menses.[54] It occurs due to:

- Demise of corpus luteum results in nadir in circulating levels of estradiol, progesterone, and inhibin
- Decrease in negative feedback effect of luteal steroids and inhibin (particularly inhibin A)

- Change in pulsatile GnRH secretion toward an increasing pulse frequency which favors predominant FSH secretion.[55]

The increase in FSH is instrumental in rescuing approximately a 70-day cohort of follicles from atresia, allowing a dominant follicle to begin its emergence **(Fig. 17)**.

UTERINE OR ENDOMETRIAL CYCLE

The uterus is a dynamic structure, responding in a sensitive fashion to classic hormonal signals (the endocrine events of the menstrual cycle) (*see* **Fig. 6**). Cyclical changes in the endometrium prepare for implantation in the event of fertilization and necessitate menstruation in the absence of fertilization. The integrated evolutionary cycle of endometrial growth and regression is described in four phases:

1. Proliferative or follicular phase
2. Secretory or luteal phase
3. Preparatory phase for implantation
4. Menstrual phase or the phase of endometrial breakdown

Morphologically, the endometrium consists of an upper two-third "functionalis/functionale" layer which is the site of proliferation and secretion meant for blastocyst implantation and a lower one-third "basalis" layer serving as the source of regenerative endometrium after menstrual breakdown.

The functionalis layer is subdivided further into two parts:

- *Stratum compactum*: A superficial layer closer to the lumen, composed of gland necks and dense stromal cells
- *Stratum spongiosum*: The deeper functionale layer adjacent to the underlying basale layer contains predominantly endometrial glands, increased interstitial tissue, and less dense stroma.

The functionalis undergoes changes throughout the menstrual cycle and is shed during menstruation while the basalis remains constant during the menstrual cycle and regenerates the functionalis each month. Almost two-thirds of the functioning endometrium is shed out during menstruation. The residue is a stable, basalis component and a small, variable amount of residual stratum spongiosum **(Fig. 18; Table 6)**.

Proliferative or Follicular Phase

The proliferative or follicular phase spans from the end of the menstruation until ovulation. As estrogen secretion occurs, mitosis and pseudostratification predominate. Rapid re-epithelialization and proliferation of cells from the stumps of glands in the basalis layer, especially in the isthmic and tubal ostial sites, is initiated within 24–48 hours. By days 5 to 6, there is onset of stromal growth. There is proliferation of all elements slowly at first but later at a rapid pace. The ovarian follicular phase corresponds to the proliferative phase.

By the mid-follicular phase, increasing levels of estrogen from the growing follicle induce proliferation of the functionalis from stem cells of the basalis, proliferation of endometrial glands, and proliferation of stromal connective tissue. Endometrial glands are elongated with narrow lumens and their epithelial cells contain some glycogen. Glycogen, however, is not secreted during the follicular phase. As the glands get tubular, the epithelium becomes columnar with the nuclei placed at the base. Stromal cells, initially compact, evolve through subepithelial congestion. Spiral arteries elongate and span the length of the endometrium but remain unbranched **(Fig. 19)**.

Proliferation peaks on 8–10 days of the cycle reflecting peak estrogen receptors and concentration.[56] The thickness of the endometrium measures about 4–6 mm in the

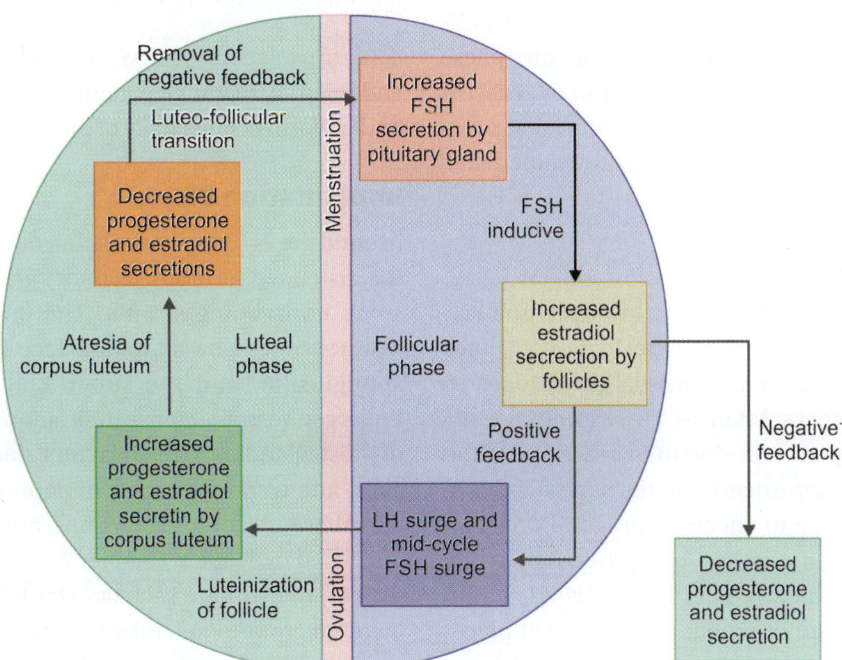

Fig. 17: Summary of ovarian events in the menstrual cycle.

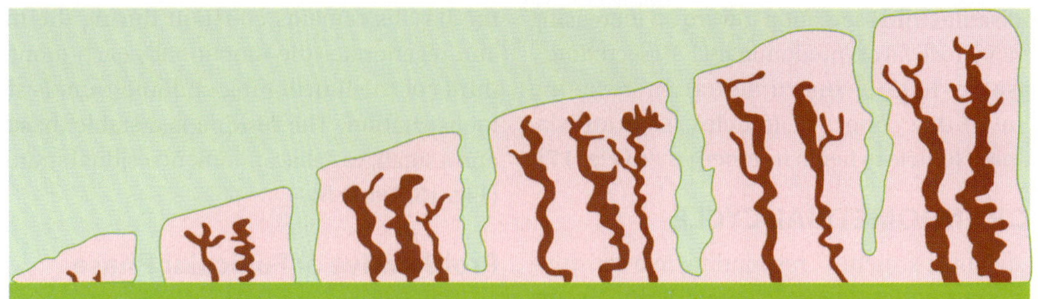

Fig. 18: Biological functions of endometrium in different stages of uterine cycle.

TABLE 6: Biological functions of endometrium in different stages of uterine cycle.

Days	*Ovarian events*	*Endometrial events*	*Hormonal dvnamics*
1–4	*Recruitment:* Cohort of follicles start growing	Endometrial lining sloughs	E2 and P4 are low FSH and LH are released from inhibition
5–7	*Selection:* A single follicle is destined to ovulate. No surrogate follicle	Endometrium proliferates	Plasma E2 rises due to secretion from selected dominant follicle
8–12	*Dominance:* • Atresia of all other follicles except dominant follicle • Dominant follicle thrives uniquely, despite the suppressive milieu	Increased E2 stimu lates the growth of glands and stroma	Increased E2 and inhibin will inhibit FSH
13–15	*Ovulation:* • Mediated by follicular enzymes and prostaglandins • Oocyte is induced to complete its first meiotic division	Transition from proliferative to secretory endometrium	LH surge induced by high plasma E2 *(Positive feedback)*
15–25	Corpus luteum forms	Secretory endometrium develops	P4 and E2 are secreted FSH and LH secretion is inhibited, so no new follicle develops
25–28	*Luteolysis:* • Corpus luteum degenerates • Recruitment of new follicles for next cycle	Endometrium begin to slough due to withdrawal of progesterone support	Plasma E2 and P4 decreases Release of hypothalamus and pituitary from negative feedback FSH begins to rise

mid- follicular phase and by the end of the proliferative phase, the mean endometrial thickness on ultrasound increases to a "trilaminar pattern" of 12 mm. Pseudostratification of the cells lining the glandular epithelium also peaks immediately before ovulation.

Secretory or Luteal Phase

The secretory, or luteal phase, begins at ovulation and lasts until the menstrual phase of the next cycle. In the early luteal phase, progesterone induces the endometrial glands to secrete glycogen, mucus, and other substances. These glands become tortuous and have large lumens due to increased secretory activity. The spiral arteries extend into the superficial layer of the endometrium. Due to effects of progesterone from the corpus luteum on an estrogen-primed endometrium, proliferation ceases and there is a decline in mitosis. Surface epithelium becomes more columnar and ciliated at places. Glands enlarge to get a corkscrew shape. Subnuclear glycogen vacuolation is an evidence of progesterone effect but does not confirm ovulation. Blood vessels undergo marked spiraling. The endometrial trilaminar pattern is lost, and there is an increased and uniform echogenicity of the endometrium **(Fig. 19)**.

Implantation Phase

Around the 7–13th postovulation day (day 21–22 of the cycle), the distended tortuous secretory glands are prominent with some intervening stroma. The endometrium gets three distinct zones—basal, middle lace-like edematous stratum spongiosum, and the superficial stratum compactum. Engorged vessels, intense infiltration of leukocytes, synthesis of prostaglandins, growth factors, decidualization of stromal cells, and a complex array of peptides and cytokines mark this phase meant to receive and nurture the blastocyst. It is discussed in detail in Chapter 7 on Implantation.

The mid-to-late secretory endometrial glands become increasingly tortuous and the stroma becomes edematous and vascular. If implantation of the blastocyst into the endometrium does not occur, and hCG is not present, the glands begin to

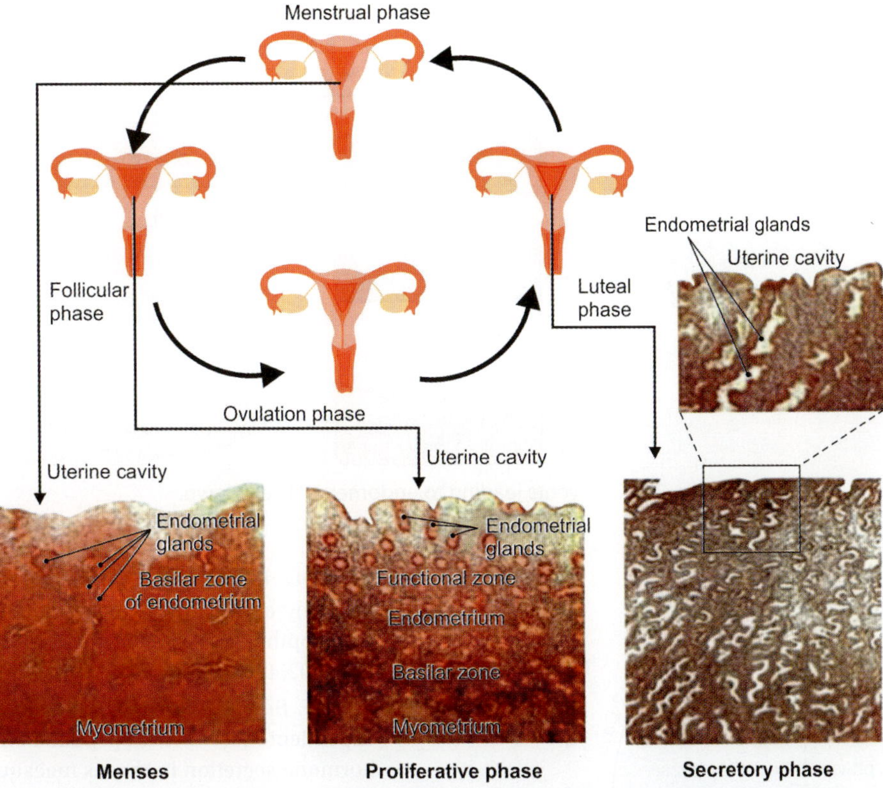

Fig. 19: Changes in endometrial histology in different stages of the uterine cycle.

fragment and collapse in the late luteal phase. In the absence of fertilization by day 23 of the menstrual cycle, the corpus luteum begins to degenerate and consequently ovarian hormone levels decrease. As estrogen and progesterone levels decrease, the endometrium undergoes involution. Days 25 and 26 of the menstrual cycle, endothelin, and thromboxane begin to mediate vasoconstriction of the spiral arteries. The resulting ischemia may cause some early menstrual cramps. By day 28 of the menstrual cycle, intense vasoconstriction and subsequent ischemia cause mass apoptosis of the functionalis **(Fig. 19)**.

Menstrual Phase or Phase of Endometrial Breakdown

In the event of nonestablishment of pregnancy, the fixed lifespan of the corpus luteum gets completed and the waning levels of estrogen and progesterone initiate important endometrial events. These events include blood stasis, arteriolar spasm, tissue necrosis, ischemia, and eventually enzymatic autodigestion caused by release of lysosomal proteolytic enzymes.[87]

The menstrual phase begins as the spiral arteries rupture secondary to ischemia, releasing blood into the uterus, and the apoptosed endometrium is sloughed off and usually lasts 4 days. Menstruation begins in different areas of the endometrium at different times. Sloughing of the endometrium occurs predominantly in the fundus and minimally in the isthmus or cornual regions, and the natural cleavage point is between basalis and spongiosum. Autolysis with subsequent desquamation of the stratum functionale layer begins. The bleeding occurs from broken arteries, veins and capillaries, and stromal hematoma. Arterial and venous blood, remnants of endometrial stroma and glands, leukocytes, and red blood cells are all present in the menstrual flow. Blood along with the superficial functional layer is shed into the uterine cavity **(Fig. 20)**.

Cessation of menstruation occurs due to a combined effect of prolonged vasoconstriction, myometrial contraction, and local aggregation of platelets with fibrin deposition. Resumption of estrogen secretion leads to repair of endometrium from the basalis layer. Regeneration of the endometrium begins 36 hours after the onset of menses at the isthmic recesses and the cornual region even as endometrial shedding continues in other areas of the uterus. Bleeding ceases usually by cycle day 5 after complete re-epithelialization of the endometrium is accomplished. Endometrial regeneration occurs in response to injury and is not hormone mediated **(Fig. 21)**.

Reproduction is affected by both the external environment and the internal environment including, among others nutrition, exposure to infections, and hormonal milieu of the individual. Endocrine disorders have a profound impact on reproduction and indeed in women. PCOS is the most common endocrine syndromic disorder affecting reproduction.

CONCLUSION

The neuroendocrinological control of menstrual cycle is of prime importance for fertility in women. As clearly evident,

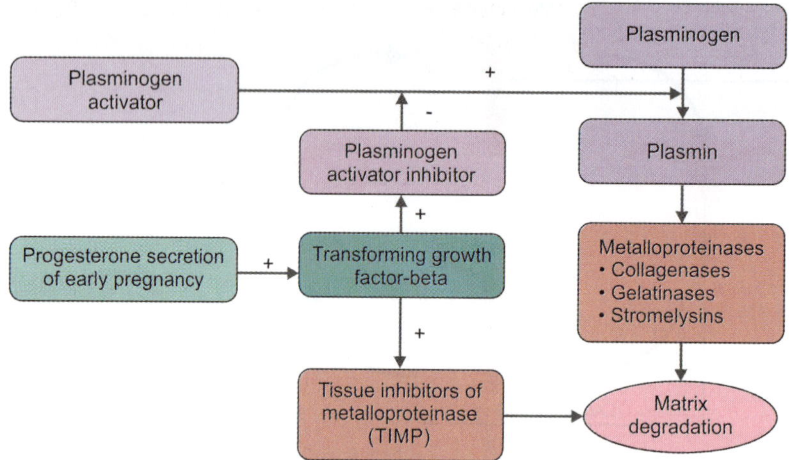

Fig. 20: Key events leading to endometrial breakdown.

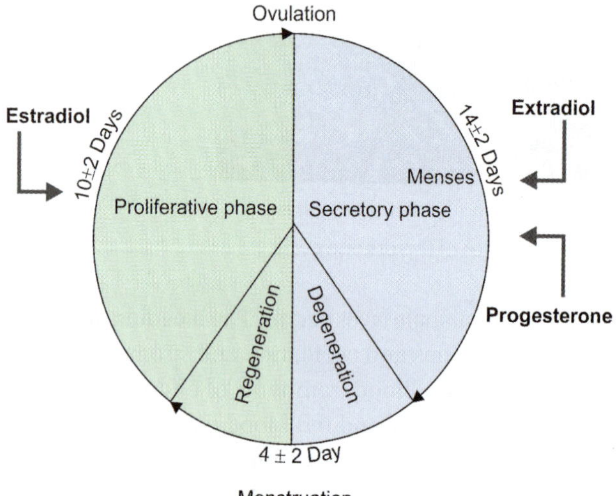

Fig. 21: Summary of ovarian and uterine events in a 28-day menstrual cycle with hormonal dynamics.

it involves a complex interplay of hormones produced by the hypothalamus, pituitary, and ovaries during the monthly reproductive cycle. The hormonal regulation of the reproductive system is complex and imperative for the proper functioning of the gonads (oogenesis and spermatogenesis), thus maintaining the vital menstrual function in the female along with fertility in both genders. Hence, it cannot be emphasized enough that the clinicians and specifically the infertility specialists need to have an in-depth understanding of the underlying physiology and neuroendocrinology for better patient care in their day-to-day practice.

REFERENCES

1. Simerly RB, Chang C, Muramatsu M, Swanson LW. Distribution of androgen and estrogen receptor mRNA-containing cells in the rat brain: an in situ hybridization study. J Comp Neurol. 1990;294:76-95.
2. Brown TJ, Hochberg RB, Naftolin F. Pubertal development of estrogen receptors in the rat brain. Mol Cell Neurosci. 1994;5:475-83.
3. Belchetz P.E, Plant T.M, Nakai Y, Keogh EJ, Knobil E. Hypophyseal responses to continuous and intermittent delivery of hypopthalamic gonadotropin-releasing hormone. Science. 1978;202(4368):631-3.
4. Pau KF, Berria M, Hess DL, Spies HG. Hypothalamic site-dependent effects of neuropeptide Y on gonadotropin-releasing hormone secretion in rhesus macaques. J Neuroendocrinol. 1995;7:63.
5. Rance NE. Menopause and the human hypothalamus: evidence for the role of kisspeptin/neurokinin B neurons in the regulation of estrogen negative feedback. Peptides. 2009;30(1): 111-22.
6. Oakley AE, Clifton DK, Steiner RA. Kisspeptin signaling in the brain. Endocr Rev. 2009;30:713-43.
7. Jayasena CN, Nijher GMK, Comninos AN, Januszewki A, Vaal ML, Sriskandarajah L, et al. The effects of kisspeptin-10 on reproductive hormone release show sexual dimorphism in humans. J Clin Endocrinol Metab. 2011; 96:E1963-72.
8. George JT, Veldhuis JD, Roseweir AK, Newton CL, Faccenda E, Millar RP, et al. Kisspeptin-10 is a potent stimulator of LH and increases pulse frequency in men. J Clin Endocrinol Metab. 2011;96:E1228-36.
9. Bauer-Dantoin AC, Wess J, Jameson JL. Roles of estrogen, progesterone, and gonadotropin-releasing hormone (GnRH) in the control of pituitary GnRH receptor gene expression at the time of the preovulatory gonadotropin surges. Endocrinology. 1995; 136:1014.
10. Blumenfeld Z. Response of human fetal pituitary cells to activin, inhibin, hypophysiotropic and neuroregulatory factors in vitro. Early Pregnancy. 2001;5:41.
11. Billestrup N, Gonzalez-M C, Potter E, Vale W. Inhibition of somatotroph growth and growth hormone biosynthesis by activin in vitro. Mol Endocrinol. 1990;4:356.
12. Corrigan AZ, Bilezikjian LM, Carroll RS, Bald LN, Schmelzer CH, Fendly BM, et al. Evidence for an autocrine role of activin B within rat anterior pituitary cultures. Endocrinology. 1991;128:1682.
13. Kaiser UB, Conn PM, Chin WW. Studies of gonadotropin-releasing hormone (GnRH) action using GnRH receptor-expressing pituitary cell lines. Endocr Rev. 1997;18:46.

14. Norwitz ER, Xu S, Jeong KH, Bédécarrats BY, Winebrenner LD, Chin WW, et al. Activin A augments GnRH-mediated transcriptional activation of the mouse GnRH receptor gene. Endocrinology. 2002;143:985.
15. Kogawa K, Nakamura T, Sugiono K, Takio K, Titani K, Sugino H. Activin-binding protein is present in pituitary. Endocrinology. 1991;128:1434.
16. Welt C, Sidis Y, Keutmann H, Schneyer A. Activins, inhibins, and follistatins: from endocrinology to signaling. A paradigm for the new millennium. Exp Biol Med (Maywood). 2002;227:724-52.
17. Menon M, Peegel H, Katta V. Estradiol potentiation of gonadotropin-releasing hormone responsiveness in the anterior pituitary is mediated by an increase in gonadotropin-releasing hormone receptors. Am J Obstet Gynecol. 1985;151:534.
18. Baker TG. A quantitative and cytological study of germ cells in human ovaries. Proc Roy Soc Lond. 1963;158:417.
19. Gougeon A. Regulation of ovarian follicular development in primates: facts and hypotheses. Endocr Rev. 1996;17:121.
20. Oktay K, Newton H, Mullan J, Gosden RG. Development of human primordial follicles to antral stages in SCID/hpg mice stimulated with follicle stimulating hormone. Hum Reprod. 1998;13:1133.
21. Hsueh AJW, Eisenhauer K, Chun SY, Hsu SY, Billig H. Gonadal cell apoptosis. Recent Prog Horm Res. 1996;51:433.
22. McNatty KP, Makris A, DeGrazia C, Osathanondh R, Ryan KJ. The production of progesterone, androgens, and estrogens by granulosa cells, thecal tissue, and stromal tissue from human ovaries in vitro. J Clin Endocrinol Metab. 1979;49:687.
23. McNatty KP, Makris A, Reinhold VN, De Grazia C, Osathanondh R, Ryan KJ. Metabolism of androstenedione by human ovarian tis sues in vitro with particular reference to reductase and aromatase activity. Steroids. 1979;34:429.
24. Hillier SG, Van Den Boogard AMJ, Reichert LE, van Hall EV. Intraovarian sex steroid hormone interactions and the regulation of follicular maturation: aromatization of androgens by human granulosa cells in vitro. J Clin Endocrinol Metab. 1980;50:640.
25. Jia X-C, Kessel B, Welsh TH, Hsueh AJ. Androgen inhibition of follicle-stimulating hormone-stimulated luteinizing hormone receptor formation in cultured rat granulosa cells. Endocrinology. 1985;117:13.
26. Andersen CY. Characteristics of human follicular fluid associated with successful conception after in vitro fertilization. J Clin Endocrinol Metab. 1993;77:1227.
27. Kobayashi M, Nakano R, Ooshima A. Immunohistochemical localization of pituitary gonadotropins and gonadal steroids confirms the two cells two gonadotropins hypothesis of steroidogenesis in the human ovary. J Endocrinol. 1990;126:483.
28. Magoffin DA. Regulation of differentiated functions in ovarian theca cells. Seminars Reprod Endocrinol. 1991;9:321.
29. Sasano H. Functional pathology of human ovarian steroidogenesis: normal cycling ovary and steroid-producing neoplasms. Endocr Pathol. 1994;5:81.
30. Schoot DC, Coelingh-Bennink HJT, Mannaerts BM, Lamberts SW, Bouchard P, Fauser BC. Human recombinant follicle-stimulating hormone induces growth of preovulatory follicles without concomitant increase in androgen and estrogen biosynthesis in a woman with isolated gonadotropin deficiency. J Clin Endocrinol Metab. 1992;74:1471.
31. Shoham Z, Mannaerts B, Insler V, Coelingh-Bennink H. Induction of follicular growth using recombinant human follicle-stimulating hormone in two volunteer women with hypogonadotropic hypogonadism. Fertil Steril. 1993;59:738.
32. Montgomery Rice V, Limback SD, Roby KF, Terranova PF. Differential responses of granulosa cells from small and large follicles to follicle stimulating hormone (FSH) during the menstrual cycle and acyclicity: effects of tumour necrosis factor-a. Hum Reprod. 1998;13:1285.
33. Zeleznik AJ, Schuler HM, Reichert LE. Gonadotropin-binding sites in the rhesus monkey ovary: role of the vasculature in the selective distribution of human chorionic gonadotropin to the preovulatory follicle. Endocrinology. 1981;109:356.
34. Schipper I, Hop WCJ, Fauser BCJM. The follicle-stimulating hormone (FSH) threshold/window concept examined by different interventions with exogenous FSH during the follicular phase of the normal menstrual cycle: duration, rather than magnitude, of FSH increase affects follicle development. J Clin Endocrinol Metab. 1998;83:1292.
35. Richards JS, Jahnsen T, Hedin L, Lifka J, Ratoosh S, Durica JM, et al. Ovarian follicular development: from physiology to molecular biology. Recent Prog Horm Res. 1987;43:231.
36. The European Recombinant Human LH Study Group. Recombinant human luteinizing hormone (LH) to support recombinant human follicle-stimulating hormone (FSH) induced follicular development in LH- and FSH-deficient anovulatory women: a dose finding study. J Clin Endocrinol Metab. 1998;83:1507.
37. Filicori M, Cognigni GE, Tabarelli C, Pocognoli P, Taraborrelli S, Spettoli D, et al. Stimulation and growth of antral ovarian follicles by selective LH activity administration in women. J Clin Endocrinol Metab. 2002;87:1156.
38. Young JR, Jaffe RB. Strength- duration characteristics of estrogen effects on gonadotropin response to gonadotropin-releasing hormone in women. II. Effects of varying concentrations of estradiol. J Clin Endocrinol Metab. 1976;42:432.
39. Cahill DJ, Wardle PG, Harlow CR, Hull MG. Onset of the preovulatory luteinizing hormone surge: diurnal timing and critical follicular prerequisites. Fertil Steril. 1998;70:56.
40. Pauerstein CJ, Eddy CA, Croxatto HD, Hess R, Siler-Khodr TM, Croxatto HB. Temporal relationships of estrogen, progesterone, and luteinizing hormone levels to ovulation in women and infrahuman primates. Am J Obstet Gynecol. 1978;130:876.
41. Fukuda M, Fukuda K, Andersen CY, Byskov AG. Right-sided ovulation favours pregnancy than left-sided ovulation. Hum Reprod. 2000;15:1921.
42. Fukuda M, Fukudu K, Andersen CY, Byskov AG. Characteristics of human ovulation in natural cycles correlated with age and achievement of pregnancy. Hum Reprod. 2001;16:2501.
43. Katt JA, Duncan JA, Herbon L, Barkan A, Marshall JC. The frequency of gonadotropin-releasing hormone stimulation deter-mines the number of pituitary gonadotropin releasing hormone receptors. Endocrinology. 1985;116:2113.
44. Adams JM, Taylor AE, Schoenfeld DA, Crowley Jr WF, Hall JE. The midcycle gonadotropin surge in normal women occurs in the face of an unchanging gonadotropin releasing hormone pulse frequency. J Clin Endocrinol Metab. 1994;79:858.
45. de Koning J. Gonadotrophin surge-inhibiting/attenuating factor governs luteinizing hormone secretion during the ovarian cycle: physiology and pathology. Hum Reprod. 1995;10:2854.

46. Christenson LK, Stouffer RL. Follicle-stimulating hormone and luteinizing hormone/chorionic gonadotropin stimulation of vascular endothelial factor production by macaque granulosa cells from pre- and periovulatory follicles. J Clin Endocrinol Metab. 1997;82:2135.
47. Golos TG, Soto EA, Tureck RW, Strauss 3rd JF. Human chorionic gonadotropin and 8-bromo-adenosine 3',5'-monophosphate stimulate [125I]low density lipoprotein uptake and metabolism by luteinized human granulosa cells in culture. J Clin Endocrinol Metab. 1985;61:633.
48. Retamales I, Carrasco I, Troncoso JL, Las Heras J, Devoto L, Vega M. Morpho-functional study of human luteal cell subpopulations. Hum Reprod. 1994;9:591.
49. Lei ZM, Chegini N, Rao CV. Quantitative cell composition of human bovine corpora lutea from various reproductive states. Biol Reprod. 1991;44:1148.
50. Brannian JD, Stouffer RL. Progesterone production by monkey luteal cell subpopulations at different stages of the menstrual cycle: changes in agonist responsiveness. Biol Reprod. 1991;44:141.
51. Lenton EA, Landgren B, Sexton L, Normal variation in the length of the follicular phase of the menstrual cycle: effect of chronological age. Br J Obstet Gynaecol. 1984;91:681.
52. Speroff L, Fritz MA. Regulation of the menstrual cycle. In: Speroff L, Fritz MA (Eds). Clinical Gynecologic Endocrinology and Infertility, 8th edition. Philadelphia: Lippincott Williams and Wilkins; 2011. pp. 199-242.
53. Bonduelle M, Dodd R, Liebaers I, Van Steirteghem A, Williamson R, Akhurst R. Chorionic gonadotropin-b mRNA, a trophoblast marker, is expressed in human 8-cell embryos derived from tripronucleate zygotes. Hum Reprod. 1998;3:909.
54. Roseff SJ, Bangah ML, Kettel LM. Dynamic changes in circulating inhibin levels during the luteal-follicular transition of the human menstrual cycle. J Clin Endocrinol Metab. 1989;69:1033.
55. Hall JE, Schoenfeld DA, Martin KA. Hypothalamic gonadotropin-releasing hormone secretion and follicle-stimulating hormone dynamics during the luteal follicular transition. J Clin Endocrinol Metab. 1992;74:600--7.
56. Bergeron C, Ferenczy A, Shyamala G. Distribution of estrogen receptors in various cell types of normal, hyperplastic, and neoplastic human endometrial tissues. Lab Invest. 1988;58(3):338-45.

LONG QUESTIONS

1. Discuss the two cell two gonadotropin theory.
2. Describe changes in the phases of the endometrial cycle and their clinical correlation?

SHORT QUESTIONS

1. Compare the various feedback mechanisms in hormonal regulation.
2. Describe the changes in the menstrual cycle.
3. Discuss the role of various neurotransmitters in neuro-endocrine axis.

MULTIPLE CHOICE QUESTIONS

1. Chronic high levels of which of the following leads to a positive feedback loop in the hypothalamo-pituitary-ovary axis?
   a. Dopamine b. Estrogen
   c. Inhibin d. Progesterone
2. Which are the hormones NOT secreted by the anterior pituitary?
   a. FSH b. LH
   c. GnRH d. TSH
3. Shortly before menstruation:
   a. Blood levels of estrogen and progesterone decrease
   b. Blood levels of estrogen and progesterone increase
   c. Blood levels of FSH stabilize
   d. The corpus luteum secretes progesterone
4. During the menstrual cycle:
   a. LH stimulates estrogen production by follicles
   b. FSH stimulates growth of the ovarian follicles
   c. LH stimulates the formation of a corpus luteum from the collapsed follicle.
   d. All of the above
5. Which of the following specifically inhibits FSH, but not LH?
   a. Progesterone b. Estradiol
   c. Inhibin d. Androgen
6. Which of the following is true?
   a. Endorphins stimulate GnRH release within the hypothalamus
   b. α endorphin is10 times more potent than morphine
   c. β endorphin is 10 times more potent than morphine
   d. Endorphin levels are lowest in the luteal phase
7. Which of the following is associated with the corpus luteum of menstruation, not the corpus luteum of pregnancy?
   a. Ovarian leuteotropins (estrogens, IGF-I, IGF-II)
   b. hCG produced by the trophoblast of the chorion
   c. LH and prolactin
   d. Corpus albicans

Answers

1. b 2. c 3. a 4. d 5. c 6. c
7. d

6.3 NORMAL MENSTRUAL CYCLE: PHYSIOLOGY AND CARE

Ameya Purandare, Ritu Hinduja

INTRODUCTION

Menstruation is the cyclical shedding of the endometrium characterized by vaginal bleeding which is a result of the hormonal interaction of the hypothalamic-pituitary-ovarian (HPO) axis. For this interaction to occur, there needs to be proper coordination of the HPO axis. Besides this, the endometrium should also respond to the estrogen and progesterone that is secreted by the ovaries and there should be no anomalies of the outflow tract.

A menstrual cycle has an average period of 28 days (normal range 21–35 days). Menarche is the beginning of menstruation and occurs at an average age of 11–15 years. Menopause is the cessation of menses with the average age being 45–50 years. There is physiological cessation of menses which occurs during pregnancy and lactation. The period of bleeding is generally about 4–5 days with an estimated blood loss of 20–80 mL. The menstrual discharge consists of dark altered blood, fragments of the endometrium, vaginal epithelial cells, mucus, enzymes, prostaglandins, and bacteria and almost 70% of it is shed in the first 2 days of the cycle itself.

The menstrual cycle is divided into the ovarian and uterine cycle. The ovarian cycle is further divided into follicular and luteal phase. The uterine cycle is divided into proliferative and secretary phase.

The five phases in a normal menstrual cycle are:[1]

1. Menstruation
2. Proliferation
3. Secretory phase
4. Preparation of implantation
5. Phase of endometrial breakdown

OVARIAN CYCLE (FIG. 1)

The ovarian cycle is under the influence of the HPO axis. The follicular phase is characterized by the rising level of follicle-stimulating hormone (FSH) and luteinizing hormone (LH).

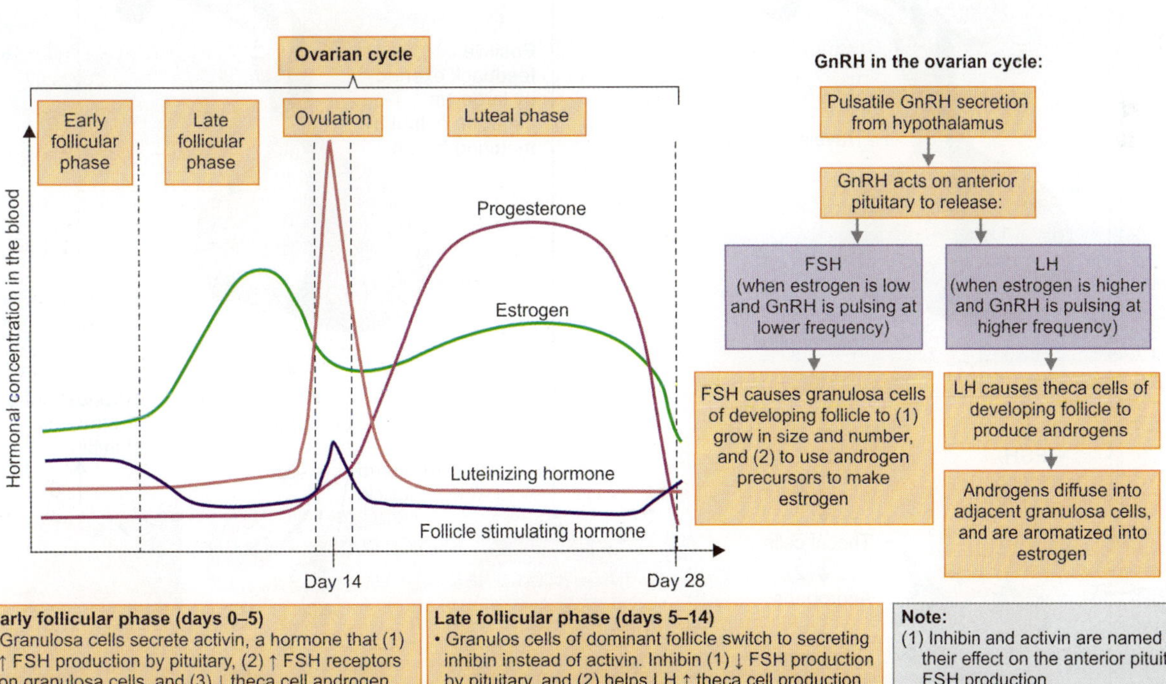

Fig. 1: Phase wise depiction of the changes that occur in the ovarian cycle.
(FSH: follicle-stimulating hormone; GnRH: gonadotropin-releasing hormone; LH: luteinizing hormone)

The ovary has a cohort of 10–20 follicles that are recruited in each phase. The rising FSH and LH levels cause all the follicles to grow but only 1 follicle is recruited as the dominant follicle. Once the dominant follicle is recruited, there is a secretion of estrogen which in turn causes the FSH levels to fall (negative feedback). The increase in estrogen levels gets accumulated in the dominant follicle and fluid-filled space is known as the antrum. The follicle then matures into a vesicular follicle. The rising estrogen levels via a positive feedback mechanism causes the LH surge. This LH surge in turn causes ovulation (release of the mature egg from the follicle). The follicle is then converted into the corpus luteum. The corpus luteum is responsible for the secretion of progesterone. If fertilization of the ova does not occur then the corpus luteum gets converted to the corpus albicans. This in turn causes the progesterone and estrogen levels to drop which causes the shedding of the endometrium and menstruation occurs. The fall in estrogen and progesterone levels via negative feedback mechanism on the HPO axis causes the FSH and LH levels to rise again **(Fig. 2)**.[2,3]

ENDOMETRIAL CYCLE (TABLE 1)[4]

The cyclic histologic changes in the endometrium occurs in an orderly manner in response to the secretion of the hormones from the ovaries **(Fig. 3)**. The histological cycling can be best viewed in two parts—the endometrial glands and the surrounding stroma. The superficial two-thirds of the endometrium is the area that proliferates and sheds with each menstrual cycle unless pregnancy occurs. The superficial two-thirds of the endometrium is known as decidua functionalism and is composed of an intermediate zone known as the stratum spongiosum and a superficial compact zone known as stratum compactum. The deep one-third of the endometrium is known as the decidua basalis. It is the source of endometrial regeneration in each menstrual cycle.

Proliferative Phase

This phase corresponds to the follicular phase of the ovary. The proliferative phase starts from menstruation to ovulation.

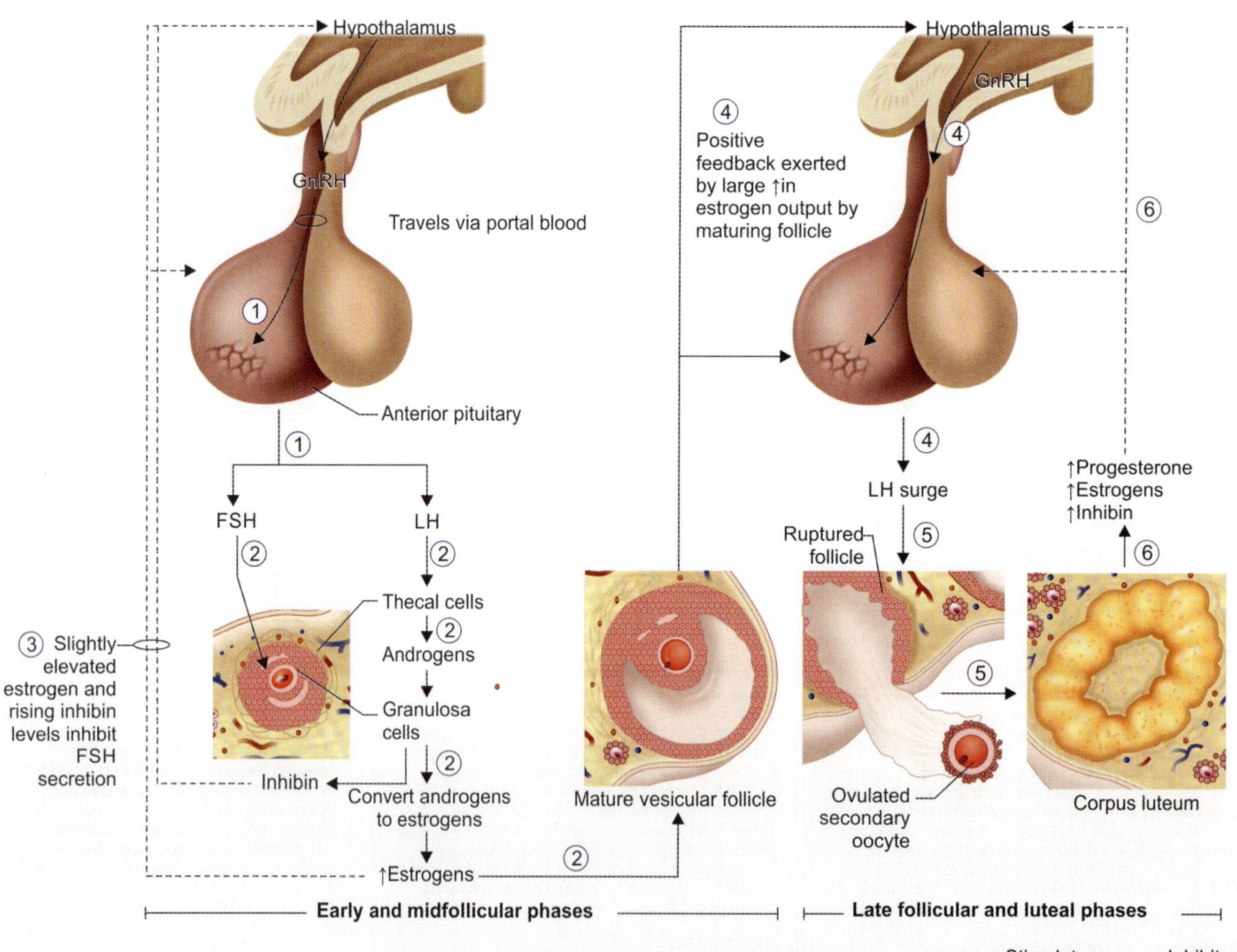

Fig. 2: Hormonal interplay involved in the execution of the ovarian cycle.
(FSH: follicle-stimulating hormone; GnRH: gonadotropin-releasing hormone; LH: luteinizing hormone)

TABLE 1: Comparison of changes in the endometrium in a 28-day menstrual cycle.

Endometrial phase				***Secretory***					
	Menstrual		***Proliferative***	***'Interval'***	***Early***		***Mid***	***Late***	
Day of 28 days cycle (ovulation on D14)		1-3	4- 15	-16	17	18	19–21	22–24	25–28
Key feature		Stromal crumbling	Mitoses	Subnuclear vacuoles, staggered with mitoses	Subnuclear vacuoles, regular with mitoses	Subnuclear and supranuclear vacuoles No mitoses	Stromal edema	Focal predecidua around spiral arteries	Predecidua involves surface
Microscopic features of functional zone	Stroma	Stromal aggregates, Blue balls hemo-rrhage	Loose stroma Mitoses	Loose stroma Mitoses	Loose stroma, scantly mitoses	Loose stroma, scantly mitoses	Stromal edema increases from D19–21	Perivascular naked nuclei (D22) from predecidual cuffs (D23) that bridge vessels (D24)	Focal (D25) then extensive (D26) surface predecidua extends downwards (D26–28) Prominent granulated lymphocytes
	Glands	Collapsed epithelium and displaced secretory glands	Straight to tightly coiled tubules Mitoses	Some staggered subnuclear vacuoles Many mitoses	Piano key subnuclear vacuoles Some mitoses	Some staggered subnuclear vacuoles No mitoses	Dilated glands with irregular outlines Luminal secretion	Saw tooth glands	Prominent saw tooth glands
Appearances									

With rising estrogen levels, the thickness of the endometrium increases resulting in a proliferative pattern. Estrogen leads to the proliferation of the stroma and glands and causes the spiral arteries to elongate.

Initially the proliferation is slow and then later the growth is rapid. The glands become tubular and lie perpendicular to the surface. The epithelium becomes columnar with the nuclei placed at the base. The epithelium of one gland becomes continuous with the neighboring gland. Mitosis is evident in the epithelial cells. The stromal cells become spindle-shaped with evidences of mitosis and are compact. The spiral vessels extend unbranched to a region below the epithelium where they form loose capillary network. There may be evidences of subepithelial congestion. The thickness measures about 3–4 mm **(Fig. 4)**.[5-7]

Secretory Phase[4]

This phase corresponds to the luteal phase in the ovary. Postovulation, progesterone levels rise. Due to this, there is secretion of glycogen and mucous. In the midsecretory phase, the endometrium is decidualized and receptive to the implantation of a fertilized embryo. If there is no pregnancy, the spiral arteries constrict, leading to involution of the endometrium and menstruation occurs. The cycle then repeats itself.

There are progesterone receptors on the endometrium which are induced by estrogen. Therefore, progesterone acts only on an estrogen primed endometrium.

This phase begins from day 15 and ceases 5–6 days prior to menstruation. The surface epithelium becomes more columnar and ciliated at places. There is an increase in size of the glands. The lining epithelium becomes taller. Vacuoles

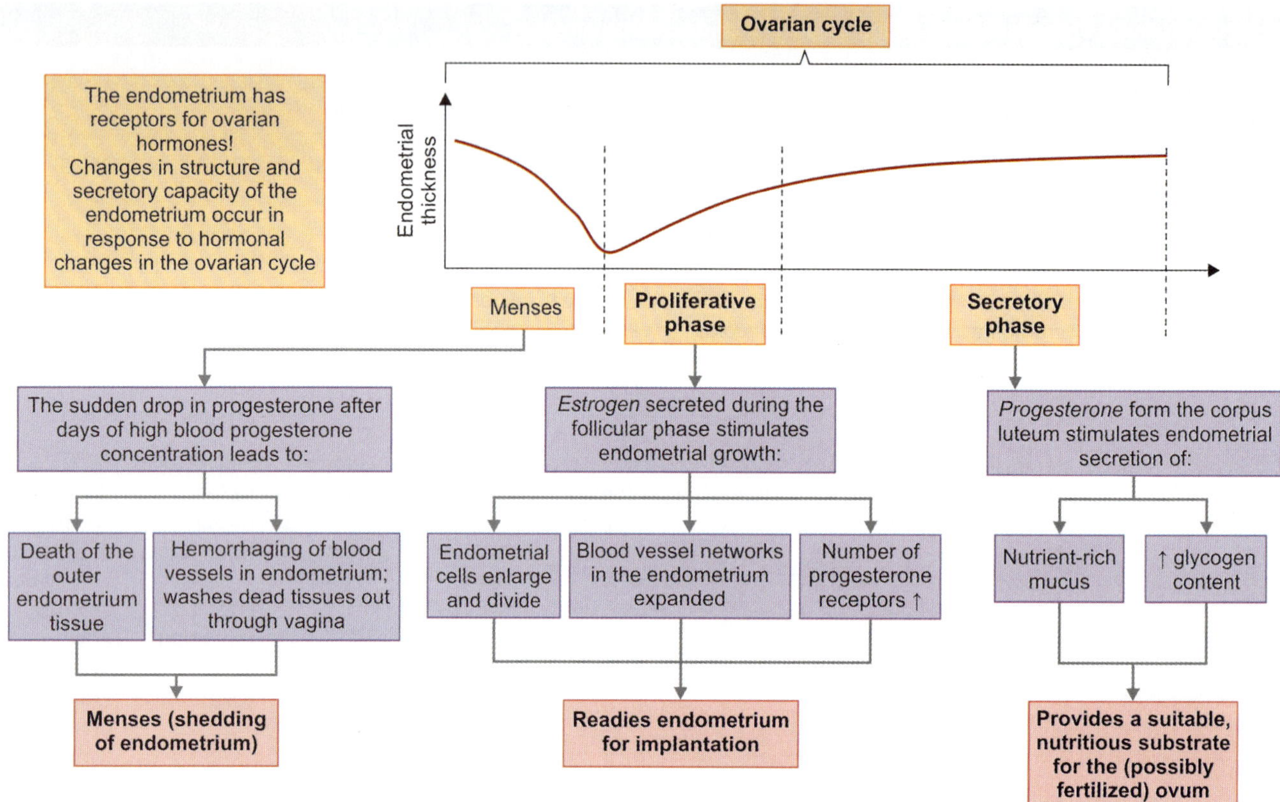

Fig. 3: Correlation of the endometrial cycle with the ovarian cycle. Changes occurring in the endometrium under the influence of the ovarian hormones.

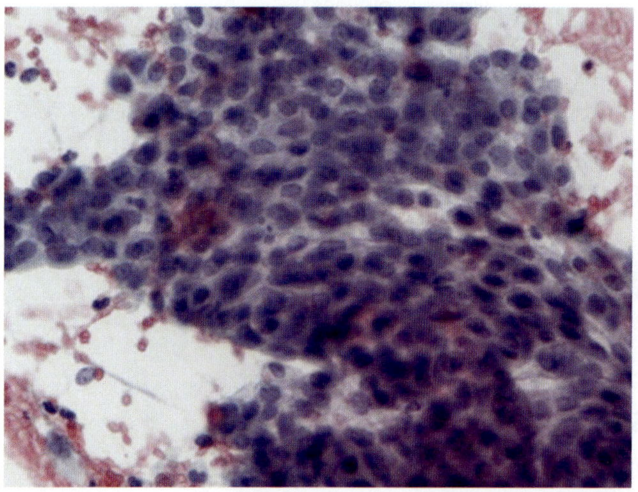

Fig. 4: Stromal cells of the endometrium; proliferative phase.

appear due to the secretion of glycogen between the nuclei and the basement membrane.

This is known as subnuclear vacuolation, which is the earliest (36–48 hours) sign of ovulation. This phenomenon persists till about 21st day of cycle. The nuclei are pushed back towards the basement membrane because of the intracellular secretion entering the grand lumina. The effect is a saw-toothed glandular epithelium. This fluid has nutritive value for an embryo reaching the uterus for implantation. The glands become corkscrew shaped. The blood vessels undergo marked spiraling.

The stromal cells swell up and become large and polyhedral. After the 21st day they become more superficial and are around the neck of the glands. The deeper spongy levels consist of convoluted glands, coiled arterioles, and few stromal cells. Histochemical studies show increase in glycogen and acid phosphatase. Histological staining is eosinophilic. The thickness of the endometrium reaches its highest (6–8 mm).

Growth of the endometrium stops 5–6 days before menstruation where pregnancy has not occurred. This phenomenon is because of the dehydration of the glands. There is engorgement of the subepithelial capillaries and spiral vessels. These regressive changes are most prominent 24–48 hours prior to menstruation. There is marked spiraling of the arterioles. Due to the withdrawal of estrogen and progesterone, there is spasm of the spiral arterioles at the basal part. This leads to stasis and tissue anoxemia. Leukocytes and monocytes infiltrate the stroma **(Figs. 5 and 6)**.[6-8]

MENSTRUAL PHASE[1]

This is the degeneration and shedding of the endometrium. The corpus luteum regresses with a decrease in estrogen and progesterone levels. This is an invariable preceding feature.

Mechanism of Menstrual Bleeding

The degeneration occurs mainly due to the vascular changes. The stasis of blood and spasm of the arterioles leads to damage

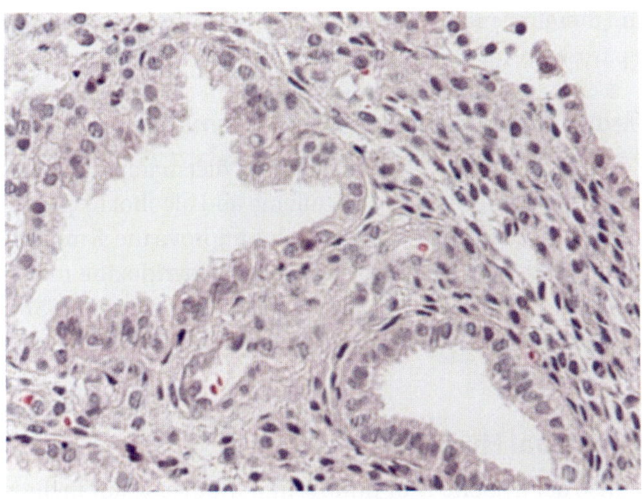

Fig. 5: Stromal cells of the endometrium; secretory phase.

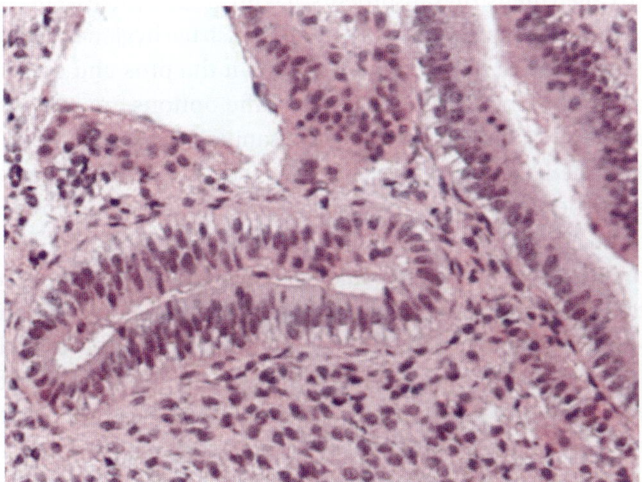

Fig. 6: Secretory phase: Histology picture showing subnuclear glycogen vacuoles and spiral arteries.

of the vessel walls. The phase of relaxation causes the blood to escape from the arterioles through the damaged walls. This process is rapid and involves the functional damaged layer. Proteolytic enzymes (released by breakdown of lysosomes) cause local tissue destruction. Therefore, enzymatic autodigestion of the functional zone occurs. Bleeding occurs from the broken arteries, veins, capillaries, and from the stromal hematoma. The superficial functional layer is shed along with the blood into the uterine cavity. The blood coagulates in the cavity but soon liquefies by plasmin. Liquefaction does not take place if there is brisk rapid bleeding. The menstrual flow stops due to prolonged vasoconstriction, myometrial contraction, and local aggregation of platelets. Endothelin and platelet activating factor are potent vasoconstrictors that are present in the endometrium. Rise in estrogen levels in the next menstrual cycle causes clot formation over the vessels. Simultaneously the endometrium is repaired.

THE MYOMETRIAL CYCLE[9,10]

Uterine muscle activity changes with the menstrual cycle. Early in the follicular phase, the muscle contracts less frequently and the response to oxytocics is limited. The contractions increase with estrogen stimulation of the approaching ovulation. In the premenstrual and menstrual phase, the contractions are less frequent but their amplitude is increased. The contractions are the strongest during menstruation possibly due to the stimulation by the release of prostaglandins.

Cyclical Changes in the Tube[11]

The muscles in the fallopian tube behave similarly to that of the myometrium that is increase movement around the time of ovulation. This is due to estrogen as it increases the activity of the tubal cilia. This occurs so as to propel the ovum towards the uterus.

The follicular phase shows slight proliferation with minimal mitotic activity of the tubal mucosa. This continues till premenstrual phase where it regresses. Once menstruation occurs, there is further regression and slight shedding of the surface epithelium. Sometimes the endosalpinx may menstruate.

THE CERVICAL CYCLE[1]

The tone of the isthmus and internal os increases due to the secretion of progesterone. This makes the cervical "sphincter" tighter and more competent during the luteal phase. During the follicular phase, the glandular elements of the cervix proliferate, and the epithelium becomes taller. Under the influence of estrogen, the glands secrete mucus which stretches into threads at the time of ovulation. This property of spinnbarkeit is the basis of the thread test for estrogen in circulation. During the follicular phase, the cervical mucus absorbs water and salts. Once dried, deposits of sodium and potassium chloride crystals form a characteristic fern pattern. The secretion is so profuse at the time of ovulation that it may be noticeable as vaginal discharge. This special characteristic of the cervix makes it easy for the sperms to penetrate.

During the luteal phase, the glands become more branched and their secretions change in physical and chemical properties. The thickness of the mucus increases formic a secure cervical plug. It is unable to stretch without breaking and does not allow sperms to penetrate. This is due to the secretion of progesterone. Progesterone also decreases the electrolyte content of the mucous, therefore ferning cannot be seen by approximately the 22nd day. During menstruation, the cervical glands collapse may show slight desquamation with loss of blood.

THE VAGINAL CYCLE[1]

Histological changes occur in the vagina as well but they are not clearly defined. The unstimulated vagina shows small basal type cells with healthy nuclei. These are intermediate basophil forms which may be seen in vaginal smears taken in the follicular phase. Once stimulated by estrogen, there is preponderance of large cornfield epithelial cells with pyknotic nuclei. During the luteal phase, there is desquamation with the cells having rolled edges. This is seen by the reappearance of clumps of intermediate cells and presence of leukocytes.

Menstrual Symptoms

Usually there are no symptoms besides bleed per vaginum. In adolescents or nulliparous women, there may be a tolerable colicky pain due to the contraction of the uterus. If the pain is excessive, where the day-to-day activity is affected, it is known as dysmenorrhea. Just prior to menses premonitory symptoms such as backache, pelvic discomfort, mastalgia, or breast discomfort may occur. Headache or depression may be present. If these symptoms are predominant, then a diagnosis of premenstrual syndrome can be made.

Treatment for Dysmenorrhea (Flowchart 1)[12]

Counseling plays an important role, if there is no pathology. Mild analgesics and antispasmodics may help reduce the symptoms **(Table 2)**. The girl should be encouraged to carry out her daily routine. Oral contraceptive (OC) pills may be given for three to six cycles which would cause anovulatory cycles and therefore make them painless. If these measures fail, then laparoscopy may need to be done to rule out endometriosis.

Flowchart 1: Algorithm for management of dysmenorrhea.

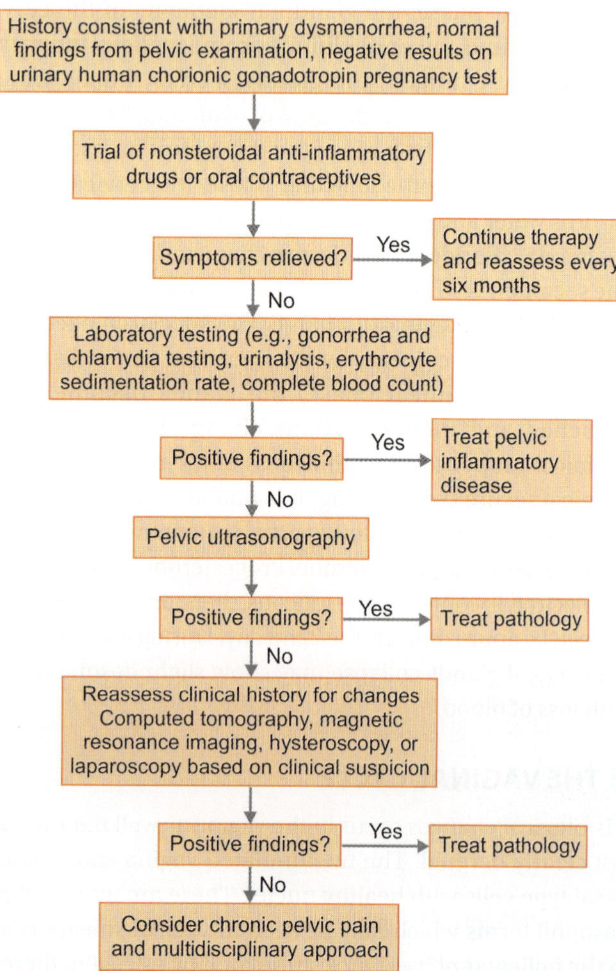

Treatment of Premenstrual Symptoms

Counselling, yoga, stress management, diet manipulation, salt restriction, and cessation of caffeine and alcohol (especially in the second half of the cycle) helps improve the symptoms. Tranquilizers, antidepressant drugs, or pyridoxine may be considered. *Selective serotonin reuptake inhibitors (SSRI****s****) and noradrenaline reuptake inhibitors (SNRI****s****)* are found to be very effective.

Menstrual Hygiene[13-15]

Menstrual hygiene is of utmost importance. It not includes access to basic sanitation facilities, soap, and water but also to so called menstrual absorbents. It is up to each adolescent and woman to choose an absorbent or menstrual hygiene product of her choice being fully aware about the pros and cons of each product **(Table 3)**. Some of the options are reusable menstrual cloth pads, disposable sanitary napkins, tampons, and menstrual cup. She should be educated to change her absorbent at regular intervals. They should be encouraged to take bath regularly, do light exercises, and continue with daily routine. Women should also be made aware of the way to dispose their absorbent. All this counselling should be done keep in perspective things that may or may not be acceptable in their culture. We need to educate the girl/woman that menstruation is a normal physiological process and equip her with strategies and methods to deal with menstruation in a dignifies manner. Also. Let them know what is normal and what is not and when do they need to seek a doctor advise. We need to counsel them about pain and management of dysmenorrhea so that it does not affect their day-to-day life **(Fig. 7)**. It is also important to make them aware about the health risks associated with unclean or unhygienic menstrual care and practices **(Table 4)**.

Menstrual Hygiene Tips

- Change your pad frequently
- Try to use good sanitary products
- Clean reusable pads properly
- Keep your vaginal area clean
- Wear comfortable and clean underclothes

TABLE 2: Nonsteroidal anti-inflammatory drugs used for the treatment of primary dysmenorrhea.

Drug	*Dosage*
Ibuprofen	200 to 600 mg every six hours
Mefenamic acid	500 mg initially, then 250 mg every six hours
Naproxen	440 to 550 mg initially then 220 to 275 mg every 12 hours

TABLE 3: Advantages and disadvantages of different sanitary protection materials.

Sanitary protection option	*Advantages*	*Disadvantages*
Natural materials (e.g., mud, cow dung, and leaves)	• Free • Locally available	• High risk of contamination • Difficult and uncomfortable to use
Strips of clothes	• Easily available in the local market • Reusable	• If old clothes are not cleaned well they can become unhygienic • Users need somewhere private, with a water supply and soap, to wash and dry the cloths
Toilet paper or tissues	Easily available in the local market	• Loses strength when wet and can fall apart. • Difficult to hold in place • May be too expensive for the poorest users
Reusable pads	• Available locally or on the internet • Income generation opportunity, if locally made • Cost effective as they are reusable • More environment-friendly than disposable pads	• Users need somewhere private, with water supply and soap to wash and dry the pads • If commercially produced, cost is prohibitive to many potential users
Tampons	Convenient and comfortable to use	• Not available in many contexts • Cost is prohibitive to many potential users • Generates a lot of waste to dispose, not environmentally-friendly • May not be culturally appropriate, particularly for adolescent girls, as need to be inserted into the vagina • Hygiene and availability of water and soap for hand-washing are particularly important, as need to be inserted into the vagina
Menstrual cups	• Reusable • Only need emptying, washing and drying	• May not be culturally appropriate for use, particularly for adolescent girls, as need to be inserted into the vagina • Hygiene and availability of water and soap are particularly important, for washing hands and menstrual cup, as need to be inserted into the vagina • Expensive first investment outlay
Panties/underwear	• Useful for keeping a sanitary product in place • Good for keeping the vaginal area hygienic	• Cost may be prohibitive to potential users • Cheap elastic can wear out relatively quickly

(*Source:* Adapted from House S, Mahon T, Cavil, S. Menstrual hygiene matters: a resource for improving menstrual hygiene around the world. London: Department for International Development; 2012.)

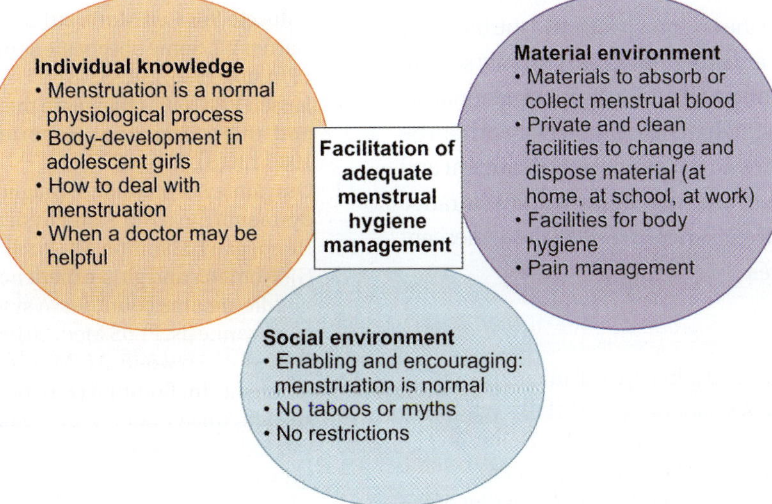

Fig. 7: Elements important for menstrual hygiene management.

TABLE 4: Potential risks to health of poor menstrual hygiene.

Practice	*Health risk*
Unclean sanitary pads/materials	Bacteria may cause local infections or travel up the vagina and enter the uterine cavity
Changing pads infrequently	Wet pads can cause skin irritation which can then become infected if the skin becomes broken
Insertion of unclean material into vagina	Bacteria potentially have easier access to the cervix and the uterine cavity
Using highly absorbent tampons during a time of light blood loss	Toxic shock syndrome
Use of tampons when not menstruating (e.g., to absorb vaginal secretions)	Can lead to vaginal irritation and delay the seeking of medical advice for the cause of unusual vaginal discharge
Wiping from back to front following urination or defecation	Makes the introduction of bacteria from the bowel into the vagina (or urethra) more likely
Unprotected sex	Possible increased risk of sexually transmitted infections or the transmission of HIV or Heptitis B during menstruation
Unsafe disposal of used sanitary materials or blood	Risk of infecting others, especially with Hepatitis B (HIV and other Heptites viruses do not survive for long outside the body and pose a minimal risk except where there is direct contact with blood just leaving the body)
Frequent douching (forcing liquid into the vagina)	Can facilitate the introduction of bacteria into the uterine cavity
Lack of hand-washing after changing a sanitary towel	Can facilitate the spread of infections such as Hepatitis B or Thrush

(*Source:* Adapted from House S, Mahon T, Cavil, S. Menstrual hygiene matters: a resource for improving menstrual hygiene around the world. London: Department for International Development; 2012.)

- Use the right washing technique
- Discard used products properly
- Consult a gynecologist if having sensitivity to any products and discontinue use immediately.

ANOVULAR MENSTRUATION[1,4]

The growth of a follicle without the recruitment of a dominant follicle and subsequent ovulation is known as an anovulatory cycle. This could be due to the imbalance between FSH and estrogen or nonresponsiveness of the hypothalamus to the rising estrogen (GnRH suppression, therefore no ovulation). The endometrium may remain in the proliferative state or sometimes in a hyperplastic state. When the estrogen falls, there is asynchronous shedding of the endometrium and the bleeding could be prolonged, heavy, and irregular. This is usually seen in adolescents, postdelivery or abortion and, in the perimenopausal period. Initial few cycles postmenarche are anovular and can be irregular, these irregular cycles do not require any treatment and only require counseling about anovular menses and assurance that eventually the cycles will regularize in most of the adolescent girls as the HPO axis matures.

REFERENCES

1. Malhotra N. Menstruation and other cyclical phenomenon. In: Malhotra N, Malhotra J, Saxena R, Bora NM (Eds). Jeffcoate's Principles of Gynaecology, 9th edition. New Delhi: Jaypee Brothers Medical Publishers (P) Ltd.; 2019. pp. 83-95.
2. Buffet NC, Bouchard P. The neuroendocrine regulation of the human ovarian cycle. Chronobiol Int. 2001;18(6):893-919.
3. Khan-Dawood FS. The ovarian cycle. In: Tulsiani DRP (Ed). Introduction to Mammalian Reproduction. Boston, MA: Springer; 2003.
4. Speroff L, Fritz MA. Clinical Gynecologic Endocrinology and Infertility. Philadelphia: Lippincott Williams & Wilkins; 2005.
5. Sturgis SH, Meigs JV. Endometrial cycle and mechanism of normal menstruation. Am J Surg. 1936;33:369-84.
6. Thiyagarajan DK, Basit H, Jeanmonod R. Physiology, Menstrual Cycle. Treasure Island (FL): StatPearls Publishing; 2020.
7. Matías J-A, Beatriz J-A. Cytology of the normal endometrium—cycling and postmenopausal. Monogr Clin Cytol. 2008;17:32-9.
8. Monard M, Marsh C, Schumacher K, Nothnick W. Secretory phase of menstruation and implantation. London, UK: IntechOpen; 2018.
9. Arrowsmith S, Robinson H, Noble K, Wray S. What do we know about what happens to myometrial function as women age? J Muscle Res Cell Motil. 2012;33(3):209-17.
10. Garrett WJ. Some observations on the human myometrial cycle. J Physiol. 1956;132:553-8.
11. Jansen RP. Cyclic changes in the human fallopian tube isthmus and their functional importance. Am J Obstet Gynecol. 1980;136(3):292-308.
12. Osayande AS, Mehulic S. Diagnosis and initial management of dysmenorrhea. Am Fam Physician. 2014;89(5):341-6.
13. Hennegan J, Shannon AK, Rubli J, Schwab KJ, Melendez-Torres GJ. Women's and girls' experiences of menstruation in low- and middle-income countries: A systematic review and qualitative metasynthesis. PLoS Med. 2019;16(5):e1002803.
14. Romm A, Hywood AJ. Menstrual wellness and menstrual problems. In: Romm A (Ed). Botanical Medicine for Women's Health. Amsterdam, Netherlands: Elsevier; 2010.
15. van Eijk AM, Sivakami M, Thakkar MB, Bauman A, Laserson KF, Coates S, et al. Menstrual hygiene management among adolescent girls in India: a systematic review and meta-analysis. BMJ Open. 2016;6:e010290.

LONG QUESTIONS

1. Define the menstrual cycle and elaborate the changes that occur in the cycle.
2. Define menstrual hygiene. How would you counsel an adolescent to maintain menstrual hygiene? What are the factors affecting women opting for menstrual hygiene products what are the advantages and disadvantages of the various products available?

SHORT QUESTIONS

1. Describe the ovarian cycle.
2. Describe the uterine cycle.
3. Describe the histological changes that occur in the endometrium during the menstrual cycle.
4. What is the cervical cycle?
5. What is 2-cell 2-gonadotropin theory?

MULTIPLE CHOICE QUESTIONS

1. How many phases are present in the reproductive cycle?
   a. 3 b. 5
   c. 2 d. 4
2. The hormones secreted during reproductive cycle are regulated by:
   a. Negative feedback system
   b. Positive feedback system
   c. Sympathetic system
   d. Parasympathetic system
3. Which of the following does not occur during ovulation?
   a. Cervical mucus becomes watery
   b. Increase body temp
   c. Atrophy of sex organ
   d. Abdominal discomfort
4. Which of the following statement is not true?
   a. The reproductive cycle occurs after every 26–30 days
   b. During ovulation, body temperature falls
   c. Proliferative phase ends when ovulation begins
   d. FSH promotes maturation of ovarian follicles
5. Which hormone stimulates the anterior pituitary for the secretion of FSH and LH?
   a. LHRH b. GH
   c. CRH d. TSH
6. Which of the following suppress the hypothalamus in order to control its regulation?
   a. Estrogen b. Progesterone
   c. FSH d. Both A and B
7. The endometrium grows and thickens during:
   a. Menstruation b. Follicular phase
   c. Luteal phase c. Ovulation
8. The follicular phase is to the ________ as the luteal phase is to the secretory phase.
   a. Postovulatory b. Menstrual
   c. Proliferative d. Myometrial
   e. Ovulatory
9. After ovulation, the follicle, under stimulation of luteinizing hormone, turns into a glandular mass of cells called the __________.
   a. Corpus cavernosum b. Corpus spongiosum
   c. Corpus glandula d. Corpus callosum
   e. Corpus luteum
10. Which hormone is produced by the corpus luteum?
   a. Estrogen b. Progesterone
   c. LH d. FSH

Answers

1.	a	2.	a	3.	c	4.	b	5.	a	6.	d
7.	b	8.	c	9.	e	10.	b				

6.4 NORMAL PUBERTY AND ADOLESCENCE: PHYSIOLOGY AND CARE

Maya Padhi, Lucy Das

INTRODUCTION

Puberty is the time in which a child's sexual and physical characteristics start to mature due to an alteration in the hormonal milieu inside the body.

Adolescence is the period between puberty and adulthood.

Puberty is, thus, the phenomenon of physical changes by which the adolescent becomes capable of reproduction while adolescence is the psychological and social transition between childhood and adulthood. Puberty and adolescence, therefore, together, constitute a phase of biologic, cognitive, and psychosocial maturation.

Adolescence refers to the interphase between childhood and adulthood and includes the psychological experiences of the child during this period. Adolescence is the period of teenage years from 13 to 18 years of age and puberty decides the onset of adolescence. During adolescence, there is progressive psychological growth and children make adjustment in their personality due to rapid physical and sexual development which occurs due to onset of puberty.

ENDOCRINOLOGY OF NORMAL PUBERTY

The understanding of the origin and development of the hypothalamic-pituitary-ovarian (HPO) axis remains the key to understanding the endocrinology of puberty. The gonadotropin-releasing hormone (GnRH) is secreted by about 1,500–2,000 specialized neurosecretory cells in the arcuate nucleus of the medial basal hypothalamus. This was described as the "hypothalamic pulse generator" by Ernst Knobil who described the rhythmic, pulsatile nature of GnRH secretion.[1] This pulsatile release of GnRH triggers the secretion of follicle-stimulating hormone (FSH) and luteinizing hormone (LH) from the anterior pituitary, also in a pulsatile manner. This rhythmic gonadotropin secretion stimulates maturation of the germinal elements of the gonads which in turn secrete sex steroids, again in a pulsatile matter.[2]

The HPO axis is active even in fetal life. GnRH secreting neurons originate in the olfactory nodule and migrate to the hypothalamus by the 6th to 9th week of intrauterine life. The gonadotropin secretion from the fetal pituitary rises progressively from 12th week and reaches a peak at 20–24 weeks.[3] Thereafter, it declines steadily, probably in response to the negative feedback of placental estrogen and progesterone.[4,5]

Following birth, the steroid levels fall sharply due to withdrawal of maternal and placental hormones. The HPO axis, consequently, regains its pulsatile nature of secretion resulting in elevated levels of FSH and LH. There is a marked sex difference here with the rise of FSH being predominant in females and that of LH being predominant in males. The FSH stimulates waves of ovarian follicular development in the females[6] while the LH is responsible for increased testosterone secretion from the testes in males. By the age of 1 year in males and the age of 2–3 years in females, the gonadotropin levels fall to the prepubertal level, indicating the activation of the normal inherent negative feedback mechanism. Thereon, the diphasic pattern of gonadotropin secretion from infancy to puberty is due primarily to a central inhibition of pulsatile GnRH secretion and, to a lesser extent, on a high sensitivity to low levels of gonadal steroid feedback **(Fig. 1)**.

In the prepubertal period, the nature of the diurnal pulse changes with the secretion of LH far exceeding that of FSH, resulting in a marked decrease in the FSH:LH ratio. There is a 10-fold increase in LH as compared to a twofold increase in the level of FSH. This marked increase in LH translates into a detectable serum concentration of serum estradiol due to a coincident increase in the latter. With the advancement of puberty, the pulsatile LH secretion increases a further 20–40 times. Inhibin B, whose levels remain low or undetectable in the prepubertal period, increase sharply in puberty indicating ovarian stimulation and subsequently fall denoting the occurrence of the luteal phase. Rising levels of inhibin A, on the other hand, start in early puberty but peak only after menstruation confirming its primary source to be the corpus luteum.[7] Inhibin has a negative feedback effect on FSH but has no effect on LH.

It is clear from the above that there exists a "neuroendocrine switch" for the GnRH pulse generator which is "on" at infancy, turns "off" in childhood and turns "on" again at puberty.

The list of central factors modulating the HPO axis (both inhibitory and excitatory) may be described as follows:[8]

- *Gamma-aminobutyric acid (GABA)*: This is an inhibitory neurotransmitter secreted by the hypothalamus. Central GABA signaling is thought to be one of the factors which keeps GnRH neuronal activity in check during childhood.
- *Neuropeptide Y*: This is also an inhibitory neurotransmitter which keeps the GnRH pulsatile release in check.
- *Glutamate*: This is an excitatory neurotransmitter secreted by the hypothalamus. It stimulates GnRH release via intermediary (N-methyl-D-Aspartate (NMDA) receptors.

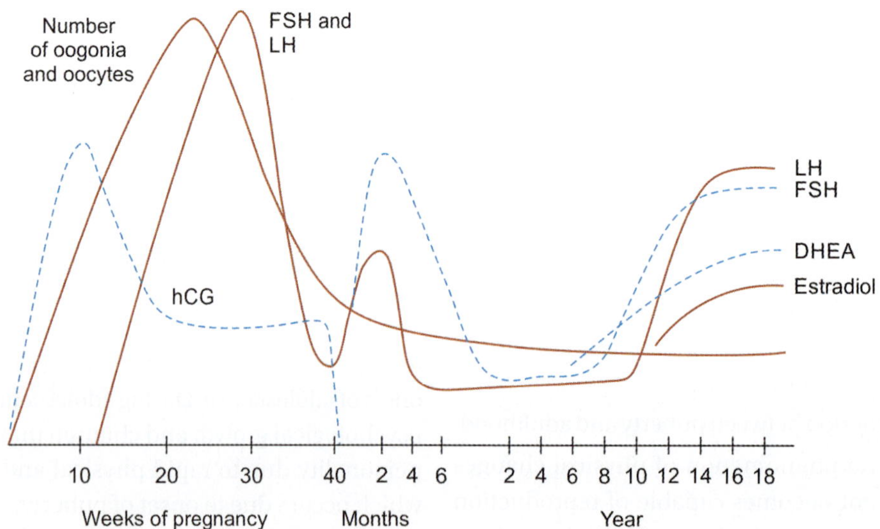

Fig. 1: Diphasic pattern of gonadotropins from infancy to puberty. (DHEA: dehydroepiandrosterone; FSH: follicle-stimulating hormone; hCG: human chorionic gonadotropin; LH: luteinizing hormone)

Source: Taylor HS, Pal L, Sell E. Speroff's Clinical Gynecologic Endocrinology and Infertility, 9th edition. Philadelphia: Lippincott Williams & Wilkins; 2019.

It probably plays a role in the resurgence of GnRH pulsatility at onset of puberty.

- *Kisspeptins*: In the past few years, kisspeptins have emerged as a primary factor regulating the pulsatile secretion of GnRH secretion. They appear to have an excitatory effect on the GnRH pulsatility by keeping it in check during childhood. Rising levels of kisspeptins at onset of puberty appear to trigger a coincident rise in the GnRH pulsatile secretion.

The most promising candidate in the peripheral signaling of the puberty mechanism appears to be leptin. It is produced by the adipocytes and serum concentrations correlate strongly with body fat. Leptin concentrations rise steadily throughout puberty in females. Leptin appears to be a somatic stimulus for the onset of puberty. Deficiency of this substance delays the onset of puberty. A study found that a 1 ng/mL increase in leptin concentration lowered the age of menarche by 1 month.[9]

Other candidates for metabolic signals proposed include ghrelin, insulin, galanin-like peptide, and free fatty acids. However, their role, if any, in the onset of puberty is yet to be established.

PHYSIOLOGY OF NORMAL PUBERTY

There appears to be a wide variation in the timing of pubertal maturation in individuals. However, the stages of pubertal development seem to follow a fairly predictable pattern. Puberty includes a series of predictable events that vary in timing, sequence, and pace. In girls, pubertal development typically occurs over 4.5 years. In general, the first sign of puberty in adolescent girls is an acceleration of growth (growth spurt) followed by breast budding (thelarche), the appearance of pubic hair (pubarche), and finally the onset of menses (menarche).

Gonadarche

This is the term used to dente the activation of the HPO axis with consequent maturation of the gonads. It is associated with increased secretion of sex steroids which in turn initiate and regulate the process of folliculogenesis and ovulation.

Adrenarche

Adrenarche is the increase in adrenal androgen production, namely dehydroepiandrosterone (DHEA) and dehydroepiandrosterone sulfate (DHEAS), which begins at 6 years of age in both boys and girls.[10,11] The primary stimulus for adrenarche is unknown though adrenocorticotropic hormone (ACTH) appears to be the most probable factor. It usually precedes activation of the HPO axis by 2–3 years. This suggests that the adrenal androgen secretion may stimulate the pubertal changes but the evidence is not conclusive. In girls, adrenarche presumably results in androgenic effects such as pubic hair, body odor, skin oiliness, and acne.[12]

Growth at Puberty

The first sign of puberty is an acceleration of growth. About 18% of adult growth is gained during puberty.[13] Distal limb growth precedes proximal limb growth and this is followed by trunk growth which primarily occurs in late puberty.[14] The pubertal growth spurt occurs approximately 2 years earlier in girls than in boys. Peak height velocity is reached approximately 6 months prior to menarche.[15] Bone mass accumulation during puberty is critical to the development peak bone mass, which is a major determinant of the risk of development of osteoporosis in later life. Peak bone mineral accretion in girls occurs at menarche, about 9–12 months after the peak height velocity is attained.[16,17]

Approximately 50% of total body calcium in females is accrued at puberty.[18,19] Although the peak bone mass is predominantly genetically determined, other factors such as nutrition and hormone exposure also contribute. During the growth spurt associated with puberty, the long bones grow in length and the epiphyses ultimately close.

Weight changes during puberty reflect the relative composition of lean body mass and fat. Adolescent girls have more body fat than boys which is mainly deposited in the upper arms, thighs and back. This body fat growth and distribution is mediated by estrogen. The body mass index (BMI) increases, initially due to an increase in the lean body mass and later due to fat.[20]

The growth rate during puberty is largely determined by the growth hormone (GH) which is secreted from the pituitary and regulated by hypothalamic GH-releasing hormone. GH is secreted in a pulsatile manner and peaks during puberty and declines with age at the rate of about 50% every 7 years.[21] The peripheral action of the GH is mediated via insulin-like growth factor-1 (IGF-1) which inhibits GH release. Nutritional factors such as fasting and high-protein diet stimulate GH secretion while hyperglycemia and leptin inhibit its release.[22,23]

The rate of increase of GH is the single most important determinant of the pubertal growth rate. Slower growing children have fewer and lower amplitude GH pulses and a more gradually increasing pattern.

Though GH and IGF-1 appear to be the predominant determinants of pubertal growth spurt, evidence suggests that sex steroids also play an important role by stimulating GH release.

Normal pubertal growth, therefore, involves the coordinated actions of GH and sex steroids.

Timing of Puberty

A number of factors seem to influence the timing of onset of puberty. Though genetic predisposition appears to be the major factor, other causes include nutritional state, general health, geographic location, social environment, environmental exposures, and psychological state **(Table 1)**.

TABLE 1: Factors influencing the onset of puberty.

Factors for early-onset puberty	Factors for late-onset puberty
Family history of early puberty	Family history of late puberty
Obesity	Lean body
Reside closer to equator	Reside further away from equator
Lower altitude	Higher altitude
Urban area	Rural area

Certain environmental toxicants which act as "endocrine disruptors" may influence the age of onset of puberty.[24] The age of onset of puberty has been slowly declining over the past decades. On an average, black American girls start puberty at 8–9 years of age and white American girls by 9 years of age. Pubertal onset in Indian girls starts at 10.3 years with an average interval of 1.5–2 years till menarche. Median age in Indian girls for thelarche is stated to be 10.8 years, that of pubarche 11.0 years, and that of menarche to be 12.4 years **(Fig. 2)**.[25]

Thelarche

This refers to the breast development in girls at puberty. The staging system for thelarche was first developed by Marshall and Tanner in 1969 **(Table 2)**.

Breast development, thus, follows a recognized sequence of events. Breast budding (Tanner stage II) is recognizable by enlargement and by widening of the areola. The breast then enlarges, becoming elevated beyond the areola (Tanner stage III). In Tanner stage IV, the breast enlarges further and a secondary mound is formed by the areola and nipple. This stage just precedes the Tanner stage V where the breast achieves the adult contour **(Fig. 3)**.

Pubarche

This term is applied to the development of pubic hair. It also includes axillary hair growth which occurs later (13 years), acne, and apocrine body odor. In most adolescents, pubarche closely follows thelarche. However, in a minority group thelarche follows pubarche. In both cases, the two are closely linked together.

The staging system used to classify the physical changes of puberty in girls were described by Marshall and Tanner in 1969.[26] This is also known as sexual maturity rating (SMR). This system classifies breast development in girls, pubic hair development in both sexes, and genital development in boys.

The development of axillary hair begins at an average age of 11.94 years, with a standard deviation of 0.93 years. The staging for development of axillary hair has been devised by the Central European study of the development of secondary sex characteristics in girls. Five stages for growth of axillary hair have been described **(Table 3)**.

Tanner Pubic Hair Staging

This is based on quantity and distribution **(Table 4)**. **Figure 4** shows the different Tanner stages of pubic hair development with stage I representing the prepubertal state and stage V representing the adult state.

Menarche

Menarche or the onset of first menstruation usually occurs at an average of 2.6 years after the onset of puberty and after the peak of growth has passed.[15,16,26] This is the most dramatic event which marks the culmination of the pubertal events. It may occur anytime between 10 and16 years, the peak time being 13 years. Ovarian estrogens induce endometrial proliferation and a temporary drop in their levels causes endometrial shedding in the form of menses. Initial anovulatory cycles persist for as much as 12–18 months and may even continue for 4 years after menarche. After menarche, growth slows down and generally does not increase >2.4 inches. The age of menarche is largely genetically determined. However, several factors such as obesity, overall health, environmental influences may affect the age at menarche.

The physical changes occurring during the process of puberty are presented in **Table 5**.

ADOLESCENCE

The word "adolescence" is derived from Latin meaning "to mature or grow up". It is a transitional period of physical and psychological development and encompasses the period from puberty to legal adulthood. This period is closely associated with the teenage years though its physical.

Adolescence can be divided into three stages:

1. *Early adolescence:* 9–13 years. This stage is characterized by growth spurt and development of secondary sexual characteristics.
2. *Mid adolescence:* 14–15 years. This stage involves psychological and emotional changes which include search for a new identity, attempt to break free from parental control, rebelliousness and aggressiveness, formation of new relationships with peer group, and experimentation. This age group also become aware of their bodily changes which may lead to shyness and clumsiness.
3. *Late adolescence:* 16–19 years. In this stage, the adolescents have fully developed physical characteristics. By this time they have usually formed a distinct identity and harbor well-formed ideas and opinions. Cognitive functions develop considerably resulting in enhanced communication skills and ability to think abstractly and critically **(Table 5)**.

Adolescence, in general, involves emotional unpredictability, oversensitivity, and an unusual vulnerability. They exhibit a desire for independence and autonomy and possess a strong desire to belong.

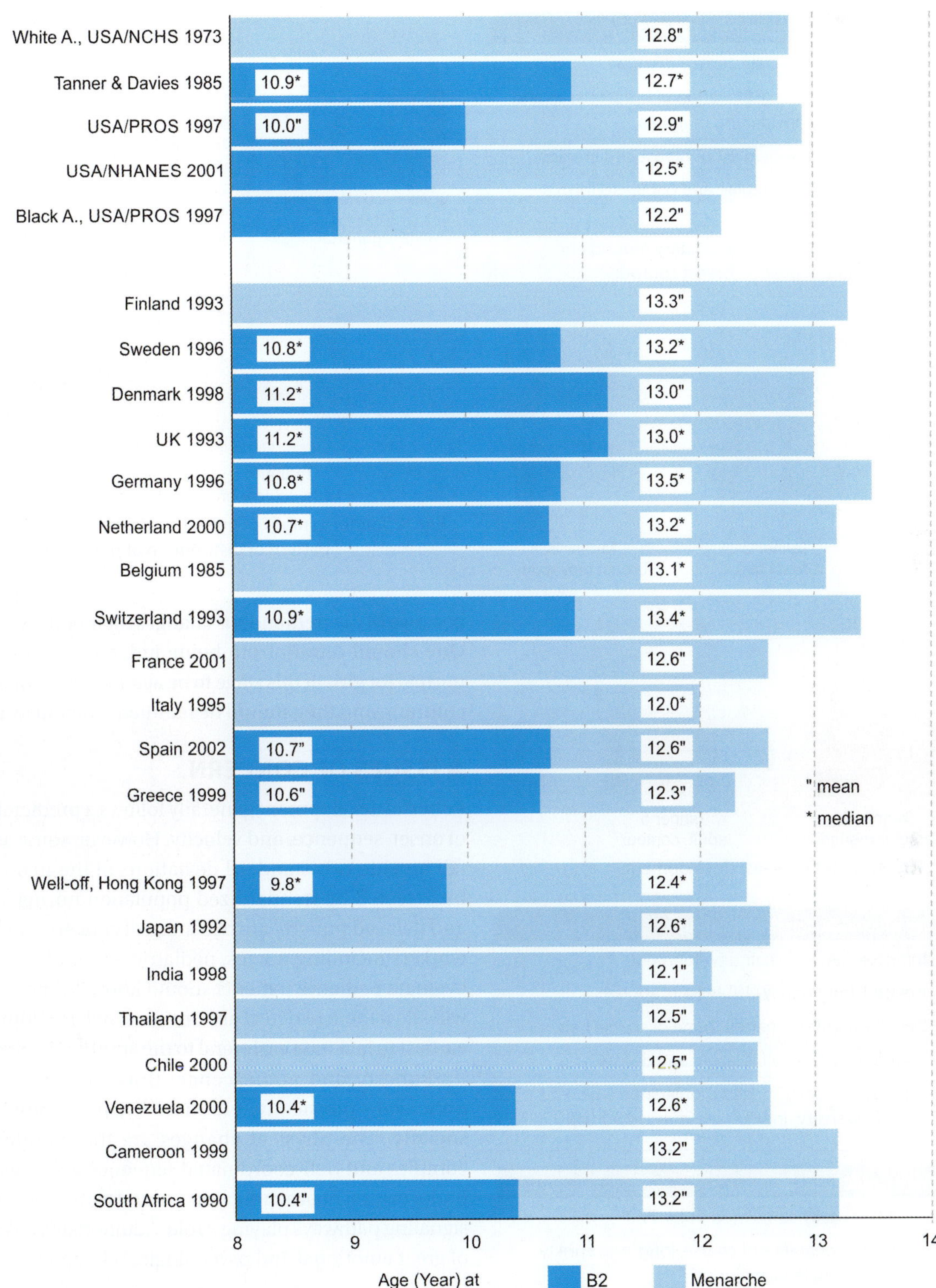

Fig. 2: Average (mean or median) ages at onset of breast development (B2) and menarche in different well-off populations around the world. *Source:* Brix N, Andreas E, Lea LB, Parner E, Støvring H, Olsen J, et al. Timing of puberty in boys and girls: a population-based study. Pediatr Perinat Epidemiol. 2019;33(1):70-8.

CARE DURING PUBERTY

This involves a multidimensional aspect and includes physical, social, emotional, and psychological parameters. Girls should be taught the basics oh hygienic practices and encouraged to inculcate them as lifelong habits. These include the following:

- Putting on clean clothes including underwear everyday
- Washing hands and face with soap and water twice daily
- Daily shower with washing all body parts and hair
- Brushing teeth twice a day
- Deodorant may be used for the body odor
- Drinking lots of clean water
- Eating healthy food

TABLE 2: Tanner's breast development staging in girls.	
Tanner stage I	***Prepubertal elevation of papilla***
Tanner stage II	Breast budding: Elevation of breast tissue and papilla and widening of areola
Tanner stage III	Further enlargement of breast and areolae
Tanner stage IV	Projection of areolae and papilla to form a secondary mound
Tanner stage V	Disappearance of secondary mound and formation of adult breast contour

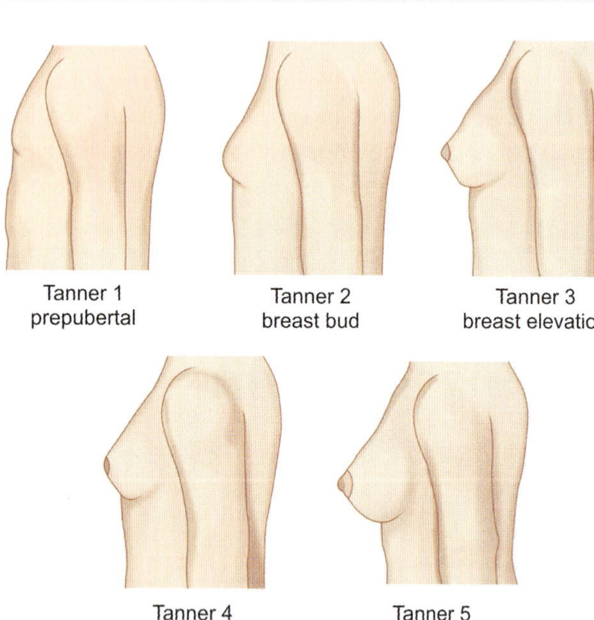

Fig. 3: Stages of breast development.

TABLE 3: Stages of axillary hair development.	
Stage A1	Infantile stage: No hair development
Stage A2	Isolated, long barely visible hairs appear
Stage A3	Development of a narrow band of sparse hair
Stage A4	Area covered by hair is larger and denser
Stage A5	Adult stage: Longish, rectangular area covered by hair of a density and texture found in adults

TABLE 4: Tanner's pubic hair staging.	
Tanner stage I	No sexually stimulated pubic hair
Tanner stage II	First appearance of coarse, long, and crinkly hair along labia majora
Tanner stage III	Coarse, curly hair extends onto the mons pubis
Tanner stage IV	Adult hair in thickness and texture but not as widely distributed in adults. Does not extend on to the inner aspect of thighs
Tanner stage V	Extension of pubic hair onto the thighs

- Maintaining menstrual hygiene in the form timely changing of pads and using clean and sterile pads.

Parents and elders should be empathetic to the adolescent girl as this is a period of great fear and insecurity for them because of the tremendous changes their body is undergoing. One should refrain from being judgmental or critical. It is normal for girls at this stage to be aggressive, inconsistent, and contrary, and they should be handled judiciously and gently.

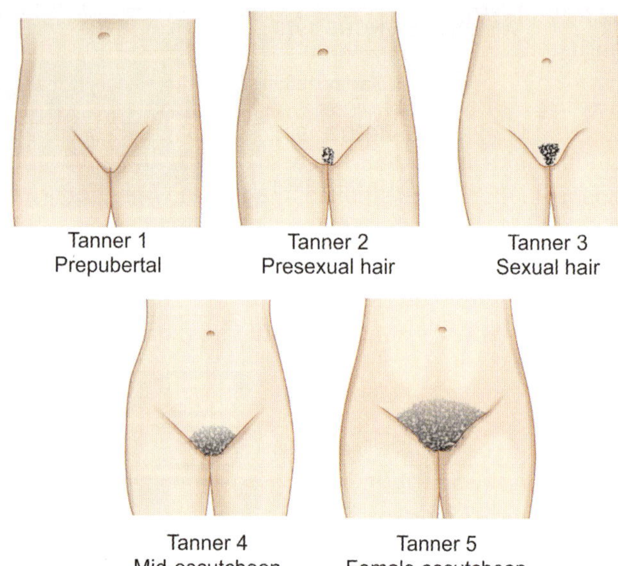

Fig. 4: Tanner's stages of pubic hair development. Escutcheon = pattern of distribution of pubic hair.

ISSUES OF CONCERN

Pubertal development generally follows a predictable pattern of onset, sequence, and velocity. However, some adolescents fall outside two standard deviations of the mean. This can be detected by standardized population norms. Precocious and delayed puberty are two areas of concern. All healthcare workers including nurses, pediatricians, and assistants who evaluate pediatric patients should know Tanner stages. This will allow them to detect abnormal sexual development at the earliest to facilitate early feral to the appropriate specialist.[26,27]

Puberty and adolescence, thus, is a period of great upheaval—physically, emotionally, psychologically, and socially. The physical changes are the culmination of a complex and well-coordinated sequence of events which are under central neuroendocrinal control with several peripheral signaling pathways playing a role. Additionally, it is also a time of great emotional and psychological change.

KEY MESSAGES

- Normal pubertal development occurs in a predictable, orderly sequence over a definite time frame.
- Transition into puberty is controlled by two physiological processes namely adrenarche and gonadarche.
- Pubertal changes occur between the ages of 8 and 13 years.
- Puberty involves a finely synchronized hypothalamic-pituitary-ovarian (HPO) axis which is largely responsible for the physical changes which occur.

TABLE 5: Physical changes at puberty in boys and girls.

Tanner staging	*Girls*	*Boys*
Tanner stage 1	• 8 years of age • Release of GnRH, FSH, and LH • No noticeable physical changes	• 10 years of age • Release of GnRH, FSH, and LH • No noticeable physical changes
Tanner stage 2	• 9–11 years • Formation of breast buds • Areola starts to expand • Uterus begins to grow • Small amounts of pubic hair appear	• 11 years • Testicles and overlying skin start to grow • Early stages of pubic hair forms at base of penis
Tanner stage 3	• 12 years • Breast buds continue to grow • Pubic hair gets thicker and curlier • Axillary hair starts forming • Acne starts to appear • Highest growth rate for height begins (about 3.2 inches/ear)	• 13 years • Testicles continue to grow, penis gets longer • Some breast tissue may start to form • Night ejaculation starts • Voice begins to change and crack • Muscles get larger • Height growth increases (2–3.2 inches/year)
Tanner stage 4	• 13 years • Breasts transition from the bud stage to take on a fuller contour • Menarche occurs (between 12 and 14 years, may occur earlier) • Height growth slows down to about 2–3 inches/year • Pubic hair becomes denser	• 14 years • Testicles, penis, scrotum enlarge, and scrotum gets darker in color • Axillary hair starts to grow • Deeper voice becomes permanent • Acne may start to appear
Tanner stage 5	• 15 years • Breasts reach adult shape and size • Periods become regular after 6 months to 2 years of menarche • Reach adult height • Reproductive organs and genitals are fully developed	• 15 years • Penis, scrotum, and testicles reach adult size • Pubic hair extends to inner thighs • Facial hair starts to grow • Growth in height slows down but muscles continue to grow

(FSH: follicle-stimulating hormone; GnRH: gonadotropin-releasing hormone; LH: luteinizing hormone)

- Several central and peripheral factors modulate the HPO axis.
- Adolescence is also a time for tremendous psychological changes which should be handled with empathy.

REFERENCES

1. Knobil E. Remembrance: the discovery of the hypothalamic gonadotropin-releasing hormone pulse generator and of its physiological significance. Endocrinology. 1992;131:1005-6.
2. Taylor HS, Pal L, Sell E. Normal and abnormal growth and pubertal development. In: Taylor HS, Pal L, Sell E (Eds). Speroff's Clinical Gynecologic Endocrinology and Infertility, 9th edition. Philadelphia: Lippincott Williams & Wilkins; 2019. pp. 304.
3. DiVall SA, Radovick S. Pubertal development and menarche. Ann N Y Acad Sci. 2008;1135:19-28.
4. Styne DM. Physiology of puberty. Horm Res. 1994;419(Suppl 2):3-6.
5. Grumbach MM. The neuroendocrinology of human puberty revisited. Horm Res. 2002;57(Suppl 2):2-14.
6. Winter JS, Hughes IA, Reyes FI, Faiman C. Pituitary-gonadal relations in infancy: 2. Patterns of serum gonadal steroid concentrations in man from birth to two years of age. J Clin Endocriol Metab. 1976;42:679-86.
7. Sehested A, Juul AA, Anderson AM, Petersen JH, Jensen TK, Müller J, et al. Serum Inhibin A and Inhibin B in healthy prepubertal, pubertal and adolescent girls and adult women: relation to age, stage of puberty, menstrual cycle, follicle-stimulating hormone, luteinizing hormone, and estradiol levels, J Clin Endocrinol Metab. 2000;85:1634-40.
8. Taylor HS, Pal L, Sell E. Speroff's Clinical Gynecologic Endocrinology and Infertility. Philadelphia: Lippincott Williams & Wilkins; 2019. pp. 306.
9. Matkovic V, Ilich JZ, Skugor M, Badenhop NE, Goel P, Clairmont A, et al. Leptin is inversely related to age at menarche in human females. J Clin Endocrinol Metab. 1997;82:3239-45.
10. Korth-Schutz S, Levine LS, New MI. Dehydroepiandrosterone sulphate (DS) levels, a rapid test for abnormal adrenal androgen secretion. J Clin Endocrinol Metab. 1976;42:1005-13.
11. De Peretti E, Forest MG. Pattern of plasma dehydroepiandrosterone sulphate levels in humans from birth to adulthood: evidence for testicular production. J Clin Endocrinol Metab. 1978;47:572-7.
12. Agarwal KN, Agarwal DK. Adolescence in Indian Children. Ann Pediatr Res. 2020;4(3):1-8.
13. Abbassi V. Growth and normal puberty. Pediatrics. 1998;102:507-11.
14. Bass S, Delmas PD, Pearce G, Hendrich E, Tabensky A, Seeman E. The differing tempo of growth in bone size, mass and density in girls is region-specific. J Clin Invest. 1999;104:795-804.
15. Biro FM, Huang B, Crawford PB, Lucky AW, Striegel-Moore R, Barton BA, et al. Pubertal correlates in black and white girls. J Pediatr. 2006;148:234-40.

16. Taranger J, Engstrom I, Lichtenstein H, Svennberg-Redegren I. Somatic pubertal development. Acta Paediatr Scand Suppl. 1976;258:121-35.
17. McKay HA, Bailey DA, Mirwald RL, Davison KS, Faulkner RA. Peak bone minimal accrual and age at menarche in adolescent girls: a 6-year longitudinal study. J Pediatr. 1998;133:682-7.
18. Lloyd T, Rolings N, Andon MB, Demers LM, Eggli DF, Kieselhorst K, et al. Determinants of bone density in young women. I. Relationships among pubertal development, total body bone mass and total body bone density in premenarchal females. J Clin Endocrinol Metab. 1992;75:383-7.
19. Magarey AM, Boulton TJ, Chatterton BE, Schultz C, Nordin BE, Cockington RA. Bone growth from 11 to17 years: relationship to growth, gender and changes with pubertal status including timing of menarche. Acta Paediatr. 1999;88:139-46.
20. Maynard LM, Wisemandle W, Roche AF, Chumlea WC, Guo SS, Siervogel RM. Childhood body composition in relation to body mass index. Pediatrics. 2001;107:344-50.
21. Giustina A, Veldhuis JD. Pathophysiology of the neuroregulation of growth hormone secretion in experimental animals and the human. Endocr Rev. 1998;19:717-97.
22. Unger RH. The hyperleptinemia of obesity–regulator of caloric surpluses. Cell. 2004;117:154-9.
23. Tanner JM. Growth at Adolescence, 2nd edition. Oxford, UK: Blackwell Scientific Publications; 1962.
24. Crain DA, Janssen SJ, Edwards TM, Heindel J, Ho S, Hunt P, et al. Female reproductive disorders: the role of endocrine-disrupting compounds and developmental timing. Fertil Steril. 2008;90:911-40.
25. Khadgawat R, Marwaha RK, Mehan N, Surana V, Dabas A, Sreenivas V, et al, Age of onset of puberty in apparently healthy school girls from Northern India. Indian Pediatr. 2016;53:383-7.
26. Marshall WA, Tanner JM. Variations in pattern of pubertal changes in girls. Arch Dis Child. 1969;44:291-303.
27. Berenbaum SA, Belt AM, Corley R. The importance of puberty for adolescent development: conceptualization and measurement. Adv Child Dev Behav. 2015;48:53-92.

LONG QUESTIONS

1. Define puberty. Discuss the physiological changes which occur at puberty.
2. Discuss the endocrinology of normal puberty.
3. Discuss the growth changes which occur at puberty.

SHORT QUESTIONS

1. Describe Tanner's staging of pubic hair development.
2. Describe Tanner's staging of breast development.
3. What is the average age of onset of puberty in Indian girls? Enumerate the factors that may influence the timing of puberty.
4. Describe the stages of adolescence.
5. List the factors which modulate the HPO axis.

MULTIPLE CHOICE QUESTIONS

1. FSH production is inhibited by:
   a. LH b. GnRH
   c. Inhibin d. LH
2. Gonadotropin secretion from the fetal pituitary reaches a peak at:
   a. 8–10 weeks b. 20–24 weeks
   c. 14–16 weeks d. 30–32 weeks
3. The key regulator of puberty is:
   a. Kisspeptin b. LH
   c. GnRH d. FSH
4. The order of pubertal development in girls is:
   a. Adrenarche-pubarche-menarche
   b. Thelarche-menarche-pubarche
   c. Pubarche-thelarche-menarche
   d. Thelarche-pubarche-menarche
5. The central factors controlling the HPO axis include all of the below, except:
   a. Kisspeptin
   b. Gamma amino butyric acid
   c. Neuropeptide Y
   d. Thyroxine
   e. Glutamate
6. The HPO axis is active in:
   a. Prepubertal period b. Intrauterine life
   c. At menarche d. 8–10 years of age
7. At puberty:
   a. Secretion of LH increases
   b. Secretion of FSH increases
   c. Secretion of both increase
   d. Secretion of both decrease

Answers

1. c 2. b 3. a 4. d 5. d 6. b
7. a

Basic Aspects of Gynaecological Care

7.1 ELICITING HISTORY AND EXAMINING GYNAECOLOGICAL PATIENTS

S Sampathkumari

INTRODUCTION

History is important not only to an archeologist to construct a linkage between the present and the past but is even more important and relevant in medical field also. It helps in avoiding incorrect diagnoses, prevents assumptions, and helps close the chasm between the actual situations and the unknown past that may or may not be the causative factor for the presenting complaints. A skip in eliciting proper information from the patient could lead to unnecessary investigations that may impact the time and money factors which patients sometimes could not afford. A casual and negligent attitude will be detrimental to the whole process and hence should be avoided.

When a little more time is spent with the patient, it not only improves the relationship with the patient but also earns the doctor trust and confidence of the patient that may continue even after the ailment is cured.

By making the patient feel at ease, handling sensitive issues deftly and asking leading questions the effort ensures that the physician diagnose properly, prescribe appropriate medication and decide the course of action that is adequate and satisfactory. A physician should deal with the patient more patiently and with care. Very often the actual cause of the complaint may lie underneath a host of unrelated, misleading complaints, and unimportant events that a patient may consider irrelevant and unnecessary.

A good gynecological diagnosis is possible by knowing the history of the patient, carrying out thorough clinical examination, and conducting relevant investigations. Rapport with the patient can be established by knowing her age, parity, and complaints. Significance of age lies in the fact that different conditions are more prevalent in different age groups. Details of patients' husband's name and address of residence will help in identification between patients having same names. Patient should be asked to state her main complaints and relate her present illness sequentially in her own words. Previous gynecological problem and treatment underwent are verified with old records to prevent missing any point and repeating a previously performed investigation.

HISTORY OF PRESENT COMPLAINTS

When the patient presents her complaint consider them by looking at the nature, onset, duration, external causes, etiology, preexisting conditions, severity, relieving factors, and the complications that are manifested by the complaint. When more than one complaint is present a careful analysis is imperative by correlating them with past history, their association with other complaints to understand the complexity, and the factors that complicate. Some examples of common complaints are:

- *Abnormal uterine bleeding*: Bleeding from vagina which patients considers as abnormal should be evaluated. Ask the patient about her menstrual pattern. Normal pattern is expressed as 4/28, meaning bleeds for 4 days once in 28 days. Normal bleeding is about 30–80 mL. bleeding before 9 years and after 52 years of age need investigation. Bleeding regularly, profuse or scanty, associated with pain or not, pain present before (congestive dysmenorrhea) or during menstruation (spasmodic dysmenorrhea), postcoital, and intermenstrual bleeding (ovulatory) are the points to be noted. History of passing clots, number of pads used to be elicited. Rule out amenorrhea as pregnancy and associated complications—ectopic, abortion, and molar pregnancy can present as heavy menstrual bleeding.
- *Abdominal pain*: Most gynecological problems are associated with abdominal pain, e.g., pelvic inflammatory disease (PID), torsion of ovarian cyst, endometriosis, and ectopic. Site of pain, onset, character, pattern of radiation, relieving, and aggravating factors provide important diagnostic clues. Acute pain followed by amenorrhea/

bleeding—ectopic, acute pain in young/old—ovarian torsion, and continuous pain during menses—fibroid/dysfunctional uterine bleeding (DUB)/endometriosis. Back pain below the first sacral vertebra—prolapse.

- *Infertility*: In cases of infertility, male factors such as occupation, alcoholic, smoking, injury, mumps, surgery for varicocele, hydrocele, undescended testis, frequency of coitus, premature and retrograde ejaculation, and any treatment taken and female factors such as menstrual cycle history, vaginismus, dyspareunia, galactorrhea, hirsutism, and mass abdomen should be recorded.
- *Vaginal discharge*: White discharge is the complaint of two-thirds gynecological outpatient. In younger age, menstrual hygiene and nutritional status are the points of vital nature. Discharge after menopause has to be investigated. Discharge before and after menstruation, during ovulation and postcoital are normal phenomena. Discharge with foul smelling and pain need evaluation. Amount, color, consistency of discharge, and itching history should be elicited. White, milky, and nonmucous—bacterial vaginosis, curdy—candidiasis, purulent—gonorrhea, malodorous—chronic infection/CA, increased discharge—chlamydia, fishy odor greenish discharge—trichomonas.
- *Abdominal mass*: Patients may miss this finding due to obesity. Onset, site of origin, and size and whether associated with pain (torsion) or painless (carcinoma) offer clue for diagnosis. History of weight reduction and loss of appetite helps in detecting malignancy. Big mass leads to pressure symptoms as change in micturition and bowel habits. Midline mass is described corresponding to uterine size in pregnancy.
- *Mass descending per vaginum*: Whether sudden onset or gradual, reducible or not give treatment clues. In this complaint obstetric history regarding delivery—place of delivery, conducted by trained person, spacing between deliveries, duration, and method of delivery are crucial. Micturition habits regarding frequency or dribbling during cough or laugh define the type of prolapse. Chronic prolapse is associated with bleeding and discharge. History of constipation, need for splinting digitations in rectal symptoms is important. Need to differentiate between prolapsed and infravaginal elongation of cervix. Examine tone of pelvic floor—levator ani and perineal body to assess need for pelvic floor repair surgery.
- *Malignancies of genital tract*: Loss of weight, loss of appetite, weight reduction, postmenopausal bleeding and discharge with purulent smell, and postcoital bleeding needs evaluation.
- *Menopausal symptoms*: Present in most of the women nearing menopause as hot flushes, increased sweating, loss of libido, dry vagina, sexual dysfunction, mental irritability, tiredness, and depression. Differentiate it from premature ovarian failure and other endocrinological disorders. History of taking any hormone replacement therapy (HRT) should be elicited, if yes, breast examination (mammogram), bone density, and lipid profile has to be evaluated.

Menstrual History

Menarche

Age at menarche, normally between 10 and 16 years. Primary amenorrhea refers to the failure of onset of menstruation beyond the age of 14 years without secondary sexual characteristics, and failure of onset of menstruation beyond the age of 16 years with well-developed secondary sexual characteristics. Evaluate other factors such as breast development, presence of axillary hair, development of pubic hair, development of external genitalia, cyclical abdominal pain, and other endocrinological factors. History of headache, visual disturbance, galactorrhea, loss of smell, height, and history of amenorrhea in siblings are elicited to evaluate pituitary, hypothalamus, and chromosomal problems. Cyclical pain, amenorrhea, and retention of urine can point to diagnosis of cryptomenorrhea.

Secondary amenorrhea is failure of menstruation for 6 months or longer in women who were previously menstruating. In such cases, history of tuberculosis (TB) exposure and bleeding following delivery should be elicited.

Irregular Bleeding

Date of last menstrual period (LMP) and previous cycle history are important. Normal bleeding is for 5 days, once in 28 days (21–35 days). Amount of flow is 30–80 mL without clots. History of amount of flow—scanty, profuse/heavy with clots to be recorded. If the flow is scanty or absent for 2 or 3 months [polycystic ovarian disease (PCOD)], factors such as obesity, facial growth in chin, jaw, upper arm, back, chest, and legs need a closer look at. If profuse and irregular—whether first time or recurrent in nature should be enquired into. Irregular bleeding could be by ovulation, hormonal fluctuation. or organic disease. PALM-COEIN classification of heavy menstrual bleeding is classified with history of bleeding type and examination (polyp, adenomyosis, leiomyoma, malignancy, coagulopathy, ovulatory dysfunction, endometrial, iatrogenic, not classified). If continuous bleeding is present, ectopic, miscarriage, and carcinoma are to be ruled out.

Menstrual Cramps

Age at onset, severity, and character of cramps and any treatment for relief, whether regular life is being disturbed is to ne noted. Primary dysmenorrhea may be idiopathic and secondary dysmenorrhea may have associated pathology.

Premenstrual history of breast discomfort, irritability, depression, back ache, and pelvic pain are also elicited.

Menopause

Cessation of menstruation for 1 year is defined as menopause, 45–50 years. Postmenopausal bleeding is evaluated for malignancy.

Marital History

Age at marriage, consanguinity, frequency of intercourse, dyspareunia, achievement of orgasm, and living with husband or partner are to be elicited. Habitual history of partners (present and past), number of partners is important to rule out infection, infertility, and carcinoma.

Contraceptive History

Record the type, method, and duration of contraception used along with attendant complications such as amenorrhea, thromboembolic disease, dysmenorrhea, heavy bleeding, pelvic infection with intrauterine contraceptive device (IUCD), and failure of contraception. History of puerperal sterilization done or not is very essential.

Obstetric History

It plays an important role in certain gynecological diagnoses to plan for treatment. History of number of deliveries, number of children alive, miscarriages, and last child birth are enquired into. Details of every pregnancy, delivery, and abortion—termination method are to be recorded chronologically. History regarding number of deliveries whether conducted by trained person or not, spacing between deliveries, duration and method of delivery, institution or home delivery, instrumental delivery, treatment or blood transfusion postdelivery [postpartum hemorrhage (PPH)], and lactation history are very important. Repeated abortion gives clues for PID and genetic problems. Parity helps in identifying risk factors for carcinoma—endometrial cancer, ovarian cancer more in nulliparous, and cervical cancer more in multiparous women.

Past History: Medical

History suggestive of TB (genital TB), asthma, and chronic cough (prolapse), diabetes and hypertension (for anesthesia), epilepsy, thyroid disorders, sexually transmitted disease (STD), human immunodeficiency virus (HIV), and history of blood transfusion must be entered. History of treatment of endometriosis is essential in cases of infertility and pelvic pain.

Obtain previous colposcopy reports and records of treatment given, follow-up details if available.

Surgical History

Any surgery underwent for present complaints (myomectomy and uterine artery embolization for fibroids, endometrial ablation for DUB, lap surgery for infertility, and sling surgeries for prolapse), history of any other surgery (nongynecologic) such as thyroidectomy, appendicectomy, any abdominal surgery (adhesions), etc., are also elicited.

Personal History

History regarding appetite, bowel habits, micturition, allergy to drugs, food and chemicals, alcohol, smoking, and tobacco chewing should also be entered.

Family History

Details of TB, diabetes mellitus (DM), hypertension, asthma, and carcinomas such as CA breast, CA ovary, and colon tumors are important.

Before going in for examination, summarize the history of relevant points for confirmation with the patient. Both the patient and the gynecologist get an opportunity to correct and add any additional information.

GENERAL EXAMINATION

General examination includes built of the body (mild/moderate/ill built), state of nutrition (cachexic or emaciated—malignancy), and state of well-being. In initial examination, mark details of height, weight, icterus, pallor, body mass index (BMI) and arm span (for endocrinological disorders). Examination of secondary sexual characters and hirsutism are needed in cases of amenorrhea and infertility. Examination should be systematic and must include the following:

- *Vital signs*: Temperature, pulse rate, and blood pressure (BP)
- *Head and neck*: Look for thyroid, supraclavicular lymph nodes, webbing of neck, and oral hygiene.
- *Cardiovascular system (CVS) and respiratory system (RS)*: Respiratory rate and CVS examined for murmurs.
- *Breast*: Very important for gynecological examination as it is the most likely site for cancer than the genitals. History of galactorrhea, bloody, or watery discharge from nipple is essential. Palpate for lump in sitting and lying posture and also educate the patient for self-examination. Tanner's staging of breast development and axillary hair to be noted in cases of primary amenorrhea **(Figs. 1A to C)**.
- *Spine*: Look for curvature of the spine (kyphosis or scoliosis) for anesthesia and to evaluate osteoporosis.
- *Extremities*: Presence of pedal edema, varicosities, cutaneous lesions, and pulsation should be noted.

ABDOMINAL EXAMINATION

Irrespective of the complaints abdominal examination is done routinely. Bladder should be emptied before examination.

Inspection

Contour of the abdomen (flat/scaphoid/protuberant), distension, movement with respiration, scars, any visible pulsation, umbilical position, presence of incisional hernia, distribution of hair and mass (size, shape, and site), and

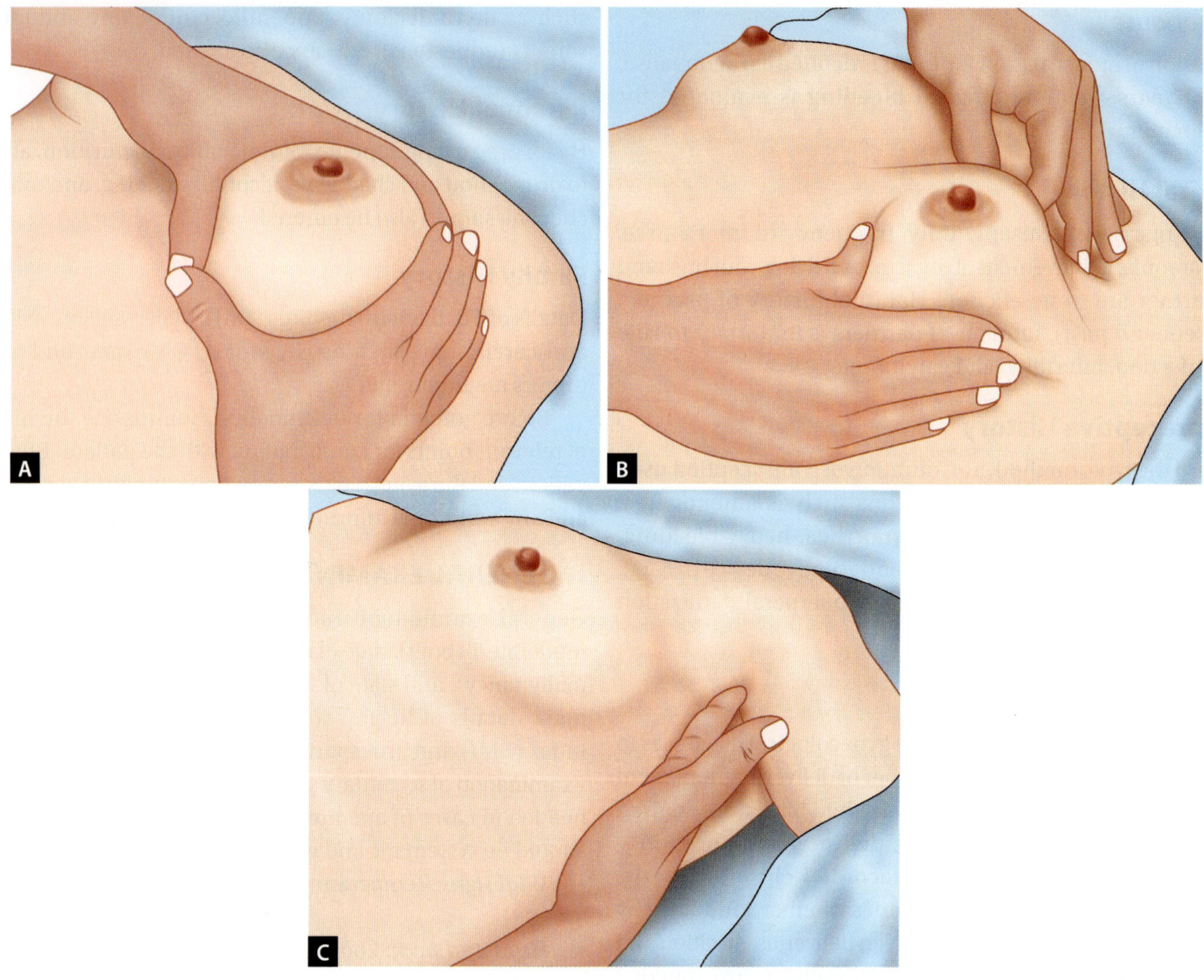

Figs. 1A to C: Breast examination.

enlarged lymph nodes are clearly noted. Any endometriotic scar and presence of Sister Joseph nodes are specifically noted—represents cutaneous deposit of CA ovary.

Palpation (Fig. 2)

Palpate by standing on the right side of the patient for any mass and note the size, shape, site, extension, margins—well-defined/ill-defined, consistency—cystic (ovarian mass) or solid (fibroid) or variable (malignant), smooth or nodular, fixed or mobile, whether associated with pain (fibroid or endometriosis), and/or ascites (ovarian malignancy). Watch the facial reaction for any tenderness, if present, look for guarding, rigidity and rebound tenderness (peritoneal irritation). Abdominal examination is incomplete without palpation of liver, spleen, para-aortic nodes, and kidneys.

Examples:

- *Uterine mass*: Mostly midline, mobile horizontally, and limited vertically. It moves with the movement of cervix.
- *Ovarian mass*: Usually in one iliac region and freely mobile, firm to hard. Large ovarian mass occupies the whole abdomen.
- *Tenderness* in both iliac fossa/hypochondrium—PID
- *Unilateral tenderness*—ectopic/torsion.

Percussion

Differentiates between solid mass, distended bowel, and free fluid in the peritoneal cavity. Large ovarian cyst—dull on percussion, distended bowel—resonant on percussion, and free fluid in peritoneal cavity—dullness in flanks which shifts. Free fluid in peritoneal cavity is elicited be following signs: puddle sign—knee elbow position (minimal), shifting dullness—midline to lateral (500 mL fluid), horseshoe—dull around flank and suprapubic region with center resonant (1,000 mL), fluid thrill—transmission of impulses (2,000 mL), gentle tap on flank while keeping palm of other hand on opposite flank—thrill is felt on palm.

Auscultation

Not routinely done in gynecological examination. Acute abdomen with bowel obstruction and postoperative paralytic ileus—bowel sound auscultated. Soufflé over tumor indicates vascularity.

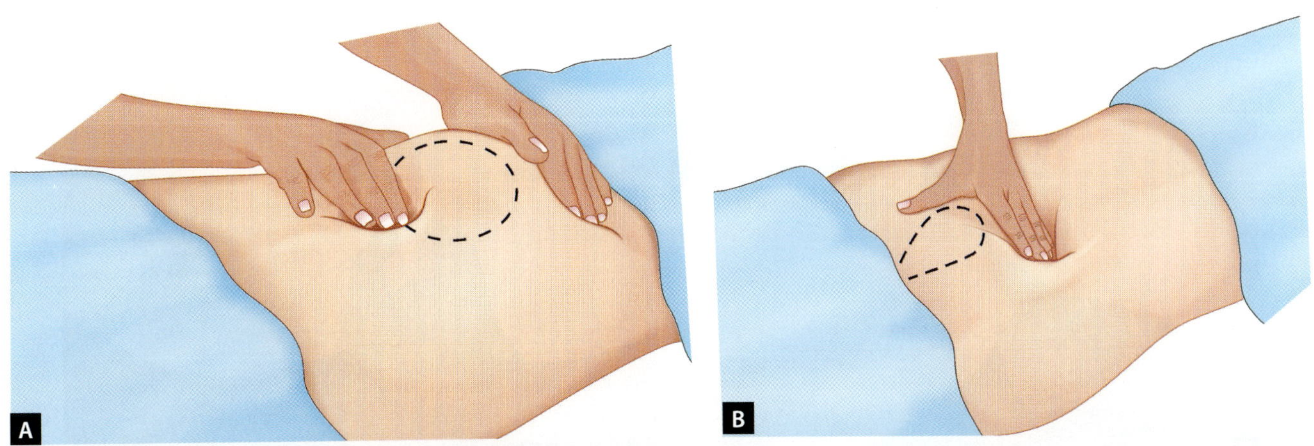

Figs. 2A and B: Abdominal palpation.

PELVIC EXAMINATION

Before pelvic examination, verbal consent of the patient is important. Explain the procedure to the patient for her to be relaxed and cooperative. Presence of chaperone and privacy is essential as are good light, glove, and lubricant jelly. Pelvic examination includes external examination, bimanual, and rectal examination.

External Examination (Fig. 3)

Patient is examined in dorsal position, look for degree of development and lesions of labia, character of hymen and introitus (virgin, nulliparous, or multiparous), and distribution of hair. Document lesions, growth, mass, and discharge at external genitalia. Specially look for clitoromegaly, Bartholin's gland (junction of anterior two-thirds and posterior one-third of labia majora), urethra, and Skene's glands for purulent exudates. Perineal relaxation and scarring are noted for history of dyspareunia and defects in rectal sphincter tone. Note down degree and reducibility of prolapse in cases of mass descending per vaginum. Document dryness, ulcer, and rugosities on mass. Other positions for examination are left lateral positions, Sims' semiprone position—good for external genitalia, cervix and vaginal wall exposing vaginal end of vesicovaginal fistula (VVF) and lithotomy position for under anesthesia examination.

To demonstrate the stress incontinence patient is asked to cough or bear down. If patient complaints of stress or urgency then she should be examined in full bladder.

Speculum Examination

Speculum should be warmed with warm water and not lubricated as it may interfere with cervical cytology reports. Cusco speculum is a bivalve; self-retaining speculum designed to open after insertion to visualize the cervix and is useful to take smear or swabs. Cervix is noted for its color, shape, centrally placed os or transverse configuration (multiparous), any discharge, any polyp, any growth, and distended nabothian follicles. Look for transformation zone (squamocolumnar junction) in perimenopausal women. Pap smear is taken by rotating spatula twice around the os at 360° and smeared. Endocervical tissue is sampled with cytobrush. If the patient is in lithotomy position at the edge of couch, speculum can be turned downwards to avoid pressure on clitoris. If lying on couch, rotate the speculum upwards. Sims' speculum needs vaginal wall retractor to visualize and another person to take smears is good for prolapse and VVF.

Bimanual Examination (Fig. 4)

Bimanual examination is done after the bladder is emptied, provides information about the cervix, uterus, and adnexa. The labia are separated and two fingers of right hand is inserted through the vaginal introitus as the left hand is placed over the abdomen (suprapubic region). The cervix is palpated by the right hand fingers for hardness and irregularity and tenderness to motion. The uterine position size, mobility, shape, and tenderness are experienced with the left hand while the right hand fingers pressing the anterior or posterior fornices. The inserted fingers in the vagina are moved to lateral fornix to palpate the adnexal mass. Normally ovaries are not palpable. Pouch of Douglas (POD) is examined for any mass and endometriotic nodule. Uterosacral ligament can be palpated in posterior fornix. In endometriosis it may be scarred or shortened. Uterine mass is differentiated by transmitted mobility with cervix and adnexal mass shows a groove between mass and uterus.

Rectal Examination

Rectal examination is performed in virgins to examine uterine and adnexal pathology and in specific conditions such as carcinoma to evaluate the extent up to parametrium and involvement of rectal mucosa. Rectal examination also differentiated rectocele and enterocele. Weakness of the pelvic floor and tone of anal sphincter are noted. Anus is noted for lesions, hemorrhoids and inflammations.

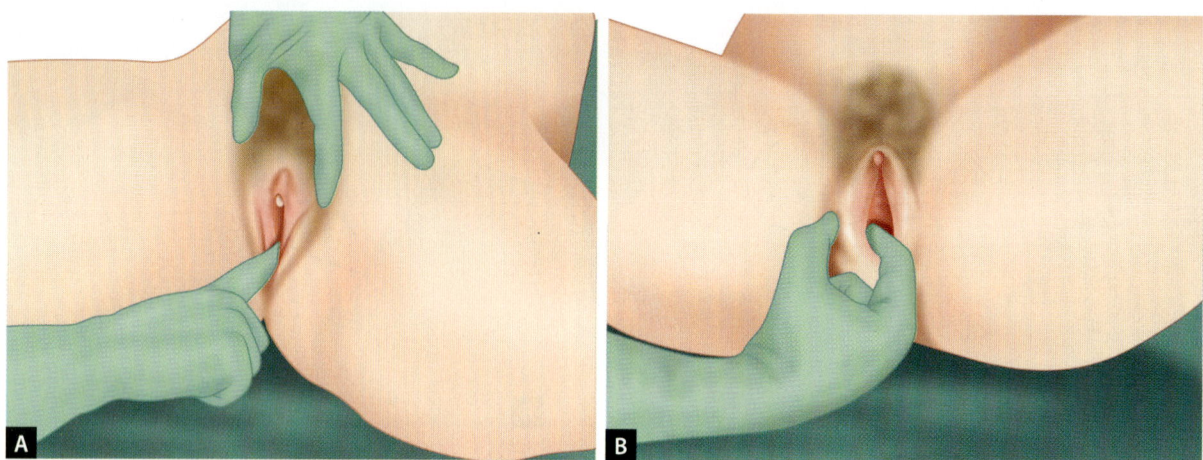

Figs. 3A and B: Examining the introitus.

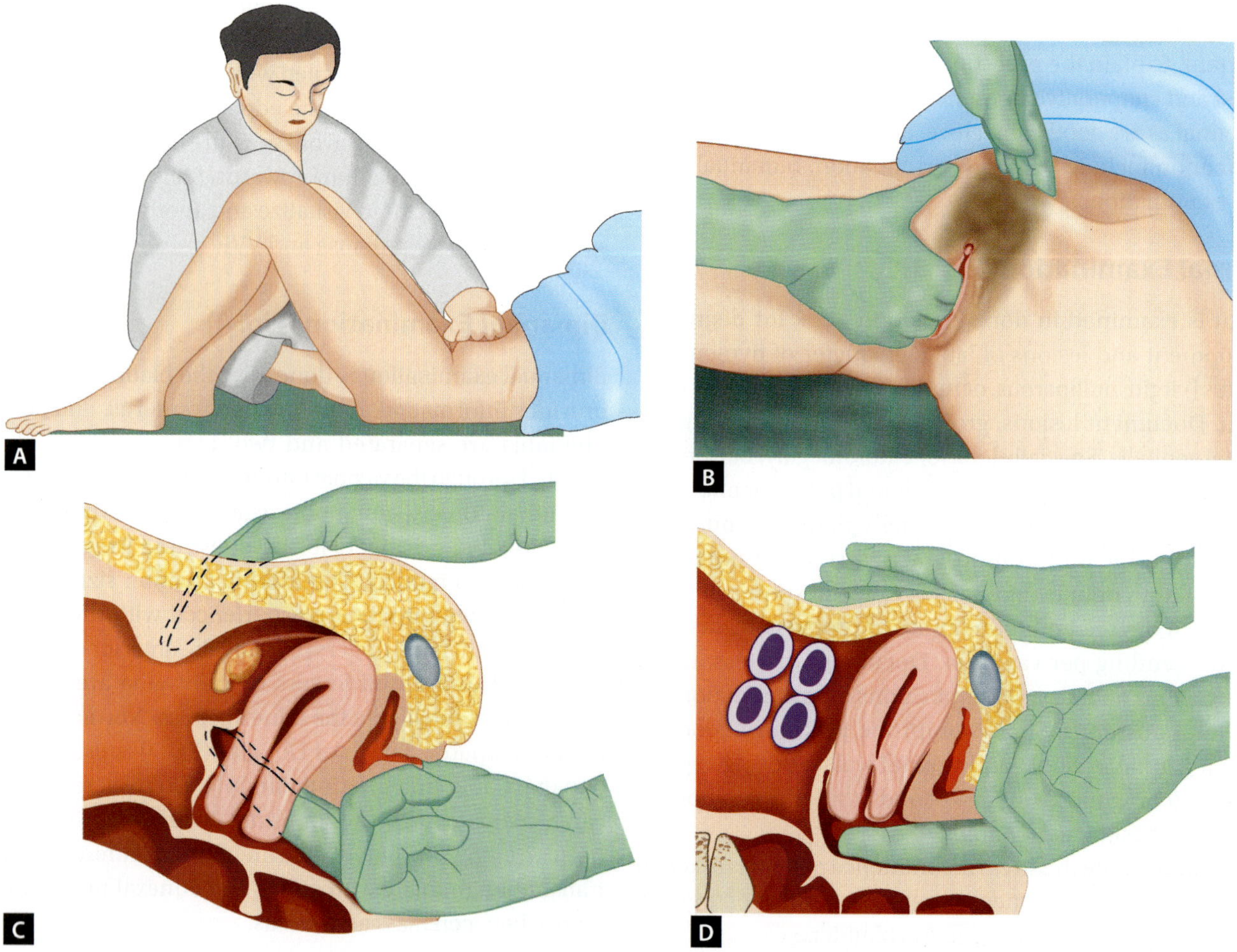

Figs. 4A to D: Bimanual abdominovaginal examination.

Rectovaginal Examination (Fig. 5)

Palpate the rectovaginal septum and malignancy involvement by right middle finger in the rectum and index finger in vagina. It is helpful in evaluating masses in cul-de-sac or adnexa. If the vagina admits only one finger, then rectal vaginal examination is useful.

Only a well-informed clinician can device an appropriate management plan. Proper assessment of information from history, physical examination, and inputs from necessary laboratory tests aid in differential diagnosis which should then be confirmed with biochemical, histologic, imaging, and other investigations.

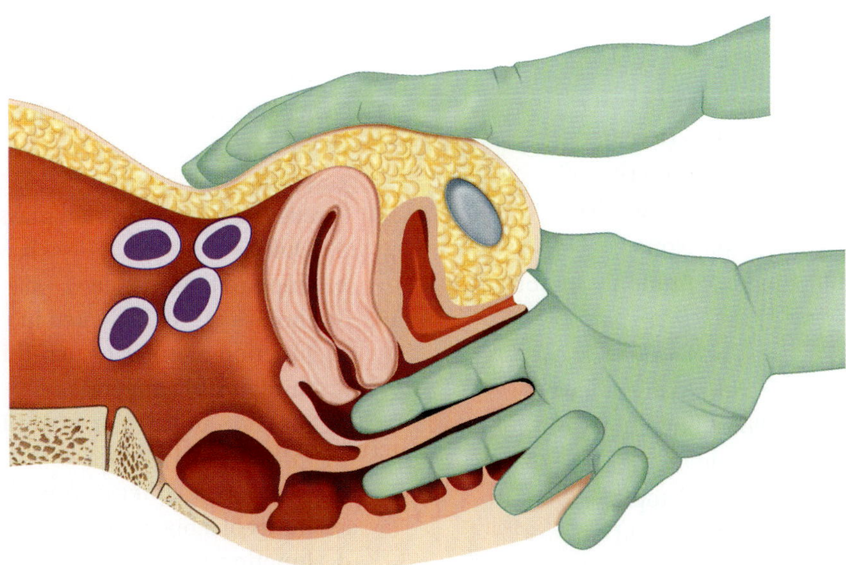

Fig. 5: Rectovaginal examination.

CONCLUSION

Detailed history taking and a thorough examination are imperative components of in the assessment of every patient. While eliciting history one should keep in mind sensitivity and confidentiality. Ensuring a comforting interaction will help in deciphering various details which the patient may not be easily reveal. All the positive points on history should be summarized before staring a clinical evaluation. Examination of every female patient should be performed in privacy in the presence of a female attendant. Adequate consent is to be obtained prior to any evaluation and all the relevant information of procedures to be performed should be told to the patient. Indeed the history taking and clinical examination require practice and skill which are acquired with experience and help in reaching the diagnosis successfully if optimally executed.

KEY MESSAGES

- Examination should be in privacy and with attendant.
- Good rapport is established by introducing and by being friendly with patient.
- History is elicited in one's own set fõrmat, not to miss any point and without haste.
- Before examination summarize the relevant positive histories.
- Explain the procedures to patient and get verbal consent.

FURTHER READING

1. Arulkumaran S, Sivanesaratnam V, Chatterjee A, Kumar P. Essentials of Gynecology, 2nd edition. New Delhi: Jaypee Brothers Medical Publishers (P) Ltd.; 2010.
2. Benson MD. OB/GYN Mentor: Your Clerkship & Shelf Exam Companion, 4th edition. Philadelphia: F.A. Davis Company; 2009.
3. Hacker NF, Gambone JC, Hobel CJ. Hacker and Moore's Essentials of Obstetrics and Gynecology, 5th edition. Amsterdam, Netherlands: Elsevier; 2009.
4. Hart DM, Norman J. Gynaecology Illustrated, 5th edition. London, United Kingdom: Churchill Livingstone; 2000.
5. Magowan B, Owen P, Drife J. Clinical Obstetrics and Gynaecology, 2nd edition. Amsterdam, Netherlands: Elsevier; 2009.
6. Malhotra N, Malhotra J. Jeffcoate's Principles of Gynaecology. 9th edition. New Delhi: Jaypee Brothers Medical Publishers (P) Ltd; 2019.
7. Monga A, Baker P. Gynaecology by Ten Teachers, 18th edition. London, United Kingdom: Hodder Education Publishers; 2006.
8. Padubidri VG, Anand E. Gynaecology: Prep Manual for Undergraduates. Amsterdam, Netherlands: Elsevier; 2005.
9. Padubidri VG, Daftary SN. Shaw's Textbook of Gynaecology, 15th edition. Amsterdam, Netherlands: Elsevier; 2011.
10. Shamsundar S. Manual of Gynaecology. New Delhi: CBS Publishers; 2007.

LONG QUESTIONS

1. A 32-year-old female married for 8 years with no child. How will you proceed with history and examination?
2. What is the importance of history taking in gynecological diagnosis?
3. How will you evaluate the history of leukorrhea?

SHORT QUESTIONS

1. Mention the types of vaginal speculums.
2. Write a short note on differential diagnosis of abdominal mass.
3. Elucidate the importance of rectal examination.
4. Discuss on Pap smear.
5. What are the types of abnormal uterine bleeding (AUB)?

MULTIPLE CHOICE QUESTIONS

1. Age of menarche is:
   a. 9–16 years b. 8–12 years
   c. <12 years d. >16 years
2. Dysmenorrhea during menstruation is:
   a. Spasmodic b. Congestive
   c. Membranous d. None
3. Postmenopausal bleeding is commonly important to rule out:
   a. Fibroid b. DUB
   c. PID d. Malignancy
4. Acute abdominal pain followed by history of 2 months amenorrhea and spotting could be:
   a. PID b. Ectopic
   c. Malignancy d. Fibroid
5. Movement of cervix is transmitted to abdominal mass in:
   a. Ovarian cyst b. Fibroid
   c. Ovarian tumor d. None
6. Mass in abdomen freely mobile in all directions:
   a. Uterine mass b. Endometriosis
   c. Ovarian cyst d. Adenomyosis
7. Low backache is the common complaint associated with:
   a. Fibroid b. Malignancy
   c. Prolapse d. PID
8. Menorrhagia is:
   a. Regular cycle b. Irregular cycle
   c. Both d. None
9. Thromboembolism is the complication of:
   a. OC pills b. Analgesics
   c. IUCDs d. All
10. Sister Joseph nodes seen around:
    a. Neck b. Inguinal region
    c. Umbilicus d. Breast
11. Gynecological examination includes:
    a. Breast b. Thyroid
    c. Spine d. All
12. Percussion note in ovarian mass is:
    a. Dull b. Resonant
    c. Impaired resonance d. Hyper resonant
13. Bartholin's gland is situated in:
    a. Junction of anterior two-thirds and posterior one-third of labia majora
    b. Junction of anterior two-thirds and posterior one-third of labia minora
    c. Junction of anterior one-third and posterior two-thirds of labia minora
    d. Junction of anterior one-third and posterior two-thirds of labia majora
14. Self-retaining speculum:
    a. Sims' speculum b. Cusco's speculum
    c. Both d. None
15. Endocervical cytology is sampled with:
    a. Ayre's spatula b. Brush
    c. Cotton swab d. None
16. Rectal mucosa involvement of CA cervix is felt by:
    a. Bimanual examination b. Pelvic examination
    c. Rectal examination
    d. Rectovaginal examination

Answers

1.	a	2.	a	3.	d	4.	b	5.	b	6.	c
7.	c	8.	a	9.	a	10.	c	11.	d	12.	a
13.	a	14.	b	15.	b	16.	c				

7.2 CYTOLOGY: CERVICOVAGINAL SMEAR AND ENDOMETRIAL BIOPSY

Anita Singh, Richa Jha

INTRODUCTION

Cervical cancer is a major public health problem in India with an incidence of 122,844 cases and mortality of 67,477 cases every year.[1-3] Carcinoma cervix is the second most common gynecological malignancy among Indian women aged 25–44 years with an incidence of 3.5% after carcinoma breast (28.6%).[3,4] The age standardized incidence rate for carcinoma cervix in Indian women is 22 per 100,000 women per year, which is the highest in South Asia, compared to 19.2 in Bangladesh and 13 in Sri Lanka. Cervical cancer mortality is 12.43/100,000 per year. Due to the lack of an organized cervical screening program, the disease burden is high in India.[5] There is an intense need to standardize the diagnosis and management of preinvasive disease of cervix.

Cervical cytology has been the mainstay of cervical cancer screening since the mid-20th century and has played an important role in defining risk thresholds for cancer cervix screening and for management of abnormal screening results. Screening with the conventional Pap test was successful in reducing the incidence of cervical cancer by 79% and the mortality by 70%. The sensitivity of cervical cytology for detection of cervical intraepithelial neoplasia (CIN) 2 or 3 ranged from 47 to 62% and specificity ranged from 60 to 95%.[6]

SCREENING OF PRECANCEROUS LESIONS

The main modalities of screening are:
- Cytology—Pap smear/liquid-based cytology (LBC)
- Human papillomavirus (HPV) testing

- Co-testing—combined HPV plus cytology
- Visual inspection of the cervix with acetic acid (VIA)
- Newer modalities of screening—dual staining, epigenetic modifications, and E6/E7 oncoprotein detection.

CERVICAL CYTOLOGY

In 1988, first National Cancer Institute (NCI) workshop held in Bethesda, Maryland, resulted in the development of the Bethesda system of cytologic reporting. The standard method of reporting cytologic findings facilitate quality assurance, and it has been updated and refined in the 2014 Bethesda System for Reporting Cervical Cytology.[7]

The 2014 Bethesda System for Reporting Cervical Cytology

Specimen Type

Indicate conventional smear (Pap smear) vs. liquid-based preparation vs. other.

Specimen Adequacy

- Satisfactory for evaluation (describe presence or absence of endocervical/transformation zone component and any other quality indicators, e.g., partially obscuring blood, inflammation, etc.)
- Unsatisfactory for evaluation . . . (*specify reason*)
  - Specimen rejected/not processed (*specify reason*)
  - Specimen processed and examined, but unsatisfactory for evaluation of epithelial abnormality because of (*specify reason*).

General Categorization (Optional)

- Negative for intraepithelial lesion or malignancy (NILM)
- *Other:* See interpretation/result (*e.g., endometrial cells in a woman ≥45 years of age*)
- Epithelial cell abnormality: See interpretation/result (*specify* "squamous" *or* "glandular" *as appropriate*).

Interpretation/Result

Negative for intraepithelial lesion or malignancy (*When there is no cellular evidence of neoplasia, state this in the General Categorization above and/or in the Interpretation/Result section of the report, whether or not there are organisms or other non-neoplastic findings*) **(Fig. 1)**.

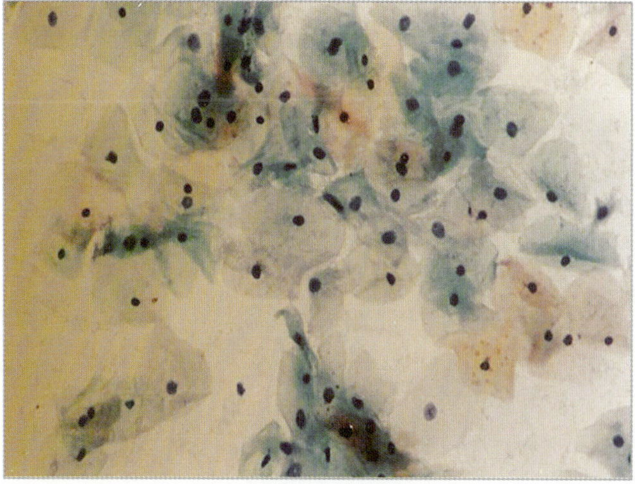

Fig. 1: Normal Pap smear.

Non-neoplastic Findings (Optional to Report; List not Inclusive)

- Non-neoplastic cellular variations:
  - Squamous metaplasia
  - Keratotic changes
  - Tubal metaplasia
  - Atrophy
  - Pregnancy-associated changes
- Reactive cellular changes associated with:
  - Inflammation (includes typical repair)
  - Radiation
  - Intrauterine contraceptive device (IUD)
- Lymphocytic (follicular) cervicitis
- Glandular cells status post hysterectomy.

Organisms

- *Trichomonas vaginalis*
- Fungal organisms morphologically consistent with *Candida* spp.
- Shift in flora suggestive of bacterial vaginosis
- Bacteria morphologically consistent with *Actinomyces* spp.
- Cellular changes consistent with herpes simplex virus
- Cellular changes consistent with cytomegalovirus.

Other

Endometrial cells (*in a woman ≥45 years of age*)
(*Specify if "negative for squamous intraepithelial lesion"*).

Epithelial Cell Abnormalities

Squamous cell:

- Atypical squamous cells (ASC)
  - Of undetermined significance (ASC-US)
  - Cannot exclude HSIL (ASC-H)
- Low-grade squamous intraepithelial lesion (LSIL) (*encompassing: HPV/mild dysplasia/CIN 1*)
- High-grade squamous intraepithelial lesion (HSIL) (*encompassing: moderate and severe dysplasia, CIS; CIN 2 and CIN 3*)
  - With features suspicious for invasion (*if invasion is suspected*)
- Squamous cell carcinoma **(Figs. 2 and 3)**.

Glandular cell

- Atypical
  - Endocervical cells (NOS *or specify in comments*)
  - Endometrial cells (NOS *or specify in comments*)
  - Glandular cells (NOS *or specify in comments*)

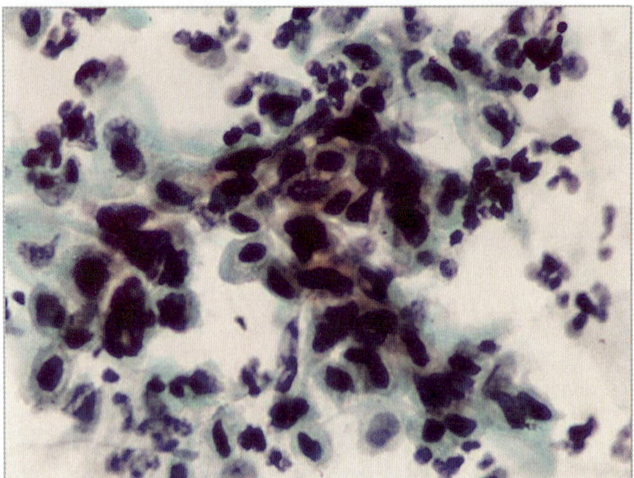

Fig. 2: Pap smear showing high-grade squamous intraepithelial lesion (HSIL).

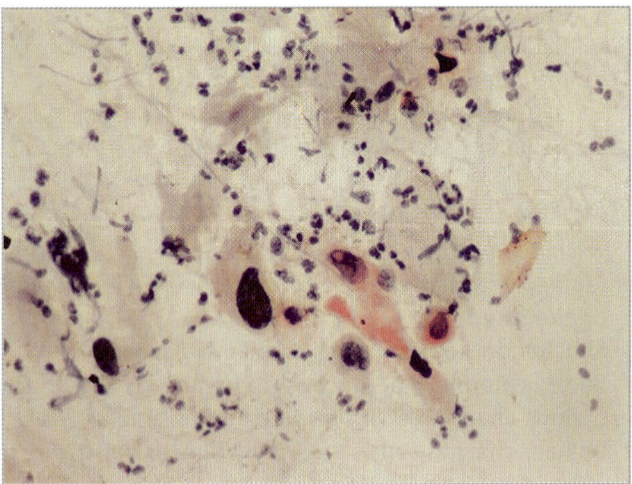

Fig. 3: Squamous cell carcinoma on Pap smear.

- Atypical
  - Endocervical cells, favor neoplastic
  - Glandular cells, favor neoplastic
- Endocervical adenocarcinoma in situ (AIS)
- Adenocarcinoma
  - Endocervical
  - Endometrial
  - Extrauterine
  - Not otherwise specified (NOS).

Other Malignant Neoplasms (Specify)

Adjunctive testing: Provide a brief description of the test method(s) and report the result so that it is easily understood by the clinician.

Computer-assisted interpretation of cervical cytology: If case examined by an automated device, specify device and result.

Educational notes and comments appended to cytology reports (optional): Suggestions should be concise and consistent with clinical follow-up guidelines published by professional organizations (references to relevant publications may be include).

Conventional cytology has been associated with a high incidence of false negative errors. Sampling errors occur because the lesion is too small to exfoliate cells or the device did not pick up the cells and transfer them to the fixation media. Preparation errors occur due to poor fixation on the glass slide, leading to air drying of the slides. The slide preparations could be too thick and obscured by vaginal discharge, blood or mucus. These problems were obviated by the wide spread use of LBC. The ubiquitous use of liquid-based media to collect and preserve the collected cervical cells significantly decreased specimen sampling and preparation errors.[6,7]

With this technique, liquid samples are processed to provide a uniform, thin layer of cervical cells without debris in a glass slide. The cell sample is collected with the endocervical brush used in combination with a plastic spatula. The sample is rinsed in a vial containing liquid alcohol-based preservative. With this technique, 80–90% of the cells are transferred to the liquid media, as compared to 10–20% transferred to the glass slide with conventional cytology. The cells are retrieved from the vial by passing the liquid through the filter, which traps the larger epithelial cells, separating them from the small blood and inflammatory cells, thereby yielding a thin layer of diagnostic cells which can be properly interpreted by the cytologist.

ADEQUACY OF THE SPECIMEN

The age and hormonal status of the patient must always be taken into account before interpreting the results. The adequacy of the specimen obtained for cervical cytology depends upon the following criteria:[8,9]

- *Minimum squamous cellularity criteria*: An adequate LBP should have at least 5,000 well-visualized squamous or squamous metaplastic cells. Endocervical cells and completely obscured cells should be removed from the estimate. Women who have had chemo/radiotherapy or postmenopausal with atrophic changes or posthysterectomy status, may have fewer than 5,000 cells.[8,9]

  An adequate conventional cervical specimen should contain 8,000–12,000 well-preserved/well-visualized squamous epithelial cells.
- *Endocervical/transformation zone component*: The presence of transformation zone component is not necessary for adequate specimen. However, the presence or absence of transformation zone must be reported.
- *Obscuring factors*: Specimens in which >75% of the squamous cells are obscured are unsatisfactory for evaluation. Presence of interfering substances such as lubricants and blood also have a significant effect on adequacy rates.[10]

- The 2012 ASCCP consensus guidelines recommend repeat cytology in 2–4 months for women with unsatisfactory cytology. High-risk human papillomavirus (hrHPV) triage is not recommended for such patients. For women with two consecutive unsatisfactory cytology tests, colposcopy should be done.

Another Food and Drug Administration (FDA) approved technology for primary screening is the automated image-guided slide screening system. This technique uses an automated microscope coupled to a special digital camera. The system scans the slide and uses computer imaging techniques to analyze each field of view on the slide. Computer algorithms rank each slide on the probability that the sample may contain an abnormality. The selected slides are reviewed by a cytotechnologist or cytopathologist.[6]

The results of cervical cytology cannot be used to make a definitive diagnosis or to initiate the treatment, unless it is HSIL. The results guide further evaluation with colposcopy and biopsy and treatment decisions must be taken on the basis of the results obtained from these tests.

TERMINOLOGY FOR SQUAMOUS ABNORMALITIES

According to the Bethesda system **(Fig. 4)**, potentially premalignant lesions fall into the following categories:

- *Low-grade squamous intraepithelial lesion*: LSIL in young women is a transient HPV infection and has relatively lesser risk of cancer progression and associated with a probable histological diagnosis of CIN 1.

LSIL on cytology is characterized by mature squamous cells with enlarged nuclei with variable chromatin and nuclear membranes. Koilocytosis or perinuclear cavitation in the cytoplasm may be present.[11,12]

- *High-grade squamous intraepithelial lesion*: HSIL is associated with a probable histological diagnosis of CIN 2/3.

The cells of HSIL are smaller and show less cytoplasmic maturity than LSIL and occur singly, in sheets or in syncytial like aggregates. Higher grade lesions contain quite small basal type cells with dense nuclear enlargement. There is marked increase in the nuclear-cytoplasmic ratio, contour of the nuclear membrane is irregular with prominent indentations and nucleoli are generally absent.

- *Atypical squamous cells*: The interpretation of ASC requires that the cells must fulfill the following criteria:
  - Squamous differentiation
  - Increased nuclear to cytoplasmic ratio
  - Minimal nuclear changes which may be hyperchromasia, chromatin clumping, irregularity, smudging, or multinucleation.

ASC is subdivided into two categories:

1. *Atypical squamous cells of unknown significance (ASC-US)*: Nuclei are 2.5–3 times the area of a normal intermediate cell, nuclear abnormalities include atypical parakeratosis and incomplete koilocytosis.
2. *Atypical squamous cells cannot exclude HSIL (ASC-H)*: Specimens containing a few cells that are suspicious for, but not diagnostic of HSIL are reported as ASC-H. Several

Epithelial cell abnormalities

Abbreviation	Terminology
NILM	Negative for intraepithelial lesion or malignancy
ASCUS	Atypical squamous cells of undetermined significance
ASC-H	Atypical squamous cells: Cannot exclude high grade squamous intraepithelial lesion
LSIL	Low-grade squamous intraepithelial lesion
HSIL	High grade squamous intraepithelial lesion
SCC	Squamous cell carcinoma

Glandular cell abnormalities

Abbreviation	Terminology
AGC	Atypical glandular cells (specify endocervical, endometrial or NOS, i.e., not otherwise significant)
AGC-FN	Atypical glandular cells: Favor neoplastic
AIS	Endocervical adenocarcinoma in situ
Endometrial cells in a woman > 40 years of age	
Adenocarcinoma	
Others	

List of other abbreviations

CIN : Cervical intraepithelial neoplasia
ECC : Endocervical curettage
HPV : Human papillomavirus
LEEP : Loop electrosurgical excision procedure
TZ : Transformation zone
VIA : Visual inspection with acetic acid

Fig. 4: The Bethesda system of reporting cytology.

patterns may include atypical immature metaplastic cells, crowded sheets of cells, markedly atypical repair, or abnormal nuclear cells with focal irregularity.

TERMINOLOGY USED FOR GLANDULAR CELL ABNORMALITIES

Benign appearing endometrial cells are reported only in women >45 years of age.[13]

- *Atypical glandular cells:*
  - *Endocervical cells: NOS*: Endocervical cells that display nuclear atypia that exceeds obvious reactive or reparative changes but lack unequivocal features of endocervical AIS or invasive adenocarcinoma.
  - *Endometrial cells: NOS*: The distinction of cytologically benign from atypical endometrial cells is based primarily on the criterion of increased nuclear size. Nuclei are enlarged and there is mild hyperchromasia and chromatin heterogenicity.
- *Atypical glandular cells, favor neoplasia (AGC-FN):*
  - *Endocervical cells:* Cell morphology, either quantitatively or qualitatively, falls just short of an interpretation of endocervical AIS or invasive adenocarcinoma or NOS is noted.
  - *Endocervical AIS:* Noninvasive high-grade endocervical glandular lesion that is characterized by nuclear enlargement, hyperchromasia, chromatin abnormality, pseudostratification, and mitotic activity.
  - *Adenocarcinoma:* Abundant abnormal cells, typically with columnar configuration, syncytial aggregates, enlarged pleomorphic nuclei, nuclear membrane abnormalities, finely vacuolated cytoplasm, and necrotic tumor diathesis.

Upon further evaluation, either high-grade squamous cells or glandular abnormalities are found in 10–39% of women of with a finding of AGC on cytology.

NON-NEOPLASTIC FINDINGS

- *Negative for intraepithelial lesion or malignancy:* Specimens for which no epithelial abnormality is identified are reported as "negative for intraepithelial lesion or malignancy (NILM)". If optional non neoplastic findings are reported, NILM should still be included as the primary interpretation to avoid ambiguity.[14]
- *Normal cellular elements:* The normal cells seen in the cervical cytology include*:*
  - *Squamous cells:* Superficial, intermediate (the nucleus of the intermediate cell serves as the basic size reference for other cells in cervical cytology) and parabasal cells.
  - *Glandular cells:* Endocervical cells and endometrial cells.
  - *Non-neoplastic cellular variations:* These can be in the form of squamous metaplasia, keratotic cellular changes (occur as a protective-reactive phenomena or in association with HPV infection), tubal metaplasia (common finding in the upper endocervical canal/ lower uterine segment) or atrophic changes.
  - *Pregnancy-associated changes:* True stromal decidual nature of the cells in pregnancy, such as smudgy chromatin with nucleolus, can be mistaken with a HSIL. Therefore, changes associated with pregnancy should be reported as a normal process.

SCREENING AGE AND PERIODICITY

- In healthcare settings with good resources, screening should begin from 21 years of age. However, in low resource settings, screening can be delayed till 30 years.
- In healthcare settings with good resources, women aged 21–65 years should undergo screening with preferably primary HPV test/co-testing with cytology every 5 years or with cytology every 3 years.
- In healthcare settings with limited resources, women aged 30–65 years should undergo cervical cancer screening with VIA every 5 years.[15-17]

AGE TO STOP SCREENING

- Women should continue to be screened for cervical cancer till 65 years of age, after which it can be discontinued in women with consistent negative results in last 15 years.
- In hysterectomized women, screening is not advised unless there was history of previous intraepithelial neoplasia. If the indication of hysterectomy is unknown, screening may be performed at clinician's discretion.
- In women who have undergone any treatment for CIN 2, screening for 20 years following the treatment is recommended.

HUMAN PAPILLOMAVIRUS TESTING AS PRIMARY SCREENING MODALITY

Human papillomavirus is the main causal factor for the development of cervical cancer. HPV testing alone for screening is recommended in women aged 30 years and older, as a negative HPV test alone provides greater reassurance against CIN 3 in the subsequent years than cytology alone. The cumulative incidence of CIN 3 in HPV negative women aged >25 years was reported to be 0.34% while in cytology negative women, it was 0.78%.[18]

The benefit of using HPV testing as a primary screening method is its high sensitivity and negative predictive value, and this allows for the prolongation of screening intervals. The *Cobas* test, which detects hrHPV and genotypes 16 and 18 are used for the primary screening in women >25 years. However, presently HPV testing is available only in good resource settings.

Following are the recommendations for management when HPV testing is used as the primary modality of screening:

- Women with positive HPV testing can be triaged with cytology, HPV genotyping or VIA depending on the availability.
- When HPV positive women are triaged with cytology, a normal cytology report should be followed by a repeat HPV test *after 1 year*. If cytology is ASCUS or above, colposcopy and directed biopsy is recommended.
- When HPV positive women are triaged with genotyping 16 and 18, a positive result must be followed by colposcopy-directed biopsy and further follow-up of such patients is needed.

HUMAN PAPILLOMAVIRUS TESTS USED IN CANCER SCREENING

Different types of HPV testing are given in **Table 1**.

CO-TESTING AS PRIMARY SCREENING (FLOWCHARTS 1 AND 2)

For women aged 30–65 years, co-testing with combined cytology and HPV testing every 5 years is the preferred method of screening presently. The negative predictive value is high when both the test results are negative and there will be very high level of reassurance that they will not be at risk of cervical cancer for a long time.

While testing with HPV is more sensitive than cytology, it is somewhat less specific. Co-testing in younger women aged <30 years would lead to an increase in the unnecessary work up procedures without a corresponding decrease in carcinoma cervix incidence because of increased probability of clearance of infection by the immune system.[19]

The following are the recommendations for screening women when using co-testing as the primary modality:[20,21]

TABLE 1: Types of HPV testing.

Test	*Technique*	*Name*
Deoxyribonucleic acid (DNA)	Direct genome detection	• Hybrid capture 2 • CareHPV test
	Amplification	• GP5+/GP6+ bio PCR-EIA • Cervista HPV HR
	Amplification and genotyping of HPV 16 and 18 Extended genotype testing–HPV 16, 18, 45, 31, 51, and 52	• Cervista HPV 16/18 • Cobas HPV test (FDA approved 2014) • Onclarity HPV (FDA approved 2018)
Ribonucleic acid (RNA)	Amplification of E6/E7 proteins	Aptima HPV assay
	Monoclonal antibodies	Avantage HPV E6 test

(FDA: food and drug administration; HPV: human papillomavirus)

- For women aged 30–65 years, co-testing is the preferred modality of treatment (Level A)
- The women with negative cytology and negative HPV test should return to routine screening with co-testing in 5 years (Level A)
- For women with positive cytology and positive HPV test, colposcopy and guided biopsy is recommended
- For women with positive cytology and negative HPV test, follow-up depends on the cytology test results:
  - If cytology is ASC-US or LSIL, repeat co-testing is advised at 1 year (Level B)
  - Women with cytology > ASCUS or HPV test positive on repeat co-testing, should be managed by colposcopy and directed biopsy
  - Women with ASC-H or HSIL on cytology and HPV test negative, should be managed by colposcopy and directed biopsy (Level A)
- The women with HPV test positive and cytology negative, should either go for repeat co-testing at one year or should go for HPV specific genotyping (Level C)
  - Women who go for genotyping, if the result is negative, should be followed by repeat co-testing after 1 year (Level B)
  - If the HPV genotype result is positive, it should be managed by colposcopy and directed biopsy (Level A).

VISUAL INSPECTION OF CERVIX WITH ACETIC ACID AS PRIMARY MODALITY OF SCREENING (FLOWCHART 3)

Visual inspection of cervix with acetic acid is used in low resource settings because it is economical and provides immediate results. When VIA-based screening is used, it is important to ensure quality control and validated training and evaluation procedures.[22]

The following are the recommendations when VIA is used as the primary screening modality:

- In limited resource settings, VIA should be done at least one to three times in a lifetime (Level B)
- Screening should not be continued beyond 50 years, especially in postmenopausal women as the transformation zone recedes into the endocervical canal and prevents it from being fully visible (Level A).

NEWER SCREENING MODALITIES

- *Dual staining*: Dual staining has emerged as a way to more accurately predict the chance that a woman with positive HPV test has precancerous cervical changes. The test measures the presence of two proteins p16, and Ki-67.

  It has been realized that most of the HPV infections are transient and can be eliminated from the body's immune system. As such, it is neither feasible nor efficient to send all HPV positive women for colposcopy. Therefore,

Flowchart 1: Screening with primary HPV testing in women aged >30 years.

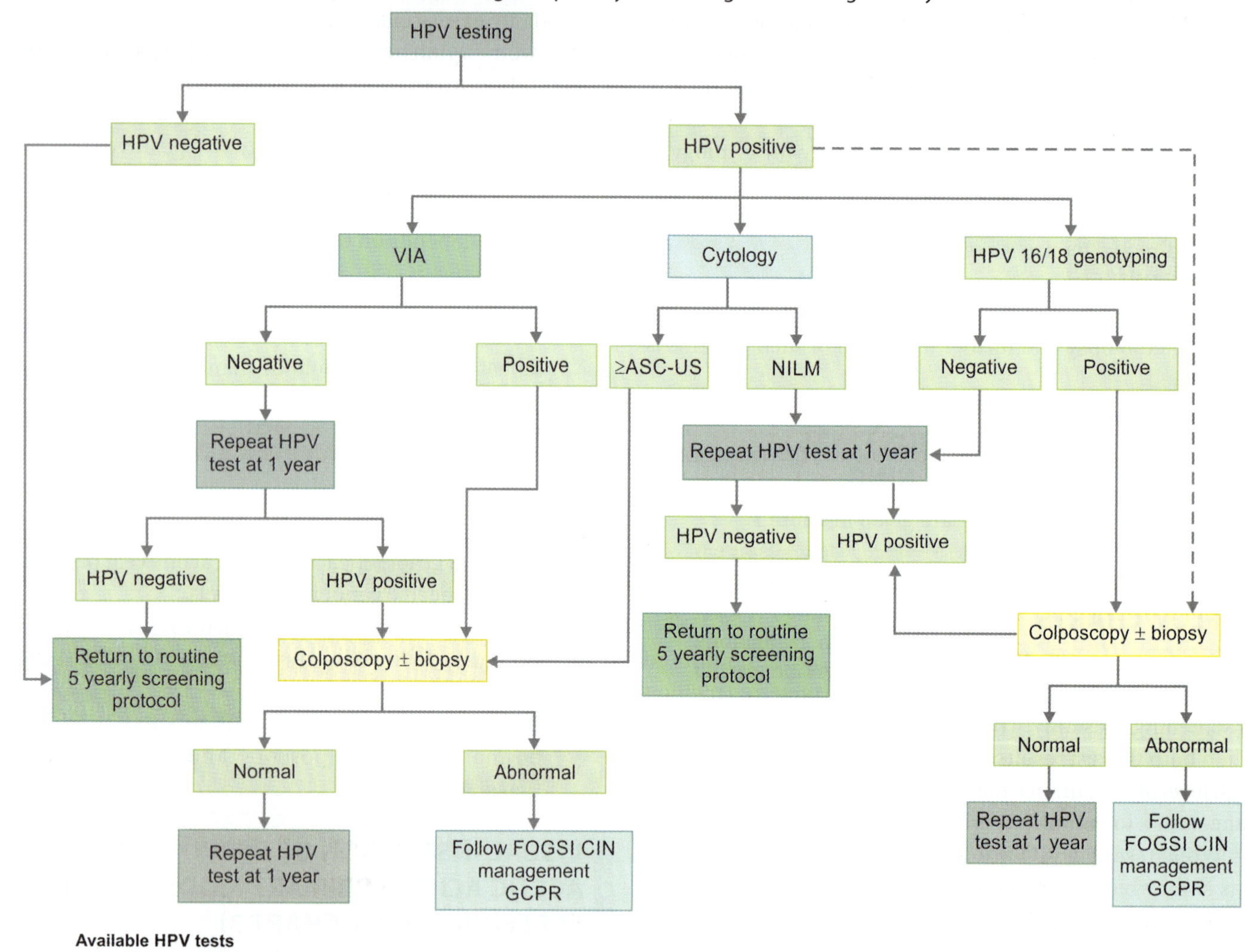

(ASC-US: atypical squamous cells of unknown significance; CIN: cervical intraepithelial neoplasia; HPV: human papillomavirus; NILM: negative for intraepithelial lesion or malignancy; VIA: visual inspection of the cervix with acetic acid)

additional triage strategies **(Figs. 5 and 6)** are needed to distinguish those who are at high risk and those who can safely return to routine screening. P16 and Ki-67 dual staining has shown promise as a new triage strategy. The simultaneous detection of p16, a cell cycle arrest protein under normal physiological conditions and Ki-67, the cell proliferator marker, within the same cervical epithelial cell indicates HPV-induced dysregulation of the cell cycle. Higher indices of these markers on immunostaining of the cervical smears have been associated with histologically poorer grades of disease.[23,24]

- *Epigenetic modifications*: Changes in deoxyribonucleic acid (DNA) methylation (hypomethylation/hypermethylation) cause defective gene expression, genetic instability through faulty condensation of chromosomes, and silencing of mobile DNAs such as jumping genes (transposons). Methylation can be measured in HPV positive cases using quantitative methylation specific-polymerase chain reaction (PCR).
- *E6 and E7 messenger ribonucleic acid (mRNA)*: In hrHPV positive women, E6/E7 RNA positivity has a higher specificity than HPV DNA testing for prediction of high-grade lesions.

FOGSI RESOURCE BASED CERVICAL CANCER SCREENING RECOMMENDATIONS

The FOGSI resource-based cervical cancer screening recommendations are given in **Table 2**.

ENDOMETRIAL BIOPSY

Abnormal uterine bleeding (AUB) is reported to occur in 9–14% women between menarche to menopause.[25] The prevalence varies in each country. In India, the reported prevalence is around 17.9%.[26] To standardize the nomenclature of AUB,

Flowchart 2: Screening with co-testing (HPV test with cytology) in women aged >30 years.

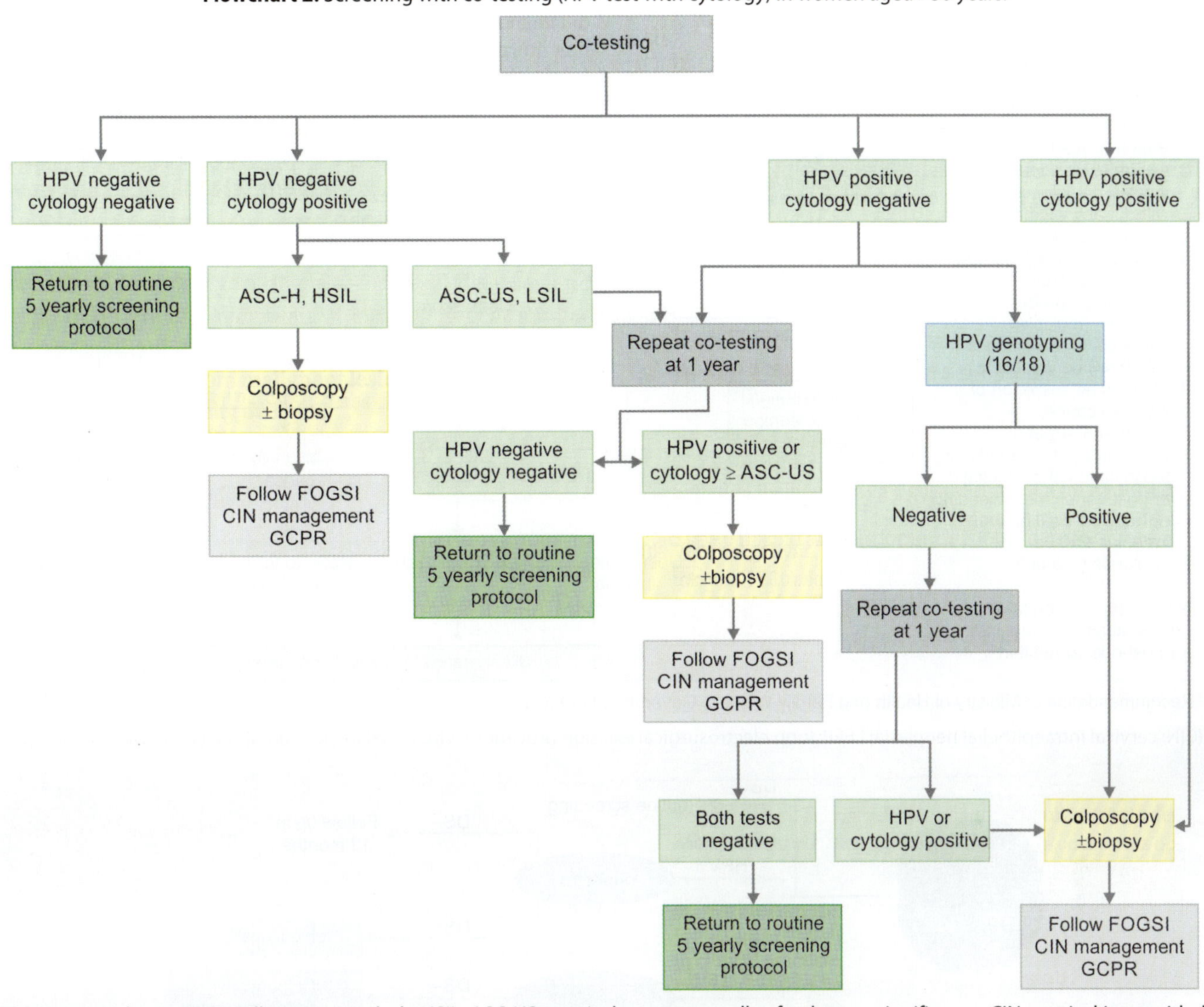

(ASC-H: atypical squamous cells cannot exclude HSIL; ASC-US: atypical squamous cells of unknown significance; CIN: cervical intraepithelial neoplasia; HPV: human papillomavirus; HSIL: high-grade squamous intraepithelial lesion; LSIL: low-grade squamous intraepithelial lesion; NILM: negative for intraepithelial lesion or malignancy)

a new system known by the acronym of PALM-COEIN was introduced in 2011 by The International Federation of Gynecology and Obstetrics (FIGO). The PALM-COEIN system is etiopathogenesis based, with PALM describing structural causes (**P**olyp, **A**denomyosis, **L**eiomyoma, **M**alignancy) and COEIN describing nonstructural causes (**C**oagulopathy, **O**vulatory dysfunction, **E**ndometrial, **I**atrogenic, **N**ot otherwise specified) of AUB.

Office endometrial aspiration biopsy is the accepted first step in evaluating a patient with AUB or suspected endometrial pathology. The diagnostic accuracy of office based endometrial biopsy is 90–98% when compared with subsequent findings at dilatation and curettage (D&C). However, despite a negative biopsy result, 2% of women will still have endometrial hyperplasia **(Fig. 7)**.

The narrow plastic cannulas are relatively inexpensive, can be used without a tenaculum, cause less uterine cramping and are successful in obtaining adequate tissue samples in >95% cases. If cervical stenosis is encountered, a paracervical block can be performed, and cervix can be dilated. Premedication with antiprostaglandin agent may reduce cramping. Endocervical curettage may be performed at the time of endometrial biopsy if cervical pathology is suspected. A Pap test is unreliable diagnostic test for endometrial hyperplasia because only 30–50% of patients with endometrial cancer have abnormal Pap test results.

Hysteroscopy and D&C should be reserved for situations in which cervical stenosis or patient tolerance does not permit adequate evaluation by aspiration biopsy, bleeding recurs after negative endometrial biopsy, or specimen obtained is inadequate to explained to explain abnormal bleeding. Hysteroscopy is more accurate in identifying polyps and submucous myomas than endometrial biopsy or D&C alone.

In evaluating an endometrial biopsy specimen, an adequate clinical history is important, including the age of the patient and the reason for the biopsy. The menopausal

Flowchart 3: Screening with VIA in women aged 30–65 years.

* Eligibility for screen-and-treat (ablative procedures)

1. Lesion should be entirely visible and occupy not more than two quadrants of cervix
2. Entire lesion should be located on ectocervix without any vaginal and/or endocervical extension
3. Lesion can be adequately covered by largest cryotherapy probe available (multiple overlapping applications with thermocoagulation)
4. There is no suspicion of invasive cancer
5. Screen-and-treat by cryotherapy is contraindicated in cases of postcoital or postmenopausal bleeding, obvious cervical growth, irregular surface or bleeds on touch

N.B. biopsy can be taken prior to ablation, if feasible, for post-hoc correlation

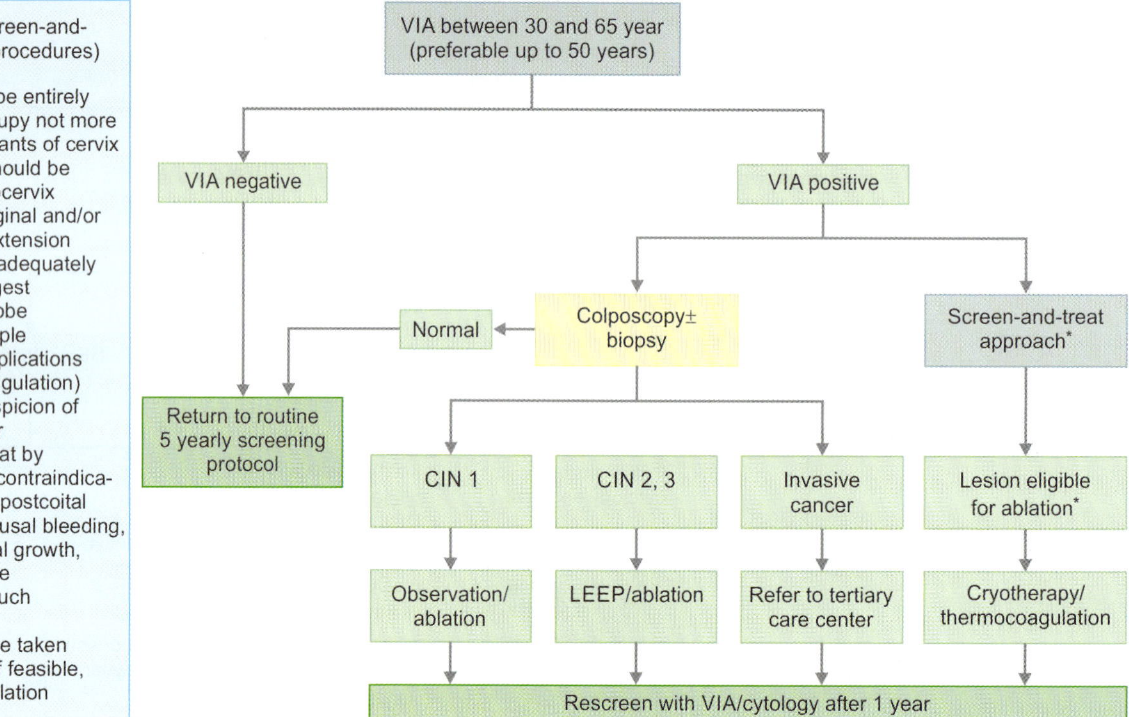

*Recommendation of Ministry of Health and Family Welfare, Government of India

(CIN: cervical intraepithelial neoplasia; LEEP: loop electrosurgical excision procedure; VIA: visual inspection of the cervix with acetic acid)

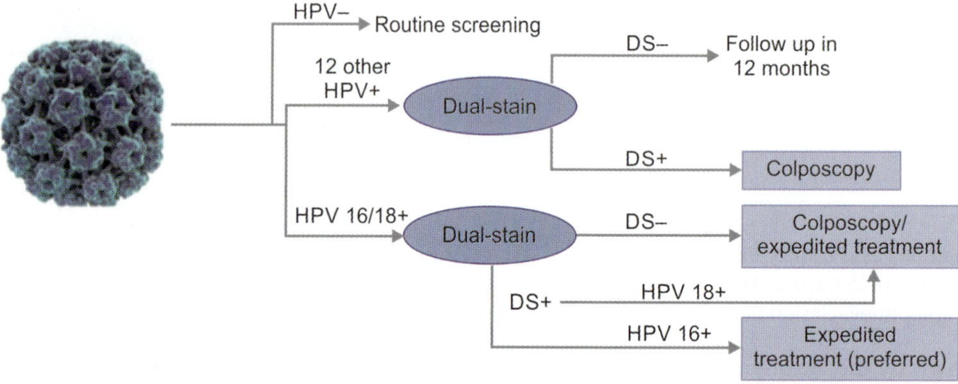

Fig. 5: Future triage algorithm of HPV positive women.
(HPV: human papillomavirus)

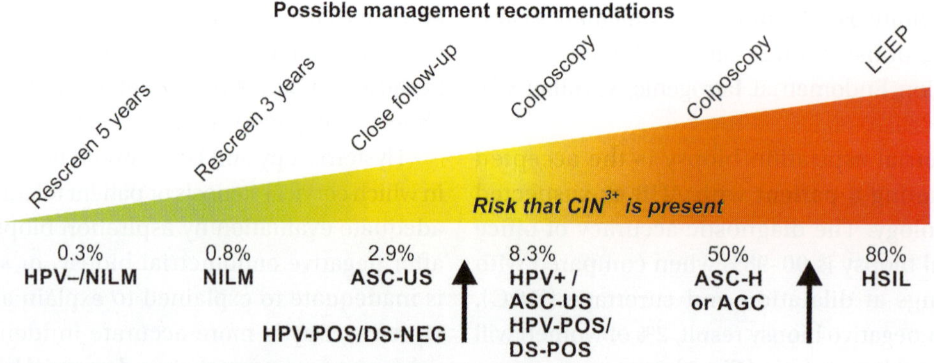

Fig. 6: Management based on risk stratification.
(AGC: atypical glandular cells; ASC-H: atypical squamous cells cannot exclude HSIL; ASC-US: atypical squamous cells of unknown significance; DS: dual staining; HPV: human papillomavirus; HSIL: high-grade squamous intraepithelial lesion; LEEP: loop electrosurgical excision procedure; NILM: negative for intraepithelial lesion or malignancy)

TABLE 2: FOGSI resource-based cervical cancer screening recommendations.

	Good resource settings	***Limited resource settings***
Modality	HPV testing • Primary HPV testing • Co-testing (HPV + cytology) Cytology Colposcopy and biopsy VIA	VIA Colposcopy ± biopsy
Target age group (years)	25–65	30–65
Age to start (years)	Cytology at 25 Primary HPV testing or co-testing at 30	30
Frequency	Primary HPV testing or co-testing—every 5 years Cytology—every 3 years	Every 5 years (at least 1–3 times in a lifetime)
Age to stop (years)	65 with consistent negative results in last 15 years (women with no prior screening should undergo tests once at 65 years and, if negative, should exit screening)	
Follow up after treatment (method and interval)	HPV testing (preferred) or cytology 12 months	VIA 12 months
Screening in hysterectomized women	• *Following hysterectomy in which cervix was removed for benign causes:* No need for screening, unless there is history of previous cervical intraepithelial neoplasia • If indications for hysterectomy are not known, screening depends on the clinician's discretion	
Follow-up in women with CIN in hysterectomy HPE report	Need to be screened with HPV at 6 months and 18 months	

(CIN: cervical intraepithelial neoplasia; HPE: histopathological examination; HPV: human papillomavirus; VIA: visual inspection of the cervix with acetic acid)

Fig. 7: Endometrial biopsy sampler (Pipelle).

status as well as the date of onset of the last menstrual period and the length of the menstrual cycle in premenopausal women should be provided. In many cases of postmenopausal bleeding, the patient is not actually postmenopausal but rather is perimenopausal, with a prolonged interval between periods. This results in the clinician and the patient assuming that the woman is postmenopausal. Before biopsy, many women with AUB are already taking exogenous hormones, especially progestogenic compounds, to control the bleeding, and this information is not always conveyed to the pathologist. Other women may be taking hormone replacement therapy (HRT) or contraceptives. These hormonal compounds may alter the morphological appearance of the endometrium and a knowledge that these, and other relevant drugs such as tamoxifen, are being taken is of paramount importance to the pathologist.

Criteria for Adequacy of Endometrial Biopsy Specimens

Previously, endometrial biopsy specimens were largely obtained by D&C carried out under general anesthesia. Most endometrial specimens are now taken at outpatient by Pipelle or other techniques, with the result that many biopsy specimens contain scant, or even no, endometrial tissue. The presence of even a minimal amount of endometrial tissue provides presumptive evidence that the endometrial cavity has been entered, although theoretically endometrial-type glands with or without stroma can be derived from tuboendometrial metaplasia or endometriosis within the cervix. It is emphasized that biopsy specimens with scant tissue, which usually comprise only superficial strips of endometrial glands, should be examined carefully under high power to look for mitotic activity (abnormal in truly postmenopausal women) and atypia **(Flowchart 4)**.[27]

Flowchart 4: Evaluation of endometrial biopsy specimen.

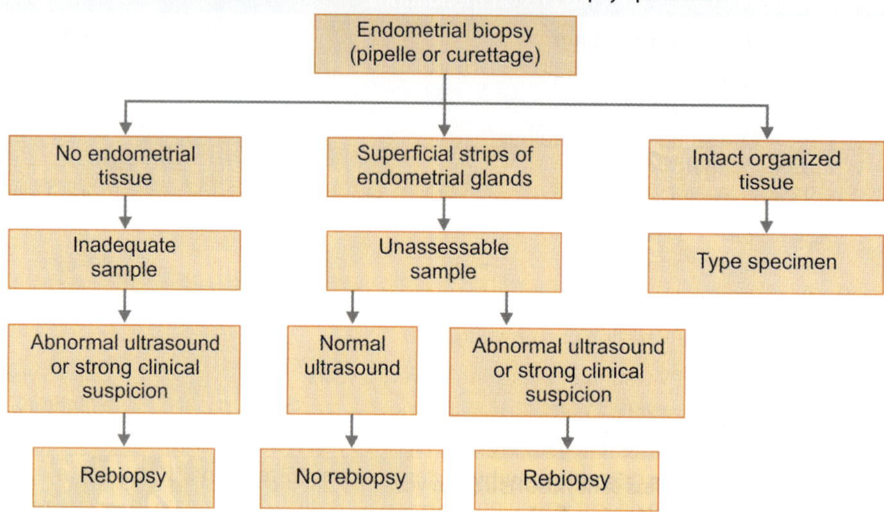

The following conditions must be considered while evaluating the biopsy reports in a patient with AUB.

Endometritis

Endometritis may result in symptoms of AUB and the pathologist should always exclude this. Lymphocytes, including natural killer cells and lymphoid aggregates, are a normal component of the endometrium, and polymorphs are characteristic of the premenstrual and menstrual phases. The presence of plasma cells is widely regarded as the most useful criterion for a diagnosis of endometritis, although these are often admixed with other inflammatory cells, both acute and chronic, and may be a minor component of the inflammatory cell infiltrate.[28,29] In endometritis, the inflammatory cell infiltrate may be focal and plasma cells just beneath the surface glands are usually most easily identified.

Endometrial Polyps (Fig. 8)

Polyps are a common cause of abnormal bleeding in premenopausal and postmenopausal women. On examination under low power, the initial clue to the presence of a polyp is often the admixture of fragments of a normal cyclical endometrium and fragments that are morphologically different.[30]

Effects of Hormones on Endometrium

Hormones have varying effects on the endometrium and it is essential that the clinician supplies details to the pathologist regarding any hormone treatment. With any unusual, noncyclical appearance of the endometrium, the pathologist should consider exogenous hormones. Some hormone preparations, especially those that contain both estrogen and progestogen (most modern hormone replacement treatment regimens), characteristically result in a weak or poorly developed secretory endometrium.[31]

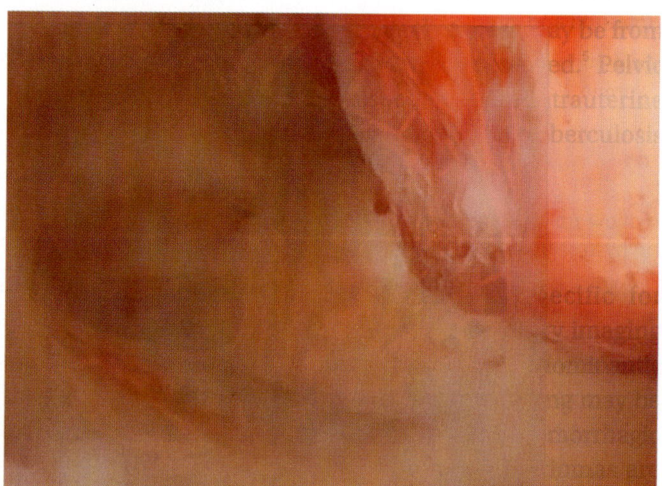

Fig. 8: Endometrial polyp on hysteroscopy.

Progestogen-only compounds result in a characteristic morphological appearance with atrophic or weak secretory-type glands set in an expanded stroma that exhibits varying degrees of pseudodecidualization. This pseudodecidualization is often most prominent just beneath the surface glands and is usually accompanied by an inflammatory cell infiltrate, largely comprising natural killer cells.

Endometrial Hyperplasia

Endometrial hyperplasia represents a spectrum of morphologic and biologic alterations of the endometrial glands and stroma, ranging from an exaggerated physiological state to carcinoma in situ. Clinically significant hyperplasias usually evolve within a background of proliferative endometrium as a result of protracted estrogen stimulation in absence of progestin influence. The classification scheme endorsed by the International Society of Gynecological Pathologists is based on the architectural and cytological features and long-term studies that reflect the natural history of the lesions **(Table 3)**.

TABLE 3: Risk of progression to cancer in endometrial hyperplasia.

Type of hyperplasia	*Progression to cancer (%)*
Simple (cystic without atypia)	1
Complex (adenomatous without atypia)	3
Atypical	
Simple (cystic without atypia)	8
Complex (adenomatous with atypia)	29

Morphological Features of Endometrial Hyperplasia

In a simple hyperplasia, the normal gland to stroma ratio is maintained or there is slight increase. The endometrium shows proliferative activity, with cystically dilated glands of irregular sizes and shapes. Some glands may exhibit "outpouchings", "infoldings", and "budding". No nuclear atypia is seen, the nuclei being oval and maintaining their orientation to the underlying basement membrane. A major problem is the distinction between simple endometrial hyperplasia and disordered proliferative endometrium, a term widely used, although the histological features are not well characterized. The morphological features of these overlap and the distinction is poorly reproducible. Disordered proliferative endometrium is common in the perimenopausal years because of anovulatory cycles **(Fig. 9)**.[32,33]

In complex hyperplasia, there is an increase in the gland to stroma ratio with glandular crowding. The glands are often closely packed, although some stroma usually remains between individual glands. The glands show proliferative activity and, by definition, there is no nuclear atypia. Simple hyperplasia is usually a generalized condition, whereas most, but not all, cases of complex hyperplasia are focal, often occurring on a background of simple hyperplasia **(Fig. 10)**.

In atypical hyperplasia, there is, by definition, nuclear atypia. Assessing nuclear atypia is one of the most subjective and problematic areas in gynecological pathology, but this assessment is crucial **(Table 3)** in the management of endometrial hyperplasia, as surgery is generally undertaken for atypical hyperplasia, whereas hormone treatment is common for nonatypical hyperplasia, although there are many exceptions. In atypical hyperplasia, the nuclear changes are often accompanied by cytoplasmic changes, such that the cells have more abundant, often eosinophilic, cytoplasm.

Endometrial Intraepithelial Lesion

Endometrial intraepithelial neoplasia (EIN) classification is based on the integration of morphological, molecular genetic, morphometric, and prognostic data. Briefly, five criteria must be fulfilled for a diagnosis of EIN:[34,35]

1. Area of glands exceeding that of stroma (volume percentage stroma <55%)
2. Cytology differing between architecturally crowded focus and background—that is, cytological demarcation
3. Maximum linear dimension of the lesion exceeding 1 mm

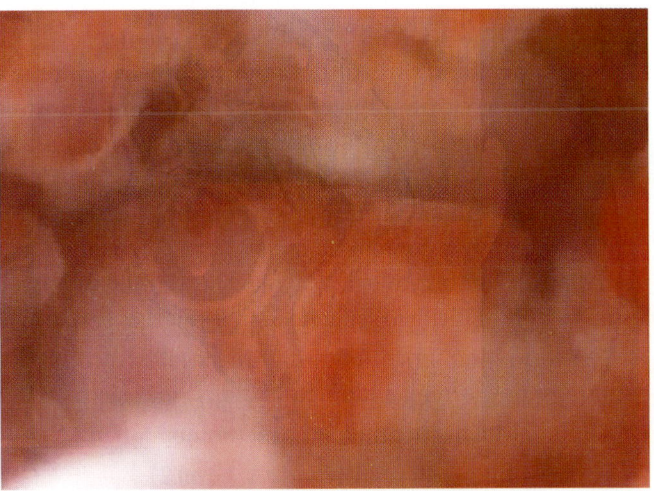

Fig. 9: Endometrial hyperplasia on hysteroscopy.

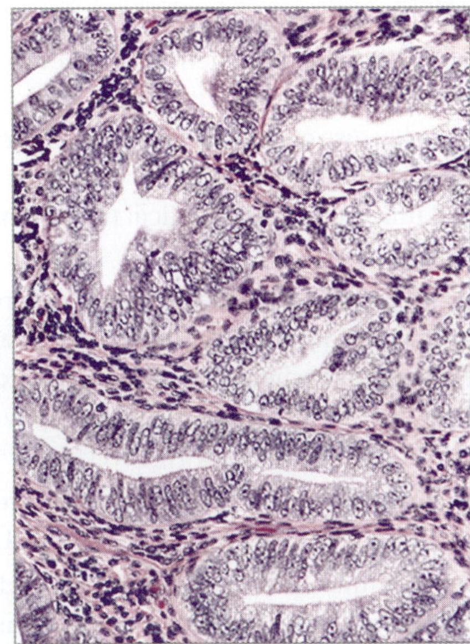

Fig. 10: Endometrial hyperplasia with atypia.

BOX 1: Histological classification of carcinoma arising in endometrium.

- Endometrioid adenocarcinoma: Variants
- Villoglandular or papillary:
  - Secretory
  - With squamous differentiation
- Mucinous carcinoma
- Papillary serous carcinoma
- Clear cell carcinoma
- Squamous carcinoma
- Undifferentiated carcinoma
- Mixed carcinoma

4. Exclusion of benign mimics
5. Exclusion of carcinoma.

Endometrial Carcinoma

The histological classification of carcinoma arising in endometrium is shown in **Box 1**.

Endometrioid Adenocarcinoma

Accounts for about 80% of the endometrial carcinomas. These tumors are composed of glands that resemble normal endometrial glands, they have columnar cells with basally oriented nuclei, little or no intracytoplasmic mucin, and smooth intraluminal surfaces. As the tumor becomes less differentiated, they contain more solid areas, less glandular formation and more cytological atypia. The well-differentiated lesions may be difficult to separate from atypical hyperplasia.[36]

Hence, to summarize, following are the latest recommendations for performing endometrial biopsy in cases of AUB:

- Endometrial histopathology is recommended in AUB:
  - In women > 40 years (Grade A; Level 2)
  - In women < 40 years who have high-risk factors for carcinoma endometrium such as irregular bleeding, obesity, hypertension, polycystic ovary syndrome (PCOS), diabetes, endometrial thickness > 12 mm on ultrasound, family history of malignancy of breast/ovary/colon, use of tamoxifen for HRT or breast cancer, hereditary nonpolyposis colorectal cancer (HNPCC), or AUB unresponsive to medical treatment (Grade A. Level 2).
- Endometrial aspiration should be the procedure of choice for obtaining endometrial samples. If endometrium is thick on imaging, but where histopathological examination (HPE) is inadequate or atrophic, hysteroscopy should be done to rule out polyps (Grade A, Level 2).
- Dilatation and curettage should not be the procedure of choice for endometrial assessment (Grade A; Level 3).
- Transvaginal ultrasound may have a role in diagnosing hyperplasia in pre- and postmenopausal women.

KEY MESSAGES

- Cervical cancer is the second most common gynecological malignancy, with incidence of around 22/100,000 women per year. Hence, there is an intense need standardize the diagnosis and management of preinvasive disease of cervix.
- Screening with conventional Pap test was successful in reducing the incidence of cervical cancer by 79%; however, due to sampling and preparation errors associated with conventional Pap test, LBC has replaced the conventional Pap test.
- An adequate specimen for cervical cytology should contain minimum 5,000 well-visualized squamous cells with minimum obscuring factors. The presence of Transformation Zone Component is not necessary for adequate specimen.
- The various squamous abnormalities on cervical cytology include LSIL (corresponding to a histological grade of CIN 1), HSIL (corresponding to a histological grade of CIN 2, 3), Atypical Squamous Cells-US and ASC-H (squamous cells that are suspicious of, but not diagnostic of HSIL).
- Specimens for which no epithelial abnormality is noted must be labeled as "NILM".
- Screening must be started from 21 years of age. Women aged 21–65 years should undergo screening with preferably HPV test/co-testing with cytology every 5 years or cytology every 3 years.
- Screening should be stopped after 65 years, if the result of the screening test has been consistently negative in last 15 years.
- HPV testing + cytology (co-testing) is the preferred method of treatment as the negative predictive value is very high when both the test results are negative.
- Newer screening modalities include dual staining, detection of epigenetic modifications (DNA methylation) and detection of E6/E7 mRNA.
- Prevalence of AUB in India is reported to be around 17.9%, and all cases of AUB must be classified according to the PALM-COEIN system, which is based on etiopathogenesis.
- Endometrial biopsy is recommended in AUB in women > 40 years of age and in those having risk factors such as obesity, hypertension, diabetes, endometrial thickness > 12 mm on transvaginal scan (TVS), cases of PCOS, having a positive family history of breast/colon/ovarian cancer, or use of tamoxifen for HRT.
- Endometrial aspiration biopsy is the first step in evaluating a patient with AUB.
- Dilatation and curettage should be reserved in cases having cervical stenosis or where inadequate specimen was obtained.
- Hysteroscopy is more accurate in identifying polyps and submucous myoma.
- Simple endometrial hyperplasia without atypia has 1% (least) and complex hyperplasia with atypia has the maximum chances (29%) to progress to malignancy.

REFERENCES

1. Rodriguez AC, Schiffman M, Herrero R, Hildesheim A, Bratti C, Sherman ME, et al. Longitudinal study of human papillomavirus persistence and cervical intraepithelial neoplasia grade 2/3: critical role of duration of infection. J Natl Cancer Inst. 2010;102(5):315-24.
2. Kaarthigeyan K. Cervical cancer in India and HPV vaccination. Indian J Med Paediatr Oncol. 2012;33(1):7-12.
3. Carter JJ, Koutsky LA, Hughes JP, Lee SK, Kuypers J, Kiviat N, et al. Comparison of human papillomavirus types 16, 18, and 6 capsid antibody responses following incident infection. J Infect Dis. 2000;181:1911-9.
4. Muñoz N, Bosch FX, De Sanjosé S, Herrero R, Castellsagué X, Shah KV, et al. Epidemiologic classification of human papillomavirus types associated with cervical cancer. N Engl J Med. 2003;348(6):518-27.

5. Bhatla N, Lal N, Bao Y-P, Ng T, Qiao Y-L. A meta-analysis of human papillomavirus type distribution in women from South Asia: implications for vaccination. Vaccine. 2008;26:2811-7.
6. Novak's Textbook of Gynaecology.
7. Nayar R, Wilbur DC. The Bethesda System of Reporting Cervical Cytology: A Historical Perspective. Acta Cytol. 2017;61(4-5):359-72.
8. Gupta S, Sodhani P, Sardana S, Singh V, Sehgal A. Clinical determinants and smear characteristics of unsatisfactory conventional cervicovaginal smears. Eur J Obstet Gynecol Reprod Biol. 2013;168:214-7.
9. Quiroga-Garza G, Saturn LS, Trujilo CJ, Mody DR, Ge Y. Common causes for unsatisfactory Pap tests in a high-risk population: insights into a yet unresolved problem in gynecologic cytology. J Am Soc Cytopathol. 2014;3:256-60.
10. Spires SE, Banks ER, Weeks JA, Banks HW, Davey DD. Assessment of cervicovaginal smear adequacy. The Bethesda system guidelines and reproducibility. Am J Clin Pathol. 1994;102:354-9.
11. Stoler MH, Schiffman M. Atypical Squamous Cells of Undetermined Significance-Low-grade Squamous Intraepithelial Lesion Triage Study (ALTS) Group. Interobserver reproducibility of cervical cytologic and histologic interpretations: realistic estimates from the ASCUS-LSIL Triage Study. JAMA. 2001;285:1500-5.
12. The ALTS Group. Human Papillomavirus testing for triage of women with cytologic evidence of low grade squamous intraepithelial lesions: baseline data from a randomized trial. J Natl Cancer Inst. 2000;92:397-402.
13. Ronnett BM, Manos MM, Ransley JE, Fetterman BJ, Kinney WK, Hurley LB, et al. Atypical glandular cells of undetermined significance (AGUS): cytopathological features, histopathological results, and human papillomavirus detection. Hum Pathol. 1999;30:816-25.
14. Colgan TJ, Woodhouse SL, Styer PE, Kennedy M, Davey DD. Reparative changes and the false positive/false negative Papanicolaou test. Arch Pathol Lab Med. 2001;125:134-40.
15. Markowitz LE, Dunne EF, Saraiya M, Chesson HW, Curtis CR, Gee J, et al. Human papillomavirus vaccination: recommendations of the Advisory Committee on Immunization Practices (ACIP). MMWR Recomm Rep. 2014;63(RR05):1-30.
16. Paavonen J, Naud P, Salmeron J, Wheeler CM, Chow SN, Apter D, et al. Efficacy of human papillomavirus (HPV)-16/18 AS04-adjuvanted vaccine against cervical infection and precancer caused by oncogenic HPV types (PAT RICIA): final analysis of a double blind, randomised study in young women. Lancet. 2009;374:301-14.
17. Kitchener H, Canfell K, Gilham C, Sargent A, Roberts C, Desai M, et al. The clinical effectiveness and cost effectiveness of primary human papillomavirus cervical screening in England: extended follow up of the ARTISTIC randomised trial cohort through three screening rounds. Health Technol Assess. 2014;18(23):1-196.
18. Couto E, Saeterdal I, Kristine Juvet L, Klemp M. HPV catch-up vaccination of young women: a systematic review and meta-analysis. BMC Public Health. 2014;14:867.
19. Roteli-Martins CM, Naud P, De Borba P, Teixeira JC, De Carvalho NS, Zahaf T, et al. Sustained immunogenicity and efficacy of the HPV-16/18 AS04-adjuvanted vaccine: up to 8.4 years of follow up. Hum Vaccin Immunother. 2012;8(3):390-7.
20. HPV and HPV Vaccine-HCP. http://www.cdc.gov/std/HPV/STDFact-HPV-vaccinehcp.htm (accessed 6 Sep2015).
21. van Aar F, Mooij SH, Van der Sande MAB, Speksnijder AGCL, Stolte IG, Meijer CJ, et al. Anal and penile high-risk human papillomavirus prevalence in HIV negative and HIV-infected MSM. AIDS. 2013;27(18):2921-31.
22. Burger EA, Sy S, Nygard M, Kristiansen IS, Kim JJ. Prevention of HPV-related cancers in Norway: cost-effectiveness of expanding the HPV vaccination program to include pre-adolescent boys. PLoS One. 2014;9(3):e89974.
23. European Centre of Disease Prevention and Control. Introduction to HPV vaccines in European Union countries—an update. Stockholm: ECDPC; 2012.
24. Fraser IS, Langham S, Uhl-Hochgraeber K. Health-related quality of life and economic burden of abnormal uterine bleeding. Expert Rev Obstet Gynecol. 2009;4:179-89.
25. Sharma A, Dogra Y. Trends of AUB in tertiary centre of Shimla hills. J Midlife Health. 2013;4:67-8.
26. NICE. Heavy menstrual bleeding. [online] Available from: http://www.nice.org.uk/guidance/QS47. [Last accessed December, 2021].
27. Buckley CH, Fox H. Inflammation of the endometrium. In: Buckley CH, Fox H (Eds). Biopsy Pathology of the Endometrium. London: Chapman and Hall; 2002. pp. 91-111.
28. Mazur MT, Kurman RJ. Endometritis. In: Mazur MT, Kurman RJ (Eds). Diagnosis of endometrial biopsies and curettings. Berlin: Springer; 2005. pp. 147-162.
29. Kim KR, Peng R, Ro JY, Robboy SJ. A diagnostically useful histopathological feature of endometrial polyp: the long axis of endometrial glands arranged parallel to surface epithelium. Am J Surg Pathol. 2004;28:1057-62.
30. Feeley KM, Wells M. Hormone replacement therapy and endometrium. J Clin Pathol. 2001;54:435-40.
31. Kurman RJ, Norris HJ. Evaluation of criteria for distinguishing atypical endometrial hyperplasia from well differentiated carcinoma. Cancer. 1982;15:2547-59.
32. Baak JPA, Mutter GL. EIN and WHO94. J Clin Pathol. 2005;58:1-6.
33. Mutter GL. Endometrial intraepithelial neoplasia (EIN): will it bring order to chaos? The Endometrial Collaborative Group. Gynecol Oncol. 2000;76:287-90.
34. Mutter GL. Diagnosis of premalignant endometrial. J Clin Pathol. 2002;55:326-31.
35. Bokhman JV. Two pathogenetic types of endometrial carcinoma. Gynecol Oncol. 1983;15:10-7.
36. Zaino RJ, Kurman RJ, Diana KL, Morrow CP. The utility of the revised International Federation and Gynecology and Obstetrics histologic grading of endometrial adenocarcinoma using a defined nuclear grading system. A Gynecologic Oncology Group Study. Cancer. 1995;75:81-6.

LONG QUESTIONS

1. Classify endometrial hyperplasia. Discuss briefly the morphological features of endometrial hyperplasia.
2. Name the various modalities for cervical cancer screening. Describe in detail the role of HPV testing as a screening modality.

3. Elaborate on the role of cervical cytology as a screening modality for cervical cancer. Discuss in detail the various premalignant lesions noted in the cervical cytology.

SHORT QUESTIONS

1. Briefly describe the criteria for assessing the adequacy of the cervical cytology specimen.
2. Write short notes on the significance of presence of ASC present in the cervical cytology.
3. Discuss on newer screening modalities for cervical cancer.
4. Discuss briefly the non-neoplastic findings found in the cervical cytology.
5. What are morphological features of endometrial intra-epithelial lesion?

MULTIPLE CHOICE QUESTIONS

1. All of the following belong to high-risk group for development of cervical cancer, except:
   a. Women with prior CIN2, CIN3
   b. Women using OCPs for >10 years
   c. Women > 70 years of age, with negative smears in the last 3 years
   d. Smokers
2. All are true regarding cervical cancer screening, except:
   a. Screening should be started at 21 years of age
   b. Conventional cytology should be done every 3 years in women between 21 and 65 years of age
   c. In women who have already undergone treatment for CIN 2, screening is not recommended
   d. High-risk group women should be screened with HPV testing combined with cytology
3. All of the following are prerequisites for adequacy for cervical smear cytology, except:
   a. Presence of >5,000 well-preserved/well-visualized squamous cells
   b. Minimal contamination by lubricants/blood/ spermatozoa
   c. Presence of endocervical/transformation zone component
   d. All of the above
4. Which of the following tests is used to detect human papillomavirus (HPV)?
   a. Hybrid capture 2 b. APTIMA assay
   c. COBAS test d. All of the following
5. Which of the following is not true regarding combined cytology and HPV testing?
   a. Recommended in women < 30 years
   b. Women with negative cytology and negative HPV test should be offered co-testing after 5 years
   c. Women with cytology report as ASCUS with negative HPV test should be offered co testing after 1 year
   d. Negative predictive value of combined testing is very high
6. The newer modalities for cervical cancer screening are:
   a. Dual test
   b. Extended genotyping of HPV
   c. Detection of DNA methylation
   d. All of the above
7. The use of regular screening with the cytology-based Pap test for triage of HPV positive women is associated with which of the following:
   a. A low rate of false positives
   b. Retesting at lower intervals
   c. A high rate of false positives, but women are retested at longer intervals
   d. A high rate of false positives, and women are retested at shorter intervals
8. Which of the following test detects an over expression of p16 protein?
   a. Extended genotyping b. Dual staining
   c. Oncoprotein testing d. Reflex cytology
9. Regarding endometrial biopsy, which of the following statements is true?
   a. Endometrial aspiration biopsy is the first step in evaluating a patient with AUB
   b. Hysteroscopy is more accurate in identifying polyps and submucous myoma
   c. While sending endometrial biopsy specimen, the date of last menstrual period and history of hormonal intake should always be conveyed to the pathologist
   d. All of the above
10. Which of the following is the characteristic morphological appearance of the endometrium induced by progesterone?
    a. Pseudodecidualization just beneath the surface glands
    b. Disordered proliferation of the glands
    c. Cystic changes in the gland
    d. Presence of plasma cells, admixed with other inflammatory cells

Answers

1.	c	2.	c	3.	d	4.	d	5.	a	6.	d
7.	b	8.	b	9.	d	10.	a				

7.3 ULTRASOUND IN GYNAECOLOGY: UTERINE DISEASE

Sonal Panchal, Chaitanya Nagori

INTRODUCTION

Uterine abnormality is the cause of majority of the gynecological complaints and ultrasound is now considered a first-line investigation for its assessment. Uterus can be visualized on ultrasound by transabdominal route as well as transvaginal route. Though the assessment by transvaginal ultrasound (TVS) is the best choice, transabdominal scan is usually preferred before the transvaginal scan if the patient is being assessed for a particular complaint for the first time. Transabdominal scan gives a better idea about the gross anatomy, but has a disadvantage of having lower resolution than the transvaginal route, due to lower frequency probe used for transabdominal scan and also due to more distance of the uterus from the probe. Therefore, for the detailed study of the intrauterine anatomy, transvaginal route is preferred. In cases when this is not possible or permissible, transrectal route may be used. Doppler is very essential for differential diagnosis of various uterine pathologies. Volume ultrasound (3D-4D ultrasound) can significantly increase to the details available and is considered essential for the diagnosis of müllerian abnormalities and endometrial pathologies of the uterus. Sensitivity of the volume ultrasonography (USG) for the detection of congenital uterine abnormalities is very high and therefore it is also known as "virtual hysteroscopy".[1] Saline infusion sonohysterography is also a useful modality for evaluation of the endometrial pathologies.

Uterine abnormalities can be divided into müllerian duct abnormalities and acquired pathologies.

MÜLLERIAN DUCT ABNORMALITIES

Uterus is formed by the fusion of the two paramesonephric (müllerian) ducts at 10 weeks of gestation followed by resorption of fused midline tissues occurring by 20th week by apoptosis **(Fig. 1)**. Arrest of these processes at different stages may result into various müllerian duct abnormalities.

- Failure of one or more müllerian duct to develop
- Failure of the ducts to canalize
- Failure to fuse or abnormal fusion of müllerian ducts
- Failure of resorption of midline uterine septum.

Incidence of müllerian duct abnormalities is 0.1–3.8% in normal fertile females but reaches 6.7% in infertile patients.[2] For the ease of differentiating and diagnosing, these abnormalities are classified into groups. In 2003, the American Fertility Society (AFS) published a classification system **(Fig. 2)**.[3]

But in 2013, European Society of Human Reproduction and Embryology (ESHRE) and European Society of Gynaecological Endoscopy (ESGE) joined together and devised a new classification system named ESHRE-ESGE classification for müllerian abnormalities **(Figs. 3A and B)**.[3] This is claimed to be more suitable classification system for the accurate and clear diagnosis and is correlated with clinical management with simple categorization of female genital anomalies. The system is based on anatomy and cervical and vaginal anomalies are classified independently into subclasses having clinical significance. It is thought to be more practical also because according to this system, the uterus's own myometrial wall thickness measurement is used as a standard to evaluate the abnormalities of the shape. This system has been developed by common working group under the name CONUTA (CONgenital UTerine Anomalies).[4,5]

This classification system can be explained as follows:[3]

Class U0 is a normal uterus. It shows a straight or convex contour of the uterine fundus and that of the endometrium also. But even when the endometrial contour is concave, if the depth of the indentation at the fundal midline does not exceed 50% of the uterine wall thickness, it is still considered a normal uterus **(Fig. 4)**. This means that when the uterus is seen in the midcoronal plane, the vertical distance between the highest point on the endometrium to the highest point on the fundus is defined as myometrial wall thickness and this distance is the standard of measurement for evaluation of any müllerian abnormality. According to this classification therefore an entity called "arcuate uterus" does not exist.

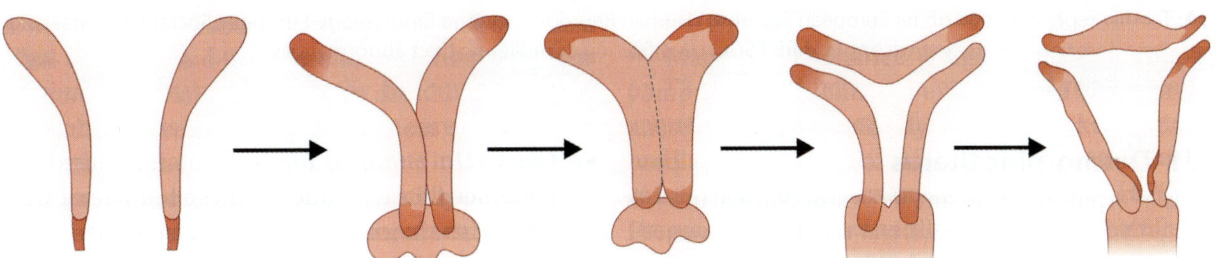

Fig. 1: Development of the uterus in utero.

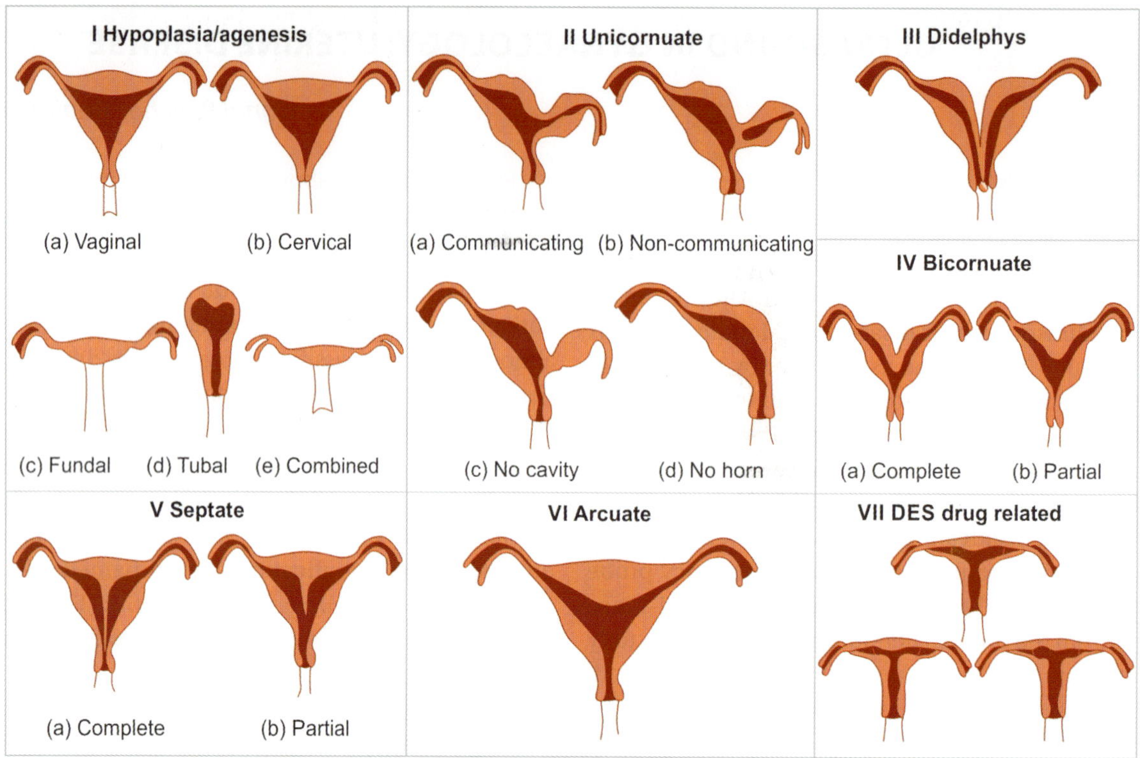

Fig. 2: Müllerian abnormalities: American Fertility Society classification.

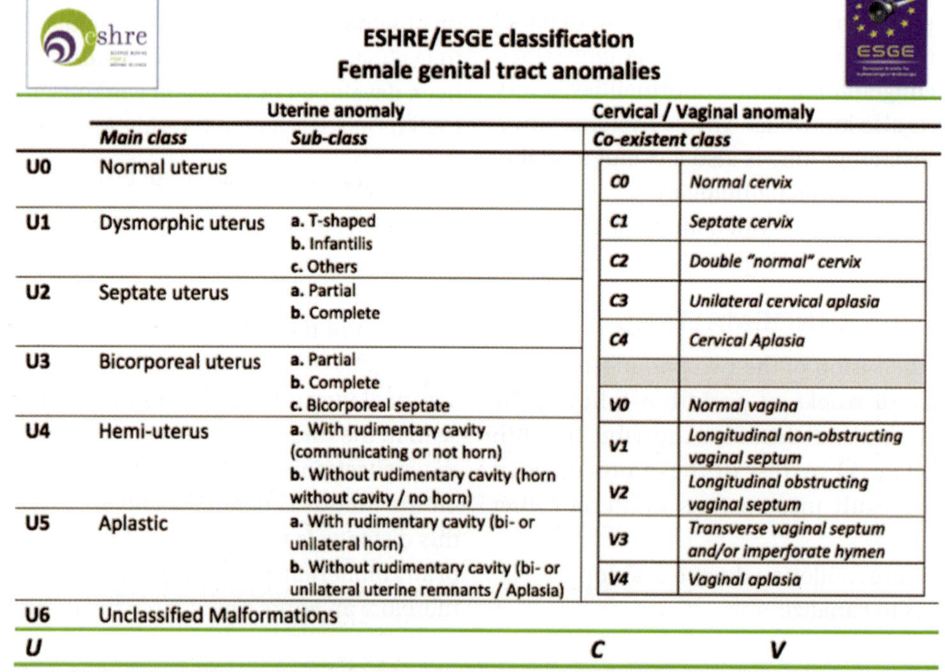

ESHRE/ESGE classification
Female genital tract anomalies

	Uterine anomaly	
	Main class	***Sub-class***
U0	Normal uterus	
U1	Dysmorphic uterus	**a.** T-shaped **b.** Infantilis **c.** Others
U2	Septate uterus	**a.** Partial **b.** Complete
U3	Bicorporeal uterus	**a.** Partial **b.** Complete **c.** Bicorporeal septate
U4	Hemi-uterus	**a.** With rudimentary cavity (communicating or not horn) **b.** Without rudimentary cavity (horn without cavity / no horn)
U5	Aplastic	**a.** With rudimentary cavity (bi- or unilateral horn) **b.** Without rudimentary cavity (bi- or unilateral uterine remnants / Aplasia)
U6	Unclassified Malformations	
U		

Cervical / Vaginal anomaly	
Co-existent class	
C0	*Normal cervix*
C1	*Septate cervix*
C2	*Double "normal" cervix*
C3	*Unilateral cervical aplasia*
C4	*Cervical Aplasia*
V0	*Normal vagina*
V1	*Longitudinal non-obstructing vaginal septum*
V2	*Longitudinal obstructing vaginal septum*
V3	*Transverse vaginal septum and/or imperforate hymen*
V4	*Vaginal aplasia*
C	***V***

Fig. 3A: Tabular representation of the European Society of Human Reproduction and Embryology-European Society of Gynaecological Endoscopy (ESHRE-ESGE) classification of müllerian duct abnormalities.

Class U1–Dysmorphic Uterus

Usually, dysmorphic uteri are smaller in size. Normal uterine fundal shape but with an abnormal shape of the endometrial cavity excluding septa. This class is further classified into three subclasses: a, b and c.

- *Class U1a-T-shaped uterus*: This is a narrow uterine endometrial cavity due to thickened lateral walls with normal uterocervical ratio (2:1). Increased lateral wall thickness is diagnosed when the lateral wall thickness is more than 1.4 times the myometrial wall thickness.

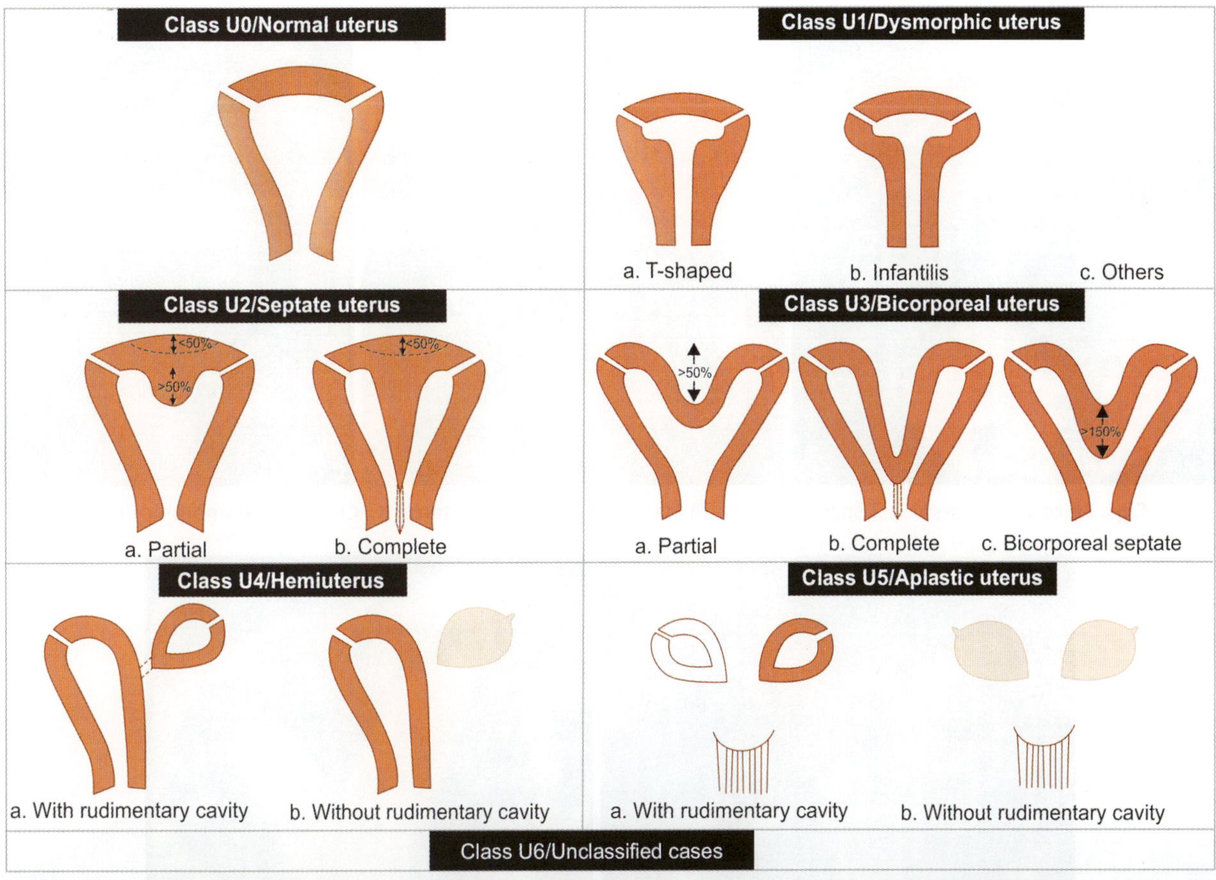

Fig. 3B: Diagrammatic representation of the European Society of Human Reproduction and Embryology-European Society of Gynaecological Endoscopy (ESHRE-ESGE) classification of müllerian duct abnormalities.

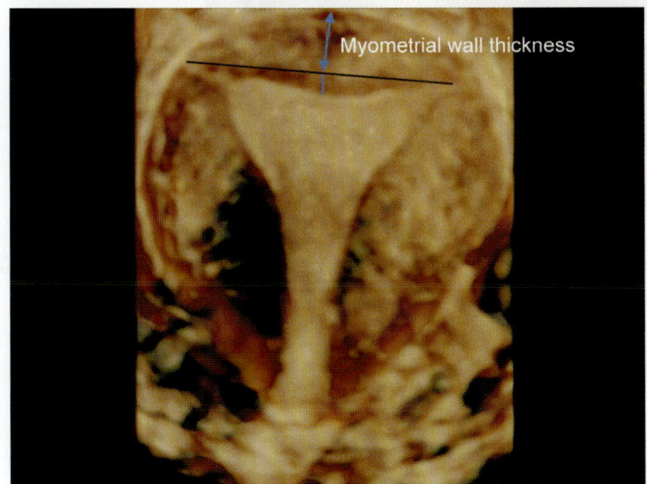

Fig. 4: 3D ultrasound image of the normal uterus (class U0) showing interostial line (black) and the two blue arrow lines, the longer one indicating uterine wall thickness.

A line is drawn from the cornu of the uterus to the internal os on the midcoronal plane of the uterus. On this line a perpendicular is drawn from the deepest point on the lateral endometrial wall. The part of this perpendicular from the cornu-internal os line to the lateral serosal wall is the lateral wall thickness **(Fig. 5A)**.

- *Class U1b*: This subclass, uterus infantilis has a narrow uterine cavity without lateral wall thickening but an inverse utero-cervical ratio **(Fig. 5B)**.
- *Class U1c*: These uteri have minor deformities of the uterine cavity including those with an inner indentation at the fundal midline level of up to 50% of the myometrial wall thickness **(Fig. 5C)**.

Class U2: Septate Uterus

Septum in the uterus is because of normal development of the uterus till the fusion of both the müllerian ducts but abnormal absorption of the midline septum. This class is identified by normal fundal outline and an internal indentation/notch on the fundus exceeding 50% of the myometrial wall thickness.

The indentation may extend up to the internal os or may end short of that and respectively then named as Class U1b (complete septum) **(Fig. 6A)**, Class U1a (partial septum) **(Fig. 6B)**. The septum may divide the cervix and/or vagina also.

On b mode it is difficult to differentiate between duplication abnormalities of uterus viz. bicornuate, septate/subseptate and arcuate. But 3D US is conclusive. Preovulatory or secretory phase are the best phases to diagnose congenital uterine abnormalities especially in 3D US. The features that diagnosed septate uterus of AFS classification were absent fundal dimple, angle of <75° between the two endometrial

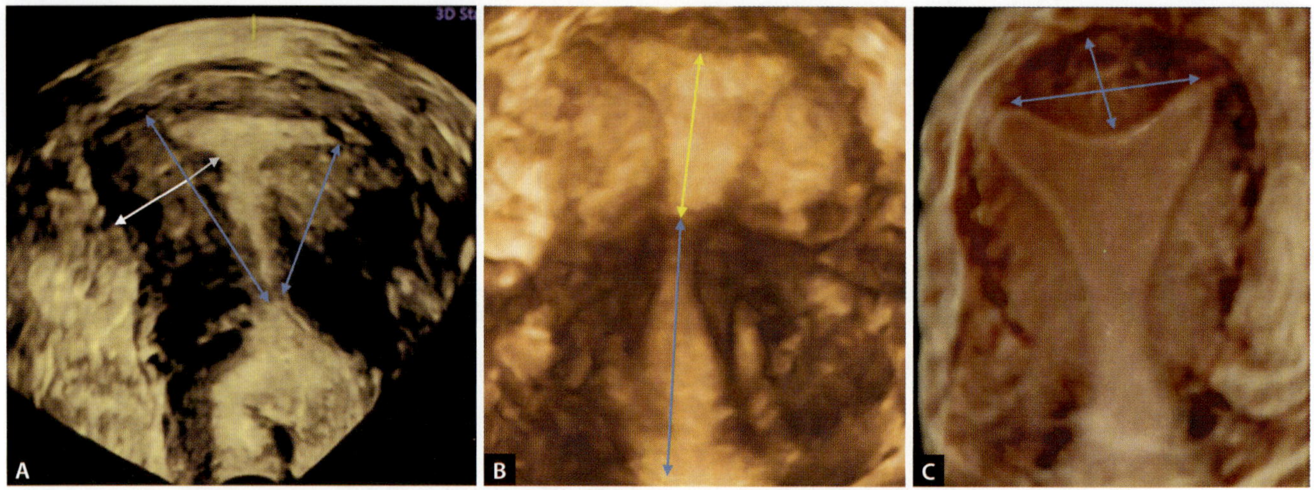

Figs. 5A to C: (A) Class U1a: T-shaped uterus; (B) Class U1b: hypoplastic uterus; (C) Class U1c: dysmorphic uterus.

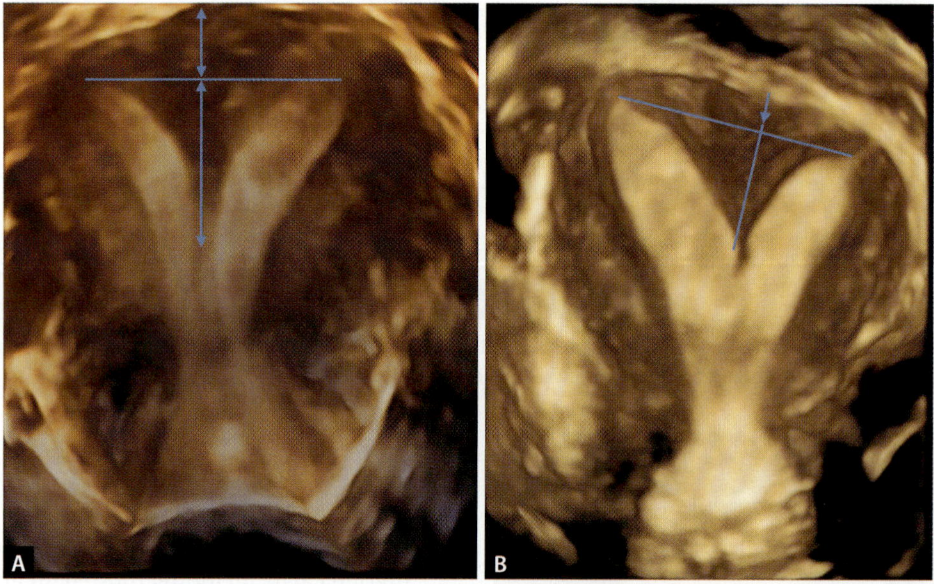

Figs. 6A and B: (A) Class U2a: complete septum; (B) Class U2b: partial septum.

cavities and at least 5 mm of uterine wall can be seen above the line joining tips of two endometrial cavities **(Fig. 7)**.

Septate uterus has maximum implications on fertility and pregnancy outcome among all müllerian duct abnormalities:[6-8]

- Infertility
- Frequency of ectopic 27.34% as compared to 13.3% otherwise
- *First trimester abortions:* 28–45%
- *Second trimester abortions:* 5%
- Premature deliveries
- Dystocia.

These may be attributed to high resistance vascularity in the septum, less development of estrogen receptors in overlying endometrium and less connective tissue in the septum to allow decidualization.

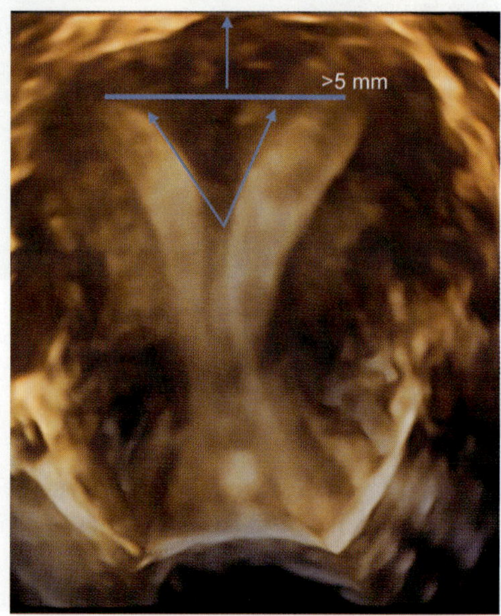

Fig. 7: Features of the septate uterus according to American Fertility Society (AFS) classification.

Class U3: Bicorporeal Uterus

The term bicornuate uterus is now changed to bicorporeal uterus. Indentation on the fundal outer surface is the hallmark of this class of abnormalities. Indentation on the external fundal outline, if it exceeds 50% of the myometrial wall thickness and the inner indentation at the midline level that divides the cavity as happens also in case of septate uterus, this is the bicorporeal uterus.

Class U3a is partial bicorporeal, when the external fundal indentation is partly dividing the uterine corpus above the level of the internal os **(Fig. 8A)**.

Class U3b is complete bicorporeal uterus, with external fundal indentation completely dividing the uterine corpus up to the level of the internal os **(Fig. 8B)**.

The third subclass in this class, Class U3c is bicorporeal septate uterus **(Fig. 8C)**. This is a result of absorption defect in addition to fusion defect. There is an indentation on the fundal wall along with the division of the endometrial cavity, but with a thick myometrial wall between the two cavities. When the distance from the endometrial dip to the fundal dip is measured, if it exceeds 150% the myometrial wall thickness then it is a bicorporeal septate uterus.

On transvaginal scan on B mode ultrasound, uterus may not be seen in the midline if the cornu are placed far from each other. Bicorporeal uterus on ultrasound shows two separate fully formed corpora as one moves the probe from one lateral wall to other in sagittal plane. But if the two corpora are closely placed, instead of midsagittal plane, parasagittal plane of the uterus is seen and on spanning the probe, both the uterine corpora can be seen. Two horns may show symmetrical or asymmetrical development. On transverse section, it typically shows figure of eight **(Fig. 9)**. Abdominal scans are essential to exclude associated renal abnormalities.

Comparing this to the AFS classification, complete bicorporeal uterus with normal double cervix was earlier named as didelphys uterus, bicorporeal uterus with septate cervix is bicornuate bicollis and that with normal cervix is what was earlier known as bicorporeal unicollis. This uterus class matches somewhat to the bicornuate group of the AFS classification and then was identified by fundal indentation, angle of >105° between the endometrial cavities, infolding of myometrium and more <5 mm distance between lowest point on the fundus and the line joining the two endometrial cavities **(Fig. 10)**.

Three-dimensional power Doppler typically shows V/Y arrangement of the blood vessels in the myometrium between the two endometrial cavities **(Fig. 11)**.

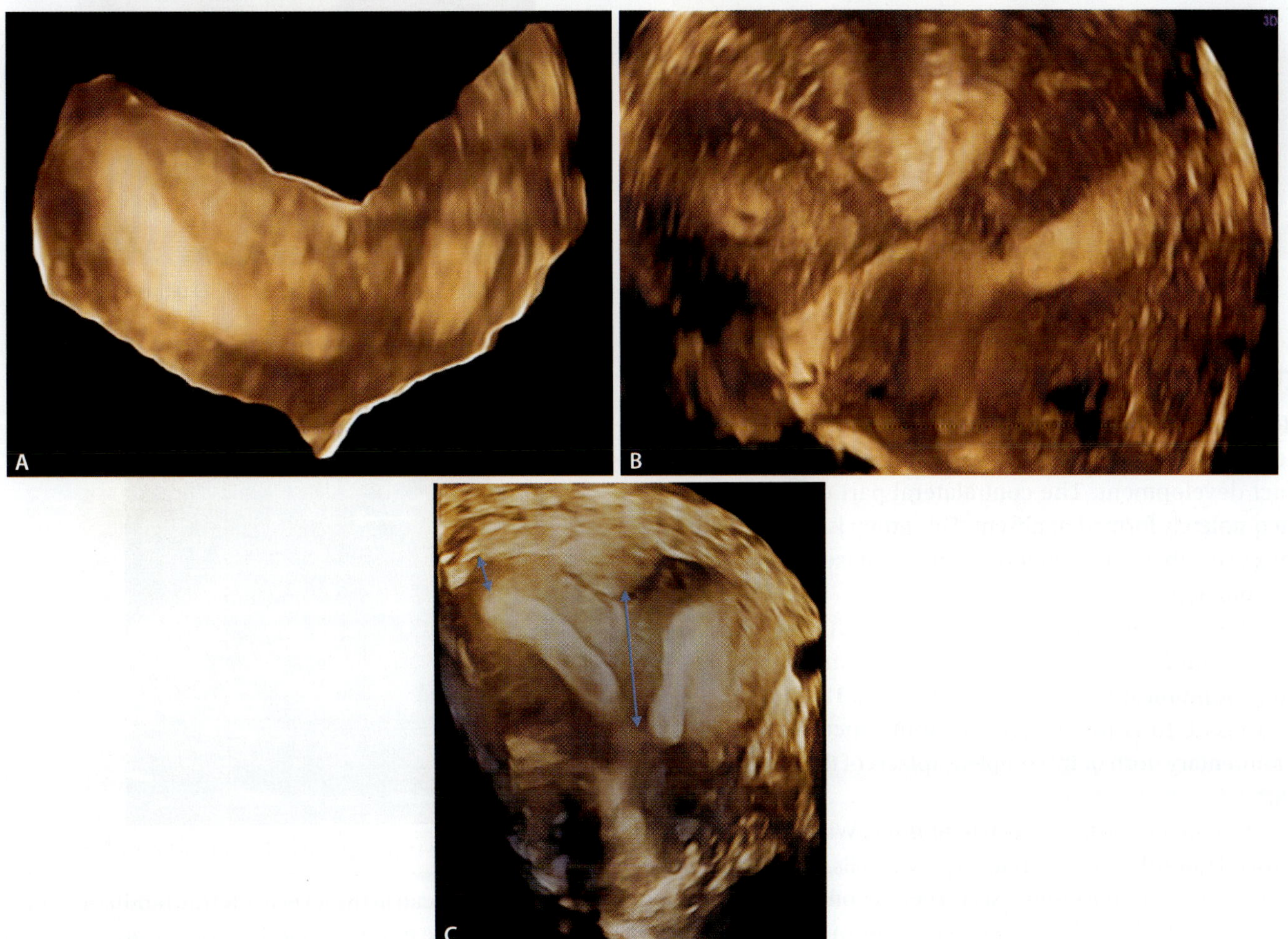

Figs. 8A to C: (A) Class U3a: partial bicorporeal uterus; (B) Class U3b: complete bicorporeal uterus as seen on 3D ultrasound; (C) Class U3c: bicorporeal septate uterus.

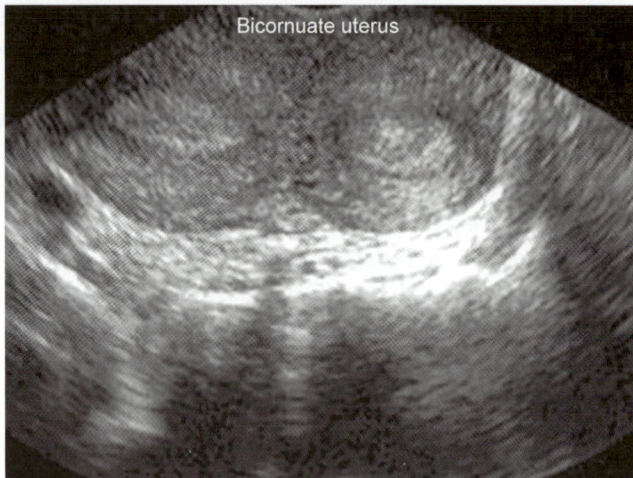

Fig. 9: Figure of eight formed by transverse section of normal double cervix.

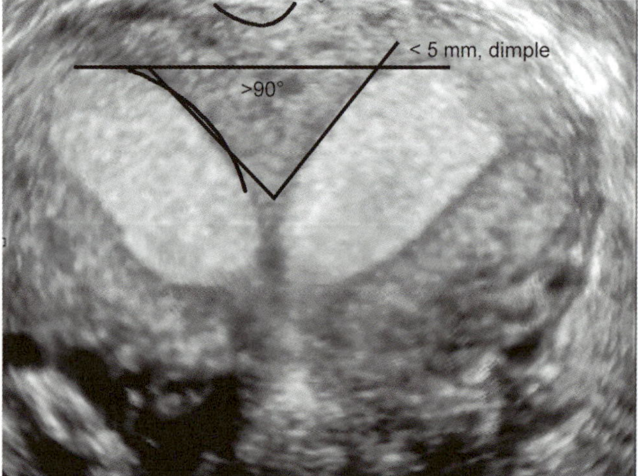

Fig. 10: Bicornuate uterus on 3D ultrasound showing diagnostic features of American Fertility Society (AFS) system.

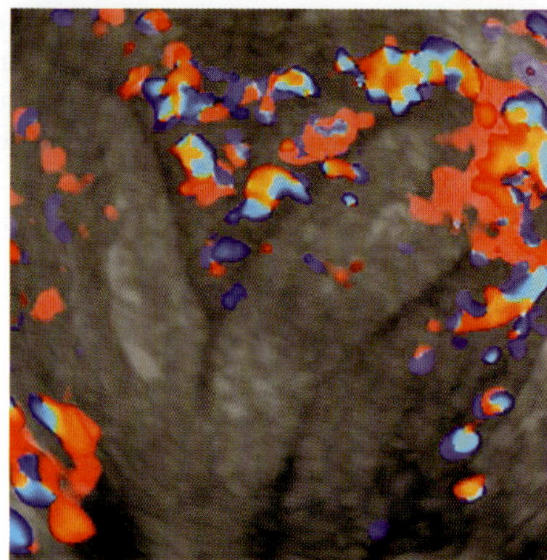

Fig. 11: 3D power Doppler image of this complete bicorporeal uterus shows typical V/Y arrangement of blood vessels.

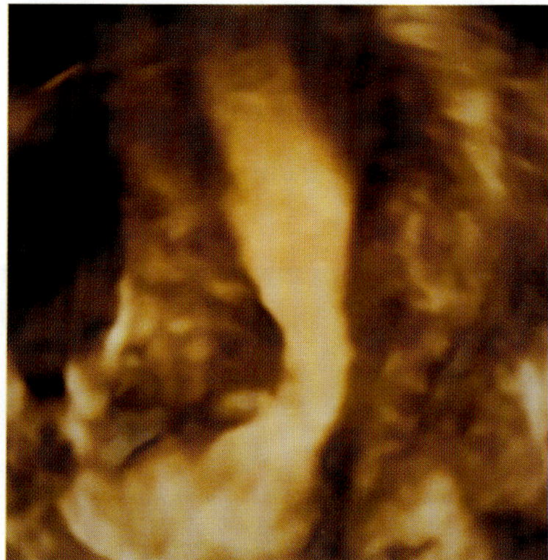

Fig. 12: Class U4: hemiuterus on 3D ultrasound.

Class U4

Hemiuterus is a term used for the old term, unicornuate uterus and it is a formation defect. It is unilateral müllerian duct development. The contralateral part could be either incompletely formed or absent. This group is further divided into two subclasses depending on the presence or not of a functional rudimentary cavity.

Class U4a is hemiuterus with a functional cavity in the rudimentary horn which may be communicating or noncommunicating with hemiuterus **(Fig. 12)**.

Class U4b is hemiuterus without functional cavity in rudimentary horn or by complete aplasia of the contralateral part.

On TVS, uterus is not seen in midline. When the probe is scrolled towards one of the lateral pelvic walls, normal looking uterine contour in its long axis is seen on one side in pelvis. No uterine shadow or only rudimentary horn is seen on other side as an isoechoic pear-shaped cavity, usually adjacent to the ipsilateral ovary **(Fig. 13)**.

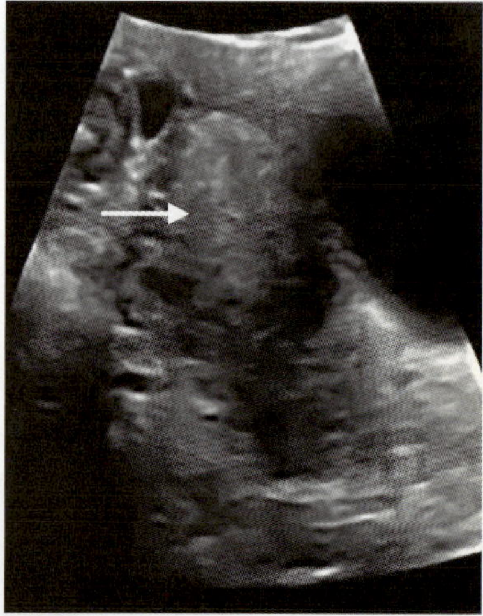

Fig. 13: B-mode image of the rudimentary horn of uterus.

On transverse scan at the level of uterine fundus a beak like projection from the endometrial shadow, cornu is seen only on one side. 3D ultrasound is diagnostic and clearly shows a banana-shaped uterine cavity **(Fig. 12)**.

Class U5: Aplastic Uterus/Uterine Aplasia

Absence of any fully developed uterine corpora. Unilateral or bilateral rudimentary horns with cavity may be seen in some, while in others there could be uterine remnants without cavity. Coexistent defects (e.g., vaginal aplasia/Mayer-Rokitansky-Küster-Hauser syndrome) are common with this group of abnormalities.

Class U5a is plastic uterus with rudimentary (functional) bilateral or unilateral functional horn. Class U5b is aplastic uterus without rudimentary (functional) cavity.

Uterine aplasia is suspected in patients with primary amenorrhea. Transabdominal scan with full bladder shows convex base with no dimple. This indicates complete absence of uterus and karyotyping is essential in these patients. Rudimentary horn is identified by pear-shaped isoechoic structures with or without thin echogenic line in the center. This echogenic line, if present, indicates a functional cavity. Ovaries may be seen in close vicinity to these horns.

Class U6: Unclassified Cases

These are infrequent anomalies, subtle changes or combined pathologies could not be allocated correctly to one of the six groups. The classification of cervical canal anomalies and vaginal anomalies is also an additional advantage.

Cervix can be classified as C0-normal cervix, C1-septate cervix, and C2-double normal cervix and can be confidently diagnosed by 3D ultrasound **(Figs. 14A to C)**. Though unilateral cervical aplasia which constitutes C3 class cannot be easily diagnosed on ultrasound. Cervical aplasia is rare.

Congenital uterine abnormalities are commonly associated with congenital renal abnormalities like ectopic kidney or unilateral absent kidney. Therefore, an abdominal scan is essential in all patients with congenital uterine malformations.

ACQUIRED UTERINE ABNORMALITIES

- Myometrial lesions
- Endometrial lesions
- Cervical lesions.

Myometrium is normally homogenously hypoechoic and serosal surface is smooth and regular. Distortion in any of these two suggests myometrial lesion. Common *myometrial lesions* are fibroids, adenomyosis, adenomyomas, and leiomyosarcomas.

Fibroid

Fibroid is a well-defined noninvasive fibromuscular mass lesion. They are found in 20–40% of women from age 30 onwards and are common in nulliparous. Fibroids may only be an incidental finding in many but may also present with dysmenorrhea, menorrhagia, metrorrhagia, infertility, or miscarriages. Fibroids affect fertility because of distortion of endometrial cavity due to submucous fibroid, pressure of the fibroid and stretching of endometrium overlying it causing atrophy of endometrial glands and stroma, and low flow due to stretching of vessels and less delivery of hormones.

On B-mode ultrasound fibroid **(Fig. 15A)** presents as a well-defined, hypoechoic, homogenous, round/oval, solid lesion, with peripheral hypoechoic rim due to displacement of myometrial fibers. Fibroids show typical vertically oriented alternating hyper and hypoechoic bands, starting from within the lesion and extending behind the lesion. These are known as "fan shadows". On both the lateral margins of the lesion, a thick hypoechoic shadow is seen and this is named as "edge shadows". Echogenicity increases with amount of fibrous tissue and vascularity. On Doppler the lesion typically shows a peripheral vascularity **(Fig. 15B)**. These vessels are vessels of displaced muscle fibers and therefore show a refractive index (RI) of 0.54 ± 0.08.[9] Resistance is higher in submucosal fibroids and deep intramural fibroids and lower in subserosal fibroids. Amount of vascularity decides the activity or growth potential of fibroid.

Fibroid may undergo a morphological change due to large size with loss of internal/central vascularity or due to alteration in morphology due to change in the hormonal environment. It thus leads to red degeneration in pregnancy, calcification

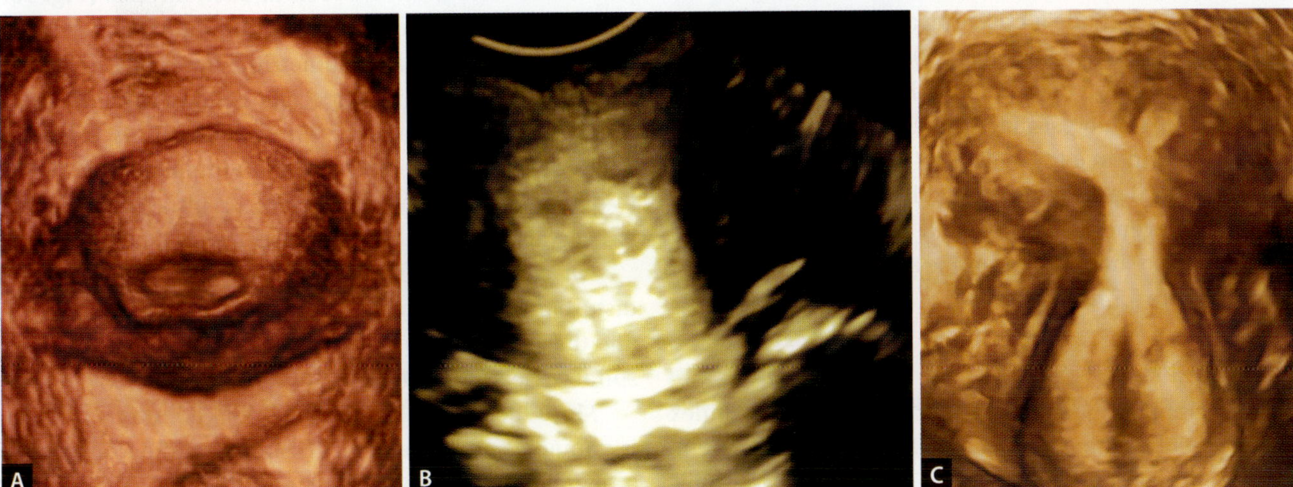

Figs. 14A to C: (A) Single normal cervix–C0; (B) Cervix with septum–C1; (C) Normal double cervix–C2.

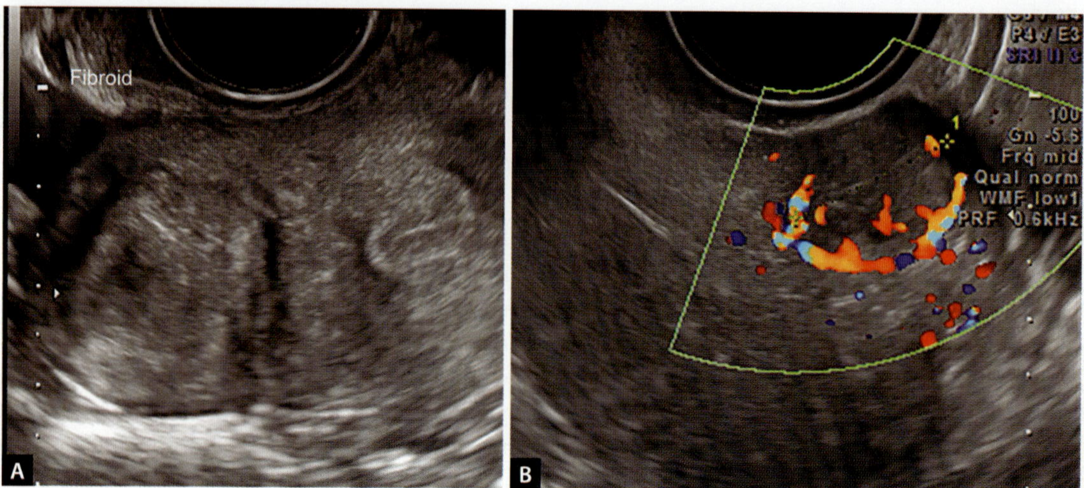

Figs. 15A and B: (A) B-mode; (B) Color Doppler image of fibroid.

or cystic change near menopause. Degeneration in fibroids causes heterogenicity of texture due to hyperechogenicity, cystic areas, or calcifications **(Figs. 16A to C)**. Red degeneration typically leads to internal vascularity in the fibroid, which is limited by the peripheral vascularity and is named as "intralesional vessels" **(Fig. 16D)**. These vessels have markedly lower resistance than that of the nondegenerated fibroid.

Fibroids are classified according to their location as **(Fig. 17)**:[10]

- *Type 0:* Pedunculated endometrial fibroid
- *Type 1:* Subendometrial lesion with >50% inside the endometrial cavity
- *Type 2:* Subendometrial lesion, <50% in the endometrial cavity
- *Type 3:* Intramural fibroid but touching the endometrium
- *Type 4:* Completely intramural fibroid
- *Type 5:* Intramural fibroid, <50% beyond the serosa
- *Type 6:* Intramural fibroid, >50% beyond the serosal margin
- *Type 7:* Pedunculated subserosal or sessile subserosal fibroid, completely beyond the serosal margin.

Malignant change is known in fibroid and this leads to a lesion named as leiomyosarcoma. It heterogeneous echogenicity on B-mode ultrasound, and low resistance flow on doppler. Resistance as low as 0.37 ± 0.03 RI with rapid growth in size and disruption of well-defined margins are typical of leiomyosarcoma. But resistance indices of vessels cannot be used as only evidence for malignant change and therefore doppler cannot be used as a reliable tool to differentiate between the degenerated fibroid and leiomyosarcoma. Uteri with fibroids also show higher uterine artery peak velocity and lower RI (mean: 0.74 ± 0.09).

Volume Ultrasound

3D power Doppler indices—vascular index (VI), flow index (FI), and vascularization flow index (VFI) are especially useful for follow-up of fibroids in patients who are on gonadotropin-releasing hormone agonist (GnRHa) therapy, menopausal, or pregnant. 3D US is also useful for the exact localization of the fibroid and precisely estimates the relationship between submucous fibroid and endometrial cavity.

Diffuse leiomyomatosis is a rare condition in which there is diffuse and uniform involvement of entire myometrium by multiple fibroids **(Fig. 18)**.

Fibroids when arise from below the internal os are cervical fibroids and show similar appearances as fibroid in the uterus.

Adenomyosis

Adenomyosis is ectopic growth of endometrium in myometrium, common in multiparous women. It is an invasive lesion with indistinct margins and may show generalized or localized involvement of the uterus.

On B-mode ultrasound it shows globular or asymmetrical thickening and heterogenicity of the myometrium due to echogenic spots/lines/islands and anechoic areas (myometrial cysts). Fan shadows as described for the fibroids are typical of adenomyosis but these are more finer than those seen in fibroids. Irregularity, interruption or inaccessibility of the junctional zone is always seen in adenomyosis **(Fig. 19A)**. Echogenic flecks may be seen at junctional zone. Reverse curvature of the fundal endometrium described as "ear sign" or "question mark sign" is especially common in asymmetrical involvement of the uterus with adenomyosis **(Fig. 19B)**. Tenderness on probe pressure is an important sign elicited by dynamic ultrasound assessment. 3D ultrasound especially is a very useful modality for assessment of junctional zone.

On color Doppler, the affected area typically shows disturbance in the normal arrangement of the spiral vessels and these vessels also show a larger caliber than the normal spiral vessels **(Fig. 19C)**.[11]

More localized and fairly defined adenomyotic lesion is named as adenomyoma. This may be often mistaken for a degenerated fibroid. The main differentiating points of adenomyoma from fibroid are absence of edge shadows,

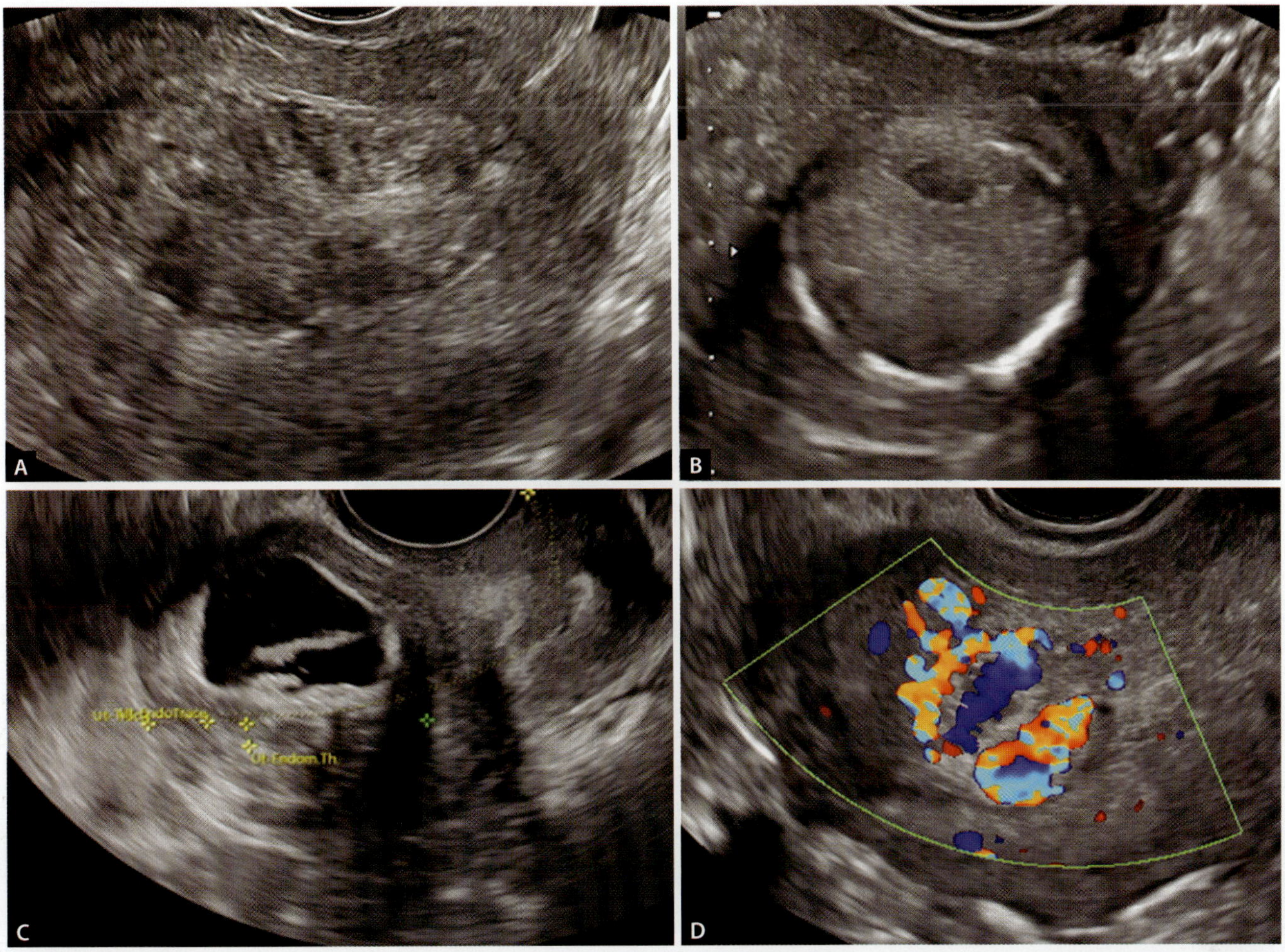

Figs. 16A to D: (A) B-mode image of hyperechoic degenerated fibroid; (B) Calcified fibroid; (C) Cystic degeneration of fibroid; (D) Peripheral and intralesional vascularity of degenerated fibroid.

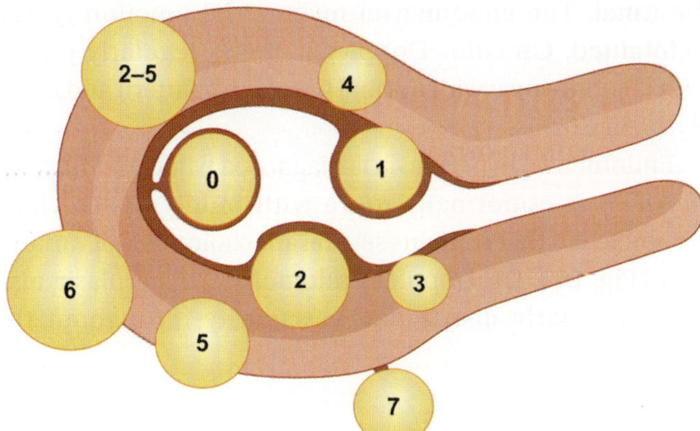

Fig. 17: Diagrammatic presentation of different types of fibroid according to FIGO-PALM-COEIN classification.

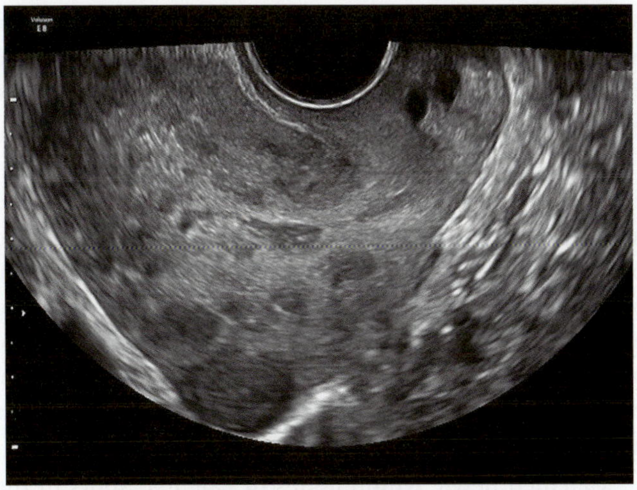

Fig. 18: B-mode image of diffuse leiomyomatosis.

absence of peripheral vascularity and altered junctional zone in the earlier.

Endometrium

Endometrium normally is pear shaped and its morphology changes with the phase of the menstrual cycle. Distortion of endometrial contour with/without alteration of junctional zone may be signs of endometrial pathologies.

Common endometrial pathologies are endometritis, polyps, endometrial hyperplasia, endometrial malignancies, synechiae, and other miscellaneous conditions with residual products of conception in endometrial cavity.

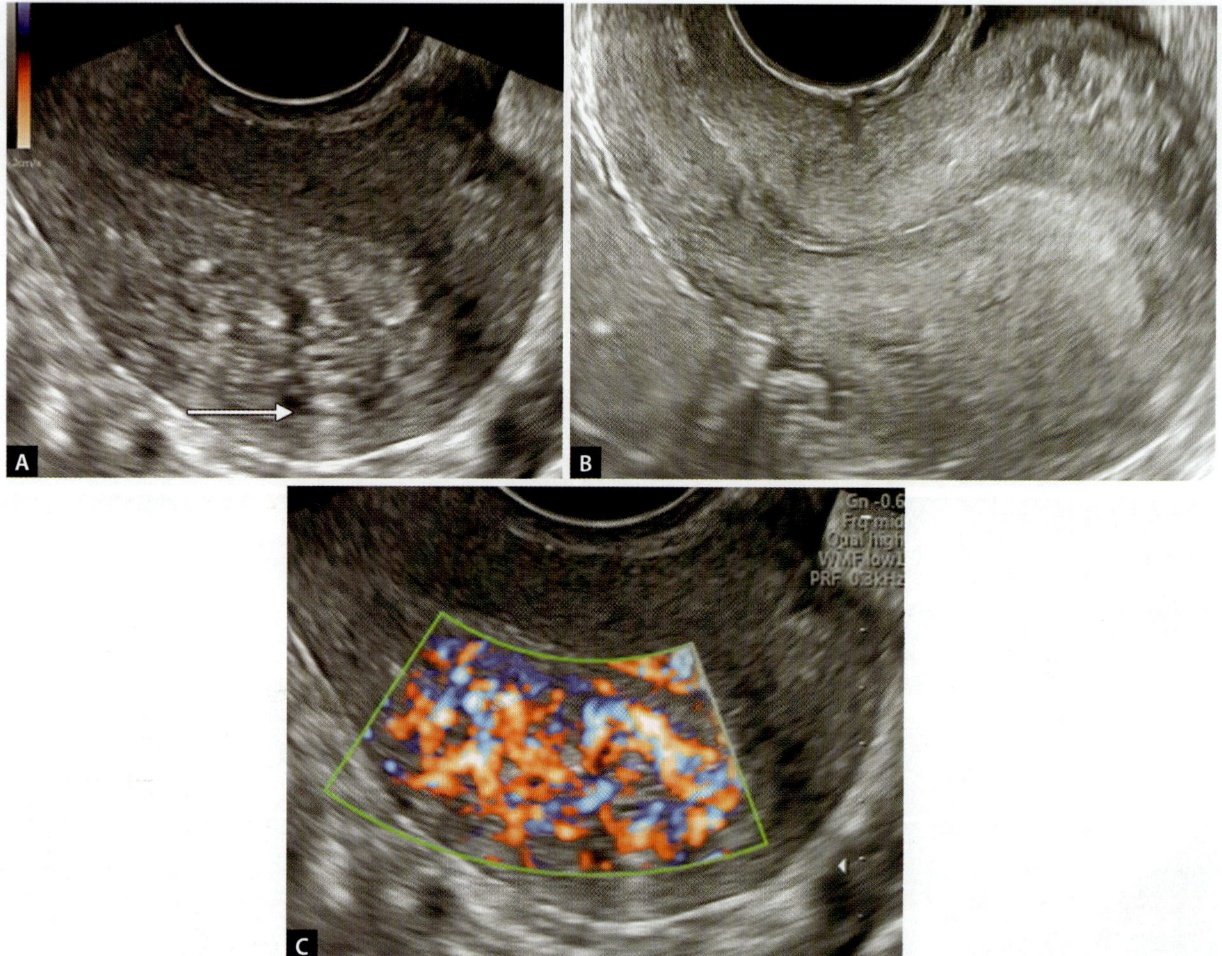

Figs. 19A to C: Adenomyosis. (A) On B-mode; (B) Ear sign or question mark sign; (C) On Doppler.

Endometritis

Acute endometritis presents as thick, isoechoic endometrium with altered junctional zone **(Fig. 20A)** and increased vascularity seen on doppler. Some fluid may be seen in the endometrial cavity.

Chronic endometritis presents as thin avascular endometrium throughout the menstrual cycle with altered junctional zone **(Fig. 20B)**. Chronic endometritis may also be due to Koch's. These uteri more commonly have vertical orientation of the interstitial part of the tube, scarred endometrial cavity, fluid in the endometrial cavity in the mid-proliferative phase with hyperechoic inner margin, endometrial, myometrial, and junctional zone calcifications and micropolyposis **(Figs. 20C to E)**.

Calcified pelvic lymph nodes or calcified spots in the adnexa may be seen in chronic inflammatory lesions.

Endometrial Hypertrophy and Hyperplasia

An overgrowth of endometrium with normal histology, presenting as thick endometrium with normal ultrasound morphology, in part or entirely is endometrial hypertrophy. Endometrial thickness >14 mm in premenopausal patient and <5 mm in postmenopausal patients may be considered abnormal. The endometrial-myometrial junction is well maintained. On color Doppler it shows regularly placed vessels supplying it with normal branching pattern and mean RI of 0.55 ± 0.05.

Endometrial hyperplasia is diagnosed when endometrial thickness is abnormally more with mildly hyperechoic endometrium that contains several anechoic areas of variable sizes **(Fig. 21)**. On Doppler endometrial, hyperplasia also shows regularly distributed vascularity throughout the endometrium.

Polyps

Endometrial polyps are solid projectile lesions from the endometrial walls into the endometrial cavity. Sonographically they are seen as solid round or oval, pedunculated or sessile echogenic lesions in the endometrial cavity **(Fig. 22A)**. When large these may fill up the endometrial cavity and look like generalized endometrial thickening.

On 2D US the polyps are best visible in the periovulatory phase. Single feeding vessel **(Fig. 22B)** is a diagnostic sign on Doppler. The vessel usually shows RI > 0.45. Infection, necrosis, or atypia may reduce resistance to 0.37.

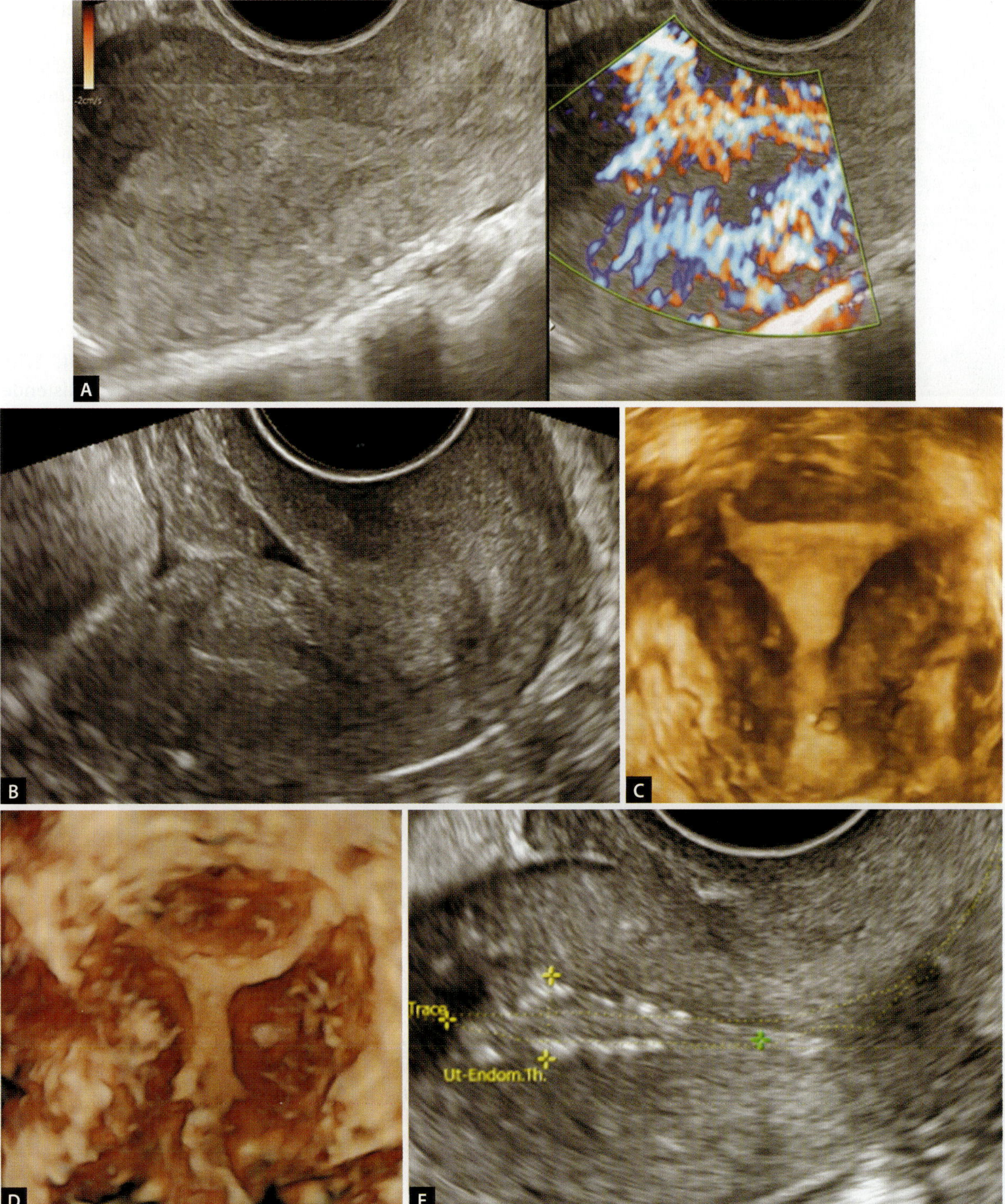

Figs. 20A to E: (A) B-mode and Doppler image of acute endometritis; (B) B-mode image of chronic endometritis; (C) Vertical orientation of cornu seen on 3D image, coronal plane; (D) Scarred endometrial cavity; (E) Endometrial calcification.

Single vessel pattern for polyp:[12]

- Sensitivity 81.2%
- Specificity 88.2%
- Positive predictive values 92.9%
- Negative predictive values 71.4%

Polyps may arise from the cervix **(Figs. 23A and B)**.

Endometrial polyps may be difficult to differentiate from type 0 fibroids. But fibroids are hypoechoic and are well demonstrated in echogenic endometrium of secretory phase and have peripheral vascularity unlike the polyps.

Saline infusion sonohysterography with B-mode ultrasound or 3D ultrasound can also be diagnostic **(Fig. 24)**.

Method

- Preferably done from day 6–10 of normal length cycle in lithotomy or lithotomy-like position.

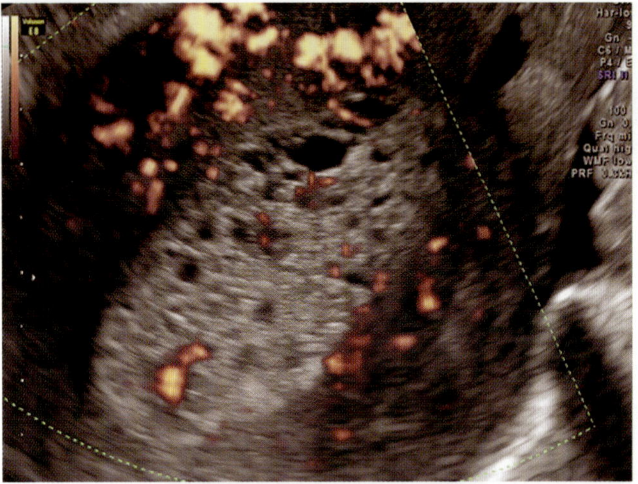

Fig. 21: Endometrial hyperplasia: B-mode and power Doppler.

- 6 Fr (external diameter 1.6 mm and internal diameter 1.1 mm) Foley's catheter is placed in cervix. Catheter balloon in cervical canal. Distend balloon with 1.5–2 mL of fluid.
- Slowly inject 5 mL of normal saline with 10 mL syringe to distend the uterine cavity.
- Remove all metal instruments and introduce the probe into the vagina with catheter in situ.
- TVS shows fluid distended endometrial cavity. Endometrial lesions will be clearly seen.

Synechiae

Synechiae are fibrous strands between the endometrial walls, due to infection or surgical insult. When the endometrium is multilayered or the cavity is distended with the fluid, synechiae are seen as lines bridging between layers

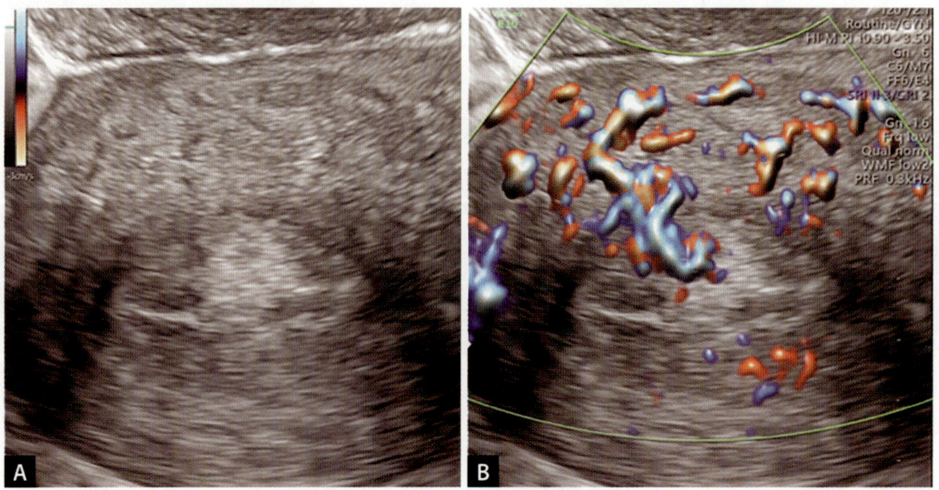

Figs. 22A and B: (A) B-mode; (B) Doppler image of polyp.

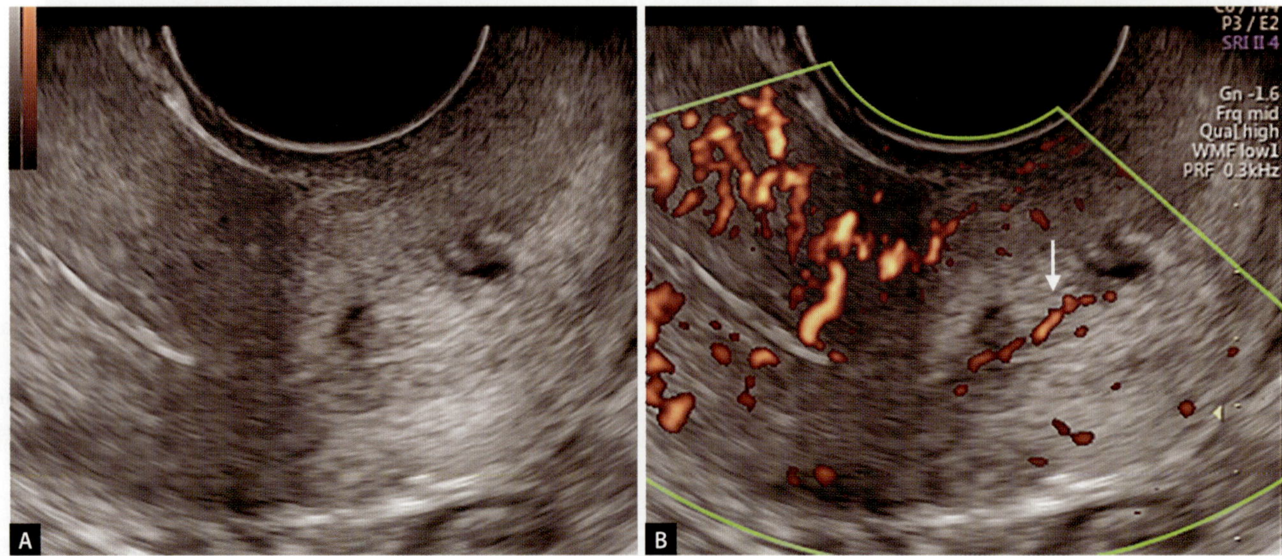

Figs. 23A and B: (A) B-mode; (B) Doppler image showing single feeding vessel of cervical polyp.

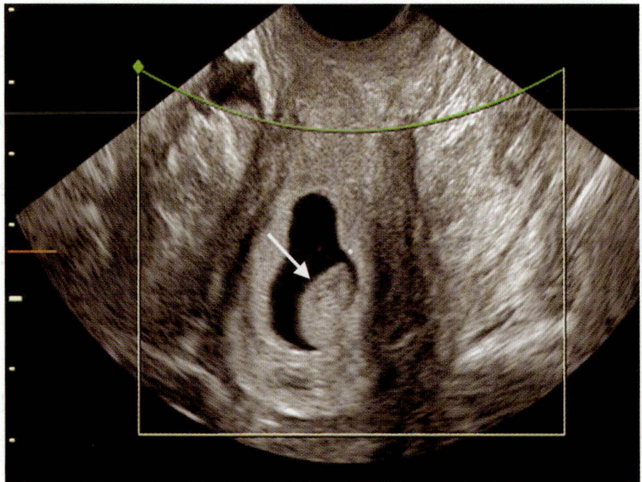

Fig. 24: Endometrial polyp on saline infusion sonohysterography.

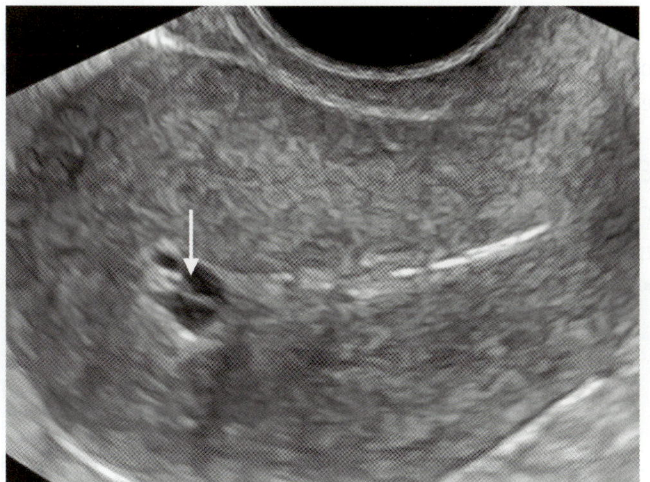

Fig. 25: B-mode image of uterine synechiae.

of endometrium **(Fig. 25)**. Sonohysterography with B-mode ultrasound or 3D ultrasound has 100% sensitivity for the differentiation of all endometrial pathologies.

There may be blood or blood products in the endometrial cavity post curettage or incomplete abortion, or in patients with hematometra due to cervical malignancies, etc. Blood in the endometrial cavity that may be partially clotted shows heterogeneous shadows filling endometrial cavity **(Fig. 26)**. Related history may correlate the finding to the cause.

Vesicular Mole

Hyperechoic endometrium with anechoic areas. This echogenicity is higher than that of a normal secretory endometrium as it is because of decidual reaction. If it becomes malignant, it would break the endometrial-myometrial interface. On color Doppler it shows low resistance and low velocity flow **(Figs. 27A and B)**. But in very early phase, Doppler will not show flow due to very low velocities. Of course, β-human chorionic gonadotropin (β-hCG) levels and its correlation with US findings are diagnostic. There is

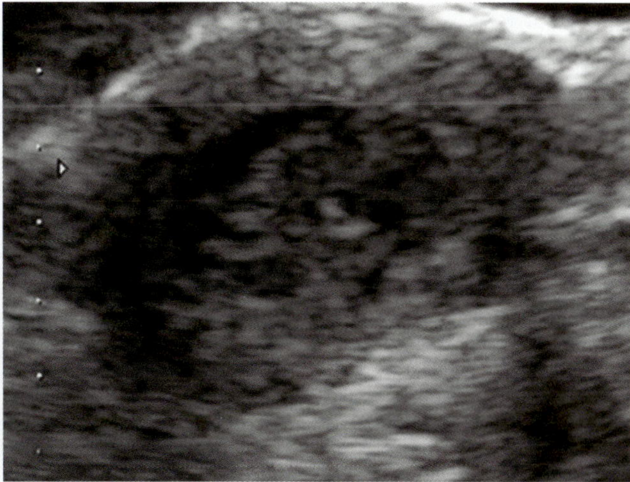

Fig. 26: Heterogeneous content (blood) in endometrial cavity.

a rare possibility of the molar tissue being coexistent with a normal gestational sac. This is partial mole. It is more difficult to suspect this diagnosis because of presence of the normal pregnancy.

In patients with missed abortion, progressive disappearance of villous vascularity after embryonic death leads to villous hydrops and this condition is known as a pseudopartial hydatidiform (vesicular) mole. This is not actually a vesicular mole.

Endometrial calcifications are common after curettage, medical termination of pregnancy **(Fig. 28)** or chronic endometritis.

Intrauterine contraceptive device (IUCD) placement can also be checked by US. It is properly placed if distance between the fundus and the tip of the IUCD < 5 mm. Even in large or very small uteri if distance from tip of IUCD to outer wall of uterine fundus ≤ (anterior wall + posterior wall)/2 × 1.33, it indicates a proper placement. For displaced IUCD, US is the investigation of choice as it determines the exact location and therefore route of removal of IUCD. 3D ultrasound is a more demonstrative and a better diagnostic modality **(Figs. 29A and B)**.

Uterine Scar

With the increase in the incidence of operative delivery, cesarean scars are seen in a huge percent of females attending the gynecologists' clinic. It may be seen as thick linear echogenic shadows traversing the whole myometrium at the level of internal os. An intact scar may also be seen as hyperechoic shadows at the serosal level with posterior acoustic shadowing. When these scars show dehiscence, a small anechoic triangle is seen with the base at the endometrium **(Fig. 30A)**. Scar thickness in nonpregnant uterus is measured as distance from the tip of the triangle to serosa. The scars sometimes are completely open and connect with the vaginal or peritoneal cavity. Fluid movement can be seen from such scar into the endometrium and may interfere

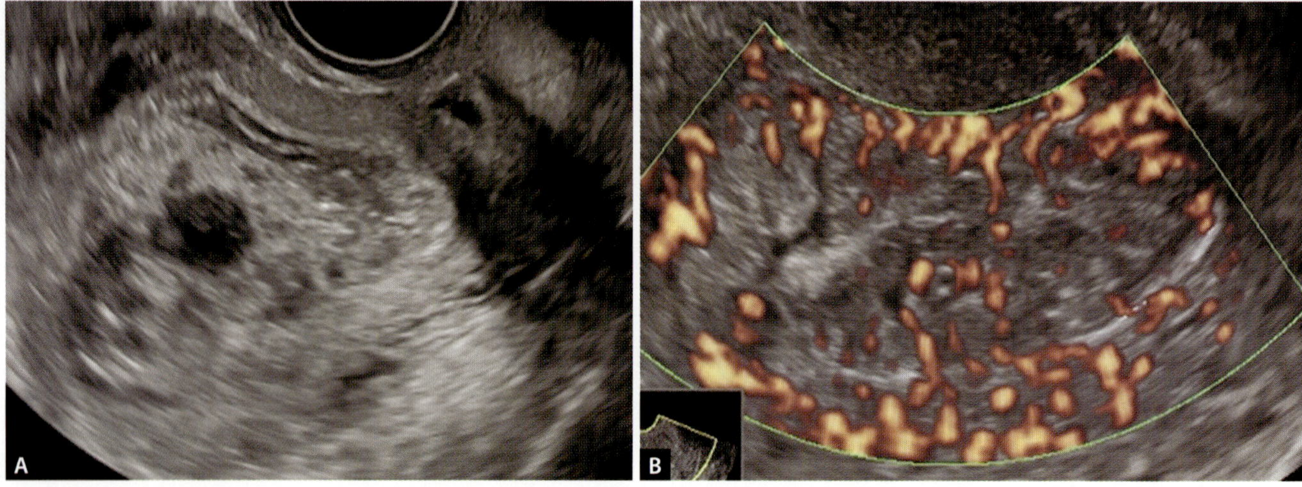

Figs. 27A and B: Vesicular mole. (A) 2D ultrasound; (B) Doppler.

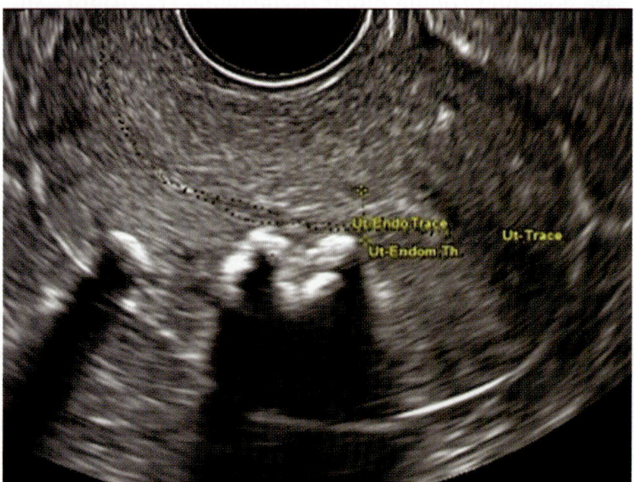

Fig. 28: Endometrial calcification on B-mode ultrasound.

with implantation **(Fig. 30B)**. 3D can be very helpful for exact assessment of the lesion.

Endometrial Malignancy

This pathology is common in postmenopausal age and may present as postmenopausal bleeding. On B-mode US, there is thickening of the endometrium, localized or generalized, with heterogeneous echogenicity **(Fig. 31A)**, interrupted endometrial-myometrial junction, with or without fluid in endometrial cavity. Though the junctional zone may be intact in early stages of the tumor. On color Doppler there is markedly increased vascularity[13] (vascularity score 4). The vessels often show low RI (< 0.45) but even higher resistance in postmenopausal age does not exclude malignancy.

With increase in size of lesion and invasion the resistance further decreases. 3D power Doppler shows dichotomous branching, intermittent narrowing and ballooning due to microaneurysms **(Fig. 31B)**. It has a sensitivity of 100%, specificity of 94.44%, and positive and negative predictive value of 83.33% and 100%, respectively.[14]

Tamoxifen has been thought to be causative of endometrial carcinoma. But this is a very late and not very common side effect of tamoxifen.

Effects of Tamoxifen on Endometrium

Changes occurring in the endometrium as a result of tamoxifen treatment are as follows:

- *Stages of endometrial metaplasia:*
  - Echogenic endometrium with good halo and homogenous structure
  - Echogenic endometrium, good boundaries with small echo free cysts
  - Echogenic nonhomogeneous, small cystic structures, and blurred boundaries
  - Echogenic nonhomogeneous endometrium, blurred boundaries, and interrupted halo
- *Endometrial cystic atrophy:*
  - Endometrial cystic atrophy mimics hyperplasia
  - Thickening of the subendometrial zone/endometrial stroma-irregular endometrial-myometrial junction
  - High resistance flow around the cyst unlike malignancy which shows increased velocity decreased resistance (0.39 vs. 0.79)
  - Increased vascularity may be seen with thinner endometrium and decreased vascularity with thick endometrium
  - lower the resistance higher chances of atypia (<0.5)
  - Uterine artery resistance >3.

Cervical Lesions

Apart from fibroids and polyps of cervix, the most common lesions in cervix are nabothian cysts. These appear as well-defined anechoic rounded lesions in cervix. These may be of infective origin, but do not have an impact on fertility.

Cervical malignancies are solid lesions in cervix and on ultrasound present as heterogeneous lesions with irregular

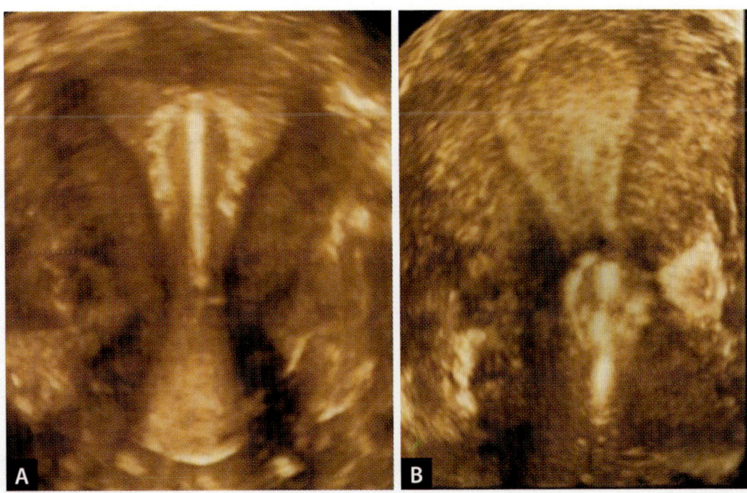

Figs. 29A and B: Intrauterine contraceptive device on 3D rendering. (A) In situ; (B) Displaced in cervix.

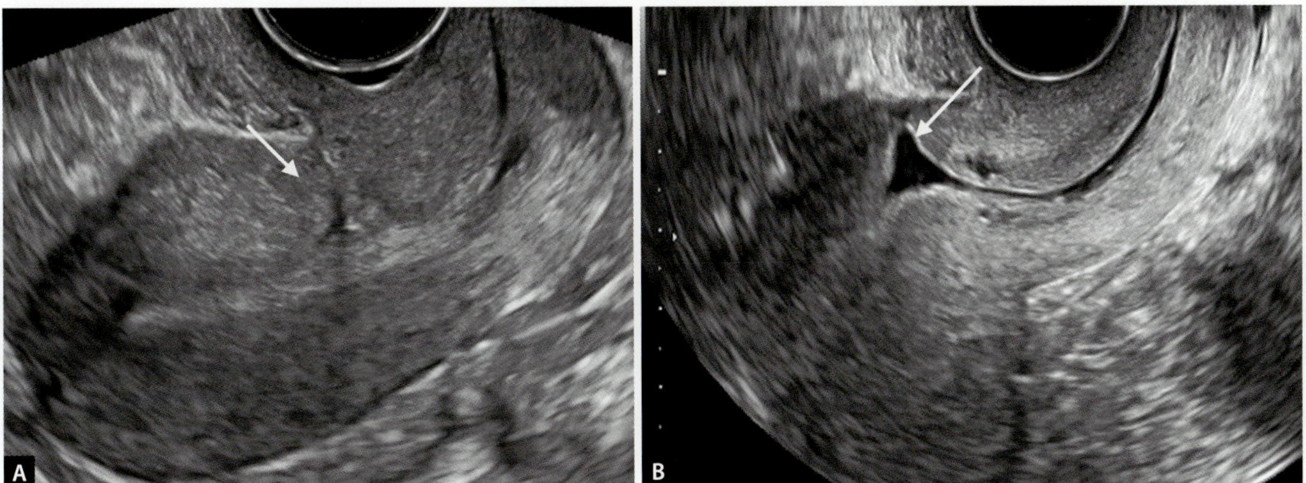

Figs. 30A and B: (A) B-mode image of the normal intact scar (arrow); (B) Weak scar seen on B-mode image (arrow).

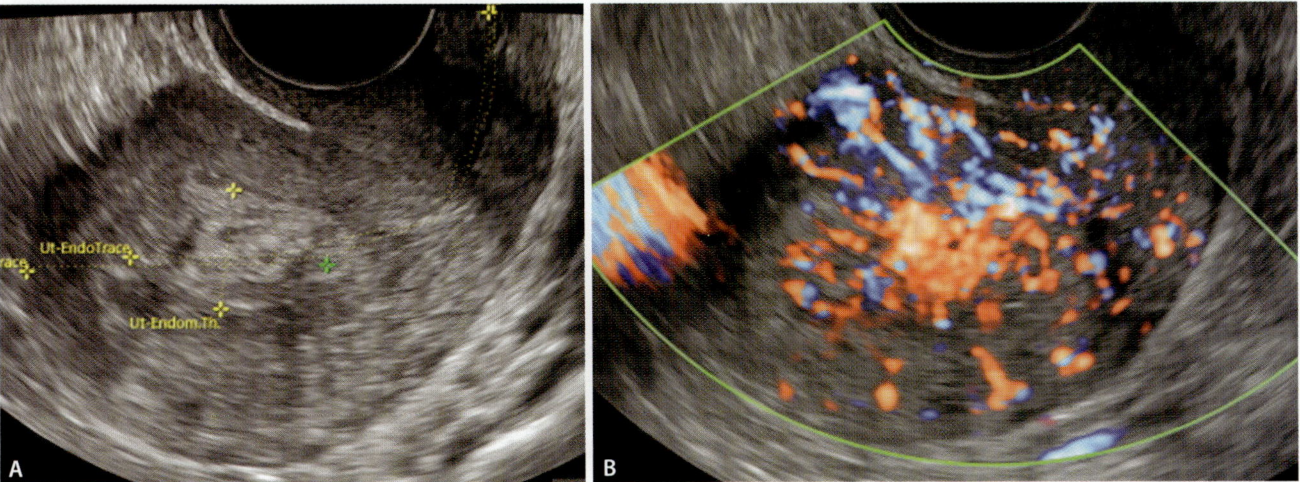

Figs. 31A and B: (A) Endometrial mass on B-mode; (B) Power Doppler (PD) showing heterogeneous vascularity.

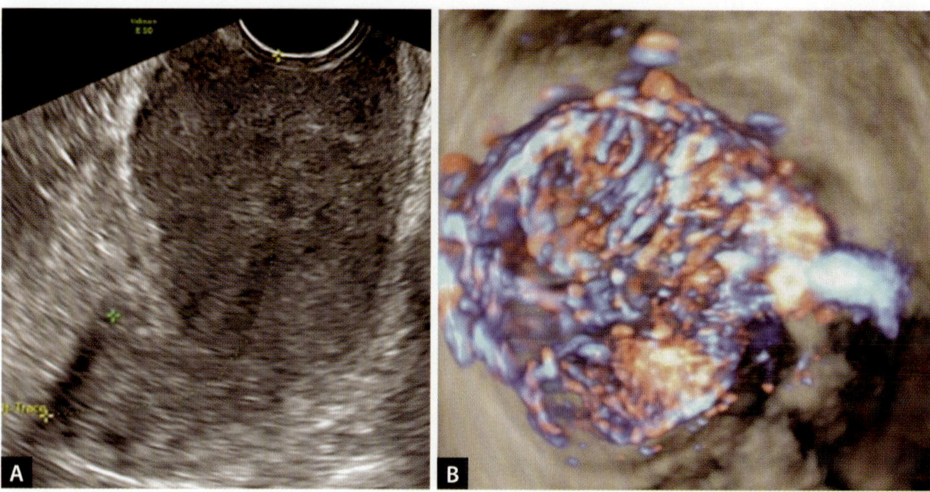

Figs. 32A and B: (A) Cervical mass possibly malignant on B-mode; (B) 3D power Doppler (PD) of the same mass with typical malignant chaotic vascularity.

margins **(Fig. 32A)**. When the lesion grows beyond the cervix, ultrasound shows broken tissue planes. Color Doppler shows significantly increased low-resistance vascularity. 3D US is an excellent tool to assess the parametrial invasion. 3D power Doppler shows typical chaotic vascular branching pattern **(Fig. 32B)**.

CONCLUSION

Ultrasound is the primary modality and modality of choice for assessment of the uterus and diagnosis of uterine abnormalities. Role of Doppler and saline infusion sonosalpingography cannot be underestimated for differential diagnosis of endometrial pathologies. 3D ultrasound is essential for differential diagnosis of müllerian abnormalities. 3D power Doppler may add to the confidence in lesions where malignancy is suspected.

KEY MESSAGES

Ultrasound is the primary modality for the assessment of the uterus. Systematic B mode assessment and dynamic assessment by transvaginal route are essential. Doppler helps in differential diagnosis of uterine pathologies due to specific vascular pattern for specific pathology, like single feeding vessel for polyp and peripheral vascularity for fibroid, etc. 3D ultrasound is indispensable for diagnosis of müllerian duct abnormalities. 3D is also an important modality for assessment of the endometrial distortion or invasion by different endometrial pathologies. 3D and 3D power Doppler add significantly to the information available by ultrasound in cases of malignancies of the uterus.

REFERENCES

1. Cossi PS, Werner H, Peixoto AB, Martins WP, Araujo Júnior E. Virtual hysteroscopy: a new noninvasive approach for the assessment of uterine cavity. Med Ultrasound. 2017;19(2):216-17.
2. Raga F, Bonilla-Mosules F, Blanes J. Congenital müllerian anomalies: diagnostic accuracy of three-dimensional ultrasound. Fertil Steril. 1996;65(3):523-8.
3. Rock JA, Roberts CP, Jones HW. Congenital anomalies of the uterine cervix: lessons from 30 cases managed clinically by a common protocol. Fertil Steril. 2010;94:1858-63.
4. Grimbizis GF, Tsalikis T, Mikos T, Papadopoulos N, Tarlatzis BC, Bontis JN. Successful end-to-end cervico-cervical anastomosis in a patient with congenital cervical fragmentation: case report. Hum Reprod. 2004;19:1204-10.
5. Grimbizis GF, Gordts S, Di Spiezio Sardo A, Brucker S, De Angelis C, Gergolet M, et al. The ESHRE/ESGE consensus on the classification of female genital tract congenital anomalies. Hum Reprod. 2013;28(8):2032-44.
6. Gaucherand P, Awada A, Rudigoz RC, Dargent D. Obstetrical prognosis of septate uterus: a plan for treatment of the septum. Eur J Obstet Gynecol Reprod Biol. 1994;54:109-12.
7. Fedele L, Arcaini L, Parazzini F, Vercillini P, Nola GD. Metroplastic hysteroscopy and fertility. Fertil Steril. 1993;59:768-70.
8. Heinonen PK, Saarikoski S, Pystynen P. Reproductive performance of women with uterine anomalies. An evaluation of 182 cases. Acta Obstet Gynecol Scand. 1982;61:157-62.
9. Kurjak A, Kupesic S, Miric D. The assessment of benign uterine tumour vascularization by transvaginal colour Doppler. Ultrasound Med Biol. 1992;18:645-9.
10. Munro MG, Critchley HO, Broder MS, Fraser IS. FIGO Working Group on Menstrual Disorders. FIGO classification system (PALM-COEIN) for causes of abnormal uterine bleeding in nongravid women of reproductive age. Int J Gynecol Obstet. 2011;113(1):3-13.
11. Perrot N, Frey I, Mergui JL, Bazot M, Uzan M, Uzan S. Adenomyosis: power Doppler findings. Ultrasound Obstet Gynecol. 2001;17(2):177-8.
12. Cil AP, Tulunay G, Kose MF, Haberal H. Power Doppler properties of endometrial polyps and submucosal fibroids: a preliminary observational study in women with known intracavitary lesions. Ultrasound Obstet Gynecol. 2010;35:233-7.

13. Leone FP, Timmerman D, Bourne T, Valentin L, Epstein E, Goldstein SR, et al. Terms, definitions and measurements to describe the sonographic features of the endometrium and intrauterine lesions: a consensus opinion from the International Endometrial Tumor Analysis (IETA) group. Ultrasound Obstet Gynecol. 2010;35(1):103-12.
14. Lee CN, Cheng WF, Chen CA, Chu JS, Hsieh CY, Hsiehet FJ. Angiogenesis of endometrial carcinomas assessed by measurement of intratumoral blood flow, microvessel density, and vascular endothelial growth factor levels. Obstet Gynecol. 2000;96(4):615-21.

LONG QUESTIONS

1. Describe the ESHRE-ESGE classification of müllerian duct abnormalities.
2. Describe the FIGO PALM-COEIN classification for myometrial lesions.

SHORT QUESTIONS

1. What is the basic difference in ESHRE-ESGE and AFS classification systems for müllerian duct abnormalities?
2. Why are patients with septate uterus are more likely to have implantation problems and miscarriages?
3. What are the signs that differentiate adenomyoma from a degenerated fibroid?
4. Describe the B mode findings in adenomyotic uterus.

MULTIPLE CHOICE QUESTIONS

1. This entity is not a part of ESHRE-ESGE classification of müllerian duct abnormalities:
   a. Septate uterus
   b. Dysmorphic uterus
   c. Arcuate uterus
2. According to the AFS classification, angle of >105? between endometrial cavities may indicate:
   a. Septate uterus
   b. Bicornuate uterus
   c. Unicornuate uterus
3. This fibroid does not affect fertility:
   a. Type 7
   b. Type 0
   c. Type 4
4. This feature indicates uterine septum:
   a. Acute angle between endometrial cavities
   b. Dimple on the fundus
   c. Infolding of myometrium
5. This ultrasound sign is not seen in adenomyosis:
   a. Edge shadow
   b. Myometrial cysts
   c. Fan shadow
6. This ultrasound sign is not seen in fibroid:
   a. Translesional vascularity
   b. Peripheral vascularity
   c. Intralesional vascularity
7. Type 0 fibroid and endometrial polyp can be differentiated by:
   a. Single feeding vessel
   b. Echogenicity
   c. Both
8. Irregular junctional zone is a feature of:
   a. Fibroid
   b. Endometritis
   c. Polyp
9. 3D ultrasound is especially of help for:
   a. Fibroid
   b. Müllerian duct abnormalities
   c. Polyp
10. This is a feature of any malignant lesion:
    a. Well-defined margins
    b. Heterogeneous echogenicity
    c. Low vascularity

Answers

1.	c	2.	b	3.	a	4.	a	5.	a	6.	a
7.	c	8.	b	9.	b	10.	b				

7.4 ULTRASOUND IN GYNAECOLOGY: ADNEXAL DISEASE

Archana Baser, Anshu Baser

INTRODUCTION

Ultrasound plays a very crucial role in diagnosis of pelvic lesions transvaginal ultrasound due to its proximity to pelvic organs is more precise in reaching close to the diagnosis, however it is important that transabdominal sonography should be performed in all cases of suspected adnexal pathologies for complete evaluation. Adnexa comprises fallopian tubes, ovaries, parametrium, cul-de-sac and structures surrounding the uterus. Ultrasound proved itself as essential modality in diagnosing pelvic masses; its origin, its morphology and its classification as benign, malignant or possibly malignant **(Fig. 1)**. Doppler plays a vital role in addition to B scan and improves the performance in diagnosis and selecting the surgical approach.[1,2]

Majority of ovarian pathologies are in form of cysts or tumors. A complete history, clinical examination, hormonal status, age, parity, biochemical markers along with a detailed scan can lead to a provisional diagnosis and management of the diseases.

In this chapter we shall be describing sonographic features of common ovarian and nonovarian lesions.

Let us first learn about sonoanatomy of ovary and adnexa.[3]

The ovaries are ellipsoid in shape usually lies lateral and posterior to either side of uterus. They are attached to broad ligament by its own mesentery; the mesovarium anteriorly and to uterus by ovarian ligament.

Sonologically, the follicles are the soft markers for ovarian identification. The medulla and stroma of ovary do not have definite borders. Medulla is identified as strong area of reflectivity whereas the stroma shows cyclical changes, depending on menstrual cycle. Stroma is identified by the echo free areas, the follicles.

Ovarian size depends on the age, menstrual status, pregnancy status, body habitus, and phase of menstrual cycle. Sonographically, we measure ovarian volume as L × B × W **(Fig. 2)**.

While transabdomen sonography (TAS) provides good information regarding relationship of ovaries with respect to adnexa, its low resolution makes it difficult for fine detailing of ovary **(Figs. 3A and B)**. Hence, transvaginal ultrasound (TVS) is tool of choice for obtaining minute details of ovary.

In TVS, to find ovaries transverse section of uterus is taken and corners of transverse scan are marked as place where tube begins. Now the tubes are followed laterally to the place where iliac vessels are seen on pelvic wall. This is the most common site where ovaries will come into view. Ovaries are scanned completely from top to bottom to obtain length and AP diameter, then transducer is rotated to 90° to get the width of ovary.

The fallopian tube is variable in length measuring 7–12 cm. It is divided into interstitial part, isthmus, ampulla and infundibulum. The sonographic appearance of the interstitial portion is that of fine echogenic line arising from endometrial canal and extending through uterine wall in transverse scan.

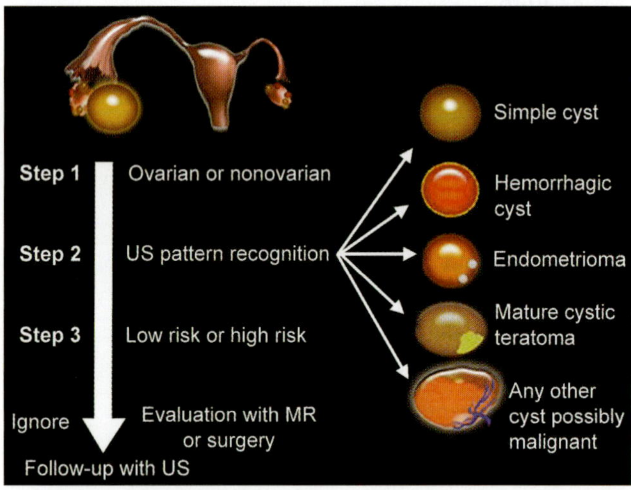

Fig. 1: Approach to adnexal pathology on ultrasound.

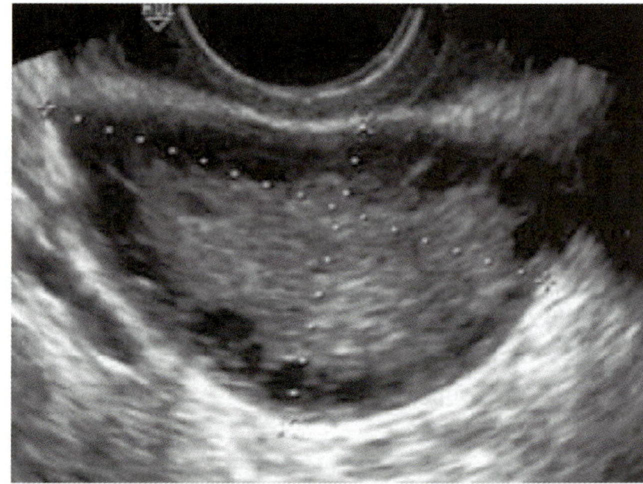

Fig. 2: Measurement of ovarian dimensions.

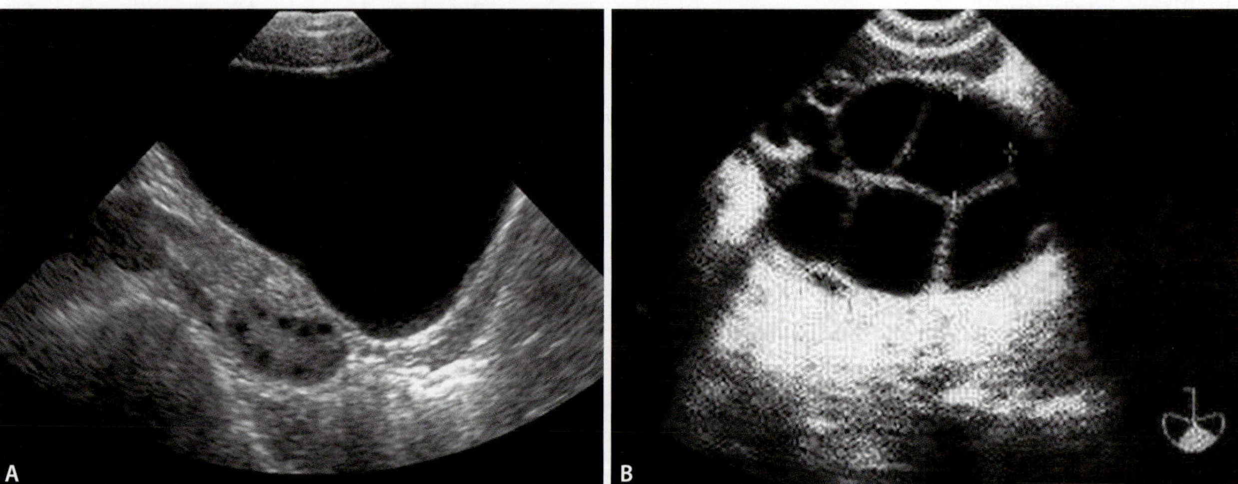

Figs. 3A and B: Comparison of ovarian imaging on transabdominal (A) and transvaginal (B) ultrasound.

The ampulla, isthmus and infundibulum are not visualized by TAS or TVS unless there is tubal pathology.

Sonographically, it is impossible to visualize a healthy fallopian tube without any intervention because there is no tissue fluid interface when tubes are healthy.

Fallopian tubes can be thus visualized when there is fluid inside the tube or there is fluid outside the tube as fluid in pelvis.

This principle is used for evaluation of tubes and commonly performed procedures to check for patency of tubes sonographically are saline infusion sonography (SIS) and Hystero-contrast sonosalpingography (HyCoSy). Its diagnostic accuracy is increased when used along with color Doppler and pulse Doppler.

Characteristic ultrasound features of diseased fallopian tube are depicted in **Figure 4** and described as:

- A sausage shaped cystic structure
- Incomplete septa inside the structure and
- Mucosal folds inside the lumen of tube in transverse section resulting in cog wheel appearance.

Timor-Tritsch IE et al.[4] defined the sonographic markers for tubal inflammation as Thickened tube wall > 5 mm, cogwheel sign, incomplete septa, beads on string appearance, TO complex, TO abscess and fluid in cul-de-sac.

OVARIAN LESIONS

Ovarian Lesions may be simple physiological cyclical changes and may appear as simple cyst. For our convenience sonographic pathologies of ovary can be classified as:

Benign Cysts

- *Functional cysts/follicular cysts:* Most common cystic masses in reproductive age group, simple fluid filled cyst with well-defined borders, hypoechoic on ultrasound, with or without fine septations **(Fig. 5)**.

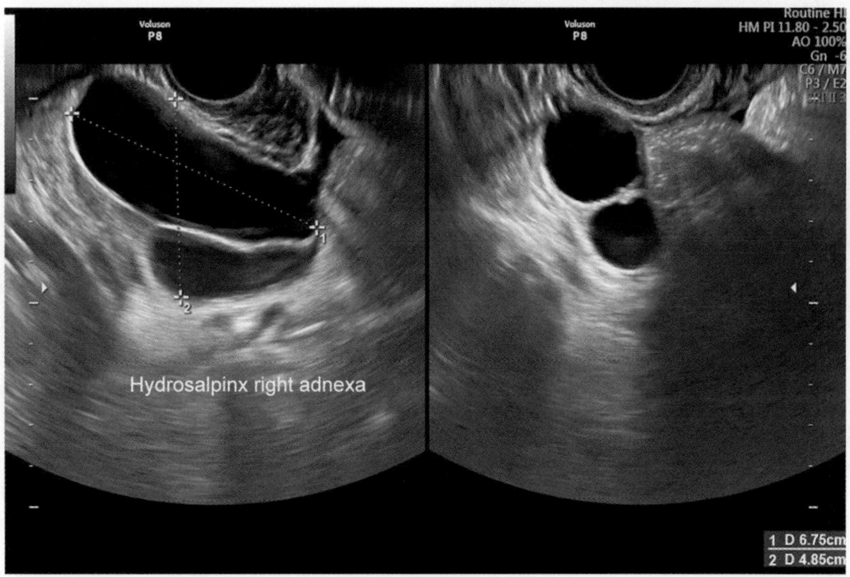

Fig. 4: Hydrosalpinx.

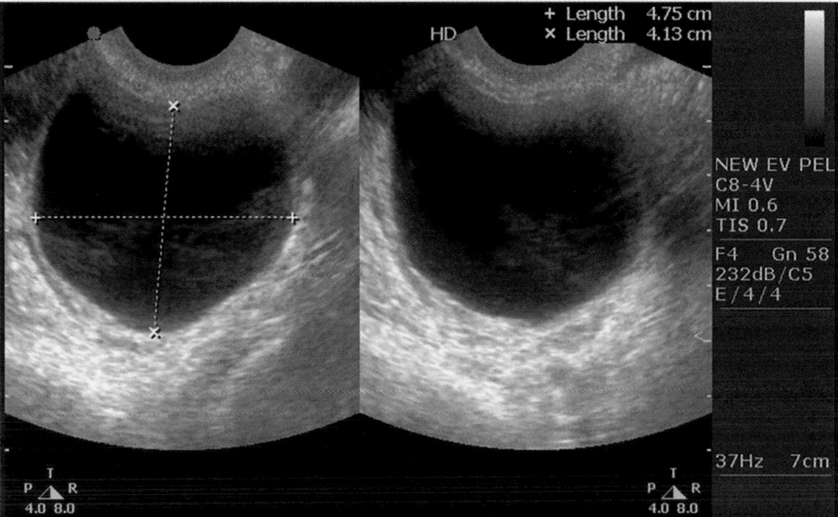

Fig. 5: Simple ovarian cyst.

- *Corpus luteal cyst:* It can be seen during pregnancy, typically resolves on its own in majority of cases in few weeks but can grow and cause pain, torsion or rupture. On color Doppler it appears like ring of fire **(Fig. 6)**.
- *Hemorrhagic ovarian cyst (HOC):* A hemorrhagic cyst can develop from hemorrhage into CL cyst. Fibrin strands are seen giving it a spider web appearance **(Fig. 7)**. Different fluid levels may be seen in HOC. It usually resolves with time.
- *Paraovarian cyst:* Paraovarian cysts (POCs) are remnants of Wolffian duct in mesosalpinx that do not arise from the ovary.

  They are hypoechoic mainly, thin walled with clear fluid inside. Sometimes papillary projections may be seen inside the POC. Malignancy may develop in such cases. POC more than 5 cm should be hence removed. They account for ~10–20% of adnexal masses. Diagnosis is confirmed if the ipsilateral ovary is visualized separately **(Fig. 8)**.

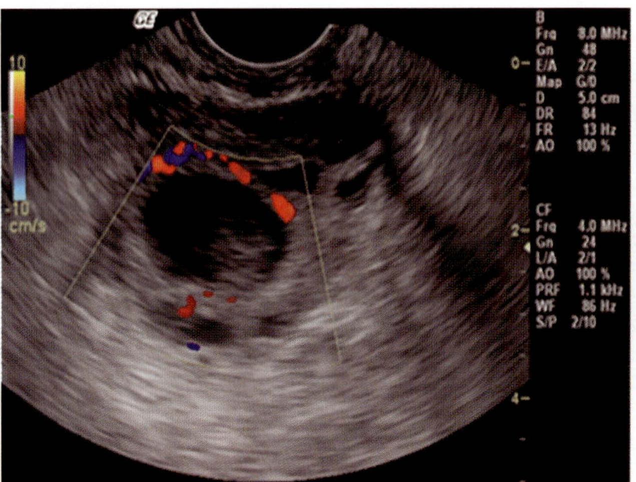

Fig. 6: Corpus luteum of the ovary with ring of fire appearance on color Doppler.

- *Postmenopausal ovarian cyst:* Cysts in postmenopausal women need to be investigated more as they are a high risk group.

  It may be simple cyst, granulosa cell tumor causing postmenopausal bleeding.
- *Polycystic ovary:* Polycystic ovaries are most frequently reported ultrasound findings in pelvic ultrasonography in reproductive age group. Currently, the sonographic assessment of ovaries is one of the obligatory criteria in the diagnosis of PCOS according to the Rotterdam consensus (2003) and Androgen Excess and PCOS Society (2006).[5,6] This criterion is determined by the presence of ≥12 follicles within the ovary with a diameter of 2–9 mm and/or ovarian volume ≥10 cm^3. Such an ultrasound image in one gonad only is sufficient to define polycystic ovaries. The arrangement of follicles can be peripheral cystic (garland like) or generalized cystic pattern **(Fig. 9)**.
  This pattern is commonly seen in subfertile, anovulatory women. It may also be an incidental finding.
- *Hyperstimulated ovaries **(Fig. 10)**:* It is one of the dreaded complications of ART. Enlarged multifollicular ovaries may be with or without ascites. If multiple follicular cysts are seen, ask history of ovulation induction.
- *Endometriotic cyst:* It is one of the common findings in subfertility patients. Possibilities of endometriotic cysts should be kept in mind even in young girls presenting with dysmenorrhea. It is challenging to see ovaries of young women as trans abdomen sonography may not reveal details of contents of cyst any persisting cyst in immediate postmenstrual phase should be looked in details and if clarity cannot be established offer pelvic MRI if symptoms are severe. The typical endometrioma is unilocular with ground glass echogenicity of the cystic fluid **(Fig. 11)**.

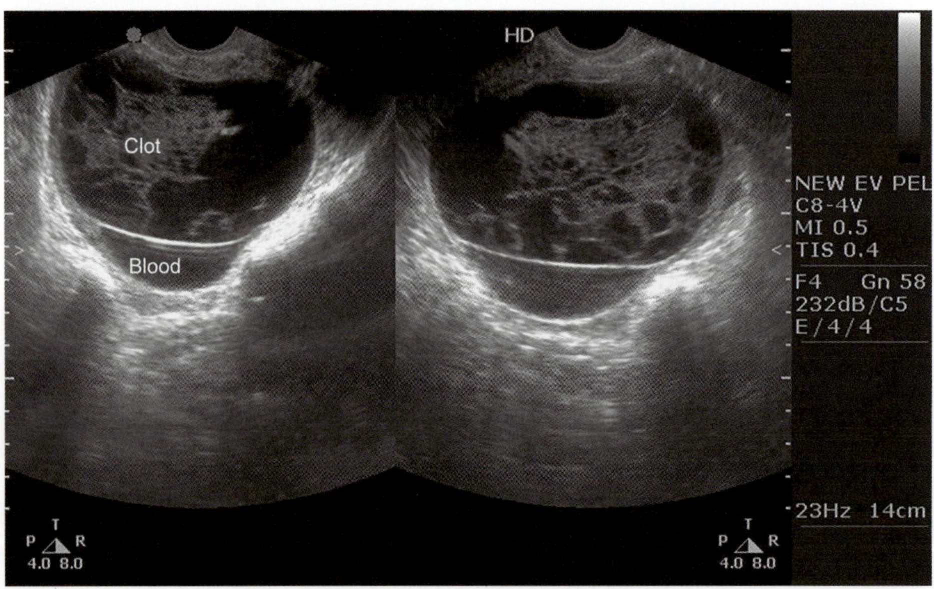

Fig. 7: Hemorrhagic ovarian cyst with spider web appearance.

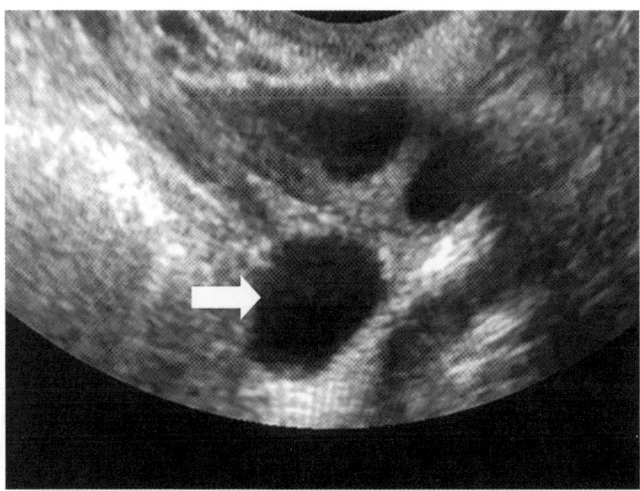

Fig. 8: Paraovarian cyst (marked with arrow) seen separate from the ovary.

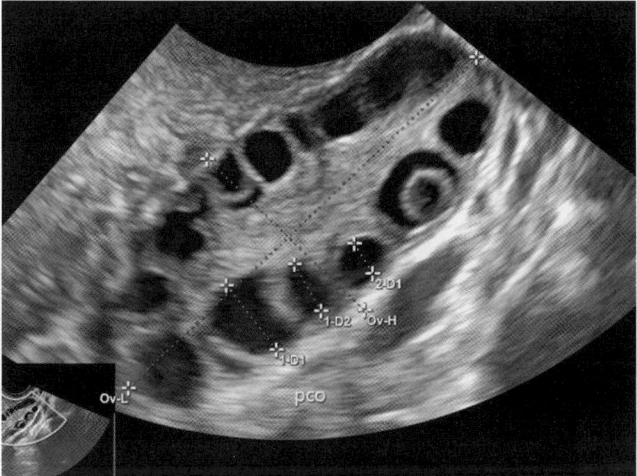

Fig. 9: Polycystic ovarian morphology on ultrasound.

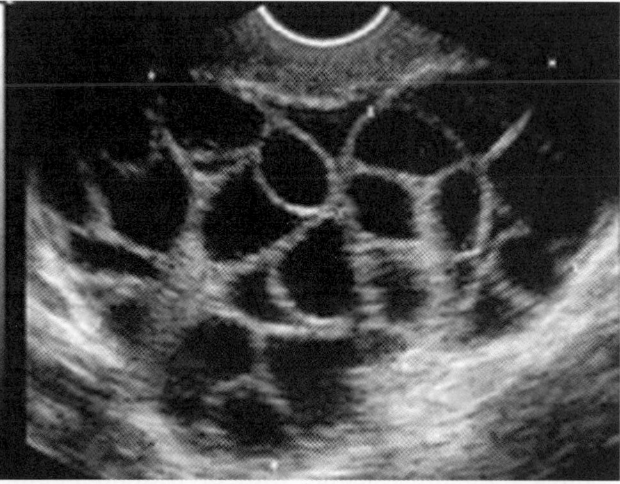

Fig. 10: Hyperstimulated ovaries.

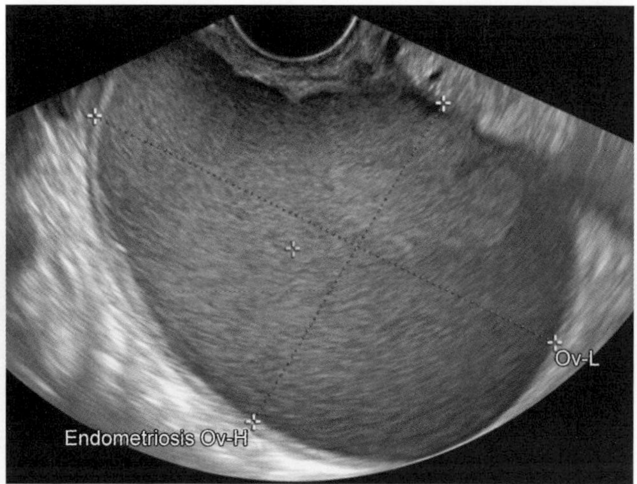

Fig. 11: Endometriotic cyst or endometrioma.

It may be multilocular, septate unilateral or bilateral presence of endometrioma suggest grade 4 endometriosis.

- *Ovarian torsion:* Ovarian torsion is a disorder with high patient morbidity. Torsion ovary though uncommon but may present during pregnancy. Patient mostly presents with pain in abdomen which may mimic other intra-abdominal pathologies. If remain undiagnosed it leads to serious consequences a young women might have to lose her ovary if there is delay in treatment. In pregnancy it may be associated with maternal morbidity and perinatal mortality. Hence a high index of suspicion should always be kept in mind when physical examination does not match with patients distress. Patient symptoms are either continuous dull aching or sudden sustained pain with or without history of ovarian pathology, nausea and occasionally vomiting. It is important not to miss diagnosis of Torsion ovary. Torsion occurs due to two main reasons (1) hypermobility of the ovary: <50%, (2) adnexal mass: ~50–80%.
  - Most lesions are dermoid cysts or paraovarian cysts
  - Large cystic ovaries, e.g., hyperstimulated ovaries
  - Masses between 5 and 10 cm are at most risk.

Radiographic Features

- The main is ovarian enlargement due to venous/lymphatic engorgement, edema and hemorrhage.
- Secondary signs include free pelvic fluid, seen in more than 80% cases with or without underlying ovarian lesion.
- Follicular ring sign can be an early sign.
- Reduced or absent vascularity.
- A twisted dilated tubular structure corresponding to the vascular pedicle.
- Doppler findings in torsion can be widely variable[7]
  - Little or no intraovarian venous flow (common)
  - Absent arterial flow (less common, but poor prognostic sign)
  - Absent or reversed diastolic flow
  - Normal vascularity does not exclude intermittent torsion.
- Whirlpool sign of twisted vascular pedicle.[8]
- Ovary tenderness to transducer pressure.

Normal Doppler flow can also occasionally be found due to dual supply from both the ovarian and uterine arteries.

Ultrasound has a sensitivity of approaching diagnosis 100% and specificity of 97%.

Benign Tumors

- *Serous cystadenoma:* It can be seen as small or large fluid filled cystic mass with a well-defined thin margins, no solid lesions, fine or thin septations with no vascularity **(Figs. 12A and B)**. Its malignant counterpart; serous cystadenocarcinoma can be seen with thick septae, internal echogenicities, solid components with or without papillary lesions and high vascularity.
- *Mucinous cystadenoma:* Mucinous cyst adenoma is characterized by small or large fluid filled mass with thick wall, thick septae with or without papillary projections. Diagnosis of any ovarian tumor is done only by histopathological examination and with tumor markers **(Fig. 13)**.
- *Germ cell tumor—teratoma (dermoids):* It constitutes second largest group of ovarian neoplasms. They contain tissues of ectodermal, endodermal or mesodermal origin (90%). Ultrasound features are presence of structures of mixed echogenicity varying from white ball (corresponding to hair and sebum), white lines (corresponding to hair), teeth, bone, Rokitansky nodule (corresponding to adipose tissue or hair or calcification) as seen in **Figure 14**.

Borderline tumors: Borderline ovarian tumors (BOT) or tumors of low malignant potential are epithelial tumors with a slow growth rate and low invasive potential. These tumors tend to occur in younger women and are often diagnosed at an earlier stage of disease than are invasive carcinomas **(Fig. 15)**.

The identification of patients with ovarian lesions suspected of being BOT may be helpful in their management. Whereas transvaginal sonography has been established as a reliable method of differentiating benign from malignant adnexal masses, little is known about sonographic features in the diagnosis of BOT.[9,10]

Tumors with papillary projections may be borderline are malignant. The simple criteria used to distinguish between

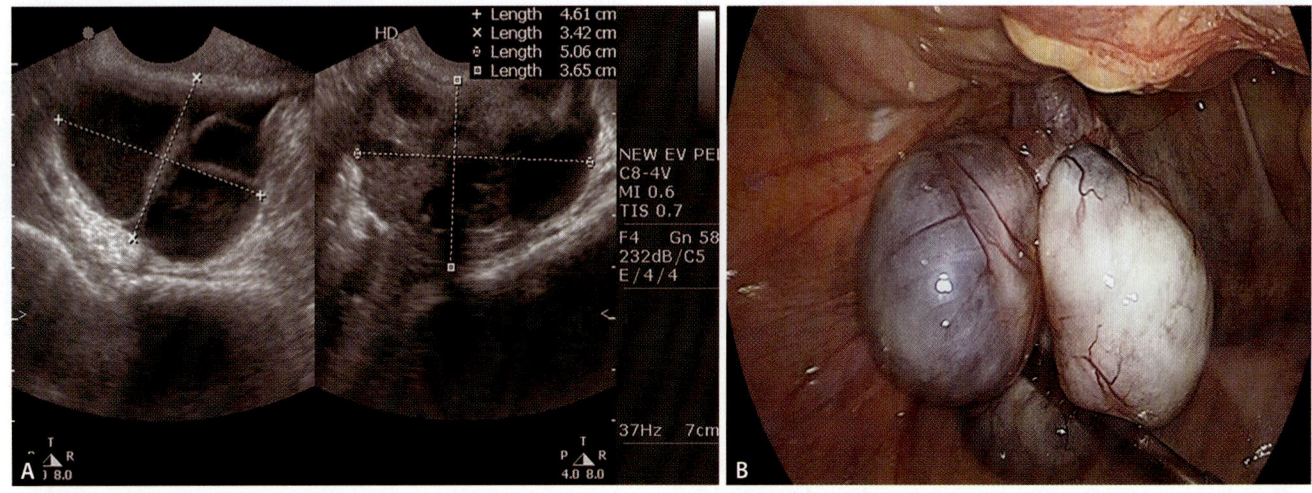

Figs. 12A and B: Serous cystadenoma. (A) Shows the ultrasound appearance; (B) Shows the clinical correlation on laparoscopy.

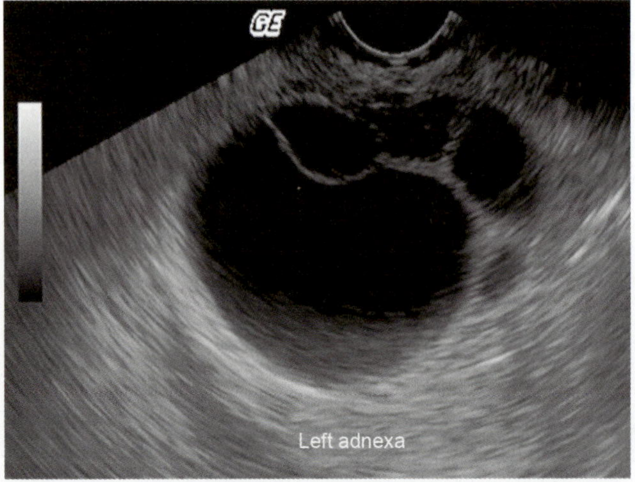

Fig. 13: Mucinous cystadenoma.

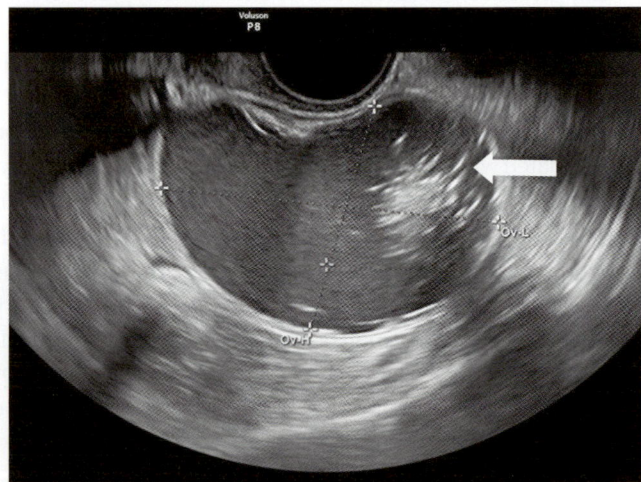

Fig. 14: Dermoid cyst or mature cystic teratoma with arrow showing the Rokitansky nodule.

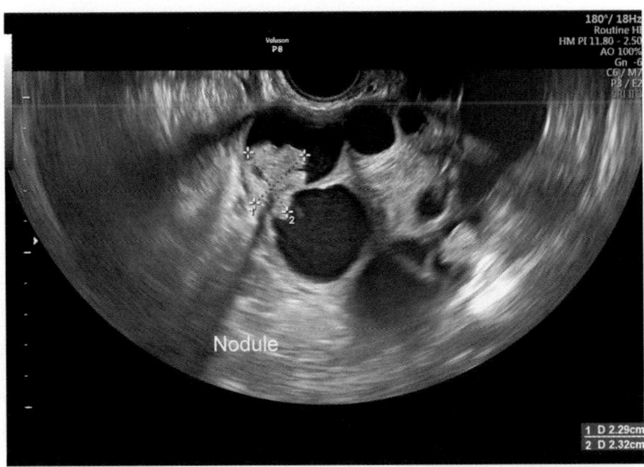

Fig. 15: Borderline ovarian tumor.

benign and malignant are based on International Ovarian Tumor Analysis (IOTA) classification.[11]

International Ovarian Tumor Analysis group ultrasound rules for ovarian masses are a simple set of ultrasound findings that classify ovarian masses into benign, malignant or inconclusive masses. These rules apply to masses that are not a classical ovarian mass (e.g., corpus luteum, endometrioma, dermoid cyst).

If an ovarian lesion has at least one of these features and no malignant features it can be confidently considered benign:

- Unilocular cyst
- Smooth multilocular tumor <10 cm
- Solid components <7 mm in diameter
- Presence of acoustic shadows
- No detectable Doppler signal.

Malignant Lesion

If an ovarian lesion has at least one of these features and no benign features it can be confidently considered malignant:

- Irregular solid tumor
- irregular multilocular-solid mass >10 cm in diameter
- ≥4 papillary structures
- Ascites
- High Doppler signal (color score 4).

IOTA suggested color score:

- *Score 1:* No detectable vascularization
- *Score 2:* Minimal vascularization
- *Score 3:* Moderate vascularization
- *Score 4:* Abundant vascularization.

There is another grading system for data reporting of adnexal masses: In this pattern recognition analysis and color Doppler blood flow location issued for determining the presumptive diagnosis. Then a system for data reporting was used. This system was called Gynecological Imaging Reporting and Data System (GI-RADS):

- *GI-RADS 1:* Definitive benign
- *GI-RADS 2:* Very probable benign
- *GI-RADS 3:* Probable benign
- *GI-RADS 4:* Probable malignant
- *GI-RADS 5:* Very probable malignant.

Patients with GI-RADS 1 and 2 were managed expectantly. All cases of GI-RADS 3, 4 or 5 tumors were removed surgically and definitive histologic diagnosis obtained. GI-RADS classification was compared with final histological diagnosis.[12]

Benign versus malignant:

- Pattern recognition in grey scale imaging is most superior way of distinguishing benign from malignant lesions than other method such as simple classification systems, scoring systems and mathematical models.
- Absence of solid components and absence of irregularities in an adnexal mass suggest benignity whereas presence of solid components or irregularity in either of outline, the cyst wall or in echogenicity of tumor suggests malignancy.
- Moreover more the irregularity in echogenicity and cyst wall outline, the greater the risk of malignancy.
- Unilocular or multilocular simple cyst without solid component are mostly benign, but some cysts with extremely large number of locules may be borderline mucinous cystadenomas of intestinal type 4.

NONOVARIAN LESIONS ON PELVIC ULTRASOUND

Commonly encountered adnexal pathology:

- *Pelvic inflammatory disease (PID):* It is most common of pathology seen in day to day practice. It can be acute or chronic depending on duration. Acute PID in initial stages can be recognized as thickened adnexa. Thickness of fallopian tube is > 5 mm in acute inflammation and its thickness decreases in chronic PID. If the inflammatory process continues, it results in collection of fluid in cul-de-sac followed by collection of fluid in fallopian tubes which can further lead to hydro-, hemato- or pyosalpinx depending on other physical factors. Fluid filled, sausage shaped, cystic structure with incomplete septae giving it cogwheel appearance or beads of string appearance. Doppler enhances diagnosis and management of patients with PID.[12] Fluid filled, sausage shaped, cystic structure with incomplete septae giving it cogwheel appearance or beads of string appearance **(Figs. 16A and B)**.
- *Tubo-ovarian abscess:* Unilocular cystic or complex multicystic structure with thick wall and thick septae, filled with homogenously echogenic material giving it typically ground glass appearance.
- *Peritoneal pseudocyst:* They are not true cysts usually formed secondary to pelvic infections or previous pelvic surgeries. They present on ultrasound as cystic mass following the contours of pelvis and ovary, often deformed suspended amongst adhesions centrally or peripherally in the cyst **(Fig. 17)**. As this fluid is not under pressure, it gets deformed with probe pressure too.

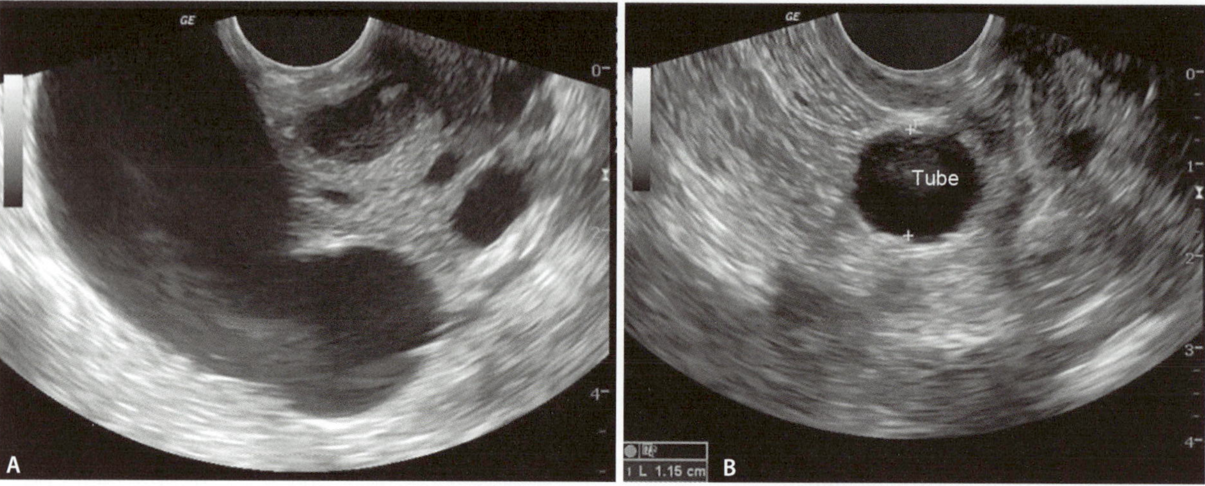

Figs. 16A and B: Ultrasound in pelvic inflammatory disease showing a retort shaped hydrosalpinx with cog wheel sign (A) and a thickened, enlarged tube (B).

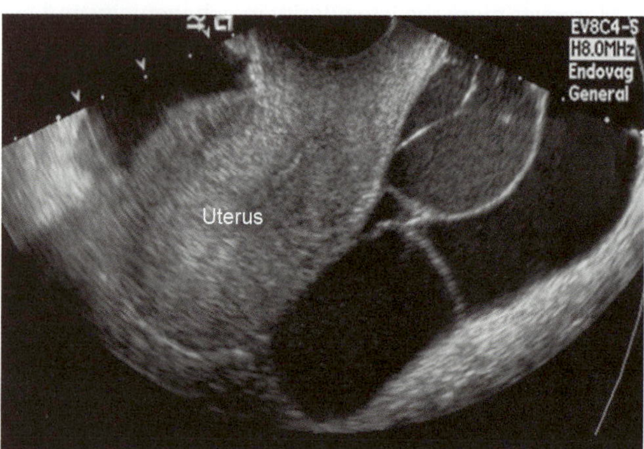

Fig. 17: Peritoneal pseudocysts.

Fig. 18: Ultrasonographic image of ectopic mass with ring of fire pattern in adnexa.

ECTOPIC PREGNANCY

The incidence of ectopic pregnancy is increasing due to increasing use of ART and also earlier diagnosis of the cases. As a matter of fact earlier diagnosis by ultrasound can prevent life-threatening complications of ruptured ectopic.

Transvaginal sonography plays a major role in diagnosis and management of ectopic pregnancy along with serial serum beta hCG levels.

High risk factors for ectopic are history of tubal surgery, previous ectopic, use of IUCD, genital infections, etc.[13,14]

Sonographic Criteria for Diagnosis of Ectopic Pregnancy (Fig. 18)[15,16]

Positive pregnancy test and no intrauterine pregnancy with:

- Extrauterine gest sac with yolk sac and embryo (with or without heartbeat)
- Adnexal ring
- Moderate to large amount of free fluid
- Decidual cast.

Endometrium may show a pseudo gestational sac (20%) in ectopic pregnancy. The hormonal change associated with ectopic pregnancy may cause fluid collection in endometrial cavity resulting in pseudo sac, which mimics a GS. It must be differentiated from early IUP. Pseudosac is ovoid in shape, centrally placed, poorly defined with no decidual reaction and single decidual layer whereas the normal early IUP is round, eccentrically placed with well-defined margins and decidual reaction, and may show double decidual sac sign.

Whenever an ultrasound is done in early pregnancy whether IUP or suspected ectopic, possibility of heterotopic pregnancy should be kept in mind. A careful evaluation of adnexa in all early pregnancy is must. Presence of intrauterine pregnancy with symptoms of ectopic calls for a follow-up ultrasound to rule out heterotopic pregnancy. A greater level of suspicion may allow early laparoscopic intervention before life threatening intra-abdominal bleeding occurs.

Non-gynecological lesions which may be present in pelvis in adnexal region:

- Appendiceal abscess
- Appendicitis
- Bladder diverticulum
- Diverticular abscess
- Nerve sheath tumor

- Pelvic kidney
- Peritoneal cyst
- Ureteral diverticulum.

CONCLUSION

An algorithm based approach in identification of adnexal lesions will be good. It is important to know about pattern recognition of adnexal masses. Solid or cystic, benign or malignant ovarian or nonovarian, acute or chronic ultrasound is a preferred modality to diagnose adnexal diseases and crucial in differential diagnosis of lesions. Recent studies have shown that US (transvaginal plus color Doppler) may differentiate benign from malignant lesions with a sensitivity of 99.1% and a specificity of 85.9%.[13]

The differential diagnosis of adnexal masses still represents a challenge in spite of the marvelous efforts that have been made to improve the sonographically based diagnosis. There were rapid technological advances in diagnostic ultrasonography in the last decade, with the recent development of three-dimensional power Doppler (3DPD).

There are several opportunity to learn ultrasound FOGSI recognized centers, online courses, conferences, workshops, PG Forums, etc. In PG curriculum Ultrasound training should be integral part. With good pelvic sonography, a confident diagnosis of adnexal diseases can be made. Keeping in mind all possible differential diagnosis but one should remember common things should be thought of first. At times to see if physiological cyst is resolving with time you may need to call patient for serial sonography. Ultrasound is definitely a good tool in hands of skilled operator. MRI may be needed to for diagnosis and staging of malignant ovarian lesions and timely referral.

KEY MESSAGES

- Adnexa comprises of fallopian tubes, ovaries parametrium and cul-de-sac.
- Adnexal diseases present in gynecology OPD as pelvic pain, pelvic mass.
- Ultrasound is an essential modality in diagnosing pelvic masses their origin, morphology and classification as benign, malignant or possibly malignant.
- It is important for Postgraduates to have a clear concept of pathologies of ovary and cyclical physiological changes in ovary. Most important thing is to learn pattern identification and diligent reporting so as to avoid scare related to cyst and adnexal masses and to prevent unnecessary surgical intervention on ovaries.

REFERENCES

1. Alcazar JL, Royo P, Jurado M, Minguez JA, Garcia-Manero M, Laparte C, et al. Triage for surgical management of ovarian tumours in asymptomatic women: assessment of ultrasound based scoring system. Ultrasound Obstet Gynecol. 2008;32: 220-5.
2. Kinkel K, Hricak H, Lu Y. US characterization of ovarian masses. A meta-analysis. Radiology. 2000;217:803-11.
3. Baser A, Dhingra H, Zaidi AK, Mahajan V, Baser A. Obstetrics and Gynaecology Ultrasound for Beginners. New Delhi: Jaypee Brothers Medical Publishers; 2019.
4. Timor-Tritsch IE, Monteagudo A, Mandville EO. Successful management of viable cervical pregnancy by local injection of methotrexate guided by transvaginal ultrasonography. Am J Obset Gynecol. 194;170(3):737-9.
5. Rotterdam ESHRE/ASRM-Sponsored PCOS Consensus Workshop Group. Revised 2003 consensus on diagnostic criteria and long-term health risks related to polycystic ovary syndrome. Fertil Steril. 2004;81:19-25.
6. The Rotterdam ESHRE/ASRM-Sponsored PCOS Consensus Workshop Group. Revised 2003 consensus on diagnostic criteria and long-term health risks related to polycystic ovary syndrome (PCOS) Hum Reprod. 2004;19:41-7.
7. Sibbal M. Follicular ring sign: a simple sign for early diagnosis of ovarian torsion. J Ultrasound Med. 2012;31(11):1803-9.
8. Vijayaragahvan SB. Sonographic whirlpool sign in ovarian torsion. J Ultrasound Med. 2004;23(12):1643-51.
9. Exacoustos C, Romanini ME, Rinaldo D, Amoroso C, Szabolcs B, Zupi E, et al. Preoperative sonographic features of borderline ovarian tumors. Ultrasound Obstet Gynecol. 2005;25:50-9.
10. Darai E, Teboul J, Walker F, Benifla JL, Meneux E, Guglielmina JN, et al. Epithelial ovarian carcinoma of low malignant potential. Eur J Obstet Gynecol Reprod Biol. 1996;66:141-5.
11. Timmerman D, Valentin L, Bourne TH, Collins WP, Verrelst H, Vergote I, et al. Terms, definitions and measurements to describe sonographic features of adnexal tumours: a consensus opinion from IOTA group. Ultrasound Obstet Gynecol. 2000; 16(5):500-5.
12. Amor F, Alcazar JL, Vaccaro H, Leon M, Iturra A. GI-RADS reporting system for ultrasound evaluation of adnexal masses in clinical practice: a prospective multicenter study. Ultrasound Obstet Gynecol. 2011;38(4):450-5.
13. Ankum WM, Mol BW, Vander Veen F. Risk factor for ectopic pregnancy: a meta-analysis. Fertil Steril. 1996;65:1093-9.
14. Tay Ji, Moore J, Walker JI. Ectopic pregnancy. West J Med. 2000;173:131-4.
15. Kupesic S, Kurjek A, Pasalic L. The value of transvaginal color Doppler in assessment of PID. Ultrasound Med Biol. 1995;21(6):733-8.
16. Turkgeldi E, Urman B, Ata B. Role of three-dimensional ultrasound in gynecology. J Obstet Gynaecol India. 2015;65(3): 146-54.

LONG QUESTIONS

1. What is the ultrasound-based classification of pathologies of ovary?
2. What are the sonographic features of torsion of ovary?
3. How to differentiate between benign and malignant adnexal mass?
4. What are the sonographic criteria for diagnosis of tubal ectopic pregnancy?
5. What are the ultrasound features of PID, to abscess, hydrosalpinx, peritoneal pseudocysts?

SHORT QUESTIONS

1. How to identify ovary on transvaginal scan?
2. Describe sonographic markers of tubal inflammation.
3. What are most frequently reported ultrasound finding of ovary in reproductive age women?
4. Describe IOTA color scoring for distinguishing benign and malignant adnexal tumors.
5. How to differentiate between pseudogestational sac and early intrauterine pregnancy?

MULTIPLE CHOICE QUESTIONS

1. Ultrasound criteria to diagnose PCO are all, except:
   a. Enlarged ovaries
   b. Peripherally arranged follicles more than 12 per ovary
   c. Must be present in both ovaries
   d. Follicle size of 2 to 9 mm
2. Ultrasound features of endometrioma are all, except:
   a. Ground glass appearance
   b. Usually unilocular
   c. Can be bilateral
   d. Ring of fire appearance on color Doppler
3. Ectopic pregnancy on USG diagnostic features are all, except:
   a. Presence of pseudogestational sac in uterus
   b. Collection in POD
   c. Adnexal mass with increased vascularity
   d. Embryo is always identifiable in adnexa
4. Typical features of a dermoid cyst on ultrasound is:
   a. Presence of nodule
   b. Ring of fire appearance
   c. Free fluid in pouch of Douglas
   d. Peripheral cystic pattern
5. The following is true about imaging of the fallopian tube on ultrasound:
   a. Hydrosalpinx has increased vascularity on Doppler evaluation
   b. A healthy tube is rarely seen on ultrasound
   c. It is diagnosed only on MRI
   d. It should be bilateral to confirm the diagnosis

Answers

1. c 2. d 3. d 4. a 5. b

7.5 CT AND MRI IN GYNAECOLOGY

Jyoti Jaiswal, Anand Kumar Jaiswal

INTRODUCTION

Imaging of the female pelvis plays a critical role in the diagnosis and evaluation of various gynecologic diseases. Typically ultrasonography (US) is used as first-line evaluation of the female genital organs. However, there are several scenarios where magnetic resonance imaging (MRI) and computed tomography (CT) are preferred for the evaluation of both benign and malignant gynecologic diseases.[1]

Magnetic resonance imaging plays a role in detecting the extent of disease and helps in local staging of gynecologic tumors. CT can be used for assessment of patients with acute pelvic pain in an emergency setting. In cases of gynecological cancer, MRI gives very good diagnostic accuracy for staging. It also defines advanced disease along with planning of radiation, monitoring treatment response, and post-treatment follow-up to detect recurrence.[2]

ROLE OF CT IN GYNAECOLOGICAL IMAGING

Imaging studies are important adjunct in the diagnosis of acute and chronic conditions. CT scan can be used for diagnosing various gynecologic disorders which include uterine disorders, ovarian disorders, endometriosis, pelvic inflammatory disease, and postoperative complications.[3]

Computed tomography is ideal for advance staging pelvic cancers because it allows for complete evaluation of the abdomen for the presence of metastatic disease in the same imaging session. In addition, evaluating peritoneal carcinomatosis, defining the origin of large pelvic masses, and differentiating uterine from adnexal masses can be easily performed on CT. It is also useful as a first-line imaging test in evaluating a wide range of etiologies of pelvic pain that may be unrelated to gynecologic issues in patients presenting to the emergency department.

Procedural Technique

In multidetector CT, multiplanar reformatted images in transaxial, coronal, and sagittal planes should be obtained using a 4–5 mm-slice thickness at 3–4-mm intervals. However, given radiation exposure associated with CT imaging, care should be taken to deliver the least amount of radiation dose possible. This includes using techniques such as automatic tube modulation and automatic current settings. Intravenous (IV) contrast is necessary, particularly for evaluation of adnexal lesions, staging malignancy, and evaluation of vascular or inflammatory disease. Ideally, a postcontrast venous phase with a 70–90-second delay should be obtained. In addition, enteric contrast should be administered to differentiate fluid-filled bowel loops from cystic adnexal lesions.

Safety

Computed tomography scan exposes to a small targeted amount of ionizing radiation and can causes slight increase in cancer risk which is higher as compared to routine X-ray. CT should not be done unless there is a clear medical benefit. The other side of the coin is that, the medical imaging including CT scan has been directly linked to a greater life expectancy and declining cancer rates. They are also generally less expensive and safer then invasive procedures.

Basic Anatomy of Genital Tract: CT Findings

The CT appearance of the normal ligamentous, vascular, and visceral anatomy of female pelvis can be confusing unless one is familiar with basic anatomy of these structures and normal variation in their appearance. The vagina appears as a thin line structure with a brightly enhancing mucosa. Cervix appears round and uterus appear as oval or triangular soft-tissue mass in cross section. The endometrium is not easily distinguished from the myometrium but can be enhanced with help of contrast medium (**Figs. 1 A to C**). The ovaries can be seen in adults, premenopausal patients as soft-tissue masses posterolateral to the uterus and their precise appearance depends on presence or absence of follicles or cysts. Postmenopausal ovaries are small and indistinguishable from surrounding structures.[4]

Uterine Fibroids and Adenomyosis

Fibroids are the most common benign lesion of the uterus. US is usually diagnostic. CT is not the primary modality for diagnosing or evaluating fibroids, but familiarity with their various CT appearances is important. The CT appearance of a myoma depends on its location and on the presence or absence of secondary changes such as hyaline degeneration, calcification, and necrosis. Most common CT finding is uterine contour deformity. When contrast enhancement is given, it appears heterogeneous. Fibroid with hyaline degeneration or necrosis gives more cystic appearance. Solid "mass-type" calcifications in a uterine mass are the most specific sign for a leiomyoma but they are not very common. Fibroids that are subserosal in location may be confused with adnexal masses (**Fig. 2**). When a leiomyoma is submucosal in location, it can

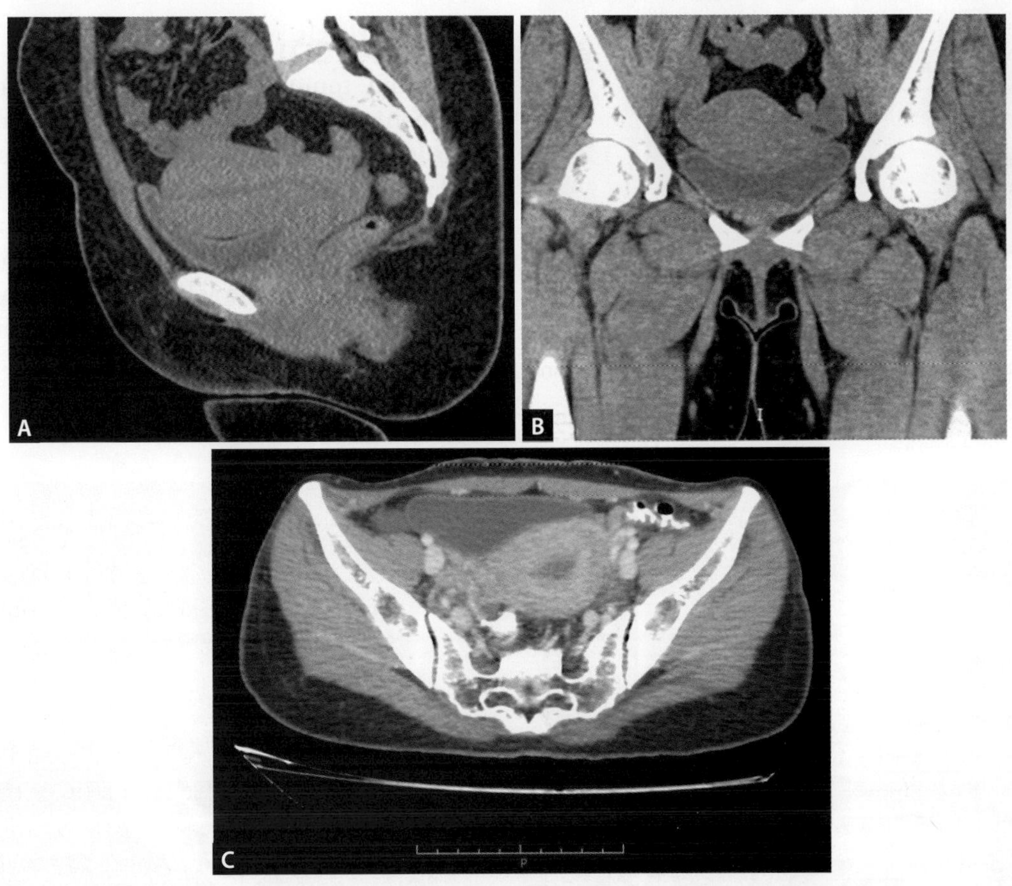

Figs. 1A to C: CT scan-anatomy of normal pelvis. (A) On sagittal view of CT pelvis showing anterior to posterior--bladder shadow with low attenuation. Behind it showing soft-tissue attenuation for uterus and cervix, only distinguishable from each other by shape (no attenuation difference). The endometrium is only slightly distinguished from myometrium; (B) On coronal section, bladder and uterine body is well differentiated but endometrium and myometrium is not easily distinguishable. Ovaries are identified better depending on presence of follicles (low attenuation) in it; (C) On axial CECT section, bladder and uterine body are well differentiated. Right ovary is identified. CE bilateral pelvic vessels seen.
(CT: computed tomography)

confuse with endometrial disease. Sonohysterography or MRI may give proper diagnosis. There may be torsion of the pedicle with subsequent infarction, degeneration, necrosis, and, potentially, infection. Lipoleiomyoma is an unusual uterine tumor containing fat and smooth-muscle elements. The CT appearance of a predominantly fatty mass containing foci of soft-tissue density is characteristic of lipoleiomyoma.[5]

Pelvic Inflammatory Disease

One of the most common causes of acute pelvic pain in women is pelvic inflammatory disease. Imaging findings vary with the stage of disease. Though US is the primary imaging modality, CT can be a helpful adjunct as it can help in assessing the extent of disease and identifying associated complications. It also helps in follow-up. In uncomplicated acute salpingitis, CT findings are usually normal or sometimes a small amount of fluid in the cul-de-sac may be seen **(Figs. 3A and B)**. In tubo-ovarian abscess **(Fig. 4)**, CT findings suggest thick-walled, low-attenuation adnexal mass with thick septa. Dilated and fluid or pus-filled fallopian tube may be seen as serpiginous structure **(Fig. 5)**.

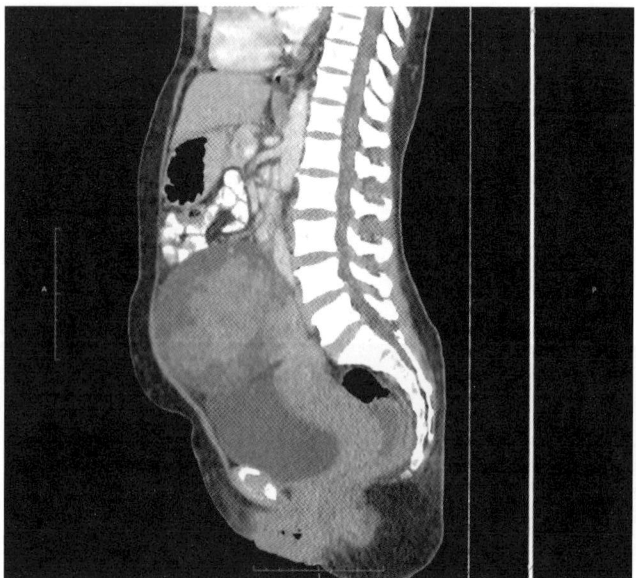

Fig. 2: CT scan—subserosal fibroid. Sagittal contrast-enhanced CT image is showing a large well-defined round pedunculated soft-tissue mass arising from posterior aspect of uterine fundus. The mass is showing similar enhancement with myometrium, and also showing area of reduced attenuation suggestive of degeneration/necrosis.

Along with imaging findings, fever, leukocytosis, and forniceal tenderness are very important clinical findings in establishing the diagnosis. The tubular nature of the mass may be better identified on reformatted images. Associated findings include thickening of the uterosacral ligaments, hydronephrosis, and indistinct margins of adjacent bowel loops. Inflammation may involve the appendix or colon and omentum. Anteriorly pushed thickened broad ligament and unclear uterine margin suggests that mass may be from adnexa so tubo-ovarian abscess can be suspected.[5] Pelvic inflammatory disease can be associated with intrauterine device also. Another condition can be genital tuberculosis with associated tubercular peritonitis.

Endometriosis

Computed tomography findings are nonspecific for endometriosis, so it is not considered as primary imaging modality. On CT, endometrioma can be seen as predominantly solid to a predominantly cystic mass. Same finding may be seen in other masses with hemorrhage such as hemorrhagic ovarian cyst. The imaging features of endometriomas are somewhat more specific at US, which is usually the first-line imaging study of choice. Sometimes endometriomas may be multilocular with thin or thick septa as well as nodularity of the wall. MRI is better for diagnosis.

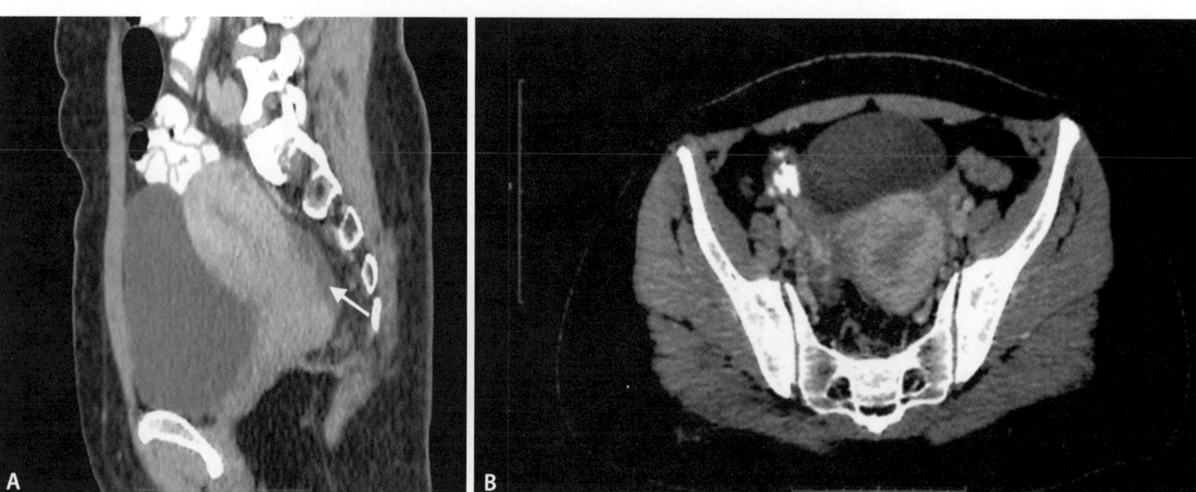

Figs. 3A and B: Pelvic inflammatory disease (PID) (CT scan). (A) Sagittal CT image of pelvis showing area of low (fluid) attenuation due to free fluid in cul-de-sac region suggestive of PID; (B) Postcontrast axial CT of pelvis engorged tortuous bilateral pelvic vessels with few fat stranding suggestive of pelvic congestion in PID.

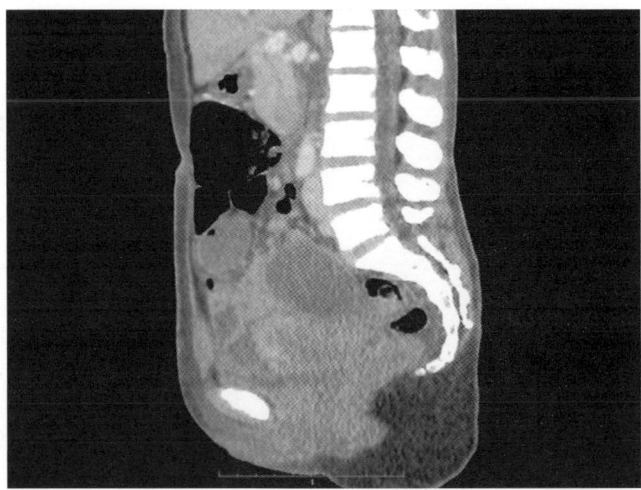

Fig. 4: Pelvic abscess (CT scan). Contrast-enhanced sagittal CT pelvis and abdomen is showing pelvic edema and thickening of uterosacral ligament and haziness of pelvic fat. There is dilation of fallopian tube demonstrating a thick-walled multicystic fluid collection.

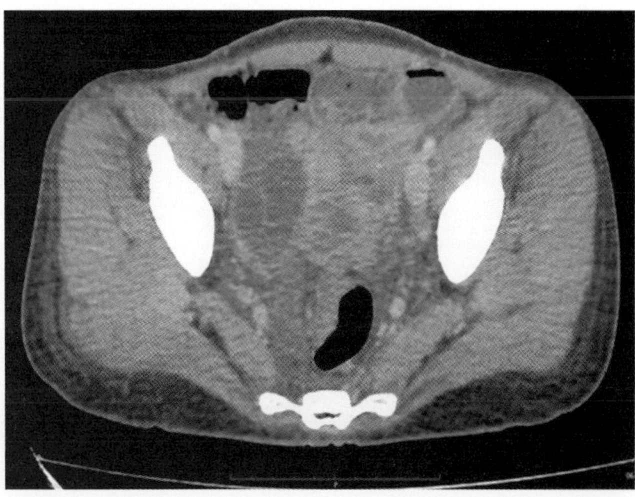

Fig. 5: Pyosalpinx (CT scan). Postcontrast axial CT of pelvis showing irregular multicystic serpiginous complex mass with enhanced incomplete septations and fluid within the mass suggestive of pyosalpinx.

Adenomyosis is also known as endometriosis interna in which endometrial glands and stroma are found within the myometrium. On CT imaging, uterus found enlarged, globular with small cystic areas in myometrium corresponding to dilated endometrial glands. MRI offers greater specificity and shows diffuse or focal thickening of the junctional zone (>12 mm), which is pathognomonic for this disorder.

Endometritis

Endometritis occurs most often after delivery or operative intervention and is the most common cause of postpartum fever. Cervical stenosis can be a cause occasionally. In endometritis, the endometrial cavity is usually thickened and distended with fluid. Presence of air in endometrial cavity can support the diagnosis. Inflammation in the parametrial soft tissues and pus collection in pelvic cavity can be found on CT scan.[3]

Endometrial Carcinoma

On CT, endometrial carcinoma typically causes a hypodense, irregular mass expanding the uterine cavity, sometimes associated with blood, fluid or pus within the cavity[4] **(Fig. 6A and B)**. Contrast enhanced CT can determine the extent of extra uterine disease. MRI is far better for staging.[6]

Torsion of Ovary

Ovarian torsion is one of the important causes of acute pelvic pain. It can be well detected by Doppler ultrasound. CT can be used in certain conditions, particularly if torsion is subacute. Torsion of ovary may occur in the slightly enlarged ovary, usually in pubertal children. In adults, there is usually an ovarian cyst or mass such as mature cystic teratoma. On CT, uterus is usually found deviated to the twisted side, ascites, obliteration of fat planes, and an enlarged ovary displaced from its normal location. Contrast-enhanced CT may show surrounding enhancing blood vessels, due to congestion. Hemorrhagic infarct may show a beaked or serpentine protrusion at the periphery of the twisted ovary, lack of enhancement and hematoma.[5,6] Sometimes, there is rotation of the adnexal mass to the contralateral side due to tortion.[3]

Hemorrhagic Cyst of Ovary

Hemorrhagic ovarian cyst may present with sudden onset of pelvic pain. USG can give a variety of picture depending upon the time of hemorrhage. On CT, there is usually a mixed-attenuation mass with a high-attenuation component in the adnexa.[6] A fluid-fluid level may be found. Hemoperitoneum may be present, if there is cyst rupture. Contrast-enhanced CT may show the cyst wall. CT is helpful in excluding other intra-abdominal diseases that can lead to hemoperitoneum.

Ovarian Malignancy

Most ovarian cancers are already advanced at the time of presentation. CT has important role in establishing staging of ovarian cancer. It can identify peritoneal and serosal deposit along with liver and nodal metastasis. Omentum may show diffuse thickening omental caking with nodular thickening of peritoneum and serosa of the bowel. CT can be used for preoperative staging and to assess tumor bulk and metastasis.

Postoperative Complications and Venous Thrombosis

Computed tomography can be used for diagnosing postoperative complications such as pelvic abscess and hematoma. One can also detect thrombosis. The right

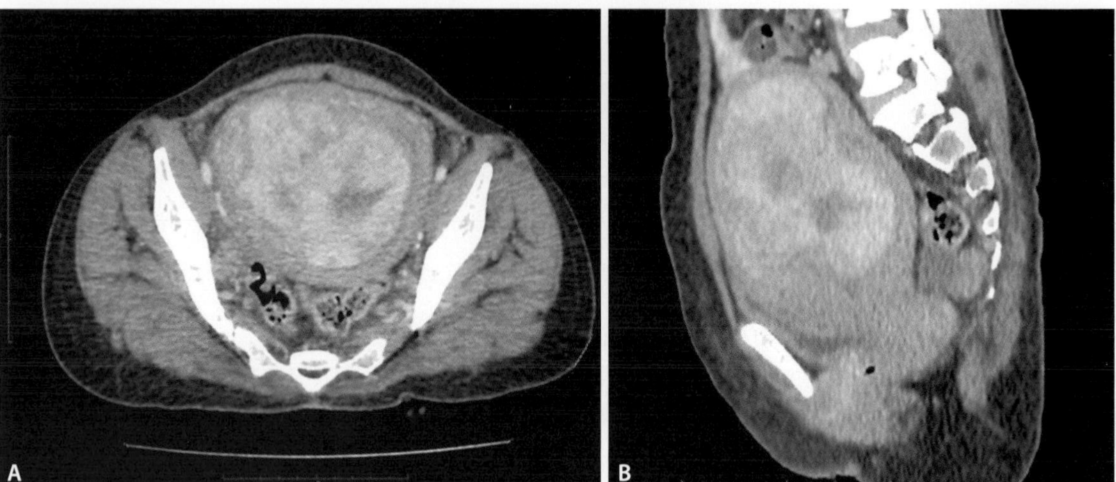

Figs. 6A and B: Carcinoma endometrium (CECT pelvis). (A) CE axial view showing large irregular enhancing mass lesion in uterus invading deep into myometrium reaching up to serosa with very small rim of remaining suggestive of carcinoma endometrium. The mass is showing area of low attenuation within it suggestive of necrosis; (B) Sagittal section shows enlargement of uterus with enhancing endometrial mass invading into almost all myometrium near fundus and anterior wall reaching near serosa except for a thin myometrial rim.

ovarian vein is commonly involved. CT findings consist of a tubular structure with an enhancing wall and low-attenuation thrombus in the expected location of the vein.

ROLE OF MRI IN GYNAECOLOGICAL IMAGING

Magnetic resonance imaging has revolutionized the imaging field. The applicability of MRI in the female pelvis has been extensively evaluated since the early 1980s. MRI has various advantages over CT and US.

Magnetic resonance imaging is particularly attractive due to its capability for multiplanar imaging. One can get transverse, sagittal, and coronal views in a short time without repositioning of the patient. Another advantage of MRI is its excellent tissue-differentiating abilities because the tissue alters the signals received during MRI. It also gives excellent tissue differentiation without the use of contrast agents. Newly developed contrast agents may further augment tissue contrast. These contrasts are much safer than the iodinated equivalents used in CT.

Magnetic resonance imaging has its intrinsic sensitivity to flowing blood so it can assess vascular abnormalities also. Additionally, biochemical states of blood also can be characterized by MRI because characteristic signals are derived from oxyhemoglobin, deoxyhemoglobin, methemoglobin, and hemosiderin in red blood cells in different stages of hematoma formation. Thus, MRI is capable of diagnosing thrombotic diseases efficiently.

Procedure

In general, the patient should be imaged in the supine position with a phased-array pelvic coil on either a 1.5- or 3-tesla magnet. The most common MRI sequences are T1-weighted and T2-weighted scans. T1WI are produced by using short TE (echo time) and TR (repetition time). The contrast and brightness of the image are predominantly determined byT1 properties of tissue. Conversely, T2 WI is produced by using longer TE and TR times. At minimum, T2 axial and sagittal imaging along with T1-weighted imaging before and after contrast administration should be performed.

Depending upon the T1 or T2 relaxation times, the appearance of an image changes markedly. On a T1WI, fat appears bright (white) and fluid appears dark. On a T2WI, fat appears gray and fluid appears bright. In majority of pathologies where water content is increased, it mimics fluid so appear dark on T1 and bright on T2WI.

T1-weighted images provide excellent differentiation between the pelvic structures and surrounding pelvic fat, allowing for detailed anatomic evaluation. Fat suppression sequences used to assist in identifying any proteinaceous or hemorrhagic material, and postcontrast imaging may be used to evaluate a variety of pathologic conditions. In addition, a partially filled bladder will also improve image quality by preventing motion artifacts and bladder contractions that may occur with a full bladder. Complete emptying of the bladder should be avoided because this may hinder evaluation of lesions in the anterior peritoneal pouch between the uterus and bladder. Endovaginal or endorectal coils may be used for detailed presurgical planning, particularly in evaluation of the female urethra. Endovaginal ultrasound gel can be applied to aid in identifying vaginal anomalies, malignant involvement, or extension into the vagina and vaginal endometriosis. Similarly, ultrasound gel can be instilled into the rectum to aid in the diagnosis of rectal wall invasion of gynecologic malignancies or rectal endometriosis. Obtaining a single large field of view, such as a T2-weighted coronal single-shot fast-spin echo (SSFSE), is useful in evaluating combined genitourinary malformations. STIR (Short Tau Inversion Recovery) is a fat suppression technique where the signal of fat is zero but limitation is that it cannot be done post gadolinium contrast. Also, the addition of diffusion-weighted imaging (DWI) uses the diffusion of water molecules to generate contrast in MRI images to highlight areas of increased cellular activities, with apparent diffusion coefficient (ADC) maps aid in evaluation of gynecologic malignancies.[1]

Safety

In general, MRI is not found to be associated with any ill effect. Heat deposition is one potential concern, but body temperature probes do not demonstrate temperature elevations.[7]

Magnetic resonance imaging is contraindicated in few conditions such as patients on pacemaker, metallic implants, etc. Any metallic/iron object is not allowed in MRI unit. Every case should be evaluated individually for safety. Few patients may have claustrophobia and may require counseling or medication support.

Normal Pelvic Anatomy on MRI

Normal female pelvic anatomy is well depicted on MRI (**Figs. 7A to C**). On T1WI, the uterus is well identified as a homogeneous structure of medium signal intensity. On T2WI, the body of uterus, isthmus, and cervix can be well differentiated. The myometrium is intermediate in signal intensity, whereas endometrium appears as high signal intensity. The myometrium and endometrium are separated by a junctional zone of low signal intensity. Hormone status markedly influences the zonal anatomy within the uterus and according to estrogen and progesterone, endometrial thickness varies. These hormones affect uterine volume also. Premenarchal and postmenopausal uterus appear similar, demonstrating both thin endometrium and small uterine volume.[7]

The cervix is easily visualized on MRI with T2WI. The normal cervix has two separate zones out of which

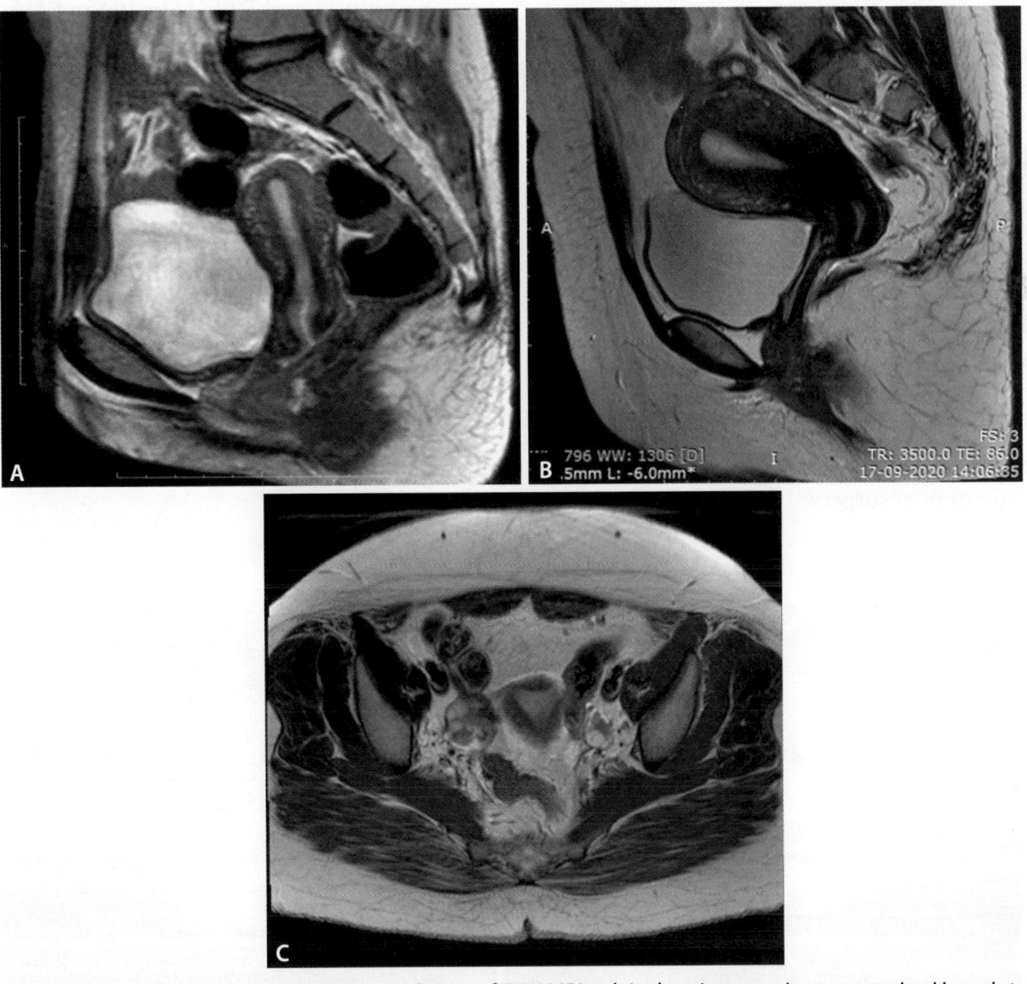

Figs. 7A to C: Normal anatomy of pelvis (MRI). (A) On sagittal view of T2W MRI pelvis showing anterior to posterior-Hyperintense shadow due to fluid suggesting bladder. Behind it showing three zones: inner hyperintense endometrium, area of decreased signal between myometrium and endometrium is called the junctional zone and outer is hyperintense myometrium; (B) Another sagittal T2W image: The cervix has less signal than uterine fundus. The vagina is apparent as thin strip of high signal intensity surrounded by linear bands of decreased signal intensity. On T2 weighted image, areas of fat is giving less signal and appeared grey; (C) On axial section, T2W image, bilateral ovarian shadow is seen showing hyperintense signals for small follicles in it. Uterine body is well differentiated. Ovaries are identified better depending on presence of follicles (low attenuation) in it.

endocervical canal is represented by high signal intensities, whereas cervical stroma gives low signal intensity.

The vagina can be identified from the surrounding structures on T2WI. Mucus in the vagina is represented as high-intensity signals in center. It can vary in thickness, being thinner in premenarchal and postmenopausal age. The vaginal wall shows low signal intensity on T2-weighted images in the early follicular phase of the menstrual cycle but increases to medium intensity in the secretory phase.[8] Transverse images can be identified posterior to bladder and sagittal image shows vaginal fornix, cervix, and rectum.

Normal ovaries usually have low-to-medium signal intensity on T1WI. On T2WI, the signal intensity increases (**Fig. 7C**). Follicular cysts may have higher signal intensity than fat, so they make easy identification of the ovaries. Ovaries are more difficult to distinguish in postmenopausal women.[9]

Identification of pelvic musculature is quite easy by MRI. As compared to fat, muscle gives low signal intensity. The vesicovaginal septum, the rectovaginal septum, and the levator ani muscle can be identified.[10] The relationship of urethra to bladder can also be identified.

GYNAECOLOGIC PATHOLOGY ON MRI

Uterus

Identification of pathologic alterations such as leiomyomas is very easy when you know normal myometrial characters (**Figs. 8A and B**). Simple myomas are usually surrounded by a capsule and gives low signal intensity regardless of the pulse sequence used.[11] MRI is very accurate in detecting the size, site, and number of leiomyomas as compared to US.[12] Before the procedure of myomectomy, MRI may help in mapping and planning the extent of surgery.

Leiomyomas may have various appearances on MRI which can depend upon the presence of hemorrhage, hyaline or cystic degeneration, and calcium deposition.[13] The degenerative area shows low signal intensity on T1WI and high signal intensity on T2WI. However, hemorrhage in the leiomyoma produces various appearances, depending on the imaging sequence used.[7]

Uterine sarcomas can also be identified with invasion of myometrium but it can give rise to confusion with endometrial carcinoma. Histopathological examination may be needed for confirmation.

Magnetic resonance imaging has been used to evaluate adenomyosis.[14,15] Uterus with adenomyosis is enlarged and have smooth external surface (**Figs. 9A to C**). Diffuse adenomyosis distorts the normal zonal anatomy of the uterus and junctional zone become enlarged. Adenomyotic areas are isointense with myometrium on T1WI and decreased in signal on T2WI but old hemorrhagic areas measuring a few millimeters in diameter are often seen as high-intensity spots on both T1 and T2WI (**Figs. 9A to C**). Adenomyosis has irregular and indistinct margins while leiomyomas have well-circumscribed margins, so in case of doubt, MRI is useful for preoperative assessment and surgical planning.[7]

Endometrium

On MRI, endometrial tissue is approximately isointense with myometrium onT1WI but appears higher in signal intensity relative to myometrium on T2WI. Endometrial polyps can either be sessile or pedunculated which can be better identified in sonohysterography or seen in direct hysteroscopy. On MRI, endometrial polyps are seen as a polypoid endometrial mass, usually with T2 hyperintense signal (**Fig. 10**). Differential diagnosis includes submucosal leiomyoma and endometrial cancer.

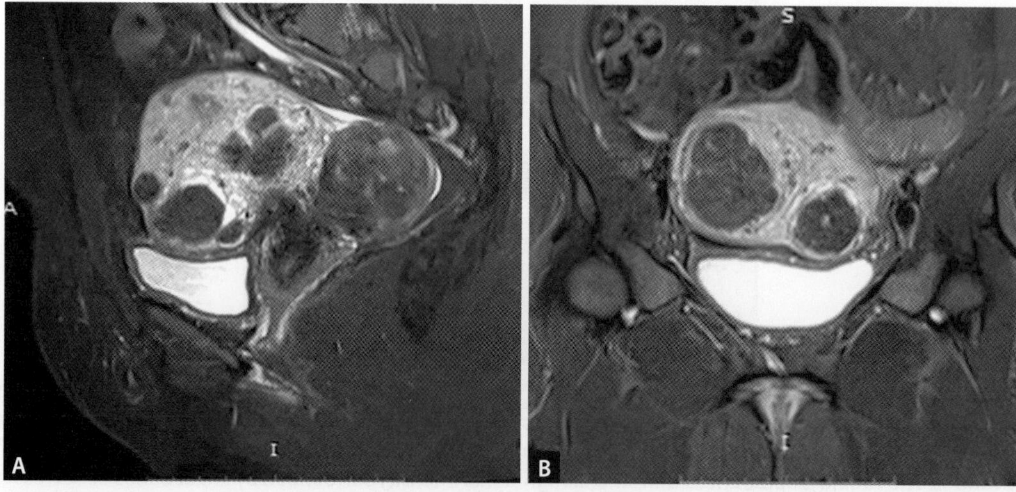

Figs. 8A and B: Multiple myoma (MRI). In a multiple leiomyomoma 39-years old patient: (A) Sagittal STIR sequence showing multiple well-defined hypointense lesions in anterior as well as posterior wall of uterus. Myoma showing multiple hyperintense areas suggestive of degeneration; (B) Axial T2W image suggesting enlarged uterine body with two large well-defined rounded hypointense areas suggestive of leiomyoma.

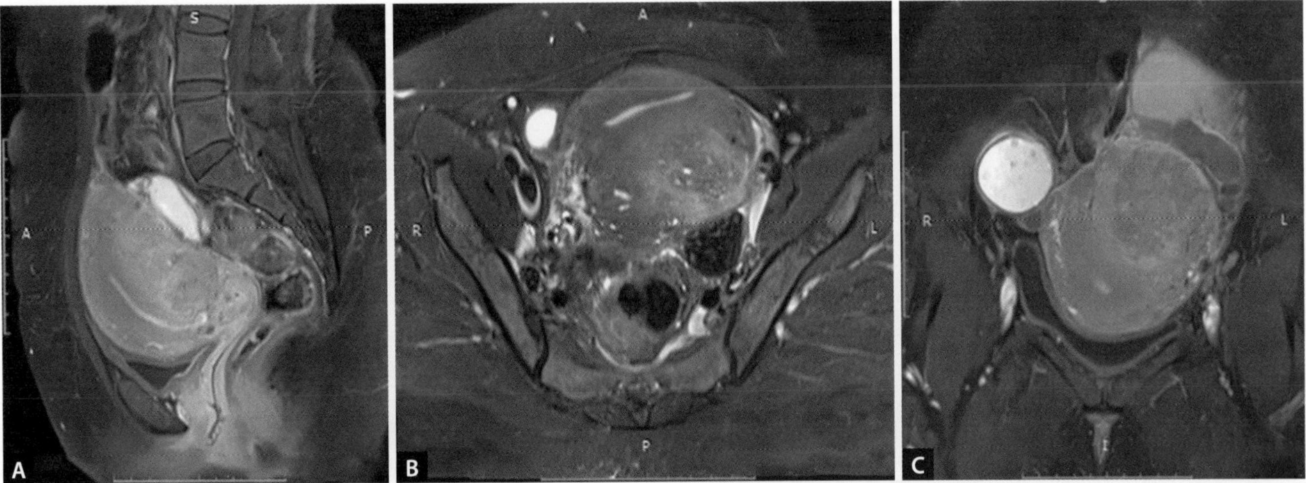

Figs. 9A to C: Adenomyosis with hematosalpinx with endometrial cyst (MRI). (A) Sagittal postcontrast T1W MRI of pelvis showing asymmetrical thickening of posterior wall of uterus involving extending down up to cervico uterine junction, sparing anterior uterine wall; (B) Axial section on STIR sequence showing few ill-defined irregular ovoid region of thickening with multiple small hyperintense cystic lesion. In right adnexa showing hemorrhagic cyst; (C) Left fallopian tube appears dilated with T1 isointense loculated collection showing left-sided hematosalpinx and on right-sided hemorrhagic cyst seen.

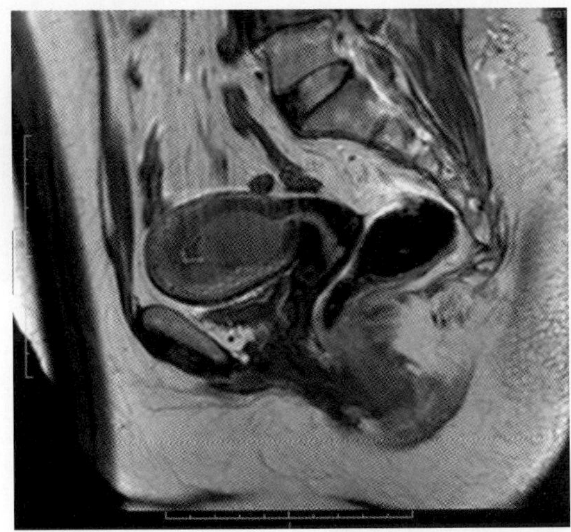

Fig. 10: MRI pelvis (endometrial polyp). A sagittal T2W image suggesting uterine cavity filled with a well-defined rounded isointense areas suggestive of endometrial polyp.

Magnetic resonance imaging is very accurate for staging of endometrial carcinoma. MRI allows good preoperative evaluation in cases of endometrial carcinoma. It can define depth of invasion of myometrium, tumor site, and cervical involvement.[16] Distorted junctional zone can be demonstrated well **(Figs. 11A to E)**. Low-intensity band between the endometrium and myometrium may become absent in deep invasion. MRI is also good to detect cervical invasion and extrauterine disease. It is highly accurate in local staging and is recommended for women in whom there is clinical suspicion of advanced disease.[17] Gadolinium enhancement with dynamic imaging has been investigated with promising results.

Cervix

On MRI, normal cervix has two distinguishable zones. The stroma gives low signal intensity on T2WI, and the endocervical canal gives high signal intensity. MRI allows excellent visualization of the cervix and the surrounding tissue, which is sometimes difficult on CT or ultrasonographic examination and MRI is now the primary technique of choice in the staging of pelvic malignancy.[4]

Advanced invasive cervical cancer has an overall poor survival. Careful clinical staging is important to differentiate between stages IB, IIA, and IIB so that the mode of treatment can be decided. CT has a limited role in this area while MRI has the widest application in cervical carcinoma out of all gynecological malignancies.[18] It can detect cervical cancer, which has increased signal intensity on T2WI in contrast to surrounding tissues; therefore, it is an important tool for clinical staging **(Figs. 12A to C)**.

Although MRI detection of parametrial involvement is excellent, no rigid criteria are currently available. Limiting factors may be distortion from hemorrhage and edema.[19] Appearance of parametrial tumor involvement may be affected by secondary infection. Overall, there is greater accuracy of MRI in parametrial assessment compared with CT scanning.

Magnetic resonance imaging staging is superior in comparison to clinical examination with or without anesthesia. MRI accurately locates the internal os so it can predict proximal extension of the tumor, thus predicting suitability for trachelectomy and fertility conserving surgery.[17] Prognostication of cervical cancer is also better as tumor volume can be accurately determined. Regarding bladder and rectal invasion of cancer cervix, one meta-analysis showed

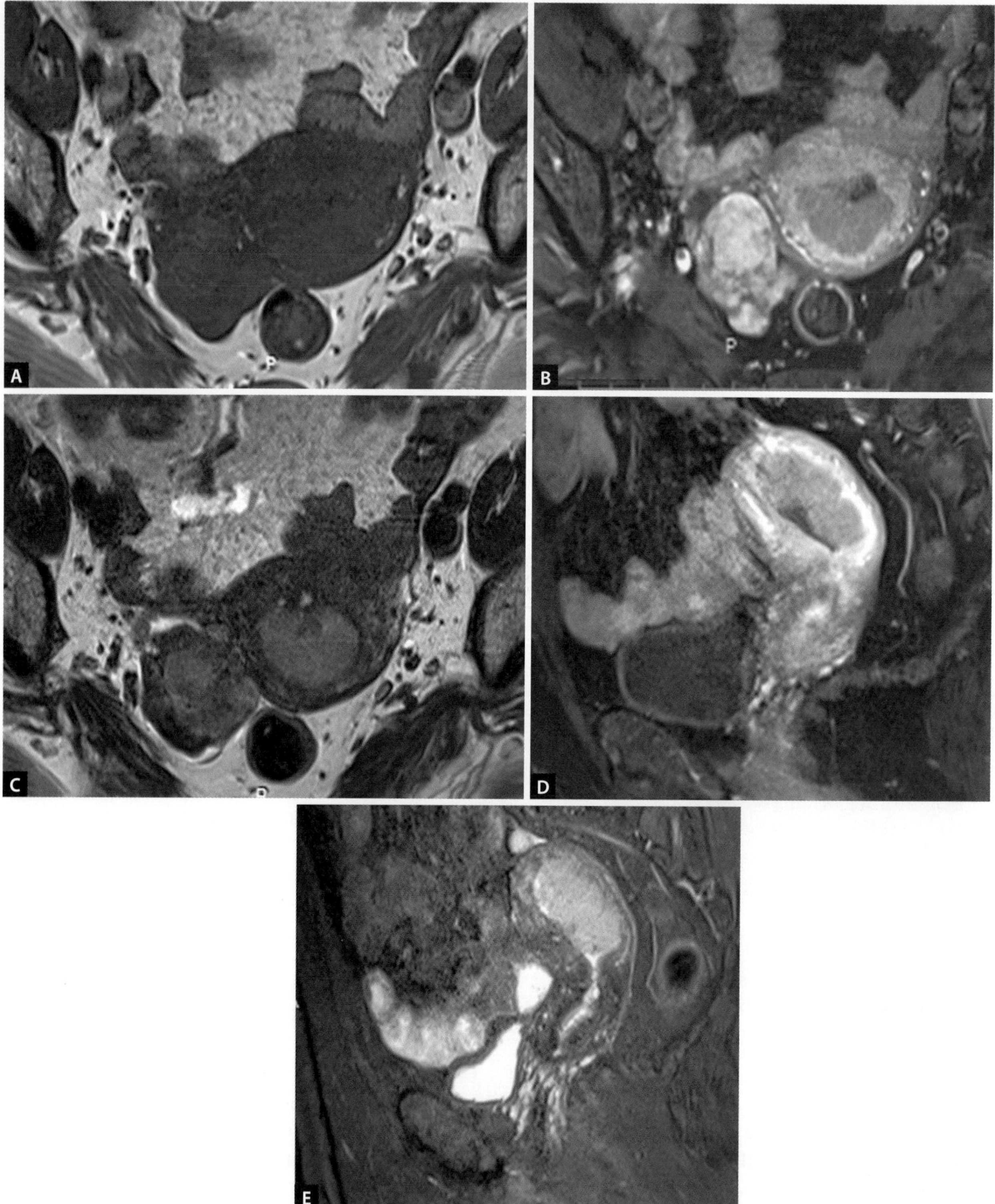

Figs. 11A to E: MRI pelvis—T1WI (A), T1W + contrast (B, D) and T2/STIR image (C, E) carcinoma endometrium: (A) T1W axial image showing relatively hypointense signal intensity area suggesting uterus. Endometrial cavity is not well depicted in T1W axial image, also showing similar hypointense mass on right side of uterus appears to be subserosal fibroid; (B) T1W axial postcontrast image showing mass in endometrial cavity hypointense as compare to myometrium. Myometrium is hyperintense after contrast. The mass is infiltrating posterior myometrium; however, overlying serosa is intact. There is minimal hypointense area in endometrial cavity suggesting fluid; (C) Axial T2W image showing irregular large area of iso-to hypointensity in endometrial cavity suggestive of endometrial mass with small hyperintense area anterior to mass lesion, suggestive of fluid in cavity; (D) T1W sagittal post contrast image showing mass in endometrial cavity hypointense as compare to myometrium. The mass is infiltrating posterior myometrium however overlying serosa is intact; (E) Sagittal (STIR) image showing irregular large area of iso-to hypointensity in endometrial cavity suggestive of endometrial mass with small hyperintense area anterior to mass lesion, suggestive of fluid in cavity.

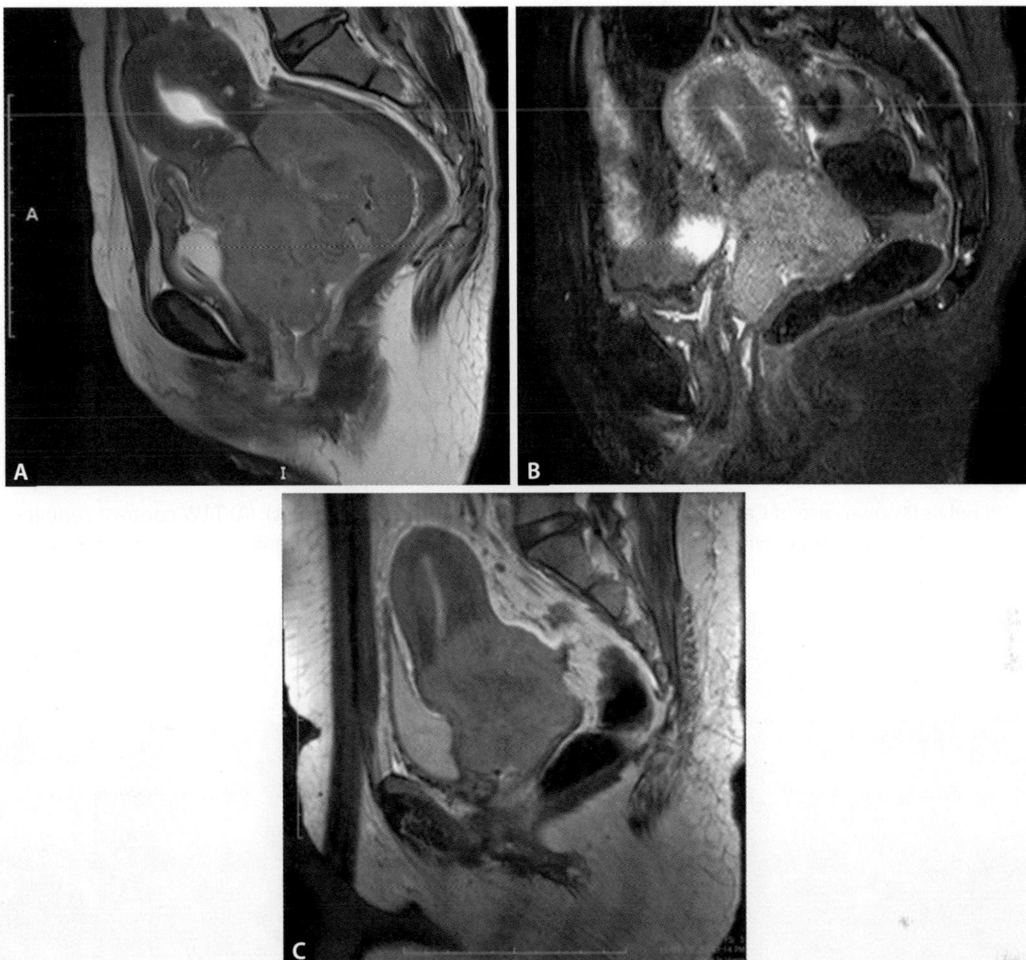

Figs. 12A to C: MRI pelvis (Ca cervix). (A) T2W- sagittal image of a known case of carcinoma cervix shows large heterogeneous hyperintense mass of cervix extending into lower part of body of uterus and upper 1/3rd of vagina and anteriorly infiltrating into posterior wall of bladder. Small amount of collection in endometrial cavity suggests hydropyometra; (B) STIR sagittal image of another known carcinoma cervix patient shows a well-defined hyperintense lesion of cervix extending into lower part of body of uterus and upper 1/3rd of vagina; (C) T2 W MRI-sagittal image of carcinoma cervix shows large heterogeneous hyperintense mass of cervix extending into lower part of body of uterus and upper 1/3rd of vagina and posteriorly infiltrating into parametrium and adjacent organ.

that MRI has a sensitivity of 91% for bladder invasion and 75% for rectal invasion.[20] Recurrent cancer of cervix can also be identified by MRI **(Figs. 13A and B)**. With recurrent tumor, signal intensity in the tumor increased as the T2 weighting increased in contrast to that seen in fibrosis, which showed decreased signal intensity when the T2 weighting increased.[21]

Characteristics of fibrotic changes vary with time. Early radiation-induced fibrosis produces high signal intensities on T2WI, while older fibrosis yields low-intensity signals **(Fig. 14A and B)**. Ongoing follow-up can be done with tumor volume assessment. Overall accuracy of MRI in the diagnosis of recurrent tumor is 78%, with higher rates of accuracy and specificity after 6 months.[22] T1 relaxation times decreased with therapy but markedly increased with tumor persistence.[23] With ongoing development of paramagnetic contrast agents, the diagnostic potential of MRI could be further extended.

Ovary

Simple ovarian cysts are unilocular and low density on CT. On MRI, they show low signal on T1WI and high signal on T2WI **(Fig. 15A and B)**. Physiologic cysts may demonstrate a thin enhancing wall on MRI, but no internal enhancement.[1] Several other types of ovarian lesions are particularly well evaluated by MRI; these include simple follicular cysts, hemorrhagic cysts, endometrial cysts, and benign teratomas. MRI can easily identify hemorrhage. However, depending on the biochemical state and age of the blood, the signal may be bright or dark on either T1 or T2 weighted images[24] **(Figs. 16A to C)**. Endometrioma tend to have adhesions on the external surface and may lack a distinct margin from the uterine body and may have multiple loculi within the cyst. Feature of shading within loculi is characteristic of endometrial cysts **(Figs. 17A to C)**. Use of fat-saturation techniques significantly increases the diagnostic accuracy of MRI for endometriomas.

Scar endometriosis is a rare cause of painful scar in which pain at incision site occurs at the time of menstruation. Here MRI acts as a most sensitive imaging modality for diagnosis **(Figs. 18A to C)**. MRI may not be very sensitive in detecting endometrial implants in peritoneal cavity rather laparoscopy

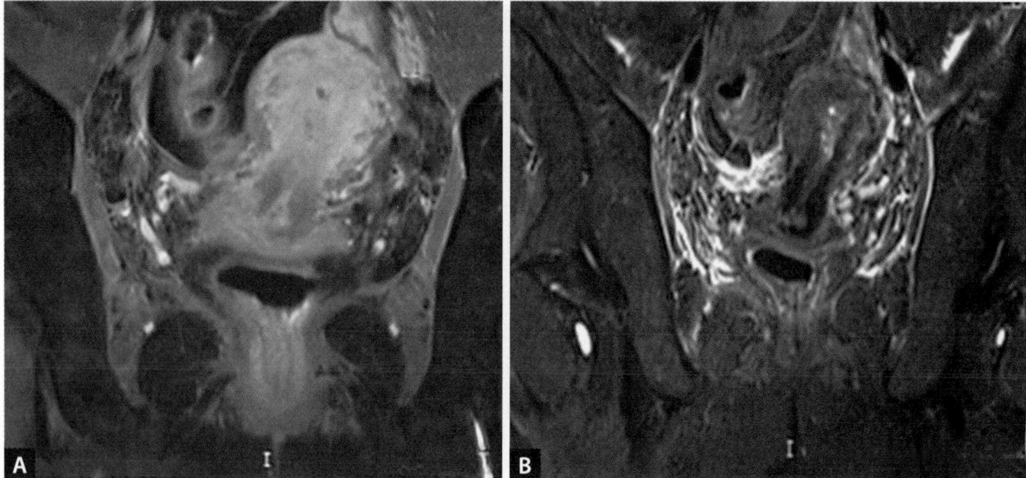

Figs. 13A and B: MRI pelvis (Known case of Ca Cx, post radiotherapy resedue/recurrence status). (A) T1W contrast sequence showing a mass lesion extending from right lateral side of cervicovaginal region; (B) STIR sequence showing heterogeneous hyperintense lesion at same place. Above finding suggestive of recurrence/residual lesion.

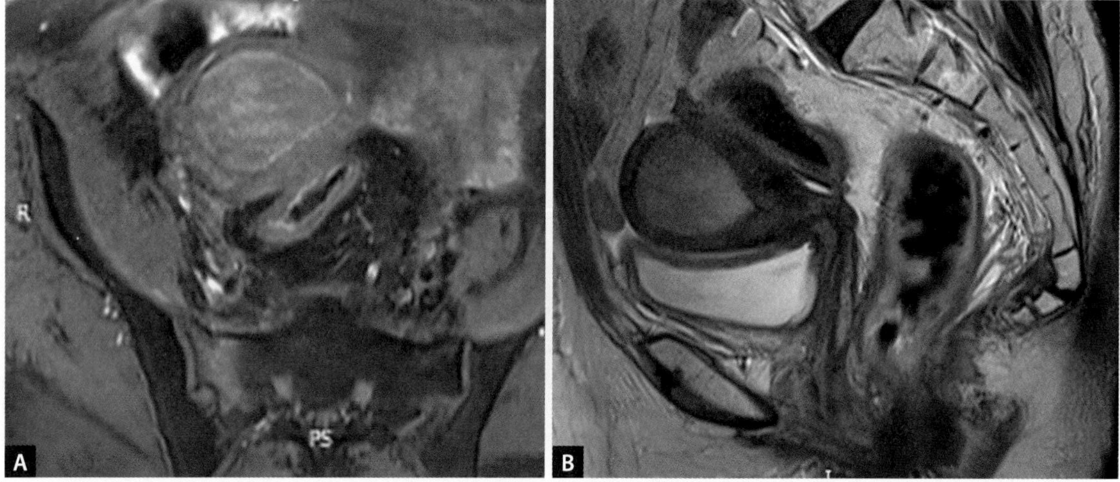

Figs. 14A and B: MRI sequence of pelvis (post radiotherapy for carcinoma cervix—cervicovaginal stenosis and fibrosis). (A) T1 W coronal image showing distended uterus with collection within the cavity with increased intensity; (B) T2W sagittal image showing hyperintense area suggestive of collection within the endometrial cavity (pyometra) with fibrosis and stenosis of cervical canal. Postcarcinoma cervix adhesion.

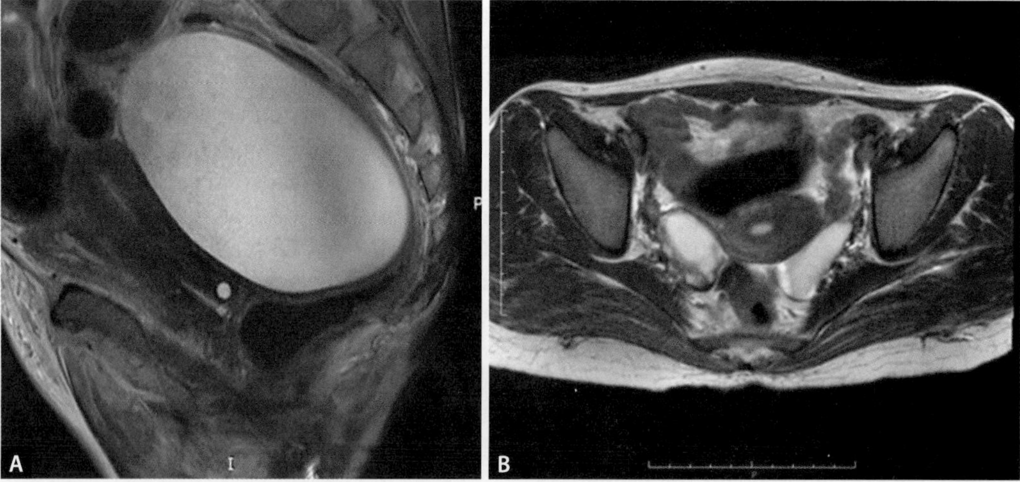

Figs. 15A and B: MRI—ovarian cyst. (A) Sagittal T2W image shows a large well-defined oval thin-walled hyperintense cystic lesion between uterus and rectum causing mass effect with significant compression of rectum up to rectosigmoid junction. A subcentimetric nabothian cyst in posterior lip of cervix also seen; (B) Axial T2 W image of pelvis shows bilateral ovaries beside uterus showing hyperintense cystic lesion within them suggesting simple ovarian cyst. All three zones of uterus—hyperintense endometrium, hypointense junctional zone and outer hyperintense myometrium—are well depicted.

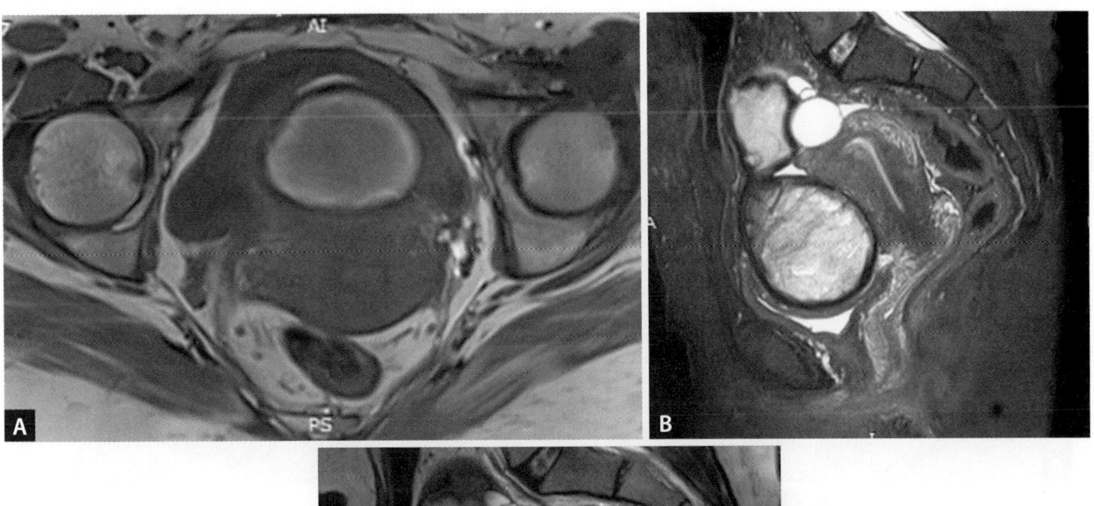

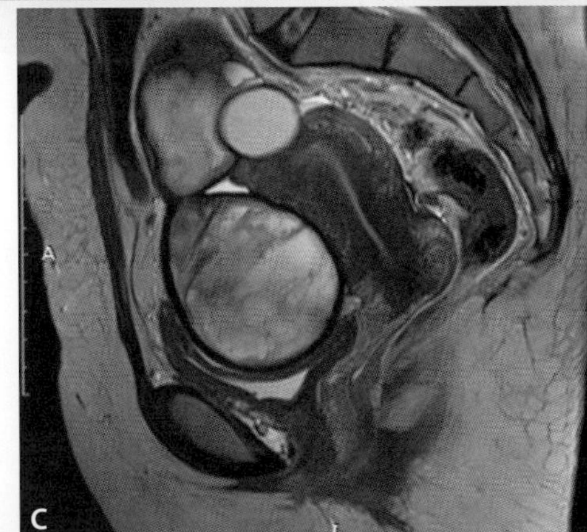

Figs. 16A to C: MRI—hemorrhagic cyst. (A) Axial T1W imaging showing a well-defined rounded hyperintense mass anterior to uterus suggesting hemorrhagic content; (B and C) Sagittal T2W imaging shows same mass with different signals of hyperintensity in that mass suggesting hemorrhage while a separate small hyperintense cyst superior to fundus is suggesting a simple cyst. Sagittal view STIR image confirming no fat content within the cystic mass.

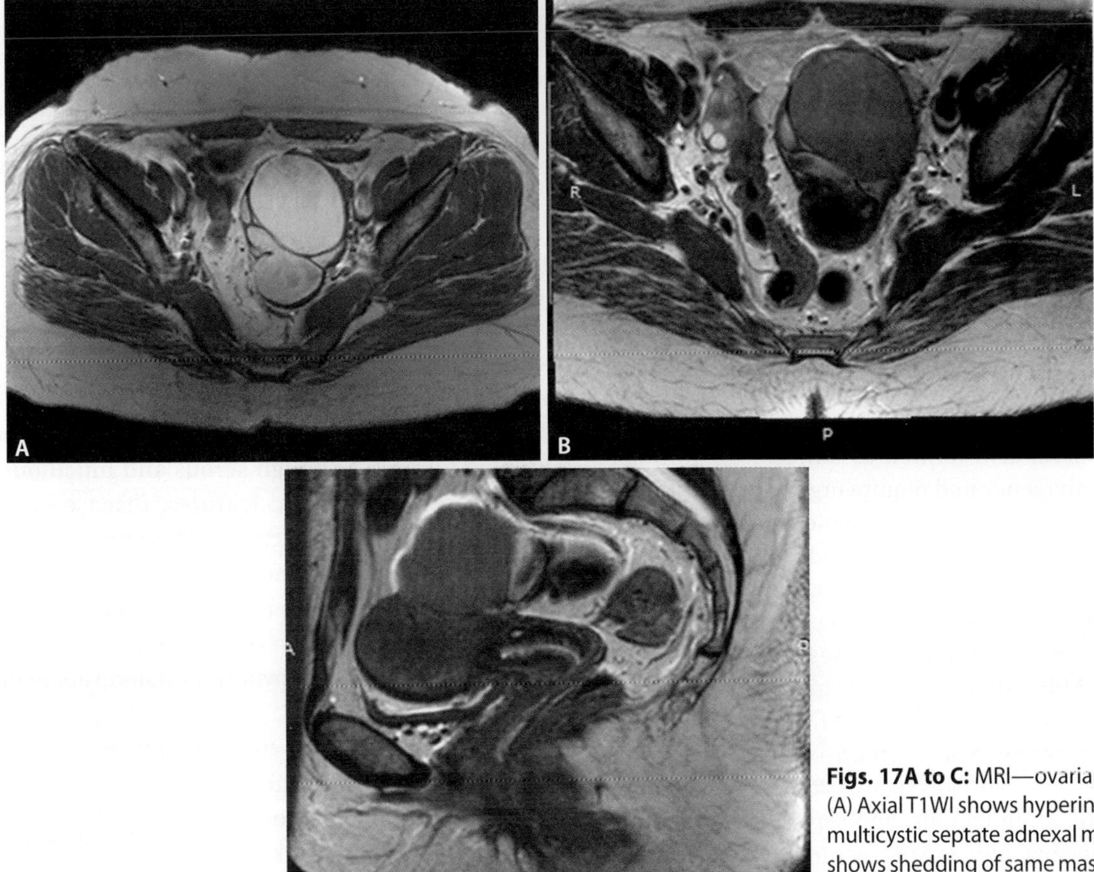

Figs. 17A to C: MRI—ovarian endometrioma. (A) Axial T1WI shows hyperintense, fairly large, multicystic septate adnexal mass; (B) Axial T2WI shows shedding of same mass; (C) Sagttal T2WI shows the endometrioma to be adherent to post wall of uterus and adjacent loop of bowel.

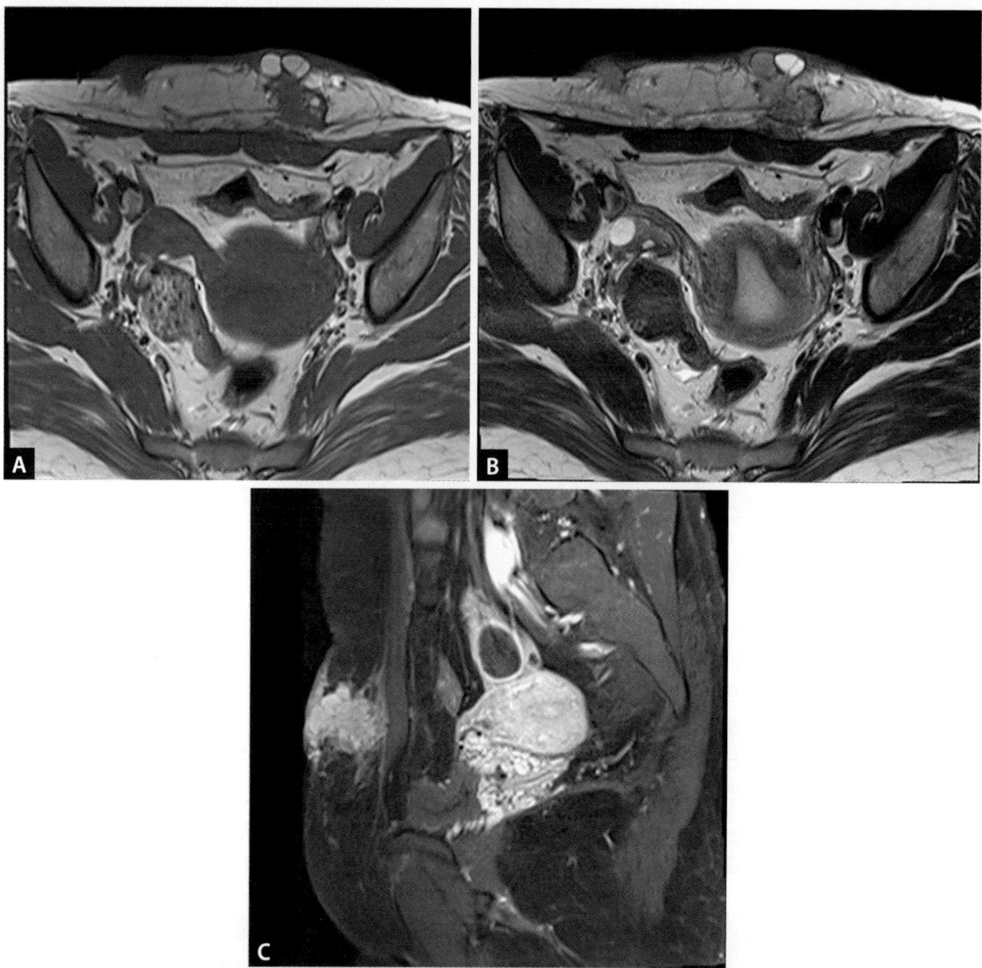

Figs. 18A to C: MRI pelvis (scar endometriosis). (A) Axial T1W imaging shows a well-defined, irregular marginated solid cystic mass lesion noted in subcutaneous plane of lower anterior abdominal wall. The solid component is T1 hypointense; (B) Same axial T2W imaging shows heterogeneously hyperintense solid area with hyperintense cystic lesions anteriorly; (C) Sagittal STIR image shows infiltration of lesion into the overlying skin. Posteriorly, there is effacement of fat plane with anterior margin of rectus muscle. Findings suggestive of scar endometriosis.

though invasive, but quite sensitive method for diagnosing endometriosis.

Not as a routine but MRI can be used to study polycystic ovarian syndrome as it provides better resolution and tissue contrast. MRI can better assess ovarian morphology and can demonstrate peripheral cysts and hyperplastic stroma.

Ovarian torsion, also termed as adnexal torsion, is a gynecological emergency and require urgent intervention. It can result in venous arterial and lymphatic stasis. Large cystic ovaries are at particular risk. Ultrasound is initial modality of choice for diagnosis and typically shows whirlpool sign in Doppler studies. MRI is not the imaging modality of choice if there is acute emergency, but in cases where there is no emergency and MRI is done, it shows thin rim of high signals without contrast enhancement on T1WI while on T2WI can have low signal due to interstitial hemorrhage **(Figs. 19A to C)**.

Various types of ovarian cysts such as simple cysts, follicular cyst, corpus luteum, mucinous, and serous cystadenomas may show somewhat similar MRI features. They show low signal intensity on T1WI and higher signal intensity on T2WI. As such signal wise no marked difference identified but morphologic criteria may provide some specificity. Solid ovarian benign and malignant tumors tend to have variable T1 and T2 values and tend to have lower signal intensities overall. Image enhancement with gadolinium can be done for better staging accuracy.

Serous and mucinous tumors are the most common epithelial tumors. Although serous and mucinous tumors have different pathologic features, disease course, and prognosis, they can be difficult to differentiate based on gross inspection and imaging findings. It is not currently possible to distinguish benign from malignant lesion based solely on the signal intensity.[25] However, imaging features can aid in differentiation as well as provide information about malignant potential.

On imaging, serous tumors may be unilocular or multilocular, with homogeneous T1 and T2 signal intensity on MRI. Thick or irregular walls, solid internal papillary projections, thick septations and large soft-tissue components with necrosis are more indicative of malignancy[1] **(Figs. 20A and B)**.

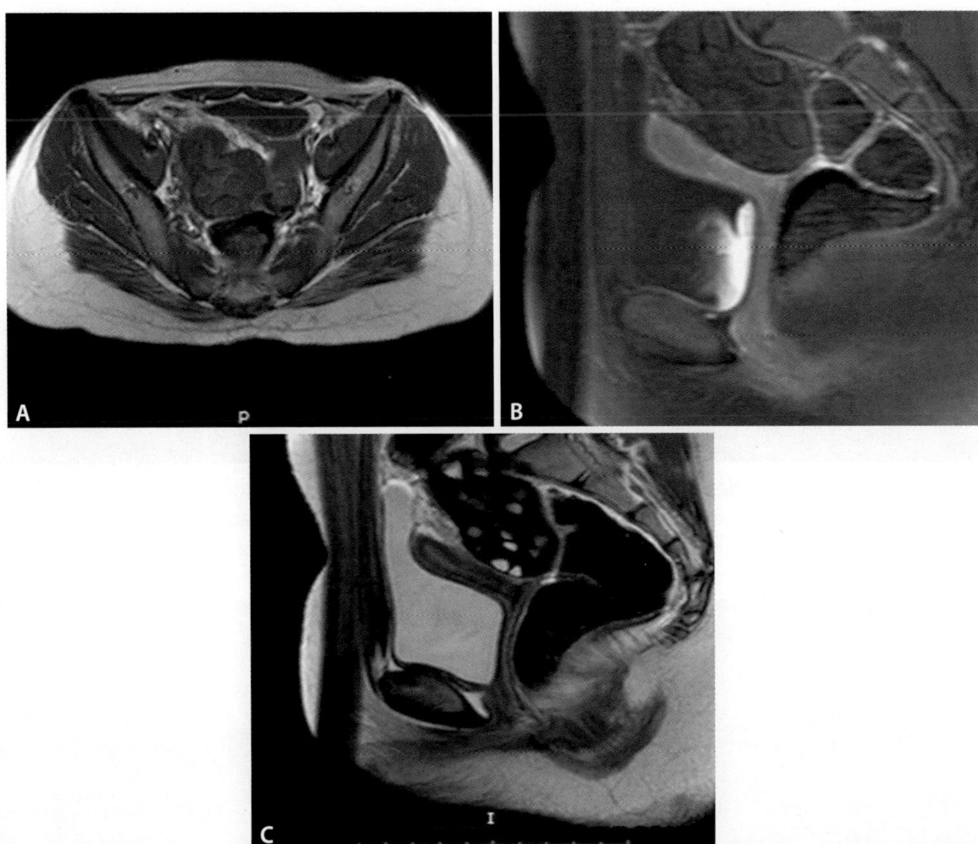

Figs. 19A to C: MRI (twisted enlarged ovary): 12-year-old girl presented with pain in abdomen. (A) Axial T1W + CE image shows marked enlarge right ovary anterior to uterus showing diffuse hypointensity with some areas of increased signals; (B) Sagittal T1W contrast enhanced image suggesting enlarged ovary with diffuse hypointense signals. No contrast enhancement seen in ovary suggesting ovarian torsion with interstitial hemorrhage; (C) On T2WI, peculiar multiple hyperintense small follicles seen with dense stroma. Uterus is showing normal anatomy.

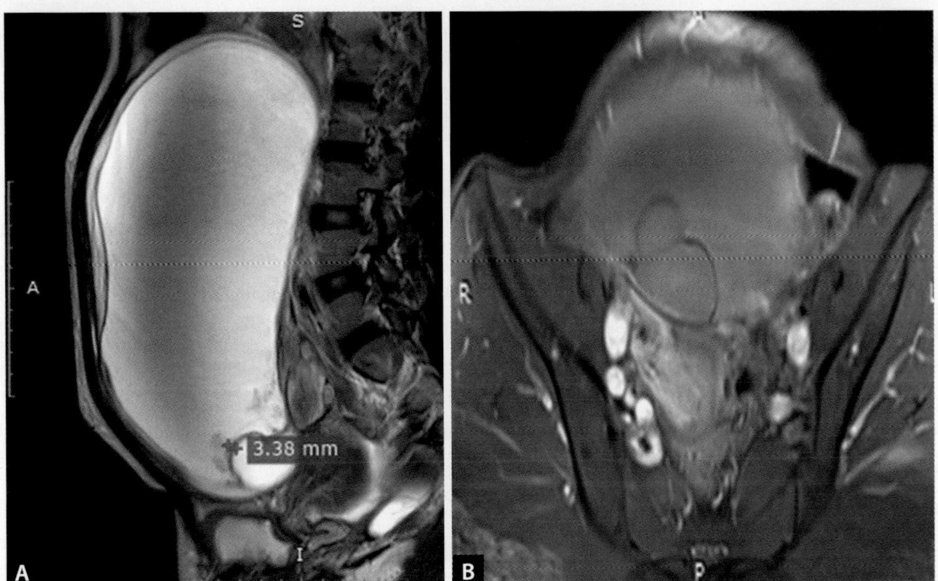

Figs. 20A and B: MRI—serous cyst adenocarcinoma. (A) T2W image sagittal image shows large abdominopelvic cystic lesion with thick septations and subtle papillary projection; (B) T1C + FS axial images show no contrast enhancement of septa. Histopathology suggestive of serous cystadenocarcinoma.

Mucinous tumors are less likely to be bilateral and tend to be larger at presentation. In neglected cases they may present as mammoth tumors. They are also more likely to be borderline malignant or malignant. Mucinous tumors are classically multilocular with mucoid material, hemorrhage, or cellular debris within the cysts. These findings result in varying

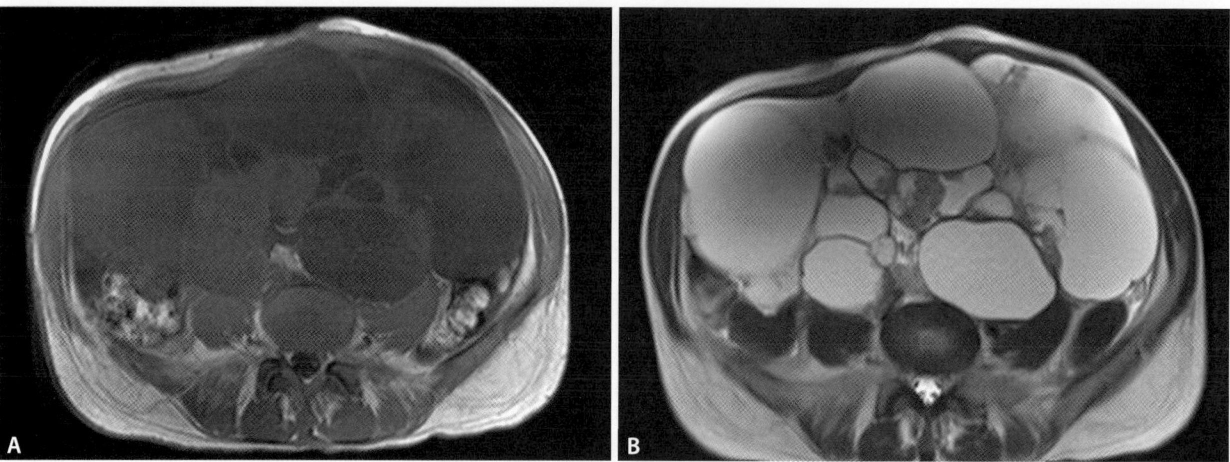

Figs. 21A and B: MRI (case of mucinous cyst adenocarcinoma). (A) Axial T1WI showing large multiloculated well-defined solid cystic mass. With predominantly cystic component with mural nodule; (B) Axial T2WI showing same large multiloculated mass. With predominantly hyperintense cystic component with mural nodule.

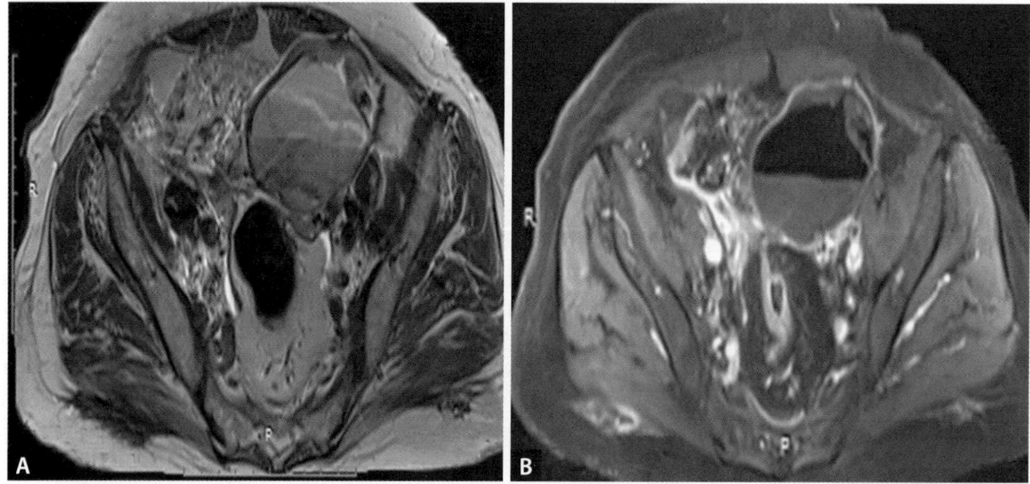

Figs. 22A and B: MRI pelvis (mature cystic teratoma). (A) Axial T2WI showing well-defined lesion with fat–fluid level and soft-tissue component; (B) T1C + FS axial image also show fat fluid level with mild enhancement of soft-tissue component and suppressed fat signal suggesting mature teratoma.

density on CT or signal intensity on MRI within the different locules such that locules with thicker mucin demonstrate increased density or increased T1-weighted signal and decreased T2-weighted signal compared to locules with more watery mucin. This is often referred to as a "stained-glass" appearance[1] **(Figs. 21A and B)**.

Germ cell tumors are the second most common type of ovarian neoplasms. The group includes mature teratoma, immature teratoma, dysgerminoma, endodermal sinus tumor, embryonal carcinoma, and choriocarcinoma. Mature teratoma is the most common of the group and the only benign neoplasm. Ovarian cystic teratomas give signal similar to the fat due to large fat content within them **(Figs. 22A and B)**. In addition to the high signal intensity due to fat, debris and nodular protrusions are seen in these tumors. Sometimes, teeth or bone are also identified as very low signals because of the high calcium. Occasionally fat/fluid levels may be seen in teratomas.

Dysgerminomas are the most malignant germ cell tumor but are rare, occurring predominately in children and young women. On CT and MRI, dysgerminomas present as unilateral multilobulated solid masses with prominent fibrovascular septa **(Figs. 23A and B)**. They demonstrate low signal on T1-weighted images and intermediate signal on T2-weighted images, with avidly enhancing fibrovascular septations and central areas of necrosis. CT may demonstrate a speckled pattern of calcification.[1]

Vagina

Vagina is easily identified by MRI. The vaginal mucosa has high signal intensity on T2WI, whereas the vaginal muscle itself has low signal intensity on both T1- and T2-weighted images.[26] The muscle is clearly differentiated from the surrounding fat. Absent vagina suggest Müllerian agenesis. Primary vaginal tumor can be identified by location, size, and extension. This growth have medium signal intensity on T1WI which is similar to the adjacent vaginal tissue.

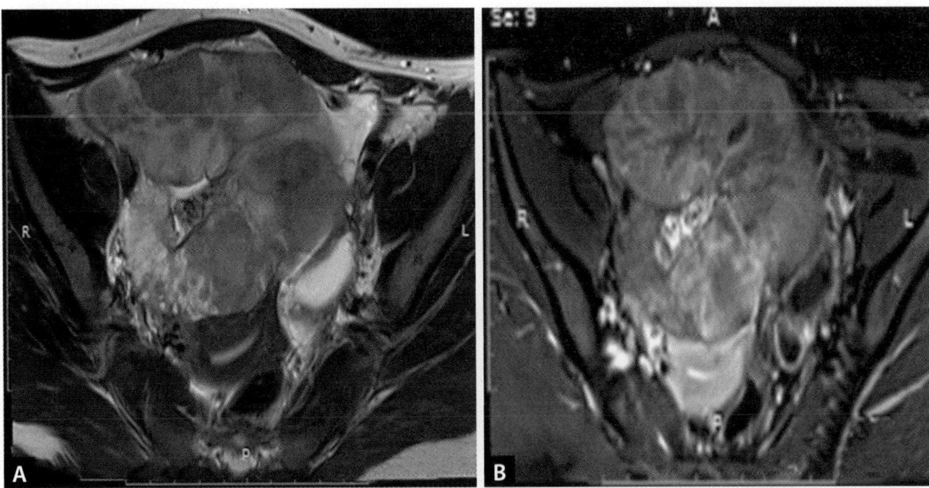

Figs. 23A and B: MRI—dysgerminoma. (A) axial T2WI showing heterogeneous multilobulated solid mass with fibrovascular septa appearing hypointense; (B) T1+C image showing heterogeneous enhancement of mass with intense enhancement of fibrovascular septa and nonenhancing necrotic areas. Histopathological examination shows nest of malignant cell separated by fibrous septa proves it to be dysgerminoma.

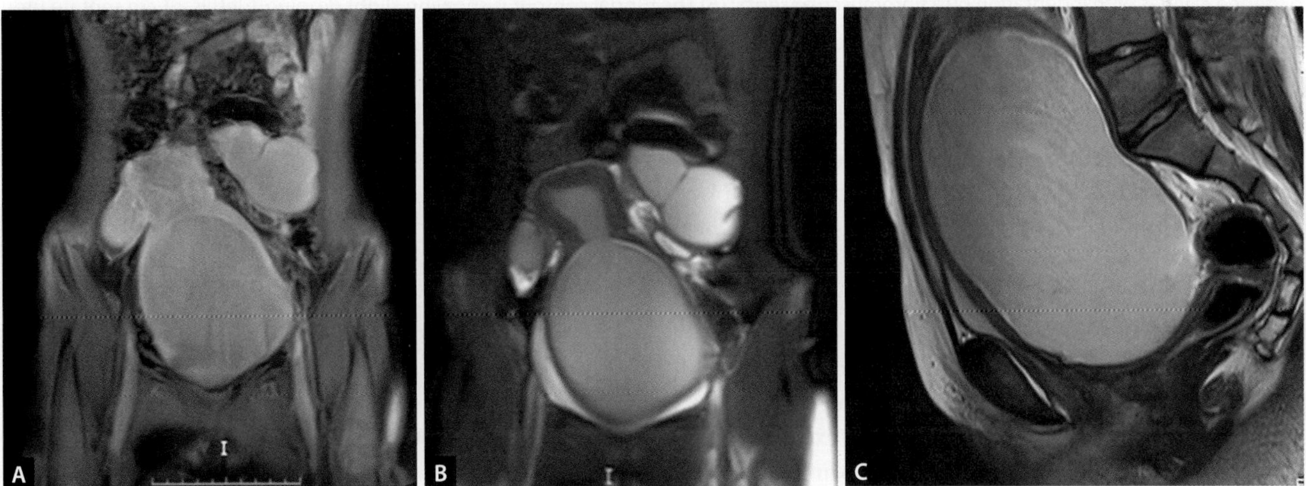

Figs. 24A to C: MRI (Mulllerian duct abnormality—atresia of lower one third of vagina). (A and B) Coronal T1W fat saturation and T2W image showing cystic ballooning dilatation of upper two third of vagina in continuity with uterine cavity. The fluid content appears hyperintense on T1, fat saturation, T2W sequence corresponding to blood products. Beside uterus, bilateral fluid-filled oval tubular structure showing hyperintense signals. Findings are suggestive of gross hematocolpos with mild hematometra and B/L hematosalpinx; (C) On sagittal T2W image showing ballooning of upper two thirds of vagina with hyperintense gross collection within it. There is nonvisualization of lower one third of vagina suggesting lower one third of vaginal atresia.

Müllerian Anomalies

Recent experience has demonstrated that MRI is the gold standard for diagnosing and can be 100% accurate in Müllerian duct anomalies and appears to be superior to endovaginal US and hysterosalpingography.[27] Pubertal or young amenorrheic patients with cyclic lower abdominal pain should be evaluated for vaginal agenesis and the presence of a hematocolpos or hematometra. Renal abnormalities should be specially checked in these cases due to high chances of associated urological anomalies.

Magnetic resonance imaging can successfully demonstrate vaginal agenesis in the absence or presence of a cervix, uterus, and ovaries.[28] MRI has been able to define the precise distance between the distal blind vaginal pouch and the upper patent vagina, so preoperative planning of reconstructive surgery can be done **(Figs. 24 A to C)**. The MRI showing a banana or a cigar shaped uterine cavity is pathognomonic of unicornuate uterine cavity. The contralateral rudimentary horn, if present, shows variable findings. It may appear as a soft-tissue lesion with the same signal intensity as myometrium, with or without the high signal intensity of normal endometrium on T2-weighted images. In obstructed rudimentary horns, central areas of high signal intensity on T1-weighted images and low signal intensity on T2-weighted images are indicative of hematometra [American Fertility Society (AFS) Class 2]. Uterus didelphys is caused by failure of two Müllerian duct anomalies (MDAs) to fuse, resulting in complete duplication of uterine corpus and cervix. Imaging finding include two

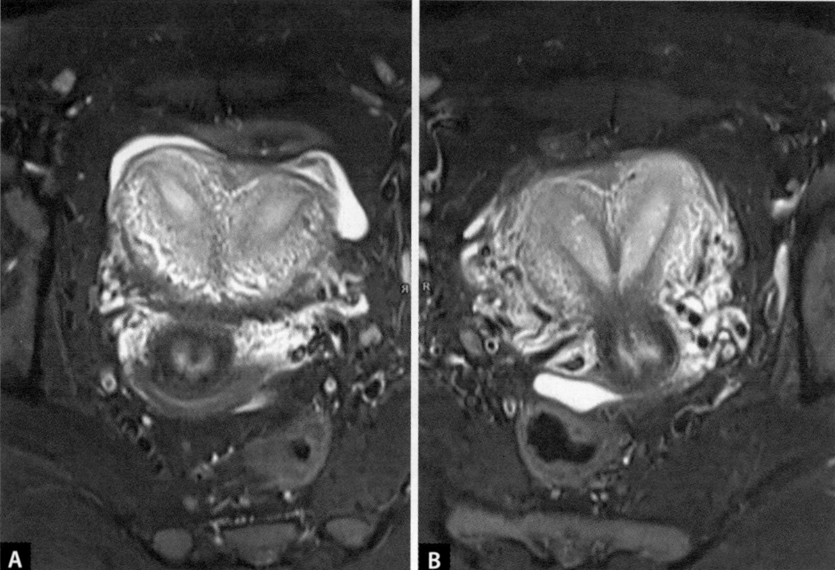

Figs. 25A and B: MRI pelvis—Mullerian abnormality Class 5 (septate uterus). (A) T2, STIR coronal image showing broadened uterine corpus with two uterine cavities with indentation by a fibromuscular septa; (B) The fundal contour is showing slight dipping. Cleft is <1 cm septate uterus.

widely separated uterine corpus with two cervices (AFS Class 3). Bicornuate uterus constitutes approximately 10% of MDAs, where two small cavities can be identified although two uterine horns are not widely separated as in uterus didelphys; there is a wide fundal cleft of >1 cm and the distance between the two uterine cornua is usually >5 cm (AFS Class 4). Septate uterus results due to incomplete resorption of median septum and it is most common type of MDA. Typical imaging feature is a uterus of normal size and normal fundal contour with duplication of endometrial cavity by a median septum (AFS Class 5) **(Figs. 25A and B)**. In arcuate uterus except for mild fundal thickening rest anatomy remains normal **(Fig. 26)**. T-shaped endometrial cavity seen in diethylstilbestrol (DES) exposure-related uterine anomalies.[1]

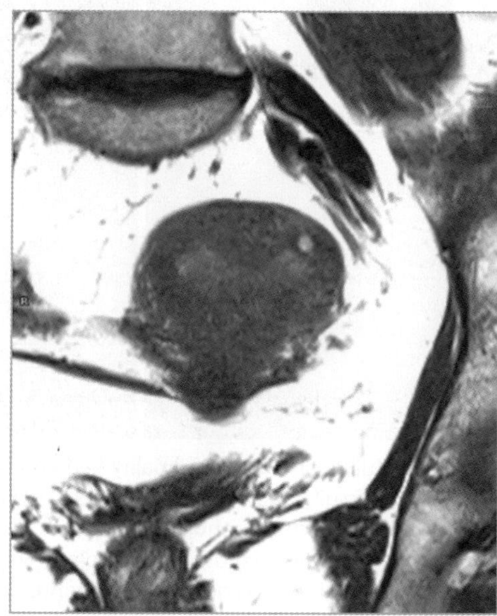

Fig. 26: MRI—MDAs class 6—arcuate uterus. In noncontrast MRI coronal sequences of T2W image shows indentation in endometrial cavity in fundal region which is of similar hypointensity with myometrium. There is fundal thickness of myometrium suggestive of arcuate uterus.
(MDA: Müllerian duct anomalies)

Lymph Node Assessment

Magnetic resonance imaging is not very sensitive or specific in the lymph node assessment for malignancies. Affected nodes tend to be brighter than muscle on T2WI but darker than fat on T1WI.[29] Nodes <2 cm in diameter tend to gives more false-negative results.

Pelvic Thrombosis

Magnetic resonance imaging can diagnose deep vein thrombosis of the lower extremities. MRI is exquisitely sensitive for detecting the presence of an intravascular clot and has a clear advantage over Doppler US.

Imaging of Pelvic Floor

Magnetic resonance imaging can be used well in urogynecology imaging. In the pelvic floor region, MRI can demonstrate uterine prolapse and pelvic floor descent. Sagittal image shows levator plate, which loses its normal anatomic relationship in presence of uterine prolapse (*see* **Figs. 7A to C**). Dynamic fast MRI and cinematic display can show prolapse of the anterior, middle, and posterior compartments during straining.[30] Such assessments may be valuable in preoperative planning and postoperative follow-up.

THE FUTURE OF GYNAECOLOGY IMAGING

Today, nearly every field of medicine is using more imaging than they used to do it before. CT and positron emission tomography (PET) scans became faster, X-rays have become sharper, MRI has developed stronger magnets, and ultrasound has become clearer and more powerful. Looking forward to the future of CT, it is expected to see faster, more automated, and easier to use scanners. This will lead to better tool with more quantification and speedy diagnosis.[31]

Future use of MRI includes further better assessment of benign and malignant disease and differentiation between them. Future researches that may have significant clinical impact include the development and use of contrast agents that should allow further tissue differentiation. MR spectroscopy may enable more accurate monitoring of tumor response to therapy. Ongoing research into imaging will get more insights into the biochemical behavior of both normal and pathologic tissue.

CONCLUSION

Computed tomography and MRI both are important imaging techniques in evaluation of pelvic pathology with their own merits and demerits and they are diagnostic gold standard in certain conditions. MRI is far superior in majority of conditions, due to its ability to obtain images with a high soft-tissue contrast resolution and discrimination in multiple planes, narrows the differential diagnosis of gynecological pathologies.

KEY MESSAGES

The role of imaging in obstetrics and gynecology has undergone a revolution over the past few decades. US has a very important role in the evaluation of gynecological conditions but additional tools such as MRI and CT for further evaluation have increased a great value. In this chapter, we will discuss about the CT and MRI as diagnostic modalities in gynecological imaging.

REFERENCES

1. Haaga J R, Boll DT. CT and MRI of the whole body, 6th edition, Vol 2. Netherlands: Elsevier; 2017. pp. 1977-2013.
2. Garcia O, Alvarez M, Nikolic O, Blanco-Lobato P, Basta-Nikolic M, de Llano-Ortega RM, et al. Role of MRI in staging and follow-up of endometrial and cervical cancer: pitfalls and mimickers. Insights Imaging. 2019;10:19.
3. Bennett GL, Slywotzky CM, Giovanniello G. Gynecologic causes of acute pelvic pain: Spectrum of CT findings. Radiographics. 2002;22(4):785-801.
4. Sutton D. Gynecological imaging. Textbook of Radiology and Imaging, 7 edition. India: Elsevier India; 2003.
5. Gross BH, Moss AA, Mihara K, Goldberg HI, Glazer GM. Computed tomography of gynecologic diseases. AJR Am J Roentgenol. 1983;141(4):765-73.
6. Iraha Y, Okada M, Iraha R, Azama K, Yamashiro T, Tsubakimoto M, et al. CT and MR imaging of gynecologic emergencies. Radiographics. 2017;37:1569-86.
7. Kay H, Spritzer C. Magnetic resonance imaging in gynecology. Glob Libr Women's Med; 2008.
8. Hricak H. MRI of the female pelvis: A review. AJR Am J Roentgenol. 1986;146(6):1115-22.
9. McCarthy S. Magnetic resonance imaging in the evaluation of infertile women. Magn Reson Q. 1990;6(4):239-49.
10. McCarthy S, Vaquero E. Gynecologic anatomy with magnetic resonance imaging. Am J Obstet Gynecol. 1986;155:255.
11. Hamlin DJ, Pettersson H, Fitzsimmons J, Morgan LS. MR imaging of uterine leiomyomas and their complications. J Comput Assist Tomogr. 1985;9:902.
12. Hricak H, Tscholakoff D, Heinrichs L, Fisher MR, Dooms GC, Reinhold C, et al: Uterine leiomyomas: correlation of MR, histopathologic findings, and symptoms. Radiology. 1986; 158:385.
13. Dudiak CM, Turner DA, Patel SK, Archie JT, Silver B, Norusis M. Uterine leiomyomas in the infertile patient: Preoperative localization with MR imaging versus US and hysterosalpingography. Radiology. 1988;167:627:1988.
14. Togashi K, Nishimura K, Itoh K, Fujisawa I, Noma S, Kanaoka M, et al. Adenomyosis: Diagnosis with MR imaging. Radiology. 1988;166:111.
15. Mark AS, Hricak H, Heinrichs LW, Hendrickson MR, Winkler ML, Bachica JA, et al. Adenomyosis and leiomyoma: Differential diagnosis with MR imaging. Radiology. 1987;163:527.
16. Powell MC, Womack C, Buckley J, Worthington BS, Symonds EM. Preoperative magnetic resonance imaging of stage 1 endometrial adenocarcinoma. Br J Obstet Gynaecol. 1986;93:353.
17. Sahdev A, Shepherd JH, Reznek RH. Magnetic resonance imaging in gynaecological malignancies. The Obstetrician Gynecologist. 2005;7(4):252-8.
18. Powell MC, Worthington BS, Sokal M, Wastie M, Buckley J, Symonds EM. Magnetic resonance imaging-Its application to cervical carcinoma. Br J Obstet Gynaecol. 1986;93:1276.
19. Togashi K, Nishimura K, Sagoh T, Minami S, Noma S, Fujisawa I, et al. Carcinoma of the cervix: Staging with MR imaging. Radiology. 1989;171:245.
20. Bipat S, Glas AS, van der Velden J, Zwinderman AH, Bossuyt PM, Stoker J. Computed tomography an magnetic resonance imaging in staging of uterine cervical carcinoma: a systematic review. Gynecol Oncol. 2003;91:59-66.
21. Ebner F, Kressel HY, Mintz MC, Carlson JA, Cohen EK, Schiebler M, et al. Tumor recurrence versus fibrosis in the female pelvis: Differentiation with MR imaging at 1.5 T. Radiology. 1988;166:333.
22. Hricak H, Swift PS, Campos Z, Quivey JM, Gildengorin V, Göranson H, et al. Irradiation of the cervix uteri: value of unenhanced and contrast-enhanced MR imaging. Radiology. 1993;189:381.
23. Santoni R, Bucciolini M, Chiostrini C, Cionini L, Renzi R. Quantitative magnetic resonance imaging in cervical carcinoma: A report on 30 cases. Br J Radiol. 1991;64:498.
24. Hamlin DJ, Fitzsimmons JR, Pettersson H, Riggall FC, Morgan L, Wilkinson EJ. Magnetic resonance imaging of the pelvis: Evaluation of ovarian masses at 0.15 T. AJR Am J Roentgenol. 1985;145(3):585-90.
25. Smith FW, Cherryman GR, Bayliss AP, Fullerton WT, Law AN, Robertson EM, et al. A comparative study of the accuracy of

ultrasound imaging, X-ray computerized tomography and low field MRI diagnosis of ovarian malignancy. MagnReson Imaging. 1988;6:225.
26. Hricak H, Chang YCF, Thurnher S. Vagina: Evaluation with MR Imaging. I. Normal anatomy and congenital anomalies. Radiology. 1988;169:169.
27. Pellerito JS, McCarthy SM, Doyle MB, Glickman MG, DeCherney AH. Diagnosis of uterine anomalies: relative accuracy of MR imaging, endovaginalsonography, and hysterosalpingography. Radiology. 1992;183:795.
28. Togashi K, Nishimura K, Itoh K, Fujisawa I, Nakano Y, Torizuka K, et al. Vaginal agenesis: classification by MR imaging. Radiology. 1987;162:675.
29. Dooms GC, Hricak H, Crooks LE, Higgins CB: Magnetic resonance imaging of the lymph nodes: Comparison with CT. Radiology. 1984;153:719.
30. Yang A, MostwinJL, Rosenshein NB, Zerhouni EA. Pelvic floor descent in women: dynamic evaluation with fast MR imaging and cinematic display. Radiology. 1991;179:25.
31. Loria K. What's Next in CT Technology. Radiology Today. 2016;17(4):18.

LONG QUESTIONS

1. Describe in detail about role of CT in gynecological practice.
2. Describe in detail about role of MRI in gynecological imaging.
3. What is the role of magnetic imaging resonance in gynecological malignancies? Describe MR findings of cervical cancers according to FIGO classification.
4. What are the types of Müllerian anomalies? Write about role of magnetic resonance imaging in evaluation of various Müllerian anomalies.

SHORT QUESTIONS

1. Describe in short about the various uterine pathologies on MR imaging.
2. Describe MRI imaging findings in carcinoma endometrium.
3. Write a short note on human safety concerns for CT and MR imaging.
4. Write down normal anatomic description of female genital organs on T1W and T2W MRI.
5. Describe findings of mature cystic teratoma on CT scan and MRI.

MULTIPLE CHOICE QUESTIONS

1. Most common disorder of uterus is:
   a. Adenomyosis b. Fibroid
   c. Leiomyosarcoma d. Müllerian anomalies
2. Fibroid that have undergone hyaline degeneration or necrosis have all findings on CT imaging, except:
   a. Cystic appearance
   b. Increased contrast material enhancement
   c. Area of low attenuation
   d. After giving contrast, the enhancement remain same
3. Best imaging modality for diagnosis of endometrioma is:
   a. NCCT
   b. MRI
   c. 2D-USG
   d. Contrast-enhanced CT
4. The best imaging modality for twisted ovarian cyst is:
   a. USG with color Doppler b. NCCT
   c. MRI d. CECT
5. Choose wrong statement about endometrial carcinoma:
   a. MRI is able to define depth of invasion
   b. MRI can diagnose cancer in situ
   c. T2W images are better predictor then T1W image for zonal disruption
   d. At place of deep myometrial invasion, low-intensity band of junctional zone remains absent
6. In adenomyosis, the thickness of junctional zone:
   a. Decreased, measuring <5 mm
   b. Increased, measuring 5–10 mm
   c. Increased, measuring >12 mm
   d. Remains normal
7. Gold standard imaging modality for early staging of carcinoma cervix is:
   a. CE MRI b. CECT
   c. Both a and b together d. 2D+3D USG
8. Extension of cervical cancer toward the uterine body can be identified best on:
   a. USG b. CT
   c. T1W-MRI d. T2W-MRI
9. Banana-shaped uterine cavity is a sign of:
   a. MRKH syndrome b. Unicornuate uterus
   c. Arcuate uterus d. Septate uterus
10. Müllerian anomalies are usually associated with:
    a. Renal anomalies
    b. Cardiovascular anomalies
    c. Hepatic anomalies
    d. CNS anomalies

Answers

1. b 2. b 3. b 4. a 5. b 6. c
7. a 8. d 9. b 10. a

7.6 HORMONE ASSAYS: INDICATIONS, TECHNIQUES, AND INTERPRETATION

Anuradha Ridhorkar

"Hormonal assays provide useful information only when applied appropriately. Many a times they are used without a clearly thought diagnostic pathway or in response to the patients demand. In such situations, the hormone assay will at the best, be of no clinical use and at worst lead to anxiety and uncertainty.

These investigations make sense only if they are tailored to the right patient at the right situation."

WHAT ARE THE MAIN REPRODUCTIVE HORMONES?

Follicle Stimulating Hormone and Luteinizing Hormone

Luteinizing hormone (LH) and follicle stimulating hormone (FSH) are important pituitary hormones. These are required to carry out reproductive process in both the genders. LH and FSH are released by the anterior portion of pituitary in response to pulsatile release of gonadotropin-releasing hormone (GnRH) stimulation from the hypothalamus and also the negative feedback of estrogen or testosterone.

In females, the combined action of FSH and LH stimulates growth of ovarian follicles and steroidogenesis, with the production of androgens, which are eventually converted to estrogens by the action of the enzyme aromatase. A midcycle surge in LH also triggers ovulation. FSH levels usually increase during menopause, because the ovaries become less responsive to FSH, which causes the pituitary gland to increase FSH production. However, fluctuating ovarian performance, especially early in perimenopause means that FSH and estradiol levels are not reliable to predict menopause, as they are sometimes at premenopausal levels.

The reference range for FSH in adult males is 1.6–8 IU/L and for LH is 1.5–9.3 IU/L **(Table 1)**.

TABLE 1: Reference range for FSH and LH in different phases.

Phase	*FSH (IU/L)*	*LH (IU/L)*
Follicular	2.5–10.2	1.9–12.5
Midcycle	3.1–17.7	8.7–76
Luteal	1.5–9.1	0.5–17
Postmenopausal	23–116	5.0–52

(FSH: follicle stimulating hormone; LH: luteinizing hormone)

Estradiol

Estradiol is the principal estrogen in females who are ovulating and the dominant ovarian hormone during the follicular (first) phase of the menstrual cycle. The levels of estradiol fluctuate throughout the menstrual cycle. Estradiol is secreted parallel to follicular growth and peaks along with follicular maturation (prior to ovulation). Estradiol production gradually subsides, if oocyte released by the follicle remains unfertilized. Laboratory testing routinely measures E2 forms of estradiol, most of which is bound to sex hormone-binding globulin (SHBG). Estradiol concentration reduces significantly with menopause.

In males, estrogen is an essential part of the reproductive system, and is required for maturation of sperm. Primary hypogonadism (impaired response to gonadotropins including LH and FSH) can result in increased testicular secretion of estradiol and increased conversion of testosterone to estradiol. Obesity may also increase estrogen levels in males.[3] An increase in the ratio of estrogen to androgens in males is associated with gynecomastia (the development of breast tissue).

The reference range for estradiol is given in **Table 2**.

The adult male reference range for estradiol is assay dependent, so it is recommended to consult the local laboratory. An example of an adult male reference range for estradiol is 0–200 pmol/L.[1]

Progesterone

Progesterone is the dominant ovarian hormone secreted during the luteal (second) phase of the menstrual cycle. Its primary function is to prepare the uterus for implantation of an embryo, in the event of fertilization occurring during that cycle. If pregnancy happens, human chorionic gonadotropin (hCG) is released which maintains the corpus luteum, which in turn maintains progesterone concentration. At approximately 12 week's gestation, the placenta begins to release progesterone in place of the corpus luteum. Progesterone concentration declines after delivery and during breastfeeding. Progesterone levels are low in women after menopause.

TABLE 2: The adult reference range for estradiol.

Phase	*Estradiol (pg/mL)*
Early follicular	20–150
Mid-cycle	150–750
Luteal	30–450
Postmenopausal	<20

N.B.: Estradiol levels are usually undetectable in females using estrogen-containing oral contraception as this suppresses estradiol production from the ovary. Estradiol levels in females taking some forms of hormone replacement therapy (e.g., estrogen valerate) will be high.

TABLE 3: Reference range for progesterone.

Phase	*Progesterone (ng/mL)*
Follicular	<0.3
Mid-cycle	0.1–1.5
Luteal	6.7–22.2
Postmenopausal	<0.2

In males, almost all progesterone is converted to testosterone in the testes.

Broadly in routine practice, there are no indications, other than fertility assessment in females (in some circumstances), that warrant progesterone measurement **(Table 3)**.

The reference range for progesterone in adult males is <0.4 ng/mL.[1]

Prolactin

In females, prolactin stimulates the breasts to produce milk, after estrogen priming. During pregnancy, prolactin concentrations begin to raise at approximately 6 weeks' gestation, peaking during late pregnancy.

In males and nonpregnant females, the secretion of prolactin from the pituitary gland is inhibited by the hypothalamic release of dopamine. Tumors or masses that result in compression of the pituitary stalk or drugs that block dopamine receptors, e.g., psychotropics, opiates and dopamine agonists, can cause hyperprolactinemia by reducing dopamine delivery to the pituitary. Hypothyroidism can also be associated with hyperprolactinemia if levels of thyrotropin-releasing hormone (TRH) are raised, which stimulates prolactin production.

Hyperprolactinemia is the most common endocrine disorder of the hypothalamic-pituitary axis and causes infertility in both males and females. Prolactin-secreting tumors (prolactinomas) are the most commonly encountered pituitary tumors. These are usually small tumors (microprolactinomas) and are characterized by anovulation or other menstrual irregularities, galactorrhea (milk secretion from the breast), and sexual dysfunction. Rarely, these lesions may be large (macroprolactinomas) and present with compressive symptoms such as headaches and bitemporal hemianopia (missing vision in the outer halves of the visual field).

N.B.: Galactorrhea can occur in males, but is a much less common symptom of high prolactin in males.

Reference range: There is a diurnal variation in prolactin levels and these levels are the lowest approximately 3 hours after waking. Samples are best collected in the afternoon.[1] Stress or illness can also lead to raised prolactin, so ideally patients should be well and not taking medicines that can interfere with prolactin assay such as psychotropics, opiates, or dopamine agonists.

Reference ranges are assay-specific so it is recommended to consult the local laboratory for their reference range. An example of a reference range for prolactin is 50–650 mU/L for adult females and 50–450 mU/L for adult males.[1]

In approximately 10% of patients, raised total prolactin can be due to prolactin binding to another serum protein (macroprolactin).[1] In these patients if the small biologically active prolactin is within normal limits, the raised prolactin can generally be regarded as a laboratory artefact. Laboratories usually test for this possibility in new patients presenting with unexplained hyperprolactinemia.

Increased prolactin levels are usually associated with decreased estrogen or testosterone levels.

Testosterone

Testosterone is the primary androgen responsible for the development and maintenance of male sexual characteristics. It also stimulates anabolic processes in nonsexual tissues. In males, LH stimulates the Leydig cells in the testes to produce testosterone. A little amount of testosterone in males is produced by the adrenal glands.

In females, the majority of testosterone is produced by peripheral conversion of androgen precursor steroids to testosterone, with the remainder produced in the ovaries and adrenal glands. Circulating levels of testosterone fluctuate with the menstrual cycle, and raising during pregnancy. Serum levels of testosterone remain relatively unperturbed during and after menopause.[4] Polycystic ovary syndrome (PCOS) is the most common cause of hyperandrogenism (increased testosterone levels) in females. Rarer causes include Cushing's syndrome, congenital adrenal hyperplasia, and androgen-secreting tumors.

Reference range: The reference range for total testosterone in adult males differs between laboratories. An approximate range is 8–35 nmol/L. If a single early morning testosterone level is clearly within the reference range (e.g., >15 nmol/L) then no further testing is required. If a low or borderline result is obtained, a confirmatory early morning test (when the patient is well) should be carried out.

Testosterone reference ranges for females are also assay-specific. An example of an adult female reference range for total testosterone is 0.5–2.5 nmol/L.[1] Modern second generation testosterone assays generally have lower ranges in females, due to less interference from other steroids such as dehydroepiandrosterone sulfate (DHEAS).

Free testosterone can be calculated from total testosterone and SHBG. However, SHBG testing is only ever rarely required, such as when abnormalities of sex hormone binding (e.g., hyperthyroidism, anticonvulsant use, severe obesity) can cause total testosterone levels to be misleading. Discussion with an endocrinologist is recommended before requesting SHBG.

Human Chorionic Gonadotropin

Human chorionic gonadotropin is structurally and functionally analogous to LH, apart from its beta chain, therefore it is often referred to as beta-hCG (or β-hCG).

Human chorionic gonadotropin is released by trophoblast cells during pregnancy. These cells form the outer layer of the developing blastocyst following conception and embryonic implantation. hCG stimulates progesterone production by the corpus luteum and increases vascularity between the trophoblast and the uterus wall. It is detectable approximately 3 days after implantation of the embryo, which occurs approximately 6–12 days following ovulation and fertilization. During a normal pregnancy hCG levels usually double approximately every 2 days, then plateau and begin to decrease at 8–10 weeks, but will remain elevated throughout pregnancy.[5] Women with twin pregnancy typically produce higher levels of hCG than those with single embryos; however, these elevated hCG levels cannot be reliably used to predict this.[6]

Urine or serum hCG measurement can be used to confirm early pregnancy (urine hCG is adequate in most cases). Serum hCG can also be useful as an initial investigation in women who have symptoms that may suggest ectopic pregnancy, miscarriage, or trophoblastic disease. Transvaginal ultrasound can be used after approximately 5 weeks gestation, or hCG levels >1,000–2,000 IU/L, to detect signs of pregnancy.[7]

A nonviable pregnancy may be indicated by a reduced or plateau in hCG levels in early pregnancy (remembering that hCG decreases in normal pregnancies after approximately 9–10 weeks' gestation). However, hCG alone is not a reliable predictor of ectopic pregnancy as there is no particular pattern of decrease or increase.[8] Following miscarriage it may take 3 or 4 weeks for hCG levels to return to nonpregnant levels (<5 IU/L).[7] In incomplete miscarriage, hCG levels can remain elevated and surgical intervention may be required.

In males, hCG is produced by some testicular tumors, and it is therefore used as a serum tumor marker for some forms of testicular cancer.

Reference range: There is a wide range of variability of hCG levels during early pregnancy. The rate of increase, i.e., doubling time, gives more useful information than the actual levels. Most urine tests turn positive with hCG levels >20–25 IU/L. Serum hCG <5 IU/L is considered negative for pregnancy.[1]

Excessively high hCG levels, e.g., >100,000 IU/L may be suggestive of gestational trophoblastic disease, e.g., molar pregnancy.

Anti-Mullerian Hormone

In recent years anti-Mullerian hormone (AMH) also known as Mullerian-inhibiting substance (MIS) has become a marker of promise in ovarian reserve assessment. Serum levels are proportional to number of antral follicles in the size range of 1–8 mm and indirectly represent pool of primordial follicles.

Serum AMH levels are increased in PCOS because of the increased number of small growing follicles . In PCOS, there also appears to be resistance to the inhibitory effect of AMH on follicular recruitment, in part due to stimulation of recruitment by ovarian androgen excess. However, AMH elevation is in part independent of ovarian hyperandrogenism, suggesting the same is true of folliculogenesis.

WHEN SHOULD REPRODUCTIVE HORMONES BE INVESTIGATED?

There are multiple indications for measuring reproductive hormones, however, in routine practice, the most common reasons are for investigating primary or secondary amenorrhea or oligomenorrhea in females, investigating hypogonadism in males, confirming pregnancy, and some aspects of investigating fertility. Measuring hormones in women with typical symptoms of menopause is usually not necessary.

Medical practitioners are not expected to investigate and diagnose every endocrine dysfunction. The role of the practitioner is often needs to segregate the patients who require referral for further assessment and individualized care.

Investigating Primary Amenorrhea (Delayed Puberty)

A possible scenario is for mothers to bring their daughters in for a consultation as they are concerned that their "menstrual cycle" has not begun, and other girls in their peer group are already started menstruating.

In most cases, reassurance and watchful waiting is all that is required. However, if there is no sign of breast development (the first demonstrable sign of puberty in girls) by age 12–14 years, or menstruation has not begun by age 16 years in a female with otherwise normal pubertal development, investigation needs to be started.

A common cause of primary amenorrhea is weight loss, dieting, or excessive exercise (known as hypothalamic amenorrhea). Rarer causes include pituitary or thyroid disease, anatomical abnormalities (e.g., Mullerian agenesis), and congenital abnormalities (e.g., Turner's syndrome, Kallmann syndrome).

Laboratory investigations may be considered if concerns persist, despite a period of watchful waiting. Appropriate tests include FSH, LH, estradiol, prolactin, testosterone, thyroid stimulating hormone (TSH), and FT4. It can be difficult to interpret the significance of abnormal results, so consultation with, or referral to an endocrinologist or gynecologist for further investigation and diagnosis is recommended.

Estradiol levels can indicate whether there is absolutely no evidence of ovarian estrogen activity, or whether levels have started to rise from prepubertal levels, indicating that gonadal activity may be starting. Low estradiol in association with low LH is suggestive of hypothalamic amenorrhea.

Low levels of FSH and LH (<5 IU/L) suggests hypogonadotropic hypogonadism, of which causes include Kallmann syndrome and space-occupying pituitary tumors. High levels of FSH (>20 IU/L) and LH (>40 IU/L) are suggestive of primary hypogonadism, which may be suggestive of Turner's syndrome.[10]

Raised prolactin levels and/or TSH and FT4 abnormalities may indicate pituitary etiology.

Although more commonly associated with secondary amenorrhea, PCOS can sometimes be a cause of primary amenorrhea. A raised testosterone level may be suggestive of this.

Normal hormone levels in a female with primary amenorrhea, but otherwise normal development, may suggest an anatomical abnormality such as an imperforate hymen or Mullerian agenesis (a congenital malformation that results in an absent uterus and fallopian tubes). Further investigation is required if this is suspected.

Precocious Puberty

Precocious (early) puberty is generally defined as the appearance of secondary sexual characteristics in girls aged under 8 years or in boys aged under 9 years. It is a much rarer presentation than delayed puberty and investigation of precocious puberty in children is complex. Any child with early signs of secondary sexual characteristics should be referred to an endocrinologist for detailed assessment. Prompt management is important, as precocious puberty results in accelerated skeletal development and impaired final adult height.

INVESTIGATING SECONDARY AMENORRHEA AND OLIGOMENORRHEA

Secondary amenorrhea (cessation of menstruation in a female who was previously menstruating) or oligomenorrhea (irregular menstruation with intervals between them consistently greater than 35 days or less than nine periods per year) is most commonly caused by hypothalamic amenorrhea, PCOS, or premature ovarian failure (after first excluding pregnancy).

Initial investigations include FSH, LH, and estradiol. Other tests will depend on the suspected cause. Add prolactin and TSH if hyperprolactinemia is suspected - this may be associated with galactorrhea or symptoms of thyroid disease.

A serum FSH level >20 IU/L and low estradiol in a female aged <40 years suggest that premature ovarian failure has occurred (or early menopause in a female aged <45 years).

Low LH and estradiol suggest a hypothalamic cause for amenorrhea (e.g., weight loss, excessive exercise, or stress).

Hyperprolactinemia

Stress, medicine use, and hypothyroidism need to be considered as causes of hyperprolactinemia. Macroprolactin, an inactive form of prolactin, can be a benign cause of raised prolactin levels - this can be detected by laboratory analysis. Once other possible causes of prolactin elevation have been excluded, imaging of the pituitary (MRI or CT) for prolactinoma may be considered in secondary care.

Polycystic Ovarian Syndrome

Diagnostic Criteria have been Developed for PCOS

Polycystic ovarian syndrome is a syndrome, so there is no single diagnostic test. Diagnostic criteria have been developed **(Box 1)** and widely adopted internationally. However, diagnosis can be difficult due to the variation in presenting symptoms and because symptoms differ with age at presentation and change over time.

Presenting Features of PCOS

Although presenting features **(Box 2)**, age of presentation, and severity of PCOS vary, a common presentation may be of a woman with a history of gradually worsening hirsutism and irregular periods, which goes back for some years. For many women however, failure to conceive may be the initial reason for presentation.

A full history is needed: It is important when taking the history to include questions about:

- Reproductive health (menarche, past and present cycle, oligo-/amenorrhea, menorrhagia, miscarriage, infertility)

BOX 1: Rotterdam consensus on diagnostic criteria for PCOS.

Two out of three of the following:

1. Oligo- or anovulation
2. Clinical and/or biochemical signs of hyperandrogenism*
3. Polycystic ovaries**

and exclusion of other etiologies (congenital adrenal hyperplasia, androgen-secreting tumors, Cushing's syndrome)

*Hirsutism, acne, male pattern baldness, elevated total or free testosterone

**On ultrasound, ≥12 follicles of 2–9 mm diameter and/or increased ovarian volume (>10 mL).

(PCOS: polycystic ovarian syndrome)

BOX 2: Presenting features of PCOS.

Presenting features (% affected):

- Hyperandrogenism (hirsutism 70%, acne 30%, alopecia 10%, but not virilization*)
- Menstrual disturbance 60–70%
- Infertility 70%
- Obesity, particularly truncal 35–50%
- Polycystic ovaries visible on ultrasound in asymptomatic woman 22–33%
- Acanthosis nigricans 1–3%**

*Rapid development of virilization signals a need for investigation to rule out the presence of an androgen secreting tumor.[8,15]

**A brown-discolored "velvety" texture to the skin typically in the region of the axillae and the back of the neck, often considered to be the cutaneous manifestation of insulin resistance (or hyperinsulinemia)

- Presence of androgenic symptoms (acne, hirsutism, alopecia of the scalp)
- Lifestyle factors (changes in body weight, eating and exercise habits, alcohol, and smoking history)
- Family history of PCOS, diabetes, obesity, hirsutism, and premature male baldness.

Examination includes General as well as Reproductive Features

Examination of a woman with suspected PCOS should include an assessment of:

- Weight (both BMI and hip/waist ratio)
- Acne and hirsutism
- Blood pressure.

Additional examination depending on the presenting features may include breast, abdominal, and pelvic exam. The presence of abdominal striae could indicate weight change or Cushing's syndrome. A bimanual examination may identify ovarian enlargement, although clinical pelvic examination is a poor predictor of polycystic ovaries, especially if the BMI is high. The presence of features of virilization (which may include frontal balding, deepening of the voice, broadening of the shoulders, breast atrophy, clitoromegaly and loss of vaginal rugae) may raise concerns about other serious conditions **(Box 3)**.

Investigation of PCOS

A clinical or biochemical finding of increased androgen levels along with either menstrual abnormalities or polycystic ovaries on ultrasound will satisfy the current diagnostic criteria (*see* **Box 1**). The initial tests recommended for diagnosis are outlined in **Table 4**. While not essential for diagnosis, some clinicians still suggest testing LH/FSH. Once the diagnosis is established, fasting glucose and lipids[11] are recommended. Other tests may be required depending on clinical suspicion, to exclude other conditions **(Table 5)**.

Investigating Menopause

Since menopause is a clinical diagnosis, endocrine testing is usually not necessary for diagnosing menopause (**Boxes 4 and 5**).

In women aged over 45 years with typical symptoms of menopause, hormone testing is not routinely recommended in clinical practice, since hormones tend to fluctuate significantly over this period, and the likelihood of menopause is higher in this age group. Usually age and 1 year history of amenorrhea are sufficient for a diagnosis.

BOX 3: Role of insulin – to test or not to test?

Fasting serum insulin is a poor measure of insulin resistance. Although used widely in large population-based epidemiological studies, it is not recommended for use in a general practice setting. It is more useful to identify the risk factors that are associated with insulin resistance (and often therefore identify metabolic syndrome and PCOS). These risk factors include raised fasting glucose and lipid levels, high blood pressure, and central obesity.

Source: Samaras K, McElduff A, Twigg SM, Proietto J, Prins JB, Welborn TA, et al. Insulin levels in insulin resistance: phantom of the metabolic opera? Med J Aust. 2006;185(3):159-61.

TABLE 4: Recommended investigations for aiding diagnosis of PCOS.

Investigation	*Expected finding in PCOS*	*Comment*
Investigations for diagnosis		
Exclude pregnancy	————	Most common cause of amenorrhea
Pelvic ultrasound	*Polycystic ovaries*	Important as part of the diagnostic criteria but not a "must do" if diagnosis is made on clinical and biochemical grounds
Free testosterone	Usually increased	More sensitive for identifying physiologically active androgens. This is calculated from total testosterone and SHBG. Very high levels of total testosterone require further investigation to rule out other causes such as late-onset congenital adrenal hyperplasia, Cushing's syndrome, adrenal or ovarian tumor. SHBG levels are decreased in PCOS
Investigations after diagnosis		
Glucose		To check for glucose intolerance or diabetes. If fasting level >5.5 mmol/L or random >7.7 mmol/L then a glucose tolerance test is recommended
Lipids	Usually high triglycerides, lower HDL and mildly elevated LDL	A fasting level may be useful in establishing cardiovascular risk
Other tests to consider		
LH/FSH ratio	LH will often be increased, FSH usually normal, giving an increased ratio	While not essential for diagnosis, some clinicians remain convinced of the value of LH testing in predicting future complications of PCOS

(FSH: follicle stimulating hormone; LH: luteinizing hormone; PCOS: polycystic ovarian syndrome; SHBG: sex hormone-binding globulin)

TABLE 5: Tests to exclude other conditions (depending on clinical suspicion).

Test	*Reason*	*Clinical signs*
Prolactin	Very high levels may suggest a pituitary cause or medication use (especially antipsychotic medications)	Galactorrhea Irregular or absent menstruation
TSH	To exclude thyroid abnormalities as a cause of menstrual irregularity	Menstrual changes associated with other thyroid symptoms (either hypo or hyper)
Estradiol + FSH	To help exclude premature ovarian failure (low estradiol, very high FSH)	Menopausal symptoms and signs in women less than 40 years
17-OH Progesterone	To help exclude late-onset or non-classic congenital adrenal hyperplasia (very rare)	Difficult to distinguish clinically from PCOS. However there may be a family history of CAH, less menstrual disruption or history of early growth of pubic hair
DHEAS	A marker for adrenal androgen production, very high levels may be associated with an adrenocortical tumor	Rapid onset of virilizing features
Androstenedione	A marker for ovarian androgen production, very high levels may be associated with an ovarian androgen secreting tumor[15]	Rapid onset of virilizing features
Cortisol	Increased in Cushing's syndrome	Typical Cushingoid features, e.g., central obesity, moon face, thinning of skin, striae, excessive sweating

(CAH: congenital adrenal hyperplasia; DHEAS: dehydroepiandrosterone sulfate; FSH: follicle stimulating hormone; LH: luteinizing hormone; PCOS: polycystic ovarian syndrome; TSH: thyroid stimulating hormone)

BOX 4: Summary of endocrinology in PCOS.[6-8,10]

There are multiple biochemical changes in women with PCOS. The key feature is the increased level of serum androgens which are responsible for most of the common presenting features:

- Increased androgens [testosterone, androstenedione and dehydroepiandrosterone sulfate (DHEAS)]
- Increased luteinizing hormone (LH)
- Decreased sex hormone binding globulin (SHBG)
- Increased prolactin
- Increased estradiol
- Increased insulin

BOX 5: Conditions for early referral to a fertility specialist.

Early referral to a fertility specialist or relevant specialist should be offered if:

- The female partner is aged more than or equal to 35 years
- The female partner has amenorrhea/oligomenorrhoea
- The female partner has a history of abdominal or pelvic surgery
- The female partner has an abnormal pelvic examination
- The female or male partner has a history of sexually transmitted infection (including pelvic inflammatory disease)
- The male partner has an abnormal semen analysis
- The male partner has undescended testes or other urogenital pathology
- The male partner has a history of urogenital surgery
- The male partner has a varicocele
- The couple are very concerned and would be reassured by a consultation

Follicle stimulating hormone testing may be beneficial in skeptical scenarios like determining the cause of oligomenorrhea and fertility potential in a younger woman (age <45 years), or when oligomenorrhea is not a presenting symptom of menopause, such as in a woman who has recently stopped taking oral contraceptives, or who has had a hysterectomy.[12] FSH should typically be repeated at least once (e.g., in 6 weeks) to confirm the result.[2]

N.B.: FSH does not reliably predict menopause in women using combined oral contraceptives.[2]

There is no benefit in measuring estradiol levels to titrate doses of hormone replacement treatment.[12] Estradiol measurement is also not useful in assessing postmenopausal fracture risk.

Investigating Hypogonadism in Males

Delayed Puberty

The first sign of puberty in males is an increase in the size of the testes, which normally occurs around age 12 years. Conventionally most common cause of delayed puberty in males is constitutional delay in growth and puberty. This is more common in boys with a family history of delayed puberty. Catch-up growth, onset of puberty, and the pubertal growth spurt occur later than average, but eventually result in normal adult stature, sexual development, and fertility.

If clinical signs of puberty are not present by approximately age 16 years, clinical examination and investigation may be considered. Initial laboratory evaluation should include FSH, LH, testosterone, prolactin, TSH, and FT4. It is highly recommended that results should be discussed with an endocrinologist, and the patient is referred for further investigation and diagnosis if deemed necessary.

Elevated FSH and LH suggest primary hypogonadism. Low or normal FSH and LH levels suggest secondary hypogonadism, which in rare cases can be due to hypothalamic dysfunction, hypopituitarism, hypothyroidism, or hyperprolactinemia. Constitutional delay in puberty is also associated with low FSH and LH.

Gynecomastia

Gynecomastia is a benign enlargement of the breast tissue in males, which indicates an imbalance between estrogen and androgens. It is important to distinguish true gynecomastia, which is felt as a concentric, rubbery or firm mound of tissue around the nipple, from an accumulation of adipose tissue.

Gynecomastia is quite common during mid-to-late puberty, when relatively higher levels of estrogen is synthesized from the testes and peripheral tissues, before testosterone reaches adult concentrations. In almost all cases, this resolves within 1–2 years. The incidence of gynecomastia rises again in older males, possibly related to a reduction in free testosterone levels.

In adult males presenting with gynecomastia, after eliminating causes such as medicines (e.g., antiandrogens, tricyclic antidepressants, metronidazole, spironolactone, calcium channel blockers, and cimetidine) or concurrent illness (e.g., cirrhosis), consider testing testosterone levels (followed by LH if low), estradiol, and hCG. hCG is measured because in rare cases, hCG production by a testicular tumor (or other ectopic hCG-secreting tumor), can lead to excessive estrogen levels, manifesting as breast tissue enlargement.

Late-onset Hypogonadism

In an adult male with clinically significant signs and symptoms of hypogonadism (e.g., reduced libido, absent early morning erection), at the outset clinician should consider testing testosterone levels. The sample should be collected during the early morning, e.g., 8 AM, as afternoon and evening levels may be significantly lower.

If a single early morning testosterone level is clearly within the reference range (e.g., >15 nmol/L), then no further testing is required. If a low or borderline testosterone level is detected, a confirmatory early morning test should be conducted (when the patient is well) and a concurrent LH measurement made to differentiate possible primary from secondary hypogonadism. If LH levels are low, prolactin may be added to investigate hyperprolactinemia.[13] FSH only needs to be added if investigating fertility.

High serum LH (and FSH if measured) and a low or borderline testosterone are consistent with primary hypogonadism. Low or inappropriately normal LH levels in combination with low testosterone are consistent with secondary hypogonadism.

Sex hormone-binding globulin, for measurement of free testosterone, is only rarely required, such as where abnormalities of sex hormone binding (e.g., hyperthyroidism, anticonvulsant use, severe obesity) can cause total testosterone levels to be misleading. Discussion with an endocrinologist may be helpful in such cases.

Investigating Subfertility

There is a 20–25% chance of a healthy couple of reproductive age becoming pregnant each reproductive cycle.[14] This rises to 60% within 6 months, 84% in the first year, and 92% within the second year.[14]

If a couple presents with fertility concerns, first give reassurance and advice about the fertile phase of the menstrual cycle and optimal frequency of intercourse, i.e., every 2–3 days. Temperature charting is not helpful and should not be recommended. Lifestyle factors that affect fertility, such as BMI <18 or >30 and smoking, should be addressed.

Investigations may be considered if pregnancy is not achieved after 12 months in a woman aged <35 years or after 6 months in a woman aged >35 years. Both partners should be assessed and examined. Initial investigations in primary care include establishing whether the female is ovulating, and whether the male has a normal semen analysis.

In a female with regular menstrual cycles, it can be presumed that ovulation is occurring. However, if there is doubt (i.e., pregnancy has not occurred within an expected time frame), progesterone can be measured 7 days before the expected date of menstruation, e.g., on day 21 of a regular 28 day cycle, to test if ovulation has occurred - ovulation is likely if progesterone is >25 nmol/L. In women with prolonged cycles, progesterone may be tested on day 21 of the cycle, then repeated every 7 days until menstruation occurs (or just 7 days prior to expected menstruation if cycles are prolonged but regular).

Follicle stimulating hormone, LH and estradiol should be checked in early phase of menstrual cycle (day 2–6, where day 1 is the first day of menstruation). Elevated FSH suggests reduced ovarian reserve and the possibility of impending premature ovarian failure.

Females with absent or irregular cycles should be investigated as for secondary amenorrhea.

If the male partner has an initial abnormal semen analysis, repeat 6 weeks later for confirmation. Further investigation of underlying causes of an abnormal semen analysis is usually carried out in secondary care. However, testosterone, FSH and LH may be investigated if there is suspicion of hypogonadism.

The criteria for assessment of subfertility in females[9] are:

- BMI 18–32
- Nonsmoker or ex-smoker for >3 months
- Age <40 years
- Less than two children from current relationship

- At least 2 years subfertility or 1 year if age <35 or 6 months if age >35, with anovulation, azoospermia, oligospermia, bilateral salpingectomy, tubal obstruction, oophorectomy, or premature ovarian failure.

Androgen Resistance

Estradiol measurement is recommended in males with a finding of high serum testosterone and LH levels, along with features of under masculinization (e.g., sparse pubic, facial or body hair, underdeveloped scrotum, penis, and testes) as this is suggestive of androgen resistance.

Investigating Early Pregnancy

A random urine hCG test can be used in primary care to diagnose early pregnancy. A positive urine test is possible on the first day of a missed period, however, delaying the test decreases the likelihood of a false-negative result. A false-negative result can occur if the urine test is performed too soon after implantation of the embryo, especially if the urine sample is dilute. If there is suspicion of pregnancy despite a negative test, the test should be repeated after 1 week. Depending on the type of test kit used, hCG levels >20–25 IU/L will show a positive result. Most brands of home pregnancy tests have a similar threshold for detection, and are considered reliable when used according to manufacturer's instructions. A positive or negative result from a home pregnancy test should usually be confirmed by a clinician, to ensure that correct sampling technique was implemented.

Females of reproductive age that present with lower abdominal pain should be offered a urine hCG test to exclude the possibility of pregnancy.

A serum hCG test can detect hCG at lower levels than a urine test to confirm pregnancy, however, there is no need to request this if there is a positive urine hCG test. It is not recommended that serial hCG tests are used in a general practice setting to ensure that a pregnancy is progressing normally, as this may cause unnecessary anxiety for the patient. If there are any clinical concerns about the viability of a pregnancy, the patient should be referred to an early pregnancy clinic or gynecology department for further investigation and ultrasound. Common causes for lower abdominal pain or vaginal bleeding, such as urinary tract infection or constipation, should first be excluded.

Table 6 summarizes the recommended hormone investigations for some of the more common endocrine-related clinical scenarios seen in daily practice.

TABLE 6: Hormonal evaluation in various gynecological conditions.

Clinical scenario	*FSH*	*LH*	*Estradiol*	*Prolactin*	*Testosterone*	*hCG*	*Notes*
Primary amenorrhea	Yes	Yes	Yes	Yes	Yes	May be	Also TSH and FT4. First exclude pregnancy where appropriate
Secondary amenorrhea or oligomenorrhea	Yes	Yes	Yes	May be	May be	Yes	First exclude pregnancy. Tests dependent on suspected cause, may add TSH, FT4
Menopause	May be	Not usually required	Not usually required	Not usually required	Not usually required	Not usually required	Only consider if age <45 years, hysterectomy or recently stopped OCP
Delayed puberty in males	Yes	Yes	Not usually required	Yes	Yes	Not usually required	Also TSH and FT4
Late-onset hypogonadism in males	May be	May be	May be	May be	Yes	May be	Add LH if low testosterone. Add FSH only if fertility concerns. Tests dependent on suspected cause. Add estradiol and hCG if gynecomastia is suspected
Fertility in females with regular menstruation	Yes	Yes	Yes	Not usually required	Not usually required	Not usually required	May add day 21 progesterone. If irregular menstruation, investigate as per secondary amenorrhea
Fertility in males	May be	May be	Not usually required	Not usually required	May be	Not usually required	Following abnormal semen analysis. Add testosterone if hypogonadism suspected, followed by LH and FSH if low
Confirming pregnancy	Not usually required	Not usually required	Not usually required	Not usually required	Not usually required	Yes	Urine test usually sufficient

(FSH: follicle stimulating hormone; human chorionic gonadotropin; LH: luteinizing hormone; OCP: oral contraceptive; TSH: thyroid stimulating hormone)

REFERENCES

1. Erickson GF, Magoffin DA, Dyer CA, Hofeditz C. The ovarian androgen producing cells: a review of structure/function relationships. Endocr Rev. 1985;6(3):371-99.
2. Abraham GE, Odell WD, Swerdloff RS, Hopper K. Simultaneous radioimmunoassay of plasma FSH, LH, progesterone, 17-hydroxyprogesterone and estradiol-17 during the menstrual cycle. J Clin Endocrinol Metab. 1972;34:312-8.
3. Crosignani PG, Rubin BL. Optimal use of infertility diagnostic tests and treatments. The ESHRE Capri Workshop Group. Hum Reprod. 2000;15(3):723-32.
4. Hull MG, Cahill DJ. Female infertility. Endocrinol Metab Clin North Am. 1998;27(4):851-76.
5. Balen A. The current understanding of polycystic ovary syndrome. Obstet Gynaecol. 2004;6:66-74.
6. The Rotterdam ESHRE/ASRM-sponsored PCOS consensus workshop group. Revised 2003 consensus on diagnostic criteria and long-term health risks related to polycystic ovary syndrome. Fertil Steril. 2004;81(1):19-25.
7. Ehrmann DA. Polycystic ovary syndrome. N Engl J Med. 2005;352:1223-36.
8. Fraser IS. Current recommendations for the diagnostic evaluation and follow-up of patients presenting with symptomatic polycystic ovary syndrome. Best Pract Res Clin Obstet Gynaecol. 2004;18(5):813-23.
9. National Health Service. Clinical Knowledge Summaries. Polycystic ovary syndrome. [online] Available from: http://cks.library.nhs.uk/. [Last accessed December, 2021].
10. Smith G. Investigation and Diagnosis of Polycystic Ovary Syndrome. Path Rev. 2007.
11. Meyer C, McGrath P, Teede HJ. Effects of medical therapy on insulin resistance and the cardiovascular system in polycystic ovary syndrome. Diabetes Care. 2007;30:471-8.
12. Jameson JL, Groot LJD. Endocrinology adult and pediatric, 7th edition. Philadelphia, Pennsylvania: Saunders; 2016.
13. Fritz MA, Speroff L. Clinical Gynecologic Endocrinology and Infertility, 8th edition. Philadelphia, Pennsylvania: Lippincott/Williams & Wilkins; 2010.
14. Melmed S, Polonsky KS, Larson PD, Kornenberg HM. William's Textbook of Endocrinology, 13th edition. Gurugram, India: Elsevier; 2015.

LONG QUESTION

1. How will you evaluate a case of 23 years old lady with primary infertility due to PCOS?

SHORT QUESTION

1. Write short note on:
   i. Evaluation of primary amenorrhea.
   ii. Evaluation of premature ovarian failure.

MULTIPLE CHOICE QUESTIONS

1. During reproductive age, principle estrogen in females is:
   a. Estradiol b. Estrone
   c. Estriol
2. Main site of testosterone production in females:
   a. Ovary b. Adrenals
   c. Pituitary d. Peripheral conversion
3. FSH is a reliable predictor of perimenopause:
   a. True b. False
4. Increased estrogen in male is seen in all conditions, except:
   a. Gynecomastia b. Primary hypogonadism
   c. Azoospermia d. Obesity
5. Commonest cause of hyperandrogenism in female:
   a. Cushing syndrome
   b. Adrenal tumor
   c. PCOS
   d. Cong adrenal hyperplasia
6. Hyperprolactinemia is seen in all, except:
   a. Hyperthyroidism b. Prolactinoma
   c. Antipsychotic drugs d. Hypothyroidism
7. Fasting insulin is a poor measure of insulin resistance:
   a. True b. False
8. Diagnostic hormone evaluation for late onset CAH:
   a. DHEA b. Cortisol
   c. 17 OH Progesterone d. Androstenedione
9. Polycystic ovaries on USG show all, except:
   a. 12 follicles b. 2–9 mm diameter
   c. Decreased stroma d. Increased volume
10. The hormone used for estimation ovarian reserve is:
    a. AMH b. Progesterone
    c. β-hCG d. LH
11. The all of the following hormones are useful in a case of androgen excess, except:
    a. Testosterone b. DHEAS
    c. 17-OH Progesterone d. Insulin
12. The hormone elevated in subclincal hypothyroidism is:
    a. T4 b. T3
    c. TSH d. TRH
13. The all of the following hormones are used as tumor markers, except:
    a. Testosterone b. CA125
    c. Estradiol d. β-hCG
14. The all of the following hormones are used as tumor markers, except:
    a. Testosterone b. CA125
    c. Estradiol d. β-hCG

Answers

1.	a	2.	d	3.	b	4.	c	5.	c	6.	a
7.	a	8.	c	9.	c	10.	a	11.	d	12	c
13.	b	14.	b								

7.7 PREOPERATIVE CARE AND PREPARATION

Gokul Das, Shehla Jamal

Patients can't measure the quality of clinical care. But they can measure the quality of experience.

INTRODUCTION

The importance of preparation before surgery cannot be overemphasized. It is an essential component of patient safety and good clinical practice. Successful surgical outcomes of operative gynecological procedures occur as a result of several factors in addition to good surgical skills, techniques, and technology. The important factors that contribute to this are:

- Making the correct diagnosis in the context of the woman's general health status
- Good selection of patient, procedure and route
- Establishing expectations from the surgery and its after effects and recovery
- Team work with a wide variety of care providers who will be involved in the pre- and postoperative care of the woman
- In settings where women would bear the cost partly or wholly, there is also a consideration of financial counseling.

Perhaps the single most important factor in patient selection is a woman satisfied with an adequate exploration of the possible nonsurgical options, their merits, demerits, and comparison to surgery. A surgeon and a patient, who is thus convinced, commit themselves fully to the procedure.

CORNERSTONES OF PREOPERATIVE CARE

The three cornerstones on which preoperative care rests are shown in **Figure 1**.

- Establishing a diagnosis is based on history, examination and supported by investigations. Investigations should be used rationally. They are not a replacement for the clinical evaluation. The purpose of the clinical evaluation goes beyond establishing a diagnosis as it forms the nidus of counseling and setting the expectations of the patient. The full details of taking a gynecological history and examination are covered in another chapter in the textbook. We will emphasize some important points in the subsequent sections.
- Counseling and consent are very important aspects of patient care. Counseling has been discussed in another chapter of the textbook. This chapter will discuss consent in further detail.
- Preoperative interventions are meant to optimize surgical conditions and outcomes. These include skin preparation, bowel preparation, preoperative diet, and antibiotic prophylaxis amongst other aspects. These may appear simple, but it is often an aspect of care that is most removed from evidence and steeped in dogma. There is a need to rationalize these interventions to prevent harm and optimize ease in the lead-up to the surgery.

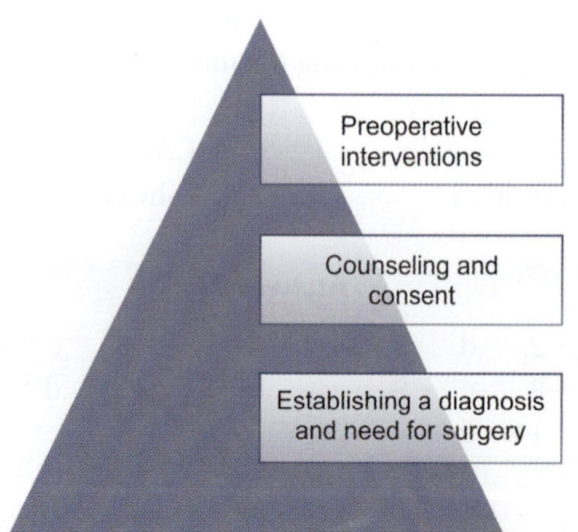

Fig. 1: The cornerstones of preoperative care.

CLINICAL EVALUATION BEFORE GYNAECOLOGICAL SURGERY

Gynecological electives should be planned only after one has obtained a meticulous history and related information. The aim of evaluation is to garner medical history and facts, thorough physical examination, and an in-depth assessment of the goals from surgery.

Maintaining highest standard of medical conduct and respecting a patient's dignity are important elements in the clinical evaluation. The initial evaluation should be performed in person, with the patient fully clothed. Direct questions can be put forward as they elicit history and confirm medical facts while communicating appropriate regards for the patient's perceptions and concerns, and they give the physician valuable insight into the patient's persona and their perspective of the gynecological problem.[1]

The evaluation should include:

- A complete history and chronological progress of the presenting symptom.
- Health aspects and background medical history that may directly or indirectly affect the anesthetic or surgical outcomes (coronary artery disease, pulmonary disease, epilepsy, psychiatric conditions). Some of these may be concealed due to social stigma.
- The drug therapy that is ongoing for the medical disorders should be enlisted. Certain agents such as anticoagulants will have to be stopped before surgery. The risk of bleeding from continuing these agents should be weighed against the risk of possible cardiovascular or cerebrovascular risk that stopping these agents may pose. The dose of steroids will need to be increased in the immediate perioperative

period. Oral contraceptives should be stopped around the time of major gynecological surgery.

- Body mass index (BMI) can be taken as a direct indicator of the nutritional status. Specific nutritional deficiencies should be ruled out. There are a number of nutritional indices available to direct interventions that may improve postoperative outcomes for women who are undergoing major surgery.[2]
- History of allergies to medications (penicillin, sulfa), foods, latex and other common allergens should be noted and mentioned. If obesity is present then sleep apnea must be ruled out. History of asthma and medications for same must also be looked for.
- Any previous surgery (for similar or different indications) should be known. Important things to note are bleeding, wound complications, prolonged hospital stay, usage of higher antibiotics and blood transfusions. It is always wise to ask for the documents of the previous surgery.
- Family history of bleeding disorders, thromboembolism, hereditary G6PD deficiency and other genetic disorders should be obtained.
- Any current intake of medications including non-prescription drugs, alternate medicine preparations, herbal preparations should be carefully elicited.
- Physical examination must be entailed to rule out gross deformities especially in spine (regional anesthesia), legs and pelvis (for lithotomy position).
- Psychological assessment should always be done, especially about her expectations from the corrective surgeries.
- Systems should be examined meticulously to avoid surprises on operation table.
- Gynecological workup should include complete genitourinary examination to look for incontinence and dysfunction of the urinary and anorectal tracts.
- A speculum examination and bimanual pelvic examination should never be underestimated, as yields valuable information about orientation of the organs, size, mobility, inflammation, and serves as a guide to decide the route of the surgery.

The operating surgeon should make every effort to perform the clinical evaluation herself. If this is not possible in the clinic, it should be done on the preoperative day. A handy mnemonic to summarize the most important aspects can be remembered as HEATS illustrated in **Figure 2**.

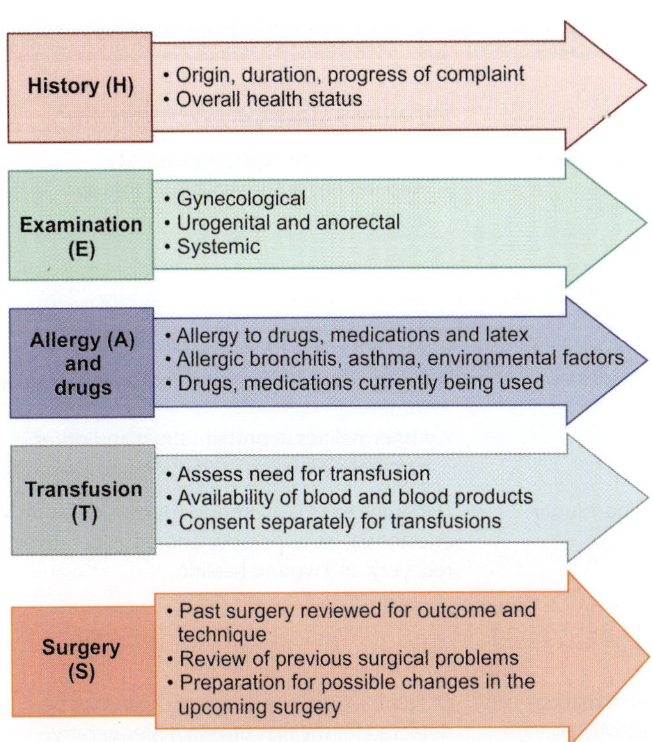

Fig. 2: HEATS tool for preoperative assessment.

IMAGING

The most popular and widely available tool for gynecological diagnosis is ultrasound. Some conditions warrant a CT scan or MRI. The purpose of imaging is to support the clinical diagnosis, uncover confounding pathologies, and rule out malignant conditions with reasonable certainty. Imaging may influence the decision of the route of surgery. These techniques have been discussed in detail in other chapters of the textbook. Some relevant and important points are:

- Imaging should be used as a support to the clinical diagnosis. It should not be the primary modality for evaluation.
- Ultrasound is a user-dependent tool. An experience operator and a discussion when there is a diagnostic dilemma can be useful to exchange insights and get better diagnosis.
- Imaging reports should not be relied on without seeing the images themselves in the form of plates, printouts or soft copies.
- The imaging should be reasonably recent.
- Other investigations such as urography, colonoscopy, endoscopy, barium studies are done under special circumstances only.

LABORATORY WORK UP

The common tests that are usually performed before gynecological surgery are discussed in **Table 1**.[3,4] These are almost regimental and are institutionalized in practice. The rationale for performing them varies from case to case. There are arguments against routine testing.[5] However, in the face of setting standards for clinical practice and medicolegal implications, laboratory workup is part of the preoperative care of women undergoing gynecological surgery. In certain clinical situations, a more elaborate preoperative work up is needed **(Table 2)**. In most hospitals, blood is usually grouped and cross matched when a woman is undergoing a

TABLE 1: Basic preoperative laboratory work up for gynecological surgery.

Test	*Importance in preoperative assessment*	*Steps to be taken if result is out of range (correction, deferring surgery, etc.)*
Hemoglobin	• Optimal oxygen carrying capacity • Preparation for surgical blood loss and transfusion	• Defer elective surgery in case of Hb is below 9 g/dL • Build Hb to a range of 10–11 g% by oral or parenteral iron supplementation. Both routes take about 20–30 days to show risk of Hb. Parenteral iron assures compliance. In case of oncological surgery, one may consider packed red cell transfusion
Urine routine and microscopy	• Rule out coexisting urine infections which are of importance especially for urogynecological surgery • Abnormalities in protein, sugar and other parameters may point to undiagnosed pathology	Treat urine infection before surgery. This would also rule out conditions where symptoms may be due to infection rather than gynecological pathology
Blood sugar	Hyperglycemia is an important consideration for anesthesia, intraoperative and postoperative care, recovery, and wound healing	Optimize glycemic control. If there is no emergent condition, defer surgery. Oral hypoglycemic agents may need to be shifted to insulin in the perioperative period for major surgeries. This is not always necessary for surgeries where the glycemic control is good and where the period of remaining without oral intake is short
Viral markers (HIV, HBsAg, HCV)	Occasionally, the presence of these may be detected for the first time in a preoperative evaluation. These should be managed with due counseling	• If surgery is planned for an individual with HIV infection, immune status should be assessed with further tests (CD4, viral load) • Universal precautions are to be taken routinely and biowaste management should be done appropriately
Chest X-ray PA view	This is a gross assessment of the pulmonary condition. Arguably, a test which may not have a high index of detection. Old lesions of tuberculosis, COPD may be picked up	The chest X-ray, if abnormal should prompt further pulmonary imaging (HRCT chest) or pulmonary function tests. Where needed lung function should be optimized before planned surgery and consideration should be given to regional anesthesia in such cases
ECG	This is the most basic objective assessment available for cardiac function. It may not always have a high index of detection	Deviations in the ECG should be investigated further and cardiac status should be optimized before planned surgery

(COPD: chronic obstructive pulmonary disease; HRCT: high-resolution CT)

TABLE 2: Advanced preoperative laboratory work up for gynecological surgery.

Test	*Indication*	*Comments*
Full liver and renal profile	• Suspected end organ damage • On medications which may affect liver or kidney function	• These tests are routinely done in some institutions before major surgery • In case of abnormalities in hepatic function, one may consider deferring surgery if the possible. Coagulation should be assessed in these situations • In case of abnormalities in renal function, dose of anesthetic agents, antibiotics and analgesics should be altered according to level of renal function
Coagulation parameters (PT, PTT, INR, d-Dimer)	• Major gynecological surgery • Oncosurgery • Obesity • Suspected coagulation abnormalities from previous history	Preoperative correction or preparation with blood and blood products may be needed
Pulmonary function test	• Abnormal respiratory examination or chest X-ray	Preoperative optimization with inhalers or other agents is desirable. These women will benefit from postoperative chest physiotherapy
2D echocardiography, stress test	• Abnormal ECG • Undiagnosed cardiac pathology	

major gynecological surgery. This is a prudent step. It should definitely be done when intraoperative bleeding is expected such as oncological surgery or when the woman has a large fibroid.[6]

ANESTHESIA ASSESSMENT AND SCORING

The preanesthesia check is an important screening step where another set of eyes (besides the surgical team) can assess the fitness of the woman. The goals of this assessment are:

- To ensure patient is in best/optimal state.
- Anesthetic drugs, technique, and duration have profound effect on human body, so a detailed major organ system assessment is performed.
- To assess airway, as incidence of difficult intubation is 1.6–5.9%.[7] Various techniques such as the Mallampati score can be used to make this preoperative assessment. Difficult intubation can be anticipated when mouth opening is less than 3 cm. Three finger breadth, obesity, restricted neck movements and mucosal fibrosis.
- To assess peripheral venous access.
- To examine spine/other regions specific to regional anesthesia.

American Society of Anesthesiologists physical status score system is used to quantify the risk associated with anesthesia and surgery **(Table 3)**.[8] Usually, women for gynecological surgery do not have a high ASA score. This tool is a good counseling tool for assessing and explaining risk before anesthesia and surgery. Other risk assessment scores such as Revised Cardiac Risk Index (RCRI) for women with a history of cardiac events[9] or Surgical Risk Preoperative Assessment System (SURPAS)[10] may be used in selected clinical situations or for research.

TABLE 3: American Society of Anesthesiologists (ASA) physical status classification system.

ASA score	*Medical status*	*Mortality risk*
ASA-1	Healthy, without organic, biochemical or psychiatric illness	0.06–0.08%
ASA-2	Mild systemic illness having no major or significant impact on daily activity, e.g., controlled hypertension, overweight	0.27–0.4%
ASA-3	Severe systemic disease limiting activity, e.g., COPD, prior myocardial infarction and sequale	1.8–4.3%
ASA-4	Incapacitating illness that is a constant threat to life, e.g., CHF, unstable angina, renal failure, etc.	Major impact 7.8–23%
ASA-5	Moribund patient, not expected to survive beyond next 24 hours, e.g., ruptured aneurysm	9.4–51%
ASA-6	Brain dead	

Add E to the emergency situation

(COPD: chronic obstructive pulmonary disease; CHF: congestive heart failure)

PREOPERATIVE COUNSELING

Gynecologic surgery involves a variety of psychological and emotional issues in women. In addition to the usual concerns surrounding any other surgical procedure (pain, disfigurement, debility, outcome), gynecologic surgery is accompanied by the specter of loss of fertility, femininity, sexuality, and attractiveness.[1] Counseling should aim at identifying the psychosocial goals of the patient too.

Several "red flags" which should prompt a clinician to refer the patient for a psychiatric evaluation have been proposed by Stockholm *viz.* numerous previous surgeries, chronic pelvic pain, a history or current evidence of a psychological disorder, and multiple indications for surgery. These issues should be addressed in a realistic way, and counseling regarding recurrence rates, failed procedures should also be explained.

The more detailed aspects of counseling are covered in another chapter of the textbook.

CONSENT

In elective or planned surgery, and in most emergency surgeries, consent is mandatory. In today's times, for surgical interventions, the standard of care is a written, informed consent. Documentation is essential. Verbal consents are not medicolegally tenable. The written document should be preserved for the appropriate duration after surgery (usually 7 years).

Informed consent is the process in which a surgeon educates a patient about the risks, benefits, and alternatives of a given procedure or intervention.[11,12] This information is provided under the light of existing clinical practice guidelines and facts. The patient must be competent to make a voluntary decision about whether to undergo the procedure or intervention. Informed consent should be considered as both an ethical and legal obligation. The following are the required elements for documentation of the informed consent discussion:

- Nature of the problem and its implications for health
- Nature of the proposed operative procedure
- Purpose and benefits of the operative procedure and the expected outcomes
- Risks of the procedure
- Other alternative forms of treatments and a comparison of the risks and benefits of the alternatives.

For consent to be considered valid, it should meet the following conditions:[13]

- Consent should be given by an adult or by the adult guardian of a child
- The patient should have the mental and physical capacity to give consent

- Consent should be obtained from the individual undergoing the procedure (except when the individual is a child or does not have capacity to give consent). There is no value of obtaining the consent from the spouse or other family members in the absence of consent from the patient.
- Consent should be obtained voluntarily without coercion or other undue influences (including preanesthesia medications).
- The patient must comprehend the discussion. If language is a barrier, a translator should be used. If the patient has hearing or speech impairments, sign language should be used.
- In case the patient is not literate and cannot read and/or write, the consent and thumb impression of the patient should be taken. This should be witnessed by a person that the patient appoints. This should also be documented. The consent and the process should be verified by an attendant and member of the surgical team.

Some new developments regarding consent are:

- Separate consents should be taken for high risk factors, anesthesia, and blood transfusion.
- Procedure specific consents should be obtained with details as far to the evidence as possible. FOGSI will be releasing a guidebook for consents in near future for easy reference.

Video consents: Videography for consents can be taken, but caution has to be practiced as whatever is spoken will be taken as evidence and whatever is *not spoken* can be the point of contention.

PREOPERATIVE CHECKLISTS

The preoperative preparation for the theater and personnel should be considered. The planned surgery should be booked with adequate time allotted to it with the right members of the surgical team being informed in advance and relevant instruments checked the day before surgery and being available in working condition. For long surgeries, it is useful to start as the first case of the day. The anesthesia and surgical team should be briefed preoperatively, especially for unusual or complex cases. In the immediate preoperative period, the WHO Safe Safety Checklist is an invaluable tool to prevent missteps and errors **(Fig. 3)**.[14,15] It should be included in routine perioperative care of the patient.

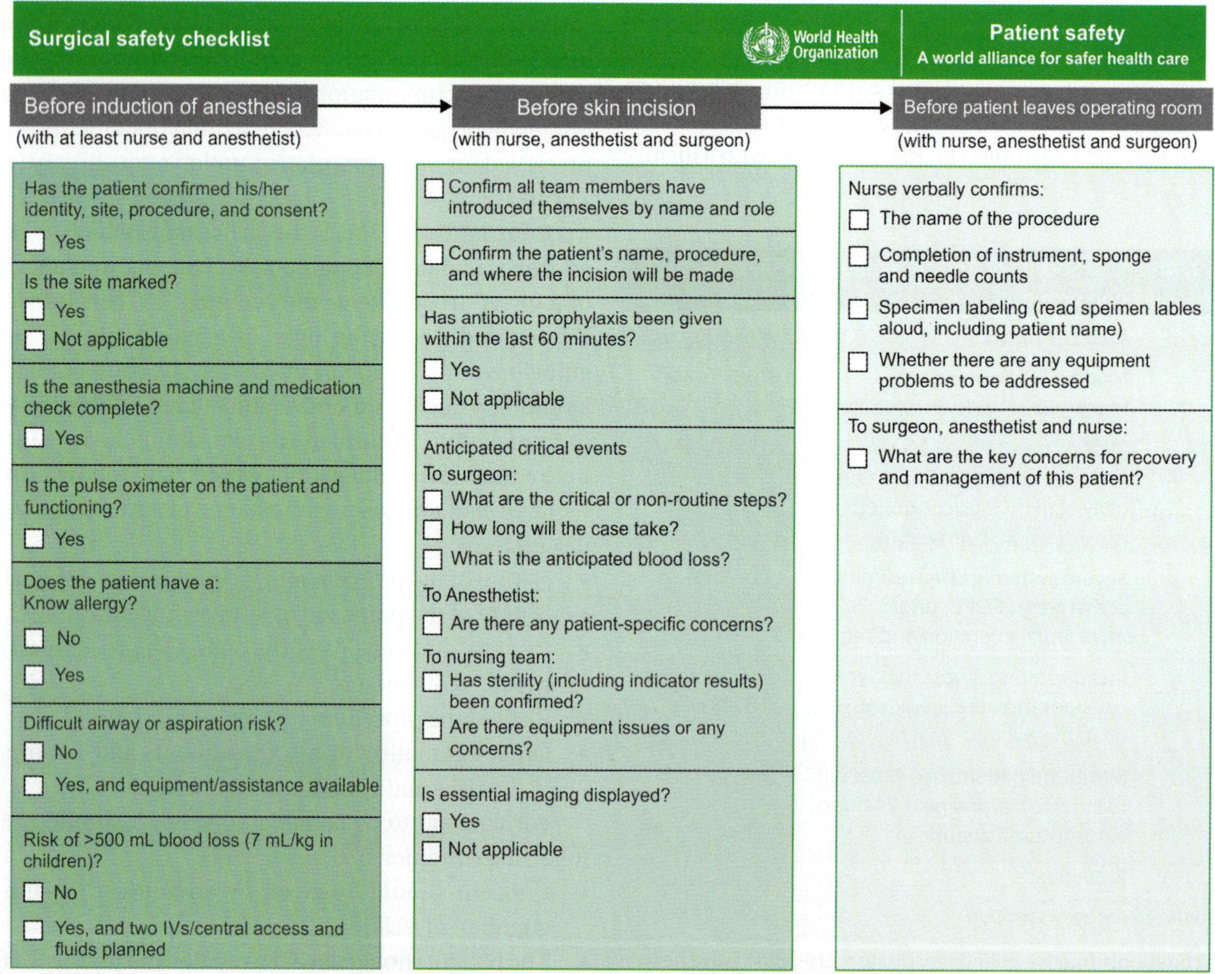
Surgical safety checklist

World Health Organization | Patient safety | A world alliance for safer health care

Before induction of anesthesia (with at least nurse and anesthetist)	Before skin incision (with nurse, anesthetist and surgeon)	Before patient leaves operating room (with nurse, anesthetist and surgeon)
Has the patient confirmed his/her identity, site, procedure, and consent? ☐ Yes	☐ Confirm all team members have introduced themselves by name and role	Nurse verbally confirms: ☐ The name of the procedure ☐ Completion of instrument, sponge and needle counts ☐ Specimen labeling (read speimen lables aloud, including patient name) ☐ Whether there are any equipment problems to be addressed
Is the site marked? ☐ Yes ☐ Not applicable	☐ Confirm the patient's name, procedure, and where the incision will be made	To surgeon, anesthetist and nurse: ☐ What are the key concerns for recovery and management of this patient?
Is the anesthesia machine and medication check complete? ☐ Yes	Has antibiotic prophylaxis been given within the last 60 minutes? ☐ Yes ☐ Not applicable	
Is the pulse oximeter on the patient and functioning? ☐ Yes	Anticipated critical events To surgeon: ☐ What are the critical or non-routine steps? ☐ How long will the case take? ☐ What is the anticipated blood loss? To Anesthetist: ☐ Are there any patient-specific concerns? To nursing team: ☐ Has sterility (including indicator results) been confirmed? ☐ Are there equipment issues or any concerns?	
Does the patient have a: Know allergy? ☐ No ☐ Yes	Is essential imaging displayed? ☐ Yes ☐ Not applicable	
Difficult airway or aspiration risk? ☐ No ☐ Yes, and equipment/assistance available		
Risk of >500 mL blood loss (7 mL/kg in children)? ☐ No ☐ Yes, and two IVs/central access and fluids planned		

Fig. 3: World Health Organization (WHO) surgical safety checklist.

BOWEL PREPARATION

The purposes of bowel preparation before gynecological surgery are:

- The stomach should be empty to reduce the risk of aspiration and lung complications, especially when general anesthesia or sedation is used.
- The bowel should empty or nearly empty to facilitate handling and keeping away from the site of surgery, namely the pelvis.
- In case bowel injury is anticipated or where bowel is intended to be opened for resection, the risk of contamination of the peritoneal cavity should be minimized.

The duration of keeping the patient nil by mouth has been generally ordered as "from midnight". This usually means duration of 8–10 hours depending on when the woman has her last meal, sleeps, and the timing of the surgery. If there are some delays, the duration is extended further. These practices are not evidence based. A long duration of remaining on an empty stomach are associated with dissatisfaction, delayed bowel function and hypovolemia. The current recommendation is that women can ingest solid food till 6 hours before surgery and clear liquids till 2 hours before surgery.[16] There is some evidence that carbohydrate loading till 3 hours before surgery may reduce metabolic disturbances and enhance recovery. This can be done in the form of liquids such as a clear fruit juice.

For long, it was believed that mechanical bowel preparation helps in the ease of handling the bowel and facilitating a clear pelvic field for surgery. However, the current evidence does not support this. A number of agents have been studied in a wide variety of clinical situations (obesity, risk of bowel injury, endometriosis, cancer) and for open or laparoscopic surgery. The evidence is clear that mechanical bowel preparation does not help in any aspect of bowel handling or ease of surgery. Furthermore, even when the bowel is opened (accidentally or intentionally) at gynecological surgery, mechanical bowel preparation does not confer any degree of safety or advantage in terms of reducing infection risk or reducing the chances of an anastomotic leak. There could be problems associated with mechanical bowel preparation such as dehydration, dyselectrolytemias and edematous or friable bowel wall due to the agent used. The current evidence, therefore, does not favor the use of mechanical bowel preparation or enemas.[16-18] If the woman is constipated or has difficulty with bowel movements, simple tablets of bisacodyl or any such simple laxatives may be used for 2–3 days before surgery is planned. A low residue diet for a day or two before the surgery is a less invasive and safer way of preparing the bowel.

Oral antibiotics may be prescribed for bowel preparation where there is an anticipation of bowel injury or where the bowel is to be resected as a part of a gynecological surgery. This is associated with a reduction in the risk of infection and anastomotic leak.[19]

PART PREPARATION

Traditionally, the skin was prepared the day before surgery by shaving. This practice was in routine use based on the belief that there is cleanliness in the operative field, reduction in infection rates and better skin approximation. Moreover, hair in perineal area was presumed to be nest of bacteria, and blood clots would lodge in them. After surgery, dressing application was less troublesome and painful, if hair was shaven. However, none of these beliefs holds true. Current evidence does not favor the routine shaving or epilation of the surgical field. Shaving actually increases the risk of perioperative staphylococcal skin infection. If hair has to be removed, it may be done with electric clippers with a single-use head on the day of surgery.[20] On the night before surgery and morning of surgery, the patient should bathe with a medicated soap preferably one containing chlorhexidine.[16]

A number of agents have been used for cleaning the skin before surgical incision. These include quaternary compounds, povidone-iodine based scrubs, and solutions, chlorhexidine solutions and these are combined with an alcohol based agent such as isopropyl alcohol or surgical spirit **(Table 4)**. The combination of 2% chlorhexidine solution with 70% isopropyl alcohol is currently favored for preincision skin cleaning.[16]

ANTIMICROBIAL PROPHYLAXIS

Incidence of surgical site infection (SSI), is the indicator of the level of care at any center. In low- and middle-income countries, it is reported that 11% of patients who undergo surgery are infected in the process of surgery and postoperative stay. SSIs are primarily caused by bacteria entering through incisions made during surgery and secondarily after surgery. While some may involve only skin and subcutaneous tissue, others are more serious and might involve muscle, fascia, organ spaces or implanted material or foreign bodies. The

TABLE 4: Agents for skin preparation before surgical incision.

Alcohol based	***Concentration***	***Type of surgery***
Chlorhexidene	0.5% in 70% alcohol	Minor
Chlorhexidene	2% in 70% alcohol	Major
Povidone-Iodine	10%	If allergy or contraindication of above two
Aqueous based	***Concentration***	***Type of surgery***
Chlorhexidene	4%	• Elective routine • When surgical site is in proximity to mucous membranes
Povidone-Iodine	7.5% 10%	When all the above preparations are contraindicated or un suitable

TABLE 5: World Health Organization (WHO) recommendations on surgical antimicrobial prophylaxis.

Consideration	*Recommendation*
Choice of agent	• The antibiotics selected for prophylaxis must cover the expected pathogens for that operative site. For gynecological surgeries the agents of first choice are first or second generation cephalosporins such as cefazolin or cefuroxime • In case of an expected contaminated field, a combination of amoxicillin and clavulanic acid can be used • In case of allergy or other contraindications, a combination of clindamycin and gentamycin can be used
Timing of the dose	Not earlier than 1 hour before the surgical incision. May be given at the time of induction of anesthesia or latest at the point of skin incision
Number of doses	• Single dose is adequate. *Exceptions:* • Surgical time is more than 3 hours – a repeat dose should be given • Excessive blood loss and transfusions – repeat dose and continue cover for 48 hours • Contaminated field or evidence of underlying sepsis – as per the clinical situation
Route	Intravenous

recommendations for surgical antimicrobial prophylaxis from the WHO are in **Table 5**.[21]

Thromboprophylaxis has been covered in the chapter on postoperative care.

CONCLUSION

Preoperative care is a phase of great importance for good surgical outcomes. It is a period where the communication should be a basis of bonding between the woman and the surgeon and the surgical team. Patient education, counseling, and consent should be meticulously performed. The important aspects of team and facility preparation should be in place. Medical interventions such as preparation of the bowel, skin and antibiotic use should be rationalized. Planning for the best and being prepared for the worst is the dictum that should be followed while working up of a patient planned for surgery.

REFERENCES

1. Dresner, N, Kurzman, A. Preoperative evaluation and preparation of the gynecologic patient. Glob Libr Women Med. 2008;10423.
2. Kuzu MA, Terzioğlu H, Genç V. Preoperative Nutritional Risk Assessment in Predicting Postoperative Outcome in Patients Undergoing Major Surgery. World J Surg. 2006;30:378-90.
3. Shields J, Lupo A, Walsh T, Kho K. Preoperative evaluation for gynecologic surgery: a guide to judicious, evidence-based testing. Curr Opin Obstet Gynecol. 2018;30(4):252-9.
4. Muñoz M, Laso-Morales MJ, Gómez-Ramírez S, Cadellas M, Núñez-Matas MJ, García-Erce JA. Pre-operative haemoglobin levels and iron status in a large multicentre cohort of patients undergoing major elective surgery. Anaesthesia. 2017;72(7):826-34.
5. Smetana GW, Macpherson DS. The case against routine preoperative laboratory testing. Med Clin North Am. 2003;87(1):7-40.
6. Chee YL, Crawford JC, Watson HG, Greaves M. Guidelines on the assessment of bleeding risk prior to surgery or invasive procedures. British Committee for Standards in Haematology. Br J Haematol. 2008;140(5):496-504.
7. Detsky ME, Jivraj N, Adhikari NK, Friedrich JO, Pinto R, Simel DL, et al. Will This Patient Be Difficult to Intubate?: the Rational Clinical Examination Systematic Review. JAMA. 2019;321(5):493-503.
8. American Society of Anesthesiologists. ASA Physical Status Classification System. [online] Available from: https://www.asahq.org/standards-and-guidelines/asa-physical-status-classification-system. [Last Accessed November, 2021].
9. Tateosian VS, Richman DC. Preoperative Cardiac Evaluation for Noncardiac Surgery. Anesthesiol Clin. 2018;36(4):509-21.
10. Lambert-Kerzner A, Ford KL, Hammermeister KE, Henderson WG, Bronsert MR, Meguid RA. Assessment of attitudes towards future implementation of the "Surgical Risk Preoperative Assessment System" (SURPAS) tool: a pilot survey among patients, surgeons, and hospital administrators. Patient Saf Surg. 2018;12:12.
11. Overcarsh P, Arvizo C, Harvey L. Informed consent in gynecologic surgery. Curr Opin Obstet Gynecol. 2019;31(4):240-4.
12. Jain R, Saraogi R, Sahetya R, Association of Fellow Gynecologists (AFG). Manual on Informed consent For Gynaecologic and Obstetric Surgical Procedures. Mumbai: AFG; 2014.
13. Kapoor L. Better safe than sorry. Medicolegal Do's and Don'ts. Association of Medical Consultants (AMC), Mumbai. 2005.
14. Haynes AB, Weiser TG, Berry WR, Lipsitz SR, Breizat AH, Dellinger EP, et al. Safe Surgery Saves Lives Study Group. A surgical safety checklist to reduce morbidity and mortality in a global population. N Engl J Med. 2009;360(5):491-9.
15. World Health Organization (WHO). Implementation Manual WHO Surgical Safety Checklist 2009. [online] Available from: https://www.who.int/publications/i/item/9789241598590. [Last accessed November, 2021].
16. Kalogera E, Nelson G, Liu J, Hu QL, Ko CY, Wick E, et al. Surgical technical evidence review for gynecologic surgery conducted for the Agency for Healthcare Research and Quality Safety Program for Improving Surgical Care and Recovery. Am J Obstet Gynecol. 2018;219(6):563.e1-e19.
17. Arnold A, Aitchison LP, Abbott J. Preoperative mechanical bowel preparation for abdominal, laparoscopic, and vaginal surgery: a systematic review. J Minim Invasive Gynecol. 2015;22:737-52.
18. Suadee W, Suprasert P. Appropriate bowel preparation for laparotomy gynecologic surgery: a prospective, surgeon-blinded randomized study. Gynecol Obstet Invest. 2017;82:287-93.
19. Nelson G, Altman AD, Nick A. Guidelines for pre- and intra-operative care in gynecologic/oncology surgery: Enhanced Recovery after Surgery (ERAS) Society recommendations part I. Gynecol Oncol. 2016;140:313-22.
20. Shi D, Yao Y, Yu W. Comparison of preoperative hair removal methods for the reduction of surgical site infections: a meta-analysis. J Clin Nurs. 2017;26(19-20):2907-14.

21. World Health Organization. Antibiotics of choice for surgical antibiotic prophylaxis. Essential Medicine List Guidance on SAP. [online] Available from: https://www.who.int/selection_medicines/committees/expert/22/applications/s6.2_surgical-antibiotic-prophylaxis.pdf. [Last accessed November, 2021].

LONG QUESTIONS

1. What is informed consent? What are the components of written informed consent and its importance in gynecological surgeries?
2. What is surgical site infection (SSI)? Enumerate causes for SSI and steps taken to reduce the incidence.

SHORT QUESTIONS

1. What are the psychological implications of gynecological surgery that should be considered in preoperative planning?
2. What are the recommendations for bowel preparation before gynecological surgery?
3. Describe imaging and its importance in preoperative preparation before gynecological surgery.
4. What is the HEATS tool for preoperative assessment?
5. What is the importance of a preoperative checklist?

MULTIPLE CHOICE QUESTIONS

1. The contributing factors for good preoperative care are all the following, except:
   a. Good patient selection
   b. MRI pelvis for all major surgeries
   c. Team approach
   d. Patient education
2. The following are all considerations for deciding the route of surgery, except:
   a. Nature of pathology
   b. Patient's choice
   c. Surgeon's training
   d. Directives from the hospital administration
3. The following drugs should be stopped before a major gynecological surgery, except:
   a. Oral contraceptive pills
   b. Antiepileptic medications
   d. Estrogen tablets for hormone therapy
   d. Warfarin
4. If a woman has been taking the following drug on a long-term basis, the dose will have to be increased before gynecological surgery:
   a. Warfarin b. Thyroxin
   d. Antifungal agents d. Corticosteroids
5. The Mallampati score is used to assess the following aspect of risk:
   a. Mortality b. Cardiovascular events
   c. Difficult intubation d. Thromboembolism
6. Consent is valid if:
   a. It is given by a 15-year-old woman
   b. It is given by the patient's husband
   c. It is obtained after sedation
   d. It is an informed consent
7. The following is true about preoperative bowel preparation:
   a. Keeping the patient nil by mouth for at least 12 hours is advisable
   b. Oral antibiotics reduce risk of surgical infection if there is bowel injury
   c. Mechanical bowel preparation reduces operative time in laparoscopy
   d. High protein diet is recommended 2 hours before surgery
8. The following is the agent of choice to prepare the skin before incision:
   a. Medicated soap b. Quaternary compounds
   c. Povidone iodine d. Chlorhexidine
9. The following is true about surgical antimicrobial prophylaxis, except:
   a. The drug of choice is cefuroxime
   b. The route of choice is intravenous
   c. The dose should be given 4 hours before surgical incision
   d. More than one dose should be given if the surgery lasts for more than 3 hours

Answers

1.	b	2.	d	3.	b	4.	d	5.	c	6.	d
7.	b	8.	d	9.	c						

7.8 POSTOPERATIVE CARE IN OBSTETRICS AND GYNAECOLOGY

Kavita V Kapadia, Vaibhav V Kapadia

"He will manage the cure best who has foreseen what is to happen from the present state of matters."

—Hippocrates

INTRODUCTION

The care of the surgical patient requires an accurate understanding of the pathophysiological changes that occurs perioperatively. During this period the body tries to maintain systemic homeostasis despite all the iatrogenic induced alterations.

GOALS OF POSTOPERATIVE CARE

1. Good postoperative care should be directed toward enhancing and maintaining patient safety, comfort, and recovery.
2. It provides an opportunity to detect complications at an early and remediable stage.
3. This is an opportunity to address and debrief the patient.
4. Complete postoperative care should include documentation for follow-up and medicolegal purposes.
5. In the long term, some patients will need prolonged care especially those operated for malignancies.

The intensity of postoperative care depends on the individuals' presurgical health, type of surgery and the geographical location.

POSTOPERATIVE MONITORING

The first postoperative assessment should take place immediately after surgery and also on return to the ward. It provides a baseline against which the patient's condition may subsequently be assessed and identifies any problems that may have occurred.

The first postoperative assessment should determine **(Table 1)**:

- Intraoperative history and postoperative instructions
- Circulatory volume and respiratory status
- Mental status.

In general, monitoring regimens for the first few hours after surgery, should include:[1] Temperature, pulse rate, blood pressure, respiratory rate, pain assessment, urine output and peripheral oxygen saturation. Monitoring will be frequent initially (every 15 minutes for the first hour), becoming less frequent over time (every 30 minutes for the next 2 hours, and hourly for a period thereafter).

The doctor completing the initial postoperative assessment should consider the monitoring regimen and appropriate level of care required for the next 24 hours in collaboration with the nursing team.

Additional monitoring may be required in certain high-risk patients which may include ECG, hourly urine volumes, arterial blood pressure, central venous pressure, arterial blood gases, drainage from wounds, hematology and biochemistry.

TABLE 1: Postoperative monitoring.

Parameter	*Acceptable range*
Temperature	>36°C
Pulse	Approximate preoperative values or at a level commensurate with the surgery
Respiration	10–20 breaths per min, SpO_2 >90
Blood pressure	Approximate preoperative values
Level of consciousness	Fully conscious, responding to light touch, able to maintain clear airway

When the patient is shifted from the recovery room to the wards or the hospital room, it is essential that the patient is stable and the basic reflexes have recovered.[2]

Invasive circulatory monitoring may help in assessing fluid balance status in high risk patients. This is done by central venous pressure (CVP) or in certain cases pulmonary capillary wedge pressure (PCWP). CVP is measured by a catheter placed in one of the large intrathoracic veins which reflects the pressure in the right atrium. The normal CVP is between 5 and 12 cmH_2O. In patients with cardiac disease the PCWP using the Swan Ganz catheter may be a more accurate way of determining the volume status. Invasive monitoring, especially that of PCWP comes with its own set of risks and complications. It is recommended for women who have had massive blood loss and are being transfused with large volumes of blood or fluid, women with preeclampsia/eclampsia with pulmonary involvement and in women with low ejection fractions undergoing major surgery.

ANALGESIA

Pain is the most urgent and most common concern that the patient will voice after surgery. Effective pain control is an essential part in the postoperative care. Inadequate pain control is inhumane and may lead to increase morbidity and mortality. Good pain control results in earlier mobilization of the patient and hence low chances of thromboembolism and respiratory complications. Some emerging concepts that should be kept in mind in providing analgesia after gynecological and obstetric surgery are **(Table 2)**:

- The use of multiple agents and modalities should be rationalized to target pain at central and peripheral mechanisms. After obstetric surgery, the agents that are used should have minimal passage into breast milk.
- *Preemptive analgesia:* This is the administration of analgesics prior to onset of noxious stimuli. Preemptive analgesia modifies peripheral and central nervous system processing of noxious stimuli, thereby reducing hyperalgesia, and allodynia.[3-5] Preemptive analgesia reduces postoperative opioid use and opioid side effects.
- *Patient-controlled analgesia (PCA):* PCA pump is the preferred mode of administering opioids for severe postoperative pain after radical pelvic surgery or surgery involving large abdominal incisions. Morphine, hydromorphone and fentanyl can be used for PCA.[6]

Analgesia can be administered parenterally in the immediate postoperative period by intravenous, intramuscular, rectal or epidural routes. The various agents used commonly in Obstetrics and Gynecology surgery are:

Nonsteroidal anti-inflammatory drugs (NSAIDs): Paracetamol, diclofenac, ketorolac.

TABLE 2: Analgesia used in gynecological and obstetric surgery.

Agent	*Mechanism of action*	*Dose and route*	*Side effects*	*Precautions and contraindications*
Tramadol	Centrally acting opioid analgesic, NMDA receptor antagonist, serotonin-norepinephrine reuptake inhibitor	100 mg IV bolus followed by 5–100 mg IV 4–6 hourly, maximum dose 600 mg/day 50-100 mg orally every 4–6 hours	Nausea, constipation, dizziness vertigo, diarrhea, fatigue	Kidney or liver failure, elderly patients, children and pregnant women
Pentazocine	Mixed opioid agonist and antagonist	75 mg IV/IM every 4 hourly, maximum of 600 mg per day	Increased heart rate, elevated blood pressure, respiratory depression, psychomimetic effects	Hypersensitivity to naloxone
Diclofenac	NSAID acts by inhibiting the enzyme COX, that is responsible for inflammation	• 50–75 mg IM 8 hourly or as an IV infusion • 50-75 mg orally every 8 hours.	Diarrhea, nausea, vomiting, constipation, skin rash	Sensitivity or anaphylaxis to other NSAID, liver or kidney disease.
Paracetamol	inhibition of COX, COX 2 > COX1	1,000 mg IV every 6 hours or 650 mg every 4 hours, maximum dose 4,000 g/day[6] 325–500 mg every 4 hours	Used with caution in alcoholics and people with hepatic dysfunction	Skin reactions use with caution is asthmatics. overdose can cause liver failure
Ketorolac	COX-1 inhibitor	30 mg IV[6]	Nausea, vomiting, constipation, dizziness, gas	Used with caution in people with peptic ulcer, liver disease, hypertensives and renal dysfunction

(NMDA: N-methyl-D-aspartate; NSAID: nonsteroidal anti-inflammatory drugs)

Opioids: Tramadol, pentazocine.

If the woman has an epidural catheter in place, its use can be extended to the postoperative period for very effective analgesia. A combination of a local anesthetic (bupivacaine, ropivacaine) and opioid (fentanyl, tramadol) is administered via a patient-controlled epidural pump (PCEA). This combination lowers the dose requirements for each drug, as well as lowers the frequency of side effects.[7-9]

Local infiltration of the incision site with 50 mL of 0.5% ropivacaine decreased postoperative pain.

Pain must be assessed by both verbal and visual methods. Patients must be asked to grade their pain on a scale between 0 and 10 (0 being no pain and 10 being the maximum pain). The surgeon on rounds can assess the patient's demeanor; a smiling patient indicates that the pain control is good.

For the postoperative period beyond the first day, choices include:

- Acetaminophen [325–1,000 mg orally (or rectally) every 4–6 hours, to a maximum dose of 4 g/day]
- Ibuprofen (300–800 mg orally three or four times per day)
- Tramadol (50–100 mg three times a day)

There should be a consideration for the addition of an effective antacid if prolonged use of NSAIDs is anticipated.

FLUID AND ELECTROLYTE BALANCE

The basal requirements for young adults are approximately 30 mL/kg/day of water, 1.0–1.4 mmol/kg/day of sodium and 0.7–0.9 mmol/kg/day of potassium.[1] Crystalloid solutions are preferred over colloid solutions for perioperative fluid replacement. Ringer lactate solution is preferred because its composition closely resembles the extracellular component. High sodium containing fluids are reserved for special indications.

The standard principles of fluid balance in the postoperative patient are:

1. To correct any preexisting deficit
2. To supply basal needs
3. To replace unusual losses (from the preexisting surgical problem, surgical drains, pyrexia)
4. To use the oral route where possible

Guidelines for fluid replacement:

- To avoid problems of fluid therapy prolonged fasting in the preoperative period must be avoided.
- In patients who are euvolemic and hemodynamically stable, a return to oral administration must begin.[10]
- In patients requiring fluid maintenance the fluid used should be sodium poor and of low volume.[10]
- Patients with epidural catheters should be checked for signs of hypovolemia prior to labeling it as post epidural hypotension.
- Hypovolemia due to blood loss should be treated with a balanced crystalloid solution or suitable colloidal solution till blood is made available.
- High risk cardiac patients may have certain dopaminergic agents in the fluid replacement to meet with the oxygen demands postoperatively.
- When hypovolemia is suspected and central venous pressure does not reflect it, a 200 mL fluid challenge may

be administered and the response should be assessed using cardiac output, stroke volume measured by flow based methods when available and alternatively by pulse, blood pressure, capillary filling time and CVP.
- It is important to make changes in fluid therapy based on changing parameters of individual patients

BLADDER CARE

Monitoring urine output is an important tool in postoperative care. In case of minor procedures, catheters are not used, however it is important to ensure that the patient can pass urine freely, prior to discharge.

Indwelling catheters are a part of routine postoperative bladder care in most major gynecological or obstetric surgeries. The following functions are achieved by a catheter:
- Allows monitoring of the urine output accurately
- Drains the bladder and allows it to rest and/or heal
- Prevents bladder distension, which can hamper uterine contractility after a cesarean birth.

Oliguria is defined as a urine output of less than 0.5 mL/kg/h for two consecutive hours. A blocked catheter should be ruled out. If there are signs of hypovolemia they should be corrected. Diuretics should only be used in case of suspected fluid overload or as a therapeutic challenge. In such cases, a dose of 40 mg of Furosemide is used. Dopamine can be used cautiously.

The timing of catheter removal depends on the type of surgery, if any injury was sustained to the urinary system and on the patient's general recovery. Usually, once a patient has tolerated orals and is ambulatory, the catheter can safely be removed. This usually happens within 24 hours post-surgery. The bladder may be drained for longer periods when there has been an injury (intraoperative) and repair (intraoperative bladder repairs, fistula repair), enervation and vascularity could have been compromised at surgery (radical pelvic surgery) or if the bladder neck has been repaired. In such case using an inert silicon catheter is useful in preventing infection and irritation.

PREVENTION OF SEPSIS AND ANTIBIOTICS (TABLE 3)

The principles of prophylactic administration of antibiotics to surgical patients are to **(Box 1)**:
- Reduce the incidence of surgical site infection
- Use antibiotics in a manner that is supported by evidence of effectiveness and minimize the effect of antibiotics on the patient's normal bacterial flora
- Minimize adverse effects
- Cause minimal change to the patient's host defences[11]

It is important to emphasize that surgical antibiotic prophylaxis is an adjunct to, not a substitute for good surgical technique. Antibiotic prophylaxis should be regarded as one component of an effective policy for the control of healthcare associated infection. Most gynecological surgeries belong to Class II (clean contaminated wound).[12]

TABLE 3: Antimicrobial prophylaxis in gynecologic surgery.

Procedure	*Antibiotic*	*Dose*
Vaginal/abdominal hysterectomy/ laparoscopic hysterectomy/pelvic reconstruction/ slings/colporrhaphy	Cefazolin Cefoxitin Cefotetan Metronidazole Clindamycin Ampicillin-sulbactam	1 or 2 single dose IV 2 g single dose IV 1 or 2 single dose IV 500 mg single dose IV 900 mg single dose IV 3 g IV
Laparoscopy	None	–
Hysteroscopy	None	–
Hysterosalpingogram	Doxycycline	100 mg b.d/5 days orally
IUD insertion	None	–
Endometrial biopsy	None	–
Induced abortion/ D&C	Doxycycline Metronidazole	100 mg orally 1 hour before procedure and 200 mg orally after the procedure 400 mg thrice daily for 5 days
Oocyte retrieval	None	–
Urodynamics	none	–

BOX 1: Patients at risk of surgical site infection.

- *Poor glycemic control:* Perioperative serum glucose greater than or equal to 180–200 mg/dL
- Smokers
- Obese patients (BMI >30)
- Depth of subcutaneous tissue >3 cm
- Coexistent infection at a remote body site (e.g., skin, urinary tract)
- Malnourished patients
- Immunodeficient patients (chronic steroid use, chemotherapy)

(BMI: body mass index)

The antibiotics selected for prophylaxis must cover the expected pathogens for that operative site. The choice of antibiotic should take into account local resistance patterns. Single standard therapeutic dose of antibiotic is sufficient for prophylaxis under most circumstances. For surgical procedures, intravenous prophylactic antibiotics should be given within 60 minutes before the skin is incised[12]and as close to time of incision as practically possible.

In women undergoing cesarean section, advice on the timing of administration of prophylactic antibiotics may be better at the time of cord clamping rather than prior to incision because of perceived concerns about unnecessary exposure of the fetus to these agents.

Penicillin and cephalosporin antibiotics are often the cornerstone of antibiotic prophylaxis.[13,14] These are highly effective against staphylococcus and streptococci which are the normal bacteria found on skin. In case of allergy to beta lactams, clindamycin or vancomycin may be used. In patients with cardiac diseases requiring prophylaxis against infective endocarditis, appropriate antibiotic cover should be used. Patients with BMI > 30 should receive twice the dose of the antibiotic. In surgeries lasting more than 4 hours[12] and blood loss of greater than 1,500 mL repeat dose of antibiotic may be administered.

In practice in our setup it may not always be possible to follow the above guidelines. In India we tend to use Cefuroxime(1.5 g IV) or Cefotaxime (1 g IV) in cases of major surgery such as cesarean section, hysterectomies, laparotomy. Also in place of a single dose of IV antibiotic, we use intravenous antibiotic for first 24 hours and then convert it to oral antibiotics till a period of 5 days.

In high risk patients, e.g., diabetes, prolonged surgery we may add aminoglycosides such as gentamicin (1.5 mg/kg every 8 hours) In patients with preexisting renal conditions we may add a fluroquinolone (500 mg IV 12 hourly).

NUTRITION

Oral intake should be commenced as soon as possible after surgery. Patients should not be fasted for any longer than necessary, either for investigations or surgery.

Most surgeons wait for the return of bowel function before starting oral diets for their postoperative patients. The return of bowel function may be assessed by presence of bowel sounds, passage of flatus or subjective feeling of hunger. Literature suggests that this might not be necessary. Early postoperative feeding appears to be safe and, according to some studies, beneficial. Allowing patients more control over their diet likely contributes to overall patient satisfaction and reduces hospital length of stay, thus decreasing medical costs. For the average patient coming from home to the hospital for elective surgery, early postoperative feeding may be an ideal treatment strategy.

Energy and protein requirements depend on body composition, clinical status, and mobility. An estimation of requirements is

- 25–30 kcal/kg/day (including protein)
- 0.8–1.5 g protein/kg/day for the average patient
- 30–35 mL fluid/kg
- Few patients require more than 2,200 kcal/day.[1] Additional calories are unlikely to be used effectively and may constitute a metabolic stress.

Screening for malnutrition must be carried out as patients who are malnourished are at high risk of developing postoperative complications. Nutritional support must be considered in people who are malnourished and at a high risk of developing refeeding syndrome[15] (severe electrolyte imbalance leading to fatal complications). The following patients are at high risk for refeeding syndrome:

- Patients with low BMI (<16)
- Poor intake or low intake of food in the last 10 days
- Weight loss or more than 15% in the last 3–6 months
- Alcoholics.

Malnourished cancer patients should be considered for nutritional advice and oral supplements in the postoperative period and for a period following discharge.

Generally, if oral nutrition is not re-established within 5–7 days postoperatively, enteral (nasogastric tube feeds for 4–6 weeks or gastrostomy/jejunostomy for longer durations) or parenteral feeding should be considered.

BOWEL CARE

There is usually a physiological ileus post operatively which may last for a period of up to 48 hours in the colon. Most patients should therefore have a bowel activity on the third postoperative day if no bowel complications have occurred, an enema may be administered if patient is unable to pass stools on the third postoperative day. Preoperative chewing of gum has shown to help in postoperative return of bowel function. However, in the case of bowel injury or anal sphincter repair the enema must be withheld.

PREVENTION OF DEEP VEIN THROMBOSIS

Prevention of deep vein thrombosis remains the most effective tool in prevention of venous thromboembolism (VTE), a possibly fatal postsurgical complication. Several clinical factors are known to identify the patient with an increased risk for VTE. We may use the Caprini VTE risk assessment model **(Annexure 1)**. The treatment protocols for the different risk groups are described in **Table 4**.

Strategies to prevent DVT can be grouped as:

- *Mechanical:* Early mobilization, physiotherapy, compression of the lower limbs
- *Pharmacological:* Heparin

Early mobilization is the simplest, risk free intervention which will not only prevent DVT, but contributes to the overall wellbeing and has a positive impact on all aspects of postoperative care. The patient should be encouraged to move her limbs even while supine. She should be mobilized with some encouragement as soon as pain is controlled.

Stockings for compressing the lower limbs minimize stasis. Simple stockings or pneumatic stockings can be used.

Heparin in a dose equivalent to 40–80 mg of Enoxaparin or 5,000–10,000 units of unfractionated heparin can be used to prevent DVT. Patients should be selected using a guideline or scoring system established as per local guidelines. Prophylaxis should commence 12 hours before surgery and continued as recommended by risk calculation. Complications such as postoperative bleeding due to thrombocytopenia and allergic reactions are rare.

The treatment of DVT is directed toward preventing further clots, pulmonary embolism and preventing long-term complications such as iliofemoral thrombosis and chronic

TABLE 4: Venous thromboembolism prophylaxis in at-risk patients.[16]

VTE risk level	*Low VTE risk (Caprini score 1–2)*	*Moderate VTE risk (Caprini score 3–4)*		*High VTE risk (Caprini score 5 or more)*	
Prophylaxis		High bleeding risk	Low bleeding risk	High bleeding risk	Low bleeding risk
	Start IPC on admission or GCS	Start IPC on admission	After surgery, use: LMWH dalteparin 5,000 units subcut once daily *Or* enoxaparin 40 mg subcut once daily *or* IPC	Start IPC on admission after surgery, reassess (and document) risks. When bleeding risk decreases, add pharmacological prophylaxis	Start IPC or GCS on admission AND after surgery, use LMWH: dalteparin 5,000 units subcut once daily *or* enoxaparin 40 mg subcut once daily
Moderate risk: Minor surgery in patients with additional risk factors non-major surgery in patients with additional risk factors; major surgery in patients <40 year with additional risk factors		10–20	2–4	1–2	0.1–0.4
Duration	Continue until mobility has returned to an anticipated or clinically acceptable level			Treat for 5–10 days β or until mobility has returned to an anticipated or clinically acceptable level or when the patient is discharged from hospital	

(GCS: graduated compression stockings; IPC: intermittent pneumatic compression; LMWH: low-molecular-weight heparin; subcut: subcutaneous)

venous insufficiency. If suspected, treatment should be initiated with high dose heparin (intravenous unfractionated heparin is preferred) to achieve a prolongation of APTT and INR of 1.5–2. Diagnosis should be confirmed with a color Doppler.

WOUND MANAGEMENT

In non-complicated cases the abdominal wound of the caesarean section or hysterectomy is usually closed with subcuticular stitches or staples. The wound is usually checked on the 5th day post-surgery and if there is no evidence of infection, no further dressing needs to be done.

Surgical site infection occurs in about 4% of clean wounds and 35% of grossly contaminated wound. Diagnosis of wound infection is clinical. Symptoms include localized erythema, induration, warmth, and pain at the incision site. Purulent wound drainage and separation of the wound may occur. Some patients will have systemic evidence of their infection such as fever and leukocytosis.

Necrotizing fasciitis, perhaps the most serious wound infection, is a rare, potentially lethal surgical emergency. It is characterized by a copious dishwater-like drainage, dusky and friable subcutaneous tissue, and pale, devitalized fascia.

Treatment

Infected wounds are opened, explored, drained, irrigated, debrided, and dressed open. If fascial disruption is suspected, drainage should be performed in the operating room. Once the infection has cleared and granulation tissue is apparent, the wound can be closed secondarily. The need for antibiotic therapy is determined by the extent of the infection, presence of systemic manifestations, and comorbidities of the patient.

Wound Dressings

Dressings that maintain moisture and warmth facilitate healing.[17] Retention of moisture is important because wound fluids contain tissue growth factors that facilitate reepithelialization and promote autolytic debridement. Once necrotic tissue has been removed and the wound is granulating, these dressings can be changed once a day or every other day in order to avoid disturbing the healing process.

The ideal dressing for healing wounds by secondary intention should absorb exudate without leakage, be impermeable to water and bacteria, lack particulate contaminants that could be left in the wound upon removal, and is not traumatic to granulation tissue.[18]

USE OF DRAINS

Prior to closure, it may be necessary to place temporary drainage systems. The primary indication of placing a drain is to prevent fluid collection and hence infection. Drains are categorized as passive relying on gravity (Penrose drain, Foley catheter, Word catheter, and Malecot catheter) or active drains that rely on negative pressure suction. Care in the postoperative period includes measures to prevent kinking and blockage and maintaining aseptic conditions to prevent the drain from becoming an infection site. Drains are removed when there is no output, usually on day 3 or day 4 of surgery.

SPECIAL SITUATIONS

Post cesarean section, there is an additional requirement of meeting up with the needs of the neonate. Additional support must be provided to the mothers to help breastfeed the neonates in the first few hours postoperatively to enhance bonding and also the milk let down.

DOCUMENTATION

It is important for the surgeon to make notes of the intraoperative period, mention any complications, and also give written instructions to the nursing staff regarding the postoperative monitoring schedule and drug schedule. Diagrams, photos and videos are helpful for future reference. The documentation should be complete by the time the patient reaches the postoperative ward.

DISCHARGE

Depending on the type of surgery and the recovery of the patient, the number of days spent in the hospital varies. In case of minimally invasive surgery, patient may go home the same evening or after 24 hours postoperatively. In cases of major surgery such as hysterectomy and cesarean section, patients are usually discharged after wound check, which is usually on day 5 post operatively. In case of complication, the stay may be prolonged.

Discharge Card

All patients must be given a discharge card which mentions the indication, type of surgery done, complication if any, unusual finding in the intraoperative period. Instructions regarding level of activity, diet, degree of pain, what to expect and follow up visits must be explained or patient information leaflets handed out. It is important to include contact information for emergencies.

FOLLOW-UP VISIT

The first follow-up visit is a great opportunity for the surgeon to assess if the patient is recovering well, is compliant with treatment and also helps to focus on certain measures which need to be discussed, reemphasized or taken such as:

- Contraception following medical termination of pregnancy
- Leuprolide or Mirena® insertion following surgery for endometriosis
- Hormone therapy after hysterectomy
- Radiation or chemotherapy after oncological surgery.

KEY MESSAGES

- Postoperative monitoring of vital parameters is the cornerstone of postoperative care.
- Multimodal methods of pain management are preferred as this decreases the need for opioid and hence minimizes respiratory depression.
- Fluid therapy must be individualized, sodium poor fluids must be used unless specified.
- Oral intake must begin as soon as possible.
- Early mobilization and identification of patients at high risk of VTE. Adequate measures to prevent must be applied.
- Appropriate antibiotic prophylaxis with beta lactam antibiotics when required.
- Adequate drainage of bladder for first 24 hours of major surgery.
- Ileus resolves after 48 hours of major surgery.

REFERENCES

1. SIGN. Postoperative management in adults: a practical guide to postoperative care for clinical staff. Edinburgh: Scottish Intercollegiate Guidelines Network; 2004.
2. The Association of Anaesthetists of Great Britain and Ireland. Immediate postanaesthetic recovery. London: AOA; 2002.
3. Kelly DJ, Ahmad M, Brull SJ. Preemptive analgesia I: physiological pathways and pharmacological modalities. Can J Anaesth. 2001;48:1000.
4. Woolf CJ, Chong MS. Preemptive analgesia—treating post-operative pain by preventing the establishment of central sensitization. Anesth Analg. 1999;77:362.
5. Suzuki H. Recent topics in the management of pain: development of the concept of preemptive analgesia. Cell Transplant. 1995;4(Suppl 1):S3.
6. Garimella V, Cellini C. Postoperative pain control. Clin Colon Rectal Surg. 2013;26(3):191-6.
7. Niiyama Y, Kawamata T, Shimizu H. The addition of epidural morphine to ropivacaine improves epidural analgesia after lower abdominal surgery. Can J Anaesth. 2005;52:181.
8. Wu CL, Hurley RW, Anderson GF. Effect of postoperative epidural analgesia on morbidity and mortality following surgery in medicare patients. Reg Anesth Pain Med. 2004;29:525.
9. de Leon-Casasola OA, Karabella D, Lema MJ. Bowel function recovery after radical hysterectomies: thoracic epidural bupivacaine-morphine versus intravenous patient-controlled analgesia with morphine: a pilot study. J Clin Anesth. 1996;8:87.
10. British Association for Parenteral and Enteral Nutrition. British Consensus Guidelines on Intravenous Fluid Therapy for Adult Surgical Patients (GIFTASUP). 2011:1-50.
11. Scottish Intercollegiate Guidelines Network (SIGN). Antibiotic prophylaxis in surgery. Edinburgh: SIGN; 2008.
12. Salkind AR, Rao KC. Antibiotic prophylaxis to prevent surgical site infections. Am Fam Physician. 2011;83(5):585-90.
13. ACOG. Prevention of Infection after Gynecologic Procedures. Chicago: ACOG; 2018.
14. Centers for Disease Control and Prevention. Guideline for the Prevention of Surgical Site Infection, 2017. Atlanta: CDC; 2017.
15. NICE. Nutrition support for adults: oral nutrition support, enteral tube feeding and parenteral nutrition. London: NICE; 2006.

16. Guideline for the prevention of Venous Thromboembolism (VTE) in adult hospitalised patients. Queensland: Queensland Health; 2018.
17. Ovington LG. Hanging wet-to-dry dressings out to dry. Home Healthc Nurse. 2001;19:477.
18. Sharp CA, McLaws M. Wound dressings for surgical sites [protocol]. In: The Cochrane Library. Chichester, UK: John Wiley and Sons Ltd.; 2002.

LONG QUESTIONS

1. How can one prevent postoperative complications in gynecological surgery?
2. Describe the diagnosis and management of post-operative complications due to injury to pelvic organs during gynecological surgery?

SHORT QUESTIONS

1. A 45-year-old diabetic woman is undergoing abdominal hysterectomy for fibroid uterus. What are the specific measures that should be taken postoperatively in this case?
2. A 23-year-old woman underwent a cesarean section for fetal distress and has returned with complaints of fever on 7th day postoperatively. What are the possible causes of fever?
3. How will you manage the above patient?
4. How will you manage a case of sudden hypotension in a 21-year-old woman who has just undergone D&E?
5. Discuss the various options for postoperative analgesia with their pros and cons.
6. Discuss the various methods of preventing thrombo-embolism in a moderate to high risk patient undergoing abdominal hysterectomy.
7. Discuss the basic principles of fluid replacement therapy in patient who has undergone laparoscopic hysterectomy which has last approximately 2 hours.
8. A 45-year-old lady who has undergone mitral valvotomy in the past is going to undergo vaginal hysterectomy. What special postoperative care should be taken?

MULTIPLE CHOICE QUESTIONS

1. The following is true regarding CVP:
   a. Measured by catheter placed in intrathoracic vein
   b. Measured by catheter placed in right atrium
   c. Normal CVP is between 12 and 18 cm of water
   d. CVP is more accurate than PCWP in patients with cardiac disease
   e. CVP is noninvasive form of monitoring
2. The following is true about analgesics:
   a. The use of multiple agents is condemned
   b. The use of multiple modalities have a synergistic effect
   c. Preemptive analgesia increases opioid side effect
   d. Tramadol is a mixed opioid agonist antagonist
   e. Diclofenac is a specific COX-2 inhibitor
3. The following is true for fluid and electrolyte therapy:
   a. Basal requirements of young adults in 30 mg/kg/day of water
   b. Colloids are preferred for perioperative fluid replacement
   c. Ringer's Lactate is the preferred solution as it closely resembles intracellular fluid
4. Antibiotic prophylaxis:
   a. Should be given within 90 minutes of skin incision
   b. Is not required for hysterosalpingogram
   c. Is required after an induced abortion/D&E
   d. Commonly used drugs are fluoroquinolones
5. Following are true about postoperative wounds:
   a. Infected wounds are never left open
   b. Drainage of infected wound is performed in the operating room
   c. Dressings that do not allow moisture to pass are preferred
   d. Necrotic tissue should ideally be removed
6. Postoperative ileus (non-obstructive):
   a. Usually occurs on day 5 to day 7 post-surgery
   b. Often associated with nausea and vomiting
   c. Abdominal radiographs show multiple loops of distended bowel with air fluid levels
   d. Bowel sounds are high pitched with borborygmi
7. Regarding DVT-VTE:
   a. Between 5 and 45% gynecological surgery patients develop DVT in their legs
   b. Deficiency of protein C and protein S does not increase risk of thromboembolism
   c. Postoperative mobility increases risk of VTE
   d. Unfractionated heparin requires APTT monitoring when used for treatment of VTE
8. Refeeding syndrome is commonly seen in:
   a. Women with BMI > 20
   b. Women with BMI < 16
   c. Weight loss of more than 20% in last 10 days
   d. Nonalcoholics
9. In case of allergies to beta lactam group of antibiotics the following may be administered:
   a. Aminoglycosides   b. Clindamycin
   c. Cotrimoxazole   d. Doxycycline
10. The discharge summary should not mention which of the following:
    a. Intraoperative complication
    b. Treatment given
    c. Follow up instructions
    d. None of the above
    e. All of the above

Answers

1.	a	2.	b	3.	c	4.	c	5.	d	6.	b
7.	d	8.	b	9.	b	10.	d				

ANNEXURE 1: Caprini's risk assessment model[11] for surgical patients.

Apply 1 point for each of the following statements that apply now or within the past month	Apply 2 points for each of the following statements	Apply 3 points for each of the following statements	Apply 5 points for each of the following statements that apply now or within the past month
Age 41–60 years	Age 61–74 years	Age 75 years or older	Elective major lower extremity arthroplasty
Minor surgery (less than 45 minutes) planned	Arthroscopic surgery	History of DVT or PE	Hip, pelvis or leg fracture within the last month
History of major surgery (longer than 45 minutes) within the last month	Malignancy (present or previous)	Family history of thrombosis	Stroke within the last month
Varicose veins	Major surgery (longer than 45 minute)	Positive factor V Leiden	Multiple trauma within the last month
History of inflammatory bowel disease	Laparoscopic surgery (longer than 45 minutes)	Positive Prothrombin 20210A	Acute spinal cord injury (paralysis) within the last month
Swollen legs (current)	Confined to bed for at least 72 hours	Elevated serum homocysteine	
Obesity (BMI 25 kg/m^2 or greater)	Immobilizing plaster cast less than 1 month	Positive lupus anticoagulant	
Acute myocardial infarction	Central venous access	Elevated anticardiolipin antibodies	
Congestive heart failure within the last month		Heparin-induced thrombocytopenia (HIT)	
Sepsis within the last month		Other congenital or acquired thrombophilia	
Serious lung disease (including pneumonia) within the last month			
Abnormal pulmonary function (e.g., chronic obstructive pulmonary disease)			
Patient currently at bed rest			
Oral contraceptives or hormone replacement therapy			
Pregnancy or postpartum less than 1 month			
History of unexplained stillborn infant, recurrent spontaneous abortion (3 or more), premature birth with toxemia or growth restricted infant			
Other risk factors			
Total points:	Total points:	Total points:	Total points:
Total score:			

SECTION 8 Puberty and Adolescence

8.1 AMENORRHEA: EVALUATION AND MANAGEMENT

Rajrani Sharma, Ameya Purandare, Parikshit Tank

INTRODUCTION

Menses is a cardinal event in every woman's life. Hence, the absence of menses at the usual time every month or delay in the occurrence of the first menses both cause concern which results in a gynecological referral.

Regular and spontaneous menstruation requires: (1) an intact hypothalamic–pituitary–ovarian endocrine axis; (2) an endometrium competent to respond to steroid hormone stimulation; (3) an intact outflow tract from internal to external genitalia.

The human menstrual cycle is susceptible to environmental influences and stressors. Missing a single menstruation rarely reflects a significant pathology. However, prolonged or persistent absence of menses may be one of the earliest signs of neuroendocrine or anatomic abnormality.

DEFINITION AND INCIDENCE

Amenorrhea is defined as the absence of menses.

Primary amenorrhea, seen in approximately 2.5% of the population, is clinically defined as the absence of menses by age 13 years in the absence of normal growth or secondary sexual development; or the absence of menses by age 15 years in the setting of normal growth and secondary sexual development.

Traditionally, evaluation was usually initiated by age 16 years if normal growth and secondary sexual characteristics were present, and at age 13 years if absent. However, because of secular trends toward earlier menarche over the past half century, the evaluation should begin at age 15 years, the age when > 97% of girls should have experienced menarche.

Secondary amenorrhea is clinically defined as the absence of menses for more than three cycle intervals, or six consecutive months, in a previously menstruating woman. The incidence of secondary amenorrhea can be quite variable, from 3% in the general population to 100% under conditions of extreme physical or emotional stress.

ETIOLOGY

The causes of different types of amenorrhea are described in **Boxes 1 and 2**.

It is important to precisely diagnose and treat amenorrhea as the implications for future fertility; risks of unopposed estrogen, including endometrial hyperplasia and neoplasia; risks of hypoestrogenism, including osteoporosis and urogenital atrophy; and impact on psychosocial development significantly affect the woman's overall health and wellbeing.

PATHOGENESIS

Pregnancy is the most common cause of amenorrhea and must be considered in every patient presenting for evaluation of amenorrhea.

BOX 1: Causes of primary amenorrhea.

- Hypothalamic-pituitary abnormalities
- Constitutional delay of puberty
- Isolated GnRH deficiency
- Eating disorder
- Stress/exercise
- Central lesions (tumors, hypophysitis, granulomas)
- Hyperprolactinemia
- Gonadal abnormalities
- Chromosomal abnormalities
- Euchromosomal gonadal agenesis or dysgenesis
- Ovarian resistance syndrome
- Abnormal gonadotropin function
- Autoimmune gonadal failure
- Idiopathic gonadal failure
- Anatomic abnormalities
- Imperforate hymen
- Transverse vaginal septum
- Congenital absence of the cervix
- Müllerian agenesis (Mayer-Rokitansky-Küster-Hauser syndrome)

BOX 2: Causes of secondary amenorrhea.

Common
- Pregnancy and lactation
- Hypothalamic amenorrhea
- Androgen disorders: Polycystic ovarian syndrome, congenital adrenal hypreplasia
- Galactorrhea-amenorrhea syndrome

Less common
- Premature ovarian failure
- Asherman's syndrome
- Sheehan's syndrome
- Tuberculosis

Rare
- Diabetes
- Hyperthyroidism or hypothyroidism
- Cushing's syndrome or Addison's disease
- Cirrhosis
- Malnutrition
- Irradiation or chemotherapy
- Surgery

Hypothalamic Defects

Gonadotropin-releasing hormone (GnRH) secreting neurons of the hypothalamus originate in the olfactory bulb and migrate along the olfactory tract into the mediobasal hypothalamus and the arcuate nucleus. Normally, the arcuate nucleus releases pulses of GnRH into the hypophyseal portal system every hour. Discharge of GnRH releases LH and (FSH) from the pituitary; LH and FSH, in turn, stimulate ovarian follicular growth and ovulation. The ovarian hormones estradiol and progesterone stimulate the development and shedding of the endometrium culminating in the withdrawal bleeding.

Anovulation and amenorrhea occur due to:
- Interference with GnRH transport
- Defects in GnRH pulse discharge
- Congenital absence of GnRH (Kallmann's syndrome).

Any of these situations leads to hypogonadotropic hypogonadism.

Defects of GnRH Transport

Interference with the transport of GnRH from the hypothalamus to the pituitary may occur with pituitary stalk compression or destruction of the arcuate nucleus. Pituitary stalk transection from trauma, compression, radiation, tumors (craniopharyngioma, germinoma, glioma, teratomas), and infiltrative disorders (sarcoidosis, tuberculosis) may cause destruction of the hypothalamus or obstruct the transport of hypothalamic hormones to the pituitary.

Defects of GnRH Pulse Production

Reduction in the normal GnRH pulse frequency or amplitude results in little or no LH or FSH release, with the result that there is no ovarian follicular development, absence estradiol secretion, finally resulting in amenorrhea.

This is the biochemical status in normal prepubertal girls and those with constitutional delayed puberty, such as in anorexia nervosa, severe stress, extreme weight loss, or prolonged vigorous athletic exertion, and in hyperprolactinemia. Amenorrhea in such cases may also be idiopathic.

Congenital GnRH Deficiency

It is called idiopathic hypogonadotropic hypogonadism when it occurs as an isolated phenomenon and Kallmann's syndrome when it is associated with anosmia.

These patients lack GnRH secretion, and express low, prepubertal levels of serum gonadotropins. Follicular recruitment and ovulation do not occur. Although more than 60% of cases are sporadic, congenital GnRH deficiency can also be inherited in an autosomal or X-linked pattern.

More common in boys with delayed puberty, constitutional delay of puberty is an uncommon etiology of primary amenorrhea in girls. Patients demonstrate delayed adrenarche and gonadarche, but ultimately go on to have normal, although delayed, pubertal development.

Functional or Hypothalamic Amenorrhea

This results from abnormal hypothalamic GnRH secretion in the absence of pathologic processes. There are decreased gonadotropin pulsations, absent follicular development and ovulation, and low estradiol secretion. Serum FSH levels are usually in the normal range; the setting of high FSH:LH ratio is consistent with prepubertal patterns.

It is associated with a number of environmental stressors such as eating disorders and physical or psychological stress. Weight loss, of at least 10% below ideal body weight, and excessive exercise are also associated with hypothalamic amenorrhea. The female athlete triad syndrome is characterized by amenorrhea, eating disorder, and osteopenia or osteoporosis.

Pituitary Defects

Pituitary causes of amenorrhea are rare; most are secondary to hypothalamic dysfunction. However, acquired pituitary dysfunction can ensue from previous local radiation or surgery. Excess iron deposition due to hemochromatosis or hemosiderosis may destroy gonadotropes. Congenital absence of the pituitary is a rare and lethal condition.

Sheehan's syndrome, characterized by postpartum amenorrhea, results from postpartum pituitary necrosis secondary to severe hemorrhage and hypotension.

Surgical ablation and irradiation of the pituitary as management of pituitary tumors also can cause amenorrhea.

Iron deposition in the pituitary may result in destruction of the cells that produce LH and FSH. This occurs only in patients with markedly elevated serum iron levels (i.e., hemosiderosis), usually resulting from extensive red cell destruction like in thalassemia major.

Pituitary microadenomas and macroadenomas also lead to amenorrhea because of elevated prolactin levels. Isolated hyperprolactinemia in the absence of adenoma is an uncommon cause of primary amenorrhea. However, the diagnosis is strongly suggested by a history of galactorrhea. Diagnosis is readily made by evaluating a serum prolactin level. Hypothyroidism may also lead to elevated prolactin levels and thereby lead to amenorrhea.

Ovarian and Ovulatory Dysfunction

Several gonadal disorders can cause amenorrhea. *The most common cause of primary amenorrhea is gonadal dysgenesis.* This group of disorders is usually associated with sex chromosomal abnormalities, resulting in streak gonads, premature depletion of ovarian follicles and oocytes, and absence of estradiol secretion.

Patients present with hypergonadotropic amenorrhea regardless of degree of pubertal development.

- *Primary ovarian failure* is characterized by elevated gonadotropins and low estradiol (*hypergonadotropic hypogonadism*) **(Box 3)**.
- *Secondary ovarian failure* is usually caused by hypothalamic dysfunction and is characterized by normal or low gonadotropins and low estradiol (*hypogonadotropic hypogonadism*) **(Box 4)**.

BOX 3: Causes of primary ovarian failure (hypergonadotropic hypogonadism).

- Gonadal dysgenesis
  - Turner's syndrome (45,XO)
  - Turner variants
  - Pure gonadal dysgenesis (Swyer's syndrome) (46,XX and 46,XY)
- Idiopathic premature ovarian failure
- Steroidogenic enzyme defects
- Testicular regression syndrome
- True hermaphroditism
- Mixed gonadal dysgenesis
- Ovarian resistance syndrome (Savage's syndrome)
- Autoimmune oophoritis
- Postinfection (e.g., mumps)
- Postoophorectomy
- Postirradiation
- Postchemotherapy

BOX 4: Causes of hypoestrogenic amenorrhea (hypogonadotropic hypogonadism).

Hypothalamic dysfunction
- Kallmann's syndrome
- Tumors of hypothalamus (craniopharyngioma)
- Constitutional delay of puberty
- Anorexia nervosa
- Severe weight loss
- Severe stress
- Exercise

Pituitary disorder
- Sheehan's syndrome
- Panhypopituitarism
- Isolated gonadotropin deficiency
- Hemosiderosis (primarily from thalassemia major)

Ovarian Dysgenesis

If the primitive oogonia do not migrate to the genital ridge, streak gonads develop resulting in primary amenorrhea. Two intact X chromosomes are required to maintain normal oocytes. Cytogenetic abnormalities of the X chromosome account for the majority of abnormal ovarian development and function. Fetuses with 45,X karyotype demonstrate normal oocyte number at 20–24 weeks' gestation, but there is accelerated atresia resulting in absence of oocytes at birth. Similarly, women with deletions in either the long or short arm of one X chromosome also develop either primary or secondary amenorrhea.

1. *Gonadal dysgenesis with No Y chromatin:* Turner's syndrome (45,XO or 45,XO,XX mosaics) and 46,XX gonadal dysgenesis are the most common karyotypes. Patients with Turner's syndrome usually present with primary amenorrhea. However, some patients with mosaic abnormalities may menstruate briefly and rarely some have even conceived.
2. *Gonadal dysgenesis with Y chromatin:* Normal female sexual differentiation does not occur in the presence of testicular secretion of anti-Müllerian hormone (AMH) by Sertoli cells and testosterone by Leydig cells. AMH causes regression of Müllerian structures, whereas testosterone and dihydrotestosterone (DHT) promote differentiation of male internal and external genitalia, respectively. A variety of disorders can result in amenorrhea in phenotypic females possessing Y chromatin material.

   Ullrich-Turner syndrome, which presents as a form of early onset vanishing testes syndrome, results from a deletion mutation in the TDF region of Y chromosome. These patients have the 46,XY genotype but do not secrete testosterone or AMH, resulting in feminization of internal and external genitalia. Patients present with primary amenorrhea and gonadal failure. The syndrome is diagnosed by DNA hybridization studies showing abnormality in the short arm of the Y chromosome.

Premature Ovarian Failure

Premature ovarian failure is defined as the occurrence of menopause before age 40 years of age. This is because the ovaries fail secondary to depletion of ova. It is characterized by amenorrhea, increased gonadotropin levels, and estrogen deficiency.

Steroid Enzyme Defects

Genetic females with steroid enzyme defects have normal internal female genitalia and 46,XX karyotype. However, they cannot produce estradiol and thus they fail to menstruate or have breast development.

Congenital adrenal hyperplasia describes one of fifteen known defects in the steroidogenic acute regulatory (STAR) protein, which facilitates cholesterol transport from the outer to the inner mitochondrial membrane. This enzyme catalyzes an early, rate-limiting step in tropic hormone-stimulated steroidogenesis. Patients thus present with hyponatremia, hyperkalemia, and acidosis in infancy. Both XX and XY individuals are phenotypically female. These patients can survive into adulthood given appropriate glucocorticoid and mineralocorticoid supplementation. XX patients may exhibit some secondary sexual characteristics at puberty, but present with amenorrhea and premature ovarian failure due to intraovarian accumulation of cholesterol.

Ovarian Resistance (Savage's Syndrome)

Savage syndrome is characterized with elevated LH and FSH levels, and the ovaries contain primordial germ cells. A defect in the cell receptor mechanism is the thought to be the cause.

Polycystic Ovary Syndrome

Polycystic ovary syndrome (PCOS) is one of the most common causes of secondary amenorrhea. PCOS is the most common cause of ovulatory dysfunction in reproductive-age women.

Diagnosis is based on the presence of at least two of the following characteristics: (1) oligo- or anovulation; (2) clinical and/or biochemical signs of hyperandrogenism; (3) polycystic ovaries; (4) exclusion of other etiologies (congenital adrenal hyperplasia, androgen-secreting tumors, Cushing's syndrome).

Although the exact mechanism is unknown, it appears that insulin resistance and hyperinsulinemia play an important role. Abnormally elevated insulin levels lead to increased androgens via decreased sex hormone-binding globulin, and stimulation of ovarian insulin and insulin-like growth factor-I (IGF-I) receptors.

UTERINE ABNORMALITIES ASSOCIATED WITH AMENORRHEA

The main uterine abnormalities associated with amenorrhea are described in **Table 1**.

TABLE 1: Müllerian abnormalities associated with amenorrhea.

Uterine abnormality	*Comments*
Müllerian agenesis	• Mayer-Rokitansky-Küster-Hauser syndrome • Congenital absence of the uterus and the upper two-thirds of the vagina • 46,XX karyotype • Normally functioning ovaries • Renal and vertebral abnormalities
Vaginal agenesis	Failure of the vagina to develop
Transverse vaginal septum	Failure of fusion of the Müllerian and urogenital sinus-derived portions of the vagina
Imperforate hymen	• If the hymen is imperforate, menstrual efflux cannot occur • An adolescent presents with complaints of primary amenorrhea and cyclic pelvic pain • It may present as back pain or difficulty with defecation or urination secondary to mass effect from vaginal distention • Inspection of the vulva may reveal a purplish-red hymenal membrane bulging outward as a result of accumulation of blood above it (hematocolpos) • Blood may fill the uterus (hematometra) and spill through the fallopian tubes into the peritoneal cavity • Endometriosis and vaginal adenosis are known but not inevitable complications
Asherman's syndrome	• Amenorrhea is caused by intrauterine synechiae • These synechiae develop following the overzealous dilatation and curettage (D&C) or infected products of conception (septic or unsafe abortions) • In our country we must keep in mind the important and still frequent cause of tuberculous endometritis resulting in endometrial cicatrization

AMENORRHEA IN WOMEN WITH 46,XY KARYOTYPE

The sexually undifferentiated male fetal testis secretes Müllerian-inhibiting factor (MIF) and testosterone. MIF promotes regression of all Müllerian structures: the uterine tubes, the uterus, and the upper two-thirds of the vagina. Testosterone and its active metabolite DHT are responsible for embryonic differentiation of the male internal and external genitalia.

Testicular Feminization Syndrome

In testicular feminization, all Müllerian-derived structures are absent. The external genital anlagen and mesonephric ducts cannot respond to androgens because of androgen receptors sensitivity. Affected individuals are therefore phenotypic females lacking a uterus and a complete vagina. They produce some estrogen, develop breasts, and are reared as girls, and therefore present with primary amenorrhea.

Pure Gonadal Dysgenesis

If the primitive germ cells do not migrate to the genital ridge, a testis will not develop, and a streak gonad will be present. Affected individuals have normal female internal and external genitalia, as neither MIF nor androgens are secreted by the streaks. Because these individuals produce no estrogen, they will not develop breasts. They are reared as girls and present clinically with either delayed puberty or primary amenorrhea.

Anorchia

If the fetal testes regress before 7 weeks' gestation, neither MIF nor testosterone is secreted, and affected individuals will present with a clinical picture identical to that of pure gonadal dysgenesis. Individuals whose testes regress between 7 and 13 weeks' gestation present with ambiguous genitalia.

Testicular Steroid Enzyme Defects

A testis with defective enzymes will produce MIF but not testosterone. Affected individuals have female external genitalia and no Müllerian structures. They will be reared as girls and present clinically with either delayed puberty or primary amenorrhea.

DIAGNOSIS

It is absolutely essential to determine, which organ is dysfunctional and then to establish the precise cause so that specific treatment can be advised. Any patient with amenorrhea who has a uterus pregnancy should be first ruled out and serum levels of thyroid-stimulating hormone (TSH) and prolactin estimated. Galactorrhea should be identified by clinical examination.

Diagnosis of Primary Amenorrhea

Flowchart 1 outlines the diagnostic scheme for primary amenorrhea.

Pelvic examination should be done to note the presence of a vagina and uterus and no vaginal septum or imperforate hymen that might result in the failure of appearance of menses. Because pelvic examination of an adolescent girl may be difficult, pelvic ultrasound or examination under anesthesia may be required to establish the presence of a uterus.

If no uterus is present, serum testosterone levels should be measured and karyotyping done to differentiate between Müllerian agenesis and testicular feminization.

Diagnosis of Amenorrhea not Associated with Galactorrhea-Hyperprolactinemia

These patients are evaluated according to the scheme outlined in **Flowchart 2**.

The first step is the progestin challenge, which determines whether the ovary is producing estrogen but not ovulating, hence not producing progesterone. If the endometrium has been primed with estrogen, exogenous progestin will produce menses. Give either medroxyprogesterone acetate, 10 mg orally daily for 5 days, or progesterone, 100–200 mg intramuscularly as a single dose. If vaginal bleeding follows, the ovaries are secreting estrogen. If it does not, it can be concluded that there is no estrogen or that the patient has Asherman's syndrome.

Asherman's syndrome can be ruled out by the estrogen-progesterone challenge test, i.e., administration of conjugated estrogen, 2.5 mg orally daily for 25 days, plus medroxy-progesterone acetate, 10 mg orally on days 16 through 25. Patients with Asherman's syndrome do not bleed following this regimen. Hysterosalpingography and hysteroscopy also help in diagnosing Asherman's syndrome.

In a patient who does not have Asherman's syndrome and who does not respond to the progestin challenge, ovarian dysfunction may be of hypothalamic or ovarian origin.

Flowchart 1: Work-up for primary amenorrhea.

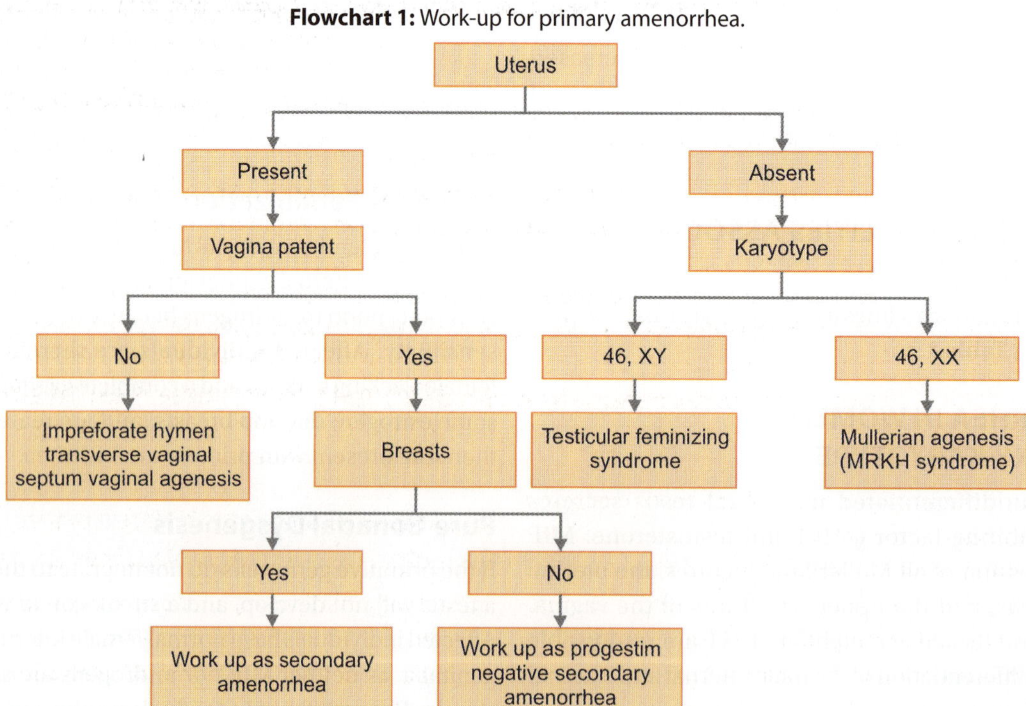

Flowchart 2: Work-up for secondary amenorrhea.

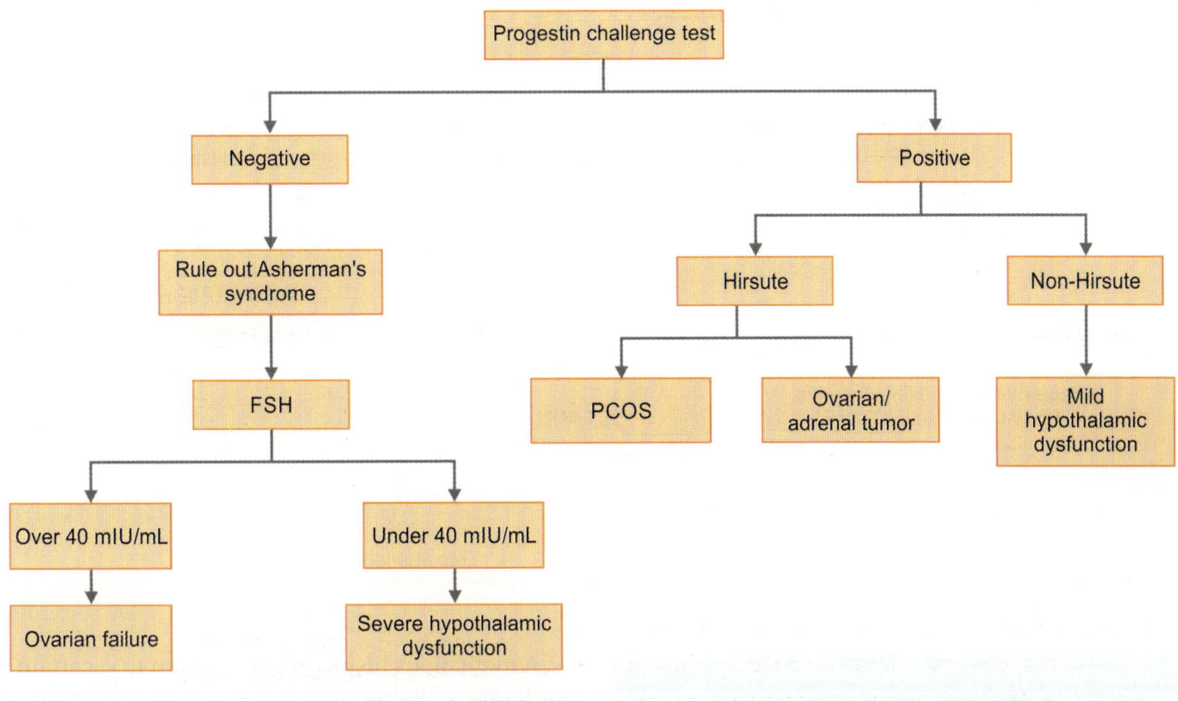

The distinction is based on the FSH level. Primary ovarian dysfunction resulting in low estradiol secretion is associated with high serum FSH.

Diagnosis of Amenorrhea Caused by Primary Ovarian Failure

Karyotyping is indicated for all women who present with premature menopause, particularly if their amenorrhea is primary. Patients with primary amenorrhea may have a steroid enzyme defect. Autoimmune oophoritis is a reversible cause of ovarian failure that must be investigated. **Box 3** lists the causes of primary ovarian failure.

Diagnosis of Amenorrhea Associated with Hypothalamic–Pituitary Dysfunction

Box 4 summarizes the differential diagnosis of hypoestrogenic amenorrhea. The category includes amenorrhea associated with athletic activity, weight loss, or stress.

Differentiation of hypothalamic from pituitary dysfunction can be achieved by giving GnRH, If there is a significant history consistent with Sheehan's syndrome, pituitary function testing is indicated in order to determine the functional capacity of the gland—particularly the integrity of the pituitary–adrenal axis.

Patients who bleed in response to the progestin challenge (i.e., whose ovaries are secreting estrogen) fit into one of four categories: (1) virilized, with or without ambiguous genitalia; (2) hirsute, with polycystic ovaries, hyperthecosis, or mild maturity-onset adrenal hyperplasia; (3) nonhirsute, with hypothalamic dysfunction; or (4) amenorrheic secondary to systemic disease **(Box 5)**. Clinical examination and transvaginal ultrasound may be helpful in making the diagnosis of PCOS. However, 25% of normal patients have polycystic ovaries; consequently, ultrasound cannot be the sole criterion for diagnosis.

BOX 5: Causes of eugonadotropic eugonadism (progestin-challenge positive).

Mild hypothalamic dysfunction
- Psychological disorder
- Emotional stress
- Weight loss
- Obesity
- Exercise induced
- Idiopathic

Hirsutism-virilism
- PCOD
- Ovarian tumor
- Adrenal tumor
- Cushing's syndrome
- Congenital and maturity-onset adrenal hyperplasia

Systemic disease
- Hypothyroidism
- Hyperthyroidism
- Addison's disease
- Chronic renal failure

Diagnosis of Amenorrhea Associated with Galactorrhea-Hyperprolactinemia

Flowchart 3 outlines the diagnostic work-up of patients with galactorrhea or hyperprolactinemia.

Box 6 summarizes the differential diagnosis of galactorrhea-amenorrhea.

Flowchart 3: Work-up for amenorrhea–galactorrhea–hyperprolactinemia.

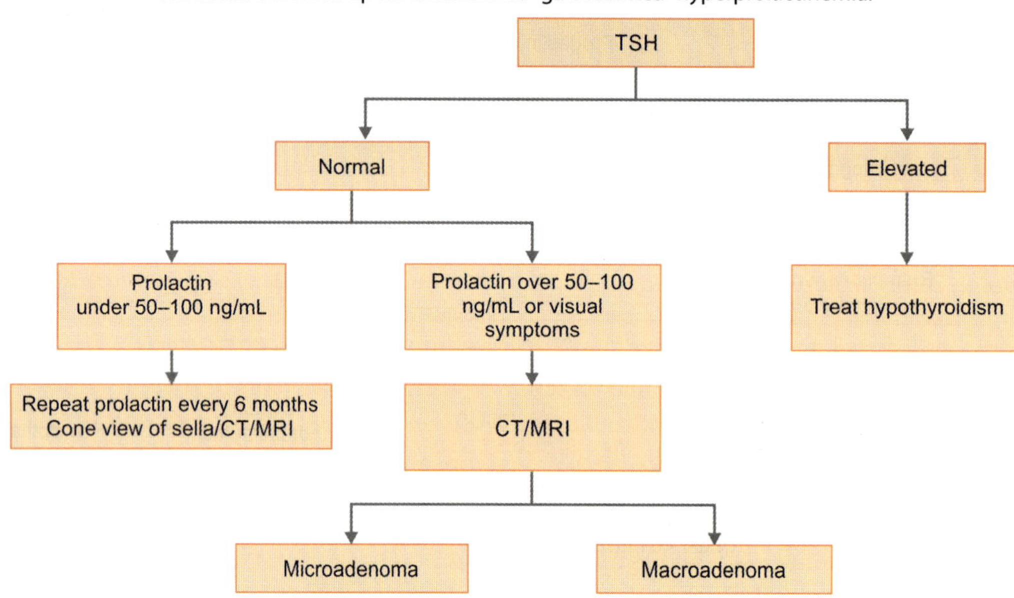

BOX 6: Causes of galactorrhea-hyperprolactinemia.

Pituitary tumors secreting prolactin:
- Macroadenomas (>10 mm)
- Microadenomas (<10 mm)

Hypothyroidism

Idiopathic hyperprolactinemia

Drug-induced hyperprolactinemia
- Dopamine antagonists
  - Phenothiazines
  - Thioxanthenes
  - Butyrophenone
  - Diphenylbutylpiperidine
- Catecholamine-depleting agents
- False transmitters—methyldopa

Interruption of normal hypothalamic–pituitary relationship
- Pituitary stalk section

Peripheral neural stimulation
- Chest wall stimulation
- Nipple stimulation
- Spinal cord lesion

Central nervous system disease
- Encephalitis
- Craniopharyngioma
- Pineal tumors
- Hypothalamic tumors
- Pseudotumor cerebri

Patients with primary hypothyroidism have elevated thyroid-releasing hormone (TRH) levels. TRH acts to stimulate the release of prolactin and may thereby lead to galactorrhea-amenorrhea syndrome. TSH is also elevated and as it is easier to measure, it is the screening test for hypothyroidism.

If prolactin remains elevated or is initially higher than 50-200 ng/mL, the patient should be further studied via cone view of the sella, or computed tomography (CT) or magnetic resonance imaging (MRI) scan of the sella, to rule out pituitary micro- or macroadenoma.

A meticulous history must be taken to ascertain whether the hyperprolactinemia is caused by ingestion of drugs. Prolactin secretion is inhibited by dopamine and stimulated by serotonin and TRH. Any drug that blocks the synthesis or binding of dopamine will increase the prolactin level. Prolactin is increased by serotonin agonists and decreased by serotonin antagonists.

TREATMENT

Management of Patients Desiring Pregnancy: Ovulation Induction

- *Ovulation induction in patients with primary ovarian failure:* Patients with primary ovarian failure can be made to ovulate only under very rarely. Patients with reversible ovarian failure due to autoimmune oophoritis, can be treated with corticosteroids. Otherwise, almost all patients with primary ovarian failure fall into the category of idiopathic premature ovarian failure and cannot be made to ovulate. In vitro IVF with oocytes donation is the only option by which they can have children.
  Any patient with a Y chromosome should undergo oophorectomy to prevent tumor development.
- *Ovulation induction in patients with hypoestrogenic hypothalamic amenorrhea (progestin-challenge negative):* In these patients with low estrogen levels, the pituitary does not release high quantities of LH and FSH.
  Injection of exogenous gonadotropins [human recombinant follicle-stimulating hormone (hrFSH) or human menopausal gonadotropin (hMG)] is usually first-line therapy. Patients showing some ovarian stimulation by clomiphene can be treated with a combination of clomiphene and hMG—the advantage being a reduction in the amount of hMG required and thus a substantial

cost reduction. Ovulation induction with gonadotropins must be carefully monitored with serial ultrasound and estradiol determinations to avoid hyperstimulation.

If a potentially reversible cause of amenorrhea can be identified like marked weight loss, it should be corrected.

- *Ovulation induction in patients who bleed in response to progestin challenge:* Most of these patients respond to clomiphene citrate. The starting dose is 50 mg orally daily for 5 days. This can be increased to a maximum of 250 mg orally daily in 50-mg increments until ovulation is induced. This medication is FDA-approved for use up to 150 mg/d. Ovulation occurs 5–10 days after the last dose.

  Patients with elevated androgens may not respond to clomiphene citrate may respond to combined treatment with an oral hypoglycemic agent (metformin) and clomiphene. If clomiphene therapy with or without metformin is ineffective, gonadotropin therapy may be attempted. Care must be taken in using FSH in these patients, as they are likely to become hyperstimulated.

  Laparoscopic ovarian drilling (LOD) is a surgical method of ovulation induction in PCOS patients. LOD involves electrocautery or laser drilling of the ovarian cortex, with the goal of creating foci of laser or thermal damage in the cortex and ovarian stroma. The mechanism of action may involve destruction of androgen-producing stromal cells, a sudden drop in ovarian androgen levels, improved follicular microenvironment, or increased gonadotropin secretion. This procedure may cause postoperative pelvic adhesions, resulting in tubal compromise.
- *Ovulation induction in patients with amenorrhea-galactorrhea with pituitary macroadenoma:* Dopamine agonist drugs such as cabergoline and bromocriptine are the first-line treatment of hyperprolactinemia of any cause, including macroadenomas. These drugs can decrease prolactin secretion and tumor size. Surgical therapy, trans-sphenoidal or frontal removal of the pituitary adenoma or the entire gland, may be required if tumor size or secretion are resistant to dopamine agonists; the lesion is rapidly enlarging or causing symptoms such as visual changes or headaches; or in women with giant adenomas (>3 cm) who wish to discontinue agonist treatment for conception and the duration of pregnancy.
- *Ovulation induction in patients with amenorrhea-galactorrhea without macroadenoma (including patients with microadenomas):* These patients ovulate readily in response to dopamine agonist treatment, with dose titrated until serum prolactin is normal. Patients are maintained on the lowest dose. Once pregnancy has been achieved, the agent can be discontinued. Patients with macroadenomas may need to continue therapy throughout pregnancy to avoid further growth of the lesion.

  Patients taking drugs that raise the prolactin level should discontinue them if possible, but continued use of such drugs is not a contraindication to therapy.
- *Ovulation induction in patients with hypothyroidism:* Amenorrheic patients with hypothyroidism respond to thyroid replacement therapy.

Management of Patients not Desiring Pregnancy

Patients who are hypoestrogenic must be treated with a combination of estrogen and progesterone to maintain bone density and prevent genital atrophy. Oral contraceptives are effective replacement therapy for most women.

Combinations of 0.625–1.25 mg of conjugated estrogens orally daily on days 1 through 25 of the cycle with 5–10 mg of medroxyprogesterone acetate on days 16 through 25 are an alternative. Calcium intake should be 1–1.5 g of elemental calcium daily.

Patients who respond to the progestin challenge require progestin administration to prevent the development of endometrial hyperplasia and carcinoma. Oral contraceptive pills may be used for regularization of the menstrual cycle. Alternatively, medroxyprogesterone acetate, 10 mg orally daily for 10–13 days every month or every other month, is sufficient to induce withdrawal bleeding and to prevent the development of endometrial hyperplasia.

Patients with hyperprolactinemia need periodic prolactin measurements and radiographic cone views of the sella turcica to check for the development of macroadenoma.

Management of Uterine Causes of Amenorrhea: Surgical Treatment

The surgical treatment of uterine causes of amenorrhea is given in **Table 2**.

SEQUELAE

The complications of amenorrhea can be numerous, ranging from infertility to psychosocial developmental delays with lack of normal physical sexual development. Hypoestrogenic patients can develop severe osteoporosis and fractures. The complications associated with amenorrhea in patients who respond to progestin challenge are endometrial hyperplasia and carcinoma resulting from unopposed estrogen stimulation.

CONCLUSION

The overall prognosis for amenorrhea is good. One must remember and reiterate to the patient and her relatives that it is usually not a life-threatening clinical event and with proper evaluation the precise etiology can be diagnosed and treated.

Many patients with hypothalamic amenorrhea will spontaneously recover normal menstrual cycles. Virtually all amenorrheic women who do not have premature ovarian failure can be made to ovulate with a dopamine agonist, clomiphene citrate, insulin-sensitizing agents, and gonadotropins.

TABLE 2: Surgical treatment of uterine causes of amenorrhea.

Uterine abnormality	*Surgical treatment*
Müllerian agenesis	• Treatment should be offered when the patient is contemplating sexual activity involves creation of neovagina • Nonsurgical creation of a vagina using serial vaginal dilators (Franks/Ingrams) • McIndoe procedure involves the creation of a cavity by dissection between the urethra and bladder anteriorly and the perineal body and rectum posteriorly. The cavity is lined by a split-thickness skin graft overlying a plastic or soft silicone mold • Laparoscopic vaginoplasty (Vecchietti procedure)
Vaginal agenesis	Same as Müllerian agenesis
Transverse vaginal septum	• If the diagnosis of a complete septum is established prior to menarche, it should be incised, creating an aperture to allow drainage • Incision of a complete septum is most easily accomplished when the upper vagina is distended and the membrane is bulging, reducing the risk of injury to adjacent structures • Surgical correction of vaginal narrowing should be performed only when the patient is contemplating initiation of sexual activity • End-to-end reanastomosis of the upper and lower vaginal mucosa, which may be accomplished with the aid of a Lucite bridge
Imperforate hymen	Hymenectomy involving a cruciate incision on the hymenal membrane to drain the collected menstrual blood and maintain patency of the vaginal tract
Asherman's syndrome	Hysteroscopic adhesiolysis with postprocedure estrogenic stimulation of the endometrium

FURTHER READING

1. Aloi JA. Evaluation of amenorrhea. Compr Ther. 1995;21(10):575-8.
2. American College of Obstetricians and Gynecologists. ACOG Practice Bulletin. Clinical management guidelines for obstetrician-gynecologists: number 41, December 2002. Obstet Gynecol. 2002;100:1389-402.
3. American College of Obstetricians and Gynecologists. Amenorrhea (ACOG Technical Bulletin 128). Washington, DC: ACOG; 1989.
4. Anasti JN. Premature ovarian failure: an update. Fertil Steril. 1998;70:1-15.
5. ASRM. Practice Committee of the American Society for Reproductive Medicine. Current evaluation of amenorrhea. Fertil Steril. 2004;82(Suppl 1):S33-9.
6. Folch M, Pigem I, Konje JC. Müllerian agenesis: etiology, diagnosis, and management. Obstet Gynecol Surv. 2000;55:644-9.
7. Laufer MR, Floor AE, Parsons KE, Kuntz KM, Barbieri RL. Hormone testing in women with adult onset amenorrhea. Gynecol Obstet Invest. 1995;40:200-3.
8. McIver B, Romanski SA, Nippoldt TB. Evaluation and management of amenorrhea. Mayo Clin Proc. 1997;72:1161-9.
9. Pickett CA. Diagnosis and management of pituitary tumors: recent advances. Prim Care. 2003;30:765-89.
10. Pletcher JR, Slap GB. Menstrual disorders. Pediatr Clin North Am. 1999;46:505-18.
11. Speroff L, Fritz MA. Amenorrhea. In: Clinical Gynecologic Endocrinology and Infertility, 7th edition. Philadelphia: Lippincott Williams and Wilkins; 2005. pp. 401-64.

LONG QUESTIONS

1. Enumerate the causes of primary amenorrhea and discuss how you would go about managing such a case?
2. Describe the surgical management in case of primary amenorrhea.

SHORT QUESTIONS

1. What are secondary sexual characters and how does one assess them?
2. Discuss the evaluation and management of a case of Mullerian agenesis.
3. Describe the events leading to menarche.
4. What is ovarian dysgenesis and how to manage it?

MULTIPLE CHOICE QUESTIONS

1. All are causes of primary amenorrhea, except:
   a. MRKH syndrome
   b. Turners syndrome
   c. Androgen insensitivity syndrome
   d. Sheehan's syndrome
2. All are features of Turner's syndrome, except:
   a. Webbed neck b. Enlarged breasts
   c. Cubitus valgus d. Aortic coarctation
3. The karyotype in testicular feminization syndrome is:
   a. 46XX b. 46XY
   c. 45XO d. 47XXY
4. All are features of normal female puberty, except:
   a. Growth spurt b. Thelarche
   c. Adrenarche d. Menarche
   e. Pubarche
5. Cryptomenorrhea is associated with:
   a. Bicornuate uterus b. Hypoplastic uterus
   c. Imperforate hymen d. Arcuate uterus

Answers

1. d 2. b 3. b 4. c 5. c

8.2 PCOS IN ADOLESCENCE

Ameet Patki, Mrinmayi Dharmadhikari

INTRODUCTION

Polycystic ovary syndrome (PCOS) is one of the most common endocrine disorders in women. It is a complex trait arising from an interaction of heritable influences and environmental factors. PCOS in adolescents should be considered a separate entity altogether and controversy continues about the etiopathogenesis, diagnostic criteria and recommendations for PCOS in adolescents. This is primarily because the diagnostic criteria and pathological and clinical features of PCOS used for diagnosis in adult women overlap the normal pubertal physiological events. It is important to distinguish between the two entities in adolescents before diagnosing one with PCOS. In recent times, these deficiencies have been recognized and a number of evidence-based expert recommendations have become more available to guide clinicians. It is of utmost importance that clinicians be cognizant of the fact that PCOS is associated not only with metabolic but also psychological comorbidity. These issues should be addressed in a holistic manner.

Physiological pubertal changes and etiopathogenesis of PCOS in adolescence: The pathogenesis of PCOS **(Flowchart 1)** can be explained as a "two-hit" hypothesis. Hereditary predisposition being the "first hit" with manifestation in the presence of a stimulatory factor, which is the "second hit".[1]

While diagnosing PCOS in adolescents, it is important to keep in mind the normal physiological changes that take place in puberty as many features of PCOS are very similar to normal pubertal changes. Onset of puberty begins with the maturation of the hypothalamopituitary-ovarian (HPO) axis. This results in the release of gonadotrophin-releasing hormone (GnRH) in a pulsatile manner. The activity of this hormone is suppressed during childhood and it appears that puberty is restrained by certain higher central nervous system controls. With the release of GnRH hormone, varying GnRH pulse frequencies act on the pituitary gland triggering the release of luteinizing hormone (LH) and follicle-stimulating hormone (FSH). These in turn stimulate the ovarian theca and granulosa cells, respectively. Gonadal steroids are produced as a response to increased gonadotropin stimulation accompanied by secondary sexual development, which follows a well-described pattern of changes. The pubertal growth spurt is due to an increased growth hormone production, which is initiated by sex steroids in consortium with the local production of growth factors. Menarche is the result of a positive feedback mechanism taking place by mid-puberty or later. Production of dehydroepiandrosterone (DHEA) and dehydroepiandrosterone sulfate (DHEAS) is by the adrenal gland and typically increases around age 6–7 years. It takes place independent of thelarche and menarche. DHEA and DHEAS influence pubic as well as axillary hair development as a part of secondary sexual characteristics.

The central cause of PCOS is androgen excess as a result of functional ovarian hyperandrogenism (FOH). Increased androgen levels, primarily by the ovaries, interfere with hypothalamic sensitivity to negative feedback from the ovary in turn increasing GnRH pulse frequency.[2] This persistently rapid pulse frequency of GnRH favors increased LH secretion,[3] which in turn stimulates the ovarian theca cells to produce more androgens. The relative decrease in FSH secretion leads to less aromatization of androgens to estradiol and impaired follicular development, resulting in the prolonged periods of oligomenorrhea that are the characteristic of PCOS.

The major features of the syndrome, i.e., hirsutism, anovulation, and polycystic ovaries on ultrasound are usually an effect of hyperandrogenism, which leads to all these features in an interlinking fashion.

In addition, certain metabolic changes that are associated with PCOS are also seen physiologically during puberty. For instance, hyperinsulinemia is seen in healthy adolescents. The insulin sensitivity decreases by about 50% in adolescence with a compensatory rise in insulin secretion, which later returns to prepubertal levels in adulthood.[4,5] However, both insulin resistance and hyperinsulinemia are more severe in adolescents with PCOS as compared to adolescents without PCOS.[6] Insulin stimulates ovarian theca cells to synthesize androgens[7] and inhibits hepatic production of sex hormone-binding globulin.[8] Collectively, these effects result in increased circulating free androgens, thus perpetuating the underlying pathophysiology of PCOS. In addition, insulin resistance promotes release of non-esterified fatty acids (NEFA) from the liver and adipose tissue due to decreased lipoprotein lipase activity, which results in the dyslipidemia that is associated with PCOS.

DIAGNOSTIC CRITERIA

Polycystic ovary morphology (PCOM) is one of the major diagnostic criteria of PCOS in adults. However, it is currently not recommended for the diagnosis of PCOS in adolescents. As such, the diagnosis of PCOS in adolescents currently is based on evidence of ovulatory dysfunction and androgen excess **(Box 1)**.

Ovulatory dysfunction incorporates a number of menstrual abnormalities in adolescents. All the following are manifestations of ovulatory dysfunction:

- Oligomenorrhea with menstrual intervals >90 days even in the first postmenarcheal year

- Two or more years after menarche, if menstrual intervals are persistently less than 21 or more than 45 days 2 or more years after menarche
- Absence of menarche by 15 years of age or 2–3 years after thelarche.

Androgen excess in PCOS in adolescents is evidenced by:
- Hirsutism (moderate to severe)
- Persistent acne, which is unresponsive to topical therapy.
- Persistent elevation of serum total and/or free testosterone level.

These adolescent-specific diagnostic criteria are important because the diagnostic criteria for PCOS used in adults have been problematic when applied to adolescents. This is because first, anovulatory cycles are frequent in adolescents especially just after menarche. This is due to the progressive maturation of the HPO axis. Hence, menstrual irregularity is also a common feature in adolescents. Second, the common signs of hyperandrogenism in adults are less reliable as far as adolescents are concerned, because hirsutism is a developmental phase feature and so is acne vulgaris. Third, measurement of testosterone concentrations in adolescents is problematic due to increase in their levels during anovulatory cycles, which are normally seen in pubertal years till complete maturation of the HPO axis. Normal androgen levels in adolescent girls have not yet been reliably established. Also, the extent to which adolescent hyperandrogenism predicts adult hyperandrogenism is not clear. Fourth, PCOM by adult standards is common in adolescents. This calls for different diagnostic criteria for PCOS in adolescents.

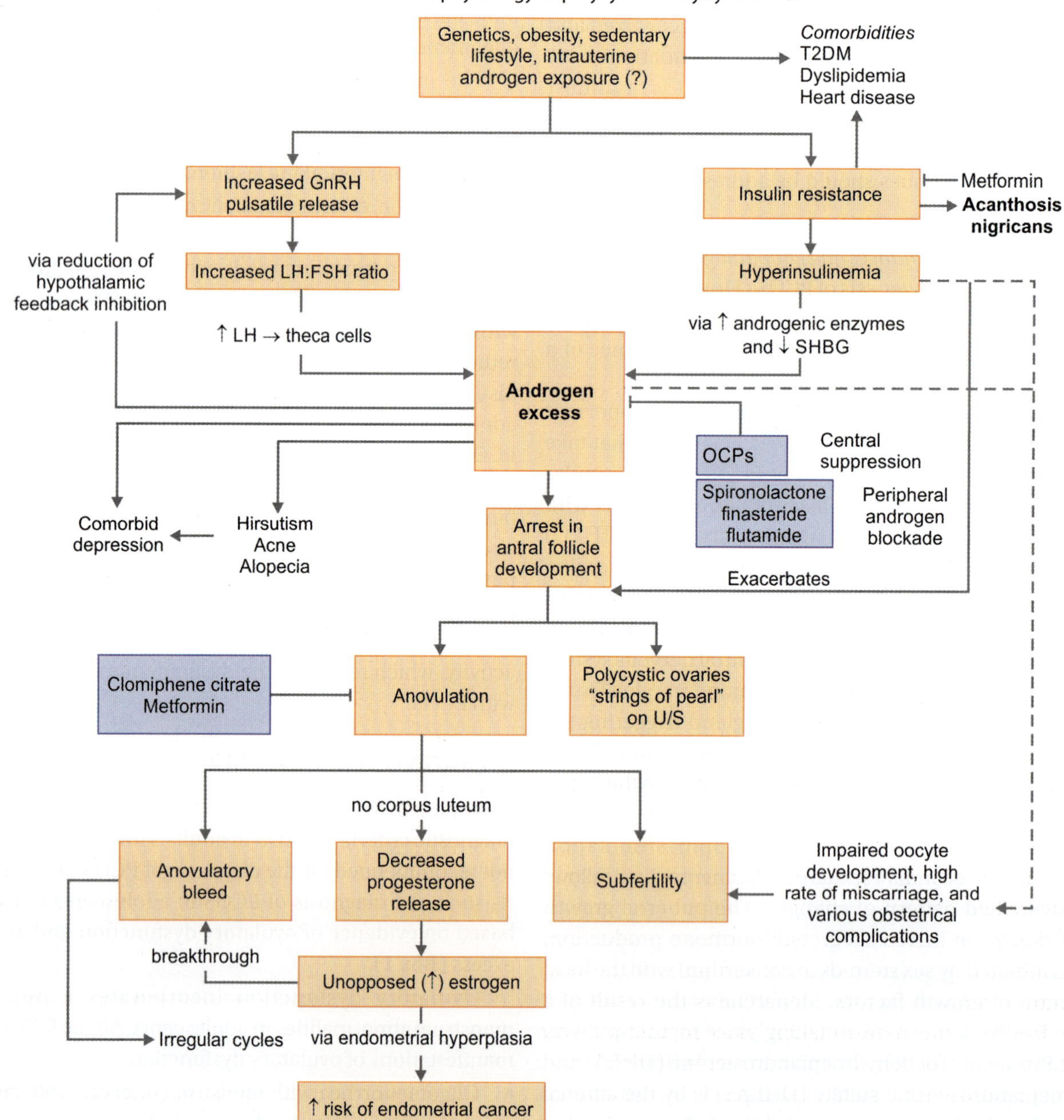

Flowchart 1: Pathophysiology of polycystic ovary syndrome.

BOX 1: Diagnostic criteria for PCOS.[9]

Adult diagnostic criteria (Rotterdam)

Otherwise unexplained alternative phenotypes:

- Phenotype 1 (classic PCOS)[a]
  - Clinical and/or biochemical evidence of hyperandrogenism
  - Evidence of oligoanovulation
  - Ultrasonographic evidence of a polycystic ovary
- Phenotype 2 (Essential NIH Criteria)*
  - Clinical and/or biochemical evidence of hyperandrogenism
  - Evidence of oligo-anovulation
- Phenotype 3 (ovulatory PCOS)*
  - Clinical and/or biochemical evidence of hyperandrogenism
  - Ultrasonographic evidence of a polycystic ovary
- Phenotype 4 (nonhyperandrogenic PCOS)
  - Evidence of oligo-anovulation
  - Ultrasonographic evidence of a polycystic ovary

Adolescent diagnostic criteria

Otherwise unexplained combination of:

- Abnormal uterine bleeding pattern
  - Abnormal for age or gynecologic age
  - Persistent symptoms for 1–2 years
- Evidence of hyperandrogenism
  - Persistent testosterone elevation above adult norms in a reliable reference laboratory is the best evidence.
  - Moderate-severe hirsutism is clinical evidence of hyperandrogenism

*AE-PCOS recognizes only hyperandrogenic phenotypes

CLINICAL PRESENTATION

Major clinical manifestations include:

- Abnormal uterine bleeding–irregular cycles/ heavy menstrual bleeding
- Cutaneous hyperandrogenism–Primarily hirsutism and persistent acne
- Obesity and insulin resistance.

Ovarian Findings

Anovulation: In adolescents, the distinction between abnormal and physiologic anovulation is often delayed because patients, families, and clinicians alike often are unsure approximately the normal range of menstrual cycle variation. There is very slight variation in normal adolescent menstrual cycles and menstrual cyclicity in reproductive-age adults. Cycles shorter than 19 days or longer than 90 days are abnormal at any stage; 75% of menstrual cycles range from 21 to 45 days during the first postmenarcheal (gynecologic) year, and 95% of girls achieve 21–40-day adult menstrual cyclicity by their fifth gynecologic year.[9-11]

Physiologic adolescent anovulation presents a paradox: the proportion of cycles that occur at regular intervals is substantially greater than mature ovulatory cycles.[12] This means that "adolescent anovulation" is asymptomatic, with cyclic menstrual bleeding occurring at regular intervals even in the first postmenarcheal year.[9] This is due to immature cyclic ovarian function. Immature cyclic follicular development is occurring in theses cycles, however, corpus luteum formation is inadequate to produce serum progesterone levels sufficient to support implantation and pregnancy.[12]

The following menstrual abnormalities suggest an ovulatory dysfunction in adolescents.[9,11]

- Primary amenorrhea: Absence of onset of menses by 15 years of age (or by 15 years bone age, if puberty onset was early) or more than three years after thelarche.
- Secondary amenorrhea: Interval of > 90 days between two menstrual periods after menarche.
- Oligomenorrhea: During the first five postmenarcheal years, the definition of oligomenorrhea varies:
  - *Postmenarcheal year 2:* Fewer than four periods in the year (average cycle length >90 days between menstrual periods).
  - *Postmenarcheal year 2:* Fewer than six periods in the year (average cycle length >60 days).
  - *Postmenarcheal year 3-5:* Fewer than eight periods per year, i.e., missing more than four periods per year (average cycle length >45 days).
  - *Postmenarcheal year 6 and after:* Fewer than nine periods per year, i.e., missing more than three periods per year (average cycle length >38–40 days). This is the adult criterion.
- *Excessive uterine bleeding:* Interval of less than 21 days (or 19 days in year 1) between two menstrual cycles or excessive amount of bleeding (i.e., bleeding lasting more than 7 days or complete soakage of a pad or tampon every 1–2 hours).

Polycystic ovary syndrome is the most common cause of excessive uterine bleeding[13] due to a hyperplastic endometrium exposed to insufficient progesterone and excess estrogen. It is commonly termed "anovulatory" uterine bleeding. However, endometrial biopsy in the broader population of patients with excessive nonstructural bleeding demonstrates that very few are completely acyclic and often shows evidence of diverse types of ovulatory dysfunction, including secretory changes consistent with luteal insufficiency and sometimes cystic glandular hyperplasia, which is a direct effect of androgen excess.[14]

Symptomatic adolescent anovulation manifesting as irregular menstrual cycles is almost always the result of anovulatory cycles. This, if persistent can lead to PCOS in adulthood.

Anovulatory adolescents with hyperandrogenemia are at a greater risk for persistent anovulation and menstrual dysfunction. The nonhyperandrogenemic ones transient cases of menstrual irregularities due to physiologic anovulation. The hyperandrogenemic cases of anovulation, which persist are mostly PCOS, and the nonhyperandrogenic cases, which are persistent have some form of hypogonadism.

Hyperandrogenic adolescents should be labeled as having PCOS, if the menstrual abnormality has persisted for 2 years or more. It was recommended that those with ongoing menstrual abnormality that has not yet persisted for 2 years be assigned the provisional diagnosis, "at-risk for PCOS", to avoid misdiagnosing physiological pubertal changes as PCOS. Frequent longitudinal re-evaluations of these patients were recommended.[15] These recommendations emphasize on the accuracy of diagnosis than on early diagnosis. However, earlier initiation of diagnostic testing is advisable in cases of irregular cycles wherein treatment is to be initiated either for regularization or for the management of comorbidities associated with PCOS (e.g., development of hirsutism, moderate inflammatory acne resistant to topical therapy, and acanthosis nigricans). This is because delaying diagnosis also delays control of symptoms and increases the risk of developing endometrial hyperplasia and carcinoma. In cases of excessive uterine bleeding there may be a need for emergency evaluation earlier in the course. Primary amenorrhea should be evaluated when recognized.

In adolescents in whom a provisional diagnosis of PCOS has been made, the recommendation for longitudinal re-evaluation requires withdrawing oral contraceptive pills for approximately three months once the patient is gynecologically mature to determine persistence of hyperandrogenic anovulation.

While PCOS often begins during adolescence, it sometimes cannot be definitively diagnosed because the menstrual abnormality does not become apparent until 3 years or more after the onset of menarche.[9,16]

Polycystic ovaries: In adults, PCOM has been defined as an ovary with a volume >10.0 mL by a simplified formula or a small antral follicle (2–9 mm diameter) count ≥ 12 per ovary on ultrasound examination.[17]

Adult PCOM criteria cannot be applied reliably for diagnosing PCOS in adolescents; one of the reasons, being need for abdominal ultrasound approach in virginal adolescents. Hence, an accurate analysis of antral follicle count cannot be made.[18] Even if a precise follicle count is obtained by other imaging modalities like MRI, it is not a reliable parameter for diagnosis of PCOM in adolescents as the adult criteria for PCOM overlaps with the criteria for multifollicular ovaries. Multifollicular ovaries are defined by the presence of ≥6 follicles of 4–10 mm diameter but without an increase in ovarian volume. It is a normal variant not related to hyperandrogenism.[15]

Ovarian volume is slightly larger in adolescents than in adults.[15,19] Hence, if adult criteria for PCOS was to be applied to adolescents, one-third to half of normal adolescents would meet adult criteria for PCOM.[20] To avoid incorrect diagnosis, current evidence suggests that a mean ovarian volume >12 cc (or single ovary >15 cc) should be taken as enlarged ovaries in adolescents.[15,19,20]

Therefore, due to the lack of appropriate criteria for PCOM in adolescents, it is not recommended as a diagnostic criterion in adolescent PCOS.

Hirsutism is defined clinically as an abnormal amount of sexual hair appearing in a male distribution pattern.[22] Ferriman-Gallwey classification system **(Fig. 1)** quantitates the extent of hair growth in the most androgen-sensitive areas and is used for grading hirsutism.

Hypertrichosis, on the other hand, is the generalized excessive growth of vellus hair distributed in a nonsexual pattern. Excess androgen secretion, though not a cause of hypertrichosis, can aggravate this condition. This is sometimes hereditary or seen in patients taking certain drugs like glucocorticoids, phenytoin, diazoxide, or cyclosporine. Most hyperandrogenic females have hirsutism or some pilosebaceous unit response to excess androgen ("hirsutism equivalent"), like acne. In some, however there is insensitivity of the pilosebaceous unit to androgens and hirsutism does not occur. Though hirsutism is a manifestation of hyperandrogenism it may occur in the absence of excess androgens. This is called idiopathic hirsutism.[21]

Acne: Acne vulgaris is a variably expressed manifestation of hyperandrogenemia in adolescents. This again is a pubertal, physiological manifestation in adolescent girls, especially comedonal acne. Acne severity can be graded on the basis of number of lesions. Hyperandrogenemia should be suspected in the presence of moderate (>10 facial lesions) or severe inflammatory acne in adolescent girls in the perimenarcheal years.[10,22] There is consensus that acne vulgaris that is moderate-to-severe inflammatory and is poorly responsive to topical or oral antibiotic treatment is an indication to test for hyperandrogenemi.[15]

Others: Balding is an unusual manifestation of hyperandrogenemia in adolescents. Other uncommon manifestation include seborrhea, hyperhidrosis, and hidradenitis suppurativa.

Frank virilization should urge investigations for other causes of hyperandrogenemia. Clinical features include rapid onset or progression of hirsutism, temporal hairline regression, increased muscle bulk, voice deepening and clitoromegaly.

Associated metabolic features: The other metabolic manifestations associated with PCOS should also be dealt with. These include obesity, insulin resistance and its associated manifestations like acanthosis nigricans. These are strongly associated with PCOS; however are not a part of the diagnostic criteria. Other comorbidities include metabolic syndrome, sleep-disordered breathing, and nonalcoholic fatty liver disease. Insulin resistance plays a key role in the pathogenesis of PCOS due to dysregulated steroidogenesis and excessive androgen production.

Adolescents with PCOS are at increased risk of a number of comorbidities in later years. These include impaired glucose intolerance and can lead to diabetes mellitus (type 2) later on.

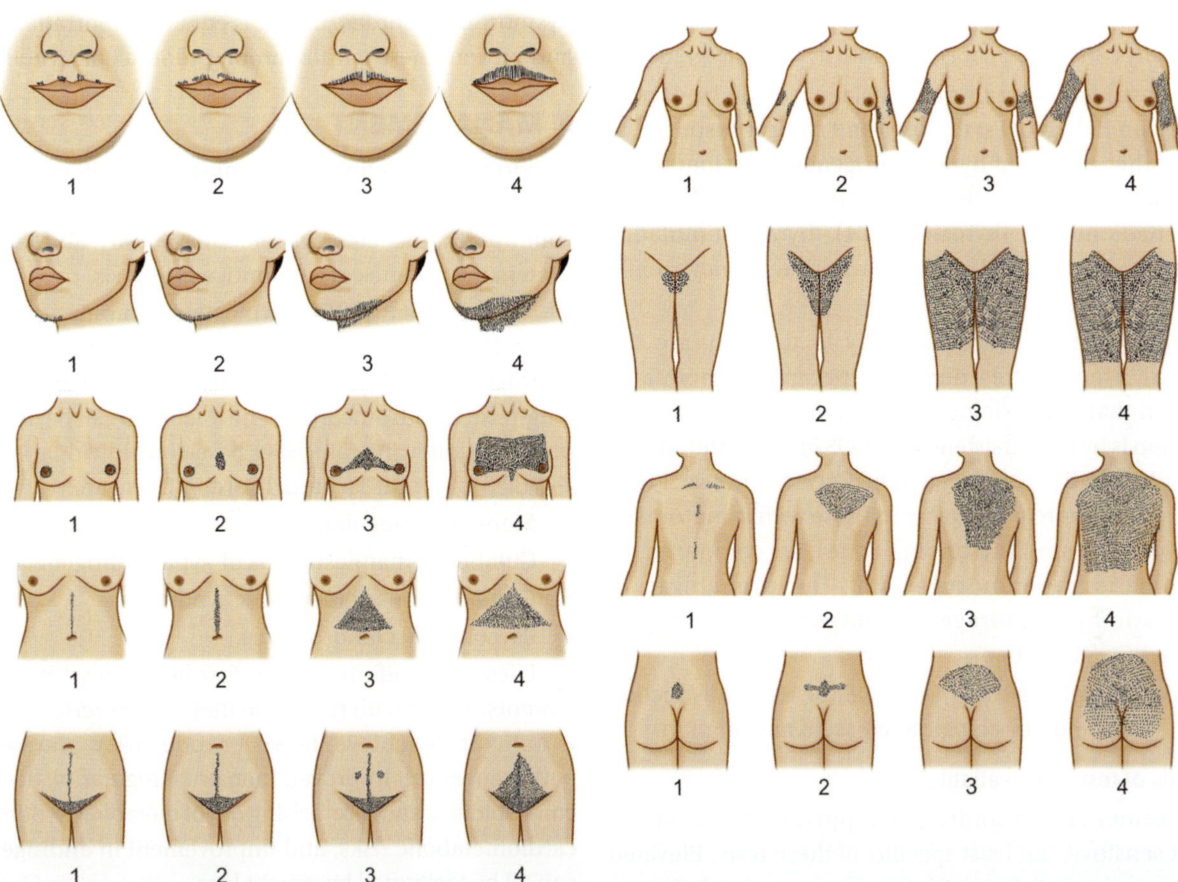

Fig. 1: The Ferriman-Gallwey scale for hirsutism. A score of 1 to 4 is given for nine areas of the body. A total score less than 8 is considered normal, a score of 8 to 15 indicates mild hirsutism, and a score greater than 15 indicates moderate or severe hirsutism. A score of 0 indicates absence of terminal hair.

Approximately 10% of women with PCOS will have type-2 diabetes mellitus by 40 years of age.[23-25]

LABORATORY EVALUATION AND DIFFERENTIAL DIAGNOSIS

The most important differential diagnosis of PCOS in adolescents is physiologic adolescent anovulation which causes confusion and delay in early diagnosis of PCOS in adolescents. Other causes are relatively rare. Screening for nonclassic congenital adrenal hyperplasia (NCCAH) is recommended as it is the most common pathological disorder which closely mimics PCOS. It, however, accounts for only ~5% of anovulation due to hyperandrogenism.[15] Other endocrine disorders like hypothyroidism and hyperprolactinemia should also be ruled out. Other than menstrual abnormalities, central obesity, and hirsutism, commonly associated with PCOS can mimic Cushing's syndrome.

The approach to the differential diagnosis of menstrual disorders due to anovulation in adolescents:

- Thorough medical history and physical examination
- Urine pregnancy test in cases of amenorrhea to rule out pregnancy
- Laboratory tests such as LH, FSH, TSH, prolactin.

Determination of the serum gonadotropins LH and FSH helps in the diagnosis of hypogonadotropic hypogonadism of neuroendocrine origin(low LH, FSH) whereas high FSH, LH suggests primary gonadal failure and a further screening for associated causes of primary ovarian failure.

Hyperandrogenism investigations include serum total and free testosterone, DHEAS and serum 17-hydroxyprogesterone (17-OHP) level. Over and above this the workup is individualized depending on clinical suspicion.

Serum testosterone (total and/or free) levels are slightly raised in PCOS. However, levels more than 200 ng/mL should provoke a further investigation to rule out adrenal and ovarian androgen producing tumors (USG pelvis, CT/MRI).

DHEAS levels may also be slightly raised in PCOS. However, levels more than 8 ng/mL should raise suspicion of adrenal gland tumors. A screening for the same should be performed (CT/MRI).

A17-OHP level should ideally be performed at 8 AM due to diurnal variation. A 17-OHP level > 200 ng/dL (6.0 nmol/L) is suggestive of nonclassical congenital adrenal hyperplasia. An ACTH test is advised to confirm the diagnosis in such cases.

Measurements of total and/or free testosterone have been the most recommended hormone determinations to document hyperandrogenemia.[26-28] In assays using an extraction step, total testosterone concentrations >55 ng/dL are generally considered consistent with hyperandrogenism.[29]

Additional laboratory workup as needed can be carried out based on individual symptoms and clinical suspicion to rule out other causes of hyperandrogenemia or menstrual irregularity. Generally, this work up includes: 17-OHP, androstenedione, free thyroxine (FT4), thyroid-stimulating hormone (TSH), LH, FSH, and prolactin. Pregnancy should be ruled out in all patients.

Currently, the only certain way to differentiate the menstrual irregularities due to hyperandrogenemia of PCOS from that of physiologic hyperandrogenic adolescent anovulation is by the persistence of PCOS into adulthood. The latter resolves with two postmenarcheal years, however, PCOS persists. This is more predictable in those with symptomatic hyperandrogenism (hirsutism, acne) as compared to asymptomatic hyperandrogenism. The probability of symptomatic hyperandrogenic adolescents resulting in persistent PCOS is higher.

By diagnosing FOH it may be possible to make a distinction between PCOS and physiologic adolescent anovulation.

Two kinds of tests are available

1. A dexamethasone androgen-suppression test is the most sensitive, but least specific, of these tests: Elevated testosterone post-dexamethasone suppression indicates a non-adrenal source, which is usually ovarian indicative of FOH pointing toward PCOS as the likely cause.
2. The more specific test involves administering either a test dose of GnRH agonist or of human chorionic gonadotropin and determining the 17-OHP level 20–24 hours later. Hyper-response of 17-OHP is indicative of FOH.

EVALUATION OF COMORBIDITIES

Polycystic ovary syndrome is associated with a significant metabolic and psychological morbidity. As already discussed this includes

- Insulin resistance and hyperinsulinemia
- Overweight and obesity
- Metabolic syndrome, impaired glucose tolerance, and type 2 diabetes.

The glucose level measured 2 hours after an oral glucose challenge test is reliable screening test for impaired glucose tolerance.

Lifestyle counseling, which includes dietary modifications and exercise goes a long way in the management of these patients.

Appropriate counseling with respect to diet is important as many adolescents fall prey to eating disorders and associated complications (anorexia nervosa, bulimia nervosa) due to weight gain and obesity.

Increased prevalence of depression and anxiety has been documented attributed to obesity, acne, hirsutism, body dysmorphic disorders, and it is equally important to identify and prevent these entities among adolescents with PCOS.

MANAGEMENT

Importantly, a definitive diagnosis of PCOS is not needed to initiate treatment. Treatment may decrease risk of future comorbidity (diabetes, dyslipidemia, obesity, and subfertility) even in the absence of a definitive diagnosis.

The treatment of PCOS is mostly symptomatic and hence, individualization is important. Goals of treatment are to improve the quality of life and to reduce adverse effects on long-term health outcomes. The treatment can be undertaken under the following categories based on individual symptoms as PCOS is a multi-faceted disorder. These are:

- Menstrual irregularities
- Cutaneous manifestations of hyperandrogenemia
- Comorbidities of metabolic syndrome
- Psycological comorbidities.

Lifestyle modification is the first-line management in these patients. This is with respect to diet and exercise. Weight loss is difficult to achieve, however motivation plays a role in persistent effort. Improved menstrual regularity, decrease in comorbidities and risks arising out of metabolic syndrome like cardiometabolic risks, and improvement in androgen levels can all be facilitated by weight loss.

COCs-Cyclic administration of estrogen-progestin in the form of combined oral contraceptive pills is the first-line pharmacotherapy of most adolescents for regularization of menstrual cycle. These inhibit the endogenous HPO axis and normalize the ovarian and endometrial cycle. This provides protection against the ill-effects of continuous unopposed estrogenic action, which can result in endometrial hyperplasia leading to heavy menstrual bleeding after months of amenorrhea as well as endometrial carcinoma due to hyperestrogenemia in anovulatory cycles. These also inhibit ovarian function and increase the sex-hormone binding globulins thereby decreasing androgen levels in the body. These actions make them optimal both for treating menstrual irregularities and as adjuncts treatments for hirsutism and acne. Progestin monotherapy is an alternative to COCs for the control of menstrual irregularity for those in whom estrogen is contraindicated (e.g., those at a risk of thromboembolism). Progestins alone, however do not have a significant effect on hyperandrogenic manifestations.

Antiandrogens: Spironolactone is a potent antiandrogen that can be used in conjunction with COC or metformin in cases of hyperandrogenism. It also has a positive effect on menstrual irregularities. A contraceptive method is indicated in sexually active adolescents while using spironolactone as it is potentially teratogenic. COCs containing cyproterone acetate and drospirenone as components further help in the hyperandrogenic manifestations besides regularizing the menstrual cycle. In a pilot study, intermittent low-dose oral finasteride was reported effective for treatment of hirsutism in adolescent girls with PCOS or idiopathic hirsutism.[30] Cosmetic methods of hair removal like electrolysis and laser hair removal therapies have also become more prevalent over recent times due to their affordability. Eflornithine cream for hair removal either alone or in conjunction with laser hair removal is also used in cases of hirsutism.

Insulin-sensitizers: Metformin has been recommended in women with PCOS along with impaired glucose tolerance or type 2 diabetes with no improvement with diet and exercise alone. Metformin was found to be as effective as COC for treatment of hirsutism in adolescents with PCOS in a recent meta-analysis of RCTs comparing metformin and COCs as pharmacotherapies in management of adolescent PCOS. Metformin was found to be superior to COC for weight reduction and improved dysglycemia especially when combined with diet and exercise. For menstrual irregularities COCs are preferred. The authors however emphasized that further studies are needed to better understand and formulate recommendations for the treatment of PCOS in adolescents.[31]

Lipid lowering medications like statins and fibrates are used in cases of dyslipidemia.

CONCLUSION

Polycystic ovary syndrome has long-term effects especially due to its association with the metabolic syndrome. This calls for a complete evaluation in adolescent girls though an absolute diagnosis of PCOS in adolescents is difficult. It may be prudent to define adolescent PCOS according to the AE-PCOS Society criteria as hyperandrogenism is most often a common finding in this adolescent patient group. The future implications of PCOS including risks associated with diabetes mellitus, dyslipidemia, obesity, subfertility, pregnancy complications, and even endometrial hyperplasia and carcinoma as well as effects on the mental health underlines the importance of early diagnosis and treatment of PCOS. This makes adolescent PCOS an important entity. In adolescents where the diagnosis is still in doubt, it is preferable to follow the symptoms and repeat the evaluation in 6–12 months. Symptomatic treatment can be started even without a definitive diagnosis, especially with severe symptoms. In addition, in cases with well-defined hyperandrogenemia, a complete workup is essential to rule out all the major hyperandrogenic disorders mimicking PCOS. Lastly, mental health is as important as physical health in these individuals and clinicians should provide for a holistic approach to treatment with early identification and support through counseling and even drugs, if required.

KEY MESSAGES

- Adolescent PCOS should be considered a separate entity.
- An absolute diagnosis of PCOS in adolescents is difficult as a number of normal physiological changes in this age group overlap features of PCOS.
- Adult diagnostic criteria cannot be reliably applied to PCOS in adolescents and this calls for a separate diagnostic criteria for PCOS in this age group.
- It may be prudent to define adolescent PCOS according to the AE-PCOS Society criteria as hyperandrogenism is most often a common finding in this adolescent patient group.
- PCOS is associated with a number of comorbidities with long-term implications which makes this entity in adolescents important. This is why clinicians should be aware of the intricacies and characteristics of this syndrome in adolescents.
- Lifestyle modification remains the first line management.
- Combined hormonal contraceptive pills remain the first line pharmacotherapy.
- Mental comorbidities associated with PCOS should also be dealt with especially in this age group and clinicians should be cognizant of the same.

REFERENCES

1. Rosenfield RL, Ehrmann DA .The pathogenesis of polycystic ovary syndrome (PCOS): the hypothesis of PCOS as functional ovarian hyperandrogenism revisited. Endocr Rev. 2016;37(5):467.
2. Waldstreicher J, Santoro NF, Hall JE, Filicori M, Crowley Jr WF. Hyperfunction of the hypothalamic-pituitary axis in women with polycystic ovarian disease: indirect evidence for partial gonadotroph desensitization. J Clin Endocrinol Metab. 1988;66:165-72.
3. Venturoli S, Porcu E, Fabbri R, Magrini O, Gammi L, Paradisi R, et al. Longitudinal evaluation of the different gonadotropin pulsatile patterns in anovulatory cycles of young girls. J Clin Endocrinol Metab. 1992;74:836-41.
4. Caprio S, Plewe G, Diamond MP, Simonson DC, Boulware SD, Sherwin RS, et al. Increased insulin secretion in puberty: a compensatory response to reductions in insulin sensitivity. J Pediatr. 1989;114:963-7.
5. Hannon TS, Janosky J, Arslanian SA. Longitudinal study of physiologic insulin resistance and metabolic changes of puberty. Pediatr Res. 2006;60:759-63.
6. Lewy VD, Danadian K, Witchel SF, Arslanian S. Early metabolic abnormalities in adolescent girls with polycystic ovarian syndrome. J Pediatr. 2001;138:38-44.
7. Nestler JE, Jakubowicz DJ, de Vargas AF, Brik C, Quintero N, Medina F. Insulin stimulates testosterone biosynthesis by human thecal cells from women with polycystic ovary syndrome by activating its own receptor and using inositolglycan mediators as the signal transduction system. J Clin Endocrinol Metab. 1998;83:2001-5.
8. Nestler JE, Powers LP, Matt DW, Steingold KA, Plymate SR, Rittmaster RS, et al. A direct effect of hyperinsulinemia on serum sex hormonebinding globulin levels in obese women with the polycystic ovary syndrome. J Clin Endocrinol Metab. 1991;72:83-9.
9. Rosenfield RL. The diagnosis of polycystic ovary syndrome in adolescents. Pediatrics. 2015;136:1154-65.
10. Ibáñez L, Oberfield SE, Witchel S, Auchus RJ, Chang RJ, Codner C, et al. An International Consortium Update: pathophysiology, diagnosis, and treatment of polycystic ovarian syndrome in adolescence. Horm Res Paediatr. 2017; 88:371.

11. ACOG Committee Opinion No. 651: Menstruation in girls and adolescents: using the menstrual cycle as a vital sign. Obstet Gynecol 2015; 126:e143. Reaffirmed 2019.
12. Rosenfield RL. Clinical review: Adolescent anovulation: maturational mechanisms and implications. J Clin Endocrinol Metab. 2013; 98:3572.
13. Maslyanskaya S, Talib HJ, Northridge JL, Jacobs AM, Coble C, Coupey SM. Polycystic ovary syndrome: an under-recognized cause of abnormal uterine bleeding in adolescents admitted to a children's hospital. J Pediatr Adolesc Gynecol. 2017; 30:349.
14. Futterweit W, Deligdisch L. Histopathological effects of exogenously administered testosterone in 19 female to male transsexuals. J Clin Endocrinol Metab. 1986; 62:16.
15. Witchel SF, Oberfield S, Rosenfield RL, Codner E, Bonny A, Ibáñez L, et al. The diagnosis of polycystic ovary syndrome during adolescence. Horm Res Paediatr. 2015;83(6):376-89.
16. Ibáñez L, de Zegher F, Potau N. Anovulation after precocious pubarche: early markers and time course in adolescence. J Clin Endocrinol Metab. 1999; 84:2691.
17. Rotterdam ESHRE/ASRM-Sponsored PCOS Consensus Workshop Group. Revised 2003 consensus on diagnostic criteria and long-term health risks related to polycystic ovary syndrome. Fertil Steril. 2004;81:19-25
18. Dewailly D, Lujan ME, Carmina E, et al. Definition and significance of polycystic ovarian morphology: a task force report from the Androgen Excess and Polycystic Ovary Syndrome Society. Hum Reprod Update. 2014;20(3):334-52
19. Rosenfield RL. The polycystic ovary morphology-polycystic ovary syndrome spectrum. J PediatrAdolesc Gynecol. 2015; 28(6):in press
20. Kenigsberg LE, Agarwal C, Sin S, Shifteh K, Isasi CR, Crespi R, et al. Clinical utility of magnetic resonance imaging and ultrasonography for diagnosis of polycystic ovary syndrome in adolescent girls. Fertil Steril. 2015;104(5):1302-9.e1-4.
21. Martin KA, Anderson RR, Chang RJ, Ehrmann DA, Lobo RA, Hassan M, et al. Evaluation and treatment of hirsutism in premenopausal women: an endocrine society clinical practice guideline. J Clin Endocrinol Metab. 2018; 103:1233.
22. Lucky AW, Biro FM, Simbartl LA, Morrison JA, Sorg NW Predictors of severity of acne vulgaris in young adolescent girls: results of a five-year longitudinal study. J Pediatr. 1997; 130:30.
23. Ehrmann DA, Barnes RB, Rosenfield RL, Cavaghan MK, Imperial J. Prevalence of impaired glucose tolerance and diabetes in women with polycystic ovary syndrome. Diabetes Care. 1999; 22:141.
24. Legro RS, Kunselman AR, Dodson WC, Dunaif A. Prevalence and predictors of risk for type 2 diabetes mellitus and impaired glucose tolerance in polycystic ovary syndrome: a prospective, controlled study in 254 affected women. J Clin Endocrinol Metab. 1999; 84:165.
25. Kahn SE. Clinical review 135: The importance of beta-cell failure in the development and progression of type 2 diabetes. J Clin Endocrinol Metab. 2001; 86:4047.
26. Azziz R, Carmina E, Dewailly D, Diamanti-Kandarakis E, Escobar-Morreale HF, Futterweit W, et al. Androgen Excess Society. Positions statement: criteria for defining polycystic ovary syndrome as a predominantly hyperandrogenic syndrome: an Androgen Excess Society guideline. J Clin Endocrinol Metab. 2006;91:4237-45.
27. Martin KA, Chang RJ, Ehrmann DA, Ibanez L, Lobo RA, Rosenfield RL, et al. Evaluation and treatment of hirsutism in premenopausal women: an endocrine society clinical practice guideline. J Clin Endocrinol Metab. 2008;93:1105-20.
28. Escobar-Morreale HF, Carmina E, Dewailly D, Gambineri A, Kelestimur F, Moghetti P, et al. Epidemiology, diagnosis and management of hirsutism: a consensus statement by the Androgen Excess and Polycystic Ovary Syndrome Society. Hum Reprod Update. 2012;18:146-70.
29. Carmina E, Oberfield SE, Lobo RA. The diagnosis of polycystic ovary syndrome in adolescents. Am J ObstetGynecol 2010;203:201. e1-5.
30. Tartagni MV, Alrasheed H, Damiani GR, Montagnani M, De Salvia MA, De Pergola G, et al. Intermittent low-dose finasteride administration is effective for treatment of hirsutism in adolescent girls: a pilot study. J Pediatr Adolesc Gynecol. 2014;27:161-5.
31. Al Khalifah RA, Florez ID, Dennis B, Thabane L, Bassilious E. Metformin or oral contraceptives for adolescents with polycystic ovarian syndrome: a meta-analysis. Pediatrics. 2016;137(5):e20154089.

LONG QUESTIONS

1. Elaborate the need for having adolescent PCOS as a separate entity.
2. Management of adolescent PCOS.

SHORT QUESTIONS

1. Diagnostic criteria of PCOS in adolescents.
2. Differential diagnosis of PCOS in adolescents.
3. Clinical features of PCOS in adolescents.

MULTIPLE CHOICE QUESTIONS

1. All of the below feature(s) make ultrasound diagnosis of PCOM challenging in adolescents, except:
   a. Lack of normative data on ovarian morphology
   b. Poor image quality provided by transabdominal ultrasound
   c. Polycystic morphological changes of the ovaries not beginning in adolescence
   d. The difficulty of differential diagnosis from the multicystic ovaries
2. Which of the following should be included in the differential diagnosis of hyperandrogenism?
   a. Hypogonadotropic hypogonadism
   b. Androgen-secreting neoplasms
   c. Cushing's disease
   d. Idiopathic hirsutism
3. Which of the following should be considered as first line treatment for hirsutism in adolescent PCOS?
   a. Hormonal contraceptives
   b. Insulin sensitizers
   c. 5α-reductase agonists
   d. Glucocorticoids

4. The following is/are the criteria required to diagnose polycystic ovarian syndrome in adolescents:
   a. Obesity
   b. Insulin resistance
   c. Elevated low-density lipoprotein cholesterol
   d. Ovary volume > 10 cm^3 on USG
   e. Abnormal uterine bleeding
5. Which of the following is not linked to adolescent PCOS?
   a. Acanthosis nigricans
   b. Obesity
   c. Androgen secreting ovarian tumors
   d. Impaired glucose tolerance
6. Symptoms of adolescent PCOS includes all, except:
   a. Amenorrhea b. Acne
   c. Clitoromegaly d. Hirsutism
7. Which of the following is not included in management of adolescent PCOS?
   a. OCPs b. Metformin
   c. Glucocorticoids d. Weight loss
8. Which of the following is true about adolescent PCOS?
   a. Diagnosis is easy due to associated pubertal changes
   b. PCOM on ultrasound is a major diagnostic criteria
   c. Frank virilization is always seen
   d. The diagnostic criteria are different from adult PCOS due to physiological changes of puberty clouding the diagnosis
9. All are comorbidities associated with PCOS, except:
   a. Endometrial carcinoma
   b. Impaired glucose tolerance
   c. Eating disorders
   d. Ovarian carcinoma
10. Most effective agent for menstrual regularization in adolescent PCOS is:
   a. Metformin
   b. Spironolactone
   c. Combined oral contraceptive pills
   d. Myo-inositol

Answers

1. c 2. b 3. a 4. e 5. c 6. c
7. c 8. d 9. d 10. c

8.3 DEVELOPMENTAL ABNORMALITIES OF GENITAL TRACT

Ragini Agrawal, KV Divya

INTRODUCTION

Congenital abnormalities of the female genital tract are anomalies which usually present during childhood or adolescence. On the other hand, ambiguous genitalia is one such abnormality which tends to be diagnosed at birth requiring a multidisciplinary approach for management. They are defined as any deviation from normal anatomy resulting from maldevelopment of embryo. Those anomalies presenting with menstrual abnormalities or fertility concerns are mostly encountered by gynecologist. The prevalence of Müllerian anomalies in the general population is 4.3%.[1] The cause of the anomalies is idiopathic. Some of the anomalies are hereditary; others are due to random gene mutation or developmental defect. Environmental and genetic factors are other proposed, unproven causes. Isolated Müllerian anomalies do not carry risk of offspring transmission as per current literature.[2]

EMBRYONIC DEVELOPMENT OF THE FEMALE GENITAL TRACT

The differentiation and further developmental course of the indifferent gonad depends on the presence or absence of sex-determining gene (SRY) and anti-Müllerian hormone as shown in **Figure 1**.

Defect in the fusion and canalization process leads to anomalies. Müllerian anomalies are associated with concomitant renal (40%) anomalies such as unilateral agenesis, a horseshoe kidney or a pelvic kidney and spinal (10–20%) anomalies. Multiple classification systems have been developed owing to the wide variation in anomalies.

The one devised by the American Society of Reproductive Medicine (ASRM) is shown in **Figure 2**.

The findings of magnetic resonance imaging (MRI) of pelvis are used for diagnosis in ASRM classification and they are:

- External fundal dipping greater than 10% or 1 cm indicates a possible diagnosis of uterine didelphys or a bicornuate uterus.[3] Two separate uterus with preserved myoendometrium zonal widths, two cervices and two vagina are observed in uterine didelphys.[4] The lower uterine segment is fused in bicornuate uterus.
- Bicornuate is characterized by an intercornual angle of >105° and external fundal dipping.[5]
- Septate uterus has flat fundal dipping and an acute intercornual angle. The septum can be muscular or fibrous.[6]
- In an arcuate uterus, myometrial dipping is seen in the inner aspect with a convex or flat outer fundal contour.[7]
- Zonal anatomy and endometrial-myometrial differentiation is maintained in unicornuate uterus.[8]
- There is loss of myometrial-endometrial differentiation in hypoplastic uterus.[9]

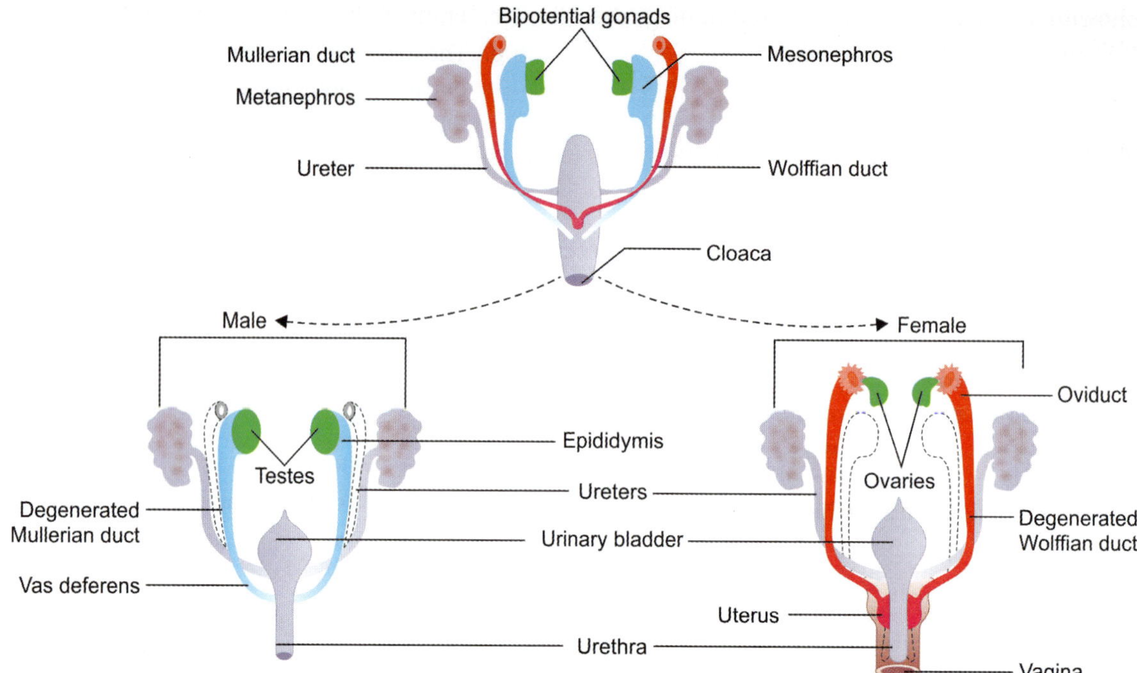

Fig. 1: Female genital tract differentiation.

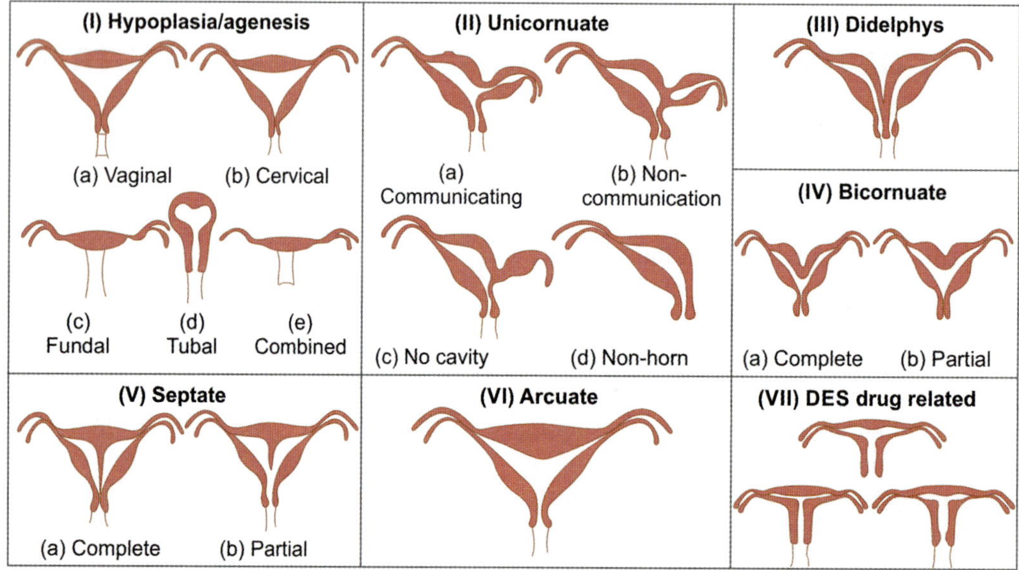

Fig. 2: ASRM classification: Müllerian anomalies.

The other classification is proposed by European Society of Human Reproduction and Embryology (ESHRE) and European Society of Gynaecological Endoscopy (ESGE) as in **Table 1**.

The diagnostic aspects of the ESHRE and ESGE classification are:

- Bicorporeal uterus includes bicornuate and didelphys uterus of the previous ASRM classification which is subcategorized as 3a and 3b, respectively. A dysfused septate uterus is 3c.
- Unicornuate uterus is classified under hemi-uterus U4.
- Septate uterus has a fundal midline indentation of >50% of the uterine wall thickness.[6]
- Arcuate uterus (type VI of ASRM) has been removed, as it is considered as almost normal variant rather than an anomaly.[10]
- This classification is more comprehensive compared to ASRM classification and it classifies 38 of the 39 congenital anomalies of the female genital tract.[10]
- Uterine, cervical and vaginal anomalies are classified independently and it is very useful, especially in cases of obstructive cervical or vaginal malformations with a normal uterus.[10]
- This classification includes associated anomalies of non-Müllerian origin as part of its system to accommodate

TABLE 1: ESHRE and ESGE classification of Müllerian anomalies.

Uterine anomaly			Cervical/vaginal anomaly	
	Main class	Sub-class	Co-existent class	
U0	Normal uterus		C0	Normal cervix
U1	Dysmorphic uterus	• T-shaped • Infantilis • Others	C1	Septate cervix
			C2	Double 'normal' cervix
U2	Septate uterus	• Partial • Complete	C3	Unilateral cervical aplasia
			C4	Cervical aplasia
U3	Bicorporeal uterus	• Partial • Complete • Bicorporeal septate		
			V0	Normal vagina
			V1	Longitudinal non-obstructing vaginal septum
U4	Hemi-uterus	• With rudimentary cavity (Communicating or not horn) • Without rudimentary cavity (horn without cavity/no horn)	V2	Longitudinal obstructing vaginal septum
U5	Aplastic	• With rudimentary cavity (bi-or unilateral horn) • Withour rudimentary cavity (bi-or unilateral uterine remnants/aplasia)	V3	Transverse vaginal septum and/or imperforate hymen
			V4	Vaginal aplasia
U6	Unclassified malformations			
U			C	V

the renal tract malformations, which are commonly associated.

- The embryological origin of the anomalies can be easily identified.

CLINICAL PRESENTATION

Clinical presentation has obstructive or nonobstructive pattern. Obstructive ones present with primary amenorrhea, dysmenorrhea.

The most common obstructive anomaly is an imperforate hymen. These patients will present with pain secondary to a hematometra/hematocolpos and with urinary retention or bowel complaints in severe cases.[11] Transverse vaginal septum is another obstructive anomaly which is rare with obstruction at any level along the vagina, most commonly (40%) in the upper third of the vagina.[2]

Non-obstructive Anomalies

Asymptomatic nature of nonobstructive anomalies leads to their delayed diagnosis when they present with primary amenorrhea, dyspareunia, recurrent miscarriage or pregnancy complications.

Pregnancy complications can also occur with Müllerian anomalies as shown in **Table 2**.

TABLE 2: Pregnancy complications of Müllerian anomalies.[12,13]

	Pregnancy complications	Rate
Unification errors		
Unicornuate, bicornuate, didelphys uterus	Malpresentation	25–50%
	Preterm birth	33–50%
	Fetal growth restriction	18–50%
	Cesarean section	64%
Communicating horns	Rupture of rudimentary horn	67%
Canalization error		
Arcuate	Nil	
Subseptate/septate uterus	First trimester abortions	44%
	Malpresentation	16%
	Preterm birth	25%
	Fetal growth restriction	6–12%
Longitudinal vaginal septum	Second stage dystocia/laceration/ bleeding from septum	

DIAGNOSIS

Varied clinical presentation of Müllerian anomalies may need more than one imaging modality for diagnosis outlined in **Table 3**. Hysterosalpingography (HSG) has been traditionally used for evaluation of cervix, uterus and Fallopian tubes with variable diagnostic accuracy. HSG helps in the evaluation of tubal patency, uterine septum, intrauterine adhesions, submucous fibroids, and endometrial polyps.[14] But it cannot identify external surface anomalies of uterus and also cannot be performed in patients who are not sexually active and also carry risk of radiation exposure, dye allergy, uterine perforation, and infection. Ultrasonography is another imaging modality used extensively in the diagnosis of Müllerian anomalies. Transvaginal ultrasound can provide further details about endometrial cavity, and cervix. But the sensitivity and specificity varies depending on various factors such as type of anomaly, radiologist experience, resolution of machine, transducer type. The specificity of TVS for detection of Müllerian anomaly has been reported from 85 to 92%.[7,15,16] Three-dimensional ultrasonography has been used

TABLE 3: Investigations for Müllerian anomalies.[7,14,15]

Investigation	*Rationale*
Pelvic ultrasound	Assess presence of pelvic organs
MRI pelvis	To confirm anatomy
Renal ultrasound	For associated renal anomalies
Hormonal profile	Assess gonadal function
Karyotype	To exclude complete androgen insensitivity syndrome or gonadal dysgenesis
Vertebral X-ray/ cardiac screening	Assessing for associated complications if symptomatic

extensively. The 3D ultrasound provides detailed information of uterine pathology with spatial orientation and has high specificity (96.9%) and sensitivity (86.6%) in evaluations of all uterine anomalies.[17] MRI is currently considered the best imaging modality for Müllerian duct anomaly. There is no radiation risk and provides better delineation of both the internal and the external uterine anatomy. The specificity of MRI is high for diagnosing Müllerian malformations.[18]

MANAGEMENT

There is potential risk of complications in patients with obstructive Müllerian anomalies which can be reduced by prompt treatment. Medical management can be done with hormonal suppression till an accurate diagnosis is made and a definitive surgical management is planned. Surgery is indicated in nonresponsive cases.

The treatment for Müllerian anomalies varies according to the specific type of malformation with surgical management being the mode of treatment.

Müllerian Aplasia (Vaginal Agenesis)

The surgical management of the above condition is by vaginoplasty, in which a space between the bladder and the rectum is developed.

Serial Dilatation

Serial dilatation and vaginoplasty, both can be used for treatment of vaginal agenesis. Vaginal mechanical dilatation should be the first choice. ACOG says vaginal dilatation has low complications and high success.[19] The most common method is Frank technique consists of daily self-application of rigid vaginal dilatators with progressive increase in the length and diameter.

Vaginoplasty

Vaginoplasty is an alternative approach. The most commonly used technique is by McIndoe which utilizes an autologous skin flap in latex mold placed after the tunneling of the vagina.[20] Other described techniques are Davydov's technique and Vechitti's technique in which through laparoscopic peritoneal coverage of vaginal walls is carried out,[21] and Baldwin's technique which uses a segment of the intestine for creation of the neovagina.[22]

Unicornuate Uterus

Women with unicornuate uterus are not the candidates for reconstruction metroplasty.

Uterus Didelphys

Surgical correction is necessary to improve reproductive outcome and to prevent complications. The recommended procedure is the Strassmann metroplasty. This method unifies the uterine cavities at the fundus, while the cervices are left intact. Full excision and marsupialization of the vaginal septum is the preferred approach in those with associated vaginal obstruction.

Surgical Techniques for Bicornuate Uterus

The surgical treatment of choice is by Strassmann metroplasty. Laparoscopic route is a feasible and better alternative to abdominal metroplasty. There is better magnification, lower tissue damage, less infections, lesser adhesions, shorter hospital stay, and enhanced postoperative recovery with laparoscopic method.

Septate Uterus

The surgical procedure of choice is hysteroscopic metroplasty or hysteroscopic transcervical division of the uterine septum. The procedure may be combined with laparoscopy as laparoscopy reduces the risk of uterine perforation and also ensures adequacy of the procedure.

Arcuate Uterus

Only selected patients who present with poor reproductive outcome are offered surgical correction.

CONCLUSION

Congenital abnormalities of the female genital tract are anomalies which are rare, present during childhood or adolescence. Most of them are asymptomatic or they present with menstrual, fertility issues. The definitive management has to be planned after taking a detailed history, examination, and appropriate investigations. Obstructive anomalies should be treated urgently to prevent future complications. Appropriate psychological counseling has to be done while disclosing the diagnosis of Müllerian agenesis or androgen insensitivity syndrome. Pregnancy in these patients is high risk and has to be managed in well-equipped tertiary care center with multidisciplinary approach.

KEY MESSAGES

- Congenital anomalies of the female genital tract usually present in adolescent population and are rare anomalies. However, some may be evident at birth.

- Most of them are asymptomatic or they present with menstrual, fertility issues.
- The definitive management has to be planned after taking a detailed history, examination and appropriate investigations.
- Obstructive anomalies require urgent management to reduce the risk of complications.
- Müllerian anomalies require multidisciplinary approach for management to improve reproductive outcome.

REFERENCES

1. Grimbizis GF, Camus M, Tarlatzis BC, Bontis JN, Devroey P. Clinical implications of uterine malformations and hysteroscopic treatment results. Hum Reprod Update. 2001:161-74.
2. Dietrich JE, Millar DM, Quint EH. Obstructive reproductive tract anomalies. J Pediatr Adolesc Gynecol. 2014;27:396-402.
3. Mueller GC, Hussain HK, Smith YR. Mullerian duct anomalies: Comparison of MRI diagnosis and clinical diagnosis. AJR Am J Roentgenol. 2007;189:1294-302.
4. Behr SC, Courtier JL, Qayyum A. Congenital pelvic abnormalities; imaging of Müllerian duct anomalies. Radiographics. 2012;32:233-50.
5. Saleem SN. MR Imaging diagnosis of uterovaginal anomalies: current state of the art. Radiographics. 2003;23(5):2-9.
6. Reuter KL, Daly DC, Cohen SM. Septate versus bicornuate uteri: errors in imaging diagnosis. Radiology. 1989;172(3):749-52.
7. Pellerito JS, McCarthy SM, Doyle MB, Glickman MG, DeCherney AH. Diagnosis of uterine anomalies: relative accuracy of MR imaging, endovaginal sonography, and hysterosalpingography. Radiology. 1992;183(3):795-800.
8. Carrington BM, Hricak H, Nuruddin RN, Secaf E, Laros RK, Hill EC. Mullerian duct anomalies: MR imaging evaluation. Radiology. 1990;176(3):715-20.
9. Grimbizis GF, Gordts S, Sardo A. Reply: Are the ESHRE/ESGE criteria of female genital anomalies for diagnosis of septate uterus appropriate? Hum Reprod. 2014;29:868-69
10. Di SpiezioSardo A, Campo R, Gordts S. The comprehensiveness of the ESHRE/ESGE classification of female genital tract congenital anomalies: a systematic review of cases not classified by the AFS system. Hum Reprod. 2015;30(5):1046-58.
11. Morcel K, Guerrier D, Watrin T, Pellerin I, Levêque J. The Mayer-Rokitansky-Küster-Hauser (MRKH) syndrome: clinical description and genetics. J Gynaecol Obstet Biol Reprod. 2008:37(6):539-46.
12. Dietrich JE, Millar DM, Quint EH. Non-obstructive Müllerian Anomalies. J Pediatr Adolesc Gynecol. 2014;27:386-95.
13. Fox NS, Roman AS, Stern EM. Type of congenital uterine anomaly and adverse pregnancy outcomes. Journal of maternal-fetal and neonatal medicine. 2014;17(9):949-53.
14. Zafarani F, Ahmadi F, Shahrzad G. Hysterosalpingographic features of cervical abnormalities: acquired structural anomalies. Br J Radiol. 2015;88(1052):20150045.
15. Doyle MB. Magnetic resonance imaging in müllerian fusion defects. J Reprod Med. 1992;37(1):33-8.
16. Ozsarlak O, De Schepper AM, Valkenburg M, Delbeke L. Septate uterus: hysterosalpingography and magnetic resonance imaging findings. Eur J Radiol. 1995;21(2):122-5.
17. Moini A, Mohammadi S, Hosseini R, Eslami B, Ahmadi F. Accuracy of 3-dimensional sonography for diagnosis and classification of congenital uterine anomalies. J Ultrasound Med. 2013;32(6):923-7.
18. Pui MH. Imaging diagnosis of congenital uterine malformation. Comput Med Imaging Graph. 2004;28(7):425-33.
19. ACOG. Müllerian Agenesis: Diagnosis, Management, and Treatment. ACOG clinical opinion. Chicago: ACOG; 2019.
20. Keser A, Bozkurt N, Taner OF, Sensöz O. Treatment of vaginal agenesis with modified Abbe-McIndoe technique: long-term follow-up in 22 patients. Eur J Obstet Gynecol Reprod Biol. 2005;121:110-6.
21. Willemsen WN, Kluivers KB. Long-term results of vaginal construction with the use of Frank dilation and a peritoneal graft (Davydov procedure) in patients with Mayer-Rokitansky-Küster syndrome. Fertil Steril. 2015;103 (1):220-7.
22. Vecchietti G. Neovaginanella syndrome di Rokitansky-Kuster-Hauser [Neovagina in Mayer-Rokitansky-Küster-Hauser syndrome]. Attual Obstet Ginecol. 1965;11:131-47.

LONG QUESTION

1. Classify Müllerian anomalies and discuss the management of each of them.

SHORT QUESTIONS

1. Discuss the embryology of the urogenital tract.
2. Discuss the management of uterine septum.
3. What are complications encountered in pregnant patient with a uterine anomaly?

MULTIPLE CHOICE QUESTIONS

1. The uterus develop from the:
   a. Wolffian duct b. Müllerian duct
   c. Bartholin duct d. Cloacal duct
2. The incidence of Müllerian anomalies are associated with concomitant renal anomalies is:
   a. 20% b. 40%
   c. 60% d. 80%
3. Second stage dystocia in labor is associated with the following anomaly:
   a. Arcuate uterus
   b. Longitudinal vaginal septum
   c. Uterine didelphis
   d. Subseptate uterus
4. Currently the best imaging modality for precise diagnosis of Müllerian duct anomaly is:
   a. TVS b. HSG
   c. MRI d. CT
5. The surgical procedure of choice for septate uterus is:
   a. Strassmann metroplasty
   b. McIndoe vaginoplasty
   c. Hysteroscopic metroplasty
   d. Hymenectomy

Answers

1. b 2. b 3. b 4. c 5. c

8.4 DISORDER OF SEX DEVELOPMENT IN AN ADOLESCENT GIRL

Kunal Thakkar, Vijaya Sarthi, Nalini Shah

INTRODUCTION

Disorders/Differences of sex development (DSD) is an umbrella term, used to congenital conditions in which development of chromosomal, gonadal, or anatomical sex is atypical. This along with many other terminologies such as "intersex", "hermaphrodite", which were once used, have been revised after the DSD classification system proposed at the Chicago consensus meeting in 2006. The summary of these new terminologies is provided in **Table 1**. There is an ongoing debate for many conditions whether these belong to this umbrella term "DSD". Particularly this also applies to structural anomalies such as bladder exstrophy or cloacal anomalies. Severe degree of hypospadias is commonly recognized as DSD, with widespread genetic testing allowing recognition of variations in androgen production or action. However, whether relatively less severe hypospadias (distal and mid-shaft) should be included in this term or not is still debatable.

Understanding physiologies of gonadal and genital development as well as adrenal/gonadal steroidogenesis pathways are of paramount importance to effectively evaluate and manage a patient with DSD.

SEX DETERMINATION AND DIFFERENTIATION

The type of developing gonad in an embryo determines the phenotypic sex of an individual and the sex chromosome complement determines the type of gonad. Humans have 22 pairs of autosomes and one pair of sex chromosomes; females have two X chromosomes (46 XX) while males have one X and one Y chromosome (46 XY). The development of reproductive system begins at 4–5 weeks after conception, whereby primitive gonad arises from urogenital ridge along with adrenal primordium **(Fig. 1)**. This primitive gonad remains bipotential (undifferentiated) until 6 weeks after conception, when expression of several important genes leads to its further development. This process whereby the bipotential gonad develops into a testis or an ovary is known as sex determination. The production of peptide hormones and sex steroids from the developing gonads leads to development of internal and external genitalia, the process known as sex differentiation. In the typical male, production of anti-Müllerian hormone (AMH) at around 7–8 weeks from sertoli cells of testis leads to regression of Müllerian structures, production of testosterone from leydig cells at around 8–11 weeks leads to stabilization of Wolffian structures (development of seminal vesicles, vas deferentia, and epididymis), while formation of dihydrotestosterone (DHT) from testosterone leads to androgenization of external genitalia (formation of penis and scrotum). Testes descend from their original abdominal position to base of scrotum, process starting as early as 8 weeks of gestation and completing by the middle of third trimester. Initial trans-abdominal phase of testicular descent (8–15 weeks) is mediated by insulin-like factor 3 (INSL3) secreted from testis itself, while later inguinal phase of descent is mediated by androgens secreted from testis. Ovarian hormonal secretion has practically no role in sex differentiation in a female fetus. Absence of AMH and lack of androgenization due to absence of testosterone and DHT production as in case of fetus with XX chromosomal complement, leads to female internal and external genitalia formation. Similarly when testosterone, DHT and/or AMH production or action is defective, atypical or female internal or external genitals develop in XY fetus.

TABLE 1: Summary of new terminologies that arose from Chicago consensus meeting 2005.

New term	*Previous term*
Disorders of sex development (DSD)	Intersex
46 XY DSD	Male pseudohermaphrodite, Undervirilized male Under masculinized male
46 XY DSD	Female pseudohermaphrodite Virilized female Masculinized female
Ovotesticular DSD	True hermaphrodite
46 XX testicular DSD	XX male, XX sex reversal
46 XY complete gonadal dysgenesis	XY sex reversal

Source: Adapted from Hughes IA, Houk C, Ahmed SF, Lee PA, LWPES Consensus Group; ESPE Consensus Group. Consensus statement on management of intersex disorders. Arch Dis Child. 2006;91:554-62

The primitive structures, which develop into female and male external genitalia in absence and in presence of testosterone/DHT, respectively are listed in **Table 2** and shown in **Figure 2**.

Gonadal and adrenal production of sex steroids and other steroid hormones from cholesterol is as indicated in **Flowchart 1**.

Overproduction of androgens in XX fetus (congenital adrenal hyperplasia, aromatase deficiency, ovotesticular DSD) leads to androgenization of urogenital sinus and external genitalia, hence leading to varying degrees of atypical genitalia in female fetus (isolated mild clitoromegaly in mild cases to complete labioscrotal fusion and male-like genitals in most severe cases). On the other hand, defective production or action of androgens in XY fetus also leads to varying degrees

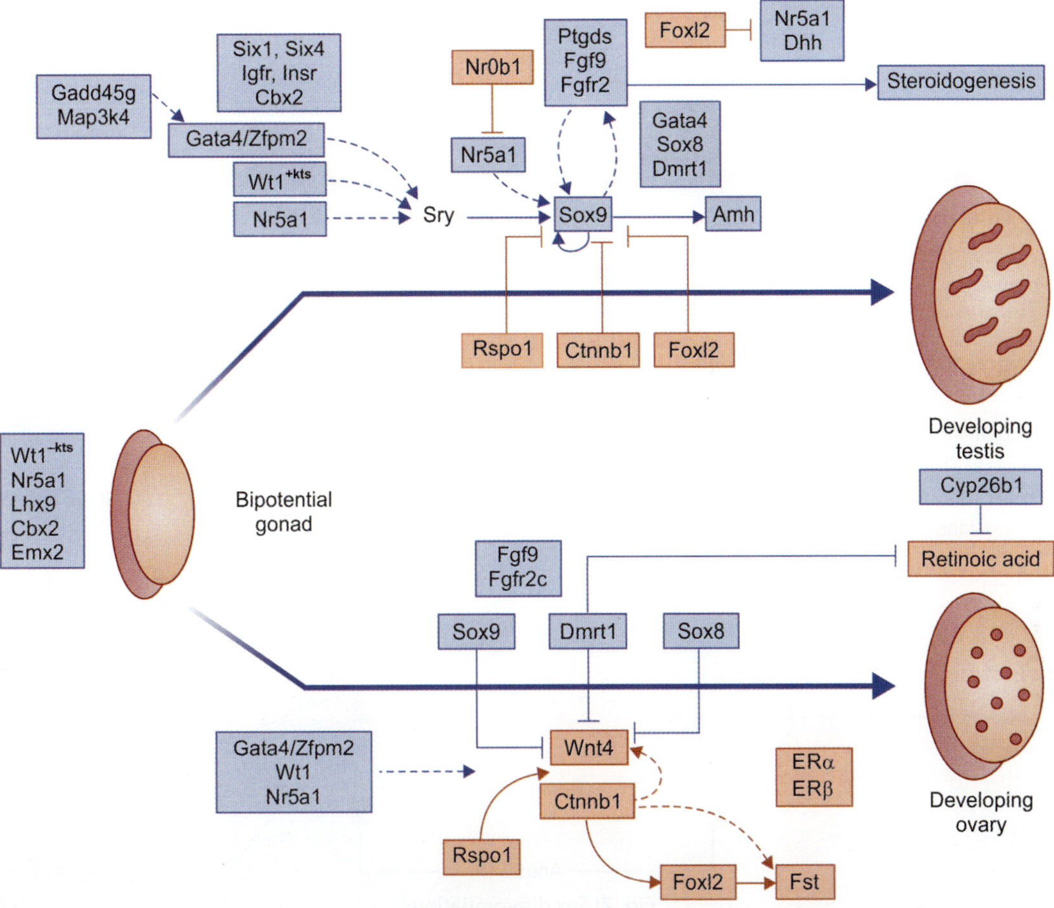

Fig. 1: Sex determination.

TABLE 2: Primitive structures that develop into male or female external genitalia.

Structure	***Male***	***Female***
Genital tubercle	Glans penis	Clitoris
Urethral (urogenital) folds	Shaft of penis	Labia minora
Labioscrotal (urogenital) swelling	Scrotum	Labia majora
Urogenital sinus	Prostate, prostatic urethra	Urethra, lower one third of vagina

of atypical genitalia (isolated hypospadias in mild cases to complete female phenotype in most severe cases).

This particular chapter is limited to approach, evaluation, and management of DSD conditions in adolescent female, while neonatal and childhood concerns of DSD and atypical genitals are out of scope of this chapter.

DSD IN AN ADOLESCENT FEMALE

Most cases of DSD present at birth or in infancy due to atypical genitals. Some may present in later childhood or early adolescent period with multiple and varying presenting features. The various presentations of DSD at puberty in an adolescent phenotypic female along with possible differential diagnosis are depicted in **Table 3**. Conversely, the clinical features in a pubertal girl with various causes of DSD are depicted in **Table 4**.

Herein, we are going to discuss these presenting clinical features of DSD in an adolescent girl in some detail.

Precocious Puberty

Precocious puberty (PP) can be due to numerous disorders of hypothalamo-pituitary-gonadal axis, but we focus on those conditions where atypical sexual development is associated. The most likely condition is congenital adrenal hyperplasia (CAH) with minimal virilization in a girl (46 XX). CAH due to 21 α hydroxylase deficiency is the most common cause of 46 XX DSD. More severe salt wasting form of CAH is usually diagnosed in neonatal or infantile period due to adrenal crisis. The delayed presentation of CAH in later childhood or early adolescence is more likely with less severe variant of simple virilizing CAH, where the minor genital differences went unnoticed at birth (prader 1,2) and patient presents with PP. It is important to note that PP here in these cases is always heterosexual PP (associated with virilization in a girl). CAH due to mutation in 11 β hydroxylase deficiency in cortisol biosynthesis pathway is a less common cause of DSD with PP in girls (46 XX) and is associated with hypertension in many patients due to excessive mineralocorticoid precursors.

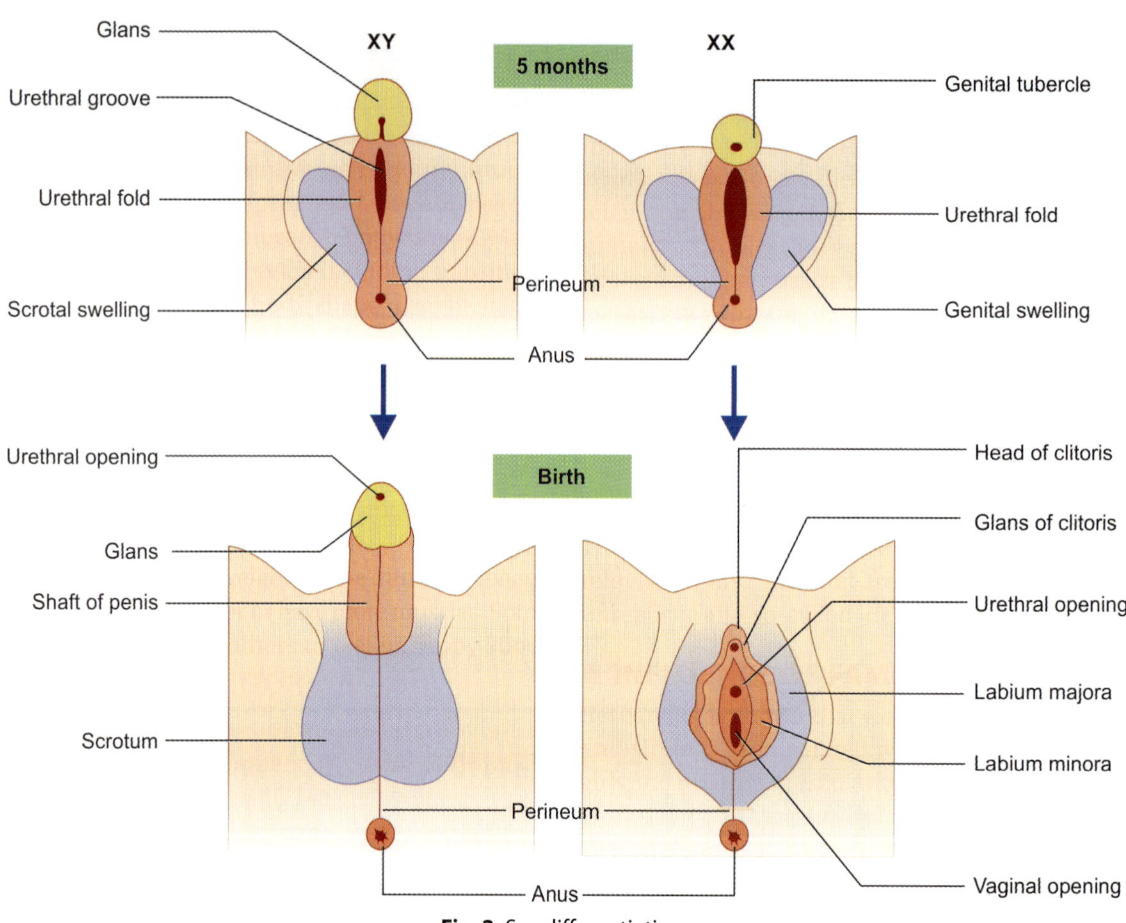

Fig. 2: Sex differentiation.

Flowchart 1: Adrenal/gonadal steroidogenesis pathway.

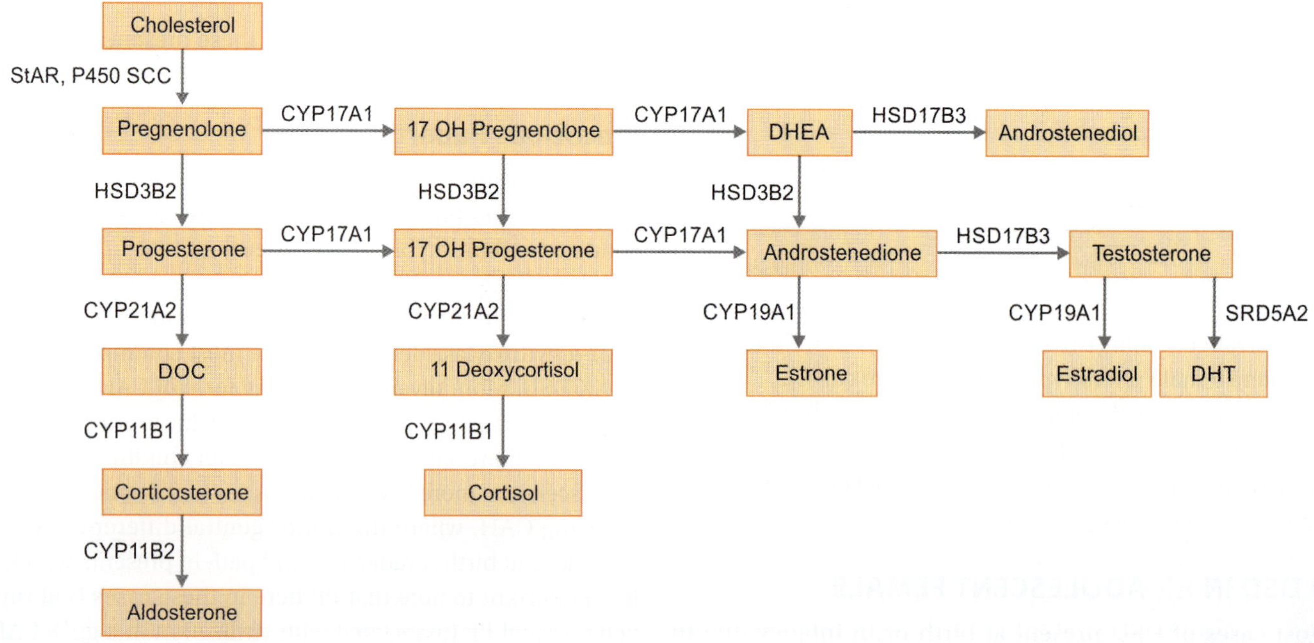

(StAR: steroidogenic acute regulatory protein; P450 SCC: side chain cleavage enzyme; CYP17A1: 17 alpha hydroxylase; CYP21A2: 21 alpha hydroxylase; CYP11B1: 11 beta hydroxylase; CYP11B2: aldosterone synthase; CYP19A1: aromatase; HSD3B2: 3 beta hydroxysteroid dehydrogenase type 2; HSD17B3: 17 beta hydroxysteroid dehydrogenase type 3; SRD5A2: 5 alpha reductase type 2)

Virilization at Puberty

The certain clinical features either in isolation or in combination indicate virilization in a female: clitoromegaly, deepening of voice, severe hirsutism and acnes, increased muscle mass and scalp hair loss. There are many conditions, which can lead to virilization in a girl at puberty. However, certain conditions such as nonclassical CAH, ovarian hyperthecosis, ovarian or adrenal androgen producing tumors are not associated with atypical sexual development and are not discussed here. Other than CAH, aromatase deficiency is one such condition where a girl (46 XX) is born with varying degrees of atypical genitals (varying from prader 1–4). Aromatase (CYP19A1) is the enzyme that leads to conversion of androgens to estrogens, deficiency of which is associated with excess androgen and low estrogen production. If mild degrees of atypical genitals went un-noticed at birth then such girl may present at puberty with signs of progressive virilization and hypergonatropic hypogonadism.

Usually however the term "virilization at puberty" in a girl with DSD is more commonly used and observed in individuals with certain forms of 46 XY DSD. These conditions include: Partial androgen insensitivity syndrome (PAIS), 17 β hydroxysteroid dehydrogenase 3 (17βHSD3) deficiency, and 5 α reductase type 2 (SRD5A2) deficiencies. The phenotype in these conditions varies from isolated hypospadias in phenotypic male to only minimal virilization in phenotypic female depending on the severity of mutation and enzyme dysfunction. In severe forms of these conditions, female sex is usually assigned at birth due severe under-virilization prenatally in 46 XY fetus. PAIS is an X-linked recessive condition due to mutation in androgen receptor (AR), leading to partial biologic response to androgens. It is generally diagnosed in infancy due to atypical genitals, but mild genital virilization might have gone un-noticed,

TABLE 3: Presentations of DSD in an adolescent girl.

Clinical scenario	*Likely DSD*
Precocious puberty	Untreated CAH (46 XX)
Virilization at puberty	46 XX: CAH, aromatase deficiency 46 XY: PAIS, 17βHSD3 deficiency, 5αRD2 deficiency
Groin lump	Enlarging inguinal testis in 46 XY DSD: common in CAIS and 17βHSD3 deficiency. Sometimes in PAIS, 5αRD2 deficiency
Delayed puberty	Gonadal dysgenesis (46 XX or 46 XY), Enzyme defects in proximal pathway of androgen synthesis (46 XY)
Primary amenorrhea	CAIS, Müllerian agenesis
Abdominal/pelvic mass or pain	Development of gonadoblastoma or other malignant germ cell tumor from dysgenetic or normal undescended gonad (46 XY)

TABLE 4: Clinical features in various DSD conditions in an adolescent girl.

Karyotype	*DSD condition*	*External genitalia*	*Müllerian structures*	*Clinical features*
46 XX	CAH	Atypical	Present	Precocious heterosexual puberty, virilization, primary amenorrhea, hyperpigmentation, short final height
	Aromatase deficiency	Atypical	Present	Virilization, tall stature with enuchoidism
	Ovo-testicular DSD	Atypical	May be present (hemiuterus)	Sometimes virilization, cyclic abdominal pain, if Müllerian structures not properly developed
46 XY	Complete gonadal dysgenesis	Female typical	Present	Delayed puberty with primary amenorrhea, tall stature with enuchoidism, rarely abdominal/pelvic tumor
	Complete androgen synthesis defect (defect in StAR, SCC, 3βHSD2)	Female typical	Absent	Delayed puberty with primary amenorrhea, tall stature with enuchoidism Salt wasting (adrenal insufficiency)
	Complete androgen synthesis defect (17α hydroxylase deficiency)	Female typical	Absent	Delayed puberty with primary amenorrhea, tall stature with enuchoidism Hypertension with hypokalemia
	Partial androgen synthesis defect (17βHSD3 deficiency)	Female typical to atypical	Absent	Virilization at puberty, primary amenorrhea, inguinal lump, gender dysphoria, enuchoidism +/–
	Partial androgen synthesis defect (5α reductase deficiency)	Atypical	Absent	Virilization at puberty, primary amenorrhea, inguinal lump, gender dysphoria
	Partial androgen insensitivity (PAIS)	Atypical	Absent	Primary amenorrhea, some pubic/axillary hair, inguinal lump, virilization at puberty
	Complete androgen insensitivity (CAIS)	Female typical	Absent	Primary amenorrhea, inguinal lump

(CAH: congenital adrenal hyperplasia; StAR: steroidogenic acute regulatory protein; SCC: side chain cleavage enzyme; 3βHSD2: 3β hydroxysteroid dehydrogenase type 2 enzyme; 17βHSD3: 17β hydroxysteroid dehydrogenase type 3 enzyme)

consistent with female sex of rearing, who then present at puberty with some further clitoral enlargement. 17βHSD3 enzyme catalyzes the conversion of androstenedione to testosterone in androgen biosynthesis pathway, its deficiency leads to low-testosterone and high-androstenedione levels. Most affected 46 XY children have female typical genitalia at birth while some have atypical genitals. In such cases, pubertal virilization is usually the presenting features and adolescent girls present with clitoromegaly, deepening of voice, hirsutism and muscle development. This occurs because of extraglandular conversion of excess levels of androstenedione to testosterone, possibly by other isoenzymes of 17βHSD family (17 βHSD5). Enzyme 5 α reductase type 2 catalyzes conversion of testosterone to its more bioactive form dihydrotestosterone (DHT). It is this more bioactive androgen (DHT), that is responsible for androgenization of external genitalia and development of prostate in 46 XY fetus. Most individuals affected by this mutation present usually in infancy and genital ambiguity is generally more than those with 17βHSD3 deficiency. Although male sex assignment is more likely with 5 α reductase type 2 deficiency, there may be female sex of rearing in some cases due to severe under-virilization. Such phenotypic females (46 XY) develop striking degree of virilization at puberty (increase in clitoral size, scrotalization of labial folds, deepening of voice, muscle development), although they rarely develop acnes and temporal hair recession despite high testosterone levels.

It is important to note here that in addition to above features, primary amenorrhea is consistent feature in all these cases of 46 XY DSD girls as Müllerian structures are absent due to normal secretion of AMH from sertoli cells prenatally. Breast development is spontaneous in most cases of PAIS, some cases of 17βHSD3 deficiency and none with 5 α reductase type-2 deficiency.

Approach to a girl with pubertal virilization is depicted in **Flowchart 2**.

Groin Lump

Testes are descended to scrotum or outside the external inguinal ring at birth in most children. Individuals (46 XY) with defective androgen synthesis or action commonly have undescended testis in inguinal canals as inguinal phase of testicular descent is androgen driven. Enlargement of testicular size at puberty in these cases may lead to pain, tender lump in inguinal region, and may be mistaken for incarcerated inguinal hernia. Presence of some genital ambiguity or clitoral enlargement with or without abnormal secondary sexual characteristics should alert to the diagnosis. It is more commonly a presenting feature in individuals with complete androgen insensitivity (CAIS) or 17βHSD3 deficiency as they have more female typical external genitalia while girls with other diagnosis (PAIS, 5 α reductase type 2 deficiency) usually have more genital ambiguity and may be diagnosed early.

Delayed Puberty and Primary Amenorrhea

All girls (46 XX and 46 XY) with DSD conditions have primary amenorrhea but development of other secondary sex characteristics varies with the diagnosis. Girls with

Flowchart 2: Approach to pubertal virilization in a girl with DSD.

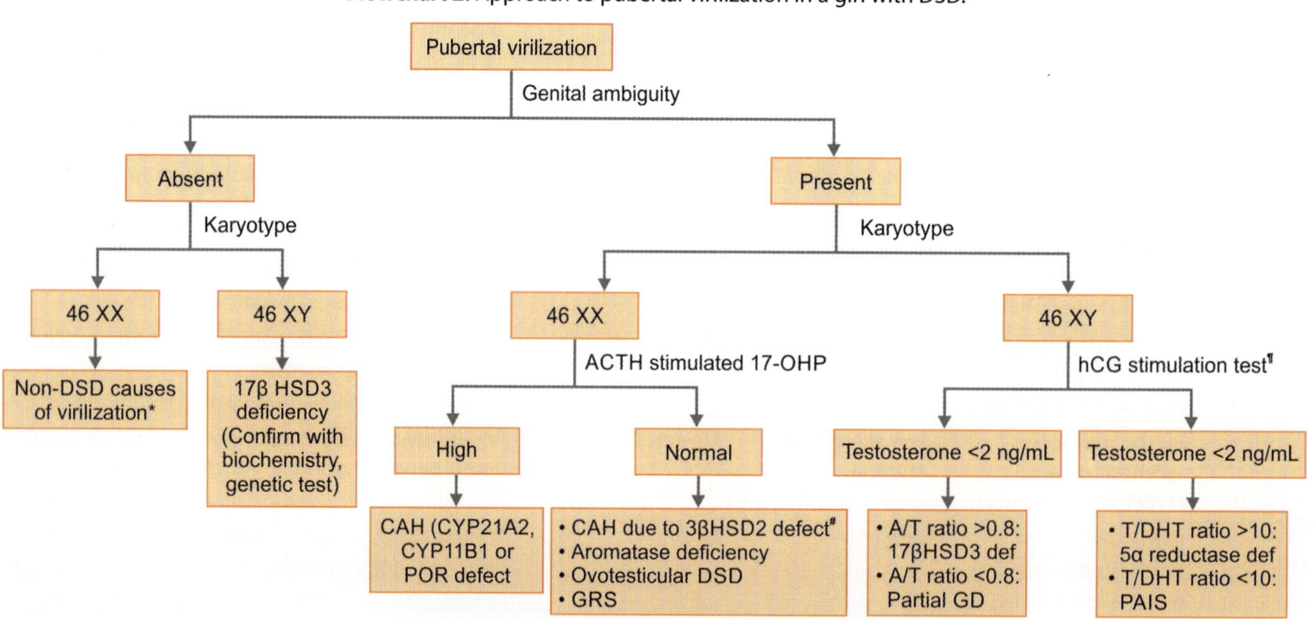

* Non-DSD causes of virilization include late onset CAH, ovarian hyperthecosis, adrenal or ovarian tumor etc.
# some cases of 3βHSD2 deficiency CAH have elevated 17-OHP levels due to peripheral conversion of excess 17 hydroxypregnenolone to 17 OHP by 3βHSD1 enzyme
¶ Ratios provided do not have good sensitivity and specificity, these are just rough guides

(A/T: androstenedione to testosterone ratio; CAH: congenital adrenal hyperplasia; CYP21A2: 21α hydroxylase; CYP11B1: 11β hydroxylase; GD: gonadal dysgenesis; PAIS: partial androgen insensitivity syndrome; POR: P450 oxidoreductase; T/DHT: testosterone to dihydrotestosterone ratio; 3βHSD2: 3β hydroxysteroid dehydrogenase; 17-OHP: 17 hydroxyprogesterone; 17βHSD3: 17β hydroxysteroid dehydrogenase)

complete gonadal dysgenesis (46 XX, 46 XY, or 45 XO) present with complete lack of pubertal changes (absent breast development, no pubarche, and primary amenorrhea). There are many genetic and inherited causes of 46 XX gonadal dysgenesis, distinction from premature ovarian insufficiency (POI) is difficult and evaluation is needed including testing for Fragile-X syndrome and autoantibodies. Turner syndrome (45 X) has similar presentation with delayed puberty associated with short stature and specific characteristic features. Although considered as sex chromosomal DSD, Turner syndrome requires a dedicated discussion and is not discussed here. All these individuals with 46 XX and 45 X gonadal dysgenesis have presence of uterus and other Müllerian structures on ultrasound or MRI, although these are hypoplastic due to lack of estrogen exposure.

Girls with 46 XY complete gonadal dysgenesis (Swayer syndrome) do not have atypical genitals at birth due to inability of dysgenetic gonads to produce testosterone and hence severe under-virilization in 46 XY individuals, leading to female sex of rearing. Although Müllerian structures are present in these individuals, they usually present at puberty with lack of secondary sexual characteristics and primary amenorrhea (hypergonadotropic hypogonadism) as functioning gonads are lacking. To the contrary, partial gonadal dysgenesis can be associated with phenotypes ranging from isolated hypospadias in male typical external genitals to mild clitoromegaly in female typical external genitals depending upon gonadal function present during organogenesis (8–12 weeks intrauterine). Not very rarely do these girls present with abdominal or pelvic mass associated with pain due development of gonadoblastoma or other malignant germ-cell tumors. Y chromosome cell line containing dysgenetic streak gonads are prone to develop gonadoblastoma and transformation to malignancy. There are some single gene mutations described in patients with various degrees of 46 XY gonadal dysgenesis and many remain unknown, as genetic diagnosis can be arrived in approximately 20–40% of such individuals.

CAIS is an X-linked condition resulting from mutation in AR leading complete resistance to androgen action. Girls with CAIS (46 XY) typically present in adolescence with primary amenorrhea. As described above, some may even present in late childhood to early adolescence with inguinal lump. These girls usually have normal breast development as excess testosterone gets converted to estradiol. Girls with Müllerian agenesis (MRKH) have similar presentation to those with CAIS: primary amenorrhea with normal breast development. Absent or scant pubic and axillary hair favors CAIS over MRKH, although 46 XY karyotype and high testosterone levels confirm diagnosis of CAIS.

Defect anywhere in the pathway of androgen synthesis in 46 XY individuals is associated with varying degree of external genitals, with more proximal enzyme pathway defects (steroidogenic acute regulatory protein, P450 side chain cleavage enzyme, 3β hydroxysteroid dehydrogenase type 2, 17α hydroxylase) also lead to defective cortisol synthesis and hence CAH. All these proximal pathway defects usually are associated with female typical genitals in 46 XY individuals and present at pubertal age with absence of secondary sexual characteristics and primary amenorrhea (hypergonadotropic hypogonadism). 3β hydroxysteroid dehydrogenase type 2 (3βHSD2) deficiency is an exception in that patients with this defect have more atypical genitals, although it ranges from female typical genitals with clitoromegaly to male typical genitals with isolated hypospadias due to partial androgenization from extragladular conversion of excess dehydroepiadrosterone (DHEA) to androstenedione by 3βHSD1. It is also important to note here that 3βHSD2 deficiency can lead to mild atypical genitals (isolated clitoromegaly to posterior labial fusion) in 46 XX individuals as well due to same mechanism (excess DHEA converted to androgens by 3βHSD1 in skin, placenta). All these proximal pathway defects may be associated with enuchoid habitus due to lack of continuous growth of long bones in absence of estrogen. Patients with 17α hydroxylase deficiency can have hypertension at presentation or later due to excessive mineralocorticoid precursors while other proximal pathway defects are associated with salt wasting.

Approach to a girl with primary amenorrhea is depicted in **Flowchart 3**.

GENDER IDENTITY AND GENDER DYSPHORIA

The term "Gender identity" refers to the self-identification by a person as male, female, or a nonbinary gender. Gender role indicates sex typical behaviors, e.g., preferences of clothes, physical aggression, choices of activities, and occupation, etc. It is possible for an individual with particular gender identity to possess gender role of opposite sex. Distress resulting from incongruence between expressed gender and assigned gender or dissatisfaction with assigned sex is known as gender dysphoria, and is the reason for sex change at puberty in some patients with DSD. In most individuals gender identity develops in accordance with physical gender characteristics. However in individuals with DSD, increasing recognition of dissatisfaction with assigned sex or gender dysphoria in some cases has questioned old theory that gender identity develops in accordance with assigned sex at birth provided the child is reared unambiguously and required surgeries have been done early in keeping with assigned sex. There are still debates about the relative contributions of chromosomes, hormones, brain structures, and societal influences on development of gender identity and gender dysphoria. Although girls with CAH (46 XX) have more masculine interests and male typical behaviors as a consequence of exposure of brain to high-androgen levels, their gender identity continues to remain as female and rarely they develop gender dysphoria. These studies on patients with CAH led to focus on chromosomal influence as predominant factor on gender identity. To the

Flowchart 3: Approach to a girl with primary amenorrhea in setting of DSD.

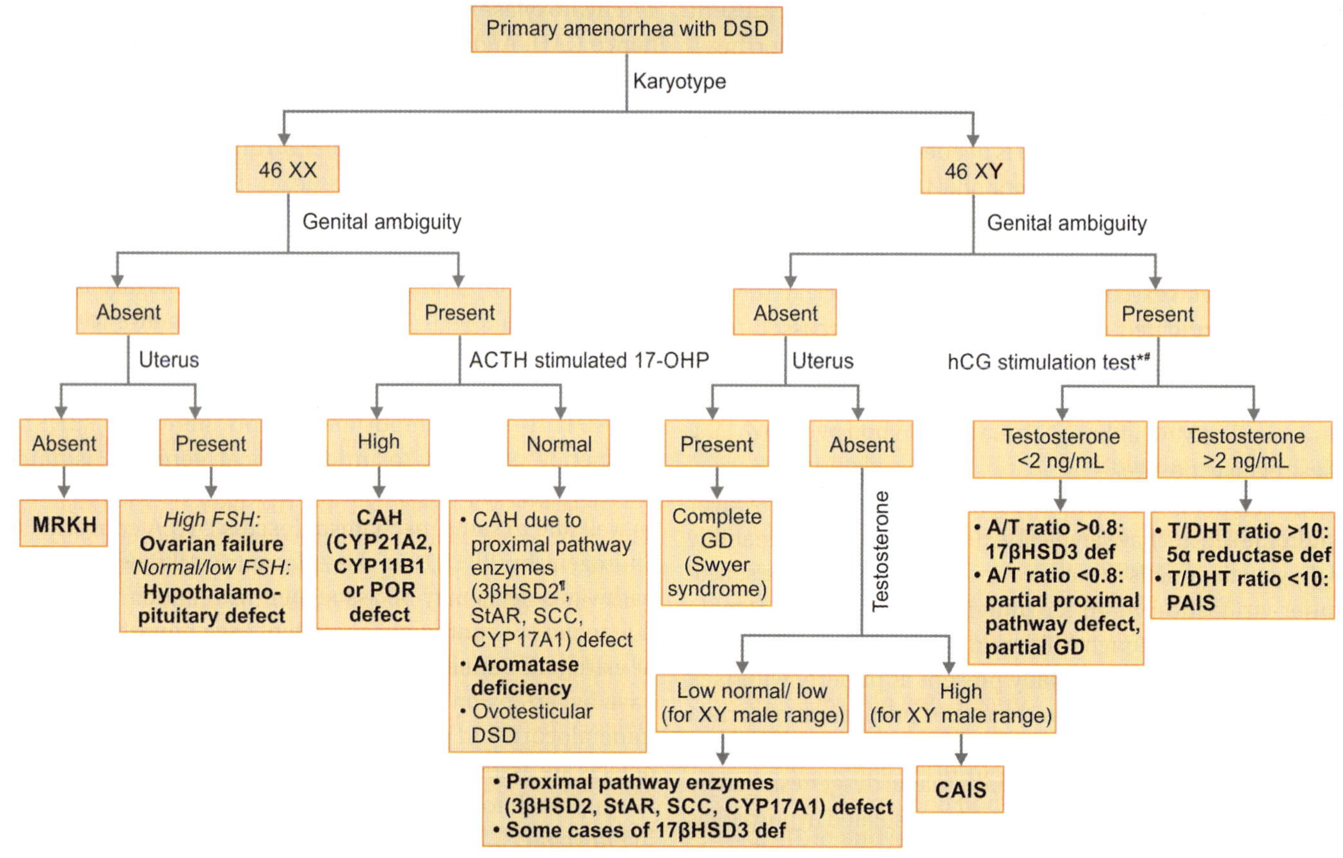

* Baseline FSH, LH and testosterone levels are important

¶ Some cases of 3βHSD2 deficiency CAH have elevated 17-OHP levels due to peripheral conversion of excess 17 hydroxypregnenolone to 17 OHP by 3βHSD1 enzyme

Ratios provided do not have good sensitivity and specificity, these are just rough guides

[A/T: androstenedione to testosterone ratio; CAH: congenital adrenal hyperplasia; CAIS: complete androgen insensitivity syndrome; CYP21A2: 21α hydroxylase; CYP11B1: 11β hydroxylase; CYP17A1: 17α hydroxylase; GD: gonadal dysgenesis; MRKH: Mayer-Rockitansy-Kuster-Hauser syndrome (Müllerian agenesis); PAIS: partial androgen insensitivity syndrome; POR: P450 oxidoreductase; StAR: steroidogenic acute regulatory protein; SCC: side chain cleavage enzyme; T/DHT: testosterone to dihydrotestosterone ratio; 3βHSD2: 3β hydroxysteroid dehydrogenase; 17-OHP: 17 hydroxyprogesterone; 17βHSD3: 17β hydroxysteroid dehydrogenase]

contrary, girls and women with CAIS (46 XY) possess female gender identity and gender role. This argument holds for greater role of androgens and lesser of Y chromosome in gender identity/gender dysphoria. However, in individuals with 46 XY karyotype and partial androgen exposure (PAIS, deficiency of 17βHSD3 and 5 α reductase type 2), prediction of long-term gender identity is difficult. In individuals PAIS (46 XY), gender dysphoria develops in approximately 25% of cases at puberty whether they are reared as a boy or a girl. However, a significant percentage of individuals with deficiency of 17βHSD3 and 5 α reductase type 2 (46 XY) and reared as girl, experience gender dysphoria at puberty to the extent that they decide to live as boys/men, particularly if the gonadectomy is not done early and pubertal virilization develops.

From above studies, it can be said that prenatal androgen exposure to brain can lead to development of male typical behaviors/male gender role but its influence on gender identity development is more complex, where chromosomal and societal factors may also be important contributors in addition.

MANAGEMENT

Taking decisions about management of children and adolescents with DSD is socially and ethically complex and medically challenging. The following ethical principles are important to consider while taking management decisions in individuals with DSD especially infants and young children.

- Minimizing physical risk to individual
- Maximizing psychosocial well-being
- Preserving potential for fertility
- Reserving ability to have satisfying sexual experiences
- Leaving options open for future
- Respecting the parents' wishes and beliefs
- Consider the views of the child/adolescent.

It is not always possible to fulfill all these principles in every individual with DSD but in general these provide a systematic approach to decision making in medically complex field.

The management of DSD conditions varies with the particular diagnosis, sex of rearing, and age at presentation. It is best possible with multidisciplinary team consisting of endocrinologist, gynecologist, urologist, and psychologist. Overall management strategies for above described DSD conditions in an adolescent female is described here.

46 XX DSD

CAH

Management of adrenal insufficiency and prevention of adrenal crisis is of utmost importance in management of an individual with CAH. Replacement of glucocorticoids and mineralocorticoids is not only lifesaving but also halts the progression of precocious puberty in children and virilization in adolescents and adults. By reducing adrenal androgen secretion optimal medical management helps to normalize hypothalamo-pituitary-ovarian axis and hence normalizes menstrual cycle and fertility. Patients with CAH due to 11β hydroxylase deficiency or 17α hydroxylase deficiency have increased mineralocorticoids at baseline and require only glucocorticoid replacement, sometimes with anti-mineralocorticoid to treat hypertension. Surgical management (feminizing genitoplasty) depends on the prader stage of external genitalia and the following principles should be considered:

- Creation of typical female looking introitus with labia majora and minora
- *Vaginoplasty:* to provide functional and adequate opening in the introitus for vagina
- *Clitoroplasty:* reduction of the size of enlarged phallus with preservation of glans and its neurovascular supply.

There is extensive debate on the appropriate timing of surgical repair in these patients. We suggest children (46 XX) reared as female with confirmed diagnosis of CAH, should be subjected to surgical repair of external genitals before 3 years of age or whenever they present later. Adequate glucocorticoid and mineralocorticoid replacement should be ensured prior to surgery and stress cover should be provided perioperatively to prevent adrenal crisis.

Aromatase Deficiency

Girls with aromatase deficiency require treatment with gradually increasing dose of oral/transdermal estrogen for pubertal development. Replacement of adult dose of estrogens usually reduces the elevated gonadotropin levels and consequently androgen levels and ovarian cyst size. However some girls and women may require treatment with anti-androgens (spironolactone, eplerenone) to reduce virilization/hirsutism. Same surgical principles as described above, apply to these patients as well.

46 XY DSD

Surgical Management

Surgical management in girls with 46 XY DSD consists of performing gonadectomy and feminizing genitoplasty. The extent of surgical intervention for genitoplasty depends upon the baseline androgenization of external genitals. While the principles of feminizing genitoplasty remain the same as described above, some highlights of gonadectomy are discussed here.

Gonads containing Y chromosome cell line are prone to dysplastic changes and at risk of development of malignant germ cell tumors if these are dysgenetic and/or are intra-abdominal. Girls with complete gonadal dysgenesis usually have presence of streak gonads in abdomen and bilateral laparoscopic gonadectomy should be carried out as soon as diagnosis is confirmed. The appropriate timing of gonadal surgery is debated in girls with CAIS. As there is very little risk of gonadal malignancy before puberty in girls with CAIS, it is suggested to postpone gonadectomy till pubertal age for allowing normal breast development. To the contrary, there is risk of pubertal virilization in girls with PAIS, hence gonadectomy should be carried out early (before pubertal age) in these girls. It is very important to be certain of diagnosis of PAIS as there is significant overlap in clinical features and biochemical test results with 5α reductase type 2 deficiency. Although girls with 5α reductase type 2 deficiency and 17β HSD3 deficiency commonly have pubertal virilization, if gonads are in situ, performing gonadectomy before pubertal years is ethically more challenging. Many of these girls may develop gender dysphoria in puberty even after gonadectomy and may prefer to change gender. Therefore, it is also a reasonable approach to delay the gonadectomy and even genitoplasty till adolescence to allow the young person is involved in decision making and also allowing more time to the individual and family to consider the options and gender is clearer.

Medical Management

Other than cases of 46 XY DSD with associated adrenal insufficiency (CAH, some genetic forms of gonadal dysgenesis), medical management is usually not required till the age of puberty. Thereafter the medical management protocols vary depending upon some factors, e.g., underlying diagnosis, status of gonads, serum levels of sex hormones, status of Müllerian structures and importantly individual's psychosexual development. Girls with 46 XY complete gonadal dysgenesis and with proximal pathway enzyme defects in androgen synthesis, lack spontaneous onset of puberty, and need to be started on gradually increasing doses of oral/transdermal estrogens for pubertal induction. Uterus grows with estrogen therapy in girls with complete gonadal dysgenesis and subsequently cyclical progesterone can be added after 2 years of estrogen therapy or when she bleeds for the first time whichever is early. Spontaneous breast development and height spurt at puberty is present in girls with CAIS, if the gonads are not removed earlier. The more challenging is managing girls with 17β HSD3 deficiency, 5α reductase deficiency, and PAIS having partial androgenization of external genitalia. Although the definitive strategy to prevent or to treat virilization is performing gonadectomy, it can be temporarily prevented by blocking androgen receptors with anti-androgens or by delaying puberty with GnRH analogues in some cases where gonadectomy is delayed for ethical reasons as stated above. All these girls should be replaced with physiological doses of oral/transdermal estrogens after gonadectomy. As Müllerian structures are absent in girls with 46 XY DSD due to androgen synthesis defect or androgen insensitivity, treatment with progesterone is not required. Appropriate counseling regarding the expectations is very important prior to starting any medical therapy.

ROLE OF GENETIC TESTING AND GENETIC COUNSELING IN DSD

Genetic Testing

Genetic testing is now a routine part of clinical practice and plays a key role in management of patients with DSD. It falls under two categories:

1. *Cytogenetics:* Cytogenetic analysis, particularly information about the sex chromosomes is among one of the very initial investigations in a case of DSD. It can be carried out rapidly by using X or Y chromosome specific probe in a process called fluorescent in situ hybridization (FISH). On the other hand microscopic or more recently molecular karyotyping allows for detection of mosaicism by looking at multiple cells as well as detection of major deletions, duplications, and translocations in addition to assessment of sex chromosomes.
2. *Gene testing:* Genetic testing for a number of DSD genes is now available on clinical basis and this number is also increasing rapidly as new genes are identified and linked to DSD. There is significant overlap in clinical features and biochemical test results among various DSD conditions, making confirmative diagnosis very difficult. Detection of a specific gene variant can help by confirming and refining clinical diagnosis, clarifying the inheritance pattern if any and hence risk to other family members and providing the opportunity for molecular pre-natal diagnosis in future pregnancies. Testing for a single gene is now mostly limited to cases where there is strong suspicion of pathogenic variant in a particular gene based on clinical or biochemical evaluation (e.g., CAH). A preferable approach is to use next generation DNA sequencing (NGS), which enables testing of a large number of DSD genes at a relatively low cost. The individual and the families however should be aware that genetic testing does not provide clear answers in all cases. In the setting of 46 XY DSD, testing a panel of 64 DSD genes has been shown to make a molecular diagnosis in about one third of individuals tested.

Genetic Counseling

Genetic counseling is an important component in management of individuals with DSD and their families. Genetic counseling for DSD can take place at any stage of life and in various clinical settings (e.g., a couple with personal or family history of DSD and planning pregnancy, prenatal diagnosis of DSD, following diagnosis of DSD in a neonate, an adolescent or young adult with DSD seeking information about one's own diagnosis, etc.). It is important for individual's primary healthcare provider to have adequate knowledge about intricacies of genetic tests and counseling, otherwise it should be carried out by genetic counselors or clinical geneticists. Genetic counseling is a complex process to define it in a single sentence. However, listed below are, to varying degrees, some of the major elements of genetic counseling:

- Diagnostic and clinical aspects
- Documentation of family and pedigree information
- Recognition of inheritance pattern and risk estimation
- Effective communication
- Providing information on available options
- Providing support in decision making.

KEY MESSAGES

- Understanding physiologies of gonadal and genital development in human embryo as well as adrenal/gonadal steroidogenesis pathway are of paramount importance to effectively diagnose and manage patients with DSD.
- Individual's psychosexual preferences should be given due consideration while taking management decisions.
- Dysgenetic and intra-abdominal gonads containing Y chromosomal cell line carry a significant malignancy risk and should be excised at the earliest.
- Genetic testing and genetic counseling has now become an integral part of management of an individual with DSD.
- Evaluation and management of individuals with DSD requires a multidisciplinary team consisting of endocrinologist, gynecologist, urologist, psychologist, and clinical geneticist.

FURTHER READING

1. Baxter RM, Arboleda VA, Lee H, et al. Exome sequencing for the diagnosis of 46,XY disorders of sex development. J Clin Endocrinol Metab. 2015;100:333-44.

LONG QUESTIONS

1. Describe the evaluation and management of an adolescent girl with disordered sexual development.
2. Describe the process of normal sexual differentiation and etiopathogenesis of disorders of sexual development.

SHORT QUESTIONS

1. What is the form and role of testosterone in sexual differentiation?

2. What is the differential diagnosis of a groin lump in an individual with DSD?
3. What are the characteristic features of complete gonadal agenesis?

MULTIPLE CHOICE QUESTIONS

1. Clitoris develops from which of the following primitive structure in a human fetus?
   a. Urogenital folds
   b. Genital tubercle
   c. Urogenital sinus
   d. Urogenital swelling
2. Determination of bipotential gonad into either testes or ovary occurs during which phase of intra-uterine life in a fetus:
   a. 3–4 weeks
   b. 5–6 weeks
   c. 8–11 weeks
   d. 16–18 weeks
3. Which of the following is a sign of prenatal virilization in a girl with 46 XX DSD?
   a. Posterior fourchette fusion (posterior labial fusion)
   b. Clitoromegaly
   c. Increased male type muscle mass
   d. All of the above
4. All of the following are causes of 46 XX DSD in an adolescent girl, except:
   a. Congenital adrenal hyperplasia (CAH)
   b. Glucocorticoid resistance syndrome (GRS)
   c. Complete androgen insensitivity syndrome (CAIS)
   d. Aromatase deficiency
5. 16-year-old, relatively short girl presents with virilization starting at 7 years age a/w primary amenorrhea. She has genital ambiguity present on examination. Which investigation will you perform first?
   a. Cortisol
   b. ACTH
   c. 17 hydroxyprogesterone (17 OHP)
   d. Testosterone
6. 16-year-old girl presents with primary amenorrhea, normal breast development and no genital ambiguity with serum testosterone level 12 ng/mL, what is the most likely diagnosis?
   a. Müllerian agenesis-MRKH (46 XX)
   b. Complete androgen insensitivity syndrome (46 XY)
   c. Swayer syndrome-complete gonadal dysgenesis (46 XY)
   d. 17α hydroxylase deficiency CAH (46 XY)
   e. 21α hydroxylase deficiency CAH (46 XX)
7. All of the following conditions may be associated with pubertal virilization in a girl with DSD, except:
   a. 5α reductase type 2 deficiency
   b. 17β HSD3 deficiency
   c. 17α hydroxylase deficiency
   d. Partial androgen insensitivity
8. Development of gender dysphoria leading to change of sex from female to male at puberty is more common with which of the following DSD condition?
   a. Congenital adrenal hyperplasia (CAH)
   b. Complete androgen insensitivity syndrome (CAIS)
   c. 5α reductase type 2 deficiency
   d. 46 XY complete gonadal dysgenesis (Swayer syndrome)
9. Which of the following test is confirmative of 17β HSD3 deficiency in a girl with 46 XY DSD?
   a. High FSH and LH with low testosterone
   b. Testosterone/Androstenedione ratio <0.8
   c. Heterozygous mutation in HSD17B3 gene
   d. Homozygous mutation in HSD17B3 gene
10. Bilateral gonadectomy should be carried out as soon as possible after diagnosis, in girls with complete gonadal dysgenesis, because of the fear of:
    a. Development of malignancy
    b. Development of virilization
    c. Development of torsion
    d. All of the above

Answers

1.	b	2.	b	3.	a	4.	c	5.	c	6.	b
7.	c	8.	c	9.	d	10.	a				

8.5 BODY ISSUE IMAGES IN ADOLESCENTS

Reeti Dutta Mehra

INTRODUCTION

Body image is how and what one thinks and feels about one's body. Body image can change through one's lifetime. A positive or healthy body image is feeling happy, satisfied and comfortable with one's body and accepting the way you look. A negative or unhealthy body image is feeling unhappy with the way you look. A positive body image is reflected by good self-esteem and mental health as well as a balanced attitude to eating and physical activity. A healthy body image in childhood and adolescence can lay the foundations for good physical and mental health later in life whereas an unhealthy body image can have long-lasting consequences. Low self-esteem and poor body image are risk factors for the development of risky weight loss strategies, eating disorders, and mental health disorders such as depression.

INCIDENCE

Body image dissatisfaction as calculated by the silhouette scale has been estimated to be between 56 and 75% in different studies and is no longer a western concept and affects Indian adolescent girls to a great extent. Indian Studies, though few have shown an incidence of about 77–81% in Indian adolescents with a higher preponderance in girls as compared to boys and more in the urban and higher socioeconomic strata.

During puberty, the body and mind is going through lots of changes. Adolescence represents a pivotal stage in the development of positive or negative body image. Many influences exist during the teen years including transitions (e.g., puberty) that affect one's body shape, weight status, and appearance. Fitting in and looking attractive becomes of paramount importance to adjust well with the peers. Body image is also influenced by many other factors including family environment, ability or disability, the attitudes of peers, social media, cultural background and more.

Boys, girls, can all be affected by body image issues, but in different ways. For example, teenage girls who do not like their bodies often want to lose weight and be thinner. Teenage boys want to lose weight, be taller or have more muscles. Some children are more likely than others to feel unhappy about their bodies.

The higher risk children may:
- Feel pressure from family, peers or media to fit into a narrow idea of beauty
- Have a different body shape or weight from their peers or from "ideal" shapes in the media
- Be perfectionists
- Look at themselves from the "outside" and worry about how others see them
- Compare themselves to others
- Have low self-esteem or experience symptoms of depression
- Belong to a friendship, sport or dance group that emphasizes a certain body type
- Have physical disabilities.

Negative body image can harm the adolescents' nutrition and lead to eating disorders (spectrum of disorders ranging from anorexia to bulimia) that are known to have grave consequences including mortality. They may skip meals or take diet pills. Some children especially girls might try to control their weight by smoking or changing their appearance by buying beauty products or getting cosmetic surgery. Having a negative body image might affect a girl's comfort with her sexuality or reproductive body functions, such as menstruation or breastfeeding, as she gets older. Spending time worrying about their bodies and how they measure up can also take away from girls' ability to concentrate on other pursuits.

Body image has become a popular topic over the past 35 years. In fact, 90% of body image studies have been published since 1980. Interest in this area parallels growing public health concerns about weight status, physical inactivity, obesity, eating disorders, and the associated spectrum of health consequences. This chapter will discuss the relevant literature on factors affecting body image issues, the consequences of an unhealthy body image and intervention strategies that address adolescent body image.

SOCIAL MEDIA AND BODY IMAGE

Groesz et al. found that the greatest decline in body satisfaction occurred in girls under the age of 19 following exposure to overtly thin media images. Recent studies indicate that current diet, exercise, and beauty trends displayed in reality television shows and social media outlets can contribute to unhealthy adolescent body perceptions. For girls, cultural expectations emphasize being thin and lean with large breasts as seen in print media, television, and online. Tiggemann and Slater later found that among 13–15-year old girls, body image concerns increased with time spent on the Internet and Facebook usage. Meier and Gray further identified that the time spent on Facebook was less important than the degree of exposure to appearance-specific media such as photo sharing, which was positively associated with body image concerns. These findings suggest that in addition to print media, current television, and Internet trends are sources of promoting unrealistic and so-called ideal images to adolescents.

INFLUENCE OF FAMILY AND PEERS

Research has shown that weight-based teasing from parents and siblings is associated with body dissatisfaction among girls and drive for muscularity among boys in eighth and ninth grade. Encouragement from parents to control weight was also linked to heightened weight concerns among high school girls and boys. Dieting among family members, especially from mothers who serve as role models for body image, has been shown to be related to body image concerns and disordered eating behaviors in adolescent girls. Peers have also been identified as a prominent source of weight-and appearance-based pressure by. Appearance-based teasing and criticism, modeling and discussing appearance concerns, making appearance comparisons, judging the appearance of friends, and social conflict or exclusion all lead to a negative body image. Body dissatisfaction among tenth grade girls is strongly predicted by the belief that thinness was critical to their attraction to boys. Further, 85% of boys did indeed perceive thinness as an attractive quality in girls.

PUBERTY AND ITS CHANGES

Changes associated with puberty, such as increases in adiposity and widening of the hips, may be perceived negatively and seen as incongruent with the prototypical and societally valued "thin ideal". Early maturing girls in particular, who are prone to greater puberty-related weight gain, have reported a greater drive for thinness and stronger preference for a slender figure than their later maturing counterparts. This finding suggests that early maturing girls may be especially vulnerable to developing a negative body image when they perceive their changing bodies to be misaligned with cultural ideals. Although evidence indicates that adolescent boys report greater weight and appearance esteem than girls, boys are not immune to body image concerns during adolescent development. Specifically, increases in height and muscle mass associated with puberty moves some boys closer to cultural expectations to be tall and muscular. Late-maturing boys specifically, who have not achieved socially constructed body ideals for men, report greater body dissatisfaction than their early maturing counterparts. Thus, the perception of physical changes in a sociocultural context plays a critical role in shaping body image throughout adolescence.

OBESITY AND BODY IMAGE

Distortion and dissatisfaction with body image may form a link between overweight and obesity, as excessive preoccupation with appearance and unremitting pursuit of the perfect, lean body can generate negative feelings and devaluation, resulting in change in the eating behavior, leading to overweight or the development of ED. The inverse also being true and obesity may be the etiology of the negative body image.

The percentage of obese adolescents has quadrupled over the past 30 years. Recent estimates indicate that ~17% youths ages 2–19 years are obese in the US, with higher prevalence rates found among Hispanic youth (22.4%), followed by non-Hispanic black (20.2%), white (14.1%), and Asian youth (8.6%). A study published in the Lancet analyzed weight and height in nearly 130 million people, including 31.5 million children aged 5–19 years of age. The number of obese children and adolescents rose from 11 million in 1975 to 124 million in 2016. Globally, in 2016, over one in six adolescents aged 10–19 years was overweight. Prevalence varied across World Health Organization (WHO) regions, from lower than 10% in the WHO South-East Asia region to over 30% in the WHO Region of the Americas.

The areas of the world with some of the largest increase in the number of obese children and adolescents were East Asia, Middle East and North Africa. Research consistently shows that greater body mass index (BMI) is associated with heightened weight concerns in both adolescent girls and boys. Childhood obesity can profoundly affect children's physical health, social, and emotional well-being, and self-esteem. It is also associated with poor academic performance and a lower quality of life experienced by the child. Overweight and obese youth are more likely to be the targets of weight-related bullying. Many comorbid conditions like metabolic, cardiovascular, orthopedic, neurological, hepatic, pulmonary, and renal disorders are also seen in association with childhood obesity. In the Indian study by Subhashini Ganesan et al. from Coimbatore, 67% of participants who were dissatisfied with their body image were adopting one or more weight control measures while in the satisfied group 57.5% had adopted weight control measures.

PHYSICAL INACTIVITY

Overweight and obese youth, especially those who have body- and appearance-related concerns, are likely to avoid physical activity. For example, Neumark-Sztainer et al. in a study of 2,516 adolescents found negative associations between body satisfaction and physical activity. The intersectionality of weight, feelings about one's body, and barriers to activity were highlighted in a systematic review of 15 qualitative research studies focused on physical activity. Specifically, common themes reported across studies indicated that overweight and obese youth perceive individual barriers (e.g., lack of fitness associated with excess weight), social barriers (e.g., exclusion and teasing), and environmental barriers (e.g., lack of privacy in gym changing rooms). Physical inactivity may further cause the children not to participate in sports, peer activities thereby leading to social exclusion, depression, low self-esteem and further obesity and related conditions.

EATING DISORDERS

Body dissatisfaction among adolescent samples has been consistently shown to be the strongest predictor of disordered eating behaviors and clinical eating disorders Eating disorders are common and serious conditions affecting up to 4% of the population. The mortality rate is high. Negative body image has been a central diagnostic feature for all clinical eating disorders (i.e., anorexia nervosa, bulimia nervosa, binge eating disorder). Anorexia nervosa involves the severe restriction of food intake to unhealthy levels that results in caloric deprivation. By contrast, bulimia nervosa is characterized by binge episodes of overeating followed by compensatory purging, such as vomiting, laxatives use, diuretics, or obligatory exercise to counteract excessive caloric intake. This obligatory exercise goes beyond what is considered "healthy exercise" and features feelings of compulsion, guilt, and rigidity. This exercise may serve as a way to compensate for the negative body image. Finally, binge eating disorder, a new classification in the Diagnostic and Statistical Manual of Mental Disorders, Fifth Edition (DSM-5), features binge episodes without an accompanying purging method. Shame and harsh self-criticism have been identified as underlying mechanisms for binge eating behavior.

Adolescents who experience guilt following a binge episode may impulsively respond by vomiting, excessively exercising, or using laxatives. Adolescents who view purging behavior as a "workaround" for dietary setback may experience the addictive quality of the purge when they feel temporary emotional relief. This "temporary solution" can ultimately reach clinical levels if the behavior continues for several months on a consistent basis. Disordered eating is often distinguished from clinical eating disorders as being pathological while not meeting all of the DSM-5 criteria. Eating disorders represent the highest mortality rate of adolescents among all psychiatric conditions, eating disorders can also be associated with increased suicide risk and self-harming behaviors. Purging behaviors such as repetitive vomiting can place excessive strain on the esophagus, larynx, or voice box resulting in bleeding, tearing, or a ruptured esophagus. Other physical complications include cardiovascular problems, amenorrhea (i.e., absence of menstrual cycle), gastrointestinal problems, tooth decay, reduced bone density, and impaired colon function. Electrolyte imbalances create an additional risk for individuals with eating disorders and may result in hospitalization.

Unfortunately, the intended goal of achieving one's body ideal and feeling satisfaction is never actualized, as adolescents often find themselves obsessively consumed with the next bodily flaw or losing the next 5 pounds. Although exercise addiction is estimated to be around 3% of the general population, this prevalence increases to 30–70% among clinical samples, and is estimated to range from 33% to almost 100% of inpatient eating disorder clients. Dysfunctional exercise is associated with physical and psychological health consequences, including poor concentration, fatigue, mood disturbances (e.g., depression, irritability), overuse injuries (e.g., stress fractures, pressure sores), social isolation, and impaired relationships.

CLINICAL APPLICATION

The importance of developing a healthy body image during adolescence should be emphasized given the associated health consequences. In light of the rising obesity rates among adolescents and the attention given to obesity as a public health priority, schools and communities tend to focus on obesity prevention and weight loss alone and many obesity interventions reinforce and normalize body dissatisfaction because of being overweight. Hence, programs are needed to emphasize a healthy life style that equally promotes a healthy body. Interventions aimed to improve physical activity should avoid strategies that may have a negative impact on the body image of adolescents, such as unrealistic weight goals, critical weight-related comments, and weigh-ins. Instead, physical activity promotion should additionally include a means of increasing body satisfaction, and improving body perceptions versus weight status alone.

CLINICAL MANAGEMENT

Addressing the problem: The question that most parents have is, whether it is normal for the child to be conscious of her body and want to lead a healthy lifestyle. But parents have to be warned of some signs if the child is focusing too much on his body. The child might seem to have *anxiety* and *stress* about how he looks. He might show this by:

- Criticizing his body, e.g., he might say he's ugly
- Continually comparing his body with others
- Not wanting to leave the house because of the way he looks
- Not doing activities or trying new things because of the way he feels about his body
- Obsessing about losing weight, or about specific parts of his body, such as his face or legs
- Spending lots of time looking in the mirror or taking photos and looking for changes or imperfections
- Linking food with feelings of guilt, shame or blame.

If parents think that the child is experiencing any of these signs, they should start by talking with him/her about the concerns. If things do not change and they are still worried, they should consider talking to their GP or another health professional. The treatment has to be:

- Family-based treatment
- Cognitive behavioral therapy
- Dialectical discussions
- Use of therapeutic drugs if severe condition.

Treatment is mainly psychosocial counseling and guidance by parents. Teachers, friends and counselors may be roped in. They must focus on the child's natural talents and encourage and improve the child's self-esteem. Relentless nagging by mothers and social comparisons should be discouraged. A healthy life style must be promoted by modifying diet and improving physical activity. Media time should be restricted by promoting hobbies. Idolizing famous people for their achievements rather than looks also promotes a healthy body image among both adolescent boys and girls.

Importance of interventions at school that target the psychological correlates of poor body image cannot be undermined. Multisession interventions targeted toward younger adolescents between 12 and 13 years of age that focus on media literacy, boosting self-esteem, and building peer support should be encouraged. Teachers should be instructed to reduce social comparisons, and address the influence of traditional gender roles on body image development. Also appropriate interventions such as life skills education and media literacy to minimize body image issues are advocated. In addition, information regarding normal growth and its variations should be provided to adolescents.

The WHO recommends for adolescents to accumulate at least 60 minutes of moderate- to vigorous-intensity physical activity daily, which may include play, games, sports, but also activity for transportation (such as cycling and walking), or physical education. Globally, only 1 in 5 adolescents are estimated to meet these guidelines. Prevalence of inactivity is high across all WHO regions, and higher in female adolescents as compared to male adolescents. To increase activity levels, countries, societies and communities need to create safe and enabling environments and opportunities for physical activity for all adolescents.

Talking about Body Image: May be Done by Parents or Counselor

Talking about body image with adolescents can make them comfortable in their own skin. When discussing body image, one might:

- *Explain the effects of puberty:* Make sure the child understands that weight gain is a normal part of development, especially during puberty.
- *Talk about media messages:* Television programs, movies, music videos, websites, magazines and even some toys might send the message that only a certain body type is acceptable and that maintaining an attractive appearance is the most important goal. Check out what the teens are reading or watching and discuss it. Encourage them to question what they see and hear.
- *Monitor Internet use:* Teens use social networking sites and services to share pictures and receive feedback. Awareness of others' judgments can make teens feel self-conscious

about their looks. Set rules for Internet use and talk about what they are posting and viewing.

- *Discuss self-image:* Offer reassurance that healthy body shapes vary. Ask them what they like about themselves and explain what the parents like about them too. Parents acceptance and respect can help build self-esteem and resilience.
- *Use positive language:* Rather than talking about "fat" and "thin," encourage to focus on eating a healthy diet and staying physically active. Discourage family and friends from using hurtful nicknames and joking about people who are overweight.

Other Strategies to Promote a Healthy Body Image

In addition to talking about a healthy body image, one might:

- *Team up with your family doctor:* Family doctor can help set realistic goals for BMI and weight based on her personal weight history and overall health.
- *Help establish healthy eating habits:* Offer healthy meals and snacks.
- *Counter negative media messages:* Expose children to people who are famous for their achievements—not their appearance. For example, read books or watch movies about inspiring women/men.
- *Praise achievements:* Help them value what they do, rather than looks. Look for opportunities to praise their efforts, skills and achievements.
- *Promote physical activity:* Participating in sports and other physical activities — particularly those that do not emphasize a particular weight or body shape — can help promote good self-esteem and a positive body image.
- *Encourage positive friendships:* Friends who accept and support can be a healthy influence.
- *Set a good example:* Remind the children that exercise and healthy eating is important for their health, not just to look a certain way. Also parents must lead by example and be careful of what they read and watch as well as the products they buy and the message their choices send.

WHEN TO CONSULT A DOCTOR

If the adolescent is struggling with a negative body image, consider professional counseling. Additional support might give the child the tools she needs to counter social pressure and feel good about her body. Eating disorders or morbid obesity associated with clinical depression in particular may need drug therapy.

KEY MESSAGES

- Body image is how and what one thinks and feels about one's body. Body image can change through one's lifetime. A healthy body image in childhood and adolescence can lay the foundations for good physical and mental health later in life. Indian studies, though few have shown an incidence of about 77–81% in Indian adolescents with a higher preponderance in girls and more in the urban and higher socioeconomic strata. Programs are needed to emphasize a healthy life style that equally promotes a healthy body. Good counseling of the adolescents, helping to establish healthy eating habits, countering negative media messages, praising achievements, promoting physical activity and encouraging positive friendships would help towards building a positive body image.
- Set a good example.
- Praise achievements. Help them value what they do, rather than looks. Look for opportunities to praise their efforts, skills and achievements.
- Promote physical activity. Participating in sports and other physical activities—particularly those that do not emphasize a particular weight or body shape—can help promote good self-esteem and a positive body image.
- Encourage positive friendships. Friends who accept and support can be a healthy influence.

FURTHER READING

1. American Psychiatric Association. Diagnostic and Statistical Manual of Mental Disorders, 5th edition. Washington, DC: American Psychiatric Association; 2013.
2. Arenas JJS, Martínez AOR. Relationship between self-esteem and body image in children with obesity. Revista Mexicana de Trastornos Alimentarios. 2015;6(1):38-44.
3. Ashikali EM, Dittmar H, Ayers S. The effect of cosmetic surgery reality TV shows on adolescent girls' body image. Psychol Pop Media Cult. 2014;3(3):141-53.
4. Burt NM, Boddy LE, Bridgett DJ. Contribution of temperament to eating disorder symptoms in emerging adulthood: additive and interactive effects. Eat Behav. 2015 Aug; 18():30-5
5. Cecon RS, Franceschini SDCC, Peluzio MDCG, Hermsdorff HHM, Priore SE. Overweight and Body Image Perception in Adolescents with Triage of Eating Disorders. Scientific World J. 2017;2017:8257-329
6. Deshmukh VR, Kulkarni AA. Body Image and its Relation with Body Mass Index among Indian Adolescents. Indian Pediatr. 2017;54(12):1025-8
7. Doornwaard SM. Sex-related online behaviors and adolescents' body and sexual self-perceptions. Pediatrics. 2014;134:1103.
8. Duarte C, Pinto-Gouveia J, Ferreira C. Escaping from body image shame and harsh self-criticism: exploration of underlying mechanisms of binge eating. Eat Behav. 2014;15(4):638-43
9. Ganesan S, Ravishankar SL, Ramalingam S. Are body image issues affecting our adolescents? A cross-sectional study among college going adolescent girls. Indian J Community Med. 2018;43(Suppl 1):S42-S46.
10. Groesz LM, Levine MP, Murnen SK. The effect of experimental presentation of thin media images on body satisfaction: a meta-analytic review. Int J Eat Disord. 2002;31(1):1-16.
11. Lofrano-Prado MC, Prado WL, De Piano A, Dâmaso AR. Obesidade e transtornos alimentares: a coexistência de comportamentos alimentares extremos em adolescentes. Con Scientiae Saúde. 2011;10(3):579-85

12. McCabe MP, Ricciardelli LA. A longitudinal study of pubertal timing and extreme body change behaviors among adolescent boys and girls. Adolescence. 2004 Spring; 39(153):145-66.
13. Meier EP, Gray J Facebook photo activity associated with body image disturbance in adolescent girls. J Cyberpsychol Behav Soc Netw. 2014;17(4):199-206.
14. Myers TA, Crowther JH. Social comparison as a predictor of body dissatisfaction: a meta-analytic review. Abnorm Psychol. 2009;118(4):683-98.
15. Nanu C, Tăut D, Băban A. Appearance esteem and weight esteem in adolescence. Are they different across age and gender? Cogn Brain Behav. 2013;17(3):189-200
16. Neumark-Sztainer D, Paxton SJ, Hannan PJ, Haines J, Story M. Does body satisfaction matter? Five-year longitudinal associations between body satisfaction and health behaviors in adolescent females and males. J Adolesc Health. 2006; 39(2):244-6.
17. Ogden CL, Carroll MD, Kit BK, Flegal KM Prevalence of childhood and adult obesity in the United States, 2011-2012. JAMA. 2014;311(8):806-14.
18. Paxton SJ, Norris M, Wertheim EH, Durkin SJ, Anderson J. Body dissatisfaction, dating, and importance of thinness to attractiveness in adolescent girls. Sex Roles. 2005;53(9-10): 663-75.
19. Quick V, Eisenberg ME, Bucchianeri MM, Neumark-Sztainer D. Prospective predictors of body dissatisfaction in young adults: 10-year longitudinal findings. Emerg Adulthood. 2013;1(4):271-282.
20. Schaefer MK, Blodgett Salafia EH. The connection of teasing by parents, siblings, and peers with girls' body dissatisfaction and boys' drive for muscularity: the role of social comparison as a mediator. Eat Behav. 2014;15(4):599-608.
21. Sharpe H, Naumann U, Treasure J, Schmidt U. Is fat talking a causal risk factor for body dissatisfaction? A systematic review and meta-analysis. Int J Eat Disord. 2013;46(7):643-52
22. Voelker DK, Reel JJ, Greenleaf C. Weight status and body image perceptions in adolescents: current perspectives. Adolesc Health Med Therapeut. 2015;6:149-58.
23. Yager Z, Diedrichs PC, Ricciardelli LA, Halliwell. What works in secondary schools? A systematic review of classroom-based body image programs. Body Image. 2013;10(3):271-81.

LONG QUESTIONS

1. Discuss the factors that play a role in creating body image issues.
2. What are different effects of body image issues on adolescent health?
3. Write a note on how to tackle an adolescent with body image issues.
4. Explain eating disorders and body image issues.
5. Discuss obesity and body image issues.

SHORT QUESTIONS

1. Write a note on: What types of adolescents are prone to body image issues?
2. Write a short note on: Role of media on body image issues.
3. Elaborate the role of parents and teachers on body image issues.
4. Write a short note on: Counseling of an adolescent with body image issues.
5. Short note on: Role of exercise in body image issues.

MULTIPLE CHOICE QUESTIONS

1. The following is false about body image issues:
   a. Body image issues can lead to eating disorders
   b. Positive body image is reflected by good mental health
   c. Body image issues are seen in girls only
   d. Adolescents with physical disabilities are more prone to body image issues
2. Negative body image can lead to all, except:
   a. Anorexia b. Bulimia
   c. Depression d. Psychosis
3. Adolescents with body image issues are not prone to:
   a. Alcoholism b. Smoking
   c. Cosmetic surgery d. Binge eating
4. Factors that affect body image issues are all, except:
   a. Internet
   b. Television and theatre
   c. Parents and teachers
   d. Academic performance at school
5. Perception of good body image among boys is:
   a. Thin and lean b. Tall, broad and muscular
   c. Short and heavy d. Tall and heavy
6. Perception of good body image in women is all, except:
   a. Tall and heavy b. Heavy breasted
   c. Small breasted d. Thin and fair
7. Childhood obesity is associated with:
   a. Metabolic syndrome in later life
   b. Body image issues
   c. Eating disorders
   d. All of the above
8. Which of the following is true for obese adolescents?
   a. They try to avoid physical activity
   b. They perform poorly in academics
   c. They have a tendency to be unhygienic
   d. They have a higher tendency for alcoholism
9. Which of the following is true for body image issues?
   a. It is seen more in girls
   b. Onset of pubertal changes may bring forth body image issues
   c. Those with body image issues tend to avoid socialization
   d. All of the above
10. Body image issues are adjudged by:
    a. Satisfaction scale b. Silhouette scale
    c. Pain scale d. Weighing scale

Answers

1.	c	2.	d	3.	a	4.	d	5.	b	6.	c
7.	d	8.	a	9.	d	10.	b				

8.6 EATING DISORDERS IN ADOLESCENCE

Nirmala Sharma, Anand Sharma, Neha Seehara

INTRODUCTION

Eating disorders are complex biopsychosocial disorders with their onset during adolescence. when the responsibility for the food intake shifts from parents to child, multiple factors such as knowledge of food, accurate recognition and acceptance of hunger and satiety, awareness of food hygiene and handling, learning the food texture, smell and nutritional needs are involved in this phase of transition.[1] The Diagnostic and Statistical Manual of Mental Disorders, 5th edition (DSM-V) defines eating disorders as a "persistent disturbance of eating or eating related behavior that results in the altered consumption or absorption of food and that significantly impairs physical health or psychosocial functioning."

HISTORY

The earliest historical descriptions of people experiencing symptoms of modern-day eating disorders date back to Hellenistic (323 BC–31 BC) and Medieval times (5–15th century AD). Deprivation of food was seen as spiritual practice and women were disproportionately burdened. Some contemporary authors have dubbed these fasting habits as "Holy Anorexia". Two cases of "nervous consumption" were reported by an English Physician, Richard Morton in 1689. 200 years later in 1873, Sir William Gull coined the term "Anorexia Nervosa". In contrast to Anorexia nervosa, Bulimia Nervosa appeared to be a more modern development. In 1979, British psychiatrist, Gerald Russell first described it as a variant of Anorexia nervosa.[2]

Eating disorders have been reported across the world, cultural variation may contribute to different presentations of eating disorder symptoms. Even celebrities are untouched by these difficult and sometimes life-threatening conditions. Andrew Morton's book "DIANA: HER TRUE STORY, 1992 revealed bulimia as Princess Diana's secret disease". As Princess Diana took courage to conflict her eating disorder, many other people have also confronted their problem, and sought treatment, this movement has come to be known as the "Diana effect".

EPIDEMIOLOGY

In the late 1800s, Anorexia nervosa was accepted as a psychological disorder. In 1952 Diagnostic and Statistical Manual of Mental Disorders (DSM-I) mentioned anorexia nervosa in its publication. In the DSM-III (1980), eating disorders debuted as a diagnostic category under the rubric of disorders of infancy, childhood or adolescence. The current form of bulimia nervosa was represented with the publication of DSM-IV (1994). DSM-V (American Psychiatric Association 2013) in their revised classification of eating disorders recognized binge eating disorders as an independent diagnosis.

Literature and researches regarding newer criteria are still limited, however in a recent US study, as per DSM-V criteria following is the reported prevalence of 0.8% for anorexia nervosa, 2.6% for bulimia nervosa, 2.8% for atypical anorexia nervosa, 3% for binge eating disorders, 3.4% for purging disorders, 3.6% for subthreshold binge eating disorders and 4.4% for subthreshold bulimia nervosa.[3] As per DSM-IV criteria the lifetime prevalence of anorexia nervosa in adolescent females is 0.3–0.6% with a higher prevalence rate in males than females. The prevalence of Bulimia nervosa in adolescent is ≈1–2% for females and 0.5% for males.[4]

ETIOLOGY

Interplay of following risk factors seems to contribute to these disorders:

- *Biological factors:* Growing body of twin studies confirmed the undeniable link between genetic factors and eating disorders.[5] The incidence of anorexia nervosa is more in families with one affected member as well as a higher concordance is found in monozygotic twins over dizygotic twins.[6]
- *Neurobiology:* Serotonin (5HT) seems to involve in appetite regulation and mood regulation. The altered 5HT1A and 5HT2A receptor activities, 5HTT (5HT transporter)and CSF 5HIAA levels are involved in eating disorders as depicted by several studies.[7]
- *Body image disturbance:* Body image misperception is common among general population. The culture of assessing over body image against the "Ideal body type" by individuals result in determination of body satisfaction and dissatisfaction.[8] A prospective study on college women found an association between the figure dissatisfaction, ineffectiveness and public subconsciousness with the symptoms of eating disorders.[9]

  The trend of self-induced malnutrition is commonly seen among young ballet dancers and gymnastics due to the intense fear of obesity. The nutritional retardation seen in this population is secondary to the reduced caloric intake as much as 40% of required one.
- *Childhood sexual abuse:* It is a topic of debate among clinician and researchers, while some studies showed strong relationship between childhood sexual abuse and eating disorders, some others strongly refuse to accept this relationship. It could be due to nonuniformity in the definition of childhood sexual abuse.[2]

- *Sociocultural factors:* Eating disorder is more common in culture where food is available and thinness is idealized. The desire to adopt a perfectionist attitude toward the body, relentless pursuit of thinness and tendency to have slim body seems secondary to exposure of the western culture is increasing the trend of eating disorders worldwide.

Countries such as Japan, Iran, Singapore, rate of eating disorders increases continuously among women who have been influenced by western culture of being slim either through short time vacation or through mass media.[10,11]

Female Athlete Triad

It is relatively common among young women participating in sports, the interrelationship of following components are seen:

- Menstrual dysfunction
- Low energy availability (with or without eating disorders)
- Decreased bone density. However, all the three components do not need to be shown by the individuals to manifest the female athlete triad.[12]

CLINICAL FEATURES (TABLE 1)

- *Anorexia nervosa:* Patients with anorexia nervosa have abnormally low body weight with intense fear of gaining weight. These patients in their mid to late adolescence rarely complain of hunger or fatigue and put extreme efforts on exercise. Just in order to prevent weight gain they tend to become socially withdrawn and increasingly committed to work or study, dieting and exercise.[5] Due to altered regulation of endocrine system, these women may present with hypothalamic amenorrhea.
- *Bulimia nervosa:* This disorder tends to start in late childhood or early adulthood. Characterized by episodes of binge eating followed by 5–10 times purging.

TABLE 1: Common characteristics of anorexia nervosa, bulimia nervosa and binge eating disorder.[5]

Clinical characteristic	*Anorexia nervosa[a]*	*Bulimia nervosa*	*Binge eating disorder[b]*
Onset	Mid-adolescence	Late adolescence/early adulthood	Late adolescence/early adulthood
Female: Male	10:1	10:1	2:1
Lifetime prevalence	1% of women	1–3% of women	4% of men and women
Weight	Markedly decreased	Usually normal	Usually obese
Menstruation	Absent	Usually normal	Usually normal
Binge eating	25–50%	Required for diagnosis	Required for diagnosis
Mortality	5% per decade	Low	Low
	Physical and laboratory findings		
Skin/extremities	• *Lanugo* • *Acrocyanosis* • *Edema*	*Callus/abrasion on dorsum of hand*	
Cardiovascular	• Bradycardia • Hypotension		
Gastrointestinal	• Salivary gland enlargement • Slow gastric emptying • Constipation • Elevated liver enzymes	• Salivary gland enlargement • Dental erosion	
Hematopoietic	• Normochromic normocytic anemia • Leucopenia		
Fluid/electrolyte	• Increased BUN, creatinine • Hypokalemia • Hypophosphatemia • Hypomagnesemia	• Hypokalemia • Hypochloremia • Alkalosis	
Endocrine	• Hypoglycemia • Low estrogen/testosterone • Low LH and FSH • Low-normal thyroxin • Normal TSH • Increased cortisol		
Bone	Osteopenia		

[a]Patients with anorexia nervosa who frequently induce purging may also exhibit the physical and laboratory findings associated with bulimia nervosa.
[b]Obese patients with binge eating disorder are at the risk for complications of obesity.

The self-imposed caloric restriction leads to increased hunger followed by overeating, then these patients try inappropriate way to lose weight like vomiting, use of laxatives or diuretics, enemas or engages in some other forms of compensatory behavior. Menstrual problems such as oligomenorrhea and amenorrhea are more frequent in these women than among women without eating disorders.[5] An association between bulimia nervosa and polycystic ovarian syndrome also has been suggested.

- *Binge eating disorders:* A common association is found between patients of binge eating disorder and obesity. It is accompanied by a feeling loss of control followed by frequent episodes of binge eating. An inappropriate behavior to compensate the binge eating is not seen in these patients. BED occurs more frequently than anorexia nervosa and bulimia nervosa in general population.
- *Other specified feeding or eating disorders (OSFED):* The "not otherwise specified" category of DSM-5 has been given two different categories. The first category OSFED incorporates specific eating disorder includes atypical AN, subthreshold BN, subthreshold binge eating disorders, purging disorders and night eating syndromes. The second category, unspecified feeding or eating disorder is intended for cases where insufficient information is available to make a specific eating disorder diagnosis or where symptoms genuinely unspecified and do not fit with other diagnostic examples.[13.]

DIAGNOSIS

Eating disorders diagnostic criteria is as follows:

Anorexia Nervosa

1a. BMI < 10th percentile for age/sex
2a. Fear for weight gain ≥2
3a. Body image disturbance:
- Importance of weight ≥2
- Importance of shape ≥2
- Feeling of fatness ≥2

1b. BMI <3 percentile for age/sex
2b. Fear of weight gain ≥1 and trying to restrict food intake ≥1
3b. Body image disturbance.

Bulimia Nervosa

- Objective binge eating. Eating an unusually large amount of food ≥1 + loss of control over eating ≥1.
- Compensatory behaviors
  - Self-induced vomiting ≥1
  - Laxative/Pill use ≥1
  - Hard exercise ≥2
- Over evaluation of weight and shape
  - Importance of weight ≥2
  - Importance of shape ≥2
- BMI >10th percentile of age/sex.

Binge Eating Disorders

- Objective binge eating. Eating an unusually large amount of food ≥1 plus loss of control over eating ≥1
- Distress over binge eating. concern over loss of control
- Over evaluation of weight/shape
  - Importance of weight ≥2
  - Importance of shape ≥2
- BMI > 10th percentile for age/sex
- No self-induced vomiting or pill/laxative use
- Hard exercise for weight control ≤1.

Other Specified Feeding or Eating Disorders

Purging disorder:
- Purging behavior
  - Self-induced vomiting ≥1 or
  - Laxative/Pill use ≥1
- Over evaluation of weight /shape
  - Importance of weight ≥2
  - Importance of shape ≥2
- BMI > 10th percentile for age/sex
- No objective binge eating.

Atypical Anorexia Nervosa

- BMI >10th percentile despite significant weight loss[1]
- Fear of weight gain ≥2
- Body image disturbance
  - Importance of weight ≥2
  - Importance of shape ≥2
  - Feeling of fatness ≥2.

Note: A score of 1 equates to symptoms occurring once per week/a few times a month, and a score of 2 equates to symptoms occurring a few times a week.

BMI: Body mass index.

Pica

- Eating nonnutritive, nonfood substances for at least 1 month
- Symptoms are developmentally inappropriate
- Not part of culturally supported or socially normative practice.

Rumination Disorder

- Repetitive regurgitation of food for at least 1 month
- Rule out gastrointestinal or other medical condition
- Does not occur exclusively with another eating disorder.

Avoidant Restrictive Food Intake Disorder

- Avoidance or restriction of food intake resulting in failure to meet nutritional or energy needs. Associated with one

[1]Significant weight loss is defined as a reduction in percentage ideal body weight (% IBW) that is 2 standard deviations of the cohort mean for change in % IBW, between age 10 and 14, age 14 and 17, or age 17 and 20 years.[4]

(or more) of the following—significant weight loss or inadequate weight gain with age; significant nutritional deficiency; dependence on feeding tube or supplements; or marked interference with psychosocial functioning.
- Unrelated to cultural practices or food availability.
- Not because of excessive concern about body weight or shape.
- Not explained by medical or mental disorders.

MEDICAL COMPLICATIONS

Although classified under psychiatric conditions, the eating disorders are often linked to significant morbidity and mortality. The medical complications involving different organ systems are tabulated in **Table 2.**[14]

The Role of Obstetrician-Gynecologist

For obstetrician and gynecologists it is crucial to have knowledge about eating disorders. Although amenorrhea is no more a part of the diagnostic criteria for any eating disorders.[15] These disorders also known to cause menstrual irregularities, disrupted reproductive health and low bone mineral density (BMD). As diagnosis and treatment of eating disorders are complex and demands multidisciplinary approach, it is presumed that it is out of the scope of practice for most of obstetrician and gynecologists. However, the healthcare provider must be able to recognize and screen adolescents at risk as delay in diagnosis and treatment may result in growth restriction, pubertal arrest, increased fracture risk, structural brain changes, and death.[16]

MANAGEMENT

This complex illness demands a multidisciplinary approach. An argument sometimes arises over which to address first: the emotional symptoms or the eating behavior. Management of these patients is notoriously difficult. A team comprising the psychiatrist, clinician, and nutritionist is effective to deal the situation. Among any psychiatric disorder, anorexia nervosa has the highest mortality. Deaths are often sudden and unexpected due to hypoglycemia and electrolyte imbalance.[17]

Initial Assessment

An imperative role is played by the physician in early identification, diagnosis and management of eating disorders as adolescent with a suspected eating disorder often first present to them. Timely intervention is crucial as association found between the improved outcome and the shorter duration of illness.[18] To screen for eating disorders, Screening tools like SCOFF questionnaire have been developed **(Box 1)**. The medical provider needs to identify the abnormal eating attitudes and behavior, recognize aberrations in weight, height, and sexual development and should plot it in growth charts. Patients should be screened for other mental health disorders (depression and anxiety) and should be questioned about suicidal thoughts.

TABLE 2: Medical complications of eating disorders.[14]

Fluid and electrolyte imbalance	• Hypokalemia • Hyponatremia • ↑Blood urea nitrogen • ↓Glomerular filtration rate • Ketonuria • Hypochloremic alkalosis
Cardiovascular	• Bradycardia • Arrhythmia • Orthostatic hypotension • ECG changes • Low voltage • Prolonged QT interval • T wave abnormalities • Conduction defects • Mitral valve prolapse • Pericardial effusion • Congestive heart failure
Gastrointestinal	• Constipation • Delayed gastric emptying • Intestinal atony • Bloody diarrhea • Esophagitis • Mallory-Weiss-tears • Perforation/rupture of stomach • Barrett esophagitis • Fatty infiltration of liver • Acute pancreatitis • Gallstones
Dermatologic	• Brittle hair and nails • Hair loss • Russell sign (callus over the knuckles) • Pitting edema • Acrocyanosis • Yellow dry skin (hypocarotenemia)
Endocrine	• Growth retardation and short stature • Delayed puberty • Amenorrhea • Partial diabetes insipidus • Hypercortisolism
Skeletal	• Osteopenia • Fractures
Hematologic	• Bone marrow suppression • Mild anemia • Leukopenia • Thrombocytopenia • Low sedimentation rate • Impaired cell mediated immunity
Neurological	• Seizures • Myopathy • Peripheral neuropathy • Cortical atrophy

- *Outpatient management:* Family based treatment (FBT) is an outpatient based intervention with the strongest evidence of effect in adolescents with anorexia nervosa.[19] FBT comprises three phases with distinct goals:

BOX 1: The SCOFF questions.

- Do you make yourself **S**ick because you feel uncomfortably full?
- Do you worry you have lost **C**ontrol over how much you eat?
- Have you recently lost more than **O**ne stone (14 pounds) in a 3 month period?
- Do you believe yourself to be **F**at when others say you are too thin?
- Would you say that **F**ood dominates your life?

One point of every yes; a score of ≥2 indicates a likely case of anorexia nervosa or bulimia

Source: Reprinted from Morgan JF, Lacey JH. The SCOFF questionnaire: a new screening tool for eating disorders. West J Med. 2000;172:164-5.

- *Phase I:* Restoring the patients weight
- *Phase II:* Returns command over eating back to the adolescent
- *Phase III:* Adolescent development and treatment termination.

The physician plays an important role in FBT by communicating between patient and family members apart from being a primary therapist who monitor and manage the medical status of adolescent.[20]

Cognitive behavioral therapy (CBT) is a short-term (4–6 months) psychological treatment that focuses on the intense concern with shape and weight, the persistent dieting, the binge eating and purging. Patients are directed to monitor the circumstances, thoughts and emotions associated with binge/purge episodes, to eat regularly and to challenge their assumptions linking weight to self-esteem. CBT produces symptomatic remission in 25–50% of patients.

Inpatient Medical Management

A team comprising experienced physician, psychiatrist, nutritionist, and nursing staff to deal with the hospitalized adolescent with eating disorders is required. Treatment of adolescent under the above team along with the standardized refeeding protocols, cardiac monitoring is a key to successful management. During early stages of treatment, patients may experience "refeeding syndrome" occasionally which is characterized by hypophosphatemia, hypomagnesemia and cardiovascular instability. Fluid retention, peripheral edema may occur but generally do not require specific treatment in absence of cardiac, hepatic, renal dysfunction **(Box 2)**.

The primary goal is to safely restore physiological stability through nutritional rehabilitation **(Fig. 1)**.[21] In contrast to old recommendation of "start low and go slow" the recent research supports initiating higher caloric prescription on admission, 1,400–2,100 kcal/day with close monitoring.[22] These studies indicate that such practices shorten hospital stay and increases rate of weight gain.[23,24] Weight gain of 1–2 kg/week normalizes cardiovascular instability.[25] But the time required for all physiological parameters to normalize is highly variable.

Management of Low Bone Mineral Density

In patients with anorexia nervosa with low BMD current recommendations are to restore body weight along with the resuming the spontaneous menses. An optimal intake of calcium of 1,300 mg/day and vitamin D (600 IU/day) is required to treat vitamins deficiency. In view of increased fracture risk, dual-energy X-ray absorptiometry scans should be offered whenever amenorrhea is present for 6 months or more.[23]

BOX 2: Indications supporting hospitalization.[3]

- <75% median BMI for age/sex
- Dehydration
- Electrolyte imbalance
- ECG abnormalities
- Physiological abnormality
  - Severe bradycardia
  - Hypotension
  - Hypothermia
  - Orthostatic changes
- Arrested growth and development
- Failure of outpatient treatment
- Acute food refusal
- Uncontrollable binging/purging
- Acute medical complications of malnutrition
- Comorbid psychiatric and medical conditions that limits OPD treatment

Psychiatric Support

Psychiatric treatment focuses primarily on two issues—first, patients require much emotional support during the period of weight gain. Second, patients must learn to base their self-esteem on the development of satisfying personal relationship and the attainment of reasonable academic and occupational goals.

Amenorrhea and Contraception

In agreement with the American Academy of Pediatrics and the Society for Adolescent Health and Medicine, The American College of Obstetrician and Gynecologists recommends against the use of combined oral contraceptive pills solely for the treatment of amenorrhea associated with eating disorders. Sexually active patients require individualized counseling for contraception.[16]

The principle of care is comprehensive with multi-disciplinary approach. It demands a close collaboration of multiple streams of medicine while imposing a great burden over sibling/parent/care taker of the patient simultaneously. We should encourage the adolescent to develop healthy attitudes about their weight, body image and self-esteem and to ameliorate the sociocultural influence that promotes the eating disorders. We need to realize an adolescent with eating disorder that treatment may be challenging and complicated but the recovery is possible.

CONCLUSION

Eating disorders are complex biopsychosocial disorders with onset during adolescence. Interplay of genetic, neurological,

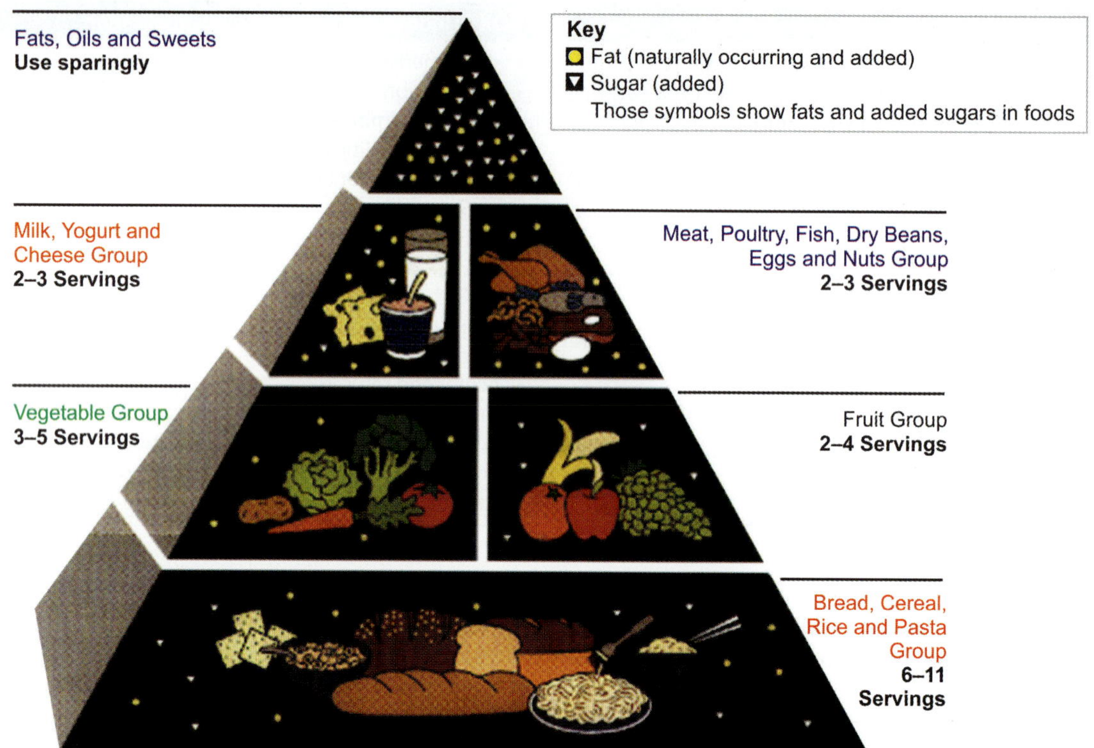

Fig. 1: Food pyramid with 35–40% fiber rich carbohydrates, 35% fruits and vegetables, 20% proteins, 5–10% fats.

sociocultural, and environmental factors seems to cause these complicated disorders. People of all races, ethnicities, genders, socioeconomic status are affected by this illness. Their diagnosis and treatment is complex and health care provider should be able to recognize and screen the "at risk patient". A multidisciplinary approach is essential involving clinician, psychiatrist, nutritionist, and parents. Treatment can be long and complicated but recovery is possible.

REFERENCES

1. Nicholls D, Barrett E. Eating disorders in children and adolescents. Cam J. 2015;21(3):206-16.
2. Verywell Mind. Are eating disorders a modern illness? History of eating disorders, Histories and Biographies. [online] Available from: https://www.verywellmind.com/history of eating disorders. [Last Accessed November, 2021].
3. Stice E, Marti CN, Rhode P. Prevalence, incidence, impairment and course of proposed DSM-5 eating disorder diagnosed in an 8 year old prospective community study of young women. Journal Abnorm Psychol. 2013;122:445-57.
4. Golden NH, Katzman D, Sawyer SM, Ornstein RM, Rome ES, Garber AK, et al. Update on the medical management of eating disorders in adolescents. J Adolesc Health. 2014;56:370-5.
5. Rikani AA, Choudhry Z, Choudhry AM, Ikram H, Asghar MW, Kajal D, et al. A critique of the literature on etiology of eating disorders. Ann Neurosci. 2103;20(4):157-61.
6. Walsh BT, Attia E. Harrison's Principle of Internal Medicine, 18th edition. New York: The McGraw Hill Companies/Cenveo Publisher Services; 2012. pp. 637-41.
7. Kaye WH, Frank GK, Bailer UF, Henry SE. Neurobiology of anorexia nervosa: clinical implications of alterations of the function of serotonin and other neuronal systems. Int J Eating Disorder. 2005;37(Suppl)S15-9.
8. Leon GR, Fulkerson JA, Perry CL. Prospective analysis of personality and behavioural vulnerabilities and gender influences in the later development of disordered eating. J Abnorm Psychol. 1995;104:140-9.
9. Cooley E, Toray T. Disordered eating in college freshman women: a prospective study. J Am Coll Health. 2001;49(5):229-35.
10. Nobakht M, Dezhkam M. An epidemiological study of eating disorders in Iran. Int J Eating Disorder. 2000;28(3):265-71.
11. Ung EK. Eating disorders in Singapore: a review. Ann Acad Med Singapore. 2003;32(1):19-24.
12. Female Athlete Triad. Committee Opinion No. 702. American College of Obstetricians and Gynaecologists. Obstet Gynecol. 2017;129:e160-7.
13. Allen KL, Byrne SM, Wendy H. Oddy, Crosby RD. DSM-IV-TR and DSM-5 Eating Disorders in Adolescents: Prevalence, Stability, and Psychosocial Correlates in a Population-Based Sample of Male and Female Adolescents. J Abnorm Psychol. 2013;122(3):720-2.
14. Fischer M, Golden NH, Katzman DK, Kreipe RE, Rees J, Schebendach J, et al. Eating disorders in adolescents: a background paper. J Adolesc Health. 1995:420-37.
15. American Psychiatric Association. Feeding and eating disorders. In: Diagnostic and Statistical Manual of Mental Disorders, 5th edition. Washington DC: American Psychiatric Publishing; 2013. pp. 329-54.
16. American College of Obstetrician and Gynecologists. Gynecologic care for adolescents and young women with eating disorders. ACOG committee opinion no. 740. Obstet Gynecol. 2018;131:e205-13.
17. Rebar RW, Paupoo AA. Berek and Novaks Gynecology, 15th edition. Philadelphia: Lippincott Williams and Wilkins; 2012. pp. 1014-6.

18. Forman SF, Grodin LF, Graham DA. An eleven site national quality improvement evaluation of adolescent medicine-based eating disorder programs: predictors of weight outcomes at one year and risk adjustment analyses. J Adolesc Health 2011;49:594-600.
19. Agras WS, Lock J, Brandt H, Bryson SW, Dodge E, Halmi KA, et al. Comparison of 2 family therapies for adolescent anorexia nervosa: a randomized parallel trial. JAMA Psychiatr. 2014;71(11):1279-86.
20. Katzman DK, Peebles R, Sawyer SM, Lock J, Le Grange D. The role of the pediatrician in family-based treatment for adolescent eating disorders: Opportunities and challenges. J Adolesc Health. 2013;53(4):433-40
21. Kohn MR, Madden S, Clarke SD. Refeeding in anorexia nervosa: Increased safety and efficiency through understanding the pathophysiology of protein calorie malnutrition. Curr Opin Pediatr. 2011;23(4):390-4. 19.
22. Garber AK, Mauldin K, Michihata N, Buckelew SM, Shafer MA, Moscicki AB. Higher calorie diets increase rate of weight gain and shorten hospital stay in hospitalized adolescents with anorexia nervosa. J Adolesc Health, 2013;53(5):579-84.
23. Golden NH, Abrams SA, Committee on Nutrition. Optimizing bone health in children and adolescents. Pediatrics. 2014;134(4):e1229-43.
24. Leclerc A, Turrini T, Sherwood K, Katzman DK. Evaluation of a nutrition rehabilitation protocol in hospitalized adolescents with restrictive eating disorders. J Adolesc Health. 2013;53(5):585-9.
25. Shamim T, Golden NH, Arden M, Filiberto L, Shenker IR. Resolution of vital sign instability: an objective measure of medical stability in anorexia nervosa. J Adolesc Health. 2003;32(1):73-7.

LONG QUESTIONS

1. Describe medical complications of eating disorders.
2. Management of eating disorders in adolescence.
3. Diagnostic criteria for eating disorders in adolescence.
4. Describe etiology, clinical features, diagnosis and management of Anorexia nervosa.
5. Bulimia nervosa - diagnosis and management.

SHORT QUESTIONS

1. Describe the diagnostic criteria for anorexia nervosa.
2. Describe avoidant restrictive food intake disorders.
3. Write short note on female athlete triad.
4. Write short note on cognitive behavioral therapy.
5. What are the indications of hospitalization of a patient with eating disorders?
6. Role of family based therapy in eating disorders.

MULTIPLE CHOICE QUESTIONS

1. Which neurological transmitter is not involved in mood regulation?
   a. Norepinephrine b. Glutamate
   c. Serotonin d. GABA
2. Term "Anorexia Nervosa" coined by:
   a. William Gull b. Richard Mortan
   c. Gerald Russel d. Andrew Morton
3. Indications for hospitalization of a patient with eating disorder are all, except:
   a. Dehydration
   b. Acute food refusal
   c. <80% median BMI for age/sex
   d. Arrested growth and development
4. PICA-pick the false statement:
   a. Symptoms are developmentally inappropriate
   b. Increased risk of gut injuries, nutritional deficiency
   c. Not a part of culturally supported practice
   d. Eating nonnutritive substances for at least 3 months
5. Which one is correct statement for Rumination disorder:
   a. Repetitive regurgitation of food for at least 3 months
   b. Doesn't occur exclusively with other eating disorder
   c. Caused by a medical condition, gastrointestinal disorder
   d. Usually respond to treatments for GERD/acid reflux
6. As per DSM-5 criteria the life time prevalence of anorexia nervosa is:
   a. 2.8% b. 2.2%
   c. 0.8% d. 1.8%
7. Eating disorders are associated with following factors, except:
   a. Altered level of 5HT1a and 5HT2A
   b. Genetic factors not involved
   c. Distorted view of body image
   d. Exposure to western culture
8. Following statement is not true for bulimia nervosa:
   a. Callus on dorsum of hand
   b. Increased hunger and overeating observed
   c. Typically seen in childhood/early adolescence
   d. Binge eating/purging reported 5–10 times a week
9. Anorexia nervosa—correct statement:
   a. Typically begins in mid adolescence
   b. Rarely complain of hunger/fatigue
   c. BMI<10th percentile for age/sex
   d. All of the above
10. Which one is the false statement:
    a. Anorexia nervosa was reported in 1st edition of DSM-I
    b. ARFID introduced in DSM-IV
    c. BED got independent diagnosis in DSM-5
    d. DSM-III debuted eating disorders under the rubric: disorders of infancy, childhood or adolescence
11. Refeeding syndrome—all are true, except:
    a. Hyperphosphatemia
    b. Fluid retention
    c. Cardiovascular instability
    d. Hypomagnesemia

12. Female athlete triad includes all, except:
    a. Menstrual dysfunction
    b. Athletes with optimal energy availability
    c. Low energy availability with disordered eating
    d. Low energy availability without disordered eating
13. Endocrinal abnormalities in eating disorders are all, except:
    a. Growth retardation b. Precocious puberty
    c. Amenorrhea d. Hypercortisolism
14. Fluid and electrolyte imbalance results in all, except:
    a. Hypokalemia b. Hyponatremia
    c. Ketonuria d. Acidosis
15 All are the features of OSFED, except:
    a. Purging behavior
    b. Over evaluation of weight/shape
    c. BMI<10th percentile for age/sex
    d. No objective binge eating

Answers

1.	b	2.	a	3.	c	4.	d	5.	b	6.	c
7.	b	8.	c	9.	d	10.	b	11.	a	12.	b
13.	b	14.	d	15.	c						

8.7 PRECOCIOUS PUBERTY

Surveen Ghumman, Rajal Thaker

INTRODUCTION

Puberty is the impressionable age at which disorders can have deep seated effects not only on physical appearance but also psychologically. Precocious puberty is puberty occurring at an earlier age than normal. The main impact is on height and most therapies are centered on taking care of that. It can be central where the hypothalamus pituitary ovarian axis is affected. History and examination is vital. Serum follicle stimulating hormone (FSH), luteinizing hormone (LH) estradiol and thyroid function tests are recommended. Central precocious puberty is treated by gonadotropin-releasing hormone (GnRH) analogs. It could be peripheral where external hormones from tumors or exogenous intake can cause puberty to occur. Estradiol in these cases would be raised. Here treatment of the cause would resolve the condition. These children also need counseling and psychological care.

Puberty is a period that links childhood to adulthood. It includes physical, endocrinological, psychological changes which accompany the increasing levels of sex steroids. There is rapid growth of bones and muscles, changes in body shape and size and development of the body's ability to reproduce. It usually occurs between 10 and 16 years in girls. The determinants of puberty are geographic location, general health, nutrition, psychological factors and excessive exercise.

Usually age at which changes begin can vary but order remains the same. Common order of development is listed in **Box 1**.

BOX 1: Order of development in puberty.

- Beginning of growth spurt is the first sign
- *Thelarche:* Breast budding (8–11 years)
- *Adrenarche:* Pubic and axillary hair growth (adrenarche) (9–14 years)
- Peak growth in height
- *Menarche:* Menstruation occurs 2.5 years after onset of thelarche (10–16 years)
- Mature sexual and breast growth

DEFINITION

Precocious puberty (PP) is defined as children attaining puberty more than 2.5–3 standard deviations (SD) earlier than the median age, or before the age of 8 years in girls and 9 years in boys.[1]

The decline in age at puberty in the general population has been paralleled by an increase in the number of girls referred for evaluation of precocious puberty. In 1999, The Lawson Wilkins Pediatric Endocrine Society recommended a lowering of the age limit for evaluation of PP in girls. However, the limited evidence on which these recommendations were based led many experts to question these new suggestions. The emergence of new European pubertal timing data evaluated by robust clinical as well as biochemical markers has broadened our insight on how to interpret the recent pubertal changes. The recent pubertal trends have resulted in a concomitant lowering of the lower limit of normality of the pubertal onset. However, evidence suggests that age at the gonadotropin and sex steroid surges have not changed. Thus, it looks as if an increasing proportion of contemporary early pubertal girls may experience isolated gonadotropin-independent thelarche rather than central precocious puberty (CPP) which may not be discernible on pubertal examination alone. Thus, the population-based limits of normality should not be directly translated into revision of age limits for evaluation of precocious puberty due to the risk of misdiagnosing rapid progressive precocious puberty as well as intracranial and other underlying pathology.[2]

INCIDENCE

The incidence of precocious puberty is 1 in 5,000 to 1 in 10,000 children in North America, prevalence being 10 times higher in girls.

SIGNS AND SYMPTOMS

Signs and symptoms of precocious puberty include development of the following before age 8 in girls **(Figs. 1A and B)**.

- Breast growth and menarche in girls
- Pubic or underarm hair
- Rapid growth in height
- Acne
- Adult body odor
- Precocious puberty can make a child fertile when very young, with the youngest mother on record being Lina Medina from Peru (who was born September 23rd, 1933) and who gave birth on May 14, 1939 at the age of 5 years, 7 months and 17 days.[3]

How early can they present? Cases of 11-month-old and 16-month old female infants have been reported who had presented with vaginal bleeding and rapidly progressive secondary sex characteristics from the age of 6 months. Both were diagnosed with CPP and were later diagnosed to have hypothalamic hamartoma.[4,5]

CLASSIFICATION OF PRECOCIOUS PUBERTY

Precocious puberty may be classified into central and peripheral.

Central precocious puberty (CPP): Central precocious puberty involves the hypothalamic pituitary ovarian (HPO) axis.

Peripheral precocious puberty (PPP): The peripheral precocious puberty is independent of GnRH and is due to peripheral causes or exogenous hormones.

Isosexual and Heterosexual Precocious Puberty:

Isosexual precocious puberty: In isosexual precocious puberty feminizing signs in girls and masculinization in boys is seen.

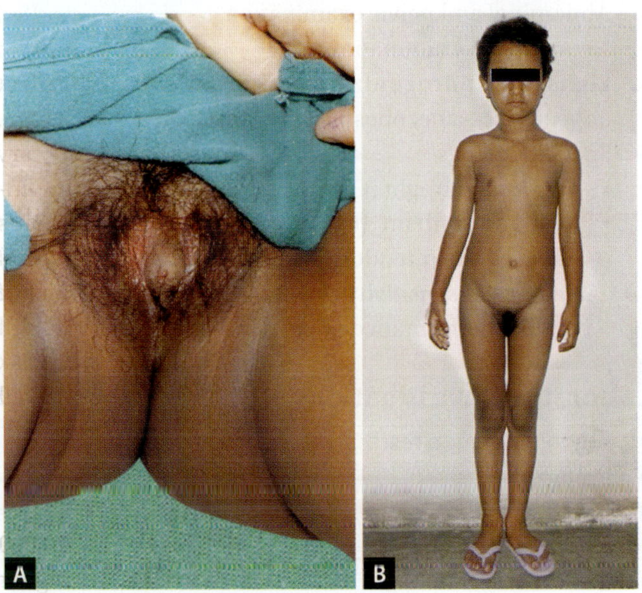

Figs. 1A and B: Adrenarche in a young girl.

Heterosexual precocious puberty: In heterosexual precocious puberty masculine characteristics in girls and feminine characteristics in boys are seen.

Central Precocious Puberty (Complete/True/GnRH Dependent)

In central precocious puberty, there is early activation of the pulsatile GnRH secretion. The puberty process starts too soon as there is early maturation of HPO axis. The pattern and timing of the steps in the process are otherwise normal. In most cases (approximately 90%), it remains unexplained and in majority there is no underlying medical problem and no identifiable reason (idiopathic).[6]

Causes of Central Precocious Puberty

Causes of CPP are listed in **Box 2**.

Peripheral Precocious Puberty (Incomplete/Pseudo/GnRH Independent GIPP)

Peripheral precocious puberty is less common. It occurs without the involvement of GnRH and there is no activation of the HPO axis. Secondary sexual characteristics result from high circulating levels of estrogens or androgens, without activation of the hypothalamic-pituitary axis because of pathology in the ovaries, adrenal glands, or there may be pathology in thyroid.

Causes of Peripheral Precocious Puberty

Causes of PPP are enlisted in **Box 3**.

RISK FACTORS

There are some children at higher risk than others:

- *Gender:* More common in girls.
- *Race:* More common among African-American.
- Family history of GnRH-dependent precocious puberty
- *Genetic mutations:* Mutations in the *kisspeptin—KISS1* (involved in GnRH secretion and puberty onset) are also thought to be the cause of idiopathic CPP.[8]
- Conditions such as McCune-Albright syndrome, congenital adrenal hyperplasia, hypothyroidism.

BOX 2: Causes of central precocious puberty.

- Unexplained
- Organic brain disease
- CNS tumor such as hamartoma, gliomas, germinomas, and adenomas
- Neurofibromatosis (NF) is a genetic disorder with highly variable manifestations, which can affect many body systems[7]
- Brain surgery
- Head trauma
- Hydrocephalus
- CNS infection (abscess, encephalitis, meningitis)
- Radiation to the brain or spinal cord

BOX 3: Causes of peripheral precocious puberty.

- Congenital adrenal hyperplasia
- Tumor of adrenal gland
- Ovarian cysts, ovarian tumors
- *Primary hypothyroidism:* It is felt to be mediated by TSH stimulation of the FSH receptor, but frequently manifests as growth delay in the setting of premature menarche; this is also referred to as Van Wyk-Grumbach syndrome[7]
- *McCune-Albright syndrome (MAS):* This is a genetic disorder affecting the skin color and bones and causes hormonal problems
- *Exposure to external sources of estrogen:* Ingestion of oral contraceptives/other estrogen containing agents, estrogen contaminated food/water, topical use of estrogen (creams or ointments)

- History of radiation treatment.
- *Obesity:* Obese children have high levels of the protein *leptin* (which regulates fat storage in body), which through a complicated chain involving the hypothalamus and pituitary gland, can stimulate the release of GnRH, LH and FSH.[9]
- *Endocrine disruptors:* Chemicals that mimic estrogen and change our hormonal balance are now everywhere. These endocrine-disruptors are found in hand soap, shampoos, and cosmetics, cleaning products and in plastics. A 2012 Centers for Disease Control and Prevention study found dichlorobenzene; a solvent used in mothballs, solid block toilet bowl deodorizers and air fresheners is linked to precocious puberty. Dichlorobenzene is a common indoor contaminant and its residue has been found in most people and it can be transmitted vertically and it is also secreted in breast milk.[9]
- *Hormone-raised meat:* Estradiol, progesterone, testosterone, zeranol, trenbolone acetate, and melengestrol are the hormones that are used in dairy and meat industry. A 2010 study in Public Health Nutrition of 3,000 girls found that girls who ate eight portions of meat a week by age three, and 12 portions of meat a week by age 7 were likely to have an early start of menstruation.[10]

COMPLICATIONS

Possible complications of precocious puberty include following:

- *Short height:* Children with precocious puberty may grow quickly at first and be tall, compared with their peers. But, because their bones mature more quickly than normal, they often stop growing earlier than usual. This can cause them to be shorter than average as adults.
- *Social and emotional problems:* Girls who begin puberty long before their peers may be extremely self-conscious about the changes occurring in their bodies. This may affect self-esteem and increase the risk of depression or substance abuse.[11,12]
- *Cancers in later life:* There is a 30% increased risk for breast cancer when a woman experiences her first period at a younger age. For each year that age of menarche was delayed, the risk of premenopausal *breast cancer* was reduced by 9% and risk of postmenopausal breast cancer was reduced by 4%. Early breast development also opens the door to *reproductive tract cancers* as estrogen, especially when combined with stress hormones, is a known cancer-causing agent.[13]
- *Hyperinsulinemia, hypertension and heart disease:* There is a higher risk of obesity, hyperinsulinemia, hypertension, and heart disease in later life.[9]

PREVENTION

Factors such as race and sex cannot be avoided, but we can keep girl child away from external sources of estrogen such as estradiol creams, endocrine disrupters and maintain ideal weight.

DIAGNOSIS

The nature of precocity dictates certain diagnostic priorities. We need to rule out life-threatening disease. This includes neoplasms of CNS, ovary and adrenals. We also need to define velocity of the disease progress and see if it is progressing or stabilized.

History and Physical Examination

- Age at onset
- Past history of CNS infection, headache, visual disturbance, seizures
- Family history
- Record of growth, by height and weight and compare with percentile charts
- Tanners staging for breast development
- Abdominal and pelvic examination
- Neurological examination
- Signs of androgenization (hirsutism, masculine appearance, acne, obesity, oligomenorrhea)
- Special findings
  - McCune Albright (Café au-lait spots)
  - Hypothyroidism (enlarged thyroid, bradycardia, delayed deep tendon reflexes, fatigue, sluggishness, increased sensitivity to cold, constipation, a drop in school performance or pale, dry skin).

Laboratory Investigations

- Thyroid function test
- Prolactin
- LH, FSH
- Testosterone
- DHEAS
- 17-hydroxyprogesterone

- GnRH stimulation test to diagnose whether precocious puberty is GnRH dependent or GnRH independent: Leuprolide acetate 10–20 µg/kg subcutaneously is given and LH, FSH and estradiol are measured at 0, 1, and 2 hours. At 24 hours post leuprolide, estradiol may be measured to improve sensitivity of the test. In GnRH-dependent precocious puberty, gonadotropin responses are pubertal. In GnRH-independent precocious puberty, gonadotropin responses to leuprolide are prepubertal[14]
- *Serum estradiol:* Estrogen exposure; if markedly elevated [> 100 pg per mL (367 pmol per L)], evaluate for ovarian tumor, especially if luteinizing hormone is suppressed[15]
- *Radiological investigations:*
  - X-ray hand and wrist for bone age
  - Basal skull bone scan for lytic bone lesions (McCune–Albright)
  - MRI/CT Scan of brain
  - MRI, CT or USG abdomen, pelvis or adrenal gland
- *Genetic testing* may be considered in familial cases of GnRH-dependent precocious puberty, but this remains controversial.[14]

TREATMENT

Precocious puberty must be treated adequately and timely. The main concern in these cases is gain of height. Also, these young children may develop psychological issues which need to be identified and addressed. Treatment for central and peripheral precocious puberty is different.

Central Precocious Puberty: Treatment

The cause of CPP is usually idiopathic. It leads to early epiphyseal fusion and a smaller height.

Aim:

- Preservation of height potential. This can be achieved by keeping estradiol levels low by giving GnRH analogs.
- Amelioration of the psychosocial consequences of unrealistic adult expectations.

  Treatment depends on following factors—rate of progression of disease and age of onset of symptoms.
  - *Progression of disease*: As progression of disease is variable and non-predictable it is often better to wait and see. If it is a fast progression treatment must be initiated immediately. Disease which progresses slowly may not require any intervention.
  - *Age of onset of symptoms*: The impact on height also depends on what age the precocious puberty changes started. In girls where puberty started before 6 years there was a higher gain in height with treatment compared to those where it started after 6 years. Beyond 8 years treatment is not advised as it does not affect height much.

GnRH Agonist

GnRHa is the recognized treatment of choice for precocious puberty. It can be given as a monthly or 3 monthly depot injection

Mechanism of action: It provides a stable level of GnRH which downregulates the GnRH agonist receptors decreasing GnRH activity It acts by downregulating and suppressing hypothalamic pituitary gonadal axis. One can use leuprolide as a monthly 3.75 mg injection or a three monthly 11.25 mg injection. The 3-monthly 11.25 mg leuprolide injection is generally preferred due to ease of frequency of administration in these children. Since they are depot preparations they are given deep intramuscular. Sometimes pain at injection site and abscess formation is reported. In case an abscess formation occurs one can switch to daily subcutaneous injections.[16]

Treatment is continued until the progress of puberty is age appropriate.

After discontinuation of treatment resumption of puberty occurs and precedes at a normal pace.

Histrelin implant: A new formulation of GnRH agonist in the form of a subcutaneous implant has been tried. Histrelin implant can be placed on the inner side of the arm subcutaneously. It was initially used for prostate cancer. For CPP dose required is 65 µg/ day. FSH and LH were suppressed with this dose. Clinical response in terms of reduction in breast development and bone age was seen. A single implant of 50 mg can be used for 2 years. There can be breakage of implant if left for long periods. Difficulty in localization while removing can be a problem and ultrasound is helpful. Local reaction, sterile abscess formation, keloids, site infection, and implant extrusion may occasionally occur. To insert or remove implant local anesthesia with sedation is given in OPD setting.[17-20]

Newer preparations like a 6 monthly depot preparation of triptorelin is being considered with the advantage of less number of injections to be administered or for those who do not want to undergo the procedure for insertion of a subcutaneous implant.[21]

Nonaromatizable Anabolic Steroids

A stimulatory effect on growth is needed for children in whom there is severe suppression of growth by GnRH agonist. This might improve the final height. Oxandrolone has been tried but requires more studies.

Growth Hormone

Addition of growth hormone to GnRH agonist has shown to improve the final height but more randomized controlled trials are needed.[22]

Aromatase Inhibitors

Since aromatase inhibitors prevent conversion of androgens to estrogens the early closure of epiphysis which is estrogen dependent may be delayed. This has been shown in a small study using letrozole and will need larger studies.[23]

Follow-Up

A regular follow-up is required to assess if treatment is effective. The follow-up is clinical and biochemical.

Clinical follow-up includes the following:

- Tanner staging
- Determination of growth velocity
- Assessment of skeletal maturation via bone age radiographs.

Laboratory testing includes:

- GnRH- or leuprolide-stimulated peak LH: Proper suppression is shown by LH <4 IU/L
- Random serum gonadotropin levels should be at level seen before puberty (LH <0.3 IU/L). However, LH values are not reliable and this value being used for monitoring is questionable.

On cessation of treatment girls menstruate after 18 months on an average. However, those who had menarche before start of treatment menstruate earlier.

Impact on bone mineral density: It is seen that the bone mineral density of these girls is lower than their peers during treatment but after cessation of treatment it catches up and is normal for that age.

Future fertility: Studies have shown that majority of women (80%) resume normal menstrual function. Furthermore, pregnancies have been reported but there is no data on onset of menopause in these women.[24]

Free alpha subunit increases with suppression of hypothalamic pituitary gonadal axis. On discontinuation of treatment there is rapid fall of alpha subunit. Hence, this marker can be used for rapid assessment of hypothalamic pituitary gonadal axis.[25]

To avoid the surge created by GnRH agonist which sometimes causes bleeding in these prepubertal girls one can give a GnRH antagonist. Kisspeptin agonist and antagonist would have similar results. They may have a more physiological outcome.[26]

Peripheral Precocious Puberty: Treatment

Treatment of PPP depends on the cause. Peripheral precocious puberty is independent of GnRH and may have genetic or acquired causes which may occur due to hormone produced by cyst or tumor in the ovary or adrenal gland. It may occur because of pseudoprecocious puberty in severe hypothyroidism or could be because of intake of exogenous hormones. The genetic causes in females are McCune-Albright syndrome (MAS), and congenital adrenal hyperplasia.

In contrast to CPP, treatment of PPP depends on the cause. If there is an ovarian tumor or an adrenal tumor it needs to be removed. Hypothyroidism will require treatment.[27]

- Testolactone, an aromatase inhibitor, inhibits conversion of testosterone to estrogen 35 mg/kg/D three divided doses
- Ketoconazole inhibits steroid biosynthesis in a dose of 200 mg TDS.

Treatment options for PPP - MAS

- *Ketoconazole:* It inhibits P450 and decreases estradiol reversing advanced bone age. There have been concerns of safety, hence its use discontinued.[28]
- *Medroxy-progesterone acetate:* It has been used because of its antiprogesterone action.
- *Aromatase inhibitors*: They inhibit the conversion of testosterone to estradiol. Letrozole, testolactone, fadrazole and anastrozole have been tried. Letrozole has been fairly successful. The drug was well tolerated and there was a decrease in bone age.[29]
- *Estrogen receptor modulators*: Tamoxifen and fulvestrant. Tamoxifen was effective but uterine volumes were unexpectedly found to increase throughout the study. Hence, ultrasound monitoring was recommended.[30] Fulvestrant is a pure estrogen receptor blocker administered parenterally. In a recent study, monthly intramuscular injections of fulvestrant were administered at a dose of 4 mg/kg. It was found to be effective.[31]
- *Cyproterone acetate*: Cyproterone acetate is a potent progestin and antiandrogen, inhibits androgens at the receptor level suppressing gonadal and adrenal steroidogenesis.

Treatment of Psychological Consequences of Precocity

Treatment of the psychological impact which precocious puberty has on the child is very important. There is stress associated with body image issues, as children of that age look different. Strong support and counseling is periodically required. Children with PP are taller and appear older than their peers leading to unrealistic expectation from parents, teachers, and others making them stressed. They perceive themselves as different but this does not have any long-term effect and they do well psychologically Sexual maturity at an immature age make them vulnerable to be victims of sexual abuse.

The data on treatment has deficiencies due to small studies which are not randomized. MAS being a rare disorder does not have too many studies on treatment efficacy and long-term data is lacking. However, it is important to put in place timely treatment as successful outcomes are known when therapy has been timely and adequate.

REFERENCES

1. Mul D, Fredriks AM, Van Buuren S, Oostdijk W, Verloove-Vanhorick SP, Wit JM. Pubertal development in the Netherlands 1965-1997. Pediatr Res. 2001;50:479-86.
2. Sørensen K, Mouritsen A, Aksglaede L, Hagen CP, Mogensen SS, Juul A. Pubertal timing: implications for evaluation and diagnosis of precocious puberty. Horm Res Paediatr. 2012;77:137-45.
3. Wikipedia. Lina Medina. [online] Available form: https://en.wikipedia.org/wiki/Lina_Medina#:~:text=Lina%20Marcela%20Medina%20de%20Jurado,seven%20months%2C%20and%2021%20days. [Last Accessed November, 2021].
4. Yoon DA, Kim JH. An 11-month-old girl with central precocious puberty caused by hypothalamic hamartoma. Ann Pediatr Endocrinol Metab. 2016;21(4):235-9.

5. Kotwal N, Yanamandra U, Menon AS, Nair V. Central precocious puberty due to hypothalamic hamartoma in a six-month-old infant girl. Indian J Endocrinol Metab. 2012;16(4):627-30.
6. MayoClinic. Precocious Puberty. [online] Available from: https://www.mayoclinic.org/diseases-conditions/precocious-puberty/symptoms-causes/syc-20351811. [Last Accessed November, 2021].
7. National Organization for Rare Disorders. Precocious Puberty. [online] Available from: https://rarediseases.org/rare-diseases/precocious-puberty/. [Last Accessed November, 2021].
8. Silveira LG, Noel SD, Silveira-Neto AP, Abreu AP, Brito VN, et al. Mutations of the KISS1 gene in disorders of puberty. J Clin Endocrinol Metab. 2010;95(5):2276-80.
9. Center for Health Journalism. Precocious puberty in girls is increasing and alarming. [online] Available from: https://centerforhealthjournalism.org/2016/06/22/precocious-puberty-girls-increasing-and-alarming. [Last Accessed November, 2021].
10. Healthy Nutrition Expert. High Meat Diet Causes Girls To Enter Puberty Early. [online] Available from: https://glyco247.wordpress.com/tag/red-meat-for-children/. [Last Accessed November, 2021].
11. Keenan K, Culbert KM, Grimm KJ, Hipwell AE, Stepp SD. Timing and tempo: exploring the complex association between pubertal development and depression in African American and European American girls. J Abnorm Psychol. 2014;123(4):725-36.
12. Hamilton JL, Hamlat EJ, Stange JP, Abramson LY, Alloy LB. Pubertal timing and vulnerabilities to depression in early adolescence: differential pathways to depressive symptoms by sex. J Adolesc. 2014;37(2):165-74.
13. Biro FM, Deardorff J. Identifying opportunities for cancer prevention during pre-adolescence and adolescence: puberty as a window of susceptibility. J Adolesc Health. 2013;52(50):S15-S20.
14. MSD Manuals. Precocious Puberty. [online] Available from: https://www.msdmanuals.com/professional/pediatrics/endocrine-disorders-in-children/precocious-puberty. [Last Accessed November, 2021].
15. Klein DA. Disorders of Puberty: an approach to diagnosis and management. Am Fam Physician. 2017;96(9):590-9.
16. Chen M, Eugster EA. Central precocious puberty: update on diagnosis and treatment. Paediatr Drugs. 2015;17(4): 273-81.
17. Hirsch HJ, Gillis D, Strich D, Chertin B, Farkas A, Lindenberg T, et al. The histrelin implant: a novel treatment for central precocious puberty. Pediatrics. 2005;116(6):e798-802.
18. Eugster EA, Clarke W, Kletter GB, Lee PA, Neely EK, Reiter EO, et al. Efficacy and safety of histrelin subdermal implant in children with central precocious puberty: a multicenter trial. J Clin En-docrinol Metab. 2007;92(5):1697-704.
19. Silverman LA, Neely EK, Kletter GB, Lewis K, Chitra S, Terleckyj O, et al. Long-term continuous suppression with once-yearly histrelin subcutaneous implants for the treatment of central precocious puberty: a final report of a phase 3 multicenter trial. J Clin Endocrinol Metab. Epub 2015 Mar 24. [PMC free article] [PubMed] [Google Scholar]
20. Chen M, Eugster EA. Central precocious puberty: update on diagnosis and treatment. Paediatr Drugs. 2015;17(4):273-81.
21. Dajani T. Efficacy, safety, and pharmacokinetics (PK) of triptorelin 6-month formulation in patients with central precocious puberty. Bethesda (MD): National Library of Medicine; 2014.
22. Pucarelli I, Segni M, Ortore M, Arcadi E, Pasquino AM. Effects of combined gonadotropin-releasing hormone agonist and growth hormone therapy on adult height in precocious puberty: a further contribution. J Pediatr Endocrinol Metab. 2003;16(7):1005-10.
23. Zhao X, Zhang Q. Clinical efficacy of letrozole in boys with idiopathic central precocious puberty. Chin J Contemp Pediatr. 2014;16(4):397-400.
24. Neely EK, Lee PA, Bloch CA, Larsen L, Yang D, Mattia-Goldberg C, et al. Leuprolide acetate 1-month depot for central precocious puberty: hormonal suppression and recovery. Int J Pediatr Endocrinol. 2010;2010:398639.
25. Hirsch HJ, Lahlou N, Gillis D, Strich D, Rosenberg-Hagen B, Chertin B, et al. Free alpha-subunit is the most sensitive marker of gonadotropin recovery after treatment of central precocious puberty with the histrelin implant. J Clin Endocrinol Metab. 2010;95(6):2841-4.
26. Pinilla L, Aguilar E, Dieguez C, Millar RP, Tena-Sempere M. Kisspeptins and reproduction: physiological roles and regulatory mechanisms. Physiol Rev. 2012;92(3):1235-316
27. Schoelwer M, Eugster EA. Treatment of peripheral precocious puberty. Endocr Dev. 2016;29:230-9.
28. Syed FA, Chalew SA Ketoconazole treatment of gonadotropin independent precocious puberty in girls with McCune-Albright syndrome: a preliminary report. J Pediatr Endocrinol Metab. 1999;12(1):81-3.
29. Feuillan P, Calis K, Hill S, Shawker T, Robey PG, Collins MT. Letrozole treatment of precocious puberty in girls with the McCune-Albright syndrome: a pilot study. J Clin Endocrinol Metab. 2007;92(6):2100-6.
30. Eugster EA, Rubin SD, Reiter EO, Plourde P, Jou HC, Pescovitz OH, McCune-Albright Study Group. Tamoxifen treatment for precocious puberty in McCune-Albright syndrome: a multicenter trial. J Pediatr. 2003;143(1):60-6
31. Sims EK, Garnett S, Guzman F, Paris F, Sultan C, Eugster EA, Fulvestrant McCune-Albright Study Group. Fulvestrant treatment of precocious puberty in girls with McCune-Albright syndrome. Int J Pediatr Endocrinol. 2012;2012(1):26.

LONG QUESTIONS

1. Describe the causes of central and peripheral precocious puberty.
2. Explain the management of central precocious puberty.
3. Describe the signs and symptoms with investigations to diagnose central precocious puberty.
4. What are the changes in normal puberty? Define and classify precocious puberty.
5. How will you diagnose and manage a case of peripheral precocious puberty?

SHORT QUESTIONS

1. Classify precocious puberty.
2. What are the complications of precocious puberty?
3. Enumerate signs and symptoms of precocious puberty.
4. Enumerate five causes of central precocious puberty.
5. Enumerate five causes of peripheral precocious puberty.

MULTIPLE CHOICE QUESTIONS

1. Height can be preserved in central precocious puberty by:
   a. Keeping estradiol levels high by giving high GnRH agonists
   b. Keeping estradiol levels low by giving high GnRH agonists
   c. Keeping estradiol levels high by giving low GnRH agonists
   d. Keeping estradiol levels low by giving low GnRH agonists
2. Histrelin implant is:
   a. Progesterone in the form of subcutaneous implant
   b. GnRH agonist in the form of subcutaneous implant
   c. GnRH antagonist in the form of subcutaneous implant
   d. Estradiol in the form of subcutaneous implant
3. Treatment in central precocious puberty should be started ideally when:
   a. Age of onset of symptoms is greater than 6 years and progression is slow
   b. Age of onset of symptoms is less than 6 years and progression is fast
   c. Age of onset of symptoms is greater than 8 years and progression is slow
   d. Age of onset of symptoms is greater than 8 years and progression is fast
4. Follow-up of treatment in central precocious puberty includes all, except:
   a. Assessment of skeletal maturation via bone age radiographs
   b. Determination of growth velocity
   c. Random serum gonadotropin levels
   d. Testosterone levels
5. Genetic causes of precocious puberty in females are:
   a. Congenital adrenal hyperplasia
   b. Sheehan syndrome
   c. Cystic fibrosis
   d. Kallmann syndrome
6. Precocious puberty is seen in:
   a. Hypothyroidism
   b. Hyperthyroidism
   c. Both hypo- and hyperthyroidism
   d. Neither hypo- nor hyperthyroidism
7. Treatment options for McCune Albright syndrome are all, except:
   a. Letrozole
   b. Medroxyprogesterone
   c. Fluconazole
   d. Fulvestrant
8. Doses of Leuprolide depot and Histrelin implants are:
   a. 3.75 mg 3 monthly and 50 mg for 2 years respectively
   b. 11.25 mg 3 monthly and 50 mg for 2 years respectively
   c. 3.75 mg monthly and 65 µg for 2 years respectively
   d. 11.25 mg monthly and 65 µgfor 2 years respectively
9. Precocious puberty is defined as child attaining puberty:
   a. Before the age of 8 in girls and 9 years in boys
   b. Before the age of 9 in girls and 8 years in boys
   c. Before the age of 8 in girls and 8 years in boys
   d. Before the age of 7 in girls and 9 years in boys
10. Possible complications of precocious puberty:
    a. Short height
    b. Social and emotional problems
    c. Cancers in later life
    d. All of the above
11. Order of development in puberty is:
    a. Menarche, Thelarche, Adrenarche
    b. Adrenarche, Menarche, Thelarche
    c. Thelarche, Adrenarche, Menarche
    d. Adrenarche, Thelarche, Menarche

Answers

1.	b	2.	b	3.	b	4.	d	5.	a	6.	a
7.	c	8.	b	9.	a	10.	d	11.	c		

General Gynaecology

9.1 PREMENSTRUAL SYNDROME

Abha Singh

Just before their periods women behave the way men do all the time! —*Robert A Heinlein*

INTRODUCTION

Premenstrual syndrome (PMS) is one of the most common disorders in women of reproductive age that has negative effects on women in terms of performance and emotion. The problems occur during the luteal phase and disappear with the onset of menstruation. However, these symptoms are usually mild and physiological. They are considered as PMS when the symptoms interfere with normal functioning and affect the quality of life (QoL) and routine work significantly.

DEFINITION

Premenstrual syndrome is a condition characterized by recurrent distressing, physical, behavioral and psychological symptoms, associated with premenstrual phase of cycle, which regress completely with the onset or by the end of menstruation, in absence of organic or underlying psychiatric disease (RCOG Green Top Guidelines No. 48).

PREVALENCE

Estimating the prevalence of PMS is a challenge due to the lack of uniformity of definitions and study methodology. PMS prevalence is widely variable and is present in women of all religions, cultures and ethnic group and geographical locations. Its prevalence is estimated to be 5–8% in moderate to severe symptoms.[1] 20% of all women in reproductive age suffer from clinically significant PMS.[2] It is more common in unmarried women, girls in initial years of menstruation (transition phase of life associated with spurt of physical, mental, emotional, and social development), women of 35–44 years of age and women of low socioeconomic group.[3] The prevalence is reported to be 20–32% in premenopausal and 30–40% in the reproductive years.[4] It is important to determine the prevalence of PMS within society and the factors influencing it, in order to plan the treatment.[5] Previous Indian studies have found a 20% prevalence of PMS in the general population.[6] Raval et al. did a study in Gujarat and found the prevalence of PMS as 18.4% and of premenstrual dysphoric disorder (PMDD) as 3.7%.[7] In a study of medical students in Delhi, about 37% of participants had PMDD.[8] The prevalence of PMS in a study in Puducherry was found to be 62.7%.[9]

Premenstrual dysphoric disorder is a severe form of PMS. It affects 2% of women and is classified as a psychiatric disorder in 5th edition of the Diagnostic and Statistical Manual for Mental Disorders (DSM-5).[10] Earlier it was called luteal phase late dysphoric disorder.

HISTORY

This entity has been known since ancient time. Hippocrates said that headaches and behavioral changes before menstruation represent anxious blood that wants to exit.[11] Later in 1953, it was suggested by Greene and Dalton that the symptoms completely disappear after menstruation.[12]

SYMPTOMS

The symptoms must be charted cyclically or daily for at least 2 months. These symptoms are the primary tool in diagnosing PMS. Sometimes they become a major hindrance to its diagnosis because not all of them may be due to PMS. Furthermore, this becomes a considerable burden to both clinicians and patients.

Premenstrual dysphoric disorder requires five of listed symptoms, including at least one mood symptom, that are severe in the luteal phase and recover with onset of menstruation, severe functional impairment, exclusion of major depressive disorder or other psychiatric disease; and prospective confirmation of the symptoms for at least two consecutive menstrual cycles.

In contrast to the specified criteria for PMDD, the World Health Organizations (WHO) International Classification of Diseases (ICD-10) broadly classifies premenstrual tension syndrome (PMTS) as a gynecological disorder but lists no symptoms and no specific criteria to guide a diagnosis.

1. Somatic/physical **(Box 1)**
2. Mood/behavioral **(Box 2)**
3. Combination of both.

Degrees of PMS

- *Mild:* Does not interfere with the personal/social and professional life of the individual.
- *Moderate:* Interferes with personal life but still the individual can interact and function.
- *Severe:* The person is unable to interact socially/professionally and withdraws herself from these activities. This form is also known as PMDD.

CLASSIFICATION

According to the International Society for Premenstrual Disorders (ISPMD), PMS is classified as:

Core: Associated with spontaneous ovulatory menstrual cycles. Presence of physical, psychological or mixed symptoms.

BOX 1: Somatic symptoms associated with PMS.

- Bloating
- Breast tenderness
- Headache
- Insomnia
- Loss of libido
- Lethargy
- Nausea
- Pain in joints /Muscular pain
- Tiredness
- Weight gain

BOX 2: Behavioral symptoms associated with PMS.

- Irritability
- Depression
- Crying without provocation
- Mood swings
- Aggressive behavior
- Reduced cognitive ability
- Suicidal tendency
- Forgetfulness
- Reduced concentration
- Anger
- Anxiety
- Food craving
- Confusion
- Social withdrawal
- Increased interpersonal conflicts

Variants: Have more complex features. It is subdivided into four categories:

1. Premenstrual exacerbation of an underlying condition
2. PMS in the absence of menstruation
3. Progestogen-induced PMS
4. PMS with anovulatory ovarian activity.

DIAGNOSIS

Depends on presence of typical symptoms, their timing (usually during the last 7–10 days of menstrual cycle) and exclusion of organic causes. There are appreciable differences among the current diagnostic approaches, as they are based on symptoms. The guidelines for PMS offered by the American College of Obstetricians and Gynecologists (ACOG) lists six affective and four somatic symptoms. At least one symptom must meet the defined cyclic pattern and confirmed by daily chart for one or more menstrual cycles, and be associated with dysfunction or impairment. Whereas, the criteria most frequently used in recent studies are those of the American Psychiatric Association (APA). These criteria define a severe form of PMS termed PMDD and are described in the Diagnostic and Statistical Manual of Mental Disorders (DSM-5).

Diagnostic Criteria for Core PMS[13]

Diagnostic criteria for core PMS are given in **Box 3**.

DIFFERENTIAL DIAGNOSIS (BOX 4)

Ideally the symptoms should be charted and their severity or disappearance or exaggeration in relation to the phase of menstrual cycle should be noted. The clusters of symptoms

BOX 3: Diagnostic criteria of core PMS.

- Precipitated by ovulation
- Typical symptoms exist but not defined
- Variable number of symptoms
- Physical/psychological/mixed symptoms
- Symptoms recur in the luteal phase
- Symptoms disappear with menstrual flow
- A symptom-free week occurs between menstruation and ovulation
- Symptoms must be prospectively rated
- Symptoms are not an exacerbation of an underlying psychological or physical disorder
- Symptoms cause significant distress and impairment of daily activities, such as work commitments, social interactions and family activities

BOX 4: Differential diagnosis of PMS.

- Psychiatric disorders
- Endometriosis and pelvic pain
- Idiopathic edema
- Anemia
- Hypo/hyperthyroidism
- Menopausal syndrome
- Obesity
- Inflammatory disease of breast/carcinoma breast

are not as important as their cyclicity. PMS is diagnosed if there is 30% increase in severity of symptoms 5 days before menses in comparison to 5 days after menses (guidelines from National Institute of Mental Health).

Diagnostic Criteria of PMDD

The diagnostic criteria of PMDD are listed in **Box 5**.

ETIOPATHOLOGY

The exact etiology of PMS/PMDD is not known. The known facts are its presence only in women of reproductive age, absence before puberty, pregnancy, after menopause and during anovulatory cycle. As most of the women suffer mild symptoms in the luteal phase, PMS must be considered more as physiological rather than pathological.[14]

Different theories that have been put forward are:

- Low progesterone levels
- Fluctuations in estrogen/progesterone levels
- Low serotonin levels
- Dysfunction of gamma aminobutyric acid (GABA) receptors
- Changes in renin-angiotensin-system
- Increased prolactin levels
- Other.

Ovarian Steroids

It was strongly suggested that if hypothalamus ovarian axis is suppressed with gonadotropins, PMS would disappear, however recent studies suggest that PMS is due to an altered response to normal cyclic changes in ovarian steroids.

Low Serotonin Levels

Evidence supports the role of low levels of serotonin in women with mood changes and that PMS/PMDD result from its increased sensitivity to ovarian steroids. Women with PMS have been found to have low concentration of serotonin on their platelets.

BOX 5: Diagnostic criteria for PMDD.

- At least 5 symptoms in the week before menses, which improve with onset of menses and become minimal post menses
- One of these symptoms present mood swings, anger/irritability, depression/hopelessness and marked anxiety/tension
- One of these symptoms (to make it 5) reduced interest unusual activities, poor concentration, lethargy, food craving, hypersomnia/insomnia, one of the physical symptoms described in **Box 1**
- Clinically significant distress,, interference with work, social withdrawal
- Exclusion of major depressive disorder
- Symptoms of diagnostic criteria should be at least confirmed by charting in 2 symptomatic cycles
- Medical conditions like thyroid disorders and substance abuse must be excluded

Gamma Aminobutyric Acid

The GABA transmitter system is an inhibitory system in the CNS. Its levels are relatively low in the luteal phase of women suffering from PMDD. Some progesterone metabolites interact with GABA receptors and have shown different responsive- ness in women with PMS. Receptor dysfunction may play a role.[15]

Changes in Renin Angiotensin System

Somatic symptoms such as breast tenderness and bloating were considered to be due to fluid retention. No evidence has been found to suggest an electrolyte shift.

Increased Prolactin

Prolactin causes electrolyte retention and breast tenderness. Current evidence does not support its role in PMS.

Other

Some theories have suggested thyroid dysfunction, genetic influence and deficiency of vitamins and mineral in the etiology of PMS but they show limited evidence.

TREATMENT

- Pharmacologic
- Alternative therapies
- Surgery.

The success of treatment depends on accurate diagnosis, which needs a documentation of symptoms in luteal phase only and exclusion of psychiatric disorders. As this occurs in the reproductive age group only, the management will require consideration for pregnancy or contraceptive.

Mild to moderate PMS can respond very well to non-pharmacological treatment like the following: Lifestyle modifications should always be considered the first-line of management before starting any medication. This includes dietary modifications, relaxation exercises, yoga and cognitive behavioral therapy (CBT). Dietary modifications include lowering caffeine, salt, sugar, alcohol and heavy fried meals. Smaller portions of simple meals should be advised. Exercise can be in the form of walking, aerobics or yoga,

Cognitive behavioral therapy is a short-term, skilled form of therapy that focuses on the interaction between thoughts, feelings, and behaviors. Repeated cycles of negative thinking magnify the symptoms and increase anxiety, depression and irritability. Cognitive therapy gives her the opportunity to be more adaptive to positive thoughts and behavior. Basically, it comprises an analysis of stress factors that trigger the symptoms, counseling sessions and relaxation therapy.

Vitamins

Pyridoxine is a cofactor that is essential for conversion of tryptophan to neuropeptides such as serotonin. So, theoretically it may have a role in depressive symptoms but RCTs as well as systematic review show limited evidence. Pyridoxine 50–100 mg /day was given in a study.[16]

Calcium

Calcium in a dose of 600 mg twice daily in the luteal phase was used in a study to reduce somatic symptoms.

Others

Evening primrose oil, magnesium, chaste berry, and vitamin D were given in different studies with poor results. Evening primrose oil has been found effective only in cyclical mastalgia. Similarly massage, acupuncture and reflexology has been studied and found ineffective.

Pharmacological Management

Progesterone

This has been the favorite treatment in the past. All doses were tried 400, 800 and 1,200 mg/day. The effects were found to be the same as placebo. Cochrane analysis done by Ford et al. in 2009 concluded that it is not an effective treatment for PMS.[17] It is not recommended in treatment of PMS.

Estrogen

It used to be given cyclically with progesterone, to prevent endometrial hyperplasia. It is no longer used now owing to its adverse effects. Long-term adverse effects on breast and endometrium are not known.

Danazol

It is a synthetic derivative of 17-alpha ethinyl testosterone which suppresses pituitary to cause anovulation. In a low dose of 200 mg, it was found to reduce severity of symptoms of PMS especially cyclical mastalgia, besides being useful in endometriosis. A woman requires contraceptive when taking Danazol as there may be virilizing effects on the female fetus. Not preferred as first-line management due to its androgenic side effects.

Combined Oral Contraceptives

The use of combined oral contraceptives (COC) was based on the fact that it delivers hormones in steady doses, and can make hormone levels more predictable and premenstrual symptoms less unpleasant. COC is the first line of management for PMS. The older ones were not much beneficial in relieving mood changes, but drospirenone, a derivative of spironolactone is found to be very effective in the dose of 3 mg along with 20 µg ethinyl estradiol (EE).[18] It was found to work better in improving social and interpersonal relations as well as productivity. However the authors concluded that it was not known if it works longer than three cycles, useful in women with less severe symptoms, or is better than other COCs. However, some recent studies show remarkable improvement in behavior and mood changes.

Spironolactone

It is a potassium sparing diuretic exhibiting anti-mineralocorticoid property. It is generally used in a dose of 25–200 mg daily in the luteal phase in women with PMS who suffer from weight gain, bloating and breast tenderness. In some studies it was found to be more effective than placebo in reducing bloatedness and breast tenderness. Also there was a significant fall in androgen levels.

Gonadotropin Releasing Hormone Agonists

These are synthetic analogs of naturally occurring gonadotropin-releasing hormone (GnRH). They act by causing anovulation by suppressing FSH and LH. They have been undoubtedly found effective in both somatic as well as psychological symptoms. Their main disadvantage is hypoestrogenic adverse effects such as hot flashes, muscle ache, headache and reduction in bone mass density (BMD). An add back therapy with 0.625 mg of conjugated estrogens or 2 mg estradiol valerate may be helpful to alleviate the postmenopausal symptoms. In addition, calcium intake should be given and promoted in diet.

When treating women with PMS, GnRH analogs should usually be reserved for women with the most severe symptoms. They are not recommended routinely unless used to treat very severe cases. Women on long-term treatment should have measurement of BMD [ideally by dual-energy X-ray absorptiometry (DEXA)] every year. Treatment should be stopped if bone density declines significantly (RCOG Green-top Guideline No. 48, 2016).

A rare use of GnRH agonists is when the diagnosis of PMS is not confirmed, despite 2 months of charting of symptoms.

Selective Serotonin Reuptake Inhibitors

Selective serotonin reuptake inhibitors (SSRIs) are used as first-line management in PMS (fluoxetine, paroxetine and sertraline). A dose of 20 mg daily has shown sustained efficacy in reducing somatic and mood symptoms. They can be used in the luteal phase or continuously. Randomized control trials were studied in a Systematic Cochrane review by Marjoribanks et al.[19] They found the evidence in favor of their use in PMS. They also commented that their adverse effects, mainly asthenia and nausea are frequent and dose dependent. Other adverse effects are loss of libido and insomnia or somnolence. SSRI should be discontinued gradually to avoid withdrawal symptoms. Only women on continuous therapy require gradual withdrawal, those in whom it is prescribed only during luteal phase do not require tapering the dose. There is a very small chance of congenital malformation as compared to general population, if the woman conceives while taking SSRI. Therefore before initiating the treatment with SSRI, preconception counseling is important.

Levonorgestrel (LNG) Intrauterine Device (IUD)

There is no evidence to support the use of the LNG-IUS 52 mg alone to treat PMS symptoms. Its role should be confined to opposing the action of estrogen therapy on the endometrium.

Alprazolam

This addictive benzodiazepine has a limited role in treating depression in PMS. Usually, used when women with anxiety are not relieved by SSRI alone.

Serotonin-Norepinephrine Reuptake Inhibitors

Serotonin-norepinephrine reuptake inhibitors (SNRIs) such as venlafaxine (50–200 mg/day) have been used off-label to treat PMDD in women with predominantly psychological symptoms. The effect is achieved over a relatively short period, 3–4 weeks, and sustained throughout subsequent menstrual cycles.

Role of Surgery

This is limited to those women with severe PMS, who do not respond to or tolerate the symptoms, despite various medical treatments. In such women hysterectomy with bilateral salpingo-oophorectomy can be done.[20] A long-term hormone replacement therapy is required after the surgery in these women. A trial of GnRH analogs for 3 months is advocated by many before going to the invasive procedure of hysterectomy if the cost is not the consideration.

CONCLUSION

A proper treatment of PMS requires a precise diagnosis which is based on charting of symptoms. So a precise diagnosis is to be made and not the woman's own diagnosis. It is mandatory to separate anxiety and depressive disorders from mild variations of physiological symptoms which require only reassurance. Treatment needs to be individualized. If it is a mild PMS with only somatic symptoms, the first line of management should include diet modification and supplementation with vitamin D and calcium, relaxation strategies and exercises like aerobics or yoga and CBT. The lifestyle interventions should be continued for life time.

If the woman wants contraception also, then the first line of treatment would be combined oral pills containing drospirenone 3 mg and EE 20 µg.

In case weight gain and bloating is more troublesome, spironolactone can be given in the luteal phase.

In women having predominant psychological dysfunction and those with established diagnosis of PMDD, SSRI or SNRI continuously or during luteal phase will be the best option. In case of no relief, alprazolam can be given.

For the nonresponders, diagnosis should be reconfirmed and major depressive disorders should be excluded.

In other words, the management will depend not only on the severity but on the predominant symptom also. Usually in moderate to severe PMS, this condition may be as debilitating as major depressive disorder. It not only affects the QoL but has a greater negative impact on interpersonal relationships and work performance. The goal of treatment should be to bring the individual back to her routine activities and promote productivity.

KEY MESSAGES

- PMS is a recurrent condition occurring during luteal phase of women of reproductive age group.
- It is characterized by somatic, psychological, and behavioral changes which may vary in severity causing deterioration in routine activity of the affected individual.
- Some degrees of premenstrual problems are experienced almost in 80% of women but its prevalence is 3–8% in moderate to severe forms.
- The symptoms appear about 1 week before the onset of menses and disappear soon after onset of menses.
- Premenstrual dysphoric disorder (PMDD) is the severe form of PMS. It affects 2% women.
- The severity of symptoms may lead to significant impairment in interpersonal relationships and work loss from school, college or office.
- The chronic nature of the condition ultimately affects the QoL.
- PMDD, as defined by the American Psychiatric Association (APA) Diagnostic and Statistical Manual, Fifth Edition (DSM-5), can be differentiated from PMS by the presence of at least five symptoms, including one affective symptom, such as mood swings, irritability, and/or depression.
- PMS is associated with an increased responsiveness to the gonadal steroids. This tendency may be inherited.
- Serotonin is an important neurotransmitter for the regulation of mood and aggression. Sex steroids modulate serotonin secretion.
- Gamma aminobutyric acid (GABA), the inhibitory neurotransmitter, also plays a role in PMDD. Low levels of GABA diminish its inhibitory effect, resulting in mood disorders.
- The diagnosis of PMS (according to ACOG criteria) and PMDD requires daily charting of symptoms over two menstrual cycles.
- The pharmacological treatment is based on the symptoms.
- The nonpharmacological/alternative management is also known to be effective. Recent studies show that a combination of both is more beneficial.
- Before beginning the management the contraceptive need and pregnancy plan should be discussed.
- COCs may be used as the first line of management. Drospirenone containing pill is found to be better tolerated and more effective.
- 17 Anxiolytics may also form the first line of management if emotional symptoms predominate.
- GnRH agonist trial should be given in case of ambiguity in diagnosis or given when COCs and antianxiolytics fail to reduce the symptoms.

- Invasive procedures such as hysterectomy with bilateral oophorectomy should be reserved only as a last resort in women not responding to any treatment. These women later require hormone therapy (estrogens).

REFERENCES

1. Yonkers KA, Shaughan O' Brien PM, Erikson E. Premenstrual syndrome. Lancet. 2008;5;371:1200-10.
2. Borenstein J, Dean B, Endicott J, Wong J, Brown C, Dickerson V, et al. Health andeconomic impact of PMS. J Reprod Med. 2003;48:515-24.
3. Cheng SH, Sun ZG, Lee IH. Perception of PMS and attitude of evaluation of work performance among incoming university female students. Biomed J. 2015;38:167-72.
4. Baker LJ, O'Brien PM. Premenstrual syndrome (PMS): a peri-menopausal perspective. Maturitas. 2012;72(2):121-5.
5. Hantsoo L, Epperson CN. Premenstrual dysphoric disorder: epidemiology and treatment. Curr Psychiatry Rep. 2015;17:87.
6. Sarkar AP, Mandal R, Ghorai S. Premenstrual syndrome among adolescent girl students in a rural school of West Bengal, India. Int J Med Sci Public Health. 2016;5:408-11.
7. Raval CM, PanchalBN, Tiwari DS, Vala AU, Bhatt RB. Prevalence of premenstrual syndrome and premenstrual dysphoric disorder among college students of Bhavnagar, Gujarat. Indian J Psychiatry. 2016;58:164-70.
8. Mishra A, Banwari G, Yadav P. Premenstrual dysphoric disorder in medical students residing in hostel and its association with lifestyle factors. Ind Psychiatry J. 2015;24:150-7.
9. Bhuvneshwari K, Ravindran P, Bharadwaj B. Prevalence of premenstrual syndrome and its impact on quality of life among selected college students in Puducherry. The National Medical Journal of India. 2019:32(1);17-9.
10. Premenstrual Dysphoric Disorder DSM-5 625.4 (N94.3)
11. Babazadeh R,Keramat A. PMS andcomplementary medicine in Iran: a systematic review.KAUM S J(FEYZ). 2011;15:174-87.
12. Zendehel M and Elyasi F. Biopsychosocial etiology of PMS: a narrative review. J Family Med Prim Care. 2018;7(2):346-56.
13. Kadian S, O'Brien S. Classification of premenstrual disorders as proposed by the International Society for Premenstrual Disorders. Menopause Int. 2012;18:43-7.
14. Rosseinsky DR, Debonnel PG. An evolutionary theory of premenstrual tension. Lancet. 1974;2:1024.
15. Girdler SS, Straneva PA, Light KC, Pedersena CA, Morrowac AL, et al. Allopregnanolone levels and reactivity to mental stress in premenstrual dysphoric disorder.Biological Psychiatry.2001; 49:788-97.
16. Williams AI, Cotter A, Sabina A, Girard C, Goodman J, Katz DL. The role of vitamin B6 as a treatment for depression: a systematic review. Family Practitioner. 2005;22;532-7.
17. Ford O, Lethaby A, Roberts H, Mol BW. Progesterone for premenstrual syndrome.Cochrane Database Systematic Review. 2009;(2):CD003415.
18. Lopez LM, Kaptein A, Helmerhorst FM. Oral contraceptives containing drosperinone for PMS. Cochrane Database of Systematic Reviews. 2008;(1):CD006586.
19. Marjoribanks J, Brown J, Shaughn O'Brien PM, Wyatt K. SSRI for PMS. Cochrane Database Systematic Review. 2013:CD001396.
20. Cronje WH, Vashisht A, Studd JW. Hysterctomy and bilateral oophorectomy for severe premenstrual syndrome. Human Reproduction. 2004;19:2152-5.

LONG QUESTION

1. Define PMS and its types. Discuss the diagnostic criteria of PMS and the management options in PMS.

SHORT QUESTIONS

1. Describe the various symptoms associated with PMS.
2. Discuss the various etiologies of PMS.
3. Discuss the various differential diagnoses of PMS.

MULTIPLE CHOICE QUESTIONS

1. PMS occurs:
   a. In absence of organic disease
   b. In presence of organic disease
   c. None of the above is true
   d. Can be in presence or absence of organic disease
2. Clinically significant PMS in reproductive age is present in:
   a. 5% b. 10%
   c. 20% d. 50%
3. Primary tool in diagnosing PMS is charting symptoms daily for:
   a. A period of 3 months
   b. A period of 2 months
   c. A period of 6 months
   d. Variable in different ethnic groups
4. Severe form of PMS is also known as:
   a. PMD b. SPMS
   c. PMS III d. PMDD
5. Etiology of PMS is:
   a. Fluctuation in estrogen/progesterone levels
   b. Dysfunction of GABA receptors
   c. Low serotonin levels
   d. All of the above
6. The first line of management in mild PMS is:
   a. Lifestyle modifications b. Evening primrose oil
   c. Acupuncture d. Reflexology
7. Danazol is not preferred as first line management due to:
   a. Virilizing effect b. Weight gain
   c. Anti-estrogenic effects d. Androgenic side effects
8. Spironolactone can be given to those who suffer from:
   a. Weight gain b. Bloating
   c. Breast tenderness d. All 3 above
9. Pre-conception counseling is important if--------- is used.
   a. Danazol b. SSRI
   c. Both d. None of the above
10. If a lady with PMS needs a contraception also, the best choice is:
    a. Progesterone only pills b. SNRI
    c. Drosperinone with EE d. LNG IUD

Answers

1. a 2. c 3. b 4. d 5. d 6. a
7. d 8. d 9. c 10. c

9.2 DYSMENORRHEA

PB Hiremath

DEFINITION

Dysmenorrhea is a cyclical pain associated with menstruation *"painful menstruation"* that significantly interferes with day to day pursuits. It is a common gynecological disorder affecting 60% of menstruating females.

Its main types are:
- Primary dysmenorrhea
- Secondary dysmenorrhea

PRIMARY DYSMENORRHEA

Primary dysmenorrhea is otherwise called as *spasmodic dysmenorrhea*. It occurs in normal ovulatory cycle without any conspicuous pelvic or uterine pathology.

Incidence

Incidence of primary dysmenorrhea is about 15–20%. It prevails mainly in adolescent girls within 1–2 years of menarche usually from opulent society, with high BMI and with familial association. Parity (mainly after vaginal delivery) appears to improve symptoms.

Pathophysiology

Mechanisms postulated in the pathophysiology of primary dysmenorrhea are:
- Psychosomatic and lifestyle factors
- Effects of prostaglandins (PG)
- Effects of autonomic nerves
- Effects of progesterone levels
- Effects of vasopressin
- Effects of endothelins, platelet activating factor (PAF), and leukotrienes
- Abnormal myometrial anatomy.

Psychosomatic and Lifestyle Factors

- Tension, anxiety and stress—lowers the pain threshold
- Long menstrual period
- Smoking, overweight and sedentary life style has its impact on primary dysmenorrhea.

Effects of Prostaglandins

Effects of prostaglandins in pathophysiology of primary dysmenorrhea is explained by, excessive or imbalanced synthesis of PGE-2 and PGF-2α or due to increased sensitivity of myometrium to normal prostaglandins during menstruation, resulting in dysperistalsis and hyperactivity of myometrium and vasoconstriction resulting in myometrial ischemia and pain.

Effects of Autonomic Nerves

This pain can be relieved by dilatation of cervix by damaging sensory nerve endings of but later may lead to incompetence. The same mechanism is explained for pain relief following vaginal delivery.

Effects of Progesterone Levels

The low levels of progesterone in the late luteal phase triggers lytic enzymatic action, resulting in a release of phospholipids with the generation of arachidonic acid and activation of the cyclooxygenase (COX) pathway.

Thus prostaglandin, thromboxane and leukotrienes are derived from arachidonic acid.

Effects of Vasopressin

Increased levels of vasopressin are noted in females with primary dysmenorrhea. It acts directly on the myometrium and causes hyperactivity, it also increases prostaglandins synthesis and in turn results in uterine hyperactivity and dysrhythmic contraction leading to ischemia, hypoxia and pain.

Abnormal Myometrial Anatomy

Abnormality in junctional zone (JZ) – subendometrial layer of myometrium such as hyperplasia, irregular thickening and less vascularity resulting in dysperistalsis and hyperactivity of myometrium causing pain.

Clinical Features

The hallmarks of primary dysmenorrhea are:
The pain of primary dysmenorrhea usually begins a few hours before or just after the onset of a menstrual period and may last *48–72 hours.*

The pain of dysmenorrhea is *spasmodic/colicky* in nature and, is relieved by abdominal massage, counter-pressure, or movement of the body. The pain is *labor-like,* with suprapubic cramping, and may be accompanied by lumbosacral backache, pain radiating down the anterior and inner thighs.

Accompanied by generalized weakness nausea, vomiting, diarrhea, vasomotor symptoms and rarely syncopal episodes.

Pelvic and bimanual examination does not reveal any pathology.

Investigations

- Investigations are done to rule out any underlying pelvic pathology

- Nucleic acid amplification test or culture for gonorrhea and chlamydia are done to rule out pelvic inflammatory disease (PID)
- Pelvic ultrasound should be done if symptoms do not resolve with nonsteroidal anti-inflammatory drugs (NSAIDs)
- Diagnosis of primary dysmenorrhea is made after considering symptoms and excluding pathologies.

Management

General considerations such as improving general health and hygiene, frequent bladder and bowel emptying and encouraging to do day to day activities and simple sport activities. Counseling and reassurance, with NSAIDs will work for most of the females.

Medical Management

Nonsteroidal anti-inflammatory agents are effective for the treatment of primary dysmenorrhea. NSAIDs—prostaglandin synthase inhibitors are effective in treatment of primary dysmenorrhea as there is strong relation of increased PGs with primary dysmenorrhea.

NSAIDs should be taken up to 1 to 3 days before or, if menses are irregular, at the first onset of even minimal pain or bleeding and then continuously every 6 to 8 hours to prevent reformation of PG by-products for 3 to 6 months.

Side effects: Nausea, dyspepsia, diarrhea, and occasionally fatigue.

Contraindication: Gastrointestinal ulcers or bronchospastic hypersensitivity to aspirin.

Selective COX-2 inhibitors have similar analgesic effect but with fewer side effects.

Commonly used oral NSAIDs in the treatment of dysmenorrhea:

- COX-2 inhibitor
- Hormonal contraceptives: Hormonal contraceptives are considered for
  - Patients who are unresponsive or have contra-indications to NSAIDs.
  - Patients who have no contraindications to hormonal contraceptive and who desire contraception.

Combined estrogen and progestin or progesterone only oral contraceptives given continuous or as cyclic regime.

Transdermal patch, vaginal ring, injectable progestin preparations, or levonorgestrel-releasing intrauterine devices (LNG-IUS) are more effective than placebo alone.

Hormonal contraceptives inhibit ovulation, decrease endometrial proliferation, and create an endocrine milieu similar to the early proliferative phase of the menstrual cycle, when PG levels are lowest. Decreased PG levels result in less uterine cramping.

GnRH agonists and androgens: The estrogen-lowering effects of these drugs lead to endometrial atrophy and diminished PG production resulting in no or less pain.

Nonpharmacologic Pain Management

Heat, acupuncture, or transcutaneous electrical nerve stimulation (TENS), may be useful but not effective as medical management.

Surgical Management

Laparoscopic procedures such as laparoscopic uterine nerve ablation (LUNA), laparoscopic presacral neurectomy (LPSN) have limited effects in primary dysmenorrhea.

Dilatation of cervical canal helps in females with primary dysmenorrhea with cervical stenosis by damaging the sensory nerve endings, still it has its risk of cervical incompetence later.

SECONDARY DYSMENORRHEA

Secondary dysmenorrhea is otherwise called as *congestive dysmenorrhea.* Secondary dysmenorrhea is cyclic menstrual pain that occurs in association with underlying *pelvic pathology.*

Incidence

It is variable and depends on the type of pelvic pathology. It is usually seen in their thirties, more often parous and not related to any socioeconomic status (SES).

Pathophysiology

In congestive or secondary dysmenorrhea the pain is due to increased pelvic tissue tension caused by premenstrual pelvic congestion or increased vascularity in pelvic organs.

Clinical Features

The pain of secondary dysmenorrhea often begins 1–2 weeks before menstrual flow and persists until a few days after the cessation of bleeding.

Pain is dull aching and mostly confined to back and not usually radiating/not associated with vasomotor symptoms.

Pelvic and bimanual examination reveals pelvic pathology.

Secondary dysmenorrhea frequently complicates or associated with endometriosis, leiomyomas, PID, adenomyosis, endometrial polyps, and menstrual outlet obstruction. And hence, it may be associated with other gynecologic symptoms, such as dyspareunia, dysuria, abnormal bleeding, or infertility.

Management

The management of secondary dysmenorrhea is mainly aimed at treatment of the underlying disorder rather than symptomatic pain relief.

The treatment depends on the type and severity of the diseases and also considering the age and parity of the patient.

OTHER CAUSES

Ovarian Dysmenorrhea

Pelvic congestion or increased blood flow in the premenstrual period resulting in marked engorgement of the vein, right ovarian vein that crosses the ureter at right angle causes pressure on the ureter, resulting in stasis–infection–pyelonephritis–pain.

FURTHER READING

1. Akerlund M, Stromberg P, Forsling MD. Primary dysmenorrheaand vasopressin. Br J ObstetGynaecol. 1979; 86:484.
2. Bergsjo P. Socioeconomic implications of dysmenorrhea.Acta Obstet Gynecol Scand. 1979;87(Suppl 1):67.
3. Chan WY, Dawood MY, Fuchs F. Prostaglandin in primarydysmenorrhea comparison of prophylactic and nonprophylactictreatment with ibuprofen and use of oral contraceptive. Am J Med. 1981;70:535.
4. Dawood MY. Dysmenorrhea and ibuprofen. Am J Med. 1984;77: 87.
5. Dawood MY. Dysmenorrhea. Clin Obstet Gynecol 1990;3:168-78.
6. Dawood MY. Hormones, prostaglandins, and dysmenorrhea. In: Dawood MY (ed). Dysmenorrhea. Baltimore: Williams & Wilkins, 1981.p 21.
7. Dawood MY. Overall approach to the management ofdysmenorrhea. In: Dawood MY, McGuire JL, Demers LM (eds). Premenstrual Syndrome and Dysmenorrhea, Baltimore: Urban & Schwarzen berg, 1985.p 177.
8. Howard FM. Chronic pelvic pain.Obstet Gynecol. 2003;101: 594-611.
9. Pickles VR, Hall WJ, Best FA, et al. Prostaglandins in endometriumand menstrual fluid from normal and dysmenorrheic subjects. J Obstet Gynaecol Br Commonw. 1965;72:185.
10. Proctor ML, Roberts H, Farquhar CM. Combined oralcontraceptive pill (OCP) as treatment for primary dysmenorrhea(Cochrane Review). In: The Cochrane Library, Issue 4, 2001. Oxford: Update Software.
11. Wesselmann U. Neurogenic inflammation and chronic pelvic pain. World J Urol. 2001;19:180-5.
12. Widholm O. Epidemiology of premenstrual tension syndromeand primary dysmenorrhea. In: Dawood MY, McGuire JL, Demers LM (eds). Premenstrual Syndrome and Dysmenorrhea, Baltimore: Urban & Schwarzenberg, 1985.p 3.
13. Wiqvist N, Lindblom B, Wilhelmsson L. The pathophysiology of primary dysmenorrhea. Res Clin Forums. 1979;1:47.

LONG QUESTIONS

1. Define and classify dysmenorrhea, discuss in detail about pathogenesis and management of secondary dysmenorrhea.
2. Define primary dysmenorrhea, discuss in detail about pathogenesis and management of primary dysmenorrhea.

SHORT QUESTIONS

1. Congestive dysmenorrhea.
2. Spasmodic dysmenorrhea.
3. Management of primary dysmenorrhea.

MULTIPLE CHOICE QUESTIONS

1. Primary dysmenorrhea is otherwise called as:
   a. Spasmodic dysmenorrhea
   b. Congestive dysmenorrhea
   c. Membranous dysmenorrhea
   d. All of the above
2. Secondary dysmenorrhea is otherwise called as:
   a. Spasmodic dysmenorrhea
   b. Congestive dysmenorrhea
   c. Membranous dysmenorrhea
   d. None of the above
3. Secondary dysmenorrhea frequently associated with all, except:
   a. Endometriosis b. PID
   c. Low prostaglandins d. A large fibroid
4. Effects of prostaglandins in pathophysiology of primary dysmenorrhea is explained by all, except:
   a. Excessive synthesis of PGE & PGF
   b. Increased sensitivity of myometrium to normal prostaglandins
   c. Myometrial ischema
   d. Increased oxytocin level
5. Increased level of vasopressin is noted in females with:
   a. Primary dysmenorrhea
   b. Secondary dysmenorrhea
   c. Ovarian dysmenorrhea
   d. All of the above
6. GnRH agonists acts by all, except:
   a. Hypo-estrogenic state
   b. Endometrial atrophy
   c. Diminished prostaglandin
   d. Altering the myometrial contractions
7. Primary dysmenorrhea prevails mainly in:
   a. Reproductive age b. Adolescent girls
   c. Premenopausal age d. All of the above
8. In primary dysmenorrhea levels of vasopressin will be:
   a. Increased b. Decreased
   c. Neutral d. Unaltered

Answers

1. a 2. b 3. c 4. b 5. a 6. a
7. b 8. a

9.3 CHRONIC PELVIC PAIN

Anupam Gupta, Shikha Singh

INTRODUCTION

Chronic pelvic pain (CPP) affects the women worldwide and of all ages. However, due to its complex nature and lack of knowledge, CPP is often neglected. It is a common debilitating condition that mostly affects women. CPP is usually diffuse and poorly defined without spatial discernment due to the varying densities of the visceral, sensory innervation, and scattering of input into the central nervous system. Diaphoresis, vital signs abnormalities, and the autonomic system including the gastrointestinal system often accompany visceral pain and may confuse the diagnosis. Patients are often focused on the viscera as the cause of pain, and therefore visceral etiology must be addressed early and often, with the assurance that these diagnoses are not being overlooked.

Chronic pelvic pain in women is defined as "persistent, noncyclical pain that is believed to occur in structures related to the pelvis and lasts for more than 6 months. Chronic pelvic pain is defined by the Royal College of Obstetricians and Gynecologists (RCOG)" as "intermittent or persistent pain in the lower abdomen or pelvis for at least 6 months", not occurring exclusively with menstruation or intercourse and is not associated with pregnancy". The American College of Obstetricians and Gynecologists (ACOG) and the ReVITALize Data Definitions initiative define CPP as, "pain symptoms perceived to originate from pelvic organs/ structures typically lasting more than 6 months and is often associated with negative cognitive, behavioral, sexual, and emotional consequences as well as with symptoms suggestive of lower urinary tract, sexual, bowel, pelvic floor, myofascial, or gynecological dysfunction". The lack of consensus on the definition of CPP has hindered efforts to understand its prevalence and the success of treatment options.

PREVALENCE

Chronic pelvic pain is more common in the reproductive and older age groups. Its prevalence in women of reproductive age is 14–24%. However, in 2006 the World Health Organization (WHO) found the prevalence to be around 2.1–24% for noncyclic pain, 8–21.1% for dyspareunia, and 16.8–81% for dysmenorrhea. The lack of consensus on the definition of CPP has hindered efforts to understand its prevalence and the success of treatment options. An updated review published in 2014 used a more stringent definition (noncyclic pain lasting at least 6 months) and estimated the prevalence to range from 5.7 to 26.6%.[1]

PATHOPHYSIOLOGY

Recent evidence supports the importance of central sensitization in maintaining chronic pain syndrome. Central sensitization occurs when peripheral pain provokes an exaggerated response by interneurons, which increases the perception of pain. The resulting pathological changes include the response of the central nervous system to noxious stimuli, activation of specific brain regions, the hypothalamic–pituitary–adrenal axis and the autonomic nervous system, all of which increase psychological distress. Central sensitization explains why patients with CPP feel pain in response to innocuous stimuli (allodynia) and an increased response to painful stimuli (hyperalgesia).[2]

Also a few numbers of mechanisms have been suggested as to the pathophysiological basis of CPP:

- An infection processes
- A neurogenic inflammation
- Hypoxia
- Weakness or cramps of the pelvic floor muscles.

CAUSES

It is quite difficult to identify a single etiology for CPP. Some important causes are:

- *Gynecological system*: Endometriosis, adenomyosis, chronic pelvic inflammatory disease, fibroids, and adhesions (secondary to infection or surgery) are common gynecological causes of CPP. Others include pelvic organ prolapse, pelvic congestion syndrome, benign tumors (uterine, ovarian), vaginal or vaginal pain syndrome, and ovarian remnant syndrome **(Figs. 1 and 2)**.

Endometriosis defined as the presence of endometrial glands and stroma outside the endometrial cavity is one of the most common causes. Typical patients are women in their thirties, anemic, involuntarily infertile with secondary dysmenorrhea, and pelvic pain. Treatment options for endometriosis include medical, surgical, and traditional pain management techniques. Conservative measures are first initiated with nonsteroidal anti-inflammatory drugs (NSAIDs), progestins, androgenic hormones, estrogen-progesterone combinations, and gonadotropin-releasing hormone agonists. The goal of hormone therapy is to lead to atrophy of the endometrial implant. Surgical treatment options include laparoscopic excision of endometrial implants, total abdominal hysterectomy with or without bilateral salpingo-oophorectomy, presacral neurectomy (PSN), and laparoscopic uterine nerve ablation. Patients also benefit from interventional pain management techniques, such as hypogastric plexus block and neuromodulation **(Flowchart 1)**.

Pelvic congestion syndrome is a disease of the childbearing years, usually in the late twenties and early thirties.

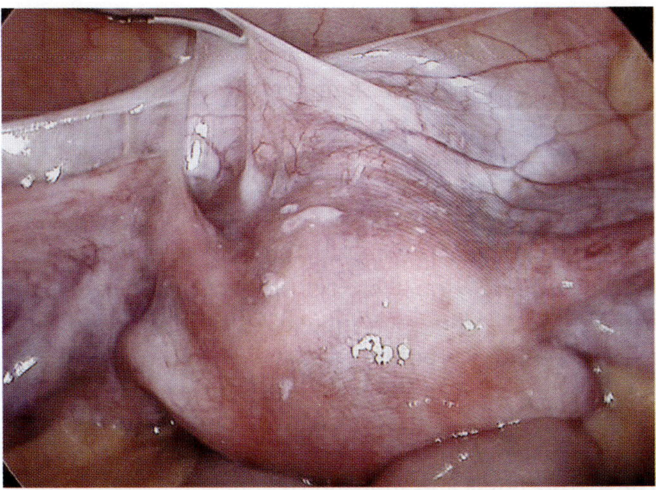

Fig. 1: Pelvic adhesions.

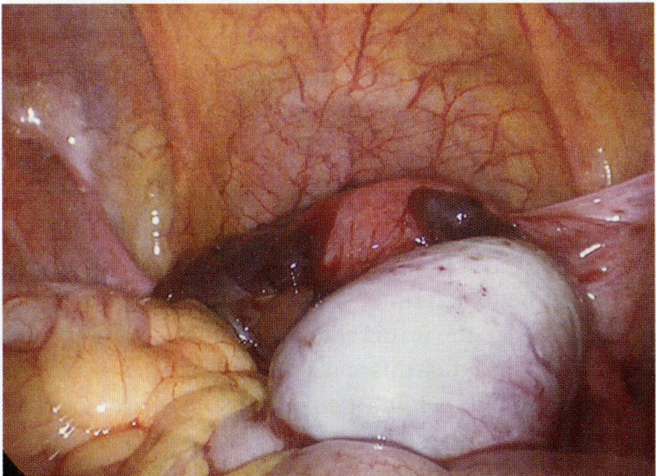

Fig. 2: Endometriosis deposits, adhesions and ovarian endometrioma.

Flowchart 1: Causes of chronic pelvic pain.

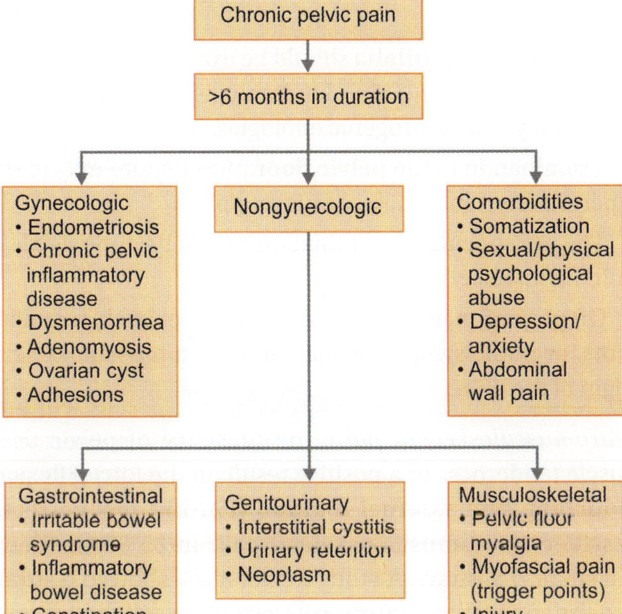

Deep dyspareunia and postcoital pain lasting from a few days to several days are hallmarks of this condition. Residual ovary syndrome—sometime after surgical removal of the ovaries and Fallopian tubes, a small piece of ovary may accidentally remain inside and a later painful cyst may develop. Removal of all ovarian tissue or suppression using a GnRH analog may provide pain relief. Vulvodynia is defined as a chronic vulvar discomfort with duration of at least 3 months. Many physicians suspect a neuropathic etiology for vulvodynia and may be related to a stretch injury of the nerve to the levator ani or pudendal nerve due to prolonged second stage of labor. Treatment strategies include oral tricyclic antidepressants (TCAs), antiseizure agents such as gabapentin, pregabalin, topical creams with estrogen or lidocaine, behavioral therapy, biofeedback, surgery (vestibuloplasty, vestibulectomy), botulinum therapy, interventional pain techniques, and therapy.

- *Gastrointestinal system:* Constipation, irritable bowel syndrome (IBS), inflammatory bowel disease, diverticulitis and diverticulosis, chronic appendicitis, or Meckel diverticulum, adhesions are important gastrointestinal system causes of CPP.
- *Urological:* Bladder pain syndrome (interstitial cystitis) (IC)—this condition affects the function of the bladder wall, accompanied by pain in the bladder with increased frequency of urination, urgency, and nocturnal without infection. Pelvic pain from IC usually refers to the lower back, buttocks, and perineal areas. In chronic cases, muscle tension in the pelvic floor can lead to myalgia. The diagnosis of IC is made based on visual observation of Hunter's cysts in the bladder mucosa and a positive potassium chloride sensitivity test. Treatment is multimodal, starting with the firstline oral agents—NSAIDs, opioids, pentane polysulfate sodium (PPS), amitriptyline, hydroxyzine and gabapentin. A PPS agent is the only FDA-approved oral agent for IC. Intravascular therapy with dimethyl sulfoxide alone or with heparin has demonstrated an efficacy of 50–90%.
- *Neuromuscular:* Trauma (secondary to vaginal delivery), surgery (cesarean section), pelvic floor muscle pain syndrome, vagal muscle spasm, neuralgia from nerve entrapment or irritation, lower back pain (sprain, strain), fracture, degenerative disease, disc lesion, sacroiliac joint dysfunction, symphysis pubis dysfunction, cerebellar pain, piriformis syndrome, myofascial pain syndrome, and abdominal migraine.
- *Psychological factors:* Depression, chronic stress, or a history of sexual or physical abuse can increase the risk of CPP. Emotional distress makes pain worse, and living with chronic pain contributes to emotional distress. These two factors often become a vicious circle.
- *Musculoskeletal problems:* Conditions affecting the bones, joints, and connective tissues such as fibromyalgia, pelvic floor muscle strain, inflammation of the pubic joint (pubic symphysis), or hernia can cause recurrent pelvic pain.

EVALUATION

Women with CPP should undergo a detailed history and physical examination for further evaluation. This includes tools for the quantification and mapping of pelvic pain, screening questionnaires, and a comprehensive review of the reproductive, urinary, and gastrointestinal systems.

HISTORY

A detailed history of CPP can identify the underlying cause:

- *Site*: Onset and if the onset was associated with a preceding event such as childbirth or surgery? Pregnancy-related pain is often musculoskeletal (peripartum pelvic pain syndrome).
- *Character*: Visceral pain is usually dull and spreads along a location that can be difficult to pinpoint. The pain of nerve damage or nerve entrapment is usually like a burning, hot, or electric shock.
- *Radiation*: Pain from vagina, cervix, or uterus often radiates to the lower back or buttocks. Pain from the ovaries or Fallopian tubes may radiate to the medial thigh.
- Relationship of pain with urination, defecation, sexual intercourse, and menstruation. Pain that accompanies the symptomatic triad of sexual intercourse, menstruation defecation may be characteristic of endometriosis.
- *Time course*: As endometriosis pain usually begins several days before menstruation and continues for the first day or two of menstruation. Pain that is worse at the end of the day and is related to posture may be due to musculoskeletal or pelvic congestion syndrome.
- Exacerbating and relieving factors, e.g., medicines or alternative treatments that can relieve pain, or life events, sleep disturbances, depression, anxiety, or stress that may exacerbate pain.

The Pelvic Pain Assessment Form published by the International Pelvic Pain Society, contains many of these assessments and is freely available for clinical use.

Menstrual Cycle

Thorough assessment of women's menstrual cycle should be done. Whether menstruation is regular, heavy or light, or associated with pain. Adenomyosis or uterine leiomyomas can cause heavy painful periods, although adenomyosis is usually more painful.

Bowel-related History

Is there any history of constipation, diarrhea or bloating? Constipation is a common contributor to lower abdominal and pelvic pain.

Bladder-related History

Bladder pain syndrome is irritation of the bladder wall in the absence of infection. It is associated with polyuria, nocturia, urgency, and pain that get worse as the bladder fills and gets better with urination. It can also be associated with pain with intercourse. Recurrent urinary tract infections should be excluded.

Sexual History

Pain on initial penetration suggests vulvodynia or vaginal/pelvic muscle spasm, deep dyspareunia is associated with endometriosis, whereas postcoital pain is characteristic of pelvic congestion syndrome.

PHYSICAL EXAMINATION

The goal of a physical examination is to identify the dermatome, tissues, nerves, muscles, and organs that produce the patient's pain in an attempt to determine the underlying cause.

The **abdomen and pelvis** should be examined for any trigger points, surgical scars, vaginal discharge, pelvic organ prolapse, uterine enlargement, or masses (**Flowchart 2**).

Abdominal examination: The Carnett test can be used to differentiate visceral pain from abdominal wall pain. In the Carnett test, the patient raises both legs off the table while lying supine. The examiner places a finger on the painful abdomen site to determine if the pain increases during the maneuver when the rectus abdominis muscle is contracted. The assumption is that this potentially exacerbates myofascial pain such as a trigger point, trapped nerve, hernia, or myositis, whereas true visceral sources of pain may be less tender when the abdominal muscles are tense **(Fig. 1)**.

A cotton swab applied to the abdominal skin can be used to identify a cutaneous source of pain. A case-control study found that a cotton-tipped applicator test had 73% sensitivity and 100% specificity to diagnose cutaneous allodynia in patients with CPP.[3]

The **external genitalia** should be examined for any signs of infection, inflammatory dermatologic conditions, vulvar malignancy, and neurogenic etiologies.

Examination of the **pelvic floor** musculature may reveal hypertonicity, tenderness, or trigger points.

The **per speculum** examination should be done slowly to limit the intensity of the pain.

On **palpation**, tenderness over the lower back, sacroiliac joints, or pubic symphysis may indicate a musculoskeletal origin of the pain.

Neuromusculoskeletal pain: the presence of pelvic floor muscle tenderness or a positive result on the forced flexion, abduction, and external rotation (FABER) test correctly classified neuromusculoskeletal pain in 85% of patients in a small U.S. study. A study in Denmark showed a strong association between CPP of myofascial origin and the presence of tenderness and hypertonicity of the pelvic floor muscles.[4]

Flowchart 2: Physical examination of chronic pelvic pain patient.

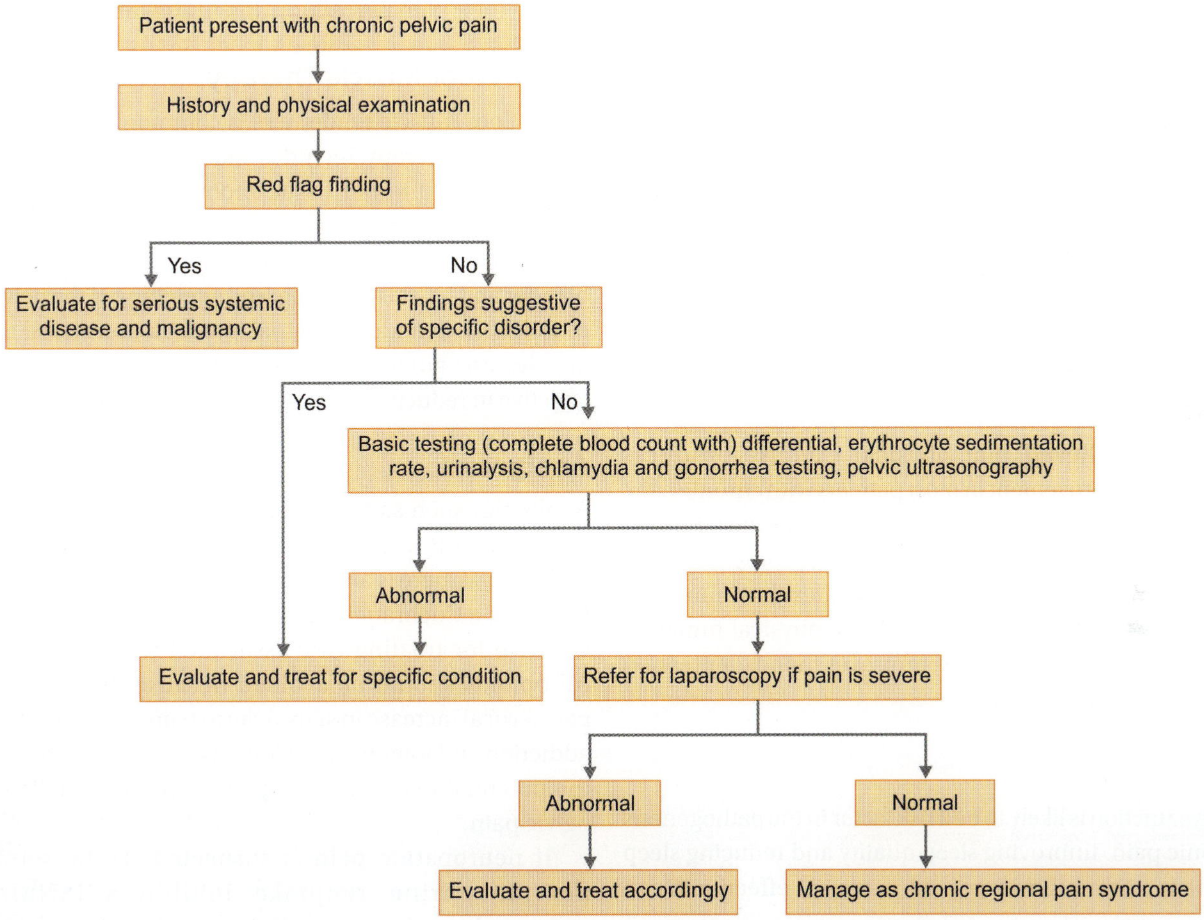

- Patient present with chronic pelvic pain
- History and physical examination
- Red flag finding
  - Yes → Evaluate for serious systemic disease and malignancy
  - No → Findings suggestive of specific disorder?
    - Yes → Evaluate and treat for specific condition
    - No → Basic testing (complete blood count with) differential, erythrocyte sedimentation rate, urinalysis, chlamydia and gonorrhea testing, pelvic ultrasonography
      - Abnormal → Evaluate and treat for specific condition
      - Normal → Refer for laparoscopy if pain is severe
        - Abnormal → Evaluate and treat accordingly
        - Normal → Manage as chronic regional pain syndrome

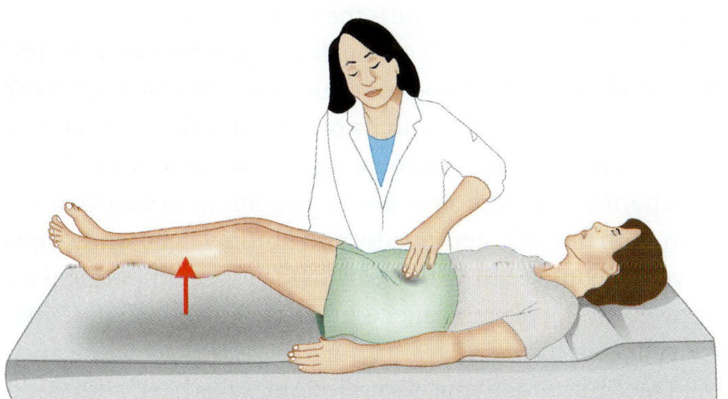

Fig. 1: Carnett test: An increase in the patient's pain during this maneuver is considered positive.

INVESTIGATIONS

Laboratory testing is of limited importance in the evaluation of women with pelvic pain.

- A complete blood count with C-reactive protein, total, and differential leukocyte count, erythrocyte sedimentation rate.
- Urinalysis for urinary tract infection.
- Swabs to remove sexually transmitted infections such as chlamydia and gonorrhea.
- Cervical smear.
- *CA 125*: This is increased in bloating, early satiety, pelvic pain, or urinary frequency or urgency.
- *Ultrasound*: Ultrasound can help to detect pelvic pathology if there is a uterine leiomyoma, ovarian tumor and endometriosis. Transvaginal sonography (TVS) is helpful in diagnosing pelvic mass and adenomyosis. It is particularly useful for detecting pelvic masses less than 4 cm in diameter, which often cannot be seen on bimanual examination. Ultrasonography is also useful for detecting hydrosalpinx indicative of pelvic inflammatory disease.
- *Magnetic resonance imaging (MRI)*: It may be considered to detect adenomyosis and other pelvic malformations but is limited in its ability to detect endometriotic deposits.
- *Diagnostic laparoscopy*: When the pain is severe, the patient should be referred for laparoscopy, if the diagnosis remains unclear. Laparoscopy may be useful to confirm and possibly treat endometriosis or pelvic/abdominal adhesions. Pain mapping can be useful while the patient is conscious and under local anesthesia during the procedure. The tissue should be examined and pulled up with surgical instruments, while the patient is asked about the severity and nature of pain. This approach may help target medical and surgical treatments.[5]

MANAGEMENT

The goal of treatment is to maximize the patient's quality of life and overall function, with an emphasis on engaging the patient in self-management. Evidence-based therapy for CPP remains limited and often focuses on symptom relief. Any obvious disease process must be treated, although even targeted treatment may not resolve the pain. Many mechanisms may be involved in the cause and outcome of pain, so a holistic approach is needed to address the physical, behavioral, psychological and sexual components of the treatment.

Lifestyle Modifications

Exercise

It is widely believed that physical exercise produces symptomatic improvement in most patients with chronic pain, yet many of these patients do not exercise because of their pain. A sedentary lifestyle also contributes to social isolation, low mood, low strength, and overall low levels of function. Exercise reduces pain, increases level of physical function, improves sleep, reduces fatigue, improves mood, depression and anxiety, reduce weight.[6]

Sleep

Sleep dysfunction is likely to be a risk factor in the pathogenesis of chronic pain. Improving sleep quality and reducing sleep disturbances through increased exercise, effective sleep hygiene.

Encourage Smoking Cessation

Smoking is also an independent risk factor for chronic pain. Smoking is associated with higher levels of physical impairment and increased pain in patients with fibromyalgia. It has its association with mood. Higher rates of depression were reported in smokers with chronic pain and those who have depression cope less well with pain.

Diet Modification

High consumption of fresh fruits and vegetables is known to reduce free-radical/oxidative stress on the body and improve immune function.[7] Reducing your intake of caffeine, citrus fruits, spicy foods, carbonated drinks, and alcohol can reduce bladder irritation. A diet rich in fruits, vegetables and fluids can reduce a woman's risk of constipation.

Cognitive Behavioral Therapy

When cognitive behavioral therapy is used in conjunction with therapy and physical therapy, it has the benefit of addressing the effects of depression and pain on relationships and other aspects of well-being. Studies of patients with other chronic pain syndromes show small-to-moderate benefits of cognitive behavioral therapy compared to no therapy. Patients learn to modify their thoughts and manipulate their environment to reduce their pain perception and improve coping skills.

Pelvic Floor Muscle Therapy

Pelvic floor muscle tenderness is commonly associated with CPP. Pelvic therapy includes manipulative treatments for external and internal tissue mobilization and myofascial release, mobilization of visceral, urogenital and joint structures; electrical stimulation; active pelvic floor retraining; biofeedback; bladder and bowel retraining; and stretching of the pelvic floor muscles.[8] In a randomized trial, pelvic floor physical therapy, and levator-guided trigger-point injections were equally effective in reducing vaginal pain and sex-related pain.

Analgesics

Analgesics such as acetaminophen and NSAIDs are widely used for CPP and may be beneficial for some women, especially if there is an inflammatory component to the pain. However, a Cochrane review concluded that NSAIDs are not effective for treating CPP associated with endometriosis. All opioids should be avoided because they can cause a paradoxical increase in sensitivity to pain, as well as the risk of addiction and tolerance. All opioids, including codeine, have the potential to cause constipation and potentially worsen pelvic pain.[9]

If neuropathic pain is suspected, TCAs, serotonin-norepinephrine reuptake inhibitors (SNRIs), or anticonvulsants (e.g., gabapentin, pregabalin) may be helpful. TCAs have a long history of use in chronic pain and may provide relief. Amitriptyline is the most frequently prescribed TCA for patients with CPP, although nortriptyline may be better tolerated. TCAs should be continued for at least 6–8 weeks as they may take some time to be of benefit. Cochrane reviews of individual antidepressants suggest that duloxetine (SNRI) is superior to placebo for the management of neuropathic pain from diabetic neuropathy and fibromyalgia, while trials of venlafaxine (SSRI with weak SNRI) for neuropathic pain showed strong placebo effects and has shown high potential for selection bias.

Once the underlying visceral etiology has been addressed and a neuropathic component of the pain syndrome has been diagnosed, there is a role for neuropathic drugs in the medical management of CPP. Gabapentin may provide analgesia more rapidly than a TCA but can cause adverse effects, such as fatigue, dizziness, nausea, and weight gain. Gabapentin is usually started at a low dose.

Clonidine is sometimes used as an adjunctive analgesic. It is usually prescribed as a transdermal patch. Clonidine can cause dry mouth, constipation, and hypotension.

Trigger point injections of saline, anesthetics, steroids, or opioids are recommended in isolation or in combination with other treatment methods to improve pain and functional ability in patients with myofascial CPP.

Botulinum toxin A injection may reduce muscle spasms in the affected pelvic floor muscles. It provides relief for about 3–6 months, sometimes longer.

If an altered sensation is displayed, daily application of topical capsaicin to the skin of the abdomen (but not the vulva) may help numb the area to the skin.

Non-pharmacological treatments such as acupuncture, transcutaneous electrical nerve stimulation (TENS), chiropractic and osteopathic manipulations may be beneficial.[10]

Hormonal Treatments

Pain produced by multiple organs may show cyclic variation and respond to hormonal treatment.

Contraceptives are effective for the treatment of dysmenorrhea associated with endometriosis, with only limited evidence that they are useful for nonmenstrual pain. A Cochrane review concluded that there is moderate evidence to support progestogen treatment for CPP (e.g., depot-medroxyprogesterone, 150 mg intramuscularly every 12 weeks).[11] If the patient has endometriosis, injectable gonadotropin-releasing hormone agonists such as goserelin depot provide longer-lasting effects than medroxyprogesterone. For many women, continued use of the combined oral contraceptive pill can be successful with minimal side effects, while others are more comfortable with progesterone preparations alone. If uterine pathology such as adenomyosis is suspected or if menorrhagia is also a problem, the levonorgestrel intrauterine system (Mirena) releasing system can be extremely effective.

An alternative approach is to use GnRH to inhibit ovarian function both clinically and reversibly. These drugs (given as monthly subcutaneous injections) cause prolonged activation of the GnRH receptor, leading to an initial worsening of symptoms ("onset flare"), followed by a decrease in gonadotrophs, as of 21 days, serum estradiol is equal to that for a postmenopausal woman and remains the same with continued dosing. The most common side effects are hot flushes and emotional symptoms, but these are usually well-tolerated when pain is relieved. Of greater concern is the loss of bone mineral density (BMD), which can be up to 6% after 6 months of treatment. If the trial is successful, treatment may be continued in addition to add-back low-dose combined (estrogen and progesterone) hormone replacement therapy (HRT). The dose of HRT should be sufficient to treat vasomotor symptoms (thus maintaining BMD) without provoking pain or bleeding. This combination has been shown to be safe and effective for up to 2 years.[12]

Physiotherapy

Dysfunction in the musculoskeletal system can be both a primary cause of CPP or secondary to pathology elsewhere.

Psychological

Psychosocial and psychological issues are often important enduring factors in CPP. Having the opportunity to explore these issues in a nonhazardous environment can improve the experience of pain and help the woman develop her own pain management plan. If negative psychological symptoms are present then more specific psychological treatments such as cognitive behavioral therapy may be used.

Surgical Interventions

Surgical intervention should be guided by the underlying diagnosis, although some options may be diagnostic. Pain is likely to improve after laparoscopic surgery to treat endometriosis. Hysterectomy is a last resort due to high morbidity and limited benefit. About half of women with uterine tenderness on pelvic examination will have improved mental health, physical health, and social functioning after hysterectomy. However, up to 40% will have persistent pain, and at least 5% will have more pain.[13]

Routine use of laparoscopic adrenolysis is not recommended for the management of CPP. Laparoscopic adrenolysis is not helpful for the treatment of CPP after visceral gynecological causes such as endometriosis, adenomyosis, and adnexal disorders have been excluded. However, the interaction findings may support the role of adhesiolysis in specific conditions such as bowel strictures and dense adhesions tethering the uterus.

Local injection of steroids may be therapeutic as well as diagnostic when peripheral nerves are involved. If the sacral nerve is involved, pain relief may be possible through a surgically implanted device with sacral nerve block or neuromodulation that stimulates the nerve with electrical pulses.

Chronic pelvic pain is common, affecting perhaps one in six adult female populations. Much is unclear about its etiology, but CPP should be viewed as a symptom and not as a diagnosis by itself, along with several contributing factors 13. As with all chronic pain, it is important to consider psychological and social factors. Several nongynecological conditions such as nerve entrapment or IBS may be relevant. Women often present because they want an explanation for their pain. The evaluation process should give the woman enough time to be able to tell her story. This in itself can be therapeutic. A pain diary can be helpful in keeping track of symptoms or activities associated with pain. Where pain is very cyclic and vaginal examination shows no abnormalities, a clinical examination of ovarian suppression may be more helpful than diagnostic laparoscopy. Other conditions, such as IBS, require specific treatment. Even if no explanation can be found for the pain initially, an attempt should be made to treat the pain empirically and develop a management plan in partnership with the woman.

There is frequently more than one component to CPP. Assessment should aim to identify contributory factors rather than assign causality to a single pathology.

At the initial assessment, it may not be possible to identify the cause of the pain.

Women with IBS or interstitial cystitis are often present with CPP. These conditions may be a primary cause of CPP, a component of CPP or a secondary effect caused by efferent neurological dysfunction in the presence of chronic pain.

If the history suggests that there is a specific non-gynecological component to the pain, referral to the relevant healthcare profession should be considered.

TVS is done most commonly to identify and assess adnexal masses, adenomyosis, fibroids .

The role of MRI in diagnosing small deposits of endometriosis is uncertain.

Women with cyclical pain should be offered hormonal treatment for a period of 3–6 months.

Women with IBS should be given antispasmodics.

Women with IBS should be encouraged to amend their diet to attempt to control symptoms. Women should be offered appropriate analgesia to control their pain. If pain is not adequately controlled, consideration should be given to referral to a pain management team or a specialist pelvic pain clinic.

KEY MESSAGES

- There is frequently more than one component to CPP. Assessment should aim to identify contributory factors rather than assign causality to a single pathology.
- At the initial assessment, it may not be possible to identify the cause of the pain.
- Women with IBS or interstitial cystitis are often present with CPP. These conditions may be a primary cause of CPP, a component of CPP or a secondary effect caused by efferent neurological dysfunction in the presence of chronic pain.
- If the history suggests that there is a specific non-gynecological component to the pain, referral to the relevant healthcare profession should be considered.
- TVS is done most commonly to identify and assess adnexal masses, adenomyosis, fibroids.
- The role of MRI in diagnosing small deposits of endometriosis is uncertain.
- Women with cyclical pain should be offered hormonal treatment for a period of 3–6 months.
- Women with IBS should be given antispasmodics.
- Women with IBS should be encouraged to amend their diet to attempt to control symptoms. Women should be offered appropriate analgesia to control their pain. If pain is not adequately controlled, consideration should be given to referral to a pain management team or a specialist pelvic pain clinic.

FURTHER READING

1. ACOG. ACOG practice bulletin number 218 on, "Chronic pelvic pain". Chicago: ACOG; 2020.
2. RCOG. Green top guideline no. 41 on, "The initial management of Chronic pelvic pain". London: RCOG; 2012.

REFERENCES

1. Ahangari A. Prevalence of chronic pelvic pain among women: an updated review. Pain Physician. 2014;17(2):E141-7.
2. Aredo JV, Heyrana KJ, Karp BI, Shah JP, Stratton P. Relating chronic pelvic pain and endometriosis to signs of sensitization and myofascial pain and dysfunction. Semin Reprod Med. 2017;35(1):88.
3. Nasr-Esfahani M, Jarrell J. Cotton-tipped applicator test: validity and reliability in chronic pelvic pain. Am J Obstet Gynecol. 2013;208(1):52-e1.
4. Loving S, Thomsen T, Jaszczak P, Nordling J. Pelvic floor muscle dysfunctions are prevalent in female chronic pelvic pain: a cross-sectional population-based study. Eur J Pain. 2014;18(9):1259-70.
5. Swanton A, Iyer L, Reginald PW. Diagnosis, treatment and follow up of women undergoing conscious pain mapping for chronic pelvic pain: a prospective cohort study. BJOG. 2006;113(7):792-6.
6. Ambrose KR, Golightly YM. Physical exercise as non-pharmacological treatment of chronic pain: why and when. Best Prac Res Clin Rheumatol. 2015;29(1):120-30.
7. Friedlander JI, Shorter B, Moldwin RM. Diet and its role in interstitial cystitis/bladder pain syndrome (IC/BPS) and comorbid conditions. BJU Int. 2012;109(11):1584-91.
8. Sharma N, Rekha K, Srinivasan JK. Efficacy of transcutaneous electrical nerve stimulation in the treatment of chronic pelvic pain. J Mid-life Health. 2017;8(1):36.
9. Engeler D, Baranowski AP, Borovicka J, Cottrell A, Dinis-Oliveira P, Elneil S. EAU guidelines on chronic pelvic pain. Netherlands: European Association of Urology; 2012.
10. Stones W, Cheong YC, Howard FM, Singh S. Interventions for treating chronic pelvic pain in women. Cochrane Database Syst Rev. 2000;(4):CD000387.
11. Cheong YC, Smotra G, de C Williams AC. Non-surgical interventions for the management of chronic pelvic pain. Cochrane Database Syst Rev. 2014;(3):CD008797.
12. Farmer JE, Prentice A, Breeze A, Ahmad G, Duffy JM, Watson A, et al. Gonadotrophin-releasing hormone analogues for endometriosis: bone mineral density. Cochrane Database Syst Rev. 2003;(4):CD001297.
13. Lamvu G. Role of hysterectomy in the treatment of chronic pelvic pain. Obstet Gynecol. 2011;117(5):1175-8.

LONG QUESTIONS

1. What are the causes of chronic pelvic pain?
2. Write a note on pelvic pain assessment form.
3. How will you investigate and manage a woman presenting with chronic pelvic pain?

SHORT QUESTIONS

1. Define chronic pelvic pain.
2. Name the gynecological causes of chronic pelvic pain.
3. Explain Carnett test.
4. What is the role of analgesics in chronic pelvic pain?

MULTIPLE CHOICE QUESTIONS

1. What is the main characteristic element of the pelvic pain syndrome?
   a. Pain, pressure, or discomfort localized in the pelvis.
   b. Pain, pressure, or discomfort related to bladder filling, relieved with urination.
   c. Pain, pressure, or discomfort related to the bladder.
   d. None of the above.
2. Which of the following conditions occur/s in the pelvic pain syndrome more frequently than in the general population?
   a. Allergies and autoimmune diseases
   b. Crohn's disease
   c. Fibromyalgia
   d. All the above.
3. In the lower urinary tract, the pain is characterized as "chronic", when lasting at least:
   a. 1 month b. 2 months
   c. 3 months d. 6 months
4. Causes of pelvic pain in a young female:
   a. Adenomyosis b. CIN
   c. PID d. Tuberculosis
5. Best investigation to establish the diagnosis of endometriosis is:
   a. Laparoscopy b. USG
   c. X-ray pelvis d. CT Scan
6. Pelvic pain congestion syndrome occurs in age group:
   a. Above 50 years b. 40–50 years
   c. 20–30 years d. 30–40 years
7. What is the FDA approved oral drug for interstitial cystitis?
   a. NSAIDs
   b. PPS (Penton Polysulfate Sodium)
   c. Gabapentin
   d. Amitriptyline
8. Carnett test is used for:
   a. Entrapped nerve
   b. Hernia
   c. Myositis
   d. All of the above.
9. Trigger point injections used in CPP consist of any of these, except:
   a. Anesthetic b. Antibiotic
   c. Saline d. Opiod
10. FABER test includes all except:
    a. Flexion
    b. Adduction
    c. External rotation
    d. Abduction

Answers

1.	c	2.	d	3.	a	4.	d	5.	a	6.	c
7.	b	8.	d	9.	b	10.	b				

9.4 HEAVY MENSTRUAL BLEEDING: APPROACH TO EVALUATION AND TREATMENT

Amala Khopkar Nazareth, Gillian Ryan, Alka Kriplani, CN Purandare

INTRODUCTION

The incidence of abnormal uterine bleeding (AUB) is 9–14% in women between menarche and menopause. This number varies in each country. In India, the reported incidence of AUB is around 17.9%. Additionally, AUB can be classified as acute or chronic. Excessive bleeding, referred to as acute AUB, requires immediate medical attention to prevent additional loss of blood. Acute AUB can occur independently or in combination with chronic AUB, which is identified as menstrual irregularity for the majority of the earlier 6 months. Approximately, 1–2% of women who have uncontrolled anovulatory bleeding may develop endometrial cancer.

The primary goal of treatment is to decrease high menstrual bleeding (HMB) while also identifying and treating the underlying cause, and the treatment strategy varies according to the patient's age and desire for immediate or long-term fertility.

PATHOPHYSIOLOGY

The uterine and ovarian arteries are the source of blood supply to the uterus. As these arteries travel through the myometrium, they branch out into arcuate arteries, which branch out into radial branches that supply blood to the functionalis and basalis layers of the endometrium. When progesterone levels fall at the end of the menstrual cycle, enzymes degrade the functionalis layer. Menstrual flow is made up of the sloughing off of the degraded functionalis layer and blood loss that occurs as a result of this breakdown. Blood loss is regulated by operating platelets and thrombin, as well as vasoconstriction of the endometrial arteries. Any uterine pathological anomaly (such as leiomyoma, polyps, adenomyosis, malignancy, or hyperplasia), clotting pathway abnormality (due to coagulopathies or iatrogenic factors), or disruption of the hypothalamic-pituitary-ovarian axis (due to ovulatory/endocrine disorders or iatrogenic factors) can alter menstruation and result in AUB.

FIGO MENSTRUAL DISORDERS COMMITTEE CLASSIFICATION SYSTEMS

To aid in the diagnosis and treatment of HMB, International Federation of Obstetrics and Gynecology (FIGO) MDC (Menstrual Disorders Committee), has proposed two classification systems that were established with the help of educators, researchers, physicians, journal editors, and investigators from around the world.

FIGO AUB System 1

Establishing parameters that characterize AUB by identifying the parameters of normal menstrual hemorrhage. Menorrhagia, oligomenorrhea, metrorrhagia, and dysfunctional uterine bleeding are all no longer used.

FIGO AUB System 2

This is also known as the PALM- COEIN system, this system categorizes the numerous possible causes or factors to the symptoms of AUB in reproductive years, providing a systematic infrastructure for research, teaching, and clinical care.

PALM-COEIN is an acronym developed by the FIGO for the purpose of classifying the underlying causes of AUB.

PALM, the first section, discusses structural/ anatomical pathologies.

COEI describes nonstructural challenges in the second section.

N is denoted by "Not otherwise classified"

- P: Polyp
- A: Adenomyosis
- L: Leiomyoma
- M: Malignancy and hyperplasia
- C: Coagulopathy
- O: Ovulatory failure
- E: Endometrial
- I: Iatrogenic
- N: Not categorized in any other category

It is broadly acknowledged that one or more of the above factors listed may contribute to an individual's irregular uterine bleeding. Likewise, certain pathological entities, such as endocervical polyps, endometrial polyps, or leiomyomas, may be clinically silent and are not the primary cause of AUB in a patient.

In the revised 2018 FIGO classification system, AUB caused by anticoagulants was recategorized as iatrogenic. Unclassified AUB can be caused by a variety of uncommon conditions, including arteriovenous malformations (AVMs), myometrial hyperplasia, and endometritis.

HISTORY TAKING AND CLINICAL EXAMINATION

History taking is the corner-stone for diagnosis in any disease. A detailed history not only guides the clinician with determining the differential diagnosis of the disease pathology but also prepares the clinician to formulate the best management protocol for that particular patient.

The following are some significant aspects of the history:

- Menstrual cycle information
- Menarche age
- Last menstrual period
- Menstrual frequency, regularity, duration, and flow volume.

  Frequency is divided into three categories: (1) frequent (< 24 days), (2) typical (24–38 days), and (3) infrequent (> 38 days).

  Regularity can be absent, regular (with a variance of ± 2 to 20 days), or irregular (with a variance of ± 2 to 20 days) (variation > 20 days).

  The duration can be classified as long (above 8 days), normal (between 4 and 8 days), or short (< 8 days) (< 4 days).

  The volume of flow might be heavy (> 80 mL), normal (5–80 mL), or light (< 5 mL of blood loss).

  Exact volume measurements are difficult to determine outside research settings and are subjective to each woman affected; therefore, detailed questions regarding frequency of sanitary product changes during each day, passage, and size of any clots, need to change sanitary products during the night, and a "flooding" sensation are important to ascertain the severity of the blood loss.
- Intermenstrual and postcoital bleeding
- History of sexual and reproductive activity
- Obstetrical history, including number of births, including still births and miscarriages and respective modes of delivery
- Desire for further fertility and history of subfertility
- Use of contraceptive methods—hormonal or nonhormonal
- Sexually transmitted infection (STIs) history
- History of PAP smears
- Associated symptoms such as
  - Weight loss
  - Discomfort and pain
  - History of bladder and bowel symptoms
- Signs and symptoms of severe blood loss - pallor, weakness - suggestive of iron deficiency anemia secondary to blood loss
- Signs and symptoms or history of underlying chronic or congenital bleeding disorders such as inherited thrombophilias, immune thrombocytopenic purpura (ITP) or other platelet functional disorders
- Infection history and symptoms, such as Dengue (causing thrombocytopenia)
- History and signs of chronic renal disease
- Signs/symptoms or history of endocrine disorders
  - Current medications
  - Family history, including questions concerning coagulopathies, malignancy, endocrine disorders

- Social history, including tobacco, alcohol, and drug uses; occupation; impact of symptoms on quality of life
- Surgical history

- *The physical exam should include*:
  - Vital signs, including blood pressure and body mass index (BMI)
  - Signs of pallor, such as skin or mucosal pallor
  - Signs of endocrine disorders
- Examination of the thyroid for enlargement or tenderness
- Excessive or abnormal hair growth patterns, clitoromegaly, acne that could indicate hyperandrogenism
- Moon facies, abnormal fat distribution, striae that could indicate Cushing's
  - Signs of coagulopathies, such as bruising or petechiae
  - Abdominal exam to palpate for any pelvic or abdominal masses
  - Pelvic exam: Speculum and bimanual
- PAP smear if indicated
- STI screening (such as for gonorrhea and chlamydia-NAAT Swab) and wet prep if indicated
- Endometrial biopsy, if indicated.

INVESTIGATIONS

A urine pregnancy test and a complete blood count should be performed in the laboratory. Additionally, ferritin, a coagulation panel, thyroid function tests, gonadotropins, and prolactin can be tested. Insulin resistance testing may also be considered for women with polycystic ovaries and AUB. Since majority of treatment protocols are hormones medications that could be potential liver enzyme inducers, it is vital to check that pharmaceutical agents administered are metabolized and the by-products are cleared by the body. Hence, liver function tests + GGT and kidney function tests, especially creatinine values are of utmost importance.

In sexually active patients, transvaginal ultrasound should be performed first, followed by MRI and hysteroscopy as necessary. Hysteroscopy can be easily performed in outpatient settings. There is no radiation exposure for the patient while using transvaginal ultrasonography to inspect the uterus and assess uterine size, shape, fibroids (leiomyomas), and endometrial thickness. AUB should be considered, if there is no other explanation for the patient's abnormal menstrual bleeding. Although MRI gives comprehensive pictures that help surgeons in the planning of therapeutic modalities, it is costly and should not be the initial imaging option for patients with AUB. In the event of endometrial polyps or submucosal myomas, that are unclear on transvaginal ultrasound pictures, hysteroscopy and sonohysterography (SHG) are useful. The more invasive hysteroscopy and SHG are regularly done in the office environment.

For individuals with an increased risk of hyperplasia or cancer, endometrial tissue sample is indicated. In postmenopausal women of 45 years of age or older who have AUB, an endometrial biopsy is considered the first-line diagnostic procedure. Women under the age of 45 years with unopposed estrogen exposure, such as obesity or polycystic ovarian syndrome (PCOS), should also have their endometrial tissue sampled. Endometrial sampling is indicated in women less than 45 years of age when transvaginal ultrasound measurement of leuteal phase endometrial thickness is more than 12 mm.[2]

EVALUATION OF INDIVIDUAL FACTORS THAT CAUSE AUB

Polyps

Polyps are abnormal proliferations of columnar epithelium that protrude into the endometrial cavity from the endometrial stroma and glands. While most of them are asymptomatic their incidences vary significantly ranging from 3.7 to 65%. They tend to coexist with fibroid uterus in women in an older age group and may be mistaken for a submucous myoma instead of a polyp in large number of cases and vice versa.

There is low prevalence of malignancy or premalignant conditions associated with polyps, however women in an older age group, particularly those that are postmenopausal, who have AUB have greater prevalence of malignancy. In such cases, these polyps need to be resected hysteroscopically and sent for histological assessment.

The clinical presentations of polyps of the endometrium are:

- *AUB*: It is the most prevalent symptom, affecting approximately 68% of females.
- *Infertility*: The association of endometrial polyps with primary infertility is in the incidence of 3.8–38.5% and with secondary infertility the incidence rates are 1.8–17%. They are one of the causative factors for recurrent implantation failures. Moreso, hysteroscopic resection of endometrial polyps seem to significantly improve fertility rates among patients with endometrial factor associated infertility irrespective of the size and number of polyps excised.
- *Malignancy*: Approximately, 1% of endometrial polyps may undergo hyperplastic transformation and develop malignancy. The most common types being endometroid adenocarcinoma and serous adenocarcinoma. There is a rise in the likelihood of malignancy in endometrial polyps with increasing age.

Diagnosis

Transvaginal ultrasound: It is a significant tool for assessment and to diagnose endometrial polyps. They appear as hyperechoic foci with regular margins and contours. Sometimes cystic glands may be well appreciated within the polyp, if large in size. These findings however may not be limited to endometrial polyps alone. submucous fibroids may also show similar sonographic appearance. To limit the possibility of false positives and negatives, it is ideal to scan the endometrium on the 10th day of the menstrual cycle, when it is at its thinnest. While transvaginal ultrasound appears to be the primary diagnostic tool for endometrial polyps, hysteroscopic evaluation of the polyp is far superior as compared to transvaginal ultrasound in diagnosing endometrial polyps.

Color Flow or Power Doppler

The addition of color flow or power Doppler to transvaginal ultrasound can improve its diagnostic capability in cases of uterine polyp. Color-flowing Doppler imaging may reveal the feeding vessel characteristic of endometrial polyps. The addition of intrauterine contrast via SHG may highlight small endometrial polyps that are missed on grey scale TVUS, thereby increasing diagnostic accuracy. Vaginal ultrasound Doppler examination with intravenous contrast may aid in the differentiation of benign endometrial polyps from cancer, but larger studies are necessary to confirm these findings.

Saline Infusion Sonography or Sonohysterography

It is a gold standard in diagnosing endometrial polyps. In this study endometrial polyps appear as smooth echogenic masses and their exact location sizes can be accurately made out using saline infusion sonography. Saline infusion SHG has been shown to be more accurate than TVS in identifying and excluding endometrial polyps, even in situations when diagnostic confidence in the presence of polyps is high. Saline infusion may still be necessary to confirm a TVS diagnosis of polyps and to minimize the frequency of negative hysteroscopies **(Fig. 1)**.

Histological Diagnosis

Endometrial polyps, the majority of which are immature endometrium, do not respond to hormone stimulation. They resemble cystic hyperplasia and appear to be unaffected by menstrual cycle hormonal stimulation, as they are not shed during the menstrual period. Endometrial polyps, which are less common, are composed of functional endometrium that undergoes cyclic histological changes.

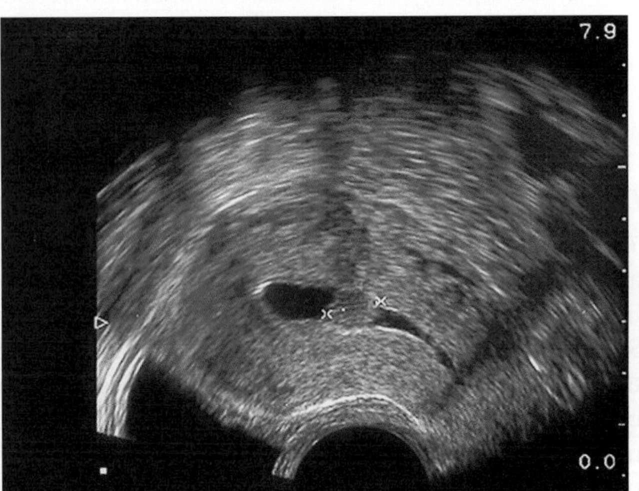

Fig. 1: Endometrial polyp on sonosalpingography.

Treatment

Small asymptomatic polyps may resolve spontaneously and may require follow-up every 6 months.

Prior to initiating management protocols for symptomatic polyps, the following assessments should be made: symptoms, risk of malignancy, and fertility concerns. Within a year of diagnosis, approximately 29% of asymptomatic polyps regress spontaneously.

Management protocols should unquestionably prioritize measures that alleviate symptoms. With the exception of women seeking treatment for infertility, the majority of endometrial polyps does not regress spontaneously and require surgical removal. Progesterone therapy following polypectomy appears to be beneficial in terms of preventing recurrence and reducing anemia caused by chronic blood loss, as well as preventing further progression to endometrial hyperplasia.

Conservative Surgery

Hysteroscopy: It remains the gold standard not only for diagnosing but also treatment symptomatic endometrial polyps. And the removal of basalis layer of the endometrial polyp prevents recurrences of the polyp. Hysteroscopy has an added edge over other imaging technologies in cases of endometrial polyps as it allows for direct sampling and removal of the polyps. It not only leads to definitive treatment of the disease, but also satisfactory results can be obtained despite the menopausal status of the patient and the size and number of the polyps.

Whether to use a resectoscope or morcellator depends on the operator. It is suggested that larger polyps more than 2 cm in diameter, especially those closer to the fundus are best removed buy a resectoscope or morcellator. Smaller polyps less than 2 cm in diameter or pedunculated polyps can be removed easily by an operating hysteroscope under direct vision using scissors **(Fig. 2)**.

Hysteroscopic polypectomy is technically feasible and has a low rate of complications and recurrence. Additionally, it is very cost effective. The complications of the procedure can result in bleeding, pelvic inflammation, infection, uterine rupture (although this is uncommon), cervix damage, and complications from the distention media.

Dilation and curettage: Dilation and curettage used to earlier be a standard method for diagnosis and therapeutic management of intra uterine polyps before hysteroscopy. However, there is a high probability for the polyps to be missed as this procedure is a blind procedure. 50–85% of polyps can be easily missed if dilation and curettage is used as a treatment modality to treat endometrial polyps.

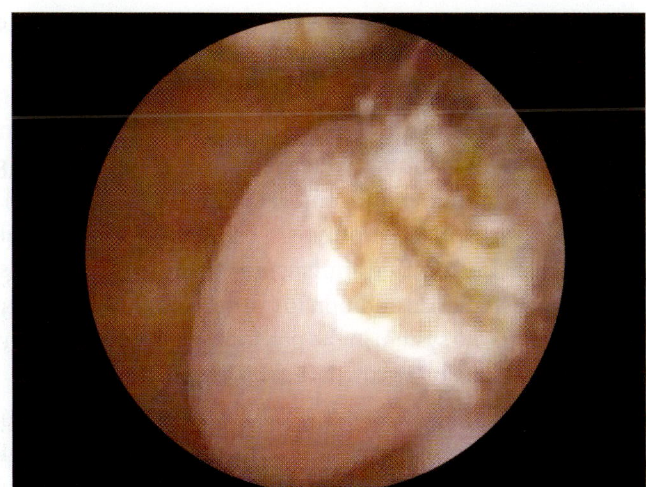

Fig. 2: Endometrial polyp (partly resected) on hysteroscopy.

Conservative Nonsurgical Management

Asymptomatic polyps less than 1 cm in size have a spontaneous regression rate within 1 year and less chance of malignancy. Such patients are ideal for conservative observational management. In postmenopausal women combined hormone replacement therapy (HRT) can be used to prevent endometrial polyps.

For symptomatic women with endometrial polyps following are the conservative nonsurgical management types.

LNG-IUS system: The levonorgestrel intrauterine system (LNG-IUS), has been successfully used for postmenopausal women on HRT and for women taking tamoxifen treatment to prevent endometrial hyperplasia and polyps.

It operates according to the following mechanism of action:

- Apoptosis and decreased cell proliferation in endometrial epithelial and stromal cells.
- Progesterone's anti-inflammatory properties, as mast cell-associated inflammation may contribute to endometrial polyp growth.
- Endometrial quiescence, maintained by stable estrogen and progesterone levels.

HRT: The efficacy of HRT may be due to reduction in endometrial thickness, resulting from estrogen suppression and thus a subsequent reduction of polyp formation. However, it has been demonstrated that HRT has no effect in reduction of polyp size due to lack of progesterone receptors in the polyp.

Desogestrel, dienogest and danazol: In a comparative study between desogestrel and danazol as preoperative therapy prior to hysteroscopic resection of submucous myomas and polyps, it was observed that desogestrel caused less side effects and favorable endometrial atrophy giving a better operative field for resection of the myoma. Dienogest, being fourth generation synthetic progesterone, seems to be more effective as a medication prior to surgical resection of submucous myomas and has been shown to have the least side effects among all progesterone preparations. Additionally, dienogest has been shown to be effective in reducing endometrial thickness, the severity of bleeding, and operative time, with fewer side effects than other pharmacological preparations or no treatment.

Gonadotropin-releasing hormone analogs: There are fewer complications when using gonadotropin-releasing hormone (GnRH) analogs before hysteroscopic myomectomy because of their reduced expense, low incidence of side effects, and lack of conclusive evidence supporting this practice. Kamath et al., carried out a systematic review of the literature to determine whether GnRH analogs were more efficacious in women with submucous fibroids than placebo/no treatment for symptom alleviation, complications, and surgery. Patients reported relief of symptoms, complete resection of fibroids, reduced operative time, and decreased complications were the outcomes. These findings support the use of GnRH agonists before hysteroscopic resection of submucous fibroids, but there is insufficient evidence to make this routine prior to the procedure. A more robust peer review is needed to make this recommendation.

Adenomyosis

Adenomyosis, also called as endometriosis interna, is a pathological condition where pockets of functional endometrium responding to hormonal stimuli, exist within the myometrium of the uterus. The modern definition of adenomyosis is "the benign invasion of endometrium into the myometrium, producing a diffusely enlarged uterus, which microscopically exhibits ectopic nonneoplastic, endometrial glands, and stroma surrounded by the hypertrophic and hyperplastic myometrium". These lesions/patches within the myometrium have no connection with the normally functioning endometrium. As these patches respond to hormonal stimulation of menstrual cycle they tend to bleed within the substance of the myometrium, leading to significant discomfort to the patient both in terms of pelvic pain and AUB. Among patients suffering from endometriosis the incidence of adenomyosis varies from 27 to 70% of cases. Despite the high prevalence of this disorder the exact pathophysiology as to why adenomyosis occurs and what are its contributing factors that trigger this pathology are not very well understood. A possible connection has been made with high estrogenic states of the body and adenomyosis.

Coexistence with Other Disorders

Adenomyosis often coexists with other gynecological disorders such as endometriosis, and fibroid uterus. Uterine leiomyomas and adenomyosis coexist in 15–57% of cases, and women who have both conditions are more likely to experience pelvic pain, infertility and AUB.

Risk Factors

Age: Around 70–80% of women, who undergo hysterectomy for adenomyosis are multiparous and in their fourth or fifth decade of life. With increasing use of MRI, several studies are now reporting adenomyosis to be a causative factor for chronic pelvic pain and severe dysmenorrhea in women in younger age group such as adolescents and women in reproductive age group. These findings suggest that the clinical age of onset of adenomyosis may be much younger than previously believed, and that early-stage adenomyosis may exhibit a clinical phenotype distinct from late-stage disease.

Multiparity: A significantly higher percentage of women suffering from adenomyosis ironically are multiparous thereby questioning the hypothesis that adenomyosis originates due to hyper estrogenic states. Pregnancy may facilitate the formation of adenomyosis by allowing for the incorporation of adenomyotic foci into the myometrium as a result of the trophoblast's invasive nature on the extension of the myometrial fibers. Additionally, it has been hypothesized that adenomyotic tissue may contain a high concentration of estrogen receptors and that the hormonal milieu associated with pregnancy may facilitate the development of these ectopic endometrial foci within the myometrium.

Previous surgeries on the uterus: There is conflicting evidence that women with adenomyosis have a significantly increased risk of prior uterine surgery. Adenomyosis occurs when endometrial glands invade the myometrial layer, with some studies indicating that surgical disruption of the endometrial-myometrial junction increases the risk of adenomyosis. There is conflicting evidence that women with adenomyosis have a significantly increased risk of prior uterine surgery. Adenomyosis occurs when endometrial glands invade the myometrial layer, with some studies indicating that surgical disruption of the endometrial-myometrial junction increases the risk of adenomyosis. It has been reported in several studies that cases of adenomyosis have increased in women undergoing surgical procedures on the uterus from dilation and curettage to both laparotomy and laparoscopic myomectomies to previous cesarean deliveries.

Depression and Use of Antidepressants

Newer studies have found an association between adenomyosis and depression and use of antidepressants, especially SSRIs, in both human as well as animal studies. Increased prolactin exposure appears to be sufficient to induce histological adenomyosis in the murine uterus and is associated with an increase in the messenger RNA for the uterine prolactin receptor. In vitro studies have demonstrated that prolactin production is found in the cells of human uterus including the endometrium and the myometrium and leiomyoma's of the uterus hypothesizing the fact that ectopic prolactin receptors present in the uterus could contribute to development of adenomyosis by acting as smooth muscle mitogen. This also proposes a theory that SSRIs taken for depression might mitigate the pre-existing adenomyosis through the dopaminergic mechanism of action of these drugs. Additionally, depression and adenomyosis may share a common pathogenic factor (i.e., inflammation). Endometriosis and adenomyosis continue to grow and progress in ovariectomized animals, according to studies. This finding suggests that, in addition to ovarian steroid hormones, the innate immune system in the pelvic environment may play a role in endometriosis growth regulation.

Treatment with tamoxifen: Tamoxifen is a selected estrogen receptor modulator that has been used as a prolonged adjuvant medication in the suppression of estrogen receptor positive breast malignancies, and it exerts its effect through its active metabolite called hydroxy tamoxifen. However, on the tissues of the uterus it acts as an estrogen agonist and can lead to reactivate pre-existing adenomyotic foci. Thus, adenomyosis maybe more common in postmenopausal women taking tamoxifen.

Diagnosis

Adenomyosis, like endometriosis, can present in a variety of ways, ranging from simple junctional zone (JZ) thickening to focal, cystic, or diffuse lesions. However, JZ thickening or hyperplasia, as well as focal lesions of the JZ, must be interpreted cautiously, as changes in the JZ can be a result of cyclic hormonal variations or aging-related JZ thickening.

Ultrasound: The accuracy of the ultrasound in the diagnosis of adenomyosis is high with a mean sensitivity of 0.72 and a specificity of 0.81, although this accuracy is operator dependent. It is advisable to scan the patient during the menstrual phase of the period to come to a correct diagnosis. Running a color Doppler during the ultrasound on adenomyotic lesions further add to the diagnosis of adenomyosis as both afferent and efferent blood vessels within lesions show a diffused pattern as opposed to a whorl like pattern in case of leiomyoma and this alone can be a key distinguishing factor between the two.

The following criteria are used to diagnose adenomyosis using transvaginal ultrasound:

- A globular or disproportionately large uterus
- Inadequate delineation of the separating line between the endometrium and the uterine muscle (myometrium)
- Thickening of the uterus's muscular layer (myometrium), particularly
  - If it is wider on one side than the other (asymmetry)
  - The junctional zone can be quantified and is more than 10 or 12 mm in thickness
- Cysts in the uterine muscle (myometrium)
- The uterine muscle component of the uterus has a distinct texture (myometrium)
- The junctional zone's blood flow is increased **(Fig. 3)**.

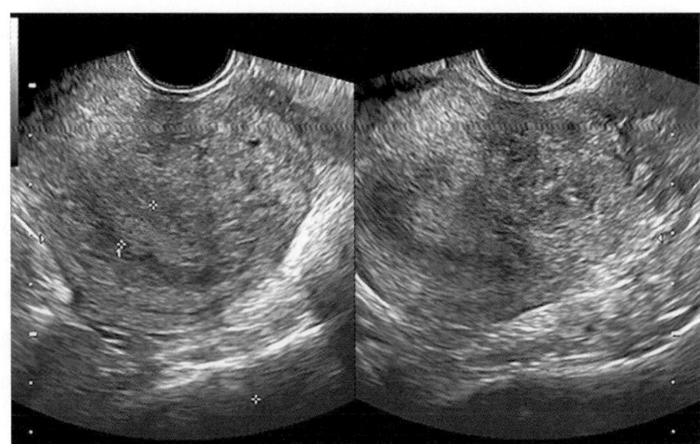

Fig. 3: Adenomyosis on ultrasound showing speckling of the myometrium and thicker posterior myometrium.

The MRI is one of the most important and definitive tools in diagnosing adenomyosis, which can be either diffuse or focal. The most characteristic feature off adenomyosis in an MRI is the thickening of the JZ exceeding 12 millimeters. High-signal intensity myometrial foci on T2- or T1-weighted images are also characteristic. MRI is characterized by diagnostic accuracy of 85%, and it adds value by verifying the diagnosis and defining the disease's features and extent, as well as the presence of other uterine lesions.

Hysteroscopy: The advantage of hysteroscopy is the direct visualization of the endometrial cavity. This important diagnostic tool sometimes becomes necessary in cases of adenomyosis seeking fertility treatments. There are many instances where other comorbidities can exist along with adenomyosis such as submucous leiomyomas and endometrial polyps.

Samples acquired through hysteroscopic biopsies confirm adenomyosis when the following features are present histopathologically—Hypervascularization, strawberry-pattern-like cell distribution, endometrial defects, and hemorrhagic cysts within endometrial tissue.

Treatment

As adenomyosis, is associated with hyper estrogenic state, the principle behind management of adenomyosis is to create a sustained progestogenic state in the body. This can be achieved in two ways; (1) During pregnancy, whereby there is a prolonged period of amenorrhea and subsequent lactation amenorrhea, causing all the ectopic endometrial foci to necrose and perish and (2) Through the creation of a pseudopregnancy like state, which can be achieved with treatment of several forms of progesterone preparations.

Adenomyosis has a negative impact on a woman's life, with high percentages of women seeking treatment throughout their reproductive age group for chronic pelvic pain an associated menstrual disorder. The appropriate treatment must be centered around the patients age, reproductive status and clinical symptoms.

Medical Management

Few clinical studies have focused on medical or surgical treatments for adenomyosis, and no medications specifically targeting adenomyosis are currently available. Nevertheless, as this disorder is found in large numbers of women in their reproductive age group medical management should be used as first line treatment.

The medications used in the treatment of adenomyosis are outlined in **Table 1**.

Surgical Management

Conservative surgical management

- *Hysteroscopic procedures*
  - *Endometrial ablation/resection procedures:* A large retrospective cohort study by Mayo Clinic researchers in Rochester, Minnesota, tracked down the long-term results and potential predictors of result for women who had thermal balloon ablation (also known as radiofrequency ablation) done to manage heavy periods.
  - The study found that women who received complete endometrial ablation and who were found to have adenomyosis with a prior ultrasound diagnosis had an increased chance of surgical failure and needed further procedures such as hysterectomy or repetitive ablation.
- *Excisional procedures*
  - *Myometrial adenoma resection and myometrial reduction:* If the location of the adenomyoma can be determined radiographically, focal excision can be performed. In comparison to myomectomy, it is more difficult to expose lesions, define margins, and ascertain the extent of disease, and thus the efficacy of excision remains low at 50%. This procedure can be achieved either through laparotomy, laparoscopy, and/or minilaparotomy. The largest study on adenomyomectomy to date enrolled 165 women who underwent surgery alone or in conjunction with medical therapy (surgery followed by 6 months of gonadotropin-releasing hormone agonist administration). Both groups of women experienced statistically significant symptom relief, and at the 2-year follow-up, all symptom scores decreased from their mean. The surgical-medical group had statistically significantly lower rates of symptom recurrence than the surgery-alone group. Additionally, 55% women became pregnant, resulting in a clinical pregnancy rate of 77.5%, and 49% women delivered successfully (69.0%). Osada et al., describe an adenomyomectomy technique in which adenomyotic tissue is excised and the uterine wall is reconstructed using a triple-flap technique. Procedure stated to result in reduction of symptoms and a low recurrence rate, as well as more than half of women who wanted to conceive successfully carried their pregnancy to term without complications.

TABLE 1: Summary of commonly used drugs in adenomyosis.

Class of compounds	*Mechanism of action*	*Effects*	*Side effects*
GnRH analogs	• Hypoestrogenic state • Anti-proliferative effects • Increased apoptosis	• Significant reduction in uterine size, bleeding and pain in short-term period • Improvement of pregnancy rates in ART cycles	• Menopausal symptoms – vasomotor symptoms, decreased bone mineral density • Consider add back therapy with estrogens if used for more than 3 months
Progestins	• Deciduation and atrophy of the endometrial tissue • Mild hypoestrogenism • Anti-proliferative effect • Anti-inflammatory effect	Significant reduction in bleeding and pain associated with adenomyosis	Breakthrough bleeding
LNG-IUS	• Endometrial atrophy • Direct local action on adenomyotic foci	• Significant reduction in menstrual blood loss increasing hemoglobin and hematocrit of the patient • Decreased uterine volume and pain symptoms	Irregular bleeding (regulated within 6 months of use) Amenorrhea
COCs	Deciduation and subsequent atrophy of the endometrium	Benefits from resulting amenorrhea	• Not well tolerated • Spotting • Headaches • Predisposition to VTE
NSAIDs	Reduced prostaglandin synthesis	Reduced pain and bleeding	Gastrointestinal side effects

(COCs: combined oral contraceptives; GnRH: gonadotropin releasing hormone; NSAIDs: non-steroidal anti-inflammatory drugs like Tranexemic acid and Mefenamic acid; VTE: venous thromboembolism)[75]

- *Other surgical procedures*
  - *Uterine artery ligation*: Only one study examined the effect of laparoscopic uterine artery ligation on symptomatic adenomyosis in 20 women. The authors concluded that the low satisfaction rate indicates that laparoscopic uterine artery ligation may not be an effective treatment option for symptomatic adenomyosis.
  - *Myometrial electrocoagulation*: The purpose of myometrial electrocoagulation of adenomyosis lesions is to cause necrosis and thus shrink the lesion. Using unipolar or bipolar electrocautery, the technique can be performed laparoscopically. However, the procedure is considered to be less precise than surgical excision due to the possibility of incomplete electrical conduction in abnormal tissue, which cannot be evaluated during surgery.
  - *Uterine artery embolization*: Numerous clinical studies examining the efficacy of UAE in the treatment of symptomatic adenomyosis have demonstrated sustained clinical and symptomatic improvement. However, none of the studies were controlled or randomized. As a result, the efficacy of UAE in adenomyosis is unknown, owing to a scarcity of high-quality data. To establish the efficacy of UAE in the treatment of adenomyosis, large-scale, randomized controlled trials with extended follow-up are required.
  - Magnetic resonance-guided focused ultrasound (MRgFUS)

MRgFUS was initially approved by the US Food and Drug Administration as a noninvasive treatment for uterine leiomyomas.

Without causing thermal damage to surrounding tissue, focused ultrasound surgery delivers a concentrated amount of ultrasound energy to deep tissue areas. Adenomyosis is caused by smooth muscle hyperplasia, and thus MRgFUS treatment is ideal for targeting such lesions. The difference between leiomyomas and adenomyosis is determined using magnetic resonance imaging, which demonstrates diffuse or focal thickening of the uterine junctional zone in the presence of adenomyosis. The positive feedback from this type of therapy was very encouraging to begin with. Despite these promising findings, further investigation is required before this treatment can be approved for women with adenomyosis in terms of safety and efficacy.

- *Radical surgical procedures*
  - *Hysterectomy*: Women who have completed their childbearing and are suffering from severe debilitating symptoms of adenomyosis, and also in whom, conservative methods, both medical as well as surgical have failed, are ideal candidates for radical management such as hysterectomy.

Leiomyomas

Uterine fibroids or leiomyoma are often benign tumors of the uterine smooth muscle. They are benign, but may lead to HMB, with resultant anemia and subfertility or fertility in some women. Uterine lipoleiomyomata, are rare benign tumors consisting of a mixture of adipocytes and smooth muscle cells, have been associated together with ovarian and other pathologies and some may undergo sarcomatous change. However, the incidence of malignant transformation of this benign condition is about 0.1%.

Epidemiology

The incidences of leiomyomas are relatively high among population belonging to Black, Asian, Middle Eastern population (BAME). By the age 50 years, close to 70% of white women and more than 80% of black women are diagnosed with leiomyomas, though the incidence of clinical symptoms in black women has been reported to be double that of Caucasian women. The use of progestin-only contraceptives and multiparity both help to reduce the risk of developing fibroids.

FIGO Classification of Uterine Leiomyoma

A uterine fibroid subclassification has been developed by FIGO and presented within the FIGO AUB classification system.

When compared to normal myometrium, leiomyomas express more estrogen and progesterone receptors. According to studies, ovarian steroids such as estradiol and progesterone promote the growth of leiomyomas, and the size of fibroids frequently decreases after menopause when those hormone levels fall.

Clinical Presentation

Clinical presentation of this condition is very varied. It ranges from an incidental finding in an asymptomatic patient to symptoms such as

- *Chronic pelvic pain*: 14.5%
- *HMB /AUB*: 59.8%
- *Poor pregnancy outcomes*: 5–21%
- *Infertility*: 5–21%
- *Constipation*: 59.3%
- *Urinary tract infection or urinary retention*: 32.6%
- *Torsion of pedunculated fibroid*: less than 0.25%
- *Degeneration of preexisting fibroids with or without infection*: 5.1%.

Clinical Evaluation

A detailed clinical history and a thorough physical examination should be performed. On physical examination the most common finding is an enlarged and abnormally shaped uterus. The bimanual per vaginal examination of the patient is necessary to distinguish this lesion from endometriosis and also to get a general size uterine enlargement. The below mentioned investigations can be used to confirm the diagnosis.

Pelvic ultrasound: Confirmation of clinical diagnosis is most easily accomplished with ultrasonography. A pelvic sonogram is a cost-effective method that allows for rapid diagnosis. The use of color Doppler alongside a pelvic ultrasound confirms the diagnosis where a typical whorl like pattern of blood flow distribution along the capsule of the fibroid is diagnostic of a leiomyoma and separates it from the appearance of endometriosis.

MRI: The use of imaging modalities such as MRI may be utilized to identify and quantify the amount of leiomyoma vascularization and degeneration. Another benefit of MRI is that it provides a more specific characterization of the interaction between the leiomyomas and the serosal and mucosal surfaces of the uterus. Whether or not these surfaces are close together often determines the modality of intervention that is indicated.

Hematological investigations: If bleeding is the primary symptom and anemia or other complications of recurrent blood loss are suspected, a complete blood count (CBC) is indicated. Additional testing for thyroid-stimulating hormone (TSH) can be performed. While the growth of the leiomyoma can be monitored, there is currently no basis for establishing a fixed time interval or establishing current guidelines for monitoring the growth. Typically, interval reassessment is triggered by changes in clinical symptoms.

Treatment/Management

Not only treatment protocols should be aimed at providing the best possible cure and care for the patient, but also at minimizing the economic burden on the health care system. Three objectives should guide treatment goals:

1. Eliminate vexing signs and symptoms
2. Decrease the size of the leiomyoma
3. Preserve or improve a woman's fertility if desired.

Medical management: Medical management is often the first line of management instituted for symptomatic fibroids. It ranges from use of hormonal therapy, both COCPs and POPs (Progesterone only Pills) to NSAIDs, and/or drugs to helps modulate the hypothalamic-pituitary-ovarian axis like GnRH analogs. Numerous medical management options are only effective for a brief period of time, and once treatment is discontinued, symptoms recur and fibroids frequently continue to grow. Systemic hormonal therapy is used only to ameliorate the menstrual symptoms of the leiomyoma. It also has no proven effect on the size of fibroids or on subfertility. Agonists of GnRH inhibit endogenous progesterone and estrogen production. Overall, the effects are comparable to menopause, resulting in amenorrhea and a subsequent decrease in uterine volume. However, these effects are transient and occur only during the course of treatment.

LNG-IUS locally releases levonorgestrel and results in improved quality of life by lowering the menstrual flow. While this may provide symptomatic relief, it has no long-term effect on reducing the overall size of the uterine fibroids; thus, it is of limited assistance with bulk symptoms. Nonhormonal options involve NSAIDs and tranexamic acid. Tranexamic acid can occasionally cause gastrointestinal upset and more seriously venous thromboembolism. NSAIDs are also useful for reducing menstrual blood loss. NSAIDs inhibit endometrial prostaglandin production, thereby inhibiting abnormal vascularization and neovascularization. While NSAIDs are effective at reducing menstrual flow, they come secondary in term of efficacy provided by tranexamic acid and LNG-IUS.

Surgical management: Surgical intervention continues to be the most effective treatment option for leiomyomas. Endometrial ablation is the hysteroscopic removal of the entire endometrium, but this procedure precludes future endometrial assessment and necessitates permanent contraception. Embolization of the uterine artery reduces blood flow to individual fibroids, thereby halting growth and alleviating symptoms. Successful myomectomy (surgical removal of only fibroids) preserves future fertility while significantly reducing the size and symptoms of fibroids; however, many women will require additional subsequent procedures to treat recurrent symptomatic fibroids. Hysterectomy is the only treatment option that is permanent.

Prognosis

The prognosis of uterine fibroids varies significantly between individuals. Numerous patients have an excellent prognosis and remain symptom-free for years, if not indefinitely. Others, depending on their desire for future fertility, may experience recurrent fibroids necessitating multiple surgeries.

Malignancy and Hyperplasia

The fourth most frequent kind of cancer among women is endometrial cancer, which resulted in around 46,470 new diagnoses and over 8,000 fatalities in 2011. Over the course of a woman's lifetime, the risk of endometrial cancer is estimated to be around 3%. A 5-year survival is now much lower for endometrial cancer patients (84% in 2006) compared to that of patients 30 years before (88% in 1975), making it one of two malignancies with a higher death rate.

Risk Factors

Certain risk factors, including those listed below, are strongly associated with the development of endometrial hyperplasia and its subsequent progression to endometrial malignancy:

- Polycystic ovarian syndrome
- Diabetes
- Hypertension
- Factors leading to exposure of the endometrium to action of unopposed estrogens such as infertility, HRT, chemoprophylaxis for breast cancer (tamoxifen) use
- Obesity.

Some of these above-mentioned risk factors, especially obesity, still have not been fully investigated yet.

Diagnosis

Endometrial cancer histopathological diagnosis can be made by an outpatient pipelle biopsy.

Indications for doing an outpatient pipelle biopsy include:

- Women in reproductive age group with AUB and an endometrial thickness of > 1 cm on USG in the luteal phase.
- Postmenopausal women complaining of bleeding PV with endometrial thickness of more than 4 mm on USG.

Additionally, ultrasonography should also be done, even if there is no vaginal bleeding, if there is an expanded endometrial thickness or intrauterine polyp noted on ultrasound then biopsy should be performed. Ultrasound is not appropriate for assessing asymptomatic individuals.

Noncancerous histological findings that are frequently encountered include simple and complex hyperplasia (both with and without atypia). If left untreated, the incidence of progression to endometrial cancer varies between 1 and 29%, depending on the type of hyperplasia (simple vs. complex) and degree of cytologic atypia. 95 Recently, many studies have noted that patients in whom a pipelle histopathology diagnosis of atypical hyperplasia was noted preoperative, 48% of these patients had endometrial carcinoma in the posthysterectomy sample.

Follow-up in Cases of Endometrial Hyperplasia

Women should be informed that the risk of endometrial hyperplasia without atypia developing into endometrial cancer is less than 5% over a 20-year period and that the majority of cases of endometrial hyperplasia without atypia will spontaneously regress during follow-up. Obesity and the use of HRT are reversible risk factors that should be identified and addressed, if possible. Observation alone with subsequent endometrial biopsies to ensure disease regression is an option, particularly when identifiable risk factors can be reversed. However, women should be informed that progestogen therapy has a higher rate of disease regression than observation alone.

To induce histological regression of endometrial hyperplasia without atypia, oral progestogens or the LNG-IUS should be used for a minimum of 6 months. If the adverse effects are tolerable and fertility is not desired, women should be encouraged to continue with the LNG-IUS for up to 5 years, as this decreases the risk of relapse and frequently alleviates AUB symptoms. After a diagnosis of hyperplasia without atypia, endometrial surveillance incorporating outpatient endometrial biopsy is recommended at a minimum of 6-monthly intervals. Individualized review schedules should be responsive to changes in a woman's clinical condition. Prior to discharge, at least two consecutive 6-monthly negative biopsies should be obtained. Women should be advised to seek additional referrals, if they experience abnormal vaginal bleeding following treatment completion, as this may indicate disease relapse or progression. Six-monthly endometrial biopsies are recommended for women at a higher risk of relapse, such as those with a BMI of 35 or greater or those taking oral progestogens. Once two consecutive negative endometrial biopsies are obtained, long-term follow-up with annual endometrial biopsies should be considered.

Surgical Management of Hyperplasia

Hysterectomy for cases of endometrial hyperplasia, when women do not wish to preserve their fertility, should be considered in the following circumstances:

- Progression to atypical hyperplasia occurs during follow-up.
- There is no regression of the disease despite 1 year of treatment with progestins.
- There is relapse of atypical hyperplasia after stopping the treatment.
- Persistence of AUB symptoms despite medical management.
- If the patient declines surveillance and refuses medical management.

Women who are postmenopausal and require surgical management for endometrial hyperplasia without atypia should be offered a bilateral salpingo-oophorectomy in addition to a total hysterectomy. The decision to remove the ovaries should be made individually for premenopausal women; however, bilateral salpingectomy should be considered to reduce the risk of future ovarian malignancy. Laparoscopic total hysterectomy is preferable to abdominal total hysterectomy because it results in a shorter hospital stay, less postoperative pain, and a faster recovery. Endometrial ablation is not recommended for endometrial hyperplasia treatment because complete and persistent endometrial destruction cannot be guaranteed and intrauterine adhesion formation may preclude future endometrial histological surveillance. Due to the risk of underlying malignancy or progression to cancer, women with atypical hyperplasia should undergo a total hysterectomy. Bilateral salpingo-oophorectomy should be offered concurrently with total hysterectomy to postmenopausal women with atypical hyperplasia.

Women with atypical hyperplasia declining hysterectomy should undergo regular surveillance with endometrial biopsy every 3 months and should continue to do so until two consecutive negative biopsies are obtained, following which they can be followed up annually. For women with evidence of histological disease regression, long-term follow-up with an endometrial biopsy every 6–12 months is recommended until a hysterectomy is performed.

Women with endometrial hyperplasia wishing to conceive should

- Have at least one negative sample on histopathology before attempting to conceive.
- Be referred to fertility specialist to discuss fertility plans for the patient and appropriate treatment should be instituted.
- Have regression of endometrial hyperplasia before attempting assisted reproductive techniques as it yields better fertility and pregnancy outcomes.

REVISED FIGO STAGING OF ENDOMETRIAL CANCER AND ITS SUBSEQUENT TREATMENT

Two subtypes of endometrial carcinomas are classified on the basis of their histology. The most common histologic subtype is endometrioid adenocarcinoma (type 1), which accounts for nearly 90% of endometrial cancers. Additional classifications are given to them according to the grade of tumor differentiation, ranging from grade 1 (highly differentiated) to grade 3 (poorly differentiated) (poorly differentiated). The endometrial carcinomas which are classified as type 2 are serous papillary and clear cell adenocarcinomas. Grade 3 endometrioid adenocarcinomas have aggressive tumor biologic characteristics and a 50% chance of being advanced or distant disease at the time of the initial test.

Treatment for endometrial cancer will depend on the FIGO staging and must involve referral to oncology unit for management and follow-ups.

Coagulopathy

Coagulopathy is reported to be involved in about 13% cases of AUB. Most commonly described is Won Villebrands disease. Systematic disorders of coagulopathies can be readily identified by proper history taking. As per new inclusions in this category, Coagulopathy is divided into two solid components.

- Coagulopathy due to inherited bleeding disorders.
- Coagulopathy due to iatrogenic causes such as drug induced.

A structure history should elicit, if any of the following are present:

- Heavy bleeding since menarche
- *One of the following*:
  - Previous PPH
  - Previous surgical site bleeding.
  - Previous bleeding associated with dental work
- *Two or more of the following*:
  - Bruising one or two times a month.
  - Epistaxis one or two times a month.
  - Frequent gum bleeding.
  - Family history of bleeding disorders
- Significant history of anticoagulant drug use such as aspirin, clopidogrel, heparin, or warfarin for underlying other pathologies.

If any of the above are present, a more thorough coagulopathy evaluation should be conducted. Anticoagulant and antiplatelet therapy have historically been included in the treatment protocol. Venous thromboembolism can occur as a result of compression of the venous system caused by a large fibroid uterus (VTE). Subsequent anticoagulation may exacerbate previous AUB-L-related bleeding, posing additional management challenges.

When a diagnosis of coagulopathy as the cause of AUB is ascertained, a referral to a hematologist is warranted and the management of the condition should involve a multidisciplinary approach. Treatments range from using tranexemic acid to desmopressin for von Willebrand disease to blood transfusion for severe anemia and should be executed after thoroughly investigating the patient and in association with the hematology colleagues.

In cases of drug induced HMB, patient management should be planned and executed involving a multidisciplinary team (MDT) comprising of an internal physician, hematologist and immunologist. Timely monitoring of APTT and prothrombin time with INR will help in monitoring the anti-coagulant therapy along with management of HMB.

An MDT management of such causes should be targeted at improving the patient's quality of life.

Ovulatory Dysfunction

Anovulatory cycles may contribute to AUB through the effect of unopposed estrogen on the endometrium, resulting in marked proliferation and thickening of the endometrium, resulting in HMB in association with an altered menstrual cycle frequency. This phenomenon has been observed at the reproductive age extremes. However, alterations of the hypothalamopituitary axis must firstly be excluded and includes:

- Polycystic ovarian disease (PCOD)
- Hyperprolactinemia
- Hypothyroidism
- Cushing's syndrome
- Congenital or adult onset adrenal hyperplasia
- Obesity
- Anorexia and weight loss
- Extreme exercise.

In this group, the majority of women have cycles that last around 38 days even more. Because dopamine levels and their associated effects on the HPO axis are affected by drugs in this category, rather than AUB-I, they currently belong in the category "dopamine-impacting drugs". Ovulatory dysfunction may complicate menstrual irregularities in women with fibroids.

Therapy for the underlying condition should be instituted first along with supportive treatment to treat the symptoms. It is observed that the moment the underlying cause is treated; there is return to ovulatory cycles and reduction in abnormal bleeding patterns.

Role of Progesterone in Managing Ovulatory Dysfunction

When ovulation does not occur on a regular basis, unopposed estrogen exposure can result in a chronic proliferative or hyperplastic endometrium. Although the exact mechanism by which ovulation disturbances result in irregular and/or HMB is unknown, it is thought to be due to local endometrial changes. Menstrual irregularity in the early years following menarche is most likely to be caused by hypothalamo-pituitary-ovarian (HPO) axis immaturity. However, in some young women, particularly those with a high body mass index, such irregular bleeding may be an early sign of PCOS.

Previously, it was believed that irregular cycles during the menopause transition were primarily caused by oligo/anovulation. However, recent data indicate that at least one-third of irregular cycles during the mid-to-late menopause transition are ovulatory but with an abnormal pattern. Due to the irregular development of a new preovulatory follicle during the prior luteal phase, these distinct endocrine disturbances have been dubbed "luteal out of phase" or "LOOP" cycles. This is frequently followed by a luteinizing hormone (LH) peak and subsequent ovulation. These LOOP cycles are most frequently observed during periods of irregular menstruation and can also result in excessive bleeding.

How progestrogens help in anovulatory HMB?

Infrequent or excessive menstrual bleeding is frequently extremely inconvenient for women. The medical management of menstrual irregularities aims to control bleeding and minimize HMB. While progestogens and estrogens, as well as progestogens in combination, are already widely used to treat irregular or heavy bleeding caused by disturbed ovulation, the regimen, dose, and type of progestogen used varies widely, with little agreement on the optimal treatment approach. The adverse effects of progestogens vary according to the type and dose of the progestogen, whether it is administered monthly (for up to 21 days in a month) or continuously uninterrupted and also vary between individuals. Progestogens frequently cause nonmenstrual adverse effects such as headaches, weight gain, and breast tenderness. Irregular bleeding and spotting are common side effects of all types and regimens of progestogens, most notably continuous low-dose preparations.

Women who experience irregular menstrual bleeding fall into three broad categories:

1. Adolescents who have not yet established regular menstrual cycles.
2. Women who experience anovulation as a result of PCOS.
3. Women who are transitioning to menopause and may experience ovulation disturbances.

Treatment protocols differ in each group. Emphasis is placed on regularizing menstruation in adolescents, assisting ovulatory menstrual patterns in women with PCO and maintaining regular bleeding patterns or amenorrhea in women with menstrual transition.

Changes in menstrual cycle length are frequently associated with disturbances of the hypothalamopituitary ovarian (HPO) axis. Due to the absence of progesterone withdrawal from estrogen-primed endometrium in irregular menstrual bleeding caused by oligo/anovulation, cycles are irregular. Prolonged estrogenaction may result in an accumulation of endometrium and irregular bleeding as it degrades and is excreted. This is why, in the second half of the menstrual cycle, cyclical progestogens are used to induce a regular withdrawal bleed. Continuous progestogen administration is intended to cause endometrial atrophy and thus inhibit endometrial proliferation stimulated by estrogen. Without progesterone, unopposed estrogen may cause the endometrium to thicken, thereby increasing the risk of developing endometrial hyperplasia or even malignancy.

Several progesterone preparations are available nowadays to the clinician and can be administered to the patient in oral, injectable or intrauterine format with or without combining with cyclical estrogens to individually cater to patient quality of life and preferences.

Endometrial

Abnormal uterine bleeding that occurs in a normal uterus with normal menstrual cycles and no evidence of coagulopathy is most likely endometrial in origin. There is a great deal of research being done to better understand the functions of the endometrium during menstruation and the causes of menstrual disorders, particularly the complex order of events that occur when progesterone levels fall (due to degradation of the corpus luteum in the absence of pregnancy). The following are significant contributors to the shedding and scarless repair of the functional upper endometrium layer: hypoxia, inflammation, hemostasis and angiogenesis, proteolysis (resulting in premature clot lysis). Although, AUB-E may be involved in the majority of women with AUB, the lack of clinically available specific tests or biomarkers precludes practical testing for such disorders. As such, diagnosis is contingent upon a thorough history taking and exclusion of other possible causes. Due to the high prevalence of endometrial dysfunction, it is highly likely that those with AUB-L will frequently have an element of AUB-E contributing to increased/abnormal menstrual blood loss, with the associated therapeutic implications. The details of diagnosis, management and follow up of AUB caused by endometrial factors, have been highlighted in the malignancy section of the chapter above.

Iatrogenic

Abnormal uterine bleeding can be due to iatrogenic causes such as exogenous therapy that may result in unplanned endometrial bleeding. Progestin therapy (systemic or intrauterine administration) or interventions that alter ovarian steroid release, such as GnRH agonists and aromatase inhibitors, are often found with continuous estrogen or progestin therapy. SERMs and SPRMs (less commonly used) can induce AUB through direct action on the endometrium. Intrauterine device (IUD) use may result in a low-grade chemical endometritis, which may contribute to AUB.

A particular mention has to be made in this category of usage of tamoxifen in patients with estrogen receptor breast cancers, who require tamoxifen as a long-term maintenance of almost 10 years to prevent recurrence of breast malignancies. Tamoxifen, being a selective estrogen receptor modulator has hyperplastic effects on the endometrium while exerting beneficial effects on the breast. These patients have to be followed up by a gynecologist annually to rule out endometrial hyperplasia. Endometrial thickness larger than 1 cm warrants a pipelle biopsy, with/without hysteroscopy to rule out atypical hyperplasia. Appropriate therapy can then be given once hyperplasia has been excluded.

Not Otherwise Classified (AUB-N)

It is certain that there will be other pathologies that will cause AUB but cannot be classified under the normal FIGO AUB classification. These pathologies are listed as under "Not Otherwise Classified" section of the classification as their occurrence is rare. These are as follows

- AVMs within the myometrium.
- Endometrial pseudo aneurysms.
- Myometrial hypertrophy
- Chronic endometritis not cause by IUD.

All of the above can be coexist with pathologies like leiomyomas and endometriosis.

A planned regular review of the FIGO PALM - COEIN Classification every 3–5 years by the committee will allow re- assessment of this category. Further areas such as of the classification might also need to be subclassified, e.g., AUB caused by polyps and endometriosis.

Role of Uterine Artery Embolization in A-V Malformations of the Myometrium

The exact incidence of AVMs is unknown, but it is a rare possibility. The diagnosis of the condition is based on exclusion. A beta hCG test differentiates it from bleeding from retained products of conception causing HMB.

AVMs are isolated vascular anomalies that occur in otherwise healthy individuals and range in size and location significantly. When a normal uterine blood vessel approaches the tissue it supplies, it divides into smaller branches. By the time it reaches the endometrium's surface, it will have branched into numerous small capillaries. Vasculature within AVM is slow and low in pressure due to the presence of numerous capillaries. Nonetheless, an AVM is defined by vascular channel proliferation, the formation of fistulas, and the interbreeding of small, capillary-like vascular channels. Congenital AVMs have multiple feeding arteries, draining veins, and an intervening nidus, whereas acquired AVMs have only a couple of feeding arteries are not supplied by extrauterine arteries, and absence of an intervening nidus. This differentiation between congenital and acquired AVMs are clearly made out upon histopathology after hysterectomy.

In the earlier days the diagnosis of AVMs was made post hysterectomy on histopathology. But currently, angiography is used as a gold standard for its diagnosis. This aids the clinician to employ conservative line of management as compared to radical management like hysterectomy giving the patient a choice of retaining her fertility and menstrual function.

Uterine AVMs can be diagnosed noninvasively by means of Doppler ultrasonography. AVMs are often diagnosed with gray-scale ultrasonography, which may be beneficial in diagnosing, but AVMs may also be mistaken for other pelvic

TABLE 2: Causes of abnormal uterine bleeding and the treatment options for each.

AUB sub-classification	*Specific treatment*
Polyps	Resection
Adenomyosis	Surgery – hysterectomy, adenomyomectomy (although not routinely performed)
Malignancy	• Surgery ± adjuvant chemotherapy • High dose progestins, if surgery not possible • Radiotherapy, palliation
Coagulopathy	• Tranexemic acid • DDVAP
Ovulation	• Lifestyle modifications • Cabergoline – Hyperprolactinomas • Levothyroxine – Hypothyroidism
Endometrial	Specific therapies await further delineation of underlying causes.
Iatrogenic	Treat underlying cause based on guidelines on problematic bleeding with hormonal contraception*
Not otherwise classified	• Antibiotics for endometritis • Embolization of A-V malformations

*This guidance provides evidence-based recommendations and examples of best practice for health professionals regarding the management of problematic bleeding in women who are currently using hormonal contraception in the world. It is intended for use by any health care professional or health service in the world that provides contraception or conception advice.[105]

structures or pathologies. That is where Doppler waveforms are used to endorse grey scale ultrasound findings.

It is preferable to perform uterine artery embolization, if the patient experiences recurring episodes of bleeding, resulting in unstable hemodynamics. Transcatheter embolization treatment of obstetric and gynecologic hemorrhages with uterine arterial embolization has proven to be extremely effective, revolutionizing the management of uterine AVMs as the underlying cause of HMB. As seen on imaging studies, the size of AVMs detected has no direct correlation with whether or not embolization is indicated. This decision is based entirely on the patient's clinical condition.

SUMMARY OF MANAGEMENT OF ABNORMAL UTERINE BLEEDING

Abnormal uterine bleeding -L management should take the patient's desire for fertility into account, as well as the impact of pressure symptoms, comorbidities, and any other AUB contributors. Each patient's treatment should be unique, and there are no "one-size-fits-all" approaches to initial and subsequent treatment options.

Although the treatment should be targeted toward individual managements, listed in **Table 2** is an overview of the selected treatments based on the pathology as per the recommendations.

CONCLUSION

Abnormal uterine bleeding can be a debilitating condition affecting the day to day activities of the patient. It must be remembered that AUB is a symptom of an underlying disease. The FIGO PALM - COEIN Classification aides the clinician to approach patients issues in a structured way and assists in determining the best possible treatment options. A detailed history and clinical examination remains a cornerstone in the approach to patients suffering from these symptoms. One should also be cognizant, that after a successful diagnosis, the treatment protocols should be individualized and implemented only after detailed counseling of the potential effects and complications of the therapy. This is of particular relevance in women of reproductive age who are planning to conceive. Outpatient hysteroscopy and the advancement of imaging technology will aid in the accurate diagnosis and treatment plan. Increased medical options have expanded women's options, and many will no longer be required to undergo potentially complicated surgery.

FURTHER READING

1. AbdollahiFard S, Mostafa Gharabaghi P, Montazeri F, Mashrabi O. Hysteroscopy as a minimally invasive surgery, a good substitute for invasive gynecological procedures. Iran J Reprod Med. 2012; 10(4):377-82.
2. Al-Jefout M, Black K, Schulke L, BerbicM, Luscombe G, Tokushige N, et al. Novel finding of high density of activated mast cells in endometrial polyps. Fertil Steril. 2009; 92(3):1104-6.
3. Alansari LM, Wardle P. Endometrial polyps and subfertility. Hum Fertil (Camb). 2012; 15(3):129-33.
4. Al Hilli MM, Stewart EA. Magnetic resonance-guided focused ultrasound surgery. Semin Reprod Med. 2010; 28(3):242-9.
5. American Cancer Society. Cancer Facts and Figures 2011. Atlanta: American Cancer Society; 2011.
6. American College of Obstetricians and Gynecologists. ACOG committee opinion no. 557: Management of acute abnormal uterine bleeding in nonpregnant reproductive-aged women. Obstet Gynecol. 2013;121(4):891-6.
7. Ascher S, Arnold L. Adenomyosis: prospective comparison of MR imaging and transvaginal sonography. Radiol. 1994;190: 803-6.
8. Babacan A, Gun I, Kizilaslan C, Ozden O, Muhcu M, Mungen E, et al. Comparison of transvaginal ultrasonography and hysteroscopy in the diagnosis of uterine pathologies. Int J Clin Exp Med. 2014; 7(3):764-9.
9. Bazot M, Cortez A, Darai E, Rouger J, Chopier J, Antoine JM, et al. Ultrasonography compared with magnetic resonance imaging for the diagnosis of adenomyosis: correlation with histopathology. Hum Reprod. 2001; 16(11):2427-33.
10. Behera MA. Abnormal (dysfunctional) uterine bleeding. Medscape.com.
11. Benagiano G, Brosens I. History of adenomyosis. Best Pract Res Clin Obstet Gynaecol. 2006; 20(4):449-63.
12. Brucker SY, Huebner M, Wallwiener M, Stewart EA, Ebersoll S, Schoenfisch B, et al. Clinical characteristics indicating adenomyosis coexisting with leiomyomas: a retrospective, questionnaire-based study. Fertil Steril. 2014; 101(1):237-41.
13. Champaneria R, Abedin P, Daniels J, Balogun M, Khan KS. Ultrasound scan and magnetic resonance imaging for the

diagnosis of adenomyosis: systematic review comparing test accuracy. Acta Obstet Gynecol Scand. 2010;89: 1374-84.
14. Cheong Y, Cameron IT, Critchley HOD. Abnormal uterine bleeding. Br Med Bull. 2017;123(1):103-14.
15. Critchley HO, Maybin JA. Molecular and cellular causes of abnormal uterine bleeding of endometrial origin. Semin Reprod Med. 2011;29:400-9.
16. Daniele A, Ferrero A, Maggiorotto F, PerriniG, Volpi E, Sismondi P. Suspecting malignancy in endometrial polyps: value of hysteroscopy. Tumori. 2013; 99(2):204-9.
17. Deligdisch L. Effects of hormone therapy on the endometrium. Mod Pathol. 1993; 6(1):94-106.
18. Di Donato N, Montanari G, Benfenati A, Leonardi D, Bertoldo V, Monti G, et al. Prevalence of adenomyosis in women undergoing surgery for endometriosis. Eur J Obstet Gynecol Reprod Biol. 2014; 181:289-93.
19. Doherty L, Mutlu L, Sinclair D, Taylor H. Uterine fibroids: clinical manifestations and contemporary management. Reprod Sci. 2014;21(9):1067-92.
20. Dreisler E, Sorensen SS, Ibsen PH. Prevalence of endometrial polyps and abnormal uterine bleeding in a Danish population aged 20-74 years. Ultrasound Obstet Gynecol. 2009;33:102-8.
21. Dueholm M, Lundorf E, Hansen ES, Sorensen JS, Ledertoug S, Olesen F. Magnetic resonance imaging and transvaginal ultrasonography for the diagnosis of adenomyosis. Fertil Steril. 2001;76:588-94.
22. El-Nashar SA, Hopkins MR, Creedon DJ, St SauverJL, Weaver AL, McGree ME, et al. Prediction of treatment outcomes after global endometrial ablation. Obstet Gynecol. 2009; 113(1):97-106.
23. Fadl SA, Sabry AS, Hippe DS, Al-Obaidli A, Yousef RR, Dubinsky TJ. Diagnosing polyps on transvaginal sonography: Is sonohysterography always necessary? Ultrasound Q. 2018; 34(4):272-7.
24. Fiçicioğlu C, Tekin HI, Arioğlu PF, Okar I. A murine model of adenomyosis: the effects of hyperprolactinemia induced by fluoxetine hydrochloride, a selective serotonin reuptake inhibitor, on adenomyosis induction in Wistar albino rats. Acta Eur Fertil. 1995; 26(2):75-9.
25. Fleischer AC, James AE, Millis JB, Julian C. Differential diagnosis of pelvic masses by gray scale sonography. AJR Am J Roentgenol. 1978;131(3):469-76.
26. Freeman SJ, Aly AM, Kataoka MY, Addley HC, Reinhold C, Sala E. The Revised FIGO Staging System for Uterine Malignancies: Implications for MR Imaging. Radiographics J. 2012;32(6).
27. FSRH Clinical Effectiveness Unit (2015). Problematic bleeding with hormonal contraception [Online]. Available from: https://www.fsrh.org/standards-and-guidance/documents/ceuguidanceproblematicbleedinghormonalcontraception/. [Last accessed on December 2, 2021].
28. Garcia L, Isaacson K. Adenomyosis: review of the literature. J Minim Invasive Gynecol. 2011; 18(4):428-37.
29. Ghosh S, Naftalin J, Imrie R, Hoo WL. Natural history of uterine fibroids: a radiological perspective. Curr Obstet Gynecol Rep. 2018;7(3):117-21.
30. Ginsburg KA, Quereshi F, Thomas M, Snowman B. Intramural ectopic pregnancy implanting in adenomyosis. Fertil Steril. 1989;51(2):354-6.
31. Giordano G, Gnetti L, Merisio C, Melpignano M. Post-menopausal status, hypertension and obesity as risk factors for malignant transformation in endometrial polyps. Maturitas. 2007; 56(2):190-7.
32. Gregoriou O, Konidaris S, Vrachnis N, Bakalianou K, Salakos N, Papadias K, et al. Clinical parameters linked with malignancy in endometrial polyps. Climacteric. 2009;12(5):454-8.
33. Grivell RM, Reid KM, Mellor A. Uterine arteriovenous malformations: a review of the current literature. Obstet Gynecol Surv. 2005; 60(11):761-7.
34. Hale GE, Burger HG. Hormonal changes and biomarkers in late reproductive age, menopausal transition and menopause. Best Pract Res Clin Obstet Gynaecol. 2009;23(1):7-23.
35. Hale GE, Manconi F, Luscombe G, Fraser IS. Quantitative measurements of menstrual blood loss in ovulatory and anovulatory cycles in middle- and late-reproductive age and the menopausal transition. Obstet Gynecol. 2011;115(2 Pt 1):249-56.
36. Hauth EA, Jaeger HJ, Libera H, Lange S, Forsting M. MR imaging of the uterus and cervix in healthy women: determination of normal values. Eur Radiol. 2007;17:734-42.
37. Hickey M, Salamonsen LA. Endometrial structural and inflammatory changes with exogenous progestogens. Trends Endocrinol Metab. 2008;19(5):167-74.
38. Hooff MH, Voorhorst FJ, Kaptein MB, Hirasing RA, Koppenaal C, Schoemaker J. Predictive values of menstrual cycle pattern, body mass index, hormone levels and polycystic ovaries at aged 15 years for oligo-amenorrhoea at aged 18 years. Human Reprod. 2004;19(2):383-92.
39. Jakab A, Ovári L, Juhász B, Birinyi L, Bacskó G, Tóth Z. Detection of feeding artery improves the ultrasound diagnosis of endometrial polyps in asymptomatic patients. Eur J Obstet Gynecol Reprod Biol. 2005; 119(1):103-7.
40. Kadir RA, Economides DL, Sabin CA. Frequency of inherited bleeding disorders in women with menorrhagia. Lancet. 1998;351:485-9.
41. Kamath MS, Kalampokas EE, Kalampokas TE. Use of GnRH analogues pre-operatively for hysteroscopic resection of submucous fibroids: a systematic review and meta-analysis. Eur J Obstet Gynecol Reprod Biol. 2014;177:11-8.
42. Kashani BN, Centini G, Morelli SS, Weiss G, Petraglia F. Role of medical management for uterine leiomyomas. Best Pract Res Clin Obstet Gynaecol. 2016;34:85-103.
43. Khan KN, Kitajima M, Fujishita A, Nakashima M, Masuzaki H. Toll-like receptor system and endometriosis. J Obstet Gynaecol Res. 2013; 39(8):1281-92.
44. Khaund A, Lumsden AM. Benign disease of the uterus. In: Edmonds K (Ed.) Dewhurst's Textbook of Obstetrics and Gynaecology, 8th edition. Hoboken, NJ: Wiley-Blackwell; 2012, pp. 715-26.
45. Kouides PA, Conard J, Peyvandi F. Hemostasis and menstruation: appropriate investigation for underlying disorders of hemostasis in women with excessive menstrual bleeding. Fertil Steril. 2005;84:1345-51.
46. Kunz G, Herbertz M, Beil D, Huppert P, Leyendecker G. Adenomyosis as a disorder of the early and late human reproductive period. Reprod Biomed Online. 2007;15:681-5.
47. Kurman RJ, Kaminski PF, Norris H. The behavior of endometrial hyperplasia. A long-term study of "untreated" hyperplasia in 170 patients. Cancer. 1985; 56(2):403-12.
48. Lacey JVJ, Chia VM. Endometrial hyperplasia and the risk of progression to carcinoma. Maturitas. 2009;63(1):39-44.
49. Laganà AS, Giacobbe V, Triolo O, Granese R, Ban Frangež H, Vrtačnik-Bokal E, et al. Dienogest as preoperative treatment of submucous myomas for hysteroscopic surgery: a prospective, randomized study. Gynecol Endocrinol. 2016; 32(5):408-11.
50. Laganà AS, Palmara V, Granese R, CianciminoL, Chiofalo B, Triolo O. Desogestrel versus danazol as preoperative treatment for hysteroscopic surgery: a prospective, randomized evaluation. Gynecol Endocrinol. 2014; 30(11):794-7.

51. Laganà AS, Vitale SG, Muscia V, Rossetti P, Buscema M, Triolo O, et al. Endometrial preparation with Dienogest before hysteroscopic surgery: a systematic review. Arch Gynecol Obstet. 2017; 295(3):661-7.
52. La Torre R, De Felice C, De Angelis C, Coacci F, Mastrone M, Cosmi EV. Transvaginal sonographic evaluation of endometrial polyps: a comparison with two dimensional and three dimensional contrast sonography. Clin Exp Obstet Gynecol. 1999;26(3-4):171-3.
53. Levgur M, Abadi MA, Tucker A. Adenomyosis: symptoms, histology, and pregnancy terminations. Obstet Gynecol. 2000; 95(5):688-91.
54. Levgur M. Therapeutic options for adenomyosis: a review. Arch Gynecol Obstet. 2007; 276(1):1-15.
55. Lieng M, Istre O, Qvigstad E. Treatment of endometrial polyps: a systematic review. Acta Obstet Gynecol Scand. 2010; 89(8):992-1002.
56. Lieng M, Istre O, Sandvik L, Qvigstad E. Prevalence, 1-year regression rate, and clinical significance of asymptomatic endometrial polyps: cross-sectional study. J Minim Invasive Gynecol. 2009;16(4):465-71.
57. Lieng M, Qvigstad E, Dahl GF, Istre O. Flow differences between endometrial polyps and cancer: a prospective study using intravenous contrast-enhanced transvaginal color flow Doppler and three-dimensional power Doppler ultrasound. Ultrasound Obstet Gynecol. 2008; 32(7):935-40.
58. Lieng M, Qvigstad E, Sandvik L, Jørgensen H, Langebrekke A, Istre OJ. Hysteroscopic resection of symptomatic and asymptomatic endometrial polyps. Minim Invasive Gynecol. 2007; 14(2):189-94.
59. Li F, Wei S, Yang S, Liu Z, Nan F. Post hysteroscopic progesterone hormone therapy in the treatment of endometrial polyps. Pak J Med Sci. 2018; 34(5):1267-71.
60. McCluggage WG, Desai V, Manek S. Tamoxifen-associated postmenopausal adenomyosis exhibits stromal fibrosis, glandular dilatation and epithelial metaplasias. Histopathology. 2000; 37(4):340-6.
61. Meresman GF, Augé L, Barañao RI, Lombardi E, Tesone M, Sueldo C. Oral contraceptives suppress cell proliferation and enhance apoptosis of eutopic endometrial tissue from patients with endometriosis. Fertil Steril. 2002; 77(6):1141-7.
62. Metello J, Jimenez J. Hysteroscopy and infertility. In: Shawki O, Deshmukh S, Pacheco LA. (Eds.). Mastering the Techniques in Hysteroscopy. New Delhi, India: Jaypee Brothers; 2017. p. 454.
63. Mittal K, Schwartz L, Goswami S, Demopoulos R. Estrogen and progesterone receptor expression in endometrial polyps. Int J Gynecol Pathol. 1996; 15(4):345-8.
64. Molinas CR, Campo R. Office hysteroscopy and adenomyosis. Best Pract Res Clin Obstet Gynaecol. 2006;20:557-67.
65. Munro MG, Critchley HOD, Fraser IS, FIGO Menstrual Disorders Committee. The two FIGO systems for normal and abnormal uterine bleeding symptoms and classification of causes of abnormal uterine bleeding in the reproductive years: 2018 revisions. Int J Gynaecol Obstet. 2018;143(3):393-408.
66. Nogueira AA, Dos Reis FJC, Silva JCRE, Manconi F. Endometrial polyps: pathogenesis, sequelae and treatment. SAGE Open Med. 2019;7:2050312119848247.
67. Novellas S, Chassang M, Delotte J, Toullalan O, Chevallier A, Bouaziz J, et al. MRI characteristics of the uterine junctional zone: from normal to the diagnosis of adenomyosis. AJR Am J Roentgenol. 2011 May; 196(5):1206-13.
68. Nowak RA, Mora S, Diehl T, Rhoades AR, Stewart EA. Prolactin is an autocrine growth regulator for human myometrial and leyomyoma cells. J Soc Gynecol Invest. 1995;2:396.
69. Osada H, Silber S, Kakinuma T, Nagaishi M, Kato K, Kato O. Surgical procedure to conserve the uterus for future pregnancy in patients suffering from massive adenomyosis. Reprod Biomed Online. 2011; 22(1):94-9.
70. O'Brien P, Neyastani A, Buckley AR, Chang SD, Legiehn GM. Uterine arteriovenous malformations: from diagnosis to treatment. J Ultrasound Med. 2006;25(11):1387-92.
71. Panganamamula UR, Harmanli OH, Isik-Akbay EF, Grotegut CA, Dandolu V, Gaughan JP. Is prior uterine surgery a risk factor for adenomyosis? Obstet Gynecol. 2004; 104(5 Pt 1):1034-8.
72. Parker JD, Leondires M, Sinaii N, Premkumar A, Nieman LK, Stratton P. Persistence of dysmenorrhea and nonmenstrual pain after optimal endometriosis surgery may indicate adenomyosis. Fertil Steril. 2006; 86(3):711-5.
73. Pepas L, Deguara C, Davis C. Update on the surgical management of adenomyosis. Curr Opin Obstet Gynecol. 2012;24(4):259-64.
74. Preutthipan S, Herabutya Y. Hysteroscopic polypectomy in 240 premenopausal and postmenopausal women. Fertil Steril. 2005;83:705-9.
75. Rackow BW, Jorgensen E, Taylor HS. Endometrial polyps affect uterine receptivity. Fertil Steril. 2011; 95(8):2690-2.
76. RCOG/ BSGE (2016). Endometrial hyperplasia, Management of (Green top Guidelines number 67) [online]. Available from: https://www.rcog.org.uk/en/guidelines-research-services/guidelines/gtg67/. [Last accessed on December 2, 2021].
77. Reslová T, Tosner J, Resl M, Kugler R, Vávrová I. Endometrial polyps. A clinical study of 245 cases. Arch Gynecol Obstet. 1999; 262(3–4): 133-9.
78. Ryan GL, Stolpen A, Van Voorhis BJ. An unusual cause of adolescent dysmenorrhea. Obstet Gynecol. 2006; 108(4):1017-22.
79. Salim S, Won H, Nesbitt-Hawes E, Campbell N, Abbott JJ. Diagnosis and management of endometrial polyps: a critical review of the literature. Minim Invasive Gynecol. 2011; 18(5): 569-81.
80. Schmandt RE, Iglesias DA, Co NN, Lu KH. Understanding obesity and endometrial cancer risk: opportunities for prevention. Am J Obstet Gynecol. 2011; 205(6):518-25.
81. Schwärzler P, Concin H, Bösch H, Berlinger A, Wohlgenannt K, Collins WP, et al. An evaluation of sonohysterography and diagnostic hysteroscopy for the assessment of intrauterine pathology. Ultrasound Obstet Gynecol. 1998; 11(5):337-42.
82. Shankar M, Lee CA, Sabin CA. von Willebrand disease in women with menorrhagia: a systematic review. BJOG. 2004;111:734-40.
83. Shokeir TA, Shalan HM, El-Shafei MM. Significance of endometrial polyps detected hysteroscopically in eumenorrheic infertile women. J Obstet Gynaecol Res. 2004; 30(2):84-9.
84. Shutter J, Wright TC. Prevalence of underlying adenocarcinoma in women with atypical endometrial hyperplasia. Int J Gynecol Pathol. 2005; 24(4):313-8.
85. Singh N, Hirschowitz L, Zaino R, Alvarado-Cabrero I, Duggan M, Ali-Fehmi R, et al. pathologic prognostic factors in endometrial carcinoma (other than tumor type and grade). Int J Gynecol Pathol. 2019;38:S93-113.
86. Stewart EA, Laughlin-Tommaso SK, Catherino WH, Lalitkumar S, Gupta D, Vollenhoven B. Uterine fibroids. Nat Rev Dis Primers. 2016;2:16043.
87. Taran FA, Tempany CM, Regan L, Inbar Y, Revel A, Stewart EA, MRgFUS Group. Magnetic resonance-guided focused ultrasound (MRgFUS) compared with abdominal hysterectomy for treatment of uterine leiomyomas. Ultrasound Obstet Gynecol. 2009; 34(5):572-8.
88. Taran FA, Weaver AL, Coddington CC, Stewart EA. Characteristics indicating adenomyosis coexisting with

leiomyomas: a case-control study. Hum Reprod. 2010; 25(5):1177-82.
89. TaranFA, Weaver AL, Coddington CC, Stewart EA. Understanding adenomyosis: a case control study. Fertil Steril. 2010; 94(4):1223-28.
90. Templeman C, Marshall SF, Ursin G, Horn-Ross PL, Clarke CA, Allen M, et al. Adenomyosis and endometriosis in the California Teachers Study. Fertil Steril. 2008; 90(2):415-24.
91. Timmermans A, Gerritse MB, Opmeer BC, Jansen FW, Mol BW, Veersema S. Diagnostic accuracy of endometrial thickness to exclude polyps in women with postmenopausal bleeding. J Clin Ultrasound. 2008; 36(5):286-90.
92. Torres WE, Sones PJ Jr, Thames FM.Ultrasound appearance of a pelvic arteriovenous malformation. J Clin Ultrasound. 1979; 7(5):383-5.
93. Tosti C, Troìa L, Vannuccini S, Lazzeri L, Luisi S, Petraglia S. Current and future medical treatment of adenomyosis. J Endomet Pelvic Pain Disord. 2016;8:127-35.
94. Urbanska E, Hirnle L, Olszanecka-Glinianowicz M, Skrzypulec-Plinta V, Skrzypulec-Frankel A, Drosdzol-Cop A. Is polycystic ovarian syndrome and insulin resistance associated with abnormal uterine bleeding in adolescents? Ginekol Pol. 2019;90(5):262-9.
95. Van den Bosch T, Ameye L, Van Schoubroeck D. Intra-cavitary uterine pathology in women with abnormal uterine bleeding: a prospective study of 1220 women. Facts Views Vis Obgyn. 2015;7:17-24.
96. van Dijk MM, van Hanegem N, de Lange ME, Timmermans A. Treatment of women with an endometrial polyp and heavy menstrual bleeding: a levonorgestrel-releasing Intrauterine device or hysteroscopic polypectomy? J Minim Invasive Gynecol. 2015; 22(7):1153-62.
97. Vannuccini S, Luisi S, Tosti C, Sorbi F, Petraglia F. Role of medical therapy in the management of uterine adenomyosis. Fertil Steril. 2018; 109(3):398-405.
98. Van Voorhis BJ, Dawson JD, Stovall DW, Sparks AE, Syrop CH. The effects of smoking on ovarian function and fertility during assisted reproduction cycles. Obstet Gynecol. 1996; 88(5):785-91
99. Venturella R, Miele G, Cefalì K, Lico D, D'Alessandro P, Arduino B, et al. Subcutaneous progesterone for endometrial polyps in premenopausal women: a preliminary retrospective analysis. J Minim Invasive Gynecol. 2019; 26(1):143-7.
100. Vercellini P, Viganò P, Somigliana E, Daguati R, Abbiati A, Fedele L. Adenomyosis: epidemiological factors. Best Pract Res Clin Obstet Gynaecol. 2006; 20(4):465-77.
101. Vogelzang RL, Nemcek AA Jr, Skrtic Z, Gorrell J, Lurain JR. Uterine arteriovenous malformations: primary treatment with therapeutic embolization. J Vasc Interv Radiol. 1991; 2(4):517-22.
102. Wang CJ, Yen CF, Lee CL, Soong YK. Laparoscopic uterine artery ligation for treatment of symptomatic adenomyosis. J Am Assoc Gynecol Laparosc. 2002; 9(3):293-6.
103. Wang PH, Liu WM, Fuh JL, Cheng MH, Chao HT. Comparison of surgery alone and combined surgical-medical treatment in the management of symptomatic uterine adenomyoma. Fertil Steril. 2009; 92(3):876-85.
104. Whitaker L, Critchley HO. Abnormal uterine bleeding. Best Pract Res Clin Obstet Gynaecol. 2016;34:54-65.
105. Wildt L, Kissler S, Licht P, Becker W. Sperm transport in the human female genital tract and its modulation by oxytocin as assessed by hysterosalpingo- scintigraphy, hysterotonography, electrohysterography and Doppler sonography. Hum Reprod Update 1998;4:655-66.
106. Wood C. Adenomyosis: difficult to diagnose, and difficult to treat. Diagn Ther Endosc. 2001; 7(2):89-95.
107. Yamashita M, Matsuda M, Mori T. In situ detection of prolactin receptor mRNA and apoptotic cell death in mouse uterine tissues with adenomyosis. In Vivo. 1999; 13(1):57-60.
108. Yu L, Wu T, Spain J, Li X, Wang W. Uterine artery embolization for the treatment of adenomyosis: questions for long-term efficacy. J Vasc Interv Radiol. 2012; 23(3):430-2.

LONG QUESTION

1. Define AUB and classify it. Discuss the evaluation and the management options in PMS.

SHORT QUESTIONS

1. Describe the PALM-COEIN classification of AUB.
2. Discuss the pathophysiology of DUB.
3. Discuss the medical management of AUB.

MULTIPLE CHOICE QUESTIONS

1. All are anatomical pathologies in the PALM-COEIN classification, except:
   a. Leiomyoma b. Endometrial cancer
   c. Coagulopathy d. Polyp
2. Unclassified AUB can be caused by a variety of uncommon conditions, except:
   a. Arteriovenous malformations
   b. Adenomyosis
   c. Myometrial hyperplasia
   d. Endometritis
3. The heavy menstrual blood flow is quantified as is:
   a. 50 mL b. >80 mL
   c. 10–80 mL d. <5 mL
4. Drug of choice for von Willebrand disease is:
   a. OCPs b. Tamoxifen
   c. Desmopressin d. IV iron
5. In relation to "luteal out of phase" or "LOOP" cycles the following statement is false:
   a. Primarily caused by oligo/anovulation
   b. Due to irregular development of a new preovulatory follicle during the prior luteal phase
   c. Occur during the mid-to-late menopause transition
   d. They are most frequently observed during periods of irregular menstruation

Answers

1. c 2. b 3. b 4. c 5. a

9.5 HEAVY MENSTRUAL BLEEDING: UTERINE CONSERVATIVE SURGERY

Anuradha Khanna, Shikha Sachan

BACKGROUND AND DEFINITION

Heavy menstrual bleeding (HMB) is the complaint of 40% of women in reproductive age group visiting a gynecological OPD and is an important cause of morbidity in women eating into their day to day life activities.[1] HMB is known to impact many women's lives as 60% of women who visit the gynecologist with this complaint will ultimately end up in hysterectomy within 5 years.[2] Medical therapy, which is safe effective and noninvasive and is often the first-line treatment started is often preferred by many women over surgery. Various options for treatment like long trusted nonsteroidal anti-inflammatory drugs, antifibrinolytics, hormones, and newer treatment options like intrauterine devices are available. The appropriate choice of medical therapy depends on age of patients, their plans for future fertility, coexisting medical comorbidities, patient preference, long-term cost of therapy.[2]

Heavy menstrual bleeding can be defined as a complaint of heavy cyclical menstrual blood loss of abnormal quantity, duration, or schedule, over several consecutive menstrual cycles in a woman of reproductive years, or more objectively, a total menstrual blood loss of > 80 mL per menstruation.[3] It can also be defined as excessive menstrual blood loss that interferes with a woman's physical, social, emotional, or material quality of life. However, the International Federation of Genecology and Obstetrics (FIGO) formally defines HMB as "the woman's perspective of increased menstrual volume, regardless of regularity, frequency, or duration", and a women intolerance to bleeding is starting point for initiation of treatment rather than objective proof of blood loss.

In 2007, FIGO introduced System 1, with standardized definitions and concise terminology for abnormal uterine bleeding (AUB). Menorrhagia, metrorrhagia, and oligomenorrhea were replaced with the nomenclature HMB, intermenstrual bleeding, and unscheduled bleeding or breakthrough bleeding (BTB) on hormone medication. The FIGO System 2 proposed the PALM-COEIN (polyp; adenomyosis; leiomyoma; malignancy, and hyperplasia; coagulopathy; ovulatory dysfunction; endometrial; iatrogenic; and not yet classified) classification system with a view to standardize methods for investigation and categorization of the various potential etiologies for AUB. The FIGO systems for nomenclature of symptoms of normal and abnormal uterine bleeding (AUB) in the reproductive years (FIGO AUB System 1) and for classification of causes of AUB (FIGO AUB System 2; PALM-COEIN) were first established together in 2011 and revised in 2018.

Abnormal Uterine Bleeding-P: Polyps

Endometrial polyps are one of the most common etiologies of abnormal genital bleeding in both premenopausal and postmenopausal women. These are usually formed due to hyperplasia of endometrial glands and stroma that project from endometrium. Women with polyps often present with HMB, intermenstrual bleeding, or postcoital bleeding. Symptoms do not correlate with the number, diameter, and site, which are further used to subclassify polyps. In premenopausal age group around 80% will have symptoms whereas usually they are symptom free in postmenopausal patient where they might be associated with cervical polyps in one fourth of the cases.

Polyps are often best diagnosed by ultrasound, saline infusion sonography, hysteroscopy, and it is often good to exclude malignancy, which is associated with 0–4.8% of cases.

Abnormal Uterine Bleeding-A: Adenomyosis

Uterine adenomyosis is a condition in which endometrial glands and its stroma are found ectopically in myometrium, which leads to myometrial hypertrophy. Some consider it as a type of endometriosis. It is one of the important causes of dysmenorrhea in late reproductive age group, with prevalence ranging from 5 to 70%. The sonographic appearance of adenomyosis is that of myometrial hypertrophy, and presence of heterotopic endometrial tissue in the myometrium. For the diagnosis of adenomyosis in PALM-COEIN classification system a sonographic criterion based on transvaginal sonography is Morphological Uterus Sonographic Assessment (MUSA) group, which suggest eight criteria for the diagnosis. Two-dimensional transvaginal ultrasonography, although considered inferior by some, has shown comparable sensitivity and specificity to MRI for the diagnosis of adenomyosis.

Abnormal Uterine Bleeding-L: Leiomyoma

Uterine leiomyomas, which are also known as fibroids or myoma are benign monoclonal tumors of smooth muscle cell. They are most common tumors of pelvis and usually present with symptoms of heavy menstrual bleeding and/or pelvic pain/pressure/backache. In the subclassification used by FIGO presence or absence of leiomyomas and their no is reflected by primary classification system, regardless of the location and size. Submucous leiomyomas (SM) being more symptomatic are differentiated from others (O) in secondary system. Categorization of the intramural and subserosal leiomyomas is included in the tertiary classification system; it also includes the category of parasitic lesion.

There was still some confusion in subclassification and hence FIGO updated 2018 guidelines, which provides more detailed and clear picture for differentiation amongst the leiomyoma subtypes. Type 0,1,2,3 are submucous leiomyomas classified according to their protrusion in endometrial cavity and their contact with endometrium, the difference between type 3 and 4 is done by hysteroscopy with lowest filling pressure. Intramural location is characteristic of types 4 and higher, with distinction between Type 4 and 5 being made by the amount of serosal distortion as seen in USG and MRI. Subclassification also describes the peduncle or stalk of Type 0 and 7 as having a stalk whose diameter is 10% or below that than the mean diameter of the leiomyoma.

Estimation of total uterine volume based on imaging (transvaginal or transabdominal or MRI) or clinical examination (if imaging is not available) as well as the number of leiomyomas (1, 2, 3, 4, or greater than 4) are used in describing leiomyomas. When TVS or MRI are available, the estimated volume of up to 4 leiomyomas and their location (anterior, posterior, left, right, or center) should be recorded.

Abnormal Uterine Bleeding-C: Coagulopathy

Systemic disorders of hemostasis, which impair coagulation, are included in this category. The presentation group for this category is usually adolescence. Most common etiologies are Von Willebrand's disease (10%) most common, platelet dysfunction, factor XI deficiency, factor X deficiency. The coagulopathy screening history incudes HMB since menarche, history of PPH, surgery-related bleeding, bleeding associated with dental work, family history of bleeding symptoms, history of epistaxis, or bruises.

Women using anticoagulants are now not included in this category but the Iatrogenic category (FIGO 2018 revision).

Abnormal Uterine Bleeding-O: Ovulatory Dysfunction

Ovulatory dysfunction occurs when a normal ovulatory cycle of a woman is disturbed with presentation ranging from minimal and less frequent ovulation, to episodes of extreme HMB which is often unpredictable and may require extreme interventions. The usual etiologies are adolescent immaturity of HPA axis, polycystic ovarian syndrome, hypothyroidism, anorexia, weight loss, hyperprolactinemia, obesity, extreme exercise, menopause transition, or mental stress.

Abnormal Uterine Bleeding-E: Endometrial

It is a diagnosis of exclusion. It is postulated that local hemostasis at the level of endometrium is disturbed with increase in local plasminogen activators and vasodilators-prostaglandin E2 and prostacyclin I2 and decreased local production of vasoconstrictors- endothelin-1 and prostaglandin F2. The condition can also be due chronic inflammation as in tubercular and chlamydial infections.

Abnormal Uterine Bleeding-I: Iatrogenic

There are many medical treatment, inert devices, which are used as a treatment for AUB due to their mechanism of action or side effects impact endometrium, blood coagulation, or disrupt ovulatory cycle. Drugs causing irregular bleeding by directly inhibiting ovulatory cycle are cyclic or continuous progesterone, OCPs, gonadal steroid therapy (e.g., gonadotropin-releasing hormone analogues, aromatase inhibitors, selective estrogen receptor modulators, selective progesterone receptor modulators). Other drugs are systemic agents that interfere with dopamine metabolism, e.g., tricyclic antidepressants (amitriptyline and nortriptyline) and phenothiazines and anticoagulation agents like warfarin, heparin, and low molecular weight heparin, rivaroxaban. Anticonvulsants and antibiotics, e.g., rifampicin and griseofulvin.

Abnormal Uterine Bleeding-N: Not Otherwise Classified

Some causes of HMB are poorly defined as arteriovenous malformations, myometrial hypertrophy, chronic endometritis. These disorders would be identified or discovered by Doppler studies or various biochemical/molecular biology assays.

MEDICAL TREATMENT

It offers the benefit of being noninvasive and not being associated with surgical morbidity and mortality. It can be individualized according to patient's needs, comorbidities and etiology. Disadvantagcs arc long-term therapy, recurrence of symptoms after stoppage, and cost of extended therapy.

Various options available are described in **Table 1**.

Medical treatment for HMB is used mostly for symptomatic relief rather than permanent cure with more propensity for side effects, and a significant number of women (approximately 60–65%) who had medical treatment would become unsatisfied and will resort to surgical treatment by 2 years. Uterine conservative surgeries offer the advantage of being less invasive, minimal side effect, preservation of uterus, and better long-term relief of symptoms.[7]

One Stop Management

This is considered beneficial for patient in terms of number of visits and compliance. It includes investigating the patient by taking key history, examination, TVS, power Doppler and hysteroscopy and planning its treatment if indicated in same visit. Most of the uterine conservative surgeries can be planned for one stop management of patients.

TABLE 1: Comparison between the benefit and side effect of various drug used in medical therapy of heavy menstrual bleeding.

Drug	*Specific benefits*	*Adverse benefits*
LNG-IUS	Contraception No need of tablets	Menstrual cramps Expulsion IMB
Oral progesterone Days 5–25	Regular cycles	Bloating, moody, PMS, nausea
Tranexamic acid	None	Nausea, diarrhea, headache
NSAIDs	Relieve dysmenorrhea, headaches	Nausea, breast tenderness, headache
OC	Contraception Relieve dysmenorrhea and PMS	Weight gain, acne, hot flushes, bloating, moody, PMS
Danazol	None	

(Guidelines for the management of heavy menstrual bleeding - New Zealand, 1998)

Various uterine conservative surgeries for treatment of HMB are:

Dilatation and Curettage

It is a very old method wherein a diagnostic procedure of endometrial biopsy was coupled with a therapeutic curettage for the relief of HMB. It is associated with risks of anesthesia and possible complications like laceration of the cervix and uterine perforation. Use of D&C as diagnostic tool has been considered questionable by many as it is a blind procedure. However, D&C is known to have a role when symptoms of HMB persist and the endometrial biopsy is in conclusive. Pipelle aspirator can be used for a less painful procedure **(Fig. 1)**.

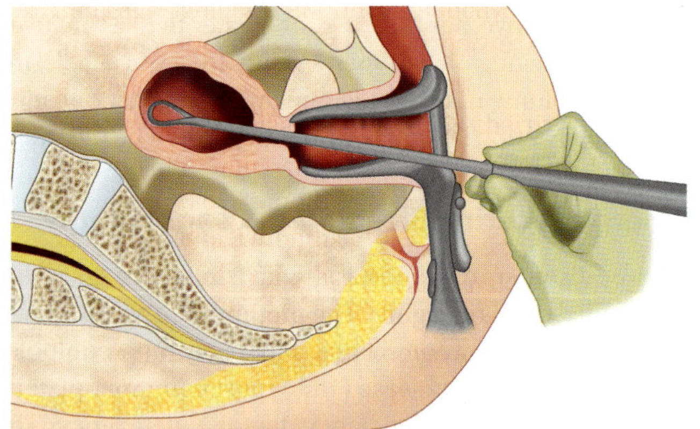

Fig. 1: Dilatation and curettage.

Endometrial Destruction or Ablation (Fig. 2)

Endometrial destruction procedures or ablative procedures best when no other gynecological condition is involved. They are more convenient and less invasive and decrease hospital stay and recovery time. The different energy sources, which are used to destroy the endometrium, are all considered equally effective in mitigating the symptoms and recurrence ranges from 0 to 38.2%, this rate was observed to be higher in women under the age 35 years when they were followed for longer duration. The first-generation techniques fare better than hysterectomy when compared in terms of cost, but the second-generation endometrial destruction techniques are costly. However, these ablative techniques have fewer incidences of intraoperative complications and take less operative time.[8]

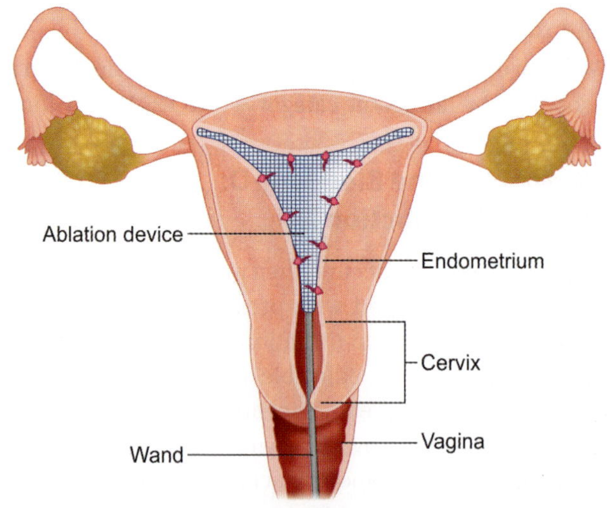

Fig. 2: Endometrial ablation.

In simple words, endometrial ablation refers to surgical destruction of the functionally active endometrium along with endometrial glands, which is approximately 4–6 mm deep, depending upon the stage of the menstrual cycle. These procedures are especially suitable for women who have no desire for future fertility, but want to preserve their uterus and want a less invasive alternative to hysterectomy. NICE recommends that in women with HMB alone who have a uterus of size 10 weeks or less, endometrial ablation should be the preferred over surgical hysterectomy. With time data from many randomized trials is now available for both first and second generation ablative techniques, making their usage in medical practice truly evidence-based. Comparisons of these techniques have been made with treatments which were earlier offered like hysterectomy, medical treatments including Mirena. Newer emerging ablative techniques require shorter time frame and sometimes do not need the prerequisite of cervical dilatation.

First-generation ablative techniques include hysteroscopic procedures where destruction or ablation of the uterine endometrium and 5 mm of the superficial myometrium is performed under direct visual guidance. A resectoscope is usually used in appropriate nonionic fluid medium (usually glycine where monopolar diathermy is used) for distension of uterine cavity. These techniques were very popular in 90s with transcervical resection of endometrium and roller ball endometrial ablation most popular techniques. The three common *first generation techniques* are discussed here:

Transcervical resection of endometrium (TCRE): TCRE involves resecting endometrium under visual guidance of an operative hysteroscope (resectoscope) using an electrosurgical loop of 3 mm. A monopolar blend current at 80–100 W is used to resect the endometrium and superficial myometrium. Inert glycine is used as distension media, which provides a clear view of the uterine cavity. Alternatively, bipolar energy source resectoscopes, which have minimum risk of transmission of current and have the advantage of using normal saline rather than glycine and thus avoiding the side effects of glycine overload and transurethral resection syndrome. However, when normal saline is used as distention media in the presence of heavy bleeding the surgical field is compromised as blood mixes easily with normal saline. As the procedure is done under visual guidance it can also be used for simultaneous treatment of polyps and fibroid and for taking endometrial biopsy if any suspicious lesion emerges. It requires a certain level of skill from surgeon to avoid complications associated with it **(Fig. 3)**.

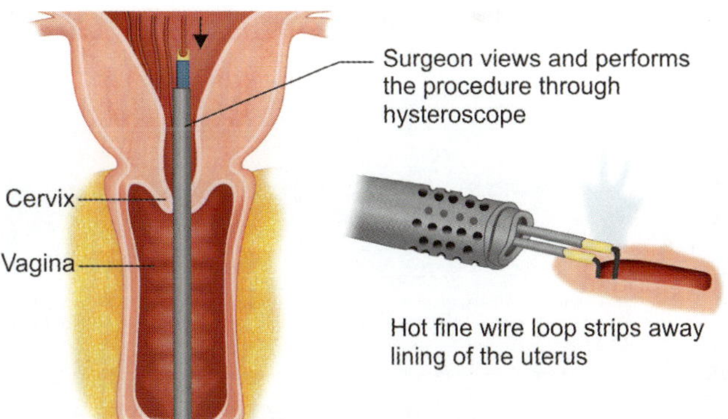

Fig. 3: Transcervical resection of endometrium.

Rollerball endometrial ablation: This procedure uses a roller ball electrode in place of a loop introduced through the resectoscope to ablate the endometrium and causes endometrial and superficial myometrial destruction up to 5 mm depth but it does not removes the tissues. The advantage of using a roller ball is that varied level of endometrium can be ablated by moving the roller ball faster or slower, so it can be safely used in areas where myometrium is relatively thin such as previous cesarean section scar or at cornua. It can be used alone or in combination with TCRE. The outcome of both TCRE and roller ball ablation are comparable but rate of complications are more with TCRE. Repeat endometrial ablations, if undertaken are recommended to be done by roller ball under direct vision **(Fig. 4)**.

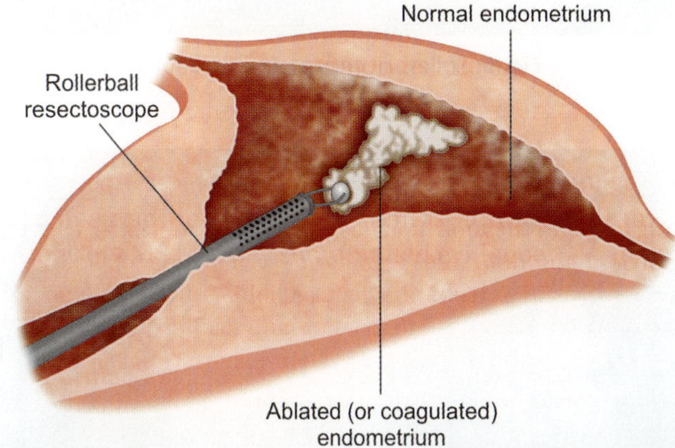

Fig. 4: Technique of endometrial ablation.

Endometrial laser ablation: In this technique Nd: YAG laser energy is used to precisely ablate the endometrium. A 600-micrometre flexible quartz fiber is inserted down the operating channel of the hysteroscope that transmits Nd: YAG laser energy to the endometrium. The power used ranges from 50 to 80 W and normal saline is used as distention media. A bare fiber dragging technique is used to draw furrows in the endometrium until the entire endometrial cavity is systematically treated.[5,6] There is high-operating cost for the procedure and it takes relatively longer operative time and hence the procedure is not widely used **(Figs. 5 to 7)**.

SECOND-GENERATION TECHNIQUES

Techniques belonging to second-generation ablation have an advantage that they do not require exceptional surgeon skill but a basic skill and are safe and easy to perform. With exception of hydrothermal ablation, they are not done under direct vision. These techniques involve destruction of endomyometrium using different energy modalities. Prerequisite for using second generation techniques are uterine size not more than 12 weeks and submucous fibroids less than 3 cm in size. A preinsertion hysteroscopy is usually performed, which documents ostia and condition of uterine cavity.

Thermal Balloon Ablation

This ablative procedure involves usage of a silicone balloon with a catheter filled with hot liquid circulating at high pressures which ablates the endometrium. There are four different choices of thermal balloon systems available:

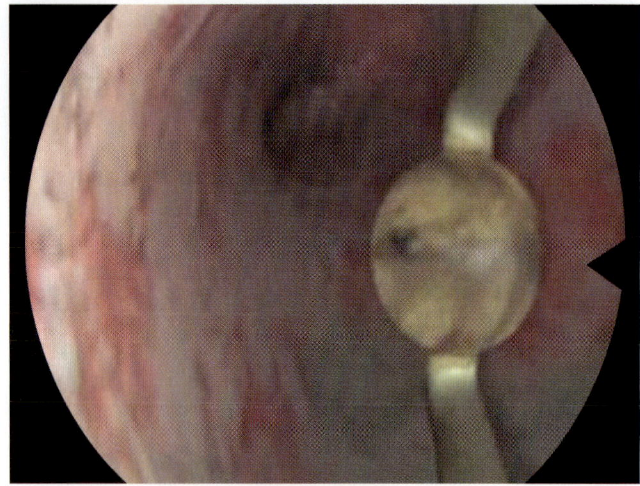

Fig. 5: Rollerball endometrial ablation.

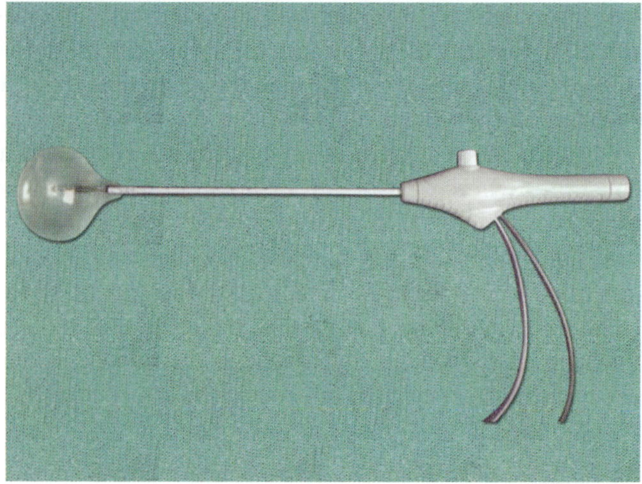

Fig. 8: Thermachoice.

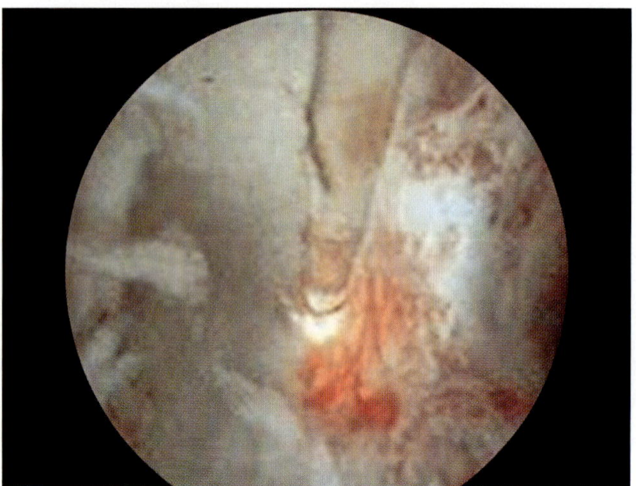

Fig. 6: Endometrial laser ablation.

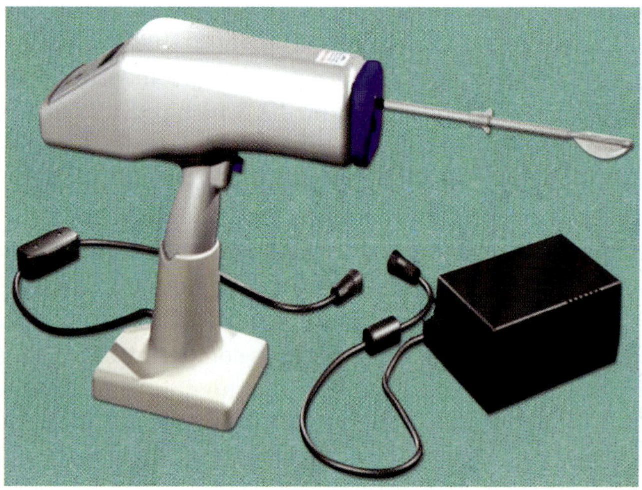

Fig. 9: Thermablate EAS.

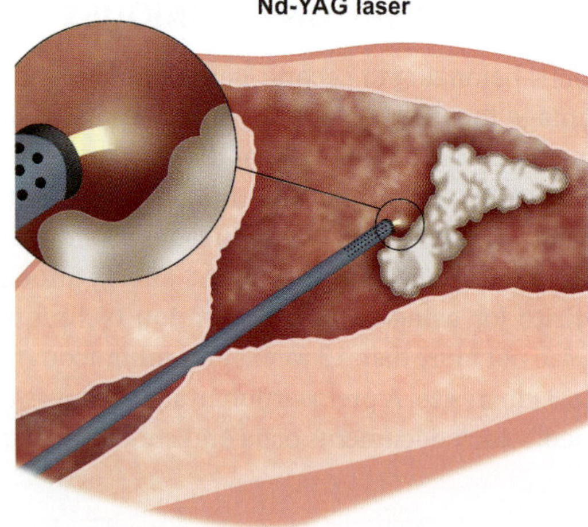

Fig. 7: Nd: YAG laser ablation of the endometrium.

1. Gynecare thermachoice[9] III Uterine Balloon Therapy System **(Fig. 8)**
2. Cavaterm™ **(Fig. 10)**
3. Thermablate Endometrial Ablation System™ (EAS™) **(Fig. 9)**
4. Menotreat balloon

Both Themachoice III and Cavaterm™ use 5% dextrose at temperatures of 87°C (pressure 160–180 mm Hg) and 78°C (pressure 230–240 mm Hg), respectively.[5,6] The Menotreat balloon is a relatively newer device that employs circulating heated saline at 85°C and a pressure of 200 mm Hg. The Thermablate EAS™ is another thermal balloon device, which uses glycerin at 173°C with pressure maintained at 220 mm Hg.[5,6] The treatment cycle for all these devices varies between 2 and 10 minutes, with the Thermablate EAS™ having the shortest treatment cycle.[5,6] The high temperature with high pressure causes immediate blistery, blanched effect leading to endovascular coagulation, followed by subsequent fibrosis and nonfunctional endometrium.[10] As the procedure involves relaxation and expansion of uterus during the treatment cycle, this decreases intra balloon pressure, which has been shown to affect clinical outcomes.[11-13] To maintain a sustained pressure

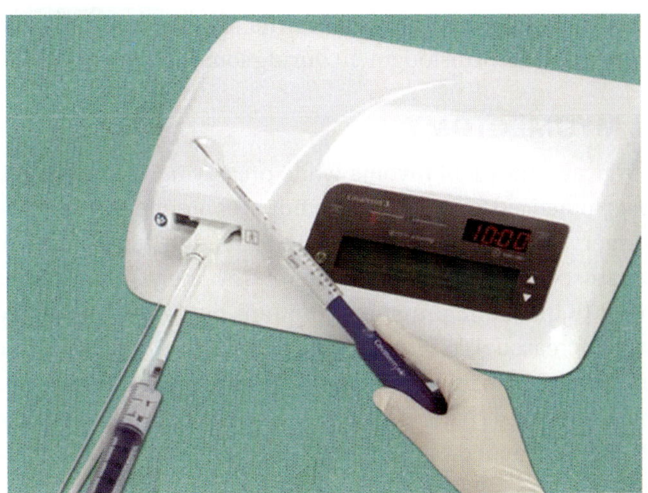

Fig. 10: Cavaterm.

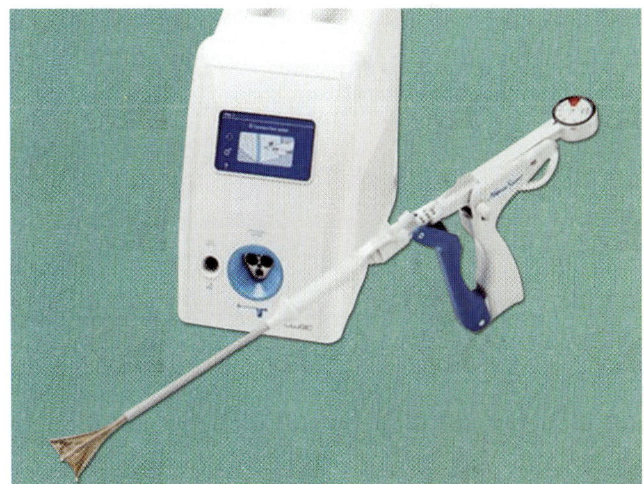

Fig. 11: Bipolar radiofrequency endometrial ablation.

therefore, additional fluid is injected. The newer devices like Menotreat and the Thermablate EAS^{TM} maintain a constant pressure through their inbuilt pressure sensors.[5,6] However, these procedures are not recommended, if there is history of previous classical cesarean section or myomectomy where endometrial cavity was breached.

Bipolar Radiofrequency Endometrial Ablation

Bipolar radiofrequency Novasure **(Fig. 11)** is known to deliver radiofrequency energy till the tissue impedance reaches 50 ohms in the endometrium. Novasure comprises of an electrode array that conforms to shape and size of uterine cavity. An inbuilt cavity integrity test is done before using carbon dioxide (CO_2) to rule out any perforation or leak. Procedure usually takes a time of 90–120 seconds.[5,6] The depth of endometrium ablated is determined by the impedance achieved by radiofrequency and it is usually up to the level of the superficial myometrium. No endometrial preparation is required bit a cervical dilatation of 8 mm is required for insertion of the device.[5,6]

Hydrothermal Ablation (Fig. 12)

It is performed under direct hysteroscopic vision. Heated saline at 90°C is circulated in the uterine cavity causing endometrial ablation. To avoid vaginal burns a tight seal at the cervix is recommended. To perform effectively uterine cavity should be from 6 to 10.5 cm. This is the only second generation, which has the advantage of being performed under direct vision and can be used to treat irregular uterine cavities with fibroids (intramural fibroids less than 4 cm or with intracavity fibroids). GnRH analogs are sometimes given before the procedure to induce endometrial thinning, which increases the cost of treatment and side effects.

Microwave Endometrial Ablation (Fig. 13)

Microwave endometrial ablation (MEA) is a 9.2 GHz, 30 watt, microwave system. After its insertion in endometrial cavity

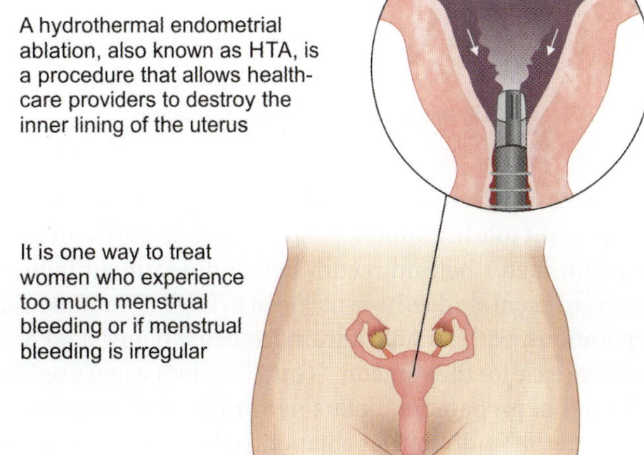

Fig. 12: Hydrothermal endometrial ablation.

it will produce a tissue temperature of 75–85°C at a depth of 6 mm. This destroys the functional endometrium but to create a uniform temperature the device is moved from cornu to cornu and across the lower uterine segment. The probe of the device is reusable. It is recommended to have a preprocedure hysteroscopic evaluation of the endometrial cavity. It was reported that microwave energy can cause bowel burn even without uterine perforation and hence it is recommended that a minimum thickness of 10 mm endometrium is necessary for the procedure.

Role of Endometrial Preparation, Preoperative Hysteroscopy, and Endometrial Biopsy

There was a time when before performing an ablative technique endometrial preparation was done by giving pretreatment with GnRH analogs, progesterone, and danazol. The idea behind it was that these treatments will thin the endometrium, which will give a better view during the procedure and will also lead to full-thickness destruction of the endometrium along with superficial myometrium till

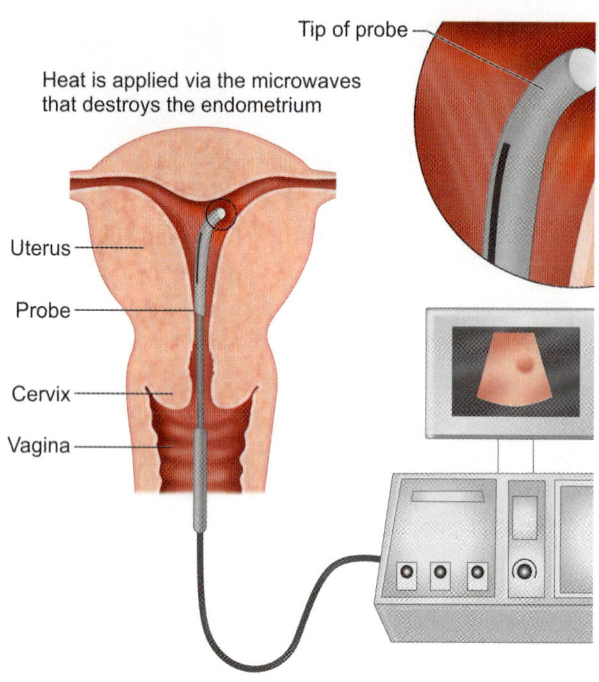

Fig. 13: Microwave endometrial ablation.

5 mm. This will destroy basal endometrial glands, which play an important role in endometrial regeneration and hence are the major factor behind recurrence and treatment failure. However, recent studies have not been in favor of endometrial preparations, with its only advantage being better field and operative ease for the surgeon.[14] GnRH analogs when used for endometrial preparation before performing first-generation techniques of endometrial ablation reduced the operating time and thus fluid absorption but increased the resistance at cervix, therefore making difficult dilatation.[15] There is not much benefit when pretreatment was used with second generation techniques albeit a higher incidence of adverse effects was noted.[14]

The biggest nightmare in a patient who undergoes ablation is when a proper workup for endometrial hyperplasia and malignancy has not been done before the procedure. Endometrial atypia has to be excluded before an ablative procedure. If not done before, a pipelle or soft suction biopsy can be done before starting ablative procedure. Curettage is not recommended for the same obtained at the time of ablation, but not by curettage. If preoperative hysteroscopy reveals suspicious endometrium, doubts about the integrity of the cavity, or if endometrial cavity is not reached, then ablative procedure is to be abandoned and if required a biopsy is taken.

Contraception after Endometrial Ablation

Pregnancy following ablation is associated with significant maternal and fetal. The incidence reported is 0.7%. Many recommend addition of tubal sterilization before the procedure but it is associated with increased surgical time and morbidity. Postprocedure permanent contraception can avoid such complications. Essure system sterilization was used in many patients 3 months prior to procedure, but it has increased risk of dislodgment during some of the procedures.

MYOMECTOMY

Surgical removal of myoma while preserving the uterus has been practiced from time immemorial as uterine conservative surgery. Myomectomy can be performed by laparotomy or laparoscopy. It leads to definite improvement in symptoms of HMB, pain and pressure symptoms but is also associated with increased risks of anesthesia and surgery. Pregnancy rate are increased in infertile women but subsequent pregnancies have increased chances of uterine rupture especially if uterine cavity is breached.

Laparoscopic Myomectomy

Laparoscopic procedures are associated with shorter hospital stay, reduced postoperative pain, and adhesions. When compared with laparotomy, it has comparable operating times and pregnancy rates with reduced febrile morbidity, decreased blood loss. Laparoscopic route is especially suitable for subserous and intramural fibroids. With time there has been improvement in laparoscopic skills of suturing, the microsurgical techniques and the development of electric morcellators, which are more efficient many big myoma can be removed by laparoscopy. However, care should be taken for complete tissue retrieval from the peritoneal cavity and the suturing of the defect left in uterine wall especially after removal of a deep intramural fibroid. Recurrence is claimed to be higher and earlier after Laparoscopic myomectomy which is due to the lack of tactile sensation during surgery and hence the small fibroids are not detected and removed. Proper patient selection, investigation and surgeon's skill can reduce this risk.

Laparoscopic-assisted Myomectomy (LAM)

Laparoscopic-assisted myomectomy involves in addition to laparoscopy a 5 cm suprapubic minilaparotomy incision, which helps in breaking up of the big fibroid and aiding its complete removal. It also offers better repair of the uterus in layers. It has all the advantages of laparoscopy with reduced operating time and better closure of uterine defect. This leads to decreased risk of uterine dehiscence in future pregnancies. Maximum benefits are in fibroids, which are greater than 5 cm in diameter, deep intramural, which require uterine closure in layers and where the primary indication for surgery is infertility.

Vaginal Myomectomy

In this procedure, depending on the position and the bulk of the fibroids an anterior or posterior colpoomy is done. The uterus is manipulated till the fibroid is approached through colpotomy site and a incision is made over it, after dissection the fibroid is removed intact or in pieces by morcellation.

The maximum number of fibroids are removed and then the uterus, which has decreased in bulk is delivered through the colpotomy incision and uterine defects are closed in layers. Blood loss is reduced due to the tourniquet effect of ante flexing or retroflexing the uterus to deliver it to the colpotomy. A higher degree of skill in vaginal surgery is required by the surgeon, to perform this procedure.

Hysteroscopic Resection of a Fibroid

Transcervical hysteroscopic resection of submucous fibroid (TCRF) is reserved for the treatment of submucous fibroids. The most important factors that influence outcome are the position of the fibroid (Type 0 are easily removed) and the size. Factors such as the age, number, and size of the individual fibroids also influence the outcome. Immediate complications of the procedure are bleeding requiring transfusions, uterine rupture, conversion to laparotomy, emergency hysterectomy, and pulmonary edema. Long term complications include formation of uterine synechiae (Aschermann's syndrome) and rarely rupture of uterus in future pregnancies. Advancement in the field like use of miniature bipolar resectoscope, which can easily negotiate the cervix without its dilation and using physiological saline as a distending medium, which reduces the chances of fluid overload. Because of its high intensity of energy, electrode tip produces vaporizing effects and no resection chips are produced.

Reduction in the Size of Fibroids

Uterine Artery Embolization (UAE)

This is a radiological procedure where under fluoroscopic guidance uterine artery is cannulated through femoral artery puncture and an embolic agent is introduced. Unilateral or both the uterine artery are embolized depending upon the site, size, and number of fibroids. Embolic agents, which have been used are polyvinyl alcohol beads, gelatin sponge and trisacryl plastic spheres. PVA particles with platinum coils have been used to prolong the duration of fibroid ischemia. This procedure involves exposure to a radiation dose of approximately 20cGy. Complications of this procedure though rare are postembolization syndrome, pain, and sepsis. Pain is the most common which responds to nonsteroidal anti-inflammatory agents, narcotic analgesia, antiemetics, and rarely requires admission. This technique however is most suitable to cases when there is a single large fibroid. Some of the late complications reported are vaginal fibroid expulsion, Laparotomy and resection of bowel due to sepsis from subserous fibroid, ovarian compromise, and amenorrhea.

Laparoscopic Bipolar Coagulation of the Uterine Blood Vessels

This procedure involves bipolar coagulation of the sites where anastomosis happens between uterine and ovarian arteries. It has been touted as an alternative to bilateral UAE with initial results showing benefits similar to UAE, but the safety and efficacy of the procedure are still being evaluated. The procedure involves isolating uterine artery from the ureter and the internal iliac artery and then desiccating it by using bipolar electrosurgery. Potential side effects are postoperative pain and infection.

Laparoscopic Myolysis (Fig. 14)

Myolysis consists of causing coagulation necrosis in the substance of the fibroid resulting in denaturation of collagen and vascular damage thereby causing shrinkage of the fibroid and reducing the chances of regrowth. Sources of energy that have been employed have been lasers, electrosurgery and cryotherapy. Myolysis can be achieved using high power, such as 80 W or low power in the region of 3–10 W. The laser fiber is introduced in to the center of the fibroid, activated, and then withdrawn to the serosal surface. This is repeated at distances of 5–7 mm. A 41% mean decrease in fibroid diameter was seen after 6 months that persisted to 1 year. The main disadvantage however of this procedure was the operating time and a 10–50% incidence of postoperative adhesions to the serosal scars many of them being dense and involving bowel. Electro surgical bipolar needles, which reduce operating time.

Cryomyolysis

Cryomyolysis is a process which consists of introducing a probe (cryoprobe) into the interstitium of fibroid and freezing it to the temperature of –180°C, this creates an ice ball in the tissues surrounding it. It is then thawed and several cycles of this are repeated. Results were not encouraging in terms of decrease in fibroid size (6%) but the decrease in size was maintained over time. Postoperative adhesions were a significant long-term complication.

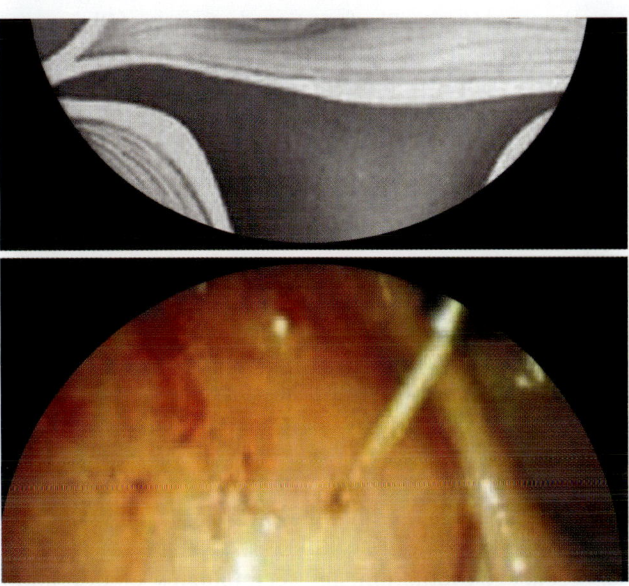

Fig. 14: Laparoscopic myolysis.

Interstitial Laser Photocoagulation

Low power (wavelength 830 nm, maximum output 20 W) laser beams, which are generated by placing laser fiber in the fibroid core. These beams generate heat in the interstitium and melt away the fibroid. Care is taken during placement and activation so as to have minimal damage to normal myometrium and serosal surface. The process professes theoretically minimal postoperative adhesion and uterine damage. Not much pain was associated with the procedure and a mean volume reduction of 47% was obtained at 1 year. Pressure effects of large fibroids were relieved by this method.

KEY MESSAGES

- Medical treatment offer symptomatic relief but have to be used for long term and also give rise to significant side effects.
- Uterine conservative surgeries offer the advantage of offering cure for long time along with minimal side effects.
- First generation endometrial ablative procedure require a skilled surgeon.
- Second generation endometrial ablative procedure take less time and can be done after a proper training.
- Preprocedure hysteroscopy should be performed before the procedure.
- Myomectomy and procedures reducing the size of myoma are the procedure to be contemplated in women having infertility in addition.
- UAE, myolysis, cryomyolysis and uterine artery coagulation are newer techniques with more researches needed to know their long-term effects.

REFERENCES

1. Vilos GA, Lefebvre G, Graves GR; Clinical Practice Gynaecology Committee Members; Reproductive Endocrinology Infertility Committee members. Guidelines for the Management of Abnormal Uterine Bleeding. Canada: Society of Obstetricians and Gynaecologists of Canada; 2001.
2. RCOG. Clinical Practice Guidelines Management of Menorrhagia. London: RCOG; 1998–2001.
3. Hallberg L, Bengtsson C, Garby L, Lennartsson J, Rossander L, Tibblin E. An analysis of factors leading to a reduction in iron deficiency in Swedish women. Bull World Health Organ. 1979;57(6):947-54.
4. Cooper K, Saraswat L. Surgical management of heavy menstrual bleeding: part 2. Obstet Gynaecol. 2017;19:101-8.
5. Saraswat L, Cooper K. Surgical management of heavy menstrual bleeding: part 1. Obstet Gynaecol. 2017;19:37-45.
6. Irvine GA, Cameron IT. Medical management of dysfunctional uterine bleeding Baillieres. Best Pract Res Clin Obstet Gynaeco. 1999;13(2):189-202 .
7. Marjori banks J, Lethaby A, Farquhar CM. Surgery versus medical therapy for heavy menstrual bleeding. Cochrane Database Syst Rev. 2003;2:CD003855.
8. Agence d'évaluation des technologies et des modes d'intervention en santé (AETMIS). Endometrial ablation techniques in the treatment of dysfunctional uterine bleeding. Report prepared by Chantale Lessard and Alicia Framarin. (AETMIS 02-04 RF). Montréal: AETMIS; 2002. pp. xxxi-166.
9. Vilos GA, Aletebi FA, Eskander MA. Endometrial thermal balloon ablation with the Therma Choice system: effect of intrauterine pressure and duration of treatment. J Am Assoc Gynecol Laparosc. 2000;7:325-9.
10. Lok IH, Leung PL, Ng PS, Yuen PM. Life-table analysis of the success of thermal balloon endometrial ablation in the treatment of menorrhagia. Fertil Steril. 2003;80:1255-9.
11. Reid PC. Endometrial ablation in England: coming of age? An examination of hospital episode statistics 1989/1990 to 2004/2005. Eur J Obstet Gynecol Reprod Biol. 2007;135:191-4.
12. Cromwell DA, Mahmood TA, Templeton A, van der Meulen JH. Surgery for menorrhagia within English regions: variation in rates of endometrial ablation and hysterectomy. BJOG. 2009;116:1373-9
13. Tan YH, Lethaby A. Pre-operative endometrial thinning agents before endometrial destruction for heavy menstrual bleeding. Cochrane Database Syst Rev. 2013;(11):CD010241.
14. Cooper KG, Pinion SB, Bhattacharya S, Parkin DE. The effects of the gonadotrophin releasing hormone analogue (goserelin) and prostaglandin E1 (misoprostol) on cervical resistance prior to transcervical resection of the endometrium. Br J Obstet Gynaecol. 1996;103:375-8.
15. Kumar V, Chodankar R, Gupta JK. Endometrial ablation for heavy menstrual bleeding. Women's Health. 2016;12(1):45-52.

LONG QUESTIONS

1. What is the FIGO classification of the etiology of heavy menstrual bleeding (HMB)? Discuss with pros and cons of the classification.
2. Discuss the first generation endometrial ablation techniques and compare them to the second generation techniques.
3. What are the surgical options for managing HMB by conservative surgery without hysteroscopy? What are the benefits and problems of the various techniques to do so?

SHORT QUESTIONS

1. What is the definition of heavy menstrual bleeding (HMB) as given by FIGO?
2. What are the structural causes of HMB?
3. What is the One-Stop concept of managing HMB?
4. What are the criteria for selecting a woman to have an endometrial ablation procedure for HMB?
5. Compare and contrast various hysteroscopy-based endometrial ablation techniques.
6. What is microwave endometrial ablation?
7. What is cryomyolysis?

MULTIPLE CHOICE QUESTIONS

1. Regarding heavy menstrual bleeding (HMB) which of the following is true?

a. Investigations should be initiated when the hemoglobin is lower than a defined value for a population
b. The definition of HMB is a loss of more than 30 mL per day
c. A woman's perception of blood loss is the main determinant of starting treatment
d. HMB is a physiological event

2. The following is true about endometrial polyps:
a. Intermenstrual or postcoital bleeding is a typical feature
b. They are malignant in 75% of women
c. They are associated with endometrial atrophy
d. All women with endometrial polyps should undergo hysterectomy

3. The following is included in AUB-N:
a. Endometrial polyp b. Adenomyosis
c. Endometrial cancer d. Myometrial hyperplasia

4. The following is true about endometrial ablation techniques:
a. The depth of endometrial destruction is 15 mm
b. First generation techniques are hysteroscopy-based techniques
c. Second generation techniques have a longer learning curve than first generation techniques
d. Hysterectomy provides a faster recovery than endometrial ablation techniques

5. Regarding transcervical resection of the endometrium (TCRE), the following is true:
a. It is a second generation ablation technique
b. Destruction of endometrium is to a depth of 4 to 6 mm
c. After the procedure, fertility is not affected
d. Monopolar current is used with normal saline distension

6. The following are types of thermal balloon ablation techniques, except:
a. Hydrothermal ablation b. Cavaterm
c. Thermachoice d. Thermablate

7. The following second generation endometrial ablation technique requires hysteroscopy:
a. Therablate b. Cavaterm
c. Novasure d. Hydrothermal ablation

Answers

1. c 2. a 3. d 4. b 5. b 6. a 7. d

9.6 FIBROID UTERUS

PC Mahapatra, Nitin Raithatha

INTRODUCTION

The uterine muscle is prone to forming benign neoplasms. This extremely common condition has been given various names such as fibroids, myomas, leiomyomas, solid uterine tumor, and many others over the years.[1] The prevalence of fibroids varies with age and ethnicity and depending on the population studied, varies from 5 to 65%. Women in the reproductive age group and of African ethnicity have a high prevalence of fibroids. Most, if not all, fibroids will regress after menopause.[2] The study of fibroids is a vast subject. Recent advances are mind-boggling when it comes to refinements in imaging, medications, minimally invasive surgery, and conventional surgery. The challenge for the clinician is to select the right approach of care for the woman that suits her medical condition and affords her choice.

ETIOLOGY

Fibroids are benign, estrogen-dependent tumors. They arise from the myometrial smooth muscles as monoclonal tumors. Over the last five decades, a number of theories have been proposed to expain their origin. In modern times, molecular studies have shown the importance of specific driver mutations and substantial changes in the microenvironment of the extracellular matrix (ECM). This is accompanied by changes in growth factors, cytokine signaling, and other biochemical and molecular variations which enhance fibroid growth.[3, 4] The etiopathogenesis is illustrated in **Figure 1**.

FIBROID GROWTH

The origin, growth rate, and symptomatology of fibroids vary from woman to woman and also from fibroid to fibroid in the same woman. Growth is hormone dependent and women in the reproductive age group will show some fibroid growth. In a majority of women, the growth is slow and most tumors remain indolent over long periods of time. Relatively rapid growth is seen in about one third of fibroids. When hormone levels decline, fibroids shrink. This occurs after delivery and after menopause. 7–40% of fibroids will regress in 3–36 months after delivery. After menopause, fibroids are expected to shrink. When the growth pattern varies (i.e., rapid growth of fibroids or a fibroid that grows after menopause), the clinician should keep the possibility of malignant change in mind. This is an extremely rare event.[4-6]

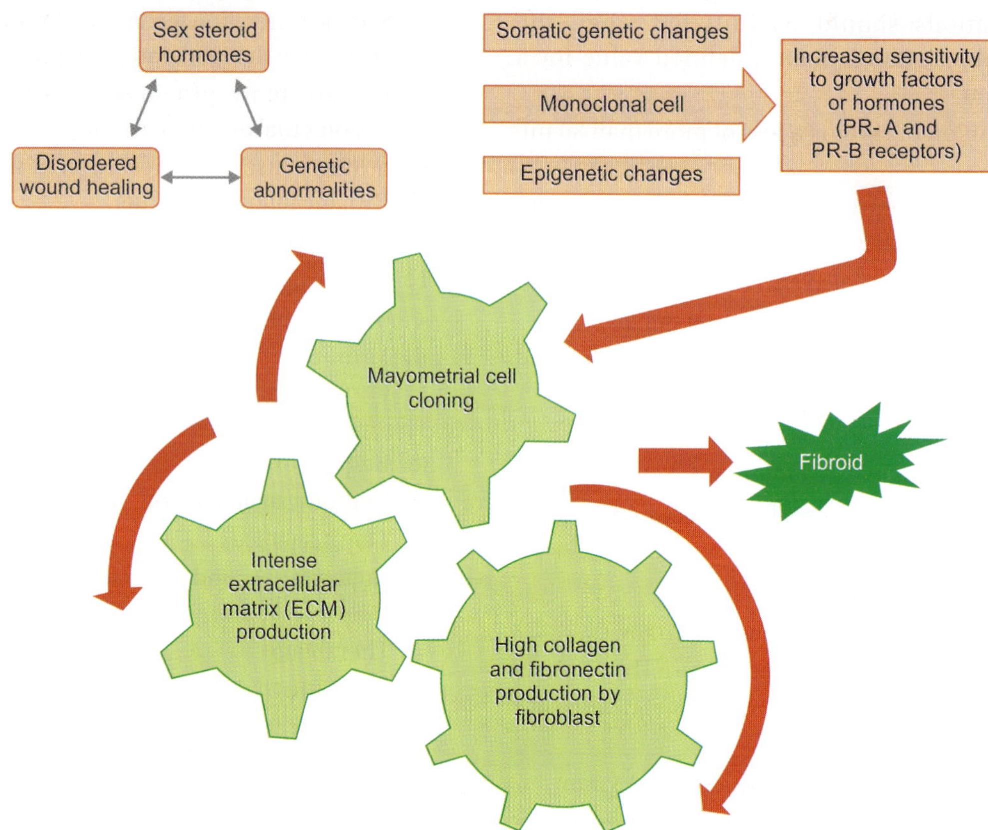

Fig. 1: Etiopathogenesis of fibroid.

The growth of the fibroid leads to an increase in volume. The available blood supply is then lower than the tissue requirement and this leads to some degenerative changes. An acute degenerative change may be seen in the form of red degeneration, necrosis, infection, and hemorrhage. Chronic degenerations are cystic, hyaline, atrophy, calcifications, fatty, or myxomatous in nature.[7,8]

EPIDEMIOLOGY AND RISK FACTORS

The prevalence of fibroids has increased over the years. This could be due to a number of factors such as:

- More estrogen exposure in the lifetime of a woman due to fewer pregnancies and childbirths
- Higher environmental estrogen exposure in modern times
- Health awareness
- Better imaging allowing higher rates of detection

It is difficult to determine the exact prevalence of a condition as ubiquitious as fibroids. Studies on epidemiology have cohorts of varying natures. Prevalence rates differ by population. These populations could be asymptomatic women undergoing health screening, symptomatic women, different diagnostic criteria and modalities, histopathological studies, or event autopsy reports.[3]

Age and race have the biggest role to play in prevalence rates. Fibroids are tumors of the reproductive age group. They are uncommon in adolescence or after menopause. Women of African origin have a higher prevalence of fibroids. They also have more and larger fibroids and the age of onset is earlier than Caucasian, Asian, or women from Latin America. First-degree relatives have a risk 2.5 times higher than the general population.[1-3] The major risk factors have been outlined in **Table 1**.[1-3, 9-12]

CLASSIFICATION

Fibroids are classified by their location in the uterus. A number of studies have been done to optimize such classification, with significant variation. The European Society of Gynecological Endoscopy (ESGE) and the Canadian Task Force have more specific classifications which directly impact management. However, they are limited in their scopes. In recent times, the FIGO (2011) classification is well-accepted globally. It is based on location, penetration of the myometrium, and encroachment of the uterine cavity. It allows for fibroid mapping and description of multiple fibroids in the same uterus. The types of fibroids are illustrated in **Figures 2A and B**.[1,3,9]

CLINICAL PROFILE

A large majority of women remain asymptomatic with myomas. They may be incidental findings on health screening or "well-woman check ups". The range of symptoms attributable to fibroids is vast, can be severe, and can affect the woman's quality of life. The symptomatology seems to depend more on location, the relationship of the fibroid to the endometrium,

TABLE 1: Risk factors for fibroids.

Age	• Higher prevalence in reproductive age group • Women younger than 35 years have faster growth of fibroids compare to those older than 45 years
Race	• African women have greater prevalence, larger fibroids, and more numerous fibroids • African women have faster growth and higher recurrence rates
Menstrual pattern	Early menarche and late menopause are associated with higher prevalence of fibroid
Obstetric history	• Late conception is associated with higher incidence • Higher the parity lower, the incidence as postpartum remodeling leads to apoptosis of small lesion
Anthropometry	Obesity—high BMI associated with increase risk of fibroid
Lifestyle	Women with sedentary lifestyles have higher prevalence than those with regular physical activity
Smoking	Reduces the risk in some studies , while other studies find no difference
Aelchohol and Caffeine	• Alchohol—particularly beer increases risk of fibroids • High consuption in younger age have minor increased risk
Diet	• Red meat increases in dietary glycemic index, porducts with marine omega 3 fatty acid increase chances of fibroids • Green vegetables, citrus food, dairy products, vitamin D-rich food reduces risk of fibroid
Endocrine abnormalities	• Prenatal exposure of DES can increase fibroid risk • Environmental estrogen exposures (phtalates, polychlorinated biphenyl, and bisphenol A) are associated with increased risk of fibroids
Contraception	• COC pills do not increase risk of fibroid if started after adulthood. Earlier consumption of COC may be associated with higher prevalence of fibroids. • Progesterone only depot preparation reducess fibroid growth
Infection	Do not play a role
Genetics	Familial tendency is associated with chromosomal mutations called chromothripsis.

(BMI: body mass index; COC: combined oral contraceptive; DES: diethylstilbestrol)

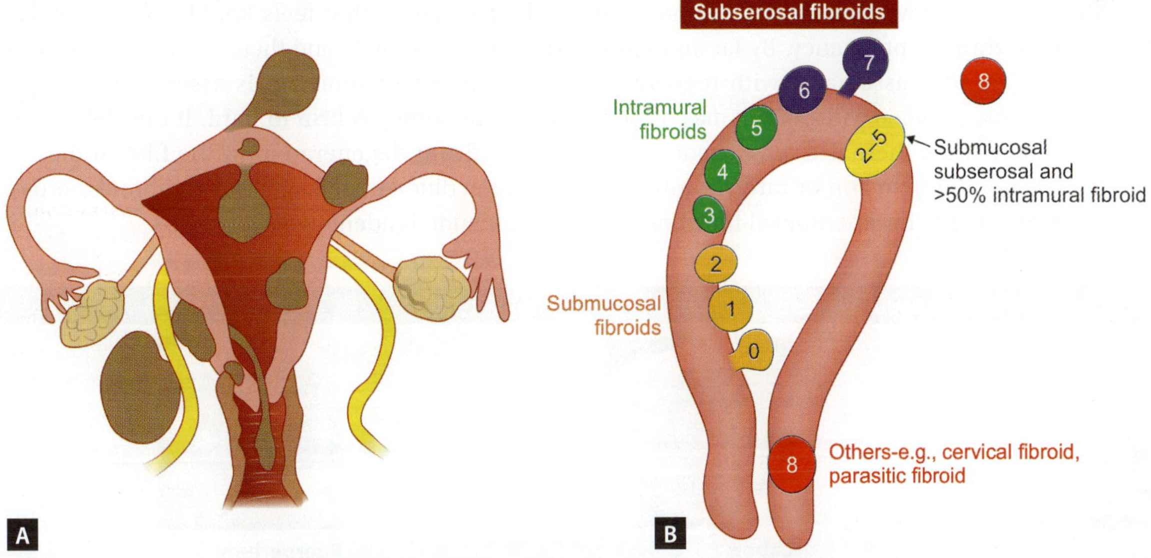

Figs. 2A and B: Types of fibroids and FIGO (2011) classification of leiomyoma. (FIGO: International Federation of Gynecology and Obstetrics)

and growth rather than size. The symptoms and their salient features are enumerated here:

- *Menstrual disturbances:* In general, these occur when the endometrium is disturbed by an endometrial polyp, submucus fibroid, or an intramural fibroid distorting the cavity. Heavy menstrual bleeding (HMB) is due to increase in vascularity and surface area as well as altered uterine contractility. Submucus fibroids may cause intermenstrual bleeding. Fibroids that are emerging out of the cervix can cause postcoital bleeding. Postmenopausal bleeding may be a presenting feature of a submucus fibroid; however, it merits investigation to rule out malignancy.

- *Lump in abdomen:* Women may present with a sense of fullness, heaviness in the pelvis, palpable mass, or bloating. This is usually seen with large subserous fibroids. Cervical and broad ligament fibroids also tend to grow to a large size.
- *Pain:* Usually, fibroids are not a painful pathology. However, a woman may experience spasmodic dysmenorrhea. The pain is cramping and of a colicky nature. Chronic pain can be due to a large fibroid, compression of other organs, or associated adenomyosis or endometriosis.
- *Pressure effects:* Large fibroids may compress the viscera, nerves, and vessels in the pelvis. Anterior fibroids may cause urinary complaints including dysuria, retention of urine, or incontinence. Posterior fibroids may occasionally cause constipation. Compression of vessels and lymphatics may result in pedal edema. Nerve compression is unusual, but may present with sharp, shooting pelvic pain.
- *Infertility:* Fibroids are an unusual cause of infertility. Unless the fibroid is very large, or distorts the endometrial cavity significantly, or is located largely in the cavity, infertility should be regarded as unrelated to the fibroid.
- *Reproductive events and fibroids:* **Table 2** shows the various effects of fibroid on pregnancy. Most fibroids do not affect the pregnancy outcome. Some complications may arise as outlined. Pregnancy may also demonstrate fibroids. Most fibroids show some initial enlargement and then stabilize through pregnancy. By far and large, the postpartum period is associated with regression. Occasionally, pregnant women with fibroids may present with an emergency when there is a red degeneration, rapid cystic degeneration, torsion or rarely, rupture of a capsular vein leading to intraperitoneal bleeding and hemoperitoneum. A submucus lower segment fibroid, especially a pedunculated one, may get expelled.
- *Associated conditions:* The woman presenting with fibroids may also have associated gynecological conditions such as adenomyosis and endometriosis. She may also have comorbidity as a result of the effects of the fibroid in the form of anemia. There is a higher prevalence of obesity and depression in these women.[10-12]

NATURAL HISTORY

The natural history of fibroids varies. Just as the symptomatology, the natural history depends to a large extent on the fibroid location.

- Submucus fibroids are more likely to be symptomatic and detected at a small size. Women present early in the course of the pathology with menstrual complaints. They are also likely to affect reproductive life. A long-standing submucus fibroid in a postmenopausal woman can cause chronic inversion. This is an uncommon event.
- Intramural fibroids usually grow to a significant size (5 cm or more) before they cause symptoms. The symptoms are usually of heavy bleeding or pain.
- Subserous fibroids usually do not cause symptoms unless they are large in size. They remain undetected and asymptomatic. for a long time.

DIAGNOSIS

Clinical examination (abdominal and pelvic) will reveal an enlarged uterus that feels knobby and irregular. Usually, the uterus is mobile and there is no tenderness unless there is significant endometriosis associated with the fibroid. The consistency is firm to hard. It may be soft when there is significant degeneration in the fibroid mass. The most common differential diagnosis of a fibroid uterus on clinical examination is adenomyosis.

TABLE 2: Effects of fibroid on reproductive life of a woman.[3,5,8]

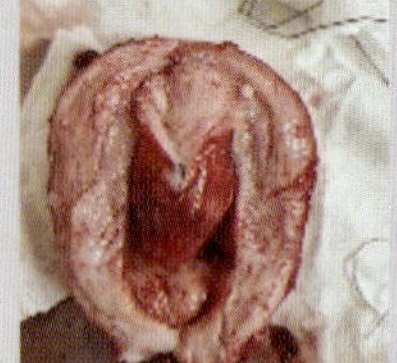	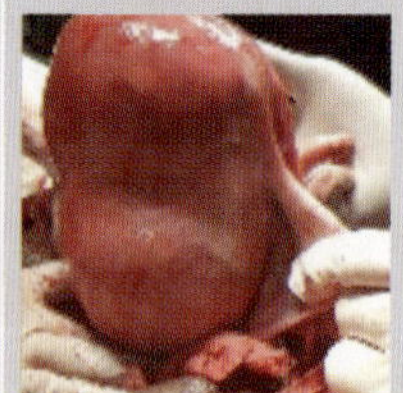	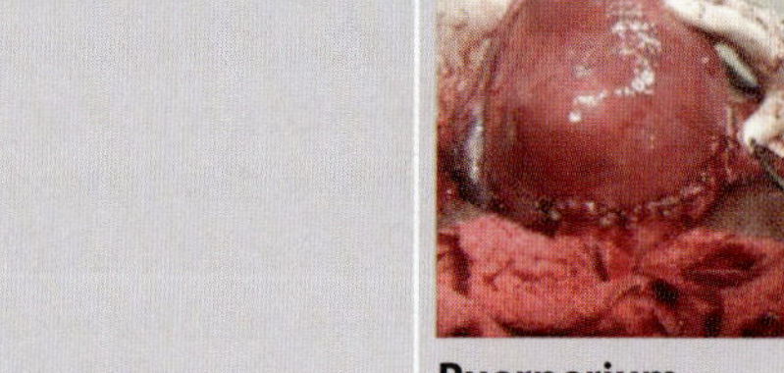
Pregnancy • Infertility • Implantation failure • Abortion • Pressure symptoms • Malpresentation • Torsion • Ectopic pregnancy • Placenta previa	**Labor** • Preterm Labor • Malpresentation • Uterine inertia • Dystocia • Obstruction • PPH • Increased operative intervention • MRP	**Puerperium** • Secondary PPH • Inversion • Subinvolution • Puerperal sepsis

(MRP: manual removal of the placenta; PPH: postpartum hemorrhage)

Imaging is widely available today and is routinely used to confirm the diagnosis. The standard imaging of choice is a pelvic ultrasound, preferably by the transvaginal route. High-end ultrasound machines are excellent tools to diagnose and characterize the fibroid. The fibroid appears as a well-defined, circumscribed, variegated mass. Depending on the type and degree of degeneration, appearances may vary. Fibroid mapping is a crucial element of planning treatment, especially surgical interventions. Characteristics that should be reported are the size, number, location, extension outside the uterus and compression of viscera, and relation to the endometrium.

There can be significant interobserver variations. Guidelines, such as the International Society of Ultrasound in Obstetrics and Gynecology endorsed the Morphological Uterus Sonographic Assessment (MUSA) consensus statement (2015), are useful to standardize reporting, improving the quality of diagnosis and enhancing counseling and surgical planning.[13] Reporting should include the above-mentioned characteristics and assessment of the size of the uterus and junctional zone are also desirable. The guideline suggests a Doppler evaluation and 3D mapping if facilities are available. Reporting with a diagrammatic representation is a useful adjunct.[14] There may be a learning curve and such detailed reporting may be tedious. However, it has an important part to play in surgical planning and preventing surprises on the operation table.

Other ultrasound-based modalities such as saline infusion sonography are simple procedures which can enhance visualization and characterization of the uterine cavity. New modalities such as strain ratio elastography (SE) may have value in understanding fibroid degeneration.[15]

In some situations, ultrasound falls short of the diagnostic standard. There may be confusion in the diagnosis. Magnetic Resonance Imaging (MRI) is useful in these circumstances. It helps to clarify the pathology when there is a difficulty in differentiating between a fibroid and an adenomyoma. Unusual tumors such as smooth muscle tumors of uncertain malignant potential (STUMP), leiomyosarcomas, and ovarian fibromas are better characterized by MRI. These tumors may be mistaken as degenerative changes in a fibroid. MRI is useful to study the relationship of the fibroid to other pelvic viscera.[16]

Hysteroscopy is the gold standard to treat endometrial and submucus fibroids. However, in modern gynecology, there is no role for only diagnostic hysteroscopy. These lesions are amenable to correction by hysteroscopic surgery and interventions should be planned accordingly.[17]

MANAGEMENT OF FIBROIDS

The management of fibroids is a complex subject due to the vast number of options available. It is useful for the practitioner to have a logical and generally conservative approach when managing this situation. There are a number of factors to be considered when treatment plans are made in the management of a fibroid **(Table 3)**.

The arrays of choices are mentioned in **Table 4**. It is unreasonable to discuss every management option with every woman with fibroids. However, the clinician should be aware of the various options. These choices should be offered with clinical judgment and with an understanding of the infrastructure and expertise at hand. In offering treatment to a symptomatic woman, it should be reasonably ascertained that the symptom is due to the fibroid and that the fibroid is not an incidental finding which may drain resources and time with no therapeutic benefit to the woman.

EXPECTANT MANAGEMENT OF FIBROIDS

It is desirable and reasonable to manage most fibroids without intervention. This is especially true for fibroids that are incidentally diagnosed. The ideal fibroids for expectant management are:

- Which do not cause symptoms or minimal symptoms that do not disrupt quality of life
- Those which are small to moderate sized
- Mural or subserous in location
- In perimenopausal women

Periodic assessment of symptoms, associated comorbidities (anemia), and fibroid characteristics (volume, location) should be done. Other modalities should be offered when there is a change in circumstances such as new-onset symptoms or significant change in fibroid size or nature.

TABLE 3: Factors to be considered in planning management of fibroids

Factors related to the woman	*Factors related to the fibroid*	*Factors related to healthcare settings*
Age	Location of the fibroid	Availability of different modalities
Desire to retain menstrual and/or reproductive function	Other characteristics such as number, degenerative changes	Surgical training and expertise
Symptoms, extent to which quality of life is affected	Associated gynecological conditions such as enometriosis	Financial considerations
General health status		
Personal choice and belief		

TABLE 4: Available options for fibroid management.[18]

Expectant management	• Suitable for a significant proportion of fibroids • Fibroids should be kept under surveillance
Medical magnagement for symptoms	• Correction of anemia • Management of pain by appropriate analgesics • Management of heavy bleeding by non hormonal medications (NSAIDs, and antifibrinolytic such astranexamic acid) or hormonal medications (progesteone, combined oral contraceptive pills, LNG IUS)
Medical magnagement that reduce fibroid size	• Androgens (danazol) • GnRH agonist depots • SPRM—selective progesteron receptor modulator- mifepristone, ulipristal acetate • SERM—selective estrogen receptor modulator • Aromatase inhibitors— letrozole and anastrazole
Interventional radiology	• Uterine artery embolization • MRgFUs/HIFU • Radiofrequency volumetric thermal ablation (RFVTA)
Surgical management	• Vaginal occlusion of uterine artery • Myomectomy—conventional, laparoscopic, hysteroscopic , robotic • Hysterectomy—conventional, laparoscopic, robotic • Laparoscopic radiofrequency volumetric thermal ablation (RFVTA) • Endometrial ablaton

(GnRH: gonadotropin-releasing hormone; HIFU: high-intensity focused ultrasound; LNG-IUS: levonorgestrel-intrauterine system; MRgFU: magnetic resonance-guided focused ultrasound; NSAIDs: nonsteroidal anti-inflammatory drugs; SERM: selective estrogen receptor modulator; SPRM: selective progesterone receptor modulator)

MEDICAL MANAGEMENT OF FIBROIDS

Fibroids can be managed medically but are usually cured only surgically. This dictum should be kept in mind when counseling and setting expectations at the initial stages of fibroid management. The rationale for medical management of fibroids to provide symptom relief is as follows:

- Fibroids are benign tumors in general and rarely cause emergency situations.
- Surgery may need to be scheduled at a later date if the woman is unfit and her medical condition needs to be optimized (treatment of anemia that results from fibroid-related bleeding or control of medical conditions that may co-exist such as hypertension or diabetes).
- Surgery may not be the optimal choice for women who have recurrent fibroids or are close to menopause.
- Some women may not want to be operated for personal reasons.

The following selection criteria are desirable in selecting women for medical therapy:

- There is a need to treat the fibroid and the symptoms are ascribable to the fibroid.
- Small to moderate sized.
- Mural or subserous location.
- The woman is counseled about the process, is compliant and can accept a failure of medical therapy as a possible outcome.

Medical Therapy to Control Heavy Bleeding

Heavy bleeding can be controlled by a number of non hormonal and hormonal medications. Each have their pros and cons. Hormonal medications can be used after ruling out contraindications for their use, particularly if the preparation contains estrogen. Most oral preparations are meant for acute control of bleeding. The usual horizon for therapy is 3–6 months. It is not possible to sustain oral medical therapy for longer periods for most women. Long-term control of bleeding can be achieved by non oral routes such as injectables [Gonadotropin-releasing hormone (GnRH analog depots, depot medroxy progesterone - DMPA depots, and levonorgestrel intrauterine systems - (LNG IUS)].

Nonsteroidal Anti-inflammatory Drug

Nonsteroidal anti-inflammatory drugs (NSAIDs) can be looked upon as sole therapy for control of pain and bleeding or as adjuvant to other medical treatment options. They inhibit the cycloxygenase enzyme and reduce prostaglandin reduction. These in turn, will reduce pain and bleeding. NSAIDs are easily available, cheap, and have a good safety profile for short-term use. Some options are mefenamic acid, ibuprofen, and naproxen. They are less effective than hormonal medications in control of bleeding. Gastrointestinal side effects are a limitation of this therapy.

Tranexamic Acid

It is nonhormonal option to control heavy bleeding related to fibroid by virtue of its antifibrinolytic activity and procoagulation property. It reduces blood loss and prevents fibrin destruction at plasminogen receptor site. According to the Cochrane review, there is a 40–50% reduction in blood loss.[19] Tranexamic acid has minimal side effects. Bleeding control effect increases when used with other medical management.

Combined Estrogen + Progesterone Therapy

It was most commonly used option to control heavy bleeding with fibroids.[20,21] Oral contraceptive pills are easily available and affordable. They also function as effective contraception if the couple so desires. Other options of route for delivering combined estrogen and progesterone are the transdermal patch and vaginal ring. Contraindications to the use of estrogen should be ruled out before embarking on treatment with this option.

Progesterone-only Therapy

Progesterone therapy is a logical step in treating an estrogen-dependent tumor such as fibroid. There is a downregulation of both estrogen and progesterone receptors in the fibroid and this leads to remodulation. Overall, there is a reduction in the endometrial thickness and reduction in blood loss, but no significant change in fibroid size. In general, progesterone has a better safety profile than combined hormonal preparations. Progesterone can be delivered orally in the form of medroxyprogesterone acetate tablets (20–30 mg/day in dividend doses) or norethisterone acetae tablets (5–15 mg/day in divided doses). It can be also administered as a depot injection of medroxyprogesterone acetate, which also provides contraception. There may be breakthrough bleeding with progesterone therapy and the woman should be duly counseled.

Levonorgestrel Intrauterine System

If there is no significant cavity distortion, the LNG IUS is a suitable choice to deliver progesterone to the uterus. The effects are mainly local in the endometrium and to some extent on the myometrium and there is negligible systemic absorption. It is very effective for the management of bleeding related to fibroids.[22] It also functions as a long-acting reversible contraceptive (LARC). Some studies show small reductions in uterine volume and fibroid size, but this is not consistent. It is a minimally invasive, long-term symptom-based solution and is a popular method.

Medical Therapy for Symptom Control and to Reduce Fibroid Size

Some medical therapy options have been studied which reduce fibroid size and control symptoms. Many authorities look upon them as a "cure" for fibroids. However, the reduction in size is usually temporary. The fibroid tends to grow back sooner or later and symptoms also return when the life of the drug runs out.

Androgens (Danazol)

Danazol is a 17-alpha ethinyl testosterone molecule. It inhibits gonadotropin release and occupies the androgen receptors. It causes a 20% shrinkage in fibroid size. It is moderately effective in symptom control. However, this option is no longer popular due to the side effects of androgenization in the woman.

Gonadotropin-releasing Hormone Analogs

Gonadotropin-releasing hormone analogs may be agonists or antagonists. The GnRH agonists are typically used in depot form for the management of fibroids. GnRH antagonists are less studied and are available only as daily preparations.

The main benefits of GnRH analogs is symptom control, improvement in quality of life, and rise in hemoglobin level. They reduce fibroid size temporarily and relieve pressure symptosm and can favorably affect the route of surgery, taking it to a less invasive option.[18, 20, 21]

They act by desensitization and downregulation of GnRH receptors. They inhibit cell proliferation and induce apoptosis. The fibroid shrinks as a result of this. The shrinkage is to the extent of 30–50%, but is temporary. Fibroids return to their earlier size within 6 months of cessation of treatment.

Gonadotropin-releasing hormone analogs are limited by their cost, side effects, and duration of usage. Side effects include sudden onset of menopause, like symptoms such as hot flushes, sweating, dizziness, and headaches. Duration is limited to 3–6 months. Long-term usage can result in bone loss. To manage side effects and avoid bone loss, add-back therapy with estrogens may be considered.

The GnRH agonist molecules are goserelin, triptorelin, and leuprolide acetate for injectable depot forms. Nasal sprays such as nafarelin and buserilin are also available for daily use but may not be practical. GnRH antagonists are used in daily injectable form of cetrorelix and ganirelix. Recently, oral GnRH antagonists have been studied. These are elagolix and relugolix. They are under research and can be options in the future with estrogen add-back therapy for long term use.

Selective Progesterone Receptor Modulators

A number of agents which block progesterone receptors are available. The ones which have been studied widely in the management of fibroids are mifepristone (RU-486, the abortion pill), ulipristal acetate (UPA), and asoprisnil.

These drugs block the estrogen and progesterone receptors in the tumor. There is a loss of cellularity and deceleration of growth. The result is a shrinkage of the fibroid and control of symptoms. There is a 30–50% shrinkage of the fibroid volume over a course of treatment of 3–6 months. The shrinkage is more sustained than that observed with GnRH agonists.[23]

The side effect profile is generally favorable and menopausal symptoms are uncommon. There is no significant reduction in bone density. The commonly reported side effects are gastrointestinal upset and bloating. Ulipristal has potential for liver toxicity. It is a rare event but may be severe enough to need a liver transplant.[24] There may be endometrial hyperplasia with long-term selective progesterone receptor modulator (SPRM) use.

Ulipristal is used in a dose of 5–10 mg. Recent studies have looked at intermittent therapy over a long term and there is a significant number of women who can avoid a hysterectomy with this approach.[23] Mifepristone is used in a daily dose of 10–25 mg for 3–6 months. The formulation has recently become available in India.

Selective Estrogen Receptor Modulators

Estrogen receptor modulation can also result in fibroid shrinkage. The options available are fulvestrant, ormeloxifene and raloxifen. Fulvestrant is less effective than GnRH agonists.[25] Most studies show some effectiveness in fibroid shrinkage and symptom control. Ormeloxifene can cause ovarian cyst formation, which are temporary and benign.

Aromatase Inhibitors

Aromatase inhibitors such as letrozole, anastrazole, and fadrazole act on aromatase P450 enzyme and prevent conversion of androgens to estrogen. This results in a hypoestrogenic environment. This could lead to fibroid shrinkage. Some trials have reported such results.[26] They may be options for medical management after more research and comparative studies.

INTERVENTIONAL RADIOLOGY FOR FIBROID MANAGEMENT

Interventional radiology has opened up a new vista in the management of fibroids. It can be looked upon as a minimally invasive option between medical and surgical therapy. The purpose of radiological interventions is to reduce or block the blood supply to the fibroid (uterine artery embolization – UAE or uterine fibroid embolization – UFE) or to ablate the fibroid tissue by delivery of focused energy to the tumor (magnetic resonance-guided high-intensity focused ultrasound – MRgHIFU or myolysis by radiofrequency volumetric thermal ablation – RFVTA). UAE has been the most studied technique in interventional radiology for fibroids. Other techniques are relatively new. They offer the advantage of minimal invasion and are suitable for women who are:

- Not fit for surgery
- Not responding to medical management
- Not agreeable to have surgery

Uterine Artery Embolization (UAE) or Uterine Fibroid Embolization (UFE)

This is a minimally invasive procedure done under light sedation. It does not require anesthesia. The procedure is conducted in a cath lab. The femoral artery is entered by percutaneous route in the groin and under radiological guidance, a catheter is passed to the uterine artery. Polyvinyl occluding particles or gel are then injected to occlude the uterine artery (UAE) or selected branches going to the fibroid (UFE). The result is an ischemia and necrosis of the fibroid. Consequently, the size decreases, cellular content reduces, and symptoms should abate.[18, 27]

Compared to a myomectomy, the procedure is less invasive and has a shorter hospital stay, pain, and blood loss. The overall procedure related risk is lower. However, pregnancy rates, fertility, and abortion rates compare adversely to myomectomy. Recurrence rates and need for repeat procedures are also higher for UAE/UFE as compared to myomectomy.

The procedure has a risk of permanent impairment of uterine and ovarian function. Postembonlization syndrome with severe pain, fever, and acute abdomen are known complications. Selective distal vessel embolization and avoiding cervicovaginal and ovarian vessels may reduce these problems. Patient selection and informed decision become crucial steps before UAE/UFE.

Focused Energy Delivery Systems

Various energy sources such as radiofrequency, laser, electricity, crayon probes, and high-frequency ultrasound waves have been used to deliver ablative focused energy to the fibroid. The advantages listed are non invasive approach, no scar, daycare procedure, short hospital stay, and early resumption of activities. However, their scope is limited by the strict inclusion and exclusion criteria, need for repeat procedures, limited availability, and questionable efficacy. Long-term outcomes have not been studied in most of these methods.

Magnetic resonance-guided high-frequency focused ultrasound delivers high-intensity ultrasound waves to the fibroid under precise MR guidance. This results in protein denaturation and irreversible cell damage. This targets the center of the fibroid, but peripheral, faster growing cells are not adequately treated. Multiple sittings are need to allow adequate tissue to be treated to become clinically significant. Only one fibroid can be treated at a time. Surrounding myometrium may be damaged. Skin, bowel, and bone injury have been reported. Recently, high-end ultrasound machines have also been used to deliver the same energy.

Originally, radiofrequency myolysis was a combination of interventional radiology with laparoscopy. At laparoscopy, a radiofrequency probe is inserted into the center of the fibroid. Recently, the probe placement has been done through a 2-mm incision using imaging to direct it to the center of the fibroid. Acessa radiofrequency volumetric thermal ablation (RFVTA) system is the Food and Drug Administration (FDA)-approved one for treatment of fibroid. Studies have shown favorable results and up to 75% reduction in volume with effective control of symptoms in daycare settings. However, failure of treatment and reintervention may be required in significant number of patients. Postprocedure pregnancy had been reported but data is limited. At presnt, it should not be recommended for patients planning for pregnancy.

SURGICAL MANAGEMENT OF FIBROIDS

The mainstay of surgical treatment options for fibroids are myomectomy (removal of the fibroids only) and hysterectomy (removal of the uterus) **(Figs. 3A and B)**. The surgical options may be required in more than half of the cases of symptomatic fibroids. The choice of procedure and surgical technique depends upon the location of fibroids, the number of fibroids, the need of fertility preservation (uterus sparing), the expertise of the surgeon, the available equipment, associated gynecological or medical comorbidities, fitness for anesthesia, and the patient's desire to undergo surgery.

Myomectomy

This is an uterus- and fertility-preserving surgery where only fibroids are surgically removed. It is most suitable for single or a less number of fibroids which are symptomatic and future fertility is desired.

The various types of myomectomy are:

- Hysteroscopic
- Laparoscopic
- Open (laparotomy)
- Vaginal
- Robotic.

Hysteroscopic Myomectomy

It is recommended for submucous fibroids distorting uterine cavity. Performed under anesthesia, an operative hysteroscope is introduced in to the uterine cavity and the fibroids are identified and removed by one of the following different approaches:

- Cutting the pedicle with electrocautery or scissor or laser with retrieval of specimen by hook or resectoscope or loop. This is most suitable for pedunculated fibroids.
- Slicing the myoma in single sitting, where with using monopolar or bipolar-embedded electrocautery, the myoma is removed in strips. It has been observed that once protruding myoma is excised in bits, there is thickening of myometrium above it and contraction pushes the remaining myoma into the cavity. Piece meal removal should be continued till the fibers of myometrium are visualized and it is considered as completion of the process. The use of the intrauterine morcellator has made this process easier especially in fibroids <3 cm.
- Two-step approach may be needed at time, where piece meal resection of the protruding part of the fibroid in the cavity is done in first step. Post procedure, the remaining fibroid is pushed out in cavity by surrounding myometrium and simultaneous thickness of myometrium also increases. This facilitates complete and safe myoma excision in second step.

Distention media-related complications such as hyponatremia, fluid overload, or embolism are known to occur in hysteroscopic myomectomy. These can be minimized by using bipolar current instead of monopolar current and changing the distention medium. If available, laser knife may also help in minimizing complications. Other complications include perforation, intraoperative hemorrhage, incomplete removal, and infection. Recurrence of symptomatic fibroids may be encountered in about 10–15% patients. The overall failure rates at 5 years range from 14.5 to 30%. Coexisting adenomyosis or endometriosis may at times contribute to treatment failure.

Myomectomy with endometrial ablation can also be done when fertility is not the question and severe HMB is presenting complain. This combined approach allows better control of symptoms.

Correct selection of patient, appropriate mapping of fibroid, expertise and experience of surgeon, upgraded equipment, good visualization, and careful selection of safe

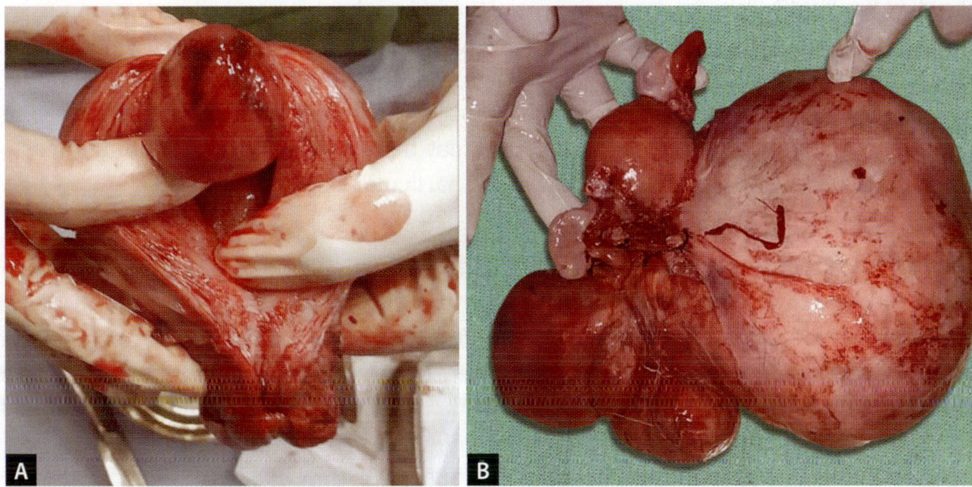

Figs. 3A and B: Post-hysterectomy specimens of the uterus showing a solitary submucus fibroid (A) and multiple fibroids (B).

distention medium and lowest distention pressure used are some of the key factors responsible for success of the treatment.[28-30]

Laparoscopic Myomectomy

Undoubtedly laparoscopic myomectomy is associated with lesser postoperative pain, faster recovery, less hospital stay, less blood loss, cosmetic advantages, and overall less morbidity compared to open myomectomy with laparotomy. The laparoscope with the attached camera is introduced via the central port and additional ports for hand instruments are placed depending on as the site and size of the fibroid as well as operative surgeon's expertise. Currently, usage of 3D cameras offer the added advantage of depth assessment during surgery.

Subserous fibroids with a pedicle are easy to handle by just coagulating and then cutting the pedicle followed by specimen retrieval. For other types of subserous fibroids, incision over uterus is first placed after infiltration with vasopressin or using vaso-occlusive methods such as clamps, clips or torniquets. A transverse incision is preferred but if required, the incision is be made depending on the position of the fibroid. The myoma is the enucleated totally as the pseudocapsule helps in easy dissection once the correct plane is identifed. The feeding vessels are coagulated. The fibroid is the removed with due care taken not to enter endometrial cavity. Hemostasis is checked and confirmed. Multilayer or single-layer suturing of the myoma bed is done. Care must be taken to avoid hematoma formation and ensuring optimum suturing with good approximation. Polyglactin (vicryl), polydioxanone (PDS), or barbed sutures can be used.

Important key surgical points:

- Patients with fibroids with size preferably <10–12 cm, number of fibroids not more than 4 and uteri of size <16 weeks are generally to be selected .
- Avoid entry in the endometrial cavity which may affect future reproductive outcome.
- Care to be taken as to not to compromise tubal patency at any stage of dissection or suturing.
- Preventive steps to minimize blood loss and operative time same as used in open myomectomy to be employed.
- Optimal suturing neither too tight to cause necrosis nor loose to cause hematoma is to be performed.
- Retrieval of specimen can be done via colpotomy or extension of one of the port
- In-bag morcellation should be considered on case to case basis.

Overall results of lap myomectomy are comparable to open myomectomy with respect to recurrence, postsurgical pregnancy as well as the risk of rupture in pregnancy and labor. In appropriately selected cases, laparoscopic myomectomy seems to be superior to open myomectomy as it is associated less operative morbidity. However entry-related complications, long learning curve, availability of upgraded equipment, identification of small fibroids, difficult excision of fibroids at abnormal locations, and finally retrieval of specimen are remain key challenges.[31]

Concerns Related to the Retrieval of the Myoma Specimen

As postoperative histopathologic evaluation may reveal occasionally an undiagnosed or unsuspected leiomyosarcoma following routine myomectomy, hence inadvertent tissue spread after morcellation has raised alarm. The FDA issued a warning for the same, particularly following the use of a power morcellator. Nevertheless, incidence of the specimen reported to have malignant potential in various studies is quite low, only about < 0.03–0.6%. Endobag morcellation and through lavage with the patient placed in Trendelenburg and anti-Trendelenburg position at the end of surgery helps in removal of most leftover pieces, which further reduces likelihood of inadvertent spread of the disease.[32-34]

Conventional Myomectomy (Figs. 4A to C)

This conventional surgical procedure has evolved and refined over time. Conventionally, myomectomy was considered lethal but with improved surgical techniques, availability of blood and blood products, preoperative fibroid mapping due to improved imaging, availability of hemostatic agents, better suture material, and better anesthesia, it is now comparatively a safer and effective surgery. Principles are similar to those discussed in laparoscopic myomectomy but advantages are open access to the myoma and quicker and easier suturing. The only probable drawbacks compared to laparoscopy are larger incisions and slower recovery. Open myomectomy can be done for fibroids of any size, any number, any location, i.e., both intramural and subserous fibroids.

Prevention of Hemorrhage in Myomectomy[27]

Several mechanical and pharmacological measures have been used for preventing or reducing hemorrhage open or laparoscopic myomectomy myomectomy and have been found to be variably beneficial as reported in literature and so may be used alone or in combination as per the need in the particular case.

Preoperatively:

- Preoperatively ensure that the hemoglobin is at least 10 g/dL and the patient is fit for anesthesia.
- Preoperative medical management with a GnRH analog for 3–6 months may reduce fibroid size and hence smaller incision may be needed and lesser blood loss may occur because of reduced vascularity and additionally the operative time is also reduced. However, few studies suggest that the its use may result in difficulties to easily

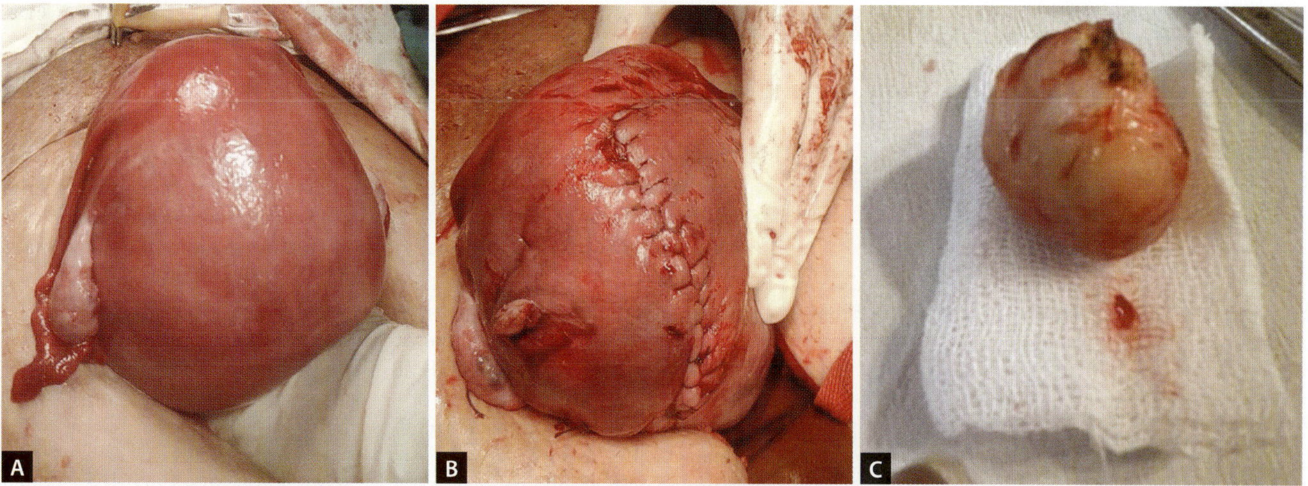

Figs. 4A to C: Conventional myomectomy. (A) Enlarged uterus with myoma; (B) Uterine incision sutured after enucleation of the myoma; (C) Myoma specimen.

obtain a plane of cleavage during enucleating the myoma from myometrium. It has also not shown any advantage for hysteroscopic myomectomy.

- Preoperative use of SPRMs such as UPA that are known to shrink the fibroid size and reduce blood loss have been proposed. However, more studies are required to demonstrate significant benefits justifying routine use.

Intraoperatively:

- Tourniquet application or uterine artery occlusion (UAO) at level of uterine isthmus results in occlusion uterine arteries and at infundibulopelvic ligament for ovarian collateral circulation with help of Bonney's myomectomy clamp, red rubber catheter through a hole in broad ligament, and specialized vascular clamp on uterine. Important point to note is that the occlusion is to be released every 15–20 minutes for some time to avoid tissue ischemia and necrosis.
- Vasopressin diluted in a dose of 10 units in 10 mL or 20 units in 20 mL of saline is to be infiltrated in fibroid boundaries or just medial to feeding vessel or uterine artery thereby reducing the blood loss by 40–50%
- Misoprostol 400 µg per rectally 30 minutes prior to surgery and oxytocin 10 units infusion pre- and intraoperatively decreases blood flow and increases myometrial contraction thereby reducing overall blood loss. This is also helpful in hysteroscopy as it causes softening of cervix for easy dilatation and minimizes the risk of perforation.
- Antifibrinolytics such as tranexamic acid 1 g IV just before onset of surgery reduce blood loss and need for blood transfusion significantly.
- Gelatin-thrombin matrix for local application as hemostatic plug over the bleeding site acts as sealant causing rapid hemostasis and reduces need of blood.

Myomectomy and Pregnancy

Postmyomectomy, different studies have described variable pregnancy rates depending on the type and methodology of the study; however, overall, a pregnancy rate of 49–57% has been documented in literature. Myomectomy is known to reduce the abortion rate, particularly in submucous fibroids. There is statistically no significant difference observed between laparoscopy versus open myomectomy in subsequent obstetric and perinatal outcomes including cumulative pregnancy rate.[35-37]

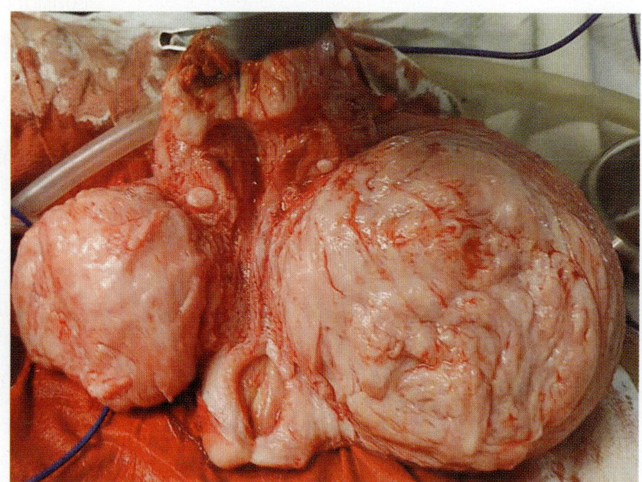

Fig. 5: Hysterectomy specimen of an enlarged uterus with multiple fibroids.

Hysterectomy (Fig. 5)

Fibroids are the one of the top three indications for hysterectomies performed worldwide. The common indications for offering an hysterectomy in symptomatic fibroids are:

- Symptomatic fibroids refractory to medical management
- Age > 40 years
- Child bearing completed and future fertility/uterus preservation not desired by patient
- Anticipated difficult compliance and follow-up

Hysterectomy is known to provide relief of symptoms and drastically improve quality of life.

TABLE 5: Treatment options of fibroids.

Type of myoma as per FIGO[39]	*First line*	*Supportive interventions*	*Remarks*
0	Hysteroscopic myomectomy		
1	• <3 cm hysteroscopic myomectomy (1 step) • >3 cm hysteroscopic myomectomy (2 steps)	• Preoperative patient fitness with anemia correction and reduction of fibroid volume with SPRMs or GnRH analogs	• 1–3 month medical therapy may convert two-step procedure to single step due to reduction in size or • No further treatment may be needed if no further symptoms
2 desiring pregnancy	• Long-term intermittent SPRM therapy	• Volume reduction > 50% and uterine cavity normal—no further treatment • Volume reduction > 25–50% and HMB controlled—no further treatment or hysteroscopic myomectomy if cavity is uneven with the possibility of interfering with pregnancy • No response or insufficient response or no relief of symptoms then consider hysteroscopic myomectomy	• Natural conception • Natural conception • If other indications or no pregnancy after initial efforts then consider IUI or IVF • Natural conception • If other indications or no pregnancy after initial efforts then consider IUI or IVF
2 not desiring pregnancy	• Myomectomy • Long-term intermittent SPRM (3-4 courses of 3 months) • If 40+ or not interested in uterine conservation and poor compliance to medical management- Hysterectomy	• Preoperative anemia correction • If good response • If inadequate symptomatic relief • Preoperative fitness and anemia correction	• No further treatment • If symptomatic or if recurrence consider myomectomy
Type 2–5 single or multiple fibroid	• Same as above	• Same as above	• Same as above
Type 6–7	• No pressure symptoms , size < 6 tcm—no treatment • If pressure symptoms or possible torsion—myomectomy • Size > 8 cm with minimal symptoms but high risk group—myomectomy	• Counselling regarding prognosis and follow up is particularly important in high risk group • If no desire for uterine preservation consider hysterectomy	
Type 8	• Asymptomatic < 6 cm—no treatment • Pressure symptoms or pain – Myomectomy / hysterectomy	• Follow-up advised • If childbearing completed or difficult myomectomy anticipated then consider hysterectomy	

(GnRH: gonadotropin-releasing hormone; HMB: heavy menstrual bleeding; IUI: intrauterine insemination; IVF: in vitro fertilization; SPRM: selective progesterone receptor modulator)

Route of hysterectomy:[38]

- Laparoscopic hysterectomy
- Vaginal hysterectomy
- Abdominal hysterectomy
- Robotic surgery.

Laparoscopy had been proved to be an effective mode of hysterectomy in fibroids with less perioperative complications and a faster recovery. However, Donnez et al. have reported statistically no significant difference between any type and route of hysterectomy.

Important key surgical points: All steps are same as any other hysterectomy; however, certain important points should be always remembered.

- Always firstly identify round ligaments to get orientation of the uterus and its relations with other organs.
- After clamping and transfixing upper pedicles, identify uterine artery and vessels feeding the fibroids. Camp and double ligate these vascular pedicles separately.
- If space is restricted, enucleation of the fibroid like in myomectomy can be done so as to allow more space and provide better orientation. After ligating the uterine and feeding vessels, subsequent myomectomy will not cause bleeding.
- Always try to restore normal anatomy, avoid torsion while handling specimen.
- When in doubt, identify the ureter and trace it down before clamping.

Generally, most patients seem satisfied postoperatively due to symptom relief and improvement in quality of life and are usually back to their normal lifestyle within 6–8 weeks postoperatively.

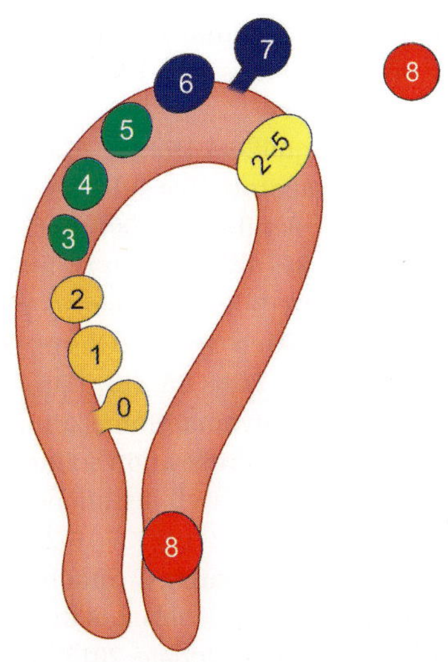

Fig. 6: FIGO classification based on location of fibroids. (FIGO: International Federation of Gynecology and Obstetrics)

Vaginal Occlusion of Uterine arteries

By using a specialized clamp which can be applied on the uterine arteries through vagina and occlusion of both the uterine arteries is achieved which leads to ischemia of the uterus and primarily the myoma. Postprocedure pregnancy outcome needs further study and hence at present is not recommended in patients a planning pregnancy. Published medical literature has shown efficacy in reduction in menstrual blood loss and shrinkage of fibroid.[27]

SUMMARY OF TREATMENT PLAN

As there are several treatment options are available, a simplified approach can be adopted using the different guidelines and FIGO classification based on location of fibroids **(Fig. 6 and Table 5)**.

CONCLUSION

An individualized approach in each patient of fibroids should be offered with the aim to provide relieve the symptoms of HMB, pelvic pressure, subfertility, and pain. Detailed evaluation of the clinical presentation, examination, and imaging are the first steps in management of fibroids. Planning of treatment offering a expectant, medical, surgical, or endoscopic option using an evidence base approach is to done after an informed decision-making session explaining the pros, cons, and limitations of all treatment options and respecting patient choices will usually lead to desired positive outcomes.

KEY MESSAGES

- Fibroids are benign tumors of the uterus.
- Clinical presentations are variable ranging from being asymptomatic to symptoms such as HMB, pain, pressure, and infertility.
- Imaging using ultrasound and MRI have greatly helped in precise fibroid mapping.
- Spectrum of treatment options is available ranging from expectant, medical, open surgery, to minimally invasive surgery.
- If selected appropriately, they result in favorable outcomes providing symptom relief and improving quality of life.

REFERENCES

1. Donnez J, Dolmans MM. Uterine Fibroid management: from present the future. Hum Reprod Update. 2016;22(6):665-86.
2. Berek JS. Uterine Fibroids. In: Berek JS (Ed). Berek & Novak; Gynecology essential, 1st Edition. Netherlands: Wolters Kluwer; 2020. pp. 138-53.
3. Giuliani E, As-Sanie S, Marsh EE. Epidemiology and management of uterine fibroids. Int J Gynecol Obstet. 2020;149:3-9.
4. Vergara D, Catherino WH, Trojano G, Tinelli A. Vitamin D: Mechanism of action and biological effects in uterine fibroids. Nutrients. 2021;13:597.
5. Tochie JN, Badjang GT, Ayissi G, Dohbit JS. Physiopathology and management of uterine fibroids. Intech Open. 2020;94162.
6. Peddada SD, Laughlin SK, Miner K, Guyon JP, Haneke K, Vahdat HL, et al. Growth of uterine leiomyomata among premenopausal black and white women. Proc Natl Acad Sci USA. 2008;105:19887-92.
7. DeWaay DJ, Syrop CH, Nygaard IE, Davis WA, Voorhis VJV. Natural history of uterine polyps and leiomyomata. Obstet Gynecol. 2002;100:3.
8. Baird DD, Garrett TA, Laughlin SK, Davis B, Semelka RC, Peddada SD. Short-term change in growth of uterine leiomyoma: Tumor growth spurts. Fertil Sterill. 2011;95:242.
9. Lasmar RB, Barrozo PRM, Dias R, de Oliveira MAP. Submucous mayoma: A new presurgical classification to evaluate viability of hysteroscopic surgical treatment–preliminary report. J Minim Invasive Gynecol. 2005;12(4):308-11.
10. Borah BJ, Nicholson WK, Bradley L, Stewar EA. The impact of uterine leiomyomas: a national survey of affected women. Am J Obstet Gynecol. 2013;209:319.e.1.
11. Stewart EA, Laughlin-Tommaso SK. (2021). Uterine fibroids (leiomyomas): Epidemiology, clinical features, diagnosis, and natural history. [online] Available from https://www.uptodate.com/contents/uterine-fibroids-leiomyomas-epidemiology-clinical-features-diagnosis-and-natural-history [Last accessed December, 2021].
12. Bonine NG, Banks E, Harrington A, Vlahiotis A, Moore-Schiltz L, Gillard P. Contemporary treatment utilization among women diagnosed with symptomatic uterine fibroids in united states. BMC women's Health. 2020;20:174.
13. Bell SW, Kempson RL, Hendrickson MR. Problematic uterine smooth muscle neoplasms: A clinicopathologic study of 213 cases. Am J Surg Pathol. 1994;18:535.
14. Daga SR, Phatak SV. Ultrasound evaluation of uterine leiomyoma in perimenopausal females with histopathological correlation. J. Evolution Med Dent Sci. 2020;9(08):562-5.
15. Van den Bosch T, Dueholm M, Leone FP, Valentin L, Rasmussen CK, Votino A, et al. Terms, definitions and measurements to describe sonographic features of myometrium and uterine masses: a consensus opinion from the Morphological Uterus

Sonographic Assessment (MUSA) group. Ultrasound Obstet Gynecol. 2015;46:284-98.
16. Bougie O, Bedaiwy MA, Laberge P, Lebovic G, Leyland N, Atri M, et al. Quality of ultrasonography reporting and factors associated with selection of imaging modality for uterine fibroids in Canada: results from a prospective cohort registry. CAMJ Open. 2020;8(3):E506-13.
17. Sasaran V, Turdean S, Gliga M, Ilyes L, Grama O, Muntean M, et al. Value of strain-ratio elastography in the diagnosis and differentiation of uterine fibroids and adenomyosis. J Pers Med. 2021;11;824.
18. Hartmann KE, Fonnesbeck C, Surawicz T, Krishnaswami S, Andrews JC, Wilson JE, et al. Management of Uterine Fibroids. Comparative Effectiveness Review No. 195; AHRQ Publication No. 17(18)-EHC028-EF. Rockville, MD: Agency for Healthcare Research and Quality. 2017.
19. Bryant-smith AC, Lethaby A, Farguhar C, Hickey M, Antifibrinolytics for heavy menstrual bleeding. Cochrane Database Syst Rev. 2018;4:CD000249.
20. Yao X, Sewart EA, Laughlin-Tommaso SK, Heien HC, Borah BJ. Medical therapies for heavy menstrual bleeding in women with uterine fibroids: a retrospective analysis of a large commercially insured population in the USA. BJOG. 2017;124:322.
21. Marsh EE, Galitsky A, Stewart EA, Kerolous M. Burden, prevalence and treatment of uterine fibroids: A survey of US women. J Women's Health. 2018;27(11)::1359-67.
22. Sayed GH, Zakherah MS, El-Nashar SA, Shaaban MM. A randomized clinical trial of a levonorgestrel-releasing intrauterine system and a low-dose combined oral contraceptive for fibroid-related menorrhagia. Int J Gynaecol Obstet. 2011;112:126-30.
23. Mahase E. Uterine fibroid drug is recalled after case of liver failure requiring transplantprompts EU review. BMJ. 2020;368:m1112.
24. Murji A, Whitaker L, Chow TL, Sobel ML. Selective progesterone receptor modulators(SPRMs) for uterine fibroids. Cochrane Database Syst Rev. 2017;4:CD010770.
25. Donnez J, Hervais Vivancos B, Kudela M, Audebert A, Jadoul P. A randomized, placebo-controlled, dose-ranging trial comparing fulvestrant with goserelin in premenopausal patients with uterine fibroids awaiting hysterectomy. Fertil Steril. 2003;79:1380-9.
26. Song H, Lu D, Navaratnam K, Shi G. Aromatase inhibitors for uterine fibroids. Cochrane Database Syst Rev. 2013;(10):CD009505.
27. Vilos GA, Allaire C, Laberge PY, Leyland N Vilos AG, Murji A, et al. The management of uterine leiomyomas. J Obstet Gynaecol Can. 2015;37:157-78.
28. Munro MG. Abnormal uterine bleeding: surgical management–part 3. J Am Assoc Gynecol Laparosc. 2001;8:18-47.
29. Loffer FD. Improving results of hysteroscopic submucusal myomectomy for menorrhagia by concomitant endometrial ablation. J Min Invas Gynecol. 2005;12:254-60.
30. AAGL Advancing Minimally Invasive Gynecology Worldwide, Munro MG, Storz K, Abbott JA, Falcone T, Jacobs VR, et al. AAGL practice report. Practice guidelines for the management of hysteroscopic distendng media. J Minim Invasive Gynecol. 2013;20:137-48.
31. Donnez O, Donnez J, Dolmans MM, Dethy A, Baeyens M, Mitchell J. Low pain score after total laparoscopic hysterectomy and same-day discharge within less than 5 hours: Results of a prospective observational study. J Minim Invasive Gynecol. 2015;22:1293-9.
32. Donnez O, Jadoul P, Squifflet J, Donnez J. Iatrogenic peritoneal adenomyoma after laparoscopic subtotal hysterectomy and uterine morcellation. Fertil Steril. 2006;86:1511-2.
33. Bojahr B, De Wilde RL, Tchartchian G. Malignancy rate of 10,731 uteri morcellated during laparoscopic supracervical hysterectomy (LASH). Arch Gynecol Obstet. 2015;292:665-72.
34. Parker WH, Kaunitz AM, Pritts EA, Olive DL, Chalas E, Clarke-Pearson DL, et al. Leiomyoma Morcellation Review Group. US Food and Drug Administration's Guidance regarding morcellation of leiomyomas: well-intentioned, but is it harmful for women? Obstet Gynecol. 2016;127:18-22.
35. Galliano D, Bellver J, Días-Garcia C, Simón C, Pellicer A. ART and uterine pathology: how revelant is the maternal side for implantation? Hum Reprod Update. 2015;21:13-38.
36. Metwally M, Farquhar CM, Li TC. Is another meta-analysis on the effects of intramural fibroids on reproductive outcomes needed? Reprod Biomed Online. 2011;23:2-14.
37. Tian YC, Long TF, Dai YM. Pregnancy outcomes following different surgical approaches of myomectomy. J Obstet Gynaecol Res. 2015;41:350-7.
38. Aarts JW, Nieboer TE, Johnson N, Tavender E, Garry R, Mol BW, et al. Surgical approach to hysterectomy for benign gynaecological disease. Cochrane Database Syst Rev. 2015;8:CD003677.
39. Munro MG, Critchley HO, Broder MS, Fraser IS. FIGO Working Group on Menstrual Disorders. FIGO classification system (PALM-COEIN) for causes of abnormal uterine bleeding in nongravid women of reproductive age. Int J Gynaecol Obstet. 2011;113:1-2.

LONG QUESTIONS

1. Discuss the management approach to a primigravida at 6-week pregnancy who presents to the clinic with an 8-cm intramural fibroid. What are the difficulties anticipated in labor and delivery with such a fibroid?
2. Discuss the pharmacological management of fibroids.
3. What is the role of radiology in the management of fibroids? Discuss the various diagnostic and therapeutic modalities.
4. What impact do fibroids have on fertility? Discuss the possible mechanisms and possible interventions.

SHORT QUESTIONS

1. What is the FIGO classification of fibroids? Why is it useful?
2. Name the indications and contraindications for myomectomy.
3. What are the pros and cons of ulipristal acetate in treating fibroids?

MULTIPLE CHOICE QUESTIONS

1. Heavy menstrual bleeding is typically associated with:
   a. Cervical fibroid
   b. Subserosal fibroid
   c. Submucosal fibroid
   d. Intramural fibroid

2. Which of the following is not a risk factor for fibroid uterus?
   a. Nulliparity b. African-American race
   c. Menopause d. Obesity
3. Which of the following options are correct? Fibroids lead to heavy menstrual bleeding because fibroids alter myometrial contractility:
   a. Both statements are true and causally related
   b. Both statements are true but not causally related
   c. First statement is true and second is false
   d. Both statements are false
4. Which is/are true about red degeneration of fibroids?
   i. Occurs in pregnancy
   ii. Occurs in menopause
   iii. Managed conservatively
   iv. Surgery is the definitive management
   a. Only i, ii and iii are correct
   b. Only i and iii are correct
   c. Only ii and iv are correct
   d. Only iv is correct
5. The most common site for fibroids is:
   a. Cervical fibroid b. Subserosal fibroid
   c. Submucosal fibroid d. Intramural fibroid
6. Which of the following fibroid is /are associated with pressure symptoms ?
   i. Cervical fibroid
   ii. Subserosal fibroid
   iii. Broad ligament fibroid
   iv. Intramural fibroid
   a. Only i, ii and iii are correct
   b. Only i and iii are correct
   c. Only ii and iv are correct
   d. Only iv is correct
7. Which type of fibroid has been associated with adverse pregnancy outcomes?
   a. Submucous Fibroid b. Intramural fibroid
   c. Subseroal fibroid d. Seedling fibroid
8. Which of the following is/are true about use of GnRH in treatment of fibroids?
   i. Reduces fibroid volume
   ii. To change the initially decided route of surgery
   iii. To improve pre operative hemoglobin
   iv. To postpone surgery and manage symptoms
   a. Only i and iii are correct
   b. Only ii and iv are correct
   c. Only iv is correct
   d. All four are correct

Answers

1. c 2. c 3. a 4. b 5. d 6. b
7. a 8. d

9.7 ADENOMYOSIS

N Sanjeeva Reddy, Radha Vembu

INTRODUCTION

Adenomyosis of the uterus is a benign disorder with pathologically demonstrated endometrial glands and stroma in the uterine myometrium. It is one of the specific entities in PALM-COEIN FIGO classification of abnormal uterine bleeding (AUB). Even though this condition was considered as a disease of multiparous women over 40 years, it is more commonly diagnosed in younger women with the advancement of imaging techniques. However, there is no clear consensus in the diagnosis and classification of adenomyotic lesion.

DEFINITION

According to histological classification, focal adenomyosis is defined as circumscribed nodular aggregates of endometrial glands and stroma surrounded by normal myometrium. Within the myometrium, when the ectopic endometrial tissue is surrounded by hypertropic myometrium, it is called adenomyoma. In diffuse adenomyosis, endometrial glands and stroma are recognized throughout the myometrium.[1]

PREVALENCE

Adenomyosis was a disease of elderly, multiparous women, but now, it is commonly diagnosed in young women, infertile patients, and women with pain or AUB or both.[2] It often coexists with other uterine lesions like fibroid and endometriosis and hence it is difficult to estimate. In women less than 45 years, it is around 31.2% and increases to 65.6% over the age of 45 years. However, among the general population, it is estimated to be present in 20–35% of women[3,4] with majority of women being postmenopausal. But age is not consistently associated with the disease. It is diagnosed in 24.4% of infertile women, especially in those with endometriosis, recurrent miscarriage, and recurrent implantation failure, and in older women seeking IVF treatment.[5] Cystic adenomyosis is seen in adult form in 5–7% of hysterectomy specimen with fibroid uterus. The juvenile form is seen in nulliparous women between 13 and 20 years of age where the true incidence is not known with only few case reports. Even though adenomyosis is rare before 20 years of age, cystic forms are reported in young women, till now less than 10 cases are reported.

RISK FACTORS

The natural history and risk factors are uncertain as the definitive diagnosis is made usually after the pathological evaluation of hysterectomy specimen. It can coexists with leiomyoma (50%), endometriosis (11%), and endometrial polyp (7%).

Age

Around 70–80% of women are in the fourth or fifth decade undergoing hysterectomy for adenomyosis. However, with the use of MRI in the diagnosis, many adolescent and younger women in the reproductive age group presenting with dysmenorrhea and chronic pelvic pain are diagnosed with adenomyosis. So, the onset of the disease might be at an earlier age with different clinical phenotype.

Multiparity

Majority of the patients are multiparous. This might be due to inclusion of adenomyotic foci by the invasion of trophoblast on the extension of myometrial fibers.[6] This adenomyotic tissue may have higher ratio of estrogen receptors and hormonal milieu during pregnancy may promote ectopic islands of endometrium.

Prior Uterine Surgery

Endometrial glands may invade the myometrium due to disruption of endomyometrial junction and increase the risk of adenomyosis. The most common surgeries observed are dilatation and curettage and cesarean section.

Smoking

The association between adenomyosis and smoking is controversial. There is decreased incidence of adenomyosis among smokers as it is estrogen dependent and there is decreased serum level of estrogen in smokers. Alternatively, some have shown no association between smoking and adenomyosis.

Ectopic Pregnancy

Women with adenomyosis are hypothesized to be at increased risk of ectopic pregnancy most commonly intramural ectopic.

Depression and Antidepressant Use

Many animal studies have shown association between adenomyosis, depression, and antidepressants, and this may be due to prolactin dynamics.

Tamoxifen Treatment

Adenomyosis is common in women treated for breast cancer with tamoxifen and may present with postmenopausal bleeding.

PATHOGENESIS

- There is diffuse or globular enlargement of the uterus due to hypertrophy and hyperplasia of the surrounding myometrium induced by the endometrial glands and stroma in the myometrium. The two theories postulated in the pathogenesis of adenomyosis are endomyometrial invagination of the endometrium or de novo from Mullerian rests.[7]
- Ultra structural changes and differential growth factor expression in the junctional zone of the myometrium also plays a key role.[8]
- Estrogen and progesterone have been postulated in the pathogenesis. It is shown that estrogen is secreted in the adenomyotic tissue and aromatase in the endometrium is normalized by GnRH agonist and danazol treatment.[9]
- Prolactin and FSH have been shown to have direct effect on the uterus in animal models.[10] This hypothesis is supported by association of depression and antidepressant use in these women.
- Growth factor dysregulation and abnormalities of angiogenesis may play a role in the pathogenesis.[11]
- According to the most common theory, adenomyosis results from the invagination of basalis into the myometrium through an altered or interrupted junctional zone (JZ).[12] So molecular alterations in eutopic endometrium might lead to this migration and survival of ectopic endometrium beyond the myometrial interface.[13]
- The role of tissue injury and repair (TIAR) as a primary mechanism for myometrial invasion has been postulated.[14] Chronic peristaltic myometrial contractions can induce micro trauma to JZ, which in turn promotes inflammation and local estrogen production and this vicious cycle continues.[15] So, this TIAR theory supports the understanding that adenomyosis is common in multiparity, previous cesarean section and prior uterine surgery.
- Chapron et al., described the "outside to inside invasion" theory suggesting the migration of ectopic endometrial cells from posterior endometriosis nodules into the myometrium. This supports the high prevalence of posterior focal adenomyosis of the outer myometrium (FOAM) and is common in patients with deep infiltrating endometriosis.[16] The intraperitoneal seedling of endometrial cells after menstruation can cause invasion of vesicouterine pouch, leading to both bladder nodule and anterior FOAM.

PATHOLOGY

Adenomyosis may be diffuse or confined to a discrete area (adenomyoma). If diffuse, uterus is uniformly enlarged and boggy. Adenomyoma can resemble leiomyoma with irregular and firm appearance but cut section of leiomyoma shows "whorled appearance".

Cross section of adenomyosis shows myometrial wall thickening with areas of hemorrhage or chocolate color representing islands of endometrial bleeding (**Fig. 1**). The term "cystic" is used to describe either diffuse or adenomyoma with cysts ≥ 1 cm on imaging studies.

The pathognomonic feature of adenomyosis is the presence of endometrial tissue in the myometrium in at least one low-power field from the endomyometrial junction **(Fig. 2)**. This endometrium usually shows immature proliferative pattern.

CLINICAL PRESENTATION

- Heavy menstrual bleeding (60%) and dysmenorrhea (25%)
- Chronic pelvic pain
- Asymptomatic (33%)
- Increased risk of preterm birth but no clinical evidence suggesting increased risk of spontaneous abortion or other obstetric outcomes
- Infertile women undergoing assisted reproductive technology (ART) (20–25%).[5]

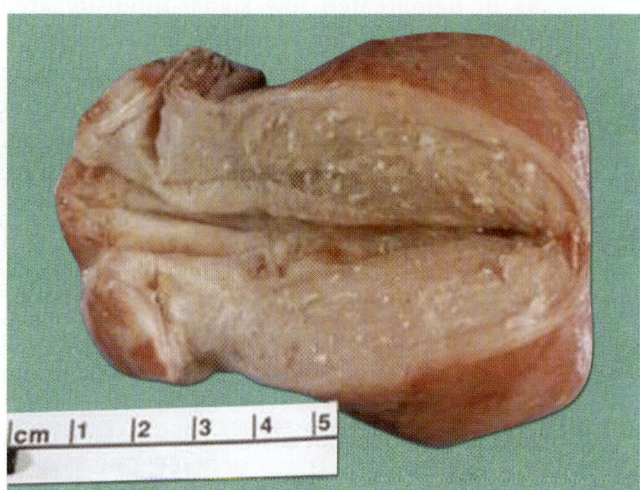

Fig. 1: Cut section of adenomyotic uterus.

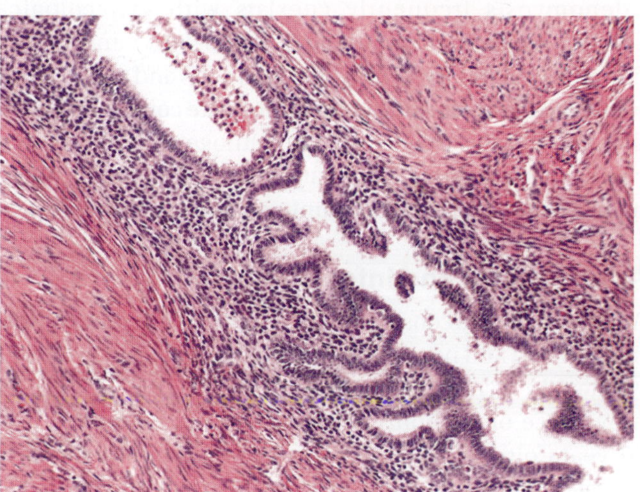
Fig. 2: Histopathology of adenomyotic lesion.

EVALUATION

This includes detailed history, pelvic examination, laboratory tests, and imaging.

- *History*: Obstetric and gynecologic history, relevant medical history.
- *Pelvic examination*: Diffusely enlarged uterus, boggy, globular rarely exceeds 12 weeks size of gravid uterus, restricted mobility, if associated with endometriosis.
- *Laboratory tests:*
  - No specific tests for diagnosis of adenomyosis.
  - Hemogram: if excessive bleeding to rule out anemia.
  - Urine or serum β hCG: to exclude pregnancy in AUB.
- *Imaging*
  - **Transvaginal scan (TVS)** is the first line imaging choice for evaluation **(Fig. 3)**. It is widely used, relatively inexpensive, and accurate if performed by trained personal. The sensitivity ranges from 65 to 81% and specificity of 65 to 100%. In a recent meta-analysis, 2D USG has a sensitivity and specificity of 83.8% and 63.9%, respectively and 3D USG, 88.9% and 56%, respectively.[17] Recently, a uniform reporting system of ultrasound findings in adenomyosis has been developed using Morphological Uterus Sonographic Assessment (MUSA) criteria.[18] The typical ultrasound features according to these criteria include
    - Asymmetrical thickening of uterine walls,
    - Intramyometrial cysts or hyperechoic islands (or both),
    - Fan-shaped shadowing of the myometrium,
    - Myometrial echogenic subendometrial lines and buds,
    - Translesional vascularity,
    - Irregular or interrupted JZ.

However, the available evidence linking the ultrasound features with histopathology is limited, even though the different sonographic characteristics may be explained by the relative proportion of endometrial glandular structures,

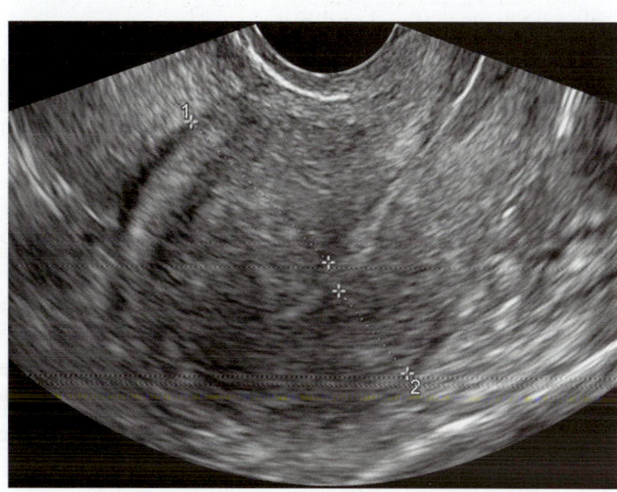

Fig. 3: Transvaginal scan image of adenomyosis.

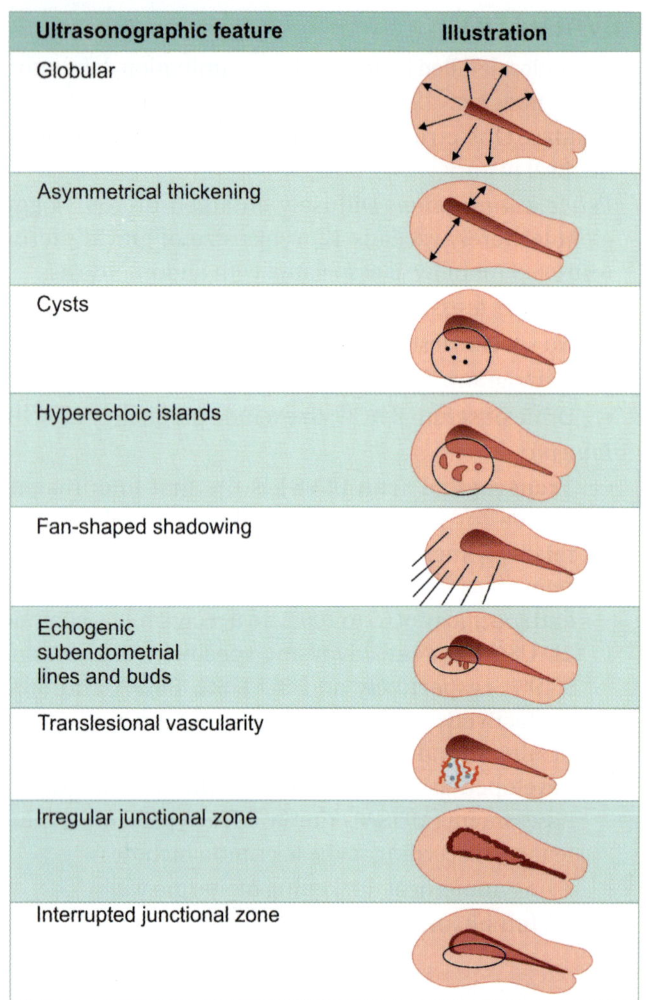

Fig. 4: Transvaginal ultrasound features of adenomyosis.
Source: Adapted from Reference 18.

endometrial stroma, and hypertrophic muscle elements.[19] The TVS images of the uterus[18] are depicted in **Figure 4**.

A new reporting system has been proposed, which includes description of:

- disease location (anterior, posterior, left lateral, right lateral, and fundal)
- classify disease (focal or diffuse)
- presence or absence of intralesional cysts
- myometrial layer involvement (JZ, myometrium, serosa)
- disease extent (< 25%, 25–50%, and > 50% of uterine volume).[2]
  - *Magnetic resonance imaging (MRI)*
    - MRI should be considered as second line imaging technique for diagnosis **(Fig. 5)**.
    - It is reserved to distinguish diffuse and focal adenomyosis from leiomyoma, if planned for conservative surgery.
    - It is essentially linked to the thickening of JZ, but also includes direct and indirect signs of presence of endometrial glands within the myometrium and smooth muscle hypertrophy.[20] The sensitivity and specificity of MRI to diagnose adenomyosis is 77% and 89%, respectively and with ultrasound is 72% and 81%, respectively.[21]
    - It is ideally done in the late proliferative phase. On T2 weighted images, typical lesions appear as ill demarcated low signal-intensity area. This indicates smooth muscle hyperplasia and heterotropic endometrial tissue. Small high signal intensity areas refer to ectopic endometrium and small intramyometrial cysts can also be detected.
    - On T1 weighted sequence, high-signal intensity foci represent areas of hemorrhage.
    - Common appearance on MRI—enlarged, asymmetric uterus when lesion is mainly in the posterior wall or at fundus.
    - JZ of 8–12 mm or maximum JZ/total myometrial ration over 40% and difference between maximum and minimum thickness of > 5 mm.[22]
    - MRI classification of adenomyosis is depicted in **Figure 6**.[23]

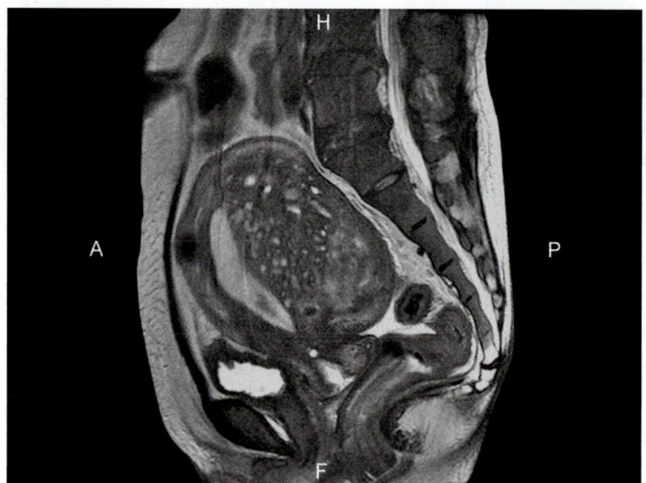

Fig. 5: MRI image of adenomyotic uterus.

COEXISTING GYNAECOLOGICAL CONDITIONS

Adenomyosis frequently coexists with gynecological conditions such as endometriosis (20–80%) and uterine fibroids (15–57%). Previously endometriosis and adenomyosis were considered as same but now, they are considered as two different entities due to specific pathogenic pathways and clinical presentations. They can present with chronic pelvic pain, dysmenorrhea, dyspareunia, and noncyclic pelvic pain.

Adenomyosis and Infertility

Adenomyosis was considered previously as a uterine condition of multipara and now, it is increasingly diagnosed in infertile women. In a cross-sectional study on infertile women, the prevalence of adenomyosis was 24.4% in women at least 40 years old and 22% in women less than 40 years. Its prevalence is increased to 38.2% in recurrent pregnancy loss and 34.7% in previous ART failure.[5]

The mechanism of infertility in these patients might be due to abnormal utero-tubal transport, which can be due to anatomical distortion of the uterine cavity, disturbed uterine peristalsis and sperm transport.[24] The JZ and the inner myometrium show dysfunctional hyper peristalsis and increased intrauterine pressure. The eutopic endometrium shows a variety of molecular alterations leading to altered receptivity. This includes sex steroid hormone pathway, increased inflammatory markers, lack of expression of adhesion molecules, and altered gene expression (HOXA 10 gene) and these can cause impairment of implantation.[25] In adenomyosis women undergoing ART, miscarriage rate is 31% which is higher than non affected women (14.1%). In a multicenter prospective study comparing clinical pregnancy rate (CPR) in patients with and without adenomyosis, there was a decrease in CPR from 42.7 to 22.7%. So the severity of the condition, which is expressed as a number of morphological features on ultrasound worsens the reproductive outcome.[26]

A recent systemic review and meta-analysis on IVF treatment outcome in adenomyosis patients showed detrimental effect on reproductive outcome. The implantation rate (IR), CPR per cycle, clinical pregnancy per embryo transfer, ongoing pregnancy, and live birth rate were significantly reduced and miscarriage rate was increased. So pretreatment down regulation with GnRH analog prior to IVF may be beneficial to pregnancy rate.[27]

MANAGEMENT OF ADENOMYOSIS

Medical Management

In the present scenario, medical therapy has shown increased efficacy for control of symptoms and fertility treatment.

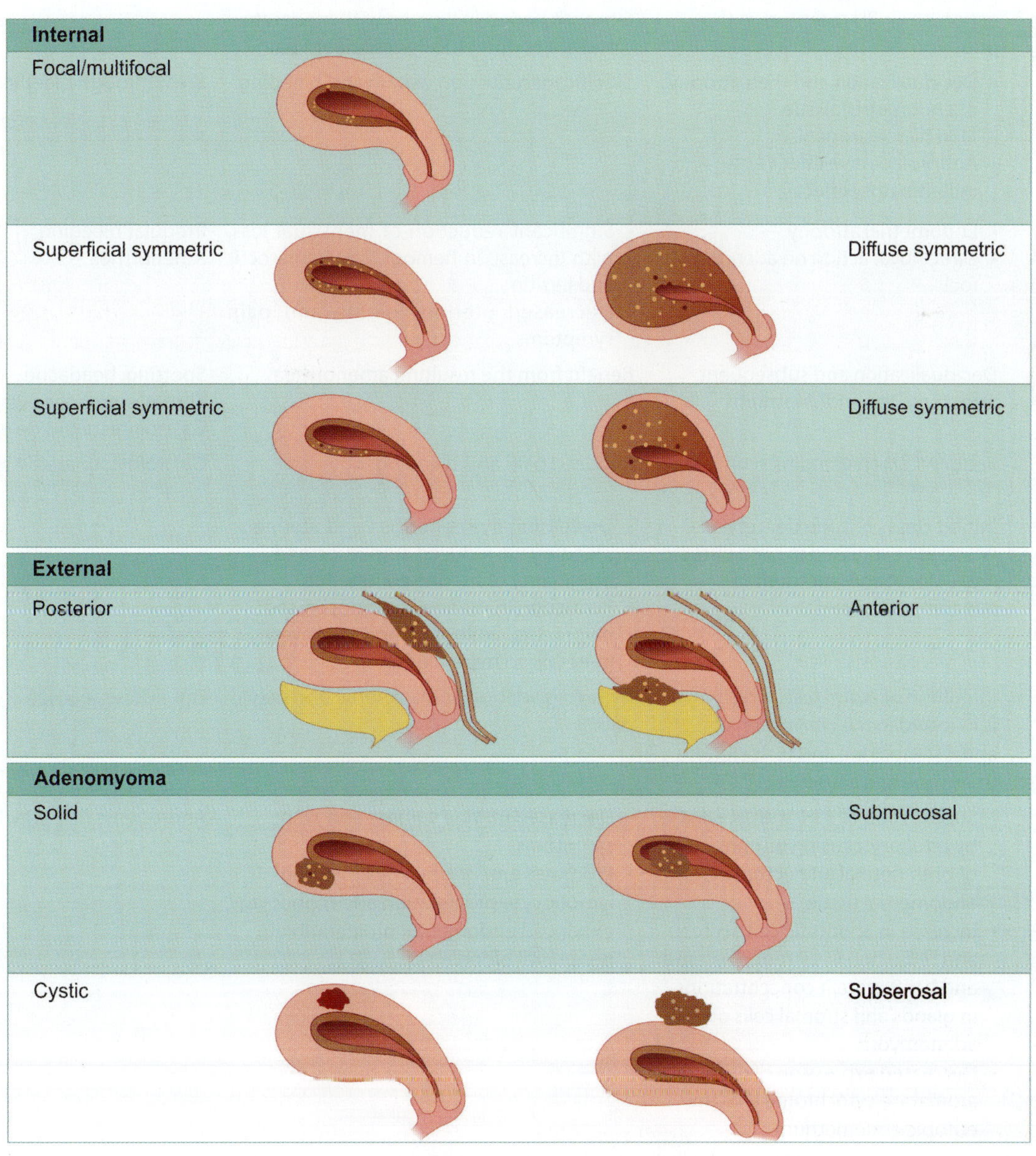

Fig. 6: MRI classification of adenomyosis.
Source: Adapted from Reference 23.

However, there are no guidelines for the management of adenomyosis. The rationale for medical therapy is based on pathogenetic mechanisms which are similar to endometriosis. The commonly used drugs in the management of adenomyosis are depicted in **Table 1**.

Newer Drugs

Selective progesterone receptor modulators (SPRM): Selective progesterone receptor modulators have been tried in hormone dependent conditions like fibroid. They exhibit progesterone agonist and antagonist activities in the endometrium

TABLE 1: Commonly used drugs for adenomyosis.[28,29]

Drug	*Mechanism of action*	*Effects*	*Side effects*
GnRH agonist	• Hypoestrogenic state Antiproliferative effect Increased apoptosis	• Reduces the size of adenomyosis • Improvement in dysmenorrhea and heavy menstrual bleeding	• Menopausal symptoms (i.e., vasomotor syndrome, reduced bone mineral density, genital atrophy, mood instability) • Need to consider add- back therapy for prolonged treatment
GnRH antagonist	Blocks secretion of gonadotropins through immediate antagonist action on GnRH receptors in the pituitary	Effective in improving dysmenorrhea and nonmenstrual pelvic pain during a 6-month period in women with moderate to severe endometriosis-associated pain	Hot flushes, nausea
Progestins	• Decidualization and then atrophy of endometrial tissue • Mild hypoestrogenism • Antiproliferative effect Anti-inflammatory effect	Significant reduction of pain and bleeding	Breakthrough bleeding
LNG-IUS	• Endometrial atrophy • Direct local action on adenomyotic foci	• Significant reduction of menstrual loss, with increase in hemoglobin, hematocrit and ferritin • Decreased uterine volume and pain symptoms	Irregular bleeding Amenorrhea
COCs	Decidualization and subsequent atrophy of the endometrium	Benefit from the resulting amenorrhea	Spotting, headache Thromboembolic events, Gastrointestinal side effects
NSAIDs	Reduced prostaglandins synthesis	Reduced pain and bleeding	Gastrointestinal side effects
Valproic acid	Inhibit class I histone deacetylase which are expressed in both eutopic and ectopic endometrium of adenomyotic tissue	• Decreasing dysmenorrhea and uterine bleeding via reduced amplitude and irregularity of uterine contractions. • Reduction in uterine size. Suppressed myometrial infiltration and improved generalized hyperalgesia	
Aromatase inhibitors	Inhibition of aromatase, which is involved in the conversion of androstenedione and testosterone to estrone and estradiol	Reducing adenomyoma volume and pelvic pain	Hot flushes, nausea
Danazol	• Suppression of FSH and LH release by pituitary, causing atrophy of both normal and ectopic endometrial tissue • Increase in apoptotic cell necrosis and reduction in estrogen receptor and bcl-2 protein concentrations in glands and stromal cells of adenomyosis • Decreased expression of aromatase cytochrome P450 in eutopic endometrium	• Decreased uterine volume and pain symptoms • Promotes amenorrhea by inhibiting lymphocyte proliferation and monocyte-enhanced endometrial proliferation in peripheral blood	Androgenic side effects

(COCs : combined oral contraceptives; GnRH: gonadotropin releasing hormone; LNG-IUS: levonorgestrel-releasing intrauterine system; NSAIDs : nonsteroidal anti- inflammatory drugs)

and hence reducing pain, bleeding, cell proliferation, and inflammation.[30] Mifepristone influences the caspase 3 expression in adenomyotic tissue and induces cell apoptosis inhibit the onset and development of adenomyosis.[31] The dose of 50 mg/day improved the pain and regression of the lesion. Other drugs like asoprisnil and telapristone have been tried. However, well-designed, large randomized controlled trial (RCT) are required to assess their clinical use and long-term effects.

Antiplatelet therapy: Emerging evidence has shown adenomyotic lesions are wounds undergoing repeated tissue injury and repair.[32] Platelets cause fibrosis by inducing epithelial—mesenchymal transition, fibroblast to myofibroblast transdifferentiation. Currently, there are no studies on the use of drugs targeting the platelets. However, in a mouse model, it is shown that thromboxane A2 synthetase inhibitor suppresses myometrial infiltration, improving hyperalgesia and reduces the uterine hyperactivity and systemic corticosterone levels. It also reduces the expression of some proteins involved in fibrogenesis and hence has shown a promising role.[33]

Medical Management of Adenomyosis in Infertile Women

Adenomyosis has been shown to have a detrimental effect on clinical outcome of an IVF program by reducing the pregnancy rate, live birth rate, and increasing the miscarriage rate. Currently, there are no consensuses on the appropriate therapeutic options in infertile women with adenomyosis. The studies have shown that GnRH agonist treatment may improve the reproductive performance by improving the uterine and endometrial receptivity.[34] The GnRH analogs were tried before and after surgical treatment of adenomyosis with relatively good results for fertility. They significantly improved chances of pregnancy in infertile women with endometriosis and adenomyosis when they are administered GnRH analogs before IVF. It has also improved pregnancy outcome in these women, if they were pretreated with GnRh analogs for a long period before frozen embryo transfer in a suppressed cycle.

A recent systematic review and meta-analysis also showed pretreatment with long-term GnRH analog or long protocol could be beneficial in improving the CPR in both symptomatic and asymptomatic patients.[27]

Surgical Management of Adenomyosis

The indications for surgical management include

- Dysmenorrhea and hypermenorrhea not responding to medical therapy
- Infertility and recurrent miscarriages
- Desire to preserve uterus or fertility.

Routes of Surgery

- *Hysterolaparoscopy*: It is suitable for focal adenomyoma. However, there is a risk of leaving behind some of the lesion unexcised.
- *Laparotomy*: It is used for diffuse adenomyosis.
- *Laparoscopy-assisted laparotomy*: When size of the lesion, area involved, and demarcation between the lesion and normal tissue is made only by palpation. This helps in excising the lesion accurately and suturing the uterine wall in layers.

Conservative Surgical Management

Partial Reduction Surgeries

Wedge resection of the uterine wall: The serosa and uterine adenomyoma is excised via a wedge resection by either laparoscopy or laparotomy and the remaining uterine wall is sutured. However, the risk of recurrence and the regression of clinical symptoms are variable.

Modified reduction surgeries: It can be done by laparoscopy or laparotomy.

- **Transverse H-incision of the uterine wall**:
  - The incision is made over the fundus using electrosurgical scalpel.
  - Uterine serosa is separated and adenomyoma is removed.
  - Using tension-free sutures myometrial edges are approximated.

In a study, among 41 patients who underwent this surgery, 38.7% achieved clinical pregnancy, 16.1% had miscarriage, and live birth was reported in 22.5%.[35]

- **Wedge-shaped uterine wall removal**

In this procedure, sagittal incision is made on the uterine wall and the adenomyoma is excised with a thin margin (wedge-shaped removal) and the layers are approximated. In a study following this procedure, among 103 patients, CPR was 30% and live birth rate was 22.8%.[36]

Complete Adenomyosis Excision

Triple -flap method: This technique is effective for both diffuse and nodular adenomyosis. In this technique, uterine wall defect is reconstructed using normal uterine muscle and there is complete extraction of adenomyosis (A and B) **(Fig. 7)** followed by wound repair to avoid suture failure and wound reopening using cold knife; reconstruction of uterine cavity to sustain subsequent pregnancy (B and C). Here endometrial muscle flap is prepared by metroplasty through opening the uterine cavity and removing the adenomyotic tissue by palpation. Uterine wall is reconstructed in such a way as to prevent rupture during pregnancy (D to F). If adenomyosis resection is performed without opening the uterine cavity and uterine wall is formed by superimposing the uterine muscle flap from the serosal side, it is called "double flap" method.[37]

Asymmetric dissection method ***(Fig. 8)****:*

- Asymmetric dissection of uterus longitudinally followed by retraction of fundus upward by silk sutures (A)

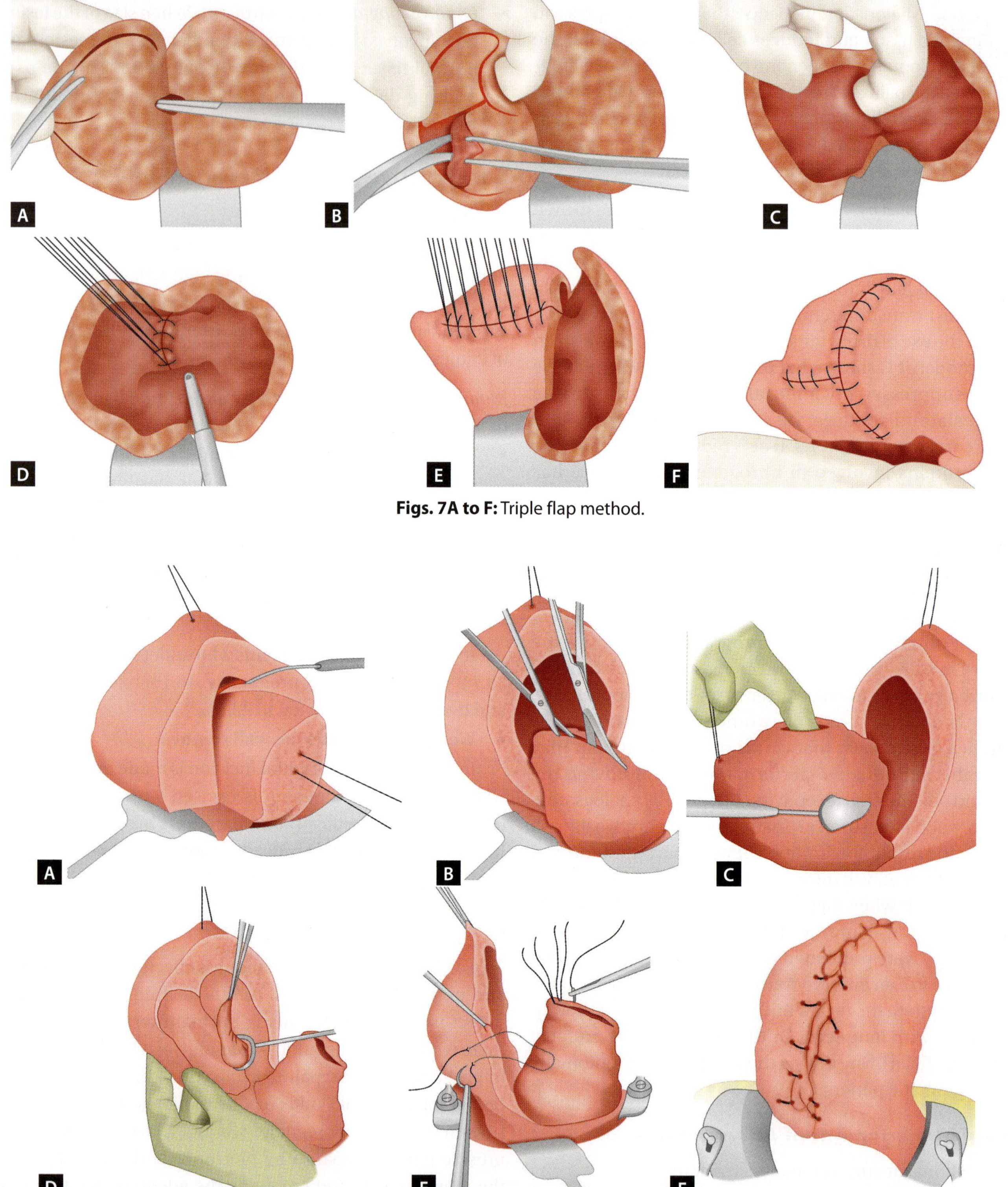

Figs. 7A to F: Triple flap method.

Figs. 8A to F: Asymmetric dissection method. (A) Dissecting the uterus; (B) Opening the uterine cavity; (C) Excising the inner side lesion; (D) Excising the outer side lesion; (E) Suturing the lesion; (F) Rejoining the uterus.
Source: Adapted from Reference 38.

- Myometrium is dissected hollowing out of the cavity and opening the uterine cavity by transverse incision (B)
- Index finger is inserted into the uterine cavity and adenomyotic lesion is excised (C)
- Lesion is excised > 5 mm of the serosal myometrium (D)
- Uterine cavity is closed followed by uterine reconstruction (E)
- Serosa is sutured with continuous suture (F).

Laparoscopic Adenomyosis Surgery

The surgical methods are limited due to restricted movements, limited instrumentation, and palpation is impossible. It is suitable for focal adenomyosis but is limited with diffuse lesions. The laparoscopic approach includes a longitudinal or transverse incision on the uterus over the adenomyoma. This is followed by excision of the lesion using a monopolar needle or laser knife and then the suturing of the endometrial cavity, if opened followed by the myometrium and serosa. The adenomyoma can be removed by morcellation or removal bag.

HYSTERECTOMY

Hysterectomy is a suitable option of treatment in women with adenomyosis who have completed the family, not responding to conservative treatment.

Surgical Alternatives

Hysteroscopic Procedures

Endometrial ablation/Resection: It is indicated in patients with adenomyosis and menorrhagia. It can be performed using yttrium garnet (YAG) laser, roller ball resection, or global balloon ablation techniques. It reduced the need of hysterectomy to 30%.

Uterine artery ligation: Bilateral uterine artery ligation can be done laparoscopically and the mean uterine volume decreased between 0.4 and 74% 6 months postoperatively. As patient satisfaction is poor, it may not be an effective option.

Myometrial electrocoagulation: Electrocoagulation shrinks adenomyosis by causing necrosis. It is used in both local and extensive disease. It is not well accepted as the electric conduction in abnormal tissue is incomplete and this cannot be evaluated during surgery.

Uterine artery embolization (UAE): UAE is a minimally invasive procedure commonly used in leiomyoma. It is cost effective, shorter recovery period, and less painful. Around 60% of the patients had long-term improvement in the symptoms and 20% had short-term decrease in uterine volume.[39] Even though UAE shows favorable outcomes, RCTs are still lacking. Currently, American College of Obstetrics and Gynecology and Society of Interventional Radiology guidelines still consider this procedure as a relative contraindication for future fertility.[40]

MAGNETIC RESONANCE-GUIDED FOCUSED ULTRASOUND

Magnetic resonance-guided focused ultrasound (MRgFUS) is a noninvasive treatment approved for leiomyoma. A prior MRI is required to demarcate leiomyoma and adenomyosis. Focused ultrasound surgery delivers a concentrated quantity of ultrasound energy to deep tissue areas without thermal effects to surrounding tissue. Patients had symptomatic relief and shrinkage of adenomyomatous tissue. However, additional studies are required comparing the safety and efficacy of MRgFUS.

Postoperative Outcomes

These patients have variable improvement in the symptoms of dysmenorrhea and hypermenorrhea. The pregnancy rate varies from 17.5 to 72.7% with a live birth rate of 29%. This can be achieved following spontaneous conception but in majority following ART.[37] These women are at increased risk of miscarriages especially in older women, placenta accreta might result in postpartum hysterectomy, uterine rupture (6%).[41] Even though there is no certain period of contraception recommended postsurgery, many prefer a period of 6–12 months.

CONCLUSION

- Adenomyosis has become a clinical entity rather than just a histological diagnosis.
- There is a need for uniform diagnostic criteria to identify adenomyosis.
- Medical treatment has a role in diffuse adenomyosis and in those requiring preservation or restoration of fertility. Further, RCTs are required to identify the effective drug.
- Focal adenomyosis can be treated by laparoscopy; however, diffuse lesion warrants laparotomy or laparoscopy-assisted laparotomy.
- Although powered instruments reduce blood loss and operative time, surgeries using scalpel has shown to have reduced chances of rupture.

KEY MESSAGES

- Adenomyosis of the uterus is a benign disorder with pathologically demonstrated endometrial glands and stroma in the uterine myometrium.
- It is one of the specific entities in PALM-COEIN FIGO classification of abnormal uterine bleeding (AUB).
- It is being more commonly diagnosed in younger women with the advancement of imaging techniques.
- There is a need for uniform diagnostic criteria to identify adenomyosis.
- Medical treatment has a role in diffuse adenomyosis and in those requiring preservation or restoration of fertility.
- Adenomyomas can be treated surgically using laparoscopy or laparotomy.

REFERENCES

1. Vannuccini S, Petraglia F. Recent advances in understanding and managing adenomyosis. F1000Research. 2019;8(F1000 Faculty Rev):283.
2. Naftalin J, Hoo W, Pateman K. Is adenomyosis associated with menorrhagia? Hum Reprod. 2014;29(3):473-9.
3. Abbott JA. Adenomyosis and abnormal uterine bleeding (AUB-A)-pathogenesis, diagnosis, and management. Best Pract Res Clin Obstet Gynaecol. 2017;40:68.

4. Vercellini P, Viganò P, Somigliana E. Adenomyosis: epidemiological factors. Best Pract Res Clin Obstet Gynaecol. 2006;20:465
5. Puente JM, Fabris A, Patel J, Patel A, Cerrillo M, Requena A, et al. Adenomyosis in infertile women: prevalence and the role of 3D ultrasound as a marker of severity of the disease. Reprod Biol Endocrinol. 2016;14:60
6. Weiss G, Maseelall P, Schott LL, Brockwell SE, Schocken M, Johnston JM. Adenomyosis a variant, not a disease? Evidence from hysterectomized menopausal women in the Study of Women's Health Across the Nation (SWAN). Fertil Steril. 2009;91:201-6.
7. Gargett CE, Schwab KE, Deane JA. Endometrial stem/progenitor cells: the first 10 years. Hum Reprod Update. 2016;22(2):137-63.
8. Ibrahim MG, Chiantera V, Frangini S, Younes S, Köhler C, Taube ET, et al. Ultramicro-trauma in the endometrial-myometrial junctional zone and pale cell migration in adenomyosis. Fertil Steril. 2015;104:1475.
9. Wang S, Duan H, Zhang Y, Sun FQ. Abnormal activation of RhoA/ROCK-I signaling in junctional zone smooth muscle cells of patients with adenomyosis. Reprod Sci. 2016;23:333.
10. Łupicka M, Socha BM, Szczepańska AA, Korzekwa AJ. Prolactin role in the bovine uterus during adenomyosis. Domest Anim Endocrinol. 2017;58:1.
11. Chen N, Du B, Zhou H, Shen F, Li J, Xie Z. Abnormal expression of Nrf2 may play an important role in the pathogenesis and development of adenomyosis. PLoS One. 2017;12:e0182773.
12. García-Solares J, Donnez J, Donnez O, Dolmans MM. Pathogenesis of uterine adenomyosis: invagination or metaplasia? Fertil Steril. 2018;109(3):371-9.
13. Benagiano G, Brosens I, Habiba M. Structural and molecular features of the endomyometrium in endometriosis and adenomyosis. Hum Reprod Update. 2014;20(3):386-402.
14. Leyendecker G, Bilgicyildirim A, Inacker M. Adenomyosis and endometriosis. Re-visiting their association and further insights into the mechanisms of auto-traumatisation. An MRI study. Arch Gynecol Obstet. 2015;291(4):917-32.
15. Shaked S, Jaffa AJ, Grisaru D. Uterine peristalsis-induced stresses within the uterine wall may sprout adenomyosis. Biomech Model Mechanobiol. 2015;14(3):437-44.
16. Chapron C, Tosti C, Marcellin L. Relationship between the magnetic resonance imaging appearance of adenomyosis and endometriosis phenotypes. Hum Reprod. 2017;32(7):1393-401.
17. Andres MP, Borrelli GM, Ribeiro J. Transvaginal ultrasound for the diagnosis of adenomyosis: systematic review and meta-analysis. J Minim Invasive Gynecol. 2018;25(2):257-64.
18. Van den Bosch T, Dueholm M, Leone FP. Terms, definitions and measurements to describe sonographic features of myometrium and uterine masses: a consensus opinion from the Morphological Uterus Sonographic Assessment (MUSA) group. Ultrasound Obstet Gynecol. 2015;46(3):284-98.
19. Van den Bosch T, de Bruijn AM, de Leeuw RA, Dueholm M, Exacoustos C, Valentin L, et al. A sonographic classification and reporting system for diagnosing adenomyosis. Ultrasound Obstet Gynecol. 2019;53(5):576-82..
20. Exacoustos C, Manganaro L, Zupi E. Imaging for the evaluation of endometriosis and adenomyosis. Best Pract Res Clin Obstet Gynaecol. 2014;28(5):655-81.
21. Champaneria R, Abedin P, Daniels J, Balogun M, Khalid S Khan KS. Ultrasound scan and magnetic resonance imaging for the diagnosis of adenomyosis: systematic review comparing test accuracy. Acta Obstet Gynecol Scand. 2010;89:1374.
22. Novellas S, Chassang M, Delotte J. MRI characteristics of the uterine junctional zone: from normal to the diagnosis of adenomyosis. AJR Am J Roentgenol. 2011;196(5):1206-13.
23. Bazot M, Darai E. Role of transvaginal sonography and magnetic resonance imaging in the diagnosis of uterine adenomyosis. Fertil Steril. 2018;109:389-97.
24. Harada T, Khine YM, Kaponis A, Nikellis T, Decavalas G, Taniguchi F. The Impact of adenomyosis on women's fertility. Obstet Gynecol Surv. 2016;71(9):557-68.
25. Yen CF, Huang SJ, Lee CL, Wang HS, Liao SK. Molecular characteristics of the endometrium in uterine adenomyosis and its biochemical microenvironment. Reprod Sci. 2017;24(10):1346-61.
26. Mavrelos D, Holland TK, O'Donovan O, Khalil M, Ploumpidis G, Jurkovic D, et al. The impact of adenomyosis on the outcome of IVF-embryo transfer. Reprod Biomed Online. 2017;35(5):549-54.
27. Younes G, Tulandi T: Effects of adenomyosis on in vitro fertilization treatment outcomes: a meta-analysis. Fertil Steril. 2017;108(3):483-90.e3.
28. Vannuccini S, Luisi S, Tosti C, Sorbi F, Petraglia F. Role of medical therapy in the management of uterine adenomyosis. Fertil Steril. 2018;109:398-405.
29. Tan J, Yong P, Bedaiwy MA. A critical review of recent advances in the diagnosis, classification, and management of uterine adenomyosis. Curr Opin Obstet Gynecol. 2019;31:212-21.
30. Wagenfeld A, Saunders PTK, Whitaker L, Critchley HOD. Selective progesterone receptor modulators (SPRMs): progesterone receptor action, mode of action on the endometrium and treatment options in gynecological therapies. Expert Opin Ther Targets. 2016;20:1045-54.
31. Wang Y, Jiang X, Wang S. The influence of mifepristone to caspase 3 expression in adenomyosis. Clin Exp Obstet Gynecol. 2014;41:154-7.
32. Ding D, Liu X, Duan J, Guo SW. Platelets are an unindicted culprit in the development of endometriosis: Clinical and experimental evidence. Hum Reprod. 2015;30:812-32.
33. Zhu B, Chen Y, Shen X, Liu X, Guo SW. Anti-platelet therapy holds prom- ises in treating adenomyosis: experimental evidence [Internet]. Reprod Biol Endocrinol. 2016;14:66.
34. Wang PH, Yang TS, Lee WL, Chao HT, Chang SP, Yuan CC. Treatment of infertile women with adenomyosis with a conservative microsurgical technique and a gonadotropin-releasing hormone agonist. Fertil Steril. 2000;73:1061-2.
35. Fujishita A, Hiraki K, Kitajima M, Matsumoto Y, Satoh H, Masuzaki H, et al. Shikyusenkinsho to shikyu no onzonchiryo. [Uterine adenomyosis and uterine preservation treatment.]. J Obstet Gynecol Prac (Tokyo). 2010;59:769-76.
36. Saremi AT, Bahrami H, Salehian P, Hakak N, Poolad A. Treatment of adenomyomectomy in women with severe uterine adenomyosis using a novel technique. Reprod Biomed Online. 2014;28:753-60.
37. Kitade M, Kumakiri K, Kuroda J, Jinushi M, Ujihira Y, Ikuma K, Ozaki R, et al. Is laparoscopic uterine preservation surgery effective against infertility associated with uterine adenomyosis?-A study of perinatal prognosis by postoperative pregnancy rate and the presence of prior surgery. J Jpn Soc Endometriosis. 2017;38:70.
38. Nishida M, Takano K, Arai Y, Ozone H, Ichikawa R. Conservative surgical management for diffuse uterine adenomyosis. Fertil Steril. 2010:94:715-9.

39. Keung JJ, Spies JB, Caridi TM. Uterine artery embolization: a review of current concepts. Best Pract Res Clin Obstet Gynaecol. 2017;46:66-73
40. Mohan PP, Hamblin MH, Vogelzang RL. Uterine artery embolization and its effect on fertility. J Vasc Interv Radiol. 2013;24:925-30.
41. Morimatsu Y, Matsubara S, Higashiyama N, Kuwata T, Ohkuchi A, Izumi A, et al. Uterine rupture during pregnancy soon after a laparoscopic adenomyomectomy. Reprod Med Biol. 2007;6:175-7.

LONG QUESTIONS

1. Discuss the etiology, pathogenesis, and diagnosis of adenomyosis.
2. Discuss the clinical features and surgical management of adenomyosis.
3. Discuss the role of imaging modalities in the diagnosis of adenomyosis.
4. Enumerate the various risk factors of adenomyosis. Add a note on adenomyosis and infertility.

SHORT QUESTIONS

1. Diagnostic criteria of adenomyosis in transvaginal scan.
2. Role of MRI in the diagnosis of adenomyosis.
3. Write briefly on medical management of adenomyosis.
4. Discuss briefly the surgical options in the management of adenomyosis.
5. Newer drugs in the management of adenomyosis.

MULTIPLE CHOICE QUESTIONS

1. The risk factors for adenomyosis includes all, except:
   a. Age b. Multiparity
   c. Previous uterine surgery d. Alcoholism
2. Adenomyosis is more common in the:
   a. Anterior wall b. Posterior wall
   c. Lateral wall d. Diffuse
3. Which of the following statement is false?
   a. It is a benign condition seen only in women over 40 years
   b. They present with chronic pelvic pain, heavy menstrual flow
   c. Can be diagnosed by imaging modalities
   d. Can be associated with infertility
4. The first line investigation of choice in the diagnosis of adenomyosis is:
   a. Transvaginal scan
   b. Magnetic resonance imaging
   c. Histopathology
   d. None of the above
5. The junctional zone thickness in adenomyosis should be:
   a. < 8 mm b. 8–10 mm
   c. 8–12 mm d. > 12 mm

Answers

1. d 2. b 3. a 4. a 5. c

9.8 ENDOMETRIOSIS

Kanthi Bansal, Anu Agarwal, Shweta Shah

INTRODUCTION

Endometriosis is one of the most commonly encountered gynecological diseases. It is very complex, least understood, and controversial disease. There is no cure for this disease till date. All the treatment modalities are only aimed at relieving the symptoms. The two main symptoms of endometriosis are pain and infertility. Endometrial glands and stroma occurring outside the uterus is the characteristic of this disease.[1]

INCIDENCE

The exact incidence is not known as yet. There are studies, which have estimated the incidence to be around 10–15% of all the women in the reproductive age group. Other study done on diagnostic laparoscopy found 10–15% endometriosis.[2] The study of only infertility cases undergoing laparoscopy found that there is 30–40% endometriosis in these cases.[3]

RISK FACTORS

There are several risk factors that are associated with endometriosis. Age of menarche,[4] if the length of the menstrual cycle is short, higher amount of estradiol and estrone in the blood, this is more common and associated with early menarche and infertile or nulliparous women.[5] The contrast is found in multiparous women and women on oral contraceptive pills. The risk is increased in women who are obese and whose BMI is higher.[6]

PATHOGENESIS

An inflammatory microenvironment is created by immune and hormonal factors, which causes persistence of endometriosis. The disease is still proposed on several theories for its origin as follows:

Retrograde Menstruation or Implantation Theory

The retrograde menstruation[7] occurs at birth[8] when there is a severe drop in hormones. The flow is not able to escape out of the cavity due to malformations or tight cervical os. The flow is then diverted to the peritoneal cavity causing implants, which are dormant initially due to lack of hormones.

Coelomic Theory

There is conversion of normal peritoneal tissue to ectopic endometrial tissue by which a coelomic invasion occurs. According to Müllerian rests theory, residual cells from the embryonic Müllerian duct migration "maintain the capacity to develop into endometriotic lesions under the influence of estrogens." [3] Modifications in endocrine system, immune system, stem/progenitor cells, and epigenetic alteration "must be considered in the context of genetic background as well as stimulus driven reprogramming of the female reproductive tract." [3] Even extrauterine stem/progenitor cells derived from bone marrow are suggested to be possible sources of ectopic endometriotic tissue.

As per evidence of the recent review article, persistence of endometriosis is facilitated by the proinflammatory microenvironment created by immune and hormonal factors causing pain and infertility. Based on this pathogenesis, new drugs are developed which can act on inflammation and endocrine functions.

Theory of Implantation

John Albertson Sampson in 1927 came up with the theory of a retrograde flow.[1] According to him, the menstrual blood flow through the Fallopian tubes into the peritoneal cavity leading to the disease. Another theory suggested that at birth first retrograde bleeding occurs as per Brosens and Benagiano.[2] Tight internal uterine cervix os, thick cervical mucus, or malformations impede the normal external drainage of that mixture, considered as a source of stem cells. This leads to first implants, which remains in the body and once the girl hit puberty and start menstruating the implants will grow casing endometriosis.

Inflammatory Disease

Pelvic inflammation has evidence that it has an increased concentration of activated macrophages and an inflammatory profile in the cytokine/chemokine axis. Stromal fibroblast of endometrium with resistant to progesterone phenotype are generate by eMSCs. Differential diagnosis between health and women with endometriosis can be known by stem/progenitor cells.

Endometriomas

The following theories for origin of endometrioma have been put forth:

- *Invagination*: These are pseudocysts formed by debris of menstrual blood with active implants at inversion.[9]
- *Coelomic metaplasia*: Invaginated ovarian coelomic epithelium is the origin of this type of endometrioma, having metaplasia of its glandular epithelium and stroma.
- *Follicle*: No evidence or explanation of how ovarian endometrioma is formed.

Aromatases

Autologous aromatase production at the site gave rise to a full-thickness infiltrating nodule from remnants or metaplastic endometrial tissues and give rise to deep infiltrating nodule (DIE).[10] I was noted that without any surgery at all, the nodule vanished after prolonged anti-aromatase treatment.

Hormonal Receptors

Distributions of progesterone and estrogen receptor are the cause of poor response to endocrine treatment in DIE.[11]

Deep Infiltrating Endometriosis

Deep infiltrating endometriosis is different type of endometriosis,[12] shared with endometriomas and peritoneal. Found at anterior compartment disease (bladder) and posterior compartment disease (vagina, uterosacral ligaments, rectum, and urethra). There is enhancement of expression of the different mechanisms of neuroangiogenesis (nerve growth factors, vascular endothelial growth) in DIE.

Epigenetic Modulators

According to Gordts, Koninckx, and Brosens a "master review", elaborate two different pathogenic hypotheses.[13]

There is a hypothesis that pathogenesis of early-onset endometriosis by neonatal uterine bleeding with the cyclic menstruation is the driving mechanism for adenomyotic nodule formation.[13]

Another hypothesis is that deep endometriosis is a specific type of abnormal endometrium-like cell benign tumor.

SYMPTOMS AND SIGNS

Endometriosis can be symptomatic or asymptomatic. When symptomatic, it is commonly seen in women of reproductive age group, presenting classically with dysmenorrhea, dyspareunia, intermenstrual pain, infertility, chronic pelvic pain, and cyclical bowel and bladder symptoms.[14] The symptoms depend upon the site of involvement.

Progressive, chronic dysmenorrhea, which begins with menses and later progressing to continuous pain, is seen commonly in these patients.[15] Diffuse, dull aching pain radiating to back and thighs and may be accompanied by rectal pressure, nausea and episodic diarrhoea.[16] The diagnosis is misleading, as these symptoms are also seen in several other gynecological and nongynecological conditions.[2,3]

Dyspareunia and painful defecation is more common when the disease is involving the cul-de-sac and rectovaginal septum.[17,18]

Most women with endometriosis have normal physical findings. But the external and internal genitalia must be observed for endometriosis. On bimanual examination, the uterus is fixed, retroverted. Women with ovarian endometriomas may have a fixed, tender adnexal mass.

The only physical finding present may include focal tenderness, nodularity, and induration of uterosacral ligaments.[19]

DIAGNOSIS

Through history and examination should raise the suspicion of endometriosis, which could be supported further by imaging modalities like transvaginal ultrasonography (TVS) and magnetic resonance imaging (MRI). Imaging is pivotal in diagnosis and mapping of extent of endometriosis, which is indispensable for appropriate surgical management of disease. However, the gold standard for diagnosis of endometriosis is laparoscopic visualization of lesions with histological confirmation.[20]

Transvaginal Ultrasonography

The European Society of Human Reproduction and Embryology (ESHRE) and The American College of Obstetricians and Gynecologists (ACOG) recommend TVS as first line imaging modality for endometriosis. TVS can reliably detect ovarian endometrioma and a deep endometriotic nodule but it has no role for peritoneal disease. However, the absence of endometriosis, TVS does not rule out presence of deep and peritoneal endometriosis and a laparoscopy should be considered, based on patient symptoms.

The typical appearance of ovarian endometrioma is described as ground glass appearance of cyst fluid, with no solid components and one to four loculi.[21]

Magnetic Resonance Imaging

Magnetic resonance imaging can detect smaller lesions and extrapelvic endometriosis[20] with greater sensitivity and specificity but it has limited role as compared to TVS and is not the first line tool for diagnosis of endometriosis. Negative MRI does not rule out peritoneal endometriosis as lesions are identified only when they are hemorrhagic, >5 mm and when associated with extensive adhesions leading to distortion of anatomy. When clinical evidence is available, deep endometriosis, ureteral, bladder or bowel, evaluation should be considered using an ultrasound, CT urogram, or MRI.

CA 125

It is neither sensitive nor specific for diagnosis of endometriosis as it is elevated in varied conditions; which is why for diagnosis no specific blood test is available till date. It has no role as a diagnostic tool when compared to laparoscopy in modern practice.[22]

Laparoscopy

It has now become the standard method of visual pelvis inspection and establishing the confirm diagnosis.[23] It involves complete inspection and palpation with blunt probe to check for nodularity as sign of deep endometriosis. The type, location, and extent of all lesions and adhesions should be documented in the operative notes; ideally, the findings should be recorded with photographs or on video.[23]

Laparoscopic findings include:

- Peritoneal lesions
- Ovarian endometriomas
- Deep endometriosis invading the peritoneal surfaces.

In deep endometriosis and ovarian endometriomas (> 4 cm), it is recommended to obtain a biopsy and send for histological evaluation to rule out malignancy in rare cases.[23]

CLASSIFICATION OF ENDOMETRIOSIS

Currently, three classification systems are available, namely

1. Revised American Society for Reproductive Medicine (rASRM)—most widely used
2. The Endometriosis Fertility Index (EFI)[24]
3. ENZIAN score.[25]

Recently, the World Endometriosis Society (WES) published a consensus statement in which they recommend that rASRM classification has to be completed for surgery, ENZIAN for DIE and EFI for fertility concerns.[26]

rASRM (Fig. 1)

1. Appearance, size, and depth of peritoneal and ovarian implants. The morphology of peritoneal and ovarian implants should be categorized as red (red, red-pink, and clear lesions), white (white, yellow-brown, and peritoneal defects), and black (black and blue lesions), according to color photographs provided by ASRM.
2. The presence, extent, and type of adnexal adhesions.
3. The degree of cul-de-sac obliteration.[27]

Based upon these findings at laparoscopy, it is classified as minimal, mild, moderate, and severe endometriosis .The disadvantage of this classification is that it is subjective and it correlates poorly with pain and fertility outcomes.[28] Despite, these shortcomings, it is recommended by WES, as it is most widely used system in clinical practice and research and it is partially incorporated in EFI and Enzian system.

EFI (Fig. 2)

It is based on two factors—historical and surgical.

Historical factors include age, years of infertility, prior pregnancies surgical factors include total ASRM score, the ASRM endometriosis score, and the least function score, which describes functionality of the Fallopian tubes, fimbriae, and ovaries.

This system is mainly described for infertility patients who have had surgical staging and treatment of their disease for predicting nonIVF pregnancy rates.[29]

American Society for Reproductive Medicine
Revised classification of endometriosis

Patient's Name ______________________ Date: ______________________

Stage I (Minimal) 1–5 Laparoscopy ______ Laparotomy ______ Photography ______

Stage II (Mild) 6–15 Recommended treatment ______________________

Stage III (Moderate) 16–40 ______________________

Stage IV (Severe) >40

Total ____________ Prognosis ______________________

	Endometriosis	<1 cm	1–3 cm	>3 cm
Peritoneum	Superficial	1	2	4
	Deep	2	4	6
Ovary	R superficial	1	2	4
	Deep	4	16	20
	L superficial	1	2	4
	Deep	4	16	20
	Posterior Cul-de-sac obliteration	Partial		Complete
		4		40
	Adhesions	<1/3 Enclosure	1/3–2/3 Enclosure	>2/3 Enclosure
Ovary	R Filmy	1	2	4
	Dense	4	8	16
	L Filmy	1	2	4
	Dense	4	8	16
Tube	R Filmy	1	2	4
	Dense	4	8	16
	L Filmy	1	2	4
	Dense	4*	8*	16

*If the fimbriated end of the fallopian tube is completely enclosed, change the point assignment to 16.

Additional endometriosis: ______________ Associated pathology: ______________

To be used with normal tubes and ovaries

L R

To be used with abnormal tubes and/or ovaries

L R

Fig. 1: A different phenotypes of the same disease.

ENZIAN (Fig. 3)

It is used for location and extent of deep endometriosis lesions and the involvement of retroperitoneal structures or other organ, which helps in planning of surgical management. It is based upon the

- Anatomic location of lesions categorized as
- Rectovaginal septum and vagina
- Uterosacral ligament to pelvic wall
- Rectum and sigmoid colon.

Depth of invasion

- Grade 1: < 1 cm
- Grade 2: 1–3 cm
- Grade 3: > 3 cm.

Invasion of distant organs

- FA: adenomyosis
- FB: Bladder
- FU: intrinsic involvement of ureter
- FI: Intestinal disease cranial to rectosigmoid junction
- FO: Other locations - abdominal wall.

SURGICAL MANAGEMENT

The goals of surgery are to excise all the visible endometriotic lesions and visible adhesions including peritoneal lesions, ovarian cyst, and deep rectovaginal endometriosis, and restore the normal anatomy.[23] Minimal invasive approach has become the standard technique for surgical management of endometriosis for advantages like shorter

Endometriosis fertility index (EFI)
Surgery Form
Least function (LF) score at conclusion of surgery

Score		Description		Left	Right
4	=	Normal	Fallopian tube	☐	☐
3	=	Mild Dysfunction			
2	=	Moderate Dysfunction	Fimbria	☐	☐
1	=	Severe Dysfunction			
0	=	Absent or Nonfunctional	Ovary	☐	☐

To calculate the LF score, add together the lowest score for the left side and the lowest score for the right side. If an ovary is absent on one side, the LF score is obtained by doubling the lowest score on the side with the ovary

Lowest score ☐ Left + ☐ Right = ☐ LF score

Endometriosis fertility index (EFI)

Historical factors			Surgical factors		
Factor	**Description**	**Points**	**Factor**	**Description**	**Points**
Age	If age is ≤35 years	2	LF score	If LF score = 7 to 8 (high score)	3
	If age is 36 to 39 years	1		If LF score = 4 to 6 (moderate score)	2
	If age is ≥40 years	0		If LF score = 1 to 3 (low score)	0
Years infertile	If years infertile is ≤3	2	AFS endometriosis score	If AFS endometriosis lesion score is <16	1
	If years infertile is > 3	0		If AFS endometriosis lesion score is ≥ 16	0
Prior pregnancy	If there is a history of a prior pregnancy	1	AFS Total score	If AFS total score is <71	1
	If there is no history of a prior pregnancy	0		If AFS total score is ≥ 71	0
Total Historical Factors			**Total Surgical Factors**		

EFI = Total historical factors + Total surgical factors: ☐ Historical + ☐ Surgical = ☐ EFI score

Estimated percent pregnant by EFI score

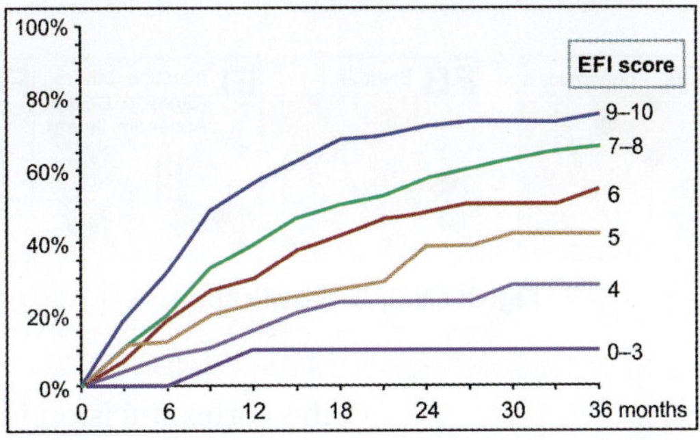

Fig. 2: Endometriosis fertility index form and score.

hospital stay, better cosmesis, less postoperative pain, quick recovery, less morbidity, less postoperative adhesions.[23]

Indications for Surgical Management[30]

- Severe incapacitating pain with significant functional impairment
- Severe and advanced endometriosis with distorted anatomy
- Failure of medical management
- Noncompliance or intolerance to medical management
- Rupture or torsion of endometrioma, obstructive uropathy, and bowel obstruction.

Type of Surgeries

This depends upon multiple factors like age of patient, desirous of fertility, symptoms relief for pain or infertility, stage of endometriosis as per rASRM classification. Two types of surgical strategies are currently followed, which are conservative and definitive.

Preoperative Preparation

This includes an informed valid consent with through counseling regarding the operative procedure, intra-operative complications, and postoperative outcomes. A multidisciplinary approach involving a gynecologists, colorectal surgeon, and urologist is recommended in advanced cases. A through preoperative evaluation and mapping of the nodules in advanced cases is a must. Bowel preparation is a prerequisite in these cases.

Conservative Surgeries

This approach aims at removing all endometriotic lesions, restoration of normal anatomy with preservation of uterus and adnexa, planned mostly for infertile patients having endometriosis.

ENZIAN Classification (DIE)
Complementary to rAFS
Anatomical Scoring for DIE
Surgical/histological staging (denoted by prefix ENZIAN) which can be provisionally based on clinical/ US/MRI + diagnostic laparoscopy, (denoted by prefix C)

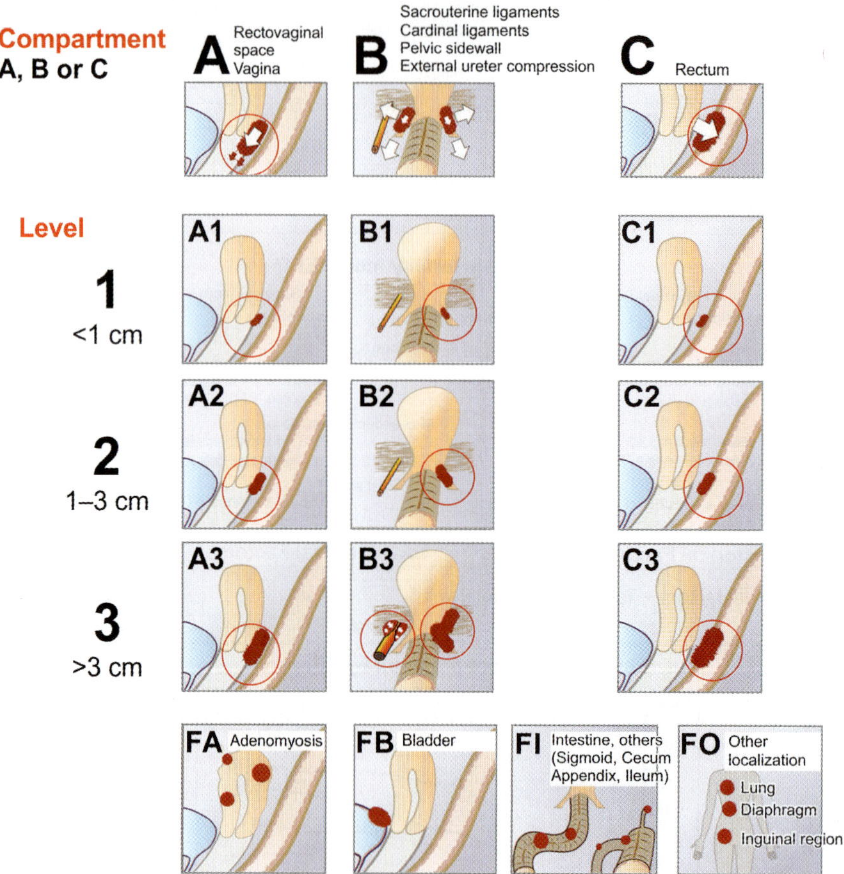

Fig. 3: ENZIAN classification.

Peritoneal Implants

During laparoscopy, these can be removed using cold scissors, bipolar coagulation or CO_2 laser. There is no evidence, to suggest, one technique is superior over other. Surgical ablation is as effective as excision, but excision is preferred as it allows histological evaluation and confirmation of endometriosis **(Figs. 4A and B)**.

Ovarian endometriosis: Surgical intervention is indicated in cases of endometriomas > 3 cm.

The standard care includes drainage and ablation of cyst wall and cystectomy. ESHRE guidelines recommend cystectomy over drainage and coagulation because a cystectomy reduces endometriosis-associated pain and has a lower recurrence rate.

Cystectomy: Cystectomy is a surgical procedure to remove the endometrioma through laparoscopy. Adhesiolysis is the first step of the procedure, this mobilizes the cyst and then with the help of forceps the cortex is hold and introduced through a second trocar. Diluted vasopressin (10 U in 100 mL) of 8–10 mL can be injected in between the cyst wall and the cortex. Incision is made with the help of scissor or laser on the antimesenteric surface, distinct as possible from the ovarian hilus. With the help of scissor, the incision is extended and the separate the cyst wall is separated from the ovarian stroma using hydrodissection. In case of spillage of cyst fluid, peritoneal irrigation must be performed, compressed by suction drainage and washed. The cyst wall is then wide open and inspected to confirm the diagnosis of an endometrioma **(Figs. 5A and B)**.

After identifying the correct plane of cleavage between the wall of the cyst and the ovarian tissue by applying opposite bimanual traction with two 5-mm grasping forceps, providing strong but nontraumatic traction, the inner lining of the cyst is stripped from the normal ovarian tissue. The bed of the cyst needs to be carefully inspected to detect possible bleeding zones that may require coagulation with bipolar forceps. The endometrioma is removed through the 10-mm trocar.

In case of very large endometriomas where excision is technically difficult without removing a large part of the ovary, a three-step procedure (marsupialization and rinsing followed by hormonal treatment with GnRH analogs and cyst

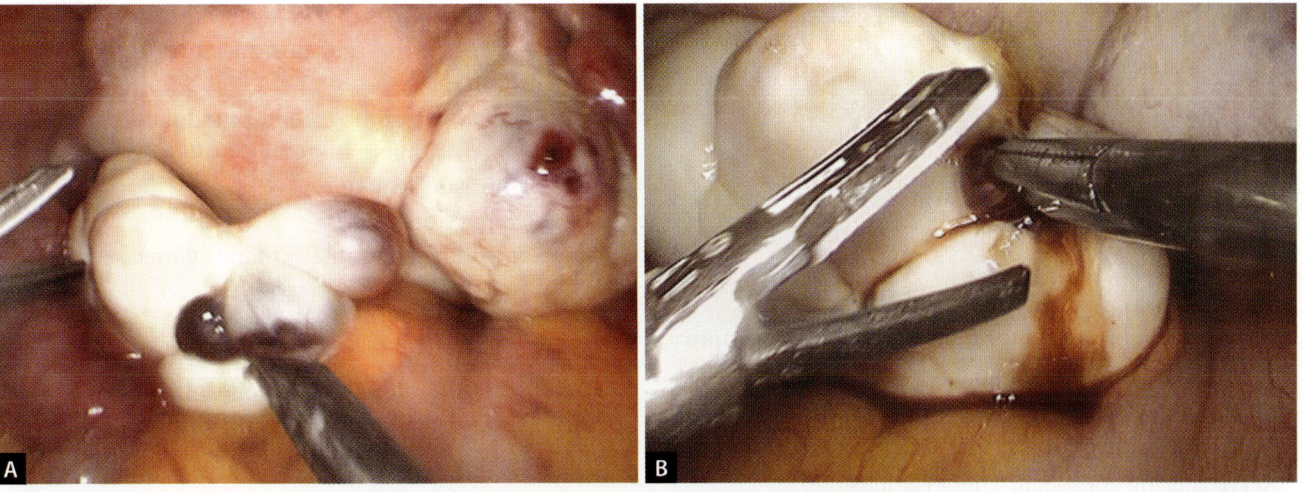

Figs. 4A and B: Laparoscopic excision of endometriotic implants.

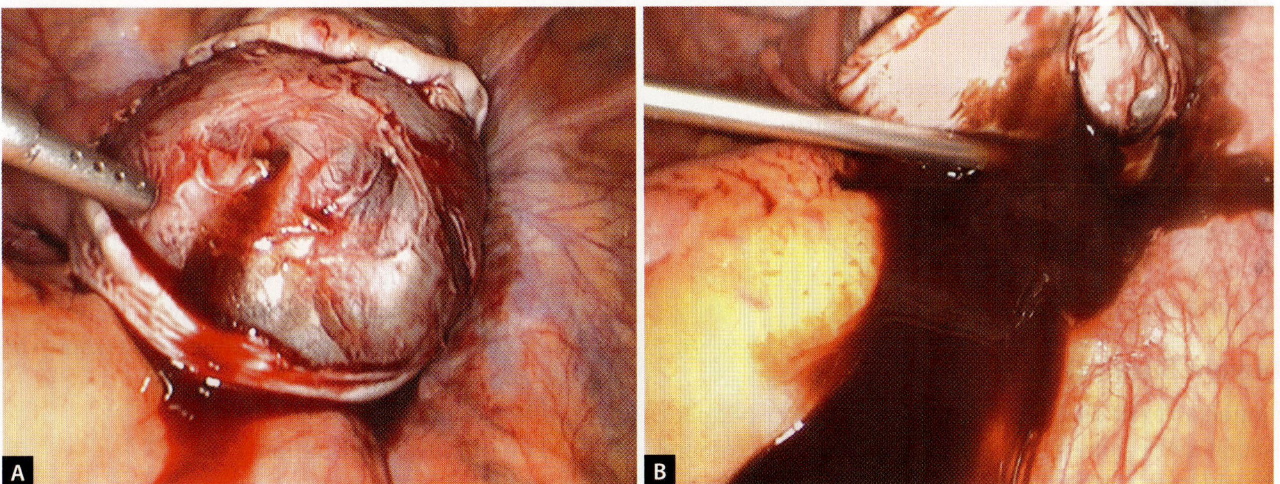

Figs. 5A and B: Laparoscopic cystectomy for ovarian endometrioma.

wall electrocoagulation or laser vaporization 3 months later) can be considered.[31]

Drainage and ablation of cyst wall: It is indicated in endometriomas < 3 cm in diameter. During drainage and ablation, the ovarian endometrioma is aspirated and irrigated. Cyst wall inspected and vaporized to destroy the mucosal lining of the cyst.

Definitive Surgery

The current definitive approach is total laparoscopic hysterectomy with bilateral salpingectomy with or without oophorectomy. The decision to perform bilateral oophorectomy at the time of surgery is dependent upon many factors, one of which is the discretion of the operating surgeon and if ovaries are clearly the cause of pelvic pain. The challenging part is most of them have undergone previous multiple surgeries in the past either open or laparoscopic for endometriosis[32] and this poses an increased risk of dense adhesions involving both the peritoneum and retro peritoneum during subsequent surgery, more so in cases where previous attempts of performing a radical surgery have failed.

The goal at hysterectomy is the same as in any endometriosis surgery, i.e., to remove all disease.

Indications: Women with symptomatic endometriosis who have completed child bearing

- With failed medical line of management
- When conservative measures have failed
- Rectovaginal endometriosis or nodule
- Recurrent disease.

Deep infiltrating endometriosis: When the lesions penetrate 5 mm or more (rectovaginal nodules, bowel invasion and constriction, bladder invasion, ureteric invasion or compression, and nerve involvement) is referred as DIE. These lesions are multifocal and are much deeper than perceived. When DIE is diagnosed during laparoscopy, it is not advised to perform immediate excision. An informed consent has to be taken along with a proper preoperative evaluation due to the complexity of the disease. Surgical treatment of DIE requires a multidisciplinary approach, gynecologists experienced in minimally invasive surgery, along with a general surgeon or urologist.

Principles of Surgery

- Identify the lesions
- Perform easy steps first, which will facilitate difficult steps
- Adhesiolysis and restoration of normal anatomy
- Free and isolate the lesions
- Start the dissection from virgin areas
- Optimize exposure by using manipulators, ovariopexy, and mobilization of sigmoid colon
- Aim for complete excision whenever feasible
- Retroperitoneal approach with development of spaces
- Nerve sparing approach, whenever feasible.

Complications

- Intraoperative hemorrhage
- Injury to vital structures like bowel, bladder, ureter
- Anastomotic leaks and stenosis, bowel obstruction
- Urinary retention
- Constipation
- Dyschezia
- Dysuria
- Recurrent disease.

Adjuvant Surgical Treatments

For intractable endometriosis associated chronic pelvic pain, presacral neurectomy (PSN), and laparoscopic uterosacral nerve ablation (LUNA) have been recommended. PSN is mainly advocated for midline pain but is associated with bladder and bowel complications. A Cochrane review suggests that LUNA did not show any significant improvement in symptoms as compared to, PSN.[33]

MEDICAL MANAGEMENT OF ENDOMETRIOSIS

Pharmacotherapy has an important role in managing patient of endometriosis. Medical management of endometriosis should be based on patient's age, her future reproductive plans, pain, and severity of disease, cost, and obviously risk benefit ratio of the drugs. Pharmacotherapy may be continued till she is desirous of pregnancy or physiological menopause. Counseling is must, that almost all the options are palliative and not curative.

Medications Used in Endometriosis

Hormonal

- Combined OCP
- Progesterone containing contraceptives
  - Oral
  - Injectable
  - Implants
  - Levonorgestrel containing intrauterine system (LNG-IUS)
- Selective progesterone receptor modulators
  - → Mifepristone
  - → Ulipristal acetate
  - →Onapristone
- Gonadotropin-releasing hormone agonist
  - Leuprolide acetate
  - Nafarelin
  - Goserelin
- Gonadotropin-releasing hormone antagonists
  - Cetrorelix
  - Elagolix.

Nonhormonal

- NSAIDs
- Aromatase inhibitors
- Danazol.

Hormonal

Combined Hormonal Contraceptives

- Most common used in first-line hormonal therapy.
- *Advantage*: Financially affordable, administration mode is easy and tolerability. It can be given cyclically or as continuous therapy. Continuous therapy has shown better pain control.[34]
- *Limiting factors*:
  - Long-term administration
  - Impaired fertility
  - Risk of thromboembolism
  - High rate of recurrence after discontinuation.
- Combination containing lower dose of ethinylestradiol (20 μg as compared to high dose 30 mg) is recommended.[35]

Progesterone Containing Contraceptives

Mode of administration:

Oral: Medroxy-progesterone acetate: 10–100 mg/day for 3–6 month[36]

Norethisterone acetate: It has been proven for the control of pain, dyspareunia, dysmenorrhea and dyschezia.

Dienogest: A 19—nortestosterone derivative.

Dose: 2–4 mg per day.

- According to studies, it can be given for 52 weeks
- Patients reported overall improvement in quality of life[37]
- Side effects: Irregular bleeding—improves with time, headache, breast tenderness, weight gain.

Injectable: Medroxy-progesterone acetate 150 mg intramuscularly every 3 months.

Side effects: Irregular menstrual bleeding, decrease bone density, if used for prolong period of time, weight gain, nausea, headache, and breast tenderness.

Levonorgestrel-containing intrauterine systems (LNG-IUS): T-shaped device that contains 52 mg of levonorgestrel, which releases 20 μg of hormone per day over a period of 5 years. Also helpful in patients with adenomyosis and deep rectovaginal endometriosis.[38]

Advantage:

- Avoid systemic side effects of progesterone
- Long-term use and lesser side effects
- Provide contraception also.

Etonogestrel implant:

- Commonly marketed as Implanon and Nexplanon
- Inserted intradermally in the arm
- Contains progestin—Etonogestril
- Used for 3 years
- Large studies are needed for its use.

Selective Progesterone Receptor Modulators (SPRMs)

- These are the agents that have effect on tissues that ranges from agonist to agonist/antagonist to antagonist.
- Mifepristone and ulipristal acetate are commonly used SPRMs.
- But studies in humans are limited.

Gonadotropin-releasing Hormone Agonists (GnRH Agonists)

- They block ovarian estrogen production, which leads to regression of endometriotic implants.
- They are available as nasal spray and injections.
- Examples are (a) Leuprolide acetate 3.75 mg monthly depots or 11.25 mg 3 monthly depots. (b) Goserelin (c) Nafarelin
- They provide good pain relief and longer symptom free period of up to 12 month.[39]

Side effects:

- Bone loss, vaginal dryness and atrophy, hot flushes, and abnormal lipid profile.
- Addition of add back therapy in the form of norethindrone acetate, low-dose oral contraceptive pill, calcium, and vitamin D provide symptomatic relief and decrease bone loss.
- They are approved for up to 6 months due to concerns for side effects.

Nonhormonal

NSAIDs

Most commonly used first-line agents for management of endometriosis associated pain and dysmenorrhea.[40]

Aromatase Inhibitors

- Letrozole, anastrozole, and exemestane.
- They are used in combination with oral contraceptive pills (OCP), GnRH agonist, or progesterone. They significantly decrease the endometriosis-associated pain, improve quality of life, and decrease size of lesion. In postmenopausal women, it can be used alone.
- *Side effects:* Ovarian follicular cyst, and bone loss with long-term use.[41]
- If used in combination with OCP, effective in preventing follicular development and decrease bone loss.

Danazol

- It is a derivative 17-alpha ethinyl testosterone.
- *Dose*: 400–800 mg per day for 6 months.
- *Side effects*: Acne, hirsutism, deepening of voice, weight gain, muscle cramps, liver dysfunction and abnormal lipid profile.
- Adverse effects related to hyperandrogenism limit their use.
- Alternative to oral route of Danazol are Danazol vaginal ring and intrauterine devices. But they are in research and studies have shown improvement in pain and better tolerability.[42]

NEWER THERAPIES

Anti-angiogenesis Factors

- *Dopamine receptor 2 agonists*: Cabergoline, Quinagolide.
- Cabergoline 0.5 mg twice weekly for 12 weeks.
- *Side effect*: nausea.
- *Other drugs*:
  - TNP 470
  - Endostatin
  - Anginex
  - Anti-VEGF-antibody (Avastin) (No human data is available).

Statins

- Statins may work by anti-inflammatory, antiangiogenic, and antioxidant properties.
- They could be used for the treatment of endometriosis.

TNF-alpha Blockers

Gonadotropin-releasing Hormone Antagonist (GnRH Antagonists)

- Compared to GnRH agonist they do not have initial flare and causes lesser hypoestrogenism, e.g., cetrorelix
- *Elagolix*: A promising oral GnRH antagonist effective for treatment of endometriosis associated pain.
- *Side effects*: Nausea, headache, and hot flushes (But less marked than GnRH agonist).
- The US food and drug administration (FDA) has approved Elagolix (ORILISSA) use.
- *ORILISSA is available in two oral doses*: The dose to be taken is 150 mg daily or 200 mg daily, it could be taken with or without food.

ENDOMETRIOMA

- Endometrioma is the presence of ectopic endometrial tissue in and on the ovary.
- They are pseudocysts.
- It is the most common form of endometriosis.
- It contains thick, brown tar-like fluid, which may be referred to as "chocolate cyst".
- The term endometrioma is used when endometriosis appears as a circumscribed mass.
- Apart from the ovaries (which is the most common site, endometrioma, can manifest as umbilical endometrioma, incisional endometrioma, etc.).

Incidence: Endometrioma is found in 17–44% patients with of endometriosis.

Accounts for 35% of all benign endometrial cysts.

Symptoms: painful periods, pelvic pain, pain with intercourse, pain with bowel movements or urination, excessive bleeding, and infertility.

Diagnosis: History and careful clinical examination.

INVESTIGATIONS

Noninvasive Techniques

Imaging Techniques

- *Ultrasound*: Readily available and inexpensive tool.
- *Transvaginal sonography (TVS)*: Has high specificity and sensitivity in the diagnosis of ovarian endometrioma.
- TVS is also helpful in diagnosing bladder lesions, deep nodules such as those in the rectovaginal septum.
- Sonographic features are:
  - Cystic lesions with diffuse low level internal echoes described as "Ground glass appearance" (95% of endometrioma having this appearance.[43-45]
  - Endometriomas are usually devoid of internal vascularity but show per cystic flow with high resistance.
  - Endometrioma show posterior acoustic enhancement.
  - Multilocularity and echogenic foci in the wall and thick wall.
  - Malignant transformation should be suspected in endometriomas that develop solid mural nodule or that typically increases in size.[46]

Differential Diagnosis

- Dermoid cyst
- Hemorrhagic cyst
- Ovarian abscess
- Ectopic pregnancy
- Neoplasm.

MRI

- Magnetic resonance imaging is very accurate, but is expensive. MRI is helpful for diagnosing deep infiltrating lesions and other unusual sites of presentation.
- MRI is most useful for ultrasonographically indeterminate pelvic masses.
- MRI is superior to ultrasound in diagnosing rectosigmoid lesion and endometriosis of bladder.

Serum Markers

- Several serum biomarkers have been investigated over the years, but none of these has shown a clinical utility.
- The more holistic biomarker consists in a panel of biomarkers.
- The use of new technologies such as genomic and proteomics may represent future perspective of endometriosis diagnosis.
- *Some serum markers are*:
  - Monocyte chemo-attractant protein
  - Migration inhibitory factor
  - Leptin
  - SCA 125: Found to be higher in women with moderate or severe endometriosis
  - SCA 125 is also elevated in most nonmutinous epithelial ovarian carcinomas and in many nongynecological conditions.
  - Human epididymis secretory protein-4 (HE4).[46]
- Could be use to differentiate border line ovarian tumors and early stage epithelial ovarian tumors from endometriomas. HE4 levels are not increased in endometriomas.[47]

Invasive Techniques

Laproscopy with histological diagnosis remains the gold standard.

TREATMENT

Medical

- Depending upon the symptoms, medical treatment can be given to patients
- OCP
- Dinogest
- Aromatose inhibitors
- Cabergoline
- GnRH agonists and antagonists.

Surgical

- Conservative surgery is very important for providing lasting relief from symptoms.
- Endometriomas > 4 cm in size can be treated surgically.
- Aim of surgical excision should be
  - Elimination of endometriotic tissue
  - Provide sufficient tissue for histological assessment
  - To preserve maximum amount of normal ovarian tissue (where fertility is desired /or risk of menopause is to be avoided).
- It has been found that surgical excision of endometrioma is associated with postoperative reduction in serum AMH (anti-mullerian hormone) levels and antral follicle count on ultrasound.

- Appropriate consent from the woman before surgery should be taken. She should be informed about potential risk of reducing ovarian reserve.
- Fertility preservation should be considered in women of reproductive age group, who is desirous of pregnancy.
- Surgery should be done by expert endoscopic surgeon.

MEDICAL MANAGEMENT

Medical management of infertility related to endometriosis in the form of hormonal suppression is ineffective and should not be offered as first line of management.[48]

CLINICAL TIPS

- Adherence to principal of microsurgery such as diligent hemostasis
- Reduced fulguration and limited use of sutures may improve fertility
- Excision is preferred over fenestration, drainage, or ablation of the cyst
- Lining for the treatment of an ovarian endometrioma
- Use of adhesion—prevention adjuncts may help reduce adhesion formation but improvement in fertility is unknown.

Role of Surgery Before IVF

Commonly in medical practice, it is found that endometriomas are present in many patients who are planning to undergo IVF. Surgical excision always carries the risk reducing the ovarian reserve by reducing the amount of healthy tissue remaining. But nonremoval of endometriomas might have certain drawback such as increasing the risk of infection, rupture, and follicular fluid contamination during oocyte retrieval. As per ESHRE and RCOG recommendation, it is advised that if the diameter of the endometrioma is more than 3 cm, it is to be surgically removed.

This may cause difficulties during oocyte pickup, whereas ASRM does not give a recommendation, but emphasizes that the benefit of such a procedure is doubtful.[49] Surgery before IVF is also needed, if there is hydrosalphinx. If salpingectomy is surgically challenging due to the extent of endometriotic disease, then proximal resection, clipping, or even aspiration at time of IVF can be the option.

Assisted Reproductive Techniques, Controlled Ovarian Stimulation, and Intrauterine Insemination

Several studies and RCTs have proven that IUI combined with COS improves the pregnancy outcome in stage I and II endometriosis.

In Vitro Fertilization

In women with stage III and IV endometriosis, presuppression with GnRH agonist depot for 3–6 months along with add back has to be advised. IVF after this will increase the pregnancy rates.[50]

BOX 1: Indications for IVF.

- Age >35 years
- Ovarian reserve
- Severe endometriosis
- Failure to conceive after surgery > 12 months
- Associated tubal/male factor ninfertility

GnRH agonists long protocol is used to prevent deleterious effect of premature LH surges in ART. Success rates are similar in both long protocol and of the patients with tubal infertility. GnRH antagonists could act as a reasonable choice for poor responder. In patient with reduced ovarian reserves GnRH antagonist may be used. ESHRE guidelines recommend that IVF treatment is suitable for endometriosis-associated infertility, particularly for cases **(Box 1)** involving impaired Tubal function, male factor infertility and/or failure of other treatments associated with lower IVF pregnancy rates than tubal infertility (recommendation Grade A, evidence level 1a). Finally, prolonged GnRHa treatment prior to IVF should be considered for cases of moderate-severe endometriosis, as it has been associated with increased pregnancy rates (recommendation Grade A, evidence level 1b).

KEY MESSAGES

- Endometriosis remains an enigma despite having been extensively studied.
- Although the exact etiology of endometriosis is unknown, several hypotheses about is origin exist.
- Newer drugs and advances in the surgical procedures have enhanced the management of endometriosis.
- There are many medical and surgical treatments for endometriosis; the knowledge about the disease is still in its fancy.

REFERENCES

1. Giudice LC, Kao LC. Endometriosis. Lancet. 2004; 364(9447): 1789-99.
2. Hasson HM. Incidence of endometriosis in diagnostic laparoscopy. J Reprod Med. 1976;16(3):135-8.
3. Burney RO, Giudice LC. Pathogenesis and pathophysiology of endometriosis. Fertil Steril. 2012;98(3):511-9.
4. Darrow SL, Vena JE, Batt RE, Zielezny MA, Michalek AM, Sharon S. Menstrual cycle characteristics and the risk of endometriosis. Epidemiology. 1993;4(2):135-42.
5. Peterson CM, Johnstone EB, Hammoud AO, Stanford JB, Varner MW, Kennedy A, et al. Risk factors associated with endometriosis: importance of study population for characterizing disease in the ENDO Study. Am J Obstet Gynecol. 2013;208(6)451.e451-11.
6. Shah DK, Correia KF, Vitonis AF, Missmer SA. Body size and endometriosis: results from 20 years of follow-up within the Nurses' Health Study II prospective cohort. Hum Reprod. 2013; 28(7):1783-92.
7. Sampson JA. Peritoneal endometriosis due to the menstrual dissemination of endometrial tissue into the peritoneal cavity. Am J Obstet Gynecol. 1927;14(4):422-69.
8. Brosens I, Benagiano G: Is neonatal uterine bleeding involved in the pathogenesis of endometriosis as a source of stem cells? Fertil Steril. 2013;100(3):622-3.

9. Rizzello F, Coccia ME: Direct shedding of endometrioma contents through the follicle rupture: insight on the pathogenesis of endometriosis. Eur J Obstet Gynecol Reprod Biol. 2018; 223:144–5.
10. Snyder BM, Beets JW, Lessey BA, et al. Postmenopausal deep iInfiltrating endometriosis of the colon: rare location and novel medical therapy. Case Rep Gastrointest Med. 2018; 2018: 9587536.
11. Brichant G, Nervo P, Albert A, et al.: Heterogeneity of estrogen receptor α and progesterone receptor distribution in lesions of deep infiltrating endometriosis of untreated women or during exposure to various hormonal treatments. Gynecol Endocrinol. 2018;34(8):651–5.
12. Tosti C, Pinzauti S, Santulli P, et al.: Pathogenetic mechanisms of deep infiltrating endometriosis. Reprod Sci. 2015; 22(9):1053–9.
13. Gordts S, Koninckx P, Brosens I. Pathogenesis of deep endometriosis. Fertil Steril. 2017; 108(6):872-85.e1.
14. Sinaii N, Plumb K, Cotton L, Lambert A, Kennedy S, Zondervan K, et al. Differences in characteristics among 1,000 women with endometriosis based on extent of disease. Fertil Steril. 2008; 89(3):538-45.
15. ACOG Practice Bulletin no. 51: chronic pelvic pain. Obstet Gynecol. 2004;103:589-605.
16. Practice Committee of American Society for Reproductive Medicine. Treatment of pelvic pain associated with endometriosis. Fertil Steril. 2008;90(Suppl 5):S260-9.
17. Fuldeore MJ, Soliman AM. Prevalence and symptomatic burden of diagnosed endometriosis in the United States: national estimates from a cross-sectional survey of 59,411 women. Gynecol Obstet Invest. 2017;82:453-61.
18. Schliep KC, Mumford SL, Peterson CM, et al. Pain typology and incident endometriosis. Hum Reprod. 2015; 30:2427–38.
19. Mounsey AL, Wilgus A, Slawson DC. Diagnosis and management endometriosis. Am Fam Physician. 2006;74(4):594-600
20. Nisenblat V, Bossuyt PM, Farquhar C, et al. Imaging modalities for the non-invasive diagnosis of endometriosis. Cochrane Database Syst Rev. 2016;2:CD009591.
21. Van Holsbeke C, Van Calster B, Guerriero S, et al. Endometriomas: their ultrasound characteristics. Ultrasound Obstet Gynecol. 2010;35(6):730-40.
22. Mol BW, Bayram N, Lijmer JG, et al. The performance of CA-125 measurement in the detection of endometriosis: a meta-analysis. Fertil Steril. 1998;70(6):1101-8.
23. Dunselman GA, Vermeulen N, Becker C, et al; European Society of Human Reproduction and Embryology. ESHRE guideline for the management of women with endometriosis. Hum Reprod. 2014;29(3):400-12.
24. Tomassetti C, Geysenbergh B, Meuleman C, et al. External validation of the endometriosis fertility index (EFI) staging system for predicting non-ART pregnancy after endometriosis surgery. Hum Reprod. 2013; 28(5):1280-8.
25. Tuttlies F, Keckstein J, Ulrich U, et al. ENZIAN-score, a classification of deep infiltrating endometriosis. Zentralbl Gynakol. 2005;127(5):275-81.
26. Johnson NP, Hummelshoj L, Adamson GD, et al. World Endometriosis Society Sao Paulo Consortium. World Endometriosis Society consensus on the classification of endometriosis. Human Reprod. 2017;32(2):315-24.
27. The American Fertility Society. Classification of endometriosis. The American Fertility Society. Fertil Steril. 1979;32(6):633-4.
28. D'Hooghe TM, Debrock S, Hill JA, et al. Endometriosis and subfertility: Is the relationship resolved? Sem Reprod Med. 2003; 21(2):243–254.
29. Adamson GD, Pasta DJ. Endometriosis fertility index: the new, validated endometriosis staging system. Fertil Steril. 2010;94(5):1609-15.
30. Bedaiwy and Liu Pathophysiology, diagnosis, and surgical management of endometriosis: a chronic disease, Sem Reprod Med. 2010;8(3).
31. Donnez J, Nisolle M, Gillet N, et al. Large ovarian endometriomas. Hum Reprod. 1996;11(3):641-646.
32. MacDonald SR, Klock SC, Milad MP. Long-term outcome of nonconservative surgery (hysterectomy) for endometriosis-associated pain in women < 30 years old. Am J Obstet Gynecol. 1999;180:1360-63.
33. Hidaka T, Nakashima A, Hashimoto Y, Saito S. Effects of laparoscopic radical surgery for deep endometriosis on endometriosis-related pelvic pain. Minim Invasive Ther Allied Technol. 2012;21(5):355-61.
34. Daniels J, Gray R, Hills RK, et al. LUNA Trial Collaboration. Laparoscopic uterosacral nerve ablation for alleviating chronic pelvic pain: a randomized controlled trial. JAMA 2009;302:955
35. Zorbas KA, Economopoulos KP, Vlahos NF. Continuous versus cyclic oral contraceptives for the treatment of endometriosis: a systematic review. Arch Gynecol Obstet. 2015; 292(1):37-43.
36. Lidegaard O, Nielsen LH, Skovlund CW, et al. Risk of venous thromboembolism from use of oral contraceptives containing different progestogens and oestrogen doses: Danish cohort study, 2001–9. BMJ. 2011; 343:d6423.
37. Moghissi KS, Boyce CR. Management of endometriosis with oral medroxyprogesterone acetate. Obstet Gynecol. 1976; 47(3): 265-67.
38. Schindler AE. Dienogest in long-term treatment of endometriosis. Int J Womens Health. 2011; 3:175-84.
39. Fedele L, Bianchi S, Zanconato G, et al. Use of a levonorgestrel-releasing intrauterine device in the treatment of rectovaginal endometriosis. Fertil Steril. 2001; 75(3):485-8.
40. Winkel CA, Scialli AR. Medical and surgical therapies for pain associated with endometriosis. J Womens Health Gend Based Med. 2001;10(2):137-62.
41. Marjoribanks J, Ayeleke RO, Farquhar C, et al. Nonsteroidal anti-inflammatory drugs for dysmenorrhoea. Cochrane Database Syst Rev. 2015; 7:CD001751.
42. Nawathe A, Patwardhan S, Yates D, et al. Systematic review of the effects of aromatase inhibitors on pain associated with endometriosis. BJOG. 2008; 115(7):818-22.
43. Igarashi M, Iizuka M, Abe Y, et al. Novel vaginal danazol ring therapy for pelvic endometriosis, in particular deeply infiltrating endometriosis. Hum Reprod. 1998;13(7):1952-6.
44. Valentin L. Use of morphology to characterize and manage common adnexal masses. Best Pract Res Clin Obstet Gynaecol. 2004;18(1):71-89
45. Patel MD, Feldstein VA, Chen DC, Lipson SD, Filly RA. Endometriomas: diagnostic performance of US. Radiology. 1999;210(3):739-45.
46. Guerriero S, Ajossa S, Mais V, Risalvato A, Lai MP, Melis GB. The diagnosis of endometriomas using colour Doppler energy imaging. Hum Reprod. 1998;13(6):1691-5.
47. Taniguchi F, Harada T, Kobayashi H, Hayashi K, Momoeda M, Terakawa N, et al. Clinical characteristics of patients in Japan with ovarian cancer presumably arising from ovarian endometrioma. Gynecol Obstet Invest. 2014;77(2):104-10.
48. Huhtinen K, Suvitie P, Hiissa J, Junnila J, Huvila J, Kujari H, et al. Serum HE4 concentration differentiates malignant ovarian tumors from ovarian endometriotic cysts. Br J Cancer. 2009;100:1315-9.S

49. Vercellini P, Somigliana E, Viganò P, Abbiati A, Barbara G, Crosignani PG. Surgery for endometriosis-associated infertility: a pragmatic approach. Hum Reprod. 2009;24(2): 254-69.
50. Leyland N, Casper R, Laberge P, Singh SS, SOGC. Endometriosis diagnosis and management. J Obstet Gynaecol Can. 2010;32(7 supple 2):S1-32.

LONG QUESTIONS

1. Discuss the theories of endometriosis causation with emphasis on newly emerging pharmacotherapy.
2. Discuss the diagnostic modalities for endometriosis with their pros and cons.
3. What is the goal of surgery in a woman with an endometrioma of 6 cm with infertility? Discuss the surgical approach and types of surgery that can be performed along with risks and benefits of these approaches.
4. What is the role of medical therapy in a woman with painful periods known to have endometriosis?

SHORT QUESTIONS

1. What is the retrograde menstruation theory of endometriosis origin?
2. Diagnostic-only laparoscopy has no role in a woman suspected to have endometriosis. Discuss this statement.
3. What is the purpose of scoring or grading endometriosis?
4. What are the important components of the revised American Society of Reproductive Medicine (r-ASRM) classification?
5. What are the indications for surgery in a woman with features of endometriosis?
6. What are the principles of surgery in a woman with deep infiltrating endometriosis?
7. Mention the indications to use medical therapy in a woman with endometriosis who is keen to conceive.
8. What are the indications for assisted reproduction in a woman with endometriosis?

MULTIPLE CHOICE QUESTIONS

1. The following is not a risk factor for endometriosis:
   a. Early age of menarche
   b. Prolonged menstrual cycles
   c. BMI < 25
   d. Premature ovarian failure
2. The following may reduce the risk of endometriosis:
   a. Sexually transmitted infections
   b. Weight gain in the postpartum period
   c. Use of oral contraceptives for contraception
   d. Alcohol consumption
3. The following is true about theories of endometriosis causation:
   a. According to coelomic theory, the origin of endometriosis depends on shedding of endometrial tissue into the peritoneum
   b. Women with endometriosis have an anti-inflammatory peritoneal response
   c. There is high aromatase activity in the tissue deposits and peritoneum
   d. Estrogen and progesterone receptors are uniformly distributed and sensitive in endometriosis
4. The following is not a common symptom of endometriosis:
   a. Dyspnea b. Dysmenorrhea
   c. Dyspareunia d. Dyschezia
5. Ultrasound features of Endometrioma are all, except:
   a. Ground glass appearance
   b. Usually unilocular
   c. Can be bilateral
   d. Ring of fire appearance on color doppler
6. The following is the gold standard of endometriosis diagnosis:
   a. Clinical examination showing nodularity in pouch of Douglas
   b. Transvaginal ultrasound showing Endometrioma
   c. MRI findings of peritoneal deposits
   d. Laparoscopic visualization of endometriotic deposits
7. The following is not a component of the revised American Society of Reproductive Medicine classification for endometriosis:
   a. History of severe dysmenorrhea
   b. Appearance of ovarian implants
   c. Adnexal adhesions
   d. Degree of cul de sac obliteration
8. For a woman with deep infiltrating endometriosis:
   a. Medical treatment produces complete cure
   b. Bowel resection may be a part of the surgery
   c. The surgical approach should be to begin with the densest lesion and move outwards
   d. Hysterectomy is mandatory
9. Which of the following statements about medical therapy for infertility related to endometriosis is true?
   a. Three doses of leuprolide acetate depot will restore natural fertility in an operated case
   b. Combined oral contraceptive pills for six months should be given before embarking on assisted reproduction
   c. Most medical therapies are contraceptive and do not enhance fertility in women with endometriosis
   d. After an Endometrioma is drained, GnRH agonist depots should be given on the day of surgery
10. The following is true about women with endometriosis undergoing assisted reproduction:
    a. Assisted reproduction is rarely needed in women with severe endometriosis
    b. Ovarian stimulation can be carried out with recombinant or urinary gonadotropins
    c. Ovarian response may be high in women who have undergone cystectomy
    d. Laparoscopy is needed for oocytes retrieval in 50% of women with endometriosis

Answers

1.	d	2.	c	3.	c	4.	a	5.	d	6.	d
7.	a	8.	b	9.	c	10.	b				

9.9 HYSTERECTOMY: CHOICE OF SURGICAL APPROACH

Shirish S Sheth, Kurush P Paghdiwalla

Man learns as he lives and experience is the greatest teacher in the world.

—Vivekananda

INTRODUCTION

Hysterectomy is the most major gynecological surgery performed in women,[1] 143/100,000 in US, 165 and 236/100,000 in Germany and Australia, respectively. UK data finds it 142/100,000.[2] The first reported elective hysterectomy was performed through a vaginal approach by Conrad Langenbeck in 1813. The first elective abdominal hysterectomy (AH), a subtotal operation (where the cervix was conserved), was performed by Charles Clay of Manchester in 1863.[3] These approaches remained the only two options until the latter part of the 20th century. It was introduction of laparoscopic hysterectomy (LH) that ignited thought provoking debates on "which hysterectomy" and place of each one. Harry Reich who gave first LH to the world distinctly said that there is no evidence to support the use of LH, if vaginal hysterectomy (VH) can be done.[4] We all should heavily respect this, exclude bias and put into action moreso, by laparoscopic hysterectomists in the best interests of patients.

WHICH HYSTERECTOMY, THEN?

Choosing between abdominal, vaginal, and laparoscopic approaches to hysterectomy is a good subject for gynecologic surgeons but unfortunately Gynecologist's personal bias prevents fair discussion. The decision is often based on the indications for surgery, acquired training and teachers preferences, uterine size, presence or absence of associated pelvic pathologies, availability of facilities, and patient's willingness. Recently, robotic technique is added but it needs large scientific studies.[5]

For choosing the route and method of hysterectomy, vital is to first consider which is ideal in the best interest of patients. In other words, technique that can be performed most safely be least invasive and cost-effective, so as to fulfill the medical needs.

Literature heavily favors that when feasible VH as the safest and most cost-effective method. However, analysis of US surgical data shows that AH is performed in 66% of cases, VH in 22% of cases, and LH in 12% of cases.[6] Incidence in UK is no less with 67% of cases undergoing AH. Generally, the rate of VH to AH varies from 1: 3 to 1: 4 or more though in experienced vaginal hands ratio is reversed to what is ideal for the patients, e.g., Kovac 90%, Hewson 80%, Hefni 65%, Magos 57%, and Querleu 77%.[7]

Evidence comes from:

- Complications,
- Morbidity/recovery,
- Time and cost,
- Invasion,
- Surgical technique,
- Randomized double blind well-controlled trials,
- Scar,
- Quality of life and satisfaction, and
- Availabilities, facilities and operator's status.

The evidence-based crystallized conclusions from various randomized controlled trials, observational studies, and meta-analyses are as follows **(Table 1)**:

- A Cochrane review of 34 randomized trials of AH, LH, and VH, including 4,495 patients, concluded that VH has the best outcomes and fewer complications of these three routes and when a VH is not possible, LH has advantages (including faster return to normal activity, shorter duration of hospital stays, lower intraoperative blood loss, and fewer wound infections) over AH.[8]

TABLE 1: Summary of meta-analysis gives crystal clear of benefits of technique used.

Measure	***Statistical significance***	***Interpretation***
Abdominal vs. laparoscopic hysterectomy		
Operating time	$p < 0.01$	LH>AH
Anesthesia time	$p < 0.01$	LH>AH
Length of stay	$p < 0.01$	LH>AH
Hospital charges	$p < 0.01$	No difference
Vaginal vs. laparoscopic hysterectomy		
Operating time	$p < 0.01$	LH>VH
Anesthesia time	$p < 0.01$	LH>VH
Length of stay	$p < 0.05$	No difference
Hospital charges	$p < 0.05$	LH>VH

(AH; abdominal hysterectomy; LH: laparoscopic hysterectomy; VH: vaginal hysterectomy)

Source: Modified from Betram DA, Kovac SR, Cruikshank SH. The role of laparoscopy in hysterectomy. J Pelvic Surg. 1997;39:147-58.

- Donnez et al.,[9] concluded that in experienced hands, total LH (TLH) is safe, cost-effective, and without any increase in major complication rates. Importantly, however, when VH can be performed safely, the laparoscopic method does not come into consideration. In other words, TLH can replace AH. Remarkably, they have reduced the incidence of AH to a paltry 3.8%.
- Likewise, (a) the EVALUATE hysterectomy study, a multicenter randomized trial in the UK showed LH was associated with a significantly higher risk of major complications and took longer time than AH.[10] (b) Magos[11] find TLH is associated with longer operating time and higher bladder and ureteric trauma. Laparoscopic-assisted VH (LAVH)/TLH is the most expensive of all three methods.
- The American College of Obstetricians and Gynecologists (ACOG) Committee concluded that VH is associated with better outcomes and fewer complications than LH or AH.[12]

Authors strongly feel that while VH is labeled as minimally invasive, one should put it as the "least" invasive as the word "least" means less than minimal, i.e., less invasive than minimally invasive LH. This is important in the best interests of practitioners.

If one was to literally go by word "invasion", truly VH is the least invasive. All that is invaded and cut for hysterectomy at VH is also cut at hysterectomy laparoscopically or abdominally but they have added invasion of one big abdominal incision or 3–5 small cuts on abdominal wall including all the abdominal layers, respectively. "Invasion" is not to be looked at through surgical cuts only but by several other factors as given in **Box 1**.

Despite such strong evidence in favor of VH and TLH, in the UK and US the most common route for hysterectomy is abdominal in 60–70%. One wonders at kindness of medico legal experts allowing gynecologists to perform what is not in the best interests of patients and instead indulging on less desirable surgery for them. Interestingly, chronic excuses come from chronic evaders of the vaginal approach and favor an AH or LH. They are:

- There is a fibroid in the uterus or the uterus is large though less than 12 weeks size
- Nullipara
- There is a history of caesarean section or pelvic surgery in the past

BOX 1: Invasion from laparoscopic hysterectomy and laparoscopic-assisted vaginal hysterectomy.[13]

- Theater occupancy
- Prolonged anesthesia
- *Abdominal wall*: multiple cuts, large portal entry wound
- *Abdomino-pelvic contents*: prolonged carbon dioxide exposure, electrosurgical, morcellator
- *Ethics*: General surgeons and nongynecological laparoscopic surgeons carrying out gynecological surgery
- Evidence-based scientific indication
- Cost and insurance company

- There may be adhesions or endometriosis
- Needs an oophorectomy.
- Narrow subpubic angle
- Obesity
- Inspection of the abdominal organs, particularly the appendix, is essential.

In actuality, none of the above is contraindication to undertake vaginal route for hysterectomy.

There is a Fibroid in the Uterus or Uterus is Large

Uterine size up to 12 weeks indicates vaginal route and alternatives come into play only when the size is greater than either 12 weeks size or uterine volume is more than 285 cm^3. Presence of fibroid does not contraindicate VH but makes it gratifying as it may offer opportunity to easily debulk as fibroid is always accessible in uteri up to 12–14 weeks size. Larger uteri need beyond VH. No doubt, as experience increases, the size that contraindicates VH becomes proportionately greater and thus reducing the number of TLH or LAVH.

Clinically measured uterine size based on gestational fundal height can easily misguide as even with the same fundal heights, uterine volumes can grossly vary[14] in two women. Therefore, it is desirable that the operator makes it a practice to depend on a reliably measured uterine volume and not go by fundal height or uterine size in weeks, moreso, when uterine size is 8–10 weeks.

For AH, The Royal College of Obstetricians and Gynaecologists (RCOG) rightly puts that AH is really indicated when uterine size is more than 18 weeks and women in UK are being "short changed".[15] In other words, we need to understand that uterine size less than 18 weeks rules out abdominal route for hysterectomy unless vaginal as well as LH are contraindicated.

The Patient is Nulliparous/There is no Uterine Descent

In actuality, VH is contraindicated in nulliparous women only when it is also contraindicated in multiparous women with identical pelvic findings.

Every nulliparous woman with normal pelvic findings will show physiological descent to permit the start of VH. Those in doubt can utilize and learn from the diagnostic hystero-laparoscopy in infertile nulligravida and confirm that nullipara do have physiological vaginal descent. Commonly, misused term "non-descent VH" as a contradiction can be misleading. In 300 women without uterine prolapse, nulliparity did not impede successful VH in 92% of planned cases as other factors played role in remaining 8%.[13] Careful clinical examination, if required in super flexed position and if still in doubt, examination under anesthesia will clear it. A trial VH, with or preferably without preceding laparoscopic evaluation can resolve apprehension and permit successful vaginal completion.

There is a History of Cesarean Section or Pelvic Surgery in the Past

History of C. section (s) in past is never a contraindication to take vaginal route for hysterectomy. It only needs extra care to separate the bladder from cervico-uterine surface. On the basis of anatomical studies in women with history of C. section, it can be said that if the bladder is adherent, it is almost always in the central 3/5ths and not the lateral 1/5th. The author has "as a rule" utilized this free lateral or "uterocervical broad ligament space" for more than last 25 years to obtain access in all cases scheduled for VH with a history of C. section without fear of bladder trauma.[7,13,16] In women with C. Section (s) in past, the same space is often utilized at abdominal hysterectomy or LH when separation of the bladder in its central portion is unfavorable.

In the absence of contraindication, vaginal route should be always considered in women with history of C. section. An earlier vaginal operation either warns the surgeon to exercise extra caution or to consider previous vaginal surgery like Fothergill's operation as a contraindication.

There may be Adhesions or Endometriosis

This can be demystified by diagnostic laparoscopy before the start of hysterectomy and finding absence of adhesions and endometriosis to permit vaginal route. A history of cul-de-sac obliteration or pelvic adhesions from endometriosis is an indication for LH rather than VH, though vaginal surgeon's hysterectomists can utilize posterior uterocervical broad ligament space—a space beginning between uterine body and cervix, in select cases of endometriosis or small to moderate sized endometrial cysts of ovary.

The Patient Needs an Oophorectomy

This does not indicate avoidance of vaginal route for hysterectomy. ACOG guideline recommends laparoscopic assistance or LAVH only when ovarian removal is difficult.[13,17] In other words, rest of times one can comfortably perform salpingo-oophorectomy, i.e., oophorectomy. Several reports favor concomitant bilateral salpingo-oophorectomy at VH. Concomitant removal of ovaries at VH is usually not difficult, with 2–3% failure rate as experienced in more than 1,500 women[7] and now in more than 2,000 women.

In women with documented BRCA 1 or 2 mutations or with family history of ovarian cancer,18 operator must go well beyond the ovarian tissue while applying clamp on infundibulo-pelvic ligament and ensure that residual ovarian tissue is not left behind. In these women, one needs to consider younger age to favor oophorectomy, may be 40 years or above.

Narrow Subpubic Angle

Quinlan[19] in South Africa has shown adequately that narrow subpubic angle did not make him change the route from VH.

The Patient is Obese

Obesity and more so, visibly morbid obesity per se should only dissuade or relatively contraindicate the abdominal route either for laparoscopy or laparotomy.[13,20] Careful clinical examination and examination under anesthesia will give crystal clear picture and convert many into VH.

Inspection of the Abdominal Organs, Particularly the Appendix, is Essential

Evaluation of pelvic and abdominal cavity has to be complete and satisfying and if suspicion or doubt appears, diagnostic or evaluatory laparoscopy can supplement the vaginal route.

WHEN LAPAROSCOPIC HYSTERECTOMY (LAVH OR TLH)?

Indications

The American College of Obstetricians and Gynecologists committee opines. The vaginal approach is preferred among the minimally invasive surgery. Only when VH is contraindicated or not feasible, LH comes into play as preferable alternative to abdominal hysterectomy. Not only that, ACOG's desired ratio of vaginal versus abdominal should be 70% versus 30%.[17] In 2019, Lee et al.,[21] find VH is surgery of choice when VH and laparoscopic are feasible. Thus, LH helps only when hysterectomy via vaginal route is contraindicated and thus spare from laparotomy or opening of the abdomen.

ACOG Guidelines recommend LAVH for following conditions:[17]

- Lysis of adhesions
- Treatment of endometriosis
- Management of uterine leiomyomata that complicate the performance of VH
- Ligation of infundibulo-pelvic ligaments to facilitate difficult ovary removal
- Evaluation of the pelvic and abdominal cavity before hysterectomy.

In other words, in absence of above indications, laparoscopic technique is not indicated.

Contraindications

- When hysterectomy is indicated via vaginal route
- Very difficult and/or high risk to bowel and/or ureter and/or large vessels.

Relative Contraindications

- Ventral scar hernioplasty
- High risk, e.g., interstitial lung disease, poor cardiac status, diabetes, and/or hypertension[13,20]
- Tuberculous abdomen
- Keloids.

They clearly discourage taking the abdominal route[22] from a larger incision and opening it.

Any patient who is not a candidate for VH should be considered for laparoscopic assistance or TLH. The general rationale for the surgery is to convert most of the AHs into VHs, in the best interest of patients and if vaginal is contraindicated switchover to the laparoscopic approach as much as possible.

WHEN ABDOMINAL HYSTERECTOMY?

- When vaginal as well as LH are contraindicated.
  - Uterus larger than 18–20 weeks size
  - Pelvic pathology that risks bowel and/or ureteric trauma with other techniques.
- Malignant conditions
  - Cancer cervix*
  - Endometrial cancer*
  - Ovarian cancer
  - Fallopian tube cancer.

As mentioned earlier Institute for Health and Clinical Excellence guidelines, (RCOG 2011), clearly advises that the only real indication necessitating total abdominal hysterectomy (TAH) is uterine size greater than about 18 weeks. States further that in UK with 67% abdominal hysterectomies women are not being offered the full range of available treatments and are being "short changed".[15] This invites good introspection globally.

Traditionally, AH has been used for gynecological malignancy. Presence of concomitant pelvic pathology, such as endometriosis or adhesions or if the uterus is unduly enlarged. AH is a final choice—only choice, especially when the vaginal or laparoscopic approach is not appropriate to manage the patient's clinical situation or when facilities cannot support a specific procedure. It remains the "fallback option", if the uterus cannot be removed by another approach.

Abdominal Hysterectomy: Contraindicated When?

- When VH or laparoscopic assisted vaginal hysterectomy (LAVH) or laparoscopic hysterectomy (LH) are indicated.

Relatively Contraindications

Same relative contraindications as for LH (Vide supra).

WHEN VAGINAL HYSTERECTOMY?

- Hysterectomy is indicated for benign conditions
- Select endometrial or cervical malignancy.

When not Vaginal Hysterectomy?

Absolute Contraindications

Common

- Uterus more than 12 weeks' size or uterine volume more than 285 cm^3;
- Restriction of uterine mobility;
- Adnexal pathology.

Uncommon

- Cervix flush with the vagina, or past Fothergill's operation makes the cervix look most unlike a cervix;
- Inaccessible cervix: Uncommonly, after C. section in past because of dense adhesions the cervix is inaccessible or accessible with difficulty with presence of cervico-fundal sign **(Figs. 1 and 2)**.[7,13,23] With a rise in the C. section rate, gynecologists should be aware of such adhesions;
- Invasive cancer cervix.

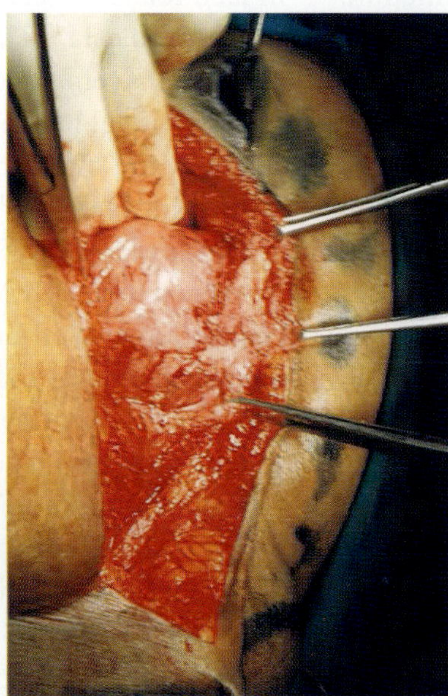

Fig. 1: Classic adhesions seen at laparotomy with a cesarean section in past. Deaver's retractor.[6]

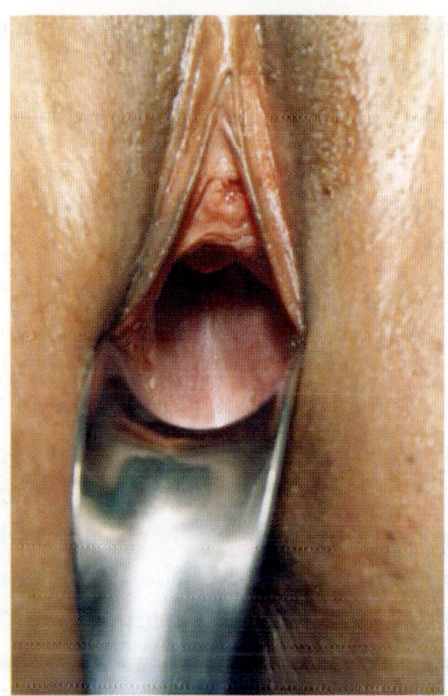

Fig. 2: Speculum examination shows a stretched and pulled up posterior vaginal wall and unseen cervix, high up behind pubic symphysis. (This should make clinician suspect adhesions as pictured in Figure 1).[6]

*Select cases can be approached vaginally and/or laparoscopically or combined.

- Repaired vesicovaginal and/or rectovaginal fistula. Though not always.

Thus, so long VH is not contraindicated, LH or AH should never come into consideration.

Only onco-surgeons, who are not familiar with vaginal route, choose to take the abdominal route either for laparoscopic or laparotomy.

TOTAL OR SUBTOTAL HYSTERECTOMY

Several prospective, randomized trials suggest that preservation of the cervix does not help bladder, bowel, and sexual function.[13,24] In fact, retained cervix can be an iatrogenic source of spotting, dysplasia, or malignancy. One wonders at laparoscopic surgeons commending subtotal hysterectomy. Is hysterectomy subtotal because of lack of surgical skill to safeguard ureters and bladder, advocating better sex life later and/or preserving uterosacral ligaments? Sounds a marketing gimmick! Howkins and Stallworthy[13] apologized for including a chapter on subtotal hysterectomy in their book Bonney's Gynecologic Surgery and later in edition of 1986, subtotal was only mentioned to say that there is no indication for it in modern surgical text.[24] We feel performing subtotal hysterectomy when not indicated reflects the lack of surgical skill or operating surgeon is subtotal surgeon. Some of the patients who choose to preserve cervix at hysterectomy can minimize the invasion by having subtotal hysterectomy performed vaginally and thus sparing the abdomen. However, this does not make VH easier unlike abdominal hysterectomy becoming easier, if subtotal.

We recommend subtotal or supracervical hysterectomy only when:

- The anesthetist requests a quick completion of surgery in interest of patient.
- Because of dense adhesions ureter and/or colon are at risk of trauma.
- The woman is keen to preserve her cervix.

Can Examination under Anesthesia Change the Decision/Choice?

The findings of an examination under anesthesia (EUA) performed just before the start of hysterectomy serves as the gold standard for a decision as to which route and technique is appropriate for hysterectomy.[7,25,26] This examination must be routine or even mandatory. When clinical examination is dissatisfying, more so, in obese and/or non cooperative women, giving super flexion position will permit satisfying examination. EUA is performed only after placing the patient in the lithotomy position and not in supine position for careful speculum examination using a vulsellum or tenaculum on the cervix and bimanual examination. This can direct the surgeon to undertake vaginal route for hysterectomy or consider Trial VH with or without diagnostic laparoscopy or omit vaginal route and undertake indicated alternative EUA guides decision making.

CAN LAPAROSCOPIC EVALUATION GUIDE THE DECISION?

Laparoscopic evaluation is indicated in patients when in doubt so as to decide trial VH or if trial fail and/or to gain confidence. When indicated it can exclude vaginal route and/or decide for alternative.[13]

TRIAL VAGINAL HYSTERECTOMY

Just as "trial of forceps" is utilized in obstetrics "trial VH" is judiciously resorted to with a facility for laparoscopic assistance and/or laparotomy kept on stand-by, if required.[13,25,26] When in doubt in select cases after careful EUA it may be felt that VH may succeed. They are:

- Enlarged uterus with a volume greater than 285 cm^3 or 12 weeks' size.
- Clinically, decent is not satisfying
- ?Adnexal pathology.

The choice of route, unfortunately, has often become more of convenience and training based in interest of operator rather than on scientific and factual data in interest of recipient/patient.

CONCLUSION

Evidence concludes that because of significantly better outcomes on all parameters, VH should be performed in preference to AH, unless it is contraindicated. There is no evidence to support the use of LH, if VH can be done safely but when VH is not possible, LH or LAVH may avoid the need for AH. Reich, who pioneered the first laparoscopic hysterectomy, recommended VH when it can be safely carried out in preference to LH.[4,13,23]

One wonders at the scientific crystallized surgical finding of only 3.7% VH incidence in Nigeria that too with uterine prolapse as the most common indication.[27] We strongly feel that it is far from what is the best in interests of patients.

Both the American College of Obstetricians and Gynecologists and the Cochrane Database have determined that VH is optimal route for hysterectomy "when technically feasible". Levy emphasizes that why, then, is so much energy being directed toward training and skill acquisition in laparoscopic and robotic surgery and so little devoted to the acquisition of fundamental skills in the procedure that is truly unique to gynecologic surgery? No wonder Levy rightly says that little is devoted to fundamental skills in the VH and so much energy directed toward training laparoscopic or robotic.[28] The use of the vaginal natural orifice

Flowchart 1: Indicated hysterectomy.

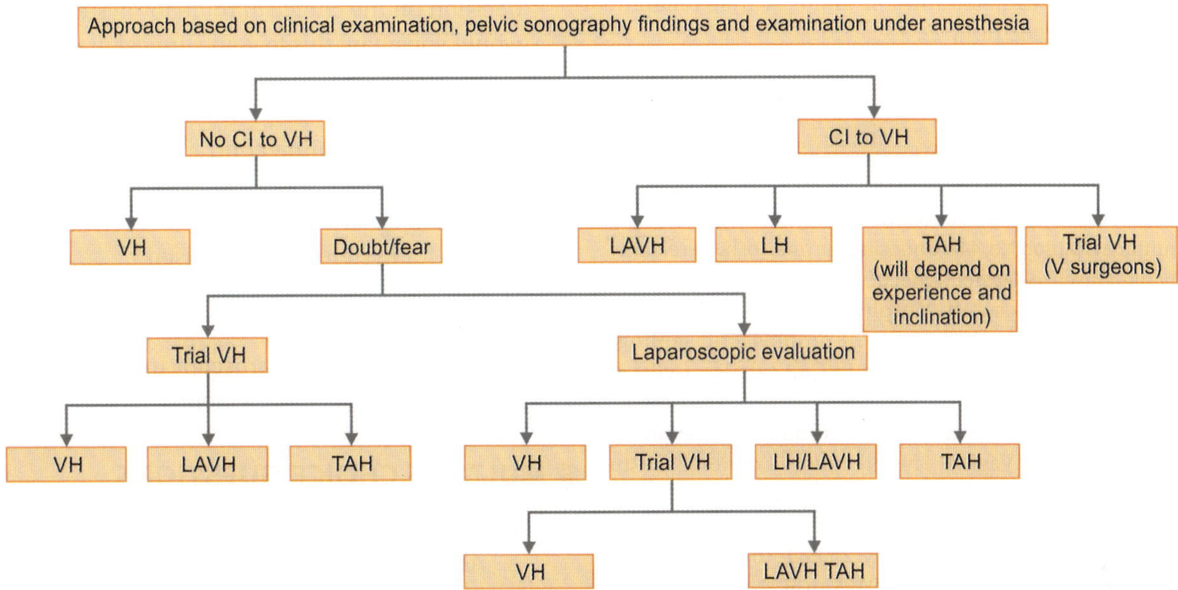

(CI: contraindication; EUA: examination under anesthesia; LAVH: laparoscopic-assisted vaginal hysterectomy; LH: laparoscopic hysterectomy; TAH: total abdominal hysterectomy; VH: vaginal hysterectomy)

gives an opportunity for gynecologists to nurture and build surgical art. Lack of availability of laparoscopes and laparoscopists in 80% of the world can easily accentuate the need for it.[13,26]

The surgical approach to hysterectomy is often be decided by the woman in discussion with her surgeon in light of the relative benefits and hazards. If one takes path of what is the best for a woman who is pinning her total faith in operating Gynecologist and scientific indications and contraindications, at least three out of four should have hysterectomy by vaginal route. The decision should be based on the holistic words of Hippocrates—*"If choicest is not chosen, it is harm".* Therefore, one must respectfully look at message broad broadcast on the BBC by Jill McGivering in 2013, which says that hysterectomy is abused in India with overwhelming number of women being subjected to the operation unnecessarily.[29]

When a hysterectomy is decided, every gynecologist should first consider using the vaginal route without any laparoscopic assistance.[13,30,31] French surgeon Doyen insisted in 1939 that no one can call himself a Gynecologist until he performed VH "in private".[32] We strongly feel that Gynecologists have to mold their skill as per patient's ideal requirement and scientific evidence and not mold the patient as per their inability.

Flowchart 1[7] can guide the course with scientifically rationale to be undertaken.

REFERENCES

1. Wiser A, Holcroft CA, Tulandi T, Abenhaim HA. Abdominal versus laparoscopic hysterectomies for benign diseases: evaluation of morbidity and mortality among 465,798 cases. Gynecol Surg. 2013;10:117-22.
2. Canadian Medical Association. OECD Health Data. Ottawa:Canadian Medical Association; 2003;pp.5-7.
3. Sutton C. Hysterectomy: a historical perspective. Ballieres Clin Obstet Gynaecol. 1997;11:1-22.
4. Reich H, Decaprio J, McGlynn F. Laparoscopic hysterectomy. J Gynecol Surg. 1989;5:213-6.
5. Schreuder HW, Wolswijk R, Zweemer RP, Schijven MP, Verheijen RH. Training and learning robotic surgery, time for a more structured approach: a systematic review. BJOG. 2012;119:137-49.
6. Wu JM, Wechter ME, Geller EJ, Nguyen TV, Visco AG. Hysterectomy rates in the United States, 2003. Obstet Gynecol. 2007;110:1091-5.
7. Sheth SS. Vaginal hysterectomy. In: Arulkumaran S (Ed). Best Prac Res Clin Obstet Gynaecol. 2005;19(3):307-32.
8. Nieboer TE, Johnson N, Lethaby A, Travender E, Curr E, Garry R, et al. Surgical approach to hysterectomy for benign gynaecological disease. Cochrane Database Syst Rev. 2009;3:CD003677.
9. Donnez O, Jadoul P, Squifflet J, Donnez J. A series of 3190 laparoscopic hysterectomies for benign disease from 1990 to 2006: evaluation of complications compared with vaginal and abdominal procedures. BJOG. 2009;116:492-500.
10. Maresh MJ, Metcalfe MA, McPherson K, Overton C, Hall V, Hargreaves J, et al. The VALUE national hysterectomy study: description of the patient and their surgery. Br J Obstet Gynecol. 2002;109:302-12.
11. Magos A. XIX FIGO World Congress. South Africa; 2009.
12. Adanu RMK, Hammoud MM. Contemporary issues in women's health. Int J Obstet Gynecol. 2010;109: 3-4.
13. Sheth SS, Paghdiwalla KP, Hajari AR. Vaginal route: a gynaecological route for much more than hysterectomy. In: Arulkumaran S (Ed). Best Prac Res Clin Obstet Gynaecol. 2011;25(2):115-32.

14. Sheth SS. Preoperative sonographic estimation of uterine volume: an aid to determine the route of hysterectomy. J Gynecol Surg. 2002;18:13-22.
15. Barton-Smith P. Clinical practice: Modernising hysterectomy surgery – is robotics the answer? RCOG – Membership Matters. 2011;1(1): 14-5.
16. Sheth SS, Malpani AN. Vaginal hysterectomy following previous caesarean section. Int J Gynecol Obstet. 1995;50:165-9.
17. American College of Obstetricians and Gynecologists. ACOG Committee Opinion No. 444: Choosing the route of hysterectomy for benign disease. Obstet Gynecol. 2009;114:1156-58.
18. Finch A, Shaw P, Rosen B, Murphy J, Narod SA, Colgan TJ. Clinical and pathologic findings of prophylactic sapling-oophorectomies in 159 BRCA1 and BRCA2 carriers. Gynecol Oncol. 2006;100:58-64.
19. Quinlan DK. Indications and contraindications. In: Sheth SS, Studd JWW (Eds). Vaginal Hysterectomy. London: Martin Dunitz Ltd.; 2002. pp. 7-14.
20. Kruschinski D. The pneumoperitoneum – a continuing mistake in laparoscopy? EndoGyn Germany. 2005; 1-16.
21. Lee SH, Oh SR, Cho YJ, Han M, Park JW, Kim SJ, et al. Comparison of vaginal hysterectomy and laparoscopic hysterectomy: a systematic review and meta-analysis. BMC Womens Health. 2019;19(1):83-94.
22. Sheth SS. Contraindicated abdominal route. In: Sheth SS, Studd JWW (Eds). Vaginal Hysterectomy. London: Martin Dunitz Ltd.; 2002. pp. 137-41.
23. Sheth SS. Newer perspectives. In: Sheth SS (Ed). Vaginal Hysterectomy, 2nd edition. New Delhi, India: Jaypee Brothers Medical Publishers (P) Ltd; 2014. pp. 225-34.
24. Miskry T, Magos A. Subtotal vaginal hysterectomy. In: Sheth SS (Ed). Vaginal Hysterectomy, 2nd edition. New Delhi, India: Jaypee Brothers Medical Publishers (P) Ltd; 2014. pp. 163-71.
25. Sheth SS. Vaginal hysterectomy. In: Studd J (Ed). Progress in Obstetrics and Gynaecology, 10th edition. London: Churchill Livingstone; 1993. pp. 317-40.
26. Sheth SS, Paghdiwalla K. Do we need the laparoscopic route? J Obstet Gynaecol India. 2001;51:25-30.
27. Atta AA. Abdullahi HI. Vaginal hysterectomy at university of Abuja teaching hospital: A 5-year review. N Niger J Clin Res. 2018;7:48-50.
28. Levy B. Experience counts (Editorial). Obstet Gynecol. 2012;119:693-4.
29. Mukhopadhaya N, Manyonda IT. The hysterectomy story in the United Kingdom. J Midlife Health. 2013;4(1):40-1.
30. Sheth SS. The scope of vaginal hysterectomy. Eur J Obstet Gynecol Reprod Biol. 2004;115:224-30.
31. Sheth SS. Vaginal or abdominal hysterectomy? In: Sheth SS (Ed). Vaginal Hysterectomy, 2nd Edition. New Delhi, India: Jaypee Brothers Medical Publishers (P) Ltd.; 2014. pp. 273-93.
32. Doyen Cited in Green-Armytage V.B. Vaginal hysterectomy: new technique – follow-up of 500 consecutive operations for haemorrhage. J Obstet Gynaecol Br Empire. 1939;46: 848-56.

LONG QUESTIONS

1. Discuss the pros and cons of various surgical routes for hysterectomy.
2. What are the features to be considered in making a decision on the choice of route for hysterectomy? How would you adapt this to your surgical practice?

SHORT QUESTIONS

1. What are the genuine contraindications for a vaginal hysterectomy?
2. Name the criteria on which the decision on route of surgery for hysterectomy be based.
3. Please summarize the evidence base on route of hysterectomy.
4. Describe the role of laparoscopy in the decision making process of route of hysterectomy.

MULTIPLE CHOICE QUESTIONS

1. The most common indications for hysterectomy are:
   a. Abnormal uterine bleeding
   b. Symptomatic uterine leiomyoma
   c. Endometriosis
   d. Prolapse
   e. All of the above
2. Laparoscopic hysterectomy is preferred over abdominal hysterectomy because of
   a. Faster return to activity
   b. Shorter duration of hospitalization
   c. Lesser intraoperative Blood loss and fewer wound infections
   d. All of the above.
   e. None of the above
3. ACOG guidelines recommend LAVH for the following conditions:
   a. Previous cesarean delivery
   b. Nondescent of uterus
   c. Obese patient
   d. All of the above
   e. None of the above
4. Relative contraindications for laparoscopic hysterectomy:
   a. Tuberculous abdomen b. Morbid obesity
   c. Ventral scar hernioplasty d. Interstitial lung disease
   e. All of the above
5. Absolute contraindications for vaginal hysterectomy are:
   a. Inaccessibility of cervix
   b. Uterus greater than 12 weeks or uterine volume more than 250 cm3
   c. Adnexal pathology
   d. Previous vesicovaginal or recto-vaginal fistula repair
   e. All of the above
   f. None of the above

Answers

1. e 2. d 3. e 4. e 5. e

9.10 TECHNICAL ASPECTS OF ABDOMINAL AND VAGINAL HYSTERECTOMY

VP Paily, Raji Raj

HISTORY

Reference has been made to hysterectomy in the 5th century BC at the time of Hippocrates. Vaginal hysterectomy was performed many centuries before abdominal hysterectomy was attempted. These early vaginal hysterectomies were done for uterine prolapse or inversion. In the 19th century, the earliest attempts to perform abdominal hysterectomy usually involved cases where large fibroids were misdiagnosed as large ovarian cysts. Almost all the mortalities following hysterectomy were due to hemorrhage. In the 20th century, with the understanding of pathophysiology and management of hemorrhage, development of blood transfusion and availability of antibiotics, hysterectomy became safer.

INTRODUCTION

Conventionally, a prolapsed uterus is removed vaginally and the nondescent uterus is removed abdominally. Today, vaginal hysterectomy is the standard procedure for removing uterus in most of the patients even without prolapse.[2,3] In benign conditions, abdominal hysterectomy should be adopted only when pathological circumstances and the patient's characteristics preclude the vaginal and/or laparoscopic route.[4-6] In this chapter, we deal with the technical aspects of abdominal and vaginal hysterectomy. Surgery for malignancy is not under the purview of this chapter.

PREOPERATIVE PREPARATION

There should be a proper indication for any hysterectomy irrespective of the chosen route. Alternative options of management, if available, should always be explained to the patient. She should be convinced that hysterectomy is the best option under the circumstances.

Consent for Surgery

Consent should be informed and in writing by the patient, after being told about the alternative options, routes, risks, and cost involved. Consent for blood transfusion is not part of routine surgery consent. It has to be taken separately. If oophorectomy is being done, it should be mentioned in the consent separately.

- Blood investigations such as hemoglobin, white cell count, group and sugar and urine investigation for sugar, protein, and microscopy should be routine. Renal function tests, ECG and chest X-ray should be done.
- It is desirable to get the details of any previous surgery especially about any distorted anatomy of bowel, bladder, ureter, etc., and adhesions at different levels.
- Clipping or cutting the hair short at the incision site is preferred over shaving. This is because shaving will predispose to microbial colonization of the minute abrasions acquired during shaving.
- Vaginal preparation with antiseptics like povidone iodine is routinely used in many centers.
- Complete mechanical bowel preparation with electrolytes solution and antibiotics is not necessary for routine hysterectomy where bowel involvement is unlikely. Enemas are optional but if it is chosen, the best time is the morning of the surgery. Instead a laxative administered the previous afternoon may suffice.
- Blood should be arranged if excess bleeding is anticipated.
- Nothing should be taken by mouth for about 6 hours prior to surgery.
- *Prophylactic antibiotics*: First generation Cephalosporin (Cefazolin) 1 g IV 30 minutes before incision and preferably one more dose after 12 hours is recommended.
- If the body weight is above 50 kg, the dose may be hiked to 2 g.

Oophorectomy at Hysterectomy

Ovaries are supposed to be functionally active even beyond menopause. There seems to be a survival advantage in conserving the ovaries up to the age of 65 years.[7] Our practice is to discuss with the patient and go as per her wish. Pros and cons of oophorectomy should be discussed with the woman. Separate consent should be there for oophorectomy.

Indications for Oophorectomy

- Carcinoma endometrium
- Endometriosis
- Ovarian pathology
- High risk factors like old Ca ovary, Ca breast, or strong family history of heritable malignancies of genital organs.

ABDOMINAL HYSTERECTOMY

Positioning

Supine position is the usual but if need for transvaginal manipulation of uterus is anticipated thighs can be flexed approximately 15 degrees and knees separated by 30 degrees with the help of stirrups so that the vagina and urethral meatus are available for instrumentation. One of the assistants can be positioned between the thighs of the patient.

Surgical Site Preparation

Skin preparation with chlorhexidine in alcohol is recommended. The painting should extend to well above the umbilicus and down to midthigh for a transverse supra pubic incision.

Incision

Pfannenstiel incision is preferred over vertical incision. Maylard (muscle cutting) or Cherney incision can be adopted in difficult cases. Vertical incision is preferred when more exposure of the upper abdomen is desired.

Technical Steps of Abdominal Hysterectomy

An indwelling Foley catheter during surgery may help to avoid a distended bladder, which may interfere with dissection.

A suprapubic muscle splitting incision is the most common incision used for abdominal hysterectomy. If there is a previous scar, the incision may be put on it unless it is thick and needs excision.

The whole abdomen is inspected/palpated for any pathology. A 15-degree head down tilt may assist to pack off the omentum and intestines. The pelvic anatomy is then delineated. If the uterus, tubes or ovaries are bound down by adhesions, it is advisable to release them and restore the normal anatomy before starting clamping and cutting. This is especially important if the adhesions involve the pelvic side walls overlying the ureters. The first step is usually to deliver the uterus out of the abdomen and applying clamps on the cornual structures is an atraumatic way to do so and give traction **(Fig. 1)**.

Round ligament can be identified without difficulty even when the pelvic anatomy is distorted because of its course to the inguinal canal. It is preferably ligated separately. This allows the leaves of the broad ligament to be delineated and dissected **(Fig. 2)**.

The direction of tying the suture is important to note. This allows the knots to be square and placed flat on the pedicle. Sutures used to ligate vascular pedicles are cut and not held.

The cornual structures or infundibulopelvic ligament should be ligated next depending on whether ovaries are to be removed or not **(Fig. 3)**. If the ovary is to be conserved the cornual ligature should be medial to them. As per the current concept, the tubes are removed with the uterus. A free tie, rather than transfixing stitch may be good enough provided there is enough tissue of the pedicle medial to it to prevent slippage. Make sure the tie is kept as clear off the ovary as possible to avoid interfering with its blood supply. Care should be taken not to cut the tissues beyond the tip of the clamp as bleeding from vessels not included in the clamp can occur.

The ureter can be as close as 1.5–2 cm to the uterine artery. So, uterovesical fold of peritoneum should be opened and the bladder pushed down before clamping the uterine vessels. Bladder should be pushed down from the cervix also. Posteriorly check for the presence of bowel. The clamp for the uterine vessels should be placed close to the side of the uterus at the level of the internal os. A practical tip is to allow

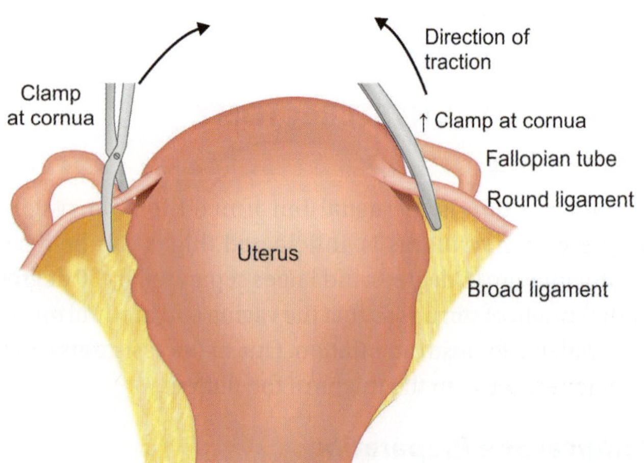

Fig. 1: Abdominal hysterectomy. Clamps on the cornual region to deliver the uterus out and provide traction.

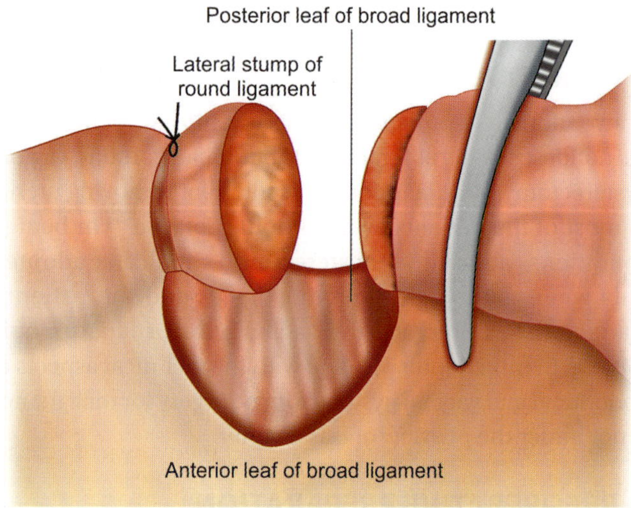

Fig. 2: Ligating and diving the round ligament at abdominal hysterectomy allows the broad ligament leaves to be dissected.

Fig. 3: Site of clamps for conservation or removal of ovary at abdominal hysterectomy.

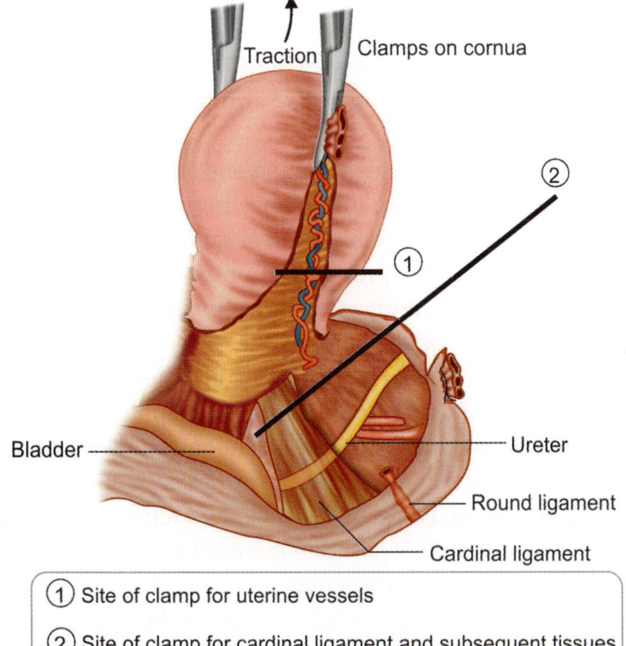

Fig. 4: Site of clamps for tackling the uterine vessels and cardinal ligaments at abdominal hysterectomy and the course of the ureter after bladder is retracted away.

the clamp slip out of the lateral uterine wall in the process of clamping, so that it does not wander laterally. The clamp may be held at 45-degree angle to the side of the uterus **(Fig. 4)**. Try to avoid too much tissue in this clamp as it is a vascular pedicle. Double clamping of the stump will help to avoid tissue receding which, if it happens, can lead to hematoma formation. An additional clamp placed medially will help to avoid backflow bleeding, if the uterus is too large.

There is no need to cut the posterior peritoneum separately unless the bowel is adherent to the cervix. This may happen in cases of pelvic endometriosis. Incision of peritoneum between the adherent bowel and the back of the cervix followed by separation of the bowel is essential before cutting the posterior vaginal wall. Before clamping the lateral angle of vagina, the authors recommend to cut open the anterior vaginal wall and to apply the clamp for the lateral cervical and uterosacral ligaments with one blade in the inner aspect.

Vault closure is recommended rather than leaving it opened. A drain can be left through the vault, if deemed necessary but in practice is seldom required. Vaginal mucosa should be included in the suturing. Bladder base and vaginal bleeders are to be tackled. Precervical fascia and Mackenrodt ligament strengthening to the vault will prevent the risk of future vault prolapse. If there is a deep cul-de-sac, it should be obliterated with circumferential running stitches from the sides and anterior surface of the rectum and posterior surface of the vagina. Failure to do this can lead to early development of vault prolapse. Cornual structures should not be used to lift up the vault as done by some.

Intrafascial and Extrafascial Hysterectomy

A lot of emphasis used to be given to the plane of dissection at the level of the vagina. The conventional recommendation was to do an extra fascial dissection for hysterectomies for malignancies and an intrafascial for benign conditions. The argument was that when an extrafascial hysterectomy is done, the lymphatic channels will also be removed. On the other hand, while removing the uterus for benign conditions, the fascia is left behind so that the vault will be stronger. The fascia referred to is the thin layer of fascia that can be identified on the anterior vaginal wall adjacent to the bladder wall. After laparoscopic hysterectomies gained popularity, this distinction into extrafascial and intrafascial is not emphasized much.

Closing the Abdomen

Mop and instrument count should be checked before closing the abdomen.

Parietal peritoneal closure is recommended, if muscle cutting incision was used. Rectus sheath is closed with delayed absorbable suture material for transverse abdominal incision. For vertical incision bulk closure with nonabsorbable suture material is recommended. Make sure that the edges of the rectus sheath are not missed. Skin closure can be with staples, adhesive tapes or subcuticular stitches. Wound dressing can be removed after 24 hours.

Suture Material

Delayed absorbable suture material like Polyglactin or Polyglycolic acid (No.1 or No.1-0) is recommended for stumps and vault of vagina.

VAGINAL HYSTERECTOMY

Surgery for prolapse uterus will be dealt with in the corresponding chapter. Here, we will consider only nondescent vaginal hysterectomy (NDVH). Preoperative preparation remains the same as for abdominal hysterectomy.

Advantages of Vaginal Over Abdominal Approach

- It is an almost entirely extraperitoneal operation. So, the chance of paralytic ileus is less.
- Abdominal incision-related morbidity in the form of infection, dehiscence, evisceration, hernia, etc.,[5] is also less.
- Early ambulation, less of analgesics, early feeding, less requirement of IV fluids, and early discharge from hospital are possible with vaginal hysterectomy.
- Postoperative adhesions are reduced.
- Simultaneous repair of pelvic floor can be done.

Contraindications for Vaginal Approach

Surgery for invasive endometrial and cervical cancers is done by abdominal route.

Extensive endometriosis, bowel adhesions, ovarian neoplasms, suspected bowel disease, etc., are all indications for the abdominal route.

Previous cesarean section is not a contraindication for vaginal hysterectomy. The vaginal approach is usually easier here as the correct plane can be identified easily. The adhesion between bladder and uterus is most dense in the midline. Planes are easier to identify on the sides (Shirish Sheth).[8] Taking advantage of this principle the dissection may be started on the sides and then preceded medially. However, there is a catch here. The uterine vessels may be more medially placed. Care should be taken to avoid injury to them. Whether approached abdominally or vaginally a scarred vesico uterine plane dissection can be difficult. The fundamental principle to follow is to dissect closer to the uterine side rather than the vesicle side. If there was more than one cesarean, there would be adhesions at different levels as the previous incisions would not have been at the same level. Care should be taken until all the scarred areas are freed and the free peritoneum or free peritoneal cavity is reached. If there is doubt about planes, inserting a metal catheter into the bladder will aid in delineating the bladder wall. Some recommend instilling methylene blue into the bladder to see, if bladder is reached or incised. The authors have not found this necessary.

Technical Aspects

Positioning: Special stirrups are available for the proper positioning of the patient giving ample space in between the legs of the patient for the assistants to occupy. Allen stirrups are ideal for this. But these are expensive. Simpler and cheaper leg support systems are available locally. In this the legs are not supported under the popliteal fossa but at the area of the calf muscle on broad canvas stirrups. This prevents pressure points and hence postoperative thromboembolic risk is reduced.

After proper positioning, cleaning, and draping, the bladder is emptied. Examination under anesthesia is a must before starting the procedure. Infiltration of saline with adrenaline (1 in 200,000) or vasopressin (20 units of vasopressin in 100 mL of saline) is useful not only to reduce the bleeding but also to define the tissue planes.

Traditionally, circular incision is made at the cervicovaginal junction. Instead, anterior and posterior colpotomy incision can be made separately. Through the anterior colpotomy incision, bladder is dissected free from the cervix, uterovesical fold of peritoneum is reached and bladder retracted **(Fig. 5)**. The uterovesical fold of peritoneum may be left unopened in the beginning to prevent omentum or bowel popping out. The vaginal incision is not extended laterally; this helps to keep the Mackenrodt's ligament attached to the vagina as a safeguard against future vault prolapse.

For the beginners, it is advisable to proceed in the traditional way of clamping cutting and ligating the Mackenrodt-uterosacral complex, uterine vessels, and upper pedicles with a delayed absorbable suture material. Holding the needle on the needle holder at a forward oblique angle helps to introduce it even in narrow vagina and tie the pedicle. For tying a pedicle we recommend passing the needle from front to back at the lower edge of the pedicle and bringing it from back to front at the upper edge of the pedicle. This helps to tie the pedicle with needle holder **(Fig. 6)**. Once uterine arteries have been tied, blood supply to the uterus is dramatically diminished (~75–80%), allowing a safe morcellation, bisection, myomectomy, or encoring without blood loss.[9]

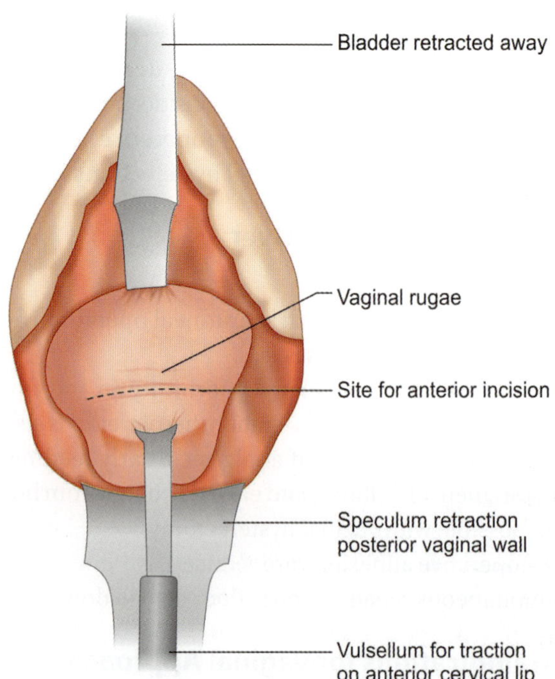

Fig. 5: Site for anterior incision at vaginal hysterectomy.

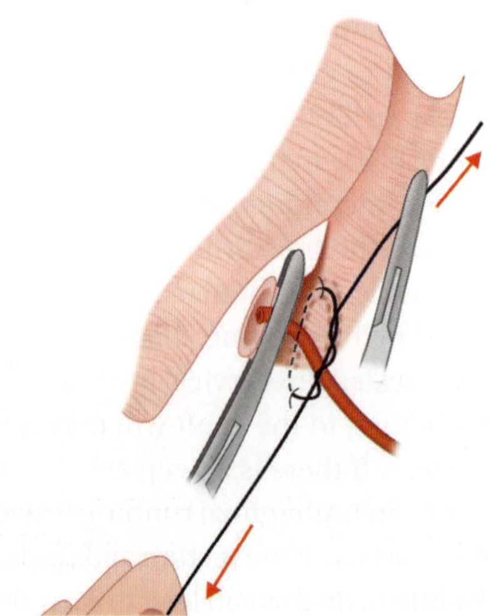
Fig. 6: Suture and knot tying technique with needle holder. Note the direction of tying and traction of the suture.

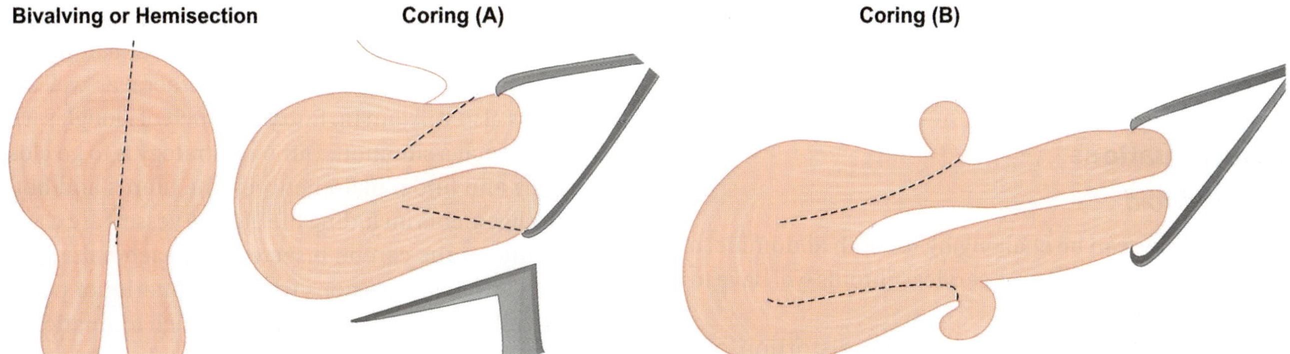

Fig. 7: Debulking techniques at vaginal hysterectomy.

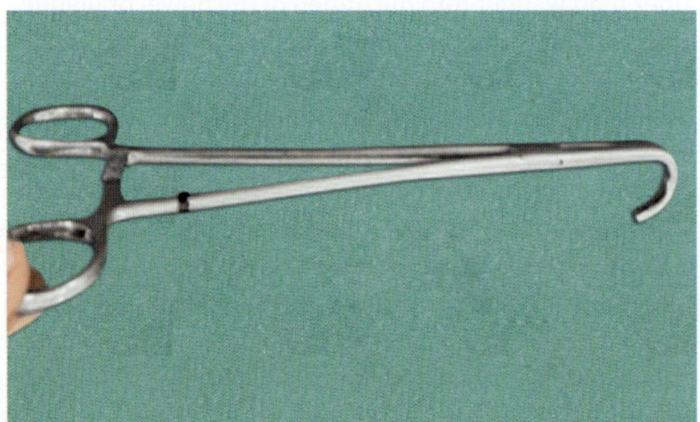

Fig. 8: Transvaginal oophorectomy clamp.

Instead of tying the pedicle, bipolar coagulation is also possible. Bipolar clamps with electronic control to shut off the electric circuit when coagulation is completed are available. Some companies have incorporated cutting blades to make the procedure easier. Even though this uses bipolar current, lateral spread of the current is possible and one has to be conscious of this risk. As a safeguard, the amount of tissue caught in the clamps should be controlled. A large pedicle may require keeping the activation of the clamp for a longer time leading to more lateral spread.

When the exposure is limited, vigorous posterior retraction is helpful. Another step that helps in increasing available space is to remove tissues as one progresses after the uterine arteries have been tied. Adenomyosis or fibroids can be removed to increase the space and to gain access to upper structures.[9] Various debulking techniques such as bivalving, coring, morcellation, or myomectomy can be used **(Fig. 7)**.

The indications for oophorectomy remain the same as for abdominal route. There are different techniques described for oophorectomy via the vaginal route. Special reverse angled clamp has been developed by the first author for the purpose of oophorectomy which helps in the proper placement of the ligature **(Fig. 8)**.

When a deep cul-de-ac or enterocoele sac is encountered, the excess peritoneum is excised and a high-internal obliteration of the pouch of Douglas is done. After closing the vaginal mucosa, the suspension of the vault with Mackenrodt–uterosacral complex (external McCall's sutures) is recommended to prevent future vault prolapse.

The preferred suture material for the McCall stitch is delayed absorbable one like No. 1 or No. 1-0 Polydioxon (PDS).

Closure of Vault of Vagina

In NDVH, some would recommend closure of peritoneum. The advantage claimed is that it provides an additional layer of support for the pelvic floor. This may help in reducing adhesions of omentum and bowel to the stumps. However, as the step is not followed in laparoscopic hysterectomy, many have stopped doing it in NDVH also.

The vault is closed horizontally. The angles are specially taken care of with separate stitches. The central part is closed with continuous or interrupted stitches. One should take care that the raw area on posterior vaginal edge from where the peritoneum is stripped off is included in the stitch so that oozing and hematoma formation can be prevented.

Postoperative Care

- *Antibiotics:* A single preoperative dose with an additional dose of first generation Cephalosporin (Cefazolin) is sufficient.
- *Thromboprophylaxis:* To be given in obese patients, long surgeries, and those with risk factors for venous thromboembolism.
- *Diet*: Patient can resume normal diet by the next day after surgery.
- *Ambulation*: She can ambulate as early as 6 hours after the procedure. For this good, 24 hour coverage of analgesics is required. It can be NSAIDs or Tramadol parenterally, orally or as suppository
- *Bath:* She can have full bath from first postoperative day itself.
- *Catheter:* Once the patient is ambulant catheter can be removed.
- *Hospital stay:* Patient can go home after 24–48 hours in otherwise uncomplicated hysterectomy.

- *Resuming work:* She can do light nonweight bearing work in the first week itself. Weight bearing work and exercise is recommended after 6 weeks.

Special Situations

Cervical Fibroid

Cervical fibroids can be challenging for both abdominal and vaginal hysterectomies. Large cervical fibroids will have to be tackled abdominally.

The main problems are due to the distortion of the anatomy. It makes it difficult to apply clamps for the ligaments as well as the uterine arteries. There is also a possibility of injury to the ureters and trigone of the bladder.

It is easier to tackle a fibroid arising from the portio vaginalis part of the cervix than the one higher up especially at the isthmus. The relation of the ureter and uterine arteries will vary depending on the exact location of origin and direction of growth. Applying clamps on the sides in fibroids expanding to pelvic side walls can be hazardous. The principle is to stay close to the fibroid, beware of the ureter, and enucleate the fibroid, if possible before proceeding with clamping the adjacent pedicles. To start with bladder may be separated and pushed down. After the round ligament is taken, the broad ligament can be opened and the ureter can be identified by dissection, which allows visualization and avoiding injury to it. One may consider placing ureteric catheter prior to the surgery and leave them in situ during the procedure.

The usual dictum is not to incise on the fibroid until the blood supply has been cut off. But in this situation, an exception should be considered. A practical way to circumvent this problem is to debulk the central part of the fibroid. If the fibroid is filling the pelvis making it difficult to clamp structures laterally, after injecting vasopressin, chunks of tissue may be removed from the central part of the fibroid. This will help to create space laterally. Once the central bulk is reduced, there will be space to work on the sides and apply clamps.

If it is possible, put clamps for the uterosacral and Mackenrodt's ligaments. If the uterine arteries are accessible clamp them. Then the fibroid can be debulked from its center. A method we have found most useful is to insert a myoma screw and cut a pyramidal part of the myoma around it. A long knife with curved handle will make it easier. Once the central part of the fibroid is removed rest of the procedure will be straight forward.

Adherent Uterus

In women with previous surgery like cesarean section or myomectomy, there is chance of adhesions to bowel, omentum, bladder, or even anterior abdominal wall. The adhesions may limit the mobility and access to the uterus. Adhesions to bladder will be dealt with separately later. Bowel adhesions usually result from surgeries other than lower segment cesarean or from endometriosis.

Endometriosis, which is the most common reason for adhesion of rectosigmoid to back of uterus, can make the uterus anchored to the thickened uterosacral as well. Often the ovaries also will join in. Entry to pouch of Douglas will be difficult in such a situation. Our own strategy is to go close to the uterus and find a plain between the uterus and bowels. Once the ligaments including the uterine vessels are clamped and cut the uterus can be bisected and each half removed separately. We had occasions when the anterior or posterior wall was adherent up to the fundus. In such a situation once the uterine arteries are tied whichever side is free may be incised up to the fundus and the opposite side released by retrograde dissection. The clue is to stay close to the uterus rather than wander into the lumen of the bowel or bladder.

If the adhesions are on the fundus, as is often the case following myomectomy some degree of descent of uterus is possible. Again, by staying close to uterus the plane of cleavage can be identified and the bowel or omentum separated.

Adhesion to anterior abdominal wall can be particularly difficult especially if a broad area is plastered to anterior abdominal wall. In such cases it may be better to have laparoscopic assistance to release the uterus or convert the vaginal to an abdominal hysterectomy. However, sometimes it may be just a fibrous band holding the fundus to the anterior abdominal wall. Often it may be possible to coagulate or cut the band transvaginally. Occasionally, laparoscopy or laparotomy may be required to severe this band of adhesion.

Previous Lower Segment Cesarean Section and Adherent Bladder

Almost invariably previous lower segment cesarean section leads to adhesions of the bladder to the isthmus of the uterus. The level at which this occurs depends on whether the previous cesarean was after the onset of labor or not. In an elective cesarean the adhesion is likely to be at a higher level compared with the one where cesarean was done in advanced labor. If there was more than one cesarean the scar may be single or multiple. Shirish Sheth has pointed out the fact that the adhesion is usually most dense at the middle and not on the sides.[8] This gives a window of free space on the sides. However, to offset this advantage there is usually a medial displacement of the uterine vessels. So, one has to tread carefully here, lest troublesome bleeding will occur. Once bladder is lifted up on the sides and the uterosacral Mackenrodt's ligaments are transected, the uterus will yield further. We have found the following technique useful in separating the bladder from the scar area. The assistant pulls the cervix down and the surgeon stretches the bladder with a tongue depressor and separates the bladder by sharp dissection. The area of scar is usually felt as a groove. However, before attempting to cut the layers of tissue above the level of the scar, one has to make sure that it is really thin as is expected of the uterovesical fold. If there is any doubt put a metal catheter into the bladder and outline its limits.

Endometriosis

The concerns are stuck ovary, adhesions to ureter, and rectovaginal endometriosis. The basic principle here is restoring the anatomy by releasing adhesions before starting the hysterectomy. In difficult cases, the uterus may be removed first and then the adnexa. Stenting or ureteric catheterization may be helpful in distorted ureteric anatomy.

Cornual Fibroid

A useful tip is to clamp the round ligament and the other cornual structures separately.

Broad Ligament Fibroid

In false broad ligament fibroids, there will not be any vessels laterally. So the fibroid can be lifted up from its bed and dealt with. In true broad ligament fibroid, the vessels and the ureter may be medial or lateral but the advantage is that rarely only they grow big. Myometrial condensation (false capsule) will be deficient for both types of broad ligament fibroids.

Subtotal Hysterectomy Followed by Removal of Cervix

Often, there may be difficulty to work in the pelvis while attempting abdominal hysterectomy of a large uterus through a transverse lower abdominal incision. A simple way to overcome this problem is to do a subtotal hysterectomy first followed by removal of the cervical stump. The parts above the isthmus can be removed by transection at the level of the isthmus after the uterine arteries are ligated. This will give adequate space to work in the pelvis and remove the cervix.

Subtotal Hysterectomy versus Total Hysterectomy

While doing hysterectomy, whether to remove the entire uterus along with the cervix or leave the cervix behind (subtotal) has been a controversial issue since the beginning of hysterectomy in the 19th century to the present day. Subtotal remained the operation of choice until 1929, when EH Richardson performed the first total abdominal hysterectomy. In 1930s, only one out of every four hysterectomies was total, primarily in an effort to reduce the risk of hemorrhage and infection. By 1950s with advances in antibiotics, blood banking, and anesthesia, total hysterectomy became the standard of care to eradicate the perceived risk of cervical stump carcinoma. The transition to total hysterectomy by the 1950s was largely motivated by a desire to decrease rates of cervical cancer, as the rate of carcinoma in the residual cervical stump was as high as 1–2%. The rationale for subtotal hysterectomy is that women may have better pelvic floor function and sexual function, if the cervix is retained. However, the theoretical advantages of subtotal hysterectomy have not been supported by randomized clinical trials.[10,11]

Cochrane review of total versus subtotal hysterectomy concluded that existing data do not support any difference in sexual, bladder, or bowel function between the two approaches.[12] The American College of Obstetricians and Gynecologists cautions that there is a lack of data to support superiority of subtotal hysterectomy and urges practitioners to carefully screen patients for cervical or uterine neoplasia prior to recommending this approach. Should a patient meet criteria and elect to retain her cervix, she should be informed of the need for continued routine cervical cancer screening following hysterectomy.[13] A further concern regarding retention of the cervix is posthysterectomy cyclic bleeding, which has been reported in 11–17% of cases.[14] Despite these issues, the subtotal hysterectomy may allow for a shorter procedure with less blood loss and faster immediate postoperative recovery. Additionally, one must consider the risk of vaginal cuff dehiscence or cellulitis when total hysterectomy is performed and the risk of injury to ureter and bladder during dissection to get the bladder separated from the cervix.

COMPLICATIONS OF HYSTERECTOMY

Urinary Injuries

All gynecological surgeons should develop the skills to diagnose and repair bladder injury sustained during the surgery. As far as possible, a bladder injury sustained during vaginal hysterectomy should be repaired vaginally. It can be done by identifying the extent of the defect and repairing with no. 2-0 Polyglactin. Watertight closure should be ensured by instilling methylene blue. Cystoscopy should be undertaken in difficult cases. The most common clinical scenario is bladder injury sustained during NDVH for previous cesarean patients. It happens while trying to separate the bladder at the scar area. Even if it happens at the early part of the procedure the recommendation is to delay the repair until the uterus is removed.

Ureteric injury: Urologist may be called in if there is difficulty in identifying and repair. If it is a low ureteric injury the same may be repaired vaginally.

Hemorrhage

Primary hemorrhage has to be tackled on the table. Close monitoring of all these patients in the postoperative period is a must. Reactionary hemorrhage is usually due to slippage of ligature and has to be tackled depending on the site and extend of bleeding. Most of the time it may be possible to tackle it transvaginally. The most difficult to tackle will be bleeding from the infundibulopelvic ligament as it may be difficult to access from below. But special long retractors and the reverse angled clamps developed by the first author will help in this. The special feature of this clamp is that it gives access to the infundibulo pelvic ligament even when it is placed high as is the case in nondescent vaginal hysterectomy especially in the postmenopausal age group. The shorter part of the blades directed toward handle (reversed) grips the infundibulo pelvic ligaments and hence prevents slippage. In the conventional clamp the thicker tissues will be close to the joint and the infundibulo pelvic vessels closer to the tip are likely to slip.

Bowel Injury

Suspected bowel injury intraoperatively or in the postoperative period may need surgeon's input. It is a serious complication and has to be tackled immediately.

Granulation Tissue

Granulation tissue at the vault can cause persistent discharge and discomfort for the patient. Removal of the tissue followed by local copper sulfate application can be a useful remedy.

KEY MESSAGES

Conventionally vaginal hysterectomy was for prolapsed uterus and abdominal hysterectomy for all other pathologies of the uterus. This trend has changed recently with vaginal hysterectomy for nondescent uterus recognized as the best and safest option.[1] In this chapter, we deal with the technical aspects of abdominal and vaginal hysterectomy. The preoperative preparation and the postoperative care are touched upon. The advantages of vaginal over abdominal route are discussed. Subtotal hysterectomy under special circumstances and the complications of hysterectomy in general are also dealt with.

REFERENCES

1. American college of obstetricians and gynecologists. Committee opinion number 701. Choosing the route of hysterectomy for benign diseases. Obstet Gynecol. 2017;129(6):e155-9.
2. Magos A, Bournas N, Sinha R, Richardson RE, O'Connor H. Vaginal hysterectomy for the large uterus. BJOG. 1996;103:246-51.
3. Darai E, Soriano D, Kimata P, Laplace C, Lecuru F. Vaginal hysterectomy for enlarged uteri, with or without laparoscopic assistance: randomized study. Obstet Gynecol. 2001;97:712-6.
4. Kovac SR. Hysterectomy outcomes in patients with similar indications. Obstet Gynecol. 2000;95:787-93.
5. Johnson N, Barlow D, Lethaby A, Tavender E, Curr L, Garry R. Methods of hysterectomy: systematic review and meta-analysis of randomised controlled trials. BMJ. 2005;330:1478-86.
6. Benassi L, Rossi T, Kaihura CT, Ricci L, Bedocchi L, Galanti B, et al. Abdominal or vaginal hysterectomy for enlarged uteri: a randomized clinical trial. Am J Obstet Gynecol. 2002;187:1561-5.
7. Shoupe D, Parker WH, Broder MS, Liu Z, Farquhar C, Berek JS. Elective oophorectomy for benign gynecological disorders. Menopause. 2007;14 (Suppl 1): 580-5.
8. Sheth S. Access to vesico uterine and rectouterine pouches. In: Vaginal Hysterectomy, 2nd edition. New Delhi: Jaypee Brothers Medical Publishers Pvt. Ltd.; 2014.
9. Mazdisnian F, Kurzel RB, Coe S, Bosuk M, F Montz F. Vaginal hysterectomy by uterine morcellation: an efficient, non-morbid procedure. Obstet Gynecol. 1995;86:60-4.
10. Thakar R, Ayers S, Clarkson P, Stanton S, Manyonda I. Outcomes after total versus subtotal abdominal hysterectomy. N Engl J Med. 2002;347(17):1318-25.
11. Learman LA, Summitt RL Jr, Varner RE, McNeeley SG, Goodman-Gruen D, Richter HE, et al. A randomized comparison of total or supracervical hysterectomy: surgical complications and clinical outcomes. Obstet Gynecol. 2003;102:453-62.
12. Lethaby A, Mukhopadhyay A, Naik R. Total versus subtotal hysterectomy for benign gynaecological conditions Cochrane Database Syst Rev. 2012;4(4):CD004993.
13. Kives S, Lefebvre G. No 238. Supracervical hysterectomy. SOGC Clin Pract Guidelines. 2018;40(7):E597-604.
14. Ghomi A, Hantes J, Lotze EC. Incidence of cyclical bleeding after laparoscopic supracervical hysterectomy. J Minim Invasive Gynecol. 2005;12:201-5.

LONG QUESTIONS

1. Explain the preoperative preparations for abdominal hysterectomy.
2. Describe the important steps of of non descent vaginal hysterectomy.

SHORT QUESTIONS

1. Enumerate any five complications of abdominal hysterectomy
2. What are the advantages of vaginal over abdominal hysterectomy?
3. What are the occasions to do oophorectomy along with hysterectomy? Justify.

MULTIPLE CHOICE QUESTIONS

1. Separate consent should be there for:
   a. Anesthesia b. Oophorectomy
   c. Blood transfusion d. All of the above
2. The prophylactic antibiotic of choice in both abdominal and vaginal hysterectomy:
   a. I generation cephalosporin
   b. III generation cephalosporin
   c. II generation cephalosporin
   d. Amoxycillin—Clavulanic acid
3. The incision used for abdominal hysterectomy:
   a. Pfannenstiel b. Cherney's
   c. Maylard d. All of the above
4. The structure which has to be clamped first during abdominal hysterectomy:
   a. Round ligament
   b. Upper pedicle
   c. Infundibulopelvic ligament
   d. UV fold of peritoneum
5. Oophorectomy is indicated along with hysterectomy in the following, except:
   a. Ca endometrium
   b. Ca cervix
   c. Post menopausal age.
   d. Endometrial hyperplasia

6. External Mc Call's sutures is to prevent:
   a. Hemorrhage b. Vault prolapse
   c. Bladder injury d. cystocele
7. Absolute contraindication for vaginal hysterectomy:
   a. Previous cesarean b. Uterus size 12 weeks
   c. Adenomyosis d. None of the above
8. In which of the following, there is an increased risk of ureteric injury?
   a. Cervical fibroid b. Endometriosis
   c. Broad ligament fibroid d. All of the above
9. The proposed advantages of subtotal over total hysterectomy are all, except :
   a. Less vault prolapse
   b. Better sexual satisfaction
   c. Better bowel and bladder function
   d. Regular menstruation
10. Injury to the bladder is repaired with:
    a. No.1 nonabsorbable
    b. No.1 delayed absorbable
    c. No. 2-0 nonabsorbable
    d. No. 2-0 delayed absorbable

Answers

1.	d	2.	a	3.	d	4.	a	5.	c	6.	b
7.	d	8.	d	9.	d	10.	d				

9.11 TECHNICAL ASPECTS OF LAPAROSCOPIC HYSTERECTOMY

PG Paul, George Paul, Sanghamitra Thakur

INTRODUCTION

Laparoscopic hysterectomy is one of the most common major gynecological surgeries in today's clinical practice. So, every gynecologist must be able to perform this surgery safely. As laparoscopic hysterectomy involves a limited number of key steps, it can be easily mastered under supervision. Aim of this chapter is to describe the steps in total laparoscopic hysterectomy (TLH) along with few tips to avoid complications.

OPERATING ROOM SETUP

A good laparoscopic surgery setup requires an operating room with adequate size (20 × 20 feet preferred). Air-conditioning should have fresh air intake for the safety of the operating team. A central suction system is preferred over a portable suction machine to avoid contamination of the operating room air with surgical smoke and aerosols. Instrument cart is placed on the right-side of the patient to allow the surgeon to see the monitor display. Video monitor should be placed just below the level of the surgeon's eye view to avoid neck strain. The operating table should allow 25–30 degrees Trendelenburg position and low-level positioning. Adequately sized (2 × 2 feet) step stool is useful for average height surgeons.

INSTRUMENTATION

Apart from standard laparoscopic surgery equipment, TLH requires only a limited number of additional instruments.

- Zero/30-degree laparoscope for large-sized uterus.
- Bipolar hand instrument for coagulation of tissues with grasping capability (e.g., Bessinger) is preferred as it can also be used for holding tissues when required without instrument change.
- Vessel-sealing instruments like Enseal (Johnson & Johnson) or Ligasure (Covidien) can coagulate and divide. These instruments are convenient and faster compared to traditional bipolar and scissors as one instrument can do both. Ultrasonic instruments like Harmonic (Johnson and Johnson) or Sonicision (Covidien) have an additional advantage of dissection apart from coagulation and division. Instrumentation cost is high for these instruments as they are mostly disposable. These are optional instruments.
- Monopolar hook or L-shaped electrode for dividing tissues (not needed, if ultrasonic instruments are used).
- One or two atraumatic graspers.
- Myoma spiral or tenaculum for manipulating large uterus.
- Uterine manipulators useful for mobilizing the uterus and to delineating the tissues to be dissected or divided. Fornix bulger or colpotomizer helps to identify the limit of bladder dissection and during the circumcision of the vagina. It also blocks the gas leak while performing the colpotomy. Several designs are available in the market. We prefer modified Clermont-Ferrand model with full round colpotomizer without silicon fins (Karl Storz).

PATIENT POSITIONING

The patient is positioned in the dorsal lithotomy position, preferably with boot stirrups rather than knee crutch stirrups. Intermittent pneumatic compression devices are preferred in all cases for DVT prevention. The table should be kept at the lowest position during the surgery for better ergonomics. The patient should be brought to the foot end of the table so that buttocks are at table margin to allow free movement of the uterine manipulator. We keep the left hand tucked on the sides, and right hand bent on the chest with the intravenous line. The patient should be stabilized during tilting, and we prefer well-padded shoulder support placed over the acromion. The bladder should be kept drained during surgery. We prefer a simple catheter fixed with a towel clip rather than Foley's catheter intraoperatively. The uterine manipulator is fixed by the nurse or assistant surgeon before the trocar introduction. Correct placement is crucial for effective use of the manipulator. Fornix bulger should be changed to a smaller one, if the vagina is narrow.

TROCAR PLACEMENTS

Good visibility and ease of surgery largely depend on the correct placement of primary and secondary trocars. The patient should be in a horizontal position during the introduction of a primary trocar. It should not be very close to the upper limit of uterus for allowing a panoramic view. We normally place primary trocar 4–5 cm above the umbilicus except in normal-sized uterus. Two secondary 5-mm trocars lateral to the right and left epigastric vessels and a median supra-pubic trocar are inserted under vision. Levels of the lateral secondary trocars are usually one-two fingerbreadths above and one finger medial to the anterior superior iliac spine. The median supra-pubic trocar should be at the same level or higher than the lateral trocars with sufficient distance in between the trocars. Position of the secondary trocars is moved higher depending on the size of the uterus. Surgeons, who prefer ipsilateral positioning, place a trocar at the level of umbilicus medial to the lower-left trocar instead of the median suprapubic trocar.

KEY SURGICAL STEPS

Most TLH can be performed in an order as described below. Rarely modification or order of steps needs to be changed when anatomical variations are encountered. An initial inspection is performed to identify the landmarks of the uterus **(Fig. 1)**.

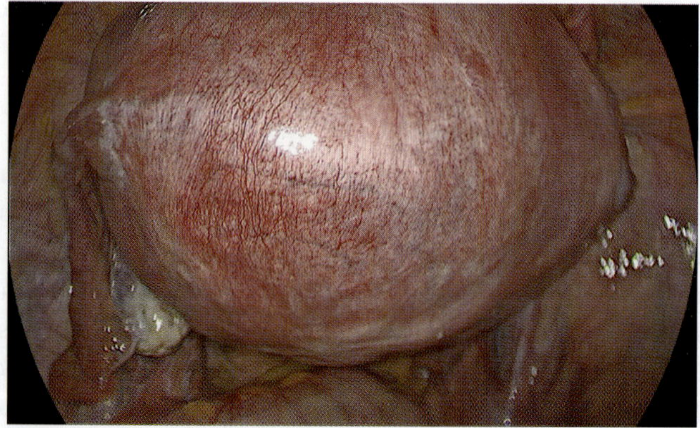

Fig. 1: Initial picture showing 18 weeks sized uterus.

Transection of Round Ligaments

Round ligaments are coagulated and divided midway with a vessel sealer **(Fig. 2A)**. Alternatively, coagulation with bipolar forceps, followed by division with scissors, can also be performed. The round ligament is kept taut during this step by moving the uterus to opposite side either with the uterine manipulator or myoma spiral fixed on the uterus. Sampson's artery, a branch of ovarian artery anastomosing with uterine artery immediately beneath the round ligament should be coagulated before division. The opened peritoneum is extended anteriorly and posteriorly for 1–2 cm **(Fig. 2B)**.

Transection of the Cornual Structures

When ovaries are preserved, the cornual structures, namely Fallopian tube and ovarian ligament, are divided after coagulation. It is a common practice to remove the tubes when ovaries are preserved (tubal origin of ovarian cancer).[1,2] So mesosalpinx is coagulated and divided starting from the fimbrial end up to its origin **(Fig. 3A)**. This is followed by division of ovarian ligament close to the ovary with the vessel sealer (Hug the ovaries!) **(Fig. 3B)**. Staying close to ovary avoids injury to the ascending uterine vessels close to the uterus. The remaining parametrium between the ovarian and the round ligament is carefully coagulated and divided avoiding injury to the parametrial veins **(Fig. 3C)**.

Transection of Infundibulopelvic Ligament

When the ovaries have to be removed, it is gently pulled away from pelvic sidewall with an atraumatic grasper, and IP ligament is divided close to the ovary after coagulation **(Fig. 4)**. Ureter should be identified before this step to ensure adequate space for safe coagulation of infundibulopelvic (IP) ligament. Excessive stretching of the IP ligament can cause premature transection causing bleeding or hematoma formation.

Bladder Flap Dissection

Identifying the upper limit of bladder is an important step, and it is clearly visible in normal cases **(Fig. 5A)**. The uterus is retroverted and pushed cephalad with the help of uterine manipulator. The loose fold of peritoneum just above the upper limit of bladder is divided with monopolar-L hook, scissors, or ultrasonic device **(Fig. 5B)**. Incision extended laterally to join the already divided round ligament without provoking bleeding **(Fig. 5C)**. The uterovesical ligament (bladder pillars) is now divided to expose the glistening cervical tissue **(Fig. 5D)**. Following this, the bladder can be easily pushed down over the vagina. Good hemostasis during this step should be maintained; otherwise, the loose areolar tissue gets stained, causing difficulty in identifying the bladder wall. The limit of bladder dissection can easily be verified now by pushing the fornix bulger of the uterine manipulator **(Fig. 5E)**. Approximately, 1.5 cm of the vagina should be free for safe colpotomy and suturing.

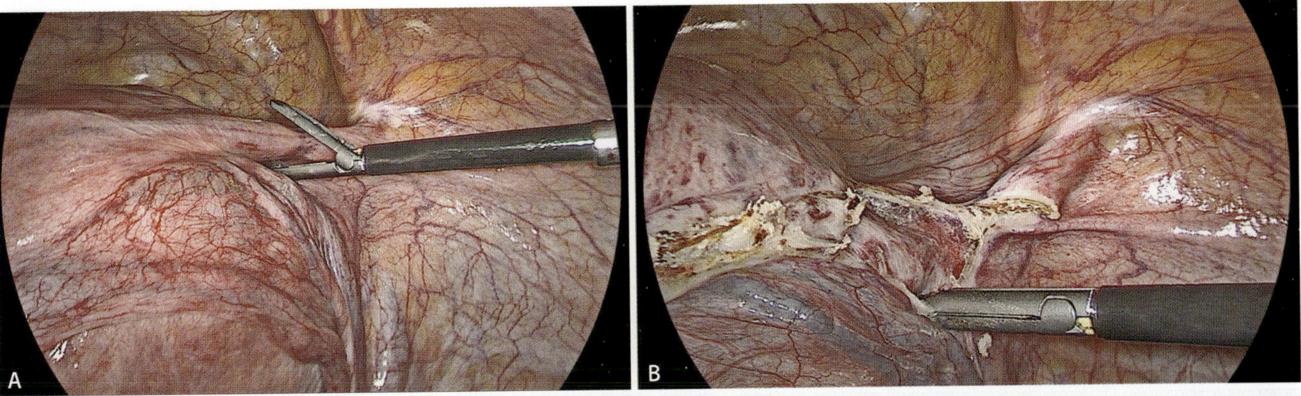

Figs. 2A and B: (A) Coagulation of right round ligament; (B) Opening the broad ligament.

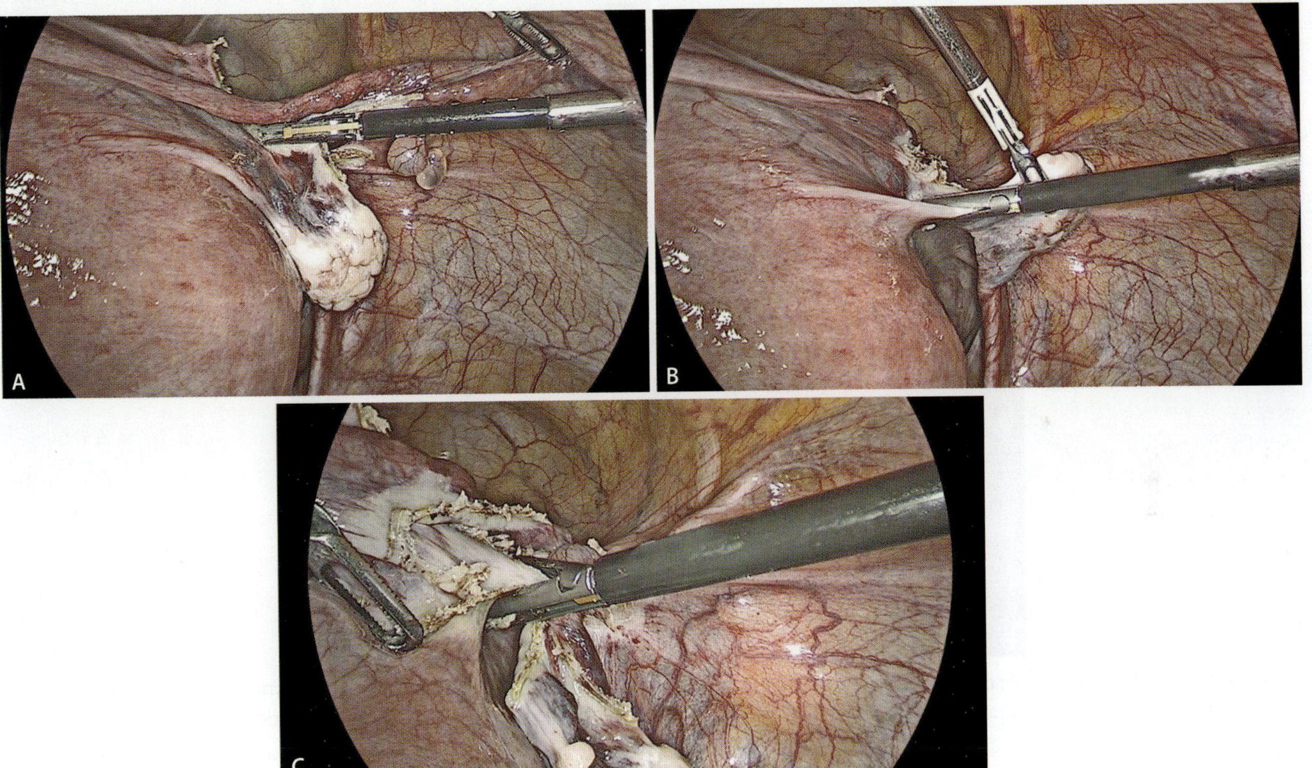

Figs. 3A to C: (A) Coagulation and division of right mesosalpinx from fimbrial end; (B) Division of right ovarian ligament; (C) Division of right parametrium.

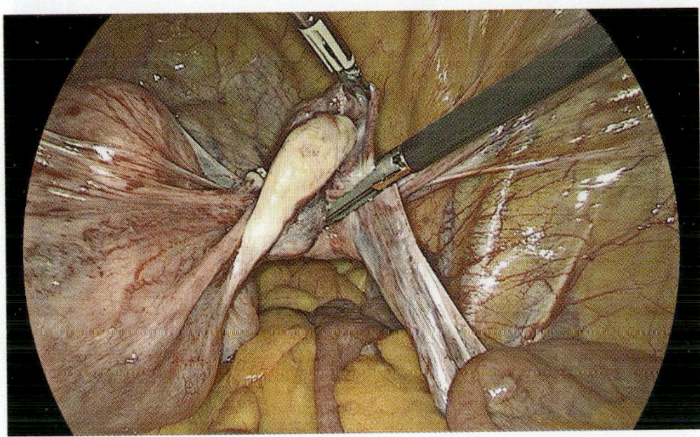

Fig. 4: Division of right infundibulopelvic ligament.

Bladder dissection in the previous cesarean section can be difficult due to adhesions. The adhesions are usually denser in the midline, so the peritoneal incision is better starting from the lateral side. It is started as a continuation of the already opened peritoneum during the round ligament division. A small window is identified over the cervix between the bladder and uterine vessels. This is further developed by sharp dissection with scissors or ultrasonic instrument **(Figs. 6A and B)**. If bladder limit is not easily identifiable, partial filling of the bladder is useful. If fat is encountered during this dissection, it indicates dissection is closer to bladder and care should be taken to avoid injury.

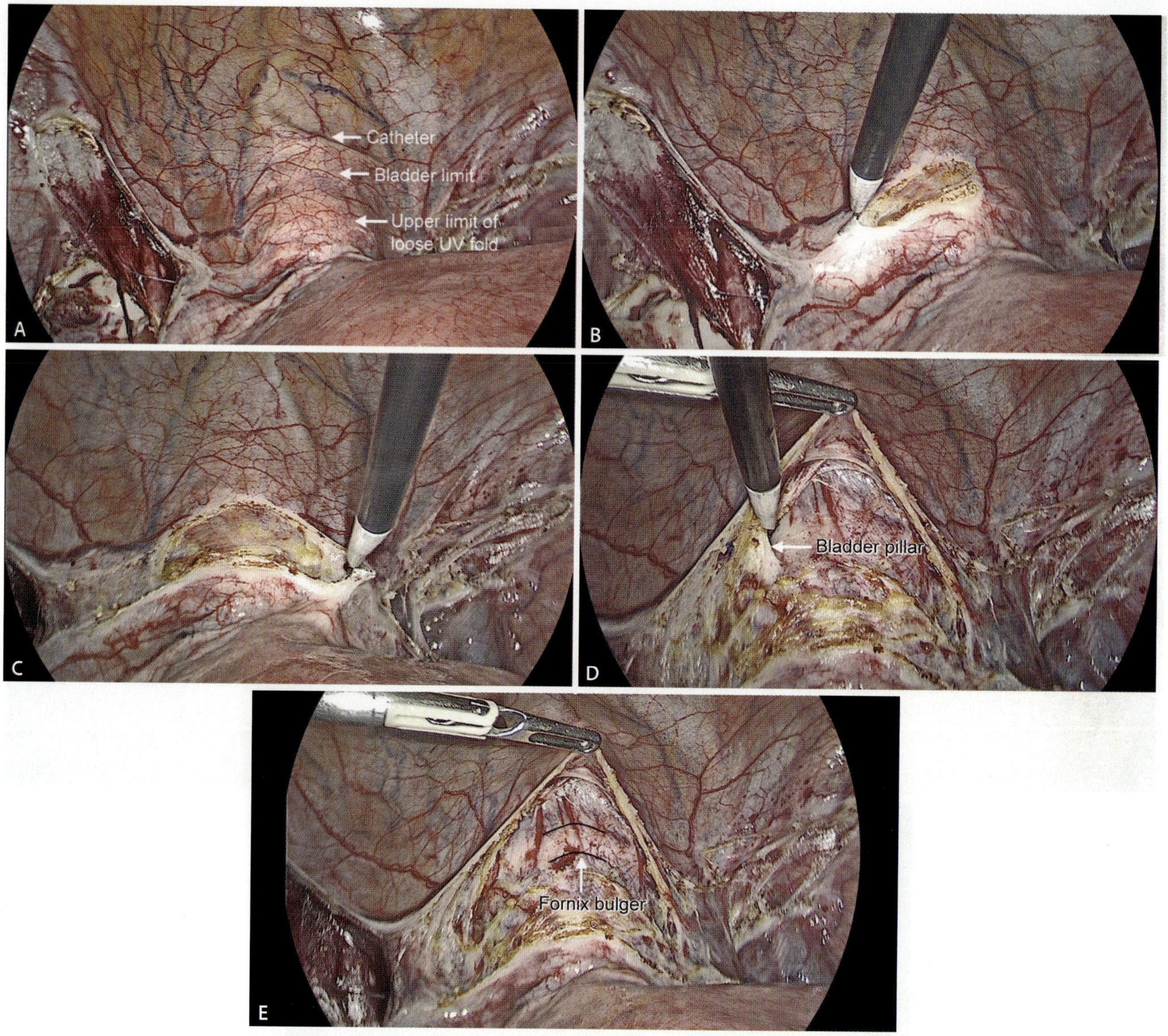

Figs. 5A to E: (A) Identification of uterovesical fold of peritoneum; (B) Division of uterovesical fold with monopolar L-hook; (C) Lateral extension of uterovesical-fold peritoneal incision; (D) Division of uterovesical ligaments; (E) Bladder dissection showing fornix bulger.

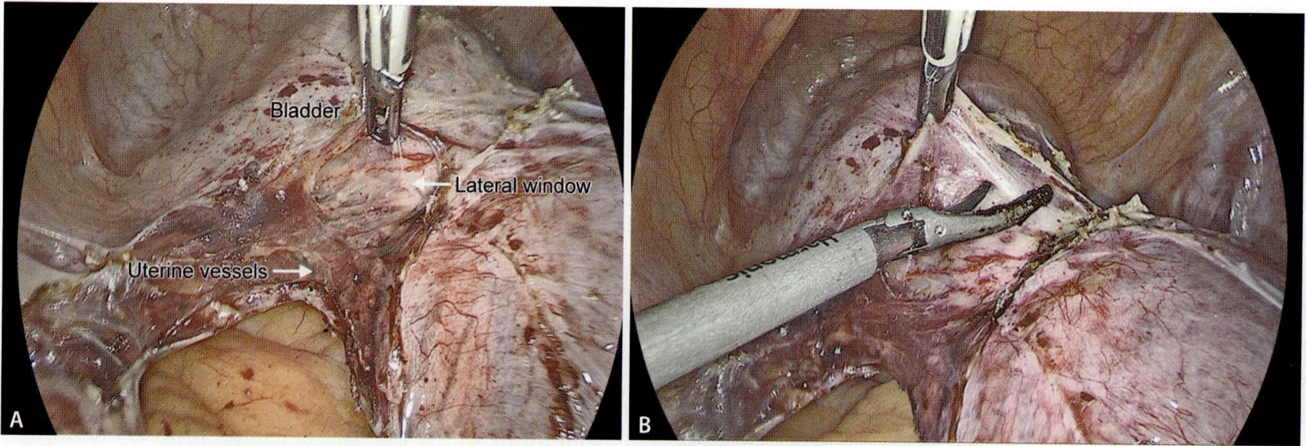

Figs. 6A and B: (A) Developing lateral window; (B) Bladder dissection starting from lateral window.

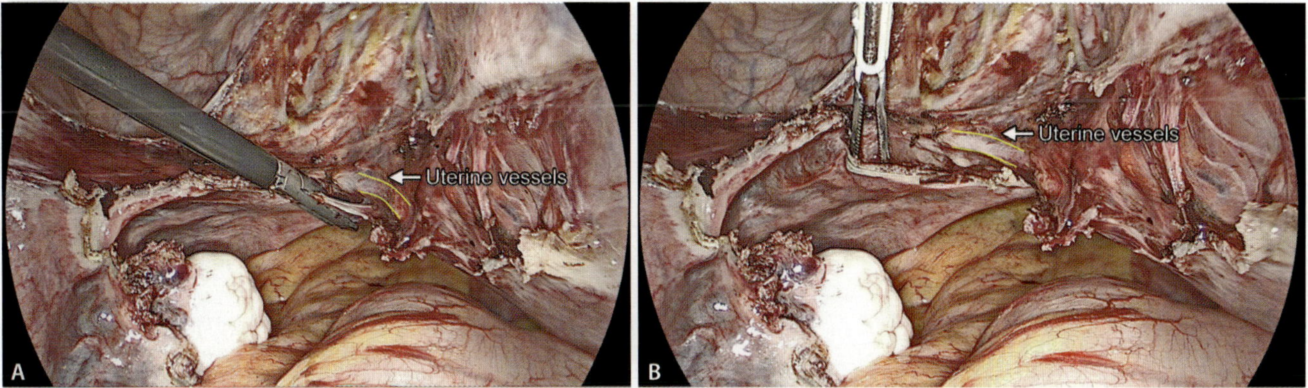

Figs. 7A and B: Skeletonization of left uterine artery.

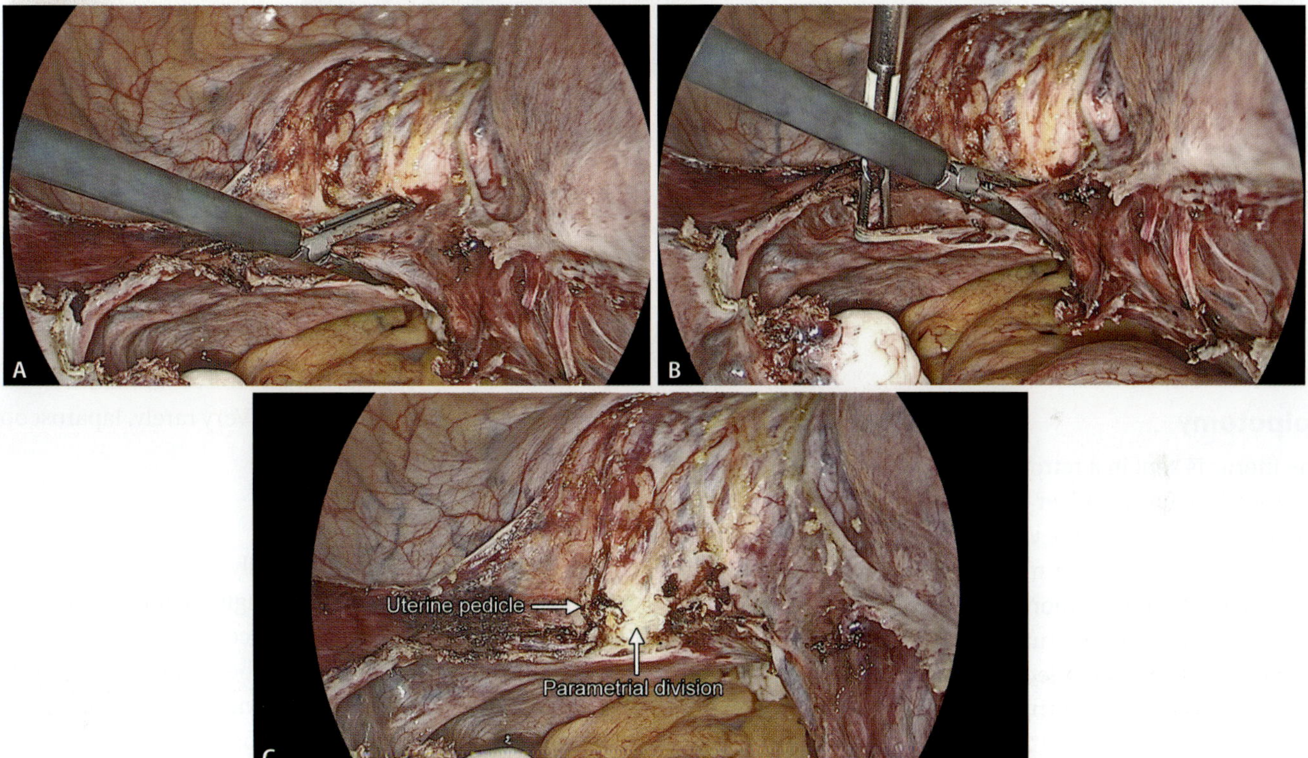

Figs. 8A to C: (A and B) Coagulation and division of left ascending uterine vessel; (C) Lateralizing the left uterine pedicle.

Securing the Uterine Vessels

The leaves of the broad ligament are divided to expose the uterine vessels **(Figs.7A and B)**. Complete skeletonization is not necessary as it can injure the veins and provoke bleeding in inexperienced hands. The ascending uterine vessels are divided at the level of internal os. We coagulate a segment of 1 cm of the uterine vessels and divide in the center with a vessel sealing instrument **(Figs. 8A and B)**. When enlarged veins are present, the vessels are compressed with a bipolar instrument inferior to the vessel sealing instrument to include the complete pedicle.

Coagulation with a bipolar instrument followed by division with scissors is also equally effective. It is performed with a lower power setting of 25–30 watts for deeper penetration of coagulation. The endpoint of coagulation is identified by the cessation of bubbles from the tissues. Division with scissors is done in small steps (coagulate more and cut less!) to avoid bleeding. Once both uterine vein and artery are divided, the parametrial tissue is cut little more to lateralize the uterine pedicle **(Fig. 8C)**. This helps in colpotomy without disturbing the coagulated pedicle. In the event of bleeding from the uterine vessels, it can be precisely coagulated without lateral damage. The uterus is maintained in a slightly anteverted position and minimally deviated to the opposite side for good visibility and to avoid rectum.

Uterine artery ligation at the origin is rarely required during routine laparoscopic hysterectomy.

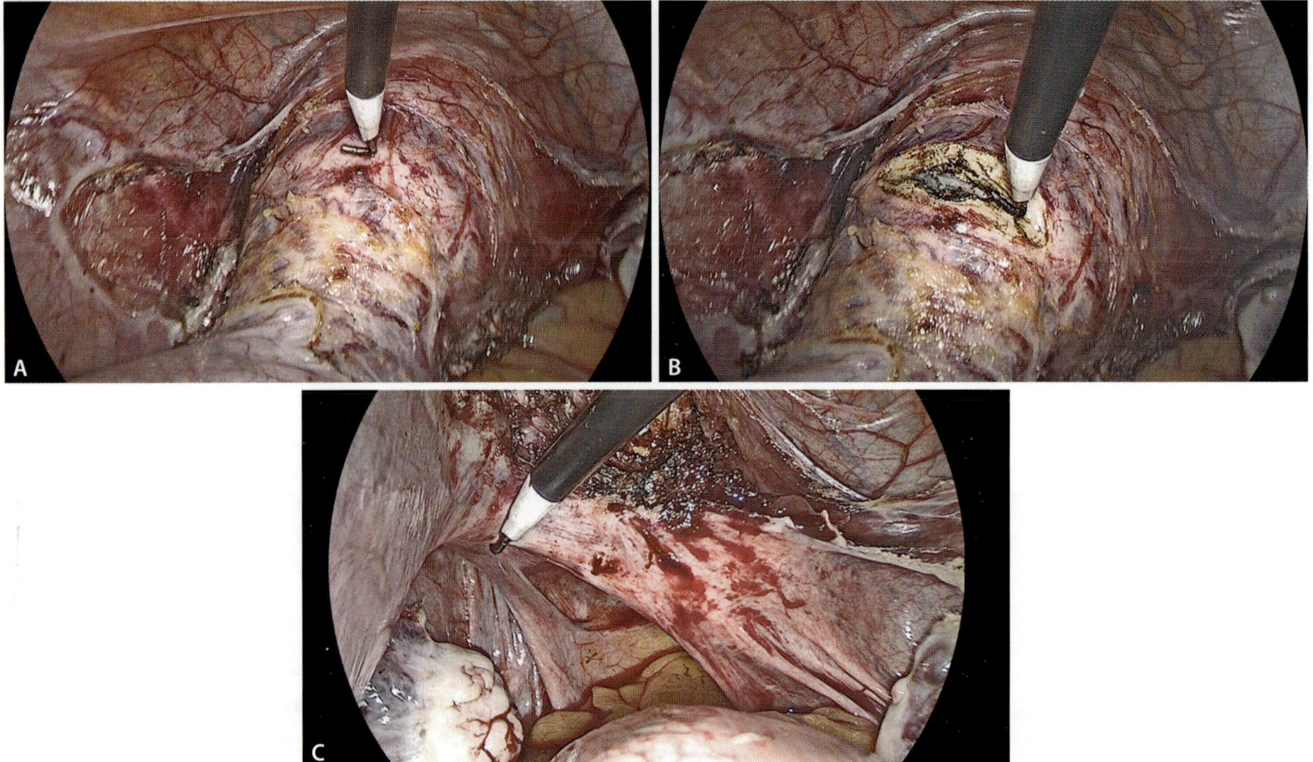

Figs. 9A to C: (A and B) Colpotomy with monopolar L-hook; (C) Colpotomy above the arch of uterosacrals.

Colpotomy

The uterus is kept in a retroverted or neutral position during this step. The fornix bulger or colpotomizer is pushed firmly over the cervix, so that the vaginal fornix is clearly visualized. It can be divided with a monopolar L-hook or ultrasonic instrument. We prefer a monopolar electrode, if we are already using a vessel sealing instrument to avoid another disposable instrument. We use blended current to reduce bleeding from small vessels during cutting. We start at 12 o'clock position and extend toward 10 and 2 o'clock, where there is minimal bleeding (**Figs. 9A and B**). Minimal coagulation with bipolar is required at 3 and 9 o'clock position before incision. During colpotomy, the diathermy pedal is activated in small bursts and movement of the electrode is kept minimum to achieve concurrent hemostasis. The posterior incision is made above the level of the uterosacral arch to preserve the pericervial ring for the support of the vagina (**Fig. 9C**).

Specimen Retrieval

Hysterectomy specimen is removed vaginally. Larger specimen requires morcellation and can be done with a scalpel. A pair of wide speculum anteriorly and posteriorly can protect the bladder and rectum during vaginal morcellation. Long tenaculum or cats-paw forceps are useful to hold the specimen firmly during morcellation. Any of the vaginal morcellation techniques can be performed for larger specimens (Helical incision technique, paper roll technique, etc.).[3,4] We perform helical incision technique. Very rarely, laparoscopic morcellation is required.

Vaginal Cuff Closure

The vaginal cuff can be closed vaginally or laparoscopically. We prefer to close vaginally when prolonged vaginal morcellation is required as a matter of convenience. Laparoscopic closure is actually faster and needs less number of sutures. Vagina has to be occluded to prevent gas leak with a blocker or a gauze-filled glove (**Fig. 10A**). It can be closed with continuous or interrupted sutures, and we prefer continuous barbed sutures. It is important to achieve good hemostasis especially from the uterine pedicles. It is not safe to coagulate after suturing the vaginal cuff as some brands of barbed sutures are heat-labile. Suturing is started from one angle, and bites are taken at least 1 cm from the vaginal cut edges (**Figs. 10B and C**). The uterosacral and Mackenrodts are incorporated in the bites for good vaginal support. Sutures are always taken medially to the uterine pedicles to avoid injury to the ureter.

At the end of the procedure, blood and clots if present are suctioned out and saline lavage is given. All the vascular pedicles are checked for complete hemostasis **(Fig. 10D)**.

POSTOPERATIVE MANAGEMENT

We give prophylactic antibiotic (Ceftriaxone 1,000 mg + Tazobactum 125 mg) before surgery, and another dose is given 12 hours after surgery. If surgery is prolonged for > 3 hours,

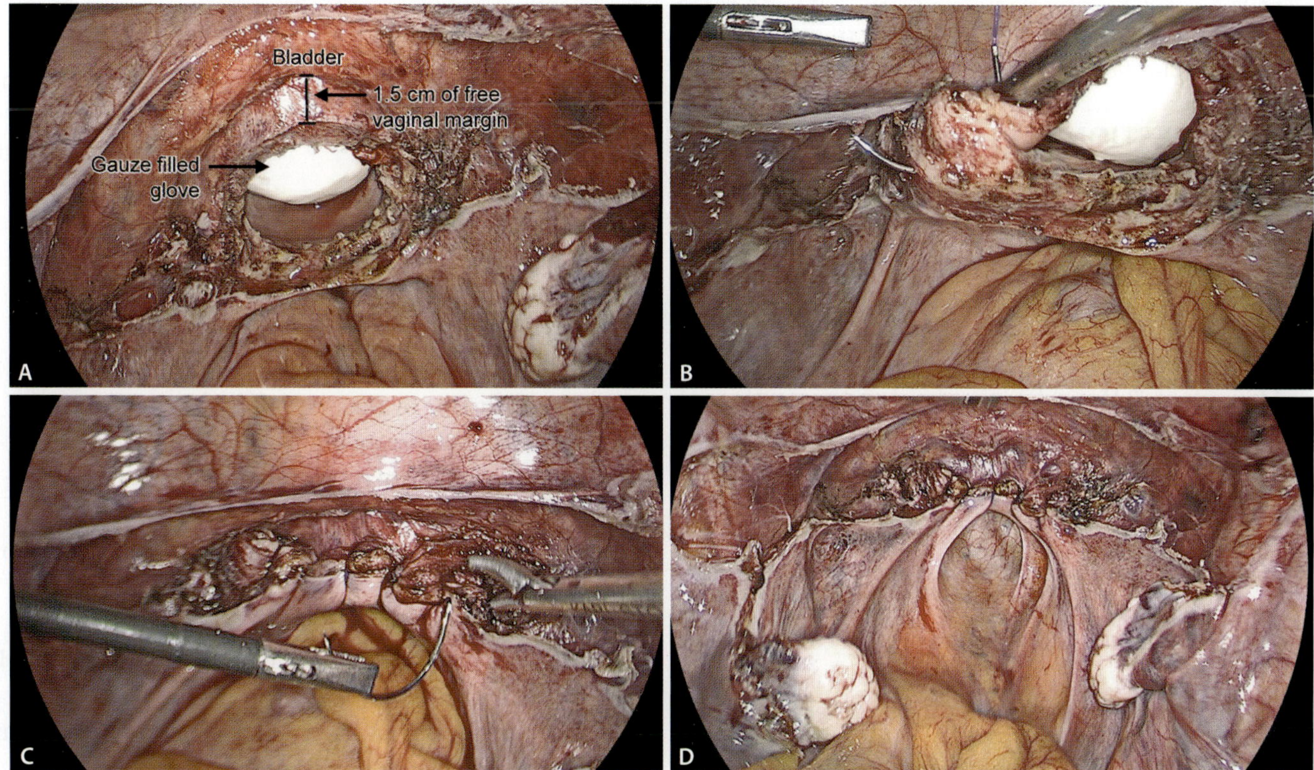

Figs. 10A to D: (A) Vaginal cuff; (B and C) Vaginal cuff suturing; (D) Final picture showing reconstructed uterosacral arch.

another dose is given intraoperatively. No oral antibiotics are given after discharge. We usually do not keep an indwelling catheter postoperatively. Patients are encouraged for early ambulation.

A diclofenac rectal suppository is given at the end of the surgery. Injectable analgesics are prescribed only on demand. Oral fluids are allowed after 4 hours, and oral analgesics are given. The patient is discharged after overnight stay (approximately 28–30 hours after admission). Advised restrict activity for 2 weeks and resume normal activities after 2–3 weeks. We advise postoperative visit after 2–4 weeks. The patient can resume sexual intercourse after 6 weeks.

CONCLUSION

Laparoscopic hysterectomy can be performed effectively and safely with limited set of instruments. Good preoperative evaluation and adhering to a systematic approach can reduce complications. It is shown that learning curve for laparoscopic hysterectomy is around 30 cases.[5]

KEY MESSAGES

- Since laparoscopic hysterectomy involves a limited number of key steps, it can be easily mastered under supervision.
- It requires only a limited number of additional instruments.
- Operating room should meet the current recommendations.
- Patient positioning is crucial.
- Initial laparoscopic inspection is important to identify any abnormalities.
- Key steps are a division of round ligament, cornual structures/IP ligament, bladder dissection, securing uterine vessels, colpotomy, specimen removal, and suturing the vault.
- Bladder dissection in previous cesarean section needs special attention and modification of the technique.
- Vaginal morcellation techniques for larger specimen.
- Vault closure can be performed vaginally or laparoscopically.
- Final inspection for good hemostasis is important.
- Only prophylactic antibiotics required in routine cases.
- Patients can resume normal activity in 2–3 weeks.

REFERENCES

1. Joseph WC, Alexander M, Elke AJ, Mana MP, Michelle SH, Lee Y, et al. Serous tubal intraepithelial carcinoma: its potential role in primary peritoneal serous carcinoma and serous cancer prevention. J Clin Oncol. 2008;26(25):4160-5.
2. David WK, Yonghee L, Alexander M, Michelle SH, Colleen F, Fabiola M. Intraepithelial carcinoma of the fimbria and pelvic serous carcinoma: evidence for a causal relationship. Am J Surg Pathol. 2007;31:161-9.
3. Wong WSF, Lee TCE, Lim CED. Novel vaginal "paper roll" uterine morcellation technique for removal of large (.500 g) uterus. J Minim Invasive Gynecol. 2010;17: 374-8.
4. Lin YS. New helical incision for removal of large uteri during laparoscopic-assisted vaginal hysterectomy. J Am Assoc Gynecol Laparosc. 2004;11:519-24.

5. Makinen J, Johansson J, Tomas C. Morbidity of 10110 hysterectomies by type of approach. Human Reprod. 2001;16(7):1473-8.

LONG QUESTION

1. Enumerate the key steps of total laparoscopic hysterectomy.

SHORT QUESTIONS

1. Technique for bladder dissection in TLH in a case of previous cesarean section.
2. Methods of TLH specimen retrieval and precautions to be taken during this process.
3. Energy sources in laparoscopy in relation to TLH and safety measures.
4. Enumerate instruments needed for TLH.
5. Preoperative and postoperative management of patient for TLH.
6. What precautions to be taken to prevent complications during TLH?
7. Explain the patient positioning and trocar placement for TLH in 18 weeks sized uterus.

MULTIPLE CHOICE QUESTIONS

1. Patient positioning during the placement of primary trocar:
   a. Trendelenburg b. Horizontal
   c. Reverse Trendelenburg d. Lateral tilt
2. Common vessel injury during the lateral trocar placement:
   a. Injury to External iliac
   b. Injury to internal iliac
   c. Injury to inferior epigastric artery
   d. Injury of circumflex iliac artery
3. An appropriate instrument for endoscopic coagulation of uterine artery is:
   a. Ultrasonic energy source
   b. Vessel sealing
   c. Bipolar
   d. All of the above
4. The following statements are true regarding the ergonomics during surgery, except:
   a. Table height b. Positioning of monitor
   c. Step stool d. Level of monitor
   e. Instrument cart
5. Equipment cart should be placed on a patient's:
   a. Right b. Left
   c. Head end d. Anywhere
6. Site of division of infundibulopelvic (IP) ligament in TLH:
   a. Close to the ovaries
   b. Close to the origin of IP ligament
   c. In the middle of IP ligament
   d. 1 cm from pelvic sidewalls
7. Extend of vaginal margin kept during bladder dissection:
   a. Half centimeter b. Two finger
   c. 1.5 cm d. Minimum
8. Where do you encounter Sampson's artery during TLH?
   a. Ovarian ligament b. Vaginal vault
   c. Round ligament d. Lateral Trocar placement
9. Steps to reduce vault prolase after TLH:
   a. Double layer suturing of vault
   b. Preserving pericervical ring
   c. Use of Barbed sutures
   d. Suturing round ligament to the vault
10. Which morcellation technique for specimen removal is preferred?
    a. Laparoscopic morcellation
    b. Minilap morcellation
    c. Vaginal morcellation
    d. All of the above

Answers

1.	b	2.	c	3.	d	4.	e	5.	a	6.	a
7.	c	8.	c	9.	b	10.	c				

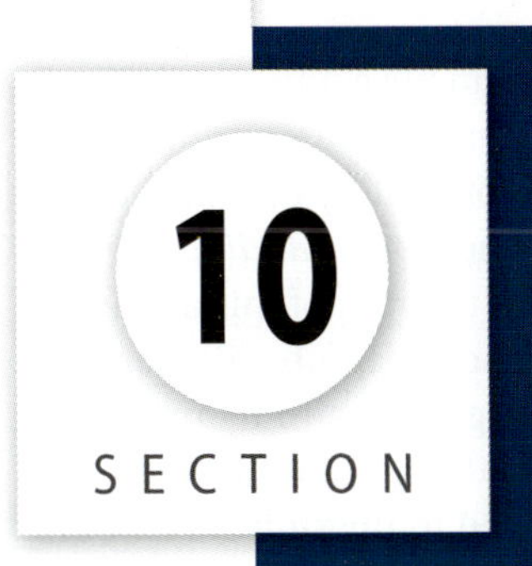

Benign Gynaecological Conditions

10.1 VAGINAL DISCHARGE

Sheela Mane

INTRODUCTION

Vaginal discharge may be considered as a healthy bodily function or a subjective complaint when secreted excessively with abnormal color, odor or texture. Even when the patient is asymptomatic with no complaints, abnormal secretions may be noted. The term *"vaginal discharge"* usually refers to any genital complaint or discomfort in patients. Vaginal discharge must be assessed if it is a normal physiologic occurrence or due to a pathological issue by preforming physical and laboratory examination to determine diagnosis and treatment.

ANATOMY AND PHYSIOLOGY OF THE VAGINA

From puberty to the menopause, human vaginal microbiota comprises mainly lactobacilli so called *Döderlein's bacilli*, including glycogen-fermenting *Lactobacillus acidophilus* and related species that inhabit the vaginal milieu. Despite the predominance of the *lactobacilli* over the vaginal microenvironment, many other beneficial microbes and opportunistic pathogens can be reported in the vaginal milieu of healthy women. These organisms alone do not trigger a pathological state; yet, once the disruption of microbial community in vagina occurs, it results gynecological diseases including vaginitis/vaginosis.[1]

The canal of the cervix uteri is in line with columnar epithelium in which branching glands lined with same epithelium ramify deeply in the fibromuscular layer of the cervix. The main role of columnar epithelium is mucus secretion, which in turn assures that the vagina is continuously lubricated and moist, assists fertility when being alkaline in reaction, and lethal to spermatozoa when it is acid, and prevents the infection.[2]

Vaginal pH

For more than a century, it is believed that high level of hydronium ions found in the vagina protected from pathogenic organisms where the pH is more acidic than interstitial fluids and blood. As a deduction, it is thought that lactobacilli are responsible for the pH and its antipathogen effect in the vagina.

Vaginal pH was the main focus in vaginal physiology and microbiology due to two factors—(1) vaginal physiology research was in the antiseptic era of the early 20th century; therefore, it was assumed that the vaginal microflora was regulated by some antiseptic substance; and (2) the development of pH paper has caused its application in pH testing of clinical specimens including vaginal secretions. In 1903, Scizly and Friedenthal[3] introduced colorimetric determination of pH with test papers for the first time. Early findings suggested that lactic acid produced by *lactobacilli was* likely antiseptic. This was presumed to be caused by the mildly acidic pH of the vagina (pH around 4.5).

Besides, vaginal flora was being studied simultaneously through microscopic examination, in which *Döderlein* theorized that the asymptomatic reproductive-age effect linked with vaginal flora was due to a single microbial entity, which became eponymically known as *Döderlein* bacillus. As a result, a microscopic observation of vaginal culture indicating only large rods (with the morphology of *Lactobacillus*) indicated a healthy vagina, whereas another containing mixed flora or absence of *Lactobacillus* morphotypes indicated an unhealthy vagina.

After the development of a morphologic scoring system based on lactobacilli morphotypes in recent decades, the Nugent scoring was developed based on the association with vaginal pH and abnormal flora.[4] Generally, the Reinheitsgrad of Döderlein became the Nugent score of the contemporary practitioner.

Due to microbiological research, and more specifically the capability of bacteria culture using artificial media and isolation of distinct species, a healthy vaginal flora was found composed of multiple species coexisting. Furthermore, the introduction of anaerobic culture technology had shed light on the presence of previously unknown anaerobic organisms in a healthy vagina **(Box 1)**. Another significant innovation, gene amplification methods used to detect microbial DNA, also revealed difficult-to-culture organisms as components of the vaginal flora.[5]

A major influence on the microbial composition of the vagina is the vaginal pH. This in turn is dependent upon the woman's hormonal status, specifically the vaginal concentration of estrogen. Estrogen stimulates glycogen deposition on the surface of vaginal epithelial cells. Both epithelial cells and microbial enzymes degrade the glycogen to glucose. Cells of the vaginal tract are abundant in number and are constantly shed into the lumen of the vagina. Once the cell autolyzes, the glucose released from glycogen is used as an energy source for bacteria known as lactobacilli. *Lactobacillus crispatus* and *Lactobacillus jensenii* are the predominant species.[6] Lactobacilli, and perhaps also the vaginal epithelium, then metabolize glucose to yield lactic acid. This causes a vaginal pH <4.5 in most asymptomatic, reproductive age women with normal menstrual cycles. The lactobacilli have a selective advantage and constitute the major microbial species under these distinctly acidic physiological conditions. It has been estimated that there are approximately 10^8–10^9 lactobacilli in the vagina of healthy cycling women. Other microorganisms, such as the yeast *Candida albicans* and aerobic streptococci, are also tolerant of this acidic pH. In addition to producing lactic acid, lactobacilli serve an important role in determining vagina health by producing hydrogen peroxide, a bactericidal when found alone and highly bactericidal when combined to physiologic amounts of myeloperoxidase and chloride. Lower-than-normal amount of *Lactobacillus*-dominated vaginal flora was found associated with higher risk of sexually transmitted exogenous infection, and endogenous infection linked to pregnancy and gynecologic surgery.[7]

BOX 1: Microorganisms detected in the vagina of healthy, asymptomatic reproductive age women.

- *Lactobacilli*: Predominantly *L. crispatus, L. jensenii*, and *L. gasseri* both producers and nonproducers of H_2O_2
- *Cocci*: *Staphylococcus aureus*, *group* B and D streptococci, peptococci, peptostreptococci
- *Bacilli*: *Gardnerella vaginalis*, *Diphtheroids*, *Escherichia coli*, *Propionibacterium*, *Clostridia*, *Bacteroides* species, *Prevotella* species, *Fusobacteria*
- *Mycoplasmas*: *Mycoplasmas hominis*, *Ureaplasma urealyticum*
- *Yeast*: *Candida albicans*
- *Virus*: *Human papillomavirus*

Defense Mechanism

- A continuous open pathway from exterior to peritoneal cavity
- Natural defense system against ascending infection
- The secretion of apocrine glands rich in undecylenic acid
- The closure of introitus by apposition of labia
- The apposition of anterior and posterior vaginal walls
- Vaginal acidity
- Vaginal flora (Döderlein bacillus)
- Closure of cervix by mucus—bacteriolytic
- Periodic shedding of endometrium
- Nonpathogenic anaerobic streptococci clearing debris after menstruation and pregnancy.

Vaginal Ecosystem (Fig. 1)

The normal vaginal flora:

- Anaerobic and aerobic bacteria
- Dominated by facultative organism
- *Lactobacillus acidophilus* "Döderlein bacillus"

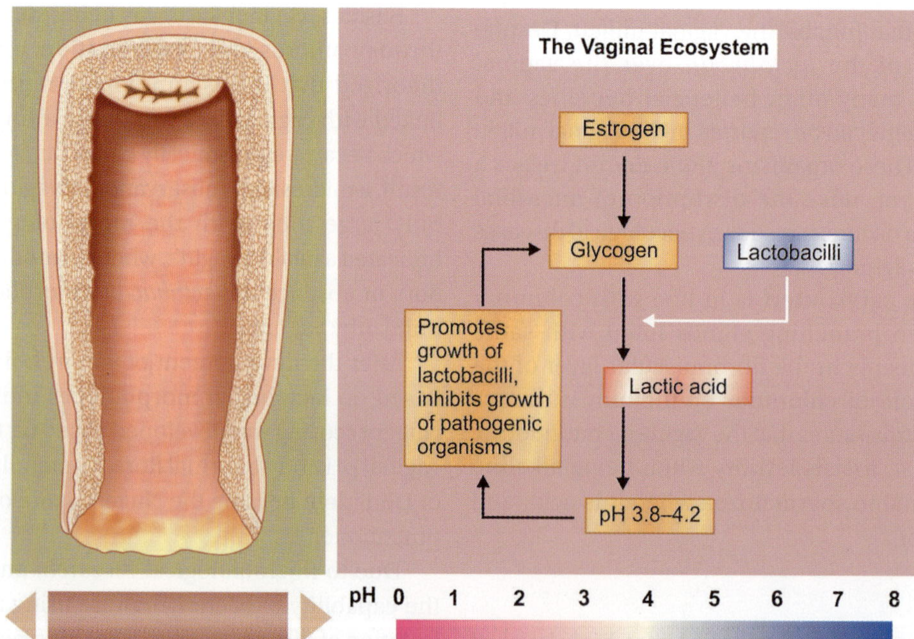

Fig. 1: The vaginal ecosystem.

- Important part of the regulatory mechanism of vaginal ecosystem.

Factors Maintaining Vaginal Ecosystem (Box 2)

- Estrogen
- Lactic acid
- Glycogen
- Role of Döderlein bacilli
- Role of pH **(Flowchart 1)**:
  - Potential hydrogen
  - Relative concentration of hydrogen atoms in the solution compared to the negative log of hydrogen ion concentration in moles/liter
  - Relative acidity or alkalinity of a solution.

DEFINITION

It is strictly defined as an excessive normal vaginal discharge.

Criteria for Defining Leukorrhea

- Excess secretion
- Need to wear a vulval pad.

BOX 2: Endogenous and exogenous factors influencing the composition of the vaginal microbial flora.

- *Vaginal estrogen*: Decreases vaginal pH and fosters lactobacilli predominance
- Concentration
- *Genetics*: Individual variations in production of immune activators or inhibitors influence the capacity of the host to eliminate specific microorganisms
- *Immune status*: Vaginal immediate hypersensitivity reactions or immune tolerance to specific microbial antigens affect the ability of the immune system to control microbial proliferation
- *Sexual activities*: Deposition of semen, saliva, or foreign objects into the vagina alters vaginal pH and immune functions and elicits the direct deposition of exogenous microorganisms. The ability of H_2O_2-producing lactobacilli to inhibit growth of *E. coli* is inhibited by semen
- *Oral or vaginal*: Alter local immune status, vaginal pH, and ability of select
- *Medications*: Microorganisms to survive and replicate (*Candida* species)
- *Vaginal blood*: Increases vaginal pH, alters microbial ecology by providing nutrients for a select group of microorganisms
- *Contraception*: Oral contraception alter vaginal estrogen levels; diaphragm and condom usage are associated with increased vaginal level of enterobacteria, intrauterine devices have been associated with increased levels of *Bacteroides* species and group B streptococci

Flowchart 1: Alteration of lactobacilli.

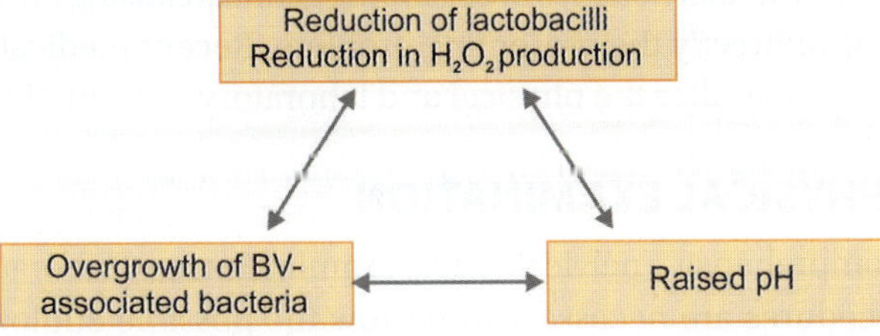

ETIOLOGY OF LEUKORRHEA

- Pregnancy and premenstrual/menstrual periods are conditions when women may present with excessive vaginal discharge **(Box 3)**.
- *Vaginal products:* Douches, deodorants, pads, and tampons can alter the vaginal ecosystem.
- Other causes of excessive vaginal discharge, congestion, and leukorrhea include—(1) pathological conditions of the female genitals, such as infection, growths and displacements, etc.; (2) chronic inflammatory process due to irritation caused by mechanical factors, such as chemical contraceptives, pessaries, and intrauterine devices; (3) psychogenic factors including stress, anxiety, overwork, and sexual excitement without fulfillment **(Box 4)**.
- More recently, endocrinal factors were found possible cause of leukorrhea where the noninfective erosion is due to excess of estrogen in the system.
- Errors in diet, excessive use of stimulants, such as tea, coffee, alcohol, and smoking are also found to produce the same phenomena.
- Finally, the constitutional cause of leukorrhea includes debilitated conditions due to anemia, tuberculosis, etc.

Leukorrhea has been described as under:

- *General causes*:
  - Malnutrition
  - Anemia
  - Sedentary habits
  - Chronic illness
  - Excess of tea and coffee
  - Alcohol
  - *Occupation:* Women serving the whole day long
  - Constipation
  - Diabetes
  - Intestinal worms in children

BOX 3: Characteristics of normal vaginal secretions.

- Heterogeneous suspension of desquamated *vaginal* epithelial cells in water
- Lactobacilli dominate the microbial *flora*
- pH 3.5–4.6
- Odorless
- Do not cause itching or irritation
- Usually do not soil underclothing

BOX 4: Characteristics of patients who present with normal vaginal secretions.

- Chronicity
- Many prior visits to healthcare practitioners
- Multiple ineffective treatments with *vaginal* and oral antimicrobial agents
- Absence of odor
- Absence of itching and irritation
- Minimal, if any, staining of clothing

- *Local causes*:
  - Gonorrhea
  - Cervical erosion
  - Displacements of uterus retroversion
  - Prolapsed of uterus
  - Cancer of all types
  - Leukoplakic vulvitis
  - Chronic salpingitis.

CAUSES OF LEUKORRHEA IN DIFFERENT AGE GROUPS

- *Before puberty*: Poor hygienic conditions, presence of worms including *Oxyuris vermicularis* or thread worms, and presence of gonorrhea infection
- *Unmarried girls after puberty*: Unhygienic conditions especially during menses, constipation, sedentary lifestyle, having chronic diseases and anemia, presence of congenital erosion of cervix
- *In the married women*: Poor hygienic conditions, presence of gonorrhea or *Trichomonas vaginalis* infections, presence of chronic diseases (including cervicitis or erosion) or cancer, chronic use of pessaries, repeated and excessive intercourse, and use of birth control measure
- *After menopause*: Presence of different types of cancer (vulva, uterus, cervix), presence of gonorrhea or *Trichomonas vaginalis*, fungus infection, and leukoplakic vulvitis. Prolapse and decubitus ulcer, and chronic diseases including chronic cervicitis.

SYMPTOMS OF LEUKORRHEA

It is manifested mostly by vaginal discharge that may be slimy, viscid to dark colored or even bloody with a foul smell.

Yet, some cases presented other accompanying symptoms including:

- GI symptoms, such as lower abdominal pain, digestive disturbances (constipation, diarrhea, and vomiting)
- Nonspecific symptoms, such as backache or leg pain (mostly in thigh and calf muscles), soreness and dryness, irritability and lack of concentration in work due to consciousness of discharges, and tiredness due to loss of vital fluids
- In the genital tract, soreness and burning, intense itching and edema of vagina, and rash and sore spots on the genitals
- Painful sexual intercourse
- Burning sensation during urination and frequent urge to pass very poor amount of urine
- *Discharge:* Strong smelling, frothy, and dark colored.

CLINICAL HISTORY

A good gynecologic history is important to understanding the cause of a vaginal discharge; therefore, particular attention must be taken into the following details:

- Age, last menstrual period, the timing and regularity of her periods, pre/post hormonal status, and birth control use
- Differentiate different types of infections according to the onset, such as yeast infections (before menses), *Trichomonas* (after menses), and gonorrhea (the upper tract post menses). Postmenopausal women are more at risk of noninfectious causes than having yeast infections, whereas pregnant women and those consuming birth control pills are more likely to present yeast infections.
  During follow-up, it is important to ask about the discharge pattern whether it is acute, chronic, or frequently recurrent. In addition, ask about the color (white, gray, yellow, or brown) and consistency of the discharge (mucoid, thick, frothy, or cheesy). For instance, grayish white and nonhomogeneous discharge indicates a possible bacterial vaginosis (BV). Chronic discharges are most probably pathological BV, or just physiologic discharges.
- Elicit the presence of pruritus, irritation, dysuria whether inside the body (internal dysuria) or on the labia (external dysuria), dyspareunia, and offensive smell. Every manifestation above suggests different etiologies; for example, internal dysuria is suggestive of urinary infection, gonorrhea, and chlamydia, whereas external dysuria indicates vulvovaginal irritation with secondary burn from urine. Pruritus also differs according to the cause; bacteria rarely cause pruritus, whereas *Trichomonas* little more, and *Candida* intensively. *Trichomonas* and BV are similar as they both result in dysuria (mostly external), yet can be differentiated throughout their odor, where BV causes a fishy smell and *Trichomonas* causes a foul one. The intense inflammatory reaction secondary to yeast infection or *Trichomonas* could result in dyspareunia whereas herpes can result in intense external dysuria and pruritus.
- Another important key-characteristic is that vaginitis must not have systemic symptoms; therefore any manifestation of fever or abdominal pain, gonorrhea, chlamydia, and upper genital tract infection, or of urinary tract infection must be looked at. Furthermore, primary herpes may present fever and malaise.
- Elicit the history of sexual activity—the gender and number of partners, recent changes or manifestations in partners. Vulvovaginal candidiasis, *Trichomonas*, BV, and herpes can all be transmitted between lesbians whereas gonorrhea rarely. These different sexually transmitted diseases have variation in prevalence according to the setting of the studied population [emergency room, office-based practice, sexually transmitted disease (STD) clinic].
- It is important to know about hygienic practices. Irritant dermatitis can be as a result of frequent douching using commercial douches or scrubbing genitals causing directly or indirectly the presenting problem. Recent medication use may alter the physical and laboratory examination.

PHYSICAL EXAMINATION

A comprehensive pelvic physical examination and laboratory procedures are necessary to narrow the possible etiologies of vaginal discharge with special consideration to herpetic vesicles and contact dermatitis on the external genitals. The evaluation of vaginal walls can reveal erythema and coating with discharge. Mucopus in the endocervix must be looked at by the right procedure—(1) clean the ectocervix using swab; (2) insert a small sterile swab in the endocervix; and (3) look for yellow pus on the swab. For better findings, a bimanual evaluation should be performed and proper laboratory specimens should be collected. When evaluating or treating vaginal discharge, the history correlates poorly with objective clinical findings.

INVESTIGATIONS

- *External examination*: Including the examination of Bartholin glands, vulva, urethra, and others.
- *Special examinations*: It includes pap smear tests from the urethra, vagina and cervix, blood and urine tests, blood pressure examination, biopsy in case of doubting any malignancy, and hanging drop method for *Trichomonas*.

DIAGNOSIS

The National AIDS Control Organization (NACO) introduced syndromic approach to treat patients with abnormal white discharge. In syndromic approach, presence of discharge (yes/no) and type of discharge (curd-like, cervical mucopus, and other abnormal discharge) is highlighted.

Many times, it is confusing to state whether it is abnormal discharge or normal physiological discharge.

In such cases, vaginal discharge was taken directly from the mid-vagina and three slides were made **(Flowchart 2)**. Two slides were used for wet mount. On one slide, one drop of saline was put and on another, a drop of 10% KOH. Both slides were covered by coverslip and examined under the microscope. Saline mount was observed for motile flagellated pear-shaped organism for diagnosis of trichomoniasis. Candidiasis was diagnosed by hyphae and budding yeast-like structure on 10% KOH mount. The third slide was fixed with ethanol and sent for Nugent's scoring. BV was diagnosed by Nugent's criteria. Nugent's score 7–10 was considered diagnostic of BV. Mixed vaginitis was diagnosed when >1 organism was found in the above mentioned tests.

Flowchart 2: Evaluation of symptomatic vaginitis.

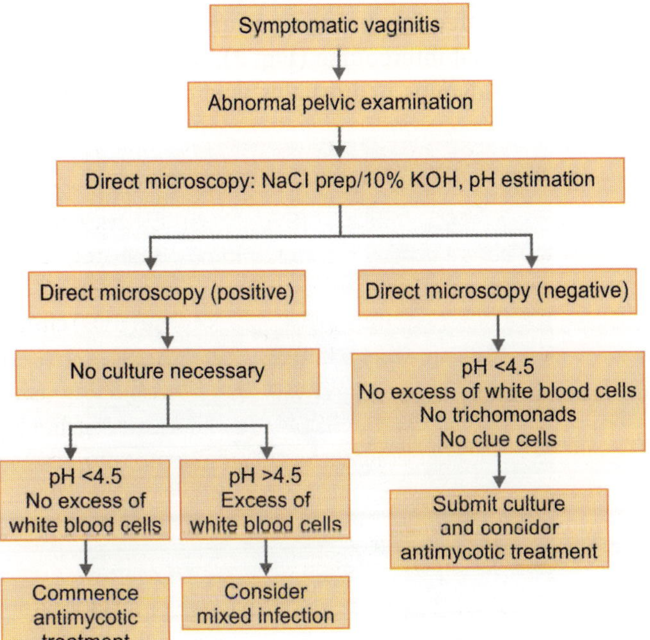

Physiological discharge was considered when pH was <4.5 and/or no above mentioned cause was found.

Cervicitis was diagnosed when there was cervical mucopus on clinical examination. Vaginal pH is the most sensitive single criterion in diagnosing BV. If pH >4.5 and Whiff test is positive, consider BV; if pH >4.5 and Whiff test is negative, consider *Trichomonas*; and if pH <4.5 and Whiff test is positive/negative, consider candidiasis.

CLASSIFICATION OF ABNORMAL VAGINAL DISCHARGE

- Noninfective—(1) physiological; (2) cervical causes; (3) vaginal causes
- Infective—(1) specific and (2) nonspecific
- Neoplasm
- Foreign body.

Noninfectious Causes

Noninfectious pathologies, such as atrophic vaginitis, contact dermatitis, malignancy, or other mechanical/chemical irritation. A foreign body, such as intrauterine contraceptive device, can result in vaginal discharge due to chronic irritant cervicitis or endometritis.

Physiologic Leukorrhea (Box 3)

- Clear white odorless discharge
- Smear contains epithelial cells, lactobacilli
- pH 3.8–4.5
- Increased with estrogen states—pregnancy, oral contraceptive pill (OCP), mid-cycle, and polycystic ovary syndrome (PCOS)
- Manifested in newborns for a week due to maternal estrogens, in teenagers during puberty after hormonal changes, and in females during ovulation, early pregnancy, and sexual excitement.

Prepubertal vulvovaginitis:

- Irritation, pruritus, discharge, and vulvar erythema
- *Etiology*: Infection caused by poor hygiene practices, sexual abuse, and proximity of the vagina to anus
- Nonspecific
- Possible risk factors include lack of estrogenization, lack of protective hair and labial fat pad, and susceptibility to chemicals, soap, and clothing
- Foreign body and enuresis.

Inflammatory leukorrhea:

Pathological leukorrhea is defined as discharge secondary to disease or disorder of the female reproductive tract.

- General ill-health and undernutrition
- Dysfunctional state in genital tract
- Psychological factors.

Cervical Causes[2]

- *Mucous polyps*: Leukorrhea is caused by cervical lesions and mostly by mucous polyps. Such a polyps protrude through the cervical canal as a bright red stalked mass with its attachment. The polyp is usually lined by columnar cervical epithelium. This secretes mucus, which is the presenting complaint in some women. In long-standing polyps, the epithelium may be of a stratified variety. It must be noted that in some cases, streaks of blood, and such may be reported after any trauma, such as coitus.
  These masses can be investigated by a speculum. As for the treatment, it consists of tumor removal under an anesthetic, histological examination. The procedure can be combined with a uterine curretage if deemed clinically necessary.
- *Erosion*: In its definition, erosion signifies a loss of surface presented by the appearance of a red and finely granular area of the cervix surrounding the external os. This surface is very susceptible to bleeding. The appearance may suggest a loss of epithelium, but this is only a perception. The epitheilium is transformed from a squamous stratified to a columnar type. Columnar epithelium covers all the granular area driving back the squamous epithelium over the surface of the portio vaginalis rather than giving place to squamous epithelium at the external. Occasional bleeding and discharge are reported because of the thinness and vascularity of the epithelium. However, the substance of the cervix underneath is not fragile and does not break down under pressure. This is a characteristic used to distinguish this condition from carcinoma. When being uncertain, the suspected area is exposed by means of a speculum and pressured by the point of a uterine sound; this point will sink into the substance of the area should it be carcinomatous. Means applied for this destruction include actual cautery, diathermy, or chemical means. Many gynecologists usually treat an erosion using deep linear cauterization by about six radial applications of the hot electrode. Possible complication, such as secondary hemorrhage, might occur 16 days post-cauterization.
- *Ectropion*: Another cervical lesion often seen during labor when the cervix is split and more specifically split bilaterally making it into a two-lipped structure. As a consequence, the mesial part of the raw surface adjoins the columnar epithelium of the cervical canal, while the peripheral part adjoins the squamous epithelium of the portio vaginalis. As a result, these epithelia will compete in which will grow the most over the raw surface and heal the tear. If the squamous epithelium succeeds, the split will be mainly covered by the same squamous epithelium that will be close to normal with some excess of secreting epithelium. On other hand, if the columnar epithelium wins in growing the most of the tear, then the owner may have the symptoms that one would expect—these are an excessive mucous discharge and less often occasional streaks of blood secondary to trauma. Healing can only occur by trachelorrhaphy.
- *Acute/chronic cervicitis*: Cervicitis can manifest in its typical acute form or a mild acute attack already described. It may occasionally appear insidiously by itself due to obstetric/gynecological event such as miscarriage, confinement, and a period with low health status in the woman's life associated with some pelvic manifestations. Chronic cervicitis can be frequently seen in the form of one of the lesions already described.

Infectious Causes

- Abnormal vaginal discharge is caused by vaginal or cervical infections.
- Causes of vaginal infections are: *Gardnerella, Trichomonas vaginalis*, and *Candida albicans*
- Causes of cervical infections are: *Neisseria gonorrhoeae, Chlamydia trachomatis,* and *Herpes simplex.*

Trichomonas Vaginitis

Trichomoniasis, caused by *Trichomonas vaginalis* (parasitic protozoan), is a frequent cause of vaginitis. *T. vaginalis* has four free flagella and one recurrent costa at the base of the undulating membrane, and an axostyle extending through the cell **(Fig. 2)**.

Symptoms vary between genders. Either gender may transmit the infection being unaware of the symptoms by penile-vaginal intercourse **(Fig. 3)**. Males can manifest urethritis, epididymitis, or prostatitis, whereas females women

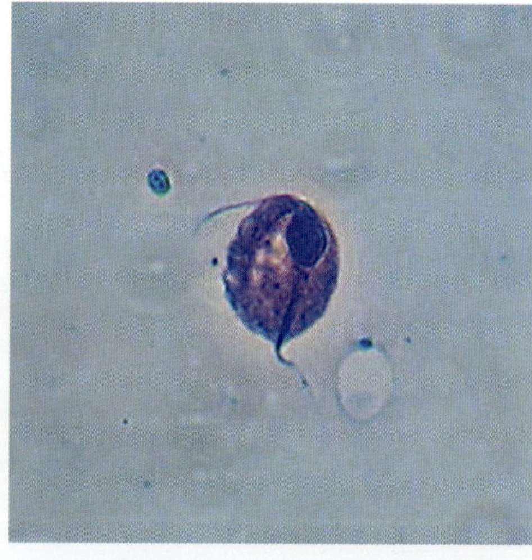

Fig. 2: *Trichomonas vaginalis.*

present vaginal discharge (diffuse, bad smell, yellow-green colored, and with/without vulvar irritation).[8] To protect from trichomoniasis, sexually active individuals must constantly use condoms and in the right way during every penile-vaginal sex.[9] Partners of men who have been circumcised have possibly lower risk of *T. vaginalis* infection.[10] It is better to avoid douching due to its effect on increasing the risk of vaginal infections, even trichomoniasis.

T. vaginalis infection can increase the risk of HIV infection by 2 to 3 folds. Preterm birth, and different pregnancy-related adverse events in pregnant females. In HIV-positive females, *T. vaginalis* infection can increase the risk for pelvic inflammatory disease (PID).[12] Due to the dangerous effect of asymptomatic trichomoniasis in HIV individuals, it is recommended to perform routine screening for *T. vaginalis* in HIV-infected patients. Furthermore, diagnostic testing for *T. vaginalis* must be performed in females complaining of vaginal discharge whereas screening must be performed in individuals treated in high-risk settings (STD clinics or correctional facilities) and in high-risk asymptomatic individuals (with multiple sex partners, exchanging sex for payment, with drug use, and history of STD).

It is still contradictory if the *T. vaginalis* infection can be found in the rectum, further research is important to explain the occasional result where contamination in 5% of people reporting recent receptive anal sex was found.[10] Besides, there is still a lack of evidence in accuracy, benefit, and cost-effectiveness of rectal screening making it not recommended for *T. vaginalis*. In addition, oral testing is still unknown for *T. vaginalis* and also not recommended.

Diagnosis: It can be performed by direct microscopic examination of the vaginal fluid. Yet, this method has low sensitivity (60%) even for skilled diagnosticians.[13] When spotting motile trichomonads, the diagnosis is confirmed. Vaginal fluid has a pH often higher than 4.5 yet can be normal (<4.5). In these cases, the *Trichomonas* are dispersed usually due to their preference of alkaline pH. Laboratory

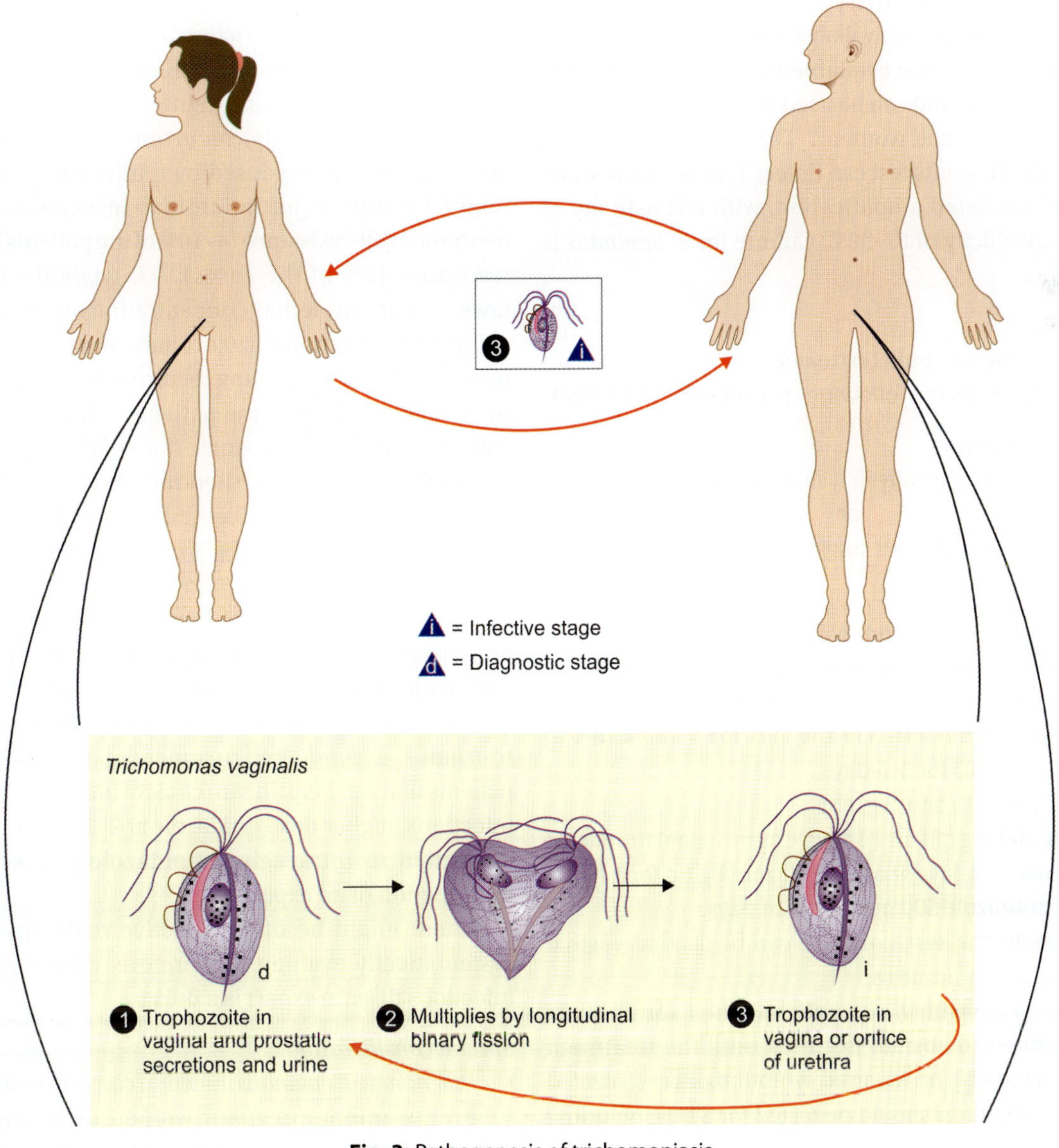

Fig. 3: Pathogenesis of trichomoniasis.

examination often reports the presence of neutrophils and altered vaginal bacteria. Culture media is commercially available and is currently the gold standard for diagnosis, yet needs incubation. Specimens can endure viability for 24 hours in various transport pre-culture media. Other high sensitivity tests (80%) are approved only for vaginal specimens, such as RNA probe semi-automated system also used in detection of candidiasis and bacterial vaginosis and a dipstick enzyme-linked immunosorbent assay (ELISA).[14] Both of these tests are better alternatives when microscopy is not available. Nucleic acid amplification tests (NAATs) are still under development with conflicted findings. Other licensed tests reported higher sensitivity (>83%) and specificity (<97%) for vaginal secretions—the OSOM Trichomonas Rapid Test and the Affirm VP III test. Amplicor, a polymerase chain reaction assay previously used for *C. trachomatis* and *N. gonorrhoeae* detection has been modified for *T. vaginalis* detection in vaginal or endocervical swabs and in urine from both genders. It reported the highest sensitivity and specificity rates with 88–97%, and 98–99% respectively.

Recently, a commercially available transcription-mediated amplification test became available in an analyte-specific reagent (ASR) format, and can be used with urine and genital specimens from men and women.[15] The Aptima *T. vaginalis* Analyte Specific Reagents test can detect *T. vaginalis* RNA by transcription-mediated amplification, with a sensitivity of 74–98% and specificity of 87–98%. Culture for *T. vaginalis* is another option.

Treatment:

- Both the partners should be treated.
- CDC recommends the following regimens for treatment.

Recommended regimen:

- *Metronidazole* (2 g) orally in a single dose

or

- *Tinidazole* (2 g) orally in a single dose

Another regimen:

- *Metronidazole* (500 mg) orally BID for 7 days
- Oral metronidazole is superior to vaginal
- FDA recommends tinidazole 2 g single dose
- *Failure:* Metronidazole 500 mg bid for 7 days or 2 g metronidazole OD for 3–5 days
- Oral intolerance IV Met 4 g/day
- Tinidazole 500 mg qid for 14 days + intravaginal tinidazole 500 mg bid for 14 days *or* oral tinidazole 1 g tid for 14 days + vaginal tinidazole 500 mg tid for 14 days.

Fenticonazole and sertaconazole can be used as vaginal tablets to treat trichomoniasis.

Patients infected with *T. vaginalis* and their sex partners are recommended to abstain from sex until the treatment course is complete with no reported symptoms. Every infected patient with *T. vaginalis* should be tested for STDs including HIV.

Follow-up advice: Evidence showed high prevalence of reinfection among females treated for trichomoniasis (17% within 3 months); therefore, it is advised to be retested for *T. vaginalis* within 3 months post initial treatment despite if their sex partners were treated. Nucleic acid amplification testing can be performed starting from 2 weeks after treatment only.

Management of sex partners: It is of great importance to treat all sex partners in order to reduce symptoms, treat and prevent the transmission and reinfections. Partners are advised to restrain from any intercourse until resolve of symptoms and the end of treatment course, in addition they should be referred for presumptive therapy to avoid reinfection. However, no one partner management intervention has been shown to be superior in reducing reinfection rates. There is a lack of information on treatment recommendations for partners of patients with persistent or recurrent trichomoniasis in whom nonadherence and reinfection are unlikely; usually both patients and partners undergo same evaluation and treatment regimen.

Persistent or recurrent trichomoniasis: There is a difference between persistent/recurrent infection due to antimicrobial-resistant *T. vaginalis* and reinfection due to an untreated sex partner. Generally, recurrent *T. vaginalis* infections are suggested to be caused by reinfection, yet, some cases might be due to antimicrobial resistance for example metronidazole resistance (4–10% of the patients) or tinidazole resistance (1% of the cases).[16] *T. vaginalis* isolates have lower minimum lethal concentrations to tinidazole when compared to metronidazole. Single-dose therapy should be prescribed only for treating recurrent trichomoniasis caused by reinfection. Firstly, the patient (and partners) is treated with metronidazole 2 g single dose, if this regimen fails and reinfection is excluded, then metronidazole 500 mg orally BID for 7 days is prescribed. Similarly, if treatment failure occurs, the patient can be treated with metronidazole or tinidazole at 2 g orally for 7 days. If several 1-week regimens have failed in a person who is unlikely to have nonadherence or reinfection, testing of the organism for metronidazole and tinidazole susceptibility is recommended.[17] CDC reported recommendations on susceptibility testing for nitroimidazole-resistant *T. vaginalis* and treatment management of infected patients that can help. In rare cases of nitroimidazole-resistant infections, higher dose tinidazole at 2–3 g for 14 days usually combined to intravaginal tinidazole is prescribed after examination of an expert.

There might be other effective regimens that are yet systematically evaluated; therefore, consultation with an infectious disease expert is a must.

Special consideration:

- *Pregnancy*: *T. vaginalis* infection can cause various adverse events among pregnant women including premature rupture of membranes, preterm delivery, and birth to a low birthweight infant.[18] Despite its antiparasite production, metronidazole has no significant effect in perinatal morbidity after treatment. Recent larger studies reported no association between metronidazole use during pregnancy and adverse outcomes of pregnancy.[19]

When infected, pregnant women are recommended to take metronidazole 2 g single dose orally. As for symptomatic pregnant women, they all should be tested and considered for treatment regardless of their pregnancy stage. Treatment of trichomoniasis will reduce vaginal discharge and lower the risk of sexual transmission to partners. Even though perinatal transmission of *T. vaginalis* infection is rare, treatment also protects the newborn from any respiratory or genital infection. Experts should advise every symptomatic infected pregnant women despite the potential risks for and benefits of treatment and the necessity of partner treatment and condom use in the prevention of sexual transmission.

Screening at the first prenatal visit and prompt treatment, as appropriate, are recommended for pregnant women with HIV infection, due to the fact that *T. vaginalis* infection increases the risk of vertical transmission of HIV.[20] After 3 months of treatment, infected pregnant women with HIV should be retested.

Although metronidazole crosses the placenta, it poses only low risk to pregnant women. Previous studies (prospective and cross-sectional) denied any evidence of teratogenicity or mutagenic effects in infants of pregnant women.[20] Metronidazole can also be secreted in breast milk. When treating the mother, breastfed newborns receive metronidazole in doses that are lower than those prescribed to treat infections in infants, although the active metabolite adds to the total infant exposure.

- *HIV*: More than half of females with HIV (53%) are also infected with *T. vaginalis*.[21] *T. vaginalis* infection in these women can increase the risk of PID, and treatment of trichomoniasis decreases significantly genital tract HIV viral load and viral shedding.[22] Therefore, all HIV-positive women should be routinely screened and promptly treated at the point of entry to care. They should be followed up annually for this.

Factors that might interfere with standard single-dose treatment for *T. vaginalis infection* in women with HIV are elevated rates of asymptomatic BV coinfections, use of antiretroviral therapy, vaginal ecology modifications, and immunity disorder.[23]

Treatment: Treatment of *T. vaginalis* infection is capable of both reducing its manifestations and its transmission. In addition, it was associated with lower risk of adverse events in women with HIV.

Treatment regimen recommended for women with HIV infection: Metronidazole (500 mg) orally BID for 7 days: Retesting for of *T. vaginalis* infection is recommended after 3 months after the initial treatment. NAAT scored higher sensitivity, therefore it is encouraged.

Bacterial Vaginosis

Many women visiting their physicians with vaginal symptoms have a specific condition, first described by Gardner and Dukes in 1955,[24] that is now referred to as BV. Inflammation and perivaginal irritation are considerably milder than in trichomoniasis or candidiasis. Dysuria and dyspareunia are correspondingly rare. Affected women are usually sexually active and often complain of vaginal odor, which frequently is described as "fishy". About 90% of patients also notice a mild-to-moderate discharge. Abdominal discomfort is occasionally present, but it is usually mild and should prompt evaluation for coincident infections such as salpingitis.

Discharge is manifested usually at the introitus and visible on the labia minora. The labia and vulva are not erythematous or edematous. On speculum examination, vaginal walls are usually uninflamed, the vagina contains a grayish, thin, homogeneous discharge (with probable pungent smell) **(Fig. 4)**. The endocervix is unaffected by the process, and any cervical discharge should be normal/physiologic. A purulent cervical discharge might be due to coincident gonococcal or chlamydial infection.[25] Unusual bimanual examination are rare in uncomplicated BV and suggestive for other pathologic processes. There is a higher risk of endometritis and salpingitis among women with BV.[26]

Other vaginal infections may resemble BV; an accurate differential diagnosis depends on laboratory examination. The pH of vaginal fluid is elevated above the normal of 4.6 in about 90% of women with BV.[27] A vaginal pH of 5 or higher strongly suggests BV.[28] A whiff test is positive.[29] BV is a syndrome characterized by a shift in the vaginal flora. It is a strong independent risk factor for adverse pregnancy outcomes, found in 9–23% of pregnant women.[30]

Bacterial vaginosis has been shown to increase the risk of gynecological morbidity and adverse obstetrical outcomes,

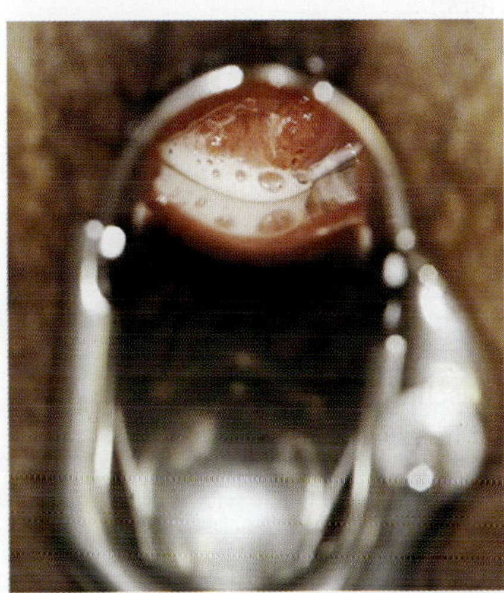

Fig. 4: Speculum examination and discharge in bacterial vaginosis.

such as preterm delivery, PID following surgical procedures, hysterectomy, and upper genital tract infections.[31]

Certain complications have been associated with BV infection, such as:

- Chorioamnionitis
- Endometritis
- Congestive dysmenorrhea
- Chronic backache.[32]

And with respect to the neonate:

- Increased neonatal intensive care unit (NICU) admissions
- Intermittent positive pressure ventilation
- Respiratory distress.[32]

Other most common complications countered with BV are:

- Preterm labor
- Infertility
- STI specifically HIV to the sexual partners
- Cervical intraepithelial neoplasms.[33]

Etiology: Gardnerella vaginalis was reported in 40–50% of vaginal secretions. It contains mostly anaerobes and produces amines. In addition, due to lower hydrogen peroxide-producing lactobacilli, vaginal pH is increased.

When amines are alkalinized by either semen, menstrual blood, or alkaline douches, or 0% potassium hydroxide, they volatilize and cause bad "fishy" smell.

- *Bacteroides* (anaerobes) species are increased 1,000× the usual concentration.
- *G. vaginalis* is 100× normal.
- *Peptostreptococcus* is 10× normal.
- *Mycoplasma hominis* and *Enterobacteriaceae* species are presented in high amount.
- Findings of DNA-based molecular methods reported new and fastidious species highly specific for BV (such as *Atopobium vaginae, novel Clostridial spp. categorized into* "BVAB1", "BVAB2", and "BVAB3").
- The spectrum of bacteria associated with BV is suggested to be far more diverse than previously thought.
- Risk factors:
  - Multiple sexual partners
  - IUDs
  - Douching
  - Lack H_2O_2-producing strains of Lactobacilli.

Symptoms:

- Foul smelling vaginal discharge
- Some women report a fish-like odor, especially after intercourse
- Color of discharge—white-gray
- Offensive fishy smelling discharge not associated with soreness, itching or irritation.

Methods for diagnosis of BV:

- *Clinical diagnosis, Amsel criteria*: Used to clinically treat patients **(Box 5)**.

BOX 5: BV diagnosis: Amsel criteria.

- Must have at least three of the following findings:
- Vaginal pH >4.5
- Presence of >20% per HPF of "clue cells" on wet mount examination
- Positive amine or "Whiff" test
- Homogeneous, non-viscous, milky-white discharge adherent to the vaginal walls

(WBC BV: white blood cell bacterial vaginosis)

- *Discharge*: It is usually white-colored and homogeneous. Before examination, the patient should avoid douching, cleansing or using microbicide/placebo gels, and it is recommended to give sufficient amount of discharge for better evaluation.
- *pH of vaginal fluid*: Using S/P pH indicator strips (3.6–6.1), the specialist touches the wall of the vagina or uses a swab to moisten the pH paper, then according to the color of chart on the container, the pH can be determined. A pH >4.5 indicates BV. Many substances found in the vagina can cause modifications in pH, such as cervical mucus, blood, and sperm, which increase the pH.
- *Amine odor*: Put vaginal fluid on a slide with 1 drop of 10% KOH prep. Amines are detected if there is a fishy smell. Put a coverslip on the slide and read for budding yeast and pseudohyphae. A possible limitation is inability to smell the odor.

Specimen collection:

- Swab the lateral or posterior fornices of the vagina.
- Transfer the swab into a sterile tube with almost six drops of saline.
- Transfer to the laboratory as soon as possible.
- *Wet mount*:
  - Put a small amount of the vaginal fluid onto a slide, and if it is too dry, add a drop of saline and then mix. Lastly, put a coverslip on the slide.
  - Firstly, read at 10X for *Trichomonas and yeast*, and then read the whole coverslip for *Trichomonas*; to differentiate epithelial cells, read at 40X.
  - It is limited by the presence of gel and reading after 1 hour.

  Wet Mount Preparation in Bacterial Vaginosis
- *Gram stain, Nugent score*: It a standard laboratory-based procedure used in clinical trials but not in clinical management **(Table 1)**.
- Gram stain for diagnosing BV **(Fig. 5)**
- Based on the quantity of three morphotypes—lactobacilli, gram variable rods, and curved rods
  - Sensitivity varies between 86% and 89%, whereas specificity between 94% and 96% higher to Amsel criteria.

Quantitation of bacterial morphotypes:

- 0–1/1,000× magnification = 1+
- 1–4/1,000× magnification = 2+

TABLE 1: Nugent scores.[25]

Score	*Lactobacillus*	*Gardnerella and Bacteroides spp morphotypes*	*Curved gram-variable rods*
0	4+	0	0
1	3+	1+	1 + or 2+
2	2+	2+	3 + or 4+
3	1+	3+	
4	0	4+	

*Morphotypes are scored as the average number seen per oil immersion field. Note that less weight is given to curved gram-variable rods.
Total score = lactobacilli + *G. vaginalis* and *Bacteroides* spp + curved rods
Quantitation: O, No morphotypes present; 1 +, <1 morphotype present; 2+, 1 to 4 morphotypes present; 3+, 5 to 30 morphotypes present; 4+, 30 or more morphotypes present

Total	Interpretation
0–3	Normal
4–6	Intermediate
7–10	Bacterial vaginosis

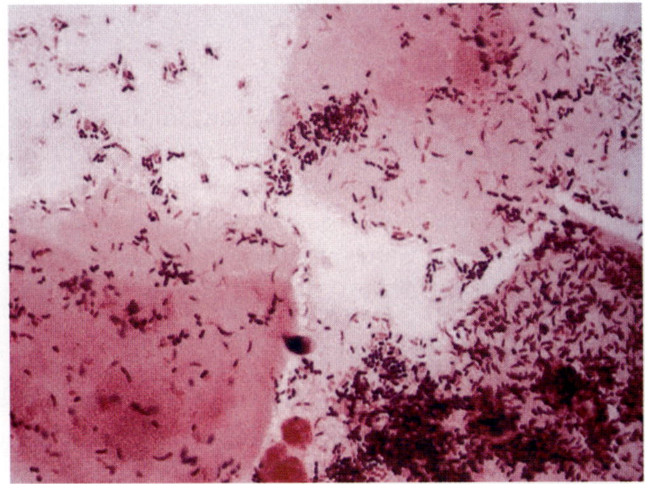

Fig. 5: Bacterial vaginosis.

- 5–30/1,000× magnification = 3+
- >30/1,000× magnification = 4+

Other diagnostic tools can be used, such as culture, DNA probe, and novel technologies, such as FemExam™ and PIP Activity TestCard.™

- *Seattle group criteria*: The presence of 3–4 of these symptoms will diagnose 90% correctly, with <10% false-positive results:
    - Thin, gray, homogeneous, malodorous discharge that adheres to the vaginal walls
    - Elevated pH >4.5
    - Positive potassium hydroxide Whiff test
    - Clue cells present on wet mount.

  Cultures are unnecessary.
  Pap smear will not identify *G. vaginalis.*
  Gram stain of vaginal secretions will reveal clue cells and abnormal mixed bacteria.
- *CDC criteria For BV:* BV can be determined through clinical criteria, such as Amsel's diagnostic criteria[29] requiring three of these signs—pH >4.5, a fishy smell (before or after the Whiff test), presence of clue cells, and thin homogeneous and white discharge on the vaginal walls.

  A Gram stain, gold standard method for BV, is used to determine different species' concentration, such as lactobacilli (long gram-positive rods), gram-negative, and gram-variable rods and cocci (*G. vaginalis*), and curved gram-negative rods (*Mobiluncus*) characteristic of BV.

  Diagnostic criteria had similar results to Gram stain.

Other tests include:
- Affirm VP III (Becton Dickinson, Sparks, MD), a DNA hybridization probe test for high concentrations of *G. vaginalis*
- The OSOM BV Blue test (Sekisui Diagnostics, Framingham, MA) detecting vaginal fluid sialidase activity has better performance characteristics than Gram stain.

Complications with BV:
- Preterm delivery
- Increased risk of PID
- Increased susceptibility to HIV acquisition/transmission
- Recurring treatment.

Morbidities associated with BV:
- Studies have found a significant association between BV and HIV infection
    - BV increases the risk of HIV transmission 2–4 folds
- Many studies have found an association between BV during pregnancy and all major adverse pregnancy outcomes (preterm labor, preterm delivery, low birth weight, premature rupture of membranes, postpartum metritis, intra-amniotic infection). Treatment with metronidazole reduces these risks.[34] The safety of metronidazole in pregnancy and lactation is now fairly established.[35,36]

Treatment:
CDC-recommended regimens:
- Metronidazole 500 mg orally BID for 7 days, *or*

- Metronidazole gel 0.75%, one full applicator (5 g) intravaginally, once a day for 5 days, *or*
- Clindamycin cream 2%, one full applicator (5 g) intravaginally at bedtime for 7 days.

Alternative regimens:[26]

- Metronidazole 2 g orally in a single dose, *or*
- Clindamycin 300 mg orally twice a day for 7 days, *or*
- Clindamycin ovules 100 g intravaginally once at bedtime for 3 days
- Metronidazole, clindamycin preparations, oral and intravaginal tablets of *Lactobacillus* are effective for BV
- Hydrogen peroxide douche and triple sulfonamide cream are ineffective.

The first or second recurrence—treat with CDC recommended regimens for a longer period.

If recurrence continues—vaginal met twice weekly for 6 months.

Screening and treatment in asymptomatic patients:

- Low-risk pregnant women screening is not recommended whereas male partners of women with BV are not advised to take treatment.
- Females before surgical abortion or hysterectomy or those partners of women with BV should be examined and treated.

Recurrence:

- BV recurs frequently.
- The persistence of BV-associated organisms and failure of *Lactobacillus* flora to recolonize may cause recurrence.
- Suppressive treatment with metronidazole gel can suppress recurrence.
- Physiological approaches, such as acidification and probiotics, have been investigated with variable results.
- Under study—vaginal suppositories containing human lactobacillus strains.

Prevention:

- Partner management:
  - After multiple occurrences, some consider empiric treatment of male sex partners to see if recurrence rate diminishes, but this approach has not been validated.
- Patient counseling and education:
  - *Nature of the disease*: Normal versus abnormal discharge (malodor), BV signs and symptoms, sexual association
  - *Transmission problems*: It is not sexually transmitted between heterosexuals, high association in female same-sex partnerships.[37]
  - *Risk reduction* by douching avoidance and lowering the number of sex partners.

Candidiasis

Candidal vaginitis known as "yeast" caused by *Candida albicans,* that is still unknown if it is a part of the vagina flora. It occurs less than what we believe. A study conducted on self-referred women with chronic recurrent yeast infections showed that only half of them had candidal vaginitis.[38,39] In addition, its pathogenicity is not associated to its abundance in the vagina where few amounts can result in severe symptoms **(Flowchart 3)**. Previous evidence revealed that healthy/normal bacterial colonization such as lactobacilli plays a major role protecting against *Candida* infection. Yet, *Candida-infected* women present predominant lactobacilli on gram stain of vaginal fluid.[40-44]

Candida vaginitis has the most characteristic history of the vaginitis, presenting pruritus in most cases, often with sparse or no discharge (similar cottage cheese). Possible erythema and swelling of the vulva and vaginal walls are reported. Diagnosis is suggested by history and confirmed through physical and laboratory examination (potassium hydroxide preparation and culture) **(Fig. 6)**. The treatment options for candidiasis are outlined in **Table 2**.

Foreign Bodies

Neglected pessary can have important implications, for example, a forgotten and retained pessary can cause profuse vaginal discharge, ulceration, and even carcinoma. In addition, a less neglected pessary results in a lesser degree of discharge seen as "whites" resulting in chronic discharge, and therefore leukorrhea.

LONG-TERM SEQUELAE

- Untreated or chronic infection can reach the cervix, uterus, fallopian tubes, and other resulting in congestion of the

Flowchart 3: Etiopathogenesis of recurrent vulvovaginal candidiasis.

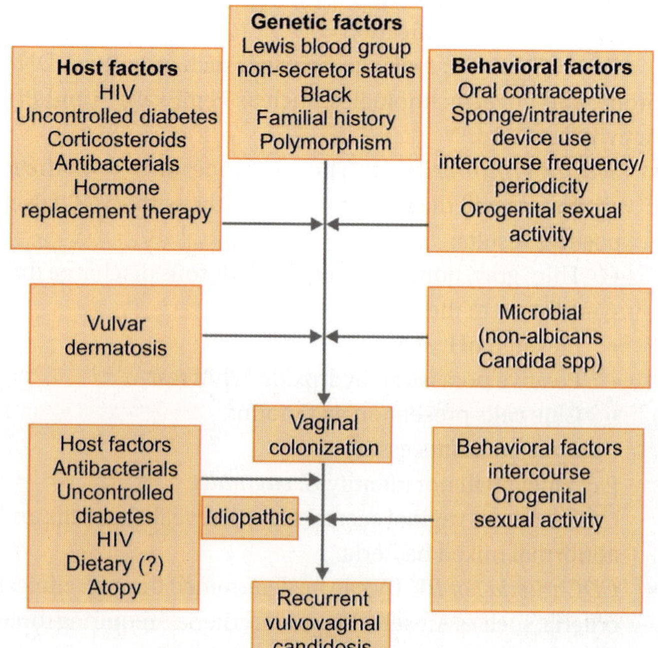

uterus or ovary or pelvis, and causing heavy menstrual flow in next period.

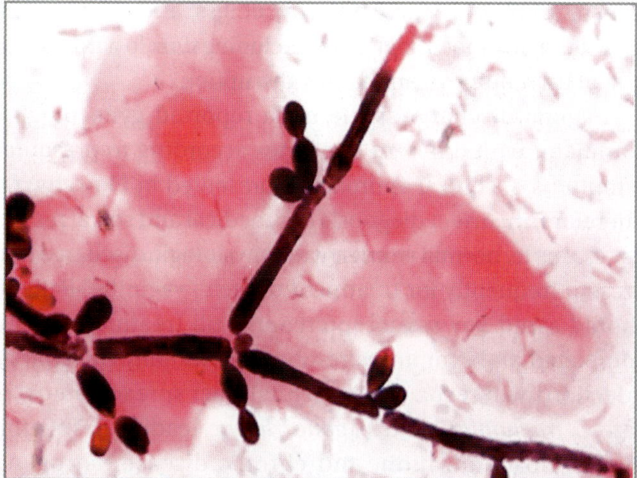

Fig. 6: Candidiasis.

TABLE 2: Therapy for vaginal candidiasis.

	Formulation	*Dosage*
Butoconazole	2% cream 2% cram (bioadhesive)	5 g per day for 3 days Single dose
Clotrimazole	1% cream 10% cream 100 mg vaginal tablet 100 mg vaginal tablet 500 mg vaginal tablet	5 g per day for 7–14 days 5 g single application One tablet per day for 7 days Two tablets per day for 3 days One tablet once
Miconazole	2% cream 100 mg vaginal suppository 200 mg vaginal suppository 1200 mg vaginal suppository	5 g per day for 7 days One suppository per day for 7 days One suppository per day for 3 days One suppository once
Econazole	150 mg vaginal tablet 150 mg vaginal suppository	One tablet per day for 3 days Single dose
Fenticonazole	2% cream	5 g per day for 7 days
Sertaconazole (Zalain)	300 mg pessary	Single dose
Ticonazole	2% cream 6.5% cream	5 g per day for 3 days 5 g single application
Terconazole	0.4% cream 0.8% cream 80 mg vaginal suppository	5 g per day for 7 days 5 g per day for 3 days One suppository per day for 3 days
Fluconazole	150 mg tablet	Single dose
Ketoconazole	200 mg tablet	Two tablets per day for 5 days
Itraconazole	100 mg tablet	Two tablets per day for 3 days

- It acts as a precursor of PID, salpingo-oophoritis (infection of fallopian tube and ovaries), which mostly result in pelvic adhesions like peritoneal adhesions and fallopian tube adhesions, which obstruct tubes and may cause infertility.
- In case of white discharges in women during late fertile period/menopause, analysis is of great importance to rule out cervix cancer (one of the most reported cancer in women).
- The infection can spread into the urinary tract, reproductive tract, and other neighboring organs given the adjacency of the urethra, vagina, and anus.

Prevention is more effective than treatment.

Proper hygiene practices must be respected, such as washing genitals every day from front to back, using clean underwear, and using a nonchemical and nonallergenic vaginal wash that maintains the pH of the vagina, such as VAGISIL.

Other precautions include avoidance of—(1) irritants such as perfumed sprays, soaps, and bath products; (2) stress (due to its association with hormonal status); (3) sharing same towels and underwear; (4) tight-fitting synthetic clothing to avoid moisture; and (4) sexual intercourse during heavy discharges or unprotected sex (without condoms while under treatment).

The treatment must be in full course even after the cessation of symptoms. No sexual intercourse through treatment course to avoid irritation of tissues, which are in the process of healing.

FACTORS ADDRESSING RECURRENT VAGINAL INFECTIONS

- Restoration of the normal vaginal flora
- Keeping proper hygiene practices
- Dietary control
- Management and avoidance of stress.

Syndrome Approach to Vaginal Discharge[45-48]

The magnitude of the problem of sexually transmitted infections has to be recognized by the World Health Organization (WHO), which has recommended the syndrome approach at community level. This is especially important for resource-poor settings.

Main Features

- Classify key-causative organisms by clinical symptoms to which they give rise
- Use flow charts to identify causes of a given syndrome
- Treat patients for all the important causes of the syndrome
- Ensure that both partners are treated.

Supplementary Elements

- Women should be advised on treatment compliance (on the right time with the right dose and until the end of the course)

- Patients educated on risk reduction
- Use condoms in sexual intercourses.

Benefits

- Accessibility
- Immediate treatment
- Effectiveness
- Efficiency
- Quality assurance/standardization.

Disadvantages of Syndrome Treatment

- Treatment failures
- Does not cover asymptomatic infection.

If the problem persists after primary management, the patient is referred to a higher center.

CONCLUSION

Vaginal discharge can occur as a normal physiologic phenomena or a secondarily due to serious systemic illness (diabetes mellitus or endometrial cancer), causing major discomfort and suffering for women. Epidemiological data revealed that 25% of primary care office visits are for vaginal discharge, and even higher number of visits to gynecologic consultations and STD clinics. Abnormal vaginal discharge can be associated with symptoms, such as pain, sexual transmission of disease, systemic illness, and even sterility in addition to other social issues including time lost from work, sexual unhappiness, and family disruption.

Vaginal discharge is the most reported gynecological complaint with different etiologies according to presented symptoms. A clinical approach is presented in **Flowchart 4**. Therefore, incorrect diagnosis has medical and social results. For example, normal women with physiologic discharge may present frequently for treatment of their "vaginitis". Patients should avoid any sexual intercourse till treatment course completed and symptoms resolved, as sexually transmitted infections will recur. Upper genital tract spread can occur with *C. trachomatis* and *N. gonorrhoeae*, leading to systemic illness, hospitalization, and chronic disease. Iatrogenic vulvovaginal candidiasis mostly presented in women during reproductive age who failed routine treatment strategies can be avoided with appropriate forethought and prescription. Unrecognized herpes simplex, vulvovaginal candidiasis, or gonococcal infection at the time of delivery can cause illness in the neonate. Referral to a gynecologist and high healthcare

Flowchart 4: Management of vaginal discharge.

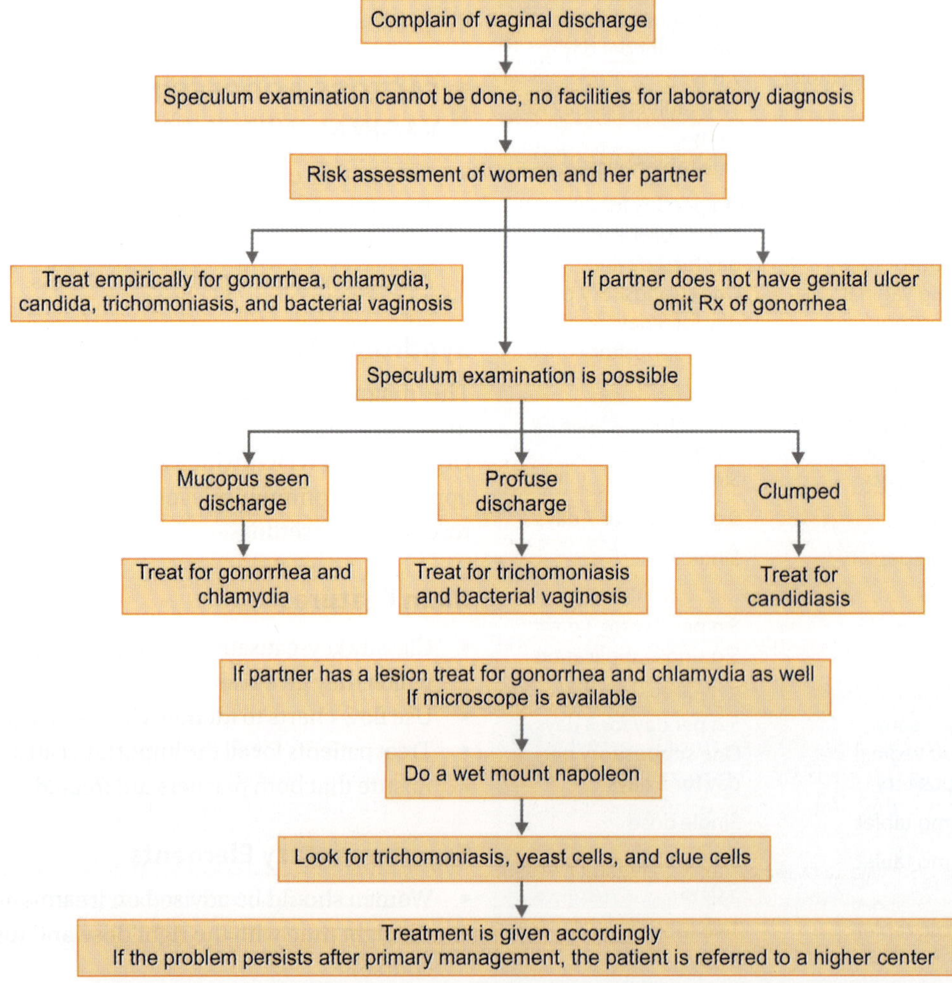

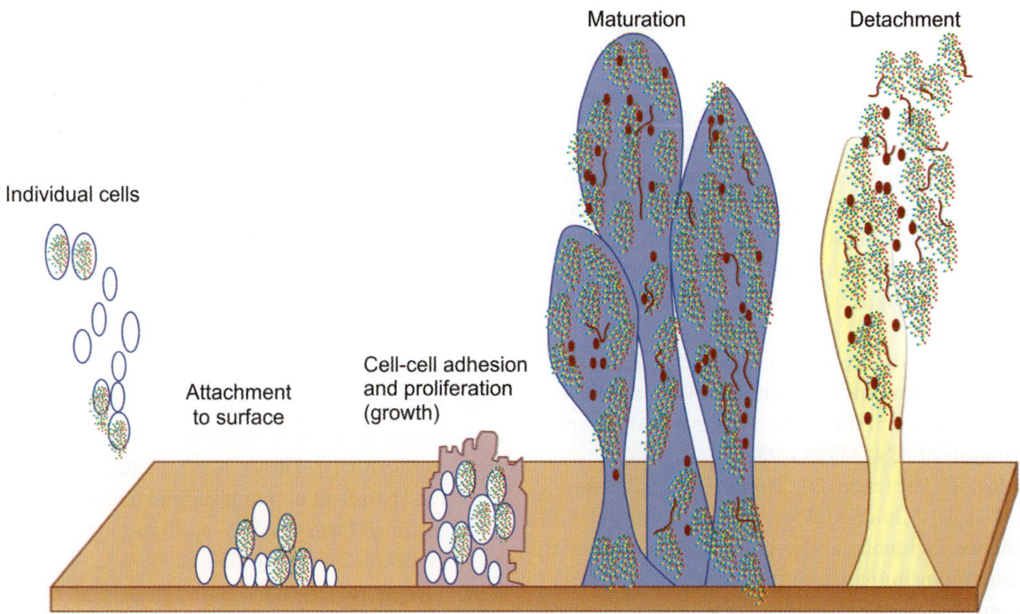

Fig. 7: The biofilm life cycle in three steps—attachment, growth of colonies (micro-colony formation and formation of three-dimensional structures) and detachment in clumps.

costs are caused by incorrect diagnoses treated by telephone or with simple physical examination **(Fig. 7)**.

Sexually transmitted diseases are continuously on the increase. Further spotlight shed on this condition and future research of vaginitis will lead to better diagnosis and treatment.

REFERENCES

1. Casari E, Ferrario A, Morenghi E, Montanelli A. Gardnerella, Trichomonas vaginalis, Candidia, Chlamydia trachomatis, Mycoplasma hominis and Ureaplama urealyticum in the genital discharge of symptomatic fertile and asymptomatic infertile women. New Microbiol. 2010;33(1):69-76.
2. Ledger WJ. Historical review of the treatment of bacterial vaginosis. Am J Obstet Gynecol. 1993;169(2 Pt 2):474-8.
3. Szabadvary F. Indicators a historical perspective. J Chem Educ. 1964;41(5):285.
4. Nugent RP, Krohen MA, Hillier SL. Reliability of diagnosing bacterial vaginosis is improved by a standardized method of gram stain interpretation. J Clin Microbiol. 1991;29(2):297-301.
5. Fredricks DN, Fiedler TL, Marrazzo JM. Molecular identification of bacteria associated with bacterial vaginosis. N Engl J Med. 2005;353(18):1899-911.
6. Vallor AC, Antonio MA, Hawes SE, Hillier SL. Factors associated with acquisition of, or persistent colonization by, vaginal lactobacilli: role of hydrogen peroxide production. J Infect Dis. 2001;184(11):1431-6.
7. Soper DE, Bump RC, Hurt WG. Bacterial vaginosis and trichomoniasis vaginitis are risk factors for cuff cellulitis after abdominal hysterectomy. Am J Obstet Gynecol. 1990;163(3): 1016-21.
8. Gray RH, Kigozi G, Serwadda D, Makumbi F, Nalugoda F, Watya S, et al. The effects of male circumcision on female partners' genital tract symptoms and vaginal infections in a randomized trial in Rakai, Uganda. Am J Obstet Gynecol. 2009;200(1):42.e1-7.
9. Crosby RA, Charnigo RA, Weathers C, Caliendo AM, Shrier LA. Condom effectiveness against nomsel rn-viral sexually transmitted infections: a prospective study using electronic daily diaries. Sex Transm Infect. 2012;88(7):484-9.
10. Peterman TA, Tian LH, Metcalf CA, Satterwhite CL, Malotte CK, DeAugustine N, et al; RESPECT-2 Study Group. High incidence of new sexually transmitted infections in the year following a sexually transmitted infection: a case for rescreening. Ann Intern Med. 2006;145(8):564-72.
11. Hughes JP, Baeten JM, Lingappa JR, Magaret AS, Wald A, de Bruyn G, et al; Partners in Prevention HSV/HIV Transmission Study Team. Determinants of per-coital-act HIV-1 infectivity among African HIV-1-serodiscordant couples. J Infect Dis. 2012;205(3):358-65.
12. Moodley P, Wilkinson D, Connolly C, Moodley J, Sturm AW. Trichomonas vaginalis is associated with pelvic inflammatory disease in women infected with human immunodeficiency virus. Clin Infect Dis. 2002 Feb;34(4):519-22.
13. Krieger JN, Tam MR, Stevens CE, Nielsen IO, Hale J, Kiviat NB, et al. Diagnosis of trichomoniasis. Comparison of conventional wet-mount examination with cytologic studies, cultures, and monoclonal antibody staining of direct specimens. JAMA. 1988;259(8):1223-7
14. Kurth A, Whittington WL, Golden MR, Thomas KK, Holmes KK, Schwebke JR. Performance of a new, rapid assay for detection of Trichomonas vaginalis. J Clin Microbiol. 2004;42(7):2940-3.
15. Nye MB, Schwebke JR, Body BA. Comparison of APTIMA Trichomonas vaginalis transcription-mediated amplification to wet mount microscopy, culture and PCR for diagnosis of trichomoniasis in men and women. Am J Obstet Gynecol. 2009;200(2):188.e1-e7.
16. Crowell AL, Sanders-Lewis KA, Secor WE. In vitro metronidazole and tinidazole activities against metronidazole-resistant strains of *Trichomonas vaginalis*. Antimicrob Agents Chemother. 2003;47(4):1407-9.

17. Nyirjesy P, Gilbert J, Mulcahy LJ. Resistant trichomoniasis: Successful treatment with combination therapy. Sex Transm Dis. 2011;38(10):962-3.
18. Cotch MF, Pastorek JG 2nd, Nugent RP, Hillier SL, Gibbs RS, Martin DH, et al. Trichomonas vaginalis associated with low birth weight and preterm delivery. The Vaginal Infections and Prematurity Study Group. Sex Transm Dis. 1997;24(6):353-60.
19. Koss CA, Baras DC, Lane SD, Aubry R, Marcus M, Markowitz LE, et al. Investigation of metronidazole use during pregnancy and adverse birth outcomes. Antimicrob Agents Chemother. 2012;56(9):4800-5.
20. Gumbo FZ, Duri K, Kandawasvika GQ, Kurewa NE. Risk factors of HIV vertical transmission in a cohort of women under a PMTCT program at three peri-urban clinics in a resource-poor setting. J Perinatol. 2010;30(11):717-23.
21. Cu-Uvin S, Ko H, Jamieson DJ, Hogan JW, Schuman P, Anderson J, et al; HIV Epidemiology Research Study (HERS) Group. Prevalence, incidence, and persistence or recurrence of trichomoniasis among human immunodeficiency virus (HIV)-positive women and among HIV-negative women at high risk for HIV infection. Clin Infect Dis. 2002;34(10):1406-11.
22. Anderson BL, Firnhaber C, Liu T, Swarts A, Siminya M, Ingersoll J, et al. Effect of trichomoniasis therapy on genital HIV viral burden among African women. Sex Transm Dis. 2012;39(8):638-42.
23. Balkus JE, Richardson BA, Mochache V, Chohan V, Chan JD, Masese L, et al. A prospective cohort study comparing the effect of single-dose 2 g metronidazole on Trichomonas vaginalis infection in HIV-seropositive versus HIV-seronegative women. Sex Transm Dis. 2013;40(6):499-505.
24. Gardner HL, Dukes CD. Haemophilus vaginalis vaginitis: a newly defined specific infection previously classified "nonspecific" vaginitis. Am J Obstet Gynecol. 1955;69(5):962-76.
25. Brunham RC, Paavonen J, Stevens CE, Kiviat N, Kuo CC, Critchlow CW, et al. Mucopurulent cervicitis--the ignored counterpart in women of urethritis in men. N Engl J Med. 1984;311(1):1-6.
26. Eschenbach DA. Bacterial vaginosis and anaerobes in obstetric-gynecologic infections. Clin Infect Dis. 1993; 16(Suppl 4):S282-7.
27. Chen KC, Forsyth PS, Buchanan TM, Holmes KK. Amine content of vaginal fluid from untreated and treated patients with nonspecific vaginitis. J Clin Invest. 1979;63(5):828-35.
28. Hanna NF, Taylor-Robinson D, Kalodiki-Karamanoli M, Harris JR, McFadyen IR. The relation between vaginal pH and the microbiological status in vaginitis. Br J Obstet Gynaecol. 1985;92(12):1267-71.
29. Amsel R, Totten PA, Spiegel CA, Chen KC, Eschenbach D, Holmes KK. Nonspecific vaginitis. Diagnostic criteria and microbial and epidemiologic associations. Am J Med. 1983;74(1):14-22.
30. Lusike DM, Waiyaki P, Kiiyukia C, Bukusi EA. Bacterial vaginosis and associated risk factors in pregnant women attending Ante Natal Clinic at Pumwani Maternity Hospital–Kenya. Afr J Health Sci. 2018;31(1):13-30.
31. Singh A, Kanti V, Dayal S. Prevalence and risk factors of bacterial vaginosis among women of reproductive age attending rural tertiary care institute of Western Uttar Pradesh. J Evolution Med Dent Sci. 2016;5(43):2695-701.
32. Ranjit E, Raghubanshi BR, Maskey S, Parajuli P. Prevalence of bacterial vaginosis and its association with risk factors among nonpregnant women: A hospital based study. Int J Microbiol. 2018;2018.
33. Durga Kumari P, G Aruna, G Naga Sugeetha. Study of association of bacterial vaginosis in preterm labor and fetal outcome. IAIM. 2015;2(4):114-8.
34. Hauth JC, Goldenberg RL, Andrews WW, DuBard MB, Copper RL. Reduced incidence of preterm delivery with metronidazole and erythromycin in women with bacterial vaginosis. N Engl J Med. 1995;333(26):1732-6.
35. Briggs GC, Freeman RK, Yaffe SJ. Drugs in Pregnancy and Lactation, 9th edition. Philadelphia, PA: Lippincott Williams & Wilkins; 2011.
36. Erickson SH, Oppenheim GL, Smith GH. Metronidazole in breast milk. Obstet Gynecol. 1981;57(1):48-50.
37. Jamieson DJ, Duerr A, Klein RS, Paramsothy P, Brown W, Cu-Uvin S, et al. Longitudinal analysis of bacterial vaginosis: findings from the HIV epidemiology research study. Obstet Gynecol. 2001;98(4):656-63.
38. Livengood CH. Bacterial vaginosis: an overview for 2009. Rev Obstet Gynecol. 2009;2(1):28-37.
39. Briselden AM, Hillier SL. Longitudinal study of the biotypes of Gardnerella vaginalis. J Clin Microbiol. 1990;28(12):2761-4.
40. Sutton M, Sternberg M, Koumans EH, McQuillan G, Berman S, Markowitz L. The prevalence of Trichomonas vaginalis infection among reproductive-age women in the United States, 2001-2004. Clin Infect Dis. 2007;45(10):1319-26.
41. Meites E, Llata E, Braxton J, Schwebke JR, Bernstein KT, Pathela P, et al. Trichomonas vaginalis in selected U.S. sexually transmitted disease clinics: testing, screening, and prevalence. Sex Transm Dis. 2013;40(11):865-9.
42. Peterman TA, Tian LH, Metcalf CA, Malotte CK, Paul SM, Douglas JM Jr; RESPECT-2 Study Group. Persistent, undetected Trichomonas vaginalis infections? Clin Infect Dis. 2009;48(2):259-60.
43. Gatski M, Kissinger P. Observation of probable persistent, undetected *Trichomonas vaginalis* infection among HIV-positive women. Clin Infect Dis. 2010;51(1):114-5.
44. Seña AC, Miller WC, Hobbs MM, Schwebke JR, Leone PA, Swygard H, et al. Trichomonas vaginalis infection in male sexual partners: implications for diagnosis, treatment, and prevention. Clin Infect Dis. 2007;44(1):13-22.
45. Tsai CS, Shepherd BE, Vermund SH. Does douching increase risk for sexually transmitted infections? A prospective study in high-risk adolescents. Am J Obstet Gynecol. 2009;200(1):e31-8.
46. Kirkcaldy RD, Augostini P, Asbel LE, Bernstein KT, Kerani RP, Mettenbrink CJ, et al. Trichomonas vaginalis antimicrobial drug resistance in 6 US cities, STD Surveillance Network, 2009-2010. Emerg Infect Dis. 2012;18(6):939-43.
47. Mann JR, McDermott S, Barnes TL, Hardin J, Bao H, Zhou L. Trichomoniasis in pregnancy and mental retardation in children. Ann Epidemiol. 2009;19(12):891-9.
48. Carter JE, Whithaus KC. Neonatal respiratory tract involvement by *Trichomonas vaginalis*: a case report and review of the literature. Am J Trop Med Hygiene. 2008;78(1):17-9.

LONG QUESTIONS

1. What is the treatment of Trichomonas vaginitis?
2. What is the treatment of candidiasis?

3. How oral contraceptive pills are responsible for increased incidence of vaginitis?
4. What is bacterial vaginosis?
5. Is bacterial vaginosis sexually transmitted?
6. What is "Nugent criteria" in bacterial vaginosis?

SHORT QUESTIONS

1. What is leukorrhea?
2. What are the types of vaginitis?
3. What are the predisposing factors for candidal vaginitis?
4. What lesions will you rule out on the cervix in case of excessive vaginal discharge?
5. What is the treatment of Chlamydia infection?
6. What is clue cell?
7. In a wet mount preparation, what is the characteristic feature of—(1) Trichomonal infection; (2) Gardnerella infection.

MULTIPLE CHOICE QUESTIONS

1. The normal ph of vagina is:
   a. 5.5–6.5 b. 3.5–4
   c. 3.8–4.5 d. 5–6
2. Strawberry vagina is seen in:
   a. Candida vaginitis b. Trichomonas vaginitis
   c. Bacterial vaginosis d. All of the above
3. Which of the following organisms does not constitute the normal flora of vagina?
   a. Lactobacillus b. Mobiluncus
   c. Gardnerella vaginalis d. Trichomonas vaginalis
4. Amsel's criteria constitute which of the following?
   a. Curdy while discharge
   b. pH <4.5
   c. Clue cells on microscopy
   d. All of the above
   e. b and c
5. Nugent criteria is based on the use of:
   a. Gram stain b. KOH mount
   c. Wet smear d. None of the above
6. What constitutes complicated candidal infection?
   a. 4 or more symptoms in one year
   b. Candidal infection present with pregnancy
   c. Infection by a species other than *Candida albicans*
   d. All of the above
7. Drug of choice for treatment of trichomoniasis is:
   a. Secnidazole b. Metronidazole
   c. Terconazole d. Ornidazole
8. Syndrome approach of WHO is:
   a. Meant to be used in all situations
   b. To be used only when testing facilities are not available
   c. Meant to be used in low-resource settings
   d. Used for quick diagnosis of STIs
9. Clue cells are seen in:
   a. Trichomonas vaginalis b. Candidiasis
   c. Gonorrhea d. Bacterial vaginosis
10. Bacterial vaginosis does not include:
    a. Profuse creamy discharge
    b. Clue cells present
    c. Positive Whiff test
    d. Absent leukocytes

Answers

1. c 2. b 3. d 4. e 5. a 6. d
7. b 8. c 9. d 10. a

10.2 SEXUALLY TRANSMITTED INFECTIONS AND HIV IN WOMEN

Atul Munshi, Munjal Pandya

INTRODUCTION

Sexually transmitted infections (STIs), along with human immunodeficiency virus (HIV), have become major healthcare issues in past few decades. STIs are usually associated with reduction in quality of life to morbidity spanning over years to even mortality in case of severe AIDS. Globally, these STIs are putting burden on many lives and healthcare system, specifically so, in developing countries. NACO (National AIDS Control Organization) has reported that around 6% of adult population gets STI every year in our country.[1]

Sexually transmitted infections can present with genital, anal, or perineal ulcers, or can present with their characteristic vaginal discharge, or their specific lesions. This chapter focuses on various STIs and their characteristic presentations, the modalities of their diagnosis, their treatment, and importance of tracking down and evaluation-treatment of their partners.

BACTERIAL VAGINOSIS

It is a condition where hydrogen-producing lactobacilli are replaced by anaerobic bacteria, *Gardnerella vaginalis, Ureaplasma, Mycoplasma*, and other anaerobes. Women with multiple partners, nonusage of barrier contraceptives are majorly affected with bacterial vaginosis (BV). Women with BV are at an increased risk of getting HIV, gonorrhea, chlamydia, and Herpes.[2-4] One of the studies suggested that treatment of male partner will not prevent recurrence.[5]

Diagnosis

Amsel's diagnostic criteria are useful for diagnosis along with Gram stain. The latter is important to know relative concentration of gram-positive rods (lactobacilli) and gram-negative and gram variable cocci and rods.[6]

Clinically, BV can be diagnosed by any 3 out of following 4 symptoms/signs:

1. Vaginal pH >4.5
2. Positive whiff test (fishy odor of vaginal discharge on addition of 10% KOH)
3. Clue cells (vaginal epithelial cells with adherent organisms, visualized on microscope) **(Fig. 1)**
4. Homogeneous white discharge, coating vaginal wall.

Gram staining of vaginal smear can add to above clinical criteria for confirmation of diagnosis.[7] Polymerase chain reaction (PCR) has been studied as one of the diagnostic tools, but its acceptance in clinical setting is still debatable. Pap smear and culture are yet nonspecific, and are having low sensitivity, thus, having no defined role as diagnostic tools.

Treatment

Women with symptoms are to be treated, mainly to relieve symptoms, as well as to reduce chances of coinfection with other organisms.

Metronidazole 200–400 mg thrice daily for 7 days orally, or metronidazole gel (0.75%) intravaginally once a day for 5 days, or clindamycin cream (2%) intravaginally one time a day for 7 days can be given.

Caution: Abstinence from alcohol is recommended to avoid disulfiram like reaction, at least till 24 hours after last dose of nitroimidazoles. Clindamycin cream may weaken latex barrier contraceptives after 5 days of use.

Usage of barrier contraception of abstinence for the period of treatment is advised.

Alternatively, tinidazole 2 g orally, one time a day, for 2 days or 1 g orally, one time a day for 5 days can be given.[8] Clindamycin can also be given orally (300 mg twice a day for 7 days) or as ovules (100 mg intravaginally once a day for 3 days).[9]

Role of intravaginal lactobacillus preparations: Till date, not much of consolidated studies have shown promising results with usage of such preparations for treatment of BV.[10]

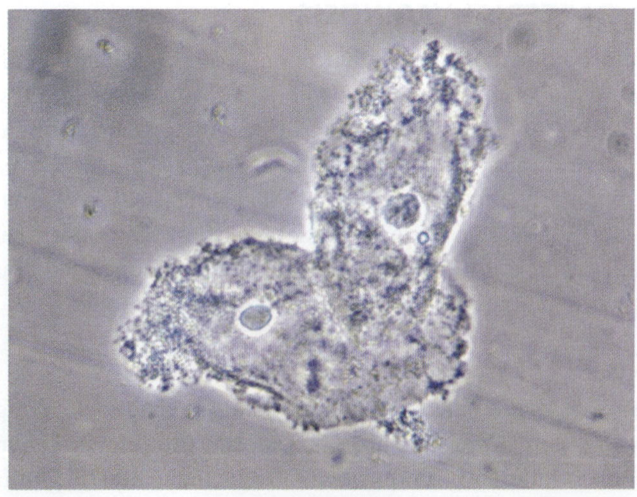

Fig. 1: Clue cells.

Persistent/recurrent BV may occur, and may need change of regimen. In cases where only one previous cycle of treatment was given, the same regimen may work effectively.[11]

Various regimens have been used with success in cases of recurrent BV. 0.75% metronidazole gel two times a week for 4–6 months has shown efficacy. One more regimen was metronidazole or tinidazole for 7 days, followed by intravaginal boric acid 600 mg daily for 21 days, followed by metronidazole gel twice weekly for 4–6 months.[12]

Oral fluconazole (150 mg) and 2 g of metronidazole once a month have been found to be effective as a tool to reduce incidence of BV.[13]

Pregnancy: BV is associated with complications, such as preterm labor, premature rupture of membranes, and chorioamnionitis. Treatment of BV can reduce vaginal symptoms. Use of antibiotics may not contribute to prevention of preterm labor, but it may help in waiting for effect of steroids on lung maturity.

Symptomatic pregnant women can be treated with metronidazole orally (250 mg regimen) or metronidazole gel with equal efficacy.[14] Oral clindamycin has also been used effectively in such cases. No adverse effect on fetus was demonstrated with use of metronidazole or oral clindamycin.

Asymptomatic pregnant patients, who are at high risk of preterm labor, might get benefited with treatment of BV.

Metronidazole is secreted in breast milk, but its level in infant remains lower than that in maternal plasma. There have been few opinions of deferring breastfeeding for at least 12–24 hours after treatment with single dose 2 g regimen.

Tinidazole has shown moderate risk in animal studies with regards to pregnancy, thus, it has to be avoided in pregnancy.[15]

Bacterial vaginosis has been found to be occurring frequently in patients with HIV.

TRICHOMONIASIS

Women infected with *Trichomonas vaginalis*, most of the times, are symptomless or have minimum symptoms (70–80%), while rest may exhibit malodourous, yellow green discharge. Condom will protect against trichomoniasis. Circumscribed men were shown to reduce chances of transmitting it.[16]

Trichomoniasis is associated with premature rupture of membranes, low birth weight, preterm labor as adverse pregnancy outcomes, as well as increased chances of HIV. In HIV-infected individuals, trichomoniasis increases chances of pelvic inflammatory disease (PID).[17] Thus, it is recommended to screen HIV-positive patients for *T. vaginalis* infection.

Diagnosis

Nucleic acid amplification test (NAAT) is the choice of investigation due to low sensitivity of microscopy **(Fig. 2)**. Culture has sensitivity of 75–95%, while specificity up to 100%,[18] the choice of sample being vaginal secretions, as

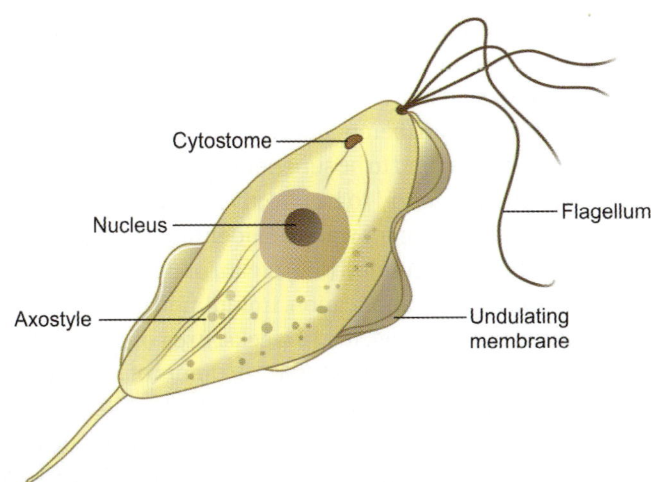

Fig. 2: *Trichomonas vaginalis.*

urine culture is less sensitive. Microscopic evaluation of wet mount preparation from vaginal secretions is of low sensitivity (50–65%), yet cheaper option. Important step in microscopic evaluation is to examine the preparation without any delay, as sensitivity declines significantly even after 1 hour of delay. Pap smear is not a preferred method, as it gives false negative as well as false positive results.

Treatment

Metronidazole 2 g orally single dose or tinidazole 2 g orally single dose can be given. Alternatively, metronidazole 200–400 mg orally three times a day can be given for 7 days. Tinidazole is having higher levels in serum and genitourinary tract, higher cure rates, longer half-life, and lesser gastrointestinal side effects, as compared to metronidazole. Metronidazole gel is not recommended as it was not found to be efficacious.

Intercourse is to be avoided till the patient and her sex partner are cured completely. It is very important to treat partner simultaneously to avoid transmission or reinfection.

Antimicrobial resistance is a possibility for recurrent infection. If single dose regimen has failed, and reinfection has been excluded, 400 mg of metronidazole thrice daily for 7 days is to be given orally. Failure of this regimen as well can be tackled by metronidazole 2 g orally for 7 days. If this fails as well, culture and sensitivity are to be checked to rule out antimicrobial resistance. One of the options in such cases will be tinidazole 2 g for 14 days, along with intravaginal tinidazole.

Pregnancy: Metronidazole is safe during third trimester of pregnancy, and it reduces chances of respiratory or genital infection of newborn.[19] Vertical HIV transmission rate is increased with presence of *T. vaginalis*, thus making it a condition mandatory to be treated.

HIV infection: Association of *T. vaginalis* with HIV was seen in around 53% of patients.[20] Treating *T. vaginalis* will lead to reduced viral load in genitourinary tract and reduced viral shedding. Regimen chosen is 400 mg metronidazole thrice a day for 7 days, as single dose regimen was less effective due to antiretroviral therapy (ART), higher rates of coinfection with BV, and impaired immunity.

CANDIDIASIS

Candida albicans is the most common *Candida* causing candidiasis, but other species can also be responsible. Symptoms can be dyspareunia, dysuria, curdy white vaginal discharge, pruritus, and vaginal soreness. It can be divided as follows:

- *Uncomplicated vulvovaginal candidiasis (VVC)*: Sporadic or infrequent VVC, mild-to-moderate VVC, in women with no immunocompromised. There will be vulvar edema, fissures, and thick curdy white discharge. Vaginal pH is normal. 10% KOH wet preparation of Gram stain will help establish diagnosis. Culture will yield yeast, which is gold standard method. In symptomatic women, if wet mounts are negative, culture is needed. In cases where there are no symptoms, yet culture is positive for candida, treatment is not recommended, as they might be physiologically present in approximately 10–20% of women.

  Treatment: Azoles are choice of drug. Clotrimazole (1% cream intravaginally for 7–14 days) or miconazole (2% intravaginally for 7 days) can be used locally. Oral fluconazole 150 mg, itraconazole 200 mg, or miconazole 200 mg in single dose is recommended. Creams are oil-based preparations, which might weaken latex barrier contraceptives. Partner can be offered treatment in case of pruritus or irritation, with topical antifungal agents. Drug interaction of azole with other drugs need to be kept in mind while prescribing. They may also elevate liver enzymes rarely.
- *Complicated VVC*: Recurrent, severe or non-albicans candidiasis, as well as candidiasis in women with diabetes, immunocompromised state fall under this category. Culture from vagina will reveal unusual species, even when pseudohyphae are not visible on microscopy.

Recurrent VVC is four or more episodes within 1 year. Antifungal regimen for 7–14 days, followed by maintenance therapy of oral fluconazole 100–200 mg weekly for 6 months.

In case of non-albicans VVC, non-fluconazole azole regimen is used. In case of recurrence, 600 mg boric acid in gelatin capsule vaginally daily for 2 weeks is recommended.

In case of pregnancy, topical azole therapy for 7 days is useful.

How to Differentiate Various Conditions of Abnormal Vaginal Discharge?

Vaginal pH is to be determined, elevated pH indicates BV or trichomoniasis. Microscopic examination of discharge after diluting in 0.9% normal saline, and second sample is to be diluted in 10% KOH. Amine odor upon KOH addition suggests BV or trichomoniasis. Microscopic examination of saline preparation suggests motile trichomonads or clue cells indicative of BV. KOH preparation will help in diagnosing hyphae of blastospores seen in candidiasis.

HUMAN PAPILLOMAVIRUS

Most of the times, human papillomavirus (HPV) infection stays asymptomatic. At least once in a lifetime, person gets HPV infection. HPV infection is perceived seriously because of its potential for contributing toward cervical, vulvar, vaginal, and oropharyngeal cancers. HPV types 16 and 18 are responsible for oncogenic infection, while types 6 and 11 are attributed to genital warts and recurrent respiratory infections.

Mode of Transmission

The mode of transmission is through anogenital contact. It can be transmitted via genital to genital contact and oral sex. Rarely, it can be transmitted to infant because of vaginal delivery.

Treatment

Subclinical HPV infections are self-limiting, not requiring any treatment. Treatment of symptomatic patients helps in treating conditions arising out of HPV infection, but cannot guarantee removal of virus.

Prevention

Condom can reduce probability of getting transmission of HPV to certain extent, but cannot completely protect against it, as HPV can affect areas not covered by condom. The most effective way can only be abstinence from intercourse.

Various vaccines are available for prevention of cancer resulting from HPV infection. Bivalent vaccine protecting against types 16 and 18 and quadrivalent vaccine protecting against types 6, 11, 16, and 18 are commercially available. 9-valent vaccine protects against five additional variants. HPV vaccine is usually given in three doses—second dose is given 1–2 months after first and third dose is given 6 months after first dose. Vaccine can be started at the age of 9 years for girls. Women between age groups of 13 and 26 years should receive vaccine if not received previously. In USA, vaccination is not recommended after the age of 26 years.[21]

Warts: Anogenital warts are majorly caused by types 6 and 11. Other types may be involved, particularly in patients with HIV. Warts can be seen around vaginal introitus and in anogenital mucosa. These warts are asymptomatic in most of the cases, they can be flat, papules or pedunculated growth. In some cases, they can be painful.

Visual inspection leads to diagnosing this condition, which can be confirmed by biopsy. Biopsy is indicated in immunocompromised patients, who do not respond to therapy. HPV testing is not recommended, as it is not confirmatory.

Warts may resolve spontaneously, or may increase in size. Spontaneous resolution may take around 1 year. Treatment is indicated for their removal as well as for relieving symptoms. Reduction of warts with therapy does not reduce HPV infectivity.

No treatment is found to be superior to any other treatment, and no treatment is found to be effective in all warts of same patient! Various location of warts are identified and patients can be prescribed imiquimod (5%) cream or podofilox (0.5%) solution or gel for local application. Imiquimod cream is to be applied three times a week for 16 weeks. Area of application needs to be washed thoroughly after 7–10 hours of application with soap and water. Podofilox can be applied twice a day for 3 days, followed by rest of 4 days, and such cycle can be repeated four times. Green tea extract preparation (sinecatechins 15% ointment) can be applied three times a day, but not >16 weeks. But, safety of this preparation is not known in pregnancy, HIV, and genital herpes cases.

In clinical settings, cryotherapy with liquid nitrogen or surgical removal or application of trichloroacetic acid (TCA) solution are the options. Cryotherapy induces cytolysis, and in case of more number of warts, local anesthesia can be used. Blistering may occur at the site of application. Surgical removal can be done by cautery, taking caution of not going deep to avoid scarring. Excision can be done by scalpel or CO_2 laser or curate. CO_2 laser is of particular use in cases of large wart and intraurethral warts. Recurrence may occur after surgical removal. TCA causes chemical coagulation of proteins. After application of TCA, the area is allowed to dry, followed by application of sodium bicarbonate, followed by washing with liquid soap to avoid damage to surrounding area. Such a course can be applied on weekly interval.

Pregnancy: Anogenital warts can proliferate during pregnancy. Removal may not heal warts completely till termination of pregnancy. Infants may be affected with respiratory papillomatosis, in case of HPV 6 and 11. Cesarean section has not been found to reduce incidence of such probability.[22] Cesarean is indicated only when there is pelvic outlet obstruction or chances of excess bleeding with vaginal delivery.

HEPATITIS B

Hepatitis B infection has incubation period of 6 weeks to 6 months. It is found in blood and body fluids, such as semen, saliva, and vaginal secretions. Infectivity of HBV is more than HIV. HBV infection can become chronic in most of the cases involving children, against only 2–6% cases in adults proceeding toward chronic infection.[23] Unprotected intercourse with infected partner, high-risk sexual behavior, sexually transmitted disease (STD), and injectable drug abuse are the risk factors.

Diagnosis

Serological testing confirms the diagnosis. IgM anti-HBc (IgM antibody to core antigen) suggests acute infection. Presence of anti-HBs suggests resolved phase and is seen in vaccinated individuals. HBsAg and total anti-HBc in absence of IgM anti-HBc suggest chronic infection.

Treatment

Only supportive treatment is given in acute HBV infection, as there is no definitive therapy. Chronic infections can be benefited by therapy by reducing HBV replication and remission of liver disease.

Prevention

Hepatitis B Ig (HBIg) along with hepatitis B vaccination are used for postexposure prophylaxis. Dose of HBIg is 0.06 mL/kg. Hepatitis B vaccination dose schedule depends on the vaccine. If the dose of vaccine is missed after first or second dose, next dose needs to be given at the earliest. Vaccine is said to be effective for 20 years after completion of schedule.[24] Before vaccination, if a person is found to be anti-HBc positive, but HBsAg negative, no action is needed. But if HBsAg is present, further management as HBsAg positive patient is needed. Post-vaccination testing is not recommended except in cases of HIV infection and in drug abusers and those having high-risk sexual behavior, to check the need for re-vaccination.

Barrier contraceptive needs to be used to prevent further spread to the partner. Infected person should cover skin lesions to avoid further spread to the contacts. Further liver damage can be prevented by avoiding or reducing alcohol consumption and vaccination against Hepatitis A.

PARASITIC INFECTIONS

Pediculosis Pubis

Lice/nits on pubic hair can be noticed by patients, along with pruritus, and is sexually transmitted. Permethrin (1%) cream is locally applied, followed by washing after 10 minutes. Resistance has been increasing to this agent. Alternatively, ivermectin 250 μg/kg orally can be given, which needs to be repeated after 14 days. But, it does not have ovicidal property, thus, it requires repeat cycle. Permethrin cream must not be applied on eyes. When eyelashes are affected, ophthalmic preparations should be used for 10 days. Clothes and bedsheets should be decontaminated. Follow-up is recommended after 1 week if there is persistence of symptoms. Partners within 1 month are to be traced and treated. Sexual activity is to be avoided till both partners are cured. Permethrin is safe to be used during pregnancy and ivermectin is safe during lactation.

Scabies

Sarcoptes scabiei sensitization takes weeks after first infection, after which pruritus develops. It is sexually transmitted in adults. Permethrin (5%) cream is to be applied all over body starting from neck and to be washed off after around 8–12 hours. Alternatively, ivermectin (200 μg/kg) orally to be repeated after 2 weeks can be used. Its intake with food increases its bioavailability. Decontamination of clothes and bedsheets is recommended.

CHANCROID

It is an infection caused by *Haemophilus ducreyi*, and is a risk factor for transmission for HIV. Clinical features include painful genital ulcer and tender suppurative inguinal lymph nodes.[25] For the purpose of diagnosis, one or more painful ulcers, genital ulcers, and lymphadenopathy, along with absence of evidences of syphilis and herpes simplex virus (HSV) infection are considered as reliable criteria. Azithromycin 1 g orally single dose or ceftriaxone 250 mg intramuscularly single dose or ciprofloxacin 500 mg orally twice a day for 3 days is the recommended treatment. Patient needs to be followed up after 3rd and 7th day of starting of therapy for symptomatic improvement. Larger ulcers require longer time for healing. Lymphadenopathy may need incision and drainage procedure even after successful correction of ulcer. Partner needs treatment if there is exposure within 10 days of onset of symptoms.

HSV INFECTION

Genital herpes is usually of HSV type 2 origin. But, in male-to-male sexual transmission, HSV type 1 involvement is also seen.[26] Majority of patients are asymptomatic, thus, are unaware of the transmission to their partners. Typical lesions would be of painful multiple vesicular or ulcerative variety, but may be absent in many cases. HSV-2 is associated with more recurrence than HSV-1 infection.[27] Type-specific investigations are needed to explain prognosis of HSV infection.

A PCR for HSV DNA is more sensitive than cell culture, latter being less sensitive. Tzanck preparation, which is cytologic detection of changes in cells, is not a reliable method. Type-specific antibodies are useful, which diagnose glycoprotein. IgM testing for HSV 1 or 2 is of no use, as it is nonspecific and might be present in recurrent infection. HSV serologic testing is needed in high-risk sexual behavior people, those having HIV, and as a part of evaluation for STD.

Acyclovir, valacyclovir, and famciclovir are drugs of choice, the latter two are having higher bioavailability after oral administration. Acyclovir 400 mg orally three times a day for 7–10 days, or valacyclovir 1 g orally twice a day for 7–10 days or famciclovir 250 mg orally three times a day for 7–10 days can be given in first episode of HSV. Recurrent episodes are mainly seen with HSV-2 infection, in which case, therapy given as suppressive for reducing frequency of episodes, or can be given episodically for reducing duration of episodes. Acyclovir can be given daily for up to 6 years as a suppressive therapy, being superior to episodic therapy with regards to quality of life. Intravenous acyclovir is indicated for severe HSV infection, 5–10 mg/kg every 8 hours for 2–7 days, followed by oral therapy to complete 10 days of therapy.

Pregnancy: Asymptomatic infection is common during pregnancy, resulting in unexpected neonatal herpes later on.[28] Transmission rate is high when active infection occurs near delivery time. Cesarean section has not been associated with complete eradication of chances of perinatal transmission, but it is indicated in cases where there is recurrent genital herpes infection. Acyclovir is safe during pregnancy.

DONOVANOSIS

It is also known as granuloma inguinale, and is caused by *Klebsiella granulomatis,* a gram-negative bacteria. Ulcers are painless, slowly progressive, located on genital and perineal area, with absence of lymphadenopathy. Vascularity is very high and can also bleed. Extension of infection can occur to abdominal and pelvic organs. Biopsy or tissue preparations may reveal dark staining Donovan bodies as diagnostic criteria. Azithromycin given 1 g once a week for 3 weeks, and continued till all lesions are healed. Healing starts from the margin and proceeds to inward. Alternatively, doxycycline 100 mg twice a day or ciprofloxacin 750 mg twice a day can be given for similar duration as mentioned above. Partners with contact within 60 days before onset of symptoms are to be examined, and to be treated if found to be symptomatic. Pregnant women can be treated with azithromycin or erythromycin.

LYMPHOGRANULOMA VENEREUM

Chlamydia trachomatis types L1, L2, or L3 cause lymphogranuloma venereum (LGV). Clinical features include unilateral inguinal and/or femoral lymphadenopathy, with self-limiting genital ulcer or papule. Proctocolitis may result in case of rectal exposure. Diagnosis can be made by culture, immunofluorescence or nucleic acid detection. Doxycycline 100 mg twice a day for 21 days cures the disease, but tissue scarring can be there. Buboes may require incision and drainage. Alternatively, erythromycin 500 mg four times a day for 21 days can be given. Persons with contact history with patient within 60 days before onset of symptoms should be examined and investigated. Erythromycin is drug of choice in pregnant women with LGV.

SYPHILIS

Treponema pallidum is the organism responsible for causing syphilis. The disease is divided in various stages—primary syphilis (ulcers/chancre), secondary syphilis (skin rashes, lymphadenopathy), tertiary syphilis (cardiac, gummatous lesions, paresis), early latent infection (syphilis without clinical manifestation within preceding year), and late latent syphilis (latent syphilis beyond the early latent phase). Central nervous system (CNS) involvement can occur at any stage of disease. Early neurological involvement in form of stroke, ophthalmic or auditory problems, meningitis, and altered mental status can occur within few months or years of infection. Late neurological sequelae (Tabes dorsalis) usually occur 10–30 years after infection.

Syphilis in early phase can be diagnosed by dark field examination and various tests. There are two types of tests available—nontreponemal tests [venereal disease research laboratory (VDRL) and rapid plasma reagin (RPR)] and treponemal tests [Treponema pallidum passive particle agglutination (TPPA)] assay, enzyme immune assay, rapid treponemal assay)]. Only one serological test may result in false negative and false positive results. Offering only nontreponemal test might lead to false positive in cases of patients having HIV, autoimmune diseases, pregnancy, and elderly age group.[29] Thus, making it mandatory to have treponemal test, when there is positive nontreponemal test result.

Treatment

Penicillin G is the treatment of choice.

Primary and secondary syphilis: Benzathine penicillin G 2.4 million units in single dose. Follow-up is to be done at 6 and 12 months.

Latent syphilis: Sexual transmission during this stage does not occur, but treatment is to be given to prevent complications and to reduce transmission to fetus from pregnant mother in latent phase. Benzathine penicillin G 2.4 million units intramuscularly in a single dose. Serological tests need to be repeated at 6, 12, and 24 months.

Tertiary syphilis: Benzathine penicillin G 2.4 million units intramuscularly at 1 week interval for three doses.

Neurosyphilis: Neurological involvement can occur at any stage of disease. Cerebrospinal fluid (CSF) examination is needed for confirmation of diagnosis in case of ocular and neurological involvement. Aqueous crystalline penicillin G 3 million units i.v. 4 hourly for 10–14 days. Follow-up CSF examinations are needed 6 monthly till cell count comes normal.

Pregnancy: Penicillin G is the only drug that can be given during pregnancy, and in cases of allergy to penicillin, desensitization needs to be done, followed by penicillin therapy.

Partners within 90 days preceding onset of symptoms need to be treated for early syphilis, even if serological findings are negative.

CHLAMYDIASIS

Asymptomatic infection is common with *Chlamydia trachomatis* infection. It has severe consequences in form of PID and its complications. Samples in form of first catch urine or vaginal/endocervical swab can be assessed. NAATs are most sensitive tests. Treatment is aimed to prevent complications and sexual transmission, and delays in treatment may lead to complications, such as PID. Pregnant women are to be treated to prevent transmission to neonate during birth. Azithromycin 1 g orally in single dose is the drug of choice. Alternatively, doxycycline 100 mg twice a day for 7 days, or erythromycin 500 mg four times a day for 7 days can be given. Sexual partners within 60 days preceding onset of symptoms are to be examined, evaluated, and treated if found to be affected. Pregnant women can be treated with azithromycin, and follow-up with NAAT is to be done after 3–4 weeks to check eradication of chlamydia to prevent maternal and neonatal complications.[30]

GONORRHEA

Neisseria gonorrhoeae infection is usually asymptomatic, but can lead to symptoms once complications of PID occur. Culture from endocervical swab and NAAT from vaginal/endocervical swab and urine can confirm diagnosis. Gram staining will reveal polymorphonuclear leukocytes with intracellular gram-negative diplococci. Ceftriaxone 250 mg intramuscularly in single dose with azithromycin 1 g orally in single dose on same day is the preferred regimen. Alternatively, injectable ceftriaxone can be replaced by cefixime tablet 400 mg orally in single dose. Sexual contacts within 60 days preceding onset of symptoms are to be traced, examined, and given presumptive therapy.

HIV

Human immunodeficiency virus (HIV) infection gradually attacks immune system, leading to reduction in CD4 T lymphocytes, and slowly progressing to AIDS, with median time of around 11 years.[31] ART helps HIV-infected patients to live a near normal life. Early diagnosis of HIV helps, as transmission of HIV in acute phase is more, due to higher concentration of virus in blood and genital tract.[32] Patients presenting with STD should be screened for HIV, as in acute phase, HIV-associated symptoms may not be present, but presence of STD may be one of the initial symptoms.

Acute HIV symptoms can present with nonspecific symptoms in initial few weeks, in form of rashes on skin, fever, malaise, and lymphadenopathy.

Informed consent must be taken before voluntary testing for HIV. Proper pre-test and post-test counselling are of immense importance and must be done, with regards to testing, results, and future implications of the results. Rapid antibody test usually gives result within 30 minutes, but may be negative in early phase of the disease. A combination of Ag-Ab immunoassay can be performed, which, if found reactive, can be subjected to differentiation immunoassay for HIV-1 and HIV-2 (**Fig. 3**).

Antiretroviral therapy in acute phase helps in reducing severity of disease, reduces viral replication, and helps in preserving immune function.[33] Positive report comes with a lot of challenges for the patient, requiring counseling, and support for psychological, behavioral, corrective, and medical aspects of the disease. Partners should be tracked down and should be offered counseling and voluntary testing option. Screening for STD needs to be performed in HIV-positive patients.

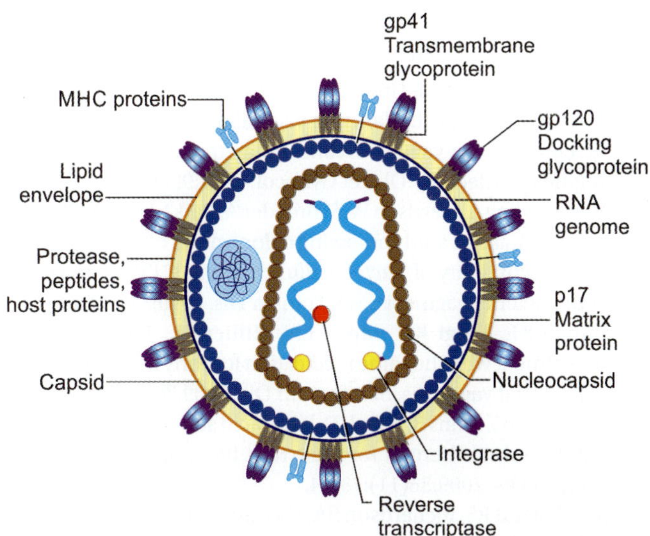

Fig. 3: Human immunodeficiency virus (HIV).

Pregnancy: Antenatal patients should be screened for HIV at their first antenatal visit. Perinatal transmission can significantly be reduced by starting ART and obstetric intervention.

REFERENCES

1. National AIDS Control Organization. Annual report 2016-17. [Online] Available from: http://www.naco.gov.in/sites/default/files/NACO%20ANNUAL%20REPORT%202016-17.pdf [Last accessed November, 2021].
2. Laxmi U, Agrawal S, Raghunandan C, Randhawa VS, Saili A. Association of bacterial vaginosis with adverse fetomaternal outcome in women with spontaneous preterm labor: a prospective cohort study. J Matern Fetal Neonatal Med. 2012;25(1):64-7.
3. Cherpes TL, Wiesenfeld HC, Melan MA, Kant JA, Cosentino LA, Meyn LA, et al. The associations between pelvic inflammatory disease, *Trichomonas vaginalis* infection, and positive herpes simplex virus type 2 serology. Sex Transm Dis. 2006;33(12):747-52.
4. Cohen CR, Lingappa JR, Baeten JM, Ngayo MO, Spiegel CA, Hong T, et al. Bacterial vaginosis associated with increased risk of female-to-male HIV-1 transmission: a prospective cohort analysis among African couples. PLoS Med. 2012;9(6):e1001251.
5. Mehta SD. Systematic review of randomized trials of treatment of male sexual partners for improved bacteria vaginosis outcomes in women. Sex Transm Dis. 2012;39(10):822-30.
6. Amsel R, Totten PA, Spiegel CA, Chen KC, Eschenbach D, Holmes KK. Nonspecific vaginitis. Diagnostic criteria and microbial and epidemiologic associations. Am J Med. 1983;74(1):14-22.
7. Schwebke JR, Hillier SL, Sobel JD, McGregor JA, Sweet RL. Validity of the vaginal gram stain for the diagnosis of bacterial vaginosis. Obstet Gynecol. 1996;88(4 Pt 1):573-6.
8. Livengood CH, 3rd, Ferris DG, Wiesenfeld HC, Hillier SL, Soper DE, Nyirjesy P, et al. Effectiveness of two tinidazole regimens in

treatment of bacterial vaginosis: a randomized controlled trial. Obstet Gynecol. 2007;110(2 Pt 1):302-9.
9. Sobel J, Peipert JF, McGregor JA, Livengood C, Martin M, Robbins J, et al. Efficacy of clindamycin vaginal ovule (3-day treatment) vs. clindamycin vaginal cream (7-day treatment) in bacterial vaginosis. Infect Dis Obstet Gynecol. 2001;9(1):9-15.
10. Hemmerling A, Harrison W, Schroeder A, Park J, Korn A, Shiboski S, et al. Phase 2a study assessing colonization efficiency, safety, and acceptability of *Lactobacillus crispatus* CTV-05 in women with bacterial vaginosis. Sex Transm Dis. 2010;37(12):745-50.
11. Bunge KE, Beigi RH, Meyn LA, Hillier SL. The efficacy of retreatment with the same medication for early treatment failure of bacterial vaginosis. Sex Transm Dis. 2009;36(11):711-3.
12. Reichman O, Akins R, Sobel JD. Boric acid addition to suppressive antimicrobial therapy for recurrent bacterial vaginosis. Sex Transm Dis. 2009;36(11):732-4.
13. McClelland RS, Richardson BA, Hassan WM, Chohan V, Lavreys L, Mandaliya K, et al. Improvement of vaginal health for Kenyan women at risk for acquisition of human immunodeficiency virus type 1: results of a randomized trial. J Infect Dis. 2008;197(10):1361-8.
14. Yudin MH, Landers DV, Meyn L, Hillier SL. Clinical and cervical cytokine response to treatment with oral or vaginal metronidazole for bacterial vaginosis during pregnancy: a randomized trial. Obstet Gynecol. 2003;102(3):527-34.
15. Briggs GC, Freeman RK, Yaffe SJ. Drugs in Pregnancy and Lactation, 9th edition. Philadelphia, PA: Lippincott Williams & Wilkins; 2011.
16. Gray RH, Kigozi G, Serwadda D, Makumbi F, Nalugoda F, Watya S, et al. The effects of male circumcision on female partners' genital tract symptoms and vaginal infections in a randomized trial in Rakai, Uganda. Am J Obstet Gynecol. 2009;200(1):e41-7.
17. Moodley P, Wilkinson D, Connolly C, Moodley J, Sturm AW. *Trichomonas vaginalis* is associated with pelvic inflammatory disease in women infected with human immunodeficiency virus. Clin Infect Dis. 2002;34(4):519-22.
18. Nye MB, Schwebke JR, Body BA. Comparison of APTIMA *Trichomonas vaginalis* transcription-mediated amplification to wet mount microscopy, culture, and polymerase chain reaction for diagnosis of trichomoniasis in men and women. Am J Obstet Gynecol. 2009;200(2):e181-7.
19. Trintis J, Epie N, Boss R, Riedel S. Neonatal *Trichomonas vaginalis* infection: a case report and review of literature. Int J STD AIDS. 2010;21(8):606-7.
20. Cu-Uvin S, Ko H, Jamieson DJ, Hogan JW, Schuman P, Anderson J, et al. Prevalence, incidence, and persistence or recurrence of trichomoniasis among human immunodeficiency virus (HIV)-positive women and among HIV-negative women at high risk for HIV infection. Clin Infect Dis. 2002;34(10):1406-11.
21. Markowitz LE, Dunne EF, Saraiya M, Chesson HW, Curtis CR, Gee J, et al. Human papillomavirus vaccination: recommendations of the Advisory Committee on Immunization Practices (ACIP). MMWR Recomm Rep. 2014;63(RR-05):1-30.
22. Silverberg MJ, Thorsen P, Lindeberg H, Grant LA, Shah KV. Condyloma in pregnancy is strongly predictive of juvenile-onset recurrent respiratory papillomatosis. Obstet Gynecol. 2003;101(4):645-52.
23. Hyams KC. Risks of chronicity following acute hepatitis B virus infection: a review. Clin Infect Dis. 1995;20(4):992-1000.
24. Poovorawan Y, Chongsrisawat V, Theamboonlers A, Leroux-Roels G, Crasta PD, Hardt K. Persistence and immune memory to hepatitis B vaccine 20 years after primary vaccination of Thai infants, born to HBsAg and HBeAg positive mothers. Hum Vaccin Immunother. 2012;8(7):896-904.
25. Lewis DA. Chancroid: clinical manifestations, diagnosis, and management. Sex Transm Infect. 2003;79(1):68-71.
26. Ryder N, Jin F, McNulty AM, Grulich AE, Donovan B. Increasing role of herpes simplex virus type 1 in first-episode anogenital herpes in heterosexual women and younger men who have sex with men, 1992-2006. Sex Transm Infect. 2009;85(6):416-9.
27. Engelberg R, Carrell D, Krantz E, Corey L, Wald A. Natural history of genital herpes simplex virus type 1 infection. Sex Transm Dis. 2003;30(2(:174-7.
28. Pinninti SG, Kimberlin DW. Maternal and neonatal herpes simplex virus infections. Am J Perinatol. 2013;30(2):113-9.
29. Nandwani R, Evans DT. Are you sure it's syphilis? A review of false positive serology. Int J STD AIDS. 1995;6(4):241-8.
30. Jacobson GF, Autry AM, Kirby RS, Liverman EM, Motley RU. A randomized controlled trial comparing amoxicillin and azithromycin for the treatment of *Chlamydia trachomatis* in pregnancy. Am J Obstet Gynecol. 2001;184(7):1352-4.
31. Smit C, Geskus R, Walker S, Sabin C, Coutinho R, Porter K, et al. Effective therapy has altered the spectrum of cause-specific mortality following HIV seroconversion. AIDS. 2006;20(5):741-9.
32. Pilcher CD, Tien HC, Eron JJ Jr, Vernazza PL, Leu SY, Stewart PW, et al. Brief but efficient: acute HIV infection and the sexual transmission of HIV. J Infect Dis. 2004;189(10):1785-92.
33. DHHS Panel on Antiretroviral Guidelines for Adults and Adolescents. (2013). Guidelines for the use of antiretroviral agents in HIV-1-infected adults and adolescents.

LONG QUESTIONS

1. HPV vaccination.
2. Differential diagnosis of genital ulcers.

SHORT QUESTIONS

1. Differential diagnosis of abnormal vaginal discharge.
2. Describe in brief treatment of scabies.

MULTIPLE CHOICE QUESTIONS

1. All of the following are part of Amsel criteria for bacterial vaginosis, except:
   a. Positive whiff test (fishy odor of vaginal discharge on addition of 10% KOH)
   b. Clue cells (vaginal epithelial cells with adherent organisms, visualized on microscope)
   c. Homogenous white discharge, coating vaginal wall
   d. Vaginal pH <4.5
2. Duration of therapy for recurrent VVC (vulvovaginal candidiasis) is:
   a. 7–14 days   b. 2 weeks
   c. 3 months   d. 6 months
3. Trichomonas vaginalis causes all of the following, except:
   a. Increased risk of PID
   b. Increased vertical transmission in pregnancy
   c. Preterm birth
   d. Intrauterine fetal death

4. Cesarean section is indicated in case of anogenital warts during pregnancy:
   a. True
   b. False
5. Following diseases can be completely prevented by use of condom, except:
   a. HIV
   b. Hepatitis B
   c. HPV
   d. Candidiasis
6. Presence of Anti-HBs antibody suggests following:
   a. Vaccinated status b. Chronic infection
   c. Acute infection d. Incubation period
7. HSV type 1 can cause genital infection:
   a. True b. False
8. Which of the following drugs used for pediculosis pubis is teratogenic?
   a. Lindane b. Permethrin
   c. Ivermectin d. Malathion
9. Unilateral inguinal lymphadenopathy with self-limiting ulcer is seen in:
   a. Primary syphilis b. Chancroid
   c. LGV d. Donovanosis
10. In case of neurosyphilis, follow-up CSF examination is to be done:
    a. 3 monthly b. 6 monthly
    c. 9 monthly d. Yearly

Answers

1.	d	2.	d	3.	d	4.	b	5.	c	6.	a
7.	a	8.	a	9.	c	10.	b				

10.3 PELVIC INFLAMMATORY DISEASE

Kusum Lata Singhal, Uma Jain

DEFINITION

Pelvic inflammatory disease (PID) is the infection of the upper part of the female reproductive system, involving one or more of the following organs—the uterus, fallopian tubes, ovaries, and inside of the pelvis.[1]

INTRODUCTION

Pelvic infection is the most common infection in the women of reproductive age group. 24–32% of women around the world are affected. It can be as mild as to go unnoticed or become a serious problem causing many complications.

EPIDEMIOLOGY

Approximately 1.5% of young women are affected with PID every year; teenagers and first-time mothers are most vulnerable. PID is the major cause of infertility affecting over 100,000 in the US each year. About 1% of young adults between 15 and 25 years of age are affected. In India and other developing countries, the incidence of PID is much higher. Multiple reasons of sexually transmitted diseases (STDs), illegal abortions, puerperal sepsis, and low awareness about contraceptive usage increase the risk of PID. Studies have reported prevalence ranging from 5.2 to 17.2% PID in various parts of the country.

Epidemiology of PID: What has Changed?

- Most of the patients do not require admission.
- With increasing awareness, patients present with less severity.
- *Chlamydia trachomatis* has become more common over the years while decreasing infections with gonococcus and others.

ETIOLOGY AND CAUSATIVE ORGANISMS

Neisseria gonorrhoeae and *Chlamydia trachomatis* infections are found in 75–90% of cases. *Mycoplasma genitalium* and *Mycoplasma hominis* are also found in few cases of PID. In some women, normal vaginal flora such as *Gardnerella vaginalis*, anaerobes, and other organisms ascend into the upper reproductive organs. In India, genital tuberculosis is also frequently responsible for PID. Many times, multiple different bacteria are involved, including certain anaerobic and aerobic bacteria, such as *Escherichia coli* and *Haemophilus influenzae*. Rarely, *Trichomonas vaginalis*, human immunodeficiency virus (HIV), cytomegalovirus (CMV), actinomycosis [usually associated with intrauterine contraceptive device (IUCD)] are responsible. If not treated, about 10% of cases with chlamydial infection and 40% of women with gonorrhea infection will develop PID. In the majority of cases, the infection is sexually transmitted.

RISK FACTORS

The ascending infections are most likely to occur in the following circumstances:

- Poor menstrual hygiene
- Following breach of the mucosa during childbirth or miscarriage
- After an invasive procedure, like surgical instrumentation through the cervix, insertion of an IUCD, hysterosalpingography, hysteroscopy, IUI including termination of pregnancy
- Bacterial vaginosis
- Young age is more prone to PID
- Vaginal douching also alters vaginal flora

- Forgotten tampons
- Young females engaged in sexual activity without methods of protection
- Multiple sexual partners and drug abuse
- Presence of sexually transmitted infections in sexual partner
- Living in an area of high prevalence of PID
- Previous history of STD or PID
- PID is not common but still has been seen in virgin females
- Infection following a burst appendix or bowel infection sometimes spreads toward the pelvis causing PID
- Lower socioeconomic status, alcohol intake, substance abuse, smoking, anemia, diabetes mellitus, and malnutrition are few other predisposing factors
- The classic high-risk patient is one who has attained menarche, <25 years of age, indulges in sex with multiple partners, not uses contraception, and belongs to a region of high endemicity for STD.

PROTECTIVE FACTORS

- *Natural defense of genital tract:*
  - *Vulva:* Labia majora, minora, Bartholin glands, high resistance of vulval and perineal skin for infections provides good defense against infection
  - *Vagina:* Well opposed, anterior and posterior walls with its transverse rugae; stratified epithelium, which is devoid of glands, maternal estrogen in the early postpartum period provide good protection against infections
  - *Cervix:* Racemose type of glands; mucus plug with its bactericidal action
  - *Uterine defense:* Regular endometrial shedding and tubal ostium closure in response to endometrial inflammation
  - Tubal epithelial cilia causing the peristalsis of the tube toward the uterine cavity
- *Contraceptive practice:*
  - Barrier methods, such as condoms and diaphragm
  - Contraceptive pills provide protection by:
    - Producing thick mucus plug preventing bacterial penetration
    - Decreasing duration of menstruation
- Having sex with a single partner that too vasectomized
- Other factors include pregnancy, tubal sterilization, menopause, and vaccines—hepatitis B and human papillomavirus (HPV).

PATHOGENESIS: ACUTE PID

Infection may reach the pelvis by one of the following routes:

- Ascending—most common **(Flowchart 1)**[2]; continuity of pathway from the vagina to the pelvic cavity through tubal infundibulum provides a pathway for pathogens to ascend to the pelvic cavity. Disturbed bacterial vaginal flora along with bacterial vaginosis also favors PID.
- Hematogenous spread, as seen in tuberculosis.
- Dissemination through parametrial lymphatics or venous spread—e.g., endometritis after abortion or labor.
- Local spread from bowel or appendix, peritoneum, etc.

Initially, the patient acquires an infection of either vagina or cervix often through sexual contact. The protective action of cervical mucus is disturbed under certain circumstances and when the efficacy of this barrier decreases and microorganisms find their way upward. These conditions can be:

- Vaginal inflammation
- Opening of the cervix during menstruation
- Hormonal changes that occur during ovulation
- Antibiotic treatment disrupts the vaginal flora causing normally nonpathogenic organisms to overgrow and ascend
- Intercourse may contribute through rhythmic uterine contractions occurring during orgasm
- Cervical dilatation for performing any uterine procedure, post-abortion or post-childbirth conditions may all facilitate microorganisms to ascend upward favoring the occurrence of PID.

This ascending infection initially involves endometrium and tubal mucosa but rapidly involves other layers too **(Fig. 1)**. The ascent of infection with *Gonococcus* and *Chlamydia* is

Flowchart 1: Pelvic inflammatory disease based on source and type of infection.[3]

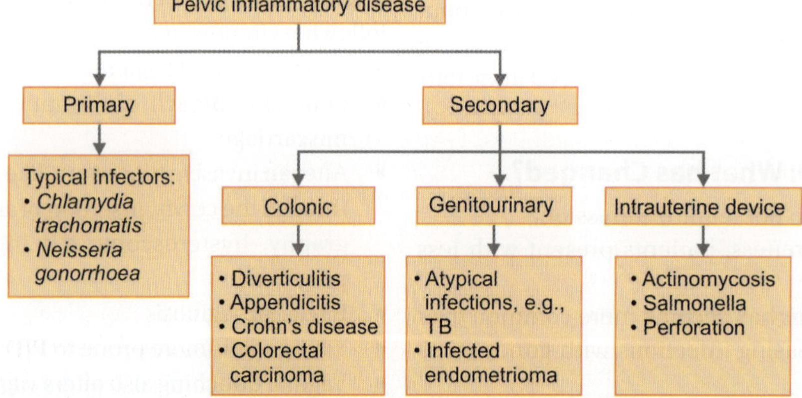

facilitated many times along with motile sperms. Therefore the gonococcal inflammatory disease is rarely seen in women whose husband is azoospermic. The ovaries are so closely placed with tubes that generally they are involved in all infections of tubes, except the involvement of ovaries in mumps without the involvement of tubes. Microbial virulence is also important in the causation of PID. Protein production by certain bacteria poses increased susceptibility. Variants in the genes that regulate toll-like receptors (TLRs) have been associated with an increased progression of infection to PID. For example, chlamydial heat shock protein 60 (CHSP60), P9Opa(b) protein by gonorrhea

- Tubes are generally bilaterally affected usually because of a lack of genital defense.
- Endosalpinx is generally the first organ where pathology begins showing salpingitis.
- The epithelial cells, microvilli, and cilia are grossly destroyed and become edematous and hyperemic if the infection is severe.[4]
- Exfoliated cells and the exudates are poured into the lumen of the tube and cause agglutination of mucosal folds. The abdominal ostium is closed by the indrawing of the edematous fimbriae and by inflammatory adhesions. The uterine end is closed by congestion. The closure of both the ostia results in the pent up of the exudates inside the tube.
- The severity of disease and virulence of organisms decides the consistency of exudates, which may be watery leading to hydrosalpinx or purulent leading to pyosalpinx.
- Penetration of exudate deeper into the tissues then causes more tissue destruction.

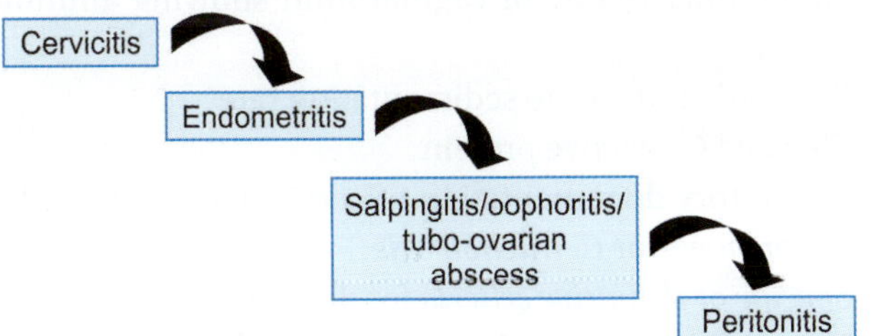

Fig. 1: Pathophysiology of ascendant infection.[2]

- Because of exudates, tubes get adherent to the surrounding structures.
- Sometimes the exudates find their way through the abdominal ostium to produce pelvic peritonitis and pelvic abscess or ovarian abscess.
- Parametrial structures including the bowel are sometimes involved with the spread of infection. Infection may extend via spillage of purulent materials from the fallopian tubes or via lymphatic spread beyond the pelvis to produce acute peritonitis and acute perihepatitis (Fitz-Hugh–Curtis syndrome).
- Post-abortal and puerperal infections generally spread from the cervix via lymphatics to the cellular tissue in the broad ligament causing cellulitis. The tube is therefore affected from outside with mucosal involvement in the end. The wall of the tube is thickened considerably with hardly any distension of lumen. Multiple intraluminal adhesions eventually block the tubes.

TYPES OF PID BASED ON SOURCE AND TYPE OF INFECTION

Pelvic inflammatory disease can be primary or secondary **(Table 1)**.[3]

CLINICAL FEATURES AND DIAGNOSTIC CRITERIA[5]

All women presenting with lower abdominal pain should be considered for other signs and symptoms of PID **(Flowchart 2)**.[6]

Symptoms

Patients may not have any symptoms or may present with:

- Lower abdominal pain, typically bilateral, sometimes unilateral
- Lower back pain
- Abnormal vaginal discharge often foul-smelling and purulent
- Fever
- Burning and discomfort during urination

TABLE 1: Forms of pelvic inflammatory disease (PID).

Subclinical PID	There is a growing body of evidence that most cases of PID are subclinical and recognized by neither the patient nor her physician. Most experts believe that subclinical PID is an often overlooked cause of infertility and is responsible for more cases of postinfectious tubal infertility than acute PID. It has long been realized that many women with tubal factor infertility have serological evidence of prior chlamydial or gonococcal infection yet do not have a history of acute PID
Atypical PID	Patients with PID may have minimal pain and atypical symptoms and remain undiagnosed, or they may be misdiagnosed as having gastrointestinal or noninfectious gynecologic illnesses
Acute PID	Acute PID means an active infection is present and causing severe symptoms
Chronic PID	Following the acute stage, the infection may completely resolve or may become chronic leaving behind few residual endosalpingeal adhesions leading to tubal occlusion, or peri-adnexal and uterine adhesions with fixed retrodisplacement of the uterus and dense bilateral tubo-ovarian masses and rarely frozen pelvis
Disseminated PID	Infection and inflammation may spread to the abdomen producing pelvic and later generalized peritonitis, including perihepatic structures (Fitz-Hugh–Curtis syndrome in 15–30% cases). Rarely, it may further lead to bacteremia, endocarditis, meningitis, and suppurative arthritis. Death from acute PID is very rare in modern gynecology, but was not that rare in the past

Flowchart 2: Practical approach to the diagnosis of pelvic inflammatory disease.[6]

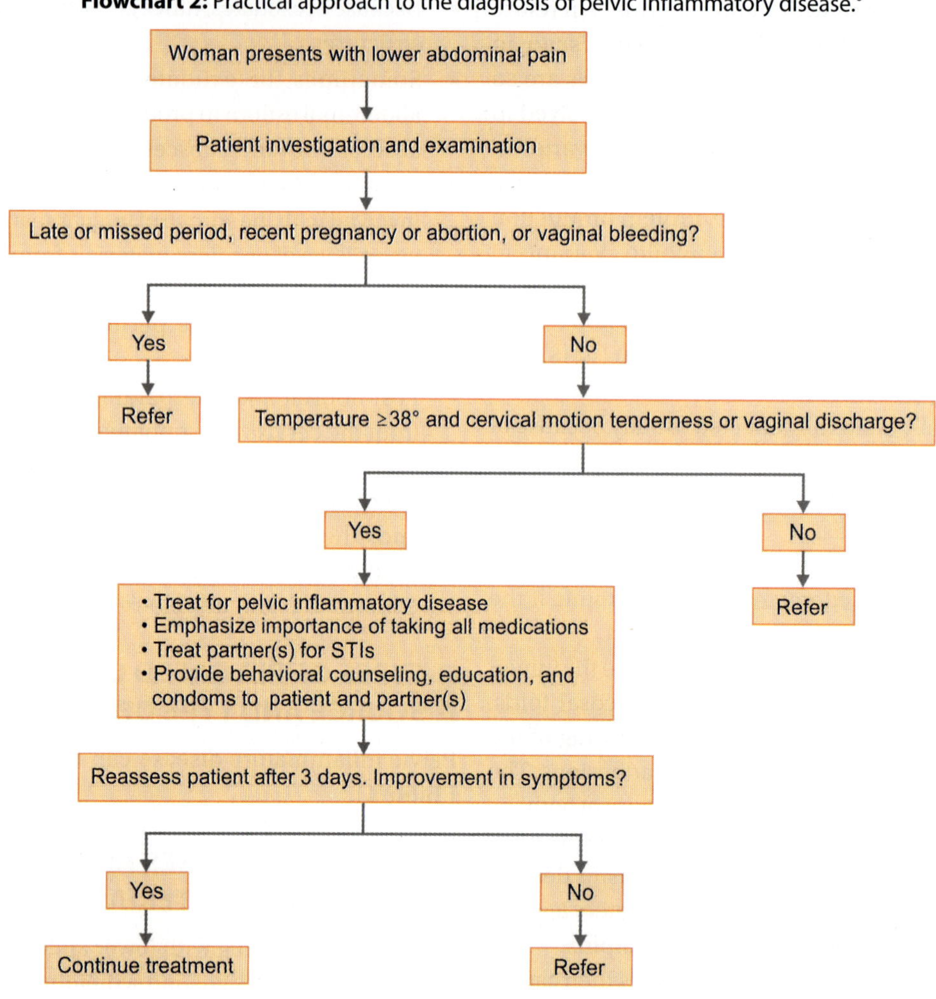

- Dyspareunia of recent onset
- Postcoital bleeding, intermenstrual bleeding, or irregular menstruation, heavy bleeding in menses
- Secondary dysmenorrhea
- Nausea, vomiting, and right upper quadrant pain in perihepatitis
- Diarrhea due to rectal irritation in pelvic abscess.

Physical Signs

CDC Minimum Criteria for Diagnosis of PID

- Lower abdominal tenderness
- Bimanual examination shows cervical motion tenderness
- Adnexal tenderness and/or fullness in fornices.

CDC Additional Criteria

All the above physical signs may not be present in all cases, therefore to increase the specificity of the diagnosis, one or more of the following additional criteria in addition to any one of the above physical signs can be used to reach a correct diagnosis.

- Fever >101°F
- Mucopurulent discharge from cervix, cervix becoming friable
- Saline microscopy of vaginal fluid showing abundant WBCs
- Elevated erythrocyte sedimentation rate
- Elevated C-reactive protein
- Laboratory documentation of cervical infection with *N. gonorrhoeae* or *C. trachomatis*

Specific or definitive criteria for diagnosing PID include:

- Histopathological evidence of endometritis on biopsy
- Imaging studies like ultrasonography (USG) or magnetic resonance imaging (MRI) showing fluid-filled tubes or TO masses
- Laparoscopic evidence of PID.

INVESTIGATIONS

- Swabs and cultures from samples from the cervix and vagina for identification of specific organism using Blood agar or McConkey agar at 37°C
- Giemsa-stained or iodine-stained cervical smears may be used to identify intracytoplasmic inclusions of *Chlamydia*
- Histopathologic evidence of endometritis in a biopsy specimen
- *Culdocentesis:* White cell count if >30,000/mL in a peritoneal fluid is pathognomonic of acute PID

- Transvaginal ultrasound (TVS) and MRI may show thickened, fluid-filled tubes, fluid in the pouch of Douglas (POD), and/or tubo-ovarian mass or Doppler studies suggesting tubal hyperemia
- Laparoscopy is not routinely recommended as a first-line investigation. But it can be advised if imaging is not conclusive, or symptomatic relief not obtained after treatment **(Figs. 2 to 4)**.

Laparoscopy in PID[7] may show edema and inflammation of the fallopian tubes, purulent exudate around tubes, peritubular adhesions, violin string adhesions characteristic of Fitz-Hugh-Curtis syndrome, and abscesses if present.

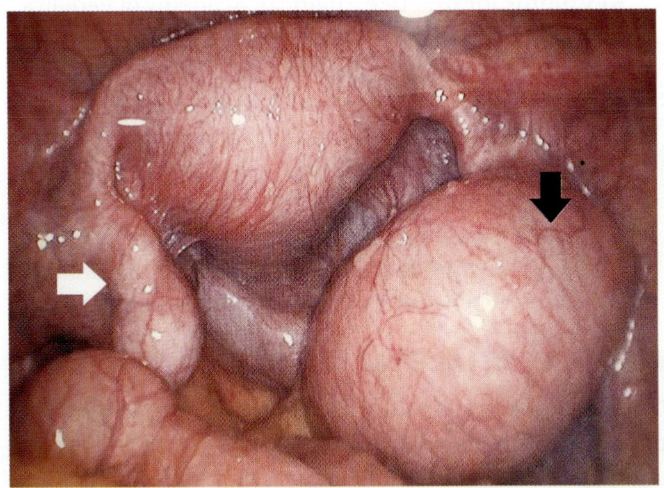

Fig. 2: Laparoscopy in Chronic PID with hydrosalpinx (white arrow) and pyosalpinx (black arrow).

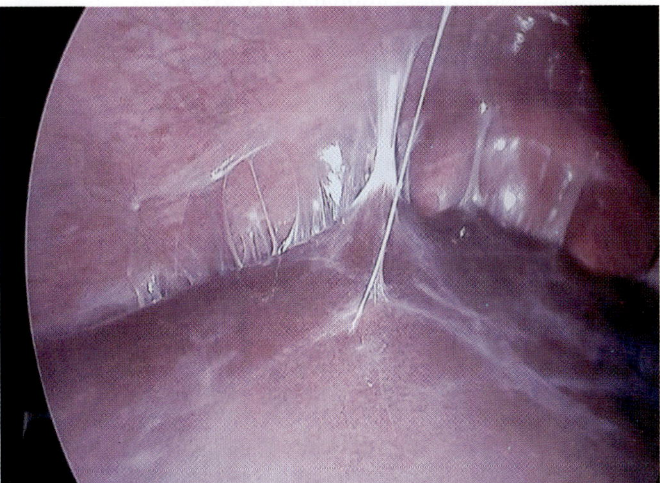

Fig. 3: Fitz Hugh Curtis Syndrome – perihepatic adhesions with pelvic inflammatory disease.

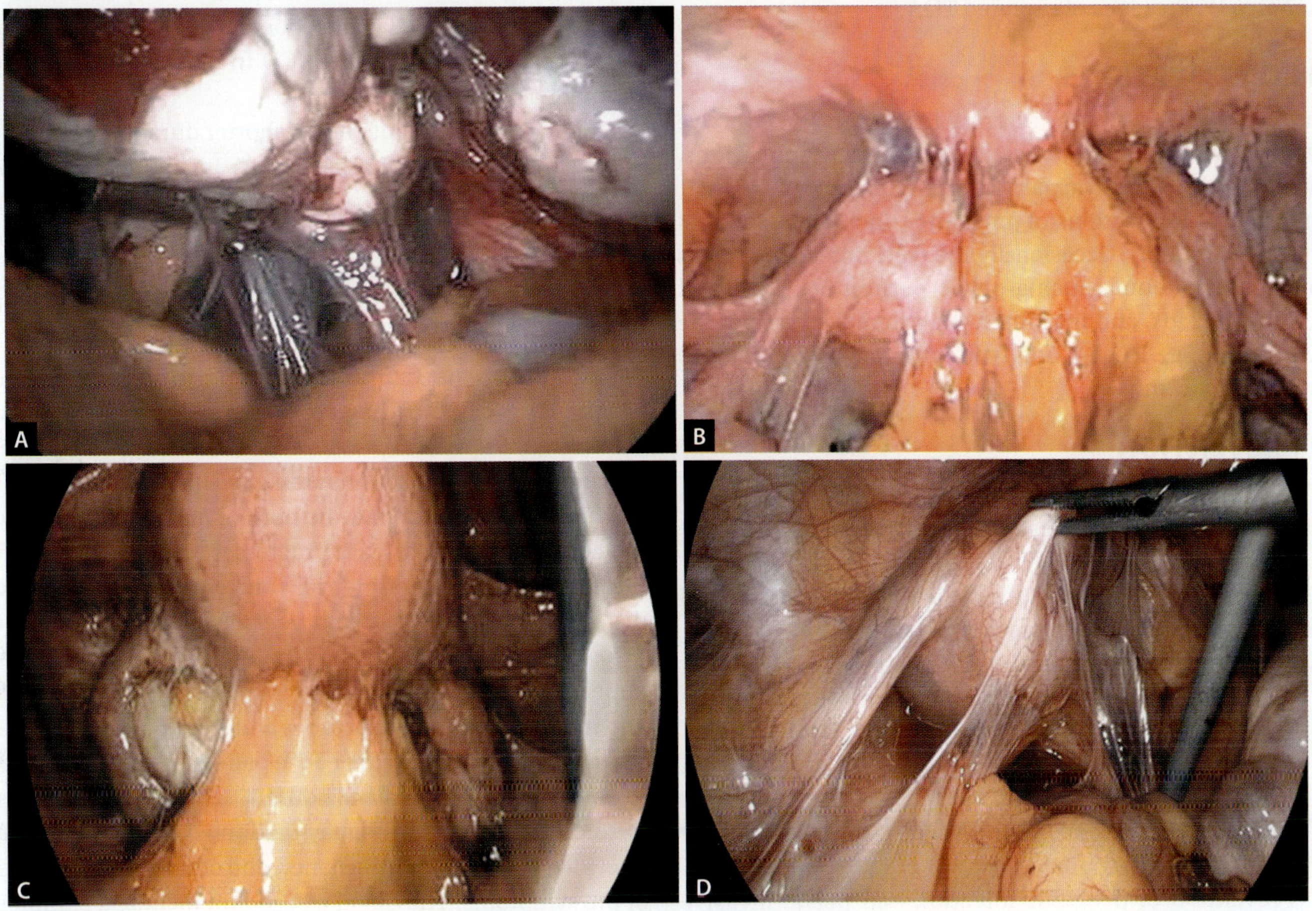

Figs. 4A to D: Tubo-ovarian and pelvic adhesions.

Laparoscopy is the confirmatory diagnostic tool for the diagnosis of PID. Drainage from tubo-ovarian abscess (TOA),[8] the culture of exudates may also be done at the same sitting. A tissue specimen may also be obtained for histopathological examination (HPE).

Specific Tests for Chlamydia and Gonorrhea

- Nucleic acid amplification tests (NAATs).
- Cell culture and DNA probes for chlamydial and gonococcal infections have a high specificity of 100%.
- Enzyme-linked immunosorbent assays (ELISAs) can identify actual pathogens present.
- Serology testing for antibodies IgG and IgM for *Chlamydia* can predict recent or long-standing infection, and is not of much use.
- Direct fluorescence tests (DFAs).

A practical approach to the diagnosis of pelvic inflammatory disease is shown in **Flowchart 3**.[9]

STAGING OF ACUTE PID

- *Stage I:* CDC major criteria along with at least one of the minor criteria, if present without overt peritonitis (which can be elicited by rebound tenderness), and absence of any prior documented STD or upper tract infections
- *Stage II:* All findings of Stage I, with peritonitis
- *Stage III:* Presence of tubo-ovarian complex or TOA
- *Stage IV:* Presence of ruptured TOA.

COMPLICATIONS

Untreated PID can cause scarring inside the reproductive system, which can later cause serious complications, including chronic pelvic pain, infertility, ectopic pregnancy, and other complications of pregnancy, including maternal and fetal morbidity. Occasionally, the pelvic infection spreads to the peritoneum causing pelvic peritonitis, TOA, and periappendicitis, and may reach the external surface of the liver causing Fitz-Hugh–Curtis syndrome. Other complications include septicemia.

PREVENTION

- Using barrier methods of contraception
- Early diagnosis and management of symptoms of PID
- Hormonal combined contraceptive pills are also protective
- If the sexual partner is suffering from STD, take medical advice and use strict protection
- Avoid intercourse, after the end of a pregnancy or after gynecological procedures, to ensure cervical closure
- Less number of sexual partners
- Monogamy
- Abstinence
- Treatment of sexual partners for suspected sexually transmitted infections.

Prevention of pyogenic infection—all pelvic invasive procedures including IUCD insertions, dilation and curettage (D&C), and labor should be carried out with strict aseptic precautions.

- Hygiene and sex counseling at schools and colleges
- Adolescent friendly clinics
- Screening and treating sexually active adolescents for chlamydial infection. Self-collected urine or vaginal swab samples may be subjected to nucleic acid amplification assays for the screening.
- **Key points for practice** American Academy of Pediatrics recommendations:[10]
    - Yearly screening of all women below 25 years every year for *C. trachomatis* and *N. gonorrhoeae* infection, with follow-up after 3 months after treatment if the screening test was positive.
    - Sex partners in the past 60 days of women with positive results should be screened for infection.
    - Sexually active males who have sex with males should also be screened every year for chlamydia and gonorrhea.

DIFFERENTIAL DIAGNOSIS

Other disorders often confused with PID include ectopic pregnancy, acute appendicitis, ovarian cyst, endometriosis and ruptured endometriotic cyst, septic abortion, irritable bowel syndrome, complications of ovarian cyst, such as rupture or torsion, urinary tract infection, peritonitis, cholecystitis-like symptoms in Fitz-Hugh–Curtis syndrome, bacterial vaginosis, and functional pain or idiopathic.

Prior history of pelvic infection, recent onset of menses, recent sexual contact or an IUCD in place or if the sexual partner has an STD suggest PID.

Right lower quadrant pain of shorter duration <21 hours, along with gastrointestinal symptoms, including nausea and vomiting, are suggestive of appendicitis; women with PID tend to have diffuse and prolonged pain of at least 48 hours duration, with fewer women having GIT symptoms.

A serum pregnancy test can be used to rule out ectopic pregnancy.

Culdocentesis can differentiate ruptured ectopic pregnancy or hemorrhagic cyst from pelvic sepsis-like salpingitis, ruptured pelvic abscess, or even ruptured appendix. Pelvic ultrasounds are a great help in the diagnosis of PID. The ultrasound may be normal in the early stages of infection, but as the disease progresses, certain nonspecific findings, such as endometrial thickening, uterine cavity distension by fluid or gas, and free pelvic fluid, may suggest the diagnosis. The borders of the uterus and ovaries may appear indistinct. Laparoscopy fails to detect endometritis and minor inflammation of tubes and should be done only if the diagnosis is not certain or if the patient has not responded to antibiotic therapy after 48 hours.

Blood and urine tests may be done to rule out urinary tract infections, ectopic pregnancy, and other potential causes of the symptoms. The blood test should include a complete blood count, sedimentation rate, and C-reactive protein.

Flowchart 3: Diagnosis of pelvic inflammatory disease.[9]

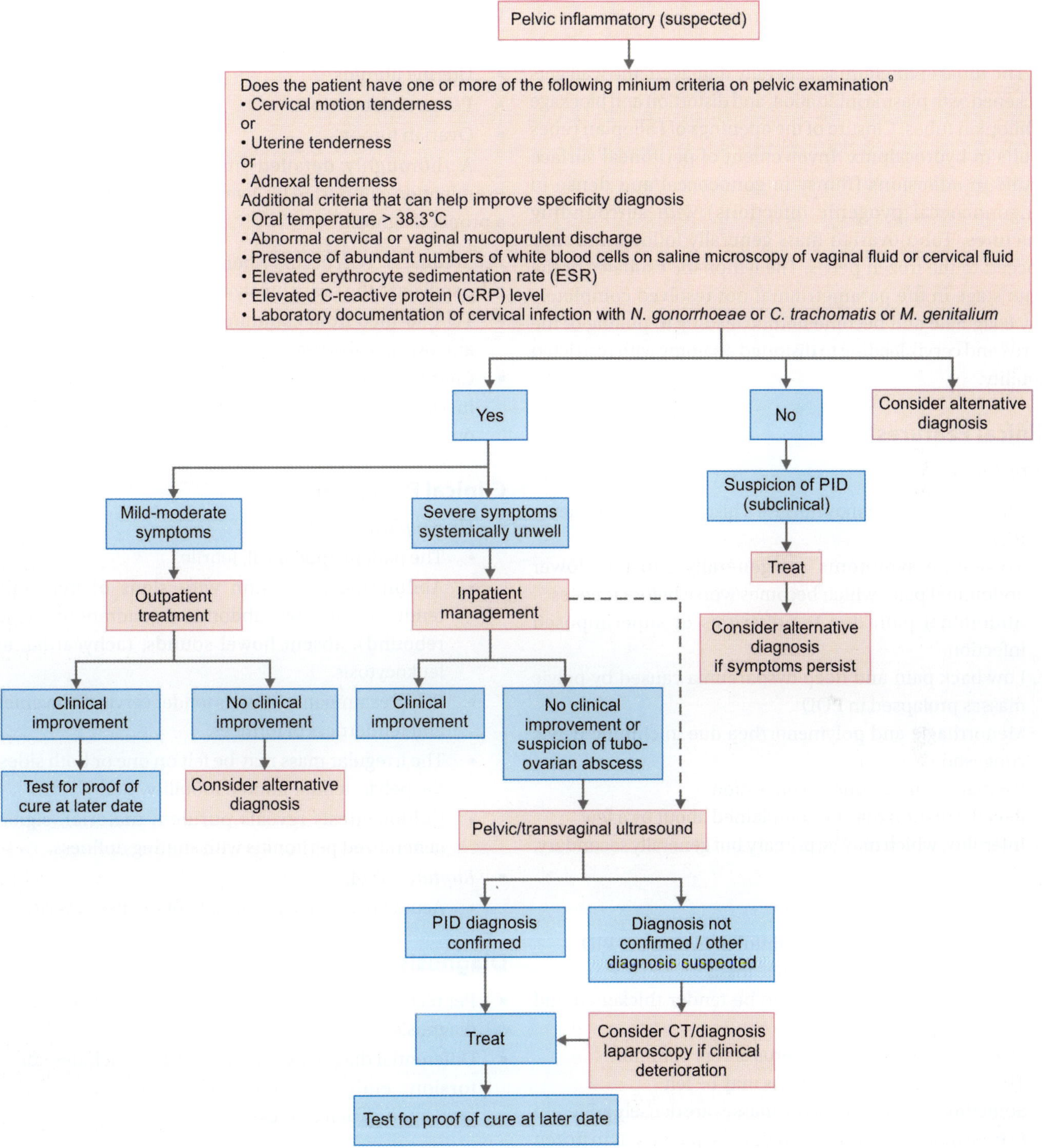

The complete blood count will normally show an elevated number of WBCs, which is an indication of infection, and the sedimentation rate and C-reactive protein elevation are suggestive of inflammation.

USG, laparoscopy, and MRI can all help in diagnosis. CT scan is less preferred.

Vaginal pH assessment: Bacterial vaginosis may be associated with PID frequently and needs to be looked for and managed. Assessment of vaginal pH with strips or pH assessment gloves give a clue to altered vaginal flora and PID. Whiff test, Nugent score, and Amsel's criteria can all help to diagnose and manage bacterial vaginosis.

CHRONIC PID

It may follow:

- Delayed or inadequate treatment of acute PID
- Low-grade recurrent infection
- Asymptomatic infection of the past which goes unnoticed.

Pathogenesis

The periodic shedding of endometrium generally spares the uterus.

The tubal epithelium is generally damaged, the wall gets thickened with plasma infiltration, and distortion and blockage of fallopian tubes. Closure of the openings of Fallopian tubes results in hydrosalpinx. Involvement of peritoneal surface results in adhesions (flimsy in gonococcal and dense in nongonococcal pyogenic infections) with surrounding structures. Tubo-ovarian mass generally follows and may proceed to the frozen pelvis. The lymphatic exudates of the acute stage in the parametrium if not resolved completely may coagulate and become fibrotic leading to pulling of the uterus and cervix leading to distorted anatomy with restricted mobility.

Clinical Features

Symptoms

- The patient may or may not give a history of previous acute PID
- Presenting symptoms are generally constant lower abdominal pain, which becomes worse before menses
- Abdominal pain due to adhesions or superimposed infection
- Low back pain and deep dyspareunia caused by pelvic masses prolapsed in POD
- Menorrhagia and polymenorrhea due to chronic pelvic congestion
- Vaginal discharge due to congestion
- Rectal irritation may be complained about by a few
- Infertility, which may be primary but generally secondary.

Signs

- Pelvic examination is less painful than in acute PID
- Tenderness in one or both iliac fossa
- The appendages are found to be tender thickened and fixed
- Fixed retroversion of the uterus is very common
- The irregular and tender mass may be felt
- Sometimes uterus and pelvic masses are densely adherent to each other and cannot be defined separately as in frozen pelvis
- The involvement of parametrium and uterosacral ligaments can be easily assessed by rectal examination.

Investigations

- Blood tests for evidence of leukocytosis, ESR, and urine examination including culture sensitivity
- Ultrasonography
- MRI
- Diagnostic laparoscopy may help in the diagnosis.

Differential Diagnosis

Conditions that mimic chronic PID include:

- Chronic ectopic
- Uterine fibroids
- Pelvic endometriosis
- Ovarian tumor.

A thoroughly detailed history followed by clinical examination, supported by investigations will help to lead to a proper diagnosis.

Pelvic abscess: TOA occurs when exudates from the fallopian tube spill onto the ovary involving the ovarian tissue

- TOA, formed from communication between pyosalpinx and ovarian abscess
- Central pelvic abscess: Pelvic peritonitis—pus collection in Douglas pouch—roofed by adherent intestine and omentum.

Clinical Presentation

- *Uncomplicated TOA:*
    - The patient appears ill, febrile.
    - Abdominal distension with signs of peritonitis, tenderness in lower abdominal quadrant (direct and rebound), absent bowel sounds, tachycardia, and leukocytosis.
    - Pelvic examination reveals tender cervical movements and tenderness of fornices.
    - The irregular mass may be felt on one or both sides of the pelvis, tender limited mobility.
    - Culdocentesis reveals purulent material, signs of generalized peritonitis with shifting dullness.
- *Ruptured TOA:*
    - Acute progressive pelvic pain of intense severity.

Diagnosis

- Per rectal examination, USG, and CT scan may clinch the diagnosis.
- Differential diagnosis of unilateral TOA includes adnexal torsion, endometrioma, leaking ovarian cyst, and periappendicular abscess.

TREATMENT

Serious complications often ensue from delayed treatment; therefore treatment should be started on clinical diagnosis, without confirmation.

The 2002 CDC guidelines state that "empiric treatment of PID should be initiated in sexually active young women and other women at risk for STDs if they experience pelvic or lower abdominal pain, one or more minimum criteria are present on pelvic examination, and no other cause for the illness can be identified."[11]

Treatment of Acute Pelvic Inflammatory Disease

Therapeutic Goal

The therapeutic goals in the management of acute PID include:
- Elimination of the acute infection and symptoms
- Prevention of long-term sequelae, such as infertility, ectopic pregnancy, chronic pelvic pain, and residue infection
- To prevent reinfection.

Principles of Management[12]

- Treatment of the acute infection and symptoms
- Treatment of partner, even if asymptomatic
- Follow-up to prevent long-term sequelae
- Counseling regarding the importance of prevention of complications and taking complete treatment
- Family planning advice.

The CDC provides definite recommendations for outpatient and inpatient treatment of PID. In 2006, the CDC published recommended treatment guidelines for the outpatient and inpatient management of acute PID, which have been periodically updated. Oral therapy can be initiated within 24–48 hours of clinical improvement. At least 24 hours of inpatient observation is recommended in women with TOA.

Criteria for Hospitalization

The decision for hospitalization is based on the clinical scenario. CDC criteria should be followed **(Box 1)**.

Associated treatment:
- Rest: In the hospital or at home
- Sexual abstinence till the complete cure is there
- Treatment with anti-inflammatory drugs
- Estrogen and progesterone for contraceptive effect.

Re-infection can be prevented by cervical mucus induced by OP.

BOX 1: Indications for hospitalization for treatment.

CDC—2015 criteria for hospitalization
- Uncertain diagnosis—surgical emergencies such as ectopic pregnancy and appendicitis cannot be excluded
- Pregnant patient
- Unresponsive to outpatient therapy for 48 hours
- Unable to follow or tolerate an outpatient oral regime
- Severe illness, vomiting, temperature >38°C
- Suspected tubo-ovarian abscess

TABLE 2: CDC recommendations for intramuscular/oral therapy.

Drug	***Dosage***
Regimen A	
Ceftriaxone plus	250 mg intramuscularly (IM) once as a single dose plus
Doxycycline *With or without*	100 mg orally twice daily for 14 days
Metronidazole	500 mg orally twice daily for 14 days
Regimen B	
Cefoxitin plus probenecid	2 g IM once as a single dose concurrently with probenecid 1 g orally in a single dose
Doxycycline *With or without*	100 mg orally twice daily for 14 days
Metronidazole	500 mg orally twice if there is evidence or suspicion of gynecologic instrumentation in the preceding 2–3 weeks
Another third-generation cephalosporin	e.g., ceftizoxime or cefotaxime plus Doxycycline 100 mg orally twice daily for 14 days with or without metronidazole 500 mg orally twice daily for 14 days
Alternative regimen	
Azithromycin	500 mg IV daily for 1–2 doses, followed by 250 mg orally daily for 12–14 days or in combination with metronidazole
Azithromycin	1 g orally once a week for 2 weeks in combination with ceftriaxone 250 mg IM single dose
Levofloxacin	500 mg orally once daily, or Ofloxacin 400 mg twice daily, or Moxifloxacin 400 mg orally once daily With Metronidazole for 14 days (500 mg orally twice daily) can be considered if the patient is allergic to the first line of drugs and the community prevalence of *Gonococcus* is low

Medical Treatment of Acute PID

The CDC recommendations for intramuscular/oral therapy can be opted for women with mild-to-moderate acute PID **(Table 2)**.[13]

Follow-up: If no clinical improvement has occurred within 72 hours after outpatient IM/oral therapy.
- *After 72 hours:* According to CDC guidelines, women should demonstrate clinical improvement in:
  - *Effervescence:* Direct or rebound abdominal tenderness reduction
  - Uterine tenderness, adnexal and cervical motion tenderness should be reduced.

If there is no clinical improvement within 72 hours after outpatient IM/oral therapy:
  - The patient should be hospitalized
  - The antimicrobial regimen should be assessed.
  - Review diagnosis
  - Diagnostic laparoscopy for an alternative diagnosis
  - Surgical modalities
- *Retesting:*[14] All diagnosed case of chlamydial or gonococcal PID should be retested 3 months after treatment, regardless of whether their sex partners were treated. If retesting at 3 months is not possible, retesting can be done after 12 months when the woman comes for medical care.

Women should be counseled for sexual abstinence during and after medical treatment and should be educated to use barrier contraception until their symptoms have fully reduced and they completed their antibiotic regime.

CDC inpatient management regimen: Currently accepted.

CDC regimen for the hospitalized patient is given in **Table 3.**[15]

Alternative parenteral regimes:

- Clindamycin in 900 mg IV every 8 hours
  plus
  Gentamicin loading dose IV or IM (3–6 mg/kg as a single daily dose with renal monitoring)
  Followed by either (clindamycin orally 450 mg every 6 hours daily to complete 14 days) or (oral doxycycline 100 mg every 12 hours plus oral metronidazole 500 mg every 12 hours to complete 14 days) (Evidence level A European guidelines).
- *Ampicillin/Sulbactam* 3 g IV every 6 hourly
  plus
  Doxycycline 100 mg oral or IV every 12 hours[16]
  If patient is having mild-to-moderate PID and unable to tolerate metronidazole, it may be discontinued.

TABLE 3: CDC inpatient management regimens.

Recommended regimen A	
Cefotetan Or Cefoxitin plus Doxycycline	2 g IV every 12 hours 2 g every 6 hours 100 mg orally or IV every 12 hours After the patient remains clinically improved, this regimen is continued for 24 hours after which doxycycline 100 mg is given orally twice daily for 14 days If a TOA is present, metronidazole or clindamycin is used with doxycycline for more effective anaerobic coverage
Recommended regimen B	
Clindamycin plus Gentamicin	900 mg IV every 8 hours Loading dose IV or 1 M (2 mg/kg body weight) followed by a maintenance dose (1.5 mg/kg body weight) Every 8 hours; single daily dosing (3.5 mg/kg) can be substituted
Alternative parenteral regimen	
Amoxycillin/ sulbactam Plus Doxycycline Levofloxacin plus Metronidazole Ofloxacin plus Metronidazole Azithromycin	3 g IV every 6 hours + Doxycycline 100 mg orally or IV every 12 hours 500 mg IV OD + Metronidazole 500 mg IV 8 hourly 400 mg IV 12 hourly + Metronidazole 500 mg IV 8 hourly Azithromycin 500 mg IV daily for 1–2 doses, followed by 250 mg orally daily for 12–14 days or in combination with metronidazole

Treatment with moxifloxacin is recommended in women who are positive for *M. genitalium*.

Management of Sex Partners According to CDC

- All men with a history of intercourse with a woman with PID in the 60 days before the onset of symptoms in her should be evaluated, investigated, and treated for chlamydia, gonorrhea, regardless of the pathogens isolated from the woman.
- If a woman had no intercourse in the past 60 days before getting symptoms of PID, the most recent partner needs to be evaluated and treated.
- In women suffering from PID caused by *C. trachomatis* and or *N. gonorrhoeae*, male partners should be treated as well irrespective of whether they have symptoms or not.
- Strict abstinence of both partners is mandatory until treatment is complete.

Surgical Treatment of Acute PID[17,18]

Indications of surgery:

- Drainage of ruptured pelvic abscess by colpotomy
- Dilatation and evacuation of septic products of conception or for hemorrhage in postabortal sepsis
- Acute spreading peritonitis not responding to a full course of chemotherapy. The presence of pockets of pus in the peritoneum mandates laparotomy
- Suspected intestinal injury in a criminal abortion
- Failed response to medical treatment in cases of tubo-ovarian masses or ruptured TOA
- Adhesions—intestinal obstruction/general peritonitis
- Uncertain diagnosis or when suspecting a malignancy
- Perimenopausal female with a history of recurrent acute exacerbations
- Cervical dilation and antibiotics in cases of pyometra.

Management of Pelvic Abscess

- The patient is admitted to the hospital for drainage when there is—(1) persistent high fever, (2) increase in the size of abscess, (3) if rupture is suspected, (4) persistent ileus, and (5) septic shock.
- Hospital management consists of:
  - Bed rest
  - Monitoring of pulse, BP, temperature, and respiration and oxygen saturations
  - Replacement of electrolytes and fluid
  - Blood parameters particularly the white cell count and the C-reactive protein levels should be checked daily
  - Nasogastric suction when indicated
  - The senior consultant should review the women at least twice every 24 hours
  - Antibiotics are the basis of medical treatment
  - Analgesics if required.

The image-guide drainage of TOAs can be performed via the transabdominal, transvaginal, transrectal or transgluteal route (Sudakoff).[37] Laparoscopy or laparotomy with drainage of the abscess, and copious irrigation of the abdominal cavity (if fertility is desired) unilateral or bilateral salpingo-oophorectomy or pelvic clearance may give good results.

Role of Laparoscopy

It is an underused but usually helpful procedure for:[19,20]

- Confirmation of diagnosis.
- Prognosis prediction
- Management can be planned:
    - Explore all the organs
    - Aspiration
    - Laparoscopic drainage of abscess with antibiotic cover
    - Laparoscopic salpingectomy or salpingo-oophorectomy
    - Peritoneal fluid to be sent for culture and sensitivity
    - Adhesiolysis pelvic and perihepatic adhesions
    - Irrigation.

Laparotomy should generally be reserved for patients with surgical emergencies such as ruptured abscesses or definitive treatment of failed medical management.

Treatment of Chronic Pelvic Inflammatory Disease

Treatment depends on symptomatology of patient and parity.

Medical Treatment

Various antibiotics used are

- *Standard:*
    - Tetracycline 500 mg QDS—7 days
    - Doxycycline 100 mg—10–14 days
    - Metronidazole 400 mg TDS—7 days
    - Norfloxacin 400 mg BD—5–7 days
    - Ciprofloxacin 500 mg BD—5–7 days
    - Pefloxacin 400 mg BID—5–7 days
    - Lomefloxacin 400 mg once a day—5–10 days
- *Newer potent antibiotics:*
    - Cefotaxime (Third-generation cephalosporin) 1–2 g 12 hourly day
    - Ceftriaxone 250 mg IM—1 day
    - Roxithromycin: 150 mg daily for 7–10 days
    - Azithromycin: 500 mg (2 capsules daily)—3 days.

Surgical Treatment of Chronic PID

The signs and symptoms of chronic PID that most often require surgical treatment include:

- Severe, persistent, progressive pelvic pain usually bilateral, although occasionally localized in one of the lower abdominal quadrants
- Repeated exacerbations of PID requiring multiple hospitalizations and recurrent medical treatment
- Progressive enlargement of a tubo-ovarian inflammatory mass, especially if it cannot be distinguished from a neoplastic tumor of the ovary
- Severe dyspareunia related to chronic pelvic infection
- Bilateral ureteral obstruction from ligneous cellulitis

  The selection of the exact surgical procedure depends on—(1) patient's age, (2) parity, (3) desire for children, (4) previous history of pelvic disease, and (5) other associated pelvic disease and symptoms
- *Conservative surgical techniques*: (1) Adhesiolysis is preferred when both the tubes are patent; (2) unilateral salpingectomy is sought when one tube is hopelessly destroyed; (3) tuboplasty is done to ensure the tubal patency; (4) Salpingo-oophorectomy, with or without hysterectomy; and (5) conservation of uterus, one adnexa and repositioning of ovaries or for future in vitro fertilization and embryo transfer as a last resort to conservatism when both the tubes are damaged. Laparoscopy is a gold standard. The nature of pathology that affects the tubes can be identified. Treatment depends upon the site of tubal blockage.

  Drainage of pyosalpinx and TOA may be required with copious irrigation of the abdominal cavity in some chronic cases.
- *Radical treatment*: Either unilateral or bilateral salpingo-oophorectomy with hysterectomy is required in chronic TO mass in peri or postmenopausal women not responding to medical treatment. Dense pelvic adhesions may render surgery difficult.

Syndromic Case Management

This management approach is based on an easily identifiable group of symptoms and signs detected during clinical examination rather than laboratory test as it provides treatment for the most common organism causing the syndrome.

Laboratory support is generally not required or minimally required. This is a client-oriented treatment approach for low-resource setting. It includes—(1) history; (2) clinical examination; (3) laboratory examination—whenever feasible; (4) treatment with drugs; (5) partner management; (6) counseling; (7) follow-up; (8) documentation of case details and laboratory results **(Flowchart 4)**.

Prevention of Re-infection

- To avoid potential hazards of re-infection, patient should be educated about healthy and safe sex.
- The patient should be counseled against multiple sexual partners.
- The patient should be educated about methods of protection and barrier contraception.
- If the sexual partner is suffering from nongonococcal urethritis, treatment with tetracycline 500 mg 6 hourly

or doxycycline 100 mg twice daily for 7 days should be initiated for him.

Management in Special Situations

- *Children*: Acute PID is rarely seen in very young girls over 12 years. Doxycycline can be safely used.
- *Pregnancy*: Pregnant women having PID should be hospitalized and treated with intravenous antibiotics to prevent maternal morbidity and preterm delivery.
- *HIV*: HIV-positive women and HIV-negative women with PID have similar symptoms and microbiological findings. Both should be treated with similar parenteral and IM/oral antibiotic regimens. Although women with HIV infection are more likely to have concomitant *M. hominis* and streptococcal infections and also are more susceptible for TOA and should be looked for and treated accordingly.
- *IUCD*: First 3 weeks after insertion are risky for PID and is uncommon thereafter. An IUCD may be left in situ in women with clinically mild PID but should be removed if there is no improvement within 72 hours of starting treatment **(Flowchart 5)**.[21,22]
- *Postmenopausal women:* Most commonly iatrogenic causes are responsible. Many times PID is a presenting feature of malignancies. Organisms causing STDs in the reproductive age group are generally not found in this group. Parenteral management is generally preferred requiring admission. Surgical exploration may be needed if there is no improvement within 48 hours. TOA is common in them requiring aggressive management to prevent morbidity and mortality.

Flowchart 4: Syndromic management for pelvic inflammatory disease (PID).

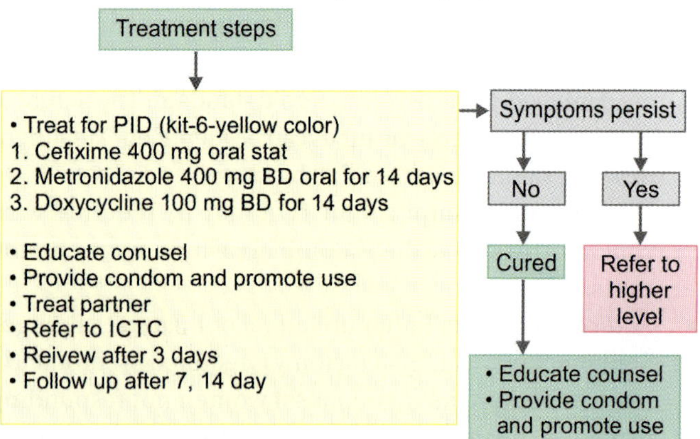

Source: Dasgupta Dr Sujoy. Management of PID (slide 42). BOGSCON 41. The Annual Conference of Bengal Obstetric and Gynaecological Society, January 2016.

PID AND ADOLESCENCE

Young age is one of the most important risk factors for PID and STDs and most women experience PID before the age of 19 years. Adolescents are at high risk of getting PID because of two factors, multiple sexual partners, and a high prevalence of sexually transmitted infections.[23] The adolescent is at higher risk of infection with sexually transmitted pathogens because of the immaturity of the epithelial lining of the cervix and lack of local immunity. In addition, behavioral factors common to adolescents, such as inconsistent use of methods of protection like a barrier or hormonal contraception, limited access to gynecologic healthcare to screen for asymptomatic infection, and fear associated of disclosure of sexual activity, lead to the high PID rate in this age group.[24]

Flowchart 5: Management of PID with IUD.[21]

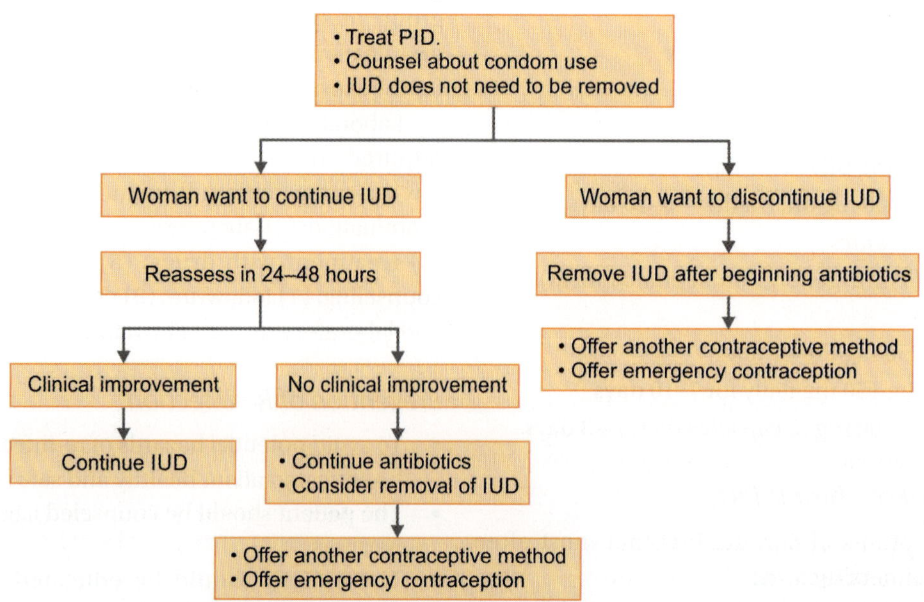

(Cu-IUD: copper-containing IUD; IUD: intrauterine device; LNG-IUD: levonorgestrel-releasing IUD; PID: pelvic inflammatory disease)
Centers for Disease Control and Prevention, Morbidity and Mortality Weekly Report. Pelvic Inflammatory Disease, Guidelines for Prevention and Management.

Because recurrent STI infection and PID lead to long-term risk for chronic pelvic pain and infertility and ectopic pregnancy in girls, that is why more aggressive prevention, counseling, and treatment of teenagers with PID is needed.

Management

Aim

Symptomatic relief:

- Treatment of the acute condition
- Prevention of sequelae

Parenteral antibiotics inpatient treatment is recommended by CDC expert for all adolescent diagnosed as having PID. Because of poor treatment compliance and their psychosocial immaturity, living circumstances and confidentiality issues in addition, the guidelines recommend risk reduction counselling and notification of sex partners for all women diagnosed as having PID.[25]

REFERENCES

1. Wikipedia. Typical Sites for Pelvic Inflammatory Disease. [Online] Available from: https://upload.wikimedia.org/wikipedia/commons/9/91/Blausen_0732_PID-Sites.png
2. Welch, Damian. Pelvic Inflammatory Disease (PID). [Online] Available from: https://slideplayer.com/slide/4445880/
3. European Society of Radiology. Flow diagram of causes of primary and secondary pelvic inflammatory. [Online] Available from: https://epos.myesr.org/posterimage/esr/ecr2018/142575/mediagallery/748954?deliveroriginal=4.
4. Wikipedia. Low magnification micrograph of acute and chronic salpingitis. [Online] Available from: https://en.wikipedia.org/wiki/File:Salpingitis_-_low_mag.jpg
5. Wikipedia. Pelvic inflammatory disease. [Online] Available from: https://en.wikipedia.org/wiki/Pelvic_inflammatory_disease
6. Fawzi, Mary Smith. Protocol for treatment of pelvic inflammatory disease PID among women in Haiti. [Online] Available from: https://www.researchgate.net/profile/Mary_Smith_Fawzi2/publication/7197625/figure/fig1/AS:601609528688673@1520446297500/Protocol-for-treatment-of-pelvic-inflammatory-disease-PID-among-women-in-Haiti.png
7. Beigi RH, Wiesenfeld HC. Pelvic inflammatory disease: new diagnostic criteria and treatment. Obstet Gynecol Clin North Am. 2003;30(4):777-93.
8. STD-Symptoms.com. Pelvic Inflammatory Disease (PID). [Online] Available from: https://std-symptoms.com/pelvic-inflammatory-disease
9. Diagnostic Imaging Pathways, Government of Western Australia. Pelvic Inflammatory Disease. [Online] Available from: http://www.imagingpathways.health.wa.gov.au/images/PID.gif
10. Am Fam Physician. 2015 May 1;91(9):652-654. [Online] Available from: https://www.aafp.org/afp/2015/0501/p652.html
11. Centers for Disease Control and Prevention. Pelvic inflammatory disease (PID) treatment and care. [Online] Available from: https://www.cdc.gov/std/pid/treatment.htm [Last accessed December, 2021].
12. Centers for Disease Control and Prevention. Sexually Transmitted Diseases Sumary of 2015 CDC Treatment Guidelines. [Online] Available from: https://www.cdc.gov/std/tg2015/pid.htm
13. uspharmacist.com. CDC-Recommended Parenteral Regimens for Severe PID. [Online] Available from: https://www.uspharmacist.com/CMSImagesContent/2016/9/USP1609-PID-T1.gif
14. Hosenfeld CB, Workowski KA, Berman S, Zaidi A, Dyson J, Mosure D, et al. Repeat infection with Chlamydia and gonorrhea among females: a systematic review of the literature. Sex Transm Dis. 2009;36(8):478-89.
15. Workowski KA, Bolan GA; Centers for Disease Control andPrevention. Sexually transmitted diseases treatment guidelines,2015. MMWR Recomm Rep. 2015;64(RR-03):1-137.
16. Jonathan Ross, Secondo Guaschino, Marco Cusini and Jorgen Jensen. 2017 European guideline for the management of pelvic inflammatory disease.
17. Kumar A, Bhatnagar G. Chronic pelvic pain. In: Kumar D, Singh N, Tempe A (eds). Evidence of Based Clinical Gynecology, 1st edition; 2017. pp. 138-50.
18. Virkud A (Ed). Modern Gynecology, 3rd edition. New Delhi: APC Publishers.
19. Sudakoff GS, Lundeen SJ, Otterson MF. Transrectal and transvaginal sonographic intervention of infected pelvic fluid collections:a complete approach. Ultrasound Q. 2005;21(3):175-85.
20. Sharma R. Tubal factor infertility and ectopic pregnancy—diagnosis and management. In: Rao KA, Divyashree PS (eds). The Infertility Manual, 4th edition. New Delhi: Jaypee Brothers Medical Publishers (P) Ltd; 2018. pp. M173-80.
21. National AIDS Control Organization. Training of Medical officers to deliver STI/RTI services: Participant's Handout. [Online] Available from: http://nhm.gov.in/images/pdf/programmes/materna-health/guidelines/Medical-Officer-Handout.pdf
22. Centers for Disease Control and Prevention. Pelvic Inflammator Disease. [Online] Available from https://www.cdc.gov/mmwr/preview/mmwrhtml/figures/r6205a7f1.gif
23. Jan E. Paradise; Linda Grant. Pelvic Inflammatory Disease in Adolescents. Pediatrics in Review. Volume 13, Issue 6. June 1992.
24. Cates W Jr. The epidemiology and control of sexually transmitted diseases in adolescents. Adolesc Med. 1990;1(3):409-28.
25. Pelvic inflammatory disease: guidelines for prevention and management. MMWR Recomm Rep. 1991;40(RR-5):1-25.

LONG QUESTIONS

1. Describe in detail pathogenesis of PID.
2. What are the clinical features and diagnostic criteria of acute PID?
3. What all conditions mimic the presentation of acute PID and how do you reach the final diagnosis?
4. Describe clinical presentation and management of pelvic abscess.
5. What are the CDC guidelines for inpatient and outpatient management of acute pID?

SHORT QUESTIONS

1. Answer in brief the following:
   a. Causative organisms of PID.
   b. What are body's natural defense against PID?
   c. Laparoscopic findings consistent with PID.
   d. Complications if PID is left untreated.
   e. What do you understand by syndromic management of PID?

MULTIPLE CHOICE QUESTIONS

1. Incidence of PID is highest in age group:
   a. 15 to 24 years b. 20–40 years
   c. Postmenopausal age d. Before menarche
2. Answer true or false: Shift in the microbial etiology of more Chlamydia trachomatis than gonococcus and others has been observed in past few years.
   a. True b. False
3. All of the following are risk factors for PID, except:
   a. Presence of bacterial vaginosis
   b. Being sexually active and under the age of 25, not using a condom during sex
   c. Invasive intrauterine procedure
   d. Pregnancy
4. In PID, following abortion and puerperium infection spreads commonly through:
   a. As ascending infection
   b. Cervix via lymphatics to the cellular tissue in the broad ligament causing cellulitis and involving tube from outside
   c. Via bloodstream
   d. Myometrium involved first leading to salpingtis
5. Most common symptom of acute PID is:
   a. Abdominal pain b. Vaginal discharge
   c. Vomiting d. Fever
6. The infection that causes more damage to the mucosa and the wall of tube leading to fibrosis and tubal occlusion is:
   a. Chlamydia infection b. Gonococca infection
   c. Mycoplasma infection d. Trichomonas infection
7. Which of the following statements is false regarding hydrosalpinx in PID?
   a. Often bilateral
   b. Histology reveals flattening of the tubal plicae and exfoliation of the lining epithelium
   c. The wall of the hydrosalpinx is thick and translucent
   d. None of the above
8. Which organism is associated with PID in women who are IUCD users?
   a. Chlamydia b. Gonococcus
   c. Staphylococcus d. Actinomyces
9. Which of the following is not included in PID?
   a. Endometritis b. Salpingitis
   c. Cervicitis d. Pelvic peritonitis
10. Best treatment option for OPD management of acute PID is:
    a. Single IM INJ OF Ceftriaxone with oral doxycycline and oral metronidazole for 14 days
    b. Oral ofloxacin and oral metronidazole for 14 days
    c. Oral azithromycin for 14 days
    d. Single injection of ceftriaxone with oral metronidazole for 14 days
11. Which of the following is a definitive criteria for PID?
    a. Cervical motion tenderness
    b. Histopathological evidence of endometritis
    c. Bilateral lower abdominal pain
    d. Temperature >38°C
12. Differential diagnosis of PID includes:
    a. Ectopic pregnancy b. Twisted ovarian cyst
    c. Endometriosis d. All of the above
13. Salpingitis is best confirmed by:
    a. MRI b. Hysterosalpingography
    c. Laparoscopy d. Sonosalpingography
14. Which of the following is most likely to cause beaded appearance of fallopian tubes, with clubbing of fimbrial end and ampulla:
    a. Tuberculosis b. Chlamydia
    c. Gonococcal salpingitis d. Candidiasis
15. During laproscopy the preferred site for obtaining cultures in a patient with acute PID is:
    a. Endocervix b. Pouch of Douglas
    c. Endometrium d. Fallopian tube

Answers

1.	a	2.	a	3.	d	4.	b	5.	a	6.	a
7.	c	8.	d	9.	c	10.	a	11.	b	12.	d
13.	c	14.	a	15.	b						

10.4 FEMALE GENITAL TUBERCULOSIS

Jai Bhagwan Sharma, Eshani Sharma, Sona Dharmendra

INTRODUCTION

Tuberculosis (TB) is a major health problem all over the world with 10 million new cases and 1.33 million deaths annually.[1] Liberal immigration, human immunodeficiency virus co-infection, and development of drug-resistant TB have fueled the epidemic of TB all over the world, but especially in Africa and Asia.[2]

Extrapulmonary TB (EPTB) is becoming more common. About 9% cases of EPTB are due to female genital TB (FGTB). FGTB is a type of EPTB that is common in developing countries, such as India, causing about 10% cases of infertility,[4] but the incidence of FGTB in infertility patients is higher in tertiary hospitals (up to 26%) due to referral and concentration of cases and still higher (up to 48%) in women referred for assisted reproduction in tertiary centers.[5-6] Mean age of presentation is 40 years in developed countries but is much less (20–30 years) in developing countries, such as India, possibly due to early marriage and childbearing.[5,7] HIV coinfection has increased the incidence of FGTB in Africa and India.[8]

ETIOPATHOGENESIS

Female genital TB is caused by *Mycobacterium tuberculosis* (rarely *Mycobacterium bovis*).[2] Predisposing factors are poverty, lack of ventilation and healthcare facilities, diabetes, drug abuse, renal disease, and HIV infection.[9,10] Genital TB usually comes from pulmonary TB through hematogenous (common) or lymphatic route or direct spread from surrounding areas (intestine) or abdominopelvic lymph nodes.[11] Various genital organs involved are as follows:

- *Fallopian tubes*: Fallopian tubes are most commonly involved genital organs (>90%) with involvement being TB endosalpingitis (inside of tube), exosalpingitis (outside of tube), interstitial TB salpingitis, and salpingitis isthmica nodosa.[4,10] In tuberculous endosalpingitis, the infection starts from inside the tube (endosalpinx) making tubes inflamed and swollen with hydrosalpinx, pyosalpinx, tubo-ovarian masses, pelvic adhesions, and risk of ectopic gestation and infertility.[2,4,10] In tuberculous exosalpingitis, infection starts from outside with congestion, adhesions or miliary tubercles or shaggy areas on the tubal surface with beading, tubo-ovarian masses, hydrosalpinx, and pyosalpinx.[2,4,10,11]
- *Endometrium*: The endometrium is involved in 70% women through hematogenous, lymphatic or direct spread. There can be focal or multiple ulcers, necrosis or hemorrhagic areas. Endometrial atrophy and adhesions (Asherman syndrome) may occur causing secondary amenorrhea and infertility.[12] On microscopy, epithelioid granulomas may be there or only focal collection of lymphocytes may also suggest FGTB.[13]
- *Ovaries*: Ovaries are involved in about 25% cases with adhesions, cysts with decrease in ovarian function, and reserve.[14,15]
- *Peritoneum*: Involvement of abdominal and pelvic peritoneum by TB causes ascites, abdominal and pelvic masses, which may be confused with ovarian cancer.[16] Various types of pelvic and abdominal adhesions can be formed in FGTB including perihepatic adhesions and hanging gall bladder sign.[17]
- *Cervix*: The cervix can be involved in 5% cases of genital TB and may resemble cervical cancer through growth or ulcer.[4,18]
- *Vagina and vulva*: The vulva and vagina are rarely involved and can cause ulcer or growth or genital fistulae.[4,18]

Infertility and Female Genital Tuberculosis

Both primary and secondary infertility are common in FGTB due to various causes, such as tubal factors (ciliary damage, blockage of tubes, hydrosalpinx, pyosalpinx), ovarian factors (anovulation, ovarian damage, decreased ovarian reserve and oocyte defect), and endometrial factors (Asherman syndrome and poor implantation).[2,4,12,14]

SYMPTOMATOLOGY

Signs and symptoms of FGTB are given in **Table 1**.

DIAGNOSIS

A high index of suspicion is needed to make the diagnosis. A careful detailed history should be taken from patient about any family history of TB or past history of tuberculosis or antituberculosis therapy in past including before marriage as quite often unmarried girls look after their parents and grandparents with TB and may acquire disease. A thorough general physical examination should be performed to get any evidence of TB elsewhere (pulmonary TB, lymph node TB, skeletal TB or abdominal TB). Abdominal, speculum, and

TABLE 1: Symptomatology and signs in female genital tuberculosis.[2,4,7,10,11]

Symptoms	*Signs*
• Asymptomatic (12%) • Constitutional symptoms – Fever – Loss of appetite – Loss of weight – Malaise • Menstrual symptoms – Abnormal or heavy uterine bleeding (in early stage) – Scanty menses (late stage) – Amenorrhea – (primary or secondary) – Painful periods • Infertility (primary or secondary) • Abdominal or pelvic lump • Abdominal and pelvic pain • Excessive vaginal discharge • Growth or ulcer on cervix • Growth or ulcer on vulva or vagina • Incontinence of urine or stool	• No sign (11%) • Raised temperature • Cervical, axillary or inguinal lymphadenopathy (in lymph nodes TB) • Crepitations on chest (Pulmonary TB) • Abdominal examination – Abdominal or pelvic mass – Ascites – Doughy feel • Vaginal examination – Enlarged uterus (pyometra) – Tenderness and induration in one or both fornices – Adnexal mass – Tenderness and induration in the pouch of Douglas • Uncommon findings – Growth on external genitalia – Ulcers on external genitalia – Vesicovaginal fistula – Rectovaginal fistula

vaginal examination for any lumps, vaginal discharge, TB lesions on cervix and vulva, vagina, and adnexal masses are done.[4,11]

INVESTIGATIONS

No single investigation is enough. Multiple tests should be done.

- Complete hemogram for anemia, leukocytosis, lymphocytosis, and raised ESR may help.
- Serological tests are banned and are not to be done.
- X-ray chest for any present or past TB lesions including hilar lymph nodes.
- Mantoux/Tuberculin test and interferon gamma release assay (IGRA) have limited sensitivity (55%) and specificity (80%) and are used with other tests.
- *Blood markers:* Many markers are being investigated but results are not promising. Cancer antigen 125 (CA 125) (normal levels <35 U/mL) is moderately raised usually <200 U/mL in FGTB (as compared to the higher rise in thousands in cancer ovary) but alone is not a reliable marker for the diagnosis of FGTB.
- *Radiological tests:* These are of use mainly in tubo-ovarian masses. Ultrasonography (USG) may demonstrate tubo-ovarian masses with calcification and fluid in the pouch of Douglas. It may also show thin endometrium, calcification or bands, and intrauterine synechiae and hydrosalpinges with free peritoneal fluid and fixed adnexal masses.[4,10] Computerized axial tomography (CAT) scan **(Fig. 1)** may demonstrate abdominal and pelvic masses with ascites, thickened and enhanced peritoneum, with lesions in the abdominal viscera and lymph nodes.[4,10] Magnetic resonance imaging (MRI) with higher resolution may demonstrate tubo-ovarian masses, hydrosalpinx, adnexal cysts or tuberculous deposits on peritoneum or hepatic surface.[19] Positron emission tomography (PET) scan may show unilateral or bilateral tubo-ovarian masses with increased fluorodeoxyglucose (FDG) uptake in TB lesions and may differentiate between abdominopelvic TB and ovarian cancer[20] **(Fig. 2)**. Hysterosalpingography (HSG), though contraindicated in active FGTB, can show internal uterine and tubal architecture with tobacco pouch, golf club, and Maltese cross appearance of tubes and shrunken uterine cavity with tubal block[21] **(Figs. 3 and 4)**.
- *Microbiological tests:* Endometrial biopsy or aspirate is done in premenstrual phase. It is homogenized and divided in two parts, one part is sent in saline for acid-fast bacilli (AFB) microscopy, AFB culture, polymerase chain reaction (PCR), gene Xpert or CBNAAT (cartridge-based nucleic acid amplification test).[4,22,23] The other part is sent in formalin solution for histology to demonstrate epithelioid granuloma of TB or even local accumulation of lymphocytes. Even loop-mediated isothermal amplification process (LAMP) assay has been used on endometrial tissue with varying accuracy.[24] Demonstration of AFB on microscopy, culture, geneXpert or histopathological demonstration of epithelioid granuloma are gold standard in diagnosis but positive PCR alone is not taken as diagnosis of TB.

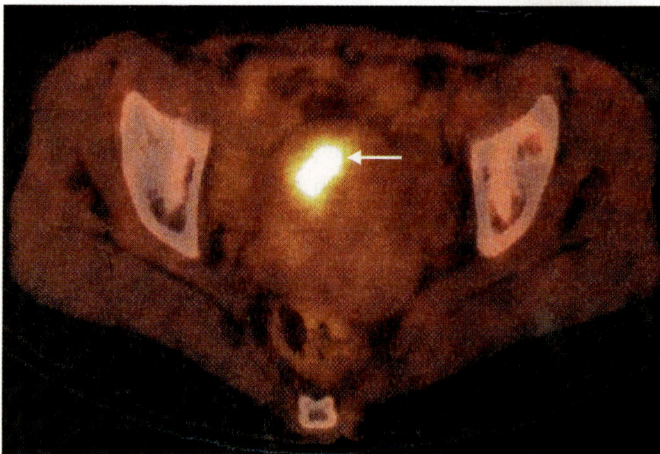

Fig. 2: PET CT of pelvis showing increased fluorodeoxyglucose uptake (arrow) in active case of female genital tuberculosis.

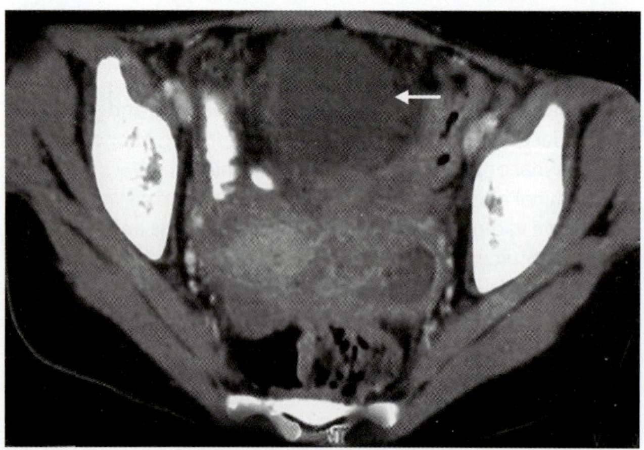

Fig. 1: CT scan pelvis showing a tubo-ovarian mass (arrow) in case of female genital tuberculosis.

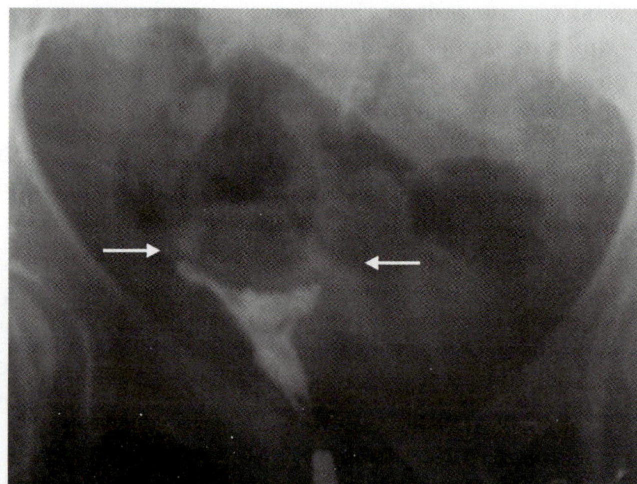

Fig. 3: Hysterosalpingography (HSG) showing bilateral corneal block with filling defect (arrows) in a case of female genital tuberculosis.

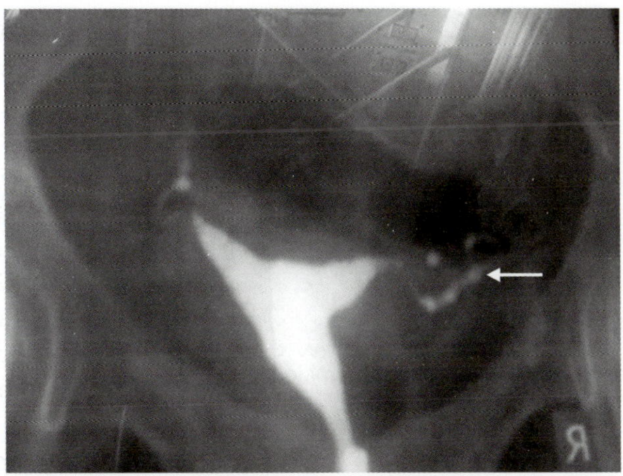

Fig. 4: Uterus showing bilateral fimbrial block with beaded tubes (arrow) in female genital tuberculosis.

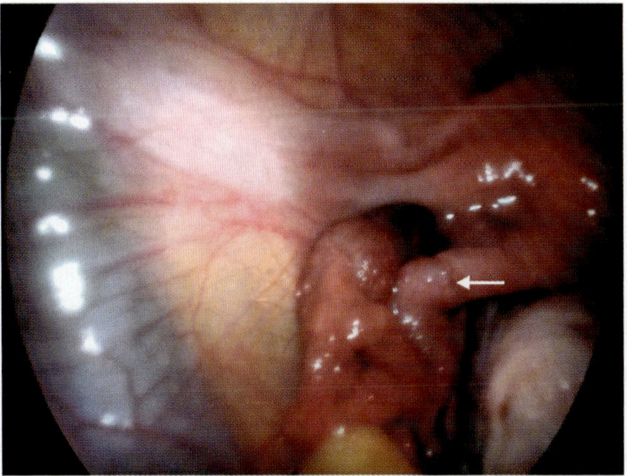

Fig. 6: Laparoscopy showing hyperemic tube with tubercles and adhesions in a case of female genital tuberculosis.

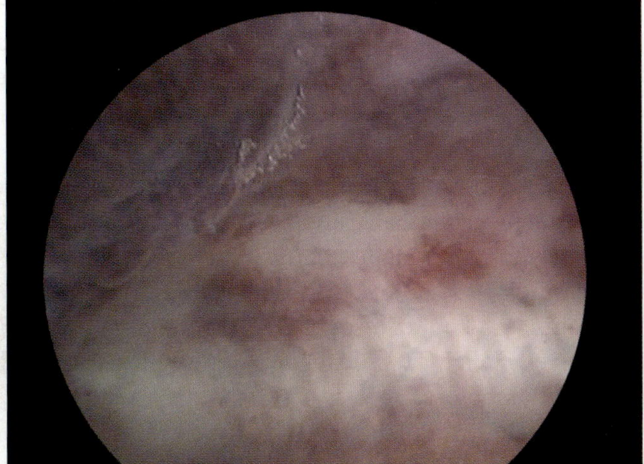

Fig. 5: Hysteroscopy showing pale cavity and grade III adhesion in female genital tuberculosis case.

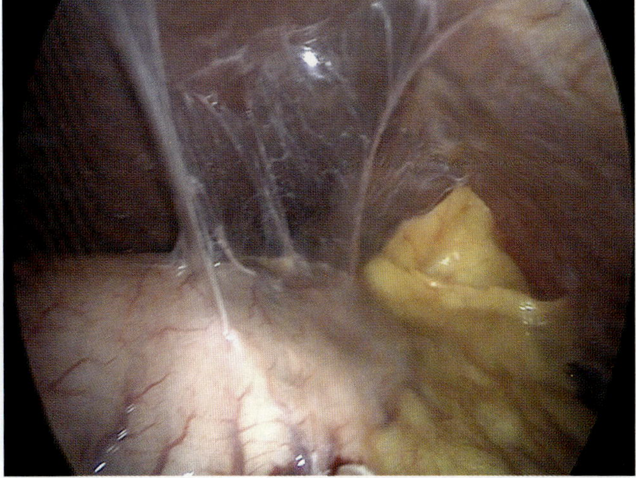

Fig. 7: Laparoscopic showing perihepatic adhesions in a case of female genital tuberculosis.

- *Hysteroscopy:* It can demonstrate pale cavity, tubercles, shaggy areas or endometrial adhesions or caseous nodules in women with FGTB[12] **(Fig. 5)**.
- *Laparoscopy:* It is a very useful modality with direct visualization of whole of pelvic or abdominal cavity for any TB lesions, such as tubercles, caseous nodules (definite findings) or pelvic or abdominal adhesions, straw-colored fluid, congested convoluted tubes, and hydrosalpinx or pyosalpinx (probable findings)[25] **(Figs. 6 and 7)**. However, performing laparoscopy or other surgery in FGTB needs expertise and is associated with increased difficulty and complications.[25]
- An algorithm has been developed for FGTB in INDEX-TB guidelines, an initiative of Central TB Division, Ministry of Health and Family Welfare, Government of India and the WHO in 2016 for the diagnosis and management of FGTB.[4,10]
- *Composite reference standard (CRS):* Currently, CRS is taken as gold standard for diagnosis of FGTB and is a combination of tests like positive AFB on microscopy or culture or histopathological demonstration of epithelioid granuloma on histology or presence of definite findings of TB on laparoscopy (tubercles, caseation or beaded tubes) or probable findings of TB (straw-colored fluid, extensive pelvic, peritubal or peri-ovarian adhesions, tubal hyperemia, mid-tubal block, tubo-ovarian mass or peri-hepatic adhesions).

TREATMENT

There have been changes in treatment policy. Categories are no longer used. All women with FGTB whether new or old cases are given daily 2 months rifampicin, isoniazid, pyrazinamide, and ethambutol (RHZE) in intensive phase followed by daily three drugs [rifampicin, isoniazid, and ethambutol (RHE)] in continuation phase **(Table 2)**.[26] In a randomized controlled trial, we confirmed that 6 months antitubercular therapy (ATT) was as effective as 9 months of ATT. Treatment is give free of cost through DOTS (Directly observed treatment, short-course) centers all over India. Patients are reported to

TABLE 2: Treatment regimen for drug sensitive TB including FGTB (WHO 2018, RNTCP 2019).

TB patients	*TB treatment regimens*	
	Intensive phase (daily)	Continuation phase (daily)
New and old smear-positive patients and defaulters. New and old smear-negative and defaulter patients of pulmonary TB with extensive parenchymal involvement. Severe concomitant HIV disease or both. New and old cases and defaulters of extrapulmonary TB (FGTB included)	2HRZE Dose Isoniazid 300 mg Rifampicin 450 (600 mg if >45 kg) Pyrazinamide 1,500 mg Ethambutol 1,200 mg for 2 months	4HRE Isoniazid 300 mg Rifampicin 450 (600 mg if >45 kg) Ethambutol 1,200 mg for 4 months

(FGTB: female genital tuberculosis; HIV: human immunodeficiency virus; HRZE: isoniazid, rifampicin, pyrazinamide, and ethambutol)

Government of India and are followed up for any complication of medicines. Liver function tests are done only if needed.[4]

Surgical Treatment

Surgery is hazardous in TB and is not usually needed.[5] Only limited surgery in the form of drainage of persistent pelvic or tubo-ovarian abscess despite medical treatment can be performed. Repeat laparoscopy and hysteroscopy should be performed after completion of a full course of ATT for prognostication and planning further treatment. Tuboplasty is avoided in case of FGTB as it does not improve the prognosis for fertility with risk of flare-up of TB and ectopic pregnancy after ATT.[4]

Assisted Reproduction in Female Genital Tuberculosis

Prognosis for fertility is poor in FGTB. If after completion of ATT on repeat laparoscopy and hysteroscopy, tubes and endometrium are normal then ovulation induction or intrauterine insemination (IUI) is done. If tubes are blocked but endometrium is normal, then in vitro fertilization and embryo transfer (IVF-ET) is done with good success.[10,11] If tubes are blocked and endometrium is blocked by severe adhesions, then surrogacy or adoption are advised.[10,11]

CONCLUSION

A high index of suspicion is needed to make the diagnosis of FGTB using CRS using endometrial sampling for AFB microscopy, AFB culture, histopathological evidence of epithelioid granuloma, and definite or probable findings of TB on laparoscopy. Antituberculosis therapy is given for 6 months. IVF-ET is a useful modality. Newer vaccines, diagnostic methods, and medicines (like bedaquiline, delamanid), and stem cell therapy are being developed to make prognosis better in future.

ACKNOWLEDGMENTS

We thank Dr SK Sachdeva, Deputy Director General, Central TB Division and MOHFW, Dr Sangeeta Sharma Professor and Head NITRD and Pawan for their help.

KEY MESSAGES

- Female genital TB is a common cause of infertility in India being responsible for about 10% cases of infertility.
- High index of suspicion is needed to diagnose FGTB from past or family history of TB or ATT in past.
- Endometrial aspiration or biopsy for AFB, microscopy, culture, and gene Xpert or presence of epithelioid granuloma on histology are gold standard in diagnosis of FGTB but are positive in few cases.
- CRS taking AFB (microscopy or culture) and histopathology with definite or probable findings of TB on laparoscopy are taken gold standard these days.
- Treatment is medical with daily 2 month therapy of rifampicin, isoniazid, pyrazinamide, and ethambutol followed by daily 4 month therapy of rifampicin, isoniazid, and ethambutol.
- IVF-ET after completing ATT is an effective method for optimum outcome for fertility.

REFERENCES

1. World Health Organization. WHO global tuberculosis report 2018. Geneva: WHO; 2018.
2. Kumar S, Sharma JB. Female genital tuberculosis. In: Sharma SK, Mohan A (Eds). Tuberculosis, 3rd edition. New Delhi: Jaypee Brothers Medical Publishers (P) Ltd; 2015. pp. 362-71.
3. Golden MP, Vikram HR. Extrapulmonary tuberculosis: An overview. Am Fam Physician. 2005;72(9):1761-8.
4. Sharma JB, Sharma E, Sharma S, Dharmendra S. Female genital tuberculosis: Revisited. Indian J Med Res. 2018;148(Suppl):S71-S83.
5. Gupta N, Sharma JB, Mittal S, Singh N, Misra R, Kukreja M, et al. Genital tuberculosis in Indian infertility patients. Int J Gynecol Obstet. 2007;97(2):135-8.
6. Singh N, Sumana G, Mittal S. Genital tuberculosis: A leading cause for infertility in women seeking assisted conception in North India. Arch Gynecol Obstet. 2008;278(4):325-7.
7. Neonakis IK, Spandidos DA, Petinaki E. Female genital tuberculosis: A review. Scand J Infect Dis. 2011;43(8):564-72.
8. Duggal S, Duggal N, Hans C, Mahajan RK. Female genital TB and HIV co-infection. Indian J Med Microbiol. 2009;27(4):361-3.
9. Ali AA, Abdallah TM. Clinical presentation and epidemiology of female genital tuberculosis in Eastern Sudan. Int J Gynecol Obstet. 2012;118(3):236-8.

10. Grace GA, Devaleenal DB, Natrajan M. Genital tuberculosis in females. Indian J Med Res. 2017;145(4):425-36.
11. Sharma JB. Current diagnosis and management of female genital tuberculosis. J Obstet Gynecol India. 2015;65(6):362-71.
12. Sharma JB, Roy KK, Pushparaj M, Gupta N, Jain SK, Malhotra N, et al. Genital tuberculosis: An important cause of Asherman's syndrome in India. Arch Gynecol Obstet. 2008;277:37-41.
13. Bazaz-Malik G, Maheshwari B, Lal N. Tuberculous endometritis: A clinicopathological study of 1000 cases. Br J Obstet Gynecol. 1983;90(1):84-6.
14. Malhotra N, Sharma V, Bahadur A, Sharma JB, Roy KK, Kumar S, et al. The effect of tuberculosis on ovarian reserve among women undergoing IVF in India. Int J Gynecol Obstet. 2012;117(1):40-4.
15. Sharma JB, Sneha J, Singh UB, Kumar S, Roy KK, Singh N, et al. Effect of antitubercular treatment on ovarian function in female genital tuberculosis with infertility. J Hum Reprod Sci. 2016;9(3):145-50.
16. Sharma JB, Jain SK, Pushparaj M, Roy KK, Malhotra N, Zutshi V, et al. Abdomino-peritoneal tuberculosis masquerading as ovarian cancer: A retrospective study of 26 cases. Arch Gynecol Obstet. 2010;282:643-8.
17. Sharma JB. Sharma's hanging gall bladder sign: A new sign for abdomino-pelvic tuberculosis: An observational study. IVF Lite. 2015;2:94-8.
18. Tripathy SN, Tripathy SN. Tuberculosis: Manual for Obstetrics and Gynaecologists, 1st edition. New Delhi: Jaypee Brothers Medical Publisher (P) Ltd; 2015. pp. 155-275.
19. Sharma JB, Karmakar D, Hari S, Singh N, Singh SP, Kumar S, et al. Magnetic resonance imaging findings among women with tubercular tubo-ovarian masses. Int J Gynecol Obstet. 2011;113(1):76-80.
20. Sharma JB, Karmakar D, Kumar R, Shamim SA, Kumar S, Singh N, et al. Comparison of PET/CT with other imaging modalities in women with genital tuberculosis. Int J Gynecol Obstet. 2012;118(2):123-8.
21. Sharma JB, Pushparaj M, Roy KK, Neyaz Z, Gupta N, Jain SK, et al. Hysterosalpingographic findings in infertile women with genital tuberculosis. Int J Gynaecol Obstet. 2008;101:150-5.
22. Thangappah RBP, Paramasivan CN, Narayanan S. Evaluating PCR, culture & histopathology in the diagnosis of female genital tuberculosis. Indian J Med Res. 2011;134(1):40-6.
23. Sharma JB, Kriplani A, Dharmendra S, Chaubey J, Kumar S, Sharma SK, et al. Role of geneXpert in diagnosis of female genital tuberculosis: A preliminary report. Eur J Obstet Gynecol Reprod Biol. 2016;207:237-8.
24. Sethi S, Dhaliwal L, Dey P, Kaur H, Yadav R, Sethi S, et al. Loop-mediated isothermal amplification assay for detection of Mycobacterium tuberculosis complex in infertile women. Indian J Med Microbiol. 2016;34(3):322-7.
25. Sharma JB, Roy KK, Pushparaj M, Kumar S, Malhotra N, Mittal S, et al. Laparoscopic findings in female genital tuberculosis. Arch Gynecol Obstet. 2008;278:359-64.
26. Sharma JB, Singh N, Dharmendra S, Singh UB, Vanamail P, Kumar S, et al. Six months versus nine months anti-tuberculous therapy for female genital tuberculosis: A randomized controlled trial. Eur J Obstet Gynecol Reprod Biol. 2016;203:264-73.

LONG QUESTIONS

1. Enumerate diagnostic methods of female genital tuberculosis (FGTB). How will you manage a 30-year-old infertility patient with FGTB?
2. Enumerate the cause of high prevalence of genital tuberculosis in India. How will you manage a case of 32-year-old infertile patient with tuberculous tubo-ovarian masses?

SHORT QUESTIONS

1. Causes of infertility in female genital tuberculosis.
2. Diagnosis of female genital tuberculosis.
3. Newer diagnostic modalities in female genital tuberculosis.
4. Laparoscopic findings in female genital tuberculosis.
5. Treatment of female genital tuberculosis.

MULTIPLE CHOICE QUESTIONS

1. All of the following are reliable tests on endometrial biopsy for diagnosis of female genital tuberculosis, except:
   a. Positive AFB on microscopy
   b. Positive AFB culture
   c. Epithelioid granuloma on histopathology
   d. Positive polymerase chain reaction
2. Newer diagnostic modality accepted and recommended by World Health Organization for diagnosing female genital tuberculosis on endometrial biopsy:
   a. Positive DNA polymerase chain reaction
   b. Positive RNA polymerase chain reaction
   c. Positive CB-NAAT (Cartridge based nucleic acid amplification test)
   d. Positive Loop-mediated isothermal amplification (LAMP)
3. Current recommendation for treatment of female genital tuberculosis:
   a. Daily 2 isoniazid, rifampicin, pyrazinamide, and ethambutol for 2 months (intensive phase), followed by isoniazid, rifampicin, and ethambutol daily for 4 months (continuation phase)
   b. Thrice weekly isoniazid, rifampicin, pyrazinamide, and ethambutol for 2 months (intensive phase), followed by thrice weekly isoniazid, rifampicin, and ethambutol for 4 months (continuation phase)
   c. Thrice weekly isoniazid, rifampicin, pyrazinamide, and ethambutol for 2 months (intensive phase), followed by thrice weekly isoniazid and rifampicin for 4 months (continuation phase)
   d. Daily isoniazid, rifampicin, pyrazinamide, and ethambutol for 3 months (intensive phase), followed by isoniazid, rifampicin, and ethambutol daily for 6 months (continuation phase)
4. All of the following are definite findings of tuberculosis on laparoscopy, except:
   a. Tubercles   b. Caseous nodules
   c. Pelvic adhesions   d. Shaggy areas

5. Common cause of Asherman syndrome in India is:
   a. Past dilatation and curettage (D&C)
   b. Past medical termination of pregnancy (MTP)
   c. Female genital tuberculosis
   d. Pelvic inflammation disease
6. Female genital tuberculosis is responsible for what percentage of cases of infertility overall in India?
   a. 5%   b. 10%
   c. 15%   d. 20%
7. Highest incidence of female genital tuberculosis in India is in which age group?
   a. Premenarchal   b. Reproductive age group
   c. Perimenopausal   d. Postmenopausal
8. Which of the genital organs are most involved in female genital tuberculosis?
   a. Fallopian tubes   b. Uterus
   c. Ovaries   d. Cervix
9. Which of the following genital organs is least commonly involved in female genital tuberculosis?
   a. Fallopian tubes   b. Uterus
   c. Cervix   d. Vulva
10. The best therapeutic modality for success pregnancy outcome with tubal disease due to female genital tuberculosis after treatment:
    a. Ovulation induction
    b. In utero insemination (IUI)
    c. Tubal surgery
    d. In vitro fertilization and embryo transfer

Answers

1.	d	2.	c	3.	a	4.	c	5.	c	6.	b
7.	b	8.	a	9.	d	10.	d				

10.5 BENIGN DISEASES OF OVARY AND FALLOPIAN TUBE

Shobhana Mohandas, Haritha C

The ovary and fallopian tube are two vital organs, situated in very close proximity by the side of the uterus in the pelvis. Diagnosis of an adnexal mass presents a dilemma to the clinician, as diseases of the ovary and fallopian tubes have similar symptoms, clinical findings, and ultrasound features. The ovary and the fallopian tube can be the seat of many physiological changes and pathological entities and a thorough knowledge of these conditions will be helpful in clearly identifying the cause of pain or distension of abdomen or incidental finding of a cyst on ultrasonography.

BENIGN DISEASES AFFECTING THE OVARY

Ovaries are affected by aberrations of hormones related to its functions, aberrations of various cells in the organ or by external factors like infections or neoplasms in adjacent organs **(Table 1)**.

Briefly, they could be classified as:[1]

- Functional cysts
- Benign neoplasms of the ovary
- *Hormonal:* Insulin resistance leading to increased androgen production by the ovary could lead to excessive development of follicles in the periphery of the ovary, called the polycystic ovarian syndrome
- Torsion of the ovary with or without a cyst in it due to various causes
- Endometrioma due to deposits of endometriotic tissue in the ovary
- Pelvic infection that could cause an ovarian abscess
- Ovarian remnant syndrome.

Functional Cysts

Follicular, corpus luteal, and theca lutein cysts are functional cysts of the ovary. Being aberrations of a physiological process, they may disappear spontaneously, unlike pathological cysts which require surgery.

Follicular Cysts

These arise from the ovarian follicle, and are commonly found in young menstruating women, although solitary cysts could

TABLE 1: Benign diseases of the ovary.

Functional cysts	*Benign neoplasms*					*Others*
Follicular	Cell of origin	Types				Torsion
Corpus luteal	Epithelial	Serous	Mucinous	Endometrioid	Brenner	PCOS
Theca lutein	Stromal	Fibroma	Thecoma	Leydig cell	Steroid cell	Infection
	Sex cord	Granulosa cell		Sertoli cell		Endometrioma
	Germ cell	Mature teratoma				Ovarian remnant
	Germ cell/sex cord		Gonadoblastoma			Hydatid cyst of Morgagni
	Mixed stromal sex cord		Sertoli Leydig cell tumor			

(PCOS: polycystic ovary syndrome)

be found even in the fetal and neonatal periods. Situated in the ovarian cortex, they are thin-walled and contain clear fluid. They are lined by granulosa cells, and majority of them disappear spontaneously by either reabsorption of the cyst fluid or silent rupture within 4–8 weeks of initial diagnosis.

Corpus Luteal Cysts

Hemorrhage into the corpus luteum with later absorption of blood could lead to a corpus luteal cyst. In most cases it is small, 3–4 cm in size. In a few cases, it may be as large as 10 cm. There may be associated prolonged secretion of progesterone. These cysts could cause a delay in menstruation.

When a corpus luteum is cut, the convoluted lining is yellowish orange, and the center contains an organizing blood clot. If this finding is found during ovarian cystectomy, one can almost guess that it is a corpus luteal cyst.

Theca Lutein Cysts

Least common of all three, they are usually bilateral and may lead to massive enlargement of the ovaries, sometimes up to 20–30 cm. The individual cysts vary in size from 1 cm to 10 cm or more in diameter. These cysts arise from either prolonged or excessive stimulation of the ovaries by endogenous or exogenous gonadotropins or increased ovarian sensitivity to gonadotropins.

The ovary may appear lobulated with hundreds of thin-walled locules or cysts, producing a honeycombed appearance. The cyst is lined by theca lutein cells with occasional granulosa cells.

Neoplasms of the Ovary

Ovarian neoplasms can be distinguished histologically depending on their cell type of origin. These are grouped as epithelial tumors, germ cell tumors, sex cord-stromal tumors, and others. Benign ovarian tumors are:

- *Epithelial*: Serous, mucinous, endometrioid, Brenner, and seromucinous
- *Stromal*: Fibroma, thecoma, Leydig cell, and steroid cell
- *Sex cord*: Granulosa cell, Sertoli cell
- *Mixed sex cord stromal tumors*: Sertoli–Leydig cell
- *Germ cell tumors*: Mature teratoma
- *Germ cell/sex cord stromal tumor*: Gonadoblastoma.

Prevalence

In one Indian[3] study of benign tumors of the ovary, on pathological specimens of benign ovarian cysts/tumors, the most common findings were of epithelial tumors (21%), followed by benign teratoma (19%).

Epithelial Ovarian Tumors

These may be serous or mucinous. Serous tumors are thin-walled and unilocular with serous fluid, while mucinous tumors are thicker walled, with mucoid containing fluid. They may be multilocular.

Teratoma

It is dealt with in the section of question and answers.

Transitional Cell Tumors: Brenner Tumors

They occur in the age group 40–60 years. They may be just discovered incidentally, or they may cause endometrial hyperplasia and later postmenopausal bleeding.

Fibroma

Fibromas comprise 5% of benign ovarian neoplasms.[2] The average size is about 6 cm. these usually occur in the perimenopausal age group. They do not elaborate hormones. Meigs syndrome is the association of an ovarian fibroma, ascites, and right sided hydrothorax. Both the ascites and the hydrothorax resolve after removal of the ovarian tumor. Meigs syndrome is rare and occurs only in <2% of ovarian fibromas. The hydrothorax develops secondary to a flow of ascitic fluid into the pleural space via the lymphatics of the diaphragm.

Torsion of the Ovary

Ovarian cysts may along with the tube undergo torsion and present with acute pain. It could happen in the adolescent age group or in a woman in her mid-20s and even in pregnancy. With torsion, initially, veins and lymphatics draining the ovary are obstructed, leading to a cyanotic edematous ovary. If no intervention is done, this may progress to arterial obstruction, and necrosis of the adnexa.

Endometrioma

It is dealt with in another chapter in this book.

Ovarian Abscess

Collection of pus in the ovary may occur as a sequela of pelvic inflammatory disease.

BENIGN FALLOPIAN TUBE PATHOLOGIES

Common pathologies that could affect the tube are salpingitis and ectopic pregnancy. Other conditions could be hydrosalpinx, torsion of the tube, singly or with the ovary, pyosalpinx, or rarely benign or malignant tumors.

- *Hydrosalpinx*: The fimbriae of the tube get adherent due to infection or endometriosis and the tube is filled with a clear fluid. The adjacent ovary may be adherent to the tube.
- *Torsion*: Torsion of the fallopian tube usually occurs along with the ovary, or along with a para-ovarian mass.
- *Pyosalpinx*: Pus can fill the fallopian tube as a result of intractable pelvic infection.
- *Benign tumors of the fallopian tube*: Fallopian tubes could rarely be affected by the mesothelioma, arising from the wall of the tube, being 1–2 cm in diameter. Even rarer, leiomyomas could also develop in the fallopian tube.

- *Salpingitis isthmica nodosa (SIN)*: SIN or tubal diverticulum is an acquired pathologic condition that results from the direct invasion of the muscularis layer by the endosalpinx in the isthmic portion of the fallopian tube for varying distances between the lumen and the serosa. It follows inflammation of the tube and occurs in young women.

Clinical Findings in Benign Diseases of the Ovaries and Fallopian Tube

- *Asymptomatic*: Most of the ovarian pathologies are asymptomatic and found incidentally on ultrasonography (USG). Fear of malignancy or surgery alarms the patient quite often with this finding.
- *Distension of the abdomen*: The patient may be able to notice the mass in her abdomen. Huge size of the tumor need not be alarming, as they are not always malignant.
- *Pain in the abdomen*: Dull aching pain in the lower abdomen may be caused by pressure of the fluid I n the cyst as in corpus luteum cysts leading to enlarged ovaries. It can be tender on palpation. Partial torsion of adnexa can also cause intermittent low-grade pain.

When severe, acute pain in lower abdomen is accompanied by vomiting or even bowel disturbance, one must suspect torsion of the ovarian cyst. The patient is quite often young, and sometimes a diagnosis of either acid peptic disease or abdominal colic is made and the patient is sent home. Routine USG can aid in diagnosis in such cases.

Tenderness in the lower abdomen may be present in ovarian torsion as well as pelvic infection or even appendicitis. In centers where the patient lands up at night and facilities for USG are not available at that point, it may be prudent to convince the patient to stay overnight till an ultrasound next day proves/disproves an ovarian pathology.

Severe abdominal pain could also be caused be caused by rupture of an ovarian cyst, which may resolve after some time. In case of corpus luteum cyst, the cyst may continue to hemorrhage, leading to hemoperitoneum, sometimes confusing it with ruptured ectopic pregnancy. USG along with clinical findings helps in reaching a diagnosis in such tricky situations **(Flowchart 1)**.

- *Menstrual disturbances*: Beside polycystic ovary syndrome (PCOS), simple ovarian cysts could also delay menstruation, and in the latter case, the patient needs to be reassured that it may disappear in the course of time. Teratomas may also be accompanied by a positive pregnancy test [due to marginally raised human chorionic gonadotropin (hCG)] and delayed periods, and therefore USG has to be done systematically to detect the typical features of a dermoid even if the cyst is small in size. Sometimes a small-sized dermoid can even mimic an ectopic pregnancy due to delayed periods, positive pregnancy test, and adnexal mass on USG.

Flowchart 1: Mechanisms of acute abdomen with ovarian cyst.

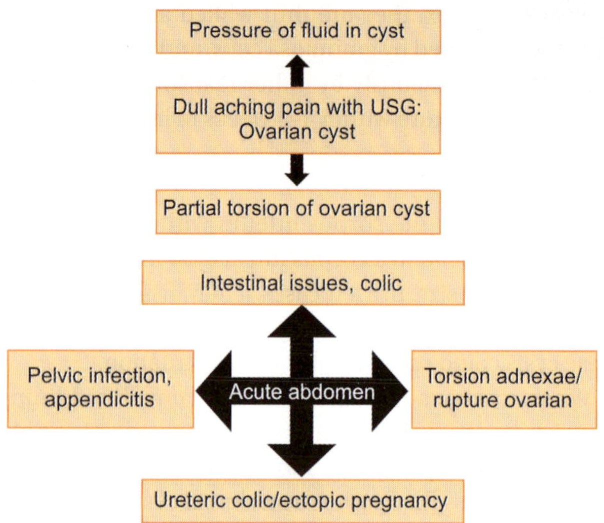

Some of the benign ovarian tumors are accompanied by endometrial hyperplasia due to excessive production of estrogen. This may cause heavy menstruation or even postmenopausal bleeding.

Physical Examination

Clinically, ovarian masses may be felt as a mass that moves separate from the uterus. Large ovarian cysts can be missed on per vaginal (PV) examination, as the cyst could have grown out of the pelvis. Per abdominal palpation is very important in such cases. The mass may be missed in obese women.

With liberal use of USG, most of the cases are diagnosed on USG. However, there is still a role for PV examination. PV may give a clue to pelvic infection when there is cervical tenderness. When one gets a report of ovarian cyst on USG, there should be a high index of suspicion of ovarian abscess, in the presence of a high count of polymorphs on blood examination, fever, and tenderness on PV. It is easy to misdiagnose it as a functional cyst leading to procrastination and progression to florid pelvic infection, which worsens in the waiting period **(Fig. 1)**.

DIAGNOSIS OF AN OVARIAN/TUBAL PATHOLOGY

To arrive at a diagnosis, the key factor is a good USG. Tumor markers, CT scan, and MRI can supplement this investigative modality. The need to use tumor markers or CT scan can be decided manly on USG findings with clinical correlation.

Ultrasound Features of Ovarian Cysts[4]

- *Follicular cysts*: Unilocular, thin-walled, with anechoic contents not larger than 8–10 cm. Lack of cyst wall papillae identifies them as simple cysts.[5]
- *Corpus luteal cysts*: Thick-walled hyperechoic cysts that typically demonstrate peripheral circumferential blood flow, sometimes known as the "ring of fire". The cyst

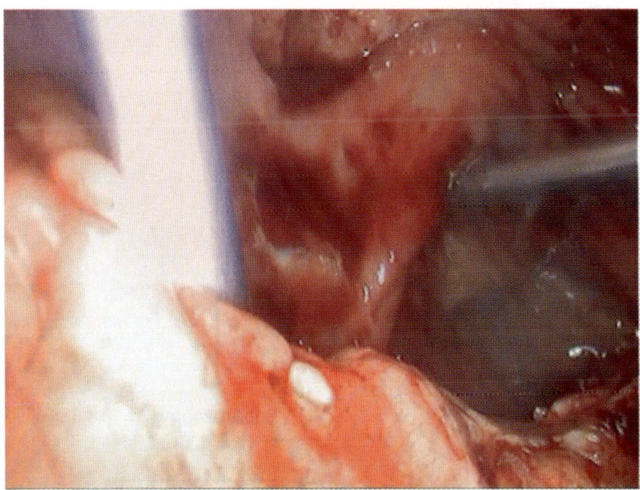

Fig. 1: Ovarian abscess bursting at laparoscopy. Patient was diagnosed with a complex 4 cm ovarian cyst. She had constant dragging pain for 4 months.

contents typically have a spider-web-like appearance due to a small amount of internal hemorrhage.

- *Serous cystadenomas*: These appear as smooth, thin-walled, anechoic, fluid-filled structures and their mean size is 5–8 cm. Persistence beyond 6–8 weeks may be the only differentiating point from functional cysts. Presence of papillae may be a pointer to cystadenoma.
- *Mucinous cystadenomas*: These are also thin-walled, but large and unilateral. However, the mucin they contain may appear as fluid with low level echogenicity.
- *Mature teratoma/dermoid cysts*: The cyst will have mixed echogenicity representing the different components of fat, bone, and fluid. A mural nodule representing areas of floating hair is a pathognomonic sign of dermoid cysts. Bright echoes and sharp acoustic shadows associated with hair or even teeth in the cyst may also be seen.
- *Ovarian fibromas and fibro thecomas*: Round or oval solid tumors with regular margins.
- *Tubo-ovarian abscess*: It appears as a complex cyst with thick walls and seemingly solid areas. When cystic areas start appearing in it, over time, percutaneous drainage may be possible in selected cases. It has to be differentiated from endometrioma or hemorrhagic cyst, and this is usually possible by corelating it with clinical findings.

Ultrasound Features of Tubal Pathology

Hydrosalpinx: The appearance on grayscale ultrasound is of a tubular and elongated cystic mass with incomplete septations or indentations along its walls ("waist sign" or "cogwheel"). In the chronic stage, small mural nodules may be noted, resembling "beads on string".

Tumor Markers Used in Detecting Malignancy in Ovarian Tumors

Cancer antigen 125 (CA125), human epididymis protein 4 (HE4), alfa-fetoprotein (AFP), hCG, lactate dehydrogenase (LDH), and inhibin are some of the tumor markers used to detect malignancy. Details are available in the chapter on ovarian malignancy.

Role of CT and MRI in the Work-up of Ovarian/Tubal Pathology

A CT scan is useful in suspected ovarian malignancy, especially to look for spread of malignancy. MRI is useful in differentiating clearly lesions, such as mature teratoma, endometrioma, and leiomyoma. These modalities along with color Doppler USG should be useful in evaluating adnexal masses diagnosed on USG.[6]

Differential Diagnosis of Ovarian/Tubal Pathologies

While diagnosing an ovarian cyst/tubal pathology, one has to keep in mind various pathologies that could mimic them. They are—hydronephrosis, hydrosalpinx, para-ovarian cyst, peritoneal pseudocyst, pedunculated leiomyoma, pelvic kidney, pelvic lymphocele, psoas abscess, abdominal abscess, ectopic pregnancy, ovarian torsion, polycystic ovarian syndrome, renal calculi, and urethral diverticulum.

Peritoneal pseudocysts are collections of peritoneal fluid trapped in adhesions usually caused by previous pelvic surgery, pelvic inflammatory disease or endometriosis. Para-ovarian cysts (*see* **Fig. 3**) arise in the broad ligament between the ovary and the fallopian tube.

Work-up of a Patient with Ovarian Pathology

When an ovarian cyst is diagnosed, several situations may arise, which can be handled, keeping in mind the age, USG findings, clinical correlation, and some blood tests **(Flowcharts 2 and 3)**. The special considerations of managing a pelvic mass in the adolescent age group is presented in **Flowchart 4**.

Cysts that can be left alone and not followed up:

- Simple cysts <5 cm in premenopausal women can be left alone as these usually resolve on their own in 2–3 cycles.

Cysts that need to be followed up:

- In postmenopausal women, even <5 cm simple cysts have to be evaluated in 4–6 months with repeat USG.
- Simple cysts, 6–7 cm in premenopausal women need to be followed up in 6 weeks' time as the difference between functional cysts and simple benign tumors, such as serous cystadenoma, may be very little on USG. In the latter, the cyst does not disappear on follow-up. If a cyst does not disappear in 10 weeks' time, a neoplastic pathology should be looked for.[2]
- Ovarian cysts in newborns are almost always functional and disappear rapidly, but should be observed for 2–4 weeks.
- Hemorrhagic cyst is a complex cyst. It should be rescanned in 6–8 weeks to differentiate corpus luteum (CL)

Flowchart 2: Management of simple ovarian cysts on USG.

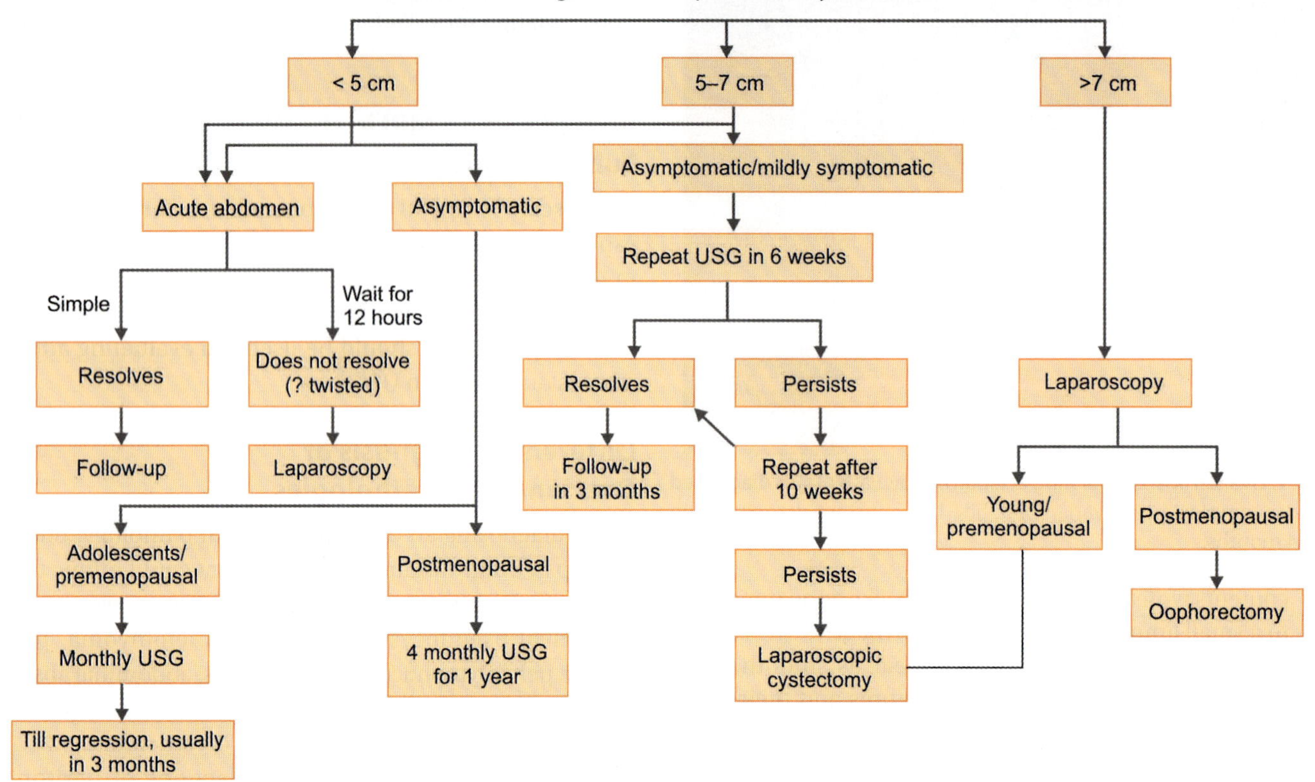

Flowchart 3: Complex ovarian cysts on USG.

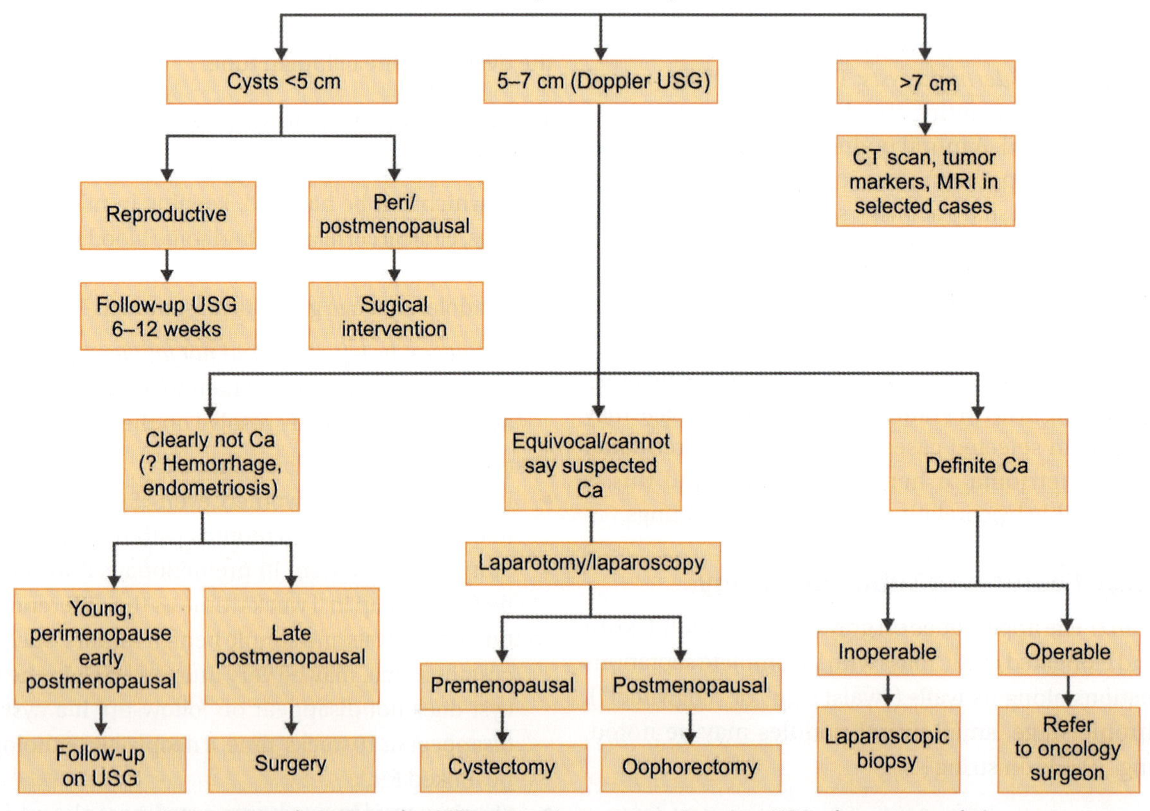

(CT: computed tomography; MRI: magnetic resonance imaging; USG: ultrasonography)

hemorrhage from endometrioma as CL hemorrhage may disappear on its own in the reproductive age group. Since early postmenopausal women also ovulate occasionally, follow-up is allowed in this group too. However, in the late postmenopausal group, a complex hemorrhagic cyst is more likely to be neoplastic and needs immediate surgical

Flowchart 4: Management of pelvic mass in adolescents.[16]

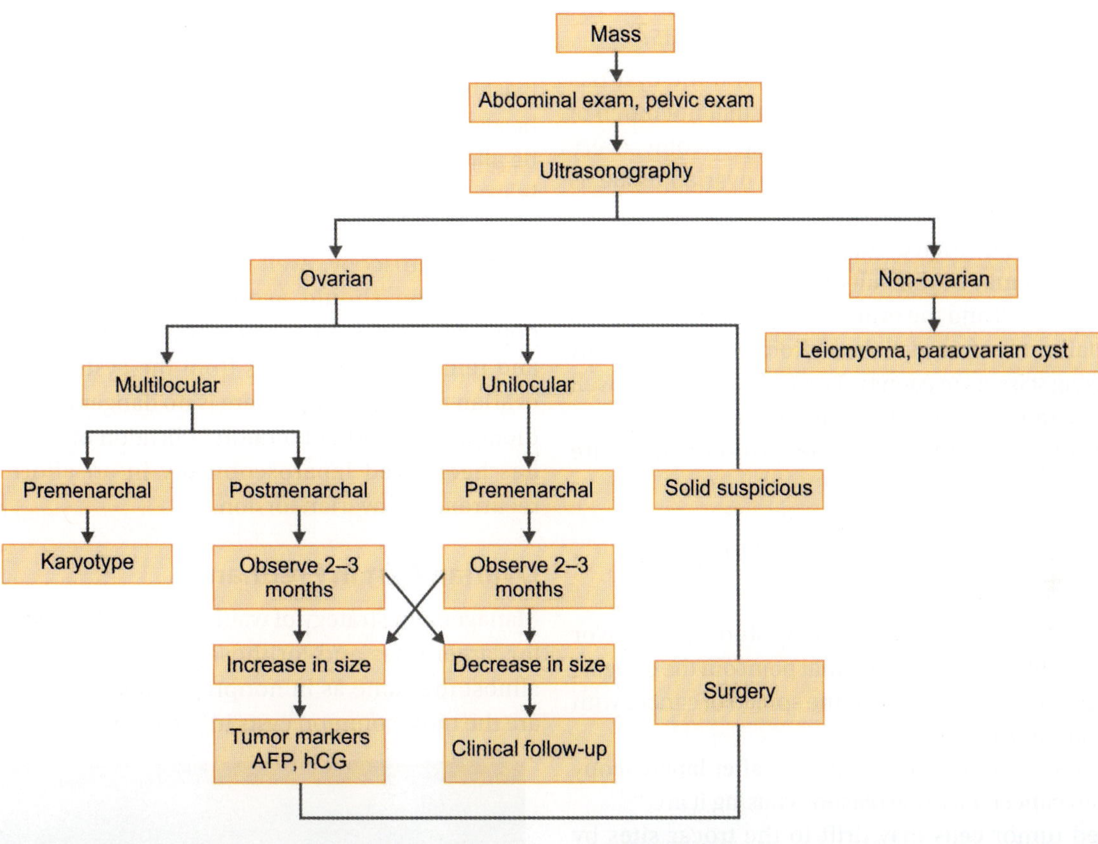

intervention as these women are not likely to ovulate compared to their younger counterparts.

- Endometriomas where surgical intervention is not done should be followed up yearly.
- Cysts that are >7 cm almost always need intervention. MRI or CT scan may be useful to give further information on these cysts, as rarely they could be large corpus luteal cysts or theca lutein cysts, which may in selected cases, be followed up without immediate surgery.

Pathologies that need surgical intervention:

- Cysts >7–8 cm where imaging modalities cannot diagnose clearly that the cyst is functional. Most often, these are benign ovarian tumors.
- Severely symptomatic cysts for large simple cysts (>5 cm), if symptoms did not resolve in 12–24 hours. Nonresolution of symptoms could be due to torsion of the cyst, which needs immediate intervention, to salvage ovarian tissue.
- Suspected tubo-ovarian abscess.
- Solid ovarian tumors.
- Dermoid tumors of any size.

Pathologies that suggests cancer, and therefore merit immediate intervention: Ovarian tumors do not have any one definite character, that can distinguish a benign tumor from a malignant tumor. Therefore, a combination of factors is taken to prognosticate the tumor as being benign or malignant. Some basic characters are seen more in malignant tumors. They are:

- Bilaterality
- Multilocularity
- Older age
- Postmenopausal status
- Thicker septae in the cyst
- Solid areas in the cyst
- Positive tumor markers
- Evidence of metastasis.

Keeping these in mind, several indices have been made, by which an ovarian tumor is evaluated, to see if it is malignant or not. The most popular among them is the risk of malignancy index (RMI). Other indices are Risk of Malignancy Algorithm (ROMA) and the International Ovarian Tumor Analysis (IOTA). Details of these indices are available in the chapter on Ovarian malignancy.

SURGICAL MANAGEMENT OF BENIGN OVARIAN PATHOLOGY

Surgical management is needed in large ovarian cysts, solid ovarian tumors, symptomatic cysts, or in ovarian cysts that do not decrease in size or disappear over time. In the premenopausal woman, where malignancy is not suspected, ovarian cystectomy, preferably by the laparoscopic approach, may be the best.[7] In postmenopausal women, ovarian function has ceased, and the chance for malignancy is higher. In this group, oophorectomy, or salpingo-oophorectomy is the surgery of choice. Solid ovarian tumors may need oophorectomy.

Gray Zones in Management

Should Cystectomy be Done in Very Large Cysts?

Large cysts are not always malignant. Even if the cyst has almost replaced the ovary, and it may seem that not much of the ovarian tissue will be left behind after cystectomy, every effort should be taken to preserve as much ovarian tissue as possible, especially in young women.

In large cysts, the ovarian tissue will be stretched so much over the cyst that it may be difficult to find the cleavage plane between the cyst wall and the ovary. In such cases, it helps to remove a small circle of ovarian tissue from the thinnest part of the cyst, using scissors or cautery. Lower down, the cyst wall will be thicker, and here it will be easier to do

Cystectomy as the cleavage planes will now be more visible.

Is Laparoscopy Safe in Women Where Malignancy Has not been Ruled Out?

This is a situation where there are many studies that favor laparoscopy and many other studies that point out the dangers of laparoscopy. Possible reasons for the spread of cancer with laparoscopy quoted are:

- Port site metastasis has been reported after laparoscopy for ovarian cancer. Possible reasons causing it are:[12,13]
  - Spilled tumor cells may drift to the trocar sites by contaminated instruments and pneumoperitoneum
  - Presence of ascites and direct contact of tumor to trocar canals
  - CO_2 and smoke from electrocautery with tumor cells implant to trocar sites when pressing out through narrow canals—the chimney effect
- Pressure of carbon dioxide used for pneumoperitoneum, acidity of the gas, combined with tumor cells falling on the peritoneum may damage the mesothelium, leading to metastasis.
- Rupture of a malignant cyst can upstage the disease to a higher grade.

In spite of reports of port site metastasis in earlier literature, several later studies have shown that in early stage of ovarian malignancy and in suspected or borderline ovarian malignancy, very good outcome is possible after laparoscopic surgery.[8-10]

Tips[11] to prevent trocar site metastasis:

- Suture of peritoneum and rectus sheath
- Excising the whole trocar site and suturing layer by layer
- Clean trocar site with povidone iodine
- Copious lavage of abdomen
- Avoid frequent removal of instruments to decrease chance for tumor infiltration.[12-15]

OVARIAN CYSTS IN SPECIAL SITUATIONS

Torsion of the Ovarian Cyst

Acute abdomen, autonomic symptoms like vomiting, and presence of ovarian cyst on USG lead to a diagnosis of torsion of ovarian cyst **(Fig. 2)** or paraovarian cyst **(Fig. 3)**. In complete torsion, unless immediate surgery is done, the ovary may undergo gangrene **(Fig. 4)**. In partial torsion, if the twist is corrected on its own or if the cyst bursts, surgery can be avoided. A reasonable time period of about 12 hours may be allowed, asking the patient to lie on the side where pain is less. If symptoms worsen, laparoscopic cystectomy should be resorted to.

At laparoscopy, even if the ovary appears gangrenous, the surgeon should avoid the temptation of doing an oophorectomy. Studies have shown that undoing the torsion and removing blood clots from the cyst can salvage some ovarian tissue **(Fig. 5)**. There is no danger in doing so as was thought of in earlier literature. Plication of ovarian ligament has been tried laparoscopically in an effort to prevent recurrence of ovarian torsion.

Ovarian Cyst in Pregnancy

Management strategy of waiting in smaller cysts and surgery for larger ones and for those that do not resolve remains almost the same as in nonpregnant state. Functional cysts are the most common cysts in pregnancy.

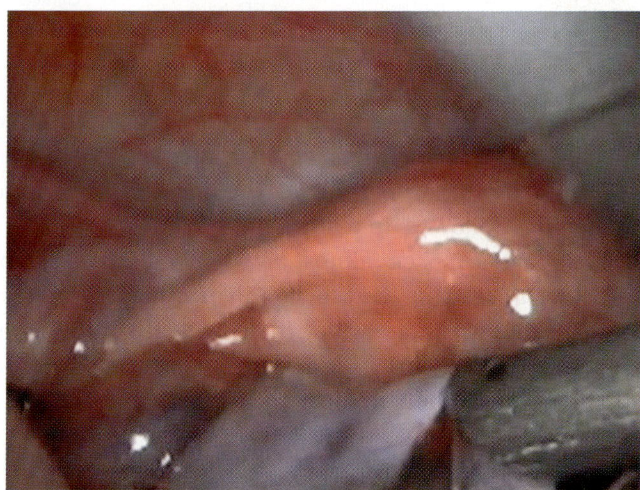

Fig. 2: Twist of twisted ovarian cyst.

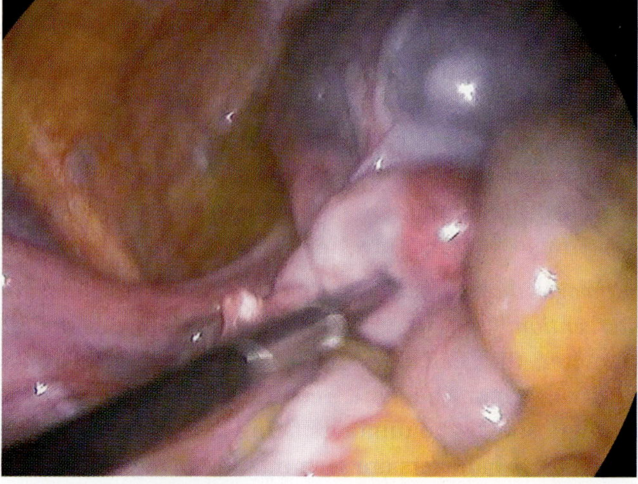

Fig. 3: Twisted para-ovarian cyst.

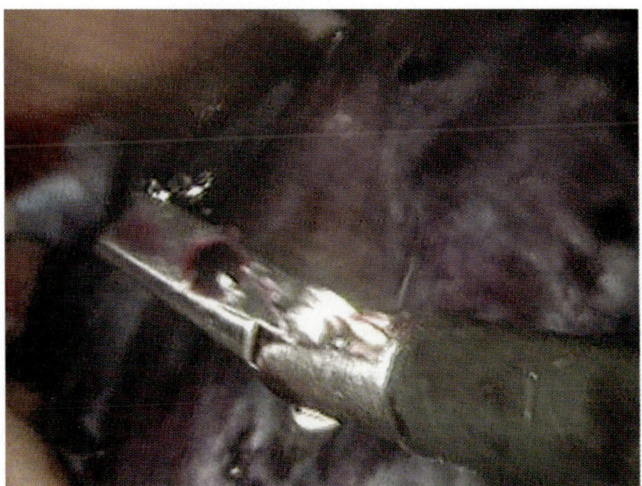

Fig. 4: Twisted gangrenous cyst in the only ovary in an unmarried lady. The other ovary had twisted ovarian cyst twice and it was removed the second time by the surgeon.

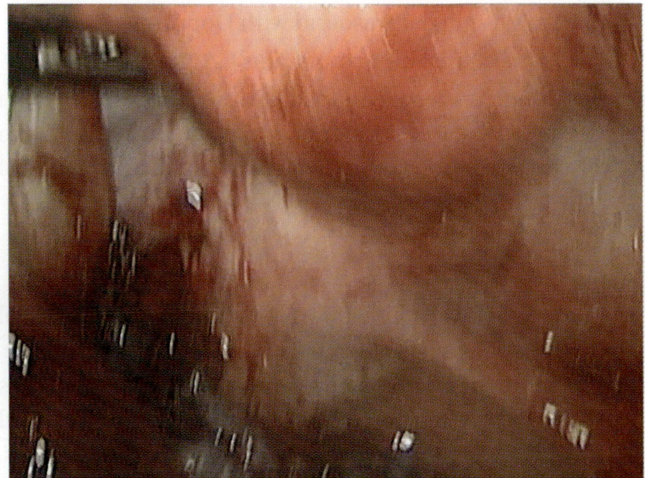

Fig. 5: A small papery thin ovarian remnant seen below after removal of clots in the case shown in Figure 2. Initially follicle-stimulating hormone rose to 65 IU, but the patient gradually got her periods and conceived. She has 2 children even with this sparse ovarian tissue in only one ovary.

If surgery has to be done, the best time is between 14 weeks and 20 weeks. Surgery in first trimester is associated with increased incidence of miscarriage and loss of luteal function due to cystectomy. Waiting into the third trimester can lead to rupture of the cyst, torsion, premature labor or progression into malignancy in suspected cases.

In expert hands, laparoscopy is safe in pregnancy. Putting a nasogastric tube to deflate the stomach may help. Primary trocar is best inserted by open laparoscopy supraumbilically. CO_2 is not detrimental to the fetus. Although data on tocolytics is not available, it is best to use them postoperatively, as manipulations on the ovary can make the uterus irritable.

Ovarian Remnant Syndrome

Sometimes after oophorectomy, some ovarian tissue may be left behind in the pelvic cavity. In some women, it may grow, undergo cystic degeneration, or hemorrhage and produce pain. The woman may present with chronic pelvic pain, dyspareunia, bowel symptoms, back pain or cyclic pelvic pain. USG may show a cystic lesion, but most often there may be no finding on USG.

In some cases, oral contraceptive (OC) pills may provide some relief, but in many cases, there may be no relief with OC pills or gonadotropin-releasing hormone (GnRh) analogs. Surgical removal, preferably using the laparoscope, may sometimes be the only way out. As ovarian tissue may be difficult to see among adhesions, it may be useful to stimulate the ovary with clomiphene citrate preoperatively, so that the ovarian tissue becomes cystic, and thus easier to locate.

The remnant is liable to be attached to vital structures like bowel bladder or even the ureter if the remnant is found in the lateral pelvic wall. Dissection of the remnant will be difficult and there may be a higher chance of bladder or bowel injuries associated with it.

CONCLUSION

Following standard guidelines in handling adnexal masses will help a lot in most situations, but there being many varied presentations for varied situations, it is necessary to innovate and decide for a particular patient after taking into consideration all risk factors.

KEY MESSAGES

- Ovarian cysts are a common finding on routine USG.
- Most of the cysts are functional.
- Distinction of an ovarian cyst from tubal cysts or hydrosalpinx is sometimes possible, but not always.
- USG is the best modality of investigating an adnexal pathology. Further delineation of the type of pathology may be done with CT scan or MRI.
- If the adnexal pathology appears to be a benign cyst, it may be prudent to wait for a few months to see if it disappears.
- If it does not disappear, cystectomy or oophorectomy has to be done.
- Every effort should be taken to determine if the pathology has borderline or overt malignancy, but quite often it is only on histopathology that it is possible to come to a final diagnosis.
- Follow-up of the case should be more diligent in the postmenopausal age group even if the cyst appears benign.
- Possibility of torsion ovary or ovarian abscess may require special decisions, like immediate surgery in selected cases, so in these situations, waiting and follow-up may not be possible.

REFERENCES

1. Hoffman BL, Schorge JO, Schaffer JI, Bradshaw KD, Halvorson LM, Corton MM (Eds). Williams Gynecology, 3rd edition. Australia: McGraw-Hill Education; 2016.

2. Katz VL (Ed). Comprehensive Gynecology, 5th edition. United Kingdom: Mosby Elsevier; 2007.
3. Yogambal M, Arunalatha P, Chandramouleeswari K, Palaniappan V. Ovarian tumours-Incidence and distribution in a tertiary referral center in south India. IOSR-JDMS. 2014;13(2):74-80.
4. Sayasneh A, Ekechi C, Ferrara L, Kaijser J, Stalder C, Sur S, et al. The characteristic ultrasound features of specific types of ovarian pathology (review). Int J Oncol. 2015;46(2):445-58.
5. Levine D, Brown DL, Andreotti RF, Benacerraf B, Benson CB, Brewster WR, et al. Management of asymptomatic ovarian and other adnexal cysts imaged at US: Society of Radiologists in Ultrasound Consensus Conference Statement. Radiology. 2010;256(3):943-54.
6. Valentini AL, Gui B, Miccò M, Mingote MC, De Gaetano AM, Ninivaggi V, et al. Benign and suspicious ovarian masses-MR imaging criteria for characterization: Pictorial review. J Oncol. 2012;2012:481806.
7. Demir RH, Marchand GJ. Adnexal masses suspected to be benign treated with laparoscopy. JSLS. 2012;16(1):71-84.
8. Ghezzi F, Cromi A, Uccella S, Bergamini V, Tomera S, Franchi M, et al. Laparoscopy versus laparotomy for the surgical management of apparent early stage ovarian cancer. Gynecol Oncol. 2007;105(2):409-13.
9. Semaan AY, Abdallah RT, Mackoul PJ. The role of laparoscopy in the treatment of early ovarian carcinoma. Eur J Obstet Gynecol Reprod Biol. 2008;139(2):121-6.
10. Mizrachi Y, Weiner E, Keidar R, Kerner R, Golan A, Sagiv R. Intraoperative rupture of benign mucinous cystadenoma does not increase its recurrence rate. Arch Gynecol Obstet. 2015;291(5):1135-9.
11. van Dam PA, DeCloedt J, Tjalma WA, Buytaert P, Becquart D, Vergote IB. Trocar implantation metastasis after laparoscopy in patients with advanced ovarian cancer: can the risk be reduced? Am J Obstet Gynecol. 1999;181(3):536-41.
12. Wang PH, Yen MS, Yuan CC, Chao KC, Ng HT, Lee WL, et al. Port site metastasis after laparoscopic-assisted vaginal hysterectomy for endometrial cancer: possible mechanisms and prevention. Gynecol Oncol. 1997;66(1):151-5.
13. Hopkins MP, von Gruenigen V, Gaich S. Laparoscopic port site implantation with ovarian cancer. Am J Obstet Gynecol. 2000;182(3):735-6.
14. Leminen A, Lehtovirta P. Spread of ovarian cancer after laparoscopic surgery: report of eight cases. Gynecol Oncol. 1999;75(3):387-90.
15. Chang WC, Lee LC, Huang SC, Sheu BC. Application of laparoscopic surgery in gynecological oncology. J Formos Med Assoc. 2010;109(8):558-66.
16. Berek JS, Novak E (Eds). Berek & Novak's Gynecology, 15th edition. Philadelphia: Lippincott Williams & Wilkins; 2012.

LONG QUESTIONS

1. What are the common benign neoplasms of the ovary?
2. Discuss the management approach to a 19-year old girl who presents with an acute abdomen to the casualty and has an ovarian cyst on ultrasound.
3. Discuss the role of laparoscopy in the management of an adnexal mass. What safety precautions to rule out malignancy should be taken when taking this approach?

SHORT QUESTIONS

1. What are functional ovarian cysts?
2. Mention the mechanisms of acute pain in an ovarian cyst.
3. What features of an ovarian enlargement favour torsion?
4. What surgical techniques can prevent recurrence of ovarian torsion?
5. What are the risks of laparoscopic surgery in ovarian borderline tumors?

MULTIPLE CHOICE QUESTIONS

1. A 64-year-old post-menopausal woman has been recently diagnosed with a 4 cm ovarian cyst on transabdominal scan. Which of the following investigations is best suited for further evaluation?
   a. CA125
   b. CT abdomen and pelvis
   c. Transvaginal ultrasound with Doppler
   d. Transvaginal ultrasound plus CA125
2. A patient undergoes laparoscopic cystectomy for a dermoid cyst and some spillage of contents occurs in to peritoneal cavity. What will be the incidence of chemical peritonitis?
   a. 5% b. 15%
   c. 25% d. 35%
3. A 32-year-old anxious lady presents with lower abdominal pain. She has a past history of irritable bowel syndrome. Pelvic ultrasound showed a 4 cm ovarian cyst which was followed up 6 months later, when the cyst was reported to be 5 cm. Serum CA125 was normal on both occasions. What is an appropriate management option?
   a. Repeat USG in 4–6 months
   b. Do nothing
   c. Laparoscopic cystectomy
   d. USG-guided cyst aspiration
4. An 18-year-old girl presents with urinary frequency. On examination she is found to have a lower abdominal mass. Ultrasound shows a 7 cm left-sided ovarian mass with mixed echogenicity. CT confirms the findings with fatty content s in the cyst but no other pathology. CA125 and carcinoembryonic antigen levels are normal. What is the appropriate management option?
   a. Diagnostic laparoscopy
   b. Laparotomy and removal of cyst
   c. Ultrasound guided cyst aspiration
   d. Repeat ultrasound in 4–6 months
5. A 29-year-old woman presents with sudden onset pelvic pain at approximately 11 weeks of gestation. She is investigated with an ultrasound scan, which confirms an intrauterine pregnancy of 12 weeks and a suspicious looking ovarian cyst 8 cm, was multicystic with some

solid areas, so some blood tests were performed. What blood tests would be most appropriate in this situation?
   a. Lactate dehydrogenase (LDH), human chorionic gonadotrophin (hCG), C-reactive protein (CRP)
   b. Lactate dehydrogenase (LDH), alfa-fetoprotein (αFP), human chorionic gonadotrophin (hCG)
   c. Lactate dehydrogenase (LDH), alfa-fetoprotein (αFP), C-reactive protein (CRP)
   d. CA125, lactate dehydrogenase (LDH), human chorionic gonadotrophin (hCG)
6. A 20-year-old woman attends the casualty with acute abdominal pain. The surgeon suspects appendicitis and performs a diagnostic laparoscopy. You are the on-call registrar for that night and the surgeon calls you to give an opinion on an incidentally found large solid ovarian mass in the right adnexa with papillary projections on the surface. There is some free fluid in the pelvis and the other ovary appears normal. What is the most appropriate next step in the patient's management?
   a. Refer to gynecology oncology center
   b. Ovarian cyst aspiration
   c. Ovarian cystectomy
   d. Staging laparotomy
   e. Oophorectomy

Answers

1. d 2. a 3. c 4. b 5. b 6. a

10.6 BENIGN LESIONS OF VULVA AND VAGINA

Rajashree Dayanand Katke, Deepti Prasad

INTRODUCTION

The aim of this topic is to know about common dermatoses seen in general practice to help in diagnosis and management.

It is non-neoplastic lesion of epithelium and mucosa of vulva and vagina.

ANATOMY

The vulva, which is visible externally, consists of mons pubis, labia majora, labia minora, clitoris, vestibule, and perineum. Bounder by mons pubis anteriorly, labia majora laterally, and perineum posteriorly.

Vagina is a fibromusculomembranous organ for copulation and parturition. It is a communicating canal between uterine cavity and exterior, providing passage for flow of secretions and menstrual blood. It has anterior (7 cm), posterior (9 cm), and two lateral walls. Its epithelium is under action of sex hormone, has stratified squamous epithelium without any gland (sweat and sebaceous) or hair follicles, from puberty till menopause.

ETIOLOGY

It is multifactorial:
- Traumatic
- *Irritation:* Cosmetic products, undergarments, perfumes, fecal, or urinary incontinence, etc.
- Allergies
- Infection
- Vitamin deficiencies
- *Systemic disorders:* Liver, hematological
- *Autoimmune conditions:* Thyroid disorder, diabetes, pernicious anemia
- *Drugs:* β-blocker, angiotensin-converting enzyme (ACE) inhibitors
- Cigarette smoking
- Personal/family history of atopy, such as eczema, hay fever, and asthma.

SYMPTOMS AND SIGNS

- Pruritus
- Pain
- Change in skin color and texture
- Dyspareunia.

APPROACH TO CASE

- Relevant history for etiology
- Investigations for thyroid, diabetes, and sexually transmitted infection (STI), if indicated
- Biopsy in nonresponsive and suspicious cases [vulvar intraepithelial neoplasia (VIN) or cancer]
- *Skin patch test:* In case of dermatitis to rule out potential contact allergens.

  Common lesions are discussed herein.
- *Lichen sclerosis*: Can present at any age but is more common in postmenopausal **(Fig. 1)**.

  Intense pruritus more at night leading to scratching causing bleeding, skin splitting, discomfort, pain, dyspareunia, also erythema and keratinization of vulval skin; figure of 8 distribution of vulval perineal region. It involves entire vulva, vestibule, clitoris, labia minora and inner labia majora, and anal skin. There may be lateral fusion of labia minora leading to difficult micturition. 40% women have or are going to have autoimmune condition. Biopsy is done to confirm diagnosis. Histology shows atrophic and flat epithelium with loss of rete ridges, and presence of hyalinized collagen tissue and chronic inflammatory cells.

  Treatment: Ultrapotent steroids; clobetasol propionate. In case of steroid resistance, calcineurin inhibitors, such as

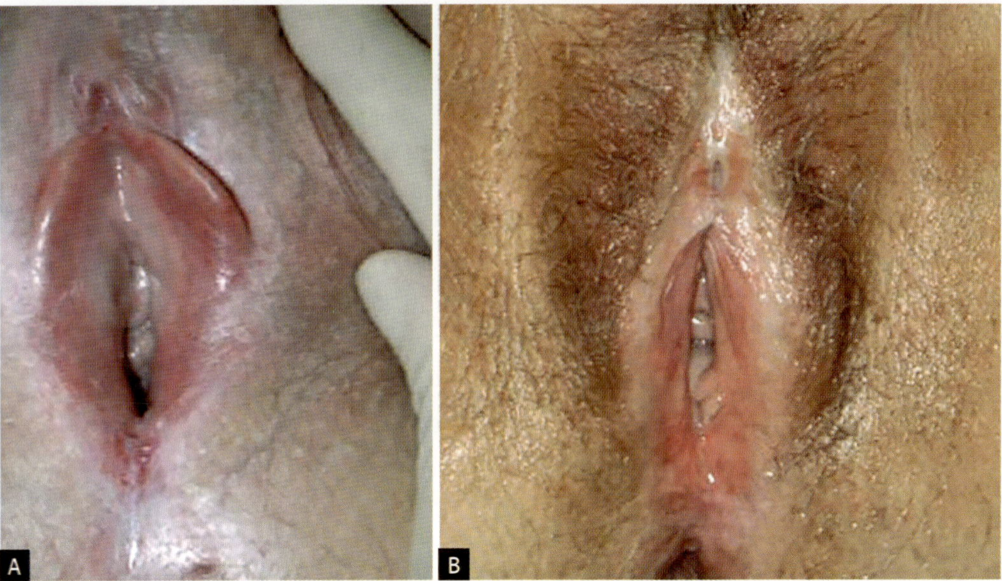

Figs. 1A and B: Lichen sclerosis.

tacrolimus and pimicrolimus, can be used. Surgery and CO_2 laser vaporization to release adhesions for urinary retention or narrow vaginal introitus.[1]

- *Lichen planus (**Fig. 2**):* It may affect skin anywhere on the body. It can affect all ages and not linked to hormonal status. It presents with polygonal flat-topped violaceous purpuric plaques and papules with fine white reticular pattern (Wickham striae).
  Treatment: Ultrapotent steroids; clobetasol propionate. In case of steroid resistance, calcineurin inhibitors, such as tacrolimus and pimicrolimus, can be used. Surgery and CO_2 laser vaporization to release adhesions for urinary retention or narrow vaginal introitus.[2]
- *Lichen simplex chronic/chronic vulval dermatitis:* It presents in women with sensitive skin, dermatitis, or eczema. Symptoms of intense itching are exacerbated by chemical or contact irritant. Serum ferritin should be checked.
  Treatment: General care of vulva, avoiding potential irritants, and use of emollients and soap substitute; antihistaminics and antipruritics; moderate or ultrapotent topical steroids.
- *Vulval candidiasis*: Irritation and soreness of the vulva and anus. Diabetes, obesity, and antibiotic may be the cause.
  Treatment: Oral or topical antifungal therapy.
- *Vulval psoriasis*: It can involve skin of the vulva but not vaginal mucosa. It often appears as smooth, nonscaly red or pink discrete lesions **(Fig. 3)**.
  Treatment: Emollients, soap substitutes, topical steroids, and calcipotriene are used for symptom control.
- *Behçet's disease:* It is a chronic multisystem disease. It presents as recurrent oral and genital ulcers involving the cervix, vagina, or vulva **(Fig. 4)**.
  Treatment: Topical or systemic immunosuppressants.
- *Extramammary Paget's disease*: It is rare, seen in postmenopausal women, and presents as pruritis. Lesions have florid eczematous appearance, lichenification, erythema, and excoriation. Underlying adenocarcinoma may be present. GIT, urinary tract, and breasts should be checked.
  Treatment: Surgical excision, photodynamic therapy, and topical imiquimod may be used.[3]

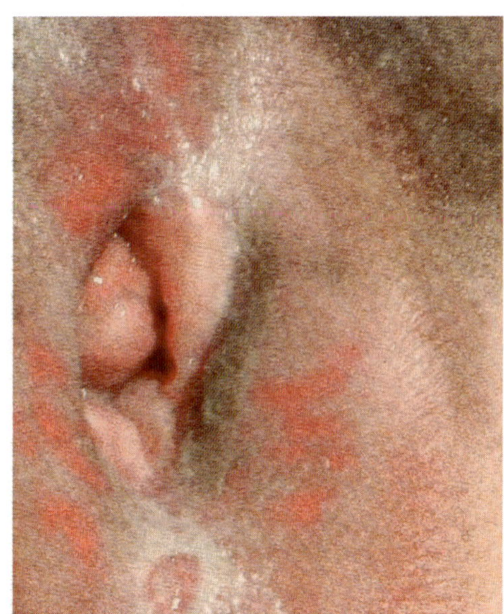
Fig. 2: Lichen planus.

- *Plasma cell (Zoon) vulvitis:* Histological diagnosis by dermal infiltration with plasma cells, vessel dilatation, and hemosiderin deposition.[4]
  Treatment: Topical ultrapotent steroids.
- *Vulval Crohn disease:* It involves the vulva by direct extension from involved bowel or metastatic granulomas **(Fig. 5)**.
  Treatment: Metronidazole and oral immunomodulators.[5]
- *Vulval cysts.*
- *Vulval varicosities*: Mostly during pregnancy; may cause pain on standing, subside following delivery.

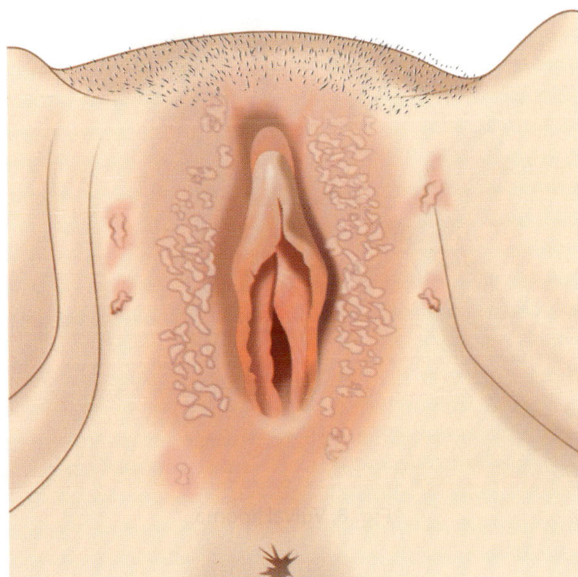

Fig. 3: Vulval psoriasis.

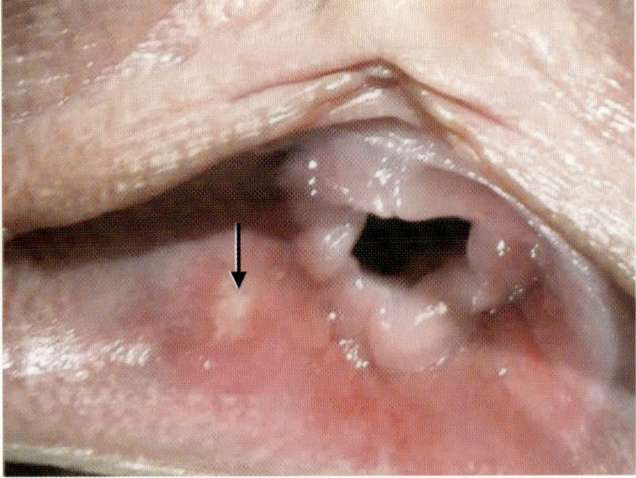

Fig. 4: Behçet's disease of the vulva.

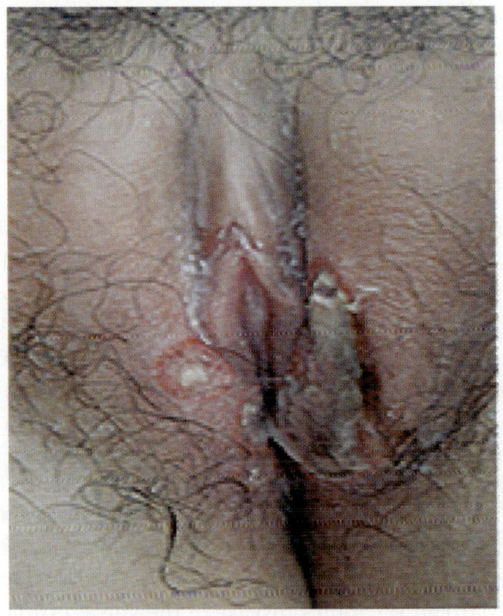

Fig. 5: Crohn disease of the vulva.

Treatment: Supporting pads, T bandage for symptom relief, sclerosing agent injection, and high ligation of long saphenous vein.

- *Elephantiasis vulvae*: Lymphatic obstruction by microfilaria.

  Treatment: Plastic surgery along with antifilarial treatment.
- *Vulval ulcers.*
- *Vulval pain syndrome*: Burning, stinging or irritation due to various causes.
- *Benign tumors of vulva*:
  - *Fibroma*: Vulval fibroma is rare and most common benign tumor that is predominantly found in women of reproductive age group. It is slow growing, arising from deeper connective tissues of labia majora and less frequently labia minora, clitoris, vestibule, and posterior commissure. In long duration, ulceration with superficial bleeding has been observed due to repeated trauma **(Figs. 6A and B)**.[6]

  Treatment: Surgical removal.[7]
- *Hidradenoma*: From vulval sweat gland, mostly in the anterior part of labia majora. Though benign lesion, its reddish look and histological complex adenomatous is confused with adenocarcinoma **(Fig. 7)**.

  Treatment: Biopsy and simple excision.[8]

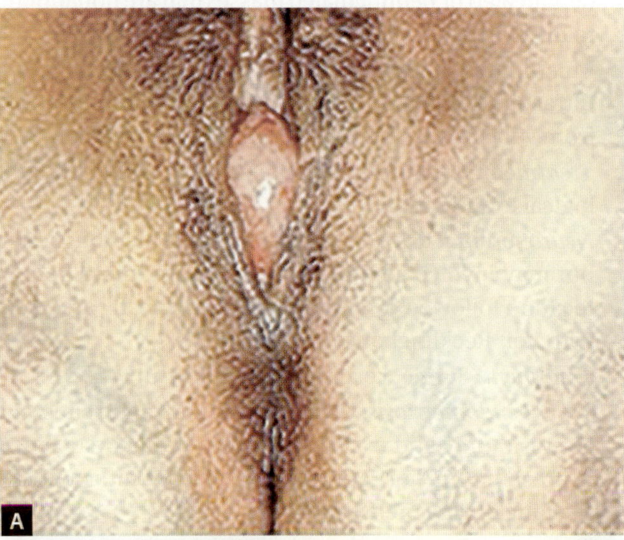

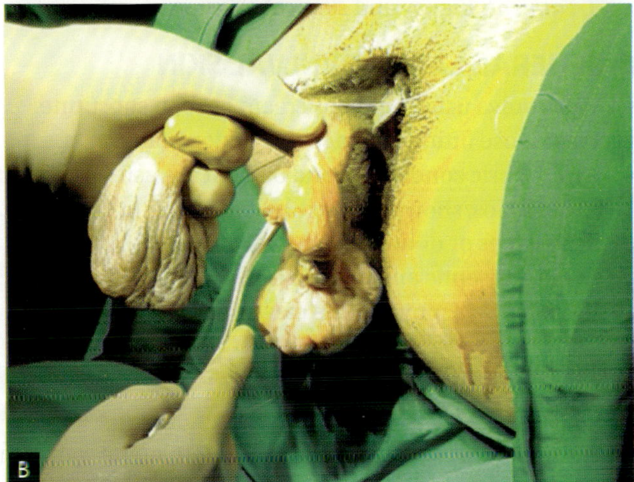

Fig. 6: Vulval fibroma.

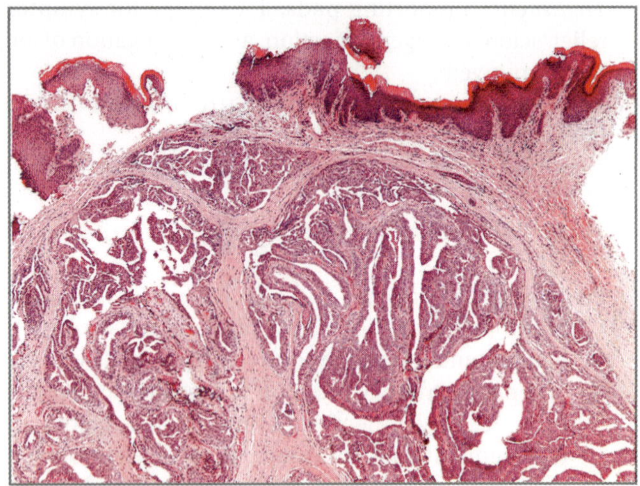

Fig. 7: Histopathology of hidradenoma vulva.

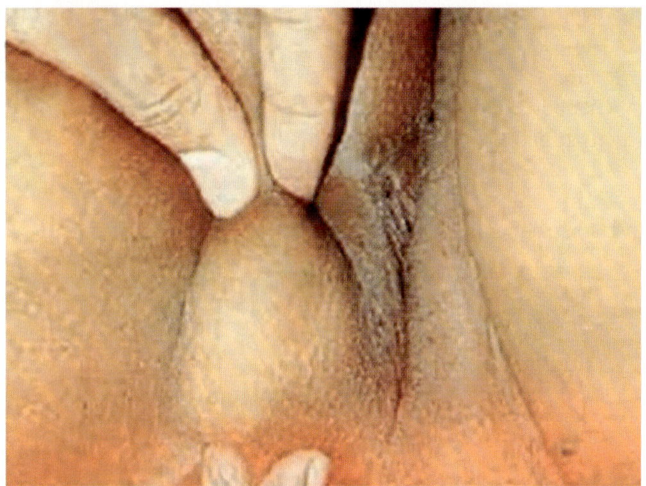

Fig. 8: Vulval lipoma.

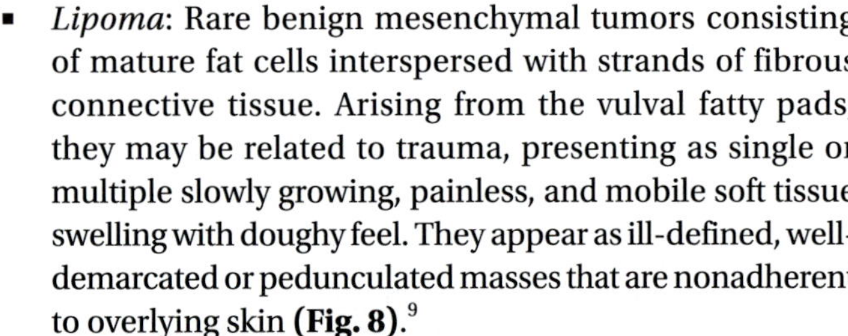

- *Lipoma*: Rare benign mesenchymal tumors consisting of mature fat cells interspersed with strands of fibrous connective tissue. Arising from the vulval fatty pads, they may be related to trauma, presenting as single or multiple slowly growing, painless, and mobile soft tissue swelling with doughy feel. They appear as ill-defined, well-demarcated or pedunculated masses that are nonadherent to overlying skin **(Fig. 8)**.[9]

  Mostly it is a clinical diagnosis, but when in doubt, ultrasound, CT, and MRI are useful in differentiating it from vulval cysts, inguinal hernias, and liposarcomas.

  Treatment: Complete surgical excision and histopathological examination.[10]
- *Neurofibroma:* It is a disease of peripheral nervous system, but may involve genital tract with vulva; most frequent location followed by clitoris and labia, mostly associated with Von Recklinghausen's disease.[11]

  Treatment: Surgical excision and follow-up.
- *Vulval endometriosis*: Usually at old laceration sites, such as episiotomy and excised Bartholin's duct cyst **(Fig. 9)**; it presents during reproductive period with pain and swelling during menstruation.

  Treatment: Biopsy and surgical excision.

GENERAL CARE OF VULVAL SKIN

- Wash vulva using aqueous cream or soap substitute
- Wear loose fitting silk or cotton underwear
- Avoid fabric conditioner and biological washing powders
- Avoid soaps, shower gel, scrubs, bubble bath, deodorants, baby wipes or douches in the vulval area
- Avoid antiseptic and colored toilet paper
- Emollients as moisturizers can be used.

BENIGN LESIONS OF VAGINA

Vaginal Wall Cysts

- *Gartner's duct cyst*: It is present in anterolateral wall of the vagina, made of columnar epithelium secreting mucinous material, which collects to form cyst.[12]

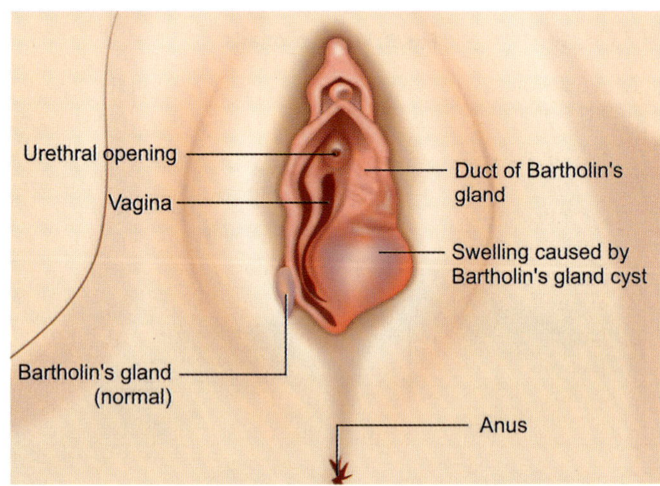

Fig. 9: Bartholin's cyst.

Treatment: Surgical excision.

- *Inclusion cyst (epithelial)*: Following traumatic injury during childbirth or surgery, healing leads to burying of epithelium under the mucosa, mostly in lower third of vagina on posterior or posterolateral wall, having stratified squamous epithelium.

  Treatment: Surgical excision.

REFERENCES

1. Khaitan BK. Nonvenreal diseases of genitalia. In: Sharma VK (Ed). Sexually Transmitted Diseases and AIDS, 1st edition. New Delhi: Viva Books Pvt. Ltd; 2003. pp. 413-21.
2. Soper DE, Patterson JW, Hurt WG, Fantl JA, Blaylock WK. Lichen planus of the vulva. Obstet Gynecol. 1988;72(1):74-6.
3. Yildiz P, Ronen S, Aung PP, Trinidad C, Kajoian A, Prieto VG. Extramammary Paget disease-A challenging case. Am J Dermatopathol. 2019;41(11):867-8.
4. Çelik A, Haliloglu B, Tanriöver Y, Ilter E, Gündüz T, Ulu I, et al. Plasma cell vulvitis: A vulvar itching dilemma. Indian J Dermatol Venereol Leprol. 2012;78(2):230.
5. Barret M, de Parades V, Battistella M, Sokol H, Lemarchand N, Marteau P. Crohn's disease of the vulva. J Crohns Colitis. 2014;8(7):563-70.

6. Najam R, Chowdhury HH, Awasthi S. A large fibroma polyp of labia majora? A case report. J Clin Case Rep. 2013;3:297.
7. Jones HW. Benign diseases of the vulva. In: HW Jones, AC Wentz, LS Burnett (Eds). Novak's Textbook of Gynecology. Baltimore: Williams & Wilkins; 1988. pp. 570-96.
8. Daniel F, Mahmoudi A, de Parades V, Flejou JF, Atienza P. An uncommon perianal nodule: hidradenoma papilliferum. Gastroenterol Clin Biol. 2007;31(2):166-8.
9. Sherer DM, Gorelick C, Wagreich A, Lee YC, Serur E, Zigalo A, et al. Sonographic findings of a large vulvar lipoma. Ultrasound Obstet Gynecol. 2007;30(5):786-7.
10. Lee JH, Chung SM. Large vulvar lipoma in an adolescent: a case report. J Korean Med Sci. 2008;23(4):744-6.
11. Gordon MD, Weilert M, Ireland K. Plexiform neurofibromatosis involving the uterine cervix, endometrium, myometrium, and ovary. Obstet Gynecol. 1996;88(4 Pt 2):699-701.
12. Hoogendam JP, Smink M. Gartner's duct cyst. N Engl J Med. 2017;376(14):e27.

LONG QUESTION

1. A 55-year old postmenopausal woman consults you for a discoloration on the vulval skin. Discuss the differential diagnosis and approach to her condition.

SHORT QUESTIONS

1. Name the common etiologies of vulval lesions.
2. What is the role of steroid treatment in vulval lesions?
3. Name the indications for surgical treatment in vulval lesions.

MULTIPLE CHOICE QUESTIONS

1. A postmenopausal women presented with florid eczematous lesion associated with lichenification and excoriation. The most probable diagnosis could be:
   a. Lichen planus
   b. Extramammary Paget's disease
   c. Lichen sclerosis
   d. Vulval psoriasis
2. Flat topped violaceous purpuric papules with white reticular pattern called Wickham's striae are seen in:
   a. Lichen sclerosis b. Lichen planus
   c. Vulval Crohn's d. Behcet's disease
3. dVIN is usually associated with which of the benign vulval condition?
   a. Vulval psoriasis b. Lichensimplexchronicus
   c. Lichen sclerosis d. Vulval cysts
4. Local steroid therapy is indicated in all the following vulval conditions, except:
   a. Vulval candidiasis b. Lichen sclerosus
   c. Lichen planus d. Bechet's disease
5. Clinically appreciable lesion is NOT seen in the following condition:
   a. Vulval cyst b. Herpes
   c. Elephantiasis vulvae d. Vulval pain syndrome

Answers

1. b 2. b 3. c. 4. a 5. d

10.7 GENITAL TRACT TRAUMA AND SEXUAL ASSAULT

Saroj Singh, Neha Agarwal

INTRODUCTION

Traumatic injuries to the genitourinary tract are seen in 2.2–10.3% of patients admitted to the emergency department.[1] One-third to two-third of these injuries are of the external genitalia.[1] Severe external genitalia trauma may also be seen in female genital mutilation (FGM) and self-mutilation in transsexuals and psychotic patients.[1]

There is higher risk in females of injuries to neighboring organs (bladder, urethra, vagina, and rectum) associated with genital trauma; therefore, it is very important to make accurate diagnosis and provide prompt and proper treatment for genital injuries. Sexual assault should always be considered in genital trauma.

DIRECT TRAUMA

Direct trauma of genital organs may include abrasions, cuts, lacerations, contusions, and hematoma of the vulva and vagina; cervical laceration or tear; uterine perforation and rupture; and broad ligament hematoma and fistula of the genital tract.

Etiology

Trauma to the vagina and vulva due to nonobstetrical causes can occur due to vigorous sexual intercourse, falling accidentally on pointed objects in the straddle position, jet skiing, water skiing, snowboarding, injury by blunt object, bull horn injury, etc.[2]

Genital trauma is quite common in girls, usually resulting from straddle injury **(Figs. 1A and B)**. Most of these straddle injuries are generally minor, still they are a cause of great anxiousness in children because of their sensitive location and concern about future sexual and gynecological development. The unestrogenized female genital tissues before puberty are friable, have good blood flow, and are nondistensibile. Therefore, even minor trauma can cause extensive injury and bleeding.

Specialized treatment is required if there are severe pelvic fractures or sexual assault and interpersonal violence. Genital trauma occurs in 20–53% of victims of sexual assault.

Presentation

Blunt trauma usually presents with blood staining of the underpants or the perineum and presence of contusions.[3]

Vaginal lacerations may be obstetric, which are sustained during childbirth, or nonobstetric, which may further be of two types.

First type is comparatively *minor* and is sustained during sexual intercourse, usually first. These lacerations generally resolve with minimal treatment.

Second type of laceration, which is usually caused due to injury or assault, is *more extensive and deeper*, and often results in *profuse vaginal bleeding* **(Figs. 2A and B)**. This requires immediate intervention as it can be a life-threatening situation.[2] These cases can have associated internal organ injury as well as injury to the lower urinary tract and urethra and classified according to severity **(Table 1)**.[1] If the associated injuries to the *urinary tract and gastrointestinal tract* remain unidentified in case of vaginal trauma, they may lead to formation of abscess, septicemia, and even death.

Perineal tears are classified according to extent of involvement **(Table 2)**.[4] Obstetric anal sphincter injuries (OASIS) mean the third- and fourth-degree perineal lacerations involving respectively, the anal sphincter and the rectal mucosa.[5]

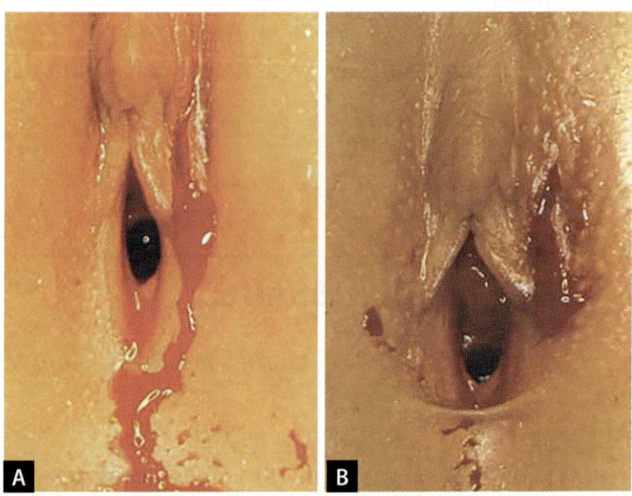

Figs. 1A and B: Straddle injury in a young girl.

Clinical Assessment

History

Detailed history is taken about the circumstances leading to the injury, the cause of injury, its timing, any first aid provided, ability to pass urine and feces normally, any other associated injuries, presence of witnesses, etc. If the history does not corelate with the injury, suspect and keep in mind a nonaccidental injury.

Examination

General assessment looking for evidence of other injuries. Examination of a child is usually done in *supine frog-legged position*. Gentle handling and explaining the process is important. Analgesia or sedation during procedure can be considered. Examination under anesthesia should be considered if the upper limit of the wound cannot be evaluated.

As it is extremely difficult to perform a thorough genitourinary examination in a child, especially if the child is anxious and uncomfortable; most of the patients are *best examined under general anesthesia in the operation theater*. Irrigation allows blood that may have collected to be washed away and the source of bleeding to be identified.

Look for any expanding hematoma or any anal, rectal or urethral involvement. *Vaginoscopy* may be needed if a more thorough evaluation of the injury is required. Illuminated nasal speculum or pediatric cystoscope may be used for visualization. A detailed description of the injury should be documented. The location of the injury can be shown by drawing a clock face in the notes **(Fig. 3)**.

May need *colposcopy, cystourethrography, proctoscopy, toluidine blue staining* **(Fig. 4)** and even laparoscopy/laparotomy for exact localization of extent and site of injury.

Management

The type of injury and its extent guides the management of female genital tract trauma. According to the severity,

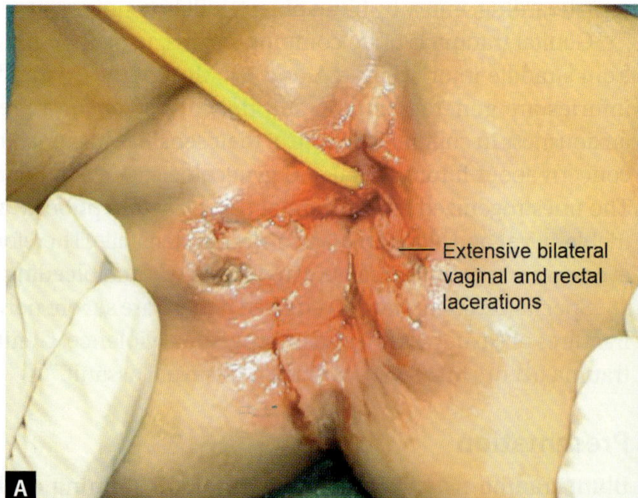

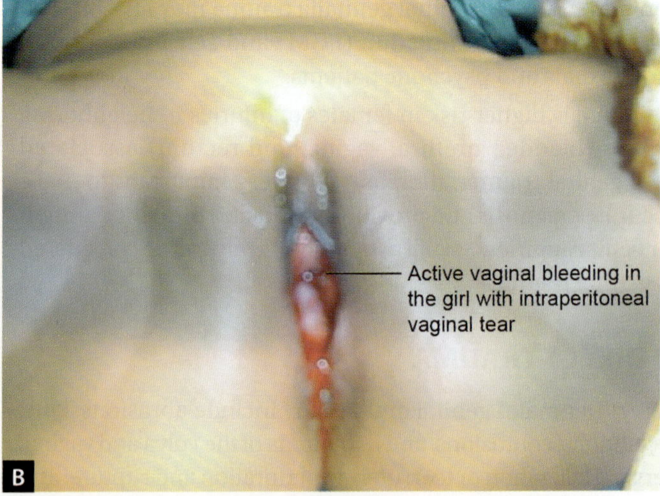

Figs. 2A and B: Extensive vaginal lacerations requiring immediate management.

TABLE 1: American Association for the Surgery of Trauma organ injury severity scale for the vagina and vulva.[1]

Grade[a]	*Description of injury*
I	Contusion or hematoma
II	Laceration, superficial (mucosa only)
III	Laceration, deep into fat or muscle
IV	Laceration, complex, into cervix or peritoneum
V	Injury into adjacent organs (anus, rectum, urethra, bladder)

[a]Advance one grade for multiple injuries up to grade III

TABLE 2: Classification of perineal tears.[4]

First-degree tear	Injury to perineal skin and/or vaginal mucosa
Second-degree tear	Injury to perineum involving perineal muscles but not involving the anal sphincter
Third-degree/complete perineal tear	Injury to perineum involving the anal sphincter complex
Grade 3a	<50% of external anal sphincter (EAS) thickness torn
Grade 3b	>50% of EAS thickness torn
Grade 3c	Both EAS and internal anal sphincter (IAS) torn
Fourth-degree tear	Injury to perineum involving the anal sphincter complex (EAS and IAS) and anorectal mucosa

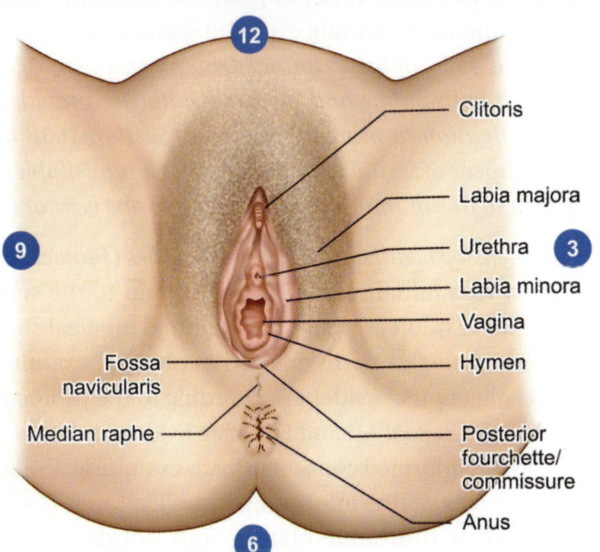

Fig. 3: A clock face can be used to describe the location of the injury.

the treatment may vary; with small hematomas needing only *conservative management* to severe injuries requiring *aggressive resuscitation and prompt surgical management.* Up to 75% of women presenting with vaginal injuries require repair. Up to 15% of the patients may present with a hemorrhagic shock.[6]

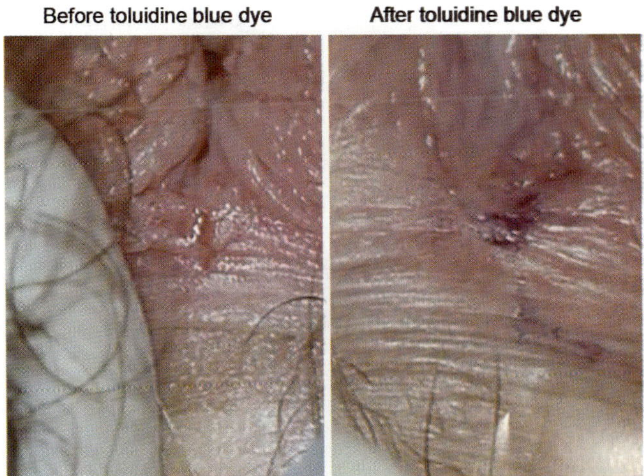

Fig. 4: Recent genital trauma better visualized after toluidine blue.

- General principles of care.
- Bleeding site to be compressed with a clean dressing pad.
- If the bleeding is from an abrasion and it is oozing, it can often be treated with ice and compression. If the oozing continues, then Gelfoam or Surgicel can be applied. A tampon or gauze can be used to pack the vagina in older adolescents if vaginal bleeding is significant.
- Ice packs can be used to decrease the swelling and bleeding, but they should not be applied directly over the clitoris.
- Review tetanus status.
- Vigorous sexual intercourse may cause vaginal *lacerations* in the distal part, which are usually 3–5 cm long. They are more common on the right side, located posteriorly. In fewer than 1% of the patients, these lacerations may extend into the peritoneal cavity.[6] Lacerations are primarily repaired after hemostasis is achieved. Absorbable sutures are used to preclude the need for removal.
- Urinary retention can occur with vulvar *hematomas.* These may require evacuation of large hematomas and insertion of a urinary catheter **(Fig. 5)**. Debridement of necrotic contused tissue is to be done. Smaller nonexpanding hematomas may be managed conservatively. Arterial embolization has also been successful in selected cases.
- *Repair of anal sphincter injuries*: The standard repair operation of perineal tear consists of *dissection of the vagina free from the rectum* and *identification of the ends of the anal sphincter*. Suturing of the tissues is then done in the following order from above downward—anal and rectal mucosa; anal sphincter; vaginal wall; levator ani muscles; superficial perineal muscles; and perineal skin.

Repair the torn internal anal sphincter (IAS) separately with mattress or interrupted sutures if it can be distinctly identified. A full thickness external anal sphincter (EAS) tear can be repaired using either an overlapping or an end-to-end approximation method with comparative outcomes. An end-to-end technique is recommended for partial thickness (all

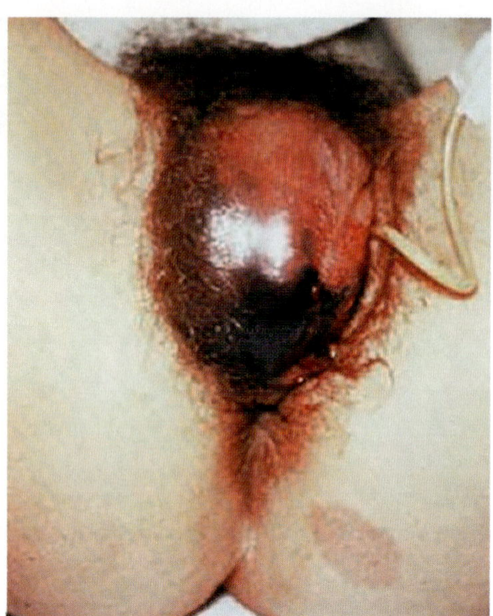

Fig. 5: A large vulval hematoma.

3a and some 3b) tears. The surgical knots should be buried under the superficial perineal muscles to reduce the risk of migration of knot and suture to the skin.[7]

Suture material: 3-0 polyglactin should be used to repair the anorectal mucosa. For the repair of the EAS and/or IAS muscle, either monofilament suture (3-0 PDS) or braided suture (2-0 polyglactin) can be used with equal outcomes.[7]

Timing: Repair of perineal tear can be done immediately after the injury is sustained or after 6–8 weeks with emergency colostomy, depending on extent and time of presentation.[8]

The results of the standard repair operation, performed at the right times, are usually satisfactory. Still, perfect sphincteric control may not be there even after anatomical success, especially in case of diarrhea.

- Surgical repair is almost always needed in case of life-threatening vaginal injury.[6]
- Always keep urological and abdominal injuries in mind.

A set protocol in place may help in a prompt evaluation and a speedy intervention. Services of pediatric surgeon/urologist/gastroenterologist may be required as per extent of injury.

SEXUAL ASSAULT

Sexual violence is defined by the World Health Organization (WHO) as "any sexual act, attempt to obtain a sexual act, unwanted sexual comments/advances and acts to traffic, or otherwise directed against a person's sexuality, using coercion, threats of harm, or physical force, by any person regardless of relationship to the victim in any setting, including but not limited to home and work."

Sexual assault is a form of sexual violence and is often used synonymously with rape. But it could include anything from touching another person in an inappropriate way without their consent to forced sexual intercourse, oral or anal sexual act, fondling, molestation of child, and attempted rape.[9]

The fourth most common crime against women in India is rape. There were 33,356 rape cases reported in our country as per the National Crime Records Bureau (NCRB) 2018 annual report. About 93.9% of these (31,320) were committed by someone who was acquainted to the victim.

In India, "rape" was recognized only as penovaginal sexual intercourse until 2012. As per section 375 of the IPC, the Criminal Law Amendment Act (CLA) 2013 has expanded the definition of "rape", to include *all forms of sexual violence—penetrative (oral, anal, vaginal) including by objects/weapons/fingers and nonpenetrative (touching, fondling, stalking, etc.) and recognized right to treatment for all survivors/victims/victims of sexual violence by the public and private healthcare facilities.*[9]

Under the law, failure to treat is now an offence. The law also does not allow any reference to be made with regards to the survivor's past sexual practices.

Role of Health Facility and Components of Comprehensive Response of Healthcare Professionals

We as health professionals have a double responsibility when responding to the survivors of sexual assault. Firstly, providing the necessary medical and surgical treatment and also psychological support. Secondly, assisting the survivors in their medicolegal proceedings by meticulously collecting evidence and documenting everything properly.[10]

Section 357C of the Criminal Law Amendment Act 2013 states that both public and private healthcare providers are under obligation to provide treatment. Section 166B makes non-treatment of sexual assault survivors a punishable act. It may lead to fine or imprisonment for up to one year or both.

*Comprehensive healthcare response includes **(Flowchart 1)**:*

- To provide initial resuscitation/first aid to the survivor of sexual assault as well as the required medical support
- To establish a uniform method of physical examination and collection of evidence according to the protocols [in the SAFE (Sexual Assault Forensic Evidence) kit]
- To obtain informed consent prior to examining, collecting evidence as well as informing the police
- To take a thorough history and conduct medical examination
- To estimate age (physical/dental/radiological)—if the investigating agency requests it
- To document and collect evidence according to the protocol
- To pack, seal, and maintain an unambiguous and proper chain of custody of medical evidence, which is handed over to police after collection
- To provide treatment of injuries

Flowchart 1: Components of comprehensive healthcare response to sexual violence.[9]

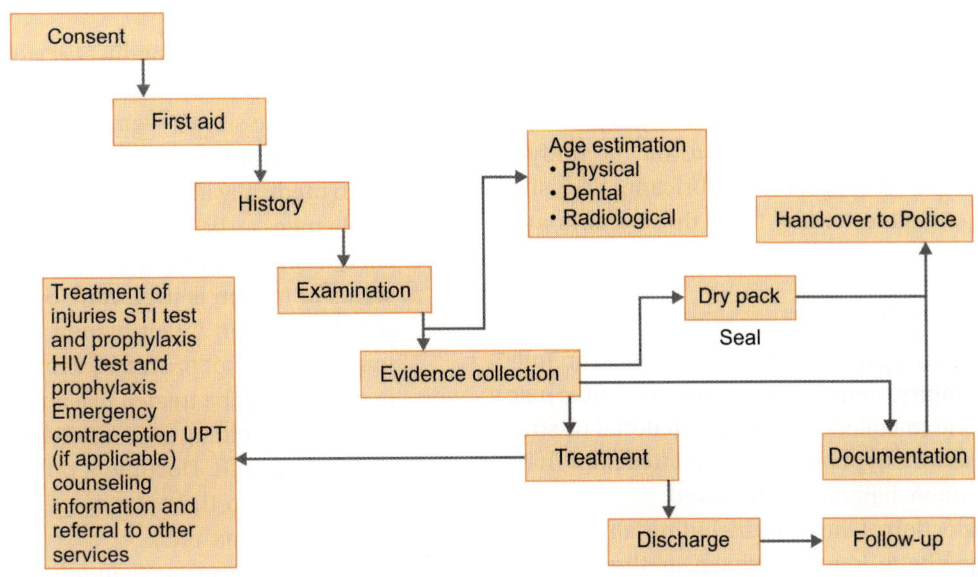

- To test or give prophylaxis for sexually transmitted infections, hepatitis B, and human immunodeficiency virus (HIV). The risk of pregnancy after rape is 10%, so emergency contraception should be given
- To provide first contact psychological support and validation
- To refer to appropriate agencies for further assistance (e.g., legal support services, shelter services, etc.).

Informed Consent

- The hospital is legally required to examine and treat with consent of the survivor or parent or guardian (according to age), if the person comes to the hospital directly without the police requisition.
- The person may or may not want to file a complaint if she has come on his/her own without FIR as she needs medical examination and treatment. The healthcare professional is required to inform the police by the law even in these cases.
- If the survivor comes with a police requisition or is stating that she wants to file a complaint later, record the details about medicolegal case *(MLC) number and police station.*
- It is not required for police personnel to be present during any part of the examination.

It is compulsory to get an informed consent or refusal for conducting examination and collecting evidence, providing treatment and informing the police in all these circumstances.

Note *two marks of identification*. Take left thumb impression in the given space.

Pertinent Surgical or Medical History

The relevant medical and surgical history should include a history of pelvic inflammatory disease, past gynecological and other surgeries and chronic medical conditions. The history should be focused and taken in a sensitive manner.

Sexual Violence History

The event of sexual violence which has brought the woman to the care provider may not be an isolated one. This may be a part of the circumstances in which a woman has to live and survive. This history may be difficult to obtain. The woman may not be forthcoming and the lack of rapport makes it difficult for her to open up to a new provider. The history may emerge later in the interaction or even at a later meeting.

General Physical Examination

- Orientation of the person to time, place, and person to be recorded and whether she is able to respond to all the questions. Note any signs of drug or alcohol intoxication by ingestion or injection.
- Record the vitals—pulse, blood pressure, respiratory rate, temperature, and state of pupils.
- Mention if the clothes are same as those worn during assault. Write down the state of clothes—if they are recently torn or have blood or semen or mud stains, etc.; describe the size, location, and color of such stains.

Examination of Injuries

- Only one-third of forced sexual intercourse cases present with injuries. Their absence does not imply consent of the survivor.
- Inspect the entire body area carefully to look for signs of physical torture, bruises, nail abrasions, teeth bite marks, cuts, lacerations, fracture, tenderness, any other injury, and lesions or discharge. The areas to be especially examined are the face, neck, scalp, shoulders, breasts, medial part of upper arms, forearms, wrists, buttocks, and thighs.
- All the injuries are to be described in detail—*the type* (abrasion, incision, laceration, contusion, etc.), site, size, color, shape, swelling, signs of healing, simple or grievous.[11]

If possible, mention the likely weapon of infliction, e.g., sharp, blunt, smooth, rough, etc.

- *All the injuries are to be marked on body charts so that they can be best represented.* Mark on the body charts with numbers and describe each in detail.
- Note down the presence of *any stains* on the body—describe their type (blood, semen, lubricant, etc.), site, size, color, etc. Collect swabs from these stains and mention their sites.

Local Genital Examination

- Examine the external genital area and perineum carefully for presence of injury, seminal stains, and stray pubic hair. Combing is done to collect any foreign material or stray hair. Preserve sample of pubic hair and matted pubic hair. Make a note if pubic hair has been shaved.
- Systematic inspection of the *vulva* including labia majora and minora, fourchette, introitus, hymen, urethral meatus, and vestibule is to be done. Look for signs of recent injury, such as bruises, bleeding, tears, abrasions, swelling, or infection and discharge. Posterior fourchette is the most common site of injury in sexual assault **(Fig. 6)**.[12]
    - Use a sterile speculum lubricated with sterile water or warm saline for examination of the *vagina* of an adult female. Inspection is done to look for redness, bruises, bleeding, and tears. These may even be extended to the perineum, especially in very young girls. If the injuries are suspected but not visible, use a good light source to look for micro-injuries. A magnifying glass or colposcope may be used if available. 1% toluidine blue stains the micro-injuries blue. All these tests should be done only after collecting swabs for trace evidence.
    - In children or young girls who do not give history of penetration and there are no visible injuries, a *per speculum examination* is not necessary. In minors, especially with severe injuries, the treatment as well as examination may have to be performed under general anesthesia.

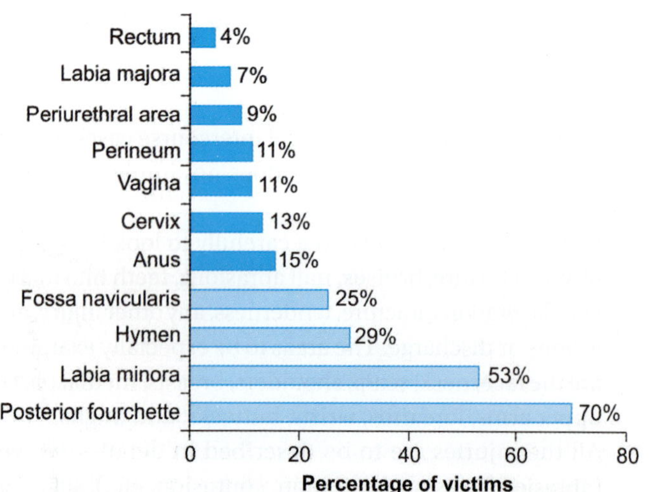

Fig. 6: Patterns of genital injury from sexual assault.[12]

Mention the color, odor, and texture of vaginal discharge, if present.

- It is not necessary to conduct *per vaginum examination* to establish rape or sexual assault. In a case of sexual violence, the size of vaginal introitus has no bearing. Do per vaginum examination in an adult woman only when medically indicated.
- The hymen can be torn during many physical activities, such as cycling, riding or masturbation, etc. So the status of hymen is irrelevant. Sexual violence is not ruled out by an intact hymen and previous sexual intercourse is not proved by a torn hymen. Therefore, hymen should be treated like any other genital organ when documenting the examination findings in cases of sexual assault. Document only those findings that are relevant to the episode of assault (fresh tears, bleeding, edema, etc.).
- *Mark and appropriately number the genital findings on body charts.*

- Document any tears, bleeding, stains, swelling, discharge or warts around the anal orifice. Carry out per-rectal examination to identify stains, tears, fissures or hemorrhoids in the anal canal and collect relevant swabs.
- Examine oral cavity for any sign of tear, bleeding, discharge, edema or tenderness.

Sample collection for hospital or clinical laboratory:

- *Radiographs of shoulders, elbow, wrist, dental examination,* etc., can be advised for estimating age if requested by police.
- Advise appropriate investigation of the relevant body part in case of suspected fracture or injury.
- The doctor on duty should perform *urine pregnancy test* and enter the report.
- Collect blood for documenting baseline *HIV status, venereal disease research laboratory (VDRL), and HbsAg.*

Sample collection of samples for central/state forensic science laboratory:

- It should be determined what evidence needs to be collected after properly assessing the case. The samples will depend on the nature of assault, duration between assault and examination, and whether she has washed herself or bathed since the violence.
- *Collect all evidence including swabs if the woman reports within 4 days (96 hours) of the assault,* according to the nature of the assault. Although the chances of finding evidence after 3 days (72 hours) are greatly minimized, it is prudent to collect evidence up to 96 hours as the survivor may not be sure about the number of hours passed since the act.
- As the spermatozoa can only be identified for 72 hours after sexual violence, in these cases, swabs should be sent only for tests for semen identification.
- The evidence on the body surface and clothing can be collected even after 96 hours.

- The survivor is requested to stand on a large sheet of paper. Any foreign materials like grass, mud, pubic or scalp hair, etc., which may have been transferred from the accused or the place of assault should be collected on it. Carefully fold this sheet of paper and preserve it in a bag that is sent for detection of trace evidence to the forensic science laboratory.
- Separately preserve the clothes that the survivor was wearing at the time of assault if they have any stains, tears or trace evidence. These are of evidentiary value.
- Properly note the presence of stains—semen, blood, foreign material, etc. If the woman has changed the clothes already then ask for the ones worn at the time of assault and preserve them.
- The samples and clothes should be air dried before storing them in labeled packets. Each piece of clothing should be packed in a separate bag, sealed, and labeled.
- *Two swabs are to be taken from the vulva, vagina, and anal opening for anogenital evidence.* If there is a history of penetration, only then collect swabs from orifices. Prepare two vaginal smears on the provided glass slide, air-dry it in the shade, and send for detection of seminal fluid or spermatozoa.
- Distilled water is provided in the kit to moisten the swab sticks for sample collection.
- It is necessary to dry the swabs to prevent degradation or decomposition of evidence. They are to be air-dried under shade, not in direct sunlight.

About 2–3 mL of saline is infused in the vagina using a small rubber catheter and a syringe. The fluid is aspirated and collected. A knot is tied over the rubber catheter and the fluid-filled syringe is sent to the forensic science laboratory.

- Check that the numbering on the requisition form and the numbering of individual packets match.

Evidence on body:

- Take swabs from the stains on the skin surfaces—blood, semen, foreign material, etc. Presence of pubic or scalp hair of the survivor on the accused's body and vice versa has evidentiary value. Collect all hair in the catchment paper and then fold it and seal it.
- In case of physical struggle during assault, the survivor and the accused may scratch one another. DNA may be found in the epithelial cells under the nails of the other. Take nail clippings and scrapings from both hands and pack them separately.
- Collect blood for grouping as well as to compare and match blood stains at the crime scene.
- Urine and blood are to be collected for detecting drugs or alcohol. The validity of consent is questioned if these substances are present.
- The likelihood of finding evidence from oral swabs is highest when they are taken posteriorly from behind the last molars.

Provisional Clinical Opinion

- Immediately after finishing the examination, corelate the history and clinical examination, and draw professional inference and note down.
- Mention the relevant points in history, clinical findings, and samples sent for analysis to laboratory in the provisional clinical opinion.

Rape and sexual violence have a major effect on public health. Women's healthcare providers, especially gynecologists, should keep a keen eye to screen all women for sexual assault. When examining and evaluating survivors of sexual assault, we have to follow certain medical and legal requirements. It is important to identify the short-term and long-term health consequences of sexual violence, such as infection, pregnancy, and mental health problems, and providing their proper management.

FEMALE GENITAL MUTILATION

The procedures involving partial or total removal of the external female genitalia as well as other nonmedical injuries to the female genital organs are included in FGM **(Table 3)**.[13]

The FOGSI accepts and supports the international consensus regarding FGM or cutting being a harmful practice and a violation of girls' and women's rights to life, physical integrity, and health. FGM in any form and to any extent is a cruel traditional practice. There are about 27 countries in which FGM is practiced by their citizens (Africa and Yemen, Asia, Middle East, few population groups in Central and South America) as well as immigrants from these countries.

The classification of FGM is based on the anatomical extent of the procedure **(Table 3)**. Clitoridectomy or excision is involved in about 90% of FGM, and infibulation in around 10%. The most severe negative consequences are seen with infibulation.

Health Consequences

There is documented medical evidence of the risk of hemorrhage, infection, and shock at the time of female genital mutilation, as also long-term physical and sexual consequences, including incontinence, infertility, obstetric

TABLE 3: Types of female genital mutilation.[13]

Type 1	*Clitoridectomy:* Partial or total removal of the clitoris and/or in very rare cases only, the prepuce
Type 2	*Excision:* Partial or total removal of the clitoris and the labia minora, with or without excision of the labia majora
Type 3	*Infibulation:* Narrowing of the vaginal opening through the creation of a covering seal. The seal is formed by cutting and repositioning the inner, or outer, labia, with or without removal of the clitoris
Type 4	*Other:* All other harmful procedures to the female genitalia for nonmedical purposes, e.g., pricking, piercing, incising, scraping, and cauterizing the genital area

complications, and psychological problems, including serious consequences for sexuality.

Management

Specialist multidisciplinary FGM services should be offered. Examination findings should be accurately recorded in the clinical records. Legal and regulatory procedures must be followed. Sexual health screening, HIV, hepatitis B and C testing as well as psychological assessment and treatment should be given to all patients.

De-infibulation should be offered after counseling to women who are likely to benefit from it, before pregnancy, ideally before first sexual intercourse. Avoid performing clitoral reconstruction because of its high complication rates. Manage labial tears in the same way as in women without FGM.

CONCLUSION

Female genital trauma is an important subject to be taken care of. Early recognition and prompt management prevents future sexual, obstetrical, and psychosocial problems. Involvement of adjoining structures needs to be excluded. Suspicion of sexual assault should always be kept in mind unless proved otherwise. Genital trauma in children and adolescent needs extra care and may require services of specialists.

KEY MESSAGES

The risk of associated injuries to neighboring organs (bladder, urethra, vagina, and rectum) after genital trauma is higher in females; thus accurate diagnosis and treatment of genital injuries are of utmost importance. Early recognition and prompt management prevent future sexual, obstetrical, and psychosocial problems. Involvement of adjoining structures needs to be excluded. Suspicion of sexual assault should always be kept in mind unless proved otherwise. Both private and public healthcare providers are obligated to provide treatment to sexual assault survivors. Genital trauma in children and adolescent need extra care and may require services of specialists.

REFERENCES

1. Berger I. Genital trauma. In: Hohenfellner M, Santucci RA (Eds). Emergencies in Urology. Berlin, Heidelberg: Springer; 2007.
2. Sloin M, Karimian M, Ilbeigi P. Nonobstetric lacerations of the vagina. J Am Osteopath Assoc. 2006;106(5):271-3.
3. Singhal VP, Neelam Ankur HK, Kaur P, Katiyar N. Traumatic massive vulval haematomas. Int J Gynae Plastic Surg. 2010;2:35-7.
4. Sultan AH. Obstetric perineal injury and anal incontinence. Clin Risk. 1999;5(6):193-6.
5. Joshi AV, Pradhan M, Gupta AS. Obstetric challenges with previous unrepaired third degree perineal tear. JPGO. 2017;4(12).
6. Jana N, Santra D, Das D, Das AK, Dasgupta S. Nonobstetric lower genital tract injuries in rural India Int J Gynaecol Obstet. 2008;103(1):26-9.
7. Royal College of Obstetricians and Gynaecologists. RCOG Green-top Guideline No. 29. (2015). The management of third- and fourth-degree perineal tears. [Online] Available from: https://www.rcog.org.uk/globalassets/documents/guidelines/gtg-29.pdf [Last accessed December, 2021].
8. Malhotra N, Malhotra J, Kumar P, Bora NM. Injuries. Jeffcoate's Principles of Gynaecology. New Delhi: Jaypee Brothers Medical Publishers; 2014.
9. Ministry of Health & Family Welfare. Government of India. (2014). Guidelines & protocols medico-legal care for survivors/victims of sexual violence. [Online] Available from: https://main.mohfw.gov.in/sites/default/files/953522324.pdf [Last accessed December, 2021].
10. ACOG Committee Opinion No. 777: Sexual Assault. Obstet Gynecol. 2019;133(4):e296-e302.
11. Roland D, Lewis G, Rowlands R, Davidson E, Davies F. Female perineal injuries in children and adolescents presenting to a paediatric emergency department. Emerg Med J. 2016;33(1):73-5.
12. Sommers MS. Defining patterns of genital injury from sexual assault: a review. Trauma Violence Abuse. 2007;8(3):270-80.
13. Royal College of Obstetricians and Gynaecologists. Green-top Guideline No. 53. (2015). Female genital mutilation and its management. [Online] Available from: https://www.rcog.org.uk/globalassets/documents/guidelines/gtg-53-fgm.pdf [Last accessed December, 2021].

LONG QUESTIONS

1. How will you manage a 9-year-old girl with bleeding per vaginum following bullhorn injury?
2. Discuss the management of a 17-year-old girl with suspected sexual assault.
3. A 5-year-old girl is brought to you with retention of urine and history of fall from bicycle. How will you manage her?
4. How will you examine a case of sexual assault? What samples will you collect?

SHORT QUESTIONS

1. What are the components of comprehensive healthcare response to sexual violence?
2. Write short note on FGM.
3. Discuss the management of:
   i. Vulval hematoma
   ii. Complete perineal tear
4. How will you classify genital injuries?

MULTIPLE CHOICE QUESTIONS

1. Sexual assault does not include:
   a. Rape
   b. Forced sexual activity that does not result in penetration
   c. Oral or anal intercourse
   d. Flashing ones genitalia at the victim
   e. Attempted rape

2. Which statistics are incorrect with regard to sexual assault?
   a. 90% of victims of sexual assault are women
   b. 98% of offenders are men
   c. 1.5% of the adult women are sexually assaulted each year
   d. 25% of sexual assault victims report the incidence to police
   e. <5% of sexual assault victims need admission to hospital
3. Most nongenital injuries of sexual assault are found on the:
   a. Head
   b. Arms
   c. Chest
   d. Back
   e. Legs
4. Which is true with regard to specimen collection of a sexual assault?
   a. Vaginal and cervical swabs are taken with a wet swab stick and plated onto slides. Both slide and swab are included for evidence
   b. Semen on the skin is collected by using a wet swab stick then a dry swab stick, both are plated onto slides and all swabs and slides are included for evidence
   c. A dry swab stick rubbed in the buccal mucosal is insufficient to gain patient DNA for comparison
   d. Patient blood collected for drug analysis put into normal hospital collection tubes but these tubes go with the police for forensic assessment
   e. Finger nails scrapings must be rubbed on a glass slide at the time of collection
5. The risk of becoming pregnant from a rape is:
   a. 15%
   b. 10%
   c. 7.5%
   d. 5%
   e. 2.5%
6. Which of the following statements is false?
   a. The likelihood of getting sperm from the vagina at 72 hours is very low
   b. Acid phosphatase is normally found in both seminal fluid and vaginal fluid
   c. Acid phosphatase can be detected in the vagina for up to 14 hours
   d. PSA can be detected in the vagina for up to 48 hours
   e. A police officer, usually female, must be present at the examination to ensure the "chain of evidence" is continued
7. How should the morning after pill be taken?
   a. Two OCP each containing ethinyl estradiol 50 μg within 12 hours of sexual intercourse and two more taken at 72 hours post sexual intercourse
   b. Two such pills taken as a single dose within 72 hours of sexual intercourse
   c. Two such pills taken within 72 hours of sexual intercourse and two more taken 12 hours later
   d. Two pills taken at 12 hours post sexual intercourse and two more taken 72 hours later
   e. Two pills taken with 12 hours of sexual intercourse does not require a second dose
8. With regards to the forensic medical examination of a sexual assault, which of the following statements is false?
   a. Photography of genitalia is not allowed routinely
   b. Each item of clothing that a person is wearing must be placed in a separate bag, they cannot be put in the same bag
   c. All clothes and specimens should be handed directly to the attending police officer
   d. The results of the forensic tests are available for the victim if they approach the medical officer
   e. Informed consent for specifically for specimen collection is required
9. Which site of bruising would make you suspicious of child abuse?
   a. Anterior shins
   b. Knees
   c. Upper arms
   d. Elbows
   e. Forehead
10. Examining a girl who is a victim of sexual assault, which of the following statements is false?
    a. They are usually examined in the frog leg position
    b. The use of a speculum is usually advocated
    c. General anesthetic should only be used if internal injuries requiring surgical repair are suspected
    d. The hymen can be best seen without instrumentation and the girl supine with her knees drawn to her chest
    e. Semen fluoresces with a Woods lamp

Answers

1.	d	2.	d	3.	a	4.	a	5.	b	6.	d
7.	c	8.	d	9.	c	10.	b				

10.8 DYSPAREUNIA AND VAGINISMUS

Shantanu Abhyankar

"The surgeon thinks of difficult coitus as a knife passed through muscles in spasm; the psychiatrist thinks of dyspareunia as a mental knot to be disentangled by analysis; the gynecologist who is weary of patching poor and late patching begins to think in terms of prevention through routine premarital examination and instruction."[1]

INTRODUCTION

Sexual medicine is a field infested with quacks, for want of physicians trained and willing to practice it and good research to support such practice. However, slowly and surely newer research has brought it into the ambit of modern, rational medicine and qualified doctors are rapidly replacing the quacks. An obstetrician-gynecologist often faces individuals/couples with sexual problems and the reactions range from awe to acute embarrassment. The person(s) seeking help are equally ill at ease. A good clinician should therefore be a good listener, be comfortable with the language used (which at times borders on the vulgar), be able to give adequate time, and be nonjudgmental and supportive.

PREVALENCE

Various studies have reported the prevalence to be between 6% and 27%.[2,3] Sporadic dyspareunia is estimated to be 4–8-fold higher.[4]

THE PROBLEM OF CLASSIFICATION

Women's sexual disorders have traditionally been classified according to the phases of the sexual response cycle; disorders of desire, arousal, orgasm, etc. This classification is now thought to be inadequate. Moreover, disorders of sexual pain (vaginismus and dyspareunia) do not fit into any one "phase" of the sexual response cycle. In fact, the assumption that vaginismus and dyspareunia are two distinct entities has been challenged.[5-9] Both seem to have the following three components to varying extent:

1. Problems of muscle tension, voluntary or involuntary; limited to the vaginal muscle or extending to the pelvic floor, at times involving the adductor muscles, back, jaw, etc.
2. Fear of sexual pain associated with genital touching or coitus; or fear of intercourse for reasons other than pain.
3. Tendency toward avoidance. Despite pain, some women continue to accept and tolerate sexual touching or even intercourse while others rabidly guard their genitalia from any type of touch.

With this background, let us now dwell on what we know of vaginismus, dyspareunia, and vulvar vestibulitis syndrome (VVS).

DEFINITIONS

Vaginismus: Vaginismus is defined as an involuntary spasm of the pubococcygeus muscles in the female when coitus or insertion of a finger or object (e.g., speculum) in the vagina is attempted.

An international committee has recently recommended the following definition[10]—"The persistent or recurrent difficulties of the women to allow vaginal entry of the penis, a finger and/or any object, despite the women's expressed wish to do so. There is variable (phobic) avoidance, involuntary pelvic muscle contraction, and anticipation/fear of experience of pain. Structural and other physical anomalies should be ruled out/addressed."

This results in difficult, often impossible, penetration. Pain, burning at the introitus, and dyspareunia with forced intromission is reported. Commonly, even a visual physical examination is refused and a lot of fuss made over separating the labia to look at the introitus.

Dyspareunia: Recurrent or persistent genital pain associated with sexual intercourse.[10] This can be subdivided into deep or superficial pain. Dyspareunia could be with or without VVS.

Vulvar vestibulitis syndrome: This includes painful penile vaginal intercourse or pain upon touching the vulvar vestibule and signs limited to variable vestibular erythema.

NEUROBIOLOGY OF THE PELVIS

Readers are referred to the textbooks of anatomy and physiology for a detailed review, but a few points of clinical significance will be covered here.

Pelvic floor is now thought to be an integrated functional structure with varied disorders of micturition, defecation, sexual and genital pain, thought to be "pelvic floor dysfunctions". There is now evidence to show that the pelvic floor, like some other muscle groups, is indirectly innervated by the limbic system, and therefore highly responsive to emotional stimuli and stress.[11-13]

The pelvis is innervated by the autonomic (sympathetic and parasympathetic), as well as somatic (sensory and motor) nerves. Odd as it may appear, it is now known that the afferent sensory nerves of the pelvis carry efferent signals as well!! Electrical stimulation of the sensory nerves near the spinal cord leads to impulses toward the spinal cord (orthodromic) as well as toward the periphery (antidromic). The antidromic impulses produce vasodilatation, edema, and hyperalgesia in the area of innervations. This is called neurogenic inflammation. This is an adaptive response in normal circumstances but can get maladaptive. This probably explains pain in interstitial cystitis, vulvodynia, and many other painful conditions of the pelvis for which no cause has been discerned.

Neuropathic pain is typically characterized by spontaneous paresthesias, dysesthesias, and evoked pain. Pain is experienced when impulses reach the brain via A delta or C fiber nociceptive afferents. Minor tissue injuries can cause reduction in the threshold for nociceptors resulting in "peripheral sensitization". This leads to responses to weak non-noxious stimuli—"allodynia". Further stimulation will lead to exaggerated pain response—"primary hyperalgesia". Allodynia can also occur due to abnormal signal amplification in the central nervous system called "central sensitization". Here the signals entering the CNS through non-nociceptive A-beta touch fibers evoke pain. The exact cause of increased descending excitatory signals and/or decreased inhibitory signals to allow this is unclear. Frequent success of therapies with tricyclic antidepressants, venlafaxine, carbamazepine or gabapentin appears to support this theory.

INDIVIDUAL PSYCHOLOGICAL AND PERSONALITY CHARACTERISTICS IN WOMEN WITH VAGINISMUS

Women with vaginismus have been noted do to have higher rates comorbid anxiety disorders like agoraphobias without panic disorder and obsessive compulsive disorder. Personality traits suggest the presence of self-focused attention and negative self-evaluation.

INDIVIDUAL PSYCHOLOGICAL AND PERSONALITY CHARACTERISTICS IN WOMEN WITH DYSPAREUNIA (AND/OR VESTIBULITIS)

In women with dyspareunia due to vestibulitis, no definite trends have been noted apart from the fact that these women have increased anxiety and depressive disorders. Attention bias of hypervigilance for pain relation stimuli has been noted.

In those without vestibulitis, signs of hostility, psychotic symptoms, erotophobia, negative/conservative attitude toward sex, and sexual aversion are common. They have more problems with experiencing sexual arousal and relationship issues are common.

MUCOUS MEMBRANES AND SEXUAL PAIN DISORDERS

Acute inflammation of the vulvovaginal mucous membrane is a common cause of dyspareunia. Often the cause is readily discernible; candidiasis, trichomoniasis, and herpes being common.

In chronic vulvovaginal pain, it is difficult to pinpoint a cause. Iatrogenic inflammation due to self-treatment is a common cause that is often missed.

There are three main types of mucous membrane diseases—chronic vulvar dermatoses, vulvar vestibular syndrome, and vulvodynias.

Chronic Vulvar Dermatoses

Lichen simplex, lichen sclerosis, and lichen planus can cause severe sexual pain. Lichen simplex is the result of the itch-scratch cycle due to chronic scratching. Topical steroids and oral antihistaminic usually help.

Lichen sclerosis is a result of extreme thinning of the epidermis leading to parchment paper appearance of the skin. Topical steroids appear to be the treatment of choice.

Lichen planus gives rise to superficial ulcers with concomitant inflammation of the vaginal mucosa and profuse discharge. Often Behçet's syndrome like picture is seen with involvement of oral, esophageal mucosa. Topical steroids for a prolonged period, interleukin inhibitors, and anti-inflammatory agents are the key to treatment.

Vulvar Vestibulitis Syndrome

The classical triad is vulvar itching, burning, and pain with sexual activity and the classical triad is vulvar itching, burning and pain. This can be with sexual activity or otherwise. Sometimes sitting or running too can be painful.

Vulvodynias (Syn: Dysesthetic Vulvodynia)

Intense burning sensation causing profound sexual and psychological distress is usually the presenting symptom. There are no positive findings at all. Culture, biopsies, etc., are negative. Topical treatment increases the pain. Oral tricyclic antidepressants or anticonvulsants offer a reduction in symptoms.

COMMON ETIOLOGIES

With the above background, **Table 1** lists the common causes of sexual pain. Many of the conditions are commonly seen and sexual pain may or may not be the presenting complaint. The onus lies on the clinician to gently probe this aspect of the problem and help the patient open out and seek more specific treatment if need be **(Fig. 1)**.

CLINICAL APPROACH TO SEXUAL PAIN

Clinicians are often perplexed about how exactly to go about asking details of sexual pain. Here is brief list of questions that will help.

Questions qualifying various aspects of the distress need to be asked.

a. Pain:
   i. Where does it hurt? How would you describe the pain?
   ii. Is it with contact with introitus? With partial entry? Full entry? Deep thrusting? With ejaculation? After withdrawal? With subsequent micturition?
   iii. Does your body tense up on attempt at insertion by partner? What are your fears and feelings then?
   iv. How long does the pain last? Does touching elsewhere in the genital area cause pain? Does it hurt when you ride a two wheeler or wear tight clothes? Do other types of penetration hurt? (Tampons, fingers)

TABLE 1: Causes of sexual pain.

Superficial	*Deep*
• VVS	• Estrogen deficiency
• Atrophy	• Vaginitis
• Vulvitis, vulvovaginitis	• Chronic PID
• Interstitial cystitis	• Fibroid uterus
• Condylomata	• Ovarian tumor
• Dermatologic diseases	• Hemorrhoids
• Noninfectious inflammations	• Fixed inverted uterus
• Episiotomy neuroma	• Ovarian remnant syndrome
• Epithelial defects	• Foreshortened vagina
• Scarring	• Endometriosis
• Size of penis	• Vaginal septum
• Urethritis	• Urethritis/cystitis
• Anatomic variations	• Chronic abdominal pain
• Hymenal remnants	• Irritable bowel syndrome
• Radiation	

(PID: pelvic inflammatory disease; VVS: vulvar vestibulitis syndrome)

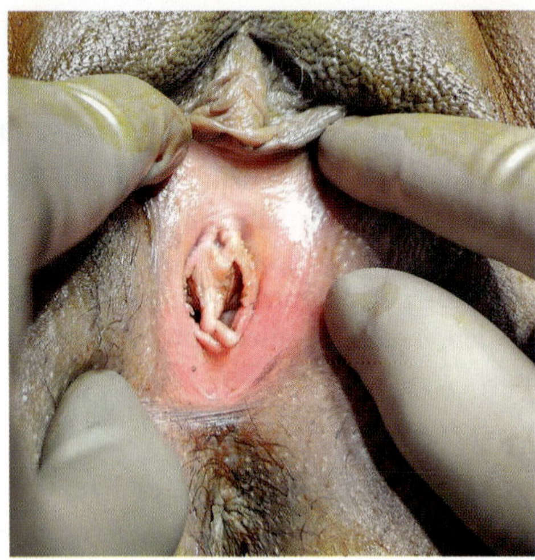

Fig. 1: Narrow introitus with longitudinal vaginal septum.

b. Pelvic floor muscle tension:
   i. Do you realize the sensation of pelvic floor muscle tension during sexual contact and/or in non-sexual situations?
c. Arousal:
   i. Do you feel subjectively aroused when sexually stimulated/does your vagina feel sufficiently moist? Do you recognize the feeling of dying up?
d. Consequences of the complaint:
   i. What do you do when you experience pain during sexual contact? (continue/stop intercourse/continue to make love without intercourse)?
   ii. Do you currently include intercourse or attempts at intercourse or do you use other ways to make love? If so, are you both comfortable with this arrangement?
   iii. What consequences does pain have on the rest of your relationship?
e. Biomedical antecedents:
   i. When and how did the pain start? What tests have been done?

EDUCATIONAL GYNAECOLOGICAL SEXOLOGICAL EXAMINATION

If conducted in a proper manner, the examination of a patient with sexual pain in itself can be diagnostic as well as therapeutic!

An educational gynecological sexological examination is different than a routine one in following aspects.

It may not be the part of evaluation in the first consultation itself. The patient and the care provider are to decide the timing, nature, and persons present during this examination. As far as possible, the participation of the sexual partner is encouraged.

There are three steps to be followed. Counseling about how and what is going to be done and about the anatomy of the genitals with the help of suitable diagrams/films, etc. Patient should be assured in advance that she has total control over the procedure and nothing will be done without her explicit consent. She is assured that during the examination, her personal boundaries will be respected. She should also be told that the use of speculum or such other means for internal examination will not be used unless she permits it. The next is the examination proper where the patient is given a hand mirror and the examiner sees, points out, explores, and examines the external genitalia while giving a running commentary about what is going on. Apart from seeking verbal approval for what is being done, a close watch is kept for nonverbal signals from the patient and her partner. If all the findings are normal, it is important to specifically state so. The patient is asked to spread the vulva herself. The vulva is carefully inspected including the labia minora, majora, the crease between the clitoral hood and clitoris, the posterior fourchette, vestibule, hymen, and hymenal edge. For women with introital dyspareunia, areas of allodynia are explored using a cotton Q tip. The skin at the openings of the Skene's ducts must also be examined as it is frequently involved. A new instrument named Vulvalgesiometer is useful in quantifying the vulvovaginal pain. By bearing down or coughing the patient will be able to see the introitus getting larger. With good rapport and gentle technique, an internal examination too may become possible. Some may even allow a transvaginal scan, which is informative in deep dysparunia.

QUESTIONNAIRE ASSESSMENT OF PATIENTS WITH SEXUAL PAIN

Questionnaires are the best way to save time, bypass embarrassment faced by the patient while narrating her complaints and get a quick overview of what is going to be said. Questionnaires administered before and after treatment can help in assessing the efficacy of treatment.

Many validated questionnaires are available in English; but in the Indian context, they need to be translated and revalidated in the local language. Cultural ethos of the subcontinent needs to be considered while translating these questionnaires.

Here is the "female sexual function index (FSFI)", which tests for several domains of female sexual dysfunction (and not just pain). The part provided here lists the questions with standard options. For scoring analysis protocols, readers are advised to visit *http://www.fsfiquestionnaire.com.*

Female Sexual Function Index

Subject Identifier ______________ Date ________________

Instructions: These questions ask about your sexual feelings and responses during the past 4 weeks. Please answer the following questions as honestly and clearly as possible. Your responses will be kept completely confidential. In answering these questions, the following definitions apply:

Sexual activity can include caressing, foreplay, masturbation, and vaginal intercourse.

Sexual intercourse is defined as penile penetration (entry) of the vagina.

Sexual stimulation includes situations like foreplay with a partner, self-stimulation (masturbation), or sexual fantasy.

Check only one box per question.

Sexual desire or interest is a feeling that includes wanting to have a sexual experience, feeling receptive to a partner's sexual initiation, and thinking or fantasizing about having sex.

1. Over the past 4 weeks, how often did you feel sexual desire or interest?
   - □ Almost always or always
   - □ Most times (more than half the time)
   - □ Sometimes (about half the time)
   - □ A few times (less than half the time)
   - □ Almost never or never
2. Over the past 4 weeks, how would you rate your level (degree) of sexual desire or interest?
   - □ Very high
   - □ High
   - □ Moderate
   - □ Low
   - □ Very low or none at all

   Sexual arousal is a feeling that includes both physical and mental aspects of sexual excitement. It may include feelings of warmth or tingling in the genitals, lubrication (wetness), or muscle contractions.
3. Over the past 4 weeks, how often did you feel sexually aroused ("turned on") during sexual activity or intercourse?
   - □ No sexual activity
   - □ Almost always or always
   - □ Most times (more than half the time)
   - □ Sometimes (about half the time)
   - □ A few times (less than half the time)
   - □ Almost never or never
4. Over the past 4 weeks, how would you rate your level of sexual arousal ("turn on") during sexual activity or intercourse?
   - □ No sexual activity
   - □ Very high
   - □ High
   - □ Moderate
   - □ Low
   - □ Very low or none at all
5. Over the past 4 weeks, how confident were you about becoming sexually aroused during sexual activity or intercourse?
   - □ No sexual activity
   - □ Very high confidence
   - □ High confidence
   - □ Moderate confidence
   - □ Low confidence
   - □ Very low or no confidence
6. Over the past 4 weeks, how often have you been satisfied with your arousal (excitement) during sexual activity or intercourse?
   - □ No sexual activity
   - □ Almost always or always
   - □ Most times (more than half the time)
   - □ Sometimes (about half the time)
   - □ A few times (less than half the time)
   - □ Almost never or never
7. Over the past 4 weeks, how often did you become lubricated ("wet") during sexual activity or intercourse?
   - □ No sexual activity
   - □ Almost always or always
   - □ Most times (more than half the time)
   - □ Sometimes (about half the time)
   - □ A few times (less than half the time)
   - □ Almost never or never
8. Over the past 4 weeks, how difficult was it to become lubricated ("wet") during sexual activity or intercourse?
   - □ No sexual activity
   - □ Extremely difficult or impossible
   - □ Very difficult
   - □ Difficult
   - □ Slightly difficult
   - □ Not difficult
9. Over the past 4 weeks, how often did you maintain your lubrication ("wetness") until completion of sexual activity or intercourse?
   - □ No sexual activity
   - □ Almost always or always
   - □ Most times (more than half the time)
   - □ Sometimes (about half the time)
   - □ A few times (less than half the time)
   - □ Almost never or never
10. Over the past 4 weeks, how difficult was it to maintain your lubrication ("wetness") until completion of sexual activity or intercourse?
    - □ No sexual activity
    - □ Extremely difficult or impossible
    - □ Very difficult
    - □ Difficult
    - □ Slightly difficult
    - □ Not difficult
11. Over the past 4 weeks, when you had sexual stimulation or intercourse, how often did you reach orgasm (climax)?
    - □ No sexual activity
    - □ Almost always or always
    - □ Most times (more than half the time)
    - □ Sometimes (about half the time)
    - □ A few times (less than half the time)
    - □ Almost never or never

12. Over the past 4 weeks, when you had sexual stimulation or intercourse, how difficult was it for you to reach orgasm (climax)?
    - ☐ No sexual activity
    - ☐ Extremely difficult or impossible
    - ☐ Very difficult
    - ☐ Difficult
    - ☐ Slightly difficult
    - ☐ Not difficult
13. Over the past 4 weeks, how satisfied were you with your ability to reach orgasm (climax) during sexual activity or intercourse?
    - ☐ No sexual activity
    - ☐ Very satisfied
    - ☐ Moderately satisfied
    - ☐ About equally satisfied and dissatisfied
    - ☐ Moderately dissatisfied
    - ☐ Very dissatisfied
14. Over the past 4 weeks, how satisfied have you been with the amount of emotional closeness during sexual activity between you and your partner?
    - ☐ No sexual activity
    - ☐ Very satisfied
    - ☐ Moderately satisfied
    - ☐ About equally satisfied and dissatisfied
    - ☐ Moderately dissatisfied
    - ☐ Very dissatisfied
15. Over the past 4 weeks, how satisfied have you been with your sexual relationship with your partner?
    - ☐ Very satisfied
    - ☐ Moderately satisfied
    - ☐ About equally satisfied and dissatisfied
    - ☐ Moderately dissatisfied
    - ☐ Very dissatisfied
16. Over the past 4 weeks, how satisfied have you been with your overall sexual life?
    - ☐ Very satisfied
    - ☐ Moderately satisfied
    - ☐ About equally satisfied and dissatisfied
    - ☐ Moderately dissatisfied
    - ☐ Very dissatisfied
17. Over the past 4 weeks, how often did you experience discomfort or pain during vaginal penetration?
    - ☐ Did not attempt intercourse
    - ☐ Almost always or always
    - ☐ Most times (more than half the time)
    - ☐ Sometimes (about half the time)
    - ☐ A few times (less than half the time)
    - ☐ Almost never or never
18. Over the past 4 weeks, how often did you experience discomfort or pain following vaginal penetration?
    - ☐ Did not attempt intercourse
    - ☐ Almost always or always
    - ☐ Most times (more than half the time)
    - ☐ Sometimes (about half the time)
    - ☐ A few times (less than half the time)
    - ☐ Almost never or never
19. Over the past 4 weeks, how would you rate your level (degree) of discomfort or pain during or following vaginal penetration?
    - ☐ Did not attempt intercourse
    - ☐ Very high
    - ☐ High
    - ☐ Moderate
    - ☐ Low
    - ☐ Very low or none at all

TREATMENT

Dyspareunia

Treatment varies as per the etiology. A lot of counseling is required for both the partners. This is not to suggest that the male partner is "causing or aggravating" the problem but certainly to mean that "he" too is affected by it.

Infective skin and mucosal lesions are best treated with appropriate antibiotics, antifungals, and antiparasitic medications. Bacterial vaginosis is best approached with ampicillin and stopping ritualistic cleaning of the genitalia that is often undertaken under the influence of modern day notions of "hygiene and cleanliness".

Pelvic infections are more difficult and dyspareunia may be due to scarring, adhesions left behind by an infection treated long ago. Active infection needs appropriate antibiotic course. Chronic effects need to be diagnosed and tackled laparoscopicaly. Endometriosis is similarly dealt with medical/surgical management. A fixed inverted uterus, fibroids, ovarian tumors, and ovarian remnant syndrome will all need appropriate surgical intervention.

Atrophy will best respond to local estrogen creams.

Condylomata acuminata will need podophyllin application and/or cautery.

Many noninfectious inflammations will regress with mild steroids, like momentasone applied locally.

Scarring resulting from genital mutilation is difficult to treat and is thankfully not a problem in this part of the world. Scarring following radiation is equally difficult and needs serial dilatation and extreme perseverance.

The size of the penis is more of an imagined problem than real. Good foreplay, copious lubrication with water-based jellies, and gentle manner should take care of the problem; whether real or imagined.

Anatomic variations are mostly iatrogenic like those after hysterectomy, anterior/posterior repairs, sling operations for prolapse in young women or those for vault prolapse. Some adjustment in diameter and depth of the vagina happens over time with regular coitus. Avoiding coitus for the fear of pain will lead to atrophy and loss of elasticity, which will compound the problem. Couples should be encouraged to have regular coital sex once the incisions have gained enough strength. This is usually after 2–3 months. Estrogen cream, lubricant jellies, good foreplay, and gentle manner are stressed. Over correction during posterior colporaphy may at times change the direction of the vagina. Apart from dyspareunia, post void dribble also happens to be a complaint in such cases. Phenton's operation, wherein a vertical incision is placed at 6 o'clock and sutured transversely, is the surgery of choice.

Naturally occurring mismatch in size may be due to vaginal septum; which may be longitudinal or transverse (termed phimosis of the cervix), absent or rudimentary vagina, or a tough hymen. Septum resection with vaginoplasty, Mc-Indoe's vaginoplasty, and releasing incisions will take care of the respective conditions. Some improvisation and surgical ingenuity will pay rich dividends.

Hymenal remnants, tags after episiotomy, and episiotomy neuromas all need to be excised surgically.

Painful anal conditions may at times cause dyspareunia. Fissures, fistulae, hemorrhoids, helminthiasis, and even irritable bowel syndrome may be cause and relevant management will bring relief.

Vaginismus

Every gynecologist should have a set of vaginal dilators. Even in routine ob-gyn practice, there is a constant trickle of women who need this therapy and I am surprised as to how a great number of doctors practice without a set of this simple yet very useful instrument **(Fig. 2)**.

Relationship issues are identified and sorted out simultaneously with the treatment. An educational sexological gynecologic examination is the most crucial part. As elaborated earlier, the anatomy is pointed out, with patient using the hand mirror to see her own genitalia and the husband present. The technique of coitus is described in detail with relevant models, charts, etc. Techniques of relaxing the muscles at will are taught. Yoga techniques are especially useful in this area. Best is to ask her to tighten the muscles first and then to let go on command.

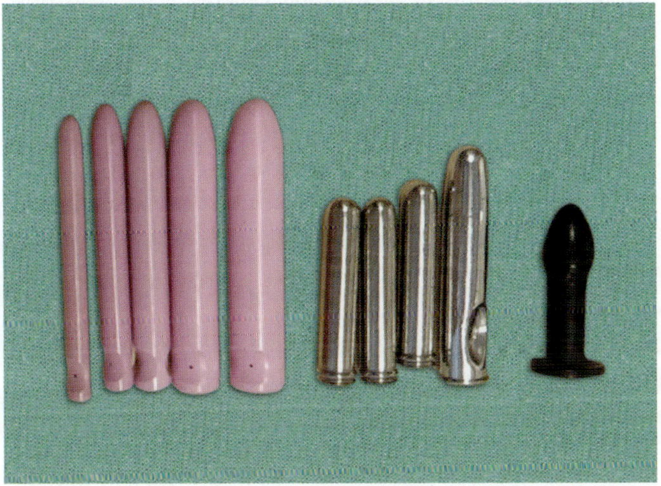

Fig. 2: Vaginal dilators.

Next would be to provide a set of plastic vaginal dilators. Fingers (her own, physician's, or partner's), cervical dilators or even a set of candles with condoms may be used. Copious anesthetic lubricant jelly is used. Patients are initially amazed to see even the small dilator getting easily inside. Soon, they are convinced that little if any harm is possible and will readily accept bigger and bigger dilators. Next would be to let her use the dilators herself, then involve the partner too, and finally give asset to be used just before coitus. The woman on top position (cowgirl position as it is called) is advisable with man asked not to thrust at all. Woman guides the penis in her vagina as she slowly sits over it. This allows her complete control over insertion. If relationships issues have been tackled, the spontaneity of the act soon takes over.

Some surgical approaches are said to be useful in extreme cases, where all else fails. Many experts feel that the surgical approach is not useful at all since the condition is one of reflex spasm. The Fenton's approach is to place a longitudinal incision over the perineum at 6 o'clock and suture it horizontally, thus widening the introitus. Only recently, Vishwaprakash et al., described a surgical technique of Z plasty of the bulbospongiosus muscle.[14] This involves:

- Developing flaps of the labia minora
- Exposing the bulbospongiosus and lengthening it with a Z plasty **(Figs. 3A to D)**
- Covering the defect with the flap.

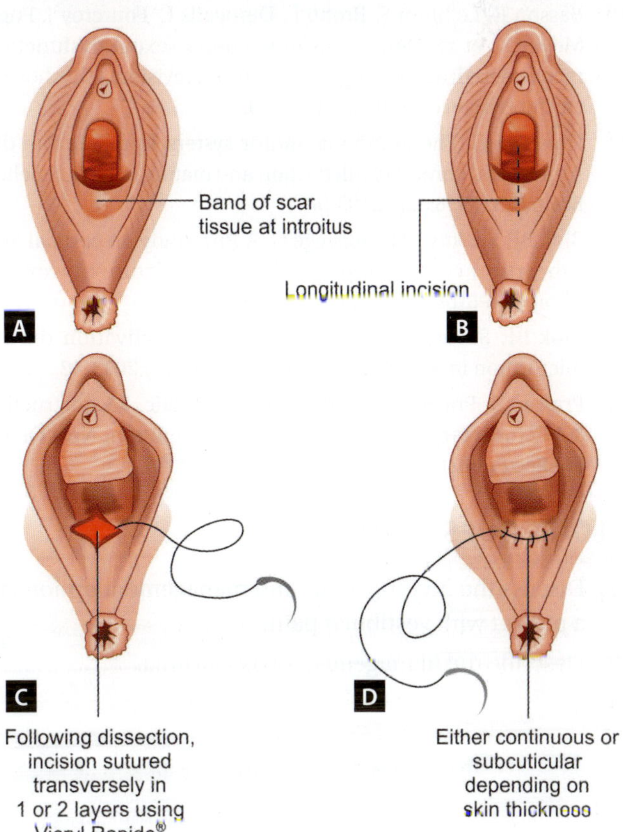

Figs. 3A to D: Z-plasty or Fenton's repair.

Vishwaprakash is of the opinion that all midline scars will give rise to dyspareunia, and hence the need for tackling the bulbocavernosus laterally and placing a flap to avoid scarring.

REFERENCES

1. Dickinson RL. Human Sex Anatomy, A Topographical Hand Atlas, 2nd edition. London: Bailliere, Tindal & Cox; 1949. p. 102.
2. Laumann EO, Paik A, Rosen RC. Sexual dysfunction in the United States: Prevalence and predictors. JAMA. 1999;281(6):537-44.
3. Safarinejad MR. Female sexual dysfunction in a population-based study in Iran: prevalence and associated risk factors. Int J Impot Res. 2006;18(4):382-95.
4. Fugl-Meyer AR, Fugl-Meyer KS. Sexual disabilities, problems and satisfaction in 18-74 year-old Swedes. Scand J Sexol. 1999;2:79-105.
5. Reissing ED, Binik YM, Khalifé S. Does vaginismus exist? A critical review of the literature. J Nerv Ment Dis. 1999;187(5):261-74.
6. Meana M, Binik YM, Khalifé S, Cohen D. Dyspareunia: sexual dysfunction or pain syndrome? J Nerv Ment Dis. 1997;185(9):561-9.
7. van Lankveld JJ, Brewaeys AM, Ter Kuile MM, Weijenborg PT. Difficulties in the differential diagnosis of vaginismus, dyspareunia and mixed sexual pain disorder. J Psychosom Obstet Gynaecol. 1995;16(4):201-9.
8. de Kruiff ME, ter Kuile MM, Weijenborg PT, van Lankveld JJ. Vaginismus and dyspareunia: is there a difference in clinical presentation? J Psychosom Obstet Gynaecol. 2000;21(3):149-55.
9. Basson R. Lifelong vaginismus; a clinical study of 60 consecutive cases. J Soc Gynecol Obstet. 1996;18(6):551-61.
10. Basson R, Leiblum S, Brotto L, Derogatis L, Fourcroy J, Fugl-Meyer K, et al. Definitions of women's sexual dysfunction reconsidered: advocating expansion and revision. J Psychosom Obstet Gynaecol. 2003;24(4):221-9.
11. Holstege G. The emotional motor system in relation to the supraspinal control of micturition and mating behavior. Behav Brain Res. 1998;92(2):103-9.
12. Blok BF, Sturms LM, Holstege G. A PET study on cortical and subcortical control of pelvic floor musculature in women. J Comp Neurol. 1997;389(3):535-44.
13. Blok BF, Sturms LM, Holstege G. Brain activation during micturition in women. Brain. 1998;121(Pt 11):2033-42.
14. Prakash V, Prakash N. Introduction to Plastic, Reconstructive & Microsurgery of Female Genitalia, 1st edition. New Delhi: PeePee Publishers and Distributors Pvt; 2005.

LONG QUESTIONS

1. Discuss the investigations and management options in a patient with vestibular pain.
2. Describe the management of dysparunia.

SHORT QUESTIONS

1. Define vaginismus.
2. What are the components common to vaginismus and dysparunia?
3. Describe the modern view of the function and dysfunction of the pelvic floor.
4. What are the common causes of sexual pain?
5. Describe the concept of an "educational gynecological sexological examination".
6. What are the advantages and disadvantages of the questionnaire approach?

MULTIPLE CHOICE QUESTIONS

1. The prevalence of persistent sexual difficulty in women is estimated to be in the range of:
   a. 5% b. 20%
   c. 50% d. 80%
2. The involuntary spasm of the pubococcygeus muscle when an attempt is made to enter the vagina is known as:
   a. Sexual pain b. Sexual tension
   c. Dyspareunia d. Vaginismus
3. The following statement about innervations of the pelvis is false:
   a. The pelvis has autonomic and somatic innervations
   b. Afferent nerve fibers carry only afferent nerve signals
   c. Antidromic nerve impulses cause vasodilation in the pelvis
   d. Pain is perceived by C type nerve fibers
4. Which of the following is not a mucous membrane related condition?
   a. Chronic vulvar dermatoses
   b. Vulvar vestibular syndrome
   c. Vulvodynias
   d. Endometriosis
5. The following are acceptable first-line treatment options for a woman with vaginismus, except:
   a. Education and counseling
   b. Dilator therapy
   c. Yoga
   d. Vaginoplasty

Answers

1. b 2. d 3. b 4. d 5. d

10.9 PREMATURE OVARIAN INSUFFICIENCY

Duru Shah, Vishesha Yadav

DEFINITION

Premature ovarian insufficiency (POI) is characterized by a triad of amenorrhea, increased gonadotropin levels, and sex steroid deficiency in women <40 years of age.

It has been defined by the European Society of Human Reproduction and Embryology (ESHRE) using three criteria:[1]

1. Presence of primaryamenorrhea/secondary amenorrhea for >4 months
2. Onset <40 years of age
3. Follicle-stimulating hormone (FSH) >25 mIU/L determined by two measurements, at least 4 weeks apart.

The ESHRE guideline group on POI defines ovarian reserve as "encompassing both the quantity and quality of primordial follicles".[1]

BACKGROUND

The number of oocytes is highest in prenatal life and diminishes gradually, falling to a critically low number around the age of 50 years. A proper diagnosis of POI is essential to differentiate women with normal menopause from women with POI, as these women have special needs and different management options.

INTRODUCTION

Premature ovarian insufficiency leads to a decrease in the residual ovarian follicles, thus causing estrogen deficiency even decades prior to the normal age of menopause. The term POI is preferred over premature menopause because this term does not mean a total shutdown of ovarian activity. This term is advocated by the National Institutes of Health because ovarian function is intermittent or unpredictable in most women.[2] Sir Fuller Albright coined the term primary ovarian insufficiency in the year 1942 to emphasize the fact that the defect lies in the ovarian function and is not a central defect.[3] Since then, there have been many variations in the terminology, such as premature/early menopause, gonadal dysgenesis, premature ovarian failure, premature ovarian insufficiency, hypogonadotropic hypogonadism, etc.

Diminished ovarian reserve (DOR) is not the same as POI. It is a term used to evaluate female infertility, referring to women >40 years of age with an abnormal ovarian reserve testing and/or a poor response to ovarian stimulation during in vitro fertilization.

PREVALENCE

There have been no recent studies estimating the prevalence of POI. In a study done by Luborsky et al., a 1.1% prevalence of POI was observed in a cross-sectional survey of women aged 40–55 years.[4] The occurrence of POI is estimated to be 1 in 100 women in <40years, 1 in 1,000 women in <30 years, and 1 in 10,000 women in <20 years.[5] Although the incidence of spontaneous POI appears to have remained stable, the rising incidence of iatrogenic POI is of increasing concern. Ethnicity and lifestyle factors play a role in determining the age of natural menopause. The incidence of POI in AfricanAmerican women is around 1.4%, around 1% in Caucasian women, and around 0.1–0.5% in Chinese and Japanese women.[4] In women with primary amenorrhea, the prevalence is 10–28%, while in secondary amenorrhea, it is 4–18%.[6]

PATHOPHYSIOLOGY

These defects can be divided into two major categories:

1. *Accelerated follicular depletion*: Due to genetic, autoimmune, iatrogenic, and environmental or toxic causes
2. *Decreased steroid production without oocyte loss:* These disorders are genetic disorders of estradiol precursor production or aromatase function, resulting in decreased estradiol and absence of normal FSH-negative feedback.

ETIOLOGY

The causes of POI stem from many probable etiologies; however, the actual cause is still a mystery. To understand the mechanisms underlying early ovarian dysfunction, it is important to divide the causes as spontaneous or as secondary to a recognized cause.

Spontaneous POI usually has an insidious onset. It occurs in almost 0.3–1.1% of reproductive aged women. It can occur due to an inherent tiny pool of ovarian reserve or due to an accelerated destruction/depletion of reserve.

Genetic Causes

Approximately 20–25% of cases are due to a genetic cause, out of which around 9–15% cases are due to the involvement of the X chromosome in the form of translocations or deletions.[7] Turnersyndrome is the most common chromosomal aberration seen in POI. About half of the patients with Turner syndrome have a mosaic genetic makeup, of which the most common is 45XO (15%), while only 6% account for 46 xxq or 46xxp deletions.[7] Partial or complete deletion of the q arm can lead to ovarian dysfunction.[8]

Fragile X syndrome, an X-linked inherited condition, is caused by a mutation of the *fragile-X mental-retardation 1 (FMR1)* gene. A full mutation refers to an allele with >200 CGG repeats. Alleles with <40 CGG are normal, while repeat lengths of 55–200 are relatively unstable and are called "premutations".[9] The full mutation can cause mental retardation but primarily in men who carry the mutation. Women who carry the premutation (55–200 repeats) have an increased risk of 13–26% to develop POI.[10] This occurs in 14–26% of women with familial POI and 2–5% of women with isolated POI.[11] Those women with either normal or full mutation are at no greater risk of developing POI than the general population. Hence, all women with POI interested in fertility should be screened for this premutation, since it can be transmitted to the conceptus.

Less common genetic mutations have been recognized, involving NOBOX, FOXO3, GDF9, and BPM15 variants.[12]These are transcription factors that regulate oocyte-specific genes. Genes encoding gonadotropin (Gn) receptors, FSH receptor (FSHR), and luteinizing hormone/human chorionic gonadotrophin receptor (LHCGR) have also been observed to have mutations causing gonadotropin resistance.[13]

However, routine screening for autosomal gene mutations in POI patients is not recommended.[1] In order to detect novel POI genes, array studies, genome-wide studies, and next generation sequencing have been used.

Autoimmune Causes

The exact mechanism of autoimmunity in the pathophysiology of this disorder remains obscure. Autoimmune conditions may be responsible for 20–30% of cases of POI.[14] The most common is the Graves or the Hashimoto's disease, responsible for almost (30%) of the cases.[15] Therefore, screening for thyroid antibodies (TPO-Ab) should be done in women with POI. In patients with a positive TPO-Ab test, thyroid-stimulating hormone (TSH) should be measured every year.[1]

Premature ovarian insufficiency of adrenal autoimmune origin is observed in 60–80% of patients with POI.[16] Circulating adrenal or ovarian autoantibodies directed to steroidogenic enzymes [steroid-cell autoantibodies (SCA)] have been found to cause selective destruction of theca cells, causing low estradiol (E2), high FSH, high inhibin B, and a gradual decline in AMH levels.[16] It is recommended that adrenocortical antibodies (ACA) and/or 21OH-Ab should be measured in every POI patient because of the possibility of latent Addison disease in POI patients.[17] If thyroid and adrenal antibodies are initially negative, there is no indication for repeat testing on a routine basis. However, if signs or symptoms develop later, a low threshold should be maintained to repeat screening for the suspected endocrinopathy.[1]

Less frequent causes include type 1 diabetes mellitus, systemic lupus erythematosus, rheumatoid arthritis, and others.[14] Diverse autoantibodies against Gn receptors and zona pellucida have been studied as markers of ovarian autoimmunity.[18] However, no confirmatory diagnosis is yet established.

Infectious Etiologies

A variety of infections, such as mumps oophoritis, tuberculosis, varicella, and cytomegalovirus have been associated with POI.[1]In the majority of cases, normal ovarian function is restored once the infection insult wanes off.[19]

Iatrogenic Causes

These include surgical oophorectomy, salpingectomy for ectopic or hydrosalpinx, excessive ovarian drilling in polycystic ovary syndrome (PCOS), removal of benign ovarian cyst, chemotherapy, and radiotherapy.

In a meta-analysis, the effect of surgery for endometriomas on ovarian reserve was studied, and it was concluded that there is a significant decline in anti-Müllerian hormone (AMH) levels after ovarian cystectomy.[20] A recently published meta-analysis on changes in AMH levels after laparoscopic ovarian drilling (LOD) concluded that LOD markedly reduces AMH levels with PCOS who have normal or low AMH levels.[21] A 2015 study established that wide excision of soft tissues adjacent to the ovary and fallopian tube does not impair the ovarian reserve in women undergoing prophylactic bilateral salpingectomy.[22] Nonetheless, the impact on in vitro fertilization (IVF) success and spontaneous pregnancy rates must be reviewed by the indication for possible salpingectomy.

With increasing incidences of cancers, more women undergo gonadotoxic therapy, leading to a rise in POI.[14] Based on recent cancer statistics, a woman's probability of being diagnosed with an invasive cancer from birth to 49 years is 5.4% (1/18).[23]

Thedegree of ovarian dysfunction depends on the woman's age at the time of the therapy and the type and dose of the gonadotoxic agent used.[24] Hence, it is crucial to counsel each patient regarding her risk of developing POI after cancer therapy.

Table 1 illustrates certain gonadotoxic drugs and their effects.

Environmental Factors

Over the last few decades, much evidence has confirmed that certain chemical, physical, and biological substances in our environment produce harmful effects on human fertility.[25] Cigarette smoking is one of the most detrimental factors causing POI. It can lead to early menopause due to the effects of the polycyclic hydrocarbons (PCH) present in them.[25] Active smoking by either partner had adverse effects, and the impact of passive cigarette smoke exposure alone was only slightly smaller than for active smoking by either partner.[26] Cigarette smoke contains >4,000 chemical substances, the main culprit being PCH. They act on the ovary via the aryl hydrocarbon receptor (AhR) present on the surface of granulosa cells, thus causing ovarian dysregulation.[27] Active cigarette smoking is associated with longer time to conceive and with decreased

TABLE 1: Gonadotoxic drugs and their effects.

Chemotherapeutic agents and class known to cause gonadotoxicity and POI risk	***Radiation dose and age of exposure as determinants of POI risk***
Alkylating agent	
Nitrogen mustard	20.3 Gy at birth
Chlorambucil	18.4 Gy at 10 years
Cyclophosphamide	16.5 Gy at 20 years
Busulfan	14.3 Gy at 30 years
Melphalan	6 Gy at age 40 or more
Anthracycline Doxorubicin	
Substituted hydrazine Procarbazine	

Source: Torrealday S, Kodaman P and Pal L. Premature Ovarian Insufficiency - an update on recent advances in understanding and management. F1000Research 2017, 6(F1000 Faculty Rev):

TABLE 2: Premature ovarian insufficiency (POI) evaluation according to ESHRE guidelines.

Genetic test	***Positive***	***Negative***
Karyotyping (for turners syndrome)	Refer to endocrinologist, cardiologist and geneticist	A second analysis of karyotype in epithelial cells if high clinical suspicion
Test for Y-chromosomal material	Discuss gonadectomy with patient	
Fragile-X	Refer to geneticist	
ACA/21OH antibodies	Refer to endocrinologist	Re-test if clinical signs/symptoms
TPO antibodies	Check TSH every year	Re-test if clinical signs/symptoms

Source: The ESHRE Guideline Group on POI, L. Webber, M. Davies et al. Human Reproduction. 2016;31(5):926-37.

results even with IVF.[28] Anderson et al., have shown that activation of this receptor could lead to a decrease in germ cells in the ovary of the human fetus.[29]

Many other environmental insults can affect ovarian function in three ways that can coexist via:

- Endocrine disrupting chemicals
- Induction of oxidative stress
- Epigenetic modifications.

Heavy metals, pesticides, and phthalates (in plastics) cause steroidogenesis disorders, thus causing alteration in reproductive functions, infertility, and POI via follicular atresia.[30] Bisphenol A (BPA), an endocrine disruptor, also present in plastics, acts like an estrogen mimicker on the estrogen receptor α.[31] It causes a decrease in the number of primordial follicles regardless of the exposure window whether it is prenatal, neonatal, or at the adult age.[32]

CLINICAL PRESENTATION

There is a variable range of symptoms in women with POI. It can include manifestations of hypoestrogenism as well as features of the causative factor of POI. The initial red flag sign of ovarian insufficiency refers to new onset menstrual irregularities before amenorrhea eventually sets in. Primary amenorrhea may be the only symptom in up to 10% of cases, especially in patients with karyotype abnormalities.[33] In majority of women, menses start and continue for varying periods following normal pubertal growth. Other alarming symptoms include hot flushes, emotional lability, fatigue, vaginal dryness, decreased libido, and sleep disturbances.

DIAGNOSIS AND EVALUATION

Diagnosis and work-up of such patients is done after a thorough clinical history, physical examination, and biochemical confirmation. This helps ruling out other conditions that might lead to amenorrhea. There are no ideal biochemical markers for the diagnosis, and the existing markers may fluctuate over time. Diagnosis is based on a triad of amenorrhea and elevated Gn levels with or without signs of hypoestrogenism. Persistent FSH rise of >25 mIU/L on two different occasions can help diagnose POI.[1] E2 levels are typically <50 pg/mL in cases of ovarian dysfunction along with suppressed AMH levels.[34] A transvaginal scan can also help confirm low antral follicle count and a persistently thin endometrium of <4 mm. However, radiological imaging is not essential to establish the diagnosis. A progesterone withdrawal test gives a false-positive result, thus delaying the actual diagnosis.

Investigating for any autoimmune conditions or endocrinopathies should be considered, after enquiring about relevant clinical symptoms.

Significance should be given to any alarming family history of mental retardation, premature menopause, recurrent pregnancy loss or any genetic disease in the family. Once the diagnosis is confirmed, one should further evaluate the cause. Chromosomal analysis, fragile X testing, and screening for thyroid and adrenal antibodies can help establish the cause.[1] If karyotyping is suggestive of the presence of a Y chromosome, gonadectomy should be done as the risk of malignancy is high these patients.

Table 2 summarizes the POI evaluation according to ESHRE guidelines.[1]

MANAGEMENT

The management of POI best involves a multidisciplinary team consisting of a gynecologist, endocrinologist, and a psychologist. It can be divided into three main components.

1. Assisting fertility

2. Hormone replacement therapy (HRT) for battling hypoestrogenism, bone health, cardiovascular health, and quality of life issues
3. Psychological support.

Assisting Fertility

The degree of residual ovarian function in women with POI varies considerably. Up to 25% of women may spontaneously ovulate and 5–10% will conceive resulting in a live birth.[14] A dual retrospective and prospective study showed that 24% of women with idiopathic POI resumed ovarian function and most of them had resumption within a year of diagnosis.[35] These pregnancies are not associated with any increased risk of adverse outcomes as compared to general population.[1]

On the contrary, women who are not interested in fertility should be recommended birth control due to the fact that spontaneous ovarian activity can resume. The disadvantage of the oral contraceptive pill is that sometimesit may fail to suppress high FSH levels, thus leading to a pregnancy. Hence, the barrier method and intrauterine device are ideal contraceptive options.[14]

Many protocols have been put forward to restore ovarian function, but in vain. A range of treatments including estrogens, gonadotropins, and corticosteroids have been studied as potential treatments to increase the chance of pregnancy. Previous studies using pretreatment with estrogen followed by Gn may allow FSH suppression, thus allowing restoration of ovarian activity.[36] More recently, the use of dehydroepiandrostenedione (DHEA) has been shown to improve the intraovarian milieu via IGF-1, thus leading to oocyte activation and increased estrogen production.[37] Few studies include the use of corticosteroids for any existing autoimmune disorders. It is thought to decrease the perifollicular inflammatory activity, thus restoring function of smaller follicles.[38]

Finally, two new promising techniques have emerged on the horizon—in vitro activation (IVA) and stem cell (SC) technology.

In Vitro Activation (IVA from Excised Ovarian Tissue)

In vitro activation involves IVA of dormant follicles in the ovarian tissue. A complete cycle consists of a laparoscopic surgery to remove the ovary, followed by vitrification of cortical ovarian strips. After thawing, the strips areincubated with P13K stimulators (Akt-P13k signal transduction pathway in cells) and then autografted through laparoscopy, post which the patient undergoes an entire stimulation cycle.[39-41] Currently, two healthy babies were delivered and two more are on the way. More controlled studies are neededbefore this procedure can be clinically used in practice.

Stem Cell Therapy or Ovarian Rejuvenation

Stem cellshave created a breakthrough for POI and poor responder patients. A recent 2018 study by Herraiz et al., showed that bone marrow-derived SCs stimulated follicular growth in poor responders leading to successful pregnancies.[42]A more recent 2019 study by Mohammad SA has established the usefulness of umbilical cord blood mesenchymal SCs to restore fertility in POI patients.[43] The transplanted SCs have been proven to differentiate into GC-like cells much more easily than into oocytes.

Oogonial stem cells (OSCs) have been detected in women and have proven to form oocyte-like structures in xenotransplant models; however, the physiological relevance of OSCs in the human females remains unclear as of now.

Assisted reproduction by IVF using donor eggs or embryos is, by far, the best option for women with POI. According to a study, the pregnancy rate after an ovum donation cycle is 40% and the cumulative pregnancy rate after 4 cycles reaches 70–80%.[44]

Table 3 lists the outcomes using donor eggs—SART DATA-2017.

Turner syndrome patients are also candidates for IVF with oocyte donation. It is known that these patients have a high rate of cardiovascular anomalies. Therefore, according to the American Society of Reproductive Medicine (ASRM), women with Turner syndrome should undergo medical and cardiovascular control before trying for pregnancy.[45] Recently, studies have demonstrated that pregnancy with donor gametes is associated with a higher rate of intrauterine growth restriction (IUGR) and pre-eclampsia.[46]

FERTILITY PRESERVATION

Oophore

Surgical transposition of ovaries prevents radiation-induced injury, thus preventing POI. During ovarian transposition, the ovaries are mobilized with their blood supply from the

TABLE 3: Outcomes using donor eggs—SART DATA-2017.

	Fresh OD eggs	*Frozen OD eggs*	*Thawed embryos with OD eggs*
No. of recipient cycles	3324	3452	14257
Mean no. of embryos transferred	1.4	1.4	1.3
eSET	60.3%	54.7%	57.4%
Live births	48.9% (47.2–50.6)	39.3% (37.7–40.9)	42.4% (41.6–43.2)
Implantation rate	54.8%	45.7%	47.0%

(Donor egg cycles: SART Preliminary Data-2017 eSET: elective single embryo transfer, OD: ovum donation)

infundibulopelvic ligament and then fixed to the anterior abdominal wall, 3–4 cm above the umbilical line. Optimal timing of oophoropexy is just before radiation.[47] A combined approach can also be implemented wherein one ovary is cryopreserved, and the other can be transposed.

Reported success rates are inconsistent, anywhere varying between 16% and 90%.[48] The failures are due to various factors, such as scatter radiation, vascular compromise, radiation dose, patient's age, and whether the ovaries are shielded during the radiation procedure.

Oocyte Freezing

It can be attempted using the Duo Stim protocol, by combining the conventional follicular phase stimulation (FPS) with luteal phase stimulation (LPS). Duo stim helps maximize the number of oocytes retrieved in a single ovarian cycle.[49] Recent studies have reported that in women with newly acquired cancer requiring urgent cancer therapy, emergency fertility preservation is possible by commencing ovarian stimulation at any time in the menstrual cycle.[50] In such patients, the premature LH surge was suppressed with either endogenously produced progesterone or exogenous use of progestational agents.

Figure 1 shows an 18-year experience of oocyte cryopreservation amongst patients in a tertiary care referral center.[51]

GnRH Analogs

Use of gonadotropin-releasing hormone (GnRH) analogs before starting chemotherapy suppresses FSH and LH levels by suspending its function temporarily. However, the ovarian follicles are still exposed to these DNA-damaging agents even though the ovarian hormone production is suppressed.[48] A recent 2018 review study including 873 patients established that GnRH agonist during chemotherapy reduces the likelihood of chemotherapy-induced POI in patients with early breast cancer.[52]

In Vitro Maturation

In vitro maturation (IVM) is indicated for patients in whom stimulation is contraindicated and gonadotoxic treatment cannot be delayed. The immature oocytes are matured in vitro either before freezing or after thawing; however, there are conflicting studies regarding the stages at which the oocyte should be vitrified. A 2016 study by Molina et al., showed that vitrifying germinal vesicle (GV)-stage oocytes seemed to be better than that of MII-stage in terms of IVM rate and embryo development.[53] Another study by Kasapi et al., observedhigher maturation rate in the group where oocytes were vitrified after IVM (82.9%) compared to oocytes vitrified at GV stage (51%).[54] A study also questioned the utility of performing IVM in very young premenarchal girls because IVM rates were particularly low for girls younger than 4 years of age.[55]

Cryopreservation of Ovarian Tissue

It involves ovarian tissue harvesting and storage for its future use. Orthotopic ovarian transplantation (OT; to remaining ovarian tissue or pelvic peritoneum) is now considered a standard clinical technique because it can possibly lead to spontaneous conception and also because of the ideal microenvironment to support the graft tissue.[24] Cryopreservation of ovarian tissue followed by heterotopic implantation (in the abdominal wall) still remains an investigational approach and is useful in

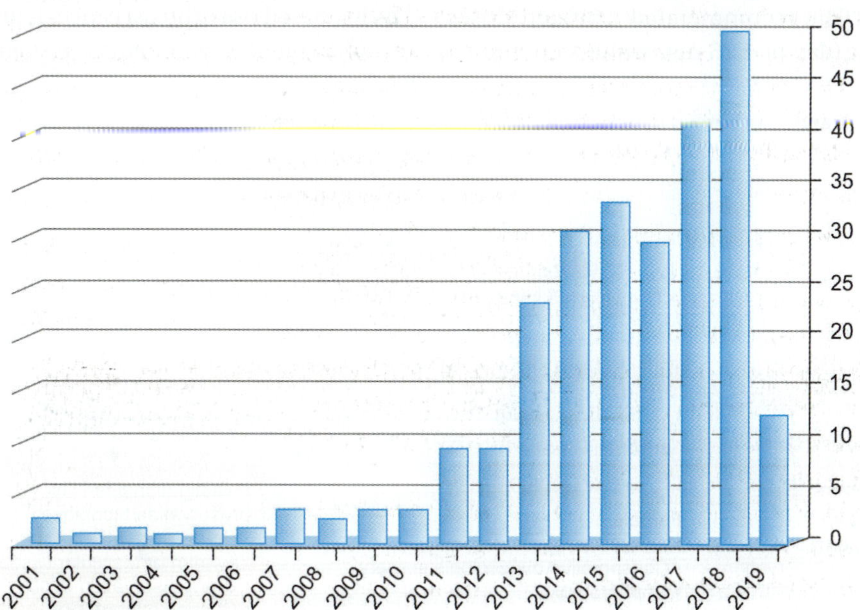

Fig. 1: An 18-year experience of oocyte cryopreservation among patients in a tertiary care referral center.
Source: Specchia C, Baggiani A, Immediata V, Ronchetti C, Cesana A, Smeraldi A, et al. Oocyte cryopreservation in oncological patients: Eighteen years experience of a tertiary care referral center. Front Endocrinol (Lausanne). 2019;10:600.

cases of pelvic adhesions. It has been observed that ovarian function lasts for up to 5–7 years after transplantation.[56] This method does not demand any initial hormonal stimulation, thus avoiding any delay in treatment. The serious concern that remains that these cells in fact could lead to primary cancer recurrence within the grafted tissue, but conclusive evidence is not present.[57]

In a 2017 meta-analysis of 19 studies on OT that included pregnancy-related outcomes, 309 OTs resulted in 84 live born children and 8 ongoing pregnancies, for cumulative clinical pregnancy and composite pregnancy rates (live birth plus ongoing pregnancy) of 57.5% and 37.7%, respectively.[58]

Flowchart 1 summarizes the recommendations by American Society of Clinical Oncology for fertility preservation.[59]

Adjuvant seroprotective agents prevent ovarian damage during gonadotoxic treatment. Pretreatment with SIP (sphingosine-1-phosphate) and GCSF (granulocyte colony-stimulating factor) helps prevent follicle loss.[60] New research also elaborates various methods of chemotherapy drug delivery, thus decreasing its field of impact.

HORMONE REPLACEMENT THERAPY

Premature ovarian insufficiency is a life-changing condition, wherein women battle with symptoms of hypoestrogenism, which include vasomotor, genitourinary, and mood symptoms. The goal of HRT in women with POI is to achieve a serum E2 level of 100 pg/mL, which should be continued till the average menopausal age.[61] The route of hormone therapy with estrogen is recommended either orally or transdermally. Transdermal estrogen avoids first-pass metabolism by the liver and achieves higher plasma levels of circulating estradiol with a lower treatment dose.[62]

Women with POI require high estrogen doses than older menopausal women. The recommended estrogen doses are 17β-estradiol 2 mg/day or 1.25 mg conjugated equine estrogen (CEE) or transdermalestradiol 75–100 µg/day or 10 µg ethinylestradiol.[63] Progesterone should be added to prevent endometrial hyperplasia, and thus minimize the risk of endometrial carcinoma. Micronized progesterone can be administered as a cyclic regimen (200 mg for 12 days each month) or as a continuous regimen of 100 mg per day, typically >2 years post final menstrual period.[63] The strongest evidence of protection of endometrium is via oral cyclic medroxy progesterone acetate.[1] Aprogestogen-releasing IUD can also provide protection from endometrial hyperplasia along with contraception.

Combined oral contraceptive (COC) pills pose as an alternative to HRT, posing less stigma to patients and increasing the compliance.

Thus, HRT helps relieve the woman of vasomotor symptoms,such as hot flushes, night sweats, vaginal dryness, joint pains, and insomnia. Local estrogen therapy is useful for vaginal symptoms. Low bone mass density can be managed effectively with HRT rather than bisphosphonates.[64] Vitamin D, calcium supplementation, and weightbearing exercises help reduce fracture risks. Androgen replacement is shown to improve fatigue and loss of libido despite estrogen replacement.[65] Women at high risk of developing thromboembolism can be treated with selective serotonin reuptake inhibitors (SSRIs).

Monitoring HRT

No specific tests are required to monitor HRT in women with POI. Routine annual checkup, mammography, and DEXA should be reviewed. Patients can be given options for change in regimens and administration routes to enhance compliance.

Risks of HRT

The increased risk of breast cancer is primarily associated with the addition of a synthetic progestogen to estrogen therapy

Flowchart 1: Recommendations by American Society of Clinical Oncology for fertility preservation.

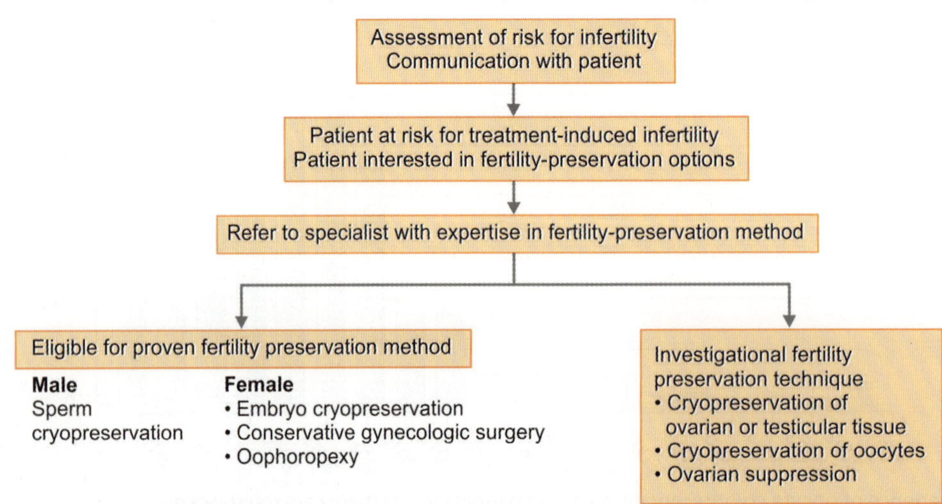

Source: Lee SJ, SchoverLR, Partridge AH, Patrizio P, Wallace WH, Hagerty K, et al; American Society of Clinical Oncology. American Society of Clinical Oncology recommendations on fertility preservation in cancer patients. J Clin Oncol. 2006;24(18):2917-31.

(CEE + MPA continuous combined therapy) and related to the duration of use. Annual mammograms should be proposed in case of high breast density in women using hormone therapy.[63] Endometrial carcinoma risk increases with estrogen only therapy, but is not true for combined regimens. Higher doses of progesterone may be needed for endometrial protection when higher doses of estradiol are used, or in women who have a high BMI.[63]Oral estrogen therapy is contraindicated in women with any history of thrombosis.In obese women suffering from menopausal symptoms, transdermal estrogen therapy should be the first choice.[63]

PSYCHOLOGICAL SUPPORT

Premature ovarian insufficiency is a very depressing condition for young women. Unexpected and sudden diagnosis leads to anxiety, depression, and reduced self-esteem among women. Therefore, they need to be meticulously counselled, given individualized treatment options and immense support. Parents of young girls should be counseled to emotionally support their daughters.[2] Help of support groups and devising coping strategies can help these women live a healthier and confident lives.

KEY MESSAGES

Premature ovarian insufficiency is defined as primary hypogonadism before the age of 40 years in women with a normal karyotype who previously had normal menstrual cycles. In the majority of the cases, the cause of POI is unknown. Certain causes, which are modifiable factors, can help prevent POI. These include avoiding iatrogenic POI, lifestyle (smoking), and gonadotoxic therapies. The diagnosis is confirmed on both symptoms and biochemical laboratory values. Egg donation is an established option for fertility in women with POI, while fertility preservation is a promising option in the future. HRT is recommended to relieve vasomotor symptoms, maintain bone health and cardiovascular health. Since the diagnosis of POI has a negative impact on the mental wellbeing, psychological support is of great importance.

REFERENCES

1. European Society for Human Reproduction and Embryology (ESHRE) Guideline Group on POI; Webber L, Davies M, Anderson R, Bartlett J, Braat D, Cartwright B, et al. ESHRE Guideline: management of women with premature ovarian insufficiency. Hum Reprod. 2016;31(5):926-37.
2. Committee opinion no. 605: primary ovarian insufficiency in adolescents and young women. Obstet Gynecol. 2014;124(1):193-7.
3. Cooper AR, Baker VL, Sterling EW, Ryan ME, Woodruff TK, Nelson LM. The time is now for a new approach to primary ovarian insufficiency. Fertil Steril. 2011;95(6):1890-7.
4. LuborskyJL, Meyer P, Sowers MF, Gold EB, Santoro N. Premature menopause in a multi-ethnic population study of the menopause transition. Hum Reprod. 2003;18(1):199-206.
5. Rudnicka E, Kruszewska J, Klicka K, Kowalczyk J, Grymowicz M, Skórska J, et al. Premature ovarian insufficiency - aetiopathology, epidemiology, and diagnostic evaluation. Prz Menopauzalny. 2018;17(3):105-8.
6. Anasti JN. Premature ovarian failure: an update. FertilSteril. 1998;70(1):1-15.
7. Qin Y, Jiao X, Simpson JL, Chen ZJ. Genetics of primary ovarian insufficiency: new developments and opportunities. Hum Reprod Update. 2015;21(6):787-808.
8. Thompson MW, McInnes RR, Willard HF. The sex chromosomes and their abnormalities. In: Thompson MW, McInnes RR, Willard HF (Eds). Genetics in Medicine. Philadelphia: WB Saunders; 1991.pp. 239-43.
9. Esther M, Azhar J, Nurit M, Arei K, JHR, Flora T. Prenatal diagnosis of fragile X: can a full mutation allele in the FMR1 gene contract to a normal size? Front Genet. 2017;8:158.
10. Wittenberger MD, Hagerman RJ, Sherman SL, McConkie-Rosell A, Welt CK, Rebar RW, et al. The FMR1 premutation and reproduction. Fertil Steril. 2007;87(3):456-65.
11. Murray A, Schoemaker MJ, Bennett CE, Ennis S, Macpherson JN, Jones M, et al. Population-based estimates of the prevalence of FMR1 expansion mutations in women with early menopause and primary ovarian insufficiency. Genet Med. 2014;16(1):19-24.
12. Fonseca DJ, Patiño LC, Suárez YC, de Jesús Rodríguez A, Mateus HE, Jiménez KM, et al. Next generation sequencing in women affected by nonsyndromic premature ovarian failure displays new potential causative genes and mutations. Fertil Steril. 2015;104(1):154-62.e2..
13. Rossetti R, Ferrari I, Bonomi M, Persani L. Genetics of primary ovarian insufficiency. Clin Genet. 2017;91(2):183-98.
14. Torrealday S, Kodaman P, Pal L. premature ovarian insufficiency - an update on recent advances in understanding and management. F1000 Res. 2017;6:2069.
15. Ayesha, Jha V, Goswami D. Premature ovarian failure: An association with autoimmune diseases. J Clin Diagn Res. 2016;10(10):QC10-QC12.
16. Silva CA, Yamakami LY, Aikawa NE, Araujo DB, Carvalho JF, Bonfá E. Autoimmune primary ovarian insufficiency. Autoimmun Rev. 2014;13(4-5):427-30.
17. Dal Pra C, Chen S, Furmaniak J, Smith BR, Pedini B, Moscon A, et al. Autoantibodies to steroidogenic enzymes in patients with premature ovarian failure with and without Addison's disease. Eur J Endocrinol. 2003;148(5):565-70.
18. Kinoshita A, Tanaka H, Komori S, Hasegawa A, Koyoma K. Autoimmunity to zona pellucida possibly causes premature ovarian failure (POF). J Reprod Immunol. 2006;71:155.
19. Ebrahimi M, Akbari Asbagh F. Pathogenesis and causes of premature ovarian failure: an update. Int J Fertil Steril. 2011;5(2):54-65.
20. Raffi F, Metwally M, Amer S. The impact of excision of ovarian endometrioma on ovarian reserve: a systematic review and meta-analysis. J Clin Endocrinol Metab. 2012;97(9):3146-54.
21. Amer SA, El Shamy TT, James C, Yosef AH, Mohamed AA. The impact of laparoscopic ovarian drilling on AMH and ovarian reserve: a meta-analysis. Reproduction. 2017;154(1):R13-R21.
22. Venturella R, Morelli M, Lico D, Di Cello A, Rocca M, Sacchinelli A, et al. Wide excision of soft tissues adjacent to the ovary and fallopian tube does not impair the ovarian reserve in women undergoing prophylactic bilateral salpingectomy: results from a randomized, controlled trial. Fertil Steril. 2015;104(5):1332-9.
23. Siegel RL, Miller KD, Jemal A. Cancer Statistics, 2017. CA Cancer J Clin. 2017;67(1):7-30.

24. Donnez J, Dolmans MM. Fertility preservation in women. Nat Rev Endocrinol. 2013;9(12):735-49.
25. Vabre P, Gatimel N, Moreau J, Gayrard V, Picard-Hagen N, Parinaud J, et al. Environmental pollutants, a possible etiology for premature ovarian insufficiency: a narrative review of animal and human data. Environ Health. 2017;16(1):37.
26. Practice Committee of the American Society for Reproductive Medicine. Smoking and infertility: a committee opinion. Fertil Steril. 2018;110(4):611-8.
27. Camlin NJ, McLaughlin EA, Holt JE. Through the smoke: use of in vivo and in vitro cigarette smoking models to elucidate its effect on female fertility. Toxicol Appl Pharmacol. 2014;281(3):266-75.
28. Sobinoff AP, Beckett EL, Jarnicki AG, Sutherland JM, McCluskey A, Hansbro PM, et al. Scrambled and fried: cigarette smoke exposure causes antral follicle destruction and oocyte dysfunction through oxidative stress. Toxicol Appl Pharmacol. 2013;271(2):156-67.
29. Anderson RA, McIlwain L, Coutts S, Kinnell HL, Fowler PA, Childs AJ. Activation of the aryl hydrocarbon receptor by a component of cigarette smoke reduces germ cell proliferation in the human fetal ovary. Mol Hum Reprod. 2014;20(1):42-8.
30. Hannon PR, Flaws JA. The effects of phthalates on the ovary. Front Endocrinol (Lausanne). 2015;6:8.
31. Richardson MC, Guo M, Fauser BC, Macklon NS. Environmental and developmental origins of ovarian reserve. Hum Reprod Update. 2014;20(3):353-69.
32. Zhang HQ, Zhang XF, Zhang LJ, Chao HH, Pan B, FengYM, et al. Fetal exposure to bisphenol A affects the primordial follicle formation by inhibiting the meiotic progression of oocytes. Mol Biol Rep. 2012;39(5):5651-7.
33. Crawford NM, Steiner AZ. Age-related infertility. Obstet Gynecol Clin North Am. 2015;42(1):15-25.
34. Visser JA, Schipper I, LavenJS, Themmen AP. Anti-Müllerian hormone: an ovarian reserve marker in primary ovarian insufficiency. Nat Rev Endocrinol. 2012;8(6):331-41.
35. Bidet M, Bachelot A, Bissauge E, GolmardJL, Gricourt S, Dulon J, et al. Resumption of ovarian function and pregnancies in 358 patients with premature ovarian failure. J Clin Endocrinol Metab. 2011;96(12):3864-72.
36. Tartagni M, Cicinelli E, De Pergola G, De Salvia MA, Lavopa C, Loverro G. Effects of pretreatment with estrogens on ovarian stimulation with gonadotropins in women with premature ovarian failure: a randomized, placebo-controlled trial. Fertil Steril. 2007;87(4):858-61.
37. Yeung TW, Li RH, Lee VC, Ho PC, Ng EH. A randomized double-blinded placebo-controlled trial on the effect of dehydroepiandrosterone for 16 weeks on ovarian response markers in women with primary ovarian insufficiency. J Clin Endocrinol Metab. 2013;98(1):380-8.
38. Badawy A, Goda H, Ragab A. Induction of ovulation in idiopathic premature ovarian failure: a randomized double-blind trial. Reprod Biomed Online. 2007;15(2):215-9.
39. Zhai J, Yao G, Dong F, Bu Z, Cheng Y, Sato Y, et al. In vitro activation of follicles and fresh tissue auto-transplantation in primary ovarian insufficiency patients. J Clin Endocrinol Metab. 2016;101(11):4405-12.
40. Kawamura K, Cheng Y, Suzuki N, Deguchi M, Sato Y, Takae S, et al. Hippo signaling disruption and Akt stimulation of ovarian follicles for infertility treatment. Proc Natl Acad Sci USA. 2013;110(43):17474-9.
41. Suzuki N, Yoshioka N, Takae S, Sugishita Y, Tamura M, Hashimoto S, et al. Successful fertility preservation following ovarian tissue vitrification in patients with primary ovarian insufficiency. Hum Reprod. 2015;30(3):608-15.
42. Herraiz S, Buigues A, Díaz-García C, Romeu M, Martínez S, Gómez-Seguí I, et al. Fertility rescue and ovarian follicle growth promotion by bone marrow stem cell infusion. Fertil Steril. 2018;109(5):908-918.e2.
43. Mohamed SA, Shalaby S, Brakta S, Elam L, Elsharoud A, Al-Hendy A. Umbilical cord blood mesenchymal stem cells as an infertility treatment for chemotherapy induced premature ovarian insufficiency. Biomedicines. 2019;7(1):7.
44. Ameratunga D, Weston G, Osianlis T, Catt J, Vollenhoven B. In vitro fertilisation (IVF) with donor eggs in post-menopausal women: are there differences in pregnancy outcomes in women with premature ovarian failure (POF) compared with women with physiological age-related menopause? J Assist Reprod Genet. 2009;26(9-10):511-4.
45. Practice Committee of American Society For Reproductive Medicine. Increased maternal cardiovascular mortality associated with pregnancy in women with Turner syndrome. Fertil Steril. 2012;97(2):282-4.
46. SavasiVM, Mandia L. Maternal and fetal outcomes in oocyte donation pregnancies. Hum Reprod Update. 2016;22(5):620-33.
47. Terenziani M, Piva L, Meazza C, Gandola L, Cefalo G, Merola M. Oophoropexy: a relevant role in preservation of ovarian function after pelvic irradiation. Fertil Steril. 2009;91(3):935.e15-6.
48. Sonmezer M, Oktay K. Fertility preservation in patients undergoing gonadotoxic treatment of gonadal resection (updated 21 July, 2017). [Online] Available from: www.uptodate.com/contents/fertility-preservation-in-patients-undergoing-gonadotoxic-treatment-or-gonadal-resection [Last accessed December, 2021].
49. Vaiarelli A, Cimadomo D, Trabucco E, Vallefuoco R, Buffo L, Dusi L, et al. Double stimulation in the same ovarian cycle (DuoStim) to maximize the number of oocytes retrieved from poor prognosis patients: a multicenter experience and SWOT analysis. Front Endocrinol (Lausanne). 2018;9:317.
50. Campos APCB, Geber GP, Hurtado R, Sampaio M, Geber S. Ovarian response after random-start controlled ovarian stimulation to cryopreserve oocytes in cancer patients. JBRA Assist Reprod. 2018;22(4):381-84.
51. Specchia C, Baggiani A, Immediata V, Ronchetti C, Cesana A, Smeraldi A, et al. Oocyte cryopreservation in oncological patients: Eighteen years experience of a tertiary care referral center. Front Endocrinol (Lausanne). 2019;10:600.
52. Lambertini M, Moore HCF, Leonard RCF, Loibl S, Munster P, Bruzzone M, et al. Gonadotropin-releasing hormone agonists during chemotherapy for preservation of ovarian function and fertility in premenopausal patients with early breast cancer: a systematic review and meta-analysis of individual patient-level data. J Clin Oncol. 2018;36(19):1981-90.
53. Molina I, Gómez J. Osmotic-shock produced by vitrification solutions improves immature human oocytes in vitro maturation. ReprodBiolEndocrinol. 2016;14(1):27.
54. Kasapi E, Asimakopoulos B. Vitrification of human germinal vesicle oocytes: before or after in-vitro maturation. Int J Fertil Steril. 2017;11(2):85-92.
55. Karavani G1, Schachter-Safrai N. In vitro maturation rates in young premenarche patients. Fertil Steril. 2019;112(2):315-22.
56. Salama M, Woodruff TK. New advances in ovarian autotransplantation to restore fertility in cancer patients. Cancer Metastasis Rev. 2015;34(4):807-22.

57. Martinez F; International Society for Fertility Preservation–ESHRE–ASRM Expert Working Group. Update on fertility preservation from the Barcelona International Society for Fertility Preservation-ESHRE-ASRM 2015 expert meeting: indications, results and future perspectives. Fertil Steril. 2017;108(3):407-415.e11.
58. Pacheco F, Oktay K. Current success and efficiency of autologous ovarian transplantation: a meta-analysis. Reprod Sci. 2017;24(8):1111-20.
59. Lee SJ, SchoverLR, Partridge AH, Patrizio P, Wallace WH, Hagerty K, et al; American Society of Clinical Oncology. American Society of Clinical Oncology recommendations on fertility preservation in cancer patients. J Clin Oncol. 2006;24(18):2917-31.
60. Chae-Kim JJ, Gavrilova-Jordan L. Premature ovarian insufficiency: procreative management and preventive strategies. Biomedicines. 2018;7(1).
61. Webber L, Anderson RA, Davies M, Janse F, Vermeulen N. HRT for women with premature ovarian insufficiency: a comprehensive review. Hum Reprod Open. 2017;2017(2):hox007.
62. ACOG committee opinion.Number 698. (2017). Hormone therapy in primary ovarian insufficiency. [Online] Available from: https://www.acog.org/clinical/clinical-guidance/committee-opinion/articles/2017/05/hormone-therapy-in-primary-ovarian-insufficiency [Last accessed December, 2021].
63. Baber RJ, Panay N, Fenton A; IMS Writing Group. 2016 IMS Recommendations on women's midlife health and menopause hormone therapy. Climacteric. 2016;19(2):109-50.
64. Goswami D, Conway GS. Premature ovarian failure. Hum Reprod Update. 2005;11(4):391-410.
65. Hewlett M, Mahalingaiah S. Update on primary ovarian insufficiency. Current Opinion in Endocrinology, Diabetes, and Obesity. 2015;22(6):483-9.

LONG QUESTIONS

1. Elaborate fertility preservation options for women with premature ovarian insufficiency.
2. Probable causes of premature ovarian insufficiency.

SHORT QUESTIONS

1. Diagnosis and evaluation for a patient suspected to have POI.
2. Hormone replacement therapy in premature ovarian insufficiency patients.

MULTIPLE CHOICE QUESTIONS

1. According to ESHRE, a diagnosis of POI is made is which age group of women?
   a. <40 years   b. < 45 years
   c. <42 years   d. <35 years
2. What is the incidence of spontaneous POI?
   a. 1–5%   b. 8–10%
   c. 0.3–1%   d. 2–3%
3. Fragile X syndrome is:
   a. X-linked dominant   b. X-linked recessive
   c. Autosomal recessive   d. Autosomal dominant
4. In order to diagnose POI in patients with a positive TPO-Ab test, TSH levels should be done every:
   a. 6 months   b. 1 year
   c. 2 years   d. No need to do the test
5. Triad of POI includes which of the following:
   a. FSH>25, E2 <100, AMH normal
   b. FSH>25, E2 <50, decreased AMH
   c. FSH<25, E2 >50, increased AMH
   d. FSH >40,E2 <50, increased AMH
6. Goal of HRT in women with POI is to achieve a serum E2 level of:
   a. 200 pg/mL   b. 50 pg/mL
   c. 100 pg/mL   d. At least 25 pg/mL
7. Best form of contraception for POI patients:
   a. Oral contraceptive pills
   b. IUD and condoms
   c. Transdermal patches
   d. Women with POI do not need any contraception
8. Current established option to overcome infertility in women with POI:
   a. Pretreatment with estrogen
   b. Microflare stimulation protocol
   c. Embryo pooling
   d. Donor eggs embryos
9. Adjuvant fertoprotective agents used for fertility preservation include:
   a. Sphingosine-1-phosphate
   b. Granulocyte stimulating factor
   c. Both of the above
   d. Intravenous Albumin
10. To rule out Addisson disease etiology in POI, which hormone should be tested?
    a. 21 OH-Ab and adrenocortical antibodies
    b. 21 OH-Ab
    c. 17 OH-Ab and adrenocortical antibodies
    d. Only adrenocortical antibodies is sufficient

Answers

1.	a	2.	c	3.	a	4.	b	5.	b	6.	c
7.	b	8.	d	9.	c	10.	a				

10.10 MENOPAUSE: PHYSIOLOGY AND ADAPTATIONS

Sheela HS, Ashwini Neelakanthi

INTRODUCTION

The word "menopause" is derived from Greek words men (month) and pausis (cessation). Menopause is defined as cessation of menses due to loss of ovarian follicular activity in women for a period of 1 year. The clinical diagnosis is retrospective. Loss of ovarian function is an essential characteristic of the concept of menopause.

Menopause is not an abrupt event. The menopause transition goes through several phases. STRAW+10 (Stages of Reproductive Aging Workshop) provides a more comprehensive basis for assessing reproductive aging in research and clinical contexts. Application of this staging system will allow comparability of studies of midlife women and facilitate clinical decision-making. The STRAW+10 staging system is applicable to women regardless of age, demographic, BMI or lifestyle characteristics.[1] There are 10 STRAW stages, which are grouped into three larger groups.[1]

1. *Reproductive group (–5, –4, –3b, –3a):* This includes categories –5 (beginning at menarche and characterized by variable to regular menstrual cycles), –4 (peak reproductive stage with regular cycles), –3b (late reproductive stage with regular cycles), and –3a (late reproductive stage with start of subtle changes in cycle length).
2. *Menopausal transition (–2, –1):* This includes categories –2 (variable length of cycle) and –1 (categorized by episodes of amenorrhea of ≥60 days). A follicle-stimulating hormone (FSH) of >25IU/L is commonly seen in late transition phase (–1 stage) and this is when vasomotor symptoms (VMS) begin to occur **(Table 1)**.
3. *Postmenopause (+1a, +1b, +1c, +2):* Stages +1a and +1b each last one year and end at the time point at which FSH and estradiol levels stabilize. VMS are most common in stage + 1a and +1b. Stage + 1a marks the end of the 12 month period of amenorrhea required to define that the FMP (final menstrual period) has occurred. It corresponds to the end of the "perimenopause", which is the time around the menopause beginning at stage –2 and ends at stage +1a (12 months after the FMP). Stage +1c represents the period of stabilization of high FSH levels and low estradiol values that is estimated to last 3-6 years. Late post-menopause stage +2 represents the period in which reproductive hormone levels reached plateauand stable. Symptoms of vaginal dryness and urogenital atrophyare more common during this period.

STRAW+10 staging of reproductive aging relevant to menopause is elaborated in **Table 1**.

TABLE 1: STRAW+10 (Stages of Reproductive Aging Workshop) staging of reproductive aging relevant to menopause.[1]

Stages	***– 2***	***–1***	***+ 1a***	***+ 1b***	***+ 1c***	***+ 2***
Terminology	Menopausal transition		Post-menopause			
	Early	Late	Early			Late
	Perimenopause					
Duration	Variable	1–3 years	1 year	1 year	3–6 years	Remaining life span
Principal criteria						
Menstrual cycle	Variable ≥7day difference in length of consecutive cycles	Interval of amenorrhea ≥60 days				
Supportive criteria						
FSH	↑ variable	↑ >25IU/L	↑ variable		Stabilizes	
AMH	Low	Low	Low		Very low	
Inhibin B	Low	Low	Low		Very low	
AFC	Low	Low	Very low		Very low	
Descriptive characteristics						
Symptoms		Vasomotor symptoms likely	Vasomotor symptoms most likely			Increasing symptoms of urogenital atrophy

(AFC: antral follicle count; AMH: Anti-Müllerian hormone; FMP: final menstrual period; FSH: follicle-stimulating hormone)

Climacteric is less precise termthat starts from the decline in ovarian activity and lasts until after the end of ovarian function. It includes perimenopause, menopause, and post-menopause.

AGE AT MENOPAUSE

Average age of menopause of an Indian woman is 46.2 years (46.2 ± 4.9) much less than their Western counterparts, which is 51 years.[2] The age at menopause appears to be genetically determined. Body fat contributes to estrogen production and so thinner women experience earlier menopause.[3] Smoking increases the risk of early menopause. There is a dose response relationship with the number of cigarette smoked per day.[4]

Premature ovarian insufficiency is defined as menopause before the age of 40 years. It occurs in approximately 1% of women. Iatrogenic menopause is permanent cessation of menses due to surgical removal of both ovaries or radiation to both ovaries before the natural age of menopause. The term should not be used to describe the cessation of menses, which follows simple hysterectomy where in ovaries are retained.

HYPOTHALAMO-PITUITARY GONADAL AXIS

Although menopause is associated with changes in hypothalamic and pituitary hormones, menopause is not a central event but primary ovarian failure. There is depletion of follicles in the ovaries most likely due to apoptosis or programmed cell death and there is resistance of ovaries to gonadotropins. Due to follicular atresia, in particular the granulosa cells, there is decreased production of estrogen and inhibin. Thus, FSH continues to rise due to absence of negative feedback from ovary. Elevated FSH level is a cardinal sign of menopause.

After menopause, there is 10–20-fold rise in FSH and 3-fold increase in luteinizing hormone (LH) reaching a peak 1–3 years after menopause, after which there is slight decline in both FSH and LH. Several months of amenorrhea along with an FSH level of 40 IU/L or more are reliableindicators that menopause is either near or already passed.[5]

Anti-Müllerian hormone (AMH) is produced in the ovary by granulosa cells of antral follicles. A good correlation has been found between AMH levels and age and also between AMH levels and the number of antral follicles.[6] The peak levels coincide with peak fertility in the mid-20s, and decline thereafter becoming undetectable at time of functional menopause.

ESTROGENS

The pathophysiologic consequences of menopause are primarily due to estrogen deficiency. There are different types of estrogens that predominate in different stages of woman's life.

- Estradiol E2—most potent(reproductive phase)
- Estrone E1—low potency (menopause)
- Estriol E3—least potent (pregnancy).

The ER-α is predominantly found in mammary gland, uterus, theca cells of the ovary, bone, male reproductive system, liver, and adipose tissue, while on the other hand, the ER-β is found for the most part in the bladder, granulosa cells of the ovary, colon, adipose tissue, skin, CVS, CNS, bones, and immune system.[7-9]

The circulating level of estrone in postmenopausal woman is more than that of estradiol. After menopause, the ovaries secrete mainly androstenedione and testosterone. The main source of estrone is peripheral conversion of androgens, which are mainly secreted by adrenals and also ovary. The trace amount of estradiol is derived from peripheral conversion of estrone and androgens **(Flowchart 1)**. Dehydroepiandrosterone (DHEA) and its sulfate (DHEA-S) originating from adrenal gland also decline with aging.

Because sex hormone-binding globulin (SHBG) declines during the menopause transition, there is likely a positive change in the free androgen index (FAI), reflecting an increase in biologically available androgen among women.[10] Late menopause may be considered as a state of relative androgen excess. The androgen/estrogen ratio changes and onset of mild hirsutism is common.

Inhibin: Inhibin A is primarily a secretory product of the dominant follicle and the corpus luteum, and inhibin B of small antral follicle. It is only those women who continue to ovulate close to the FMP contribute a significant amount of inhibin A. Inhibin in the early menopausal transition is the dominant hormone to suppress FSH. Later in the menopausal transition, E2 and also inhibin play a significant role in the ovarian hypothalamic feedback system.[11]

Intracrinology: whereby each cell of each peripheral tissue(except in the endometrium) makes a small and appropriate amount of estrogens and androgens from the inactive precursor DHEA,which then act and are inactivated locally in the same cells. This is to maintain very low and biologically inactive concentrations of estrogens and androgens in the circulation, thus avoiding biologically significant systemic exposure to active sex steroids.[12] Although determinants of ovarian reserve, including levels of AMH, cycle day-3 FSH and estradiol, and ovarian antral follicle count, are available, their clinical use is best confined to counseling women seeking fertility rather than predicting time to menopause. The diagnostic criteria for perimenopause and menopause as per NICE recommendations are given in **Box 1**.[13]

Flowchart 1: Peripheral conversion of androgens to estrogens.

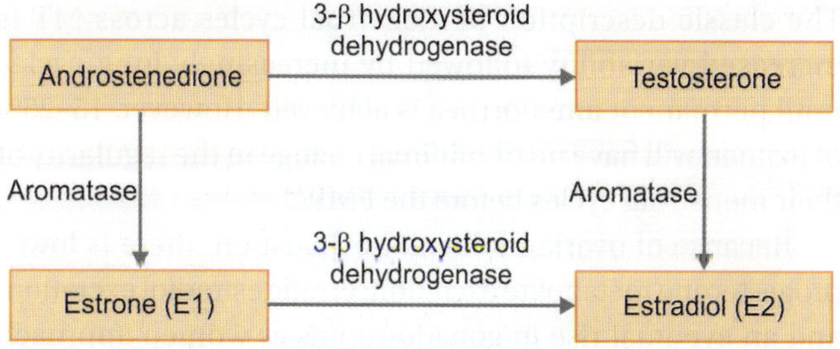

BOX 1: Diagnosis of perimenopause and menopause (NICE 2019).[13]

Consider using a follicle-stimulating hormone (FSH) test to diagnose menopause only:
- In women aged 40–45 years with menopausal symptoms, including a change in their menstrual cycle
- In women aged under 40 years in whom menopause is suspected

Diagnose the following without laboratory tests in otherwise healthy women aged over 45 years with menopausal symptoms:
- Perimenopause based on vasomotor symptoms and irregular periods
- Menopause in women who have not had a period for at least 12 months and are not using hormonal contraception
- Menopause based on symptoms in women without a uterus

Take into account that it can be difficult to diagnose menopause in women who are taking hormonal treatments, for example for the treatment of heavy periods.

Do not use a serum FSHtest to diagnose menopause in women using combined estrogen and progestogen contraception or high-dose progestogen.

Do not use the following laboratory and imaging tests to diagnose perimenopause or menopause in women aged over 45 years:
- Anti-Müllerian hormone
- Inhibin A
- Inhibin B
- Estradiol
- Antral follicle count
- Ovarian volume

SYMPTOMS

The commonly observed menopausal symptoms are abnormal uterine bleeding, hot flashes (HFs), poor sleep, adverse mood, and vaginal dryness.

Abnormal Uterine Bleeding

Women in menopausal transition period have higher overall estrogen levels due to an increased ovarian follicular reaction to the increase in FSH secretion during these years.[14] Variability in estrogen levels is characteristic of menopausal transition.

Although short bleeding and spotting episodes occur more frequently after the onset of the menopausal transition, excessive flow and prolonged menstrual bleeding are more common. Short cycles are most frequent early in the transition, whereas long cycles are most frequent late in the transition. Excessive bleeding is most often associated with ovulatory cycles during MT, although spotting and bleeding for longer than 8 days are associated with anovulatory cycles. The classic description of menstrual cycles across MT is increased variability followed by increasingly long cycles until permanent amenorrhea is achieved. However, 15–25% of women will have no or minimal change in the regularity of their menstrual cycles before the FMP.[15]

Because of ovarian follicular exhaustion, there is lower progesterone metabolite excretion, erratic estradiol excretion, and an eventual rise in gonadotropins as women approach toward FMP. The prevalence of cycles with low pregnanediol glucuronide (Pdg) excretion (i.e., cycles without evidence of luteal activity) increases rapidly in the final 3 years before the FMP and is associated with more variability in cycle length but not with large changes in bleeding duration.[16]

As many as 25% of irregular cycles with long intervals (>50–60 days) can be ovulatory.Contraception is recommended until women have experienced 12 months of amenorrhea as ovulatory cycles are present during the menopause transition.

Vasomotor Symptoms

The HF is described as a sudden onset of warmth in the face and neck that progresses to the chest, often accompanied by a visible red flush. The hands become warm and the skin of the face and neck become moist. These episodes may last for several minutes, be exceedingly uncomfortable, and are frequently associated with dizziness, nausea, headaches, palpitations, diaphoresis, and "night sweats". These symptoms can also be triggered by emotional stress, excitement, fear, or anxiety, and disappear as quickly as they appeared. It appears that hot flushes are triggered by "estrogen withdrawal" rather than by a lack of estrogen. Vasomotor instability is characterized by a rise in skin temperature, peripheral vasodilation, atransient increase in heart rate, and changes in skin impedance.[17]It is sometimes concluded by diffuse perspiration. Most importantly hot flushes can affect woman's quality of life.

Vasomotor symptoms are the primary menopausal symptom, peaking around the FMP and occurring in up to 80% of women during the menopausal transition. Occurrence is lowest prior to entering the menopausal transition, increasing in the early transition and higher still in the late transition near the FMP. Post-menopause, VMS occur in as many as 3 out of 4 women in the first 2 years post-FMP, and decline slowly afterward.

Recent research from the Study of Women's Health Across the Nation (SWAN) found that frequent VMS last a median of 7.4 years. Longitudinal analyses from SWAN found that FSH is more strongly associated with VMS than E2. SWAN data show that while greater BMI is related to less frequent VMS in the late menopause, BMI is positively related to VMS in early menopause. Thus, BMI appears to have a different relationship with VMS before and after menopause. Smoking is the primary health behavior that has been associated with VMS. SWAN has shown that both active smoking and passive smoke exposure are related to greater likelihood of VMS.[18]

Pathophysiology of VMS

- Hot flashes are triggered by "estrogen withdrawal"rather than by a lack of estrogen.
- A temporal relationship was observed between HFs and LH pulses.

- Norepinephrine (NE) plays an important role in thermoregulation acting, in part, through α2-adrenergic receptors. NE causes heat dissipation responses followed by a decline in core body temperature (Tc). Most α2 receptors in the human brain are inhibitory. Clonidine which is central alpha-2 agonist would reduce NE and reduce VMS.
- Few studies suggest that pulsatile LH secretion is modulated by a subpopulation of neurons in the arcuate (infundibular) nucleus of hypothalamus, which is mediated through kisspeptins. Kisspeptins are very potent gonadotropin-releasing hormone secretagogues,which are found to play a physiological role in development of HFs.[19]

Hot flashes are triggered by core body temperature (Tc) elevations acting within a greatly narrowed thermoneutral zone in postmenopausal women with HFs **(Fig. 1)**. An HF, consisting of sweating and peripheral vasodilation, is provoked when Tc reaches the upper threshold. Tc then declines, and when the lower threshold is crossed, shivering occurs.[20]

Genitourinary Syndrome of Menopause

The genitourinary syndrome of menopause (GSM) is a new term that replaces previous terminology"vulvovaginal atrophy". It describes various menopausal symptoms and signs associated with physical changes of the vulva, vagina, and lower urinary tract **(Box 2)**.

The GSM includes:

- Genital symptoms (dryness, burning, irritation, itching of vulva and vagina)
- Sexual symptoms (decreased lubrication, discomfort or pain during sexual activity, decreased arousal, orgasm)
- Urinary symptoms (urinary frequency, urgency, dysuria, and recurrent urinary tract infections.

These symptoms have profound impact on the quality of life of postmenopausal women by negatively affecting self-esteem and their sexual life.

Estrogen receptors (ERs; both α and β) are present in the vagina, vulva, musculature of the pelvic floor, endopelvic fascia, urethra, and bladder trigone during reproductive life; their levels decline with menopause.[21] Urethral caruncles and noninflammatory urethritis are common findings in elderly postmenopausal women.

Type I collagen provides mechanical strength to tissues while type III contributes to elasticity and regulates collagen fibril diameter during fibrillogenesis. Estrogen and progesterone hormones are required for protection against tissue deterioration and to maintain the tissue integrity. This protective effect is lost with onset of menopause. The matrix metalloproteinases (MMPs) then trigger the collagenase activity, which alters the collagen ratios, thereby decreasing the stronger and thicker collagen type I relative to weaker and distensile collagen type III. Reduced ratio of collagen types I to III leads to thinnercollagen fibrils, pathologically altered extracellular matrix (ECM). Significant reduction (68%) of total collagen in pelvic floor disorder subjects has been observed.[22]

Cognition

Neural structures in the brain that control multiple functions affected during MT are populated with estrogen receptors. Such receptors are localized to plasma membranes, mitochondria, and in the nucleus of cells, and are particularly abundant in the hypothalamus, which is the primary thermoregulatory center and regulator of sleep and circadian rhythms. Brain regions that are crucial to learning and memory, including the prefrontal cortex, hippocampus, amygdala, and posterior cingulate cortex, also contain substantial estrogen receptors.

The brain compensates for decreased estrogen and reduced receptor activity during the MT. But for some women, this adaptive compensation is diminished, lacking, or only expressed in a subset of estrogen-regulated neural networks, giving rise to the complex neurological phenotype of menopause.

Estrogenic regulation of brain glucose metabolism is dismantled during perimenopause, inducing a hypometabolic state. Hypometabolism, reduced mitochondrial function, and subsequent oxidative damage are known to promote accumulation of Aβ (amyloid beta) pathology and neuronal dysfunction, therefore increasing risk of developing Alzheimer

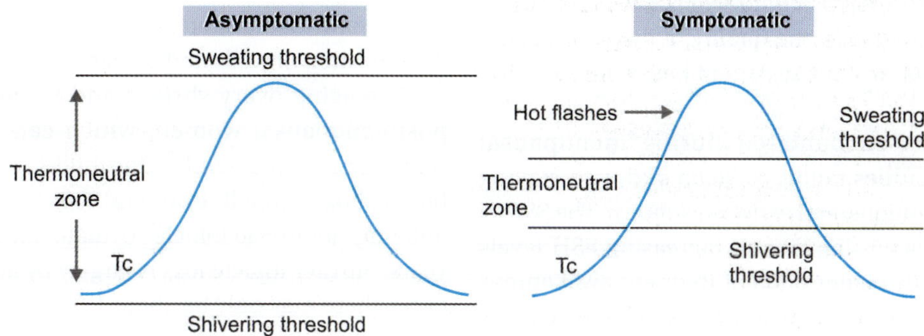

Fig.1: Relationship between core body temperature (Tc) and thermoneutral zone in symptomatic and asymptomatic postmenopausal women.[20]

BOX 2: Changes in the genitourinary tissues.[21]

- Loss of labial and vulval fullness
- Contraction of labia majora and clitoral hood
- Narrowing and stenosis of the introitus
- Loss of hymenal remnants or reduced elasticity
- Vaginal shortening and narrowing
- Prolapse
- Pelvic floor weakening
- Vaginal epithelium dry and thin with petechiae
- Loss of superficial cells and increase in parabasal cells
- Loss of vaginal rugae
- Inflamed vaginal tissues
- Alkaline pH changes the vaginal microbiome with loss of lactobacilli (vaginal pH >4.5)
- Persistent or recurrent discharge with odor (not *Candida* in post-menopause)
- Urethral meatal prominence and prolapse with thinning of the urethral epithelium
- Touch perception altered either hypersensitive or decreased feeling
- Loss of clitoral stimulation

disease later in life.[23] Estrogens are involved in a number of cellular pathways that underlie brain function. Hence, effects of reproductive aging on cognition in midlife and beyond remains a topic of great interest.

Large clinical trials, such as the Women's Health Initiative (WHI) and Women's Health Initiative Memory Study (WHIMS), exposed significant risks, including cognitive risks associated with hormone replacement therapy. In contrast, multiple previous studies revealed benefits of hormone therapy use on cognition when treatment commenced proximal to the menopause transition.

So the age of initiation of hormone therapy may be primary contributing factor to discrepancies between studies reflecting treatment benefits in cognition from those that suggested harm. That is, a critical window of treatment initiation is a key determinant in positive versus deleterious outcomes.[24]

Mood and Sleep

Perimenopausal women are more likely to develop depressive disorders even without a previous history and those who have a positive history of depression are much morelikely to relapse. There is also a correlation between VMS and depressivedisorders. Unfortunate life events, a negative mood toward menopause, lifestyle, the quality of the relationship between the partners, and surgical menopause are the other risk factors.[25]

Sleep problems encountered during menopausal transition are difficulties falling to sleep and with staying asleep, sleep interruptions, and early awakenings. The SWAN study found that decreasing E2 and increasing FSH levels were associated with higher odds of frequent awakenings across follow-ups and that a greater rate of change in FSH was associated with poorer sleep quality. Sleep problems are multifactorial, strongly associated with HFs, and depression and other factors coincident with aging, such as stress, poor health, and chronic pain.[26]

Vasomotor symptoms and adverse mood often improve after a woman is postmenopausal, whereas sleep complaints, vaginal dryness/dyspareunia, and cognitive complaints tend to persist or worsen in association with aging.[27]

Changes in Organs

Vulva: It shows features of atrophy and there is reduction in amount of glycogen in epithelial cells. Labia majora becomes smaller and pubic hair become scantier.

Vagina: Deprived of estrogen, the vagina loses collagen, adipose tissue, and the rugae progressively flatten. There is marked reduction in ratio of superficial to basal cells. The vaginal surface is friable and prone to bleeding with minimal trauma. Due to lack of glycogen in vaginal epithelium, vaginal pH becomes more alkaline. A pH >4.5 is almost always observed with estrogen deficiency.

Cervix: It often becomes flush with the apex of the vagina and the cervical os is visible as a small opening. The squamocolumnar junction moves up into the canal, which can present problems for colposcopic examination of cervical dysplasia.[17]

Uterus: The postmenopausal uterus reverts back to the prepubertal ratio—a corpus smaller than the cervix. The endometrium becomes thin and atropic. Endometrial curettings in the postmenopausal patient are usually scanty and show only superficial fragments of epithelium.[17]Endometrial thickness of 4 mm or less has a >99% negative predictive value for endometrial cancer. Transvaginal ultrasonography is a reasonable alternative to endometrial sampling as a first approach in evaluating a postmenopausal woman with an initial episode of bleeding.[28]

Ovary: Structural changes are seen in both the cortex and medulla.

In the cortex, there is—(1) reduction of its thickness; (2) epithelial inclusions forming cysts; (3) blurring the line between medulla and cortex; (4) reduction in the number of follicles; (5) tendency to fragmentation of corpora albicantia; and (6) surface epithelium invaginations.

Changes seen in the medulla—(1) fibrosis and scars in stroma; and (2) architectonical changes in blood vessels with hyalinization of walls and constriction of lumen.

The aging ovary shrinks and its volume is smaller in postmenopausal women, which can be clearly seen in transvaginal ultrasound.[29] One million oocytes are present at birth falling off rapidly to around 200,000 by the end of puberty, and only about 350 follicles ovulate during the reproductive years. Further follicle loss is largely by apoptosis. By the last cycle, there may only be about 1,000 follicles in the ovaries.[9]

Breast: During reproductive age, estrogen and progesterone exert proliferative effects on ductal and glandular structures, respectively. In a postmenopausal woman, there is significant reduction in volume and tissue density, which can be seen on mammography. Glandular tissue shrinks and loss of elasticity causes the breasts to droop and flatten. Nipples become smaller and flatter, and may lose their erectile properties.

Skin: Collagen levels in the skin, with type I (80%) and type III (15%) as the most prevalent, correlate with estrogen levels. Up to 30% of dermal collagen may be lost in the first 5 years after menopause, and collagen decreases by approximately 2.1% per year. Likewise, skin thickness decreases 1.1% per year. Estrogen helps retain and restore skin moisture through the promotion of sebum secretion. One of the first symptoms experienced is increased skin dryness, followed by decreased firmness and elasticity.[8]

Immune system: Postmenopausal women are at a higher risk of autoimmune disorders. Menopausal women have higher concentrations of cytokines such as tumor necrosis factor (TNF)-alpha, interleukin (IL)-6, and CRP and lower number of type 4 (CD4) T cells and B lymphocytes.[9] This immune senescence leads to increased susceptibility to infections and decreased response to vaccination.

Bone: Estrogen deficiency after menopause can lead to osteoporosis and an increased risk of bone fracture. Trabecular bone is more severely affected than cortical bone. Thus, bones that are rich in trabecular bone and responsible for weight bearing arc prime targets for fractures. Thus, common sites of fractures are the vertebrae, ribs, proximal femur, pelvis, and distal radius. Bone remodeling takes place by osteoblasts—the bone forming cells and osteoclasts—the bone resorbing cells.

Estrogen is protective in bone by following mechanisms:
- Represses pro-osteoclastic cytokines
- Induces apoptosis in bone resorbing osteoclasts
- Estrogen-mediated suppression of osteoclasts involves the regulation of the RANKL/(OPG) ratio
- E2 is antiapoptotic in osteoblasts.[30]

Effect on thyroid: At the menopause, thyroid uptakc of iodine decreases, leading to reduced free thyroxine (FT4) and free tri-iodothyronine (FT3), and hence the concentrations of thyroid-stimulating hormone (TSH) increase through activation of the hypothalamic–pituitary–thyroid (HPT) axis.[9]

Cardiovascular system: Estrogens can promote vasodilation through increasing plasma concentrations of endothelium-derived relaxing factor nitric oxide (NO), and can inhibit the renin angiotensin system by reducing transcription of angiotensin converting enzyme. Estrogen has favorable effects on lipids. It increases HDL and decreases total cholesterol and LDL levels.

In women, the risk of cardiovascular disease (CVD) is much lower than in men until 50 years of agebecause of protective effect of estrogen,but it rises dramatically after menopause. It has been hypothesized that lower levels of endogenous estrogens and higher endogenous androgens that occur during menopausal transition might mediate the increased CVD risk.

TABLE 2: Changes in circulating hormone levels at menopause.[5]

	Pre-menopause	*Post-menopause*
Estradiol	40–400 pg/mL	10–20 pg/mL
Estrone	30–200 pg/mL	30–70 pg/mL
Testosterone	20–80 ng/dL	15–70 ng/dL
Androstenedione	60–300 ng/dL	30–150 ng/dL

Changes in circulating hormone levels at different menopause stages are given in **Table 2.**

KEY MESSAGES

- Menopause is defined as cessation of menses due to loss of ovarian follicular activity in women for a period of one year.
- STRAW+10 (Stages of Reproductive Aging Workshop) provides a comprehensive basis for assessing reproductive aging.
- Elevated FSH level is a cardinal sign of menopause.
- The type of estrogen that predominates during menopause is estrone (E1).
- The commonly observed menopausal symptoms areabnormal uterine bleeding, hot flashes, poor sleep, adverse mood, and vaginal dryness.
- The genitourinary syndrome of menopause (GSM) is a new term that replaces previous terminologies "vulvovaginal atrophy".

REFERENCES

1. Harlow SD, Gass M, Hall JE, Lobo R, Maki P, Rebar RW, et al. Executive summary of STRAW+10: addressing the unfinished agenda of staging reproductive aging. Climacteric J Int Menopause Soc. 2012;15(2):105-14.
2. Ahuja M. Age of menopause and determinants of menopause age: A PAN India survey by IMS. J Life Health. 2016;7(3):126-31.
3. MacMahon B, Worcester J. Age at menopause. United States--1960-1962. Vital Health Stat 11. 1966;(19):1-20.
4. Midgette AS, Baron JA. Cigarette smoking and the risk of natural menopause. Epidemiol Camb Mass. 1990;1(6):474-80.
5. Taylor HS, Pal L, Sell E. Speroff's Clinical Gynecologic Endocrinology and Infertility, 9th edition. Philadelphia: Lippincott Williams & Wilkins; 2019.
6. Kruszyńska A, Słowińska-Srzednicka J. Anti-Müllerian hormone (AMH) as a good predictor of time of menopause. Prze gląd Menopauzalny Menopause Rev. 2017;16(2):47-50.
7. Leblanc DR, Schneider M, Angele P, Vollmer G, Docheva D. The effect of estrogen on tendon and ligament metabolism and function. J Steroid Biochem Mol Biol. 2017;172:106-16.
8. Rzepecki AK, Murase JE, Juran R, Fabi SG, McLellan BN. Estrogen-deficient skin: the role of topical therapy. Int J Womens Dermatol. 2019;5(2):85-90.
9. Honour JW. Biochemistry of the menopause. Ann Clin Biochem. 2018;55(1):18-33.

10. Sowers MFR, Zheng H, McConnell D, Nan B, Karvonen-Gutierrez CA, Randolph JF. Testosterone, sex hormone-binding globulin and free androgen index among adult women: chronological and ovarian aging. Hum Reprod Oxf Engl. 2009;24(9):2276-85.
11. Øverlie I, MØrkrid L, Andersson A-M, SkakkebÆk NE, Moen MH, Holte A. Inhibin A and B as markers of menopause: a five-year prospective longitudinal study of hormonal changes during the menopausal transition. Acta Obstet Gynecol Scand. 2005;84(3):281-5.
12. Labrie F. Intracrinology and menopause: the science describing the cell-specific intracellular formation of estrogens and androgens from DHEA and their strictly local action and inactivation in peripheral tissues. Menopause NYN. 2019;26(2):220-4.
13. National Institute for Health and Care Excellence. (2015). NICE guideline NG23. Summary of evidence for 2019 surveillance of menopause. [Online] Available from: https://www.nice.org.uk/consultations/672/10/overview [Last accessed December, 2021].
14. Santoro N, Brown JR, Adel T, Skurnick JH. Characterization of reproductive hormonal dynamics in the perimenopause. J Clin Endocrinol Metab. 1996;81(4):1495-501.
15. Harlow SD. Menstrual cycle changes as women approach the final menses: What matters? Obstet Gynecol Clin North Am. 2018;45(4):599-611.
16. Santoro N, Crawford SL, El Khoudary SR, Allshouse AA, Burnett-Bowie S-A, Finkelstein J, et al. Menstrual cycle hormone changes in women traversing menopause: Study of Women's Health Across the Nation. J Clin Endocrinol Metab. 2017;102(7):2218-29.
17. BuchsbaumHJ. The Menopause. US: Springer Science & Business Media; 2012.
18. Avis NE, Crawford SL, Green R. Vasomotor symptoms across the menopause transition: Differences among women. Obstet Gynecol Clin North Am. 2018;45(4):629-40.
19. Olaniyan T, Meraiyebu AK, Dare JB, Anjorin YD, Shafe MO. Kisspeptin system: A multi-homeostatic system. J Pharm Biol Sci IOSR-JPBS. 2013;5:87-101.
20. Freedman RR. Pathophysiology and treatment of menopausal hot flashes. Semin Reprod Med. 2005;23(2):117-25.
21. Kim H-K, Kang S-Y, Chung Y-J, Kim J-H, Kim M-R. The recent review of the genitourinary syndrome of menopause. J Menopausal Med. 2015;21(2):65-71.
22. Bhattarai A, Staat M. Modelling of soft connective tissues to investigate female pelvic floor dysfunctions. Comput Math Methods Med. 2018;2018:9518076.
23. Scheyer O, Rahman A, Hristov H, Berkowitz C, Isaacson RS, Brinton RD, et al. Female sex and Alzheimer's risk: The menopause connection. J Prev Alzheimers Dis. 2018;5(4):225-30.
24. Morgan KN, Derby CA, Gleason CE. Cognitive changes with reproductive aging, perimenopause and menopause. Obstet Gynecol Clin North Am. 2018;45(4):751-63.
25. Augoulea A, Moros M, Lykeridou A, Kaparos G, Lyberi R, Panoulis K. Psychosomatic and vasomotor symptom changes during transition to menopause. Prze glad Menopauzalny Menopause Rev. 2019;18(2):110-5.
26. Baker FC, de Zambotti M, Colrain IM, Bei B. Sleep problems during the menopausal transition: prevalence, impact, and management challenges. Nat Sci Sleep. 2018;10:73-95.
27. Santoro N. Perimenopause: From research to practice. J Womens Health 2002. 2016;25(4):332-9.
28. ACOG Committee Opinion No. 734: The role of transvaginal ultrasonography in evaluating the endometrium of women with postmenopausal bleeding. Obstet Gynecol. 2018;131(5):e124-9.
29. Laszczyńska M, Brodowska A, Starczewski A, Masiuk M, Brodowski J. Human postmenopausal ovary—hormonally inactive fibrous connective tissue or more? Histol Histopathol. 2008;23(2):219-26.
30. Khalid AB, Krum SA. Estrogen receptors alpha and beta in bone. Bone. 2016;87:130-5.

LONG QUESTIONS

1. Discuss STRAW +10 staging of reproductive aging relevant to menopause.
2. What are the hormonal changes seen during menopausal transition? Write a note on changes in bleeding pattern seen during this phase.

SHORT QUESTIONS

Write a short note on:

1. Vasomotor symptoms and its pathophysiology.
2. Genitourinary syndrome of menopause.

MULTIPLE CHOICE QUESTIONS

1. The time around the menopause beginning at STRAW stage –2 and ending 12 months after the final menstrual period is called:
   a. Early menopausal transition
   b. Late menopausal transition
   c. Perimenopause
   d. Early postmenopause
2. All of the following lead to early menopaiuse, except:
   a. Smoking b. Underweight women
   c. Obese women d. Chemotherapy
3. All of the following hormone levels decrease during menopausal transition, except:
   a. AMH b. Inhibin
   c. Estradiol d. LH
4. The type of estrogen which predominates during menopause is:
   a. Estradiol b. Estrone
   c. Estriol d. Androstenedione
5. Which of the following is incorrect with respect to vaginal changes during menopause?
   a. There is reduction in the ratio of superficial to basal cells
   b. Vaginal candidial infection rates decline with aging
   c. Vaginal pH becomes more acidic
   d. Vagina loses collagen and the ability to retain water
6. Menopause increases the risk of all of the following, except:
   a. Osteoporosis
   b. Cardiovascular disease
   c. Vaginal dryness
   d. Sexually transmitted diseases

7. In postmenopausal women, circulating testosterone is a precursor for which of the following steroids?
   a. Androstenedione
   b. Cortisol
   c. Dehydroepiandrosterone
   d. Estradiol
8. Which of the following enzymes converts testosterone to estradiol ?
   a. Aromatase
   b. 5 alpha reductase
   c. 17 beta hydroxy steroid dehydrogenase
   d. 11 beta hydroxylase
9. Estrogen depletion at menopause is associated with:
   a. An increase in sex hormone-binding globulin
   b. A decrease in sex hormone-binding globulin
   c. An increase in bioavailable testosterone
   d. A decrease in bioavailable testosterone
   e. b and c
10. Estrogen receptor alpha predominates in all of the following organs, except:
   a. Skin
   b. Theca cells of ovary
   c. Mammary glands
   d. Uterus

Answers

1.	c	2.	c	3.	d	4.	b	5.	c	6.	d
7.	d	8.	a	9.	e	10.	a				

10.11 IMPLICATIONS OF MENOPAUSE ON CARDIOVASCULAR AND BONE HEALTH

Revathy Janakiram, Krithika Meenakshi

INTRODUCTION

Menopause may be considered as a biological marker forcardiovascular disease (CVD).[1] Epidemiological data strongly suggests an association of increased incidence of cardiovascular events after menopause, distinct from aging factor.Framingham in a cohort of 2,083 women studied the relationship between menopause and CVD. Evidences from Framingham, Nurses' Health Study, suggestthat menopause transition accelerate long-term chronic disorders such as CVD. Postmenopausal women have double the time increased incidence of CVD than premenopausal women even after adjustments for age. Natural premature menopausal women < 35 years have 2–3 fold increase in myocardial infarction (MI) and in those with bilateral oophorectomy, younger than 35 years, there is an increase by seven times of MI. Menopause may be considered as an individual nonmodifiable risk factor other than the known common risk factors for both sexes **(Table 1)**. Hence, it is essential to understand the risk factors for CVD and institute timely primary intervention programs. There is an increased risk of cardiovascular disease mortality, with early menopause.[2,3] Every year of premature menopause increases the risk of CVDby 2%.

In women after menopause,the leading cause of death is CVD, including coronary heart disease, congestive heart failure, and stroke, compared with men oftheir age, women have a much lower risk ofcardiovascular events before menopause. The reasons for protection from CVD in premenopausal women are complex. A significant contribution can be assigned to the greater HDL levels, which is an effect of estrogen. As women enter menopause estrogen level declines. So the benefit of estrogen disappears and the risk of CVD increases exponentially. Therefore for women in menopausal transition by preventive measures we can significantly improve both their quality and quantity oflives.In postmenopausal women there is a trend for a 2–6-fold higher incidence of CVD compared with premenopausal women in the same age range. An increasedCVD is observedwith menopausal transition regardless of the age. This indicates association of withdrawal of estrogen with an increased risk of CVD.

ROLE OF ESTROGEN IN PROTECTION OF CARDIOVASCULAR HEALTH[4]

Estrogen protects cardiovascular health by the following **(Table 1)**:

- Its beneficial effecton lipids, lipoproteins, homocysteine
- Regulating coagulation andfibrinolysis
- Positive effect on endothelial cell function

TABLE 1: Risk factors for coronary heart disease are both modifiable and nonmodifiable.[5]

Nonmodifiable risks	*Modifiable risks*
Family history of MI	↑Serum cholesterol levels (>6.2 mmol/L)
Sudden death of female relative before the age of 65 years	Low plasma HDL-C levels (< 0.9 mmol/L)
Female >55 years	Obesity
Premature menopause	Hypertension
	Smoking
	Sedentary lifestyle
	Excessive alcohol intake

- Relaxation of vascular smooth muscle
- Improving glucose andinsulin metabolism
- Acting as an antioxidant.

Loss of these benefits of estrogen after menopause, alongwith other risk factors, increases the risk of CVD in menopause. In the Women's Ischemia Syndrome Evaluation (WISE) study, postmenopausal women who had used oral contraceptives in the past had less coronary artery disease. It has been found that compared with normal women, premenopausal women with coronary artery disease have lower circulating levels of estrogen. Clinical presentations of CVD in women are different in women as a result of estrogens and genetics. In men the main problem may be a blockage in the large coronary artery, which shows up on an angiogram, but women are more likely to have microvessel disease which may not be seen. This could be the reason why women with heart disease are often under diagnosed and under treated.

PATHOPHYSIOLOGY

Atherosclerosis is a chronic inflammatory disease of the arterial wall. This leads to the formation of plaques in arterial walls which narrow the arterial passage, restrict blood flow, and increase the risk of occlusion of blood flow.

There is a sequence of events leading to atherosclerosis as shown **Flowchart 1**.

Flowchart 1: Events leading to atherosclerosis.

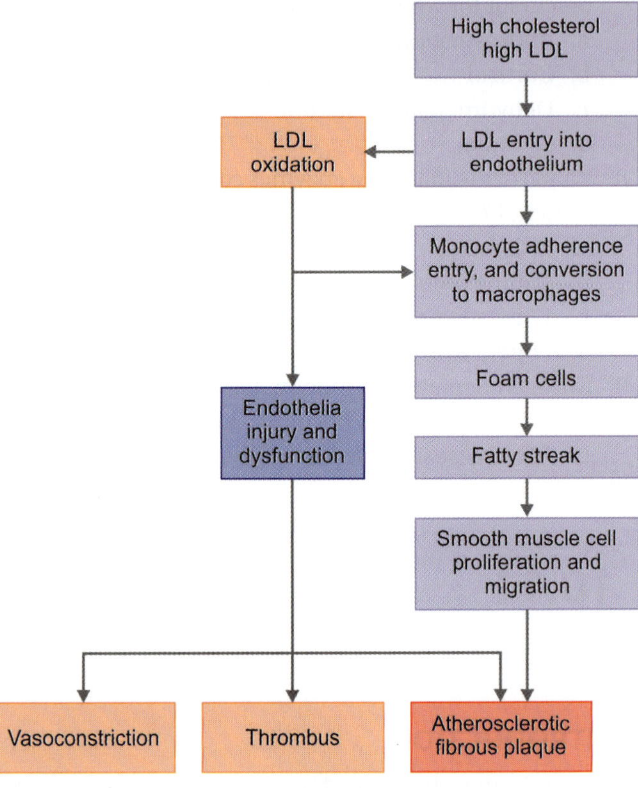

There is increased oxidative stress in atherosclerosis, which is characterized by lipid and proteinoxidation in the vascular wall **(Fig. 1)**. LDL oxidation is an early event in atherosclerosis, leading on to endothelial injury and dysfunction.Oxidized LDL (O-LDL) is one of the important contributors of atherogenesis **(Fig. 2)**. The mature atherosclerotic plaque is an acellular necrotic core that is made of cholesterol and the deadmacrophages called *foam cells*. It is encapsulated by a thin fibrous cap. These plaques become calcified subsequently. When rupture or erosion of these plaques occurs, it leads to thrombus formation. This may cause acute occlusion leading on to myocardial infarction, DVT and strokes. What causes this rupture? Factors such asinfection, physical exertion and mechanical stress, may destabilize and initiate the rupture of the vulnerable plaque and promote thrombosis.

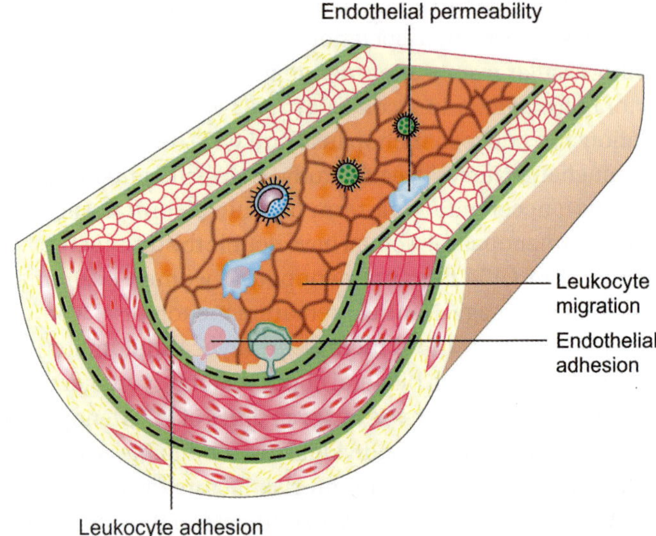

Fig. 1: Atherosclerosis.

LIPID PROFILE AND MENOPAUSE

The lipid profile is adversely altered with menopause. Total as well as LDL cholesterol levels are lower in premenopausal women. Even a 1% increase in total cholesterol levels have been shown to increase the risk of CVD significantly. At menopause HDL decreases,while the level of LDL increase. HDL is a good predictor for coronary heart disease risk in women.

Estrogen helps to maintain favorable lipoprotein profiles in women. During perimenopause period itself changes in lipid profile occur. There is elevation of triglycerides, total and LDL cholesterol levels by an absolute of 10% by 6 months before menopause. HDL concentration gradually declines about couple of years preceding menopause and thenlevels at menopause. Because ofthe reversal of HDL/LDL ratio atheromatous plaques are formed. These plaques also lead to thrombus formation and complications such as strokes.

After menopause the risk of coronary heart disease doubles for women. By theage of 60, the levels of atherogenic lipids reach greater than men. The risk of CHD is three times more in women with a total cholesterol concentration >265 mg/dL than those of women with low or normal levels. Alow HDL cholesterol is again a strong predictor of CVD in women.

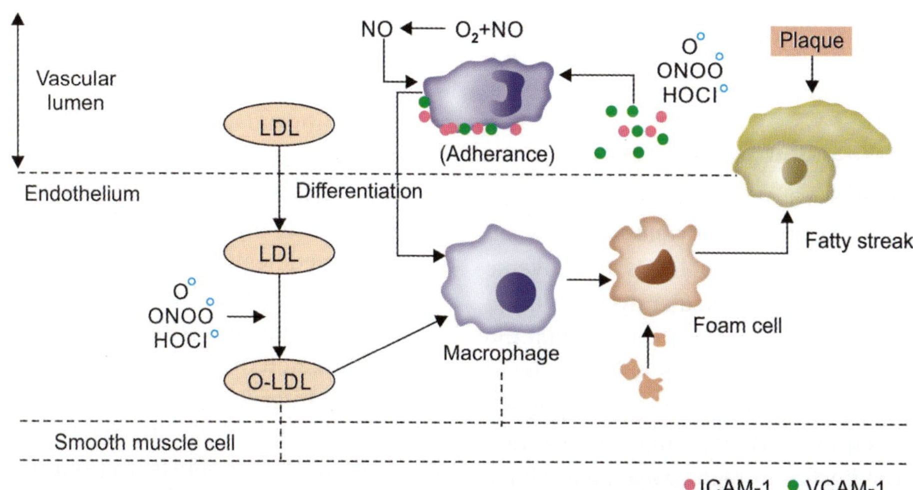

Fig. 2: Molecular changes at the endothelium. (VCAM-1: vascular-cell-adhesion molecule-1; ICAM-1: intracellular-adhesion molecule-1; LDL: low-density lipoprotein; O-LDL: oxidized low-density lipoprotein)

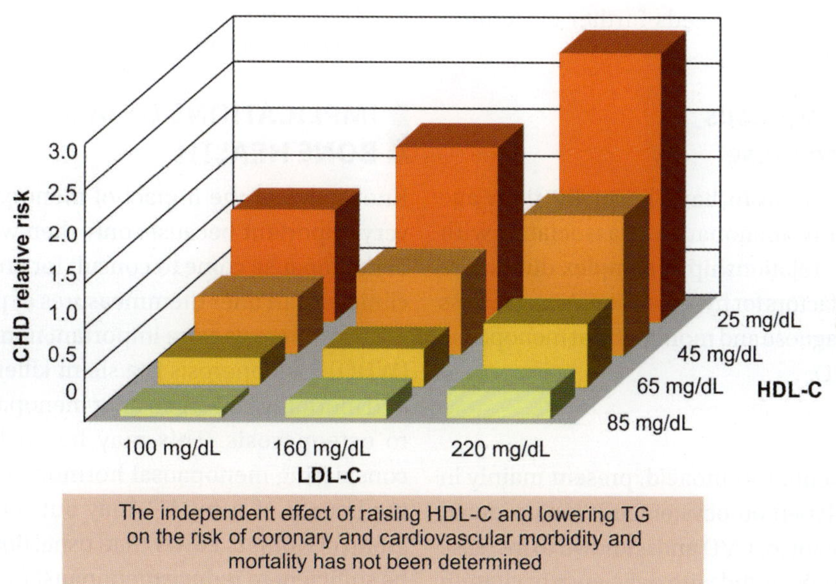

Fig. 3: Framingham heart study.

In women the average level of HDL in women is 55–65 mg/dL. A decrease of 10mg/dL HDL increases CHD risk by 40–50% **(Fig. 3)**.

Though following menopause changes in atherogenic lipids are inevitable, by dietary modifications, estrogen treatment and other lipid lowering modifications, favorable reduction in total cholesterol and LDL cholesterol can be achieved.

Endogenous Estrogens and Lipids

Study of Women's Health across Nation (SWAN) study has revealed an increase in total cholesterol and LDL specifically within a 1-year interval of the final menstrual period, independent of age, ethnicity or baseline weight. Reports from Healthy women study also state that the largest increase in the LDL and triglycerides is in the first year of menopause transition. Unlike SWAN, they also showed a decline in HDL levels during this phase. Additional prospective study from the Healthy women study indicated that premenopausal levels of lipids predict the extent of atheroma formation measured 14–20 years later by coronary artery and aortic calcium assessment with electron beam tomography. Premenopausal levels of BP, lipids and BMI, predict intima media thickness and carotid plaques measured 5–8 years after menopause. Hence, it is important to control all these well before menopause.

Weight Gain and Cardiovascular Disease in Menopausal Women

There is increasing androgen dominance as estrogen secretion declines. This is correlated with the increasing prevalence of metabolic syndrome during menopausal transition. Also a link between the magnitude of worsening in CVD and the extent of weight gained during menopausal transition has been established. Since weight gain at menopause is not an effect of hormonal changes, but only reflects exercise, diet and aging, attention to weight gain during middle age is one of the most important components of preventive health care.

Hot Flushes, Cardiovascular Disease and Endogenous Estrogens

Again SWAN heart cohort suggests a correlation between the presence of hot flushes, low estradiol levels and adverse CVD risks due to inflammation and vascular dysfunction at menopause transition. Gast et al., however, showed that the presence of night sweats but not hot flushes was associated with a higher risk of CHD. Herber-Gast in a prospective study of mid aged women in Australia, found that women who reported having hot flushes or night sweats often have an increased risk of developing CHD over a period of 14 years, even after correction for other chronic disease risk. Whether night sweats and hot flushes can be used as an objective marker for vascular dysfunction needs further evaluation and evidence.

Blood pressure, Endogenous Estrogens, and Menopause

Premenopausal women tend to have lower BP than age matched men. Premature menopause is associated with an increased BP. Yet the relationship is complex due to the coexistence of other risk factors for hypertension. Nevertheless it is more important to diagnose and monitor BP at menopause transition to prevent CVD.

Homocysteine

Homocysteieneis an essential aminoacid, present mainly in dietary animal protein. Hyperhomocysteinemia is considered as an independent risk factor for CVD and is known to increase with age, menopause, smoking and with deficiency of vitamin B6, B12, folate. Women's health study involving 28,263 healthy postmenopausal women, demonstrated a strong association between increased homocysteine levels and elevated risk of CVD. Hence, increased homocysteine at menopause could contribute to increased risk of CVD.

Summary of CVD Risk and Menopause

- Risk of CVD rises for everyone as they age, but for women symptoms can become more evident after the onset of menopause.
- Around the time of menopause some risk factors increase and a high-fat diet, smoking or other unhealthy habits begun earlier in life can also take a toll.
- Low AMH levels at younger age enable screening and prevention programs at menopause with reference to CVD, stroke, osteoporosis, cognition problems, etc.
- Postmenopausal women should understand that lipid profile for cardiac health is as important as Pap smear for cancer cervix prevention.
- Assessment of carotid atherosclerosis as a surrogate marker of general atherosclerosis by measurement of intimal medial thickness by B mode carotid sonography, may be utilized to diagnose subclinical atherosclerosis in a subset of patients.
- We have to educate women about CVD risk and should apply uniform CHD risk-reduction therapies with established health benefits in women.
- Encourage optimal blood pressure < 120/80 through lifestyle approaches. If BP 140/90 or more pharmacotherapy to be initiated to avoid end organ damage.
- Lifestyle intervention is very important. Women should take care of their heart through regular exercise and good nutrition. They should learn to eliminate unhealthy habits like smoking, which may contribute to early menopause, increase the risk of blood clots, decrease the flexibility of arteries, and lower the levels of HDL cholesterol.
- It is the duty of the clinicians to advice measures to prevent the onset of CVD to postmenopausal women.

IMPLICATIONS OF MENOPAUSE ON BONE HEALTH

Knowledge of the impact of menopause on bone health is very important because, only then whenwomen at the time of menopause come to consult for any reason, the attending clinician can offer themmeasures of preventive health care.

Osteoporosis as an important noncommunicable disease (WHO). Osteoporosis is a silent killer. The excess morbidity and mortality in women after menopause could be attributed to osteoporosis. This may be an important area, while considering menopausal hormone therapy (MHT) because the benefit of using HT may outweigh the risks in a select group of women. Lower than usual doses of estrogen seems to be sufficient to reduce menopausal symptoms and to protect bone.

Bone Remodeling (Fig. 4)

Natural bone is a dynamic tissue in the bodyand is in a continuous process of destruction and rebuilding. Microscopic damage occurs with weight bearing and daily physical activity, with simultaneous replacement also. This bone remodeling is also called bone turnover. In bone remodeling a constant resorption and reformation ofbone. The multinucleated giant cells known as osteoclasts carry out this resorption, and osteoblasts are involved in concurrent process of bone formation. The amount of bone present is the result of the balance of osteoblastic and osteoclastic activities.

It has been established that the peek bone mass in men and women is achieved in their thirties after which there is slow bone loss. This bone loss is exaggerated with menopause and estrogen deprivation. A woman might lose about 20% of her bone in the first 5–7 years after menopause while an average woman loses half her bone by the age of 70 years.

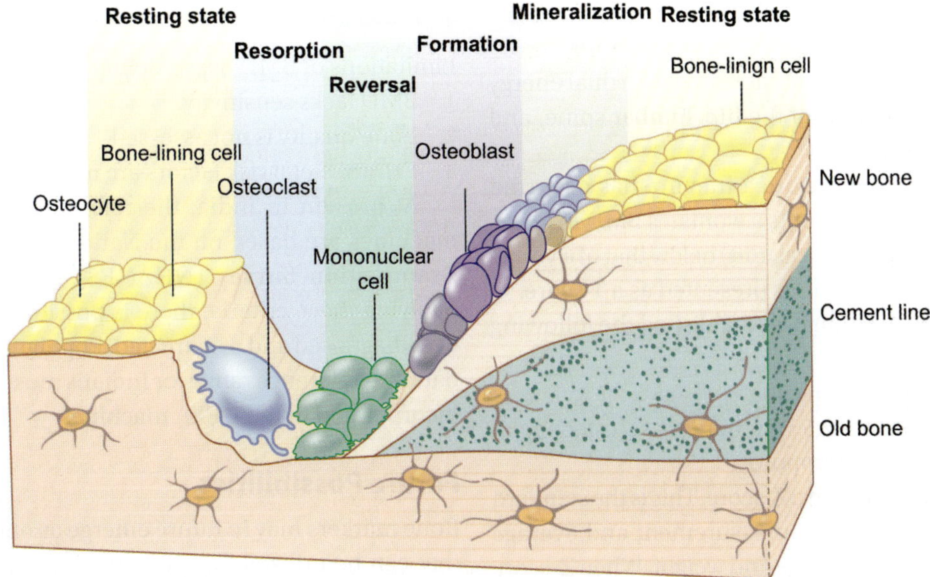

Fig. 4: Bone remodeling.

Following menopause, there is a relative increase of bone resorption, leading to thinning of bone.

Heredity and endocrine factors influence peak bone mass. Maximum bone mass in the hip and the vertebral bodies will get accumulated by late adolescence. So the years immediately following menarche (11–14 years) is very important. At the age of 25–35 years bone resorption is coupled to bone formation in such a way that positive bone balance is achieved and skeletal maturity is attained. After that, bone mass declines slowly at the rate of about 0.4% each year. At menopause, there is an increase in the rate of decline in bone mass by 2–5% per year inthe first 5–10 years. It slows down to 1% per year subsequently. The subsequent risk of fracture from osteoporosis will depend on. The bone mass at the time of menopause and the rate of bone loss following menopause decides the risk of fracture from osteoporosis.

Osteoporosis

The strength of bone is compromised in osteoporosis. So fracture risk is increased. Bone mineral density (BMD) determines the bone strength. That is why BMD measurements are effective tools to identify patients at high risk for fracture. Rate of remodeling, size and geometry, microarchitecture, mineralization, damage accumulation and matrix quality are other factors which affect the bone strength and fracture risk.

Osteoporotic fractures are important causes for increased morbidity and mortality. Compared to persons without fractures the risk of dying after clinical fracture is nearly two-fold higher.

When there is bone loss because of aging or menopausal estrogen deficiency it is referred as primary osteoporosis. The regulatory effect estrogen on bone resorption is lost after menopause, because of decline in estrogen level. There is no

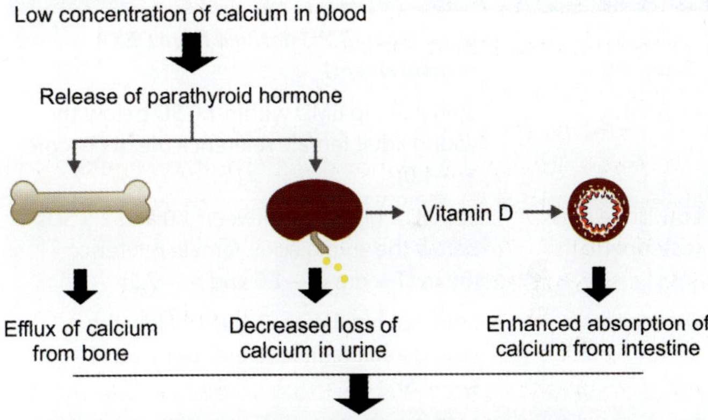

Fig. 5: Parathyroid hormone and calcium homeostasis.

compensatory bone formation to balance this effect. In the early postmenopausal year there is rapid acceleration of bone loss. Loss of estrogen in menopause, with added aging factor, increases the osteoclastic activity. Additionally the level of serum calcium decreases due to impaired absorption calcium from the gut coupled with decreased calcium intake. When serum calcium level falls, parathyroid hormone secretion is stimulated to mobilize calcium from bone as shown in **Figure 5**.

Suchchain of events result in increased serum calcium levels in a balanced way. On the contrary estrogen deficiency in menopause leads to an increased responsiveness of bone to PTH. This leads to more calcium removal from bone to rise serum calcium, ultimately leading on to lowering of PTH.

Diagnosis of Osteoporosis

Bone mineral density is the best quantifiable predictor of osteoporotic fracture **(Table 2)**. When there are other major risk factors, along with low BMD patient's risk is increased. Therefore, BMD should be routinely measured. Especially in all women more than 65 and in a woman older than 50 years with one of the other major risk factors for fracture BMD should be measured.

Bone mineral density is usually assessed with dual energy X-ray absorptiometry (DEXA) of the hip, lumbar spine, and radius **(Figs. 6A and B)**.

Diagnosis can be made before a fracture has occurred using a DEXA scan. DEXA presents a woman's BMD in terms of standard deviations (a statistical unit) below that of a young adult reference population. This is presented as a T-score.

World Health Organization has established the following guidelines:

- T-score of–1.0 or greater = normal
- T-score between–1.0 and –2.5 = low bone mass (osteopenia)
- T-score of–2.5 or less = osteoporosis.

Patients can also be assigned a Z-score. This is the standard deviation between the patient's measurement and average bone mass for a patient of same age and weight. When Z-score is lower than–2.0, it necessitates diagnostic evaluation for secondary osteoporosis.

TABLE 2: Diagnostic criteria for osteoporosis and osteopenia in postmenopausal women and men older than 50 years.

Category	*Bone mass (BMD derived from DEXA measurement)*
Normal	Spinal or hip BMD within 1.0 SD below the young adult female reference mean (T-score ≥ —1.0)
Low bone mass (osteopenia)	Spinal or hip BMD between 1.0 and 2.5 SDs below the young adult female reference mean (T-score < —1.0 and > —2.5)
Osteoporosis	Spinal or hip BMD ≥ 2.5 SDs below the young adult female reference mean (T-score ≤ —2.5)
Severe/established osteoporosis	BMD 2.5 SDs below the young adult female reference mean and the presence of one or more fragility fractures

(BMD: bone mineral density; DEXA: dual energy X-ray absorptiometry; SDs: standard deviations)
Source: Michael et al. American Family Physician. 2015.

Limitations of BMD based definitions of osteoporosis are:

1. BMD lacks sensitivity.
2. Bone quality is not assessed
3. Extra skeletal risk factors are not addressed.

At present in India, the reference range of the DEXA machines are based on the National Health and Nutrition Examination Survey (NHANES) II reference range. By applying these criteria, there is possibility of patients being over diagnosed and over treated. Population based normative data and reference range for Indians must be established and incorporated in the DEXA machines.

Future Possibilities

Bone markers may in future emerge as one of the risk factors that can be utilized for prediction of osteoporosis fracture. While BMD provides a static picture of bone, the bone markers provide a dynamic measure of bone turnover and distinguish between fast and slow bone losers at menopause transition and may aid in decision making.[6]

For bone formation, these include alkaline phosphatase, osteocalcin, procollagen peptides.

For bone resorption—pyridinoline and dexapyridinoline cross links, telopeptides of type I collagen, acid phosphatase.

For osteoporotic fractures, the risk factors are interlinked. They must be considered in the context of baseline age. For example, a 75-year-old woman with low BMD is at significantly higher risk than a 55-year-old woman with the same low BMD. Like that a woman with low BMD and a prior fragility fracture is at an increased risk than another woman with the same low BMD but no prior fracture.

Fragility Fracture

When a fracture is caused by an injury, which is not sufficient to fracture normal boneit is called fragility fracture (WHO).

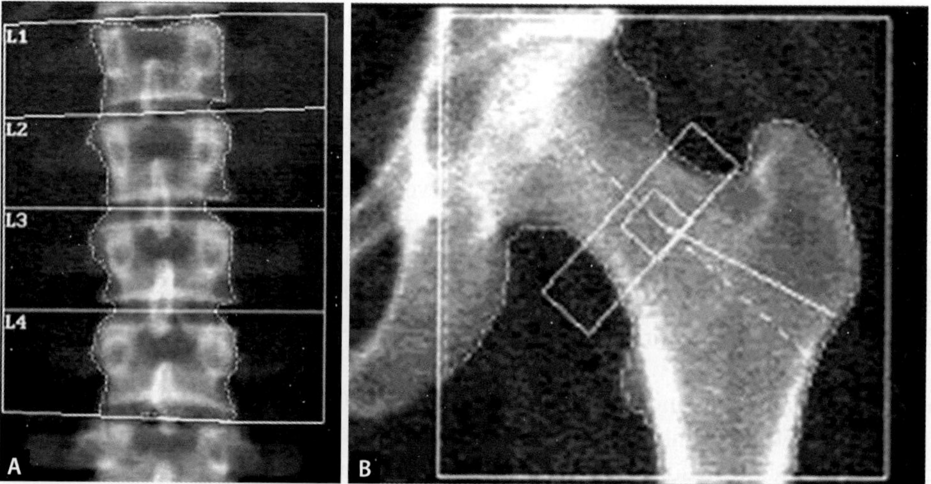

Figs. 6A and B: DEXA scan images of the vertebrae (A) and head of femur (B).

This is due to the reduced compressive and/or torsional strength of bone. Fragility fractures are responsible for 80% of fractures in women after menopause.

Prediction and Prevention

The most important predictive factors of risk of osteoporosis are bone density along with age, ethnicity, fracture history, medications, and weight loss. When a key risk factor is found it should alert clinician for further assessment. Active intervention such as calcium therapy, weight bearing exercises or pharmacologic therapy must be implemented.Prevention of postmenopausal osteoporosis include—calcium, vitamin D, vitamin K, physical activity and exercise programs, HT, selective estrogen modulators (SERM), tibolone, bisphosphonates, PTH, calcitonin and strontium ranelate.

Fall Precautions

Fractures are frequently associated with falls. Therefore history of fall should be included in risk assessment. Factors which increase rates of these accidents include—low muscle strength, impaired balance, low body mass and impaired visual acuity must be included. Alcohol use and drug abuse are additional risk factors.

KEY MESSAGES

- We should do BMD measurements in all menopausal women who
  - Are aged 65 and above
  - Have one or more risk factors for osteoporosis
  - Sustain fractures.
- If therapy to increase BMD is instituted, density should be monitored.
- As a prophylactic measure for osteoporosis, weight bearing exercises and calcium intake should begin right from adolescence itself.
- Calcium supplementation in girls before and at puberty prepubertal and at puberty improves bone accrual, which is important with long-lasting beneficial consequences.

REFERENCES

1. Fritz MA, SperoffL. Clinical Gynecologic Endocrinology and Infertility, 8th edition. Philadelphia: Lippincott Williams & Wilkins; 2010.
2. Zhu D, Chung HF, Dobson AJ, Pandeya N, Giles GG, Bruinsma F, et al. Age at natural menopause andrisk of incident CVD. Lancet. 2019;4(11):E553-64.
3. Hoffman B, Schorge J, Schaffer J, Halvorson L, Bradshaw K, Cunningham F. Williams Gynecology, 2nd edition. New York: McGraw-Hill Education/Medical; 2012.
4. Meeta M, Digumarti L, Agarwal N, Vaze N, Shah R, Malik S. Clinical practice guidelines on menopause. J Midlife Health. 2020;11(2):55-95.
5. Arulkumaran S. Essentials of Gynecology. New Delhi: Jaypee Brothers Medical Publishers (P) Ltd.; 2005.
6. Meeta M, Harinarayan CV, Marwah R, Sahay R, Kalra S, Babhulkar S. Clinical practice guidelines for postmenopausal osteoporosis. J Midlife Health. 2020;11(2):96-112.

LONG QUESTIONS

1. Describe the risk factors for cardiovascular disease in menopause and the risk reduction approaches specific to a menopausal woman.
2. What measures can be taken to optimize bone health in the menopausal woman?

SHORT QUESTIONS

1. What are the beneficial effects of estrogen on cardiovascular health?
2. Name the lipid profile alterations during menopause.
3. What is bone turnover?
4. What is a fragility fracture?
5. What are the pros and cons of BMD measurement?

MULTIPLE CHOICE QUESTIONS

1. Every year of premature menopause increases the risk of cardiovascular disease by:
   a. 2% b. 5%
   c. 10% d. 25%
2. The positive effect of estrogen on cardiovascular health is related to:
   a. Increase in platelet aggregation
   b. Higher coagulability of blood
   c. Favorable effect on lipid metabolism
   d. Increase in oxygen reactive species in the circulation
3. The following is a modifiable risk factor for cardiovascular disease:
   a. Age b. Genetic background
   c. Hypertension d. Premature menopause
4. Women achieve peak bone mass at:
   a. 15 years b. 30 years
   c. 45 years d. 60 years
5. The following is true about osteoporosis:
   a. Risk is higher in young women
   b. Risk is higher in men than women
   c. Low protein intake is a risk factor
   d. Estrogen therapy increases the risk of osteoporosis
6. The sites used to assess bone mineral density by DEXA typically are all, except:
   a. Radius b. Lumbar spine
   c. Hip d. Patella

Answers

1. a 2. c 3. c 4. b 5. c 6. d

10.12 HORMONE THERAPY IN MENOPAUSE

Suvarna Khadilkar, Madhva Prasad S

INTRODUCTION

Estrogen deficiency is linked to several symptoms and disease processes presenting after menopause. Though life expectancy has improved enormously, the average age of menopause has not changed significantly. This results in a vast majority of women spending a significant time period, almost about one-third of their lives in an estrogen deficient state. Hence, the concept of hormone replacement therapy (HRT) has been widely practiced over half a century and is important to contemporary practitioners. There have been considerable changes in the views towards HRT over the years. Absence of hormonal management of menopause, selective use of HRT, universal use of HRT, identification of HRT-related health risks, questioning the very basis of HRT and gradual selective reintroduction of HRT have been the phases in the use of HRT. Today term HRT is replaced by menopausal hormone therapy (MHT).

The possible conditions which may get benefits and possible risk which one may accrue upon usage of MHT are listed in **Box 1**. However, it should be noted that MHT has been shown to have an extremely complex pattern risks and benefits. The type of medication, duration of treatment, age at the time of initiation, time since occurrence of menopause and prior medical status are all influencing factors on the benefits and risks. Multiple studies have been done in this regarding and a brief description of few of the prominent studies which have taken place in the matter is presented.

1. The *Women's Health Initiative (WHI)* was the pathbreaking study in this topic. It was a large-scale multicentric, multi-country study involving almost 27,000 women. It had two major parts.
   a. One was the estrogen only arm compared to placebo. The average duration of active treatment in the intervention arm of the study was around 5.9 years. This part had initially reported results after a follow-up of around 7 years. In this group, among those who survived and those who consented, further results of a cumulative follow-up of around 13 years has been presented.
   b. The other part of the WHI was the combined (estrogen plus progestin) in the intervention arm. This study reported had initially reported results after a mean of 5.6 years of active treatment (intervention phase) and 2.4 years of follow-up after stoppage of intervention. Among those who survived and consented, a further follow-up was performed leading to a cumulative follow-up of around 13 years. Further follow-up results of the same cohort areexpected in regular intervals.[1]
2. The *Heart and Estrogen/Progestin Replacement Study (HERS)* was an ambitious study which attempted to study the benefits of estrogen-progestin supplementation for reduction of cardiovascular disease. However, paradoxically, it showed no benefit and rather appeared to increase the risk of cardiovascular morbidity.[2]
3. The *Effects of Postmenopausal Hormone Therapy (EPHT) trial* (HT vs. placebo) was conducted in Eastern Europe on around 1,700 patients and in 2006, published results after a follow-up of around 3.4 years.
4. *Women's International Study of Long-Duration Oestrogen After Menopause (WISDOM)* was initiated as a long-duration multicentric trial but intervention with HT was done only for 1 year and was prematurely closed due to lack of funding.
5. Initiated in the late 1990s, the *Million Women Study* prospectively recruited women to study the risk of development of various cancers in a cohort. In the initial recruitment, 33% of the recruited women were on MHT.[3]
6. *Multiple small randomized controlled trails (RCTs)* with lesser number of patients have been conducted. The combined findings of the risks and benefits of these studies have been analyzed in detail in a systematic review by Cochrane[4] and is presented here.

BOX 1: List of benefits and risks associated with menopausal hormonal therapy.

Benefits
- Hot flushes
- Pelvic organ prolapse
- Sexual function
- Urinary incontinence
- Vaginal atrophy
- Osteoporosis/ fractures
- Metabolic profile: Diabetes

Risks
- Weight and body fat distribution
- Cardiovascular disease
- Dementia and cognitive function
- Endometrial hyperplasia
- Cancer

As can be seen in **Table 1**, the usage of continuous combined hormonal therapy reduces the risk of fracture but increases the risk of various adverse events. Though the absolute risk of occurrence of any of these events is very small, the occurrence of venous thromboembolism (VTE) appears significant.

As can be seen in **Table 2**, the usage of estrogen-only hormonal therapy reduces the risk of fracture but increases the risk of various adverse events. Though the absolute risk of occurrence of any of these events is very small, the risk

TABLE 1: Risks associated with continuous combined hormonal therapy.

Event (Follow-up duration)	*Risk in general population (per 1,000)*	*Risk in treatment group (per 1,000)*	*Relative risk*
Coronary events (1 year)	2	4	1.89
Stroke (3 years)	6	8	1.46
Venous thromboembolism (1 year)	2	7	4.28
Breast cancer (5.6 years)	19	24	1.27
Death from lung cancer (8 years)	5	9	1.74
Gallbladder disease (6 years)	16	27	1.64
Fracture (5.6 years)	111	87	0.78

TABLE 2: Risks associated with estrogen-only hormonal therapy.

Event (Follow-up of 7.1 years for all)	*Risk in general population (per 1,000)*	*Risk in treatment group (per 1,000)*	*Relative risk*
Coronary events	41	38	0.94
Stroke	24	32	1.33
Venous thromboembolism	16	21	1.32
Breast cancer	25	20	0.79
Gallbladder disease	27	47	1.78
Fracture	141	103	0.73

is somewhat comparable to the risks accrued upon taking combined estrogen-progestin combination hormonal therapy.

MENOPAUSAL HEALTH CONCERNS

Vasomotor Symptoms

Hot flushes are the primary reason women seek hormone therapy. Vasomotor symptoms affect up to 75% of perimenopausal women and last for around 1–2 years in most. *Systemic estrogen therapy* is the most effective treatment for vasomotor symptoms. When systemic estrogen is not chosen or when contraindicated, progestin therapy alone *modroxy progesterone acetate (MPA) and megestrol acetate* are options. Several drugs that alter central neurotransmitter pathways, selective serotonin reuptake inhibitors (SSRIs) and SNRIs also are effective, of which *paroxetine* is the most preferred. If cessation of MHT is desired, it is important to reduce the dose slowly over several months. Stellate ganglion block has been studied, without convincing benefits.[5-8]

Urogenital Atrophy

Urogenital atrophy results in vaginal dryness and pruritus, dyspareunia, dysuria, and urinary urgency, which respond well to oral estrogen therapy. The preferred term nowadays is "*genitourinary syndrome of menopause (GSM)*". *Topical application* (estrogen cream used only one to three times weekly) is an alternative. An estradiol vaginal tablet inserted twice week and *estrogen-containing vaginal ring* (changed every 3 months) are available. Concerns regarding endometrial thickness needs to be addressed. Lubricants are nonhormonal alternatives for reducing discomfort during intercourse. *Topical androgens (DHEA)* have also demonstrated promise.[9]

Osteoporosis

Osteoporosis is an important health concern after menopause. Non-modifiable risk factors include age, Asian or white race, family history, small body frame, early menopause, and prior oophorectomy. Modifiable risk factors include decreased calcium and vitamin D intake, smoking, and a sedentary lifestyle. Medical risk factors include hyperthyroidism, hyperparathyroidism, chronic renal disease, and chronic corticosteroid use. Assessment of bone mineral density gives an indication of whether the patient falls into normal bone health, osteopenia or osteoporosis.

When combined with the history and other clinical factors, the objective Fracture Risk assessment (FRAX Scoring) can help determine whether the patient is at a low risk, moderate risk or a high risk for bone fractures in the future.[10]

- *Low risk patients* require only lifestyle advice and adequate oral calcium intake (1,200 mg) and vitamin D (800 IU)
- *Moderate risk patients* require lifestyle advice, adequate calcium and vitamin D intake and consideration for pharmacological therapy if any specific risk factors exist (as mentioned earlier)
- *High risk patients* require lifestyle advice, calcium and vitamin D intake, and pharmacological therapy.

The options are detailed in **Table 3**. Though there is a confirmed significant reduction in hip fractures in healthy women receiving MHT over 5 years, whether to give hormones only for this indication, is not clear, especially in the context of availability of non-hormonal medications for improving bone health. These are listed below and few details mentioned in **Table 3**.[11,12]

MHT and Cardiovascular Disease

To simply state that "cardiovascular disease is worsened by MHT" is a superficial oversimplification. The complex relationships between cardiovascular disease and menopause have been brought out by the detailed analyses of the WHI trial. Initially, it was shown that there is an increased risk of cardiovascular disease when MHT is given to women with menopause. Subsequently, this was questioned and further analysis showed that worsening of cardiovascular disease is a complex function of:

- Woman's age
- Time of onset of MHT with respect to occurrence of menopause
- Duration of MHT.

It should be noted that *adverse cardiovascular events among women who initiated MHT at a time period close to attainment of menopause is low*, and in younger women, probably favorable. It is clear that CVD prevention cannot be taken as an indication for initiating MHT. However, for those in early menopause and no specific contraindications, benefits of MHT slightly outweigh the cardiovascular risks.[13]

MHT and Stroke

Among postmenopausal women who are otherwise healthy, MHT increases stroke risk, mainly the ischemic subtype (approximately 2 additional events per 10,000 person-years). The age of initiating MHT or the time since menopause does not seem to have an effect on the risk of stroke. Estrogen-only and estrogen-progestin combinations have similar risks for stroke occurrence. Raloxifene and tibolone also have a propensity to increase stroke, mainly in those above 60 years. *The transdermal route does not increase the risk of stroke.*[14-17]

MHT and Breast Cancer

D'Alonzo and colleagues[18] have reviewed this complex association. The WHI initially reported an increased risk of breast cancer, which led to reduction in the usage of MHT. In an update of the WHI trial results, it was noted that there was an *increased risk of breast cancer with the usage of estrogen-progestin combination (CEE+MPA), long after stoppage of therapy also*, with continuous therapy (in comparison to intermittent) having the worst outcomes. Overall, the strength of association between MHT and breast cancer is small, with only an 8 per 1000 increase when combination MHT is used for more than 5 years. However, contrastingly, there was *a consistent reduction in the breast cancer risk with usage of CEE-only preparation* (from 25 to 20 per 1,000, 7 years follow-up), which was more prominent among hysterectomized women above 50 years of age. Those who start MHT 1 year or later after menopause had a higher risk of breast cancer. Current users of MHT are at a higher risk than past users. Bazedoxifene appears to confer a good safety profile regarding breast cancer development.

TABLE 3: Pharmacological management options for osteoporosis.

Drug group	*Dosage, Comments*
Bisphosphonates: Reduction of bone resorption by inhibition of hydroxyapatite breakdown Inhibition of osteoblast and osteoclast apoptosis Exact contribution of each component is unclear	**Alendronate:** 5 or 10 mg daily/35 or 70 mg weekly **Risedronate:** 5 mg daily/35 mg weekly/150 mg monthly **Zolendronate:** 5 mg once a year intravenous For consideration in oral therapy non-compliance Osteonecrosis of jaw is a complication
Denosumab: (Binds to receptor-activator-of-nuclear-factor-kappa-ligand (RANKL))	It is a monoclonal antibody which results in osteoclast inhibition and reduced bone resorption 60 mg subcutaneous twice a year
Teriparatide (Improves architecture of bone trabeculae)	Recombinant PTH analogue given 20 mcg subcutaneous daily cost is a prohibitive factor Should not be combined with bisphosphonates Should not be given for more than 2 years Newer formulation aboloparatide shows promise
Calcitonin (Increases bone matrix deposition)	Intranasal spray is approved for treatment Less efficacious than most alternatives Is a second line drug
Raloxifine (SERM)	60 mg oral once a day for not more than 5 years Long-term use: Thromboembolism and stroke
MHT	MHT should not be used solely for the prevention of osteoporosis. Other agents should be considered

MHT and Endometrial Cancer

The estrogen-only arm of the WHI showed an increase of endometrial cancer, which was confirmed in the Million Women Study also. Multiple reviews have been conducted in the matter, and recent review contends that in those patients with uterus-in-situ, only-estrogen regimens, tibolone and use of sequential combined therapy elevates the risk of endometrial cancer, even if the duration of MHT is < 5 years. However, *the use of continuous combined estrogen-progestin therapy gives a small reduction in the risk of endometrial cancer,* with higher beneficial effect in obese women.[18]

MHT and Ovarian Cancer

Menopausal hormone therapy may be associated with a *small but definite risk of ovarian cancer.* If a 50-year-old woman uses MHT for 5 years, the risk of developing an ovarian cancer is about 1 in 1,000 users, and a mortality risk of 1 in 1,700.[19,20]

MHT and Gastrointestinal Cancers

A definite reduction in colon cancer and liver cancer has been observed with use of MHT, mainly the combined hormonal medications. While similar results are noted for colorectal cancers also, the protection effect does not last long after discontinuation of MHT.[18]

MHT and Neurological Problems

Alzheimer's disease and Parkinson's disease are common geriatric problems coinciding with menopausal status. In the early 2000s, the WHI Memory Study (WHIMS)[21] had noted that there is an increase in the occurrence of cognitive decline in women who undergo hormonal therapy. However, the authors doubted the generalizability of those results.

Recent developments have shown the contrary picture. The Kronos Early Estrogen Prevention (KEEPS) study[22] used the Modified Mini-Mental State examination and four cognitive factors and an objective mood measure. It was noted that there was a benefit in the mood effects with four years use of CEE. However, similar benefits were noted with estradiol usage. The authors warned that these findings are limited to women who have recently attained menopause and have a good cardiovascular risk profile. A recent meta-analysis[23] which has analyzed *Estrogen replacement in Alzheimer's and Parkinson's disease shows a definite benefit.*

MHT and All-cause Mortality[24]

There is *no change in all-cause mortality, cardiovascular mortality or cancer mortality* over a cumulative 18-year follow-up, with usage of CEE plus MPA (5.6 years) or CEE alone (7.2 years)

BIOCHEMICAL CHANGES IN MENOPAUSAL TRANSITION

Menopause is characterized by a 10-fold elevation in FSH value, a reduction of estradiol upto 10–25 pg/mL, and reduction of testosterone upto 290 ng/mL. Estradiol gets replaced by estrone as the dominant estrogen and ovary gets replaced by adipose, adrenals and muscles (by aromatization of androstenedione) as the primary source of estrogens. Re-establishing physiological estrogen levels (45–65 pg) is the biochemical goal of MHT, which is presumed to alleviate the menopausal symptoms. MHT dosage should be as low as reasonably achievable, i.e., a dose which reduces symptoms but is most acceptable, with minimal side effects and shortest duration should be given.

Estrogens[25]

- Estrone (E1) is the predominant circulating type in the postmenopausal woman. Ingestion of oral estrogens (irrespective of oral preparation) also results in elevation of estrone, owing to conversion in the gut mucosa.
- Estradiol (E2) is the most physiological estrogen type since it is the predominant circulating estrogen in the premenopausal reproductive woman. Both estradiol and estrone have been demonstrated to be osteoprotective and lipid friendly.
- Estriol (E3) is a less potent estrogen which has a good local action on the genitourinary structures and is also useful for control of vasomotor symptoms. Systemic benefits are not proven.
- Estetrol (E4) is a 15-α-estriol, a molecule produced naturally only in the fetal liver. One recent RCT using estetrol for menopausal symptoms has shown safety and promise[26]

Synthetic Estrogens

Estradiol valerate is a chemically synthesized natural estrogen. It has good bioavailability, is well tolerated orally, has less metabolic liver burden and is completely hydrolyzed to estradiol. However, when taken orally it is metabolized to estrone, in which form it circulates through the body. It needs to be taken non-orally to be available in circulation as estradiol. Age-related changes in metabolism may be a concern. Non-oral form of estrogen administration is more physiological than the oral form since the estradiol/estrone ratio is preserved.[27,28]

Conjugated equine estrogens: These are a mixture of estrogens obtained from menopausal mares, containing estrone sulfate, equilin sulfate and few other compounds. These are usually sold under the brand name of Premarin. It is available as 0.3 mg, 0.625 mg and 1.25 mg.

The contraindications to MHT are presented in **Box 2**.

Some pointers toward choice of hormone replacement preparation:

- To avoid harmful effects on lipids, coagulation factors and liver enzymes, patients with hypertriglyceridemia, hypertension, past history of venous thrombotic disease and antiepileptic therapy should be considered for nonoral preparations.

- Patients with predominance of urogenital symptoms should be considered for local vaginal preparations.
- Patients with intact uterus should not be given estrogen-only preparations.

Estrogenic Side Effects

Possible side effects are leg pain, breast tenderness, headache, bloating, nausea and vaginal discharge. Approximately, 14% of women may have one or more of these side effects during therapy.

Progestins

Medroxy-progesterone acetate is the most commonly studied progestin. Possible side effects are acne, bloating, backache, breast tenderness, headache, dizziness, generalized aches and pains, greasy skin, fatigue, weight gain, backache and abdominal cramps.[29] Approximately 20% of women reported these side effects.

BOX 2: Absolute and relative contraindications to menopausal hormone therapy (MHT).

Absolute contraindications
- Active endometrial, gynecological hormone dependant cancers
- Active breast cancer: Immaterial of receptor status
- Known or suspected pregnancy
- Undiagnosed, abnormal vaginal bleeding
- Liver disease with impaired/abnormal liver function
- Increased risk of thromboembolism

Relative contraindications
- Migraine headaches
- Superficial thrombophlebitis
- Strong family history of breast cancer
- Uterine fibroids
- Endometriosis
- Gallbladder disease
- Impaired glucose tolerance
- Hypertriglyceridemia

For either estrogen/progesterone, if the effects are severe or prolonged, reduction of dosage, change of route or change to alternative preparation are options.

Types of preparations available:
- Oral preparation
- Biodegradable implants
- Transdermal patches
- Metered dose sprays
- Vaginal pessaries
- Vaginal rings
- Topical creams.

The various options are presented in **Table 4**.

Androgen Preparations

Dehydroepiandrosterone (DHEA) and its sulfate, upon their conversion, are important sources of local estrogen in the menopausal period. Local applications of intravaginal DHEA and testosterone patches have been shown to be beneficial for treatment of the genitourinary syndrome of menopause and hypoactive sexual desire disorder, respectively. However, there does not appear to be any improvement or reduction in cognitive function as demonstrated in recent studies (though it was believed to be so before).[30-32]

Tibolone

Tibolone is a steroidal molecule. It is a progestin, which has some weak selective estrogenic activity and also exhibits androgenic activity. It is effective in suppression of vasomotor symptoms. It also improves libido and mood. The recommended dose is 2.5 mg/day. It is effective against GSM but has no detrimental effect on the endometrium. It has positive effect on bone mass. However, there is a slightly increased risk stroke and breast cancer upon long-term usage. For those women who find first line hormonal therapy unsuitable, tibolone can be considered as a safe alternative for short-term usage. It can also be considered in women with premature ovarian failure and for add back therapy upon GnRH usage.[33,34]

TABLE 4: Menopausal hormonal therapy options.

Estrogen only HTs	*Continuous combined estrogen progestin replacement therapy (CCEPRT)*	*Sequential estrogen progestin replacement therapy (SEPRT)*
• Conjugated equine estrogen (CEE): 0.625 mg or 1.25 mg daily (most commonly studied): Was used in WHI (one arm) • Estradiol (17-β estradiol) : 1 mg orally • Estradiol valerate: 2 mg • Transdermal estradiol skin patches: 0.014 mg, 0.025 mg, 0.05 mg or 0.075 mg daily. • Intranasal puff of 17-β estradiol: 0.15 mg or 0.3 mg daily	• CEE 0.625 mg with MPA 2.5 mg daily : Trials in which this was used are EPHT, HERS, PEPI, WAVE, WHI (combined arm) and WISDOM. • EE 2.5 mg with MPA 10 mg daily • Estradiol 2 mg with 1 mg norethisterone daily	• Estradiol 1 mg daily with MPA 5 mg for 12 days once a year • Estradiol 1 mg daily for 4 days, estradiol 1 mg plus 0.35 mg norethindrone daily for 3 days each week • Estradiol 2 mg days 1 to 22, 1 mg days 22 to 28, with norethisterone 1 mg days 13 to 22 • CEE 0.625 with MPA 10 mg days 1 to 12 (PEPI 1995). • CEE 0.625 mg with micronized progesterone 200 mg days 1 to 12

Selective Estrogen Receptor Modulators

Raloxifene

Raloxifene is a second-generation selective estrogen receptor modulator (SERM). It has an estrogen-agonist effect on bone, and helps improve bone mineral density, thereby useful as an important agent in postmenopausal osteoporosis. It exhibits antagonist effect on the breast and uterus. Hence it can reduce the risk of breast cancer and pelvic organ prolapse in postmenopausal women. (It should not be used in those with diagnosed cancer of the breast). A small but definite increase in the risk of venous thromboembolism has also been noted. It has shown promising results in mild variants of schizophrenia. It is available as 60 mg tablets administered once a day, for not more than 5 years.[35]

Bazedoxifene

Bazeodoxifene is also an SERM with differential activity on the various estrogen receptors. One particular combination of bazedoxifene 20 mg and conjugated estrogen 0.45 mg has been designated Tissue Selective Estrogen Complex (TSEC). As reviewed by Lello et al. recently,[36] this combination appears to have many ideal properties and has demonstrated the following effects:

- It reduces vasomotor symptoms significantly
- It improves sleep quality and overall quality of life
- It is bone-protective
- It has favorable impact on GSM
- It has no stimulatory effect on breast or endometrial tissue
- It does worsen any cardiovascular risk.

Considering the favorable profile, this combination may become the first line therapy for menopause soon.

Ospemifene

Ospemifene is a recently introduced SERM available for oral administration (60 mg tablets) which is approved for management of the various symptoms of GSM (dyspareunia and vaginal dryness being most prominent). Bone protective effect and favorable profile in breast have also been noted. Hot flashes (common), vaginal discharge and hyperhidrosis are side-effects. Overall safety and acceptance are now well established. Current thromboembolic disease, severe liver disease and those using other estrogen agonist/antagonist preparation are contraindications for this preparation.[37]

DECISION MAKING REGARDING INITIATION OF MENOPAUSAL HORMONE THERAPY

Decision making for hormone therapy in menopause is complex. An approach to this is presented in **Flowchart 1**.

The patient must be clearly explained about the complex patterns of risks and benefits upon using MHT for menopausal symptoms and that the lowest possible dosage, for least possible duration will be considered. Electronic decision-making algorithms are now available.[38]

Deciding when to Stop MHT

A decision to continue MHT at any point in time should be done with due consideration to risks and benefits. Administration of MHT more than 5 years is not recommended. Abrupt

Flowchart 1: Approach to initiation of MHT.

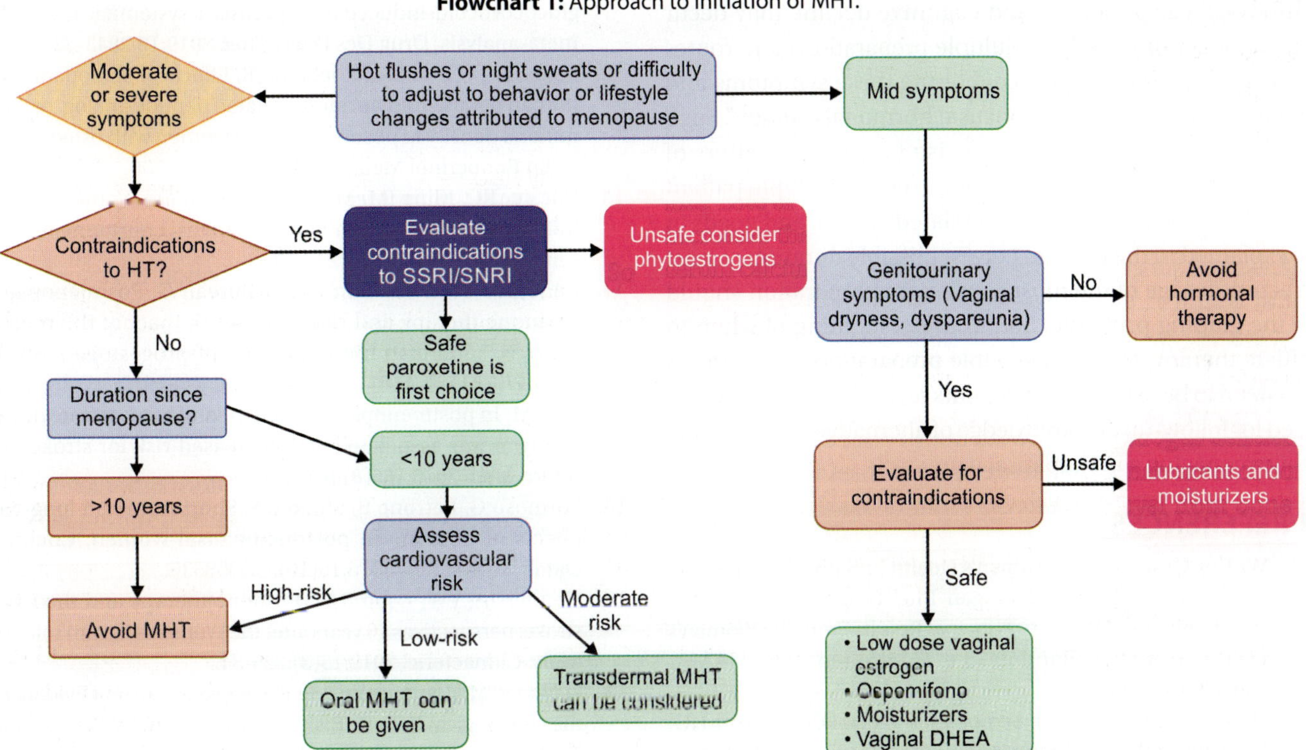

discontinuation may have some problems similar to the original conditionand weaning of medication may be considered.[39]

Nutritional Supplementation

Isoflavones (Genistin, Daidzin), Genistein, Daidzein are phytoestrogens or plant estrogens, which have shown considerable promise for management of menopausal symptoms, mainly the vasomotor. The efficacy against genitourinary symptoms is poor. Nutritional supplements provide some relief of symptoms, however, the effectiveness is not of the same order as conventional hormone therapy. For those who are reluctant to use formal hormonal therapy, these nutritional supplements are a suitable alternative.[40]

CONCLUSION

A wide range of options are now available for the administration of menopausal hormonal therapy. The benefits accrued in the prevention/management of symptoms associated with menopause must be balanced against the possible risks due to the therapy. Factors such as predominant symptom type, severity of the symptoms, age at menopause, duration since menopause, individual medical/gynecological factors should be weighed in while deciding route, dosage, and duration of therapy.

KEY MESSAGES

The quantitative reduction of estrogen and progesterone in the menopausal transition leads to multiple systemic effects. While vasomotor symptoms, genitourinary symptoms and few others may occur as acute symptoms, osteoporosis, cardiovascular problems, and cognitive decline may occur over a longer time period. Multiple preparations and routes are available for effectively countering these symptoms and come under the term "menopausal hormonal therapy". Such replacement of hormones gives rise to complex patters of risks and benefits, which are influenced on multiple patient related factors and intervention related factors, and needs to be explained to the patient. Lowest possible duration of least effective dosage of the most convenient preparation should be the guiding principle. Sound understanding of when to initiate therapy, the most suitable preparation, the pointers that need to be explained to patients regarding risks/benefits, need for follow-up and knowledge of alternatives are essential while managing a menopausal woman.

REFERENCES

1. Writing Group for the Women's Health Initiative Investigators Risks and Benefits of Estrogen Plus Progestin in Healthy Postmenopausal Women: Principal Results From the Women's Health Initiative Randomized Controlled Trial. JAMA. 2002;288:321-33.
2. Herrington DM, Fong J, Sempos CT, Black DM, Schrott HG, Rautaharju P, et al. Comparison of the Heart and Oestrogen Replacement Study (HERS) cohort with women with coronary disease from the National Health and Nutrition Examination Survey III (NHANES III). Am Heart J. 1998;136(1):115-24.
3. The Million Women Study Collaborative Group. The Million Women Study: design and characteristics of the study population. Breast Cancer Res. 1999;1(1):73-80.
4. Marjoribanks J, Farquhar C, Roberts H, Lethaby A, Lee J. Long-term hormone therapy for perimenopausal and postmenopausal women. Cochrane Database Syst Rev. 2017;1(1):CD004143.
5. Prior JC, Nielsen JD, Hitchcock CL, Williams LA, Vigna YM, Dean CB. Medroxyprogesterone and conjugated oestrogen are equivalent for hot flushes: a 1-year randomized double-blind trial following premenopausal ovariectomy. Clin Sci (Lond). 2007;112(10):517-25.
6. Goodwin JW, Green SJ, Moinpour CM, Bearden JD 3rd, Giguere JK, Jiang CS, et al. Phase III randomized placebo-controlled trial of two doses of megestrol acetate as treatment for menopausal symptoms in women with breast cancer. J Clin Oncol. 2008;26(10):1650-6.
7. Stubbs C, Mattingly L, Crawford SA, Wickersham EA, Brockhaus JL, McCarthy LH. Do SSRIs and SNRIs reduce the frequency and/or severity of hot flashes in menopausal women. J Okla State Med Assoc. 2017;110(5):272-4.
8. Walega DR, Rubin LH, Banuvar S, Shulman LP, Maki PM. Effects of stellate ganglion block on vasomotor symptoms: findings from a randomized controlled clinical trial in postmenopausal women. Menopause. 2014; 21(8):807-14.
9. Lethaby A, Ayeleke RO, Roberts H. Local oestrogen for vaginal atrophy in postmenopausal women. Cochrane Database Syst Rev. 2016;2016(8):CD001500.
10. Tella SH, Gallagher JC. Prevention and treatment of postmenopausal osteoporosis. J Steroid Biochem Mol Biol. 2014;142:155-70.
11. Yanbeiy ZA, Hansen KE. Denosumab in the treatment of glucocorticoid-induced osteoporosis: a systematic review and meta-analysis. Drug Des Devel Ther. 2019;13:2843-52.
12. Leder BZ, O'Dea LS, Zanchetta JR. Effects of abaloparatide, a human parathyroid hormone-related peptide analog, on bone mineral density in postmenopausal women with osteoporosis. J Clin Endocrinol Metab. 2015;100(2):697-706.
13. Chester RC, Kling JM, Manson JE. What the Women's Health Initiative has taught us about menopausal hormone therapy. Clin Cardiol. 2018;41(2):247-52.
14. Canonico M, Carcaillon L, Plu-Bureau G. Postmenopausal hormone therapy and risk of stroke: impact of the route of estrogen administration and type of progestogen. Stroke. 2016;47(7):1734-41.
15. Ott SM. In postmenopausal women, oral but not transdermal estrogen was associated with increased risk for stroke. Ann Intern Med. 2016;165(8):JC46.
16. Formoso G, Perrone E, Maltoni S. Short-term and long-term effects of tibolone in postmenopausal women. Cochrane Database Syst Rev. 2016;10(10):CD008536.
17. Henderson VW, Lobo RA. Hormone therapy and the risk of stroke: perspectives 10 years after the Women's Health Initiative trials. Climacteric. 2012;15(3):229-34.
18. D'Alonzo M, Bounous VE, Villa M, Biglia N. Current Evidence of the Oncological Benefit-Risk Profile of Hormone Replacement Therapy. Medicina (Kaunas). 2019;55(9):573.

19. Sjögren LL, Mørch LS, Løkkegaard E. Hormone replacement therapy and the risk of endometrial cancer: A systematic review. Maturitas. 2016; 91:25-35.
20. Collaborative Group on Epidemiological Studies of Ovarian Cancer, Beral V, Gaitskell K. Menopausal hormone use and ovarian cancer risk: individual participant meta-analysis of 52 epidemiological studies. Lancet. 2015;385(9980):1835-42.
21. Craig MC, Maki PM, Murphy DG. The Women's Health Initiative Memory Study: findings and implications for treatment. Lancet Neurol. 2005;4(3):190-4.
22. Gleason CE, Dowling NM, Wharton W. Effects of Hormone Therapy on Cognition and Mood in Recently Postmenopausal Women: findings from the Randomized, Controlled KEEPS-Cognitive and Affective Study. PLoS Med. 2015;12(6):e1001833.
23. Song YJ, Li SR, Li XW, Chen X, Wei ZX, Liu QS, et al. The Effect of Estrogen Replacement Therapy on Alzheimer's Disease and Parkinson's Disease in Postmenopausal Women: a Meta-Analysis. Front Neurosci. 2020; 4:157.
24. Manson JE, Aragaki AK, Rossouw JE, Anderson GL, Prentice RL, LaCroix AZ, et al. Menopausal Hormone Therapy and Long-term All-Cause and Cause-Specific Mortality: the Women's Health Initiative Randomized Trials. JAMA. 2017;318(10):927-38.
25. Valdes A, Bajaj T. Estrogen Therapy. Treasure Island, FL: In: Stat Pearls; 2020.
26. Coelingh Bennink HJ, Verhoeven C, Zimmerman Y, Visser M, Foidart JM, Gemzell-Danielsson K. Clinical effects of the fetal estrogen estetrol in a multiple-rising-dose study in postmenopausal women. Maturitas. 2016;91:93-100.
27. Järvinen A, Kainulainen P, Nissilä M, Nikkanen H, Kela M. Pharmacokinetics of estradiol valerate and medroxyprogesterone acetate in different age groups of postmenopausal women. Maturitas. 2004;47(3):209-17.
28. Ansbacher R. The pharmacokinetics and efficacy of different estrogens are not equivalent. Am J Obstet Gynecol. 2001;184(3):255-63.
29. Archer DF. The effect of the duration of progestogen Use on the occurrence of endometrial cancer in post-menopausal women. Menopause. 2001;8:245-51.
30. Portman DJ, Goldstein SR, Kagan R. Treatment of moderate to severe dyspareunia with intravaginal prasterone therapy: a review. Climacteric. 2019;22(1):65-72.
31. Achilli C, Pundir J, Ramanathan P, Sabatini L, Hamoda H, Panay N. Efficacy and safety of transdermal testosterone in postmenopausal women with hypoactive sexual desire disorder: a systematic review and meta-analysis. Fertil Steril. 2017;107(2):475-82.
32. Huang G, Wharton W, Travison TG. Effects of testosterone administration on cognitive function in hysterectomized women with low testosterone levels: a dose-response randomized trial. J Endocrinol Invest. 2015;38(4):455-61.
33. Fait T. Menopause hormone therapy: latest developments and clinical practice. Drugs Context. 2019;8 212551.
34. Formoso G, Perrone E, Maltoni S. Short-term and long-term effects of tibolone in postmenopausal women. Cochrane Database Syst Rev. 2016;10(10):CD008536.
35. Khorsand I, Kashef R, Ghazanfarpour M, Mansouri E, Dashti S, Khadivzadeh T. The Beneficial and Adverse Effects of Raloxifene in Menopausal Women: A Mini Review. J Menopausal Med. 2018;24(3):183-7.
36. Lello S, Capozzi A, Scambia G. The Tissue-Selective Estrogen Complex (Bazedoxifene/Conjugated Estrogens) for the Treatment of Menopause. Int J Endocrinol. 2017:5064725.
37. Kagan R, Kellogg-Spadt S, Parish SJ. Practical Treatment Considerations in the Management of Genitourinary Syndrome of Menopause. Drug Aging. 2019;36(10):897-908.
38. Manson JE, Ames JM, Shapiro M. Algorithm and mobile app for menopausal symptom management and hormonal/non-hormonal therapy decision making: a clinical decision-support tool from The North American Menopause Society. Menopause. 2015;22(3):247-53.
39. Hill DA, Crider M, Hill SR. Hormone Therapy and Other Treatments for Symptoms of Menopause. Am Fam Physician. 2016;94(11):884-9.
40. Chen LR, Ko NY, Chen KH. Isoflavone Supplements for Menopausal Women: a Systematic Review. Nutrients. 2019; 11(11):2649.

LONG QUESTIONS

1. What is menopause? What are the various menopausal health concerns?
2. List the various preparations available for menopausal hormonal therapy. Present a clinical approach to decision making regarding starting menopausal hormonal therapy in a 50-year old with no medical comorbidities with recent menopause.
3. What are selective estrogen receptor modulators? What is their role in menopausal hormonal therapy?

SHORT QUESTIONS

1. Enumerate the conditions which benefit with menopausal hormonal therapy. Enumerate the adverse health conditions which can occur or worsen with menopausal hormonal therapy.
2. Enumerate the absolute and relative contraindications to menopausal hormonal therapy
3. Enumerate the various preparations available for menopausal hormonal therapy.
4. Briefly discuss some significant clinical trials in the field of menopausal hormonal therapy.
5. Briefly discuss the various options available for prevention and management of postmenopausal osteoporosis.

MULTIPLE CHOICE QUESTIONS

1. Menopause is a not an abrupt event but a transitional phase. The menopausal transition is believed to last for how long?
   a. Less than 2 years b. About 2–4 years
   c. About 4–7 years d. Around 10 years
2. The menopausal transition is characterized by many changes. Which of the following is least likely?
   a. Urinary incontinence b. Pelvic organ prolapse
   c. Higher risk of fractures d. Vision changes

3. Which of the following biochemical changes are seen in the menopausal transition?
   a. Increase in luteinizing hormone (LH) levels
   b. Decrease in testosterone concentration
   c. Reduction in ovarian steroid synthesis
   d. All of the above
4. Regarding menopausal hormonal therapy, which of the following is correct?
   a. MHT is indicated in all women in the menopausal transition period
   b. MHT can be given for the entire duration of menopausal transition period
   c. MHT is indicated to reduce cardiovascular problems
   d. Paroxetine is effective for vasomotor symptoms
5. Regarding osteoporosis which of the following is incorrect?
   a. Estrogenic activity reduces bone resorption and improves bone health
   b. Calcium and Vitamin D intake should be encouraged in all women
   c. Calcitonin is considered the first-line therapy for women at risk of osteoporosis
   d. MHT should not be used purely for prevention of osteoporosis
6. Regarding contraindications to MHT which of the following is false?
   a. Active endometrial cancer is an absolute contraindication
   b. Gallbladder disease is an absolute contraindication
   c. Hypertriglyceridemia is a relative contraindication
   d. Though rare, pregnancy should be ruled out before starting MHT
7. Regarding raloxifene, which is false?
   a. Main indication is prevention of postmenopausal osteoporosis
   b. It exhibits estrogenic antagonistic action in the breast and reduces the risk of breast cancer when used as MHT
   c. It can be used in the treatment of breast cancer
   d. It is useful in mild cases of some psychiatric problems
8. About SERMs, which of the following is not correct?
   a. Combination of bazedoxifene and equine estrogen is designated TSEC (Tissue Specific Estrogen Complex)
   b. TSEC has a near-ideal estrogenic profile
   c. Ospemifene can be used for vasomotor symptoms such as hot flashes
   d. Ospemifene is used orally for patients with genitourinary symptoms of menopause
9. Regarding results of studies which have evaluated MHT and cancer risks, which of the following is false?
   a. Use of estrogen-progestin combination MHT increased the risk of breast cancer
   b. Use of estrogen-only MHT increased the risk of breast cancer
   c. Initiating MHT closer to menopause reduces breast cancer risks
   d. MHT is associated with a small but definite risk of development of ovarian cancer
10. Regarding initiation MHT, which is false?
   a. Those with menopause having occurred 10–12 years prior are suitable for MHT
   b. Those with predominant genitourinary symptoms are good candidates for local DHEA
   c. Those with vasomotor symptoms who have contraindications to MHT can be considered for SSRIs
   d. Transdermal preparations of estrogen largely reduce risk of cardiovascular problems

Answers

1. c 2. d 3. d 4. d 5. c 6. b
7. c 8. c 9. b 10. a

10.13 NON-HORMONAL THERAPY AT MENOPAUSE

Meeta, Akanshi Madan, Tanvir

INTRODUCTION

Menopause is a transition in life with declining estrogen levels, which may lead to undesirable symptoms and long-term health consequences. Hence, this natural phenomenon has been listed as a Disease in International Classification of Diseases. A well-managed menopause transition sets the stage for active and healthy aging.

The menopausal transition, begins on average 4 years before the final menstrual period (FMP) and is characterized by irregular menstrual cycles, endocrine changes, and symptoms may affect a woman's quality of life. It may be considered as a biological marker for chronic diseases. The biology and symptomatology of menopause is blurred due to its relationship to the underlying aging process. The symptom complex can be divided into vasomotor, somatic, urogenital, neuropsychiatric, and sexual.

In study conducted by the Indian Menopause Society (IMS), out of 1,801 women, 192 women were asymptomatic and 1,609 reported symptoms. Vasomotor symptoms (VMS) were reported by 1,211 (75.3%) women,psychological symptoms by 999 (62.01%), physical ailments by 515 (32%) and genitourinary by 250 (15.53%).[1]

INDICATIONS FOR NON-HORMONAL THERAPY

Menopausal hormone therapy (MHT) remains the gold standard and first-line therapy in the management of menopausal symptoms.[2]

Two major reasons for opting non-hormonal therapies are if the woman declines to take MHT or is contraindicated.

The absolute contraindications for MHT use are:

- Active endometrial and other gynecological hormone-dependent cancers
- Active breast cancer, estrogen-progestogen receptor-positive cancers
- Moderate and high risk for breast cancer
- Known or suspected pregnancy
- Undiagnosed, abnormal vaginal bleeding
- Severe active liver disease with impaired or abnormal liver function
- Previous personal or family history of venous thromboembolism
- Systemic lupus erythematosus
- Established cardiovascular disease (CVD) or at a high risk for (CVD).

There are various reasons for women to decline MHT. Sometimes, MHT is not tolerated. The belief that natural therapies are safe[3] and the perceived health risks associated with hormone therapy. In 2002, the initial inappropriately analyzed results of Women's Health Initiative were reported widely in the media and literature.Approximately 51% of women use complementary and alternative medicine for menopause (CAM) and more than 60% perceive it be effective for menopausal symptoms.[4] Today, the safety of MHT is established when used judiciously and individualized. The success of treatment depends on the physicians' involvement in informed and shared decision making with women regarding treatment options, including CAM, for menopausal symptoms. This type of patient-centered integrated approach can potentially reduce the risk for under treatment and adverse events. One needs to understand that any therapy claiming to reduce hot flushes must be assessed in blinded trials against placebo or a validated therapy, as placebo effects are high, with an average improvement of 40% in vasomotor symptoms due to placebo alone which may persist for several weeks[5]

NON-HORMONAL MANAGEMENT

It falls into two main categories: (1) non-pharmacological and (2) pharmacological treatment.

Non-pharmacological Treatments for Vasomotor Symptoms: Complementary and Alternative Medicine for Menopause

Complementary and alternative medicine interventions for menopause fall into 2 broad categories: mind- body practices [e.g., hypnosis, cognitive behavioral therapy (CBT), relaxation, biofeedback, meditation, and aromatherapy], and natural products (e.g., herbs, vitamins, minerals, and dietary supplements). Additionally, there are several whole system alternative medicine approaches [e.g., traditional Chinese medicine (TCM), reflexology, acupuncture, and homeopathy) that do not fit into the above categories and incorporate both mind-body practices and natural products.[6] It is important for women to be informed about the risks and benefits of CAM for menopausal symptoms.[7]

Mind and body practices including hypnosis and CBT have been demonstrated to be safe. Herbal products are frequently used. However, there is no consistent evidence to support their efficacy and safety. There is the added concern that when used in combination with other medications, some herbal products could pose serious health risks. Vitamins and minerals may be important for women who are at risk for deficiencies, may cause harm when taken beyond the recommended dietary allowances. Prescription of CAM by an allopathic doctor is legally not suggested but during counseling for options a balanced communications with evidence-based medicine is required.

Lifestyle Modifications

Lifestyle modifications to cope with VMS include dietary changes, dressing in layers, adjusting room temperature, mind-body practices, and exercises.[8] These are generally safe and may reduce stress and anxiety, improve sleep quality and quality of life, but does not appear to significantly reduce VMS.

A 2014 Cochrane meta-analysis of 5 randomized controlled trials (RCTs) with a total of 733 patients examined and concluded that the effectiveness of any type of exercise does not decrease vasomotor symptoms in perimenopausal and postmenopausal women.[9] A recent study of 15 weeks of resistance training showed a decrease in the frequency and severity of moderate and severe hot flushes among postmenopausal women could be an effective and safe treatment option to alleviate vasomotor symptoms.[10] Exercise and physical activity have a positive impact on a range of health outcomes and is an integral part in the management of menopause. A high quality large randomized control study is required before any recommendation for treatment of menopausal symptoms is made. Knowledge about adverse events, tolerability of exercise and methodology of interventions is also important.[8]

Yoga is an ancient Indian science and includes the practice of specific postures, regulated breathing, and meditation. Yoga is thought to bring back physical, mental and spiritual being back to balance.[11] Yoga appears to be safe and to improve multiple parameters of health and quality of life. A systematic review and meta-analysis including 5 RCTs concluded that there was moderate evidence for the short-term effects of yoga on psychological symptoms in menopause.[12]

Paced Respiration

Paced respirations (slow, deep breathing) with progressive muscle relaxation. An RCT comparing paced breathing with regular breathing (control) found reductions of 52% in hot flashes over 9 weeks.[13]

Cognitive Behavioral Therapy

Cognitive behavioral therapy is an action-oriented psychological intervention that has been used to treat hot flashes, depression, and other menopausal symptoms. CBT is a time-limited treatment that focuses on changing cognitive appraisals and behavior choices to alter symptoms. Mindfulness is defined as "paying attention in a particular way: on purpose, in the present moment, and nonjudgmentally." CBT may include education, motivational interviewing, mindfulness relaxation, paced breathing, and other strategies to improve symptoms.

Cognitive behavioral therapy effectively reduced the impact of vasomotor symptoms and hence improved mood, sleep and quality of life in women with and without a history of breast cancer, by an average of 50% after 8 hours of group CBT (weekly group sessions over 4–6 weeks). These benefits were maintained at 6months with no adverse effects.[14] Self-help cognitive behavior therapy (SH-CBT) booklet on hot flush and night sweat is a potentially effective management option for working women experiencing problematic VMS improvements were maintained at 20 weeks postrandomization.[15] CBT has been recommended by the North American Menopausal Society for reducing the bothersomeness of vasomotor symptoms, but not for frequency.[16]

Herbal Products, Vitamins, and Supplements

Black Cohosh (Cimicifuga racemosa): Black cohosh, is a widely studied phytopharmaceutical North American plant that has been used historically as an indigenous treatment for menopausal symptoms.

Side effects of black cohosh may include: gastrointestinal problems, rash, and acute hepatitis.

In a systematic reviewof 16 RCT son the effects of oral mono preparations of *C. racemosa* on menopausal symptoms, including VMS, sexual dysfunction, vulvovaginal symptoms, bone health, and quality of life, researchers concluded that there was insufficient evidence to support the use of black cohosh for menopausal symptoms at this time, but that there was sufficient evidence to warrant further investigations.[17]

Dong Quai (Angelica sinensis): Dong quai is a traditional Chinese herb that is most often used in combination with other herbs to treat female reproductive problems. Two trials have used *Angelica sinensis* in combination with other herbs and found a significant improvement in the frequency and intensity of hot flashes (90–96%) compared with placebo (15–20%) over the 3-month trial. However, it is difficult to determine the effects of *A. sinensis* from these 2 trials due to the use of combined preparations.[18.]

In addition, important safety concerns included interactions with other medications and herbs, photosensitization, anticoagulation, and possible carcinogenicity.[19]

Wild Yam (Dioscorea): Wild yam is a tuber that has been historically used in TCM to treat multiple symptoms, including symptoms of menopause small number of studies and insufficient information regarding long-term safety, more research is needed in order to determine the efficacy of wild yam for menopause symptoms.

Indian herbs for use in menopause are generally dietary herbs such asturmeric, ginger, fenugreek, linseed, cumin, fennel, saffron, and cinnamon. Dietary supplements like flaxseed, lycopene have been tried in managing menopause. Lycopene in the form of Lyc-o-mato at a dose of 8 mg/day has shown to be effective in reducing symptoms in up to 75% of cases by 50%—RCT by Indian Menopause Society. (In Presss).

Vitamin E: Vitamin E is thought to act as an antioxidant in the body. In an RCT comparing the effects of gabapentin to vitamin E among 115 women for VMS reduction, hot flush frequency, and score decreased by 10.02% and 7.28% respectively in the vitamin E group.[20] At this time there is an insufficient amount of empirical evidence to conclude the effectiveness of vitamin E supplementation for menopausal symptoms.

Phytoestrogens: Phytoestrogens are a group of phytochemicals from plants that exhibit weak estrogenic activity in humans byacting as natural selective estrogen receptor modulators by binding preferentially to estrogen receptor beta (SERMs), e.g., phytoestrogens. These function as proestrogen when estrogen deficiency is present and antiestrogens when excess estrogen is present:[21]

Phytoestrogens are classified into three broad groups:

1. Isoflavones (most common forms found in soybeans, lentils, chickpeas, red clover)
2. Lignans—found in flaxseed, bean sprouts, alfalfa sprouts,, sunflower seeds, spinach, clover
3. Coumestans—split peas, pinto beans, lima beans, and especially alfalfa and clover sprouts.

The most widely advertised and studied phytoestrogen is soy. Here again, there may be a difference in the effects produced by this plant because of different variables.

Source variability: The part or type of plant studied—sprout contains coumestans and beans contain isoflavones with genistein, daidzein and glycitein. The soil in which the plant is grown. Processing of the plants/beans—fermented products like tofu and miso are more efficacious.

Population variability: Phytoestrogens are active only in the form of glycosides. The aglycone form is inactive. Variability in absorption leads to differences in their bioavailability and actions. This is largely influenced by the intestinal flora of each individual and also by the ability of the individual to produce a substance called equol. It is being realized that every individual has a different capability of producing equol. For example, people eating vegetarian diets produce higher amounts of equol in their bodies and hence absorb more phytoestrogens from their diets.

Variability in the processed molecule: There is a rationale for providing active principles of phytoestrogens in the form of pills and powders. There are limitations such as the foods made from soybeans and soy protein formulations may provide other phytochemicals that enhance the effect of isoflavones. These effects could be lost when isoflavones alone are given as additives.

There is a need for regulation for purity, standardization of isoflavone extracts, the matrix in which it is delivered.

Until more studies documenting benefits and safety are conducted, it is essential for clinicians to advice their patients that whole soy foods may be better than such products as supplements or soy-enriched or soy-fortified foods. Many of these products are available, all containing differing amounts of isoflavones.

India has a high vegetarian population, and there is a high consumption of legumes and cereals, it is possible that the Indian woman may already have plasma levels of phytoestrogens equivalent to the Japanese. Indian diet contains many substances that are phytoestrogenic. This fact needs to be explored and exploited. An example is Bengal gram that has three times more estrogenic activity as compared to soy since it contains biochanins (lignans) **(Table 1)**. Common Indian dietary sources of phytoestrogens are as given in **Table 2**.

Suggested Intake of Whole Soy Foods

Optimal cholesterol reduction seems to require approximately 50 mg/day of isoflavones; this amount would be found in approximately 25 g/day of soy protein, which corresponds to the health claim allowed by the Food and Drug Administration (FDA). Most studies on hot flushes have used isoflavone amounts of 40–80 mg/day, and this amount may benefit vasomotor symptoms. These effects seem to be dose related hence the recommended intake of soy phytoestrogens is 40–50 mg/day.

Phytoestrogens are weak and of low potency **(Table 3)**.[20,21] Meta-analysis shows that phytoestrogens can be safely used for long periods without causing an increase in endometrial thickness and there is an improvement in lipid profile and vaginal maturation. The effect and potential benefits of phytoestrogens on mammographic density and testosterone levels need to be studied furthur.[23] It is prudent to be cautious for use in hormone-dependent cancers, coagulation defects as data on long-term use is lacking.

System Alternative Medicine Approaches

Eastern: TCM (China), Ayurvedic medicine, and Unani (India). Western: Homeopathy and naturopathy.

Ayurvedic medicine: Ayurveda, which literally means "the science of life", is a natural healing system developed in India. The primary Ayurvedic treatments include diet, exercise, meditation, herbs, massage, exposure to sunlight and yoga.

Homeopathy: Homeopathic practitioners (homeopaths) subscribe to the principle that "like cures like.

Acupuncture: Acupuncture techniques come from TCM and involve insertion of small needles into the skin at certain points on the body, which are called acupoints. The foundation of acupuncture is a belief that diseases and symptoms occur because of disruptions in an individual's QI, or life force energy. Two studies found no significant difference from placebo.

NON-HORMONAL PHARMACEUTICAL THERAPY

Centrally Acting Compound

Clonidine: Clonidine is a centrally active α-2 adrenergic agonist anti-hypertensive that was first proposed as a treatment for hot flushes in the 1970s. It is the only licensed

TABLE 1: Isoflavone content of pulses and legumes (mg/100 g fresh weight).

Isoflavones	*Soybean*	*Bengal gram*	*Green gram*	*Black gram*	*Red gram*
Daidzein	2.7 (49)*	5.1	80.7 (81)	88.0 (98.0)	85*
Protensin		4.8			12
Formononetin		44.1			
Biochinin A		98.6			
Genistein	2.4				
Daidzin	40.6				
Total	67.8–308.6	152.6	80.7	88.8	97

*Content on sprouting

TABLE 2: Common Indian dietary sources of phytoestrogens.

Isoflavones	*Ligors*	*Saponins*
Bengal gram	Linseed	Turmeric
Chick peas	Rye	Liquorice
Cherries	Millet	Ginger
Pareley	Bengal gram	Wild yam
Apples	All pulses	Fenugreek
Mung beans	Sesame and sunflower seeds	Beet root
Whole grains	Legumes and beans	Root vegetables
Soya		
Red clover		

TABLE 3: Potency of estradiol and phytoestrogens.

Molecule	*Relative potency*
Estradiol	100
Coumestrol	0.202
Genistein	0.084
Daidzein	0.013
Formononetin	Converted into Genistein and Daidzein
Biochanin A	Converted into Genistein and Daidzein

non-hormonal medicine for the treatment of vasomotor symptoms in the UK. A double-blind, randomized, placebo controlled trial of clonidine (0.1 mg/day) versus venlafaxine (75 mg/day extended release) versus placebo in 102 breast cancer survivors over a 12 week period showed that both clonidine and venlafaxine were superior to placebo in reducing vasomotor symptoms and, although venlafaxine worked more quickly, clonidine was more effective at 12 weeks. Side effects of clonidine include dizziness, hypotension, headache, constipation, and dry mouth.[22]

Antidepressants: Serotonin Selective Reuptake Inhibitors and Serotonin and Noradrenaline Reuptake Inhibitors

In the 1990s it was recognized that women taking selective serotonin reuptake inhibitors (SSRI) had a decrease in hot flushes. As a result of these observations, it was hypothesized that such antidepressants may have therapeutic effects on hot flushes. The SSRIs or SNRIs, clonidine, and gabapentin trials provide evidence for efficacy; however, effects are less than for estrogen, few trials have been published and most have methodological deficiencies, generalizability is limited, and adverse effects and cost may restrict use for many women. These therapies may be most useful for highly symptomatic women who cannot take estrogen but are not optimal choices for most women.[24]

Paroxetine: Paroxetine, an SSRI, was first explored as a treatment of hot flushes in a pilot trial conducted in 2000. Low-dose paroxetine 7.5 mg/day is the only non-hormonal drug approved by the US FDA for the treatment of hot flashes. Paroxetine 7.5 mg significantly reduces the number of nighttime awakenings attributed to VMS and increases sleep duration without differentially affecting sleep-onset latency or sedation.

Fluoxetine: Adouble blind randomized, crossover study of fluoxetine was performed, this trial included 81 women who were assigned to either fluoxetine 20 mg daily or placebo, after 4 weeks the groups switched. After the first treatment period, there was a 50% decrease in hot flushes scores in the fluoxetine group versus 36% reduction in placebo group. No significant adverse effects were noted in the treatment group. The recommended dose is 10–30 mg/day.

Do not prescribe paroxetine, fluoxetine to women taking tamoxifen.

Venlafaxine and Desvenlafaxine: A randomized trial comparing the SNRI venlafaxine (extended release, 75 mg/day) with 0.5 mg/day oral 17β estradiol found that both treatments were associated with a statistically significant reduction in the frequency of vasomotor symptoms of around 50% after 8 weeks of use. Desvenlafaxine 100 mg/day is the active metabolite of venlafaxine and reduces vasomotor symptoms for up to 12 months.

General consideration for prescription: The clinical response is more rapid (days) than the typical response to SSRIs for depression (weeks). Start with small dose, and needs to be evaluated periodically. One reason is to determine if it is still needed as in many women menopause-related vasomotor symptoms will improve over time.

These medications should not be taken with any other antidepressants or any substance containing St. John's Wort and discontinuation should be tapered. Do not prescribe paroxetine, fluoxetine to women taking tamoxifen. Selective serotonin reuptake inhibitors and SNRI side effects may include nausea, dizziness, dry mouth, nervousness, constipation, somnolence, and sexual dysfunction. The most common adverse effects with venlafaxine reported were insomnia or excitement. **Table 4** elaborates the medication, dose, and side effect.

According to international consensus, the discontinuity of antidepressants should be addressed at 6–18 months after symptom remission in case of anxiety and four to 12 months in case of depressive disorders.

Anticonvulsant

Gabapentin: It is an anticonvulsant also used for neuropathic pain. A systematic review of 13 RCTs including 1,714 women found that gabapentin (300 mg three times per day) reduced the severity and frequency of vasomotor symptoms in breast cancer survivors. Up to 900 mg/day gabapentin is generally

TABLE 4: Medication, dose and adverse effects of SSRIs and SNRIs.

Medication	*Dosage*	*Common adverse effects*
SSRIs and SNRIs		
Paroxetine	10–20 mg/day	Nausea, drowsiness, sexual dysfunction
Venlafaxine	37.5–150 mg/day	Nausea, drowsiness, sexual dysfunction, insomnia,excitement
Desvenlafaxine	25–150 mg/day	Nausea, drowsiness, sexual dysfunction
Fluoxetine	10-20mg/day	Nausea, drowsiness, sexual dysfunction
Anticonvulsant		
Gabapentin	100 mg at night, increase to 300 mg three times per day	Dizziness, drowsiness
Pregabalin	75 mg at night, increase to 150 mg twice daily	Dizziness, drowsiness, nausea, headache

(SSRIs: selective serotonin repute inhibitors; SNRIs: serotonin and norepinephrine reuptake inhibitors)

well tolerated, but side effects are dose related and may include somnolence, dizziness, and fatigue.

The choice of drug depends upon whether the patient is taking tamoxifen, the pattern of hot flashes, and the presence of a mood disorder or sleep problem **(Table 5)**.

Oxybutynin

Oxybutynin, an antimuscarinic, anticholinergic agent currently used to treat overactive bladder. In a 2016 trial, 73% of women taking 15 mg extended-release oxybutynin once daily experienced reduced frequency and severity of hot flashes and better sleep.

Neurokinin 3 Receptor Antagonist

The thermoregulatory center in the hypothalamus is innervated by kisspeptin/neurokinin B/dynorphin (KNDy) neurons that are stimulated by neurokinin B (NKB) and inhibited by estrogen. Neurokinin 3 receptor (NK3R) antagonists may represent a new non-hormonal approach to the management of hot flushes. However, additional trials are needed before recommending this approach.[25]

Estetrol

Estetrol (E4), a naturally occurring estrogen produced by the fetal liver. It has a long half life of 28–32 hours, and its potential mechanism may give it a different safety profile than estradiol (E2). Preliminary findings suggest it reduces vasomotor symptom severity by 44%, compared with 30% with placebo, at 15 mg.

TABLE 5: Choice of drug depending on the symptom, side effect profile.

	Gabapentin or pregabalin	*SSRI or SNRI*	*CBT or hypnosis*
VMS*	++	++	+
Sleep	+++	+/-	
Mood		+++	

*Vasomotor Symptoms
(CBT: cognitive behavioral therapy; SSRIs: selective serotonin repute inhibitors; SNRIs: serotonin andnorepinephrine reuptake inhibitors; VMS: vasomotor symptoms)

Topical Non-hormonal Treatments for Vaginal Symptoms of Menopause

Nonhormonal treatments for vaginal atrophy entail an amalgamation of protectants and thickening agents in a water-soluble base and certain other substances having maturation effect on the urogenital epithelium. They are options for women wishing to avoid hormonal therapy or in high-risk individuals with a history of hormone-sensitive malignancy such as a breast or endometrial cancer.[21]

Vaginal lubricants: Lubricants are generally used during sexual intercourse to give temporary relief from vaginal dryness and dyspareunia. There are two basic types—water and silicone based. There are several vaginal lubricants available. While they can be used to decrease immediate irritation during intercourse, there is no evidence that they have any long-term therapeutic effect. They might lead to vaginal irritation later, and importantly, Vaseline can break the latex of condoms. Women prone to yeast infections should avoid glycerin-based lubricants.

Vaginal moisturizers: Moisturizers are used on a chronic maintenance basis to replace normal vaginal secretions, whereas lubricants are specifically designed to reduce friction associated with sexual activity. Moisturizers are hydrophilic, insoluble, cross-linked polymers. They are bioadhesives; connect to mucin and epithelial cells on the vaginal wall retaining water. Their buffering properties, which lead to reduction in the vaginal pH, are the mainstay of their symptom-relieving effects. Their efficacy on vaginal symptoms is although lower than that of topical estrogen therapy. In one of the trials, which compared the efficacy of a vaginal moisturizer to vaginal estrogen cream in the symptomatic treatment of vaginal atrophy in postmenopausal women, both led to a significant improvement in the vaginal dryness index in the first week of treatment but the dienestrol was more effective than the nonhormonal preparation.

Phytoestrogens: When administered orally, phytoestrogens do not seem to have an effect on vaginal epithelium; however, intravaginal application has shown some promise. In a double-blind, randomized placebo-controlled study, the efficacy of new isoflavone vaginal gel was compared with the effectiveness of conjugated equine estrogen (CEE) and placebo in treating vulvovaginal atrophy. In this study, 90 postmenopausal women were treated for 12 weeks with either isoflavone vaginal gel 4% (1 g/day), CEE cream (0.3 mg/day) or placebo gel. Women treated with isoflavone gel showed a similar improvement to the estrogen group for vaginal dryness and dyspareunia, both of which differed significantly from the placebo group.

Laser therapy: Fractional CO_2 laser or erbium:YAG laser, has been proposed as a non-hormonal therapy for GSM. Several small studies have shown that fractional CO_2 laser therapy can restore the vaginal epithelium to a state similar to the premenopausal state, increase the amounts of *Lactobacillus* and other premenopausal flora, as well as improve the Vaginal Health Index score and subjective symptoms of GSM, including lower urinary tract symptoms. Long-term studies are awaited before this modality is recommended in routine practice.[26]

KEY MESSAGES

- Menopausal women and healthcare professionals should be involved in the care and decision making.
- Women with contraindications to MHT, or those who prefer not to use hormones, may choose to use non-hormonal medicines for relief of vasomotor symptoms. These are not as effective as MHT, nor do they have the other benefits.
- Consider cognitive behavioral therapy to alleviate low mood and anxiety in menopausal women.
- Data is insufficient for the management of moderate-to-severe VMS.
- Complementary and alternative treatments should be advised with caution.
- There is some evidence that isoflavones or black cohosh may relieve vasomotor symptoms, their safety is unknown.
- Do not routinely offer selective serotonin repute inhibitors (SSRIs) or serotonin andnorepinephrine reuptake inhibitors (SNRIs) as first-line treatment for vasomotor symptomsalone.
- Understand that there is no clear evidence for SSRIs or SNRIs to decrease low mood in menopausal women who have not been diagnosed with depression.

REFERENCES

1. Singh M. Early age of natural menopause in India a biological marker for early preventive health programs. Climacteric. 2012;15:581-6.
2. Stuenkel CA, Davis SR, Gompel A, Lumsden MA. Treatment of Symptoms of the Menopause: An Endocrine Society Clinical Practice Guideline. J Clin Endocrinol Metab. 2015;100(11):3975.
3. Santini A, Cammarata SM, Capone GE. Nutraceuticals: opening the debate for a regulatory framework. Br J Clin Pharmacol. 2018;84:659-72.
4. Posadzki P, Lee MS, Moon TW, Choi TY, Park TY, Ernst E. Prevalence of complementary and alternative medicine (CAM) use by menopausal women: a systematic review of surveys. Maturitas. 2013;75:34-43.
5. MacLennan A, Lester S, Moore V. Oral oestrogen replacement therapy versus placebo for hot flushes: a systematic review. Climacteric. 2001;4:58-74.
6. National Center for Complementary and Integrative Health. Complementary, alternative, or integrative health: what's in name? [online] Available from: https://nccih.nih.gov/health/integrative-health.[Last Accessed December, 2021].
7. Johnson A, Roberts L, MA, Elkins G. Complementary and Alternative Medicine for Menopause. J Evid Based Integr Med. 2019;24:1-14.
8. Stojanovska L, Apostolopoulos V, Polman R, Borkoles E. To exercise, or, not to exercise, during menopause and beyond. Maturitas. 2014;77:318-23.
9. Daley A, Stokes-Lampard H, Thomas A, MacArthur C. Exercise for vasomotor menopausal symptoms. Cochrane Database Syst Rev. 2014;11:CD006108.
10. Berina E, Hammar M. Resistance training for hot flushes in postmenopausal women: arandomised controlled trial. Maturitas. 2019;126:55-60.
11. Feuerstein G. The Yoga Tradition: Its History, Literature, Philosophy, and Practice, 3rd edition. Prescott: Hohm Press; 2001.
12. Cramer H, Lauche R, Langhorst J, Dobos G. Effectiveness of yoga for menopausal symptoms; a systematic review and meta- analysis of randomized controlled trials. Evid Based Complement Alternat Med. 2012;2012:863-905.
13. Sood R, Sood A, Wolf SL. Paced breathing compared with usual breathing for hot flashes. Menopause. 2013;20:179-84.
14. Mann E, Smith MJ, Hellier J. Cognitive behavioural treatment for women who have menopausal symptoms after breast cancer treatment (MENOS 1): a randomised controlled trial. Lancet Oncol. 2012;359:309-18.
15. Hardy C, Griffiths A, Norton S.Self-help Cognitive Behavior Therapy for Working Women With Problematic Hot Flushes and Night Sweats: a Multicenter Randomized Controlled Trial. Menopause. 2018;25(5):508-19.
16. NAM Society. Nonhormonal management of menopause-associated vasomotor symptoms: 2015 position statement of the North American Menopause Society. Menopause 2015;359:1155-72,
17. Leach M, Moore V. Black cohosh (*Cimicifuga spp.)* for menopausal symptoms. Cochrane Database Syst Rev. 2012;(9):CD007244.
18. Kupfersztain C, Rotem C, Fagot R, Kaplan B. The immediate effect of natural plant extract, Angelica sinensis and Matricaria chamomilla (Climex) for the treatment of hot flushes during menopause. A preliminary report. Clin Exp Obstet Gynecol. 2003;30(4):203-6.
19. Fugh-Berman A. Herb-drug interactions. Lancet. 2000;355: 134-8.
20. Biglia N, Sgandurra P, Peano E. Non-hormonal treatment of hot flushes in breast cancer survivors: gabapentin vs. vitamin E. Climacteric. 2009;359:310-8.
21. Meeta M, Digumarti L, Agarwal N, Vaze N, Shah R, Malik S. Clinical practice guidelines on menopause.Mumbai: Indian Menopause Society.2020.
22. Hickey M, Szabo RA, Hunter MS. Non-hormonal treatments for menopausal symptoms. BMJ. 2017;359:j5101.

23. Lindermann Peressoni Teixeira MJ, Colonetti Colombo C, Colonetti L, Inês da Rosa M, Colonetti T (2021): Influence of phytoestrogens on endometrial thickness: a systematic review and meta-analysis. Climacteric. DOI: 10.1080/13697137.2021.1921728
24. Nelson HD, Vesco KK, Haney E, Fu R, Nedrow A, Miller J, Nonhormonal therapies for menopausal hot flashes: systematic review and meta-analysis. JAMA. 2006;295(17):2057.
25. Crandall CJ, Manson JE, Hohensee C. Association of genetic variation in the tachykinin receptor 3 locus with hot flashes and night sweats in the Women's Health Initiative Study. Menopause. 2017;24(3):252.
26. Charity K, Vera L, Deborah F. A systematic review of laser therapy for vulvovaginal atrophy/genitourinary syndrome of menopause in breast cancer survivors. Ecancer Med Sci. 2019;13:988.

LONG QUESTION

1. What are the treatment modalities that can be offered to a woman with a history of breast cancer and suffering from severe vasomotor symptoms?

SHORT QUESTIONS

1. What are the indications of non-hormonal treatment?
2. Elaborate the absolute contraindications for menopausal hormone therapy.
3. Write a short note on cognitive behavioral therapy.
4. Write a short note on classification of phytoestrogens.
5. What is the role of non-hormonal pharmaceutical therapy for vasomotor symptoms?

MULTIPLE CHOICE QUESTIONS

1. Menopause is classified as a disease:
   a. True b. False
2. Absolute contraindications for menopausal hormone therapy:
   a. Migraine
   b. Gallbladder disease
   c. High risk for cardiovascular disease
   d. Superficial thrombophlebitis
3. Menopausal hormone therapy is safe when used judiciously and individualized:
   a. True b. False
4. Resistance exercise reduces the hot flushes in menopausal women:
   a. True b. False
5. Non-hormonal treatment includes:
   a. Cognitive behavioral therapy
   b. Medroxy-progesterone
   c. Dehydroepiandrosterone
   d. Bazedoxifene
6. Yoga does not help in:
   a. Quality of life
   b. Improves psychological symptoms
   c. Hot flushes
   d. Improves balance
7. Phytoestrogens bind preferentially to:
   a. Estrogen receptor beta
   b. Estrogen receptor alpha
   c. Both alpha and beta estrogen receptor
   d. Only to estrogen receptor beta
8. The recommended intake of soy phytoestrogens is:
   a. 40–50 mg/day
   b. 40–80 mg/day
   c. 60–100 mg/day
   d. None of the above
9. Selective serotonin repute inhibitors (SSRIs) or serotonin and norepinephrine reuptake inhibitors (SNRIs) may be offered as first-line treatment for vasomotor symptoms:
   a. True b. False
10. The time taken for antidepressants to have an effect on hot flushes:
    a. Immediate b. 1 week
    c. 3 weeks d. None of the above

Answers

1.	a	2.	c	3.	a	4.	a	5.	a	6.	c
7.	a	8.	a	9.	b	10.	b				

SECTION 11

Endoscopy

11.1 LAPAROSCOPY: SAFE ENTRY TECHNIQUE AND INSTRUMENTATION

Rajendra Sankpal, Damodar Rao

INTRODUCTION

Laparoscopy has steadily become the mode of treatment for most of the benign gynecological disease that require surgery, but entry into the abdomen in laparoscopy is one of the most challenging aspects of the entire procedure. The site, equipment, and manner of entrance are determined by the surgeon's expertise, the patient's characteristics, the available resources, and the suspected pathology.[1] Major complications associated with gynecologic laparoscopy are relatively rare and commonly occur when attempting to gain entry into the peritoneal cavity.

ENTRY TECHNIQUE (TABLE 1)

The following methods are commonly used.

- Veress needle technique
- Direct trocar insertion
- Hasson technique or open technique
- Radially expanding trocar
- Visual entry system.

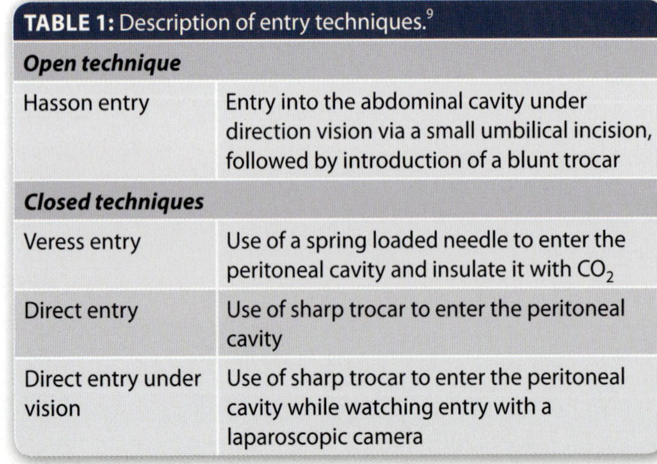

TABLE 1: Description of entry techniques.[9]

Open technique	
Hasson entry	Entry into the abdominal cavity under direction vision via a small umbilical incision, followed by introduction of a blunt trocar
Closed techniques	
Veress entry	Use of a spring loaded needle to enter the peritoneal cavity and insulate it with CO_2
Direct entry	Use of sharp trocar to enter the peritoneal cavity
Direct entry under vision	Use of sharp trocar to enter the peritoneal cavity while watching entry with a laparoscopic camera

Veress Needle

Among today's gynecologists, Veress needle is the most common and the oldest method used for creating pneumoperitoneum.

A standard Veress needle is a 12–15 cm long; hollow, with an external diameter of 2 mm containing a blunt-tipped, spring-loaded obturator. It is a blind method where the Veress needle pierces through the layers of the anterior abdominal wall. Umbilicus is the most common site for Veress needle insertion as there is absence of fat and muscle at this area **(Fig. 1)**.

Safety Test

Double Click Test

In this test, the surgeon hears two clicks that are produced when the needle pierces through the layers of abdominal wall. The first click is heard when the needle passes through the rectus sheath and a second click as it passes through the peritoneum.

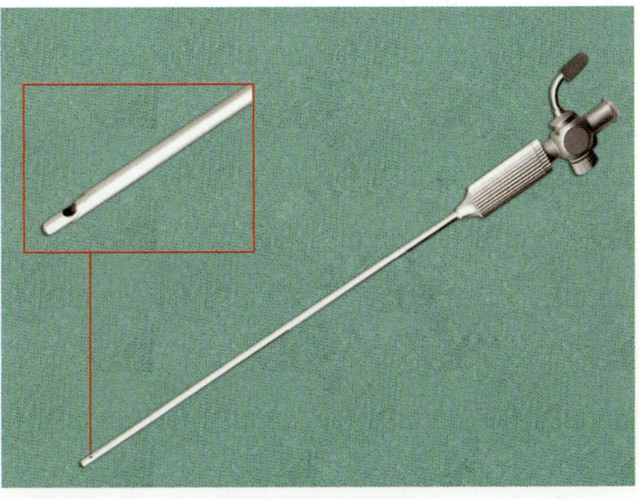

Fig. 1: Veress needle.

Irrigation and Aspiration Test

It is the most frequently used test. A syringe containing 5 mL of normal salineis attached to the Veress needle with the flow tap open.

- The first step is to aspirate, the needle should not aspirate blood, liquid, or fecal matter confirmingthe absence of any vascular injury, bladder or bowel perforation.
- The second step is to inject 2–5 mL of saline which should pass without any resistance. A simple method to ensure that no intra-abdominal viscera and adhesions are in the way.
- The injected saline is reaspirated in the third step. Reaspiration should be unattainable confirming the correct position of the Veress needle.

If fresh blood or fecal matter is aspirated, then the Veress needle should be left in its position and an emergency laparotomy should be done to identify the punctured area.

Hanging Drop Test

Raising the abdominal wall slightly, a drop of saline or distilled water should be placed over the Veress needle. Due to the negative intra-abdominal pressure, the saline should flow freely down the needle into the cavity if the needle is intraperitoneal.[2]

Gas Insufflation Test

Less than 10 mm Hg of intraperitoneal pressure at the time of gas insufflation is the most reliable test in confirming the intraperitoneal placement of Veress needle.[3,4]

Direct Trocar Entry

Direct trocar entry is faster than any other method making it the mainstay of the laparoscopic surgeon's tool kit.

Here, a skin incision is given that is slightly wider than the diameter of a sharp trocar/cannula system. By pulling on 2 towel clips placed about 2–3 cm on either side of the umbilicus, the abdominal wall is elevated slightly. To prevent sudden uncontrolled entry into the abdomen, the surgeon holds a 10-mm trocar with his index finger 3 cm away from the trocar tip. With a twisting semicircular motion, the trocar is inserted at a 90-degree angle and progressed into the peritoneal cavity in a controlled manner. After that, the laparoscope is inserted, adequate intraperitoneal insertion is confirmed, and a pneumoperitoneum is produced using high-flow insufflation. The underlying structures are then thoroughly examined for damage.[5]

THE OPEN TECHNIQUE (HASSON)

In 1971, Hasson introduced an open technique to avoid complications related to the closed techniques **(Fig. 2)**.

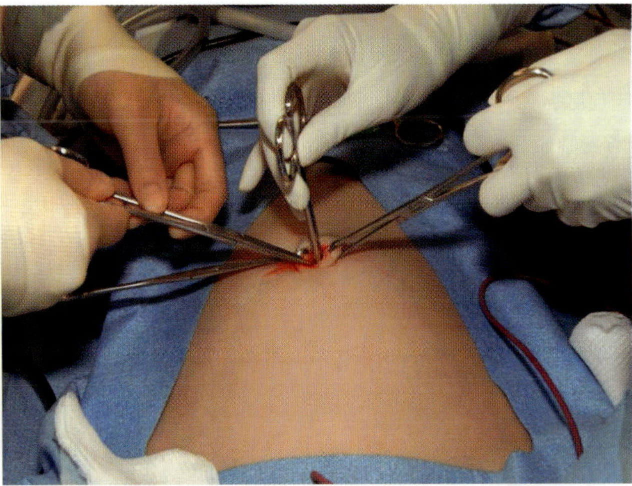

Fig. 2: Hasson technique.

Here, trocar is inserted under direct vision after meticulous dissection of the abdomen layers sometimes leading to formation of hematoma, seroma or infection. In Modified Hasson technique, we place an incision supraumbilical and reach a point of least resistance of penetration of the first trocar. The risk of excessive dissection and failure to enter the peritoneum is avoided.[6]

Advantages for the Hasson technique are:

- Preventing blind entry with a Veress needle
- Proper anatomical repair of the abdominal wall incision.

Modified Hasson technique can be used for:

- Pelvic surgeries
- Obstetric patients
- Very lean women
- Children.

Limitations:

- Time consuming
- Difficult technique
- Improper maintenance of pneumoperitoneum.[7]

Radially Expanding System

In 1994, the radially expanding access system was first implemented **(Figs. 3A to C)**. An expanding polymeric sleeve surrounds a 1.9 mm Veressneedle. The Veress is used to insufflate the abdomen first, the needle is later removed, and the outer sleeve works as a tract through the abdominal wall which can be dilated up to 12 mm by twisting motion.[8]

Visual Access Method

The optical access technique uses specialized trocars that have a transparent tipto access the peritoneal cavity, allowing the 0° laparoscope to visualize each layer of the abdominal wall as it is being traversed. Available commercially are the Optiview, Visiport and Kii optical access systems.

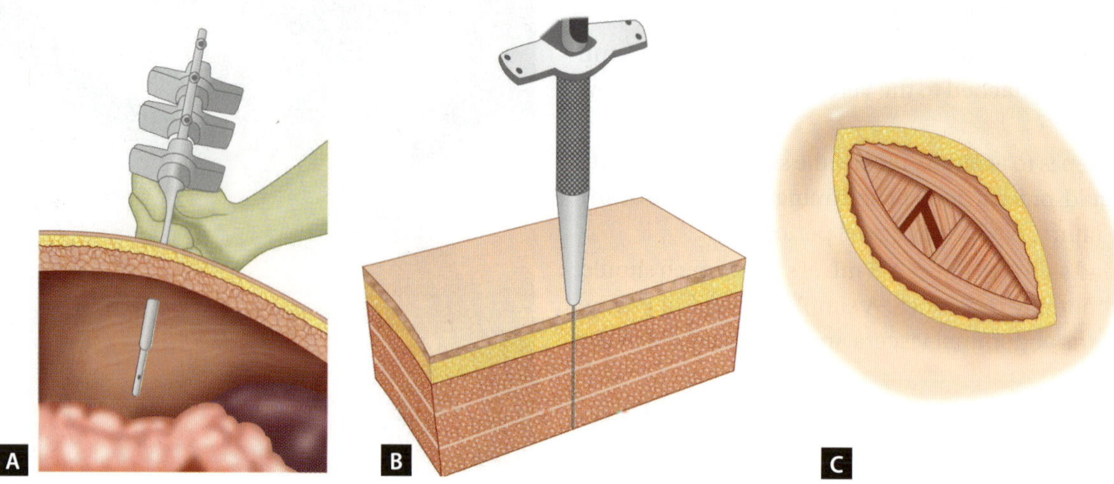

Figs. 3A to C: Radially expanding access system.

Visual access method is used for primary port placement after pneumoperitoneum is established using the Veress technique **(Figs. 4 to 10)**.

The pneumoperitoneum is first established, and then a skin incision (0.5–1 cm) at the designated port site is made. The trocar is placed at the incision with the 0° scope placed inside it. While seeing each subsequent layer of the abdominal wall, the system applies adequate downward pressure on the abdominal wall.

The right depth is attained when a rush of gas from the peritoneal cavity is heard. The telescope is then removed, with the trocar retracted slightly, and the cannula is pushed forward 1–2 cm. The telescope is reintroduced once the trocar has been removed. Visualizing the omentum ensures that the device is in the right spot in the peritoneal cavity.[7]

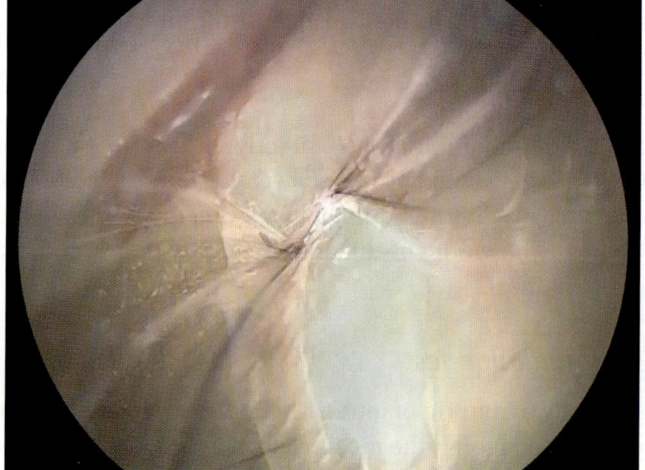

Fig. 4: Entry with optical trocar.

ACCESS LOCATION (FIG. 11)

The ideal entry site should considerthe following factors:

- Avoidance of any important structures
- Comfortable to surgeon
- Prior surgical history
- Distance from the operative site.

Umbilical Entry

Most common site is the umbilicus. Absence of the muscle and subcutaneous fat and the fused abdominal fascia result in the shortest distance from the skin to the abdominal cavity. The aorta and inferior vena cava are essential anatomic structures around the umbilicus.

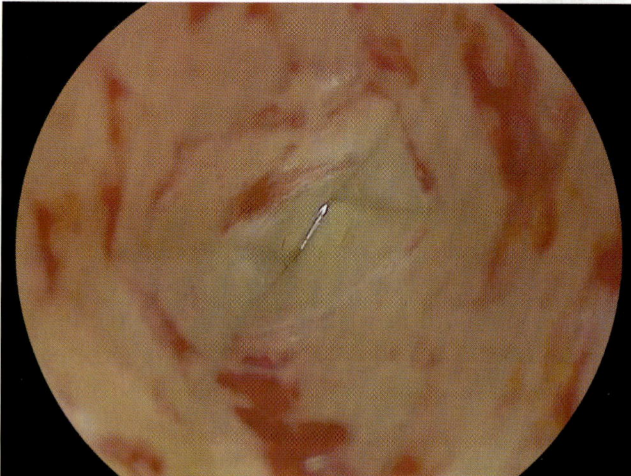

Fig. 5: Fatty layer of abdominal wall.

Advantages:

- Easy entry
- Good surgical access to the pelvic organs
- Better port movement due to less lateral resistance from adipose layers
- Cosmetically better
- Reduced postoperative discomfort.[1]

Disadvantages:

- High rate of adhesions
- History of umbilical hernia
- History of umbilical hernia repair with mesh.

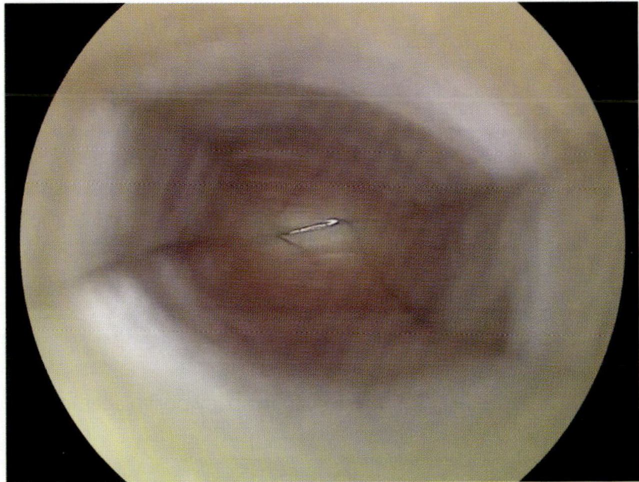

Fig. 6: Outer fascial layer and muscle layer.

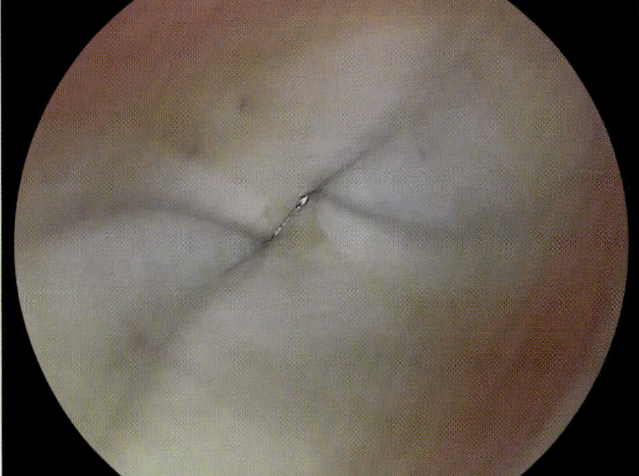

Fig. 7: Inner fascial layer.

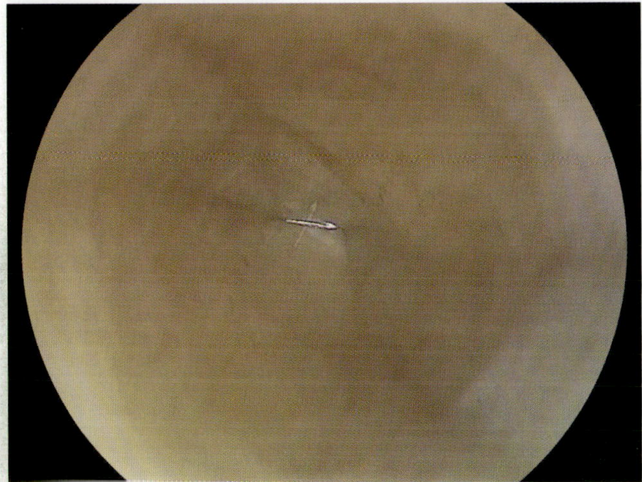

Fig. 8: Peritoneal entry.

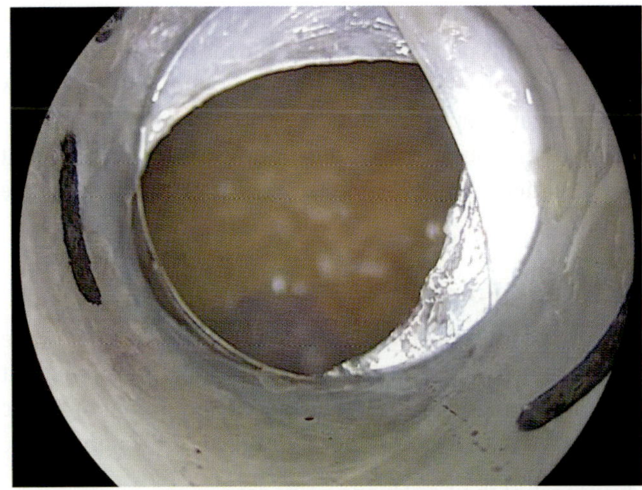

Fig. 9: Confirmation of peritoneal entry after removal of the optical trocar sheath.

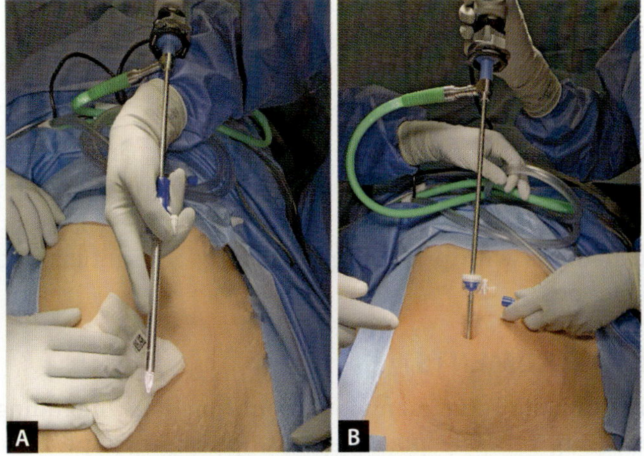

Figs. 10A and B: (A) Setup for direct trocar entry; (B) At the point of umbilicus.

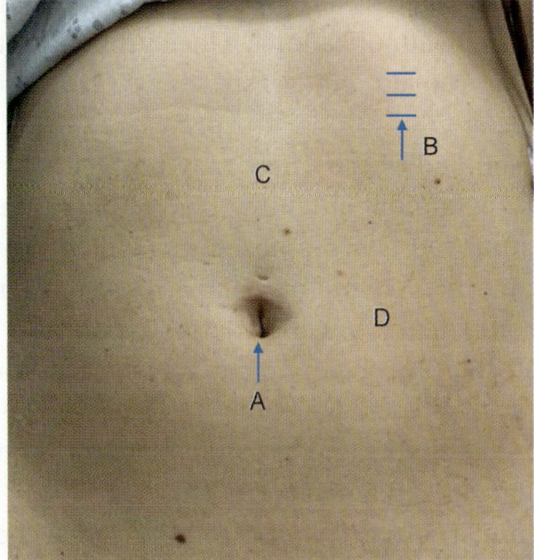

Fig. 11: Anatomical considerations for left upper quadrant entry: A. Umbilical entry; B. Palmers point; C. Lee Huang point; D. Jain point.

Palmers Point

A more usual alternative to umbilical entry in patients with previous abdominal or pelvic surgeries is the *Palmer's point.* The point is in the left midclavicular line 3–4 cm below the costal margin.

The anatomic structures that lie in close proximity to this point are the stomach, left lobe of liver and spleen. Ryles tube has to be put before the procedure for decompression of the stomach. At this point 3 clicks are heard as the needle pierces through the internal oblique, external oblique, transversus abdominis aponeuroses, and the peritoneum.

Some surgeons do prefer the routine use of palmers point even in patients without any surgical history as the first site of entry.[10]

Lee Huang Point

It is at the middle upper abdomen. It is located 10 cm below the Xiphoid or halfway between the Xiphoid and the umbilicus. It is useful in patients with past history of abdominal or pelvic surgeries with high chance of subumbilical adhesions.

Advantages of the Lee Huang point are:

- Avoid adhesions due to previous lower midline incisions and overcrowding in case of large uterus
- Higher view than common umbilical entry
- Central vision when compared to palmers point.[11,12]

Jain Point

It is located at the level of the umbilicus in the left paraumbilical area, in a straight line traced vertically upward from a location 2.5 cm medial to the anterior superior iliac spine. It is useful in patients with prior surgical history and anticipated adhesions.[12]

INSTRUMENTS

Instruments serve many important functions, including ensuring the safe placement of optical and operative equipment, administering distending gas, maintaining the operating envelope, and maintaining port competence.

These instruments consist of a removable central trocar and an outer sheath or cannula. Once inside the cavity, the trocar is removed and other instruments or telescopes can be inserted.

The distal end of the trocar may have either a conical or beveled, pyramidal or cutting blade tip. Routinely used devices employed sharp pointed tips which require less penetration force. When analyzing access, accident cause, and port competency, trocar tip design is critical.

Pointed sharp tips with no cutting edges are present in conical trocars, so more penetration force is required. Tissue layers are radially split rather than transected to accommodate the cannula's outer diameter **(Fig. 12)**.[13]

The cannula portion has valve at the proximal end to allow insertion and removal of instrument without losing insufflated gas. The trocar's outer surface is smooth, with an oblique slope or a horizontal end.

Second generation instruments are made of only a cannula without a trocar and access is visually monitored in real time. A single diagonal thread runs along the shaft's external surface, ending in a blunt notched tip **(Figs. 12 and 13)**.

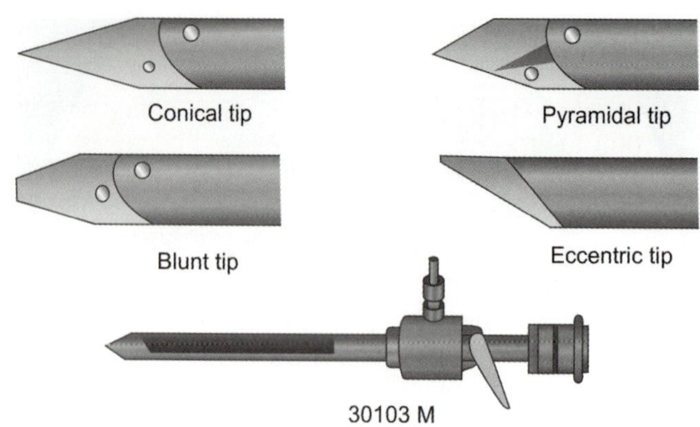

Fig. 12: Types of trocar tips for laparoscopy port placement.

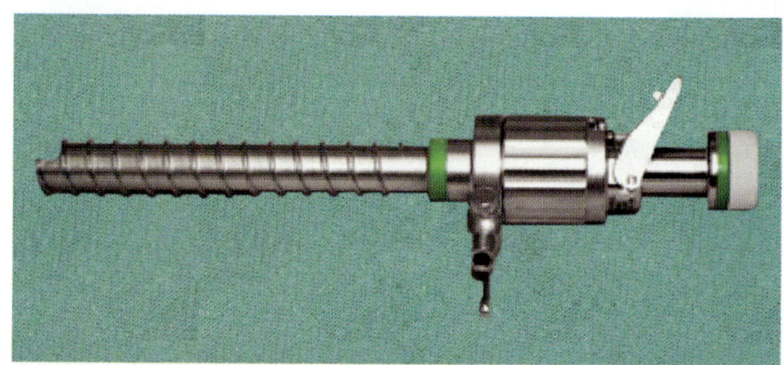

Fig. 13: Endotip.

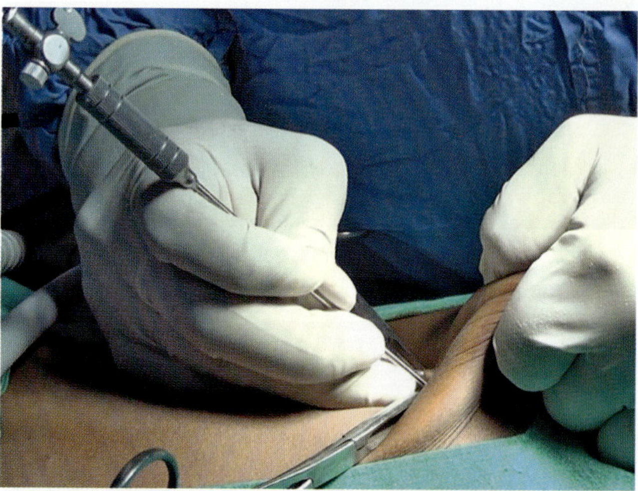

Fig. 14: Insertion of Veress needle.

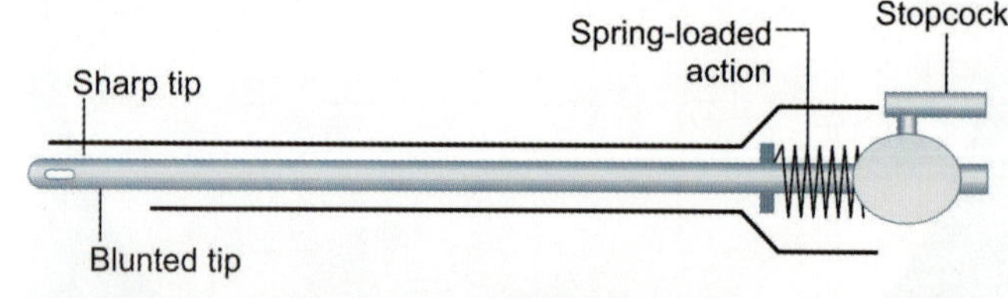

Fig. 15: Parts of Veress needle.

Veress Needle (Figs. 14 and 15)

- Initially, it was invented for penumothorax now it is used for creating pneumoperitoneum.
- The Veress needle is placed after making a small skin incision on inferior crease of the umbilicus to insufflate the abdominal cavity.

- It has two parts—an outer sharp cutting edge and an inner blunted.
- Veress needles should be examined for patency and spring action before use. By drawing the head out, you may inspect the spring action of the Veress needle.
- Insertion should be at an angle of 45° to the body of the patient, with the needle pointed toward pelvis.
- The aortic bifurcation moves more caudal as the BMI increases, the angle should increase with increasing BMI, from 60° in thin patients to 90° in people who are obese or morbidly obese.

EFFECT OF OBESITY ON LOCATION OF GREAT VESSELS (FIG. 16)

In the Trendelenburg (33%) posture, the aortal bifurcation is more caudal than in the dorsal (11%) position. The sacral promontory and vessels will be prominent in the Trendelenburg posture **(Figs. 17 and 18)**.

As a result, the patient should be placed in dorsal position and not in the Trendelenburg posture.

LAPAROSCOPY IN PREGNANCY

- Laparoscopy can be done in the first and second trimesters of pregnancy
- Depending on volume and size of the uterus, the siteof entry of first trocar is decided
- Open technique is advised after 14 weeks of pregnancy using the transumbilical or supraumbilical route
- Maximum insufflation pressure of 12 mm Hg should be maintained.

COMPLICATIONS RELATED TO ENTRY TECHNIQUE

Vascular Injury (Fig. 19)

Bladder or bowel perforation, vascular injury, surgical site infection and port site hernia are all complications involved with laparoscopic entry, regardless of the technique adopted. Veress needle insertion, primary port placement, or accessory port placement can all cause vascular injury.[14]

Most common vessels injured are the subcutaneous arteries of the anterior abdominal wall.

The inferior epigastric arteries, on the other hand, are the most common vessels that cause considerable bleeding when injured. Secondary trocar placement in the lower abdomen should be done under direct vision to prevent injury to the inferior epigastric artery.[15]

0.1–6.4 injuries per 1,000 cases of venous or arterial injuries during laparoscopic entry have been reported. Vascular injuries can be catastrophic, with 15% of them being fatal.[15,16]

Immediate identification of retroperitoneal major vascular injury is essential to prevent exsanguination and death of

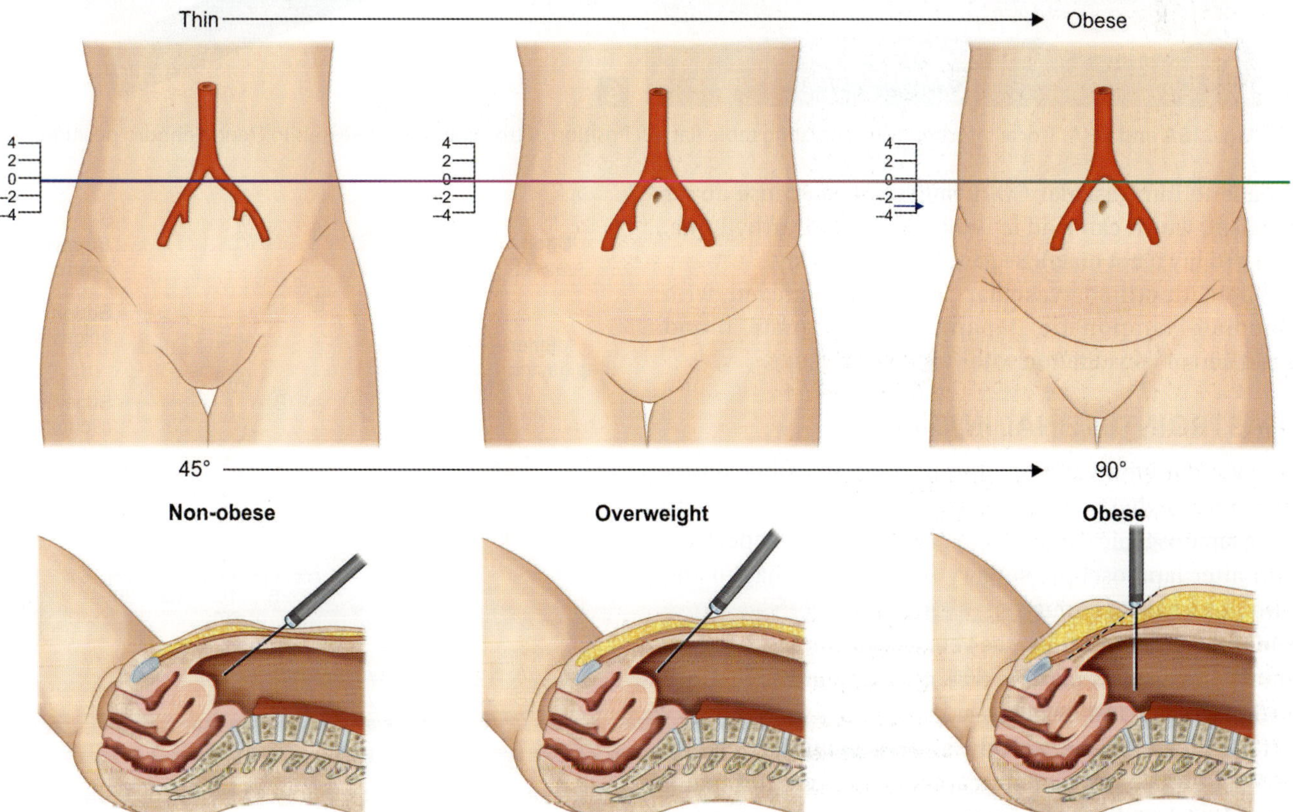

Fig. 16: Effect of body type and obesity on distance between abdominal wall and great vessels.

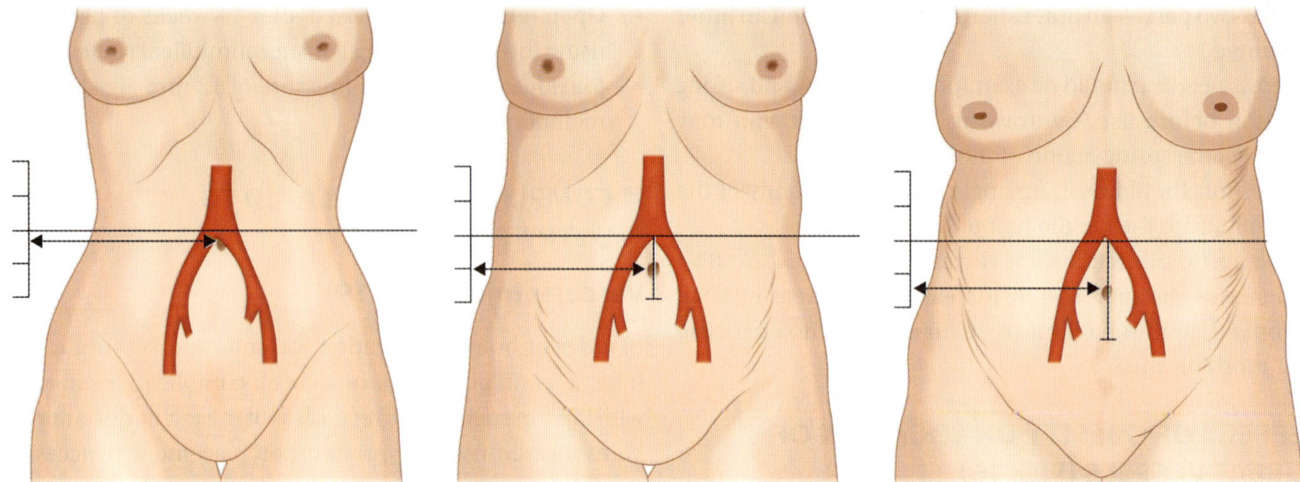

Fig. 17: Relationship of aortic bifurcation to umbilicus. In women of normal weight for height the bifurcation is, on average, 0.4 cm cephalad to and 6 cm (±3) beneath the umbilicus. For overweight women, the distances are 2.4 and 14 cm (±2), respectively. In obese women, the umbilicus is 2.9 cm inferior to the bifurcation and 13 cm (±4) anterior to the level of the aorta.

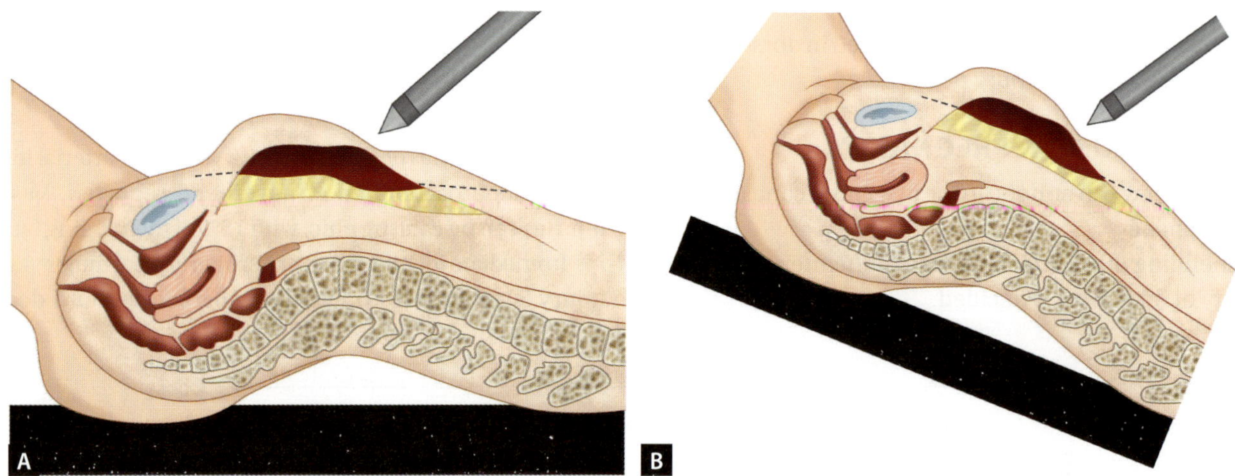

Figs. 18A and B: (A) Trocar insertion with operating table flat; (B) Position of trocar and great vessels in Trendelenburg position.

the patient. Intravascular CO_2 insufflation can cause an air embolism, which can lead to ischemia, cardiac arrhythmia, and mortality if not diagnosed and treated quickly.

When identified, vascular injury is managed with immediate tamponade, laparotomy, adequate blood transfusion or consultation with vascular surgeons.

GASTROINTESTINAL INJURY

After vascular injury and anesthesia, gastrointestinal injury is the third highest cause of serious injury and mortality during laparoscopic surgery. A major cause of postoperative death after laparoscopic surgery is a delay in diagnosing gastrointestinal tract injury.

Injuries were induced by the Veress needle in 33% of cases, primary trocar placement in 50% of cases, and secondary trocar placement in 17% of cases.[14]

If identified intraoperatively, a very small injury can be managed expectantly but bowel repair, on the other hand, can be done by either a two-layer primary repair or a bowel resection after consultation with a gastrointestinal surgeon.

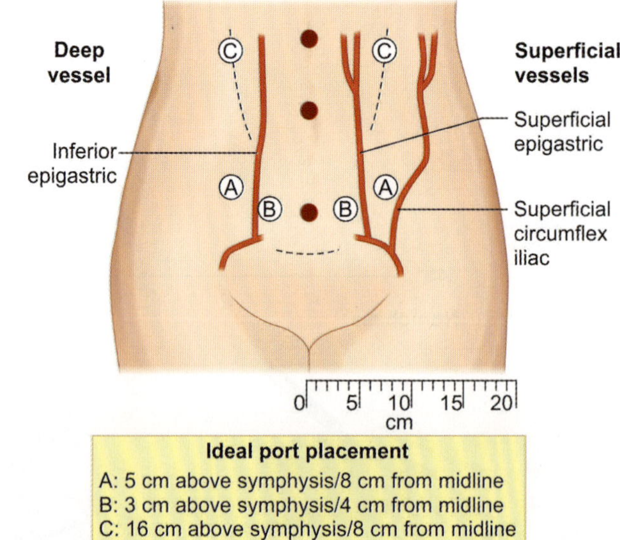

Fig. 19: Placement of secondary ports.
Source: Hurd WW, Bude RO, DeLancey JO, Newman JS. The location of abdominal wall blood vessels in relationship to abdominal landmarks apparent at laparoscopy. Am J Obstet Gynecol. 1994;171(3):642-6.

TABLE 2: Summary of Cochrane review of laparoscopic entry technique complications.[14]

Outcome	Open vs. closed (any)	Open vs. direct vision	Open vs. Veress	Closed: Direct vs. Veress	Closed: Direct vision vs. Veress
Vascular injury	Insufficient evidence	*	*	Insufficient evidence	Insufficient evidence
Visceral injury	Insufficient evidence	Insufficient evidence	*	Insufficient evidence	Insufficient evidence
Omental injury	Open favored	*	Open favored	Direct favored	*
Trocar site infection	Insufficient evidence	*	Insufficient evidence	Insufficient evidence	*
Trocar site bleeding	Insufficient evidence	Insufficient evidence	Insufficient evidence	*	Insufficient evidence
Failed entry	Insufficient evidence	Insufficient evidence	Insufficient evidence	Direct favored	*
Incisional hernia	Insufficient evidence	*	Insufficient evidence	*	*
Extraperitoneal insufflation	Open favored	*	Insufficient evidence	Direct favored	*

*Indicates no data

Warning signs of bowel injury such as difficultly in maintaining pneumoperitoneum and bubbling in irrigation fluid can be present, but could be missed if the injury is very small.

Gastrointestinal injury must be diagnosed in patients who present with high grade fever, abdominal pain, breathlessness, palpitations, nausea/vomiting, poor food intake or ileus in the postoperative period.

The summary of Cochrane review of laparoscopic entry technique complications is given in **Table 2**.

CONCLUSION

The most difficult part of any laparoscopic procedure is laparoscopic peritoneal entry. Though major complications are rare, minor complications can occur even in the best of hands but it is important that these are identified immediately and addressed. In terms of preventing serious complications, no single entry method or location has been proven to be superior to the others.

REFERENCES

1. Johnathon M, Recknagel D. Clinical Perspective Concerning Abdominal Entry Techniques. J Minim Invasive Gynecol. 2021;28(3):467-74.
2. Teoh B, Sen R, Abbott J. An evaluation of four tests used to ascertain Veress needle placement at closed laparoscopy. J Minim Invasive Gynecol. 2005;12:153-8.
3. Lacey C. Laparoscopy: a clinical sign for intraperitoneal needle placement. Obstet Gynecol. 1976;47:625-7.
4. Jacobson MT, Osias J, Bizhang R, Tsang M, Lata S, Helmy M, et al. The Direct Trocar Technique: An Alternative Approach to Abdominal Entry for Laparoscopy. JSLS. 2002;6(2):169-74.
5. Merdan I. Laparoscopic entry: a review of techniques, technologies, and complications. Basrah Journal of Surgery. 2013:19.
6. Radhakrishna V, George R. Modified Hasson technique: a quick and safe entry of first port into the abdomen. Int Surg J. 2019;6(8):2.
7. Thepsuwana J, Huangb K, Wilamartac M, Syafinaz A, Vahan A, Chyi-Long ML. Principles of safe abdominal entry in laparoscopic gynecologic surgery. Gynecol Minim Invas Ther. 2013;2(4):105-9.
8. Lam TY, Lee SW, So HS, Kwok SP. Radially expanding trocars: a less painful alternative for laparoscopic surgery. J Laparoendosc Adv Surg Tech. 2000;10(5):269-73.
9. Pepin K. Abdominal entry in laparoscopic surgery. Contempor Obstet Gyncol J. 2020;65(11):2
10. Valentine LN, Uy-Kroh MJ. Left upper quadrant entry technique. J Minim Invasive Gyneco. 2015;22(6):S133-4.
11. Lee CL, Huang KG, Jain S, Wang CJ, Yen CF, Soong YK. A new portal for gynecologic laparoscopy. J Am Assoc Gynecol Laparosc. 2001;147-50.
12. Jain N, Jain V, Agarwal C, Bansal P, Gupta S, Bansal B. Left Lateral Port: Safe Laparoscopic Port Entry in Previous Large Upper Abdomen Laparotomy Scar. J Minim Invasive Gynecol. 2019;26(5):973-76.
13. Jain N. State of Art Atlas of Endoscopic Surgery in Infertility and Gynecology. New Delhi: Jaypee Brothers Medical Publishers; 2018.
14. Fuller J, Ashar BS, Carey-Corrado J. Trocar-associated injuries and fatalities: an analysis of 1399 reports to the FDA. J Minim Invasive Gynecol. 2005;12(4):302-7.
15. Krishnakumar S, Tambe P. Entry Complications in Laparoscopic Surgery. J Gynecol Endosc Surg. 2009;1(1):4-11.
16. Up To Date. (2020). Complications of Laparoscopic Surgery. [online] Available from: https://www.uptodate.com/contents/complications-of-laparoscopic-surgery. [Last accessed November, 2021].

LONG QUESTIONS

1. Describe the construction of a Veress needle and the inbuilt safety features.
2. Discuss the tests for correct peritoneal entry with Veress needle at laparoscopy.
3. Discuss the Visual Access System for laparoscopic trocar entry.
4. Discuss vascular injury at laparoscopy entry with risk factors, preventive measures, recognition, and immediate management steps.

SHORT QUESTIONS

1. Name the commonly used entry techniques in laparoscopy.
2. What are the pros and cons of open entry technique in laparoscopy?
3. Name the sites on the abdominal wall that have been described for laparoscopy entry.
4. What are the difficulties with laparoscopy entry in obese women? What strategies should be used to make it safe?

MULTIPLE CHOICE QUESTIONS

1. What proportion of major complications in laparoscopic surgery is related to entry techniques?
   a. 10% b. 25%
   c. 50% d. 90%
2. The length of a standard Veress needle for laparoscopy entry is:
   a. 5 cm b. 12 cm
   c. 15 cm d. 20 cm
3. The Palmer's point is described as:
   a. 3–4 cm above the umbilicus in the midline
   b. 3–4 cm above the umbilicus in the right midclavicular line
   c. 3–4 cm above the McBurney's point
   d. 3–4 cm below the costal margin in the left midclavicular line
4. Nasogastric tube decompression is advisable for:
   a. Palmer's point entry by Veress method
   b. Umbilical entry by Veress method
   c. Supraumbilical entry by open technique
   d. Umbilical entry by visual access method
5. The following statement is correct regarding the construction of a Veress needle:
   a. The inner tip is sharp
   b. The outer sheath is sharp
   c. The spring has a stopcock mechanism
   d. The stopcock gives a feedback about the passage through tissue
6. The following statement is true for entry with Veress needle in Trendelenburg position:
   a. The bowel moves upwards
   b. The stomach is likely to be full
   c. The aortic bifurcation is far away from the skin surface
   d. The aortic bifurcation is more likely to be injured

Answers

1. c 2. b 3. d 4. a 5. b 6. d

11.2 HYSTEROSCOPY: INSTRUMENTATION AND DISTENSION MEDIA

Subash Mallya

INTRODUCTION

Hysteroscopy is a procedure that allows direct visualization of the uterine cavity and cervical canal. It can be used for diagnostic and therapeutic purposes and the advantage is that it is minimally invasive without incision. For performing hysteroscopy we need telescope and sheath, distension media and fluid delivery system.

INSTRUMENTS FOR HYSTEROSCOPY

Telescope: It is of two types—rigid and flexible. Rigid telescopes are the most commonly used. It is available in different diameters (2 mm, 2.9 mm, 4 mm). Telescope can be with either centered lens (0)or offset lens (12, 30, 70) with angle of view opposite the light source. Most commonly used is the 30 scope. In flexible type the tip of the hysteroscope can bend up to 110° and is usually used for diagnostic procedures for diagnostic purposes. For routine diagnostic procedures the 30° forward oblique scopes are preferred. For operative procedures involving resectoscopes where the loop is seen in the center, the 12° scope is preferred.

Telescope sheath: Telescopic sheath is different for diagnostic and operative hysteroscopy. The telescope must be fitted to a sheath through which a distending medium can be infused to provide necessary distention for panoramic viewing. Typical sheath measures 5 mm in diameter to accommodate the 4 mm telescope. A diagnostic hysteroscope consists of inflow channel only while in operative hysteroscopy inflow as well as outflow channel and channel for working element is also present. Sheath used for diagnostic purposes are smaller (5 mm) **(Fig. 1)** and for operative sheath it is about 7–10 mm **(Figs. 2 and 3)**.

The field of hysteroscopy has been revolutionized making it possible to perform a comprehensive endoscopic examination of the uterine cavity in an outpatient session, without anesthetic or dilatation of the cervical canal. The office hysteroscopy is done with a 2.9 mm scope which is fitted with fiber optic light connector and connections for irrigation. The HAMOU II 4-mm micro-hysteroscope with its examination sheath of 5 mm diameter provides a panoramic view of the entire uterine cavity. The TROPHY scope® CAMPO compact hysteroscope has a thin outer diameter of 2.9 mm and can be loaded either with a diagnostic sheath or a 4.4-mm operating sheath. The trophy scope may be used without sheath for diagnostic hysteroscopy in single-flow mode.

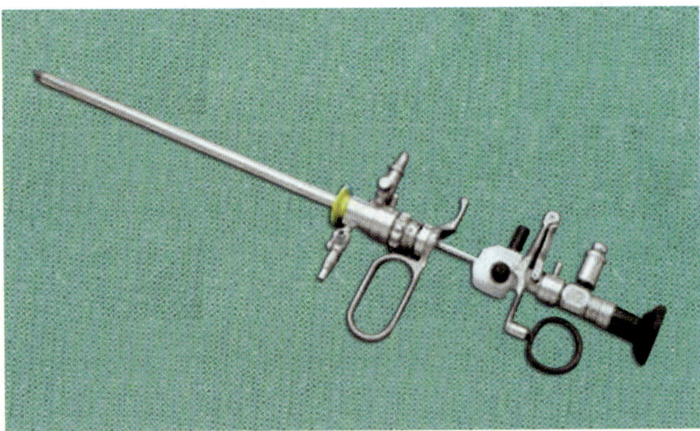

Fig. 1: Hysteroscope with sheath for diagnostic hysteroscopy.

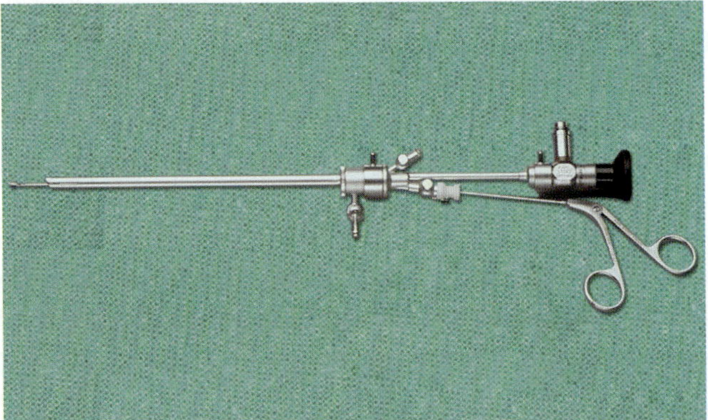

Fig. 2: Operative hysteroscopy sheath for non-electricity based procedures.

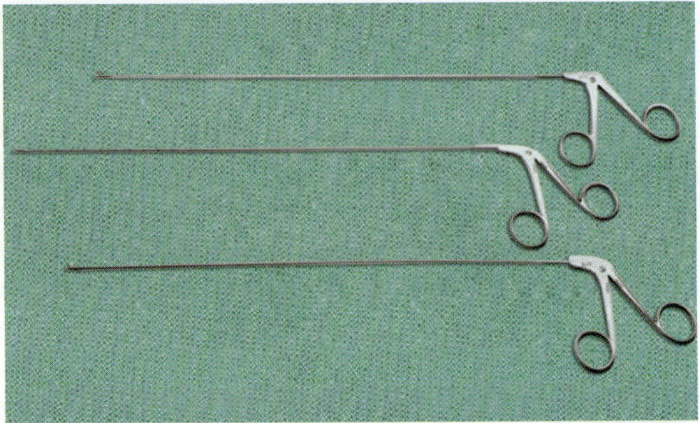

Fig. 3: Hand instruments for non-electricity based operative hysteroscopy.

Resectoscope: It is used for operative hysteroscopy. It has an inflow, outflow and channel for different electrodes which are connected to monopolar cautery. Electrodes **(Fig. 4)** include Collins knife, ball and loop electrode. There are essentially two types of resectoscopes, which differ in outer diameter: 7.3 mm (22 Fr) and 8.7 mm (26 Fr) and the type of current used (unipolar or bipolar). The resectoscope consists of a classic endoscope, with diameters ranging between 2.9 and 4 mm, preferably with a 12° viewing angle to keep the electrode within the field of view, combined with a cutting loop operated by a passive spring mechanism, and two sheaths for continuous irrigation and suction of the distension medium.

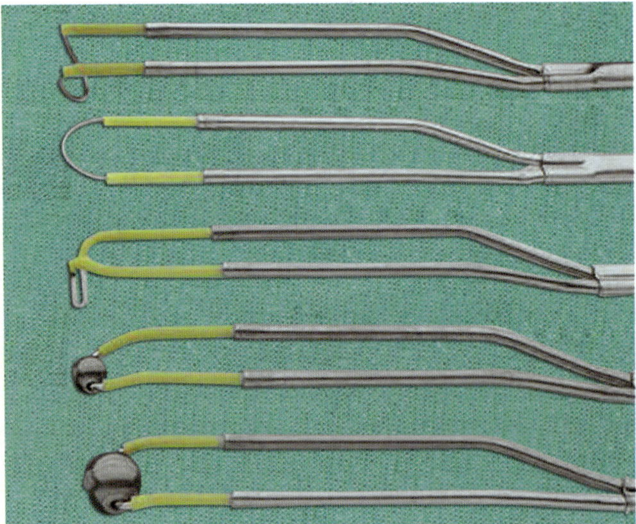

Fig. 4: Electrodes for resectoscope with hysteroscopy.

Light source: Good image quality depends on the type of light source used. A 175 watt high quality xenon light source is the preferred one and yields good results. Usually a 175 watt cold light source is sufficient, but a miniature telescopes may require up to 300 watt light source. Light is usually transmitted through fiberoptic or fluid light cables with a diameter of 2.5–4.5 mm and a length of 180–300 cm. Light cables for standard hysteroscopy are 2.5–3.5 mm in diameter and 180 cm in length are used. Light source operating at higher power levels produces more thermal energy, which causes a greater rise in temperature. Hence, due caution has to be exercised during the procedure to avoid any inadvertent thermal injury, one should keep the intensity of the light as less as possible.

Camera and Monitor

- Earlier tube cameras were used for diagnostic hysteroscopy. These were superseded by single charged coupled device (ccd) chip cameras which have now have been superseded by three-chip cameras. Modern high definition cameras offer a very high resolution and almost natural color reproduction. The camera is connected to a control unit and then to a high-resolution color monitor or medical grade monitors.
- Various types of video cameras are available. The quality of different video cameras depends on the following technical parameters: resolution (defined by number of lines or pixels), and sensitivity, high s/n ratio (signal to noise ratio)—means the change in video signal occurring in a situation like bleeding causes very minimal loss of light intensity, as well as the quality of the video images. The systems usually include facilities for storing and printing still images and video data which can be used to give a recorded data to the patients.

Sterilization of Instruments

- Thorough cleaning is an important primary step
- Essential to follow rigid protocols for instrument cleaning and sterilization

- Only well-established methods of sterilization/high level disinfection should be used
- Some current practices should be abolished like formalin chambers
- Current standard for sterilization of endoscopes is gas sterilization with ethylene oxide. Some newer telescopes may be steam autoclaved on an emergency basis without damaging the lenses.

DISTENSION MEDIA (TABLE 1)

The uterine cavity is a potential space with anterior and posterior walls in close apposition. So a minimum pressure of 40 mm Hg is needed to separate the uterine walls and visualize the uterine cavity with a hysteroscope. The distension media used is mainly of two types—gaseous and liquid media.

Gaseous Media

Carbon dioxide is a colorless gas and is the only gaseous distension media used in hysteroscopy. The CO_2 is delivered into the uterus with a hysteroscopic insufflator at a flow rate measured in milliliter per minute. The ideal flow rate is about 40–50 mL/min and it should never exceed 100 mL/min and pressure should be below 150 mm Hg. A laparoscopic insufflators should not be used as the flow rate is in liters per minute. The advantages of CO_2 as distension media is that it is inexpensive, yields a clear image of endometrial cavity, entry evaluation of endocervical canal, easy to infuse, does not foul instruments, and does not mess up the operating room. So it is ideal for diagnostic purposes. But when CO_2 flow is excess it produce bubbling which is cumbersome and may obscure the view. It also tends to flatten the endometrium and this artifact will obscure the pathology. Other severe complications include CO_2 embolism and metabolic acidosis.

Liquid Media

Fluid media can be either of high or low viscosity. The high viscosity fluid used is 32% dextran. Low viscosity fluids can be isotonic or hypotonic. Low viscosity isotonic media include 0.9% normal saline, Ringers lactate and 5% mannitol and low viscosity hypotonic fluids include 1.5% glycine, 3% sorbitol, and 5% dextrose. For operative procedures fluid media is preferred over CO_2 gas as there will be symmetric distension of uterus with fluid and is effective in flushing blood, mucus, bubbles and small tissue fragments out of the visual field.

The high viscosity fluid includes Dextran 32% which enables good visualization of the cavity in the presence of blood as it is immiscible with blood. However, it causes anaphylactic reaction, coagulopathies and crystallization within the telescope if not properly cleaned after the procedure. Dextran also causes disproportionate intravascular expansion and cardiac failure. It is rarely used nowadays for diagnostic and operative hysteroscopy.

The low viscosity fluids used can be isotonic or hypotonic. The choice of fluid used depends on the energy used for the procedure. Isotonic fluids which contain electrolytes such asnormal saline and ringer lactate are used with bipolar energy and with mechanical procedures like morcellation of submucous fibroids. Hypotonic fluids, which are electrolyte free like glycine, areused when monopolar energy is used. Normal saline is not recommended with monopolar energy as it disperses electric current without having any surgical effect on the tissue.

Distension media is delivered using simple gravity by instilling fluid under constant hydrostatic pressure by hanging a 3L bottle of fluid 1–1.5 meter above the operating table or by using blood pressure cuff around the fluid bag or by electronic suction irrigation pump **(Fig. 5)**.

The complications of distension media depend on the type of medium used and complexity of surgery performed. The main complication is due to excessive vascular absorption of these fluids which lead to hypervolemia and electrolyte imbalance like hyponatremia which can be severe and even life threatening. Absorption of the distension media into the

TABLE 1: Different types of distension media and their use in hysteroscopy.

Liquid distension media	*Osmolality*	*Electrolyte free*	*Procedure*	*Energy*
Normal saline 285 mOsm/L	Isotonic	No	Diagnostic and operative	Mechanical, bipolar, laser
Ringer lactate 279 mOsm/L	Isotonic	No	Diagnostic and operative	Mechanical, bipolar, laser
5% Mannitol 274 mOsml/L	Isotonic	Yes	Operative	Monopolar
1.5% Glycine 200 mOsm/L	Hypotonic	Yes	Operative	Monopolar
3% Sorbitol 165 mOsm/L	Hypotonic	Yes	Operative	Monopolar
5% Dextrose	Hypotonic	Yes	Operative	Monopolar
Dextran 32%	Hypertonic	Yes	Operative	Monopolar

Note: Normal osmolality of plasma is about 285 mOsm/L

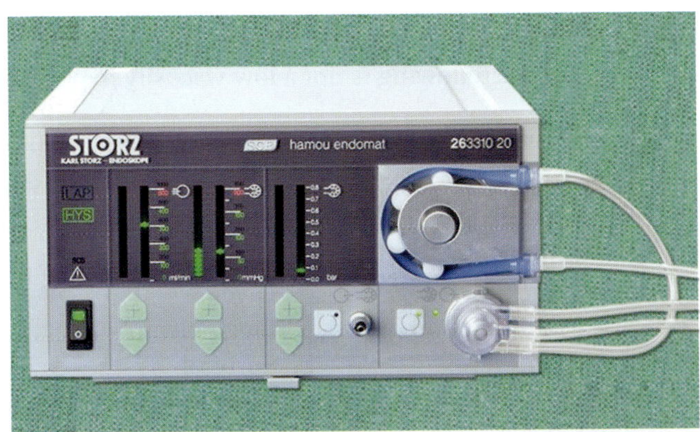

Fig. 5: Electronic suction irrigation pump for distension at hysteroscopy - Endomat.

systemic circulation occurs by retrograde passage of fluid through the fallopian tube, through the endometrium, and via opened blood vessels and sinus. The factors which influence the absorption of fluid media are:

- Intrauterine pressure
- Mean arterial pressure
- Depth of myometrial penetration
- Duration of surgery
- Size of uterine cavity.

While using liquid distension media, volume of fluid instilled, volume of return fluid and fluid deficit must be calculated. Fluid deficit is calculated by the amount of fluid infused into the uterine cavity minus fluid returned from the outflow channel and fluid leaking through cervix. Significant fluid deficit of about 1.5 liter with saline and 500 mL with glycine should warn the surgeon to discontinue the procedure.

Fluid overload is defined as fluid deficit of more than 1,000 mL when using hypotonic solutions and 2,500 mL when using isotonic solutions in healthy women of reproductive age group. In the elderly and women with cardiovascular, renal or other comorbidities the upper limits are 750 mL for hypotonic and 1,500 mL for isotonic solutions. Even with these cut-off values depending upon the clinical condition of the patient these upper limits may be reduced.

Fluid Overload with Hypotonic Fluid Media

1.5% glycine and 3% sorbitol are the most commonly used hypotonic distension media. Vascular absorption causes hypervolemia and dilutional hyponatremia with moderate fluid overload. When more than 1,000 mL of hypotonic fluid was absorbed during surgery, the serum sodium concentration fell by 10 mmol/L. Symptoms usually develop when serum sodium concentration drops below 125 mmol/L. The most frequent symptoms are headache, nausea, vomiting, and weakness. Further fluid intravasation causes reduction of blood osmolality creates an osmotic gradient between circulating blood and brain cellsthat moves water into the interstitial and intracellular spaceleading to brain edema and raised intracranial pressure. The cerebral edema presents as agitation, confusion, weakness nausea, vomiting, visual disturbances, blindness and headache. A further fall in sodium level below 120 mmol/literlead to confusion, lethargy, seizures, coma, arrhythmias, bradycardia and respiratory arrest. As glycine is metabolized to ammonia, it also causes hyperammonemia and neurological damage. So, early detection and treatment is the key to prevent cardiovascular and neurological complications. Sorbitol in addition to these may cause hyperglycemia and hypocalcemia.

Fluid Overload with Isotonic Fluid Media

Normal saline is the most common isotonic fluid media used in bipolar electrosurgery and diagnostic procedures. Isotonic fluid media reduces the risk of hypo-osmolality and hyponatremia but excessive vascular absorption causes hypervolemia leading to congestive cardiac failure and pulmonary edema.

MANAGEMENT

Early detection and rapid initiation of treatment is undertaken. Fluid intake should be restricted. Urinary catheter must be inserted and urine output is measured. Urea, creatinine and electrolytes is checked. A loop diuretic like furosemide is given intravenously. Patient should be closely monitored for signs and symptoms of pulmonary edema.If serum sodium falls below 120 mmol/L, consider hypertonic 3% saline and multidisciplinary team involvement and care in a high dependency unit.

PREVENTION

Gonadotropin-releasing hormone (GnRH) pretreatment, intracervical vasopressin injection, least minimum intrauterine pressure which should be kept below mean arterial pressure. Fluid deficit should be monitored by a dedicated theater staff assigned for it and it should be accurately checkedat least every 10 minutes and at the end of usage of each fluid bag. Trendelenburg position should be avoided and surgery time to be minimized.

KEY MESSAGES

For performing hysteroscopy we need telescope and sheath, light source, camera and monitor, distension media and fluid delivery system. Distension media is of 2 types-gaseous and liquid. Liquid distension media can be high or low viscosity. Most commonly used low viscosity isotonic fluid is 0.9% normal saline and hypotonic fluids is 1.5% glycine. Isotonic fluids are used with bipolar energy and hypotonic fluids like glycine are used with monopolar current. Fluid overload is defined as fluid deficit of >1000 mL with hypotonic solutions and >2500 mL with isotonic solutions. Fluid overload with normal saline causes hypervolemia and with glycine causes hypervolemia and dilutional hyponatremia. For prevention of complications fluid deficit should be monitored accurately.

FURTHER READING

1. AAGL practice guidelines for the management of hysteroscopic distending media - hologic education [Internet]. [cited 2021 Jan 9]. Available from: https://hologiced.com/library/aagl-practice-guidelines-for-the-management-of-hysteroscopic-distending-media/
2. Craciunas L, Sajid MS, Howell R. Carbon dioxide versus normal saline as distension medium for diagnostic hysteroscopy: a systematic review and meta-analysis of randomized controlled trials. Fertility and Sterility. 2013;100(6):1709-14.e4.
3. Garry R, Hasham F, Kokri MS, Mooney P. The effect of pressure on fluid absorption during endometrial ablation. J Gynecol Surg. 1992;8(1):1-10.
4. Imasogie N, Crago R, Leyland NA, Chung F. Probable gas embolism during operative hysteroscopy caused by products of combustion. Can J Anesth. 2002;49(10):1044-7.
5. Istre O, Bjoennes J, Naess R, Hornbaek K. Postoperative cerebral oedema after transcervical endometrial resection and uterine irrigation with 1·5% glycine. The Lancet. 1994;344(8931):1187-9.
6. Umranikar S, Clark TJ, Saridogan E, Miligkos D, Arambage K, Torbe E, et al. BSGE/ESGE guideline on management of fluid distension media in operative hysteroscopy. Gynecol Surg. 2016;13(4):289-303.
7. Witz CA, Silverberg KM, Burns WN, Schenken RS, Olive DL. Complications associated with the absorption of hysteroscopic fluid media. Fertility and Sterility. 1993;60(5):745-56.

LONG QUESTIONS

1. Discuss the pros and cons of various distension media in hysteroscopy.
2. Management of complications due to distension media in hysteroscopy.

SHORT QUESTIONS

1. Name the types of distension media in hysteroscopy.
2. What are the complications of glycine as distension media in hysteroscopy?

MULTIPLE CHOICE QUESTIONS

1. Which of the following is not a low viscosity hypotonic fluid?
   a. 1.5% glycine b. 5% mannitol
   c. 3% sorbitol d. 5% dextrose
2. Which of the following is a high viscosity fluid?
   a. Mannitol b. Sorbitol
   c. Dextran 32% d. Glycine
3. Choice of distension media in bipolar electrosurgery:
   a. Glycine b. Sorbitol
   c. CO_2 d. Normal saline
4. Choice of distension media in monopolar electrosurgery:
   a. Glycine b. Ringerlactate
   C. CO_2 d. Normal saline
5. In healthy women of reproductive age group, fluid overload is defined as fluid deficit of more than .... mL when using hypotonic solutions:
   a. 1000 mL b. 1500 mL
   c. 2000 mL d. 2500 mL
6. Which of the following is not a complication related to glycine toxicity?
   a. Hyperammonemia b. Hypervolemia
   c. Hyponatremia d. Hypokalemia
7. Which of the following distension media has the risk of hyperglycemia on fluid overload?
   a. 1.5% Glycine b. 3% Sorbitol
   c. 5% Mannitol d. Dextran 32%
8. Flow rate of CO_2 when used as distension media:
   a. 50 mL/min b. 1 L/min
   c. 2 L/min d. 3 L/min
9. Intrauterine pressure to be maintained while performing hysteroscopy:
   a. 70–100 mm Hg b. 120–130 mm Hg
   c. 140–150 mm Hg d. 150–160 mm Hg

Answers

1. b 2. c 3. d 4. a 5. a 6. d
7. b 8. a 9. a

11.3 ROBOTIC SURGERY IN GYNAECOLOGY

Seema Singhal, Alka Kriplani

INTRODUCTION

The surgical practice in gynecology has been revolutionized with the technological innovations in last few decades. Minimally invasive surgery (MIS) is now the standard of care for most of the gynecological conditions. Development of robots in 1980s has led minimally invasive surgery to a new dimension.[1] The limitations of laparoscopy including limited range of motion, sense of depth perception, surgeon's fatigue and longer learning curve are well addressed by robot. Initially it was perceived that surgeons well versed with the art of laparoscopy should do robotics, but now surgeons at all levels of surgical learning curve can switch to robotic surgery.[2] Use of robotic platform has increased worldwide with the use of 645 da Vinci system in use to more than 3,500 units in 2014, indirectly reflecting the surgeon's comfort and precision with the use of robotic platform.[3]

Robotic surgery platform was used initially for benign procedures and has been in practice for removal of myomas, hysterectomies, removal of benign adnexal masses. However, with further development it is now being used for a number of malignant procedures too, which include surgery for endometrial cancer, staging for early stage ovarian cancer and also for lymphadenectomy procedures required for staging and removal of bulky nodes in recurrent settings.[4] The robotic surgery is being adopted by surgeons and patients for management of number of conditions as it imparts all the benefits of MIS including less blood loss, reduced pain, faster recovery, and lesser work time loss without compromising the outcome but its cost, availability and expertise are the main limiting factors. The present chapter highlights the use of robotic surgery in the field of gynecology.

AN INTRODUCTION TO ROBOTIC TECHNOLOGY (DA VINCI ROBOT)[5,6]

The modern da Vinci robotic system consists of a 3-dimensional high definition camera, robotic platform, wristed instruments, and surgeon console. There are four robotic arms in the robotic platform that hold the camera and instruments. The surgeon practically sits at the console away from the actual theater and manipulates the finger graspers for controlling the endowrist instruments. In addition, there are foot pedals and clutch for controlling the camera and activation of energy sources **(Figs. 1A to F)**.

For surgery, initially pneumoperitoneum is created and then the robot platform is docked by one of the members of surgical team. Trocars are then inserted, usually 4–5 ports are made. One 12 mm camera port and the other additional ports are used for passing other instruments. One arm is not controlled by robot and is kept for assistant. Assistant uses this port for tissue manipulation, inserting needle holders and for suction and irrigation during the surgery.

Presently there are three models available for robotic surgery; the Si–e (2 arms), the Si, and the newest version, the Xi system. The newer versions of robot are incorporated with advanced technology and provide a computerized docking assistant, new patient-side cart orientation and a provision for using camera from any of the ports for enabling difficult dissections with ease. Additional benefit is provision of assistant console to facilitate training.[6]

ROBOTIC-ASSISTED SURGERY VERSUS LAPAROSCOPY

Apart from the conventional benefits of MIS over open surgery which include the quick postoperative recovery, early discharge from hospital and cosmetic benefits, robotic platform has several advantages. The limitations of laparoscopy are well addressed by robot. The camera control which is in assistant hands during laparoscopy is well addressed by robot and provision of fixed camera reduces dependence on assistant and provides a stable field of vision without unexpected movements. The freedom of seven degrees of wrist movements make surgical experience imitate open surgery and contribute to shorter learning curves even for novice. The provision of ergonomic consoles facilitates performance of longer procedures without fatigue and dual consoles facilitate hands on training under direct guidance. However, robotic experience is limited by lack of haptic feedback and this may lead to initial learning difficulty for senior surgeons, however with technological development of 3-dimensional spatial view and visual cues this problem is also reduced.[4-6]

ROBOTIC SURGERIES IN GYNAECOLOGY: AN OVERVIEW

The da Vinci robotic surgical system was approved by US Food and Drug Administration (FDA) in the year 2005 for application in gynecological procedures.

Robotic-assisted Surgeries for Benign Gynaecological Procedures

The uptake of robotic platform for performance of benign gynecological condition has substantially increased worldwide from 0.5% in 2007 to 9.5% in 2010 and is further increasing.[7] Hysterectomy is the most commonly performed gynecological surgical procedure done by MIS and several studies have confirmed the feasibility of robotic approach for conducting hysterectomy.[7-10] **Table 1** lists the comparison of laparoscopic and radical hysterectomy in terms of outcome, complications and cost. Although, robotic surgical procedures take longer OT time because of equipment set up and docking but for cases with obesity, dense and extensive adhesions, e.g., advanced endometriosis, robotic platform is better with reduced operating time, lower surgeon fatigue, better surgical experience and lower conversion rates than conventional laparoscopy. The only pitfall with robotic surgery has been relatively higher risk (3%) of vault dehiscence in robotic hysterectomy cases than with laparoscopic hysterectomy or open surgery. This is probably because of increased use of monopolar diathermy for colpotomy and resultant loss of vascularity in the tissues. However, with increasing use of barbed sutures for vault closure, closure of vault through vagina and conscious efforts to take adequate bites of healthy tissues these rates may be reduced.[11,12]

Myomectomy is another one of the most commonly done benign surgical procedures through MIS because of numerous benefits including lesser probability of adhesion formation than open approach. Several studies have compared the outcome of myomectomy with robotic, laparoscopic, and open approach and found similar results except difference in the OT time. Gobern et al.[13] in their retrospective analysis observed that surgical time was more with robotic myomectomy than laparoscopic or open approach (140 min vs. 70 min vs. 72 min respectively; $p < 0.005$). Similar findings are confirmed by

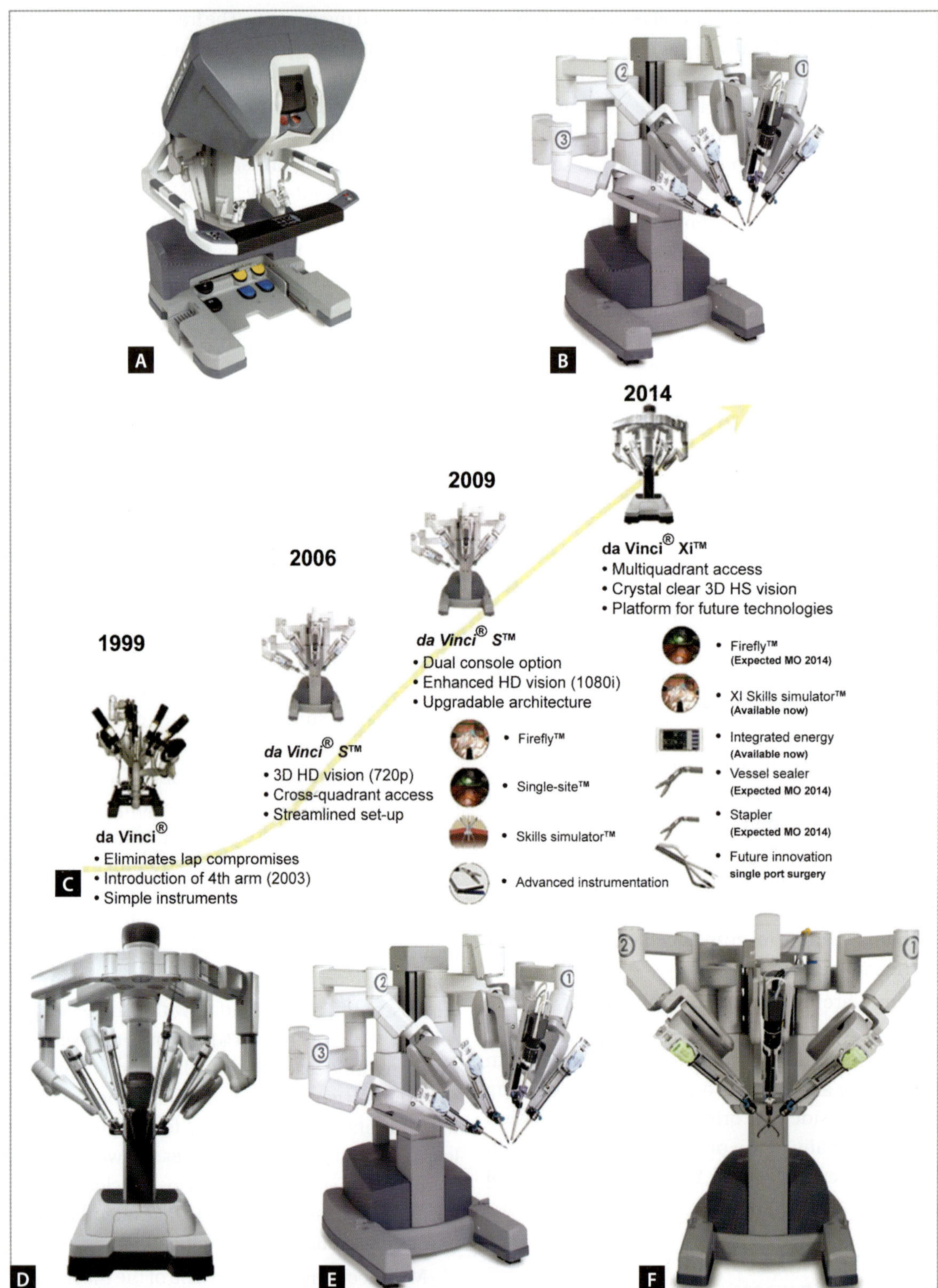

Figs. 1A to F: Components of surgical robot.

other authors too.[14] Hence, overall the robotic surgery does not offer confer additional benefits for myomectomy, but this is limited by lack of good quality evidence. However, the benefits of robot for management of fibroids in obese women and at unfavorable sites require further exploration.

As previously stated, robot has a great potential to facilitate complicated dissections in deeper tissue planes to excise the extensive grade 4 and deep infiltrating endometriosis. But for other less extensive endometriosis, robotic platform does not confer any additional advantage than laparoscopy with a

TABLE 1: Review of studies showing comparison of robotic assisted versus laparoscopic hysterectomy done for benign disease.

Study	*Interpretation*
Carcinoma cervix	
Puntambekar et al. 2012[21]	Compared the RRH with TLRH and it was observed that RRH was associated with longer OT time (95–300 min vs. 65–120 min) and higher blood loss (50–100 mL vs. 150–500 mL). The lymph node yield was higher with robotics (30 vs. 18)
Asciutto KC et al. 2015[22]	Compared RRH with ORH and confirmed the benefits of MIS approach with RRH. The complication rates (p = 0.03) were higher in open surgery group. However, robotic approach led to better the lymph node yield (31 vs. 24, p < 0.001)
Sert BM et al. 2015[23] Retrospective multicenter study	Compared the RRH with ORH and found longer OT time (220 vs. 156 min, p < 0.001), but lesser blood loss (49 vs. 97 mL, p < 0.001) with RRH
Carcinoma endometrium	
Somashekhar SP et al. 2014[25]	Compared the robotic approach with that of open surgeries. Robotic surgery conferred all the benefits of MIS with lesser OT time, lower blood loss (81.28 mL vs. 234 mL; p < 0.001), and reduced hospital stay (1.94 vs. 5.54 days; p < 0.001)
Saskia et al. 2015[26]	Compared the robotic arm with open approach. No difference in complication rates, and lymph node yield with added benefits of MIS in robotic arm. [Shorter operative time (p < 0.0001); lower blood loss (p<0.0001); shorter time to resume activities (5-days vs. 14-days, p < 0.0001)]
Carcinoma ovary	
Magrina JF et al. 2011[27]	Compared robotic vs. lap vs. open approach and found 11 months inferior survival in robotic arm than open surgery and with a high OT time (314.8 min vs. 260.7 min vs. 253.8 min; p < 0.05)

(ORH: open radical hysterectomy; MIS: minimally invasive surgery; RRH: robotic radical hysterectomy; TLRH: laparoscopic radical hysterectomy)

limitation of cost and extra OT time and therefore not a cost effective option.[15] Similarly other benign surgical procedures which are less complex, e.g., salpingectomy, ovarian cystectomy, tubal ligation, etc., are not cost-effective with a robotic approach and should be done with laparoscopy only.[12]

Other procedures where robotic approach has been found useful are robotic cerclage, robotic tubal anastomosis, and robotic sacrocolpopexy.

The feasibility of robotic cerclage has been investigated and it was found to be feasible with a good pregnancy outcomes.[16] One study, evaluated interval robotic cerclage in 24 nonpregnant women and found that the procedure had a benefit of quicker recovery. However, a long term follow up for evaluating pregnancy and delivery rates is warranted.[17] Similarly, robotic tubal anastomosis was found to be a feasible option with better conception rates than open approach (62.5% with robotic and 50% with open technique).[18] However, the cost and OT time remained the main limitations.[17,18]

Laparoscopic sacrocolpopexy for vault prolapse has not gained much popularity owing to technical difficulties. Robotic platform might be useful to address this problem. Robotic sacrocolpopexy was found to be a viable option. Although, for initial cases the mean operating time was more (197.7 minutes) but after performing 10 cases it reduced by 25.4%.[19] Other outcomes such as blood loss, perioperative complication rates, hospital stay, postoperative pain were same as that of laparoscopic surgery. The anatomical cure, functional activity and quality of life were also similar in the two groups.[20] Robotic surgery has been found feasible for sacrohysteropexy, which is done for POP in women desirous of pregnancy.[5]

To summarize we can say that currently evidence does not support robotic assisted surgical approach for simple benign gynecological procedures but it is a more viable option for complex cases.

Robotic-assisted Surgery for Malignant Gynaecological Procedures

For Carcinoma Cervix

The first robotic radical hysterectomy was conducted in the year 2008 and since then many retrospective and observational studies have been conducted to compare its outcome with laparoscopic and open surgical approach.[21-23] Overall robotic surgery confers all the benefits of MIS but for cancer surgeries oncological outcome remain the major concern. The initial studies suggested that there was no difference in recurrence (p = 1.00) and mortality rates (p = 0.48) between RRH and ORH in women with cervical cancer.[23] In 2018 a phase 3 randomized control trial LACC trial was conducted to confirm the safety of MIS in cancer cervix stage IA to IB1, the results of this trial raised questions on the safety of MIS approach in cancer cervix. In the MIS group, laparoscopy was done in 84.4% and robot-assisted surgery was done in 15.6% cases. The median follow up was 2.5 years. The rate of disease-free survival at 4.5 years was lower in the MIS group than the open surgery group (86.0% vs. 96.5%; difference, –10.6 percentage points; 95% CI: –16.4 to –4.7; p = 0.87). This inferiority was consistent in both laparoscopic and robotic surgery cohort. Similarly, a lower 3-year DFS was seen in MIS group than open surgery (91.2% vs. 97.1%; HR for disease relapse or mortality from cervical cancer, 3.74; 95% CI, 1.63-8.58). The overall survival (OS) was lower with MIS than open surgery (3-year rate, 93.8% vs. 99.0%; HR for death from any cause, 6.00; 95% CI, 1.77–20.30), an increased mortality from cervical cancer (3-year rate, 4.4% vs. 0.6%; HR: 6.56; 95% CI, 1.48–29.00), and increased probability of locoregional relapse (3-year rate of locoregional relapse-free survival, 94.3% vs. 98.3%; hazard ratio for locoregional relapse, 4.26; 95% CI, 1.44–12.60). In ORH, 43% of recurrences were isolated vault recurrences, as opposed to only 15% in LRH arm. Multiple sites of recurrences were seen in 29% and 37% of ARH and LRH arms respectively. Hence, use of MIS for doing radical hysterectomy in women with cervical cancer is associated with inferior survival than open approach.[28] This could be due to routine use of a uterine manipulator leading to tumor fragmentation along with the impact of pneumoperitoneum on tumor-cell spread or growth. Following publication of this trial several studies evaluated the safety of MIS in cervical cancer, but results have been inconsistent. Hence, currently it is preferred that MIS can be used for selected cases of carcinoma cervix with early stage disease (<2 cm growth) after informed counseling in research setting.

For carcinoma endometrium, robotic surgery has gained popularity than open[24-26] approach and is now a standard of care **(Table 2)** because of inherent benefits of MIS including wound complications, especially in obese women. The oncological outcome and lymph node yields are comparable with gold standard open surgery. Recently, robotic optical system with near-infrared fluorescent imaging and indigo cyanine green fluorescence dye has been used for sentinel lymph node mapping in early stage carcinoma endometrium with detection rates as high as 90%.[29]

There is not enough evidence available to establish the role of robotics in management of carcinoma ovary. The available studies have raised questions on oncological safety of MIS in management of advanced ovarian cancer.[29] Therefore, minimal invasive approach in the management of ovarian malignancy islimited to primary tumor excision and staging but for cases needing more than two additional procedures, open surgical approach is the preferred modality.[29] However, for women with previous incomplete surgery with no evidence of obvious disease, robotic platform may be used for completion of staging surgery. Similarly, for lymphadenectomy or removal of bulky lymph nodes, robotic platform is a viable option.

Recently robotic-assisted video endoscopic inguinal lymphadenectomy has been done in carcinoma vulva and is evolving with a potential to reduce the surgical morbidity associated with the procedure.[30]

Overall robotic-assisted surgery is feasible and safe in women with endometrial cancer with all the benefits of minimally invasive surgery. The main advantage of robotics is improved precision, which makes it suitable for complicated oncologic procedures. Its applications in cervical and ovarian carcinoma are yet to be established.[4]

ECONOMIC IMPACT OF ROBOTIC SURGERIES

The use of robotic-assisted surgery has gained wide popularity not only in gynecology but also in other surgical fields. However, the cost remains the main concern precluding its application in LMICs. The initial cost for setting up a robotic unit and the recurring costs concerning service contracts and robotic instruments remain out of pocket for most. The initial investment is approximately $2 million and service contracts afterwards confer an extra cost of $100,000–$170,000 each year.[31] Furthermore, the robot needs to be replaced every 10 years, similarly majority of ports and instruments are for one-time use. Although one may use the instruments number of times after appropriate sterilization, but the robot needs to

TABLE 2: Role of robotic surgery in malignant gynecological procedures: An overview.

Study	*Findings*
Puntambekar et al. 2012[21]	Compared the RRH with TLRH and it was observed that RRH was associated with longer OT time (95–300 min vs. 65–120 min) and higher blood loss (50–100 mL vs. 150–500 mL). The lymph node yield was higher with robotics (30 vs. 18)
Asciutto KC et al. 2015[22]	Compared RRH with ORH and confirmed the benefits of MIS approach with RRH. The complication rates ($p = 0.03$) were higher in open surgery group. However, robotic approach led to better the lymph node yield (31 vs. 24, $p < 0.001$)
Sert BM et al. 2015[23] Retrospective multicenter study	Compared the RRH with ORH and found longer OT time (220 vs. 156 min, $p < 0.001$), but lesser blood loss (49 vs. 97 mL, $p < 0.001$) with RRH
Somashekhar SP et al. 2014[25]	Compared the robotic approach with that of open surgeries. Robotic surgery conferred all the benefits of MIS with lesser OT time, lower blood loss (81.28 mL vs. 234 mL; $p < 0.001$), and reduced hospital stay (1.94 vs. 5.54 days; $p < 0.001$)
Saskia et al. 2015[26]	Compared the robotic arm with open approach. No difference in complication rates, and lymph node yield with added benefits of MIS in robotic arm [shorter operative time ($p < 0.0001$); lower blood loss ($p < 0.0001$); shorter time to resume activities (5-days vs. 14-days, $p < 0.0001$)]
Magrina JF et al. 2011[27]	Compared robotic vs. laparoscopy vs. open approach and found 11 months inferior survival in robotic arm than open surgery and with a high OT time (314.8 min vs. 260.7 min vs. 253.8 min; $p < 0.05$)

(ORH: open radical hysterectomy; MIS: minimally invasive surgery; RRH: robotic radical hysterectomy; TLRH: laparoscopic radical hysterectomy)

be replaced after 10 years. The extra cost of robotic surgery was attributed to the fixed cost of the robot in a recent study and even the savings due to reduced hospital stay could not compensate the higher cost but reduction in laparotomies could neutralize some what the costs involved.[32] Therefore, developing cheaper models is the need of hour. Recently a new such robotic system named as SPORT surgical system (Single Port Orifice Robotic Technology) has been developed by Titan Medical Inc. and has unparalleled efficiency at a lower cost. The unique features are multiarticulate instruments, 3D high visualization, ergonomic open workstation and a single arm mobile patient cart. The robotic technology is rapidly improving and recently robotic endoscope holder (ViKY) has been developed which offers a third hand to the surgeonduring laparoscopy.[33]

ROBOTIC SURGICAL TRAINING AND LEARNING CURVE OF ROBOTICS

The robotic platform is easier to learn and practice because of surgeon friendly ergonomics but it has its own learning curve, which is definitely faster than laparoscopy even for a novice.

Approximately 25–50 cases may be required to be performed, to be proficient in the robotic surgery, however this may vary depending on surgical performance and complexity of the procedure.[34] Although robotic surgery initially takes more time, approximately 245 minutes in first five cases but as one gets more experience with docking and equipment, the time gradually reduces from 245 to 175 minutes in next 10 procedures. Furthermore, as surgical technology is mastered the surgical time further reduces from 175 to 142 minutes for another 10 procedures.[35] Similarly, the cost for a robotic assisted surgery also depends upon the number of cases done at the center. One study analyzed the cost of robotic radical hysterectomy with respect to the surgeon's learning curve. It was observed that the initial costs were higher but as one performed more cases the cost was same as that of open procedures. The mean cost was $18,382 for first 30 cases and it was $12,759 for next 30 cases. The costs further reduced as one performed more cases and after 90 cases it was same as that of open radical hysterectomy, i.e., $12,986. Hence, at high volume centers OT time is likely to be lesser and thus overall cost may be lower.[35] Thus, increased use of robotic platform will further improve the cost effectiveness of robotic surgery.

The major concern with robotic-assisted surgery remains equipment failure and higher costs of disposables. Although the probability of equipment failure is as low as 0.2–0.4%, but even these low rates may not be acceptable. These rates may be further reduced by proper training of all the members of surgical team including OT technicians andnurses in docking and common trouble shooting. For robotic surgeons a minimum 30 hours training is mandatory according to European Society of Robotic Gynecological Surgery (SERGS).[2]

Therobotic training is incorporated in curricula of minimally invasive and gynecologic oncology fellowship programs[31] as the provision of dual console enables the smooth learning experience for the mentee and touch screen robotic illustrators provide visual cues intraoperatively by their trainers. The mentor and mentee can sit by side and can share the controls.[4-6] There is a need to incorporate robotic training in the surgical and gynecological curriculum of medical schools in India. Better learning opportunities are likely to enhance use of robotic technology by gynecologists and increasing use is likely to reduce the current costs in India.[4]

CONCLUSION

The robotic-assisted surgery in gynecology is evolving and is beneficial. It enables gynecologists to perform more difficult and challenging cases endoscopically with considerable ease. The concerns about its cost, availability, and outcomes are to be further investigated in clinical trials. However, the available evidence suggest that majority of benign procedures can be performed through robotic approach. The role of robotics in gynecological oncology is well established in carcinoma endometrium.

REFERENCES

1. Bouquet de Joliniere J, Librino A, Dubuisson JB, Khomsi F, Ben Ali N, Fadhlaoui A, et al. Robotic Surgery in Gynecology. Front. Surg. 2016;3:26.
2. Madhuri TK, Butler-Manuel S. Robotic surgery in gynaecology/gynaecological oncology. Obstet Gynaecol Reprod Med. 2017;27(2):65-7.
3. Kim YT, Kim SW, Jung YW. Robotic surgery in gynecologic field. Yonsei Med J. 2008;49:886.
4. Singhal S. Robotic assisted surgery in Gynecologic Oncology: Hype or Hope. Indian J Gynecol Oncol. 2017;15:43.
5. Nair R, Killicoat K, Thomas EJ. Robotic Surgery in Gynecology. Obstet Gynecol. 2016;18:221-9.
6. Simpson KM, Advincula AP. The Essential Elements of a Robotic-Assisted Laparoscopic Hysterectomy. Obstet Gynecol Clin N Am. 2016;43:479-93.
7. Wright JD, Ananth CV, Lewin SN. Robotically Assisted vs Laparoscopic Hysterectomy Among Women With Benign Gynecologic Disease. JAMA. 2013;309(7):689-98.
8. Patzkowsky KE, As-Sanie S, Smorgick N, Song AH, Advincula AP. Perioperative outcomes of robotic versus laparoscopic hysterectomy for benign disease. JSLS. 2013;17:100-6.
9. Rosero EB, Kho KA, Joshi GP, Giesecke M, Schaffer JI. Comparison of robotic and laparoscopic hysterectomy for benign gynecologic disease. Obstet Gynecol. 2013;122:778-86.
10. Albright BB, Witte T, Tofte AN, Chou J, Black JD, Desai VB, et al. Robotic versus Laparoscopic Hysterectomy for Benign Disease: a Systematic Review and Meta-Analysis of Randomized Trials. J Minim Invas Gynecol. 2016;23(1):18-27.
11. Cronin B, Sung VW, Matteson KA. Vaginal cuff dehiscence: Risk factors and management Am J Obstet Gynecol. 2012;206(4):284-8.
12. Robotic surgery in gynecology. Committee Opinion No. 628. American College of Obstetricians and Gynecologists. Obstet Gynecol. 2015;125:760-7.
13. Gobern JM, Rosemeyer C, Barter JF, Steren AJ. Comparison of robotic, laparoscopic, and abdominal myomectomy in a community hospital. JSLS. 2013;17:116-20.

14. Pluchino N, Litta P, Freschi L, Russo M, Simi G, Santoro AN, et al. Comparison of the initial surgical experience with robotic and laparoscopic myomectomy. Int J Med Robot. 2014;10:208-12.
15. Nezhat C, Lewis M, Kotikela S, Veeraswamy A, Saadat L, Hajhosseini B, Nezhat C. Robotic versus standard laparoscopy for the treatment of endometriosis. Fertil Steril. 2010;94:2758-60.
16. Cronin C, Hewitt M, Harley I, O'Donoghue K, O'Reilly BA. Robot-assisted laparoscopic cervical cerclage as an interval procedure. Gynecol Surg. 2012;9:317-21.
17. Moore E, Foster T. McHughK, Addleman R, Sumners J. Robotic-assisted transabdominal cerclage (RoboTAC) in the non-pregnant patient. J Obstet Gynaecol. 2012;32:643-7.
18. Patel SPD, Steinkampf MP, Whitten SJ, Malizia BA. Robotic tubal anastomosis: surgical technique and cost effectiveness. Fertil Steril. 2008;90:1175-9.
19. Akl MN, Long JB, Giles DL, Cornella JL, Pettit PD, Chen AH, et al. Robotic-assisted sacrocolpopexy: technique and learning curve. Surg Endosc. 2009;23:2390-4.
20. Hallock JL, Fitzgerald J, Chen CCG. Update on Robotic Versus Laparoscopic Sacrocolpopexy: outcomes and costs. Curr Obstet Gynecol Rep. 2014;3:252-64.
21. Puntambekar S, Agarwal G, Joshi SN, Rayate NV, Puntambekar SS, Sathe RM. Robotic oncological surgery: our initial experience of 164 Cases. Indian J Surg Oncol. 2012;3(2):96-100.
22. Asciutto KC, Kalapotharakos G, Löfgren M, Högberg T, Borgfeldt C. Robot-assisted surgery in cervical cancer patients reduces the time to normal activities of daily living. Acta Obstet Gynecol Scand. 2015;94:260-5.
23. Sert BM, Boggess JF, Ahmad S, Jackson AL, Stavitzski NM, Dahl AA, et al. Robot-assisted versus open radical hysterectomy: a multi-institutional experience for early-stage cervical cancer. Euro J Surg Col. 2016;42(4):512-22.
24. Krill LS, Bristow RE. Robotic surgery: gynecologic oncology. Cancer J. 2013;19(2):167-76.
25. Somashekhar SP, Jaka RC, Zaveri SS. Prospective Randomized Study Comparing Robotic-Assisted Hysterectomy and Regional Lymphadenectomy with Traditional Laparotomy for Staging of Endometrial Carcinoma–Initial Indian Experience. Indian J Surg Oncol. 2014;1;5(3):217-23.
26. Eklind S, Lindfors A, Sjöli P, Dahm-Kähler P. A prospective, comparative study on robotic versus open-surgery hysterectomy and pelvic lymphadenectomy for endometrial carcinoma. Int J Gynecol Can. 2015;25(2):250-6.
27. Magrina JF, Zanagnolo V, Noble BN, Kho RM, Magtibay P. Robotic approach for ovarian cancer: perioperative and survival results and comparison with laparoscopy and laparotomy. Gynecol Oncol. 2011;121:100-5.
28. Ramirez PT, Frumovitz M, Pareja R, Lopez A, Vieira MA, Ribeiro R. Phase III randomized trial of laparoscopic or robotic versus abdominal radical hysterectomy in patients with early-stage cervical cancer: LACC Trial. Gynecol Oncol. 2018;149:245.
29. Minig L, Iserte PP, Zorrero C, Zanagnolo V. Robotic surgery in women with ovarian cancer: surgical technique and evidence of clinical outcomes. J Minim Invas Gynecol. 2016;23(3):309-16.
30. Jain V, Sekhon R, Giri S, Hassan N, Batra K. Robotic-Assisted Video Endoscopic Inguinal Lymphadenectomy in Carcinoma Vulva: our Experiences and Intermediate Results. Int J Gynecol Cancer. 2017;27:159-65.
31. Finan MA, Rocconi RP. Overcoming technical challenges with robotic surgery in gynecologic oncology. Surg Endosc. 2010;24:1256-60.
32. Marino P, Houvenaeghel G, Narducci F. Cost-effectiveness of conventional vs robotic-assisted laparoscopy in gynecologic oncologic indications. IntJ Gynecol Can. 2015;25(6):1102-8.
33. Maheshwari M, Ind T. Concurrent use of a robotic uterine manipulator and a robotic laparoscope holder to achieve assistant-less solo laparoscopy: the Double ViKY. J Robot Surg. 2015;9:211-3.
34. Yim GW, Kim SW, Nam EJ, Kim S, Kim YT. Learning curve analysis of robot-assisted radical hysterectomy for cervical cancer: initial experience at a single institution. J Gynecol Oncol. 2013;24(4):303-12.
35. Reynisson P, Persson J. Hospital costs for robot-assisted laparoscopic radical hysterectomy and pelvic lymphadenectomy. Gynecol Oncol. 2013;130:95-9.

LONG QUESTION

1. Discuss in detail the equipment, technique, indications and challenges of robotics in gynecology.

SHORT QUESTIONS

1. Compare robotic surgeries vs laparoscopic surgeries.
2. What are the advantages of robotic surgeries?

MULTIPLE CHOICE QUESTIONS

1. The limitations of laparoscopy surgery which are well addressed by the robot include all, except:
   a. Limited range of motion
   b. Sense of depth perception
   c. Surgeon's fatigue
   d. Early discharge
2. The number of robotic arms used to hold the camera and instruments are:
   a. 1 b. 2
   c. 4 d. 8
3. The only pitfall with robotic hysterectomy has been relatively higher risk of:
   a. Bladder trauma b. Vault dehiscence
   c. Pelvic hemorrhage d. Bowel injury
4. The robotic platform does not confer any additional advantage than laparoscopy in the following indications, except:
   a. Myomectomy
   b. Salpingectomy
   c. Deep infiltrating endometriosis
   d. Tubal ligation
5. For robotic surgeons training is mandatory according to European Society of Robotic Gynecological Surgery of a minimum of at least:
   a. 10 hours b. 30 hours
   c. 100 hours d. 200 hours

Answers

1. d 2. c 3. b 4. c 5. b

11.4 COMPLICATIONS OF GYNAECOLOGICAL LAPAROSCOPY

Sunita Tandulwadkar, Abhishek Chandavarkar, Rohan Krishnakumar

INTRODUCTION

Laparoscopy surgery is frequently used and preferred to treat various conditions more so in the last decade, hence the dramatic rise in the number of laparoscopically performed procedures. Undoubtedly, almost all laparoscopic surgery is able to achieve the same goals as the open approach while offering the patient distinct advantages such as reduction of perioperative morbidity, length of hospital stay, and convalescence. Nevertheless, there are also few disadvantages associated with laparoscopy namely long learning curves for and few potential complications associated with these procedures. The much experienced open surgeons, may find it challenging to instantaneously acquire skills in endoscopic techniques.

Complications in laparoscopy, may encompass those associated with open surgery in addition a number of complications that are specific to the endoscopic approach. Knowledge about these complications is essential for their prevention. Timely recognition, aids the surgeon in managing these complications even laparoscopically and as result preserving the benefits of the minimally invasive approach. This section focuses on the recognition, the management, and the prevention of acute intraoperative and postoperative complications that may be encountered in laparoscopic surgery **(Table 1)**.

COMPLICATIONS RELATED TO ANESTHESIA AND PATIENT POSITION

Nerve Injury

Transient nerve injuries may occur due incorrect positioning, affecting brachial plexus, common peroneal nerve, and also the saphenous nerve. Most common nerve injury in gynecological laparoscopic procedures in common peroneal nerve, due to the low lithotomy position given.[1]

Cardiac Arrhythmias

Heart rate abnormalities such as bradycardia, sinus tachycardia, ventricular tachycardia, and arrest related to anesthesia have been reported during laparoscopy. In one series, cardiac arrest occurred in one (0.02%) patient and respiratory arrest in another (0.02%).[1]

ACCESS-RELATED COMPLICATIONS

Establishing a pneumoperitoneum and gaining entry access to the abdomen are the primary steps in laparoscopic surgery. These can be at times challenging and may result in peculiar complications. The overall incidence of access-related injuries is relatively small.

Injury to major blood vessels is probably the most feared complication of gaining laparoscopic access. Recognition of this complication usually is not a problem. However, in many of the less spectacular complications of trocar placement, the intraoperative recognition of the injury, which is crucial for an optimal management of the situation, may not be easily accomplished. In their review of 594 laparoscopic entry access injuries, Chandler and colleagues found that nearly 50% of both large and small-bowel injuries remained at unrecognized for at least 24 hours.

Entry into Peritoneum

If the pneumoperitoneum is established via a Veress needle, correct positioning of the needle should be verified prior to carbon dioxide (CO_2) insufflation. An irregular finding on aspiration, irrigation, respiration, or drop test indicates incorrect positioning of the needle and may lead to the suspicion of an injury to an intra-abdominal organ. If the intra-abdominal pressure reading at the beginning of the insufflation is not below 8–10 mm Hg, incorrect needle position or at least contact of the needle tip with intra-abdominal structures must be suspected and the needle should be repositioned. It is particularly important to communicate constantly with the anesthesiologist during the phase of initial CO_2 insufflation so that close monitoring can be performed. Any sudden change in the hemodynamic of the patient or end-tidal CO_2 reading should warrant a stoppage in insufflation.[3]

If a complication from the insertion of the Veress needle is suspected, the needle should be withdrawn and the pneumoperitoneum should either be established by introducing the Veress needle at a different site or by open insertion of a trocar by Hasson technique **(Fig. 1)** or by Optiview technique **(Fig. 2)**.

Carbon Dioxide Embolism

Embolization of CO_2 to the right sided chambers of heart, a very rare but potentially catastrophic situation that results from inadvertent insufflation of gas into the bloodstream, which leads to a sudden and sharp decrease in end-tidal CO_2 and oxygen saturation as well as low-output heart failure.[5,6] Transesophageal echocardiography if available in the operating room, this may aid in the visualization of the gas embolus in the right heart and make the correct diagnosis.

Once the camera is introduced, a cursory inspection of the peritoneal cavity should be performed in every procedure. In case an access injury is suspected, meticulous inspection is mandatory to verify or rule out any intra-abdominal lesion. Majority of access-related injuries are from the primary entry port.

TABLE 1: Summary or complications or laparoscopic gynecologic surgery.

Complication	*Rate (%)*	*Cause of complication*	*Clinical presentation*	*Management*
Abdominal wall vascular injury	0.5	Entry related	• Intraoperative blood dropping to operation field • Postoperative hemorrhage and hematoma	• Coagulation • Tamponade • Suturing
Intestinal injury	0–0.5	• Entry related (laceration) • Operative (thermal)	Usually diagnosed postoperatively with peritonitis-like findings	• Most cases required conversion to laparotomy • *Thermal injury:* Bowel resection • *Trocar injury:* Primary repair or resection related with localization, extension and bowel preparation • *Veress injury:* It can be managed expectantly
Ureteral injury	0.025–2	• Electrocautery (leading cause) • Other (i.e., trocar, laser, dissection, staples, suturing)	• Intraoperative diagnosis is very rare • Presentation may be delayed by the several weeks especially in thermal injury. Symptoms are variable	• *Intraoperative diagnosed patients:* Intraoperative laparoscopic repair, double J-shaped catheter for focal injury • *Postoperative diagnosed patients:* Laparotomic end-to-end anastomosis, ureteral implantation, ureteral reconstruction or ureteroneocystostomy
Bladder injury	0.02–8.3	• Entry related • Thermal • During dissection	Most of cases diagnosed intraoperatively. Abdominal discomfort and oliguria are major findings postoperatively	• Based on localization extension and type of injury • Conservative management • Surgical repair
Major vascular injury	0.04–0.5	• Entry related • Energy source • Operative	• Bleeding from trocar or veress • Observation via laparoscope • Retroperitoneal hematoma	• Laparotomic vessel repair without removing veress or trocar • Laparoscopic repair also reported
Hernia at trocar site	0.17–0.2	Entry related	• Bowel obstruction findings • Incarceration	Bowel resection in incarcerated cases
Subcutaneous emphysema	2.3	CO_2 presence in subcutaneous tissue	Subcutaneous emphysema	Resolve spontaneously
Hypcrcarbia	5.5	• Longer operative times • High end-tidal CO_2 • Older patient age	Acidosis	Ventilation
Cardiac arrhythmia	27	–	Sinus tachycardia, bradycardia, ventricular, tachycardia, and asystole	• Stopping gas in-flow • Anticholinergic agent for bradycardia • Reinsufflation after the arrhythmia settles down
Pneumothorax/ pneumomediastinum	0.2–1.9	• Pneumoperitoneum • Diaphragmatic defect	Respiratory related symptoms	• Discharging CO_2 from peritoneal cavity • Inhalation with 100% O_2 • Thorax tube
Port-site metastasis	1.1–2.3	Pneumoperitoneum and CO_2 related	Postoperative port-site tumor	Resection, chemotherapy, radiotherapy

Once the camera is introduced, the suspected intra-abdominal needle injury must be verified or ruled out. Injuries caused by the 14-gauge Veress needle can usually be managed laparoscopically even if a major vessel or a parenchymatous organ is involved. If a blood vessel has been punctured by the Veress needle, the bleeding following the withdrawal of the needle is usually not excessive and can be managed by applying pressure for a couple of minutes as well as a oxidized regenerated cellulose and fibrin glue if necessary. Puncture injuries of the liver and the spleen can be managed in the same way or they can be cauterized with the argon beam coagulator. Simple punctures of the bowel or the bladder by the Veress needle do not require any treatment.[7,8]

Carefully performed surgical technique and appropriate and optimally functioning equipment are essential for a safe laparoscopic access. None of these techniques or instruments

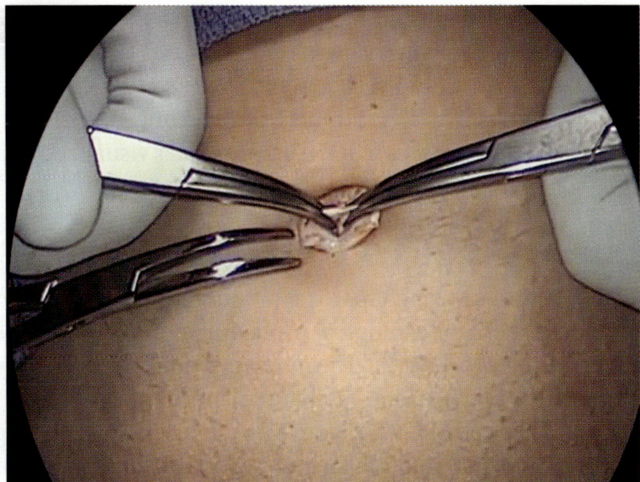

Fig. 1: Hasson technique.

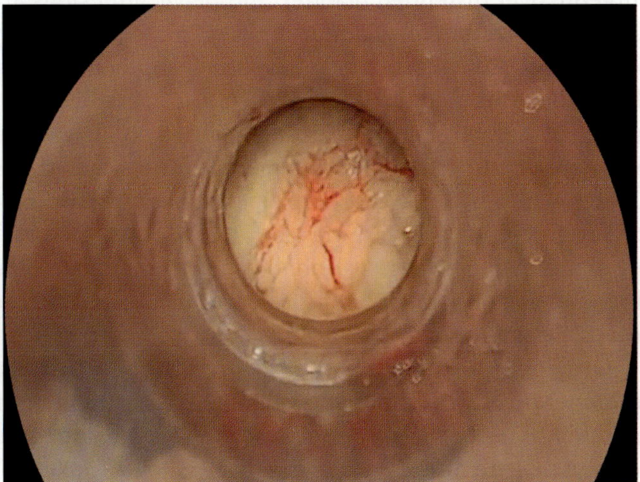

Fig. 2: Optiview entry.

is full proof and none has been able to eliminate access complications in laparoscopic surgery. Also, no particular method of access has convincingly been shown to be superior over the other.[9,10]

In order to reduce the risk of port-site hernias, all fascial defects >10 mm (5 mm in children) need to be closed at the end of the procedure.[1] If a trocar <10 mm in diameter is extensively manipulated during the operation, widening of the respective fascial defect may occur and primary closure should also be considered.[12]

INTESTINAL INJURY

The incidence of bowel injury is reported to be 0–0.5%.[13] About half of bowel injuries occur during entry **(Fig. 3)**, and the rest occur during the operation. Entry-related bowel injuries are mostly lacerations, and intraoperative injuries are usually from the thermal energy source. Unfortunately bowel injuries are may not be diagnosed during surgery. Delayed intervention may be life-threatening. Hence, this complication is reported to be the most common cause of laparoscopy-related mortality.[14]

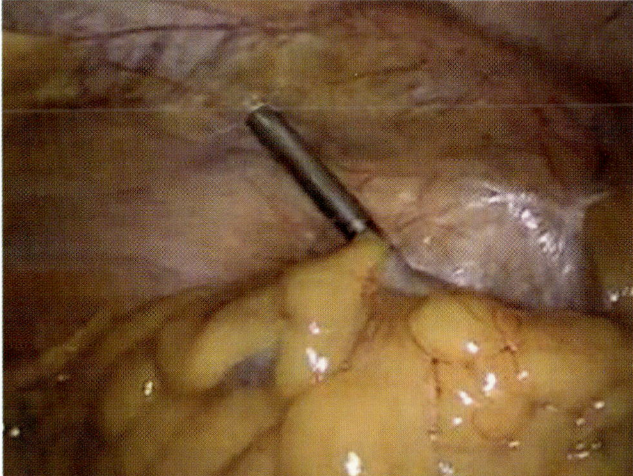

Fig. 3: Trocar entry into the bowel.

Soderstrom reviewed 66 cases of missed intestinal perforation and concluded that if the diagnosis is delayed >72 hours, the mortality rate significantly increases.[15] In a review, less than half of 363 bowel injury cases were diagnosed intraoperatively.[13] Rates of small and large bowel injuries were similar, 46.9% and 40.2%, respectively. The mean time from operation to diagnosis was 4.4 days, but recognition of thermal injury may lag behind 10 days.

When bowel is entered via Veress needle or trocar, bowel content or gas passage may be observed, or may be controlled with a syringe if suspected. A laparoscope will show bowel lumen in such a case **(Fig. 4)**. If intraoperatively unrecognized, patients present with nonspecific complaints, not exactly pointing to peritonitis, such as mild abdominal pain, fever, diarrhea, and abdominal distension, further delaying the diagnosis.[16] Late consequences may be generalized peritonitis, abscess formation, and septic-shock.

Manipulation with instruments outside this field (e.g., during instrument changes) is prone to inadvertent violation of bowel and other intra-abdominal structures. If a lesion cannot be seen directly, free intestinal contents are proof of a bowel laceration. Additionally, the escape of fecal smell through an opened port valve must lead to a search for a bowel injury.

If such a lesion is strongly suspected, the entire length bowel has to be inspected meticulously. Between 52.4 and 90.0% of intestinal injuries can be successfully repaired via laparotomy.[17,18]

Injury caused by the Veress needle may be managed expectantly. However, trocar injuries deserve laparotomic repair according to the size and location of the injury. Primary closure in two layers is recommended in small bowel injuries. If the large bowel is involved, the treatment options include primary repair, colostomy, or segmental resection. Resection is mandatory in thermal injuries.

Intraoperative lacerations may be repaired laparoscopically **(Fig. 5)** according to the size of the lesion, surgeon's experience, and preoperative bowel preparation.[19] The laceration should be sutured in one or two layers if small bowel is involved.

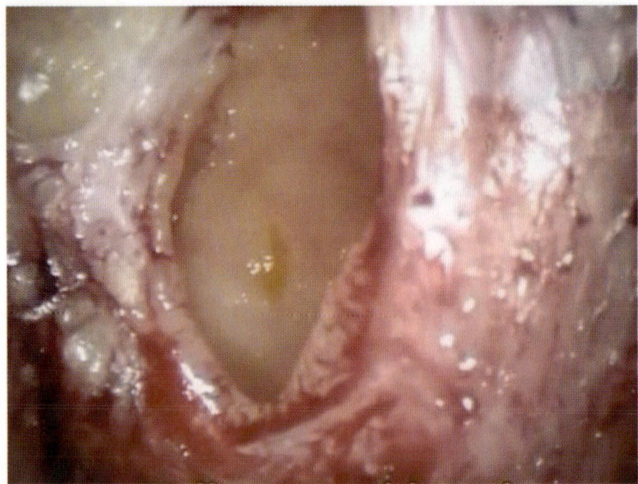

Fig. 4: Bowel mucosa popping out.

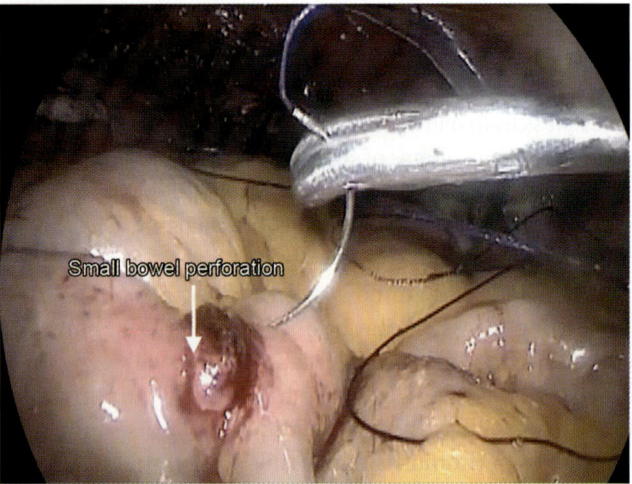

Fig. 5: Small bowel perforation being sutured laparoscopically.

Lesions of the colon and the rectum should always be closed in two layers. In simple lesions, it is usually not necessary to resect the injured bowel segment. It is advisable to also suture the small serosal abrasions, since these minor lesions can cause major postoperative complications if they are left unattended during the initial laparoscopic procedure.[20] If more than half of the circumference of the bowel segment is involved, the respective segment needs to be resected and an end-to-end anastomosis should be performed. In injuries that are caused by monopolar electrocautery, on the other hand, the extension of the tissue damage is underestimated. Therefore, any monopolar electrothermal lesion necessitates resection and end-to-end anastomosis of the involved bowel segment.

Regular use of a nasogastric tube to deflate the stomach reduces the risk of injury to the stomach. Also, preoperative bowel preparation may reduce inadvertent intestinal trauma by increasing intraperitoneal free space and by facilitating operative maneuvers.[22]

All laparoscopic instruments must be checked for insulation leaks or damage prior to their use to prevent thermal injury. Bipolar electrocautery should be used whenever possible and all diathermy must be avoided close to the bowel. Monopolar electrocautery should not be used to take down bowel adhesions. The lowest possible power setting should be used at all times. The electric energy should only be activated when the entire active part of the instrument is visualized and the tip of the instrument is in contact with the target.[23]

BLADDER INJURY

Bladder injuries during laparoscopic surgery are most often associated with gynecological procedures. Incidence rates range from 0.02 to 8.3%.[25,26] The most common type of urinary injury during laparoscopy is bladder perforation **(Fig. 6)** with an incidence of 0.02–8.3%.[24] Most injuries occur during hysterectomy operations. Pillet et al. reported the incidence of bladder injury during laparoscopic hysterectomy to be around 1%.[26] Endometriosis, previous surgery, an inexperienced surgeon, over distended bladder, and pelvic adhesions are known risk factors for bladder injury. Bladder injury may occur during insertion of trocars, especially suprapubic ones, dissection of the bladder during gynecologic operations, or as a result of thermal energy. Of bladder injuries, 90% have been reported to occur at the bladder dome, and the rest at the base. Of these injuries, 33% were sharp electrocautery dissections, 21% were blunt, 30% were via laser, and 15% by scissors.[25] 5% of thermal injuries may lead to fistula formation.[26] More than half of trocar-related injuries occur via 5-mm and the rest via 10-mm trocars.

Only 9.2% of bladder injuries were not recognized intraoperatively, in contrast to ureteral injuries; therefore, morbidity is lower.[24] In suspected cases, the bladder is to filled with methylene blue dye to dye leakage is to be looked for to establish the diagnosis. Patients with unrecognized cases usually present with abdominal discomfort and oliguria. According to type, size, and localization of injury, conservative or surgical management via laparoscopic **(Fig. 7)**, laparotomic, or vaginal approaches may be considered.

Prevention of bladder injuries can be achieved by some of the following steps during surgery:

1. Perform a very careful dissection of the vesicovaginal pouch and use uterine cannulation.
2. Fill the bladder with a methylene blue dye solution to visualize its limits in case of difficult dissection, such as previous surgery (cesarean delivery, endometriosis surgery, conization, and others).
3. Perform very careful and restricted use of bipolar coagulation in the vesicovaginal space for hemostasis.
4. Follow the safety rules of introduction, in particular avoiding the Pfannenstiel scar.

URETERIC INJURY

Pelvic surgery is the most common cause of iatrogenic ureteral injury. The incidence is rising due to the increasing number of laparoscopic hysterectomies and retroperitoneal laparoscopic procedures that are being performed. The majority of patients

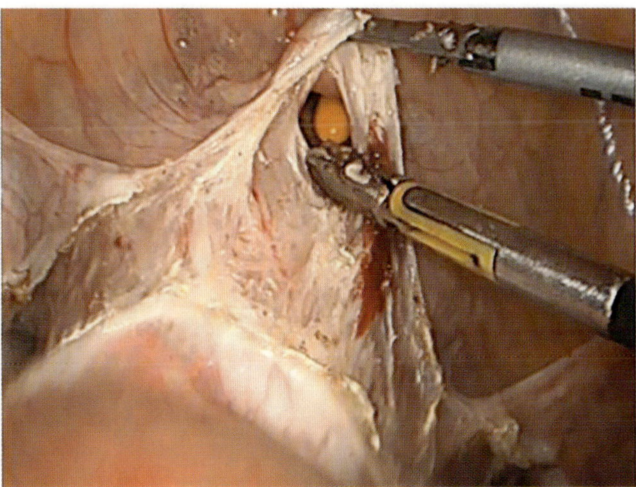

Fig. 6: Bladder injury: Foley's tip.

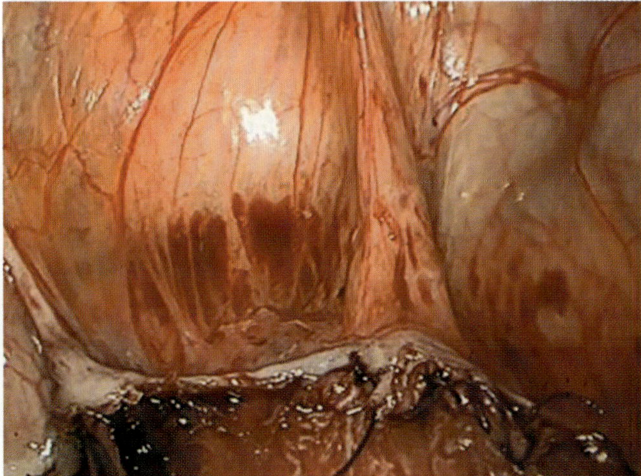

Fig. 7: Bladder sutured in two layers.

with ureteral injuries have no identifiable predisposing risk factors. Estimated incidence of ureteral injury during laparoscopic hysterectomy is 2.6–35 times more common (0.2–6.0%) than in abdominal hysterectomy.[27] Ureteral injury accounted for 4.3–7% of the total laparoscopy complications.[28,29] Overall ureteral injuries were identified with incidence rates ranging from 0.025 to 2%.[29,30]

Electrocautery (unipolar or bipolar) was identified as the leading cause of laparoscopic ureteral injury. Injuries with loop suturing, trocars, laser devices, staples, and sharp dissection have also be described.

Ureteral injury during laparoscopic surgeries is usually noted at the two following locations:

1. Pelvic brim—where the ureters lie beneath the insertions of the infundibulopelvic ligaments
2. Deep ovarian fossa where the ureter passes ureteral canal.[31]

In 44 patients with known injury site, the most common site of injury was near the infundibulopelvic ligament (29.5%), followed by injury near the uterosacral ligaments (18.1%) and uterine artery (9.9%), and below the uterine vessels (4.5%). Injuries may include transection, ligation, avulsion, crush injury, devascularization, resection, fulguration, and perforation. In a review, 20% of ureteral injuries occurred during laparoscopic-assisted vaginal hysterectomy, 11% during oophorectomy, 10% during laparoscopic pelvic lymphadenectomy, 7% during laparoscopic sterilization, and 7% during excision of endometriosis, 6% during endometriosis ablation, and 4% during each of the following: drainage of lymphoceles, electrocoagulation, and laparoscopic adhesiolysis.[30]

When dissecting a ureter, great care must be taken to preserve its blood supply and not to disrupt or interrupt it. To avoid electrothermal injury, monopolar current should never be used close to the ureter. Furthermore, routine preoperative ureteral stenting has been advocated in cases where a difficult pelvic dissection is expected.[32]

These injuries are frequently undetected due to the failure to recognize anatomic disruption **(Fig. 8)** as the surgeon does not suspect a ureteral injury. Depending on the type of injury, patients may present in the early postoperative period (first 3 days), or presentation of the thermal or laceration injuries may be delayed by several days or weeks. Only 9% of ureteral injuries were diagnosed intraoperatively, 70% postoperatively, and in 21%, the time of ureteral injury was not specified.

Hurt et al. and Li et al, propose five methods for identifying ureteral injury:

1. Retrograde ureteral dye injection;
2. 5–10 mL intravenous indigo carmine injection;
3. Intraoperative ureteral catheterization;
4. Intravenous excretory urography;
5. Dissection of the ureter.[33,34]

A coagulated or ligated ureter may not demonstrate an intraperitoneal urine leak when tested intraoperatively. The lack of a ureteral jet at cystoscopic examination will indicate the problem clearly in such a case.

Postoperative presentation is variable and nonspecific, such as acute pelvic pain, nausea, vomiting, malaise, leakage of fluid via the trocar sites, abdominal distension and an inflammatory reaction in the serum [elevated C-reactive protein (CRP) and leukocytosis], elevated creatinine level, costovertebral angle tenderness, ileus, fever, flank pain, and ileus peritonitis.[35] X-ray of the abdomen may reveal a ground-glass appearance indicative of fluid collection. A computed tomography (CT) scan revealed the presence of urine in the peritoneal cavity after intravenous contrast medium injection.[36] Ligation of the ureter, for example, with stapling or stricture resulting from thermal injury may lead to obstructive uropathy and superimposed pyonephrosis. The diagnosis should be confirmed by an intravenous urogram.

Laparoscopic repair is frequently used in cases recognized intraoperatively, while the laparotomic approach is performed in patients diagnosed postoperatively. Focal ureteral injuries can be treated using a double J-shaped catheter allowing for spontaneous healing.

However, more extensive damage may require laparotomy with the need to perform an end-to-end anastomosis or ureteral implantation. In experienced hands, this can be

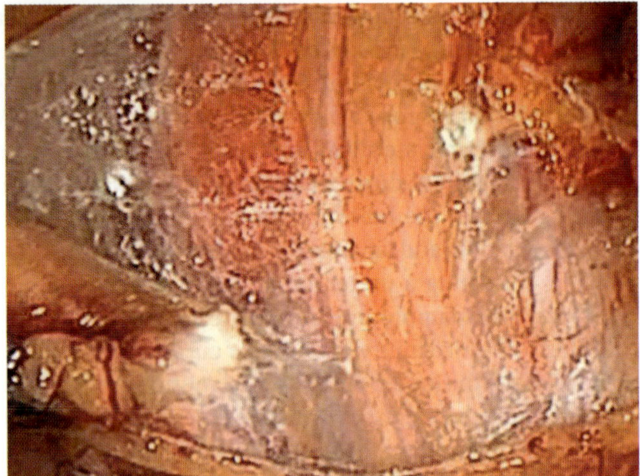

Fig. 8: Transection of ureter.

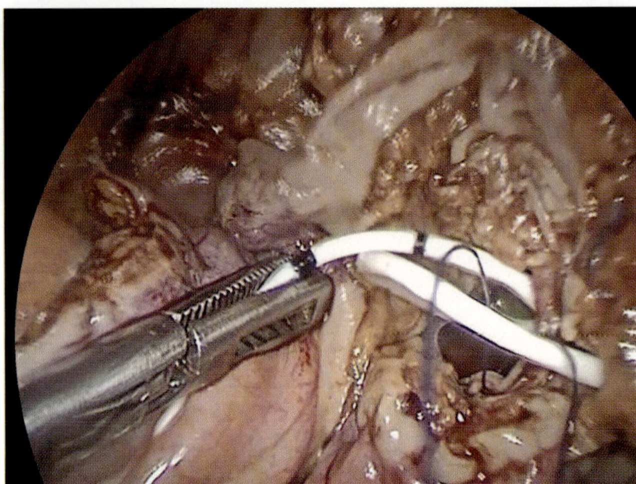

Fig. 9: Ureteric stent.

performed by the laparoscopic route **(Figs. 9 and 10)**. In delayed recognition of ureteral injury, initial treatment with ureteral stenting may not be useful and an early open repair (ureteral reconstruction, and ureteroneocystostomy) for these injuries is advocated.[37]

To minimize ureteral injury, use of sutures should be preferred instead of staplers or electrocautery in close proximity to ureters. Visualization of ureters during the operation, use of ureteral catheters, and creating hydroprotection by injection of saline to parietal peritoneum are the other protective measures.

ABDOMINAL WALL VASCULAR INJURY

High index of suspicion is needed throughout the entire laparoscopic procedure to recognize these injuries intraoperatively. Especially venous lesions can be missed intraoperatively because the pressure created from CO_2 insufflation may compress the injured vein and prevent one from locating the site of oozing blood. Therefore it is advisable to deflate the pressure and inspect the operative field prior to the completion of any laparoscopic operation.

Inferior epigastric vessel injuries are the most common type of vascular complication. The incidence of abdominal wall bleeding is 0.3–0.5%.[38] Epigastric and less commonly muscular vessels may be the origin of bleeding. These injuries usually occur in relation to the positioning of accessory ports, used principally to allow the insertion of the hand instruments necessary for dissecting and manipulating tissue. Blood dripping into the operative field may indicate intraoperative bleeding **(Fig. 11)**, but postoperatively diagnosed massive bleeding is also a possibility. Postoperative hematoma and abscess formation due to secondary infection of the hematoma are the sequelae in these cases. Whereas in access-related vascular injuries it is recommended to convert to open surgery in order to control the bleeding, vascular injuries that occur during dissection after all the ports have been placed may be dealt with laparoscopically.

Epigastric Artery Injury

The most rapid and efficient technique for achieving hemostasis is coagulation **(Fig. 12)**. If bleeding is not controlled

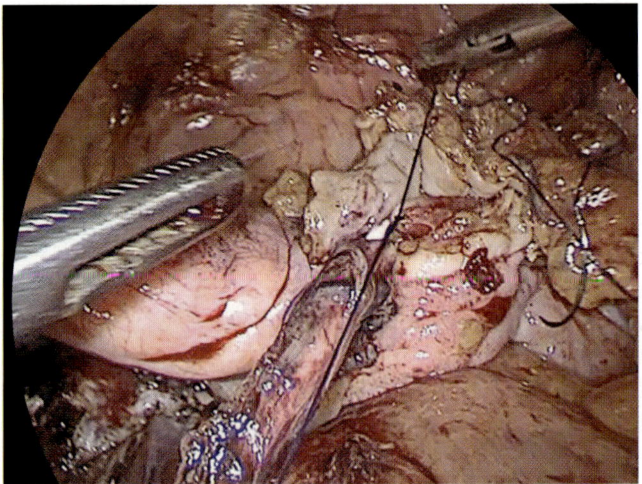

Fig. 10: Ureteric reimplantation.

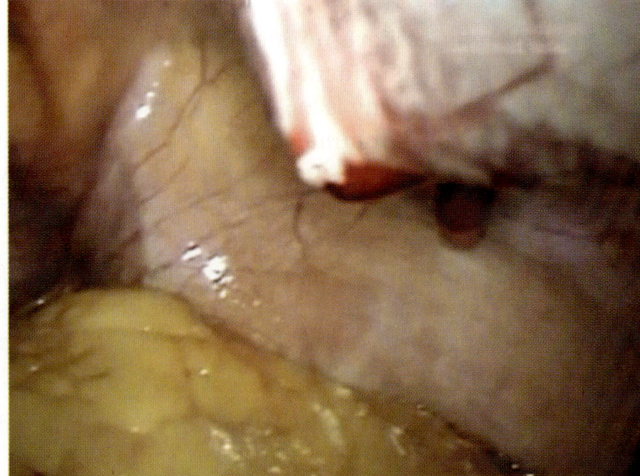

Fig. 11: Inferior epigastric artery injury.

then tamponade and suturing may be used. Suturing is done either laparoscopically or through an enlarged incision at the trocar site. Minilaparotomy may also be used. The site of bleeding should be re-evaluated under low pneumoperitoneal pressure after coagulation, tamponade, and suturing. Transillumination of the anterior abdominal wall, insertion of the trocar lateral to the sheath of the rectus muscle, and use of smaller trocars in lateral ports may help to avoid vascular injury. It is good practice to inspect all secondary trocar sites for active bleeding before the laparoscope is finally withdrawn.

In a minor vascular injury, application of pressure for a couple of minutes alone may solve the problem. In addition, hemostatic agents such as oxidized regenerated cellulose and fibrin glue may be applied alone or in combination. If there is adequate exposure of the injured vessel, electrocautery or application of clips can be enough to control the bleeding.

If the vessel needs to be repaired, endoscopic suturing of the laceration may be possible but should only be attempted by the highly experienced laparoscopic surgeon. The placement of additional ports can be helpful in such a situation, as it creates an opportunity to optimize distance and angle of the instruments toward the site of the lesion. In most cases of major vascular injury, however, it is advisable to convert to an open procedure and consider the involvement of a vascular surgeon.

MAJOR VASCULAR INJURY

Injuries of the major retroperitoneal vessels are serious complications and may due to the Veress needle, trocar, or energy source. Of the cases reported, approximately 20% of the major vascular injuries result in mortality. The incidence is estimated to range from 0.04 to 0.5%.[40,41] Most injuries were entry related and independent of the complexity of the surgery.[42] In this situation, either the aorta, vena cava, or, more commonly, the common iliac vessel have been known to be injured. Bleeding from the Veress and trocars at the entry site may be an alert. Also, intra-abdominal or retroperitoneal visualization (generally as a hematoma) with a laparoscope is possible **(Fig. 13)**. Therefore, visualization of the peritoneal cavity immediately after entry prevents any delay in diagnosis. Evident shock may develop due to abundant blood loss. Patients with anatomic distortions and retroperitoneal manipulations are more prone to energy source injuries. Such injuries may also occur at the time of pelvic lymph node dissection or when an attempt is made to dissect the lateral pelvic wall to expose the origin of the uterine artery **(Fig. 14)**. Major vascular injuries may rarely remain unrecognized intraoperatively.[43] The removal of the Veress needle or trocars in case of a vascular injury may result in abundant bleeding and the inability to locate the site of bleeding because of a retroperitoneal hematoma. Through midline incision, access to the bleeding site should be achieved before these instruments are removed, and injury should be repaired.

PNEUMOPERITONEUM-RELATED COMPLICATIONS

Hypercarbia and resultant acidosis develop in 5.5% patients due to absorption of CO_2 especially in operations with prolonged duration of surgery.[44] Subcutaneous emphysema, pneumomediastinum, and pneumothorax may result from preperitoneal insufflation or leakage of CO_2 around the cannula sites. Prolonged operations, higher maximum measured end-tidal CO_2, a greater number of surgical ports, and older patient age increase the risk. Subcutaneous emphysema is defined as the presence of CO_2 in the subcutaneous tissues.

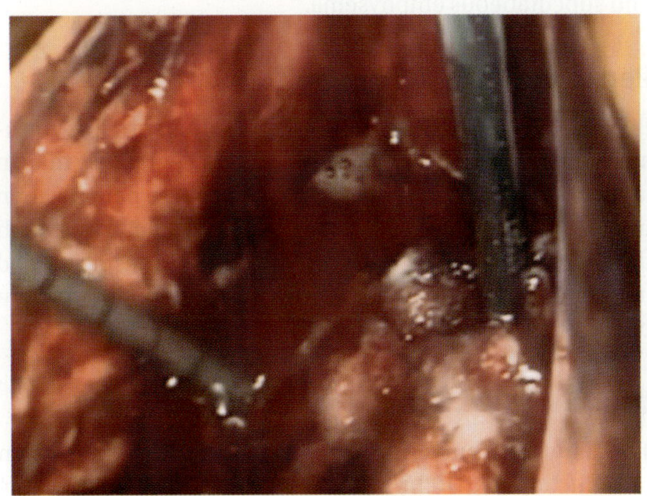

Fig. 13: Aortic injury.

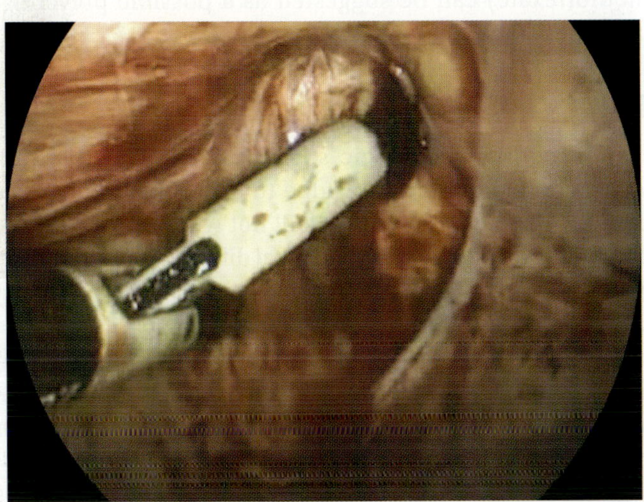

Fig. 12: Management of inferior epigastric artery injury.

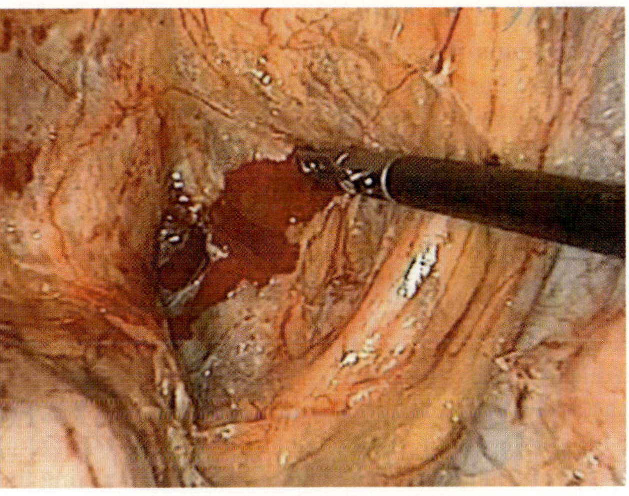

Fig. 14: Internal iliac vein injury.

Its incidence is 2.3%.[4] Generally, it has no significant adverse clinical outcome and resolves spontaneously. Subcutaneous emphysema rarely may be extensive involving the extremities, the neck, the mediastinum, and even the pericardium, and in such cases can result in hypercapnia and cardiovascular collapse. Preperitoneal emphysema results from preperitoneal insufflation, especially in obese patients when the Veress needle cannot reach the peritoneal cavity. The Veress needle can be inserted at a 90° angle in obese patients. However, this application may increase the risk of other complications. Alternatively, open-entry may be preferred. Some authors advocate direct trocar entry that may prevent preperitoneal emphysema without increasing other complications.

Pneumomediastinum results from migration of preperitoneal gas to the mediastinum. In the presence of a congenital diaphragmatic defect or intraoperative diaphragm injury, pneumomediastinum and pneumothorax may occur. The incidence is 0.2–1.9% for pneumothorax/pneumomediastinum.[44,45] Inhalation of 100% O_2 and application of a thorax tube after discharging CO_2 from the peritoneal cavity must be done. Pneumopericardium has been reported to occur in association with pneumomediastinum and subcutaneous emphysema.[45]

Persistence of Pneumoperitoneum

Because CO_2 is more rapidly absorbed than air, less intra-abdominal air persistence is observed postoperatively than in laparotomic operations. It is even less in obese patients than in lean patients. Generally, it does not persist after the seventh day. Therefore, when there is a lack of clinical suspicion and increments in serial X-rays, this finding does not point to an organ perforation.

GAS EMBOLISM

This is a rare but critical complication. It results from introduction of CO_2 through the Veress needle into the large veins. Its earliest sign is a drop in end-tidal CO_2 concentration, due to diminished blood flow to the lungs. Indicative features include sudden circulatory collapse, cyanosis, and raised jugular venous pressure. Blood coming from the Veress needle is an alert, and the needle should not be removed. It necessitates cardiopulmonary resuscitation. The patient lies on her left side. Aspiration of intracardiac gas may be tried. To prevent room-air embolism, which is more dangerous than CO_2, the air in the insufflation tube should be flushed out.

POSTOPERATIVE SHOULDER PAIN

Secondary to irritation of the diaphragm, shoulder pain is felt due to the noxious stimuli carried via the phrenic nerves. Also a stretched falciform ligament due to the Trendelenburg position adds to the shoulder pain. Careful discharge of intraperitoneal gas after the operation and counseling the patient is minimizes the discomfort.

VULVAR EDEMA

This occurs especially in patients in whom adhesion barrier solution is used; therefore, its leakage to the vulva is thought to be the cause. The method of the leakage could be either a patent canal of Nuck, as supported by the Adhesion Study Group, or a fistulous tract originating in a lower trocar puncture wound and dissecting downward subcutaneously by the force of gravity, as supported by others.[46,47]

OTHER COMPLICATIONS

Venous Thrombosis

Prolonged surgical time and the restricting effect of intraperitoneal pressure on venous return may lead to venous embolism.

Port-site Metastasis

The rate of port-site metastases in patients with gynecological malignancies is 1.1–2.3%.[48,49] Contrary to general belief, this rate is similar to the rate of wound metastasis seen in laparotomic gynecologic malignancy operations.[50]

Possible risk factors for port-site metastasis include:

- Aggressive disease
- CO_2 compared with other insufflating agents is associated with significantly increased tumor growth
- Pneumoperitoneum increases risk compared with gasless laparoscopy
- High efflux of gas from the abdominal cavity through the space around the trocars
- Decreased influence of the local immune system during laparoscopy.

The risk of port-site metastases is highest in patients with recurrence of ovarian or primary peritoneal malignancies with ascites.[49] The lavage of port-sites with cytotoxic agents (heparin, taurolidine, combination of heparin and taurolidine, 5-fluorouracil, doxorubicin, Povidone-iodine solution, and methotrexate) can be suggested as a possible preventive measure.

CONCLUSION

Laparoscopic gynecologic surgery is associated with a lower rate of complications due to extensive training and better instrumentation but is still not without risk. Certain conditions result in greater technical difficulty during surgery which are the risk factors associated with a higher frequency of complications. Hence, each patient should be evaluated thoroughly, and surgeons should perform the appropriately selected procedure carefully to prevent complications as far as possible. Complications should be identified as early as possible and must be duly managed as to minimize serious sequelae. Accurate documentation and timely communication will help in minimizing medicolegal issues.

KEY MESSAGES

- Laparoscopic gynecologic surgery is associated with a lower rate of complications due to extensive training and better instrumentation but is still not without risk.
- Each patient should be evaluated thoroughly, and surgeons should perform the appropriately selected procedure carefully to prevent complications.
- Complications should be identified as early as possible and must be duly managed as to minimize serious sequelae.
- Accurate documentation and timely communication will help in minimizing medicolegal issues.

REFERENCES

1. Gupta SP. Experience in 4500 cases of laparoscopic sterilization. Int Surg. 1993;78:76-8.
2. Chandler JG, Corson SL, Way LW. Three spectra of laparoscopic entry access injuries. J Am Coll Surg. 2001;192:478; discussion 490.
3. Porter JR. Management of intra- and postoperative complications. In: Cadeddu JA (ed) Laparoscopic urologic oncology. Humana Press, Totowa, 2004.p. 329.
4. Hasson HM. A modified instrument and method for laparoscopy. Am J Obstet Gynecol. 1971;110:886.
5. Lantz PE, Smith JD. Fatal carbon dioxide embolism complicating attempted laparoscopic cholecystectomy–case report and literature review. J Forensic Sci. 1994;39:1468.
6. Wolf JS Jr, Stoller ML. The physiology of laparoscopy: basic principles, complications and other considerations. J Urol. 1994;152:294.
7. Bateman BG, Kolp LA, Hoeger K. Complications of laparoscopy–operative and diagnostic. Fertil Steril. 1996;66:30.
8. Gill IS, Kavoussi LR, Clayman RV, Ehrlich R, Evans R, Fuchs G, et. al. Complications of laparoscopic nephrectomy in 185 patients: a multi-institutional review. J Urol. 1995;154:479
9. Gettman MT. Complications of laparoscopic access. In: Ramakumar S, Jarrett T (eds) Complications of urologic laparoscopic surgery. Taylor and Francis, Boca Raton, 2005. p. 13.
10. Moberg AC, Montgomery A. Primary access-related complications with laparoscopy: comparison of blind and open techniques. Surg Endosc. 2005;19:1196.
11. Colegrove P, Ramakumar S, Hernia. In: Ramakumar S, Jarrett T (eds) Complications of urologic laparoscopic surgery. Taylor and Francis, Boca Raton, p. 115.
12. Kulacoglu IH. Regarding: small bowel obstruction and incisional hernia after laparoscopic surgery: should 5-mm trocar sites be sutured? J Laparoendosc Adv Surg Tech A. 2000;10:227.
13. Magrina JF. Complications of laparoscopic surgery. Clin Obstet Gynecol. 2002;45:469-80.
14. Peterson HB, DeStefano F, Rubin GL, et al. Deaths attributable to tubal sterilization in the United States, 1977 to 1981. Am J Obstet Gynecol. 1983;146:131-6.
15. Soderstrom RM. Bowel injury ligation after laparoscopy. J Am Assoc Gynecol Laparosc. 1993;1:74-7.
16. Bishoff JT, Allaf ME, Kirkels W, et al. Laparoscopic bowel injury: Incidence and clinical presentation. J Urol. 1999;161:887-90.
17. Chapron C, Querleu D, Mage G, et al. Complications of gynaecologic laparoscopy. Multicentric study of 7,604 laparoscopies. J Gynecol Obstet Biol Reprod. 1992;21:207-13.
18. Jansen FW, Kapiteyn K, Trimbos-Kemper T, et al. Complications of laparoscopy: A prospective multicenter observational study. Br J Obstet Gynaecol. 1997;104:595-600.
19. Reich H, McGlynn F, Budin R. Laparoscopic repair of full-thickness bowel injury. J Laparoendoscopic Surg. 1991; 1:119-122
20. Bishoff JT, Allaf ME, Kirkels W, Moore RG, Kavoussi LR, Schroder F. Laparoscopic bowel injury: incidence and clinical presentation. J Urol. 1999;161:887.
21. Abdel-Meguid TA, Gomella LG. Prevention and management of complications. In: Smith AD, Badlani GH, Bagley DH, Clayman RV, Jordan GH, Kavoussi LR, Lingeman JE, Preminger GM, Segura JW (eds) Smith's textbook of endourology. Quality Medical, St. Louis, 1996.p. 851.
22. Li TC, Saravelos H, Richmond M, Cooke ID. Complications of laparoscopic pelvic surgery: recognition, management and prevention. Hum Reprod Up+date. 1997;3:505.
23. Saye WB, Miller W, Hertzmann P. Electrosurgery thermal injury. Myth or misconception? Surg Laparosc Endosc. 1991;1:223.
24. Hasson HM, Parker WH. Prevention and management of urinary tract injury in laparoscopic surgery. J Am Assoc Gynecol Laparosc. 1998;5:99-114.
25. Ostrzenski A, Ostrzenska KM. Bladder injury during laparoscopic surgery. Obstet Gynecol Surv. 1998;53:175-80.
26. Pillet MCL, Leonard F, Chopin N. Incidence and risk factors of bladder injuries during laparoscopic hysterectomy indicated for benign uterine pathologies: a 14.5 years experience in a continuous series of 1501 procedures. Hum Reprod. 2009;24:842-9.
27. Tanaka Y, Asada H, Kuji N, et al. Ureteral catheter placement for prevention of ureteral injury during laparoscopic hysterectomy. J Obstet Gynaecol Res. 2008;34:67-72.
28. Saidi MH, Vancaillie TG, White AJ, et al. Complications and cost of multipuncture laparoscopy: a review of 264 cases. Gynecol. Endosc. 1994;3:85-90.
29. Härkki-Siren P, Sjoberg J, Kurki T. Major complications of laparoscopy: A follow-up Finnish study. Obstet Gynecol. 1999;94:94-8.
30. Ostrzenski A, Radolinski B, Ostrzenska KM. A review of laparoscopic ureteral injury in pelvic surgery. Obstet Gynecol Surv. 2003;58:794-9.
31. Gordon AG, Lewis BV. Complications of laparoscopy. In: Gordon AG, Lewis BV, DeCherney AH (eds.) Atlas of Gynecologic Endoscopy. New York: Mosby-Wolfe; 1995:136-42.
32. Leff EI, Groff W, Rubin RJ, Eisenstat TE, Salvati EP. Use of ureteral catheters in colonic and rectal surgery. Dis Colon Rectum. 1982;25:457.
33. Hurt WG, Jones CM III. Intraoperative ureteral injuries and urinary diversion. In: Nichols DH, (ed.) Gynecologic and Obstetric Surgery. Baltimore: Mosby; 1993:900-10.
34. Li TC, Saravelos H, Richmond M, et al. Complications of laparoscopic pelvic surgery: recognition, management and prevention. Hum Reprod Update. 1997;3:505-15.
35. Chan JK, Morrow J, Manetta A. Prevention of ureteral injuries in gynaecologic surgery. Am J Obstet Gynecol. 2003;188:1273-7.
36. Donnez O, Jadoul P, Squifflet J, et al. A series of 3190 laparoscopic hysterectomies for benign disease from 1990 to 2006: evaluation of complications compared with vaginal and abdominal procedures. BJOG. 2009;116:492-500.
37. Oh BR, Kwon DD, Park KS, et al. Late presentation of ureteral injury after laparoscopic surgery. Obstet Gynecol. 2000;95:337-9.
38. Zaki H, Penketh R, Newton J. Gynaecological laparoscopy audit: Birmingham experience. Gynaecol Endosc. 1995;4:251-7.
39. Kavoussi LR. Complications of laparoscopic surgery. In: Bishoff JT, Kavoussi LR (eds) Atlas of laparoscopic retroperitoneal surgery. Saunders, Philadelphia, 2000.p. 237.
40. Munro MG. Laparoscopic access: complications, technologies, and techniques Curr Opin Obstet Gynecol. 2002;14:365-74.
41. Aksu T, Coskun F. Complications of gynaecological laparoscopy—a retrospective analysis of 3572 cases from a single institute. J Obstet Gynaecol. 2004;24: 813-6.

42. Vilos GA, Ternamian A, Dempster J, et al. Laparoscopic entry: a review of techniques, technologies, and complications. The Society of Obstetricians and Gynaecologists of Canada. J Obstet Gynaecol Can. 2007;29:433-65.
43. Leron E, Piura B, Ohana E, Mazor M. Delayed recognition of major vascular injury during laparoscopy. Eur J Obstet Gynecol Reprod Biol. 1998;79(1):91-3.
44. Murdock CM, Wolff AJ, Van Geem T. Risk factors for hypercarbia, subcutaneous emphysema, pneumothorax, and pneumomediastinum during laparoscopy. Obstet Gynecol. 2000;95:704-9.
45. Kalhan SB, Reaney JA, Collins RL. Pneumomediastinum and subcutaneous emphysema during laparoscopy. Cleve Clin J Med. 1990;57:639-42.
46. Adhesion Study Group. Reduction of postoperative pelvic adhesions with intraperitoneal 32% dextran 70: a prospective, randomized clinical trial. Fertil Steril. 1983;40:612-9.
47. Pados G, Vavilis D, Pantazis K, et al. Unilateral vulvar edema after operative laparoscopy: a case report and literature review. Fertil Steril. 2005;83:471-3.
48. Childers JM, Aqua KA, Surwit EA, et al. Abdominal-wall tumour implantation after laparoscopy for malignant conditions. Obstet Gynecol. 1994;84:765-9.
49. Nagarsheth NP, Rahaman J, Cohen CJ, et al. The incidence of port-site metastases in gynaecologic cancers. JSLS. 2004;8:133-9.
50. Ramirez PT, Frumovitz M, Wolf JK, et al. Laparoscopic port-site metastases in patients with gynaecological malignancies. Int J Gynecol Cancer. 2004;14:1070-7.

LONG QUESTIONS

1. What are the methods of reducing entry related complications in laparoscopy?
2. Discuss the features and management of suspected bowel injury on day 4 of laparoscopy.

SHORT QUESTIONS

1. What are the features that point towards the possibility of bladder trauma during laparoscopy?
2. How should ureteric integrity be tested during laparoscopy?
3. What are the complications related to patient position during laparoscopy?
4. What are the complications related to creation of pneumoperitoneum?
5. Mention the initial steps in the management of major vascular trauma at laparoscopy.

MULTIPLE CHOICE QUESTIONS

1. All of the following are complications of trocar introduction, except:
   a. Vascular injury b. Bladder injury
   c. Intestinal injury d. None of the above
2. Complications due to pneumoperitoneum during laparoscopy:
   a. Subcutaneous emphysema
   b Pneumomediastimum
   c Pneumothorax
   d All of the above
3. Which of the following is earliest sign of gas embolism?
   a. Tachycardia
   b. Cyanosis
   c. Drop in $ETCO_2$ concentration
   d. Raised jvp
4. Which of these is more common vascular complication during laparoscopy?
   a. Inferior episgastric vessel injury
   b. Superior epigastric
   c. Both
   d. None of the above
5. Which is leading cause of laparoscopic ureteral injury?
   a. Trocar injury b. Laser device injury
   c. Staple injury d. Electrocautery
6. Which is not a common site of ureteric injury during gynecologic laparoscopy?
   a. Near uterosacral ligament
   b. Above pelvic brim
   c. Near infundibulopelvic ligament
   d. Near uterine artery
7. Identifying bladder injury during laparoscopy is by:
   a. foley's bulb seen b. Air in Urine bag
   c. Haematuria d. All of the above
8. Lower bowel injury during laparoscopy can be managed by:
   a. Primary closure b. Colostomy
   c. Either 1 or 2 d. None of the above
9. Which gas is used for pmeumoperitoneum during laparoscopy?
   a. N_2O b. CO_2
   c. helium d. none of the above
10. Postoperative shoulder pain is felt through:
    a. Intercostal nerves b. Phrenic nerve
    c. Sympathetic plexus d. Vagus nerve
11. Nerve injuries caused due to incorrect positioning during laparoscopy:
    a. Common perineal nerve b. Brachial plexus
    c. Saphenous nerve d. All of the above
12. Most common nerve injury in gynecological laparoscopic procedures:
    a. Common perineal nerve b. Brachial plexus
    c. Saphenous nerve d. Sciatic nerve
13. Type of ureteric injury during gynecological laparoscopic surgery:
    a. Transection b. Avulsion
    c. Crush injury d. All of the above
14. Ureteric injury can be managed by:
    a. Ureteric reimplantation b. Boari flap
    c. Psoas Hitch for bladder d. All of the above

Answers

1.	d	2.	d	3.	c	4.	a	5.	d	6.	d
7.	d	8.	c	9.	b	10.	b	11.	d	12.	a
13.	d	14.	d								

11.5 SURGICAL TRAINING IN GYNAECOLOGICAL ENDOSCOPIC SURGERY

Pragnesh Shah, Foram Vora

INTRODUCTION

This chapter provides guidelines for practicing gynecologist and residency training program stake holders where training and exposure to advanced gynecological endoscopy training may be limited. The goal is that university residency program reformers and the practitioners review this chapter and determine independently which gynecological endoscopic procedures with preoperative selection criteria, potential advantages, availability of endoscopy instruments, OR set up in the department, safety measures, cost of the procedure and maintenance cost involved, skills necessary to perform a particular operation, gynecologist with adequate training to perform the procedure, identify the risks and complications of each procedure.

The reader should appreciate the need of learning and overall benefits gained by providing a particular endoscopic procedure to your patient. There is technological explosion in gynecological endoscopy, energy sources, 3D-HD camera system, Robotic surgery, etc., in last two decades but the cost of the procedure, patient's affordability and research is required to be critically reviewed and assessed in many areas of gynecological endoscopy by concerned stake holders and all of us.

Today following endoscopic training/curriculum are available in the different places:

- Apprentice-tutor (see one, assist one and do one) model
- Attending 1/2/3/5/7 days endoscopic training course
- Attending 1/2-day live workshop followed by hands on pelvic-trainer and hysteron-trainer
- 7 day and 15 days course in Gynecological Endoscopy
- 1/2/3 months course in Gynecological Endoscopy
- 6/12 months course in Gynecological Endoscopy
- 1/2 years Fellowship in Gynecological Endoscopy
- Video curriculum for Gynecologic Surgery
- Online curriculum for Gynecological Endoscopy
- Laparoscopic tubal ligation surgeon starts doing endoscopic surgery without any training
- Comprehensive structured gynecological endoscopic training of sufficient duration covering most of the important components.

Today training and education in endoscopic surgery has been critically reviewed.[1] Gynecologists who perform endoscopic surgery without proper training of the specific psychomotor (hand eye coordination) skills can leads to higher risk to increased patient morbidity and mortality.[1] Although the apprentice-tutor (see one, assist one and do one) model has long been a successful approach of training of surgeons, recently, clinicians have realized that endoscopic surgery requires an important training period outside the operating theater on simulator-pelvi-trainer-hystero-trainer/in pig/in cadaver before actually doing endoscopic surgery on patient.

Uniform structured curriculum[2] for gynecological endoscopic training is lacking despite the established value of simulators in surgical education.[2] Our primary objective is to develop comprehensive chapter for gynecological endoscopic training levels 1-2-3 which includes structured training/curriculum[1-3] reflecting different practice patterns at diverse institutions which includes cognitive knowledge-base-didactic lectures, practice exercises on simulator for technical skills development and assessment tasks for defining various well-defined benchmarks (tasks) on simulator for optimum outcome in patient following gynecological training.

Postgraduate residency program must include endoscopic training program in the department and practicing gynecologists should go to specialized centers for endoscopic training.

In all instance, ideal endoscopic training should include both theoretical background, practical preparations[1-4]—endoscopic psychomotor skills such as endoscopic camera navigation,[1] hand eye coordination, bimanual coordination on 2D screen and counter-intuitive movements for manipulating instruments,[1] assessment, credentialing and monitoring for quality control/validation and accreditation process.

THEORETICAL PREPARATIONS

The physician should have sound knowledge of obstetrics and gynecology before opting for endoscopic training. The aim of teaching theoretical knowledge is to offer in depth background information, recent development and understanding to prepare the trainee to perform sound, safe and effective endoscopic surgery. Theoretical teaching[1,2,4] should include:

- Knowledge of the abdomen and anterior abdominal wall, retroperitoneal spaces and pelvic anatomy.
- Knowledge of pathology of gynecological pelvic organs and gynecological conditions.
- Knowledge of various surgical techniques, suturing, hemostasis and dissection techniques.
- Knowledge of basic anesthesia techniques, muscle relaxants, pain killers, gas, multipara monitoring during endoscopic surgery, fluid balance, electricity, biochemical alterations.
- Detail knowledge about all laparoscopic and hysteroscopic instruments, indications and technique of relevant endoscopic procedure for the optimum performance.
- *Data entry:* Use of software for data entry and operative notes with documentations in the form of photos and

video recording, editing, auditing our data and Power Point (ppt) preparations in future.

PRACTICAL PREPARATIONS

Teaching should include didactic courses, lectures, videos, ppts, online or computer-generated programs. This should be followed by hands on practice[1-4] on pelvic-trainer, simulator, pig, cadaver for different level tasks and exercises to develop hand-eye coordination skills on non-tissue model and tissue models. From basic to more and more complex tasks-surgeries-exercises are designed to develop different types of skills required are listed in the chart of assessment. Practicing on pig or cadaver, assisting during endoscopic surgery and actually performing initial surgery in the presence of preceptor will definitely help in doing advanced endoscopic surgeries confidently and safely and will help in credentialing your surgical level and ultimately it will help in developing quality control and uniform accreditation process.

TODAY'S SCENARIO

Endoscopic surgery—laparoscopy and hysteroscopy—has become common place in recent gynecological surgical practice. It provides many advantages to the patients as a keyhole surgery as it involves minimally invasive surgery as a diagnostic or therapeutic-operative surgical procedure at many places. Today many diagnostic and therapeutic procedures in infertility, pain in abdomen, menorrhagia, painful menstrual periods, recurrent pregnancy loss, pelvic floor defects, etc., as the cause of it can be viewed and therapeutic procedure can be performed in pelvis, abdomen or uterine cavity without being commonly performed conventional laparotomy. Despite many advantages it provides, it should not be considered a panacea, as it is a like any surgical procedure and it has also the risk of complication as every procedure and because of endoscopic surgery itself and if selection of patient and proper training is not taken adequately.

Very commonly feared first entry of Veress needle and trocar insertion for pneumoperitoneum creation is blind which can sometimes leads to accidental complication of vascular and intestinal injury due to improper selection of patient, preoperative assessment, preoperative counseling, faulty technique and injury not detected and managed timely leads to morbidity and even mortality. Complication of first blind entry is not associated with surgery performed by laparotomy. So here lies the importance of proper training before trying complication free endoscopic surgery on patient.

Why Surgical Training in Gynaecological Endoscopic Surgery is Advisable Today for Every Gynaecologist?

Today many classical gynecological surgeries are replaced by endoscopic surgery such as tubal ligation, adnexal surgery, ectopic pregnancy, myomectomy, hysterectomy, endometriosis surgeries, infertility surgeries, cancer surgeries, septum, endometrial polyp, Asherman's syndrome, etc., because of obvious advantages of the procedure itself, no inconvenience of a large incision, there is less disfigurement, often less expense, faster recovery and resuming to work earlier, better outcome, even the possibility of less extensive postoperative adhesions and its sequalae, video recording of the procedure, difficult and complex surgeries can be performed better and safely after appropriate training.

Because of advantages of endoscopic surgeries are very much popular, many times patient demands endoscopic surgery from the gynecologist. With advent of more and more conferences, workshop, CMEs, webinars we are also exposed to many new procedures and we feel that we should learn, do and should be introduced into our practice.

Gynecologist should have learned endoscopic surgery during residency but at residency programs limitations are:

- Residents often do not get exposure, experience, opportunity of assisting and viewing endoscopic surgery during residency.
- Residency training programs do not have appropriately trained teachers for endoscopic surgery.
- Attending 1 day, 2 days, 3 days course may not qualify anyone for anything.
- Performing laparoscopy for tubal ligation, cauterize minimal endometriosis, to lyse a few adhesions, hysteroscopic removal of small polyp does not prepare a gynecological surgeon to perform advanced operative laparoscopic or hysteroscopic procedures.

The basis of endoscopic training is practicing on simulator before doing on patient: Pelvic trainer **(Fig. 1)**, hystero-trainer **(Fig. 2)**, with various tissue and non-tissue training models **(Fig. 3)** have been shown to be the most significant contributor to laparoscopic and hysteroscopic training because of 3D pelvic and abdominal organs trainee has to see/view in 2D monitor

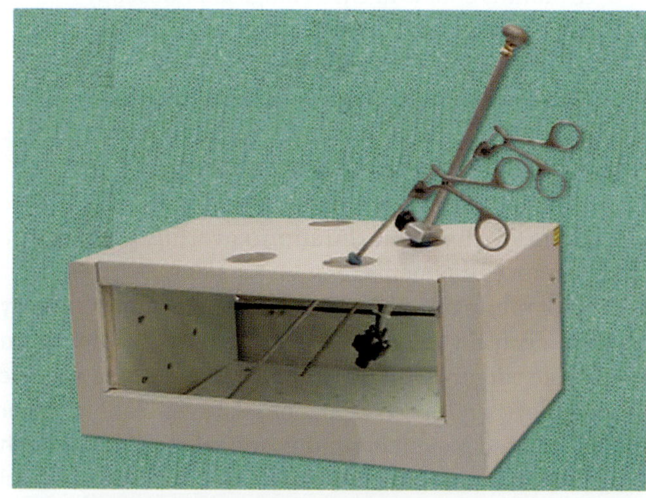

Fig. 1: Pelvic-trainer: Simulator for laparoscopic practical training practice.

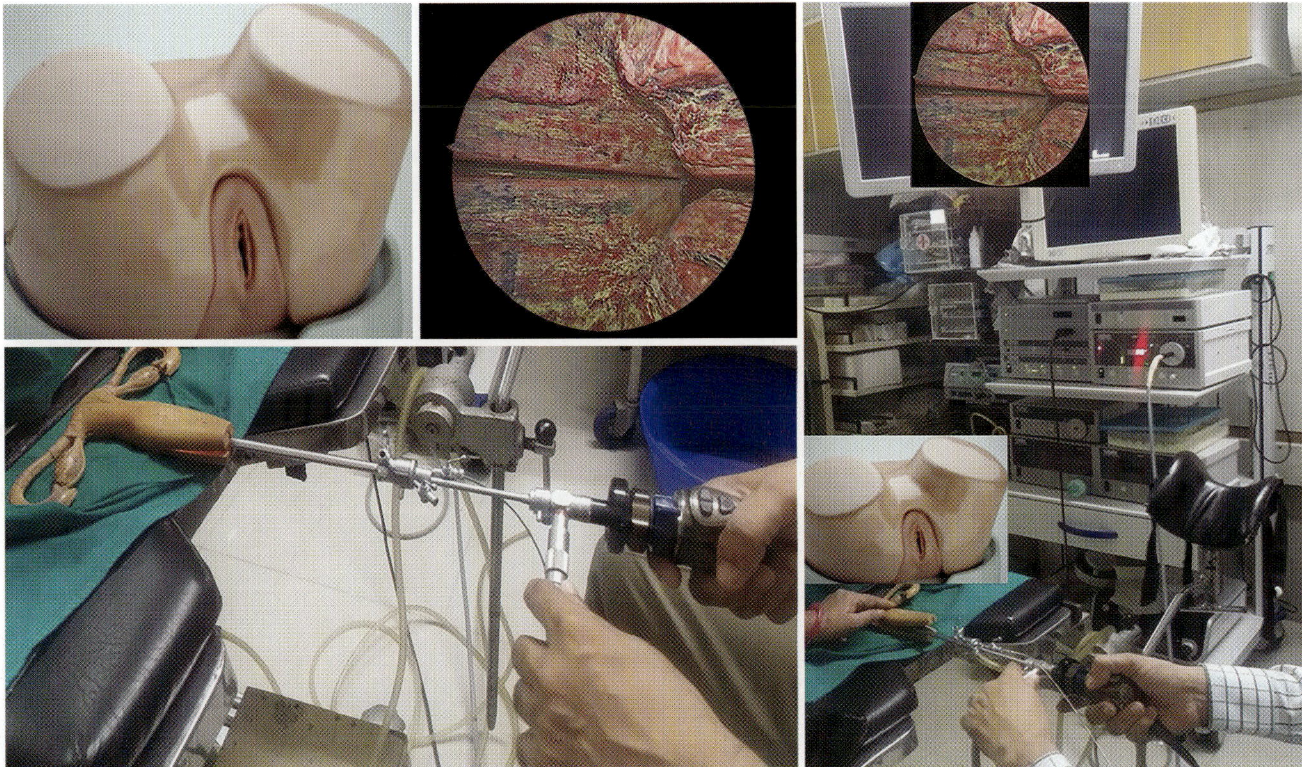

Fig. 2: Hystero-trainer: Simulator for hysteroscopic training practice.

with loss of depth perception and operate. Pelvic-trainer box **(Fig. 4)** and virtual reality simulators **(Fig. 5)** allow novice trainee to progress along the steep part of the learning curve before actually doing on patient in operating room. Various organizations,[1,4,5] also emphasize that training in laparoscopic and hysteroscopic surgery should take place in a simulated environment before the learner seeks experiences on a patient. The value of simulators may be enhanced through achievable proficiency benchmarks (various tasks to be performed on simulator) for level-1/level-2/level-3, i.e., basic/intermediate/advanced laparoscopic/hysteroscopic surgeries for assessment to validate proficiency-based skills on them.

STRUCTURED TRAINING/CURRICULUM

Comprehensive training/curriculum is necessary for teaching gynecological endoscopy by Delphi consensus.[2] Proficiency-based training[2] and structured curriculum[2] is the need of hour in current educational standards[4,5] to deliver patient safety and reducing morbidity and mortality following improper laparoscopic surgical skills. The use of checklists before planning an endoscopic surgery **(Box 1)** and in the operation theater **(Box 2)** are useful to achieve this goal.

Different curriculum for basic, intermediate and advanced level following classroom/online lectures are required before practicing tasks/exercises on simulator. Following are mandatory lectures:

- Designing a structured laparoscopy curriculum[2] for gynecology endoscopy **(Tables 1 to 3)**
  - For
    - Basic level
    - Intermediate level
    - Advanced level
    - *Procedure specific:* Cancer/retroperitoneal dissection/tubal anastomosis, etc.
  - *For cognitive items:*
    - Preoperative counseling and procedure specific consent
    - Laparoscopic and hysteroscopic instruments—information, identification, use, care, sterilization and maintenance
    - Needles and sutures used in pelvic trainer and patients
    - Understanding principals of different energy sources in endoscopic surgeries
    - Anterior abdominal wall and pelvic anatomy
    - Preoperative patient assessment, selection and preparations
    - Operating room (OR) checklists and intraoperative considerations
    - Specific requirements in specific laparoscopic surgeries
    - Anticipation and avoidance of intraoperative near miss complication
    - Postoperative complication and management
    - Achieving hemostasis with different techniques in gynecological endoscopy
    - Medicolegal issues.

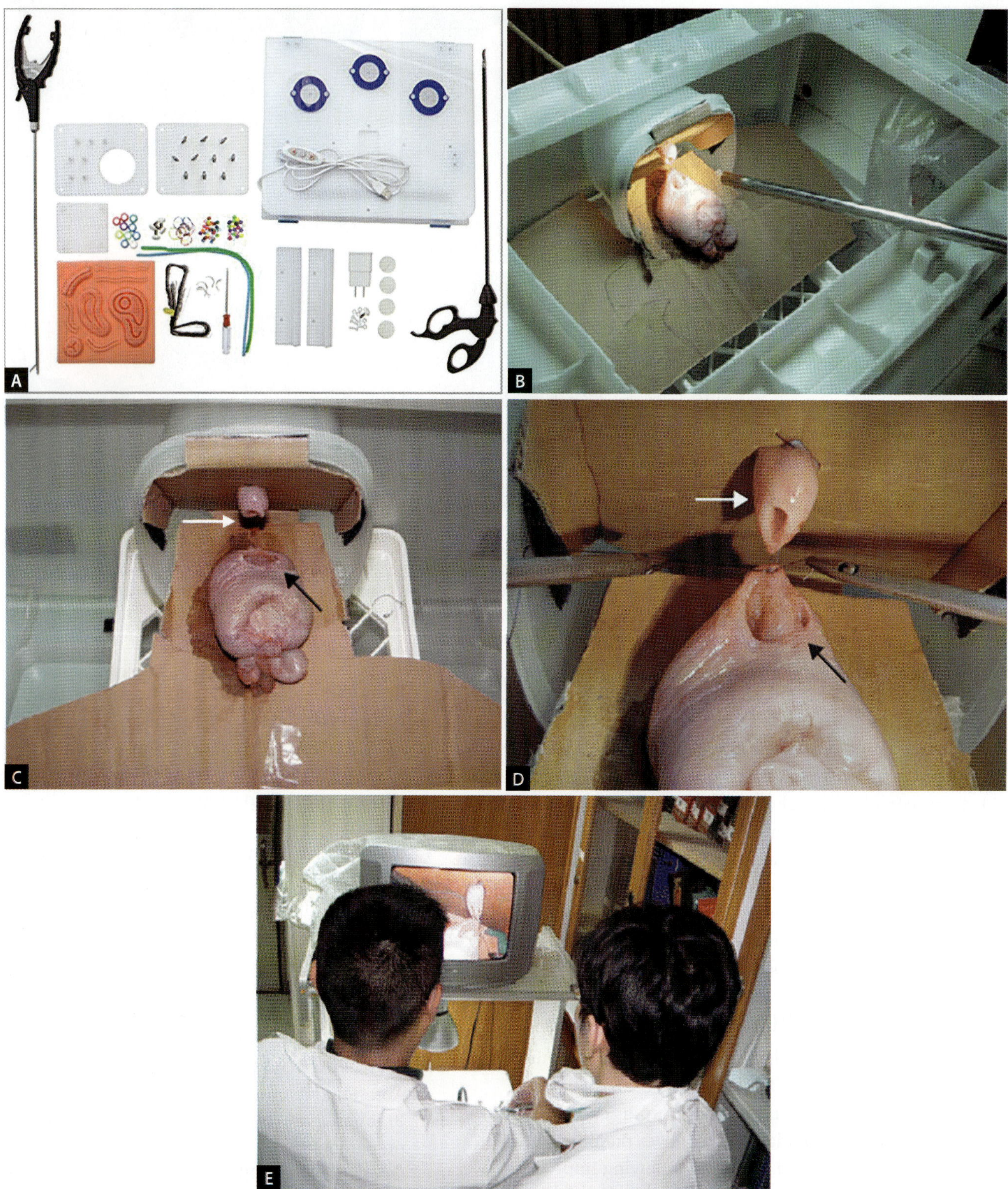

Figs. 3A to E: Various non-tissue and tissue models for different defined benchmark tasks/exercises for level 1/2/3 laparoscopic and hysteroscopic training.

- *For technical items:*
    - Laparoscopic primary and alternative entry techniques-in normal patient, obese patient and previous surgery patient
    - *Hand-eye coordination:* Instruments maneuvering in pelvic trainer/simulator
    - Laparoscopic tubal ligation/salpingectomy
    - Laparoscopic ovarian cystectomy
    - Diagnostic hysteroscopy and tubal cannulation on hystero-trainer
    - Ectopic pregnancy
    - Fibroid – Laparoscopic and hysteroscopic

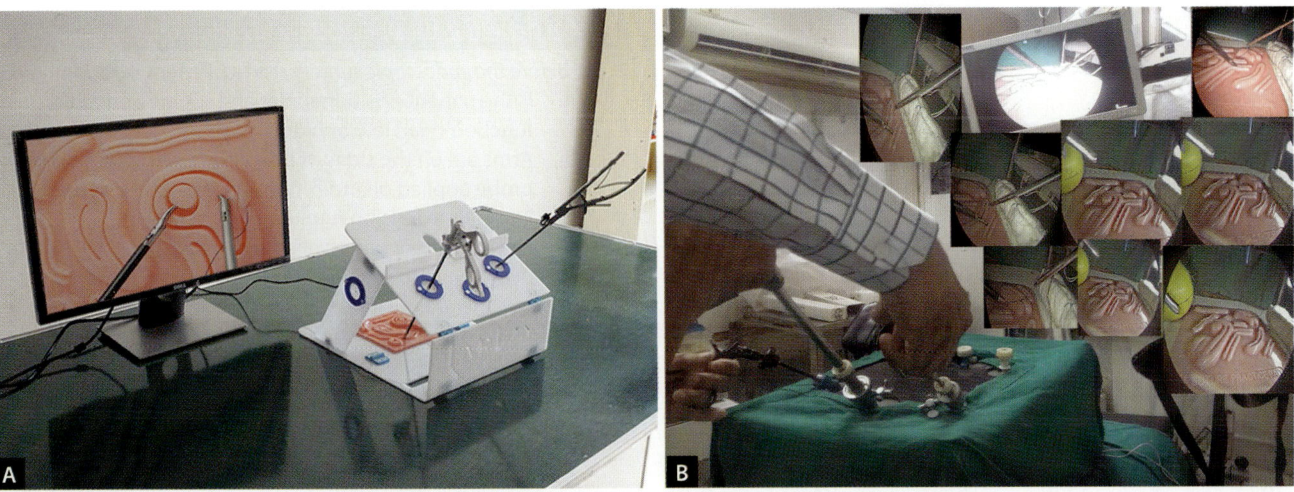

Figs. 4A and B: Laparo-pelvic trainer and various tools for exercises.

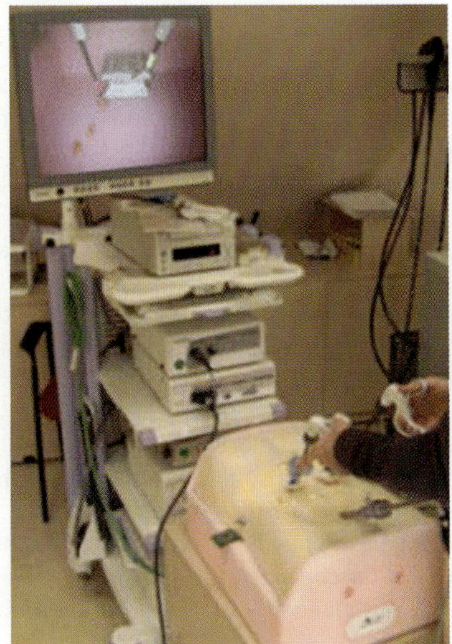

Fig. 5: Simulator.

- Total laparoscopic hysterectomy
- Endometriosis
- Adnexal mass/TO mass/ovarian cysts/tumors
- Pelvic floor defects, vault and nulliparous prolapse
- Burch's procedure and lateral cystocele repair
- Laparoscopic vaginoplasty in MRKH syndrome
- Laparoscopic and hysteroscopic surgeries in Müllerian malformations
- Endometriosis of rectovaginal and rectosigmoid part
- Urinary tract endometriosis
- Fertility enhancing surgeries and PCOD
- Endoscopic surgeries in recurrent pregnancy loss
- Adhesions prevention during laparoscopic/hysteroscopic surgeries
- Extracorporeal suturing
- Intracorporeal suturing
- Continuous running suture and shoe less suture

- *For non-technical items:*
  - Ergonomics of operation theatre in endoscopy theater
  - Ideal practice scenario
  - Crisis scenario.

- *Theoretical part:* The above detail didactic theoretical lectures can be learned from textbook, online, classroom lectures with active interaction with expert knowledgeable faculty in classroom or virtual class room to understand better and clarify any quarry or clarification.
- Practicing on non-tissue/pelvic-trainer/simulator/Pig/Cadaver
  Laparoscopic/hysteroscopic procedure specific procedures can be practiced on:
  - Lapro-pelvic trainer, hystero-trainer
  - On placenta in pelvic trainer-effect of monopolar and bipolar
  - In hysteron-trainer and mirchi-model for small polyp and septum practice
  - In pig, Veress needle, trocar insertion, tubectomy, anastomosis, retro-peritoneal dissection, bladder and intestinal repair, etc.
  - Cadaver dissection: Veress needle, trocar insertion, tubectomy, anastomosis, retroperitoneal dissection, bladder and intestinal repair, etc.

Comprehensive structured training/curriculum for basic, intermediate and advanced levels which includes topics and time duration for different levels: Following different lectures, OR and instrumentation orientations, pelvic-trainer and hysteron-trainer orientation, practicing different tasks daily with increasing complexity and procedure specific exercises, video ppt of procedures demonstrating different dissection technique, actually doing procedure specific live surgery in pig, cadaver, patient in advanced endoscopic surgery gives best hands on, training and practice under the guidance of expert faculty/preceptor.

BOX 1: Preoperative checklist before laparoscopic surgery.

1. *Preoperative investigations:* Blood and urine for major surgery with electrolytes
2. Preoperative Covid-19 test and if positive contact history with cough/fever-CT-X-ray chest
3. Preoperative physician fitness/checkup for major surgery
4. Preoperative 2D Echo and X-Ray- chest- if age more than 50 years or h/o dyspnea
5. *Bowel preparation:* Liquid diet on previous day of endoscopic surgery and Peglac on previous day evening or 6 hours prior to endoscopic surgery
6. Do not take any food drink (even water) after midnight prior to the day of surgery
7. Stop taking aspirin 3 days prior to surgery if you are taking regularly
8. Do not forget to take tablet Thyroxin or antihypertensive tablet early in the morning on the day of surgery
9. Do not wear jewelry or metallic ornaments
10. Remove nail polish before surgery
11. Any prior history of medical disorder/anesthesia/allergy of any medicines in the past
12. Latest sonography/CT/MRI report available
13. Is the indication endoscopic surgery correct?
    i. Any doubt about the diagnosis
    ii. Have you offered alternative treatment/therapy/ intervention to the patient
14. Is the endoscopic surgeon being ok with proposed planned intervention?
    i. Have you acquired the skills for proposed endoscopic surgery?
    ii. What are my personal experience and results about the proposed endoscopic procedure?
    iii. Discussed about the same procedure by laparotomy—pros and cons
    iv. Your past complicated assessed and audited for the proposed endoscopic surgery
    v. Issue of removal of ovary discussed and counseling about menopause.
15. Is the OR set up and environment OK?
    i. Who is going to assist—complicated/difficult surgery requires experienced team?
    ii. PPE kits, filters for aerosol contamination, headshield—required preparations
    iii. Checking endoscopic tower and electrocautery
16. Is the patient had asked for video recording registration?
    i. Patient's relative seeing the live video during endoscopic surgery
    ii. Recorded video given to the patient for future prospects and helps in redo surgery in future
    iii. Video registration is a strong assurance that the surgeon feels confident.
17. Need for GI surgeon or urologist or multidisciplinary approach required/counseled:
    i. Anticipation of GI and urological complication in complicated cases counseled
    ii. Tentatively booked GI surgeon or urologist during proposed timing of the operation
18. Endoscopic procedure explained well with all potential complications
19. Endoscopic procedure specific consent taken in patient's language
20. Anesthetist have done patient's preoperative checkup

BOX 2: Operation theater checklist in endoscopic surgery.

1. *Before the endoscopic surgery started:* Patient positioning:
    i. Is the patient positioned flat and supine and table function-head low or high?
    ii. Arms are on the sides of the patient with pulse oximetry probe applied on index finger and BP cuff applied and IV line with extension functioning smoothly.
    iii. Electrocautery pad applied over muscular part and not over bony prominent parts
2. *Before the endoscopic surgery started:* Instruments check:
    i. Video monitor functioning
    ii. Video monitor appropriately positioned for hysteroscopy/ laparoscopy
    iii. Check CO_2 cylinder/tank/central line adequately filled and valves opened
    iv. Is the endo camera and light source functioning correctly?
    v. Are laparotomy instruments being ready and available in OT?
    vi. Are the electric codes, adaptors, forceps checked and functions normally?
3. *Before incision:*
    i. Verification of OT table, adequate lithotomy position with soft pads under popliteal fossa and bony prominence to prevent nerve pressure injury
    ii. Connecting with electrocautery, grounding, connecting cords, checking functioning
    iii. Properly placing monopolar and bipolar pedal at surgeon's feet
    iv. Tubing's with Luer's lock connected with suction machine-functioning and attached to suction and irrigation cannula
    v. Verification of monitor, camera, light source cable—positioning and functioning.
    vi. Verification of CO_2 insufflator connecting with filter, tubing and checking functioning
    vii. Checking Veress needle, hand instruments and trocars for specific endoscopic surgery
    viii. Checking other energy sources and their probe functioning
    ix. Checking necessary instruments on vaginal end-dilators, manipulator, RT cannula, etc.
    x. Emptying bladder and stomach in complicated cases to avoid accidental injuries

- *Assessment and progress:* Assessment should be done by expert preceptor from the observation of various assessment components/tasks for different levels 1/2/3. For different level endoscopic surgeries established benchmarks/tasks in simulator, online software program, computer generate program, live surgery in pig, live surgery in cadaver, during assisting surgery in OR, actually doing surgery in OR from the basis of—*how trainee does/ performs camera navigation, instrument navigation, target navigation, associating during endoscopic surgery.*
  Many organizations insist on quality of logbook-daily work record during training period-seeing video recording of individually performed endoscopic surgeries and directly observing - especially in robotic endoscopic surgery training - how confidently he can perform for accreditation process **(Tables 4 to 6)**.[1,4,5]

TABLE 1: Proposed training/curriculum for basic course in endoscopy surgery for 6 weeks.

1st week	*2nd week*	*3rd week*	*4th week*	*5th week*	*6th week*
Introduction to laparoscopy- didactic lecture: 1 hour	Principals of Electrosurgery: 2 hours	Lecture on selection of patient and preoperative assessment 1 hour	Lecture on female anatomical considerations—pelvic and abdominal wall	Lecture on OR checklist, OR ergonomics	Lecture on complications
Laparoscopy instruments: 1 hour	Hysteroscopy instruments: 1 hour	Live surgery Assisting vaginal end	Live surgery-assisting	Live surgery	Live surgery
Pelvic-trainer simple exercises with one hand camera and another hand instrument- 2 hours	Skill station on pelvic-trainer -6 tasks 3 hours	Skill station on pelvic-trainer 6 tasks 3 hours	Skill station Pelvic trainer 6 tasks 3 hours	Skill station Needle and suture grasping, holding, passing	Skill station Intracorporeal knot tying
Pelvic-Trainer – Two hands peg transfer: 2 hours	Skill station on hystero-trainer – 2 hours	Skill station on hystero-trainer-1 hour	Skill station hystero-trainer-1 hour	Pelvic-trainer Extra-corporeal knot tying	Skill station—coordination, precision and speed
Circle cutting -2 hours	Skill station	OT notes and video editing	Video and ppt. Preparation-ectopic	Video ppt Specific procedure-adhesiolysis	Video ppt Specific procedure-septum
Live surgery in OR watching	Live surgery in OR watching	Live surgery assisting	Live surgery or Video discuss-polyp	Video ppt Specific procedure-PCOD	Exam-assessment
Logbook filling	Logbook filling	Logbook filling	Logbook filling	Log book filling	Logbook filling

TABLE 2: Proposed training/curriculum for Intermediate course in endoscopy surgery for 3 weeks.

1st week	*2nd week*	*3rd week*
Lecture on laparoscopic and hysteroscopic instruments	Lecture on fibroid	Lecture on endometriosis
Live surgery and assisting	Live surgery-assisting	Live surgery-assisting
Lecture on TLH	Lecture on consent and medicolegal aspect	Lecture on GI and intestinal complications
Lecture on hysteroscopic complications and safety-distention medium	*Skill station:* Pelvic-trainer-procedure specific exercises	*Skill station:* Pelvic-trainer-procedure specific exercises
Skill station: Pelvic-trainer-procedure specific exercises	*Skill station:* Hystero-trainer-procedure specific exercises	*Skill station:* Hystero-trainer-procedure specific exercises
Skill station: Hystero-trainer-procedure specific exercises	Video ppts-procedure-Hyst Surgeries-Tubal cannulation	Exam-assessment
Video ppts-procedure: Ovarian mass	Video ppts-procedure-Hysteroscopic complications	Exam-assessment
Logbook filling	Logbook filling	Logbook filling

- *Accreditation/credentialing of basic/intermediate/advanced training privileges:* Adequate credentialing of basic, intermediate and advanced laparoscopic and hysteroscopic levels with help of established tasks/exercises/benchmarks on pelvic trainer/simulator and during live surgery will help trainee in developing confidence of doing independent and safe endoscopic surgery and serves the purpose of adequate endoscopic training.[1,4,5]
- *Enhancing the advanced and future training in professional growth[4] can be monitored[4] by:* Monitoring[4] and skills improvement can be achieved by applying to professional body/organization for renewal of accreditation on the basis of following points for offering best performance in advanced endoscopic surgeries and better patient outcome:
  - Successfully attending relevant masterclass and examinations for specific advanced endoscopic procedure.
  - Attendance at workshops, CMEs, updates and postgraduate courses approved by reputed organizations.

TABLE 3: Proposed curriculum for advanced course in endoscopy surgery for 2 weeks.

Day-1	Laparoscopic port entry with previous surgeries	Live surgery	Prevention of adhesions in endoscopic surgeries	Video ppt Pelvic and retroperitoneal anatomy	Specific instruments requirements in specific surgery	Medico legal consideration and preoperative counseling	Logbook filling
Day-2	Lecture on advanced laparoscopic surgery	Live surgery	Video ppt Fibroid Previous-adhesions	Video ppt Fibroid-large size	Video ppt Fibroid-multiple	Video ppt Fibroid-soft-degenerated	Logbook filling
Day-3	Lecture on pelvic floor defects/ prolapse	Live surgery	Video ppt Nulliparous prolapse	Video ppt Vault prolapse	Video ppt Lateral cystocele repair	Video ppt Burch's colposuspension	Logbook filling
Day-4	Lecture on hysterectomy	Live surgery	Video ppt TLH Previous-CS	Video ppt TLH Large uterus	Video ppt TLH Rectovaginal endometriosis	Video ppt Prolapse UT	Logbook filling
Day-5	Lecture on lap. TO mass and ovarian mass	Live surgery	Video ppt Obese patient	Video ppt Fibroid-cervical fibroid	Video ppt Broad ligament fibroid	Video ppt TOT	Logbook filling
Day-6	Lecture on fertility enhancing surgeries	Live surgery	Video ppt On PCOD	Skill station-fibroid model	Skill station-fibroid model	Skill station-fibroid model	Logbook filling
Day-7	Lecture on advanced hysteroscopic surgery	Live surgery	Video ppt. Asherman's syndrome	Skill station Practice on hysteron-trainer	Skill station Practice on hysteron-trainer	Skill station-Laparoscopic hysterectomy model	Logbook filling
Day-8	Lecture on endoscopic management of Müllerian malformations	Live surgery	Video ppt Laparoscopic vaginoplasty	Skill station Practice on hysteron-trainer	Skill station-Laparoscopic model	Skill station-Laparoscopic model	Logbook filling
Day-9	Lecture od redo laparoscopic surgery	Live surgery	Video ppt Laparoscopic Chocolate cysts	Skill station Practice on hysteron-trainer	Skill station-Laparoscopic model	Skill station-Laparoscopic model	Logbook filling
Day-10	Lecture on severe endometriosis	Live surgery	Practice on Pig-advanced retroperitoneal dissection	Practice on Pig-advanced retroperitoneal dissection	Practice on Pig-advanced retroperitoneal dissection	Practice on Pig-advanced retroperitoneal dissection	Logbook filling
Day-11	Lecture on cancer and lymphadenectomy	Live surgery	Practice on Pig-advanced retroperitoneal dissection	Practice on Pig-advanced retroperitoneal dissection	Practice on Pig-advanced retroperitoneal dissection	Practice on Pig-advanced retroperitoneal dissection	Logbook filling
Day-12	Lecture on tubal anastomosis	Live surgery	Practice on pig/ cadaver	Practice on pig/ cadaver	Practice on pig/ cadaver	Practice on pig/ cadaver	Logbook filling
Day-13	Lecture on rare surgeries	Video ppt rare surgery	Video ppt Rare surgery	Video ppt Rare surgery	Video ppt Rare surgery	Video ppt Rare surgery	Logbook filling
Day-14	Exam theory	Exam theory	Assessment on skill station	Assessment on pelvic-trainer	Assessment on pelvic-trainer		

- Acceptance and auditing of our cases, indications, results and sending to it for accreditation process
- Sending and compiling list of endoscopic procedures performed, complications in a year
- Involving in quality control and auditing activities by professional bodies
- Sending list of research studies done, paper published during year
- Participation in multicenter various studies every year.

TABLE 4: For basic course skills assessment: Preceptor gives marks from 1 to 10 in every box for scoring purpose.

Task	***In pelvic trainer – assessed by faculty***	***In computerized simulator assessed by computer***	***Online software available for practice***	***In patient done/assisted assessed by surgeon in OR***
Camera navigation	1–10	1–10	1–10	1–10
Target navigation				
Instruments navigation				
Coordination with primary surgeon/ assistant				
Grasping-suture/needle				
Cutting round circle on paper and suture				
Clip applying on tubular structure				
Peg transfer				
Lifting and grasping				
Precision and speed				
Gently handling intestines				
Endoloop				
Tubal occlusion				
Salpingectomy				
Salpingostomy				
Lap TL-Falope ring				
Diagnostic laparoscopy				
Diagnostic hysteroscopy and Cu-T removal				
Hysteroscopic tubal cannulation				
Total assessment				

TABLE 5: For intermediate course assessment: Preceptor gives marks from 1 to 10 in every box for scoring purpose.

Task	***In pelvic trainer– assessed by faculty***	***In computerized simulator assessed by computer***	***In pig or cadaver assessed by faculty***	***Online software available for practice***	***In patient done/assisted assessed by surgeon in OR***
• Camera navigation • Target navigation • Instruments navigation • Coordination with primary surgeon/assistant • Hemostasis help	1–10 1–10 1–10 1–10 1–10				
Laparoscopic Myomectomy					
Laparoscopic surgery for endometriosis					
Lap. surgery for adnexal mass					
Total laparoscopic hysterectomy					
Laparoscopic adhesiolysis					
Laparoscopic hemostasis					
Hysteroscopic septum excision					

Contd...

Contd...

Task	*In pelvic trainer–assessed by faculty*	*In computerized simulator assessed by computer*	*In pig or cadaver assessed by faculty*	*Online software available for practice*	*In patient done/assisted assessed by surgeon in OR*
Hysteroscopic small polyp/fibroid					
Hysteroscopic adhesiolysis for mild adhesions					
Laparoscopic ovarian cystectomy					
Laparoscopic salpingo-oophrectomy					
Laparoscopic suturing					
Total assessment					

TABLE 6: For advanced course assessment: Preceptor gives marks from 1 to 10 in every box for scoring purpose.

Task	*In pelvic trainer—assessed by faculty*	*In computerized simulator assessed by computer*	*In Pig or cadaver assessed by faculty*	*Online software available for practice*	*No. of procedures done/assisted assessed by surgeon in OR*
• Camera navigation	1–10				
• Target navigation	1–10				
• Instruments navigation	1–10				
• Co-ordination with primary surgeon/assistant	1–10				
• Hemostasis help	1–10				
Difficult TLH					
Large uterus TLH					
Large fibroid surgery					
Bladder and ureter injury and repair					
Tubal micro surgery					
Retroperitoneal dissection					
Gyne-cancer surgery					
Redo endometriosis surgeries					
Hysteroscopic submucous fibroid resection					
Hysteroscopic adhesiolysis					
Laparoscopic suturing					
Total assessment					

(TLH: total laparoscopic hysterectomy)

CONCLUSION

After standardized endoscopic training[5] there was improvement in laparoscopic and hysteroscopic skills. Many organizations can replicate[5] the endoscopic training format partly or completely described with the objective of enhancing and assessing the skills from the basis of established benchmark tasks/exercises on different platforms.

KEY MESSAGES

Today many classical gynecological surgeries are replaced by endoscopic surgery. Because of advantages of endoscopic surgeries are very much popular. Laparoscopy and hysteroscopy has become common place in recent gynecological surgical practice. Today training and education in endoscopic surgery has been critically reviewed. Gynecologists who perform endoscopic surgery without proper training of the specific psychomotor (hand eye coordination) skills in OR are at higher risk to increased patient morbidity and mortality. Uniform structured comprehensive curriculum training is necessary for teaching gynecological endoscopy by proficiency-based training assessment, validation, credentialing, accreditation process, and monitoring every 3 years for professional development and quality.

REFERENCES

1. Campo R, Wattiez A, Tanos V, Di Spiezio Sardo A, Grimbizis G, Wallwiener D, et al. Gynaecological endoscopic surgical education and assessment. A diploma programme in gynaecological endoscopic surgery. Gynecol Surg. 2016;13:133-7.
2. Shore EM, Lefebvre GG, Husslein H, Bjerrum F, Sorensen JL, Grantcharov TP. Designing a Standardized Laparoscopy Curriculum for Gynecology Residents: a Delphi Approach. J Grad Med Educ. 2015;7(2):197-202.
3. Levinson CJ, Kaufman RH. Learning, certification and credentialing for endoscopic surgery. In: Sanfilippo JS, Levine RL (Eds). Operative Gynecologic Endoscopy. London: Springer; 1996. pp. 435-41.
4. Chapron C, Devroey P, Dubuisson JB, Pouly JL, Vercellini P. ESHRE guidelines for training, accreditation and monitoring in gynecological endoscopy. Hum Reprod. 1997;12(4):867-8.
5. Fernandes CFK, Ruano JM, Kati LM, Noguti AS, Girão MJ, Sartori MC. Assessment of laparoscopic skills of Gynecology and Obstetrics residents after a training program. Einstein (São Paulo). 2016;14(4):468-72.

LONG QUESTIONS

1. How gynecologist should plan and learn endoscopic training?
2. Why structured gynecological endoscopic training in necessary today?
3. Describe the various methods of assessment of gynecological endoscopic skills.
4. Describe the preoperative checklists before endoscopic surgery.
5. Describe the checklist in operation theater before incision kept on patient.

SHORT QUESTIONS

1. What is simulator?
2. Which are the advantages of gynecological endoscopic surgery?
3. Why gynecological endoscopic surgery is becoming popular today?
4. Which are the components used for credentialing gynecological endoscopic skills?
5. Which are the components used for monitoring of advanced endoscopic skills and professional growth?

MULTIPLE CHOICE QUESTIONS

1. What is the best way of gynecologic endoscopy training?
   a. Online web-based training
   b. Attending 1/2/3 days endoscopic training course
   c. Video curriculum for gynecologic endoscopic training
   d. Structured proficiency-based training on simulator
2. Following different simulators for gynecologic endoscopic training are used, except:
   a. Pelvitrainer
   b. Hystero-trainer
   c. Computer-based exercises on desktop/laptop
   d. Suture practice pad
3. Complications can be reduced in gynecological endoscopic surgery by:
   a. Trying laparoscopic surgery after doing many laparoscopic tubal ligation operations
   b. Attending laparoscopy and hysteroscopy workshop and trying in our OT
   c. After attending online lecture course
   d. After attending comprehensive gynecological endoscopic training for sufficient duration
4. Advanced laparoscopic training requires minimum exposure of:
   a. Taken basic and intermediate levels of training and individually done level-1/2 surgeries
   b. Web-based training
   c. Simulator based practice on non-tissue model
   d. Above all plus assisting and doing advanced surgery under the guidance of preceptor-minimum 10–15 cases
5. Who can take Gynecological endoscopic training?
   a. MBBS Doctor
   b. MS, General Surgeon
   c. First year resident
   d. Gynecologist with postgraduate qualifications

Answers

1. d 2. c 3. d 4. d 5. d

11.6 ENERGY SOURCES IN ENDOSCOPIC SURGERY

Prakash Trivedi, Soumil Trivedi

Nothing is permanent except change in medical practice. However, every change is not progress. Any progressive change has to benefit patient.

In knowledge-based society, knowledge and skill will be power only if wisdom is used along with out of the box thinking.

PRINCIPLES OF SURGERY

We all learnt surgery by Halstedstein principles of surgery: Dissection for safe access, resection and reconstruction to optimize wound healing.

Hippocrates suggested, "fire succeeds when all methods fail". The basis of using "fire" is ancient. Today's modern surgical equipments allow us to achieve a balance of cutting and coagulation.

Is Electrocautery and Electrosurgery Same?

In electrosurgery, the body forms a part of the electrosurgical circuit. A high frequency alternating current is passed through living tissue. There is a manipulation of electrons to produce heat within the cells to destroy tissues.

On the other hand, in electrocautery, the body is not part of the circuit. There is a direct current which passes through a high resistance metallic conductor. The surgical process is therefore, not as precise as with electrosurgery.

HISTORY

The use of electrical energy during surgery was first described by William Bovie in the 1920s. Further adaptations for practical use came from a neurosurgeon, Harvey Cushing at about the same time. These were the first monopolar grounded electrosurgical units (ESU) **(Fig. 1)**. In earlier days, all ESUs were grounded. This means the dispersion of current was to the ground. In modern practice, ESUs are isolated, i.e., the dispersion of current is to the ESU and not to the ground.

Further, Cushing also realized that the frequency of electrical current during surgery has to be above 100 kHz to prevent stimulation of nerves and muscles. In households, the frequency of electrical current is 60 Hz. Electrical current at this frequency can cause neural and muscular stimulation - in common language, this is an electric shock. This frequency cannot be used for electrosurgery.

William Green (1946), again, a neurosurgeon introduced the concept of bipolar cautery. This was further refined by Kleppinger, a gynecologist who devised an instrument which would achieve bipolar cautery with less compression and tissue trauma.

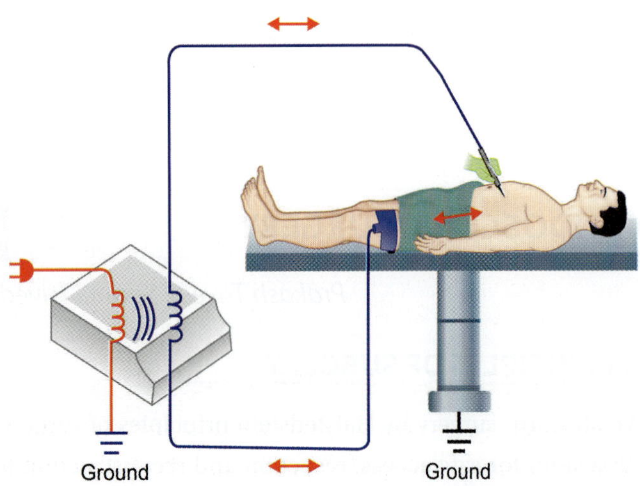

Fig. 1: Electrosurgical units (ESU) are grounded.

BASIC PRINCIPLES AND PROPERTIES OF ENERGY USE IN SURGICAL PRACTICE

In modern surgical practice, energy can be delivered to the tissue in various forms such as:

- Electrical (or more correctly, electromagnetic) energy which could be monopolar or bipolar. Bipolar devices could be basic or advanced (with vessel sealing properties)
- Light energy in the form of LASER (Nd:Yag, CO_2, Argon)
- Mechanical energy in the form of ultrasonic waves used in the Harmonic scalpel
- Radiofrequency waves
- Hybrid devices such as Thunderbeat which combine advanced bipolar and ultrasonic energies.

The purpose of all energy devices is to produce thermal effects in the tissue to cause dissection and more importantly, hemostasis. There are alternate ways of achieving hemostasis such as ligating the pedicle or the use of mechanical devices such as clips or staples. The latter need special skills or instruments and there are issues with re-usability and financial burden. Due to this, in modern endoscopic practice, energy devices have become the first choice to achieve hemostasis.

Tissue Effects of Energy and Temperature

Tissue effects depend on the nature of tissue, duration of application of energy and instrument. But the greatest determinant is the temperature achieved in the tissue. The tissue effects seen at various temperatures are as follows:

- > 37–43°C leads to preventable tissue damage
- > 43–45°C retraction
- > 50°C reduction of enzyme activity
- > 45–60°C leads to irreversible tissue damage – protein denaturation and coagulation
- > 90–100°C drying
- > 100°C (boiling point of water), destruction of cell membrane and dessication
- > 150°C carbonization charring
- > 300°C vaporization
- > 500°C burning.

Properties of Electricity and other Energy Sources

Electrical energy and its tissue effects are governed by certain important principles which are outlined below and illustrated in **Figure 2**.

- Electrical current is the flow of electrons during a finite period of time. It is measured in Amperes. It is designated by the letter I.
- Voltage is the force pushing the electrons across a given distance or tissue. It is measured in Volts. It is designated by the letter V. This is an important determinant of thermal spread in tissues.
- Impedance or Resistance (designated by the letter R) is the obstruction to the flow of electrons. It is measured in Ohms.

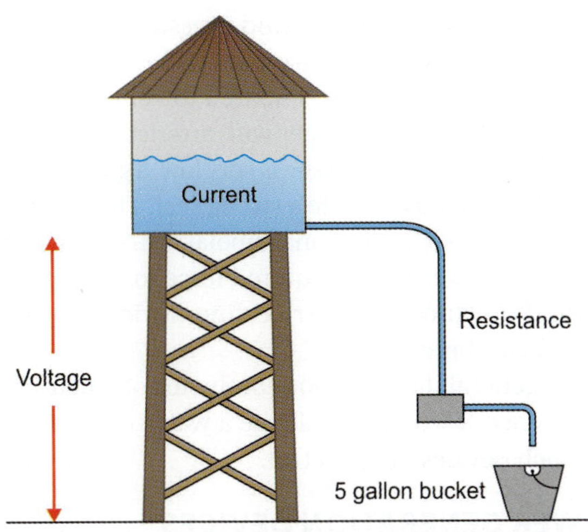

Fig. 2: Principles of current, voltage and resistance.

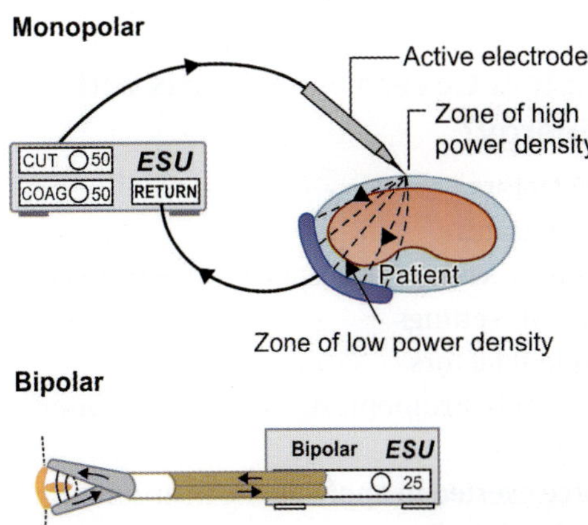

Fig. 3: Traditional bipolar and monopolar isolated.

It follows the Ohms law that states that resistance is directly proportional to voltage and inversely proportional to current. Mathematically, it can be stated as R = V/I.

- Power (P) is measured in Watts and is expressed as P = V × I. Power of the current is directly proportional to voltage and magnitude of the current.
- Mechanical energy or ultrasonic energy is measured in oscillations in thousands per second.

Properties of Conventional Monopolar

- Current < 1 amp
- Interrupted (coagulation) waveforms
- Coagulation voltage 3000–9000 V
- Continuous (cut)
- Cut voltage 1350–4000 V
- Disadvantages: Bad coupling and capacitance coupling.

Properties of Conventional Bipolar (Fig. 3)

- Continuous or interrupted waveforms
- Current < 1 amp
- Voltage 300–1200 V
- Hand instruments such as Kleppinger, Bissinger with spring action are generally used in laparoscopic surgery.

Lateral spread from bipolar is due to the spread of intracellular heat and steam. It can be limited by:

- Terminating the cautery when the tissue turns white
- Terminating the cautery when bubbles stop
- Keep tips slightly apart
- Using intermittent current.

In traditional bipolar instruments, there is low tissue compression and tissue jumps are fewer than in monopolar current use.

Properties of Advanced Bipolar (First or Second Generation) or Vessel Sealing Device

Conventional monopolar and bipolar energy sources have some drawbacks. They require longer application time to achieve tissue effects and hemostasis. This can cause more charring, tissue injury and lateral spread. Due to tissue injury, there can be tissue tearing causing to loss of hemostasis. Conventional energy sources do not have any function to cut the tissue. Advanced bipolar systems have been devised and used to overcome these drawbacks to varying degrees of success.

In general, advanced bipolar systems have device intelligence. There is no passage of current when tissues become dry. This limits the spread of energy. Also, there is a good compression effect, leading to sealing of blood vessels. Tissue cutting is achieved by a separate inbuilt mechanical device or by the energy system itself.

- In first generation advanced bipolar devices, there is a concentric spread of electrons and lateral spread of current is minimized. Compression effects at the tip of the instrument tend to be less.
- In second generation advanced bipolar devices, the current remains almost entirely within the jaws of the device and there is a more even compression from the base to the tip of the instrument.

Properties of Radiofrequency Energy Sources

Radiofrequency ablation is based on the principle of passing electrical current in the radiofrequency range (450–500 kHz) between the electrode and the grounding pads placed on the patient. The tissue effect is to generate heat and this thermal energy results in tissue effects. Ultimately, there is tissue caramelization of sugars, denaturation of protein and tissue charring. Radiofrequency energy requires specialized generators which are usually not found in most gynecological operation theaters. They are used in a limited manner.

HEMOSTASIS AND ENERGY SOURCES

Hemostasis is an important consideration for safe surgery. Energy devices are one of the primary means of achieving hemostasis in endoscopic surgery. Achieving hemostasis is primary. But safety of tissues adjacent and in the vicinity of the hemostasis is also crucial for a safe surgical outcome.

What Factors Govern Hemostasis with Use of Energy?

- Source factors
  - Temperature
  - Current, Voltage, Resistance - these are controlled by the ESU settings
- Instrument factors
  - Type of instrument, surface area in contact with the tissue
  - Force exerted in applying the instrument
  - Angle of application on vessel
- Tissue factors
  - Collagen/Elastin ratio - Artery/Vein
  - Diameter of the vessel
  - Protein denaturation
  - Platelet aggregation
  - Clot formation.

Mechanism of Hemostasis

The basis of hemostasis in electrosurgery is the formation of a coagulum. This coagulum is not the conventional blood clot, but a surgically manufactured seal on blood vessels. The coagulum is generated from denaturation and coagulation of the proteins in the vessel wall and is aided by the physiological mechanism of platelet aggregation and clot activation.

An important concept in hemostasis is the burst pressure. The burst pressure is the pressure that can be withstood by a sealed vessel before it bursts open and hemostasis is lost. Burst pressure depends on:

- Blood pressure and flow across a vessel
- Diameter of the vessel
  - Monopolar current can seal vessels up to 2 mm in diameter
  - Conventional bipolar is effective till vessel diameters of 5 mm
  - Advanced bipolar sealing devices can tackle blood vessels up to 7 mm in diameter
  - The usual diameters of uterine vessels in the non-pregnant state are 3 to 5 mm
  - The diameter of a vessel is affected by the angle at which the energy source instrument is applied. A vertical application effectively reduces the vessel diameter whereas an oblique application increases the diameter.
- Strength of the seal
  - This depends on the collagen:elastin ratio. Higher collagen content gives rise to a stronger seal and higher burst pressure.
  - Collagen: Elastin ratios are better predictors of burst pressure than vessel diameter.
  - Arteries have higher blood pressures. They need to have a stronger seal. Fortunately, they also have higher collagen content as compared to veins. The surgical seal is therefore stronger with arteries than veins.
  - When the collagen tissue is very low, a greater force has to be applied to create a strong seal. This is needed in lymphatics. Conventional bipolar instruments may not be able to exert the required force to seal lymphatics and advanced bipolar sealing devices have better efficacy here.
  - In general, fat is a poor conductor of electricity and energy. It would literally be a waste of energy to use such devices to dissect fat.

NEWER GENERATION DEVICES

Ultrasonic Energy and the Harmonic Scalpel (Figs. 4 and 5)

- Mechanical energy is a means to generate thermal effects in tissue. A simple day to day example of mechanical

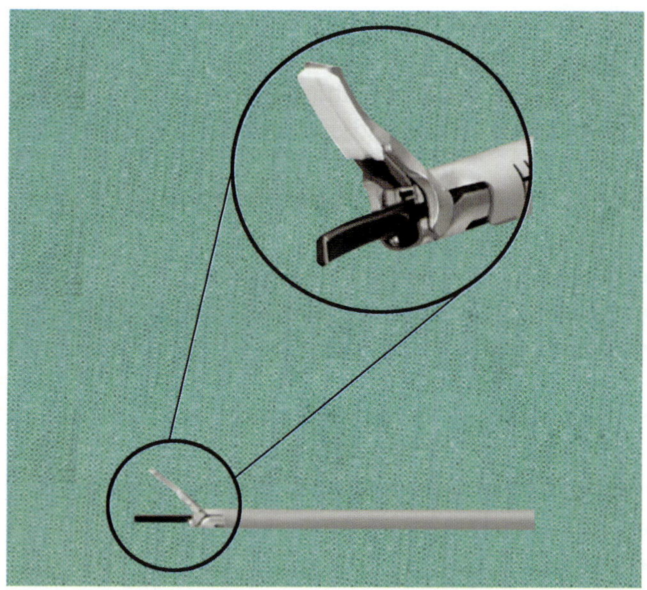

Fig. 4: Harmonic scalpel.

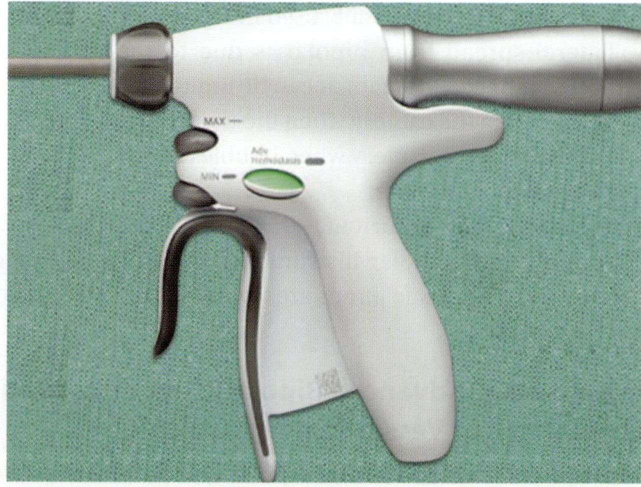

Fig. 5: Harmonic hemostasis.

energy generating heat is rubbing one's hands. When the frequency of rubbing increases, the temperature is higher. Using this principle, Pears and Jacks (1990) and Marc Davidson and Joe Emerald introduced Harmonic device.

- The Harmonic Scalpel has an active blade, which moves at 55,000 oscillations/second (55 kHz). The mechanical vibrations are produced by the piezoelectric transducers embedded in the tools which convert the applied electrical energy to mechanical vibrations which are then transferred to the active blades for cutting or coagulation.
- There is a passive blade coated with Teflon lining which reduces spread of heat. The vibrations generate thermal energy and tissue effects thereof.
- The tissue effects are mainly seen as protein denaturation causing the formation of a coagulum. The friction that is generated by the blades leads cutting and cavitational effects.
- The effect of the Harmonic scalpel varies between hemostatic and cutting. The following factors will cause a cutting effect
  - Increased tissue tension (tissues are kept under stretch)
  - Blade sharpness
  - Vertical placement of the blades
  - Strong grip force.
- The opposite factors, i.e., less tissue tension, dull blades, oblique application of blades and light grip force produce more of a hemostatic effect.
- The effects of the Harmonic scalpel are by oscillation and not by electrosurgery. There is therefore no neuromuscular stimulation. Tissue sticking is less as compared to bipolar instruments. The instrument is a good dissector and is quite sturdy.
- The disadvantage of the Harmonic scalpel is that the coagulation effect is slower than with ESU based methods.

Vessel Sealing Device

These devices represent the second generation of bipolar electrosurgery. In general, they use a high current of 4 amperes and a low voltage of about 180 V. A wide variety of devices are available in the market today and are described here.

Gyrus PKS (Fig. 6)

- The plasma kinetics (PKS) Gyrus works on the basis of a high density of electrons oscillating in an electromagnetic field. When they reach the tissue, there is a transfer of energy to the tissue and consequently coagulation occurs. When the electron burst moves away, the tissue is allowed to cool. The delivery of energy is in pulses.
- This delivers a high current, low voltage energy to the tissues. There is continuous impedance monitoring a tissue temperature generally remains below 100°C. The effects are therefore seen mainly by protein denaturation and there is less tissue charring.

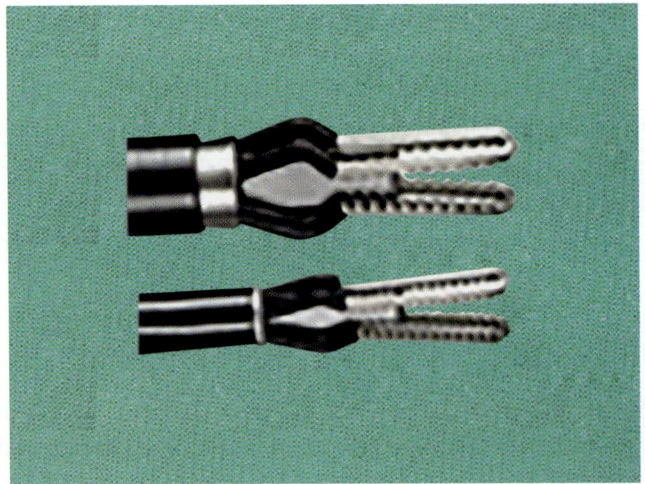

Fig. 6: Gyrus PKS.

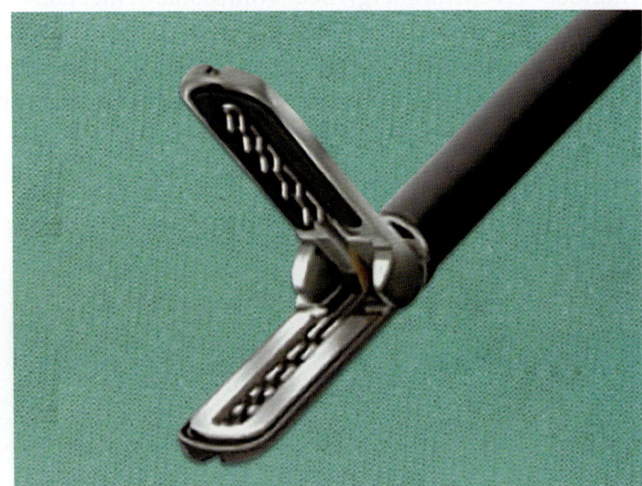

Fig. 7: Enseal.

- But the unprotected 10 mm tip can lead to more lateral spread than with other instruments.

Enseal

- The hand instrument is a tissue forceps with thermo-sensitive material containing embedded nanoparticles on the grasping surfaces **(Fig. 7)**. These nanoparticles measure impedance in the tissue and there is a continuous feedback. The delivery of energy to the tissue is therefore, finely regulated and precise.
- The outer margin conducts electricity into tissue and the inner surface acts as a return electrode with virtually no current dispersion.
- There is minimal power input and no carbonization or sticking. It generates little or no smoke and there is no disturbance in the vision.
- The surgical seal that is generated is from a fusion of the vessel walls and does not depend on the proximal thrombus. The burst pressure is very high and these vessels can withstand seven times the systolic pressure.

- Cutting of the tissue has to be carried out by an inbuilt blade which cuts the tissue after sealing is achieved. This has to be activated manually using the thumb.
- Newer modifications of the device are
    - Enseal PTC (Positive Tissue Coefficient) which reduces stickiness and thermal spread
    - Hand instruments with curved wide jaws **(Fig. 8)** and an articulating tip **(Fig. 9)**.

Thunderbeat

The characteristic elements of the Thunderbeat are the use of synergistic energy, wiper jaw mechanism, probe design and coating **(Fig. 10)**.

The name itself suggests the synergistic energy use (Thunder - Electrical energy, Beat - Ultrasonic or mechanical energy). The device uses bipolar energy and ultrasonic energy to create tissue effects. The mechanical component is responsible for efficient and quick dissection while the electrical component gives reliable vessel sealing.

The wiper jaw mechanism allows for uniform pressure on the grasped tissue **(Fig. 11)** and the jaws also have an anti-stick insulation coating. The jaw design has been modified to give better grasping capability, finer insulated tip **(Fig. 12)** and less cavitation.

It is a versatile instrument and gives fast cutting, easy dissection, widest grip, a secure hemostatic seal and a good tissue grasp.

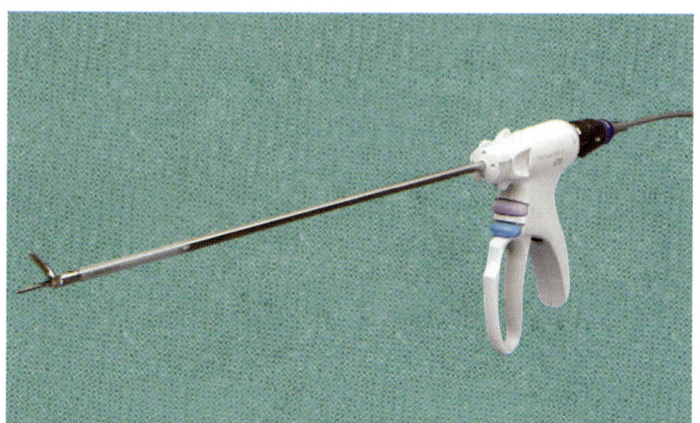

Fig. 10: Thunderbeat.

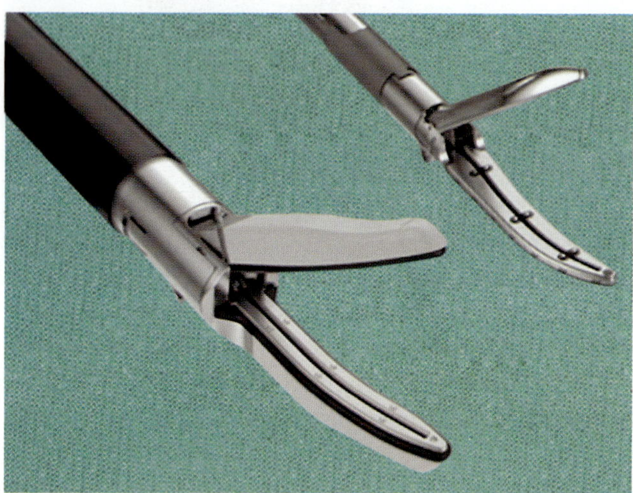

Fig. 8: Enseal curved and large jaw.

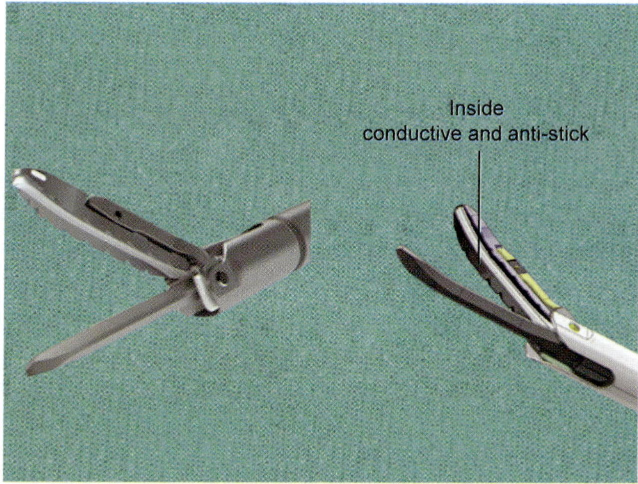

Fig. 11: Wiper jaw mechanism.

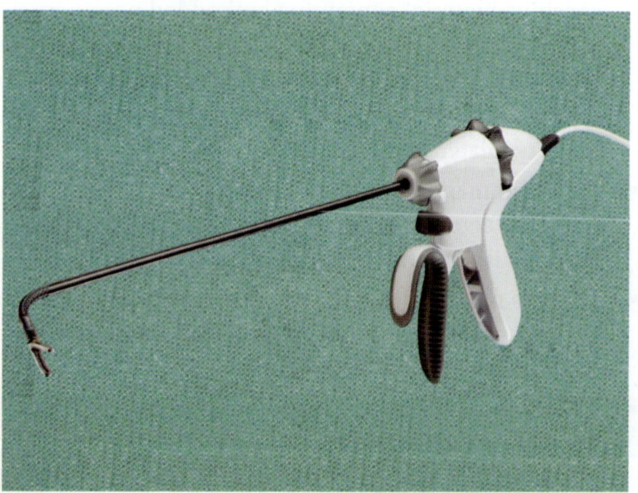

Fig. 9: Articulative Enseal.

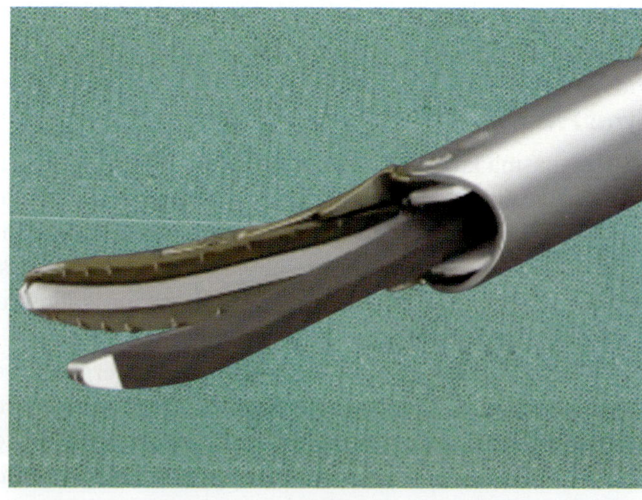

Fig. 12: Insulation coating on tip.

Thermal Ligating Shears: LigaSure (Fig.13)

The device works by delivering a high current, low voltage radiofrequency generated energy to the tissue. The energy is regulated by a feedback control response system which senses tissue impedance. The delivery of energy is stopped depending on the nature and impedance of tissue.

There is a modified mechanical compression of the tissue. The heating effect causes the denaturation of the tissue and formation of the seal. The active element is the nichrome wire which is thermally insulated in the grasping element. It reaches temperatures of 300 to 400°C. During the cooling phase, there is a crosslinking of the fibers leading to a sturdier seal. The insulated cut is bigger at 1/1000th of a mm (about 500 microns).

The jaws close over a silicone boot. This creates a good grip and a narrow high temperature cut zone flanked by a low temperature coagulation zone and very little lateral spread.

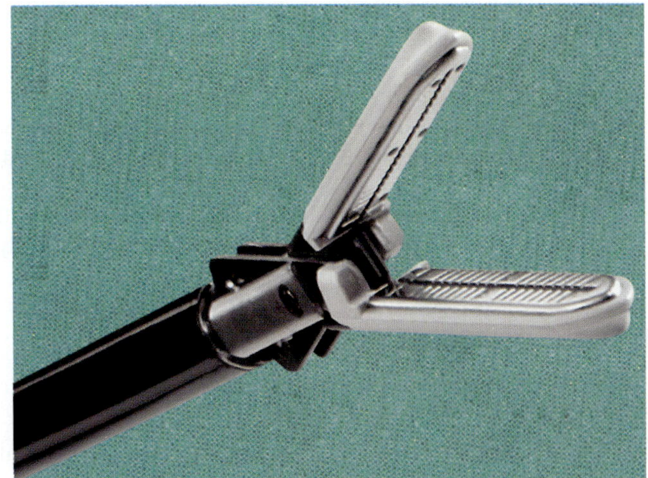

Fig. 13: Thermal ligating shears: LigaSure.

Ideal Energy Source

There is no ideal energy source that is suitable for every surgeon, every healthcare setting and every surgery on every tissue. Most units will have a range of devices to allow a surgeon to work with what is best in a given situation **(Fig. 14)**.

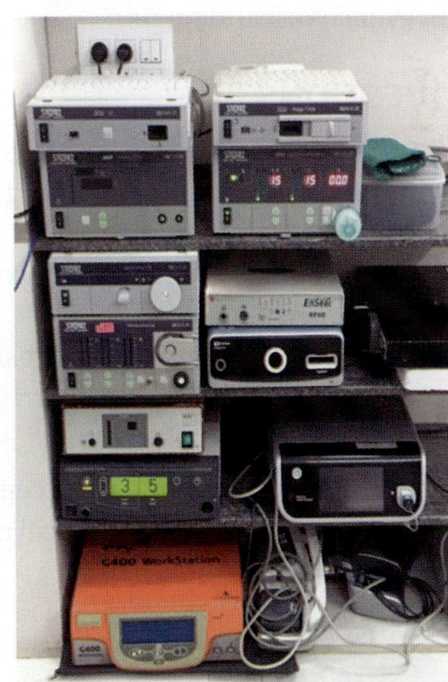

Fig. 14: Ideal energy sources.

CURRENT SETTINGS IN HYSTEROSCOPIC SURGERY

For resectoscopic procedures, electrosurgical energy is necessary. This may be delivered by a monopolar current or a bipolar current.

Monopolar current should only be used with non-ionic liquid media such as 1.5% glycine. 100 Watts pure cut or 50 Watts coagulation current should be used. Blends should be avoided. Monopolar current results in faster surgery and clean tissue cuts. However, the disadvantages of glycine overload (besides those of fluid overload in general) are hyponatremia, convulsions, glycine-ammonia toxicity and hepatic failure, and death.

Bipolar current can be used with any liquid media. Usually normal saline is used. The least amount of pure cut current should be used. Various modified electrodes, Versapoint and Gyrus PKS are available. These are not necessarily superior, but they avoid the use of glycine and give some safety. The other risks of fluid overload, gas embolization and cardiac arrest do exist with bipolar current as well.

LASERs with Nd: YAG diodes can also be used for hysteroscopic surgeries.

CONCLUSION

Newer electrosurgical units (advanced bipolar, vessel sealers, harmonic) have become widely available and economically viable. This has lead to an illusion that the device performs the surgery. The untrained hand holding these devices is the root cause of genesis of phenomenal morbidity and mortality. The simplicity, ease and expertise of the skilled hand are enhanced by these devices and they lend speed and comfort to the surgeon.

Knowledge comes but wisdom lingers, technologies come but skills persist.

FURTHER READING

1. Ayroza P, Abdalla E. Use of electricity in laparoscopy. In: Mencaglia L, Minelli L, Wattiez A (Eds). Manual of Gynecological Laparoscopic Surgery. Straub Bruck + Medien AG, Schramberg, 2013. Available at: https://cdn.websurg.com/web/img/winners/ WeBSurg_Winners_34_1.pdf
2. Kathopoulis N, Protopapas A, Xatzipapas, Antsaklis P, Zacharakis D, Samartzis K, et al. Energy sources in gynecologic laparoscopic surgery. HJOG. 2019;18(4):117-30.
3. The SAGES Manual on the Fundamental Use of Surgical Energy (FUSE). In: Feldman L, Fuchshuber P, Daniel B (Eds). Jones. Springer, New York, 2015. https://doi.org/10.1007/978-1-4614-2074-3

4. Trivedi P, D'Costa S, Shirkande P, Wahi M, Kumar S. Do new vessel sealing devices and harmonic ace increase ureteric injury in total laparoscopic hysterectomy?. J Gynecol Endosc Surg. 2009;1(2):83-88.
5. Trivedi PH (Ed). Minimal Access Surgery and Endoscopy for all Gynecologists. Jaypee Brothers Medical Publishers Pvt Ltd, 2019.
6. Vilos GA, Rajakumar C. Electrosurgical generators and monopolar and bipolar electrosurgery. Journal of Minimally Invasive Gynecology. 2013;20(3):279-87.

LONG QUESTIONS

1. Enumerate various energy sources used in endoscopic surgery.
2. Describe the principles of energy sources in gynecological surgery and their various uses.
3. Describe the precautions to be taken while using energy sources in gynecological surgeries.

SHORT QUESTIONS

1. Differentiate between electrocautery and electrosurgery.
2. What are the advantages and disadvantages of sealing devices as compared to bipolar cautery?
3. What are the complications of energy source use in gynecological surgery?
4. What factors govern hemostasis in electrosurgery?

MULTIPLE CHOICE QUESTIONS

1. The features of electrosurgery are all, except:
   a. The body forms part of electrosurgical circuit
   b. High frequency alternating current through living tissue
   c. Direct current through a high resistance metallic conductor
   d. Manipulation of electrons to produce heat within the cells to destroy tissues
2. The following temperature and tissue effect are matched correctly:
   a. >43–45°C leads to tissue charring
   b. >50°C causes reduction of enzyme activity
   c. >45–60°C leads to charring
   d. > 90–100°C leads to tissue burning
3. The following is a second generation electrosurgical device:
   a. Monopolar hook b. Bipolar scissor
   c. Kleppinger's forceps d. Enseal
4. The voltage used for conventional bipolar surgery is:
   a. 60 V to 100 V b. 300 V to 1200 V
   c. 2000 V to 3500 V d. 5000 V to 10000 V
5. Correct use of bipolar electrocautery is seen as all the following, except:
   a. Tissue turns white
   b. There is tissue charring
   c. Bubbles stop
   d. No blood flow in the tissue

Answers

1. c 2. b 3. d 4. b 5. b

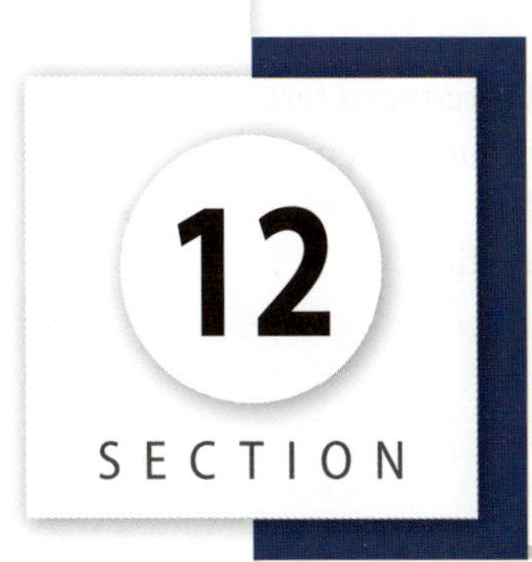

Reproductive Endocrinology and Infertility

12.1 INFERTILITY: ETIOLOGY AND CLINICAL EVALUATION

Charmila Ayyavoo, Sunil Shah

INTRODUCTION

The failure of a couple to become pregnant even after a year of regular and unprotected sexual intercourse is defined as infertility.[1]

The prevalence in India ranges from 8.9 to 12.6%.[2] The principle causes of infertility are disorders of ovulation (25–30%), tubal damage (20%), male factors (30%), peritoneal and uterine disorders (10%).[3] In about 25%, the reason for infertility is unexplained.[4,5]

Evaluation is advisable in both partners simultaneously to identify the cause. There is a 40% chance of infertility due to reasons in both the partners.[3]

MALE INFERTILITY

Etiology[4]

Male infertility may result from various causes such as:

- Disorders in the hypothalamic-pituitary system
- Disorders in the testis (primary cause)
- Disorders of sperm transport.

Hypothalamic Pituitary Causes

A disorder of the central axis which can cause deficiency of gonadotropic releasing hormone (GnRh) or gonadotropins can result in infertility. The following are the central causes:

- Idiopathic isolated gonadotropin deficiency
- Kallmann syndrome
- Tumors of the hypothalamus or pituitary such as craniopharyngioma, macroadenoma
- Diseases which are infiltrative such as sarcoidosis, hemochromatosis, histiocytosis
- Hyperprolactinemia
- Drugs such as steroids, estrogen supplements, androgens, etc.
- Infections
- Obesity.

Primary Testicular Disorders

- Klinefelter syndrome
- Single gene mutations
- Polymorphisms of the androgen, estrogen or follicle stimulating hormone (FSH) receptor
- Y chromosome deletions
- Cryptorchidism
- Varicoceles
- Infections
- Radiation
- Drugs such as antiandrogens, cimetidine
- Environmental toxins such as heat, smoking, pesticides
- Chronic illness.

Disorders of Sperm Transport

- Obstruction of the epididymal ducts
- Congenital bilateral absence of the vas deferens (CBAVD)
- Infections such as chlamydia, gonorrhea
- Vasectomy
- Kartagener syndrome
- Ejaculatory dysfunction.

Disorders of the Hypothalamic-Pituitary Axis

The most common congenital cause is Kallmann syndrome. It is due to the mutation of the genes encoding receptors needed for the migration of GnRh neurons from the olfactory placode to the site of the hypothalamus. In affected men, there will be sexual infantilism due to isolated gonadotropin deficiency because of the defective GnRh secretion. There may be associated anosmia, neurosensory hearing loss or midline facial defects.

Obesity in men can lead to infertility.[6] Free testosterone levels are reduced independent of sex hormone binding globulin (SHBG) concentrations.

Primary Testicular Causes

It is hypergonadotropic hypogonadism type of gonadal failure. Klinefelter syndrome is a cause of primary testicular failure due to sex chromosome aneuploidy. An extra chromosome is found and karyotype is 46XXY. Men affected by this syndrome have small testes, severe oligospermia and reduced virilization. There is evidence of damage to both seminiferous tubules and Leydig cells.

Y chromosome deletions can result in severe oligospermia and azoospermia. The Y chromosome has the Yq11 region called the azoospermia factor or AZF. AZF has three regions as AZFa, AZFb and AZFc. Deletions in a and b region can cause azoospermia while a defective c region causes severe oligospermia. Y chromosome abnormalities can affect the male offspring. Hence men undergoing ICSI as treatment while suffering from Y chromosomal abnormalities should be offered genetic counseling.

Cryptorchidism is the failure of the testes to descend in fetal life. The descent depends on androgen levels and men with testosterone deficiency such as Kallmann syndrome and defective testosterone synthesis can suffer from cryptorchidism. These men are prone for testicular tumors.

Varicoceles occur due to the dilatation of the pampiniform plexus of the spermatic veins. The relationship between varicoceles and male infertility is not established. The proposed mechanism of testicular damage is increased heat, hypoxia, stasis and a delay in the removal of toxins from the circulation.

Infections affecting the testes and causing infertility are mumps orchitis, gonorrhea, chlamydia, tuberculosis, leprosy, and human immunodeficiency virus.

Causes of Sperm Transport

Epididymal obstruction, congenital bilateral absence of the vas deferens (CBAVD), infections of the ducts and vasectomy are reasons of infertility due to transport defects. Kartagener syndrome affects ciliary function and can cause oligoasthenospermia. There are associated recurrent respiratory infections, bronchiectasis and situs inversus. In another syndrome called Young syndrome, there is obstructive azoospermia due to inspissated secretions in the vas deferens and epididymis.

Evaluation of Male Infertility

The evaluation of the male and female have to be done simultaneously when there is no pregnancy even after 1 year of unprotected, regular intercourse. There are indications when the evaluation can start earlier.

- There is an obvious reason for reduced fertility
- The partner is more than 35 years of age.

The evaluation starts with a comprehensive history elicitation and a physical examination.

History Taking

- Age and years of infertility
- Past fertility history
- Childhood history of illnesses
- History of surgeries and intake of medications for systemic illnesses
- Occupation history with history of exposure to heat
- History of sexually transmitted infections
- History of usage of alcohol, recreational drugs and tobacco
- Past treatment history and old reports.

Examination

- Secondary sexual characteristics noted. Hair distribution, body habitus and breasts examination done
- Penis examination with location of urethral meatus
- Testes examination
- Testicular size, consistency checked. Testicular size is estimated using Prader orchidometer. Normal size is from 12 to 30 mL
- Bilateral examination of epididymis and vas
- Examination for varicocoele is done in the standing position. There are three grades: palpable only with usage of Valsalva maneuver, palpable without the maneuver and seen by direct examination
- Per rectal examination of prostate and seminal vesicles.

Tests of Male Infertility

Semen analysis: The basic test for male infertility is a semen analysis. The examination is done with a Makler's chamber or a Neubauer chamber.

It is done after abstinence for 2–5 days. The report is compared to the World Health Organization (WHO) reference values **(Table 1)**. Another test is repeated after 3 months to confirm the diagnosis.[7]

TABLE 1: Reference values—the WHO reference values are accepted for evaluation of semen.[8]

Volume	***More than 1.5 mL***
pH	More than 7.2
Sperm concentration	More than 15 million/mL
Total sperm number	More than 39 million/ejaculate
Percent motility	More than 40%
Progressive motility	More than 32%
Morphology (normal)	More than 4%
Vitality	More than 58%

The instructions for semen collection are given to the couple before collection. The semen is collected by masturbation directly into a wide mouthed clean container. The male partner is given privacy for collection. The sample is collected totally. The couple should inform if there is any spillage. The sample is examined within one hour after liquefaction of the sample. The sample is always labeled with the couple's details.

The ejaculatory volume depends on the secretions by the seminal vesicles. The seminal vesicle secretions are alkaline and have fructose. The prostate gland produces acidic secretions.

A reduced ejaculate indicates:
- No emission
- Spillage during collection
- Bilateral obstruction of the ducts
- Hypogonadism
- Retrograde ejaculation.

The causative factor can be identified with additional information from pH and fructose concentration.

If the volume is low, pH is acidic and there is no fructose in semen, it can indicate CBAVD or ejaculatory duct (formed by vasa deferens and seminal vesicle ducts) obstruction. When there is CBAVD, there is hypoplasia of the seminal vesicles. Hence the semen ejaculated is acidic due to the contribution by the prostate alone.

In hypogonadism or testicular failure due to primary or secondary cause, there is a low volume ejaculate.

A factor of retrograde ejaculation is considered if the volume is low and all other factors are ruled out. A urine analysis is done after ejaculation to test for presence of sperms. A centrifugation of the post ejaculatory sample at 300 g for 10 minutes and a microscopic examination of the pellet can be added for confirmation.

Azoospermia[9]

The absence of sperms in the sample indicates azoospermia. Two samples need to be checked in separate occasions to report as azoospermia. The semen sample is centrifuged at 3,000 g for 15 minutes and the pellet is examined in high power magnification before a final report of azoospermia is given. It is cryptozoospermia if semen is identified in the centrifuged sample. Azoospermia may be due to obstruction of the ducts or may be due to nonobstructive causes.

Evaluation of Azoospermia

The differentiation is to be done as:
- *Pretesticular causes:* Endocrine dysfunction causing secondary testicular failure
- *Testicular causes:* Primary testicular failure
- Post testicular causes which can be due to ejaculatory dysfunction or duct obstruction

The differentiation between obstructive azoospermia and non-obstructive azoospermia is done by:
- Assessment of semen volume
- Serum FSH
- Serum testosterone estimation
- The testicular volume, karyotyping, and testing for Y chromosome microdeletion are done as per indications.

If the semen volume is less than 1.5 mL with normal FSH and testosterone levels, post-ejaculatory urine analysis is done to rule out retrograde ejaculation. A sample collection error is also ruled out. It indicates obstructive azoospermia.

An examination of the testes and vas and pH estimation is done. If there is palpable vas, absent fructose and pH is less than 7.2, transrectal ultrasound is done to rule out ejaculatory duct obstruction.

If there is normal semen volume and pH with normal FSH and testosterone levels, a testicular biopsy is done. If there is normal spermatogenesis, a scrotal exploration and vasogram is done. If there is a correctable obstruction, it is done at the same setting.

If there is normal semen volume with a decrease in serum FSH and testosterone levels, serum LH, prolactin estimations and MRI are done to rule out a pituitary tumor.

If there is elevation in serum FSH levels and there is a normal or raised testosterone levels, exogenous testosterone administration needs to be ruled out. If serum FSH, karyotyping, and Y chromosome microdeletion testing are normal, obstructive causes should be looked for.

If there is elevated serum FSH level with normal genetic testing, it is idiopathic spermatogenetic failure. If there is abnormal genetic testing, genetic counseling is needed.

Indications for Testicular Biopsy

To differentiate between obstructive and non-obstructive causes of azoospermia when there is confusion.

There is a palpable vas and a low ejaculated semen volume.

Oligospermia

Sperm concentration less than 15 million/mL is oligospermia. It is due to hypogonadism, varicocele or some forms of Y chromosome microdeletions.

Motility of sperms in a sample is examined. It is graded as rapidly motile, nonmotile and immotile. Sperm vitality testing is done when there is increase in non-motile sperms. Fresh semen is mixed with a dye like eosin Y or trypan blue. The sperms with intact membrane do not take up the stain.

Sperm viability testing is done with hypo-osmotic swelling (HOS) test . In these sperms are incubated in a hypo-osmotic solution. If there are normal functioning sperms, their tails swell and coil as the fluid can be transported across the membrane.

Morphology of sperms is examined for identification of anomalies in head, neck, mid-piece, and tail.

According to WHO, normal morphology of around 4% is considered satisfactory.[8]

If round cells are more than 5 million/mL, peroxidase test is done to identify leukocytes. If leukocytospermia is present, semen culture is done. Before collecting the sample for culture, the penis is cleaned with betadine to avoid skin flora contamination.

Specialized Tests

Antisperm antibodies: The clinical utility is not proved. They can be identified in the serum, seminal plasma or sperms. They do not form a part of the routine evaluation.

Indications:

- Previous sexually transmitted infections
- Duct obstruction
- History of torsion testis or trauma
- Vasectomy reversal surgeries
- Clumping of sperm in semen analysis
- Unexplained infertility.

Sperm penetration assay: This test is done to evaluate sperm capacitation, acrosome reaction, fusion with the oolemma and decondensation within the oocyte cytoplasm. The test is not widely done because it is expensive, difficult to do and not freely available.

Human zona binding assay: In this procedure, bisected zona derived from human oocytes which are not exposed to sperms are used. There is a comparison in the binding capacity of the test subject against fertile control sperms. It is not widely used as there is a limited availability of human oocytes.

Computer Assisted Semen Analysis

It is used for an objective evaluation of sperm characteristics and motility features. It is expensive and is not of much use if there is no standardized sample preparation, frame rate and sperm concentration.

Acrosome reaction: The sperms of infertile men are exposed to calcium ionophore. If there is spontaneous acrosome loss and decreased acrosome reactivity, it indicates a poor sperm penetration capacity. The clinical use is not validated.

DNA Fragmentation Testing in Sperms

If there is damage in sperm DNA integrity, it can cause poor semen parameters. The tests are:

- *SCSA test:* Sperm chromatin structure assay
- *TUNEL assay:* Terminal deoxynucleotidyl transferase mediated dUTP nick-end labeling
- *COMET assay:* Single-cell gel electrophoresis.

Biochemical tests: The tests such as sperm creatine phosphokinase and reactive oxygen species estimation are investigational.

Ultrasound

Ultrasound of the scrotum for evaluation of pathologies in scrotum and inguinal region and transrectal ultrasound for evaluation of prostate, ejaculatory ducts and seminal vesicles are done.

Endocrine Blood Tests

Serum FSH, serum testosterone estimations are commonly done for evaluation. In necessary patients, serum prolactin, luteinizing hormone (LH) and thyroid stimulating hormone (TSH) levels are estimated.

Genetic Tests

Karyotyping is indicated in azoospermia and severe oligospermia. Y chromosome microdeletion is also done in similar circumstances.

FEMALE INFERTILITY

The main causes of female infertility are ovulatory dysfunction, uterine anatomic and functional disorders, tubal factors which can be tubal occlusion or adnexal adhesions, cervical factors and unexplained causes.[7]

Ovulatory Causes

These disorders are an important cause of female infertility and contribute to 18–25%[5] of cases. These patients have irregular, unpredictable menstruation. The ovulatory disorders are classified by WHO into three groups.[10]

- *Group 1: Hypogonadotropic hypogonadism*: This group accounts for 5–10% of anovulatory causes. There is abnormal or absent GnRH secretion or pituitary insensitivity to GnRH. Causes can be hypothalamic due to emotional stress, weight loss, excessive exercise, and anorexia nervosa. Other causes are Kallmann syndrome, isolated gonadotropin deficiency or a pituitary mass.
- *Group 2: Normogonadotropic normogonadism:* This is the largest group accounting for 80% of the causes. The most common cause is polycystic ovarian syndrome (PCOS).
- *Group 3: Hypergonadotropic hypogonadism:* This group contributes to 10–20% of anovulation. The most common cause is premature ovarian insufficiency.

There is a fourth specific group which is hyperprolactinemic anovulation. About 5–10% of women have this problem.

Uterine Factor

Uterine factors contributing to female infertility are not common. The factors which can cause infertility are congenital uterine malformations, fibroids, polyps in the endometrium, intra uterine adhesions, and endometritis. Uterine anomalies can result in poor pregnancy outcome rather than infertility.

Tubal Factors

Pathology in the tubes and peritoneum can result in 25–35% of the causes of infertility.[11] Pelvic inflammatory disease (PID) is the major cause of tubal infertility. It is due to ascending infection. The other causes are due to endometriosis, inflammatory bowel disease or surgical trauma.

Cervical Factor

The cervical cause of infertility is very rare. Chronic cervicitis and cervical stenosis resulting from cervical conization can impair sperm mucus interaction.

Unexplained Infertility

The incidence may vary from 10 to 20% of causes.[12] The diagnosis is made by a normal semen analysis, normal uterine cavity, no ovulatory dysfunction, and the establishment of patency in at least one tube.

Evaluation for Female Factor

Evaluation of a couple is usually done when no conception happens after 1 year of unprotected, sexual intercourse. An earlier evaluation is advised if the female partner is over the age of 35 years or there are risk factors.[13] The risk factors which warrant an earlier evaluation are:

- Irregular menstruation
- PID with sequelae
- Any history of genital surgery
- Endometriosis
- Male partner with poor semen parameters.

An evaluation includes careful history taking and a thorough physical examination.

History

- *Menstrual history:* Age at menarche, number of days of flow, cyclicity, associated pain, change in menstrual pattern are elicited
- *Marital history:* Partner history, any history of sexual dysfunction, history of dyspareunia
- Duration of infertility and history of past treatments
- *Past obstetric history:* Parity, gravidity, pregnancy events, abortions either spontaneous or induced, trimester of loss, any associated medical or surgical problem
- Previous history of sexually transmitted diseases
- Past medical and surgical history
- Family history of medical illnesses, genetic problems
- Occupational history
- History of allergies
- History of usage of tobacco, alcohol and recreational drugs
- History of galactorrhea, hirsutism, abdominal or pelvic pain.

Physical Examination

- Height, weight and body mass index (BMI)
- Blood pressure estimation
- Presence of hirsutism, acne
- Thyroid gland enlargements
- Breast examination
- Per abdomen examination for mass, tenderness
- Per speculum examination for vaginal or cervical lesions, vaginal discharge characteristics
- Per vaginal examination for uterine size, position, contour, mobility and tenderness; for adnexal and pouch of Douglas (POD) mass and tenderness.

Screening tests: Before evaluation for infertility in a female, the following screening tests are done.

- Pap smear—to rule out cervical cancer changes
- Blood grouping and Rh typing of the couple: If she is Rh negative and the partner is Rh positive, an antibody test is done
- *Complete blood count:* To identify anemia and other blood disorders
- If there is a family history of genetic disorders, appropriate tests are done and genetic counseling offered
- If there is no history of vaccination against rubella, immune status is identified. If needed, rubella vaccine is given. She will need to avoid pregnancy for 1 month after the vaccination
- If there is a high risk for sexually transmitted infections (STD), screening for syphilis, hepatitis B and human immune deficiency virus 1 are done.

Ultrasound

A transabdominal and transvaginal ultrasound (TVS) are mandatory for a basic evaluation of female factor of infertility.

Tests for Female Infertility

Ovarian Factor

Ovulation can be assessed for women with irregular menstrual cycles. Women having menstruation once in 21–35 days are considered to have a regular cycle which is considered as evidence of ovulation.[14]

Tests of Ovulation

- Basal body temperature (BBT) charts were historically used
- Urinary LH kit to identify the mid-cycle LH surge
- Endometrial biopsy to date the endometrium is abandoned now
- The most common test used is the mid-luteal estimation of serum progesterone levels. Levels more than 3 ng/mL are considered as presumptive evidence of ovulation. It is usually performed 1 week before menstruation
- Serial ultrasound measurements of follicular growth with subsequent development of corpus luteum and changes in the endometrium are evidences for ovulation
- NICE guidelines advise that mid luteal estimation of serum progesterone should be done in all women undergoing

infertility evaluation even if they have regular menstrual cycles.[7]

Other Endocrine Tests

In order to differentiate between the three WHO groups of anovulation, serum FSH and serum estradiol (E2) are done initially. In group 1, both hormones are low. In group 2, both are in the normal range. In group 3, serum FSH is high and estradiol is low.

Thyroid dysfunction, hyperprolactinemia, late onset congenital adrenal hyperplasia, Cushing syndrome, and androgen secreting tumors need to be ruled out with appropriate tests in Group 2 WHO anovulatory dysfunction.

- *Thyroid disorders:* Serum TSH, free thyroxin (T4) levels
- *Hyperprolactinemia:* Serum prolactin levels
- If hyperandrogenism, serum testosterone, androstenedione, dehydroepiandrosterone and 17 hydroxyprogesterone are done.

Ovarian Reserve Estimation

It is done to evaluate the fertility capacity and to predict the response to ovarian stimulation. The tests are:

- Anti-Müllerian hormone (AMH)
- Antral follicle count (AFC)
- Day 3 serum FSH and estradiol.

The other tests which are done but not to be found as useful as the above are serum inhibin B, isolated E2, ovarian volume, ovarian blood flow estimation, and clomiphene challenge test.

Interpretation of Ovarian Reserve Tests

Anti-Müllerian hormone is produced in the ovaries by the preantral follicles and small antral follicles. Cyclic variations do not happen. Levels above 3.5 ng/mL predict high response and when below 0.75 ng/mL predict a low response.[7]

Antral follicle count is the number of follicles of 2–10 mm size in the largest diameter of the ovary measured using a transvaginal ultrasound in the early follicular phase. An AFC more than 16 is a predictor of a hyper-response to ovarian stimulation and a level less than 4 is indicative of a poor response.[7]

Cervical Factor

There are no tests to identify cervical factor as the cause for infertility in present times. Post coital test (PCT) done previously is abandoned now. Cervical chlamydia testing is advised before any instrumentation in the genital tract.

Uterine Factor

A transvaginal ultrasound is used for evaluation presence of fibroids, endometrial polyps, adhesions and uterine septum which may lead to infertility. Fibroids location and size are noted as submucus fibroids can cause infertility.

Hysterosalpingography (HSG) is used to evaluate uterine cavity. Hysterosonography is the infusion of saline into the uterine cavity and the cavity is evaluated using an ultrasound. It helps to delineate the cavity and is more useful than USG and HSG. It is very precise in identifying intrauterine lesions such as polyps and submucosal fibroids. Three dimensional (3D) hysterosonography is comparable to hysteroscopy in evaluation. Hysterosalpingo-contrast sonography (HyCoSy) is a test done with the usage of contrast medium.

The gold standard for the evaluation of the uterine cavity is hysteroscopy. It cannot be used to evaluate the uterine contour. For the diagnosis of congenital uterine anomalies, 3D-USG is done in the luteal phase as there is better visualization. Magnetic resonance imaging (MRI) and laparoscopy are expensive investigations for evaluation of uterine factor.

Tubal Factor

Hysterosalpingography: It is done by using water based or oil-based contrast media and visualizing the uterine cavity and the fallopian tubes. It is done in the early follicular phase for better visualization. It is not to be done if there is allergy to the contrast medium, pregnancy or acute infections in the pelvic cavity.

HyCoSy is done to evaluate tubal factor. Contrast medium is injected into the uterine cavity and the uterine cavity and tubes are evaluated using ultrasound.

Laparoscopy is the golden standard for evaluation of fallopian tubes. It is an invasive test and is expensive. It is done when there is a suspicion of endometriosis, adhesions in the pelvic cavity or PID.

Tests of Doubtful Utility in Infertility Evaluation

Tests which are now not considered useful in the evaluation of female factor are BBT charts and PCT.

Basal body temperature charts were used to predict ovulation. Daily temperatures in early morning are noted. In women who are ovulatory, there is a biphasic pattern. It is low in the follicular phase and starts increasing in the luteal phase due to the thermogenic nature of progesterones. It falls before the onset of menstruation. It is abandoned as it does not predict ovulation accurately. It is tedious and is stressful to the patient.

Postcoital tests are performed to identify cervical factor and male factor infertility. In this test, cervical mucus is checked for sperms after intercourse in the periovulatory period. The mucus is checked for its characteristics, for the number and motility of sperms. The test is a poor predictor of pregnancy. It is proved that cervical factor is not the sole cause of infertility. PCT is a tedious procedure with no utility. Hence it is abandoned.

CONCLUSION

Infertility is a problem which has both health and socioeconomic implications. A comprehensive evaluation of all etiological factors of infertility in both partners with timely interventions will help many a suffering couple achieve their dream of having a child.

KEY MESSAGES

- Basic investigations for a couple are done if there is no pregnancy after 1 year of unprotected sexual intercourse.
- Both the partners are evaluated simultaneously.
- Evaluation is started with a comprehensive history taking and a detailed physical examination.
- The basic fertility investigations are evaluation of the uterine cavity, ovarian function and reserve testing, tubal patency tests and a semen analysis.

REFERENCES

1. Melodie VB, Christine W. Fertility and infertility: definition and epidemiology. Clin Biochem. 2018;62:2-10.
2. Katole A, Saoji AV. Prevalence of primary infertility and its associated risk factors in urban population of central India: a community-based cross-sectional study. Indian J Comm Med 2019;44(4):337.
3. Thonneau P, Marchand S, Tallec A, Ferial ML, Ducot B, Lansac J, et al. Incidence and main causes of infertility in a resident population (1,850,000) of three French regions (1988-1989). Hum Reprod. 1991;6(6):811-6.
4. Krausz C. Male infertility: pathogenesis and clinical diagnosis. Best Pract Res Clin Endocrinol Metab. 2011;25(2):271-85.
5. Hull MG, Glazener CM, Kelly NJ, Conway DI, Foster PA, Hinton RA, et al. Population study of causes, treatment, and outcome of infertility. Br Med J (Clin Res Ed). 1985;291(6510):1693-7.
6. Kahn BE, Brannigan RE. Obesity and male infertility. Curr Opin Urol. 2017;27(5):441-5.
7. NICE. Fertility problems: assessment and treatment; Clinical guideline (CG156). London: NICE; 2017.
8. World Health Organization. WHO laboratory manual for the examination and processing of human semen, 5th edition. Geneva: World Health Organization; 2010. pp. 271.
9. Hwang K, Smith JF, Coward RM, Penzias A, Bendikson K, Butts S, et al. Evaluation of the azoospermic male: a committee opinion. Fertil Steril. 2018;109(5):777-82.
10. WHO. Agents stimulating gonadal function in the human. Report of a WHO scientific group. World Health Organ Tech Rep Ser. 1973;514:1-30.
11. Honore GM, Holden AE, Schenken RS. Pathophysiology and management of proximal tubal blockage. Fertil Steril. 1999;71(5):785-95.
12. Isaksson R, Tiitinen A. Present concept of unexplained infertility. Gynecol Endocrinol. 2004;18(5):278-90.
13. Practice Committee of the American Society for Reproductive Medicine. Diagnostic evaluation of the infertile female: a committee opinion. Fertil Steril. 201;103(6):e44-50.
14. Münster K, Schmidt L, Helm P. Length and variation in the menstrual cycle—a cross-sectional study from a Danish county. BJOG. 1992;99(5):422-9.

LONG QUESTIONS

1. Evaluate the causes of male infertility.
2. Evaluate the causes of female infertility.
3. Classify the types of azoospermia and differentiate between nonobstructive and the obstructive causes of azoospermia.

SHORT QUESTIONS

1. Classify the causes of male infertility and enumerate in each classification.
2. How is the health of semen evaluated?
3. What are the WHO reference values of semen analysis?
4. What are the causes of female infertility?
5. What are the tests for ovarian reserve?

MULTIPLE CHOICE QUESTIONS

1. Infertility is inability of the couple to conceive after 1 year of marriage:
   a. True b. False
2. The prevalence of infertility in India is:
   a. 15–18% b. 8–13% c. 20–25% d. 5–10%
3. The most common cause of female infertility is:
   a. Uterine factor b. Tubal factor
   c. Ovarian factor d. Peritoneal factor
4. The most common central cause of male infertility is:
   a. Kallmann syndrome b. Klinefelter's syndrome
   c. Young syndrome d. Kartagener's syndrome
5. The tests done for evaluating sperm DNA fragmentation are all, except:
   a. SCSA test b. Acrosome reaction test
   c. TUNEL assay d. COMET assay
6. Semen analysis is ideally done after how many days of abstinence:
   a. 1–2 days b. 2–3 days c. 2–5 days d. 2–7 days
7. The causes of anovulatory dysfunction are all, except:
   a. Kallmann syndrome
   b. Stein-Leventhal syndrome
   c. Asherman syndrome
   d. Cushing syndrome
8. The most common cause of infertility due to fibroids are because of:
   a. Subserosal fibroids b. Intramural fibroids
   c. Broad ligament fibroids d. Submucosal fibroids
9. Ovarian reserve testing is by all, except:
   a. AMH b. AFC
   c. Day 3 FSH d. Day 3 LH
10. Tests of female infertility not performed now are:
    a. PCT b. HyCoSy
    c. MRI d. Endometrial biopsy

Answers

1.	b	2.	b	3.	c	4.	a	5.	b	6.	c
7.	c	8.	d	9.	d	10.	a				

12.2 INVESTIGATIONS FOR THE MALE PARTNER

Fessy Louis T, Parvathy T

INTRODUCTION

Couples who are unable to achieve pregnancy within the first year of attempting, should only be diagnosed as infertile after 1 year of regular sexual activity without using a contraceptive method. Investigation is to be initiated earlier when risk factors are present, including advanced maternal (>35 years) or paternal age (>45 years), a history of urogenital surgery, cancer, cryptorchidism, varicocele, orchitis, use of gonadotoxins or genital infections, among others.[1]

The field of male infertility has achieved important advances with respect to diagnosis and treatment recently. Genetic tests have made it possible to correctly classify cases of nonobstructive azoospermia (NOA) previously believed to be idiopathic. With the introduction of microsurgery the success rates of reproductive tract reconstruction and sperm retrieval either from the testicle or the epididymis have been made possible. Gamete micromanipulations have helped the previously infertile men with severe oligozoospermia or azoospermia the chance to father children of their own.

Infertility is a common scenario of reproductive age group and when they seek medical attention for infertility problems, the male partner have to be systematically evaluated in every investigation of an infertile couple.[2] Whenever possible the clinician is responsible for diagnosing, counseling, and treating the underlying cause. Better late than never, it is the responsibility of treating physician to refer a patient to specialized assisted reproductive techniques (ART) center when there is no specific treatment for him or her.

CAUSES OF MALE INFERTILITY/SUBFERTILITY

Any process that affects sperm production and quality is potentially harmful to male fertility. The major causes for male infertility include varicocele, testicular failure, genital tract obstruction, cryptorchidism, idiopathic, genetic conditions, hormonal dysfunction, infections, immunological conditions, ejaculatory/sexual dysfunction, systemic diseases, and cancer.[3]

Signs

A couple who are sexually active and not using any contraceptive methods but are unable to achieve pregnancy is the typical clinical presentation of an infertile couple within the reproductive age. In general, the female partner has been evaluated by a gynecologist who orders a semen analysis for the male. With an abnormal semen analysis result, male infertility is suspected.

POSSIBLE CONFOUNDING CAUSES

In male infertility approximately 1% cases may be the clinical presentation of a more serious or potentially fatal disorder such as testicular or brain cancer, medullary spinal cancer, endocrinopathies, systemic disease, genitourinary malformation, and genetic syndromes. Infertile men has 50% more chance of harboring testicular cancer.[4] Thus the clinician have to keep in mind that the infertility may be the initial manifestation of a more severe medical condition.

The infertility history should include a detailed study of the patient's reproductive and sexual history, developmental, family, medical, and surgical history. The information to be included in each portion of the history is detailed here.

Reproductive and Sexual History

For the reproductive history, any prior conceptions for the male with present or past partners, details of any prior difficulty achieving conception, evaluations, and treatments done in the past for infertility, and previous contraceptive history should all be recorded, along with the timing and frequency of intercourse with the man's current partner. Information about erectile and ejaculatory function and frequency of masturbation should all be requested, including the timing of first masturbation and intercourse.[5]

Developmental History

A history of specific childhood illness or conditions may be informative. For example, a significant decrease in spermatogenesis can occur due to bilateral cryptorchidism, but unilateral cryptorchidism has much less impact usually. Inspite of performing orchidopexies at an earlier age, improved fertility rates have yet to be demonstrated with this approach. On the other hand, testes that are remaining undescended after puberty do not function, and fertility rates are not improved by postpubertal repair.[5] Any history of torsion or testicular trauma should be noted, since both may result in atrophic testes.[6] Pubertal development timing should also to be noted. Significantly incomplete or delayed development may suggest an endocrinopathy. Mumps either unilateral or bilateral can cause severe testicular damage.[7]

Medical History

Diabetes may alter erectile and/or ejaculatory function, and any systemic illness accompanied by fever or viremia can lead to impaired testicular function impairment, although the effects may not be measurable for approximately for 1–4 months in the ejaculate.[8] History of pyospermia or prostatitis should be noted, although both are very much uncommon and neither is proved to cause infertility.[9] Immotile cilia syndrome (also known as primary ciliary dyskinesia), which should be suspected when there is a history of chronic upper respiratory infections, causing severe defects in sperm motility. Kartagener syndrome is a condition when immotile cilia syndrome is associated with situs in versus, which might be a rare cause of male infertility.[10] Frequent respiratory infections associated with azoospermia raise the possibility of Young syndrome, in which epididymal obstruction has been caused by the inspissation of secretions.[11] Neurologic issues can also lead to male infertility as a variety of hormonal abnormalities including thyroid disorders, hyperprolactinemia, and raised estrogen levels. Lastly, any history of sexually transmitted disease or urinary tract infection should be recorded, especially if associated with epididymitis, as these conditions can lead to epididymal obstruction.

Past Surgical History and Cancer Treatments

All details of past surgeries have to be obtained. Pelvic and retroperitoneal surgery may impair the ejaculatory function. Patients with testicular cancer can present with infertility either before or after treatment. Approximately 50% of testicular cancer patients have subnormal sperm densities prior to chemotherapy itself.[12] Following cisplatinum-based chemotherapy for testicular cancer, mostly patients will develop azoospermia. However, most of them will recover sperm production within 4 years.[13] Most patients with lymphoma, leukemia or sarcoma become permanently sterile after chemotherapy.

Medication and Drug Use

A detailed medical treatment history should be obtained. Unfortunately for many substances, data detailing potential effects on male fertility are not fully known. Exogenous androgens are well-known to induce hypogonadotropic hypogonadism, which may be induced directly by testosterone or indirectly by synthetic anabolic steroids. The subsequent suppression of endogenous testosterone production usually results in azoospermia, which is a reversible condition over a span of 3–6 month period. But importantly, some patients do not recover normal pituitary function as well.

Lifestyle Exposure

Exposure to potential environmental toxins including pesticides, arsenic, mercury, cadmium, and hydrocarbons can impair spermatogenesis. In particular, the soil fumigants, amebicide and nematocide, and 2-bromopropane (a substitute for chlorofluorocarbons) can cause decreased spermatogenesis.[14] Testicular atrophy is frequently associated with alcohol dependency, but moderate alcohol consumption does not appear to impair fertility.[15] The real effect of cigarette smoking on male infertility remains still controversial, with some studies showing decreased semen health and while others showing no effect.[16] However, the sum of the accumulating evidence suggests that cigarettes smoking can mostly impact male fertility.

PHYSICAL EXAMINATION

The physical examination for male infertility should be mainly focusing on identifying abnormalities that could affect fertility. Endocrine disorders should be suspected in cases of abnormal androgenization. Gynecomastia can result from excessive estrogens, an altered estrogen-androgen ratio, or due to elevated prolactin levels. Penile curvature, angulation, and the location of the urethral meatus should be assessed vigilantly. The scrotum should be carefully palpated in standing position, with a note on the size and consistency of the testicles; and the room should be kept warm for this examination.

Orchidometer must be used to measure the size of testicle. This measurement is important because in impaired spermatogenesis there will be often a small-volume testes. The normal volume is approximately 20 mL.[17] The Asian men typically have smaller testes than men of other races. The epididymis should be examined carefully, noting the presence of the caput, corpus and cauda, as well as whether the epididymis feels indurated or full. Fullness can be due to obstruction of the genital ducts. During palpation of the spermatic cords, the clinician should note whether the vas deferens is absent or present and has to note any vasal atrophy or nodularity, or the presence of a varicocele within the spermatic cord and surrounding the testicle. An enlarged venous diameter of varicocele can be detected with the patient performing the Valsalva maneuver. Varicoceles are graded as small (grade I) if palpable only when the patient performs the Valsalva maneuver, moderate (grade II) if palpable when the patient is standing position but does not perform the Valsalva maneuver, and large (grade III) when veins can be seen through the scrotal skin without any manipulations. Varicoceles size decreases when the patient is in the supine position.[5]

ENDOCRINE EVALUATION

Endocrine evaluation has to be suggested when the following scenarios are present: (1) a sperm concentration <10 million/mL; (2) history of erectile dysfunction; (3) hypospermia (volume of semen measuring <1 mL) or (4) signs and symptoms of endocrinopathies or hypogonadism. The minimal evaluation includes the assessment of serum follicle-stimulating hormone (FSH) and testosterone levels, reflecting the germ cell epithelium and Leydig cell status respectively. If the testosterone level is low, a second collection is recommended along with free testosterone, LH and prolactin measurements. Isolated FSH elevation is usually indicative of severe germ cell epithelium damage. Highly elevated FSH and LH levels when associated with low-normal or below normal testosterone levels, suggest diffuse testicular failure and may have either a congenital (e.g., Klinefelter syndrome) or acquired cause. Concomitant low levels of FSH and LH may implicate hypogonadotropic hypogonadism. This condition may be congenital or secondary to a prolactin-producing pituitary tumor.[18]

Gonadotropin values within the normal range suggest an extraductal obstruction in azoospermic males.[18] Serum estradiol levels should be determined in patients presenting with gynecomastia. Infertile patients with a testosterone to estradiol ratio less than 10 can has significant but reversible seminal alterations.[19] Serum prolactin levels should be determined in infertile men with a complaint of concomitant sexual dysfunction or when there is clinical or laboratory evidence of pituitary disease; however, hyperprolactinemia rarely causes infertility in healthy men.[20]

ROUTINE SEMEN ANALYSIS

The most important diagnostic tool in the initial investigation of male fertility is the analysis of freshly ejaculated semen. Semen is a mixture of secretions from several components of the genital tract. Only 5% of the semen volume is contributed from testis with sperms in it. During ejaculation, this fluid moves up through the epididymis and vas. Most of the seminal fluid is produced from the seminal vesicles and prostate present at the base of the bladder. The proper assessment of semen quality is essential in the diagnosis of several treatable disorders of male fertility. In many of the cases of male factor infertility, no specific treatment is available to improve semen quality, in which case the semen analysis provides basic information about the prospects for natural pregnancy and the need for assisted reproduction. The semen analysis provides an indication of male fertility, but is not an absolute and confirmatory test for fertility because it is not assessing important aspects of sperm function, for example, the ability of the sperm to locate and penetrate an egg. The finding of poor semen quality points to a reduced chance of pregnancy, however natural conception may still occur in some cases. However the more severe the semen defects, lower the chances.

Collection of the Semen Sample

The specimen is best collected by masturbation into a wide mouthed sterile container. The sample is best collected in the facility provided at the laboratory, however collection at home is acceptable provided the sample is rapidly transported (within 1 hour of masturbation) and kept at body temperature. Semen collected by coitus interruption is not favored as it has the risk of losing of sample, particularly the first fraction of the ejaculate. Semen should never be collected into an ordinary condom, which contains substances that is spermicidal. If religious or personal practices prohibit masturbation, a special condom (SCD) can be used with no spermicidal substance that does not affect the sperm quality and collected by intercourse.

The analysis: Laboratories vary widely in their ability to provide high quality analyses. Semen analysis is best performed in a specialized laboratory with extensive experience using the approved methods of the World Health Organization. Analysis of the ejaculate includes the characteristics of the seminal fluid (volume, pH, liquefaction, viscosity) and of the sperm themselves including the number of sperm (called sperm "count" or concentration), their movement (motility) and shape (morphology). Careful mixing of seminal fluid must be done before its examination to avoid the common problem of generation of artifacts due to poor mixing. It is frequently forgotten that mixing of the components of seminal fluid occurs only after ejaculation, and in the collection of a semen sample, that can only occur in the semen container. Agglutination of spermatozoa in an ejaculate is not an uncommon finding.[21,22] Normal volume of ejaculate is 2–7 mL but usually we see around 2–4 mL. Volume is important, because a large volume may increase the total number of sperms being delivered but small reported volumes are sometimes misleading as spillage might have occurred during collection.

The normal ranges for various parameters of semen quality are shown here:

Normal values of semen variables:[23]

- Standard tests volume >1.5 mL
- Sperm concentration >15 million sperm/mL
- Sperm motility >40% with progressive + nonprogressive motility
- Sperm morphology >4% normal forms
- White blood cells <1 million cells/mL.

Sperm count: It is important to understand that an individual's semen quality can vary from sample to sample, even in men with normal semen parameters. As a result at least two, and occasionally three, semen analyses are needed, each several weeks apart, in order to get a good idea of an individual's average semen quality. It is well recognized that sperm count can be adversely affected by illness, especially fevers, which may temporarily negative effect on sperm count in normal men for the several months. In this case, the semen analysis has to be delayed for several weeks.

The finding of no sperm in the ejaculate (called "azoospermia") suggests either an absence of sperm production or obstruction to sperm outflow. It is most important that an azoospermic semen sample is centrifuged down to carefully examine whether the ejaculate contains even a few sperms. If a few sperm can be found, the technique of single sperm microinjection into ovum [also called intracytoplasmic sperm injection (ICSI)] by ART may be successful. In these severely infertile men sperm may be appearing only intermittently requiring the need for several semen analyses.

Sperm motility (movement): Along with a low sperm count, sperm motility is often impaired in men with "idiopathic" (meaning the cause unknown) poor sperm production. However there are other important conditions which predominantly effect sperm motility, such as sperm autoimmunity, a condition accounting for about 6% of male infertility. Immotile sperm, (sperm showing no movement) may be due to structural problems in the sperm tail or be due to death of sperm (necrospermia). Such couples have an exceedingly low chance of natural fertility but ICSI may provide an alternative.

Sperm morphology (shape): Sperm shape is an important predictive indicator of sperm fertilizing ability. Compared with other species the human has a relatively small percentage of sperm showing a "normal" morphology (actually defined as being ideally shaped). Fertility declines as this percentage falls, particularly in men with ejaculates with less than 4% normal-shaped sperms. This assessment requires great skill and experience. Sperms are especially stained and viewed under a microscope, with assessment of the head, middle and tail regions and positively identify white blood cells. Many structurally abnormal sperm have many defects, which may affect all regions of the sperm.

Other assessments: The percentage of sperm that are alive (sperm vitality) is noted because this declines in association with genital tract infections and disorders of sperm transport through the genital tract. The white blood cell count is also an indicator of possible genital tract infections. Even in the absence of a relevant history or symptoms, the finding of a high white cell count may prompt investigation of infection and may warrant a course of appropriate antibiotic therapy. Such infections may contribute to sperm damage and is a easily treatable condition.

Sperm autoimmunity: The immune system produces antibodies as part of the normal defense against foreign substances and organisms. Sperms are normally protected from exposure to immune system. However, some men produce sperm antibodies following surgery (e.g., vasectomy) or trauma to the testicles. In other men there is no apparent cause for the development of antibodies.[21] The antibodies get attached to the surface of the sperm and thus reducing their life span, impairing sperm motility and ability to penetrate the partner's cervical mucus. Finally antibodies located on the sperm head may prevent the sperm fertilizing the egg. Assessment for sperm antibodies is an essential initial test in suspected impaired fertility. The immunobead technique is a simple test that can be used to detect antisperm antibodies in blood or semen.

Ultrasonography

Scrotal ultrasound are very much helpful in the assessment of testicular size, in finding signs of obstruction, such as dilatation of the rete testis, enlarged epididymis with cystic lesions and absence of the vas deferens. Also to exclude signs of testicular dysgenesis such as inhomogeneous testicular architecture and micro calcifications and in the assessment of reflux of blood in men with a varicocele. Transrectal ultrasound (TRUS) can be performed on patients with a low seminal volume and in whom distal obstruction is suspected, if possible with high resolution and high frequency (7 MHz) biplane transducers. Seminal vesicle enlargement (anterior-posterior diameter 15 mm) and seminal vesicle roundish anechoic areas are the TRUS findings more often associated with ejaculatory duct obstruction, especially when the semen volume is less than 1.5 mL. Other known anomalies in cases of obstructive azoospermia are Müllerian duct cysts or urogenital sinus/ejaculatory duct cysts and ejaculatory duct calcifications, which are rare.[22]

Testicular Biopsy

A diagnostic testicular biopsy may be performed in men with azoospermia, with normal testicular volume and normal FSH, to differentiate between obstructive and NOA. Testicular biopsy can also be performed as part of a therapeutic process in patients with clinical evidence of NOA, who decide to undergo ICSI. About 50–60% of men with NOA have some seminiferous tubules with spermatozoa that can be used for ICSI.[22]

GENETIC EVALUATION

Male infertility can be associated with various genetic factors, including chromosomal aberrations, genetic alterations, and Y chromosome microdeletions. Chromosomal aberrations are assessed through G-band karyotyping. Genetic mutations and Y chromosome microdeletions may be also assessed by the analysis of the peripheral blood as such or by DNA amplified by the polymerase chain reaction (PCR) biomolecular technique.

Computer Assisted Sperm Analysis

Computer assisted sperm analysis (CASA) was developed with an intention to establish an accurate automated and objective method for evaluation of sperm concentration and motion characteristics (velocity and head movement). The technology behind CASA is employing highly sophisticated instruments for generating video image for analysis. The accuracy however depend on the method of sample preparation, frame rate and sperm concentration.

Sperm DNA Damage

Men with normal semen profiles are not necessarily fertile, which may be due to abnormal sperm DNA. Sperm DNA damage contributes to around 80% of couples diagnosed with unexplained infertility. Sperm DNA damage is associated with poor fertilization rates and lower live birth rates even following IVF.[24] The tests for sperm DNA damage include COMET assay, TUNEL, sperm chromatin structure assay (SCSA), acridine orange test and sperm chromatin dispersion test. Sperm DNA damage more than 25–27% has been associated with poor reproductive outcome.[25] Indications for sperm DNA Fragmentation Index (DFI) are prolonged idiopathic infertility, low fertilization rates in IVF, repeated abortions, varicocele patients and cancer patients.

SPECIALIZED TESTS

Inspite of great advancements in the field of infertility, there are not many specialized tests and procedures demonstrating the sperm functions namely evaluation of sperm attachment to zona pellucida, penetration of oocyte membrane and the release of acrosomal enzymes. Some of the sperm function tests which are available are mentioned here.

Sperm Penetration Assay

In this assay, zona free eggs which are collected from the superovulated golden hamsters are incubated with washed human sperms. The proportion of eggs penetrated or the number of sperm penetrations per egg by the sperms of the test is compared with a known fertile individual. This test evaluates the capacitation, acrosome reaction, fusion with oolemma and decondensation within the egg cytoplasm.[26] The disadvantage of this test include nonstandardization, not correlation with sperm morphology, cumbersome, costly, time consuming and not widely available.

Human Zona Binding Assay

In this assay, it assesses the ability of sperms to bind to and penetrate the zona pellucida. Here bisected zona derived from human oocytes not previously exposed to sperms and compares the binding of test subject and fertile control sperms. This test has been used to predict the fertilization in vitro.[27] The disadvantage of the test includes the limited availability of human zona and the technical aspects of the test effectively preclude its application beyond as an investigative tool.

Acrosome Reaction

The acrosome reaction involves the fusion of the acrosome and the plasma membrane, followed by the release of the acrosomal enzymes and exposure of the sperm head, which must occur after sperm binding to the zona pellucida. In infertile men it has been noted that, there is an increase prevalence of spontaneous acrosome loss and decreased acrosome reactivity in response to treatment with a calcium ionophore.[28,29] However, the clear cut relevance of these tests in infertility is yet to be established.

FINAL CONSIDERATION

Male infertility may be responsible for 40–60% of cases where a couple is unable to conceive and must not be underestimated. A clear and detailed medical history, physical examination, semen analysis and complementary tests as appropriate, are the key to obtaining a correct diagnosis and to determining the best treatment strategies. **Flowchart 1** depicts algorithms that may aid in the initial assessment of the infertile male and **Flowchart 2** in azoospermia. Semen parameters within the reference interval do not guarantee fertility, nor do values outside those limits necessarily imply male infertility or pathology. They must be interpreted within the context of the patient's clinical information. The reference limits provided by the WHO manual are derived from semen samples used to initiate natural conceptions; they may indicate a need for infertility treatment but not the nature of that treatment **(Table 1)**.

When no clear cause of infertility can be determined, additional tests including genetic testing, sperm DNA fragmentation, and antisperm antibody have to be considered. Novel molecular sperm function tests are emerging in the field of andrology. Genetic evaluation is recommended in cases of severe oligozoospermia and azoospermia, as this analysis may aid in identifying cases in which sperm retrieval is actually possible and may also help in counseling couples about their potential offspring.

TABLE 1: Reference values for semen values (World Health Organization).

Semen parameters	*WHO, 1992*	*WHO, 1999*	*WHO, 2010*
Volume	≥2 mL	≥2 mL	≥1.5 mL
Sperm concentration/mL	≥20 × 10^6/mL	≥20 × 10^6/mL	≥15 × 10^6/mL
Total sperm concentration/ejaculate	≥40 × 10^6	≥40 × 10^6	≥39 × 10^6
Total motility (PR + NP%)	50%	50%	40%
Progressive Motility (PR%)	25% (grade a)	25% (grade a)	32% (a + b)
Vitality (% alive)	75%	75%	58%
Morphology (normal forms %)	30%	14%	4%
Leukocyte count	<1 × 10^6/mL	<1 × 10^6/mL	<1 × 10^6/mL

Flowchart 1: Initial assessment of the infertile male.

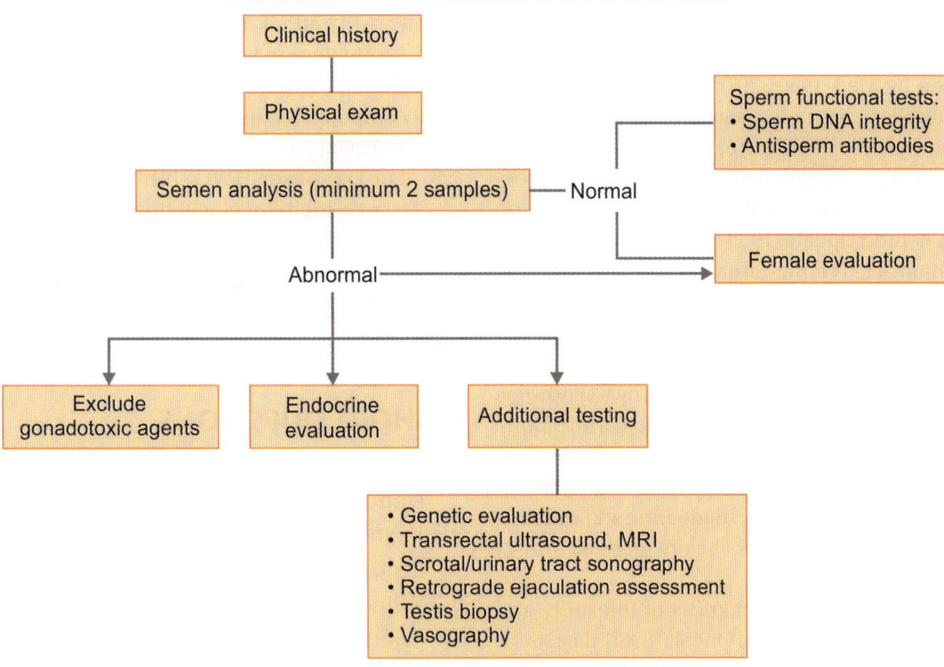

Flowchart 2: Assessment of the infertile male in azoospermia.

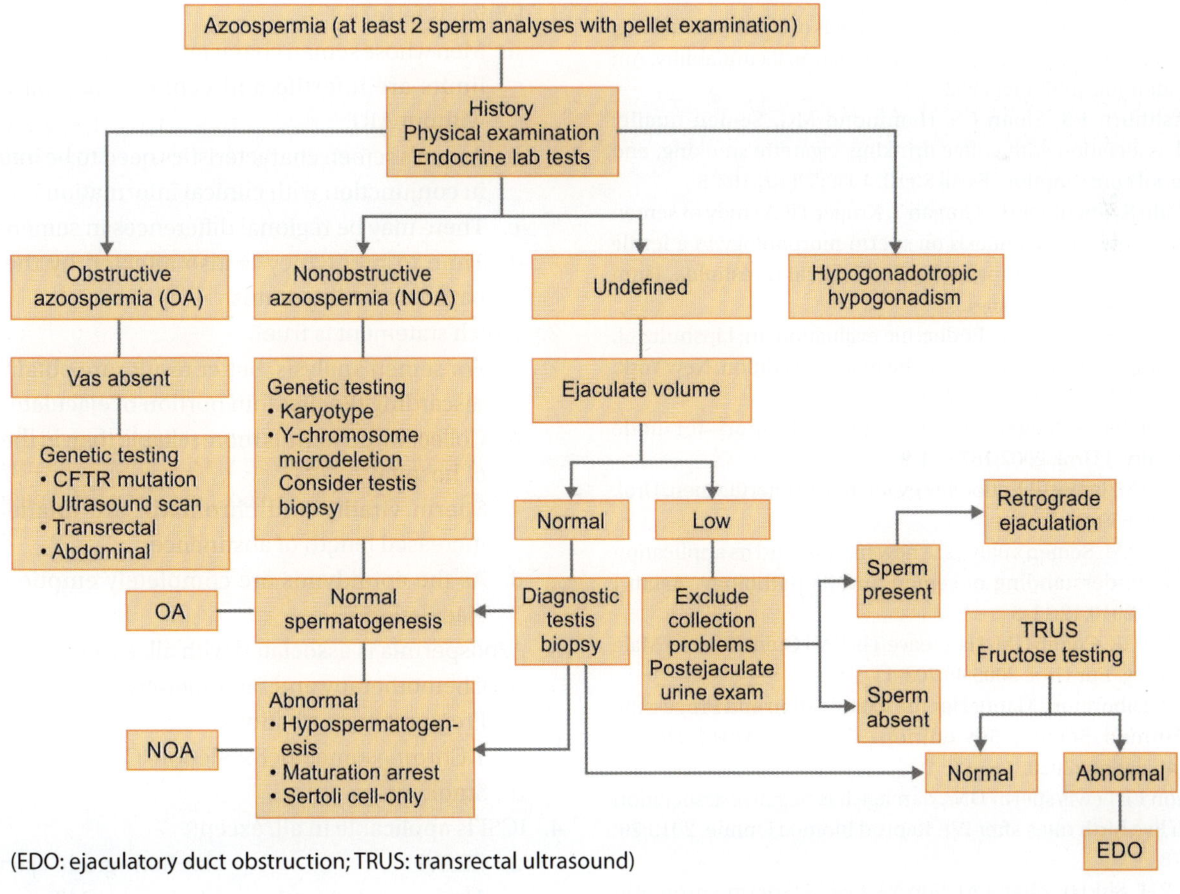

(EDO: ejaculatory duct obstruction; TRUS: transrectal ultrasound)

REFERENCES

1. Lipshultz I, Howards LI, Niederberger CS. Infertility in the Male, 4th edition. Cambridge: Cambridge University Press; 2009.
2. Robaire B, Chan P. Handbook of Andrology, 2nd edition. East Dundee, IL: The American Society of Andrology; 2010.
3. Esteves SC, Ricardo Miyaoka I. An update on the clinical assessment of the infertile male. Clinics. 2011;66(4):691-700.
4. Shefi S, Turek PJ. Definition and current evaluation of subfertile men. Int Braz J Urol. 2006;32:385-97.
5. Hideyuki K, Koichi N, Koichi N. Focus issue on male infertility. Adv Urol. 2012;823582:1-6.

6. Anderson JB, Williamson RC. Fertility after torsion of the spermatic cord. Br J Urol. 1990;65(3):225-30.
7. Werner CA. Mumps orchitis and testicular atrophy; a factor in male sterility. Ann Int Med. 1950;32(6):1075-86.
8. Greene LG, Kelalis PP. Retrograde ejaculation of semen due to diabetic neuropathy. J Urol. 1967;98(6):696.
9. Weidner W, Krause W, Ludwig M. Relevance of male accessory gland infection for subsequent fertility with special focus on prostatitis. Hum Reprod Update. 1999;5:421-32.
10. Wilton LJ, Teichtahl H, Temple-Smith PD, de Kretser DM. Kartagener's syndrome with motile cilia and immotile spermatozoa: axonemal ultrastructure and function. Am Rev Respir Dis. 1986;134(6):1233-6.
11. Wilton LJ, Teichtahl H, Temple-Smith PD. Young's syndrome (obstructive azoospermia and chronic sino bronchial infection): a quantitative study of axonemal ultrastructure and function. Fertil Steril. 1991;55(1):144-51.
12. Carroll PR, Whitmore Jr WF. Herr HW. Endocrine and exocrine profiles of men with testicular tumors before orchidectomy. J Urol. 1987;137(3):420-3.
13. Ohl DA, Sonksen J. What are the chances of infertility and should sperm be banked? Semin Urol Oncol. 1996;14(1):36-44.
14. de Celis R, Feria-Velasco A, Gonz'alez-Unzaga M. Semen quality of workers occupationally exposed to hydrocarbons Fertil Steril. 2000;73(2):221-8.
15. Curtis KM, Savitz DA, Arbuckle TE. Effects of cigarette smoking, caffeine consumption, and alcohol intake on fecundability. Am J Epidemiol. 1997;146(1):32-41.
16. Marshburn PB, Sloan CS, Hammond MG. Semen quality and association with coffee drinking, cigarette smoking, and ethanol consumption. Fertil Steril. 1989;52(10):162-5.
17. Gunalp S, Onculoglu C, Gurgan T, Kruger TF. A study of semen parameters with emphasis on sperm morphology in a fertile population: an attempt to develop clinical thresholds. Hum Reprod. 2001;16(1):110-4.
18. Sokol RZ, Swerdloff RS. Endocrine evaluation. In: Lipshultz LI, Howards SS (Eds). Infertility in the male, 3rd edition. New York: Churchill Livingstone; 1997. pp. 210-8.
19. Raman JD, Schlegel PN. Aromatase inhibitors for male infertility. J Urol. 2002;167:624-9.
20. Sigman M, Jarow JP. Endocrine evaluation of infertile men. Urol. 1997;50:659-64.
21. Jequier AM. Semen analysis: a new manual and its application to the understanding of semen and its pathology. Asian J Androl. 2010;12:11-3.
22. Dohlea GR, Colpib GM, Hargreave TB. EAU Guidelines on Male Infertility. Eur Urol. 2005;48:703-11.
23. WHO. Laboratory Manual for the Examination and Processing of Human Semen, 5th edition. Geneva: World Health Organization; 2010.
24. Simon LJ. Lewis sperm DNA damage has negative association with live birth rates after IVF. Reprod Biomed Online. 2013;26: 68-78.
25. Niu ZH, Shi HJ, Zhang AJ, Sun YJ, Lee JS. Sperm chromatin structure assay results after swim up are related only to embryo qulaity but not to fertilization and pregnancy rates following IVF. Asian J Androl. 2011;13:862-6.
26. Smith RG, Johnson A, Lamb D, Lipshultz LI. Functional tests of spermatozoa. Sperm penetration assay. Urol Clin North Am. 1987;14:451.
27. Coddington CC III. The hemizona assay (HZA) and considerations for its use in assisted reproductive technology. Semin Reprod Endocrinol. 1992;10:1.
28. Barratt CL, Tomlinson MJ, Cooke ID. Prognostic significance of computerized motility analysis for in vivo fertility, Fertil Steril. 1993;60:520.
29. Liu DY, Baker HWG. Inhibition of acrosin activity with a trypsin inhibitor blocks human sperm penetration of the zona pellucida. Biol Reprod. 1993;48:340.

LONG QUESTION

1. How will you evaluate male factor in infertility?

SHORT QUESTIONS

1. What are the normal values of semen variables by WHO standard?
2. Write a short on the importance of testicular biopsy in azoospermia.
3. What is the significance of hormonal evaluation in evaluating male factor infertility?

MULTIPLE CHOICE QUESTIONS

1. Which is false?
   a. Men whose semen characteristics fall below the lower limits are infertile and cannot enjoy parenthood without ART
   b. A man's semen characteristics need to be interpreted in conjunction with clinical information
   c. There may be regional differences in semen quality
   d. Time to pregnancy is also affected by the female partner's fertility status
2. Which statement is true?
   a. For semen analysis, better results are obtained after discarding the first thin portion of ejaculate
   b. Collection at home is more reliable than in the vicinity of hospital
   c. Sperm vitality and chromatin are unaffected by increased length of abstinence
   d. As the epididymis are completely emptied by one ejaculation
3. Azoospermia is associated with all, except:
   a. Chemotherapy and radiotherapy
   b. Frequent masturbations
   c. Y Chromosome microdeletion/*CFTR* gene defects
   d. Smoking
4. ICSI is applicable in all, except:
   a. CBAVD b. Retrograde ejaculation
   c. Undescended testis d. Severe OAT
5. While evaluating the male partner:
   a. Supine position is preferred
   b. Testicular USG has no role
   c. Delayed sexual development with anosmia can be Klinefelter syndrome

d. Chronic respiratory infections with azoospermia raise suspicion of Young syndrome

6. Which one is true?
   a. Testicular size 20 mL is hydrocele and must be operated
   b. It is a good practice to rule out Y-microdeletions and CFTR in azoospermic patients
   c. Ipsilateral, dull, pulling pain may be of varicocele hence should be operated immediately to improve sperm count
   d. ASA antibodies must be seen in every male
7. For a tall, infertile azoospermic man with a history of poor grades at school with surgery for enlarged breasts, following is false:
   a. Most likely the karyotype would reveal the extra X chromosome and the diagnosis Klinefelter syndrome
   b. Small testis and small penis is expected at clinical examination
   c. The endocrinology value will have low FSH, low LH and high testosterone
   d. Such patients are prone to other medical conditions like SLE and osteoporosis
8. Drugs that can impair semen quality are all, except:
   a. Cardiac drugs like digoxin, thiazide diuretics and β blockers
   b. Antiepileptics like phenytoin
   c. Antibiotics like erythromycin and gentamycin
   d. Antiestrogens like clomiphene
9. Lower reference limit (World Health Organization 2010): Total sperm number (106 per ejaculate)/Total motility (PR + NP, %)/Vitality (live spermatozoa, %)/Sperm morphology (normal forms, %) is:
   a. 39/40/58/4
   b. 50/45/39/5
   c. 20/40/40/15
   d. 40/20/19/25
10. Regarding varicocele, all are true, except:
    a. More common on left side as left cremasteric vein it directly inserts into renal vein
    b. Associated rise in scrotal temperature and effect of toxic metabolites of left renal/adrenal vein is the suspected pathophysiology
    c. Despite the frequent use of surgery, its benefits related to infertility are still controversial
    d. Small varicocele diagnosed on USG, not clinically felt do not need any treatment
11. Azoospermia associated with high FSH is seen in:
    a. CBAVD
    b. Varicocele
    c. Seminoma
    d. Post-sterilization
12. Regarding hypogonadotropic hypogonadism all are true, except:
    a. Also called pre-testicular azoospermia
    b. Low FSH, low LH and low testosterone is characteristically seen
    c. hCG + HMG is the effective treatment with dose titrated to keep testosterone and estrogen levels normal
    d. Testosterone is given externally to improve the sperm count
13. While discussion with the couple about male factor it is wrong to state that:
    a. Male factor is cause in 20% infertile couples
    b. 10–20% azoospermic or severely oligospermic men carry Y microdeletions
    c. An abnormal semen analysis means the impotence or absolute infertility
    d. Cessation of smoking improves the count

Answers

1.	a	2.	c	3.	b	4.	c	5.	d	6.	b
7.	c	8.	d	9.	a	10.	a	11.	c	12.	d
13.	c										

12.3 INVESTIGATIONS FOR THE FEMALE PARTNER

Rishma Dhillon Pai, Meenu Handa

INTRODUCTION

Infertility still remains a huge social and distressing situation for many couples worldwide. Infertility is defined as a disease of the reproductive system wherein there is a failure to achieve pregnancy after 12 or more months of regular unprotected intercourse.[1] It is estimated that around 85% of couples conceive by the end of first year and up to 90% at the end of 24 months of regular unprotected intercourse. The rate of conception does not seem to increase significantly thereafter, hence the cutoff of 12 months has been taken by WHO. It is imperative to ascertain the etiology of infertility before proceeding for any management strategy. In around 20–25% of the couples, ovulatory dysfunction is the main cause, tubal factor, and peritoneal pathology in another 35–40% and male factor responsible in the rest 30–40% of the infertile couple **(Fig. 1)**. Unexplained infertility compromises for around 10% of the total causes in an infertile couple. In women, tubal and pelvic pathology compromises around 35–40% cases, ovulatory disorders for 40% cases, unexplained infertility for the rest 10%. Rare causes such as immunological factors, cervical factor and infectious diseases account for less than 5% of the cases.[2]

It is also being recognized that apart from the above known causes there can be numerous undetectable defects that can

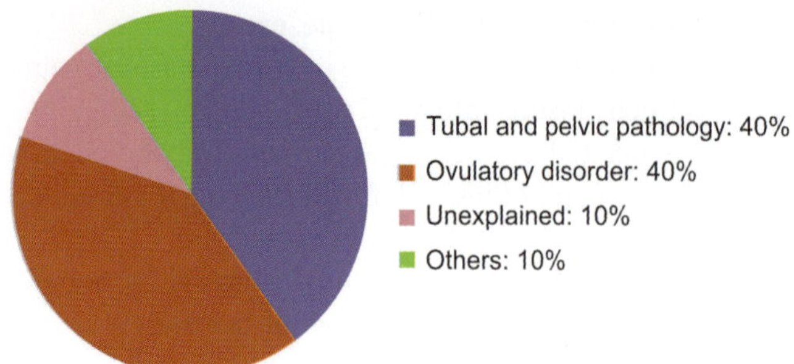

Fig. 1: Causes of infertility in women.

hinder the fertility of a couple. Factors which remain elusive from the routine investigations available today and which can hinder the fertility potential can be the factors involved in the fertilization and post fertilization processes.

There has been an increase in the need for infertility treatment as the prevalence of infertility has shown an upward trend in the last few decades worldwide. The prevalence range of infertility in developed countries varies from 3.5 to 16.7% while it is around 6.5 to 9.3% in the developing nations.[3] Numerous reasons have been accounted for the increased trend of infertility in this era. One of them is delayed child bearing of women. In one of the studies it was found that the mean age of childbearing is currently around 29.5 years in comparison to 25 years two decades earlier.[4] Age is one of the most crucial prognostic parameters of fertility index. With advancing maternal age not only there is difficulty to conceive but also the risks of complications in pregnancy increases drastically.

COUNSELING

A clear investigative and treatment protocol should be initially discussed with the couple in which thorough counseling which takes care of the emotional need of the couple should be addressed. Social factors also contribute to the heightened stress of the couple undergoing infertility treatment. If not addressed simultaneously then these patients show varied degrees of anxiety related problems, depression and helplessness due to the sense of loss of control over their life. Every assisted reproductive technology (ART) clinic should provide counseling to their patients with the aid of a trained counselor.

In one of the recent randomized controlled trials (RCT) where women with less than 2 years of infertility duration provided with adequate psychological help like cognitive behavioral therapy and support there was increase in the pregnancy rates. (55% in a cognitive behavioral therapy group vs. 54% in a support group vs. 20% in a routine care group).[5] Many couples feel that they benefit psychologically if some kind of support and counseling is provided to them at all stages of infertility investigations and treatment.

To guide infertility patients smoothly through their journey, the Human Fertilisation and Embryology Act (HFEA) Code of Practice[6] in 2008 came up with three distinct types of counseling:

1. *Implication counseling:* It aims to make the patient understand the implications of proposed treatments and consequent actions for themselves, their families and for any children born as a result of the infertility treatment given and anyone else affected by the donation or treatment.
2. *Support counseling*: It aims to give emotional support at times of stress (before, during or after the treatment). In particular times when there is a need of specific counseling like failure to achieve a pregnancy. The need of the support to the patient is identified and provided clearly.
3. *Therapeutic counseling:* It aims to help people understand and cope with the consequences of infertility and treatment, resolve any issues which these may cause and also to make adjustments to their expectations so that they can realistically and practically cope with the outcome of the treatment.

To a certain extent psychological issues related to stress and anxiety can be alleviated by providing the patient with clear written information about all aspects of investigations and management plan. All patients should be able to make informed decisions with due respect to their treatment options available with the help of information based on the current evidence. Verbal information should be well supported with written information as well.

HISTORY

Any management of an infertile couple begins with a comprehensive medical and surgical history of both partners to help develop a clear investigative and treatment protocol individualized to meet the couple's need.

Before proceeding with the history it is pertinent that one is aware of the epidemiology of infertility. The history of the female includes current history regarding her age and occupation (helps to know if an occupational hazard is present), any current medical history, menstrual history with its pattern and changes, obstetric, contraceptive, and sexual history **(Box 1)**. It is important to inquire about coital frequency and timing, sexual dysfunction, and possible use of lubricants that may be spermicidal. Questions can be directed to know the endocrinologic etiologies of infertility, including galactorrhea, weight fluctuations, frontal balding, and recent onset of acne facial hair. The male partner's history should include known prior fertility and sexual history. History should also look into previous fertility treatment taken along with previous investigations if done any.

It is imperative to guide the couple regarding optimization of their health before initiating infertility treatment plan **(Box 2)**. This is should go along with the investigations as well.

BOX 1: History taking for infertile women.

History of (H/O) infertile female:
- Current history
  - Age, occupation
  - Recent Pap smear findings
  - H/O any breast secretions
  - H/O excessive hair growth on face with or without acne
- Menstrual history
  - Age of menarche, cycle characteristics
  - H/O of painful menstruation, intermenstrual bleed
  - H/O of primary/secondary amenorrhea
- Obstetric history
  - Previous pregnancy if any and its outcome
  - H/O abortions (induced/spontaneous)
  - H/O recurrent pregnancy losses
  - H/O Post abortion/puerperal sepsis
- Contraceptive history
  - Previous history of contraception (especially intrauterine device)
  - Any history related to associated problems if any
- Sexual history
  - Coital frequency and its timing with fertile period
  - H/O difficulty/painful coitus
  - H/O loss of libido
  - H/O use of vaginal lubricants
- Past history
  - H/O any medical disorder
  - H/O surgery (tuberculosis, endometriosis)
  - H/O sexually transmitted disease
- Family history
  - H/O any medical disorder
  - H/O any genetic disorder
  - H/O consanguinity

INVESTIGATIONS

Once an elaborate history has been taken, physical examination of the endocrine and gynecologic systems should be performed thoroughly. The main causes of female infertility can be divided into ovulation disorders, tubal abnormalities along with peritoneal pathology, uterine abnormalities. Cervical pathology and immunological factors are rare causes of female fertility.

General Investigations

General health screening including body mass index (BMI), blood pressure, cervical cytology, and check for sexually transmitted diseases is recommended **(Box 3)**.

OVARIAN FACTOR

Ovulatory Disorders

Ovulatory dysfunction compromises for 40% cases in women leading to inability to conceive. WHO classifies ovulatory disorders into three groups: Group I is caused by hypothalamic pituitary failure also known as hypogonadotropic hypogonadism. This group accounts for 10% of the ovulatory disorder. Group I is characterized by low gonadotropins, low estrogen and normal prolactin. Group II is caused by hypothalamic pituitary dysfunction. This group accounts for over 85% of the ovulatory disorders. This group of disorders results in anovulatory oligo/amenorrhea, predominately involving women with polycystic ovaries. Group III is caused by ovarian failure. It is characterized by high gonadotropins levels with hypogonadism and low estrogen and this group accounts for around 5% of ovulatory disorders. A thorough history taking of the menstrual cycle can point toward ovulatory dysfunction to quite an extent. Regular menstrual cycles in the range 26–36 days are usually indicative of ovulation. A number of direct and indirect tests are available which help to determine ovulation.

BOX 2: Optimizing health conditions.

- Maintain normal BMI
- Moderate exercise – 40 minutes daily
- Restrict alcohol < 1–2 units/week
- Stop smoking
- Optimize preexisting medical conditions (HTN, DM, neurological disorders, renal disorders)
- Avoid teratogenic drugs
- Folic acid supplementation 0.4 mg/day (5 mg/day with previous H/O NTD, DM or taking antiepileptic medication)
- Rubella vaccination if seronegative
- Treat any psychosexual problem if present

(BMI: body mass index; DM: diabetes mellitus; HTN: hypertension; H/O: history of; NTD: nueral tube defect)

BOX 3: Examination for female partner during infertility workup.

- BMI
- Blood pressure
- *Signs for endocrinopathies:*
  - Acanthosis, acne, hirsutism, balding
  - Visual field defects
  - Goiter (neck swelling), signs of thyroid ds
  - Galactorrhea/any breast lump
- *Abdominal examination:* Lump, scar, striae
- *Pelvic examination:*
  - Uterine mobility, cervical tenderness/adnexal mass
  - Vaginal nodule/developmental anomaly
- Cervical smear if required
- Blood for sexually transmitted diseases (HIV, HBsAG, HCV, VDRL)
- *Endocrine profile:* TSH, serum prolactin, serum FSH, serum LH
  - *PCOS patients:* Glucose tolerance, androgen levels
- *Rubella status:* IgG rubella

(BMI: body mass index; HIV: human immunodeficiency virus; HCV: hepatitis C virus; FSH: follicle stimulating hormone; LH: luteinizing hormone; TSH: thyroid stimulating hormone; PCOS: polycystic ovary syndrome; VDRL: venereal disease research laboratory)

Indirect Methods

Indirect methods rely on measuring the ovarian or the pituitary hormones or at times their biological effects. As the secretion of estrogen increases by the dominant follicle, there is an luteinizing hormone (LH) surge due to the positive mechanism which is succeeded by the ovulation 36–38 hours later (post ovulation).

Serum progesterone levels: During the follicular phase progesterone levels generally remain below 1 ng/mL, then rise slightly on the day of the LH surge (1–2 ng/mL) and peak 7–8 days after ovulation, and decline again over the days preceding menses. A progesterone concentration less than 3 ng/mL implies anovulation, except when drawn immediately after ovulation or just before the onset of menses and levels more than 30 ng/mL are almost suggestive of ovulation. A day 21 progesterone levels can be done if a patient has regular 28 day cycles.[7] For patients who have cycles ranging from 25 to 35 days then it is advisable to measure the serum progesterone levels approximately 1 week before the expected periods. Though there is no consensus to the minimum level of progesterone which gives evidence of normal luteal function. A mid luteal serum progesterone of more than 10 ng/mL is suggestive of ovulation.[8]

Urinary LH: Commercially available urinary kits can detect mid cycle LH surge. The main advantage of using these urinary kits to detect ovulation is that it is not only simple, cost effective, cheap, can be done effortlessly by the patient but also noninvasive and does not need the patient to visit the hospital. The mid-cycle LH surge is a relatively short event lasting only for around 48–50 hours. As LH has a short half-life and cleared very rapidly in the urine, it is important to detect LH surge reliably. It should be tested daily, beginning 2–3 days before the surge is expected depending upon the overall menstrual cycle. Once the test is positive then the period of maximum fertility is on the day of the surge detected followed by the next 2 days. It should be kept in mind that women with PCOS and basal high serum LH levels can give high false positives results which can be around 7%.

Serum follicle stimulating hormone: A baseline serum follicle stimulating hormone (FSH) optimally performed during the first 3 days of the cycle helps to differentiate between different WHO groups of ovulatory disorders. A high serum FSH level (more than 30–40 IU/L) with a low estradiol level can distinguish WHO group III-Ovarian failure from WHO group I-Hypothalamic pituitary failure, which typically reveals a low or normal FSH level (less than 10 IU/L) and a low estradiol level. At times findings with high FSH level (10–20 IU/L) along with decreased anti-Müllerian hormone (AMH) can be marker of diminished ovarian reserve.[9]

The imprecise tests such as basal body temperature, cervical mucus test and endometrial biopsy is no longer recommended in clinical practice.

Direct Methods

Transvaginal ultrasound: This allows the direct visualization of the collapse of the dominant follicle with appearance of free fluid in the pouch of Douglas.[10] The preovulatory follicle grows at a steady rate of 1-3 mm/day, hence with serial ultrasound monitoring it is possible to track down the exact date of ovulation. This method of detection of ovulation is invasive and also expensive. Patients who require ovarian stimulation and the ones where the kits have failed to show mid cycle LH surge consistently will benefit from TVS. Finally, the method chosen to document ovulation should be the one which best suits an individual patient.

Ovarian reserve tests: The number of ovarian follicles remaining in the ovaries plays a significant role in determining the future fertility of a woman. During the reproductive age there is a steady decline of ovarian follicles till the menopause. It has been shown by the studies that with increasing age, both the number and the quality of the ovarian follicle diminish. Hence at any given time the age remains the most important prognostic factor for fertility. Additional ovarian reserve tests include measurement of serum FSH levels, serum AMH and determining the antral follicle count (AFC).[11] Other tests such as serum inhibin levels, ovarian blood flow, and volume are not routinely recommended as they have low level of predictability for ovarian function.[12]

Antral follicle count: With the help of transvaginal ultrasound of the pelvis, antral follicles can be easily accessed. It has been now shown that the number of small antral follicles (2–6 mm diameter) decline significantly with increased maternal age with little change in the larger follicles (7–10 mm).[13] Infact the smaller antral follicles 2–6 mm are the ones who will get recruited and respond to exogenous stimulation. According to the NICE 2012 update total AFC less than or equal to 2 predicts low ovarian response to gonadotropin stimulation in IVF cycles while AFC greater than 16 predicts a high response.[12]

Serum FSH: At times findings with basal high FSH level (10–20 IU/L) along with decreased AMH can be marker of diminished ovarian reserve. The NICE 2012 recommended that basal follicle-stimulating hormone taken postmenstrually till day 3 cycles greater than 10 IU/L predicts for a low ovarian response to gonadotropin stimulation in IVF cycles and less than 4 IU/L for a high response.

Serum AMH: Anti-Müllerian hormone is a dimeric glycoprotein and a member of transforming growth factor (TGF-beta) superfamily which is known for its role in inhibiting the Müllerian structures. AMH is produced in the preantral and small antral follicles of the granulose cells in the females and shows little cycle to cycle and also intracycle variation.[14] The studies now have shown that AMH levels of less than or equal to 5.4 pmol/L predict for a low ovarian response and greater than or equal to 25.0 pmol/L for a high response.

The current guidelines do not recommend the use of serum inhibin levels, serum estradiol levels, ovarian flow and volume as well as "ovarian challenge tests" to be used as ovarian reserve tests any more in the clinical practice.

TUBAL FACTOR

Tubal factor along with peritoneal pathology accounts for around 35–40% infertility cases. Few women have higher risks for tubal pathology such as women with previous history of ectopic disease or pelvic inflammatory disease and endometriosis.

Hysterosalpingography

Infertile women with no clear risk of tubal obstruction should be offered hysterosalpingography (HSG) as the preliminary tubal testing to screen for tubal occlusion and structural uterine abnormalities **(Table 1)**. HSG is minimally invasive tests that delineate both the uterine cavity along with tubes well. It can be done within 10 days of menstrual cycle as an outpatient procedure with few complications.[15]

TABLE 1: Hysterosalpingography (HSG) findings with probable causes of tubal occlusion.

HSG finding	*Cause*
Normal finding	Triangular smooth uterine cavity delineation with B/L free tubal spill
Small filling defects	Air bubbles/small polyps
Large convoluted/ retort sacculations	Hydrosalpinges (HS)
Convoluted distal tube	HS/Peritubal adhesions
No dye in the tubes/ cornual block	Spasm/obliterative fibrosis/ salpingitis isthmica nodosa (SIN)
Multiple small diverticula of the proximal 2 cm of the tube	SIN
Rigid tube ("pipe-stem" appearance)/beaded tube	Tuberculosis

The cannula is to be inserted into the cervical canal and the contrast media is gently injected. There can be variety of cannula used such as metallic Leisch-Wilkinson, Green-Armytage cannula or the plastic/balloon catheters. There are two types of contrast medium used —water soluble and another oil-based contrast media. Water soluble contrast medium is well absorbed and well tolerated by the patients. In a meta-analysis of 20 studies comparing HSG and laparoscopy for tubal patency it was found out that sensitivity of HSG was 0.65 and specificity 0.83 (95% CI 0.77–0.88).[16] If on HSG a tubal block is found then it is actually reconfirmed in only 38–40% cases on laparoscopy while if the tubes are patent then it is actually open in around 92–94% cases **(Figs. 2A to C)**.

Oil based contrast media though are less favored due to the risk of venous intravasation of the dye but studies favoring the oil based media have shown that they tend to "unblock/ dissolve" the tubal plugs. A meta-analysis of 10 studies comparing the oil based contrast media and water soluble contrast showed that spontaneous pregnancy rates were significantly higher after oil based contrast media.[17]

Hysterosalpingo-contrast Sonography

The advantage of doing HSG using ultrasound contrast media containing galactose microparticles (Echovist) is the

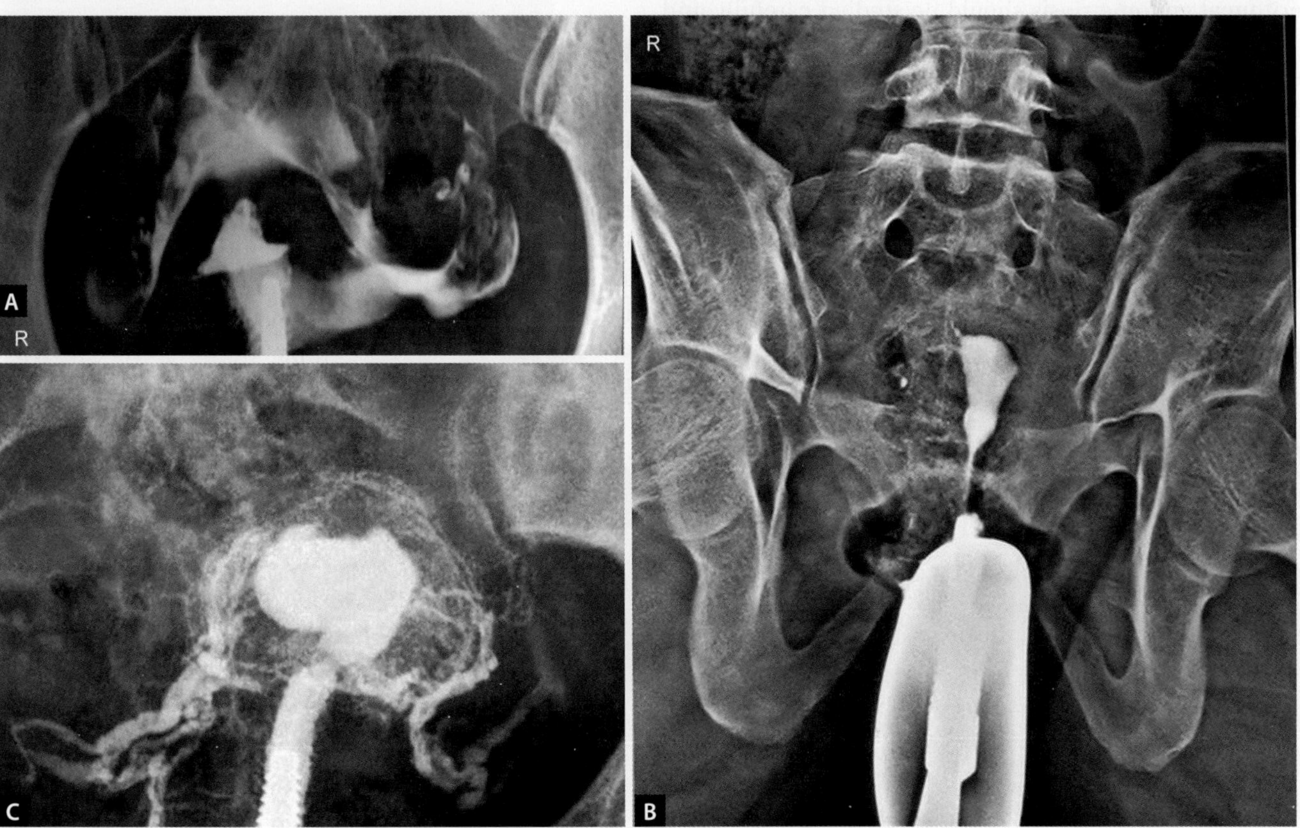

Figs. 2A to C: Hysterosalpingography. (A) Normal uterus and open tubes; (B) Normal uterus and bilateral tubal block; (C) Venous intravasation.

elimination of risk of radiation. Also one can evaluate the pelvis for uterus, adnexa and the ovarian morphology. It also has a high concordance rate of 80–90% with laparoscopy. Some studies have shown that saline used as ultrasound contrast media has similar success rate as galactose microparticles. When saline is used, 3-D imaging of the uterine cavity can also be done at the same sitting.[18] The main limitation using hysterosalpingo-contrast sonography (HyCoSy) is the need of trained personnel at all times and the additional time taken to do the pelvic assessment **(Fig. 3)**.

Laparoscopy

Laparoscopy provides detailed information about the pelvic anatomy that HSG cannot, including adhesions, endometriosis, and ovarian pathology. A laparoscopy is preferred when there is a probability of pelvic pathology which would also need "see and treat" approach. Infertile women with history of previous abdominal surgery, history suggestive of endometriosis, recurrent pelvic inflammatory disease (PID) can benefit from laparoscopy. Laparoscopic assessment of the pelvis should include careful panoramic inspection of the uterus, tubes, ovaries, peritoneal surfaces, bladder, and the bowel. Methylene blue dye is injected transcervically (chromotubation) and the fimbrial ends of the fallopian tube observed for spill.

Past infections of PID are characterized by pelvic adhesions, perihepatic adhesions (chlamydial/gonococcal infections) known as "Fitz-Hugh-Curtis syndrome". Signs of peritoneal endometriosis should be studied carefully and it is now recommended by ESHRE 2014 guideline that any peritoneal implant seen on diagnostic laparoscopy should be treated. The ablative therapy is found to significantly increase the spontaneous pregnancy rates in these infertile women.[19]

UTERINE FACTOR

Uterine abnormalities are a relatively uncommon cause of infertility, but should always be considered. About 10–15% women coming to the fertility clinic present with uterine abnormalities. The anatomic uterine abnormalities that can adversely affect fertility compromise congenital uterine malformations, fibroids, endometrial polyps, and intrauterine adhesions. The main investigations which can easily diagnose Uterine cavity can be assessed by HSG, transvaginal ultrasonography (TVS) or saline sonohysterography, and hysteroscopy. Hysteroscopy is recognized as the "gold standard" test for identifying uterine abnormalities as it allows direct visualization of the uterine cavity.[20]

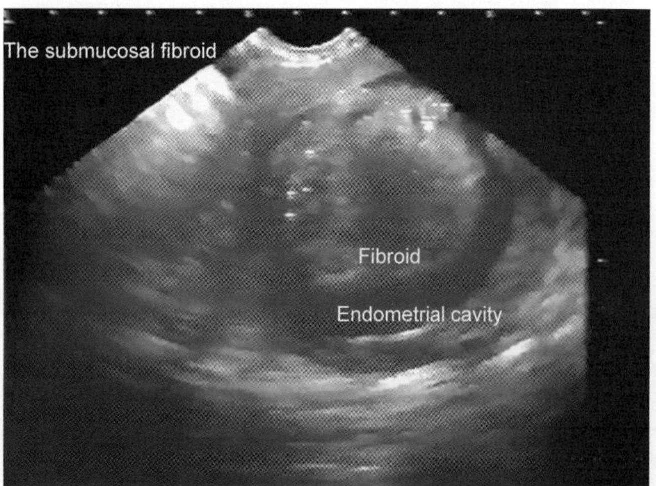

Fig. 3: Sonosalpingography or HyCosY can be used for tubal testing and defining the endometrial cavity.

Transvaginal Ultrasound

Transvaginal ultrasound is recommended as the first line of investigation to study the pelvic anatomy to with more accuracy and reliability with no radiation exposure. TVS can be used in the evaluation of pelvic pathology, such as leiomyoma, endometrioma, uterine polyp, adnexal pathology. HSG is the conventional method for testing the tubes but also gives information regarding the uterine cavity.

Hysterosalpingography (Table 2)

The accuracy of HSG for detecting intrauterine pathology in infertile women varies with the nature of the abnormality. HSG has around 75% sensitivity for detection of intrauterine adhesions and only 50% sensitivity for detection of endometrial polyps.[7]

Hysteroscopy

Hysteroscopy is recognized as the "gold standard" test for identifying uterine abnormalities as it allows direct visualization of the uterine cavity. As it is an invasive procedure and many times it is done along with diagnostic laparoscopy if required during the workup of the infertile women. Women should not be offered hysteroscopy on its own as part of the initial investigation unless clinically indicated because the effectiveness of surgical Investigation on improving pregnancy rates has not been established.[12]

TABLE 2: Hysterosalpingography (HSG) findings with probable causes of uterine pathology.

HSG findings	*Causes*
Grossly irregular cavity contours and filling defects	Intrauterine synechia/ Asherman's syndrome
Opacification of a single uterine cavity and single fallopian tube	Unicornuate Uterus
Opacification of two symmetric fusiform uterine cavities (horns) and fallopian tubes. Common lower segment with Y-shaped configuration	Bicornuate uterus/septate uterus
Small filling defects	Air bubbles/small polyps

REFERENCES

1. Zegers-Hochschild F, Adamson GD. International Committee for Monitoring Assisted Reproductive Technology (ICMART) and the World Health Organization (WHO) revised glossary of ART terminology, 2009. Fertil Steril. 2009;92:1520-4.
2. Jaffe SB, Jewelewicz MR. The basic infertility investigation. Fertil Sterili. 1991;56(4): 599-613.
3. Boivin J, Bunting L, Collins JA. International estimates of infertility prevalence and treatment seeking: potential need and demand for infertility medical care. Hum Reprod. 2007;22:1506-12.
4. ESHRE Capri Workshop Group. Fertility and Ageing. Human Reprod Update. 2005;11:261-76.
5. Domar AD, Clapp DE. Impact of group psychological interventions on pregnancy rates in infertile women. Fertil Steril. 2000;73:805-11.
6. Human Fertilisation and Embryology Authority. Code of Practice, 6th edition. London: HFEA; 2004.
7. Marca A Fritz, Leon Speroff. Clinical Gynecologic Endocrinology & Infertility. 8th Edition. Chapter 27. Female infertility;1149-1190.
8. Practice Committee of American Society for Reproductive Medicine. Diagnostic evaluation of the infertile female: a committee opinion. Fertil Steril. 2012;98(2):302-7.
9. Nelson LM. Clinical practice. Primary ovarian insufficiency. N Engl J Med. 2009;360(6):606-14.
10. Branstromm M, Zackrisson U. Preovulatory changes of blood in different regions of the human follicle. Fertil Steril. 1998; 69:435-42.
11. Broekmans FJ, Kwee J. A systematic review of test predicting ovarian reserve and IVF Outcome. Human Reprod Update. 2006;12(6):685-718.
12. National Collaborating Centre for Women's and Children's Health. Fertility: assessment and treatment for people with fertility problems. London: National Institute for Health and Clinical Excellence (NICE); 2013. pp. 1-63.
13. Haadsma ML, Bukman A. The number of small antral follicles (2-6 mm) determines the outcome of endocrine ovarian reserve tests in subfertile population. Hum Reprod. 2007;22: 1925-31.
14. La MarcaA. Volpe A. Anti-Mullerian hormone in female reproduction:is measurement of circulating AMH a useful tool? Clin Endocrinol. 2006;64:603-10.
15. Luttjeboer F, Harada T, Hughes E, Johnson N, Lilford R, Mol BW. Tubal flushing for subfertility. Cochrane Database Syst Rev. 2007;(3):CD003718.
16. Swart P, Mol BW. The accuracy of hysterosalpingography in the diagnosis of tubal pathology: a meta-analysis. Fertil Steril. 1995;64:486-91.
17. Watson A, Vanderkerckhove P. A meta-analysis of the therapeutic role of oil soluble contrast media at hysterosalpingography: a surprising result? Fertil Steril. 1994;61:470-7.
18. Balen FG, Allen CM, Gardener JE. Three dimensional reconstruction of the ultrasound images of the uterine cavity. Br J Radiol. 1993;66:588-91.
19. Dunselman GA, Vermeulen N, Becker C. ESHRE guideline: management of women with endometriosis. Hum Reprod. 2014;29(3):400-12.
20. Golan A, Eilat E, Ron-El R, Herman A, Soffer Y, Bukovsky I. Hysteroscopy is superior to hysterosalpingography in infertility investigation. Acta Obstet Gynecol Scand. 1996;75:654-6.

LONG QUESTIONS

1. Describe in detail regarding the ovulatory disorders and the ovarian reserve tests.
2. Describe in detail regarding the investigations used for assessing tubal pathology.

SHORT QUESTIONS

1. Describe in short the role of counseling in the management of infertile female.
2. Describe in short the different types of ovulatory disorders.
3. Describe in short regarding AMH.

MULTIPLE CHOICE QUESTIONS

1. The percentage of infertile couple having ovulatory disorder:
   a. 10% b. 5% c. 25% d. 70%
2. The percentage of infertile couple having tubal disorder:
   a. 40% b. 15% c. <2% d. 7 %
3. The gold standard investigation in evaluating uterine pathology is:
   a. HSG b. TVS
   c. Hysteroscopy d. None of the above
4. In how many cases immunological factors are the cause of infertility:
   a. 5% b. 25% c. 30% d. 55%
5. The sensitivity of HSG for tubal patency is:
   a. 0.15 b. 0.65 c. 0.93 d. 0.10
6. AMH is secreted from:
   a. Small preantral follicles
   b. Large antral follicles
   c. Preovulatory follicle
   d. None of the above
7. Serum progesterone is best done on:
   a. Day 11 b. Day 21
   c. Day 13 d. None of the above
8. Prevalence of infertility in developing nation is around:
   a. 6–9% b. 15–20% c. 30–40% d. 50–60%
9. HyCoSy has concordance with laparoscopy of around:
   a. 50% b. 15%
   c. 80% d. None of the above
10. Multiple small diverticula seen at the proximal 2 cm of the tube is seen in:
    a. SIN b. Tuberculosis
    c. Polyp d. Synechia

Answers

1.	c	2.	a	3.	c	4.	a	5.	b	6.	a
7.	b	8.	a	9.	c	10.	a				

12.4 MALE INFERTILITY: ETIOLOGY AND MANAGEMENT

Ajay S Shetty, Rupin Shah

INTRODUCTION

Of the 15% of couples that are unable to conceive after 1 year of unprotected intercourse, the male partner is either solely or significantly responsible for the infertility of the couple in approximately 50% of cases. With the advent of assisted reproductive techniques (ART) and the tremendous success it has enjoyed in the treatment of infertile couples, the evaluation of the male partner, and an attempt at curative treatment is often overlooked. Though, there have been no major advances in the ability to improve spermatogenesis, there are many cases where the fertility and chances of a natural pregnancy, and the self-esteem of the male partner, can be improved with appropriate therapy. Further, (and this is a point that is often ignored) even when the male cannot be helped and ART is inevitable, it is still necessary for the male to feel that he has been properly evaluated and that no stone has been left unturned in seeking a cure for his infertility. This helps the man to accept his infertility and seeking alternative solutions. Finally, with greater understanding of genetic causes of male infertility, there is a need for proper evaluation and counseling for the male partner before beginning ART.

GOALS OF EVALUATION OF THE SUBFERTILE MALE

Every male partner of a couple having difficulty in conceiving should be evaluated for the following:

- Male fertility potential
- Sexual dysfunction leading to infertility
- Semen collection problems.

If subfertility is found then it is important to:

- Look for reversible causes, the correction of which would improve fertility.
- Identify past illnesses that could have caused irreversible damage. In such cases semen will not improve with medical/surgical therapy, and ICSI or alternatives like donor insemination/adoption will be required.
- Check for any underlying medical pathology.
- Identify associated genetic abnormalities that may have implications for the patient and/or offspring.

EVALUATION OF THE SUBFERTILE MALE

Semen Analysis

The first step in the evaluation of an infertile *couple* is the semen analysis. Often, the female partner is extensively evaluated without checking the male partner, only to find out later, after a lot of time and money has been spent, that the male partner is azoospermic!

The cornerstone of the evaluation of the subfertile male remains the completion of at least 2–3 semen analyses (preferably from the same lab to establish comparison).

Even a well done semen analysis is only 60% accurate in predicting fertility. In the first 3–4 years of marriage, semen analysis will not predict, which couples will get pregnant. Men with poor quality semen may impregnate their wives especially when the duration of infertility is short. On the other hand, men with seemingly normal semen parameters may fail to achieve a pregnancy despite many years of trying. Therefore, when assessing the male fertility potential, it is important to consider the duration of infertility in addition to the semen quality.

The WHO norms for semen analysis are given in **Table 1**.

A diagnosis of pyospermia is often incorrect because it is very easy to confuse the other round cells in the semen (spermatocytes and macrophages) with leucocytes. Only if the seminologist is aware of the distinction between these various round cells and uses a phase contrast microscope or appropriate stains, will he be able to give a reliable report of pyospermia. Many men receive prolonged antibiotics for treatment of refractory seminal infection that never gets cured because they did not have an infection to start with!

Once the semen analysis is done, the male partner can be categorized as follows:

- *Aspermia:* Unable to give a semen sample.
- *Hypospermia:* Low volume of ejaculate.
- *Azoospermia:* Complete absence of any mature sperm. Several semen samples over a period of time must be analyzed to label a patient azoospermic. In addition, the semen sample must be centrifuged and the sediment should be examined for sperm. If even a few sperm are found this completely changes the diagnosis (to severe oligozoospermia) and the further management.
- *Oligoasthenozoospermia (OAS):* Reduction in total number (or concentration) and percentage of progressively motile spermatozoa, below the lower reference limits.
- *Isolated oligozoospermia:* Reduction in total number (or concentration) of spermatozoa, below the lower reference limits. Motility and morphology are normal.
- *Isolated asthenozoospermia:* In these cases the count is normal, but there is a reduction in the percentage of progressively motile spermatozoa below the lower reference limits. The degree of asthenozoospermia can be further graded as total (no motility), severe (< 10% motile), moderate (>10 % motile, but only sluggish), and mild (>30% motile, few showing progressive motility).
- *Teratozoospermia:* Percentage of morphologically normal spermatozoa below the lower reference limit.

TABLE 1: WHO norms for semen analysis.

Parameter	*Lower reference limit (WHO 1999)*	*Lower reference limits (WHO 2010)*	*Comments*
Volume	≥2.0 mL	≥1.5 mL	
Sperm concentration	≥20 million sperm/mL	≥15 million sperm/mL	Many laboratories still use old norms, giving normal reference range as 50–150 million/mL; this misleads the doctor and stresses the patient
Total sperm count per ejaculate	≥40 million sperm	≥39 million sperm	
Motility	≥50% with grade A+ B motility or ≥25% with grade A motility	≥40% with grade A+B motility or ≥32% with grade A motility	The latest norms do not distinguish between rapid progressive and slow progressive motility. This has come in for criticism
Morphology (Normal forms %)	≥15% by strict criteria	≥4% by strict criteria	Thus, a normal semen report from a good laboratory may show 95% abnormal sperm and this should not worry the clinician
Viability	≥75% of sperm viable	≥58% of sperm viable	
Other consensus threshold values			
pH	≥7.2	≥7.2	
Peroxidase positive leukocytes	<1 million/mL	<1 million/mL	Most reports of "pyospermia" are incorrect because other round cells in the semen have been wrongly counted as leucocytes. It is very important to look at a stained slide to identify true leucocytes

Usually occurs in association with OAS when it indicates severe testicular impairment, or as an isolated problem (e.g., all sperm with pin-heads or round heads) when it indicates a congenital sperm structural defect. The better the laboratory, the higher is the percentage of abnormal sperm detected even in a fertile sample.

- *Apparently normal:* There may still be a physiological sperm defect that impairs fertilization.

History

Once the semen analysis is done, the history—taking is guided by the semen report.

- *Azoospermia:* History of hernia/hydrocele surgery, vasectomy, venereal diseases, or a scrotal abscess could indicate obstructive azoospermia. History of mumps orchitis or surgery for cryptorchidism, suggests testicular failure. History of delayed puberty or use of hormones to induce puberty would indicate hypogonadotropism.
- *Oligoasthenozoospermia:* History of potential gonadotoxic factors, including occupational history, may identify reversible causes. History of recent febrile illness is relevant as it can adversely affect spermatogenesis temporarily. Enquire about consumption of any medications that interfere with spermatogenesis. History of treatment taken helps avoid repetition of therapy and plan further course of action. For example, if someone has already taken empirical medical therapy for an adequate duration and has tried intrauterine insemination (IUI) 3–4 times, then one would directly advise in vitro fertilization (IVF).
- *Asthenozoospermia:* Prolonged abstinence could cause low motility. Ask for history of recurrent respiratory tract infections (suggestive of primary ciliary dyskinesia), and recurrent genital tract infections.
- *Necrozoopermia:* Enquire if the collection was done by coitus using a condom. Also, confirm that the semen was collected in a bottle provided by the laboratory, and that no lubricant was used (soap or jelly can immobilize sperm).
- *Low semen volume:* Enquire about adequate abstinence (was there sleep emission the previous night?); spillage during collection; urinary infection.
- *Normal semen parameters:* Sexual history to rule out penetration problems, lubricant use (may be spermicidal) or sexual dysfunction (failure of intercourse due to erectile dysfunction or severe premature ejaculation). The frequency and timing of intercourse and knowledge regarding the "fertile period" must also be assessed.

Physical Examination

A general examination helps identify hypogonadism (poor secondary sexual characteristics, gynecomastia), obesity, disorders of the thyroid, and certain congenital syndromes associated with infertility, e.g., midline defects are associated with Kallmann syndrome. Local examination of the genitalia can give very useful diagnostic and prognostic information. Examination of the penis must be done to rule out anatomical abnormalities such as small penile size, curvature, or proximal hypospadias, which can result in improper placement of the ejaculate within the vaginal vault. In azoospermic men, the size of the testes (using an orchidometer), consistency of the testis (soft or firm), the feel of the epididymis (flabby or turgid), and the quality of the vas (absent, thick, or nodular) help judge whether the azoospermia is due to obstruction or testicular failure. In men with OAS, relevant findings include presence of varicocele, cord thickening indicating chronic funiculitis, adherent enlarged epididymis (chronic epididymitis), testicular size, or scrotal thickening due to chronic fungal infection.

Investigations

- *Sperm DNA fragmentation index (sDFI) testing:* With the advent of intracytoplasmic sperm injection (ICSI), a fundamental role in determining sperm competence is currently attributed to DNA integrity. Both *in vitro* and *in vivo* studies have shown that elevated-sDFI may affect fertility by hindering fertilization, early embryo development, implantation, and pregnancy.

  Sperm DNA fragmentation index represents the population of sperms with DNA damage. Abnormal sDFI, is characterized by more than 15% (fair sperm DNA integrity) to more than 30% (poor sperm integrity) fragmented DNA in ejaculatory sperm.

  Presently, the major sperm DNA testing methods are sperm chromatin structure assay (SCSA), terminal deoxynucleotidyl transferase dUTP nick-end labeling (TUNEL) assay, sperm chromatin dispersion (SCD) assay, in situ nick translation (ISNT), and COMET assay.

  Based on the TUNEL testing, a threshold of more than 20% sDFI indicates the presence of infertility with a high sensitivity of 79% and specificity of 86%.

  While TUNEL is believed by many to be the gold standard for sDFI testing, it lacks strict standardization, which makes comparison between laboratories more difficult and explains why many clinical thresholds exist. Of these, the SCSA is considered the most reliable test, if the flow cytometry instrument and skilled technicians are available. This can be performed on both fresh and frozen samples.

  Currently, there seems to be insufficient evidence to support the routine use of SDF in male factor evaluation, nevertheless the importance of DNA fragmentation in spermatozoa has been acknowledged in the latest American Urological Association (AUA) and European Association of Urology (EAU) guidelines on male infertility.

  Clinical indications of sDFI testing in the current era:

- *Unexplained recurrent miscarriage:* Losing three consecutive pregnancies, either natural or after IUI, prior to 20 weeks from the last menstrual period. SDF evaluation can help to choose the most appropriate type of ART including IUI, traditional IVF, intracytoplasmic sperm injection (ICSI) or intracytoplasmic morphologically selected sperm injection (IMSI) in this group of patients (Grade C recommendation).
- *Unexplained recurrent IVF/ICSI failures:* When ejaculatory sperms have a high level of sDFI, usage of testicular sperms for ICSI or performing IMSI on ejaculatory sperms may be a solution. (Grade B-C recommendation).

  Algorithm for clinical use of sDFI in unexplained recurrent miscarriage and recurrent IVF failures have been depicted in **Flowchart 1**.

- In patients with unexplained infertility with no male or female factors, there may be a role for sDFI testing to predict the likelihood of natural pregnancy or use of ART (Grade C recommendation).
- *Modifiable lifestyle factors:* Smoking, obesity, occupational, or environmental exposure to toxins have been linked to oxidative stress-induced SDF. The sDFI test can help reinforce the importance of lifestyle modification (e.g., cessation of cigarette smoking, antioxidant therapy), predict fertility and monitor the patient's response to intervention (Grade C recommendation).
- *Endocrine evaluation:* Although male reproductive function is critically dependent on endocrinologic control, less than 3% of infertile men have a primary hormonal etiology. Clinical interpretation of various hormonal profiles is summarized in **Table 2**.

The most common hormonal abnormality detected on routine testing of infertile men is an elevated serum FSH. FSH assay is clinically indicated in patients with azoospermia or OAS with sperm counts less than 10 million/mL.

Some facts about FSH:

- FSH is an indicator of spermatogenesis. Generally, it is assumed that normal FSH indicates normal spermatogenesis. However, almost 40% of azoospermic men with normal FSH will be found to have maturation arrest. Therefore, it is important to bear in mind that in an

Flowchart 1: Flow diagram showing utility of sDFI testing in unexplained recurrent miscarriages (A) and recurrent IVF/ICSI failures (B).

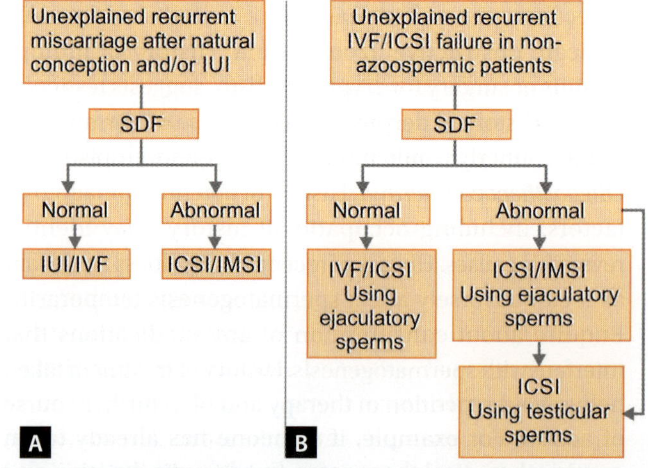

(ICSI: intracytoplasmic sperm injection; IMSI: intracytoplasmic morphologically selected sperm injection; IUI: intrauterine insemination; IVF: in vitro fertilization; SDF: sperm DNA fragmentation)

TABLE 2: Clinical interpretation of various hormonal profiles.

Clinical status	FSH (mIU/mL)	LH (mIU/mL)	Testosterone (ng/dL)
Normal men or obstruction	Normal	Normal	Normal
Isolated spermatogenic failure	↑	Normal	Normal
Testicular failure	↑	↑	Normal or ↓
Hypogonadotropic hypogonadisn[1]	↓	↓	↓

azoospermic man, normal FSH does not guarantee normal spermatogenesis (obstructive azoospermia).

- Elevated FSH indicates testicular failure. However, occasionally men with normal spermatogenesis will have mild elevations in FSH levels. Hence, only levels above twice the upper limit of normal are considered diagnostic of primary testicular failure.

In an azoospermic patient, normal FSH does not guarantee normal spermatogenesis (obstructive azoospermia).

FSH level more than twice the normal is considered diagnostic of primary testicular failure.

Elevated FSH does not preclude Focal Spermatogenesis Testicular sperm extraction TESE + ICSI may still be possible.

FSH and LH are interpreted in reference to the testosterone level. Thus, a man with low normal FSH and LH and low testosterone is a candidate for hormone therapy, while another man with similar low levels of FSH and LH but with high-normal testosterone needs no treatment since his FSH and LH are low due to feedback from the high testosterone level. In the evaluation of normally androgenized men with small testes, especially when cost considerations are important, FSH alone may suffice to confirm the diagnosis of testicular failure.

In men, unlike in women, elevated prolactin is rarely the cause of sub-fertility and routine prolactin testing is not indicated. Assay prolactin levels in an infertile male patient only if there is loss of libido and erectile dysfunction, or symptoms like severe headaches, visual field abnormalities and galactorrhea, which are clinical indicators of hyperprolactinemia. Mild elevation (< twice normal) is not significant and may be stress- or drug-induced.

Other hormones should be assayed, if there is clinical evidence to suggest a relevant problem. Thyroid profile should be done if there is clinical evidence of hypo- or hyper- thyroidism, or if hyperprolactinemia has been detected; Adrenal androgens should be assayed, if there is unexplained hypogonadism.

- *Scrotal ultrasound:* Scrotal ultrasound is routinely performed in many centers but, its clinical utility is limited. A good clinical examination is usually enough to diagnose a clinical varicocele. Subclinical varicoceles do not contribute significantly to the patient's infertility and hence there is no need for USG to look for a varicocele when there is no clinical suspicion. USG can be used to confirm the clinical diagnosis of a varicocele before surgery, and in obese patients with short scrotums in whom clinical examination is difficult. It also is useful to screen the testis for early testicular malignancy in men with testicular failure.
- *Transrectal ultrasound of prostate (TRUS):* TRUS has a significant role to play in the diagnosis and treatment of ejaculatory duct obstruction (EJDO). This has to be ruled out in patients with azoospermia or severe OAS associated with low semen volume and absent fructose or palpable abnormalities detected on Digital Rectal Examination (DRE). Seminal vesicle width greater than 1.5 cm or ejaculatory duct diameter greater than 2.3 mm on TRUS, particularly when combined with a cyst or calcification along the duct helps confirm the diagnosis. There are two types of EJDO - cystic and fibrous. The cystic type is often congenital, and TRUS may reveal a congenital intra-prostatic utricular cyst, dilated seminal vesicles (>1.5 cm) and enlarged ejaculatory ducts (diameter >2.3 mm)—this is amenable to surgical cure by trans-urethral resection (TUR) of the obstruction. Fibrous EJDO occurs after infection, especially tuberculosis, and is common amongst our patients. In these cases the seminal vesicles and ejaculatory duct will not be dilated and TRUS may appear normal. These cases are not amenable to TUR and need sperm aspiration and ICSI.

In men with vas aplasia (VA), TRUS will reveal bilateral absence of the seminal vesicles. However, in 15% of cases of VA, TRUS will demonstrate "seminal vesicle like cystic" structures. Hence, relying on TRUS to diagnose VA can lead to confusion and unnecessary exploration.

- *Testicular biopsy:* Testicular biopsy is an essential part of the evaluation and therapy of patients with azoospermia. It is used diagnostically to distinguish between obstructive and nonobstructive azoospermia, and to identify focal spermatogenesis in men with testicular failure. Therapeutically, it is used to obtain sperm for ICSI. Not all men with azoospermia need a biopsy. An azoospermic man with small testes and high FSH clearly has primary testicular failure: he does not need a biopsy to establish the diagnosis. Biopsy would be needed only for sperm extraction, if he was planning ICSI—in that case multiple micro-biopsies would be planned. Biopsy may be open or percutaneous. In our practice, most of the biopsies are needle aspiration biopsies, which yield good amount of tissue with minimal trauma. FNAC of the testis is may be used as an alternative to a tissue biopsy but may fail to detect focal sperm production in men with non-obstructive azoospermia.

ETIOLOGY

History, physical examination, and laboratory testing allows the clinician to place the patient into a diagnostic classification. It must be remembered however, that a significant percentage of patients fall into the idiopathic category (25%). Etiology may be classified as under:

Pre-testicular Causes (Endocrine)

- *Hormone deficiency:*
  - *Pituitary:* Surgery, radiation, tumors
  - *Hypothalamus:* Hypogonadotropic hypogonadism (Kallmann syndrome, idiopathic)
- *Hormone excess:*
  - *Androgen:* Congenital adrenal hyperplasia, anabolic steroid use, virilizing adrenal or testicular tumors.
  - *Estrogen:* Feminizing adrenal or testicular tumors.
  - *Prolactin:* Pituitary adenoma (Prolactinoma), stress, medications, idiopathic.
  - *Glucocorticoids:* Cushing's syndrome, exogenous steroid use.
- *Androgen receptor abnormality:* Androgen insensitivity syndrome.

Testicular Causes

- *Disorders of spermatogenesis:*
  - *Chromosomal causes:* Klinefelter's syndrome, Y-chromosome microdeletions.
  - *Cryptorchidism:* Unilateral or bilateral
  - Varicocele
  - Postorchitis
  - Postchemotherapy or radiation
  - *Gonadotoxin exposure:* Heat, drugs, alcohol, cigarettes.
- *Disorders of sperm function:*
  - *Immunologic:* Antisperm antibodies
  - *Ultrastructural defects:* Primary ciliary dyskinesia (Kartagener's syndrome).

Post-testicular Causes

- Congenital bilateral absence of Vas deferentia (CBAVD)
- *Ductal obstruction:* (unilateral or bilateral, single or multiple locations)
- *Vas deferens:* Postvasectomy status, iatrogenic (postinguinal hernia or hydrocele surgery).
  - Epididymis: Infection, iatrogenic, or idiopathic
  - Ejaculatory duct: Congenital or acquired
- *Ejaculatory disorders:*
  - Retrograde ejaculation
  - Anejaculation.

Idiopathic

Abnormal semen analysis for which no cause is identified. It accounts for 25% of cases of male subfertility.

MANAGEMENT

Based on the results of the history, physical examination, and laboratory studies, the physician should place the patient into an etiologic category. The clinician is then faced with three potential management options.

1. The first option is to improve the fertility potential of the male partner by either correcting the underlying abnormalities or utilizing empirical therapies.
2. The second is to improve the odds of conception without altering the male partner's fertility status through the use of ART.
3. The third option is to bypass the male partner completely by utilizing donor sperm or adoption.

As a general rule, it is preferable to treat the male to improve his fertility status whenever possible rather than ignore the male factor and use high-cost advanced ART, which places the burden of treatment and risk on the female partner for a male problem. On the other hand, it is often not possible to improve spermatogenesis or attempted treatment may fail. In addition, there may be a concomitant female factor that requires treatment with ART. In these instances, it is appropriate to proceed directly to ART. These two management approaches are not mutually exclusive, and some couples may choose to treat the male concurrently with utilization of the ART. This more aggressive approach may be used in the older couple when the female's reproductive potential is diminishing because of age. Finally, couples should be counseled on both donor insemination and adoption as alternatives.

- *Aspermia:* Failure to collect a semen sample could be situational or total. Situational anejaculation could occur in some situations (in the clinic, not at home) or on some occasions (at the time of ovulation when there is a pressure to perform). Men with total anejaculation are not able to collect a semen sample either during intercourse or with masturbation.

  Most common cause of total anejaculation is failure to reach a climax or orgasm, which is referred to as *anorgasmic anejaculation*. Such men have never had conscious ejaculation; however nocturnal involuntary emissions usually occur, and their occurrence rules out a physical problem. If an individual reaches orgasm but does not ejaculate, this is called *orgasmic anejaculation*, and is due to an organic defect. The causes of orgasmic anejaculation are failure of emission, retrograde ejaculation or anterior urethral obstruction.

- *Azoospermia:* The differential diagnosis of azoospermia are the following:
  - *Obstructive azoospermia*
  - *Nonobstructive azoospermia*
  - *Hypogonadotropic hypogonadism.*

  The diagnosis is arrived through history, physical examination, endocrine evaluation, and a testicular biopsy, if necessary.

  Hypogonadotropic hypogonadism is a rare cause of azoospermia. Patient who desires fertility will need to be counseled about the need for gonadotropin replacement (HCG + HMG), costs involved (2–3 lakh ₹) and the duration of therapy necessary (0.5–3 years) before venturing into therapy. If the patient is not motivated enough or does not have the financial support, then it is prudent not to waste their precious resources and refer the patient for donor insemination or adoption.

  In patients with obstructive azoospermia, evaluation is necessary to identify the location and extent of obstruction and potential for reversibility by microsurgical reconstruction. Keeping these factors in mind and after discussion with the couple, a decision needs to be taken whether surgery [vaso-epididymal anastomosis (VEA) or vaso vasal anastomosis (VVA)] or Percutaneous Epididymal Sperm Aspiration with intracytoplasmic sperm injection, i.e., PESA-ICSI is the best way ahead.

  For men with nonobstructive azoospermia, the only hope was donor insemination or adoption. But now with the advent of ICSI, a new ray of hope has emerged.

  It is now recognized that nonobstructive azoospermia is a heterogeneous entity. While most of these men will have no sperm at all, many (20–50%) will have focal areas of spermatogenesis. Thus, even in men with maturation arrest, Sertoli cell syndrome only, or even testicular atrophy, a few sperm may be recoverable from the testicular tissue, especially if multiple biopsies are done by microdissection TESE. These sperm can be used for ICSI and will lead to viable pregnancies. Prior to sperm retrieval and ICSI, the man must undergo genetic tests for karyotyping and Yq microdeletions. Karyotyping is relevant when testes size is very small and will reveal Klinefelter's syndrome in the majority of cases (sperm may still be retrieved in 20% of such cases). Yq microdeletion testing is more useful when testes size is good. If YqA or YqB deletion is present then no sperm can be retrieved. If there is YqC microdeletion then there is a 20–50% chance of finding sperm, but if a male child is born he will inherit the same abnormality.

  Algorithmic practical management of the azoospermic male is depicted in **Flowcharts 2 to 5.**
- *Oligoasthenozoospermia:* OAS is the most prevalent cause of male infertility and the management of this very common problem appears complicated due to various factors:
  - Numerous etiological factors
  - No identifiable cause in 25%
  - Several empirical medical therapies available (none proven)
  - Varying degrees of severity of OAS
  - Few correctable reversible causes of OAS.

  Various treatment options available for management of OAS are:
- *Surgery*: Varicocele ligation in the treatment of OAS should be considered in patients with clinically obvious varicoceles in whom medical therapy has failed and wife is

Flowchart 2: Practical management of the azoospermic male: Part 1.

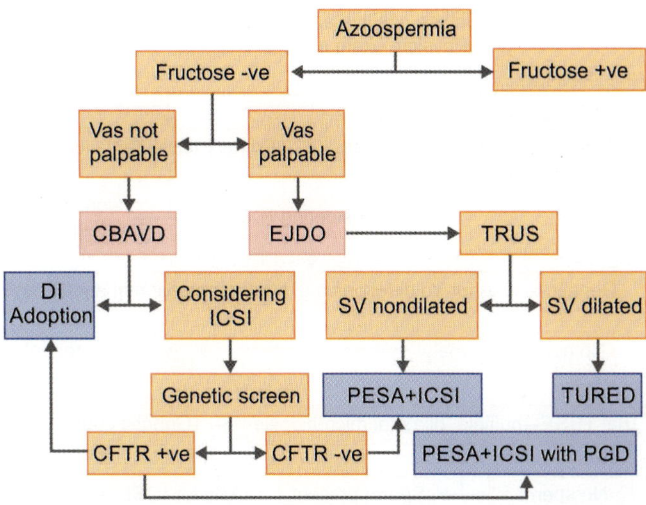

(ICSI: intracytoplasmic sperm injection; CBAVD: congenital bilateral absence of vas deferens; TRUS: transrectal ultrasound of prostate; EJDO: ejaculatory duct obstruction; PGD: preimplantation genetic diagnosis; PESA: percutaneous epididymal sperm aspiration; DI: donor insemination)

Flowchart 3: Practical management of the azoospermic male: Part 2.

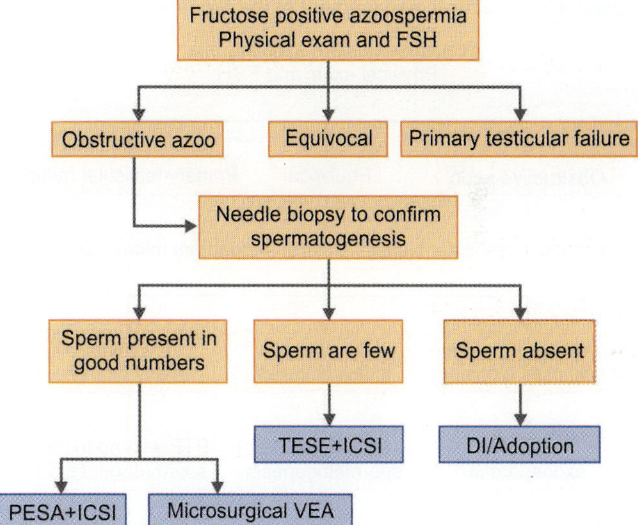

(ICSI: intracytoplasmic sperm injection; FSH: follicle stimulating hormone; PESA: percutaneous epididymal sperm aspiration; VEA: vasoepididymostomy; TESE: testicular sperm extraction; DI: donor insemination)

Flowchart 4: Practical management of the azoospermic male: Part 3.

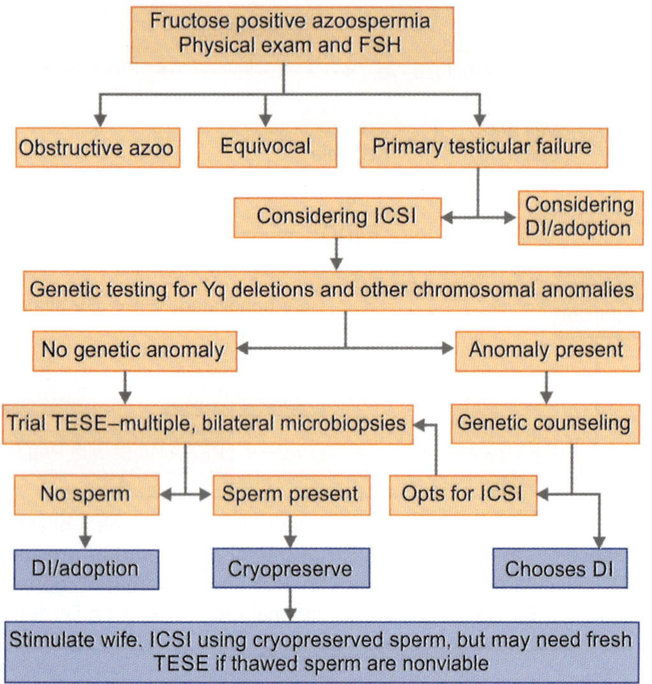

Flowchart 5: Practical management of the azoospermic male: Part 4.

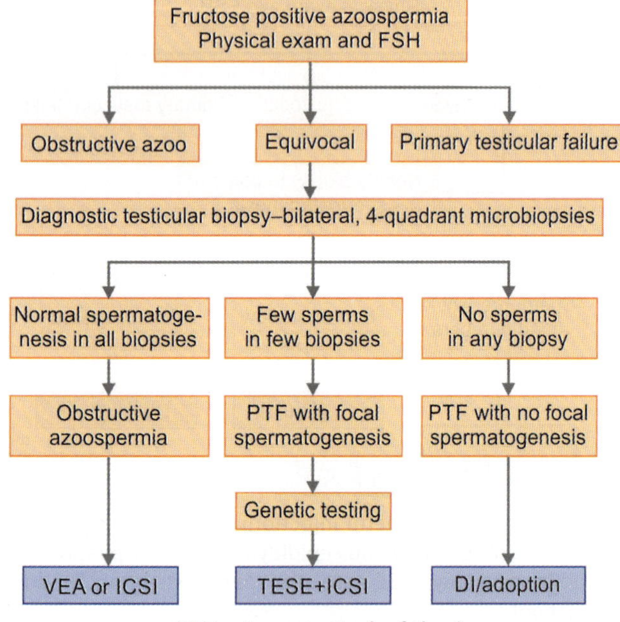

(PTF: primary testicular failure)

normal or has a correctable factor. 60% of those operated have good improvement in semen parameters.

- *Specific medical therapy:*
    - *Chronic scrotal fungal dermatitis:* Treat with antifungal topical and oral therapy. As the skin becomes normal and thin, local temperature will drop, thus improving spermatogenesis.
    - *Genital tract infection:* For proven seminal infection, treat with doxycycline 200 mg/day, fluoroquinolones 0.5–1 g/day, cotrimoxazole (sulfamethoxazole 800 mg, trimethoprim 160 mg) or erythromycin 1.5–2 g/day. These drugs are administered for 2–3 weeks. Further therapy would be determined by semen culture.
    - *Immunologic infertility:* The diagnosis of immunological infertility needs to be carefully established using Immunobead or MAR tests, which identify antibodies (type and location) on the sperm surface. Most laboratories test for sperm antibodies using an ELISA-based assay of serum levels—this is of no clinical relevance. Therapy with short course of low dose oral prednisolone can be considered; however, its efficacy is disputed and many centers prefer to proceed to IUI or ICSI. High doses of steroid should be avoided due to the risk of necrosis of the femur head.
- *Empirical therapy:* Numerous agents are available for empirical medical therapy (Hormonal agents, Antioxidants, Sperm vitalizers, Nutritional supplements, and a range of herbal preparations). *Treatment should last at least 3 months to incorporate a full 74-day spermatogenic cycle.* While small studies with these agents have often shown benefit, this has not been confirmed during larger studies. However, they are useful as supportive therapy during the initial period of conservative management and sometimes seem to produce significant improvement.
- IUI is a very commonly practiced option in the treatment of men with OAS. However, the success rate is low, 8–10% per cycle, and 16–25% cumulative over 4 cycles, and that too provided at least 1 million active sperm can be harvested. There is no point in trying IUI, if the semen sample is very poor.
- ICSI is the only option for a patient with severe OAS.

The factors that have to be kept in mind when planning therapy for men with OAS has been outlined here:

- *Age of the couple and duration of infertility:* A young couple with a short "trying time" has a fair chance of natural conception despite sub-normal semen. They can be offered various medical therapies in order to buy time to achieve a natural pregnancy. On the other hand, an older couple with a much longer trying time need to move towards ART and should not lose precious time trying medical therapy.
- *Severity of OAS and realistic chances of improvement expected:* a patient with severe OAS (less than 5 million/mL with very poor progressive motility) with no obvious reversible factors should be directed more toward ART.
- *Is there anything in the patient's history that would suggest irreversibility?* For example, a patient who has testicular atrophy following mumps orchitis or has had chemotherapy. Such a patient would not be expected to improve after medical therapy and should proceed for ART.
- *Are there any reversible correctable gonadotoxic factors?* For example, occupational exposure to gonadotoxins, smoking, genital infections; such patients can be given

medical therapy to buy time for improvement of semen parameters once the gonadotoxic factors are eliminated/ modified.

- Treatment history is imperative. It is important to know what medicines the patients has tried in the past (whether they were effective or not) so that there is no repetition. If he has already received a variety of medicines it is time to move on to ART.
- Socioeconomic status of the couple should also be considered before offering them therapy as some of the empirical medicines which are prescribed empirically are rather expensive.
- Psychosocial pressures on the couple play a major role in decision making. In a couple who is socially hard-pressed for a baby, less time should be spent on medical therapy.

Flowchart 6 summarizes a practical approach to management of asthenozoospermia.

- *Isolated oligozoospermia:* is uncommon. Since the motility is good, a satisfactory harvest can be obtained and IUI has a good chance of success.
- *Isolated asthenozoospermia:* Mild to moderate asthenozoospermia could occur as a result of accessory gland infection, varicoceles, antisperm antibodies, defective transport through genital ductal system. Occasionally, a course of antibiotics for accessory gland infection, steroids for antisperm antibodies, varicocele surgery, or antioxidant therapy might improve the sperm motility.

If these measures fail, the split ejaculate should be collected directly in beakers containing 5 mL of medium each; this results in immediate dilution of the seminal plasma. The sample is centrifuged and the pellet is resuspended in medium and processed for IUI. Since, this technique avoids incubation of sperm in the seminal plasma it is useful in those

Flowchart 6: Practical management of asthenozoospermia.

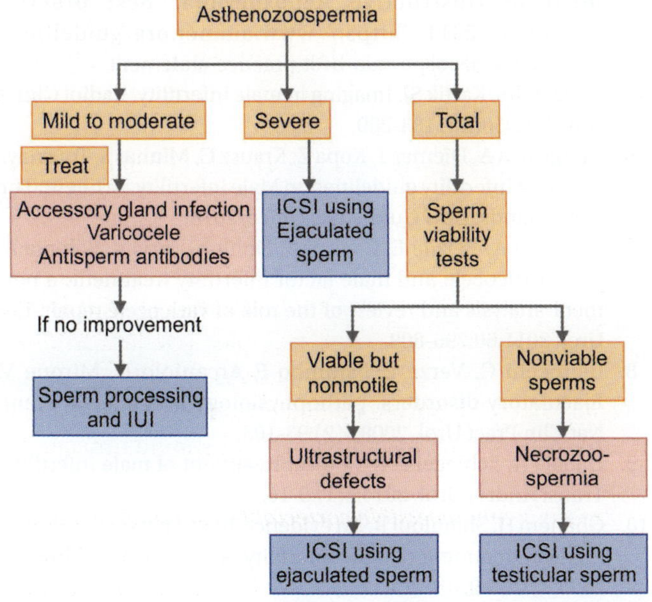

cases where sperm immobilizing substances are present in the seminal plasma. If none of these measures help, then ICSI will be required.

In severe asthenozoospermia, therapy will not improve motility - ICSI should be advised. In Total asthenozoospermia, the clinician must differentiate between nonmotile but viable sperm (due to ultrastructural defects as in Kartagener's syndrome) and nonmotile nonviable sperm (necrozoospermia) using the sperm viability tests. Both conditions cannot be treated medically and ICSI is mandatory. If the sperm are viable then these ejaculated sperm can be used for ICSI even though non-motile. If, however, the sperm are dead then it would be preferable to use testicular sperm for ICSI.

Practical management of oligoasthenozoospermia is outlined in **Flowchart 7**.

- *Isolated teratozoospermia:* This has been reported increasingly with the application of "strict" criteria. Increasingly, many of the men diagnosed with isolated teratozoospermia achieve pregnancy naturally or by IUI, if count and motility are normal, suggesting that the criteria have become over-strict. The majority of the cases are idiopathic; varicocele and gonadotoxic factors may play a role. Round-headed sperm (globozoospermia) have an absence of acrosome; they may be treated with ICSI, but pregnancy rates are low. Pinheads are actually headless sperm and cannot be used for ICSI as they have no genetic material.
- *Sexual dysfunction:* contributes to infertility in a variety of ways:
  - Non-consummated marriage due to erectile dysfunction
  - Periovulatory erectile dysfunction
  - Partial penetration with extravaginal ejaculation
  - Premature ejaculation
  - Anejaculation
  - Infrequent intercourse
  - Improper coital techniques
  - Use of spermicidal lubricants (petroleum-based jelly like K-Y jelly) for intercourse.

  Often proper counseling and sexual education regarding the right techniques and reassurance will work wonders. With the help of PDE5 Inhibitors like Sildenafil (50–100 mg, 1–2 hours before intercourse) or Tadalafil (10–20 mg, 2–3 hours before intercourse), many of the patients with psychogenic ED can consummate their marriages and impregnate their wives. The patients who do not respond to these measures should be referred to the specialists without wasting precious time with the expectation that "things will work out." The longer the duration of sexual dysfunction, more the psychological consequences and more difficult the therapy.
- *Apparently normal:* If the semen appears to be normal then the wife will have to be evaluated in detail. The sexual

Flowchart 7: Practical management of oligoasthenozoospermia.

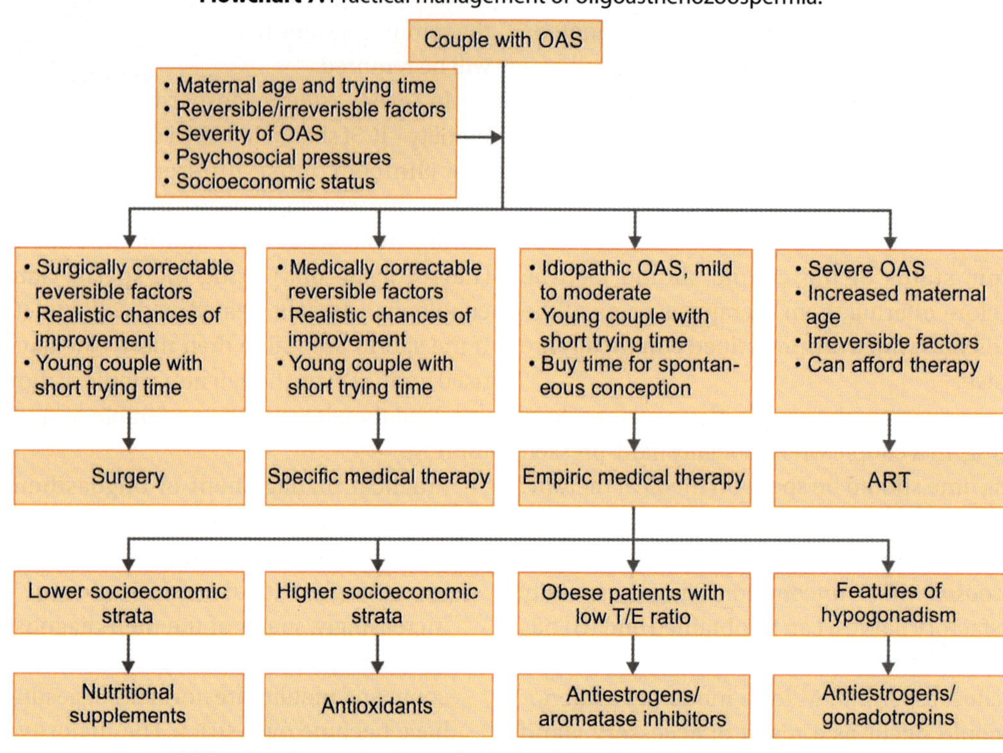

(ART: assisted reproductive techniques; OAS: oligoasthenozoospermia)

history also assumes greater importance. If no abnormality is found the couple is classified as having idiopathic infertility. In many of these cases the sperm is at fault; this can be revealed by special sperm function tests. However, with the advent of ICSI these tests are irrelevant to the clinician since ICSI bypasses most of the routine steps of fertilization and thus allows dysfunctional sperm to produce a viable pregnancy as long as the sperm nuclear chromatin is intact.

CONCLUSION

When an infertile couple comes for treatment, the first step in their evaluation should be a semen analysis. If the male partner has been found to be contributing to the infertility, then one must proceed with a semen analysis-guided history, physical examination and simple cost effective investigations to come to an etiological diagnosis. At the conclusion of the evaluation, the Urologist and reproductive medicine specialist must work hand in hand to achieve the goal of pregnancy (either naturally or through ART). Despite the advent of ICSI, the male partner should not be ignored and must be given due consideration and attention.

FURTHER READING

1. Agarwal A, Majzoub A, Esteves SC, Edmund Ko E, Ramasamy R, Zini A. Clinical utility of sperm DNA fragmentation testing: practice recommendations based on clinical scenarios. Transl Androl Urol. 2016;5(6):935-50.
2. American Urologic Association and the American Society of Reproductive Medicine (2011): Optimal Evaluation of the Infertile Male, Best Practice Statement [online]. Available from: https://www.auanet.org/guidelines/male-infertility-optimal-evaluation-best-practice-statement. [Last accessed December, 2021].
3. American Urologic Association and the American Society of Reproductive Medicine (2011). Report on the Varicocele and Infertility, Best practice statement 2011 [online]. Available from: www.auanet.org/guidelines/main_reports/varicoceleinfertility.pdf [Last accessed December, 2021].
4. American Urologic Association and the American Society of Reproductive Medicine: Report on Management of Obstructive Azoospermia, Best practice statement 2011. https://www.auanet.org/guidelines/obstructive-azoospermia-best-practice-statement.
5. Arsalan RS, Kartik SJ. Imaging in male infertility. Radiol Clin N Am. 2012;50(6):1183-200.
6. Aungwirth A, Diemer T, Kopa Z, Krausz C, Minhas S, Tournaye H. EAU e Infertility guidelines on Male infertility. Arnhem, The Netherlands: EAU Guidelines Office; 2018.
7. Baazeem A, Belzile E, Ciampi A, Dohle G, Jarvi K, Salonia A, et al. Varicocele and male factor infertility treatment: a new meta-analysis and review of the role of varicocele repair. Eur Urol. 2011;60:796-808.
8. Bettocchi C, Verze P, Palumbo F, Arcaniolo D, Mirone V. Ejaculatory disorders: pathophysiology and management. Nat Clin Pract Urol. 2008;5(2):93-103.
9. Dabaja A, Schlegel PN. Medical treatment of male infertility. Transl Androl Urol. 2014;3(1):9-16.
10. Ghanem H, Shamloul R. An evidence-based perspective to the medical treatment of male infertility: a short review. Urol Int. 2009;82:125-9.

11. Halpern JA, Brannigan RE, Schlegel PN. Fertility-enhancing male reproductive surgery. Glimpses into the past and thoughts for the future. Fertil Steril. 2019;112(3):426-1.
12. Jarow JP. Effects of varicocele on male fertility. Hum Reprod Update. 2001;7(1):59-64.
13. Kumar R, Shah R. Varicocele and male infertility: current status. J Obstet Gynecol India. 2005; 55(6):505-16.
14. Mirzazadeh M, Sadri-Ardekani H. Implications of ejaculatory sperm DNA fragmentation on male infertility management. Transl Androl Urol. 2017;6(Suppl 4):S402-4.
15. Mittal PK, Little B, Harri PA, Miller FH, Alexander LH, Kalb B, et al. Role of imaging in the evaluation of male infertility. Radiographics. 2017;37:837-54.
16. Pagani RL, Ohlander SJ, Niederberger CS. Microsurgical varicocele ligation: surgical methodology and associated outcomes. Fertil Steril. 2019;111(3):415-9.
17. Pan MM, Hockenberry MS, Kirby EW, Lipshultz LI. Male infertility diagnosis and treatment in the era of In vitro fertlisation and Intra cytoplasmic sperm injection. Med Clin North Am. 2018;102(2):337-47.
18. Schiff JD, Ramírez ML, Bar-Chama N. Medical and surgical management male infertility. Endocrinol Metab Clin North Am. 2007;36(2):313-31.
19. Shah R. Surgical sperm retrieval: techniques and their indications. Indian J Urol. 2011;27:102-9.
20. Shah RS, Malhotra V. Ejaculatory failure. In: Rao KA, Srinivas MS (Eds). Laboratory Manual in Assisted Reproductive Technology. New Delhi: Jaypee Brothers Medical Publishers Pvt Ltd.; 2006. pp. 130-5.
21. Shridharani A, Owen RC, Elkelany OO, Kim ED. The significance of clinical practice guidelines on adult varicocele detection and management. Asian J Androl. 2016;18(2):269-75.
22. Sigman M, Lipshultz LI, Howards SS. Office evaluation of the subfertile male. In: Lipshultz LI, Howards SS, Niederberger CS. Infertility in the Male. 4th edition. Cambridge: Cambridge University Press; 2010. pp. 153-76.
23. World Health Organization. WHO laboratory manual for the examination and processing of human semen. 5th edition. Geneva: World Health Organization; 2010.

LONG QUESTIONS

1. Define male infertility and explain etiology and evaluation of male infertility.
2. Discuss azoospermia and its evaluation and management.

SHORT QUESTIONS

Write short notes on:

1. WHO 2010 reference values for Semen analysis.
2. Testicular biopsy: Indications and technique.
3. Oligoasthenozoospermia - medical management.
4. Endocrine evaluation of male infertility.
5. Management of low volume, fructose negative azoospermia.
6. IUI for male factor infertility.

MULTIPLE CHOICE QUESTIONS

1. As per the WHO 2010 guidelines for Semen Analysis, the lower reference values for sperm concentration is:
   a. 20 million/mL
   b. 60 million/mL
   c. 15 million/mL
   d. 40 million/mL
2. A 25-year-old male patient presents with azoospermia, low ejaculatory volume, and a semen pH of 6.5. Post ejaculation urine is negative for sperm. The vas deferentia are palpable. What is the next test that should be done?
   a. Testicular biopsy
   b. FSH
   c. Genetic testing
   d. Transrectal ultrasound of prostate
3. A 32-year-old male patient with primary infertility is found to have a normal sperm count, but zero motility. Viability staining shows that majority of sperm are alive. Semen culture and antisperm antibody tests are negative. How do you manage this patient?
   a. ICSI using ejaculated sample
   b. Give a course of antibiotics and antioxidants and repeat Semen analysis
   c. Semen processing for IUI
   d. PESA + ICSI
4. A 28-year-old male patient, poorly androgenized, with gynecomastia and small testis, with primary infertility, is found to have very low levels of FSH, LH, and Testosterone. MRI brain is normal. What is the next step?
   a. TESE + ICSI
   b. Testicular biopsy
   c. Gonadotropin replacement
   d. Ultrasound scrotum
5. A 29-year-old male patient with Azoospermia is detected to have CBAVD. He is willing for ICSI. Prior to that, which genetic testing needs to be done?
   a. Y chromosome microdeletions
   b. *CFTR* gene mutation
   c. Karyotyping
   d. Androgen receptor gene mutations
6. A 38-year-old male patient, (wife is 33 years old) with 10 years primary infertility has been diagnosed to have Oligoasthenozoospermia (Semen count 2.5 million/mL with 20% Grade A+B motility) and gives a history of postpubertal mumps. Ultrasound reveals grade 1 varicocele bilaterally. How would you manage this patient?
   a. Bilateral microsurgical varicocelectomy
   b. Empirical medical therapy for 6 months and repeat semen analysis
   c. Testicular biopsy
   d. Recommend ICSI

7. A 32-year-old male, tall and thin, is diagnosed to have Azoospermia. Physical examination reveals bilateral small testes (6 cc volume). FSH is 26. He is unable to afford expensive therapy. How would you manage this patient?
   a. Donor insemination/Adoption
   b. Diagnostic testicular biopsy
   c. Genetic testing
   d. Multiple testicular biopsies and cryopreservation
8. Following semen parameters suggest the need for ICSI, except:
   a. Sperm count less than 2 million/mL
   b. Sperm motility grade A+B less than 5%
   c. Immuno bead test showing 90% antibody binding to head
   d. Sperm morphology showing only 14% normal forms
9. A young couple with primary infertility. The male partner has a normal physical examination and normal semen parameters. The female partner's evaluation is also normal. A post coital test on two occasions however, reveals no sperm in the cervical mucus. What is the next step?
   a. Immunobead test for antisperm antibodies
   b. Sexual history and IUI
   c. ICSI using ejaculated sperm
   d. Special sperm function tests to rule out ultrastructural defects

Answers

1.	c	2.	d	3.	a	4.	c	5.	b	6.	d
7.	a	8.	d	9.	b						

12.5 ANOVULATION: ETIOLOGY AND MANAGEMENT

Manish Banker, Jwal Banker

"Anovulation is not a disease per se, but a sign of some bigger underlying problem. Just like PCOS."

INTRODUCTION

To discuss anovulation, let us first know what causes normal ovulation. When the arcuate nucleus of the hypothalamus is stimulated, it releases gonadotropin-releasing hormone (GnRH) into the portal vessels of the pituitary stalk in a pulsatile manner. The pulsatility of GnRH stimulates the anterior pituitary gland which can cause the secretion of both follicle-stimulating hormone (FSH) and luteinizing hormone (LH). Low-frequency GnRH pulses stimulate FSH release, whereas high-frequency GnRH pulses stimulate LH. So, the pulsatility is a very important parameter in this cycle. FSH then acts on the ovaries and causes recruitment and growth of antral follicles and the selection and growth of a dominant follicle which in turn produces estrogen. The growing follicles gradually acquire the receptors to respond to LH. LH is responsible for the secretion of androgens from the theca cells of ovaries.[1]

Initially, estrogen causes a negative feedback and stops further secretion of gonadotropins, but later in midcycle, the estrogen rise suddenly causes a positive feedback and causes the LH surge. Ovulation occurs approximately after 28 hours of this surge and this releases the oocyte from the graafian follicle, which then becomes the corpus luteum. At the end of the menstrual cycle, the corpus luteum regresses and serum concentrations of estradiol, progesterone, and inhibin-A gradually go back to baseline levels. This removes the inhibitory effect on the hypothalamus and causes the release of GnRH which in turn causes release of FSH and LH from the pituitary **(Fig. 1)**. This system is very sensitive and any disturbance in this orchestration of hypothalamo-pituitary-ovarian (HPO) axis can cause anovulation.

Anovulation is quite common, and it can have variable clinical manifestations such as oligomenorrhea, abnormal uterine bleeding to even amenorrhea. It may also lead to more serious problems such as infertility and an increased risk for having endometrial hyperplasia leading to neoplasia.

Anovulation: It is the failure to release an oocyte from a mature graafian follicle during a menstrual cycle.

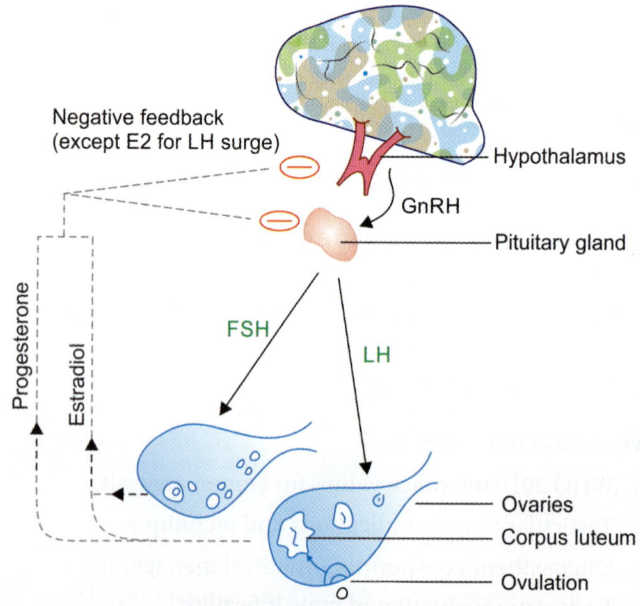

Fig. 1: Hypothalamo-pituitary-ovarian axis.
(FSH: follicle-stimulating hormone; GnRH: gonadotropin releasing hormone; LH: luteinizing hormone)

Physiologic anovulation: During menarche, there is immaturity of the HPO axis which causes altered pulsatile release of GnRH and this causes anovulation. During perimenopause, anovulation is mainly of ovarian origin, but even dysregulation of HPO axis may contribute.

When there is anovulation in between these two age groups—the perimenarchal and perimenopausal age—it causes problems.

INCIDENCE AND ETIOLOGY

The exact incidence of chronic anovulation is very difficult to estimate due to underdetection and underreporting. Yet, estimates range from 6 to 15% during their reproductive years.[2]

Anovulation and oligo-ovulation are ovulatory disorders that are estimated to cause 21% of female infertility.[3]

The World Health Organization (WHO) classified anovulation into three groups and these are still being used[4] **(Table 1)**.

Causes

WHO Group 1

- *Inherited disorders:*
  - Kallmann syndrome (X-linked, autosomal dominant, or autosomal recessive)
  - Normosmic idiopathic hypogonadotropic hypogonadism
  - Other disorders affecting genes such as *FGF8*, *NELF*, and *PROK2*
- *Acquired disorders:*
  - *Eating disorders:* Anorexia nervosa, bulimia—these affect the levels of insulin, glucagon, and catecholamines and ultimately suppress the GnRH neuronal activity.
  - *Excessive exercise:* This causes increase in B-endorphins and affects GnRH activity.
  - *Stress induced which can be traumatic or even at times positive life events:* These factors cause increase in cortisol and affect GnRH activity.
- *Anterior pituitary gland disorders:*
  - *Inherited:* Septo-optic dysplasia, mutations in genes that encode for FSH, LH subunits, or GnRH receptor.
  - *Acquired:*
    - *Pituitary adenoma and hyperprolactinemia:* These are one of the most common causes. This most commonly causes increased prolactin secretion. To control this, dopamine is secreted by hypothalamus which has an inhibitory effect. But, this dopamine causes GnRH disturbances at a central level and the cycle continues.
    - Other tumors may also exert a mass effect which can compress the gonadotropes or can damage the pituitary stalk which causes increase prolactin and dopamine.
    - Inflammatory causes, infiltrative diseases (sarcoidosis, hemochromatosis).
    - Sheehan syndrome (pan-hypopituitarism) and pituitary apoplexy.
    - *Iatrogenic:* Surgery, radiation.
    - Rare causes include AIDS, malabsorption, end-stage kidney diseases, chronic diseases—all these cause some metabolic effect which ultimately has an effect on GnRH activity.

TABLE 1: The WHO classification of anovulation.

WHO group 1: Hypothalamo–pituitary failure (10%)	It causes hypogonadotropic hypogonadism characterized by low levels of gonadotropins and low estrogen
WHO group 2: Hypothalamo–pituitary dysfunction (85%)	It is characterized by normal levels of gonadotropins and estrogen but with their asynchronicity. The clinical manifestations depend on the level of ovarian function and this happens in conditions such as PCOS
WHO group 3: Ovarian Failure (4-5%)	It causes hypergonadotropic hypogonadism

(PCOS: polycystic ovarian syndrome; WHO: World Health Organization)
(*Note:* We, the authors, could not find any reference back to the original article though many authors cite the WHO manual of 1993. In spite of that, we will use this as it is commonly being used. But we believe that a new classification system, taking into account modern methods of diagnosis and treatment, should be developed.)

WHO Group 2

- *Polycystic ovarian syndrome (PCOS):* This is the most common cause of chronic anovulation. It is not a specific endocrine disease or disorder, but it is a syndrome complex of many signs and symptoms. The brief description of the underlying pathology is shown in **Figure 2.**
- Congenital adrenal hyperplasia (late onset).
- Ovarian tumors such as granulosa cell tumor, theca cell tumor, and mature cystic teratoma. These secrete hormones and may lead to this class of anovulation.
- Causes such as hyperprolactinemia and thyroid disorders may cause hypogonadotropic or eugonadotropic anovulation. Both hyper- and hypothyroidism may affect ovulation by its metabolic effects on the sex steroids. Hypothyroidism may cause increased secretion of prolactin by the molecular similarity of thyroid-stimulating hormone (TSH), thyrotropin-releasing hormone (TRH), and other neuronal mediators such as dopamine, ultimately causing anovulation. TSH also has an effect on sex hormone-binding globulin (SHBG) levels. A specific thyroid disorder is Hashimoto thyroiditis which causes increase in TRH which causes increase in prolactin and affects GnRH.
- *Obesity:* This also may cause hypogonadotropic or eugonadotropic anovulation. Obesity affects the

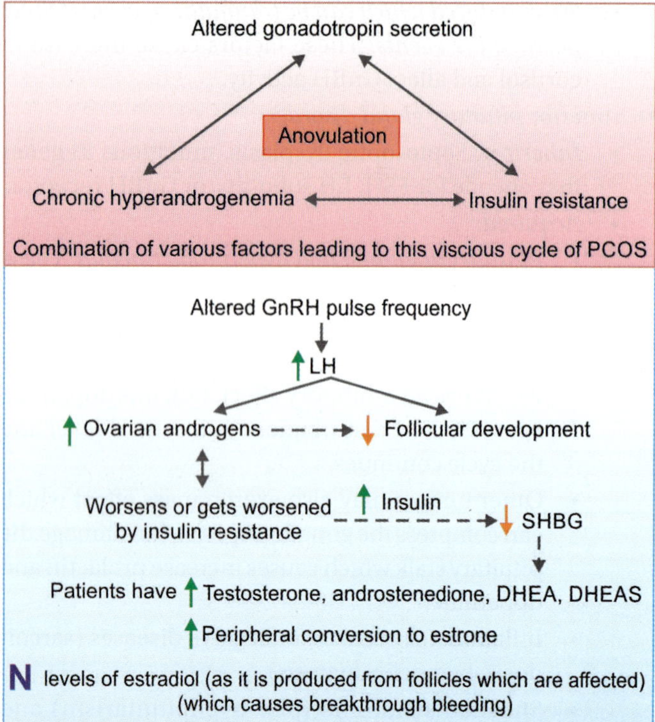

Fig. 2: PCOS—underlying pathology. (DHEA: dehydroepiandrosterone; DHEAS: sulfated form of dehydroepiandrosterone; GnRH: gonadotropin-releasing hormone; LH: luteinizing hormone; PCOS: polycystic ovary syndrome; SHBG: sex hormone-binding globulin)

metabolism in various ways and can lead to gross hormonal changes ultimately affecting the HPO axis. Adipose tissue has aromatase activity which converts the androgens to estrogen, thereby causing persistent elevated estrogen. A decrease in hepatic SHBG causes increase in peripheral free estradiol. Insulin resistance and the resultant increase in insulin levels cause increased production of androgens in the ovarian stroma, which hinders in follicular development. All these factors ultimately cause anovulation.

WHO Group 3

- Gonadal dysgenesis is the most common cause. The oocytes undergo accelerated atresia and then the ovary is replaced with a fibrous streak called as "streak ovary." So, there are no antral follicles which can secrete the sex hormones.
  - *Normal karyotype:* Pure gonadal dysgenesis (46,XX).
  - Abnormal karyotype
    - Turner syndrome (45,X)
    - Mosaics (45,X/46,XX)
  - Specific gene defects such as Fragile X syndrome and galactosemia may also cause anovulation.
- Premature ovarian failure.
- Iatrogenic causes such as surgery on ovaries (cystectomy, drilling, etc.), radiation, systemic chemotherapy.
- Autoimmune, toxins, infections, etc.

INVESTIGATIONS AND DIAGNOSIS

- *History:* A detailed menstrual history can help in knowing whether the woman is ovulating or not. A regular menstrual cycle of 21–35 days with 2–7 days bleeding usually points to ovulatory cycles. Mittelschmerz can also be present which can be of help.
- *Tests:* Many tests can be done which may help us in finding out this problem and the cause. The list is given in **Table 2**.
- Most commonly done investigation which is easy to carry out is doing serial ultrasound which can shows us the antral follicle count, the selection and growth of dominant follicle and its rupture which suggests ovulation. It can also detect polycystic or absent/streak ovaries.

Apart from this, for diagnosis of PCOS, many criteria have come up in recent times from National Institutes of Health (NIH) criteria 1990 and first Rotterdam criteria 2003. Changes have been made to the criteria and recent evidence supports the new Rotterdam Criteria which are:

Any two of the following three in adults (after excluding other pathology like adrenal hyperplasia, etc.)

- Oligo/anovulation
- Clinical and/or biochemical hyperandrogenism
- Polycystic ovaries on ultrasound.

According to the recommendations from the international evidence-based guideline for the assessment and management of PCOS, which is accepted by the American Society for Reproductive Medicine (ASRM) and the European Society of Human Reproduction and Embryology (ESHRE), the definitions should be the following:[5]

Oligomenorrhea:

- Normal in the first year post menarche as part of the pubertal transition
- 1 year post menarche: >90 days for any one cycle
- 1 to <3 years post menarche: >45 days
- 3 years post menarche to perimenopause: >35 days or <8 cycles per year
- If anovulation needs to be confirmed, serum progesterone can be done.

Biochemical hyperandrogenism: Calculated free testosterone, free androgen index, or calculated bioavailable testosterone should be used to assess biochemical hyperandrogenism in the diagnosis of PCOS with high-quality assays.

Clinical hyperandrogenism: A detailed history and physical examination should be done for all signs suggestive of clinical hyperandrogenism, including acne, alopecia, and hirsutism and, in adolescents, severe acne and hirsutism. For hirsutism, the Modified Ferriman–Gallwey score of ≥4–6 and Ludwig Visual Score for alopecia should be used.

Ultrasound for polycystic ovarian morphology (PCOM):

- Using endovaginal ultrasound transducers with a frequency bandwidth that includes 8 MHz, the threshold

TABLE 2: Investigations for evaluating anovulation.

Investigation	*Time*	*Interpretation*
BBT test	Whole cycle	A rise in temperature by 0.4–0.8°F usually suggests ovulation. Not very accurate due to user technique
Commercially available LH kits	Mid cycle	Might give an idea of LH surge
Serum progesterone	Mid-luteal phase of cycle (~ day 21)	>6–10 ng/mL usually confirms ovulation
Serum FSH	Early follicular phase (Day 2–4)	>10 IU/L indicates reduced ovarian reserve >40 IU/L indicates ovarian failure (low levels like <5 IU/L may indicate pituitary/hypothalamic problem)
Serum LH	Early follicular phase	>10 IU/L might indicate polycystic ovaries (low levels like <5 IU/L may indicate pituitary/hypothalamic problem)
Serum testosterone	Any time in cycle	>2.4 nmol/L might indicates polycystic ovaries >5 nmol/L suggests congenital adrenal hyperplasia (check DHEAS and 17-OHP levels)
Serum prolactin	Anytime in cycle (but not after exercise/stress)	>50 ng/mL indicated hyperprolactinemia. Needs further evaluation such as vision tests and MRI
Serum TSH	Anytime in cycle or with hyperprolactinemia	Normal levels : 0.70–5 mIU /L
Endovaginal scan	On visit to clinic	Serial monitoring to show growth and rupture of antral follicle Check antral follicle count and know reserve Identifying PCO
Karyotype	Primary amenorrhea and premature menopause	Identifies karyotypic abnormalities, e.g., Turner's syndrome (45,X)
Weight and BMI	Menstrual disturbances	>25: overweight then obese <18.5: underweight
Measuring insulin resistance	May help in knowing the status	HOMA-IR level measurement is not indicated
Serum AMH	May aid in diagnosing PCOS and helps in management	Routine measurement is not recommended

(AMH: anti-Müllerian hormone; BBT: basal body temperature; BMI: body mass index; DHEA-S: dehydroepiandrosterone sulfate; 17-OHP: 17-hydroxyprogesterone; FSH: follicle-stimulating hormone; HOMA-IR: homeostatic model assessment of insulin resistance; LH: luteinizing hormone; PCO: polycystic ovary; PCOS: polycystic ovary syndrome)

for PCOM should be on either ovary, a follicle number of ≥20 per ovary and/or an ovarian volume ≥10 mL, making sure no corpora lutea, cysts, or dominant follicles are present.

MANAGEMENT/TREATMENT

Managing a case of anovulation depends on various factors such as the age of the patient, body mass index (BMI), cause, other concurrent illness, and what the patient wants (fertility or normal menstrual cycles). It should be a multidisciplinary approach taking into account her present needs and future risks involved.

First step in any treatment is to sit and discuss with the patient the problem that she has. Careful counseling at this stage can go a long way. Some causes can just be cured by counseling while with others, this counseling can help her take decisions and make her more compliant in your future treatment. A suitable probable treatment plan should be discussed from this very moment. If the couple is planning for fertility treatment, a husband's semen analysis should be done so we know how to proceed.

- *For causes of WHO Group 1*:
  - Eating and stress-related disorders can be tackled with proper counseling and restoring normal status.
  - Adenomas can be managed depending on the size by medication such as cabergoline or bromocriptine or by surgery.
  - Other tumors may also need surgical removal.
  - Causes which are nonreversible such as inherited disorders or iatrogenic trauma can be helped by giving gonadotropins. Daily FSH (50–150 IU) with or without LH depending on the response may help restore ovulation. In cases where even these are not helpful, in vitro fertilization (IVF) with advanced techniques such as donor oocytes or surrogacy can help them in getting a child.
  - Thyroid disorders need supplementation according to their need and achieve a euthyroid status.

- If the patient is on other certain drugs which may cause increase in prolactin or thyroid levels, discontinuation of that drugs helps in restoring ovulation.

- *For causes of WHO Group 3:* Usually when the ovaries and affected and not producing oocytes, there is hardly anyone can do to restore ovulation. For helping them in fertility issues, IVF with donor oocytes is usually helpful.
- *For causes of WHO Group 2:*
  - Patients with nonclassical congenital adrenal hyperplasia (CAH) may benefit from replacement therapy with glucocorticoids (hydrocortisone, prednisone, and dexamethasone).
  - For hormone-secreting ovarian tumors, appropriate medical or surgical management is indicated depending on its classification.
  - *Managing PCOS:* It is responsible for around 85% of chronic anovulation and so its management is discussed in detail.

Treatment must be individualized to address the symptoms while assessing the individual's risks of near and future consequences by a personalized approach and timely intervention of preventative strategies. Long-term risks include risk for endometrial carcinoma, cardiovascular diseases, diabetes mellitus, etc. These women might come seeking help for one or more of these problems:

- Features of hyperandrogenemia
- Menstrual irregularities
- Infertility.

In any case, the first step is always *lifestyle modification.* A healthy lifestyle can help in relieving symptoms and might aid in achieving fertility. It is seen that >50% PCO women are obese and in these cases exercise and proper diet (caloric deficit) should be implemented. Even 2–5% weight reduction, mainly central abdominal fat, can help in improving systemic and reproductive functions. Weight reduction and exercise increase the amount of SHBG and decrease the insulin resistance which helps reducing the androgen levels. This helps not only in ovulation and restoring regular cycles but also in reducing the symptoms of hyperandrogenemia such as hirsutism or acne. It also reduces the risk of having cardiovascular disease (CVD) or diabetes mellitus.

- *Hyperandrogenemia*: The level of hirsutism depends on the androgen excess, the genetic sensitivity on the hair follicles and the amount of adipose tissue. Treatment should be as follows:[5]
  - If the woman does not wish pregnancy, first line of treatment is combined oral contraceptive pill (COCP). COCP blocks the endogenous LH and suppresses ovaries, thus reduces the circulating androgen levels and at the same time helps in achieving a regular menstrual cycle.
  - Antiandrogenic drugs such as spironolactone (50–100 mg twice daily) or finasteride (5 mg daily) can be given after explaining the side effects, assessing risks, and making sure that she does not get pregnant.
  - Medicated intrauterine contraceptive device (IUCD) can also be used and are better at preventing pregnancy. Flutamide use is not indicated. Newer drugs such as topical eflornithine can be used if available.
  - In spite of giving medications, we may not be able to get rid of these symptoms. In that case, the best option is to consult a dermatologist and go for the cosmetic treatments such as laser hair removal. It is the most effective way and the patient can get pregnant early if she desires so. Even for unresponsive acne, a dermatologist should be consulted.
  - For alopecia, drugs such as COCP, finasteride, spironolactone, or topical minoxidil can be tried but treatment options are limited. Final option in severe cases is hair transplantation.
  - Metformin (up to 1,500 mg daily) along with lifestyle modification can be used in women with PCOS for the treatment of weight and hormonal and metabolic outcomes. This is more effective in patients with BMI ≥ 25 kg/m^2.
  - Inositol is still considered experimental due to lack of evidence and its use is not advised.[5]
- *Menstrual irregularities*: The guidelines suggest:[5]
  - *COCP as the first line of treatment along with lifestyle changes:* There are many controversies with the use of combined pills versus progestogen-only pill (POP) but the benefits outweigh the risks in most cases. In spite of that, each case should be individualized, and the risks should be assessed before starting the COCPs. Women falling the in the WHO high-risk category such as high BMI, history of migraine, deep vein thrombosis (DVT), and CHD should be counseled and may be given POPs or offered IUCD.
  - The COCPs containing levonorgestrel, norethisterone, and norgestimate are associated with the lowest relative risk of DVT while those containing 35 µg of ethinyl estradiol and cyproterone acetate are associated with the highest risk.
  - The newer lower-dose pills can be considered by comparing the efficacy, availability and cost. Metformin can be added along with COCP in cases where the desired results are not obtained, especially in cases with a high BMI.
- *Infertility:* Treatment is complicated and should also be individualized.
  - First of all, the woman should be told counseled to optimize all modifiable risk factors such as BMI, smoking status, alcohol consumption, infections, other metabolic conditions, nutritional status, etc., as much as possible. She should also be explained that PCOS carries a higher risk of many pregnancy

complications including gestational diabetes mellitus (GDM), pregnancy-induced hypertension (PIH), preterm delivery, miscarriage rate, and also at more risk for developing ovarian hyperstimulation syndrome (OHSS), and reduced embryo implantation in case of IVF.

- A semen analysis of the husband should be done to know the status of the male partner. If normal, we can proceed further.
- A tubal patency test like hysterosalpingography, sonosalpingogram, or hysterolaparoscopy is not necessary in all cases prior to ovulation induction. It should be done in selected cases by considering the cost-benefit ratio. We recommend doing a tubal patency after one to two attempts of ovulation induction (OI).

Ovulation induction (oral drugs): If the patient's age is favorable, the first line of treatment is OI. It can be done by various drugs available such as letrozole, clomiphene, with or without metformin. Their use is off label in many countries and so it should be discussed with the patient.

- The new evidence-based guidelines suggest letrozole alone as the drug of choice as the live birth rates increase by 40–60% compared to clomiphene and a reduced rate of multiple pregnancies.[5] A more recent meta-analysis by Wang et al. also supports this finding in view of more number of live birth rates.[6]
- Second choice is using clomiphene with metformin. Clomiphene can also be used alone if required, but metformin use alone is not recommended. Metformin added to clomiphene in cases with a BMI $\geq$ 30 kg/m^2 can help improve results.

Ovulation induction with gonadotropins: The guidelines suggest gonadotropins as the second line of treatment if OI with letrozole or clomiphene fails. In this case, a specialist care with intensive monitoring should be done to avoid complications. It has better cumulative and live birth rates.

Different protocols are available for OI and they can be chosen according to the experience of the doctor. After doing OI with either oral drugs or gonadotropins, a timed intercourse can be planned. If this fails a few times, one should proceed to do an intrauterine insemination (IUI) without wasting more time. We suggest doing three to four IUIs and then stop wasting time and proceed to IVF as the patient's age is very critical to its success.

In vitro fertilization: In case OI fails or the patient is already elderly, the next step is to go for IVF or intracytoplasmic sperm injection (ICSI) . The guideline suggests the use of a GnRH—antagonist protocol versus an agonist protocol in view of reducing the chances of having OHSS. An antagonist protocol along with a GnRH agonist oocyte maturation trigger versus the conventional human chorionic gonadotropin (hCG) trigger is preferred. One might also select the option of electively freezing all embryos and transferring later in a frozen embryo transfer (FET) cycle. In case the agonist protocol is used, one has to do very vigilant so that OHSS does not occur. Metformin can be added if the agonist protocol is used.[5]

Laparoscopic electrocoagulation of ovarian surface or laparoscopic drilling (LEOS) ***(Fig. 3)****:* This is another modality in treating PCOS. It is an invasive procedure and so carries its risks. Various techniques such as using electrocautery, laser vaporization, multiple ovarian biopsies, and others are available and it is recommended by the guideline group provided that it is done in the proper way.[5] Incorrect use and overzealous surgery can reduce the ovarian reserve and patient can do into premature ovarian failure.

A summary of the treatment is given in **Figure 4**.

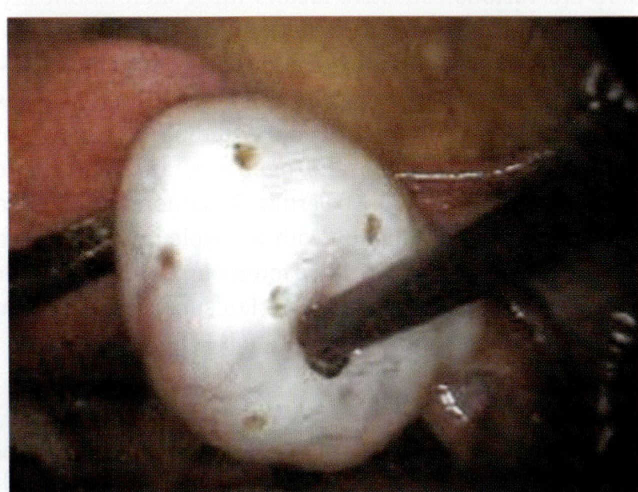

Fig. 3: Polycystic ovary drilling.

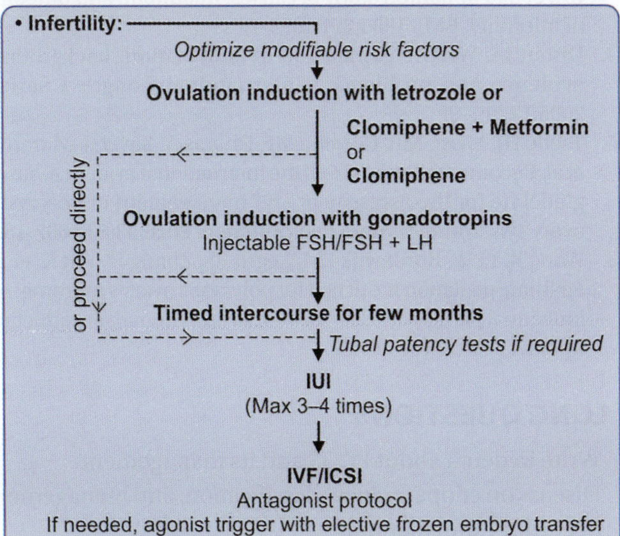

Fig. 4: Summary of treatment—PCOS.

(COCP: combined oral contraceptive pill; FSH: follicle stimulating hormone; ICSI: intracytoplasmic sperm injection; IUCD: intrauterine contraceptive device; IUI: intrauterine insemination; LH: luteinizing hormone; LOS: laparoscopic ovarian syndrome; POP: progestogen-only pill)

CONCLUSION

Anovulation needs to be evaluated thoroughly and the treatment should be according to what the patient wants. Meaningful counseling, weight reduction, exercise, and effective corrective measures without wasting time are the key to a successful treatment. The long-term complications should also be discussed, and treatment should be started accordingly.

KEY MESSAGES

Anovulation is quite a common in the reproductive age group. The WHO classifies it into three groups (hypopituitary failure, hypopituitary dysfunction, and ovarian failure) and there are various causative factors for it such as obesity, central tumors, thyroid dysfunction, hyperprolactinemia, congenital and genetic causes, and most commonly PCOS. The pathophysiology behind PCOS is complex and involves genetic and environmental factors leading to any two of oligo/anovulation, hyperandrogenism, and polycystic ovary morphology (PCOM). Fertility treatment in this case involves ovulation induction with letrozole or clomiphene with metformin along with timed intercourse or IUI. Another option is with gonadotropins. Ovarian surgery can also be done. Last but most successful option is IVF.

REFERENCES

1. Warren MP, Vu C. Central causes of hypogonadism—functional and organic. Endocrinol Metab Clin North Am. 2003;32(3): 593-612.
2. Hernandez-Rey AE. (2018). Anovulation. [online] Available from: https://emedicine.medscape.com/article/253190. [Last accessed December, 2018].
3. Hull MG, Glazener CM, Kelly NJ, Conway DI, Foster PA, Hinton RA, et al. Population study of causes, treatment, and outcome of infertility. BMJ. 1985;291:1693-7.
4. Dhont M. WHO-classification of anovulation: background, evidence and problems. . International Congress Series. 2005;1279:3-9.
5. Teede HJ, Misso ML, Costello MF, Dokras A, Laven J, Moran L, et al. Recommendations from the international evidence-based guideline for the assessment and management of polycystic ovary syndrome. Human Reproduction. 2018;33(9):1602-18.
6. Wang R, Li W, Bordewijk EM, Legro RS, Zhang H, Wu X, et al. First-line ovulation induction for polycystic ovary syndrome: An individual participant data meta-analysis. Human reproduction update. 2019;25(6):717-32.

LONG QUESTIONS

1. Write in detail about PCOS and its management.
2. Discuss on etiopathology, classification, and management of chronic anovulation.

SHORT QUESTIONS

1. Write about the HPO axis.
2. Enumerate causes and classify anovulation according to the WHO classification.
3. How does obesity cause menstrual problems?
4. Write in short about the methods of ovulation induction in patients with PCOS. Also give treatment for hyperandrogenism symptoms.

MULTIPLE CHOICE QUESTIONS

1. The increased pulsatility of GnRH leads to release of which pituitary hormone?
   a. FSH b. LH
   c. AMH d. Estrogen
2. During perimenarchal anovulation, the immaturity of what causes anovulation?
   a. Ovaries b. Uterus
   c. HPO axis d. FSH
3. WHO Class 2 of anovulation is:
   a. Hypothalamopituitary failure
   b. Hypothalamopituitary dysfunction
   c. Ovarian failure
   d. Ovarian dysfunction
4. Which thyroid dysfunction causes anovulation?
   a. Hypothyroidism b. Hyperthyroidism
   c. Both of the above d. None of the above
5. Which is not a criterion in diagnosing PCOS?
   a. Oligo/anovulation
   b. Hyperandrogenemia
   c. Polycystic ovaries on USG
   d. Reversed FSH/LH ratio
6. Serum FSH levels of > ____ IU suggest ovarian failure:
   a. 10 b. 20
   c. 30 d. 40
7. First step in management of PCOS is:
   a. Lifestyle modification b. LOS
   c. IVF d. IUI
8. Drug of choice for treating hyperandrogenemia is:
   a. Spironolactone b. Flutamide
   c. COCP d. Metformin
9. Drug of choice of OI in PCOS is:
   a. Clomiphene
   b. Letrozole
   c. Clomiphene with metformin
   d. None
10. Which IVF protocol is recommended in patients with PCOS?
    a. Agonist b. Antagonist
    c. None d. Both are same
11. PCOS patients undergoing IVF are at a higher risk of developing:
    a. Ovarian failure
    b. Pituitary failure
    c. Ovarian hyperstimulation syndrome
    d. Pituitary hyperstimulation

Answers

1. b 2. c 3. b 4. c 5. d 6. d
7. a 8. b 9. b 10. b 11. c

12.6 HORMONAL ISSUES AND INFERTILITY: THYROID, PROLACTIN AND ANDROGENS

Krishnendu Gupta, Muralidhar V Pai

INTRODUCTION

Both male and female sub-/infertility are caused by several factors such as improper gametogenesis, their faulty transport or inability to get fertilized and implanted. At all these levels, hormones play a crucial role, in that thyroid hormones, prolactin, and androgens. This chapter addresses the role of each of these hormones, their proper evaluation and interpretation, and treatment options when they are deranged.

THYROID

Although hypothyroidism is known to cause subfertility both in men and women, the controversy or confusion is with regards to definition of hypothyroidism. Most consider serum thyroid-stimulating hormone (TSH) concentration above 5 mU/L as abnormal in nonpregnant adult women. Some infertility specialists suggest that the true upper limit is only 2.5 mU/L and insist on bringing down the levels below 2.5 mU/L before inducing ovulation. A state of subclinical hypothyroidism is considered when serum-free thyroxine (T4) concentration is normal and serum TSH concentration is elevated (>5 but <10 mU/L).[1] The serum TSH levels increase with age, independent of the presence of antithyroid antibodies.[2]

The cause of subclinical hypothyroidism is same as overt hypothyroidism such as chronic autoimmune (Hashimoto's) thyroiditis with high serum concentrations of antithyroid peroxidase (anti-TPO) antibodies.

Overt hypothyroidism causes ovulatory dysfunction leading to infertility; however, the effects of subclinical hypothyroidism on reproduction are not well defined. A meta-analysis of four studies showed that the presence of thyroid autoimmunity prior to conception increased the risk of unexplained subfertility.[3]

In infertile women, the TSH cut-off range may be same as recommended for first trimester of pregnancy by the American Thyroid Association (ATA) for the Diagnosis and Management of Thyroid Disease during Pregnancy and the Postpartum, i.e., approximately 0.1–4 mU/L.[4]

As described earlier, hypothyroidism may induce hyperprolactinemia sufficiently severe to cause amenorrhea and infertility.

The serum sex hormone-binding globulin (SHBG) concentration may be low in hypothyroidism. This will lower serum total but not free sex hormone concentrations. Some men may have low serum-free testosterone concentrations but normal serum luteinizing hormone (LH) concentrations; this suggests a direct effect of hypothyroidism on the hypothalamus or pituitary, their serum-free testosterone concentrations rise with T4 treatment.[5]

A study showed decreased libido, erectile dysfunction, and delayed ejaculation in 64% of hypothyroid men.[6] In another study, sperm morphology was abnormal in 64% of hypothyroid men before treatment and 24% after T4 therapy.[7]

PROLACTIN

Prolactin is synthesized and secreted by lactotroph cells of pituitary. They are tonically suppressed by hypothalamic dopamine. Factors that induce prolactin synthesis and secretion include estrogen, thyrotropin-releasing hormone, epidermal growth factor, and dopamine receptor antagonists.

Both male and female fertility are affected by hyperprolactinemia. In females, hyperprolactinemia causes hypogonadism, which may give rise to amenorrhea, oligomenorrhea, or infertility and galactorrhea.[8] Hyperprolactinemia inhibits release of gonadotropin-releasing hormone (GnRH), thus inhibiting secretion of both follicle-stimulating hormone (FSH), and LH by pituitary giving rise to anovulation resulting in amenorrhea, oligomenorrhea, and infertility.

The best or preferred sample to evaluate serum prolactin levels is a single fasting mid-morning sample, as physiologically fasting early morning levels may be high. Serum prolactin concentration above 20 ng/mL is considered high in women of reproductive age.

- Mild degrees of hyperprolactinemia (values of 20–50 ng/mL), may cause only insufficient progesterone secretion and, therefore, a short luteal phase of the menstrual cycle and/or luteal phase defect.[9]
- Moderate degrees of hyperprolactinemia (values of 50–100 ng/mL), cause either amenorrhea or oligomenorrhea.
- Concentration greater than 100 ng/mL is associated with overt hypogonadism which not only gives rise to infertility due to anovulation; the consequent subnormal estradiol secretion induces vaginal dryness causing dyspareunia, latter being an additional cause of infertility.

Mild hyperprolactinemia can cause sub-/infertility even when there is no abnormality of the menstrual cycle, especially if it is associated with hypothyroidism; these women account for approximately 20% of those evaluated for infertility.[10]

Hyperprolactinemia in men also causes hypogonadotropic hypogonadism, which is manifested by decreased libido, impotence, infertility, gynecomastia, or, rarely, galactorrhea. Hyperprolactinemia causes erectile dysfunction by mechanisms not clearly understood but unrelated to hypogonadism as just correcting the hyperprolactinemia with a dopamine agonist drug corrects the impotence.

A number of physiological states including pregnancy, breastfeeding, stress, exercise, and sleep can influence elevation of prolactin levels. Causes of hyperprolactinemia include:

- Drugs such as antihypertensives, anticonvulsives, antihistamines, antidepressants
- Kidney disease due to decreased clearance and increased production as a result of altered central prolactin regulation
- Hypothyroidism due to pituitary hyperplasia that may mimic pituitary tumor
- Prolactin-secreting pituitary tumors and parasellar tumors.

Management

Magnetic resonance imaging (MRI) is useful to differentiate between drug-induced hyperprolactinemia and that due to pituitary tumor, and consultation with neurologists and neurosurgeon is indicated in levels above 100 ng/mL. It is worthwhile to note that 3T MRI machines with 1 mm sellar cuts provide a very high chance of diagnosing microadenomas, which hitherto may be missed by earlier generation machines and/or ≥2 mm sellar cuts.

Prolactin levels should be brought down before inducing ovulation for better yield and success. The drug-induced hyperprolactinemia is managed by temporarily suspending the drug; however, before stopping the antipsychotics, psychiatrists should be consulted.

Hypothyroidism should be corrected with administration of thyroxine which also helps in anovulation caused by the condition independent of hyperprolactinemia.

Dopamine agonist therapy may be used as first-line therapy to lower prolactin levels, decrease tumor size, and restore gonadal function for patients with symptomatic prolactin-secreting microadenomas or macroadenomas. Cabergoline (0.125–1.0 mg once/twice weekly for 12–24 months) seems to be better than other dopamine agonists (e.g., bromocriptine) because of its higher efficacy in normalizing prolactin levels. Surgery is indicated in those who have drug intolerance or resistance.[11,12]

In men, 6 months of treatment with cabergoline (0.5–1.0 mg twice weekly) restored nocturnal penile tumescence and sperm count and motility.[13]

ANDROGENS

Androgen deficiency due to GnRH or gonadotropin deficiency (hypogonadotropic hypogonadism) caused by hypothalamic or pituitary disease can render a man infertile due to reduction in sperm production. Normal sexual differentiation and spermatogenesis require testosterone and a normal androgen receptor. Mild androgen insensitivity and polymorphisms of the androgen receptor gene can cause infertility.[14]

While testosterone secretion as well as sperm production increases to near normal after replacement of LH, testosterone replacement will not restore spermatogenesis. Human chorionic gonadotropin (hCG) has longer half-life than LH and stimulates the Leydig cells of the testes to synthesize and secrete testosterone. hCG can increase intratesticular testosterone concentration 100 times that in the peripheral circulation and stimulate spermatogenesis.

In women, predominantly estrogenic intrafollicular milieu permits and favors follicular growth and development whereas androgenic milieu will lead to degeneration and atresia. In women with polycystic ovary syndrome (PCOS), there is increased androgen coming from both ovaries and adrenals due to hyperinsulinemia. The latter also causes decrease in steroid SHBG from the liver which further increases free androgens in the circulation. Preovulatory increase in androgens hampers LH surge and hence ovulation. Use of GnRH analogs or GnRH antagonists may help reduce the excessive LH and hence the androgens.

Finally, it would be worthwhile to mention that the severe acute respiratory syndrome coronavirus 2 (SARS-CoV-2) causing the coronavirus disease 2019 (COVID-19) which has been declared a pandemic by the World Health Organization (WHO) on 11 March 2020, has unveiled the multivariate pathology that this dreaded virus causes. Surprisingly, men are reportedly more vulnerable to COVID-19 even with higher fatality rate compared to women. Thus, it is crucial to determine whether SARS-CoV-2 infection can even affect male fertility as an immediate or long-term consequence of the disease. Among the discrete data available, an important finding is that angiotensin-converting enzymes 2 (ACE2) receptor, that aids the SARS-CoV-2 entry into host cells, is profoundly expressed in testicular cells. In addition, the endogenous androgen milieu and its receptors are associated with ACE2 activation reflecting that enhanced testosterone levels may trigger the pathogenesis of COVID-19. In contrary, hypogonadism has also been reported in the acute phase of some COVID-19 cases. Moreover, SARS-CoV-2 infection-induced uncontrolled inflammatory responses may lead to systemic oxidative stress (OS), whose severe disruptive effects on testicular functions are well-documented.[15]

REFERENCES

1. Biondi B, Cappola AR, Cooper DS. Subclinical Hypothyroidism: A Review. JAMA. 2019; 322(2):153-60.
2. Cappola AR. The thyrotropin reference range should be changed in older patients. JAMA 2019;322(20):1961-2.
3. van den Boogaard E, Vissenberg R, Land JA, van Wely M, van der Post JAM, Goddijn M, et al. Significance of (sub)clinical thyroid dysfunction and thyroid autoimmunity before conception and in early pregnancy: A systematic review. Hum Reprod Update. 2011;17(5):605-19.
4. Alexander EK, Pearce EN, Brent GA, Brown RS, Chen H, Dosiou C, et al. 2017 Guidelines of the American Thyroid Association

for the diagnosis and management of thyroid disease during pregnancy and the postpartum. Thyroid. 2017;27(3):315.

5. Donnelly P, White C. Testicular dysfunction in men with primary hypothyroidism; reversal of hypogonadotrophic hypogonadism with replacement thyroxine. Clin Endocrinol (Oxf). 2000;52(2):197.
6. Carani C, Isidori AM, Granata A, Carosa E, Maggi M, Lenzi A, et al. Multicenter study on the prevalence of sexual symptoms in male hypo- and hyperthyroid patients. J Clin Endocrinol Metab. 2005;90(12):6472.
7. Krassas GE, Papadopoulou F, Tziomalos K, Zeginiadou T, Pontikides N. Hypothyroidism has an adverse effect on human spermatogenesis: A prospective, controlled study. Thyroid. 2008;18(12):1255.
8. Bayrak A, Saadat P, Mor E, Chong L, Paulson RJ, Sokol RZ. Pituitary imaging is indicated for the evaluation of hyperprolactinemia. Fertil Steril. 2005;84:181.
9. Corenblum B, Pairaudeau N, Shewchuk AB. Prolactin hypersecretion and short luteal phase defects. Obstet Gynecol. 1976;47:486.
10. Shlomo M, Casanueva FF, Andrew R, Kleinberg DL, Montori VM, Schlechte JA, et al. Diagnosis and treatment of hyperprolactinemia: An Endocrine Society Clinical Practice Guideline. J Clin Endocrinol Metab. 2011;96(2):273-88.
11. Colao A, Di Sarno A, Landi ML, Scavuzzo F, Cappabianca P, Pivonello R, et al. Macroprolactinoma shrinkage during cabergoline treatment is greater in naive patients than in patients pretreated with other dopamine agonists: a prospective study in 110 patients. J Clin Endocrinol Metab. 2000;85:2247-52.
12. Molitch ME, Elton RL, Blackwell RE, Caldwell B, Chang RJ, Jaffe R, et al. Bromocriptine as primary therapy for prolactin-secreting macroadenomas: Results of a prospective multicenter study. J Clin Endocrinol Metab. 1985;60:698-705.
13. De Rosa M, Ciccarelli A, Zarrilli S, Guerra E, Gaccione M, Di Sarno A, et al. The treatment with cabergoline for 24 month normalizes the quality of seminal fluid in hyperprolactinaemic males. Clin Endocrinol (Oxf). 2006;64:307-13.
14. Gottlieb B, Lombroso R, Beitel LK, Trifiro MA. Molecular pathology of the androgen receptor in male (in)fertility. Reprod Biomed Online. 2005;10(1):42.
15. Dutta S, Sengupta P. SARS-CoV-2 and Male INFERTILITY: Possible multifaceted pathology. Reprod Sci. 2020;1-4.

LONG QUESTION

1. Discuss the role of hormones (thyroid, prolactin, and androgens) in the etiopathogenesis of sub-/infertility and their respective management.

SHORT QUESTIONS

1. Discuss the effect of hypothyroidism on sub-/infertility.
2. Discuss the effect of hyperprolactinemia on sub-/infertility.
3. Discuss the effect of hyperandrogenemia on sub-/infertility.

MULTIPLE CHOICE QUESTIONS

1. The suggested true upper limit of serum thyroid-stimulating hormone (TSH) by infertility specialists is:
   a. 5 mU/L b. 3.5 mU/L
   c. 2.5 mU/L d. 3 mU/L
2. In hypothyroidism, the concentration of serum sex hormone-binding globulin (SHBG) is usually:
   a. Unchanged b. Low
   c. High d. Very high
3. In hypothyroid men, the following symptoms and signs are true:
   a. Erectile function
   b. Decreased libido
   c. Delayed ejaculation
   d. All of the above
4. The following statements about hyperprolactinemia are true:
   a. Causes hypogonadism
   b. Stimulates GnRH release
   c. Causes menorrhagia
   d. All of the above
5. Hyperprolactinemia in men can cause:
   a. Impotence b. Galactorrhea
   c. Gynecomastia d. All of the above
6. Human chorionic gonadotropin (hCG):
   a. Has a shorter-half life than luteinizing hormone (LH)
   b. Inhibits Leydig cells of the testes
   c. Increases intra-testicular concentration
   d. All of the above
7. In males, SARS-CoV-2 causing corona disease 2019 (COVID-19), the following statements are true:
   a. Have a higher fatality rate compared to women
   b. Associated with hypogonadism in the acute phase of the disease
   c. Can cause severe disruptive effects on testicular function
   d. All of the above

Answers

1. c 2. b 3. d 4. a 5. d 6. c
7. d

12.7 TUBAL FACTOR INFERTILITY: ETIOLOGY AND MANAGEMENT

Pratap Kumar, Aswathy Kumaran

INTRODUCTION

The fallopian tubes are appendages of the uterus located on either side at the superior portion of the uterine cavity which is 10 cm long muscular tubes originating at the uterine cornua and opening distally into the peritoneal cavity. There are four parts: The proximal narrowest segment comprises the interstitium (1.25 cm long, 1 mm wide) and the isthmus (2.5 cm long, 2.5 cm wide), the ampulla, the middle segment (5 cm long, 2.5–5 mm wide) gradually widens and merges with the distal segment, and the broad funnel-like infundibulum (1.25 cm long, 6 mm wide) of the tubes. This lies in close proximity to the ipsilateral ovary. Infundibulum has fimbriae that help in capturing the cumulus oophorus complex at ovulation.

The tubes assist and modulate sperm transport, and regulate oocyte transport; the ampulla promotes fertilization, nurtures gametes and embryos, and ensures the timely passage of the embryo to the uterus.[1] The patent healthy functional tubes are hence important for fertility.

Incidence of tubal disease is approximately about 25–35% of female factor infertility and 11–30% of infertility in general depending on the population characteristics.[2,3] Salpingitis is the main cause for tubal infertility is which accounts for >50% of the cases.[2] Published literature reveals that 20–30% of women regret that they have had a tubal ligation.[4-6] Hence, prevention diagnosis and management of tubal factor-dependent subfertility is important in reproductive medicine and also proper counseling before tubal ligation is important.

CAUSES FOR TUBAL SUBFERTILITY

Congenital

Developmental/inherent anomalies of the fallopian tubes though are rare and most do not require treatment. Absence of one or both tubes is almost always associated with absence of the uterus as well as other anomalies.[7] Rudimentary oviducts, infantile ones, duplication of ostia, and accessory tubes are some other uncommon developmental anomalies.

Acquired

The most frequent cause for tubal disease is pelvic inflammatory disease. Amongst the causes, the single largest cause is *Chlamydia trachomatis* infection. Depending on the site, the problem may be categorized into proximal, mid, and distal tubal disease.

Proximal and Mid Tubal Disease

Proximal tube pathology and blockage account for 10–25% of tubal disease.[3] Pseudo-obstruction or true anatomic blockage of the fallopian tubes may the cause of proximal block[8,9] **(Table 1)**.

Salpingitis isthmica nodosa (SIN) is thought to arise from tubal inflammation of unspecified origin and affects the proximal tube prominently. Involvement of the distal tube and adhesions in pelvis and perihepatic areas, similar to pelvic inflammatory disease (PID) are also noted. Laparoscopy shows fibrosed tubal segments. Myosalpingeal hypertrophy encasing endosalpingeal diverticula is noted on histopathological examination.[8,9] Anatomic tubal occlusion by direct involvement or secondary to adhesions following PID is seen.

Distal Tubal Disease

The incidence is about 85% of tubal infertility. The distal tubal disease may cause hydrosalpinges and fimbrial phimosis. The end stage of distal tubal disease where the distal is completely occluded is the hydrosapinx, whereas a stenosed fimbrial opening due to adhesions results in fimbrial phimosis.[8,9] Causes of distal tubal disease are numerated in **Box 1**.

Iatrogenic:
- *Tubal sterilization*: Tubal sterilization causes irreversible infertility unless tubal patency restored. Thus, tubal sterilization is an iatrogenic cause of tubal infertility that needs to be addressed.

TABLE 1: Causes of proximal tubal disease.

Pseudo-obstruction	*True anatomic blockage*
Plugs of mucus and amorphous debris	Salpingitis isthmica nodosa (SIN)
Mucosal agglutination and viscous secretions	Pelvic inflammatory disease(PID)
Cornual spasm	Endometriosis
	Cornual polyps
	Intrauterine synechiae

BOX 1: Causes of distal tubal disease.

Pelvic inflammatory disease
- *85% STDs:*
  - *Neisseria gonorrheae*
  - *Chlamydia trachomatis*
  - *Mycoplasma hominis*
- 15% Iatrogenic

Tuberculosis
Peritonitis of any cause
Tubal damage from previous surgery
Endometriosis

- *Salpingectomy:* Women who have had to have bilateral salpingectomy for ectopic gestations, tubal/tubo-ovarian pathology often need assisted reproductive techniques (ART) to conceive.

EVALUATION FOR THE TUBAL FACTOR INFERTILY

Tests for tubal patency and function are recommended initially when the woman's history examinations and ultrasound evaluation is suggestive of a high risk for tubal disease. Tubal infertility should be suspected and ruled out in women with history of PID, endometriosis, prior pelvic surgery, or ectopic pregnancy. If she is considered, unlikely to have tubal pathology then evaluation of tubes are done only if she does not conceive for at least 3 months in spite of satisfactory ovulation and natural/artificial insemination around ovulation.[10] Invasive tubal patency testing should be offered depending on the treatment needs of the couple and are ideal in couples who need/opt for ovulation induction (OI), natural conception, or intrauterine insemination (IUI).

Guidelines and Recommendations

The Royal College of Obstetricians and Gynaecologists (RCOG) guidelines for investigation of suspected tubal and uterine abnormalities:[11]

Hysterosalpingography (HSG) should be offered to women with no suspicion of comorbidities (such as PID, previous ectopic pregnancy, or endometriosis) to screen for tubal occlusion.

- Where available, hysterosalpingo contrast-ultrasonography (HyCoSy) screening for tubal patency should be considered because it is an effective alternative to HSG for women who are not known to have comorbidities.

Laparoscopy and chromopertubation should be offered when comorbidities are suspected.

Hysteroscopy, as part of the initial investigation, is not needed unless clinically indicated.

The European Society of Human Reproduction and Embryology (ESHRE) recommendations:[12] The ESHRE Capri workshop in 2000 put forward three categories of test that have established association with healthy pregnancy—semen analysis, tubal patency tests by HSG or laparoscopy, and tests to detect ovulation.

- The ESHRE 2008 guidelines recommend that semen analysis and ovulation assessment before a test of tubal patency are performed. Women suspected to have comorbidities should be offered laparoscopic assessment directly so that any treatable tubal/pelvic pathology can be evaluated and managed at the same time.

The American Society for Reproductive Medicine (ASRM) recommendations:[13,14] The ASRM has suggested specific ruling out of tubal disease by tubal patency tests and *Chlamydia* antibody testing.

- Hysterosalpingography, saline infusion sonography (SIS), laparoscopy, and chromotubation, fluoroscopic/ hysteroscopic selective tubal cannulation have all been put forward as complementary and not mutually exclusive methods for evaluating tubal patency.

More than one technique often are required for accurate diagnosis and effective treatment of tubal obstruction tests for tubal function.

Ultrasound Evaluation of Fallopian Tubes

The healthy fallopian tubes are not seen on routine two/ three-dimensional (2D/3D) ultrasound (USG) imaging of the pelvis unless filled or surrounded by fluid. The tubal wall is not sonologically discernible unless thickened or distended with fluid. The characteristic retort shape pseudoseptate appearance helps us diagnose hydrosalpinx[15] **(Fig. 1)**.

The diseased distended fallopian tubes on the other hand can often be seen as adnexal masses.

The distended tubes on USG may be seen as follows:[15]

- Thin- or thick-walled (in chronic cases)
- Elongated or folded, tubular, retort-shaped fluid distended structure
- Separate the uterus and ovary.

A "cogwheel" appearance from thickened longitudinal folds in a hydrosalpinx when imaged in cross section is pathognomonic of a hydrosalpinx. It is also described as incomplete septa in an echogenic swelling in the adnexa. "Beads on a string" sign is noted when incomplete stations are present.[12]

Atypical hydrosalpinx appearance without any pseudoseptation may lead it to be mistaken for an ovarian or paraovarian cyst. Densely adherent thick multiloculated distended tubes may mimic a complex ovarian tumor.

Tubal Assessment Tests (Table 2)

Tubal testing is contraindicated with pelvic infection and active PID are absolute contraindications to performing tubal patency tests. Hence, infection locally or in the pelvis has to be evaluated. Thorough history-taking and clinical examination play an invaluable role to assess whether a patient has a high index of suspicion for pelvic infection.

Evaluating for Pelvic Infections

The Center for Disease Control (CDC) criteria to diagnose and manage PID: There is no single test or symptom that can diagnose salpingitis effectively. Even though laparoscopy was considered the gold standard to diagnose salpingitis, almost 20% of PID may show no evidence of salpingitis. The CDC criteria used to diagnose and manage PID is comprehensive and simple. PID may treated following the parenteral or oral

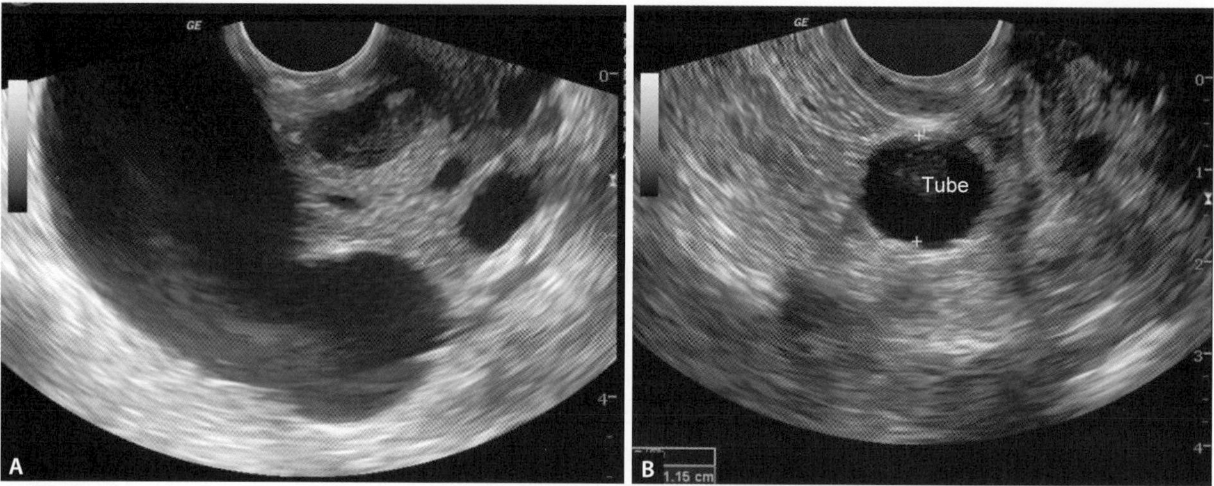

Figs. 1A and B: Hydrosalpinx USG—Retort shaped with "Cogwheel" sign.

TABLE 2: Tubal assessment tests—summary.[8]

Test	*Sensitivity*	*Specificity*	*Limitations*	*Complications*
Laparoscopy: Gold standard	Unknown (no comparator)	Unknown	• Invasive • General anesthesia • Skill requirement • Expensive	Bowel/urological/vascular injury 0.13%
Hysterosalpingography	53–65%	83–87%	• Failure to catheterize/cannulate • Leak of dye around cervix • Tubal spasm or debris causing false-positive report reporting error	Anaphylaxis PID 3.1%: Radiation exposure~ 2 Gray
HyCoSY	93.3%	89.7%		PID
SSTC	Unknown (lack of data)	unknown	unclear	Tubal perforation 2%
Fertiloscopy	86%	100%		Rectal injury 0.61% Uterine perforation
Chlamydia unknown antibody test	21–90%	29–100%		

(HyCoSY: hysterosalpingo contrast-ultrasonography; PID: pelvic inflammatory disease; SSTC: salpingography and tubal catheterization)

treatment regimens suggested by the CDC as described in the chapter on PID or may be managed in India following the syndromic management approach for sexually transmitted diseases (STD).[16]

Chlamydia antibody test (CAT):[15,17] Chlamydial infection is the most common infective cause of tubal disease. The detection of antibodies to *C. trachomatis* has been associated with tubal pathology.[15,17]

The *CAT* has sensitivity of only 40–50% and PPV of 60%, but high negative predictive value (NPV) of 80–90% for detection of distal tubal disease compared to laparoscopy.[15,18,19] The infection can be treated by treating the couple with a 14–21-day course of doxycycline.

Testing for tuberculosis (in endemic countries): Female genital tuberculosis (FGTB) is an undisputed cause for subfertility in countries like India where tuberculosis is endemic (incidence up to 16% in subfertile women).[20] It causes extensive tubal and endometrial damage. The fallopian tubes are involved in 90–100% cases. Ruling out tuberculosis and curative treatment when diagnosed should be done prior to tube testing is ideal in women with hypomenorrhea, thin endometrium, or features of chronic PID. FGTB often coexists with other causes of PID such as *Chlamydia* and gonorrhea.

Premenstrual endometria aspiration/biopsy and nucleic acid amplification (NAA) [TB Polymerase Chain Reaction (PCR)] allows for rapid diagnosis and help detect mycobacterial DNA in 80.9% of genitourinary tuberculosis (GUTB)-suspected patients.[21] However, the PCR cannot differentiate between active and latent infection and may be unreliable in identifying the cases that actually requite treatment. Hence, endometrial sampling and TB stain, BACTEC culture, and histopathological examination for tubercles diagnostic laparoscopy is used in conjunction with TB PCR to diagnose genital TB. The new self-contained cassette-based analysis (GeneXpert) is faster than PCR and helps identify rifampicin-resistant tuberculosis also.[21] Tuberculosis when diagnosed has to be treated with appropriate antitubercular agents for 9 months.

Laparoscopic diagnosis and grading of salpinitis:[22]

Jacobson and Weström laparoscopic criteria to diagnose and grade salpingitis:	
Minimum visual criteria to diagnose salpingitis	• Pronounced tubal surface hyperemia • Tubal wall edema • Presence of exudates on tubes and from fimbriae when parent
Mild salpingitis	• Minimum visual criteria • Mobile tubes • Patent ostia
Moderate salpingitis	• More evident inflammation • Patchy fibrin deposits on tubes • Loose tubal and pelvic adhesions • Tubes not freely mobile
Severe salpingitis	• Intense congestion • Dense adhesions to pelvic structures • Pyosalpinx • Tubo-ovarian masses
Each adnexa should be graded separately	
The overall grade is that of the more severe pathology	

Tubal Patency Tests

The various tests used to assess tubal patency and functional integrity are enumerated below in the order of their coming into vogue.

Laparoscopy and Chromopertubation

Laparoscopy is considered to be the gold standard for diagnosing tubal patency and inflammation. It allows diagnosis assessment and management of peritubal disease, adhesions, and endometriosis. Laparoscopy enables biopsy of suspicious lesions for further evaluation.

Laparoscopy is a better predictor of fertility prognosis compared to other tubal tests such as HSG and hence, the performances of other tests are compared to those of laparoscopy.[23,24]

Falloposcopy introduced by Kerin is hysteroscopic proximal fallopian tube endoscopic examination using a flexible microendoscope (0.5 mm dm, 1.73 mm length, 50X magnification), and guided catheterization.[25,26]

Hysterosalpingography

Hysterosalpingography is an inexpensive and widely available screening test to rule out unilateral or bilateral tubal block and provide a permanent visual record of the uterus and tubes.

It involves instillation of approximately 10 mL water-soluble radiocontrast transcervically and serial X-ray imaging of the pelvis to visualize the uterine cavity, delineate the tubes, and to assess peritoneal spill. Cornual tubal spasm is the main reason for lower accuracy of this diagnostic imaging technique. Gentle handling and administration of an antispasmodic tablet or injection prior to the procedure tackles this problem effectively. HSG ideally performed in the late follicular phase (day 7–12) following a normal menstrual cycle. Performing the HSG with an oil-based radiopaque dye has been associated with increased live birth rates. In spite of this, water-based dye is preferred due to better image quality and safety.[27]

Hysterosalpingography has a low sensitivity of 53–65% and a high specificity of 83–87%, positive predictive value (PPV) 38% of and NPV 94%, i.e., HSG is reliable indicator of tubal patency if bilateral spill is noted on evaluation.[13,28]

An abnormal HSG helps predict proximal tubal blockage and hydrosalpinges with moderate accuracy while it very inaccurate in diagnosing or ruling out distal tubal obstruction and peritubal adhesions. Although an HSG might look normal hydrosalpinges remain undiagnosed.[24] If in doubt, a laparoscopic evaluation is needed **(Fig. 2)**.

Advanced HSG may be done with using fluoroscopic guidance, manipulation, tubal cannulation, and tubal pressure to yield more information and increase reliability of testing.[9]

The tubes are categorized into three as given in **Table 3**.

Selective Salpingography and Tubal Catheterization/ Ultrasound or Hysteroscopy-guided Tubal Cannulation

Fluoroscopy guided transcervical proximal tubal cannulation, and selective salpingography and tubal catheterization (SSTC) to identify and dislodge proximal tubal block was introduced by Corfmann and Taylor in 1966. Later, hysteroscopic and ultrasound guided proximal tubal cannulation[29,30] became more commonly used modalities to identify and tackle proximal tubal obstruction due to spasm, plugs, and adhesions.

Sonohysterosalpingography

Sonohysterosalpingography is a test to determine tubal patency using transcervical fluid instillation, the filling

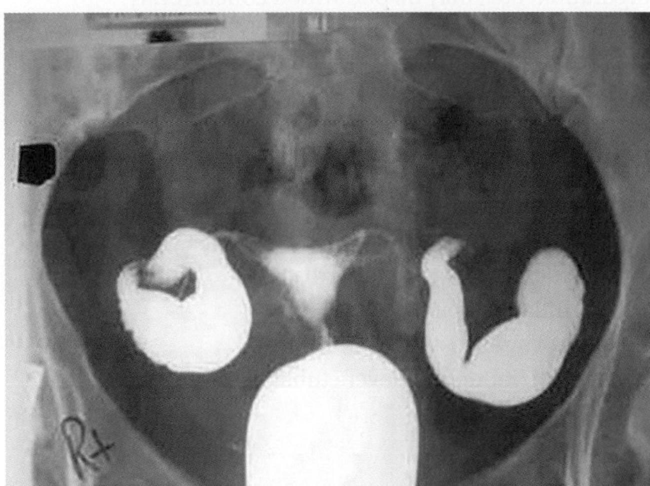

Fig. 2: Hysterosalpingography showing bilateral hydrosalpinx.

TABLE 3: The three HSG-based categories of tubal patency.[9]

Category 1: Normal	*Category 2: Patent tube with tubal disease*	*Category 3: Patent or blocked tubes, severe tubal disease*
Patency with free spill Preserved distal tubal folds	Patency with good spill Almost fully preserved distal tubal folds	Patent/blocked tubes Loss of distal tubal folds
Normal proximal, mid, distal tubal dimensions and appearance	Normal to slightly altered tubal dimensions	Altered proximal, mid, distal tubal dimensions and appearance with dilatation/narrowing/scarring/tubal rigidity
No fimbrial end clumping	+/–Fimbrial end clumping	Fimbrial end dilatation/narrowing with clumping present
No detected peritubal disease normal tubal pressures with free flow Lack of sharp pain on forceful flushing	+/– Peritubal disease Normal or elevated tubal pressures	Peritubal disease may or may not be seen Usually elevated tubal pressures but may be normal

and flow of which is monitored by transvaginal ultrasound monitoring. Although tubal patency can be observed by the appearance of fluid in the cul de sac with the saline infusion, the test does not differentiate between unilateral or bilateral patency.[13]

The uterine cavity is insufflated slowly with about 300 mL plain saline after catheterizing the cervix with a narrow (no.8 Foleys) catheter.

Where available sonohysterosalpingography is a better alternative to HSG as it has higher sensitivity and specificity of 93.3% and 89.7%, respectively.[8]

Transvaginal Hydrolaparoscopy and Fertiloscopy

Transvaginal hydrolaparoscopy (THL) involves small diameter endoscopic visualization of the pelvis after instillation of 500 mL of a fluid medium through a needle inserted through posterior vaginal fornix. When hysteroscopy, falloposcopy, and distal tubal salpingoscopy are done along with THL, it is termed fertiloscopy.[31] Fertiloscopy provides a wealth of information although consensus guidelines on how to interpret and put the findings into use has not yet been laid.

Fertiloscopy may be done in an outpatient procedure under local anesthesia. Minor adhesiolysis, endometriosis fulguration, etc., may be performed concurrently.[31]

The risk of bowel injury is much higher compared to laparoscopy and THL is not useful in evaluating women with obliterated pouch of Douglas.

MANAGEMENT OF TUBAL INFERTILITY

Deciding the management for tubal factor infertility depends on:

- Site and extent of the tubal disease:
  - Unilateral/bilateral
  - Proximal/distal
  - Mild/moderate/severe tubal disease
- Age of the patient
- Duration of fertility
- Ovarian reserve
- Prior fertility
- Presence of other infertility factors
- Experience of the surgeon if tubal surgery is planned
- Success rates of the in vitro fertilization (IVF) program/ restorative surgery.

In Vitro Fertilization for Tubal infertility

In vitro fertilization was originally developed to allow couples with tubal infertility to conceive and enjoy the joys of parenthood. Thus, IVF and embryo transfer (ET) remain ideal therapeutic options to achieve intrauterine pregnancy in women with tubal infertility. Also, IVF is the treatment modality to be opted when there are other problems such as male factor infertility, and resistant anovulation, contributing to infertility.

The ideal management of severe tubal disease especially with hydrosalpinges and severe fimbrial phimosis are always IVF and ET after salpingectomy/occlusion of hydrosalpinges.[32]

However, IVF is an expensive treatment modality, and for some unacceptable. IVF is also associated with complications ovarian hyperstimulation syndrome (OHSS), multiple pregnancies that cause significant morbidity and expenses. Women with mild/unilateral tubal disease may benefit with treatment approaches such as intrauterine insemination (IUI)/tubal reconstructive surgery. Tuboplasty may be tried in women cannot accept/afford IVF. The 2017 Cochrane review found that well-controlled RCTs or high-quality evidence comparing the post tuboplasty reproductive outcomes for diseased tubes with IVF are not available yet.[33]

Ovarian stimulation with IUI may be offered initially to patients with unilateral proximal tubal occlusion often obtaining satisfactory results. However, in women with mid-distal or distal tubal occlusion on HSG, the IUI after ovarian stimulation is ineffective. They require laparoscopic evaluation and often IVF.[34]

On the other hand, tubal reanastomosis for infertility due to tubal sterilization offers a cumulative pregnancy rate, i.e., comparable or even higher than IVF although the per cycle pregnancy rate is higher in IVF.[32] Sterilization reversal was the most cost-effective approach for most women younger than 41 years, while IVF remained the best approach for women more than 41 years of age.[35]

Reconstructive Surgery for Tubal Infertility

Tubal surgery to overcome infertility is becoming an attractive option to many as the benefits obtained from tubal surgery would potentially be sustained many years and may allow conception though intercourse or IUI. However, tubal surgery requires specialized skill development.[33] Its efficacy has to be weighed against the cons of expenses, risk of tubal ectopic pregnancy (7–18%), reocclusion and failure to conceive.[8]

Microsurgical Techniques[36]

Microsurgery was introduced into gynecology specifically to improve tubal reconstructive surgery outcomes. The microsurgical techniques should be applied universally for all tuboplasty irrespective of the approach (laparoscopy/laparotomy). The microsurgical principles include:

- Surgery under magnification using a binocular microscope (20X) and/or loupe magnifier (6X)
- Gentle handling of tissues
- Use of light-weight microsurgical instruments (13–15 mm length)
- Use of fine sutures (7–0 to 10–0)
- Use of fine tapered needles (135° curvature, 50–150 µm diameter)
- Meticulous hemostasis with electrocautery devices have microelectrodes, fingertip controls, and lowest current setting
- Copious irrigation
- Sharp precise dissection by an experienced surgeon who is ideally seated on the opposite site to the tube being operated on.

Surgery for Proximal Tubal Disease

Proximal Tubal Cannulation

Hysteroscopic proximal tubal cannulation or fluoroscopic selective salpingography and proximal tubal catheterization are effective modes to assess and treat proximal tubal obstruction due to tubal debris, sludge, intraluminal adhesions. Proximal tubal cannulation may be done under sonological guidance too.[30] Ideally, proximal tubal cannulation is done after confirming that the distal tube is normal using prior laparoscopic evaluation. Gentle pressure and flushing by the cannula inserted through the cornuotubal ostia is enough to overcome mechanical obstruction of the proximal tube.[3,10] Tubal perforation may occur in 3–11% cases but does not cause any clinical consequences. Tubal cannulation relieves obstruction in approximately 85% and around half the patients conceive.[3,10]

Tubal Resection and Reanastomosis

Proximal tube disease such as salpingitis isthmica nodosa causes extensive intraluminal and mesenchymal damage of proximal tube. IVF and ET are the best treatment option. Where IVF not acceptable or possible; diseased proximal tubal resection and reanastomosis of tubes are the best option as it is associated with higher pregnancy rates compared to expectant management or proximal tubal cannulation.[37]

Surgery for Distal Tubal Disease

Surgical reconstruction for damaged distal tubes may be offered in mild-to-moderate disease where at least 50% of the endosalpinx and tubal wall is healthy.

Extent of tubal mucosal damage and increase in wall thickness are the most important determinants and are inversely related to successful tubal restorative surgery outcomes.[38]

The best prognosis is seen in patients with mildly dilated tubes (<3 cm) having thin and pliable walls, undamaged endosalpinx with intact mucosa and only filmy adnexal adhesions. Neosalpingostomy: The opening of a blocked distal tube and fimbrioplasty where the stenosed distal tube ostia is widened are the two commonly employed methods. Salpingo-ovariolysis that involves the release of adhesions binding the tubes and ovaries restoring the normal tubo-ovarian relation is done alongside the above two options.[39,40]

The ASRM recommends that the reconstructive surgeries be done laparoscopically as they are less risky, less invasive and associated with the same treatment outcomes as in laparotomy.[37]

Laparoscopic opening of mild or even moderately diseased tubes offers a satisfactory pregnancy outcome in comparison with IVF.[38]

Intrauterine and ectopic pregnancy rates after neosalpingostomy for mild hydrosalpinges range from 58 to 77% and from 2 to 8%, respectively. For severe disease, these values were 0–22% and 0–17%, respectively.[13,38,41]

Sterilization Reversal

Tubal sterilization reversal may be accomplished by opening the occluded ends of the proximal and distal segments and anastomosing them with fine nonreactive sutures using nonmicrosurgical or magnification and microsurgical techniques.[13] Microsurgical techniques require training and experience so that the gynecologist can operate using binocular or loupe magnification allowing precise placement of fine sutures (7–0 to 10–0) as well as undistorted and tension free approximation of tissue edges.

Tubal reanastomosis success depends on multiple factors including the woman's age, ovarian reserve, the sterilization procedure she underwent as well as the endoluminal, and surface integrity of the tube left behind.

The age of the woman is the most important predeterminant for pregnancy rates following tubal reversal. The younger the woman, the better the pregnancy rates. Women <40 years have cumulative intrauterine pregnancy rates as high as 70% and 90%, respectively, following nonmicrosurgical and microsurgical reversal of tubal sterilization.[42] Another study noted that significantly higher cumulative pregnancy rates obtained and lesser cost per delivery incurred following tubal reanastomosis compared to IVF in women younger than 37 years.[43] The rate of ectopic pregnancy following tubal reanastomosis is 2–10%, compared to 2% for IVF.

Isthmus to isthmus reanastomosis and longer final tubal lengths are generally thought to yield higher success rates. Traditionally tubal reanastomosis is done via laparotomy as it is an easier approach to implement microsurgical tubal reanastomosis effectively. Laparoscopic microsurgical tubal reanastomosis requires good laparoscopic suturing skill and experience but have comparable outcomes to laparotomy sterilization reversal.[13] Recently, robotic laparoscopic tubal reconstruction is also being applied.

Destructive Tubal Surgery Followed by IVF: For Severe and Bipolar Tubal Disease, Hydrosalpinx

Tubal reconstruction is not beneficial for women with severe and/or bipolar (both proximal and distal) tubal disease. The presence of unresolving hydrosalpinx is pathognomonic of severe tubal disease and is associated with poor ART outcomes. In such cases salpingectomy/tubal occlusion/clipping followed by IVF is the preferred treatment to conceive. All sonologically detectable hydrosalpinges should be removed/occluded prior to applying ART **(Table 4)**.

In vitro fertilization was developed primarily to allow pregnancy in women with tubal infertility but paradoxically, it was noted that IVF outcomes were poorer in women with extensive tubal disease as in hydrosalpinges. Poor implantation rates and higher miscarriage rates were noted.[44-46] Randomized clinical trials (RCTs) have reported that IVF and ET following salpingectomy restores the rates of pregnancy and live birth to levels similar to those of women without hydrosalpinx who were treated with IVF.[47,48]

It is believed that the hydrosalpinges adversely affect the various embryo endometrial interactions involved in implantation. At the molecular level, hydrosalpinges have been associated with reduced $\alpha_v\beta_3$ integrin and LIF (leukemia inhibitory factor) expressions as well as decreased *HOXA* (*homeobox* gene) 10 expression in the endometrium that hamper implantation.[49]

The hydrosalpingeal fluid is considered as a main culprit for deleterious IVF outcomes though why it is so is still unclear. It contains various cytokines and growth factors which may be toxic to gametes or embryos.[50] Bathing of the endometrial cavity in hydrosalpinx fluid may hinder embryo endometrium crosstalk and cause potential embryo toxicity.[51,52] The mechanical effects exerted by hydrorrhea through the uterine cavity may cause changes in endometrial peristalsis that may washout or hinder implantation of the transferred embryo.[46] Furthermore, the hydrosalpinges provide unfavorable environment for early follicular recruitment.

The best method to detect hydrosalpinges is by routine 2D transvaginal sonography (sensitivity 84.6%, specificity 99.7%). HyCoSy is ideal to assess the uterine cavity and tubes in women with two more unexplained implantation failures as sonography distending and visualizing the tubal and uterine lumen will reveal pathologies such as intrauterine polyps/adhesions and hydrosalpinges that were not detected on routine evaluation.[8]

The less invasive laparoscopic salpingectomy is the preferred approach. The tube is delinked by coagulating and dividing the proximal tube close to the cornua. The mesosalpinx is then serially coagulated and cut staying close to the tube to avoid compromising the ovarian blood supply **(Fig. 3)**.[13,37]

A Scandinavian RCT published in 1999 that included 141 women showed that salpingectomy prior to IVF in all transvaginal ultrasound detectable hydrosalpinges improved IVF outcomes in terms of increased pregnancy and delivery rates. The histopathological examination of the tubes showed that >90% of the tubes showed pathology that could not be corrected by restorative tubal surgery.[53] Thus, hydrosalpinges that are detectable on ultrasound almost always represent dysfunctional and uncorrectable tubal pathology.

Strandell et al. in 2001 provided reassuring evidence that the salpingectomy prior to IVF does not compromise

TABLE 4: Surgical management for hydrosalpinges.[32]

Method	*Advantages*	*Disadvantages*
Salpingectomy (laparoscopic)	Total removal of chronically inflamed tissue	Invasive procedure, difficult if tube buried in adhesions
	No further risk of abscess formation or torsion	Interstitial/cornual pregnancy and rupture may rarely occur
	Increased the accessibility of the ovary for oocyte pick up	may hamper with ovarian vascularity and function
		All chances of spontaneous conception lost
Tubal occlusion: • *Electocautery* • *Clips* • *Hysteroscopic Essure microinsert*	Less invasive Easier than salpingectomy when dense adhesions are present	Risk of abscess formation or torsion
Aspiration (Transvaginal/laparoscopic)	Less invasive, easy Tube retained	May flare up infection Recurrence of hydrosalpinx
Salpingostomy	Less invasive, easy	Recurrence of hydrosalpinx Increased risk of tubal ectopic pregnancy

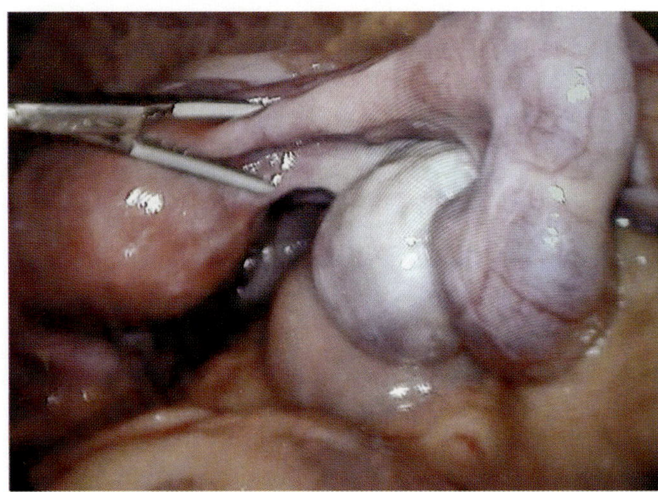

Fig. 3: Hydrosalpinx being delinked during laparoscopy.

ovarian function.[54] Salpingectomy for hydrosalpinges also does not adversely influence the response to ovarian stimulation or alter IVF parameters.[54]

The 2010 Cochrane on surgical treatment of tubal disease for IVF reviewed five RCTs including 646 women. Outcomes following laparoscopic salpingectomy, laparoscopic tubal occlusion, and USG-guided aspiration were compared. They found that the ongoing pregnancy rates and clinical pregnancy rates were increased with laparoscopic salpingectomy prior to IVF while laparoscopic tubal occlusion was associated with significant increase in clinical pregnancy. IVF outcomes following salpingectomy and tubal occlusion were similar.[55] The adverse effects following the different surgical techniques were not significantly different.[32]

They concluded that both laparoscopic salpingectomy and tubal occlusion (electrocautery delinking/proximal tubal clipping prior to IVF improved pregnancy rates). Hence, the less invasive laparoscopic occlusion may be considered as an alternative to salpingectomy.[32] Dreyer K et al. (2016) noted that the ongoing pregnancy rates were significantly lower in assisted reproductive technology (ART) cycles following hysteroscopic occlusion compared to laparoscopic salpingectomy.[56]

From the above discussion, it is clear that hydrosalpinges left unattended prior to IVF is associated with poorer pregnancy rates. So all hydrosalpinges detected prior to IVF should ideally be occluded/removed. Concurrent transvaginal aspiration of hydrosalpinges noted during oocyte pickup reduces their presence at the time of ET but whether it improves clinical outcomes is still under debate.[32]

KEY MESSAGES

- Pelvic inflammatory disease causing salpingitis and tubal infertility should be diagnosed early and treated following the CDC guidelines.
- HSG is recommended first-line test to assess tubal patency, but where available sonohysterosalpingography using saline/contrast to visualize the uterine cavity and tubes is preferred.
- Laparoscopy and chromopertubation are the current gold standard to assess tubal patency and should be offered as first-line test for women with history of pelvic comorbidities such as endometriosis and PID.
- Microsurgical tubal sterilization reversal is recommended in women younger than 40 years as the subsequent cumulative pregnancy rates are comparable if not higher than IVF pregnancy rates. It is also more cost effective.
- IVF and ET are the best option to achieve per cycle intrauterine pregnancy in severe tubal disease.
- IVF is also the best option for tubal infertility when associated with other factors such as abnormal semen parameters, anovulation, and rapidly declining ovarian reserve.
- Laparoscopic salpingectomy or proximal tubal occlusion is recommended prior to IVF in all cases of sonologically detected hydrosalpinges and severe tubal disease to improve IVF pregnancy rates.
- Tubal cannulation is recommended for proximal tubal obstruction in young women with isolated tubal factors as it restores patency in most of the cases.
- *Tubal reconstructive surgery:* Laparoscopic neosalpingostomy or fimbrioplasty improves fertility in young women with isolated tubal factor infertility due to mild distal tubal disease (hydrosalpinges/fimbrial phimosis).
- PID causing salpingitis and tubal infertility should be diagnosed early and treated following the CDC guidelines.
- HSG is recommended it is and tubal infertility should be diagnosed early and treated following the CDC guidelines.

REFERENCES

1. ESHRE Capri Workshop Group. Diagnosis and management of the infertile couple: missing information. Hum Reprod Update. 2004;10(4):295-307.
2. Evers JL. Female subfertility. Lancet. 2002;360:151-9.
3. Honore GM, Holden AE, Schenken RS. Pathophysiology and management of proximal tubal blockage. Fertil Steril. 1999;5:785-95.
4. Borrero SB, Reeves MF, Schwarz EB, Bost JE, Creinin MD, Ibrahim, SA. Race, insurance status, and desire for tubal sterilization reversal. Fertil Steril. 2008;90:272-7.
5. Schmidt JE, Hillis SD, Marchbanks PA, Jeng G, Peterson HB. Requesting information about and obtaining reversal after tubal sterilization: Findings from the U.S. Collaborative Review of Sterilization. Fertil Steril. 2000;74:892-8.
6. Chi IC. Jones DB. Incidence, risk factors, and prevention of poststerilization regret in women: an updated international review from an epidemiological perspective. Obstet Gynecol Surv. 1994;49:722-32.
7. Muckle C, Feinberg E. Developmental abnormalities of the female reproductive organs. Glob Libr women's med. 2008;1756-2228.
8. Suresh YN, Narvekar NN. The role of tubal patency tests and tubal surgery in the era of assisted reproductive techniques. The Obstetrician & Gynaecologist. 2014;16:37-45.
9. Patil M. Assessting tubal damage. J Hum Reprod Sci. 2009;2:2-11.

10. Practice Committee of the American Society for Reproductive Medicine. Role of tubal surgery in the era of assisted reproductive technology: A committee opinion. Fertil Steril. 2015;103(6):e37-43.
11. National Collaborating Centre for Women's and Children's Health (UK). NICE Clinical Guideline. Fertility: assessment and treatment for people with fertility problems. London: Royal College of Obstetricians and Gynecologists; 2013. pp. 1-555.
12. European Society of Human Reproduction and Embryology. Good Clinical Treatment in Assisted Reproduction. An ESHRE position paper The Practice Committee of the American Society for Reproductive Medicine - Optimal evaluation of the infertile female. 2008.
13. Practice Committee of the American Society for Reproductive Medicine. Diagnostic evaluation of the infertile female: a committee opinion. Fertil Steril. 2015;103(6):e44-50.
14. Benjaminov O, Atri M. Sonography of the abnormal fallopian tube. AJR Am J Roentgenol. 2004;183(3):737-42.
15. Mol BW, Dijkman B, Wertheim P, Lijmer J, van der Veen F, Bossuyt PM. The accuracy of serum chlamydial antibodies in the diagnosis of tubal pathology: a meta-analysis. Fertil Steril. 1997;67:1031-7.
16. Workowski KA. Centers for Disease Control and Prevention sexually transmitted diseases treatment guidelines. Clinical Infectious Diseases. 2015;61(suppl_8):S759-62.
17. Broeze KA, Opmeer BC, Coppus SF, Van Geloven N, Alves MF, Anestad G, et al. Chlamydia antibody testing and diagnosing tubal pathology in subfertile women: an individual patient data meta-analysis. Hum Reprod Update. 2011;17:301-10 Compared with laparoscopy.
18. den Hartog JE, Morre SA, Land JA. Chlamydia trachomatis-associated tubal factor subfertility: Immunogenetic aspects and serological screening. Hum Reprod Update. 2006;12:719-30.
19. Ubaldi F, Wisanto A, Camus M, Tournaye H, Clasen K, Devroey P. The role of transvaginal ultrasonography in the detection of pelvic pathologies in the infertility workup. Hum Reprod. 1998;13:330-3.
20. Sharma JB. Current Diagnosis and Management of Female Genital Tuberculosis. Journal of Obstetrics and Gynaecology of India. 2015;65(6):362-371. doi:10.1007/s13224-015-0780-z.
21. Yadav S, Singh P, Hemal A, Kumar R. Genital tuberculosis: current status of diagnosis and management. Transl Androl Urol. 2017;6(2): 222-33.
22. Soper DE. Diagnosis and laparoscopic grading of acute salpingitis. Am J Obstet Gynecol. 1991;164(5 Pt 2):1370-6.
23. Westrom L, Mardh PA. Acute pelvic inflammatory disease (PID). In: Holmes KK, Mardh PA, Sparling PF (Eds). Sexually transmitted diseases, 2nd edition. New York: McGraw-Hill; 1990. pp. 593-613.
24. Papaioannou S, Bourdrez P, Varma R, Afnan M, Mol BW, Coomarasamy A. Tubal evaluation in the investigation of subfertility: a structured comparison of tests. BJOG. 2004;111: 1313-21.
25. Kerin J, Daykhovsky L, Segalowitz J, Surrey E, Anderson R, Stein A, et al. Falloposcopy: A microendoscopic technique for visual exploration of the human fallopian tube from the uterotubal ostium to the fimbria using a transvaginal approach. Fertil Steril. 1990;54(3):390-400.
26. Dechaud H, Daures JP, Hedon B. Prospective evaluation of falloposcopy. Hum Reprod. 1998;131815-8.
27. Luttjeboer F, Harada T, Hughes E, Johnson N, Lilford R, Mol BW. Tubal flushing for subfertility. Cochrane Database Syst Rev. 2007;(3):CD003718.
28. Broeze KA, Opmeer BC, Van Geloven N, Coppus SF, Collins JA, Den Hartog JE, et al. Are patient characteristics associated with the accuracy of hysterosalpingography in diagnosing tubal pathology? An individual patient data meta-analysis. Hum Reprod Update. 2011;17:293-300.
29. Novy MJ. Transhysteroscopic techniques for tubal catheterization. Ref Gynecol Obstet. 1995;3:67-71.
30. Rahimunnisa S, Tanwar R, Prasad S. Ultrasound versus tactile cannulation in the treatment of proximal tubal obstruction. Int J Gynaecol Obstet. 2009;106(3):216-7.
31. Watrelot A, Nisolle M, Chelli H, Hocke C, Rongières C, Racinet C. Is laparoscopy still the gold standard in infertility assessment? A comparison of fertiloscopy versus laparoscopy in infertility. Results of an international multicentre prospective trial: the 'FLY' (Fertiloscopy–Laparoscopy) study. Hum Reprod. 2003;18:834-9.
32. Johnson N, van Voorst S, Sowter MC, Strandell A, Mol BWJ. Surgical treatment for tubal disease in women due to undergo in vitro fertilisation. Cochrane Database Syst Rev. 2004;(3):CD002125.
33. Chua S, Akande VA, Mol BJ. Surgery for tubal infertility. Cochrane Database Syst Rev. 2017; 2017(1): CD006415.
34. Jacob F, Ben-Haroush A, Lande Y, Fisch B. Role of treatment with ovarian stimulation and intrauterine insemination in women with unilateral tubal occlusion diagnosed by hysterosalpingography. Fertil Steril. 2007;88(2):396-400.
35. Messinger LB, Alford CE, Csokmay JM, Henne MB, Mumford SL, Segars JH, et al. Cost and efficacy comparison of in vitro fertilization and tubal anastomosis for women after tubal ligation. Fertil Steril. 2015;104(1):32-8.
36. Siegler A. Microsurgical tubal reconstruction. Glob Libr Women's Med. 2008.
37. Gomel V, McComb PF. Microsurgery for tubal infertility. J Reprod Med. 2006;51:177-84.
38. Milingos SD, Kallipolitis GK, Loutradis DC, Liapi AG, Hassan EA, Mavrommatis CG, et al. Laparoscopic treatment of hydrosalpinx: Factors affecting pregnancy rates. J Am Assoc Gynecol Laparosc. 2000;7:355-61.
39. The Practice Committee of the American Society for Reproductive Medicine. Optimal evaluation of the infertile female. Fertil Steril. 2006;86:S264-7.
40. Bontis JN, Theodoridis, TD. Laparoscopic management of hydrosalpinx. Ann NY Acad Sci. 2006;1092:199.
41. Kim JD, Kim KS, Doo JK, Rhyeu CH. A report on 387 cases of microsurgical tubal reversals. Fertil Steril. 1997;68:875-80.
42. Nackley AC, Muasher SJ. The significance of hydrosalpinx in in vitro fertilization. Fertil Steril. 1998; 69:373-84.
43. Boeckxstaens A, Devroey P, Collins J, Tournaye H. Getting pregnant after tubal sterilization: surgical reversal or IVF?. Hum Reprod. 2007;22:2660-4.
44. Steptoe PC, Edwards RG. Birth after the reimplantation of a human embryo. Lancet. 1978;2:366.
45. Andersen A, Yue Z, Meng F, Petersen K. Low implantation rate after in vitro fertilisation in patients with hydrosalpinges diagnosed by ultrasonography. Human Reproduction. 1994;9:1935-8.
46. Strandell A, Waldenstrom U, Nilsson L, Hamberger L. Hydrosalpinx reduces in-vitro fertilisation/embryo transfer pregnancy rates. Human Reprod. 1994;9:861-3.

47. Dechaud H, Daures JP, Arnal F, Humeau C, Hedon B. Does previous salpingectomy improve implantation and pregnancy rates in patients with severe tubal factor infertility who are undergoing in vitro fertilization? A pilot prospective randomized study. Fertil Steril. 1998;69:1020-5.
48. Kontoravdis A, Makrakis E, Pantos K, Botsis D, Deligeoroglou E, Creatsas G. Proximal tubal occlusion and salpingectomy result in similar improvement in invitro fertilization outcome in patients with hydrosalpinx. Fertil Steril. 2006;86:1642-9.
49. Cakmak H, Taylor HS. Implantation failure: molecular mechanisms and clinical treatment. Human Reprod Update. 2011;17(2):242-53.
50. Chen CD, Yang JH, Lin KC, Chao KH, Ho HN, Yang YS. The significance of cytokines, chemical composition, and murine embryo development in hydrosalpinx fluid for predicting the in-vitro fertilization outcome in women with hydrosalpinx. Hum Reprod. 2002;17:128-33.
51. Akman MA, Garcia JE, Damewood MD, Watts LD, Katz E. Hydrosalpinx affects the implantation of previously cryopreserved embryos. Human Reprod. 1996;11:1013-4.
52. Mukhurjee T, Copperman AB, McCaffrey C. Hydrosalpinx fluid has embryotoxic effects on murine embryogenesis: a case for prophylactic salpingectomy. Fertil Steril. 1996;66:851-3.
53. Strandell A, Lindhard A, Waldenström U, Thorburn J, Janson PO, Hamberger L. Hydrosalpinx and IVF outcome: A prospective, randomized multicentre trial in Scandinavia on salpingectomy prior to IVF. Hum Reprod. 1999;14:2762-9.
54. Strandell A, Lindhard A, Waldenstrom U. Salpingectomy prior to IVF does not impair the ovarian response. Human Reprod. 2001;16:1135-9.
55. Hammadieh N, Coomarasamy A, Bolarinde O, Papaioannou S, Afnan M, Sharif K. Ultrasound-guided hydrosalpinx aspiration during oocyte collection improves pregnancy outcome in IVF: a randomized controlled trial. Human Reprod. 2008;23:1113-7.
56. Dreyer K, Lier MC, Emanuel MH, Twisk JW, Mol BW, Schats R, et al. Hysteroscopic proximal tubal occlusion versus laparoscopic salpingectomy as a treatment for hydrosalpinges prior to IVF or ICSI: an RCT. Human Reprod. 201619;31(9):2005-16.

LONG QUESTION

1. Discuss the various etiological factors for tubal factor in infertility and the various management options.

SHORT QUESTIONS

1. Discuss the various tubal patency tests with advantage and disadvantages.
2. Write the diagnosis and management of hydrosalpinx.
3. What are the various modalities to diagnose genital tuberculosis?

MULTIPLE CHOICE QUESTIONS

1. True anatomical block of the fallopian tube is due to:
   a. Pelvic inflammatory disease
   b. Mucous plugs
   c. Mucosal agglutination
   d. Severe corneal spasm
2. Laparoscopy and chromotubation is not indicated with:
   a. History of previous ectopic pregnancy
   b. Past history of pelvic inflammatory disease
   c. Tubo-ovarian masses
   d. No history of any pelvic problems
3. Ultrasound evaluation of the fallopian tubes can pick up:
   a. Mid tubal blocks
   b. Ciliary problems
   c. Distal tubal blocks and tubal swellings
   d. Tubal endometriosis
4. "Cogwheel appearance" is typical description of:
   a. Hydrosaplinx
   b. Endometriosis
   c. Chlamydial infection
   d. Para ovarian cyst
5. The only blood test for antibodies connected to tubal pathology is:
   a. Tuberculosis
   b. *Chlamydia trachomatis*
   c. *Staphylococcus*
   d. Gonorrhea
6. Genital tuberculosis of the uterus is best identified by:
   a. Polymerase chain reaction test
   b. Culture
   c. Symptoms only
   d. GeneXpert test
7. Severe salpingitis is considered with the following laparoscopic findings:
   a. Redness of the tubes
   b. Exudative lesions
   c. Pyosalpinx
   d. Tubes not freely mobile
8. Ideal treatment for hydrosalpinx before assisted reproduction is:
   a. Salpingectomy b. PID regimen
   c. Ignore hydrosalpinx d. Drain the fluid
9. Unilateral proximal tubal block and no other pathology, one of the treatment can be offered:
   a. Salpingectomy b. Tubal cannulation
   c. PID regimen d. Oral contraceptives
10. Best microsurgical results of anastomosis is with:
    a. Ampullary to fimbrial
    b. Ampullart to ampullary
    c. Cornual to isthmus
    d. Isthmus to isthmus

Anwers

1.	a	2.	d	3.	c	4.	a	5.	b	6.	d
7.	c	8.	a	9.	b	10.	d				

12.8 UTERINE FACTOR IN INFERTILITY: ETIOLOGY AND MANAGEMENT

Laxmi Shrikhande

INTRODUCTION

Uterus is the most crucial organ involved in the process of reproduction. There are many uterine factors which contribute significantly to female causes of infertility. Uterine factor infertility (UFI) may affect 1 in 500 women of reproductive age group.[1] The uterine causes may be due to either structural abnormalities, space-occupying lesions, or due to altered endometrial receptivity. The UFI can be broadly classified as congenital or acquired.

CONGENITAL CAUSES

Congenital Uterine Anomalies

Congenital uterine anomalies result from embryological maldevelopment of paramesonephric (Müllerian) ducts. The incidence of congenital uterine anomalies is 7–10%. Infertility, recurrent pregnancy loss, and poor pregnancy outcomes may be attributable to these anomalies in approximately 25% women.

Embryological Development

The female reproductive tract develops from the Müllerian ducts, except the ovaries which are formed separately from the germ cells of the primitive yolk sac. The uterus, cervix, and upper two thirds of vagina are derived from caudal fused portion of Müllerian ducts. Fallopian tubes form from the upper unfused portion of Müllerian ducts. The lower one third of vagina develops from urogenital sinus and sinovaginal bulbs.

The development of female reproductive tract passes through the phases of organogenesis, fusion and septal resorption.

The process of organogenesis involves the formation of the Müllerian ducts. A longitudinal elevation of intermediate mesoderm occurs on either side of aorta known as urogenital ridge. The paramesonephric ducts arise lateral to Mesonephric (Wolffian) ducts. They form as a longitudinal invagination of mesothelium on the lateral surface of urogenital ridge **(Figs. 1A to C)**. Failure in the organogenesis phase may lead to uterine agenesis or hypoplasia of uterus or unicornuate uterus.

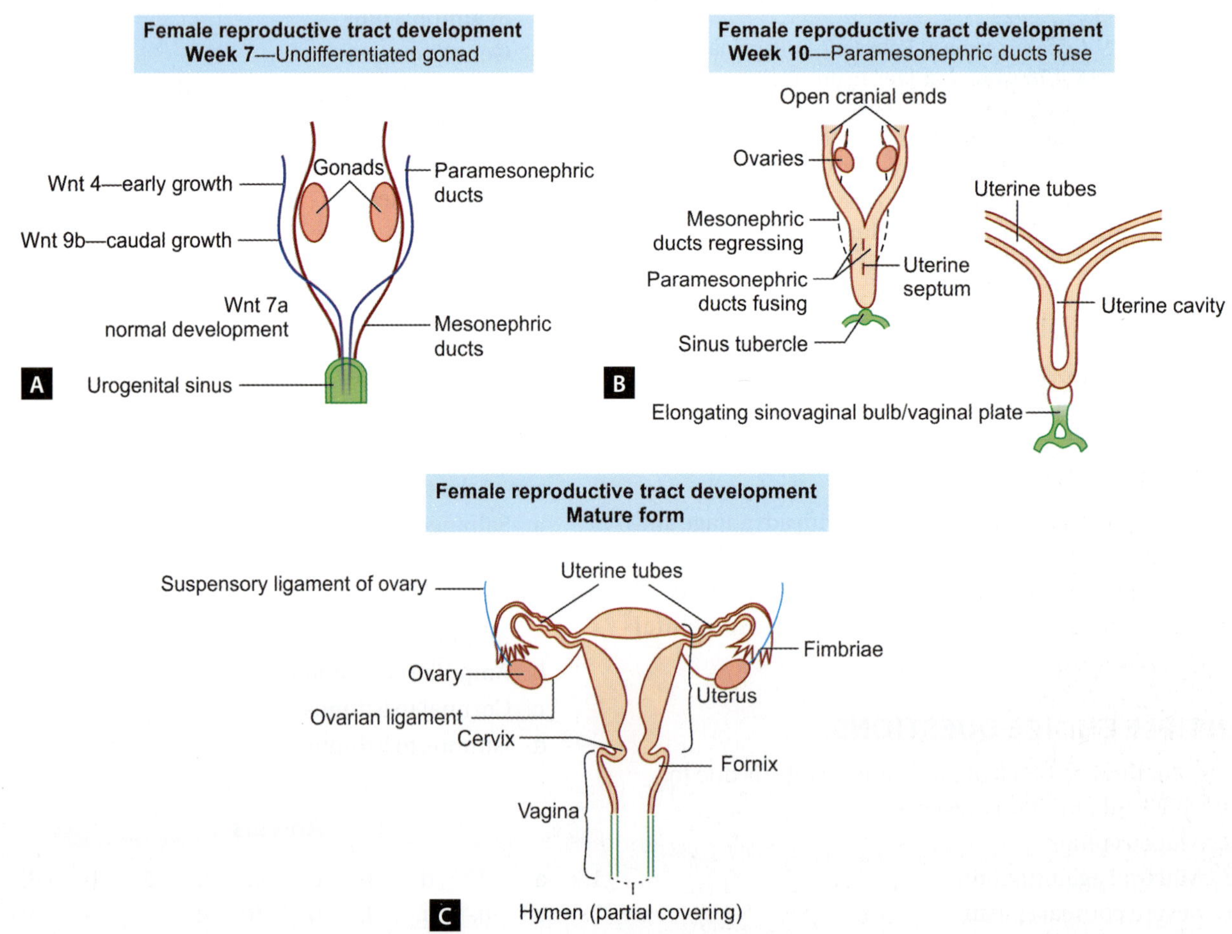

Figs. 1A to C: Normal development of female reproductive organs.

The process of fusion involves formation of the uterus, cervix, and upper part of vagina due to fusion of the ducts in the midline. The paramesonephric ducts grow caudally and cross the mesonephric ducts. They fuse in midline to form the uterovaginal canal. The lower part of uterovaginal canal connects with urogenital sinus. The fused Müllerian ducts are canalized internally forming two channels separated by a septum. Failure in the phase of fusion leads to the formation of bicornuate or didelphys uterus.

Septal resorption phase is characterized by resorption of the central septum of the fused ducts. The resorption of the septum occurs in caudal to cephalad direction around 20 weeks. Failure in the phase of resorption leads to the formation of septate or arcuate uterus.

Associated Anomalies

Congenital uterine anomalies are associated with renal, skeletal, abdominal wall abnormalities, or inguinal hernia. Associated anomalies of renal system are seen in 20–30% patients and are more common with unicornuate uterus.[2] The common associated anomalies of renal system include renal agenesis, duplicated collecting system, ectopic kidney, horseshoe kidney, and renal dysplasia.

Classification of Congenital Uterine Anomalies

The pregnancy outcomes and treatment options are different and vary widely based on the type of anomaly. So, the classification of congenital uterine anomalies is important. The widely accepted and commonly used classification system is the American Fertility Society (AFS), now known as the American Society of Reproductive Medicine **(Table 1 and Fig. 2)**.[3] This classification system only provides a framework. The limitation of this system of classification is that all anomalies do not fit completely in the categories. To overcome this, the European Society of Human Reproduction and Embryology (ESHRE) and the European Society for Gynaecological Endoscopy (ESGE) have proposed a classification system

TABLE 1: The American Fertility Society classification of Müllerian anomalies.

Class I	Hypoplasia and agenesis	(1) Vaginal, (2) cervical, (3) fundal, (4) tubal, (5) combined
Class II	Unicornuate	(1) Communicating (endometrial cavity present) (2) Noncommunicating (endometrial cavity present) (3) Horn without endometrial cavity (4) No rudimentary horn
Class III	Didelphys	
Class IV	Bicornuate	(1) Complete, (2) Partial, (3) Arcuate
Class V	Septate	(1) Complete, (2) Partial
Class VI	Arcuate	
Class VII	Diethylstilbestrol (DES) drug-related	(1) T-shaped uterus, (2) T-shaped with dilated horns

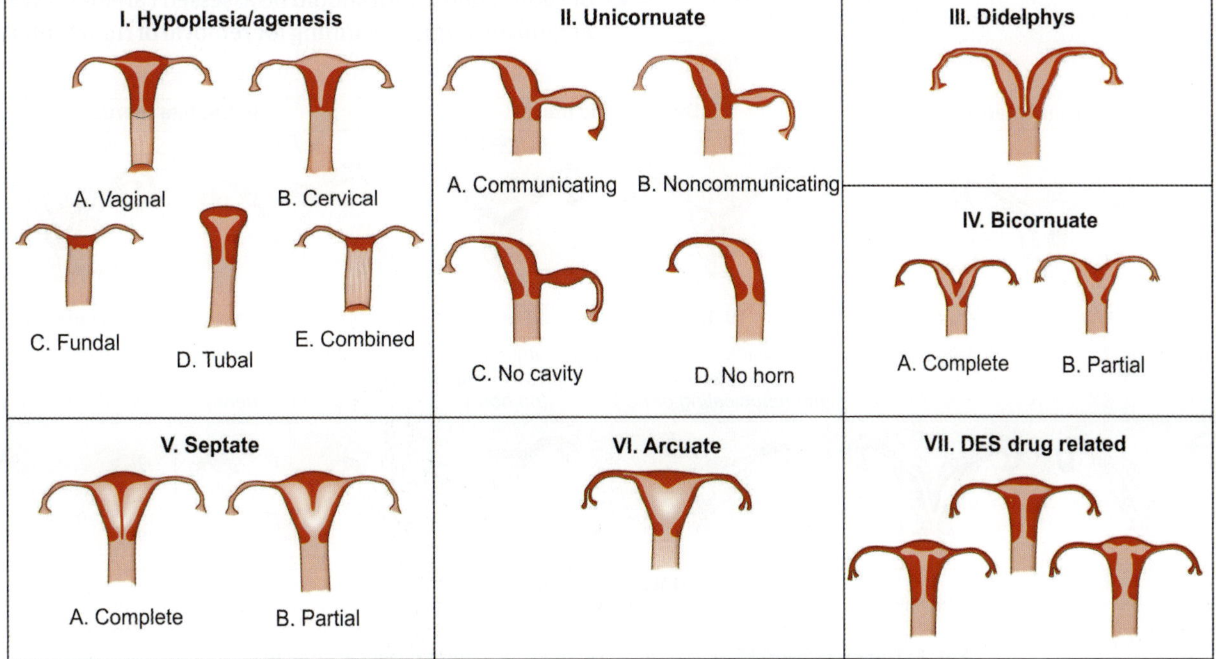

Fig. 2: The American Fertility Society classification of Müllerian anomalies.

based on the anatomy of the female genital tract. This is mainly useful for clinical orientation **(Table 2 and Fig. 3)**.[4] We will discuss the subtypes according to the most widely accepted AFS classification.

Class I: Agenesis/Hypoplasia: Small amounts of undifferentiated rudimentary tissue or no identifiable uterus characterizes uterine agenesis, while a hypoplastic uterus is a small but fully differentiated organ.

The most common presentation is the Mayer–Rokitansky–Kuster–Hauser syndrome. It is a cause of congenital absolute uterine factor infertility. The reported incidence is 1 in 4,000–5,000.[5] This syndrome is characterized by congenital absence of the upper two thirds of the vagina and an absent or rudimentary uterus. As ovaries develop separately from the primitive yolk sac, so ovarian function is preserved and karyotype is normal.

TABLE 2: The ESHRE and ESGE classification of uterine anomalies.

Main class	*Uterine anomaly*	*Subclass*
U 0	Normal uterus	
U 1	Dysmorphic uterus	(1) T-shaped (2) Infantilis (3) Others
U 2	Septate uterus	(1) Partial (2) Complete
U 3	Bicorporeal uterus	(1) Partial (2) Complete (3) Bicorporeal septate
U 4	Hemi-uterus	(1) Rudimentary horn with cavity (Communicating or not) (2) Rudimentary horn without cavity/Aplasia (no horn)
U 5	Aplastic/dysplastic uterus	(1) Rudimentary horn with cavity (bi- or unilateral) (2) Rudimentary horn without cavity (bi- or unilateral)/ Aplasia
U 6	Unclassified malformations	

(ESGE: European Society for Gynaecological Endoscopy; ESHRE: European Society of Human Reproduction and Embryology)

Most common presentation is primary amenorrhea. Rarely, it may present as subfertility and dyspareunia. It may present with cyclical abdominal pain if functioning endometrium is present. The examination shows a short, blind-ending vagina and presence of normal secondary sexual characteristics. Associated anomalies may be seen on general examination.

Two-dimensional ultrasonography (USG) confirms absence of uterus and associated renal abnormalities. Three-dimensional ultrasound is more precise in the evaluation of rudimentary uterus. Magnetic resonance imaging (MRI) is more specific and sensitive for diagnosis.

Management includes counseling and creating neovagina either by nonsurgical or surgical methods. Vaginal dilators may be used for creation of a functional vagina. Surgical treatment involves different surgical techniques for creation of neovagina and use of molds or dilators to keep the space open.

Fertility can be achieved by artificial reproduction with the woman's own eggs, as the ovaries are functioning normally, followed by surrogacy. Uterine transplantation will be useful in selected cases.

Class II: Unicornuate: Unicornuate uterus results if one of the Müllerian duct development is arrested completely or near completely. High incidence of renal abnormalities is associated with unicornuate uterus. Depending on stage of arrest of development, there are four subtypes (*see* **Table 1**). Most rudimentary horns are asymptomatic. If functional endometrium is present, that is shed cyclically. If it is noncommunicating rudimentary horn, it may lead to cyclic or chronic abdominopelvic pain.

Diagnosis is best made by three-dimensional USG showing a uterus deviated to one side of the pelvis. Noncommunicating or rudimentary horn should be assessed carefully. MRI can be helpful for surgical planning for removal of rudimentary horn.

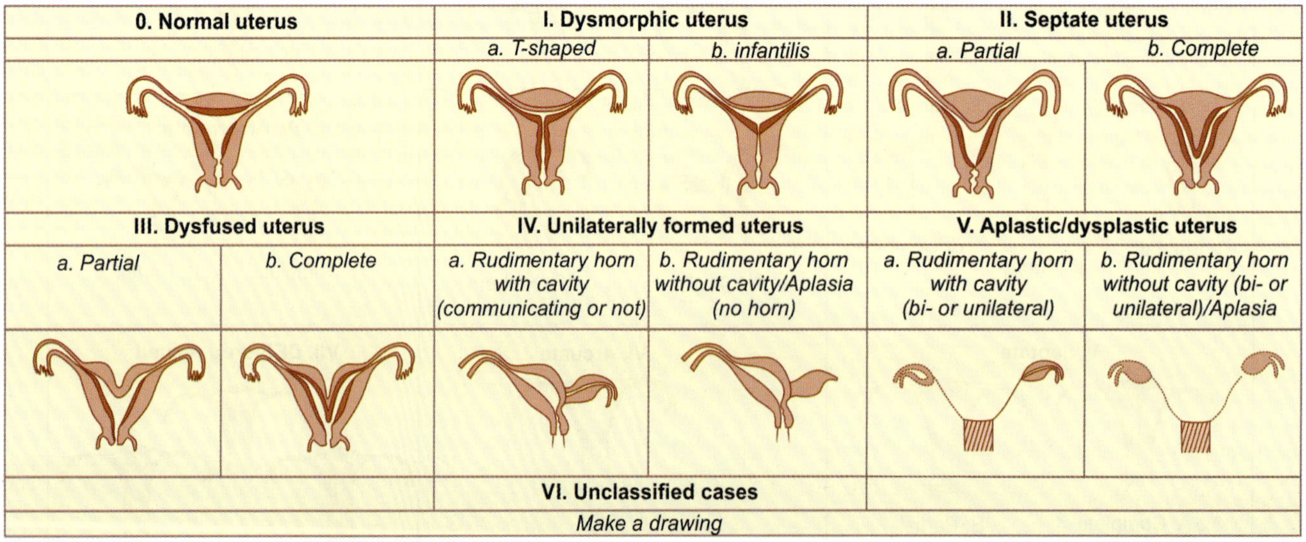

Fig. 3: The ESHRE and ESGE classification of female genital tract anomalies.
(ESGE: European Society for Gynaecological Endoscopy; ESHRE: European Society of Human Reproduction and Embryology)

This anomaly is generally associated with favorable pregnancy outcomes.[6] The surgical removal of the noncommunicating rudimentary horn with functional endometrium may be needed in symptomatic women for reducing dysmenorrhea, preventing or reducing endometriosis and avoiding a horn or tubal pregnancy.

Class III: Didelphys: Complete nonfusion of Müllerian ducts leads to formation of double uterus or uterine didelphys. The individual horns are normal in size and fully developed. Mostly, the duplication is limited to the uterus and cervix, leading to uterine didelphys—bicollis (two cervices). This may be associated with transverse or longitudinal vaginal septum.

This uterine anomaly has a relatively good prognosis for achieving pregnancy, although spontaneous abortion, preterm birth, and fetal growth restriction have been reported.[7]

Diagnosis is established by speculum examination and imaging. Examination showing two cervixes and ultrasound showing two widely separated uterine horns with a deep fundal indentation diagnoses uterus didelphys.

Metroplasty can be useful for patients with recurrent miscarriages, preterm birth, or pelvic pain.

Class IV: Bicornuate: Partial nonfusion of the Müllerian ducts results in bicornuate uterus. There is extension of central myometrium till internal cervical os (bicornuate unicollis) or external os (bicornuate bicollis) and a fundal cleft which is >1 cm deep **(Fig. 4)**. Uterus bicollis needs to be distinguished from uterus didelphys. The horns of the bicornuate uteri are smaller and not fully developed as compared to the didelphys uteri.

Most women with bicornuate uteri conceive without difficulty. These women are at increased risk of mid-trimester miscarriage and preterm birth, due to cervical insufficiency.[8] Cervical length needs to be assessed during pregnancy.

Diagnosis is by ultrasound findings, mainly three dimensional, showing two endometrial cavities which are moderately separated with an indented fundal contour. MRI is rarely needed in suspected complex anomalies with multiple system involvement.

Bicornuate uterus generally does not need surgical treatment. Transabdominal metroplasty may be considered in women with recurrent miscarriages, mid-trimester loss, or preterm birth.

Class V: Septate: This is the most common structural uterine anomaly.[8] Failure of resorption of the partition between two Müllerian ducts leads to septate uterus. The septum may be muscular, fibrous, or a combination of both. It leads to formation of uterus which is divided into two cavities—either completely due to longitudinal septum beginning at fundus and extending to vagina with two cervices or partially (subseptate uterus) with one cervix.

Septate uterus has the highest incidence of adverse pregnancy outcomes such as first- and second-trimester miscarriages, preterm birth, breech presentation, and infertility.[9]

Septate and bicornuate uterus needs to be differentiated as the reproductive outcomes and treatment options are different. Hysterosalpingography (HSG) is not useful in this differentiation, as it does not visualize the uterine fundus. Three-dimensional transvaginal USG helps in differentiating between these anomalies **(Fig. 4)**. MRI is most sensitive and can show whether the fundal contour is smooth (septate uterus) or indented (bicornuate uterus) but is rarely needed. Hysteroscopy with laparoscopy is the gold standard for diagnosis.

Operative hysteroscopy has revolutionized the management of septate uterus. The current standard treatment recommended for septate uterus is hysteroscopic metroplasty. It improves pregnancy outcome by preventing recurrent miscarriage.[10] If vaginal septum is also present, it needs to be excised with reapproximation of vaginal mucosa.

Metroplasty may be beneficial in women with a septate uterus and otherwise unexplained infertility. Metroplasty helps to improve success rate and should be considered in women with septate uterus prior to in vitro fertilization (IVF).

Class VI: Arcuate: Arcuate uterus has mild midline indentation of endometrium at the fundus leading to broad fundus due to near complete resorption of the uterovaginal septum.

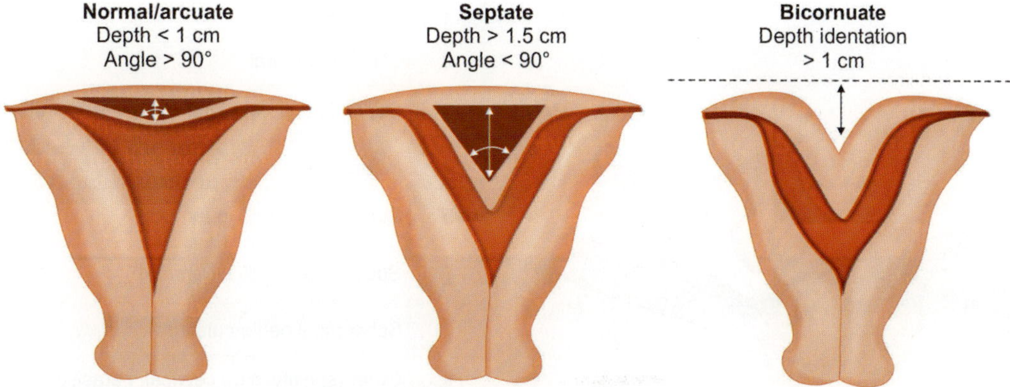

Diagrams of the ASRM definitions of normal/arcuate, septate, and bicornuate uterus based on assessment of available literature, understanding that these anomalies reflect points on a spectrum of development. Normal/arcuate: depth from the interstitial line to the apex of the indentation <1 cm and angle of the indentation >90°. Septate: depth from the interstitial line to the apex of the indentation >1.5 cm and angle of the indentation >90°. Bicornuate: external fundal indentation >1 cm. Internal endometrial cavity is similar to a partial septate uterus.

Fig. 4: ASRM definitions of septate and bicornuate uterus.
(ASRM: American Society for Reproductive Medicine)

Diagnosis is done by three-dimensional ultrasound **(Fig. 4)**. Arcuate uterus is considered as a normal variant which is asymptomatic with no fertility compromise and is not associated with adverse pregnancy outcome.

Class VII: Diethylstilbestrol related: Between 1945 and 1970, many women were treated with diethylstilbestrol (DES) for prevention of miscarriage. Uterine malformations in the form of T-shaped uterine cavity, hypoplasia, and increased risk of vaginal clear-cell carcinoma were seen in up to 15% of newborn girls exposed to in utero DES.

ACQUIRED CAUSES

Uterine Fibroids (Leiomyoma, Myoma)

Uterine fibroids are the most common benign smooth muscle tumors of the uterus. At least one fibroid is seen in 5–10% of women evaluated for infertility and in 1–2.4% of women with infertility, fibroids may be the sole etiological cause.[11] Myomas may grow in any part of the uterus. They may present as solitary or multiple lesions. Based on the location in the uterus, the International Federation of Gynecology and Obstetrics (FIGO) has classified uterine fibroids into eight subtypes **(Fig. 5)**.[12]

Most of the myomas are asymptomatic. They may present with menorrhagia, pelvic pain, infertility, recurrent pregnancy loss or bladder and bowel dysfunction due to pressure.

Effect of myomas on fertility is correlated with the number and location of myomas. Studies have concluded that fibroids that distorts the cavity (submucosal and intramural which protrude into cavity) are associated with decreased pregnancy rate. Removal of these fibroids improves pregnancy rate.[13] The effect of fibroids not distorting the endometrial cavity on pregnancy outcomes are controversial.

Treatment Options

Expectant management for myomas is acceptable in asymptomatic women planning pregnancy with myomas stable in size on serial imaging studies. It involves periodic review for any new associated symptom or any evidence of increase in size.

Medical measures such as gonadotropin-releasing hormone (GnRH) agonist, mifepristone, uterine artery embolization, and myolysis can be used to treat symptomatic fibroids or preoperatively to reduce the size of fibroid or to restore normal hemoglobin levels.[14] These medical management measures are generally not preferred for treatment of myomas in patient with infertility, as they are associated with side effects, prevent conception, and can cause rebound symptoms on discontinuation.

Surgical removal of fibroid is the standard management for fertility preservation or enhancement. Myomectomy helps to restore morphology of uterus, normalizes menstrual function, and enhances fertility. Myomectomy should be planned as close to the time of pregnancy planning as possible, as the possibility of new fibroids growth increases with time.

Myomectomy can be performed either through open incision (laparotomy) or by laparoscopy (with or without robotic assistance). The number, size, and location of the fibroids and the experience of the surgeon helps to decide on open or laparoscopic approach and it does not appear to impact live birth rate. There should be minimum no of uterine incisions and they should be planned so that multiple adjacent myomas can be removed through the same incision. Proper hemostasis with good closure of the myoma cavity is needed to improve outcome.

Hysteroscopic myomectomy is planned for submucosal fibroid or FIGO type 0, type 1, or some type 2 fibroids.

Adenomyosis

Adenomyosis is a benign condition characterized by growth of the endometrial glands and stroma within the adjacent myometrium. The myometrium responds to the intrusion by

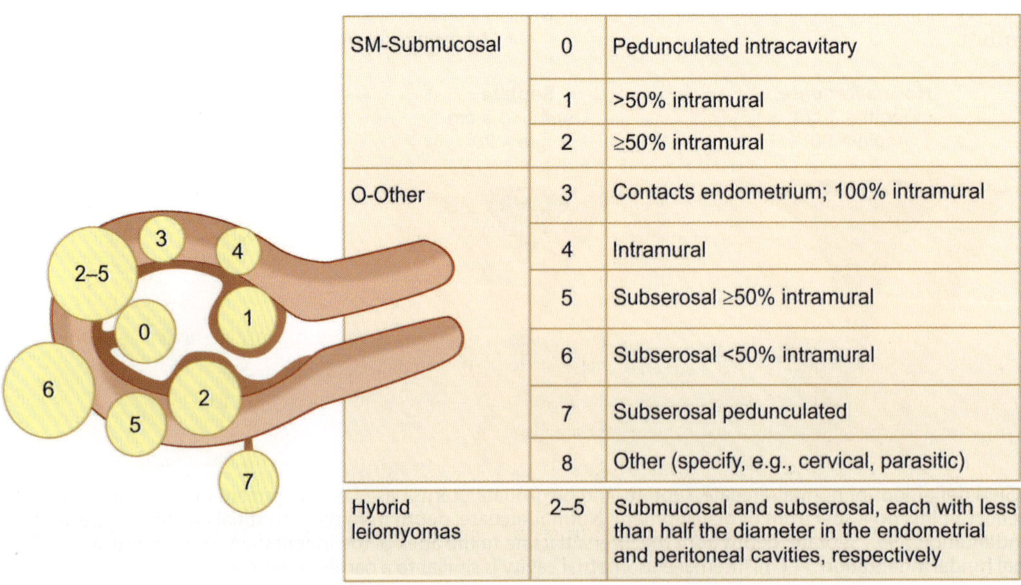

SM-Submucosal	0	Pedunculated intracavitary
	1	>50% intramural
	2	≥50% intramural
O-Other	3	Contacts endometrium; 100% intramural
	4	Intramural
	5	Subserosal ≥50% intramural
	6	Subserosal <50% intramural
	7	Subserosal pedunculated
	8	Other (specify, e.g., cervical, parasitic)
Hybrid leiomyomas	2–5	Submucosal and subserosal, each with less than half the diameter in the endometrial and peritoneal cavities, respectively

Fig. 5: The FIGO classification of uterine fibroids.
(FIGO: International Federation of Gynecology and Obstetrics)

muscular overgrowth which could be focal and localized or may be diffuse.

They may present with abnormal uterine bleeding, dyspareunia, dysmenorrhea or infertility, although majority are often asymptomatic. Transvaginal ultrasound is the imaging method of choice for diagnosis. It shows ill-defined myometrial heterogeneity with myometrial cyst. MRI may show large asymmetric uterus with thickened junctional zone and myometrial cyst.

Conservative medical management using GnRH agonist in symptomatic adenomyosis induces temporary regression of disease. Studies have shown that GnRH agonist administration prior to embryo transfer increases pregnancy rates.[15] For localized adenomyosis, excision of the focal lesion has been found to be associated with positive outcomes. Excision of adenomyoma is a challenging surgical procedure as unlike myomas, the focal adenomyotic lesion do not have well-demarcated borders and there is protrusion of the lesion into the myometrium.[16]

Endometrial Polyps

Endometrial polyps are benign, localized outgrowths of endometrium. These are commonly found during evaluation of infertility. It may be found in 6–8% women undergoing IVF.[17] The polyps may affect fertility either due to increased production of inhibitory factors or due to mechanical interference with sperm transport or embryo implantation.[18]

Hysteroscopy is the gold standard for diagnosis. It permits simultaneous polypectomy under vision. The results of impact of removal of endometrial polyp on fertility are controversial. At present, there is insufficient evidence to recommend polypectomy in infertile women.

Intrauterine Adhesions/Asherman's Syndrome

Intrauterine adhesions (IUAs) are fibrous tissue bands formed in scarred endometrial cavity. Any intrauterine procedure which can damage the basalis layer is potential risk factor for developing IUA. The most common cause is uterine curettage in gravid uterus. Uterine compression sutures such as B-Lynch suture for severe postpartum hemorrhage, myomectomy, curettage, and uterine infections, particularly genital tuberculosis, can also lead to formation of IUA. The prevalence of IUAs in general population is 1.5%.[19]

Intrauterine adhesions may range from filmy thin strings of tissue composed of endometrial tissue to dense adhesions containing connective tissue entirely. This leads to adhesions of uterine walls leading to partial or complete obliteration of uterine cavity. Endometrial damage and scarring interfere with vascularization of endometrium.

The classic clinical presentation is secondary amenorrhea or hypomenorrhea in normal ovulatory women with history of intrauterine procedure.

Intrauterine adhesions can be diagnosed by saline infusion sonohysterography, hysterosalpingography, transvaginal USG, or MRI. Duse to varied sensitivity, negative findings on these imaging do not exclude IUA. Hysteroscopy is the gold standard for diagnosis. It allows direct visualization for the presence, extent, and appearance of the IUA and also about the condition of the endometrium and allows concurrent treatment in many cases. The European Society of Hysteroscopy has classified IUA based on hysteroscopic findings **(Table 3) (Fig. 6)**.[20]

TABLE 3: European Society for Hysteroscopy classification of intrauterine adhesions.

Grade	*Extent of intrauterine adhesions*
I	Thin or filmy adhesions easily ruptured by hysteroscope sheath alone. Cornual areas normal
II	Singular filmy adhesions connecting separate parts of the uterine cavity. Visualization of both tubal ostea possible. Cannot be ruptured by hysteroscope sheath
IIa	Occluding adhesions only in the region of the internal cervical os. Upper uterine cavity normal
III	Multiple firm adhesions connecting separate parts of the uterine cavity. Unilateral obliteration of ostial areas of the tubes
IIIa	Extensive scarring of the uterine cavity wall with amenorrhea or hypomenorrhea
IIIb	Combination of III and IIIa
IV	Extensive firm adhesions with agglutination of uterine walls. Both tubal ostial areas occluded

The recommended standard management of IUA is hysteroscopic adhesiolysis. It helps in improving subsequent fertility outcomes. In order to decrease risk of reformation of adhesions, hormone therapy (estrogen with or without progestin) or intrauterine devices can be used after adhesiolysis.

Endometrial Factors

Successful implantation involves healthy embryo and a receptive endometrium along with synchronous development and interaction between these in the implantation window. Window of implantation is the time period when the endometrium is optimally receptive to blastocyst and subsequent implantation. Mostly, the implantation window starts at day 6 after ovulation and lasts for 4–5 days.[21]

The process of implantation may be classified into a series of phases starting with the hatching of blastocyst followed by apposition, adhesion, penetration, and invasion. The blastocyst is completely embedded in the stroma on day 10 after fertilization. The implantation site is covered by the growing uterine epithelium. This is followed by trophoblastic penetration and then the endometrium is decidualized.

Endometrial receptivity is a temporary dynamic unique process in which genotypic and phenotypic changes occur in the endometrial cells which makes the endometrium receptive to the embryo. There are many biochemical and morphological markers which are being evaluated for their role in endometrial receptivity.

Implantation failure can be attributed to inadequate endometrial receptivity in most of the cases and to embryo abnormalities in remaining. The causes of decreased endometrial receptivity are diverse including uterine abnormalities, hormonal disorders, immunological factors, and infections.

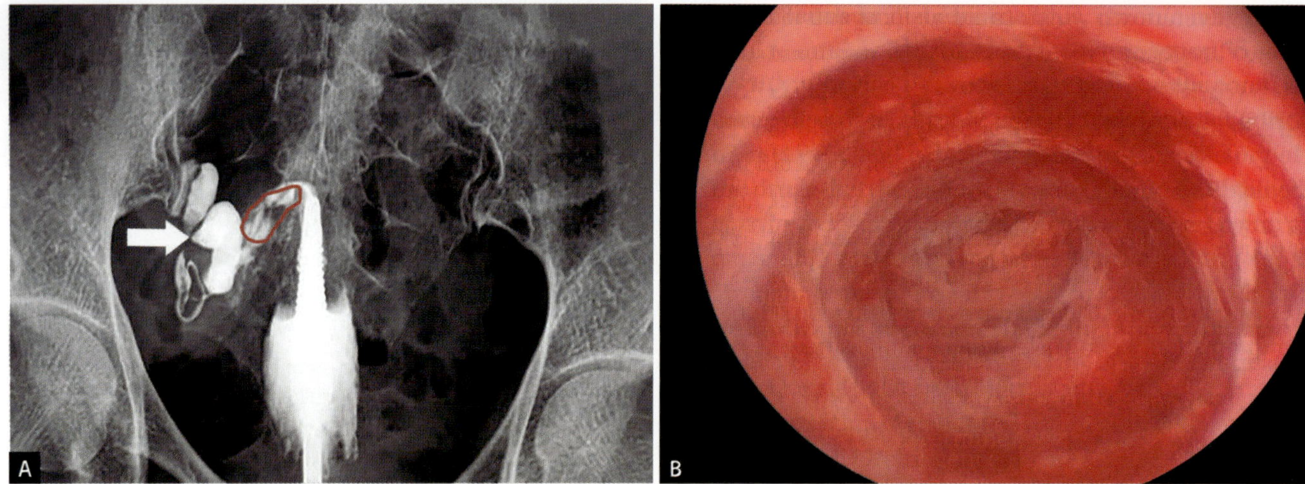

Figs. 6A and B: Asherman syndrome on HSG. (A) Showing a small cavity outlined in red and also a right hydrosalpinx (white block arrow; left tube is blocked); (B) Hysteroscopy image shows a narrow tunnel-like cavity.

Treatment of implantation failure should be targeted toward improving endometrial receptivity by using ovarian stimulation protocols which leads to minimum reduction in endometrial receptivity or by freezing all embryos and transferring them in subsequent cycles.

Certain treatments such as low-dose aspirin, L-arginine, sildenafil can help to improve uterine blood flow and improves endometrial receptivity.[21] Endometrial receptivity can be increased by treatment of luteal phase defects by exogenous progesterone, surgical removal of fibroids that distort the cavity, treatment of intrauterine adhesions, hysteroscopic metroplasty in septate uterus, salpingectomy in cases of hydrosalpinx, treatment of severe endometriosis using GnRH agonist or by use of steroids in autoantibody positive women.

Hysterectomy

Hysterectomy performed due to many indications including severe postpartum hemorrhage, premalignant or malignant lesions of the reproductive tract, and severe endometriosis with pelvic pain will lead to absolute uterine factor infertility. IVF with gestational surrogacy or uterine transplantation are the treatment modalities for fertility.

Uterine Transplantation

It is the true treatment for absolute uterine factor infertility (UFI). Remarkable progress has been made in the field of uterine transplantation over the last decade. Uterine transplantation is unique as compared to other organs transplantation, as it is only temporary for the purpose of fertility and need not remain in the recipient for rest of life. The transplanted uterus is removed once childbearing is complete and thus can limit the dose and duration of immunosuppressive medication, reducing the toxic side effects of immunosuppressive medications.

Presently, uterine transplantation is performed for absolute UFI and the recommended fertility treatment option after uterine transplant is by assisted reproduction. The American Society of Transplantation recommends delaying pregnancy for at least 1 year following uterine transplantation and there should not be any episodes of rejection in the prior 6 months before planning pregnancy.[22]

In near future, uterine transplantation may be extended to women with other causes of UFI, such as intrauterine adhesions or in those with recurrent pregnancy losses.

CONCLUSION

The prerequisite for a successful pregnancy is a healthy embryo undergoing the complex process of implantation in the receptive endometrium in anatomically normal uterine cavity. There may be failure of implantation due to congenital anomalies or acquired diseases of the uterus. These uterine factors may contribute to infertility. A detailed etiologic workup is necessary to decide the further treatment plan. Surgical treatments in selected cases can improve fertility outcomes. IVF with gestational surrogacy was the only fertility option for absolute UFI. Uterine transplant has come as a new hope in these cases of absolute UFI.

REFERENCES

1. Saravelos SH, Cocksedge KA, Li TC. Prevalence and diagnosis of congenital uterine anomalies in women with reproductive failure: a critical appraisal. Hum Reprod Update. 2008;14:415-29.
2. Oppelt P, von Have M, Paulsen M, Strissel PL, Strick R, Brucker S, et al. Female genital malformations and their associated abnormalities. Fertil Steril. 2007;87(2):335.
3. The American Fertility Society classifications of adnexal adhesions, distal tubal occlusion, tubal occlusion secondary to tubal ligation, tubal pregnancies, mullerian anomalies and intrauterine adhesions. Fertil Steril. 1988;49(6):944-55.
4. Grimbizis GF, Gordts S, Di Spiezio Sardo A, Brucker S, De Angelis C, Gergolet M, et al. The ESHRE/ESGE consensus on the classification of female genital tract congenital anomalies. Hum Reprod. 2013;28(8):2032-44.
5. Griffin JE, Edwards C, Madden JD, Harrod MJ, Wilson JD. Congenital absence of the vagina. The Mayer–Rokitansky–Kuster–Hauser syndrome. Ann Intern Med. 1976;85:224-36.
6. Acien P, Acien M, Sánchez-Ferrer M. Complex malformations of the female genital tract. New types and revision of classification. Hum Reprod. 2004;19(10):2377.

7. Ludmir J, Samuels P, Brooks S, Mennuti MT. Pregnancy outcome of patients with uncorrected uterine anomalies managed in a high-risk obstetric setting. Obstet Gynecol. 1990;75(6):906.
8. Raga F, Bauset C, Remohi J, Bonilla-Musoles F, Simon C, Pellicer A. Reproductive impact of congenital Mullerian anomalies. Hum Reprod. 1997;12:2277-81.
9. Homer HA, Li TC, Cooke ID. The septate uterus: a review of management and reproductive outcome. Fertil Steril. 2000;73:1-14.
10. Fedele L, Bianchi S. Hysteroscopic metroplasty for septate uterus. Obstet Gynecol Clin North Am. 1995;22(3):473.
11. Donnez J, Jadoul P. What are the implications of myomas on fertility? A need for a debate? Hum Reprod. 2002;17:1424-30.
12. Munro MG, Critchley HO, Fraser IS; FIGO Menstrual Disorders Working Group. The FIGO classification of causes of abnormal uterine bleeding in the reproductive years. Fertil Steril. 2011;95(7):2204-8, 2208.e1-3.
13. Fernandez H, Sefrioui O, Virelizier C, Gervaise A, Gomel V, Frydman R. Hysteroscopic resection of submucosal myomas in patients with infertility. Hum Reprod 2001;16:1489-92.
14. Lethaby A, Puscasiu L, Vollenhoven B. Preoperative medical therapy before surgery for uterine fibroids. Cochrane Database Syst Rev. 2017;11(11):CD000547.
15. Mijatovic V, Florijn E, Halim N, Schats R, Hompes P. Adenomyosis has no adverse effects on IVF/ICSI outcomes in women with endometriosis treated with long-term pituitary down-regulation before IVF/ICSI. Eur J Obstet Gynecol Reprod Biol. 2010;151:62-5.
16. Osada H. Uterine adenomyosis and adenomyoma: The surgical approach. Fertil Steril. 2018;109(3):406-17.
17. Fatemi HM, Kasius JC, Timmermans A, van Disseldorp J, Fauser BC, Devroey P, et al. Prevalence of unsuspected uterine cavity abnormalities diagnosed by office hysteroscopy prior to in vitro fertilization. J Hum Reprod. 2010;25(8):1959-65.
18. Richlin S, Ramachandran S, Shanti A, Murphy AA, Parthasarathy S. Glycodelin levels in uterine flushings and in plasma of patients with leiomyomas and polyps: implications and implantation. Hum Reprod. 2002;17:2742-7.
19. Al-Inany H. Intrauterine adhesions. An update. Acta Obstet Gynecol Scand. 2001;80:986-93.
20. Deans R, Abbott J. Review of intrauterine adhesions. J Minim Invasive Gynecol. 2010;17(5):555-69.
21. Timeva T, Shterev A, Kyurkchiev S. Recurrent implantation failure: the role of the endometrium. J Reprod Infertil. 2014; 15(4):173-83.
22. McKay DB, Josephson MA, Armenti VT, August P, Coscia LA, Davis CL, et al. Women's Health Committee of the American Society of Transplantation. Reproduction and transplantation: report on the AST Consensus Conference on Reproductive Issues and Transplantation. Am J Transplant. 2005;5(7):1592-9.

LONG QUESTIONS

1. Write in detail about congenital uterine factors contributing to reproductive outcome.
2. Discuss in detail about uterine factors contributing to infertility and their management.

SHORT QUESTIONS

1. Write in short about Mayer-Rokitansky-Kuster-Hauser syndrome.
2. Write in short about absolute uterine factor infertility.
3. Write short note on Asherman's syndrome.
4. Write short note on endometrial receptivity.

MULTIPLE CHOICE QUESTIONS

1. The most common associated anomaly with congenital uterine anomaly is:
   a. Skeletal b. Renal
   c. Inguinal hernia d. Cardiac
2. The most common uterine anomaly which has associated renal anomalies:
   a. Septate b. Bicornuate
   c. Unicornuate d. Didelphys
3. The characteristics of MRKH syndrome are all, except:
   a. Small or rudimentary uterus
   b. 46 XY
   c. Absence of upper two thirds of vagina
   d. Normal secondary sexual characteristics
4. The most common structural uterine anomaly is:
   a. Bicornuate b. Didelphys
   c. Septate d. Unicornuate
5. The gold standard for diagnosis of intrauterine adhesions is:
   a. Transvaginal Ultrasonography
   b. Hysterosalpingography
   c. Hysteroscopy
   d. MRI
6. Endometrial receptivity can be increased by all, except:
   a. Hysteroscopic adhesiolysis
   b. Myomectomy for fibroids that do not distort cavity
   c. Low dose aspirin
   d. Exogenous progesterone for luteal phase defect
7. All of the following structures develop from Mullerian ducts, except:
   a. Uterus
   b. Fallopian tubes
   c. Upper two thirds of vagina
   d. Lower one third of vagina
8. Hysteroscopic myomectomy can be performed for all of these fibroids, except:
   a. FIGO type 0 b. FIGO type 1
   c. FIGO type 2 d. FIGO type 3
9. The most common cause of intrauterine adhesions is:
   a. Uterine curettage in gravid uterus
   b. Genital TB
   c. B lynch suture for PPH
   d. Uterine curettage in non-gravid uterus
10. The acquired causes of UFI are all, except:
    a. Submucosal fibroid b. Intrauterine adhesions
    c. Subserosal fibroid d. Endometrial polyp

Answers

1.	b	2.	c	3.	b	4.	c	5.	c	6.	b
7.	d	8.	d.	9.	a	10.	c				

12.9 UNEXPLAINED INFERTILITY: TREATMENT APPROACH

Rohan Palshetkar, Nandita Palshetkar

INTRODUCTION

Unexplained infertility is a diagnosis of exclusion. The diagnosis is achieved after excluding all the identifiable causes of infertility. The three simple features considered for unexplained infertility are usually normal ovulatory function, a normal semen analysis, and patent fallopian tubes. However, in clinical practice, it is difficult to diagnose patients as unexplained infertility based on just these three criteria. Age, ovarian reserve, oocyte quality, endometriosis, uterine factors, cervical mucous factors, tubal dysfunction, immunological factors, genetic factors, coital difficulties, male factors, and failed fertilization can contribute to infertility.

Unexplained infertility management is generally empirical considering the efficiency, safety profile, costs and risks of each treatment option. Ideally, we progress from a treatment which is least invasive, least expensive followed by progression into assisted reproductive techniques. Let us discuss each of these treatment protocols individually.

EXPECTANT MANAGEMENT OF UNEXPLAINED INFERTILITY

Expectant management is generally been the first option in the treatment of unexplained infertility. This is ideal in patients with good prognosis (young couple, good ovarian reserve, patent tubes, and no male factor). Retrospective data has shown cumulative pregnancy rates (CPR) as high as 72% (over 2 years) in young women. However, CPR declines to 45% in women over the age of 35, and to 30% in couples with >5 years of infertility.[1]

Steures et al. (2006) published a multicenter trial of 253 good prognosis couples (33 years, median = 2 years infertility) (127 = immediate treatment, 126 = expectant management). They observed that patients that underwent expectant management for 6 months had 27% live birth rate (LBR).[2] Furthermore, there was no delay in time to conception when compared to the intervention group.

Bhattacharya et al. (2008) published a randomized control trial (RCT) of 580 couples (32 years, median = 2.5 years infertility). There were three arms to this trial [193 = expectant management, 194 = clomiphene citrate (CC), 193 = natural cycle intrauterine insemination (IUI)]. It was observed that LBR in expectant management group was 17%, CC group was 14%, and IUI group was 23% which was not statistically significant.[3] In 2010, Cochrane review (7 studies, 1,159 participants) suggested that there was no evidence that CC was more effective than expectant management.[4]

Aromatase inhibitors such as letrozole are also used in unexplained infertility. However, a systematic review published in 2014 compared letrozole and CC in unexplained infertility. There was no statistical significance in the results of the two drugs.[5]

Gonadotropins may also be used to stimulate the ovaries; however, there is lack of evidence to suggest gonadotropins with time intercourse. Besides this, the cost of the treatment also increases and there is an increase in chances of multiple pregnancies.

Therefore, it is recommended that patients with good prognosis, expectant treatment alone can be considered the first line of treatment.

LAPAROSCOPIC SURGERY IN UNEXPLAINED INFERTILITY

Diagnostic hysterolaparoscopy is a very common diagnostic tool in the armamentarium of a gynecologist when treating a case of infertility. However, the use of it should be judicious and recommended in cases where needed. The American Society of Reproductive Medicine (ASRM) suggests that in the absence of tubal or other pelvic pathology, laparoscopy is not required in the diagnostic workup of infertility or to diagnose unexplained infertility. However, it does recommend that there is a place of hysterolaparoscopy in young women with infertility for >3 years with no recognizable abnormalities.[6]

However, there are studies which recommended that laparoscopy should be included before diagnosing a patient as unexplained infertility. Xu XX et al. published a paper in January 2020 which included 519 patients of unexplained infertility. It showed that 89.8% of patients had pelvic pathologies or abnormalities which needed to be corrected. They reported a natural pregnancy rate within 3 years of 53.9%. They concluded that all cases of unexplained infertility should undergo hysterolaparoscopy.[7]

However, in India, with the presence of endometriosis and tuberculosis, it becomes a double-edged sword. After going through multiple articles, there is no clear evidence which suggests when endoscopy should be done in such cases. From our personal experience, we suggest diagnostic hysterolaparoscopy should be considered after trying empirical treatment or two IUIs.

INTRAUTERINE INSEMINATION

After empirical treatment, IUI is generally the next step in the treatment of unexplained infertility. IUI can be done either via natural cycle or ovarian stimulation with either oral ovulogens or with gonadotropins or a combination of oral ovulogens and gonadotropins. However, when comparing natural cycle IUI to expectant management, there is not much difference in the pregnancy rates. A high-quality RCT which included 580 couples with either unexplained infertility or couples with a mild male factor, it was seen that IUI was not more likely to achieve a live birth than those patients who underwent expectant treatment (LBR—23% vs. 17%). A further subanalysis further analyzed that natural cycle IUI and expectant management had the same live birth rates.[3] A large retrospective cohort study assessed close to 8,584 couples with unexplained infertility who underwent 14,519 cycles. They concluded that LBR was higher with ovarian stimulation and IUI rather than natural cycle IUI.[8] The American Society of Reproductive Medicine (ASRM) does not recommend natural cycle IUI for the treatment of unexplained infertility. It is less effective than ovarian stimulation with IUI and is not more effective than expectant management.[9]

Ovarian stimulation along with an IUI is a completely different story. Ovarian stimulation can be done with either CC, letrozole, gonadotropins, or a combination of letrozole or CC with gonadotropins. A network meta-analysis (26 studies, 5,316 women) published in January 2020, compares ovarian stimulation with various modalities and IUI. It was seen that IUI with gonadotropins had the highest live birth ongoing pregnancy rates. However, there was a higher rate of multiple order pregnancies as well.[10] However, in the ASRM guidelines which were published after this study, it was suggested there was insufficient data to propose that low-dose gonadotropins (<150 IU) had higher pregnancy rates than CC or letrozole. It further summated that patients of unexplained infertility with good or intermediate prognosis would have the same prognosis if they underwent expectant management or IUI with low-dose gonadotropins. There was also no difference in multiple pregnancy rates with either clomiphene, letrozole or low-dose gonadotropins. Therefore, the ASRM guidelines recommended that low-dose gonadotropins should not be used in the treatment of unexplained infertility due to its complexity and expense. Oral ovulogens would give the same result (moderate recommendation).[9] Therefore, in a country like ours, where the cost of the treatment comes completely on the patient oral ovulogens may be the first line of treatment. Oral ovulogens reduce the cost of the treatment drastically and make it feasible for patients to undergo a cycle.

Besides cost, risk of hyperstimulation is also present when ovarian stimulation is done. Therefore when stimulating, a strict cancellation policy rate should be maintained. If you have >3 dominant follicles growing, it is better to cancel the IUI cycle or step up the dosage and convert IUI stimulation to an in vitro fertilization (IVF) cycle (if the patient is willing).

IN VITRO FERTILIZATION IN UNEXPLAINED INFERTILITY

An IVF has been used as an effective treatment protocol in unexplained infertility. In fact, the international guidelines have also recommended IVF in the treatment of unexplained infertility [The National Institute for Health and Care Excellence (NICE) guidelines].[11] However, this may not be a feasible treatment option for all couples due to the cost and burden of the treatment.

There has been multiple RCTs comparing IVF to IUI with gonadotropin stimulation. However, all the data is heterogenous and cannot be compared with each other. But even then a clear benefit of IVF is seen over IUI with gonadotropins through the clinical pregnancy rate as seen in **Table 1**.[12] However, in all of these studies, adverse effects were not analyzed.

The fast track and standard treatment (FASTT) trial[13] published by Dr Richard Reindollar in 2010 demonstrated benefits in terms of time to pregnancy (8 months vs. 11 months) and cost savings of up to 9,800 dollars per delivery with immediate IVF. However, this did not take into account travel costs and time away from work.

However, another contrasting study published in November 2018 by Pham CT et al., concluded that good prognosis patients who delayed IVF for 6 months could substantially decrease out of pocket costs without compromising pregnancy.[14]

Besides cost, IVF is also seen as a benefit in reduction of multiple pregnancies with the elective selective embryo transfer. The NICE Guidelines have advised against gonadotropin stimulation with IUI and moving to IVF (elective single embryo transfer) due to risk of multiple pregnancies.[11]

However, in India, where there are no guidelines of the number of embryos that can be transferred, and the patient bearing the entire cost, it needs to be wondered whether jumping immediately to IVF is a wise option. Each case needs to be individualized and considering the financial burden on the patient, the ideal treatment needs to be given.

TABLE 1: Published randomized controlled trials comparing gonadotropin/IUI with IVF for the treatment of unexplained infertility.[12]

Reference	*Number of subjects*	*Clinical pregnancy rate*	
		Gonadotropin/IUI	*IVF*
Goverde et al., 2000	172	7.8% per cycle	12.2% per cycle
Reindollar et al., 2010	503	21.4% after three cycles	52% after three cycles
van Rumste et al., 2014	116	17.2% after three cycles	22.4% per cycle
Bensdorp et al., 2015	602	56.0% after six cycles	58.7% after three cycles
Goldman et al., 2014b	154	17.3% after two cycles	49% after two cycles
Nandi et al., 2017	207	28.7% after three cycles	33.1% per cycle

(IUI: intrauterine insemination; IVF: in vitro fertilization)

The ASRM guidelines also suggest that IVF may not be first-line therapy in patients below the age of 38 years. However, in patients above the age of 38 years, immediate IVF may be advisable as the pregnancy rates are higher and time to pregnancy is also significantly reduced. The ASRM also suggests that patients who have failed to achieve pregnancy with oral ovulogens, immediate IVF would be advisable rather than stimulation with gonadotropins and IUI. This would reduce costs and time to pregnancy while increasing the pregnancy rates.[9]

Most of the times, a patient will come to an IVF center after all empirical treatments and IUIs have already been done. So it is important for you to ensure that the past treatment history is taken to decide the treatment.

INTRACYTOPLASMIC SPERM INJECTION IN UNEXPLAINED INFERTILITY

In unexplained infertility, there is a chance of 5–10% of failed fertilization. Therefore, it begins to wonder whether it is worth considering intracytoplasmic sperm injection (ICSI) for patients of unexplained infertility.

Johnson et al. published a systematic review and meta-analysis in 2013 that suggested that routine ICSI was effective in increasing fertilization rates. However, there was no randomization in the study included and there was a high risk of potential bias. Furthermore, live birth rates were not reported in any of the studies.[15]

Another study published in 2013 by Vitek et al., concluded that IVF was preferred as the increased live birth rate with ICSI or split IVF/ICSI was not justified by the increased cost per live birth. The increase in live birth rate was 3% which was not statistically significant. However, if two cycles were needed, a split IVF/ICSI should be considered.

The ASRM 2020 guidelines also suggest that there is no difference in pregnancy rates between IVF and ICSI. However, ICSI has been associated with higher fertilization rates and also reduces risk of complete fertilization failure.

Do women with unexplained infertility have a decreased ovarian reserve?

Unexplained infertility as mentioned before is a diagnosis of exclusion, which assesses the semen analysis, tubal patency, and ovulation in a woman. However, it is important to consider the ovarian reserve as well. Should we be including women with only a decreased ovarian reserve as unexplained infertility?

A study published in 2019 by Abrahami N et al. divided 100 women into two groups. The study group included women below the age of 37 years with unexplained infertility. The control group included age-matched women with male factor infertility. The basal follicle-stimulating hormone (FSH) levels were higher and the antral follicle count (AFC) was lower in women with unexplained infertility. The number of dominant follicles is lesser in the unexplained infertility group and the dose of gonadotropins required was also more.[16]

Thus, it is worth considering that patients with unexplained infertility who have a suboptimal ovarian reserve, whether they should be considered as unexplained infertility at all!

CONCLUSION

Unexplained infertility is a common problem that affects couples all over the world. It is a diagnosis of exclusion. In all cases, the approach toward a patient should involve counseling of the couple with regards to success rates, complications and time for treatment. Each case needs to be individualized and the treatment options should be tailored accordingly. Some patients may require less invasive treatment such as expectant management while others may have to jump directly to assisted reproductive techniques.

REFERENCES

1. Hull MG, Glazener CM, Kelly NJ, Conway DI, Foster PA, Hinton RA, et al. Population study of causes, treatment, and outcome of infertility. Br Med J (Clin Res Ed). 1985;291:1693-7.
2. Steures P, van der Steeg JW, Hompes PG, Habbema JD, Eijkmans MJ, Broekmans FJ, et al. Intrauterine insemination with controlled ovarian hyperstimulation versus expectant management for couples with unexplained subfertility and an intermediate prognosis: a randomised clinical trial. Lancet. 2006;368:216-21.
3. Bhattacharya S, Harrild K, Mollison J, Wordsworth S, Tay C, Harrold A, et al. Clomifene citrate or unstimulated intrauterine insemination compared with expectant management for unexplained infertility: pragmatic randomised controlled trial. Br Med J. 2008;337:a716.
4. Hughes E, Brown J, Collins JJ, Vanderkerchove P. Clomiphene citrate for unexplained subfertility in women. Cochrane Database Syst Rev. 2010;2010(1):CD000057.
5. Liu A, Zheng C, Lang J, Chen W. Letrozole versus clomiphene citrate for unexplained infertility: a systematic review and meta-analysis. J Obstet Gynaecol. Res. 2014;40:1205-16.
6. American Society for Reproductive Medicine. Diagnostic evaluation of the infertile female: a committee opinion. Fertil Steril. 2015;103:e44-50.
7. Xu XX, Yu Q, Sun AJ, Tian QJ, Chen R. Clinical study of hysteroscopy combined with laparoscopy in the diagnosis and treatment of unexplained infertility Zhonghua Fu Chan Ke Za Zhi. 2020;55(1):15-20.
8. Huang S, Wang R, Li R, Wang H, Qiao J, Mol BWJ. Ovarian stimulation in infertile women treated with the use of intrauterine insemination: a cohort study from China. Fertil Steril. 2018;109:872-8.
9. Practice Committee of the American Society for Reproductive Medicine. Evidence-based treatments for couples with unexplained infertility: a guideline. Fertil Steril. 2020;113(2): 305-22.
10. Danhof NA, Wang R, van Wely M, van der Veen F, Mol BWJ, Mochtar MH. IUI for unexplained infertility-a network meta-analysis. Hum Reprod Update. 2020;26(1):1-15.
11. NICE Guidelines Fertility. Assessment and treatment for people with fertility problems, Clinical guideline. London: RCOG press; 2004.
12. Buckett W, Sierra S. The management of unexplained infertility: an evidence-based guideline from the Canadian Fertility and Andrology Society. Reproductive BioMedicine Online. 2019;39(4):633-40.
13. Reindollar RH, Regan MM, Neumann PJ, Levine BS, Thornton KL, Alper MM, et al. A randomized clinical trial to evaluate optimal treatment for unexplained infertility: the fast track and standard treatment (FASTT) trial. Fertil Steril. 2010;94:888-99.

14. Pham CT, Karnon JD, Norman RJ, Mol BW. Cost-effectiveness modelling of IVF in couples with unexplained infertility. Reprod Biomed Online. 2018;37(5):555-63.
15. Johnson L, Sasson IE, Sammel MD, Dokras A. Does intra-cytoplasmic sperm injection improve the fertilization rate and decrease the total fertilzation failure rate in couples with well-defined unexplained infertility? A systemic review and meta-analysis. Fertil Steril. 2013;100:704-11.
16. Abrahami N, Izhaki I, Younis JS. Do young women with unexplained infertility show manifestations of decreased ovarian reserve? J Assist Reprod Genet. 2019;36(6):1143-52.

LONG QUESTIONS

1. Unexplained infertility is a diagnosis of exclusion. Discuss and debate this statement.
2. Discuss the therapeutic approach with assisted reproduction in a couple with unexplained infertility.

SHORT QUESTIONS

1. What are the standard tests that should be in place to make a working diagnosis of unexplained infertility?
2. What is the role of expectant treatment in unexplained infertility?
3. Write a short note on the place of endoscopy in unexplained infertility.
4. What are the prognostic markers in unexplained infertility?

MULTIPLE CHOICE QUESTIONS

1. The standard tests to reach a working diagnosis of unexplained infertility are all, except:
   a. Sperm function test
   b. Semen analysis
   c. HSG
   d. Pelvic ultrasound
2. The following factors indicate a good prognosis with expectant management in unexplained infertility, except:
   a. Semen analysis shows a sperm count of 50 million per mL
   b. FSH on Day 2 of cycle is 15.5 U/L
   c. Prolactin on Day 2 of cycle is 20 ng/mL
   d. Ovaries show an antral follicle count of 12
3. The most effective method of treating unexplained infertility is:
   a. Clomiphene citrate with planned relations
   b. Letrozole with IUI
   d. Gonadotropins with IUI
   d. IVF
4. The following is true about Laparoscopy in unexplained infertility:
   a. It is mandatory to perform laparoscopy to reach a diagnosis of unexplained infertility
   b. HSG is mandatory before laparoscopy
   c. Laparoscopy should be performed before all IVF cycles for unexplained infertility
   d. Laparoscopy is the gold standard to diagnose mild endometriosis lesions
5. Which of the following is true about assisted reproduction in unexplained infertility?
   a. High dose gonadotropin stimulation is preferable
   b. ICSI gives similar live birth rates as IVF
   c. At least 4 embryos should be transferred during embryo transfer
   d. All embryos should be subjected to preimplantation genetic screening before embryo transfer

Answers

1. a 2. b 3. d 4. d 5. b

12.10 INTRAUTERINE INSEMINATION

Sudha Prasad, Aswathy Kumran, Saumya Prasad

INTRODUCTION

Infertility is defined as the inability to conceive after 1 year of regular unprotected intercourse or due to an impairment of a person's potential to reproduce either as an individual or with her/his partner. In couples with advanced female age (>35 years), it is better to start evaluation and management sooner, i.e., after 6 months.[1] About 15–30% of the over 50 million subfertile couples world over do not yield any specific cause on evaluation for their condition and are considered to suffer from unexplained infertility. Various treatment options are available to optimize fertility based on the couples/individual's pathology.

Gamete handling and assisted reproductive technology (ART) have heralded a new era in the management of infertility. Although ART by definition refers to techniques involving the handling of oocytes/embryos, e.g., in vitro fertilization (IVF) or intracytoplasmic sperm injection (ICSI); simpler procedures involving isolated sperm/semen handling such as intrauterine insemination (IUI) are considered to fall under the broad umbrella of ART; the National Institute for Health and Care Excellence (NICE) guidelines 2013 considers any treatment that helps achieve pregnancy conception other than by vaginal intercourse as ART.[2]

Intrauterine insemination is the treatment method involves the placement of laboratory processed semen (partner/donor) in the uterine cavity close to the time of ovulation. It can therefore be considered as the most basic of ARTs, John Hunter of London claims credit for the first pregnancy from intrauterine insemination achieved in the 1970s. IUI is currently considered the first-line treatment for unexplained infertility as it is less invasive and more economical compared to IVF)/ICSI.

RATIONALE OF INTRAUTERINE INSEMINATION

Intrauterine insemination increases the rate of conception by increasing the chance that maximum number of healthy sperms reaching the site of fertilization.[3]

The procedure may help in increasing the chances of pregnancy in following ways:

- Allowing sperm–ovum contact close to the date and time of ovulation
- By bringing the sperm very close to the site of fertilization and by passing the cervical factors
- Sperm preparation increases the sperm density and removes all antigens on the surface of sperm and in seminal plasma.

PRINCIPLE OF INTRAUTERINE INSEMINATION

Intrauterine insemination is the simplest of assisted reproduction procedures involving semen handling and processing, depending on a healthy and functioning female reproductive system to tackle the hurdles of conception.

Intrauterine insemination ensures the timely availability of reasonable number motile spermatozoa in the uterine cavity around ovulation. The female partner's ovulation may or may not be pharmacologically assisted but, ovulation, fertilization, embryogenesis, and implantation, take place naturally. Hence, IUI does not deviate much from natural conception.

For IUI, the semen sample is washed and processed to:

- Remove seminal plasma that can cause uterine contraction and even anaphylaxis if introduced into the endometrial cavity
- To pool the healthiest and motile spermatozoa into the small insemination volume.

Prerequisites for IUI:

- Functional ovaries capable of ovulation (natural or stimulated)
- Healthy uterus with responsive endometrium
- Patent/negotiable cervical canal
- At least one patent functional fallopian tube (preferably both)
- Total motile sperm count >10 million/mL (minimum 3 million/mL).

INDICATIONS AND CONTRAINDICATIONS

Intrauterine insemination may be homologous insemination, where the husband/partners semen is used, or heterologous/donor insemination where donor semen is prepared and inseminate **(Table 1 and Box 1)**.

TABLE 1: Indications for homologous insemination.

Coital dysfunction	*To prevent/reduce transmission of sexually transmissible disease*	*Infertility*
Erectile dysfunction	Serodiscordant couple	Unexplained
Retrograde ejaculation		Mild semen analysis defects
Hypospadias		Minimal/mild endometriosis
Vaginismus		Anovulatory infertility
Psychosexual coital dysfunction		Unilateral tubal disease
		Cervical factor

BOX 1: Indications for donor insemination.

- Testicular azoospermia
- Severe oligoasthenoteratozoospermia but not opting for IVF/ICSI
- Inheritable genetic disease in male partner
- Sexually transmissible infection in male partner
- Lesbian couple
- Single women
- Persistent failure of ICSI
- Rh Isoimmunization

(IVF: in vitro fertilization; ICSI: intracytoplasmic sperm injection)

Situations where IUI should not be done:

- Evidence of acute untreated pelvic inflammation
- Nonfunctional/blocked bilateral fallopian tubes
- Advanced endometriosis
- Diminishing ovarian reserve an advanced age (to avoid time wastage)
- Frozen pelvis/dense pelvic adhesions
- Severe oligoasthenoteratozoospermia (OATS) where IVF is feasible
- Untreated sexually transmitted diseases in couple
- Cervical stenosis/atresia.

STEPS OF AN INTRAUTERINE INSEMINATION CYCLE

- Couples are evaluated and assessed to see if IUI is the suited treatment strategy.
- Ovarian stimulation should be offered as a patient's treatment strategy.
- Transvaginal ultrasound follicular imaging should be started by day 8th or 10th to assess follicular growth and endometrial thickness.
- Ovulation is either triggered pharmacologically and IUI timed 36–48 hours later or luteinizing hormone (LH) kit is used to detect the LH surge and IUI done on second day from the start of surge.

- Ovulation is triggered when the leading follicles is >18 mm in size.

Procedure on the day of IUI:
- Informed and written consent taken
- Semen sample collected and prepared or prepared and cryopreserved semen sample warmed
- Patient placed in dorsal position with thighs flexed/ semilithotomy position with buttocks at edge of table.
- All aseptic precautions taken.
- Parts cleaned with saline, no antiseptics are to be used.
- Cusco's speculum placed and cervix visualized. If cervix is not visualized properly due to cystocele or if it's very high; Sim's speculum and retractor may be used and anterior lip of the cervix may be held gently by a long Allis forceps.
- Cervical mucus cleaned with saline.
- A few drops of sperm washing medium placed at the external os.
- 1 cc insulin or BD syringe taken, and suitable IUI catheter attached and flushed with media **(Fig. 1)**.
- The prepared sperm sample is drawn into the syringe via the catheter (the ideal inseminate volume is 0.3–0.5 mL).
- No air bubbles ensured.
- The catheter is slowly introduced into the cervix till it is just beyond the internal cervical os.
- The inseminate is instilled by pressing the syringe plunger slowly.
- Keeping the plunger pushed inward, the syringe and cannula are withdrawn.
- Patient is advised to remain recumbent for 20 minutes.
- Then patient may resume routine activity.

Couple coital restriction is not advised. If no coital dysfunction or indicated restriction for coitus, couple are encouraged to be together for 2 or 3 more days.

Luteal support/adjuvants given based on individual patient's treatment requirements.

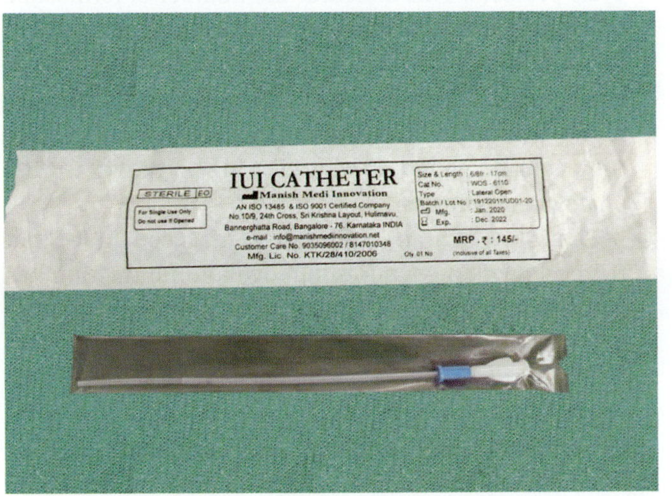

Fig. 1: Cannula for intrauterine insemination.

FACTORS DETERMINING INTRAUTERINE INSEMINATION SUCCESS

- *Duration of infertility*: The evidence available so far, suggests that the longer the duration of infertility, the lower the conception rates with IUI.
- *General health and body mass index (BMI):* Optimal BMI and health reflect better gamete quality; hence, optimizing couple health improves the fertility outcomes.
- *Age*: The female and male partner age is an important determinant of gamete quality. Clinical pregnancy and live birth rates are higher in females <35 years of age, in cases of both natural as well as assisted conception. In women >35 years, IVF would be the judicious choice in couples with unexplained infertility as is shown by the evidence in the FORT-T (Forty and Over Treatment Trial).[4]
- *Infertility etiology*: Couples who have conceived once score better than those with primary infertility. Couples with multiple causes for subfertility albeit mild have poorer IUI outcomes compared to couples with a single cause for infertility.[5]
- *Unexplained infertility*: In couples with unexplained infertility, especially if they are younger, IUI with ovarian stimulation offers better fertility outcomes compared to expectant management. IUI is the current first-line management for unexplained infertility.

  Although, the European Society of Human Reproduction and Embryology (ESHRE) workshop in 2009 had concluded that IUI was inferior to IVF in unexplained and mild male factor infertility.[3] The 2013 NICE guidelines of UK based do not recommend ovarian stimulation and IUI for unexplained infertility considering it cost ineffective.[2] Newer higher quality research evidence since then has led to the revival of IUI as an effective and less expensive management modality. Ombelet et al. in 2017 summarized that more recent good-quality randomized controlled trials (RCT) showed that IUI was indeed more effective than expectant managements in term of live birth rates.[6]

  Ayeleke RO et al. reviewed data from 15 RCTs with 2,068 women assessing fertility outcomes of IUI for unexplained subfertility and published a Cochrane review in 2020. They found moderate-quality evidence that IUI with or without ovarian stimulation improved cumulative live birth rates compared to expectant management or timed intercourse with ovarian stimulation.[7]

  All these evidence reinstate IUI as an effective and affordable first-line management strategy for unexplained subfertility.
- *Male factor infertility and semen parameters*: Infertility due to suboptimal semen parameters can be overcome by IUI in males in whom sperm count, motility, or morphology is affected moderately, while IVF-ICSI is the treatment of choice in cases where a severe defect or a combination of defects is present.

Literature reviews reveal the minimum total motile sperm count (TMSC) or number of motile spermatozoa in inseminate (NMSI) ranging from as low as one million[8] to at least 10 million[9] for satisfactory birth rates following IUI. It is reasonable to assume that IUI has maximum positive impact on fertility outcomes when the motile sperm count of the inseminate is higher. The morphological evaluation should show >4% normal spermatozoa.

DNA integrity of the spermatozoa may be assessed beforehand and gentler semen washing techniques such as magnetic-assisted cell sorting (MACS) may be used to segregate the best-quality spermatozoa for the inseminate. The male partners health needs to be optimized, any medical disorders if present well controlled, to ensure the quality of the spermatozoa. Collecting the sample after 2–3 days abstinence also improves semen parameters.

Based on the shortcomings noticed in the semen sample, individualized semen preparation techniques may be used. In mild oligoasthenospermia, a simpler technique of inseminate preparation such as swim up or simple washing and centrifuging (wash technique) may be used. But in semen samples with debris and pus cells and more abnormal spermatozoa density gradient technique of semen preparation helps in segregating higher number of healthy motile spermatozoa. In the current setting, there is paucity of good-quality evidence to suggest which semen preparation technique is better.

The 2019 Cochrane review reviewed RCTs comparing three semen preparation techniques—(1) swim up, (2) wash technique, and (3) density gradient technique. The reviewers concluded that the evidence available as of now is of very poor quality and found no significant differences in outcomes in the data that is available.[10] Hence, the semen washing techniques that is practically feasible economical, yielding the highest-quality inseminate based on the individual centers experience may be opted.

The 2016 Cochrane review states that there is still insufficient good-quality RCT evidence available to suggest that IUI is superior to expectant management, timed intercourse with or without ovarian stimulation, or IVF in mild male factor infertility.[11] Still IUI remains an in younger couples.

- *Cervical factor subfertility*: Current fertility evaluation recommendations do not suggest evaluating for cervical hostility. Hence, these couples would fall under unexplained infertility if no other causes are determined. IUI is hence the recommended first-line strategy in these patients. IUI can also help in women with negotiable cervical stenosis that can by passed by manipulating the IUI catheter.
- *Endometriosis*: Controlled ovarian stimulation (COS) with IUI is a viable treatment option in women with the American Fertility Society (AFS)/American Society for Reproductive Medicine (ASRM) Stage I and II endometriosis after laparoscopic correction of the disease.[12] In mild-to-moderate endometriosis with functioning fallopian tubes ovarian stimulation and IUI increases pregnancy and live birth rates. In severe endometriosis, IVF is the better option.
- *Anovulatory infertility*: Intrauterine insemination can be considered in women with polycystic ovarian syndrome if there is an associated male factor or in women who failed to conceive, despite successful induction of ovulation. IUI is not indicated in anovulatory infertility, yet most ovulation induction cycles are combined with IUI to obtain better results. Current recommendations suggest ovulation induction as the choice of treatment for anovulation. Lower-dose gonadotropin-induced ovulation induction is the best strategy for polycytic ovarian disease (PCOD) and should be associated with IUI may improve the results, according to the 2019 Cochrane review.[13]
- *Number of IUI cycles*: There is a general consensus in the literature that between four and six IUI cycles may be performed in appropriately selected patients. Revaluation of the patient's age, duration of infertility, pelvic factors, and semen parameters and ovarian reserve is recommended before continuing with IUI treatment beyond three to four cycles.

In a retrospective study of over 15,000 IUI cycles, the ongoing pregnancy rate per cycle decreased from 7.4% in the first cycle to 4.7% by the sixth cycle, but the cumulative pregnancy rate increased from 18.3 to 30.3%.[14]

The NICE guidelines recommend up to a year of unstimulated IUI cycles in couples with coital dysfunction as the sole cause of subfertility with evaluation to rule out other coexisting causes after failure of six IUI cycles. It also recommends IUI in stimulated cycles while waiting for IVF or when in women with patent tubes, IVF is not affordable.[2,3]

- *Ovarian stimulation and endometrial thickness*: Mid ovarian stimulation aiming for two to three dominant follicles to emerge is commonly incorporated in an IUI cycle protocol. This increases the number of fertilizable oocytes; thereby increasing the chances of conception. Letrozole, clomiphene, citrate tamoxifen, and gonadotropins (human menopausal gonadotropin urinary highly purified FSH, recombinant FSH), combination protocol, and gonadotropin-releasing hormone (GnRH) analogs, etc., are used for COS-IUI.

The 2007 Cochrane review of 43 trials concluded that IUI cycle with a gonadotropin ovulation induction has higher pregnancy rates, although multiple pregnancy and ovarian hyperstimulation syndrome (OHSS) risk were also higher.[15] Therefore, we should follow a safe and cost-effective individualized stimulation protocol for IUI cycles. Cycle cancellation strategy is to be considered if more than three follicles of 16 mm emerge to reduce the OHSS and higher order pregnancy risk. The ideal recommended endometrial thickness is >7 mm with typical triple line and adequate vascularity in midcycle.

- *Timing of IUI:* To achieve optimal success, IUI should be done as close to ovulation as possible; hence, the timing of IUI is very important. Documentation of ovulation on ultrasound before IUI is also reported to yield higher pregnancy rates.[16]
- *Ovulatory trigger:* There are multiple methods to time the IUI as close to ovulation as possible. Detection of LH surge in urine or blood and timing the IUI around 2 days afterward; administration of urinary human chorionic gonadotropin (hCG) (5,000–10,000 international units intramuscularly) or recombinant HCG (250 μg subcutaneously) or GnRH agonist (Leuprolide 1 mg/ Triptorelin 0.2 mg) or a combination of them and doing IUI on the day after are the commonly used timing schedules. According to 2014 Cochrane review that analyzed 14 RCTs, there was no difference in live birth rate between the various triggering protocols used.[17]
- *Timing of semen collection, preparation, and insemination:* The semen sample should be preferably collected at the clinic and be processed without delay. The ample should be processed within 30 minutes of ejaculation. The processed sample sound be inseminated as soon as possible. Semen preparation causes acrosomal changes and induces capacitation. Delay beyond 2 hours decreases sperm motility due to exhaustion.[5]
- *Semen parameters:* The optimal volume of inseminate should be between 0.3 and 0.5 mL.[18] Inseminate volume >0.2 mL would not be sufficient for IUI as it may not compensate for the dead space of an IUI catheter if extra air is drawn. Similarly, higher volumes of inseminate increases the chances of backspill. Also, there is no evidence that increasing inseminate volume can increase the chances of conception.
- *Number of inseminations:* Insemination is timed around ovulation and can be done once or twice. The rationale of double IUI in a multifollicular cycle and in male factor subfertility is to widen the fertilization window so as to deliver more sperm for fertilization of multiple oocytes released sequentially. The evidence is conflicting regarding double IUI to form definitive recommendations.[19,20]
- *Easy versus difficult IUI:* Difficult IUIs yield lower success rates compared to easy one.

  Use of tenaculum/Allis, uterine sound, blood on the tip of an IUI cannula, or touching the fundus while doing an IUI, back-spillage of semen, and abdominal cramps or spotting post-IUI indicates a difficult IUI.
- *Type of catheter:* Various types of catheters are available commercially, such as soft/flexible or firm/rigid, with or without stylet, curved or straight, disposable or metal. IUI catheter should be atraumatic, nontoxic, and easy to use and one that negotiates the patients cervical canal easily. The clinician may choose based on patient requirement and experience.
- *Abstinence not recommended:* Sexual intercourse around the time of IUI in couples with nonmale factor infertility is recommended. In natural intercourse, cervical crypts act as a sperm reservoir, providing a supply of sperms for up to 72 hours, but in IUI, there is no such reservoir.[5] The fertilizable life span of washed sperms is only 2–3 hours, while it is 12–24 hours for a mature oocyte. Therefore, vaginal coitus around ovulation is encouraged.
- *Immobilization post-IUI:* Sperm reaches the fallopian tubes within 5 minutes of insemination.[21] The rationale of immobilization after IUI is to prevent any leakage of semen and to compensate for the absence of sperm reservoir in cervical mucus that forms after natural intercourse. Significant improvements in ongoing pregnancy rates and livebirth rates were reported after 15 minutes of immobilization versus immediate mobilization post IUI.[22]
- *Luteal phase support:* In women with luteal phase defect and those women undergoing gonadotropin-induced IUI cycles, luteal progesterone support is recommended. In gonadotropin-stimulated IUI cycles, supraphysiologic oestradiol levels lead to luteolysis post ovulation, reducing the implantation rates. In women undergoing natural cycle IUI or IUI following oral ovulation induction, luteal support is not needed.
- *Complications:*
  - *Procedure related:*
    - Trauma
    - Infection
    - Bleeding
    - Pain and cramping
  - *Protocol related*
    - Expenses
    - OHSS risk
    - Multiple pregnancy risk
    - Faulty monitoring
  - *Remote complications*
    - Pelvic inflammatory disease
    - Psychological problems
- *Why does intrauterine insemination fail?*

The main reasons for failure of IUI treatment are:

- Poor patient selection
- Faulty technique or difficult IUI
- Poor oocyte quality/advanced age
- Nonreceptive maternal milieu
- Dysfunctional tubes though they may be patent
- Poor semen preparation technique or triple sperm defects.

CONCLUSION

Intrauterine insemination should be considered as a first-line treatment option in the management of unexplained infertility, considering its simple, patient friendly, noninvasive nature, and cost effectiveness over IVF. The approach of mild ovarian stimulation and IUI when individualized and administered is an effective approach for fertility treatment. In young couples without multifactorial causes for infertility and satisfying the prerequisites of IUI, four to six stimulated IUI cycles yield favorable fertility outcomes.

KEY MESSAGES

- Intrauterine insemination is the current first-line treatment strategy in unexplained infertility and mild male factor infertility.
- Intrauterine insemination aims to provide higher concentration of washed motile spermatozoa closer to the site of fertilization.
- Ovaries capable of satisfactory ovulation, reproductive anatomy that does not hamper natural conception, and at least one functional fallopian tube are prerequisites to be met prior too planning an IUI cycle.
- Treatment outcomes are better when the female partner is younger, i.e., < 35 years and has good ovarian reserve and response as well as healthy uterus and fallopian tubes.
- Homologous IUI is the fertility treatment of choice in otherwise normal couples with uncorrectable coital dysfunction, or where coitus is risky as in serodiscordant couples. In severe Rh isoimmunization, negative group donor semen insemination may be considered.
- Heterologous IUI offers hope for conception in couples with testicular azoospermia or severe OATS for whom IVF/ICSI is not an acceptable option.
- Careful patient selection improves the live birth rates. IUI with mild ovarian stimulation has higher pregnancy and livebirth rates compared to nonstimulated IUI cycles.

REFERENCES

1. Practice Committee of the American Society for Reproductive Medicine. Definitions of infertility and recurrent pregnancy loss: A committee opinion. Fertil Steril. 2020;113(3):533-5.
2. NICE. Nice guideline: Fertility: for people with fertility problems. 2013. NICE clinical guideline 156. 2013;1.8(1):3-4.
3. Crosignani PG. Intrauterine insemination. Human reproduction update. 20091;15(3).
4. Goldman MB, Thornton KL, Ryley D, Alper MM, Fung JL, Hornstein MD, et al. A randomized clinical trial to determine optimal infertility treatment in older couples: The Forty and Over Treatment Trial (FORT-T). Fertil Steril. 2014;101(6):1574.
5. Jain S. Intrauterine insemination: current place in infertility management. EMJ. 2018;3(1):58-66.
6. Ombelet W. The revival of intrauterine insemination: evidence-based data have changed the picture. Facts, views & vision in ObGyn. 2017;9(3):131.
7. Ayeleke RO, Asseler JD, Cohlen BJ, Veltman-Verhulst SM. Intrauterine insemination for unexplained subfertility. Cochrane Database Syst Rev. 2012;(9):CD001838.
8. Dinelli L, Courbière B, Archard V, Jouve E, Deveze C, Gnisci A, et al. Prognosis factors of pregnancy after intrauterine insemination with the husband's sperm: conclusions of an analysis of 2,019 cycles. Fertil Steril. 2014;101(4):994-1000.
9. Miller DC, Hollenbeck GD, Randolph JF, Christman GM, Smith YR, Lebovic DI, et al. Processed total motile sperm count correlates with pregnancy outcome after intrauterine insemination. Urology. 2002;60(3):497-501.
10. Boomsma CM, Cohlen BJ, Farquhar C. Semen preparation techniques for intrauterine insemination. Cochrane Database Syst Rev. 2007;(4):CD004507.
11. Cissen M, Bensdorp A, Cohlen BJ, Repping S, de Bruin JP, van Wely M. Assisted reproductive technologies for male subfertility. Cochrane Database Syst Rev. 2016;2:CD000360.
12. Practice Committee of American Society for Reproductive Medicine. Endometriosis and infertility: A committee opinion. Fertil Steril. 2012;98(3):591-8.
13. Weiss NS, Kostova E, Nahuis M, Mol BWJ, van der Veen F, van Wely M. Gonadotropins for ovulation induction in women with polycystic ovary syndrome. Cochrane Database Syst Rev. 2019;1(1):CD010290.
14. Custers IM, Steures P, Hompes P, Flierman P, van Kasteren Y, van Dop PA, et al. Intrauterine insemination: How many cycles should we perform? Hum Reprod. 2008;23(4):885-8.
15. Cantineau AEP, Cohlen BJ. Ovarian stimulation protocols (anti-oestrogens, gonadotrophins with and without GnRH agonists/antagonists) for intrauterine insemination (IUI) in women with subfertility. Cochrane Database Syst Rev. 2007;(2):CD005356.
16. Kucuk T. Intrauterine insemination: is the timing correct? J Assist Reprod Genet. 2008;25(8):427-30.
17. Cantineau AEP, Janssen MJ, Cohlen BJ, Allersma T. Synchronised approach for intrauterine insemination in subfertile couples. Cochrane Database Syst Rev. 2014;(12): CD006942.
18. Ok EK, Doğan ÖE, Okyay RE, Gülekli B. The effect of post-wash total progressive motile sperm counts and semen volume on pregnancy outcomes in intrauterine insemination cycles: a retrospective study. J Turk Ger Gynecol Assoc. 2013;14(3):142.
19. Cantineau AEP Heineman MJ, Cohlen BJ. Single versus double intrauterine insemination (IUI) in stimulated cycles for subfertile couples. Cochrane Database Syst Rev. 2003;(1): CD003854.
20. Polyzos NP, Tzioras S, Mauri D, Tatsioni A. Double versus single intrauterine insemination for unexplained infertility: a metaanalysis of randomized trials. Fertil Steril. 2010;94(4): 1261-6.
21. van der Poel N, Farquhar C, Abou-Setta AM, Benschop L, Heineman MJ. Soft versus firm catheters for intrauterine insemination. Cochrane Database Syst Rev. 2010;11:CD006225.
22. Custers IM, Flierman PA, Maas P, Cox T, Van Dessel TJHM, Gerards MH, et al. Immobilisation versus immediate mobilisation after intrauterine insemination: randomised controlled trial. BMJ. 2009;339:b4080.

LONG QUESTION

1. Define intrauterine insemination. How does it differ from IVF? What are the contraindications for IUI? Describe an IUI cycle in brief.

SHORT QUESTIONS

1. What are the indications and prerequisites for IUI?
2. What factors influence IUI outcomes?

MULTIPLE CHOICE QUESTIONS

1. Intrauterine insemination involves:
   a. Sperm handling
   b. Oocyte handling
   c. Sperm and oocyte handling
   d. None
2. Homologous insemination means:
   a. Insemination of donor inseminate
   b. Insemination with partner inseminate
   c. Insemination with cryopreserved warmed inseminate
   d. Mixing partner sperm and oocytes in lab
3. When is IUI done?
   a. Follicular phase
   b. 2 days after ovulation
   c. As close to ovulation as possible
   d. Day 21 of cycle
4. What is the ideal inseminate volume?
   a. 0.3–0.5 mL
   b. 2 mL
   c. 0.01 mL
   d. 3 mL
5. Which is not a prerequisite for intrauterine insemination?
   a. Functional ovaries
   b. Responsive endometrium
   c. Patent fallopian tubes
   d. Male factor infertility
6. Which is not an indication for donor insemination?
   a. Lesbians
   b. Male partner with HIV and high viral load
   c. Mild OATS
   d. Inheritable diseases in male partner

Answers

1. a 2. b 3. c 4. a 5. d 6. c

12.11 ASSISTED REPRODUCTIVE TECHNOLOGY

Jaideep Malhotra, Shally Gupta, Neharika Malhotra, Neerja Sachdev, Narendra Malhotra, Keshav Malhotra

INTRODUCTION

Assisted reproductive technology (ART) are procedures that involve handling of sperms, ova, and embryos outside human body.

Assisted reproductive technology is not new. Ancient Indian scriptures mention of surrogacy and artificial insemination. Certainly artificial insemination has been practiced for the last century. ART finds its roots in animal rearing and husbandry. However, in humans, Louis Brown world's first in vitro fertilization (IVF) baby in 1978 in Oldham was the first major breakthrough. In the words of Patrick Steptoe it was "the end of the beginning, not the beginning of the end".

INDICATIONS OF ASSISTED REPRODUCTION TECHNOLOGY/IN VITRO FERTILIZATION

- Infertility is defined as inability to conceive after 1 year of regular unprotected intercourse.
- Approximately, 15% of couples seek treatment for primary infertility.
- Common indications of IVF would be in female or male partner or combined.

Female Factors

These are responsible for 40% of causes of infertility and IVF:

- Tubal blockage
- Anovulation
- Uterine factors such as Asherman's syndrome, fibroids, adenomyosis
- Ovarian pathologies like endometriosis, polycystic ovarian syndrome, and decreased ovarian reserve.
- Increasing age and unexplained infertility are other common causes.

Male Problems

Oligozoospermia, azoospermia, asthenozoospermia, teratozoospermia, sexual dysfunction, and ejaculatory disorders are common indication for IVF.

About 30% of couples would have combined male factors.

Hereditary or genetic diseases may also be the problem in some partners male or female requiring IVF ART.

TECHNIQUES OF ART

- Ovulation induction
- Intrauterine insemination (IUI)
- IVF
- Intracytoplasmic sperm injection (ICSI)
- Cryopreservation of embryos
- Third-party IVF or donor IVF program
- Peri-implantation genetic testing (PGT)
- Surrogacy.

IN VITRO FERTILIZATION AND EMBRYO TRANSFER

After finding success in veterinary science, IVF was advanced for use in humans especially for women with damaged fallopian tubes. In 21st century, there are wide variety of indications, including long-standing unexplained infertility, treated endometriosis, male factor infertility, cervical hostility and, rarely, after therapy for female cancer. Today though more than 0.5 million babies have been born by IVF worldwide, it still remains a very limited service as it is expensive, very specialized and requires good laboratory infrastructure and a team of skilled scientists, doctors, and staff. Newer ART techniques have been constantly evolving defining and new developments are continually taking place.

In vitro fertilization involves four basic steps: (1) Controlled ovarian hyperstimulation (COH), (2) oocyte retrieval, (3) sperm penetration by IVF or ICSI and (4) embryo transfer (ET).

In superovulation one stimulates ovaries by the use of drugs like letrozole or clomiphene and/or gonadotropins. This leads to the formation of several ova can be retrieved or extracted also known as OVU pick up. Drugs such gonadotropin-releasing hormone (GnRH) agonists or GnRH antagonists are used to suppress the hypothalamic-pituitary-ovarian axis and stop intrinsic LH surge. They have been useful in increasing the number of oocytes retrieved, better endometrial receptivity, and higher clinical pregnancy rates with reduced cycle cancellation.

CONTROLLED OVARIAN HYPERSTIMULATION

There are a number of different ovarian hyperstimulation protocols, viz., long protocol, antagonist protocol, short protocol, ultra short protocol, and flare protocol. Choice of protocol depends on many factors including expected response of patients. The patients are categorized normal responders, poor responders, or a hyper-responders **(Box 1)**.

For normal responders, the standard long protocol is used. GnRH agonists (GnRHa) is started from middle of luteal phase of the previous cycle, as follicle recruitment for next cycle normally starts at this time in response to the increasing levels of follicle-stimulating hormone (FSH), estrogen, and inhibin. Commonly used agonists are Leuprolide 0.5 mg administered daily subcutaneously or intranasal nafarelin, administered 200 μg BD. The administration is continued throughout the follicular phase along with gonadotropin, which are started from day 2 of next cycle till human chorionic gonadotropin (hCG) is administered when the follicles have reached maturity (17–19 mm). Follicle growth is monitored by serial ultrasound, preferably transvaginal ultrasound (TVS) and hormonal profile, i.e., serum FSH, luteinizing hormone (LH), estradiol (E2), and progesterone (P4) **(Fig. 1)**.

BOX 1: Controlled ovarian stimulation protocols.

- Long agonist down-regulation with gonadotropin stimulation
- Antagonist down-regulation with gonadotropin stimulation
- Minimal stimulation protocol with gonadotropin with or without clomiphene citrate combined with antagonist

For poor responders, a microdose flare protocol can be used. Injection Leuprolide 20 μg is given subcutaneously BD from day 2 or 3 of the cycle, whereas gonadotropin is started on day 6.

In patients who are hyper-responders such as are patients with the polycystic ovary syndrome (PCOS), low-dose gonadotropins (75 IU/day) are started from day 2 or 3 of the menses. GnRH antagonist are started according to fixed protocol (day 6) or flexible protocol (DF 12–13 mm). This is known as antagonist protocol. Monitoring is done with serial hormones like in other protocols. Hyper-responders are at risk of ovarian hyperstimulation syndrome. Monitoring of the same can be done with estradiol levels.

When estradiol levels are more than 3,000 pg/mL, gonadotropin is stopped irrespective of the follicle size and GnRH antagonist is continued. hCG is administered when estradiol level falls below 3,000 pg/mL. This is called *coasting* and it prevents and decreases the incidence of ovarian hyperstimulation syndrome(OHSS) **(Figs. 2 and 3; Box 2)**. This is the key advantage of antagonist protocol over agonist protocol that it prevents this dreaded complication and therefore considered safer especially hyper-responders.

OOCYTE RETRIEVAL

Oocyte retrieval or ovum pick up is done 34–36 hours after ovulation trigger.

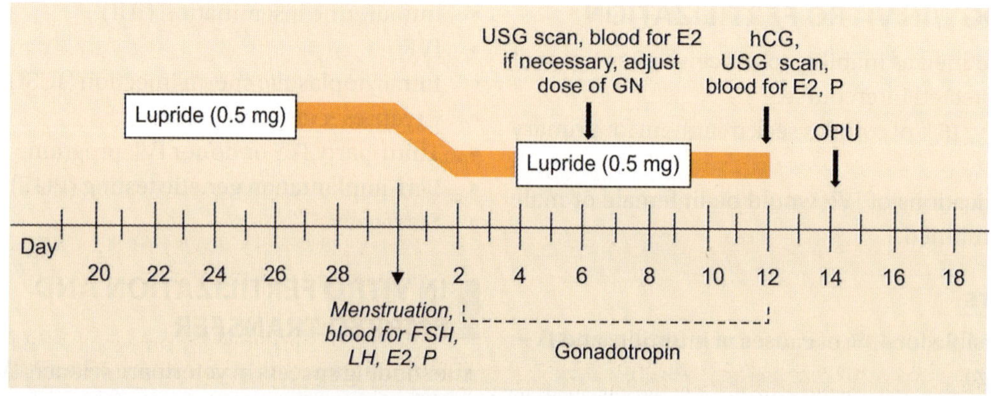

Fig. 1: Long protocol-ovarian stimulation.
(E2: estradiol; FSH: follicle-stimulating hormone; hCG: human chorionic gonadotropin; LH: luteinizing hormone; OPU: ovum pick-up; P: progesterone; USG: ultrasound)

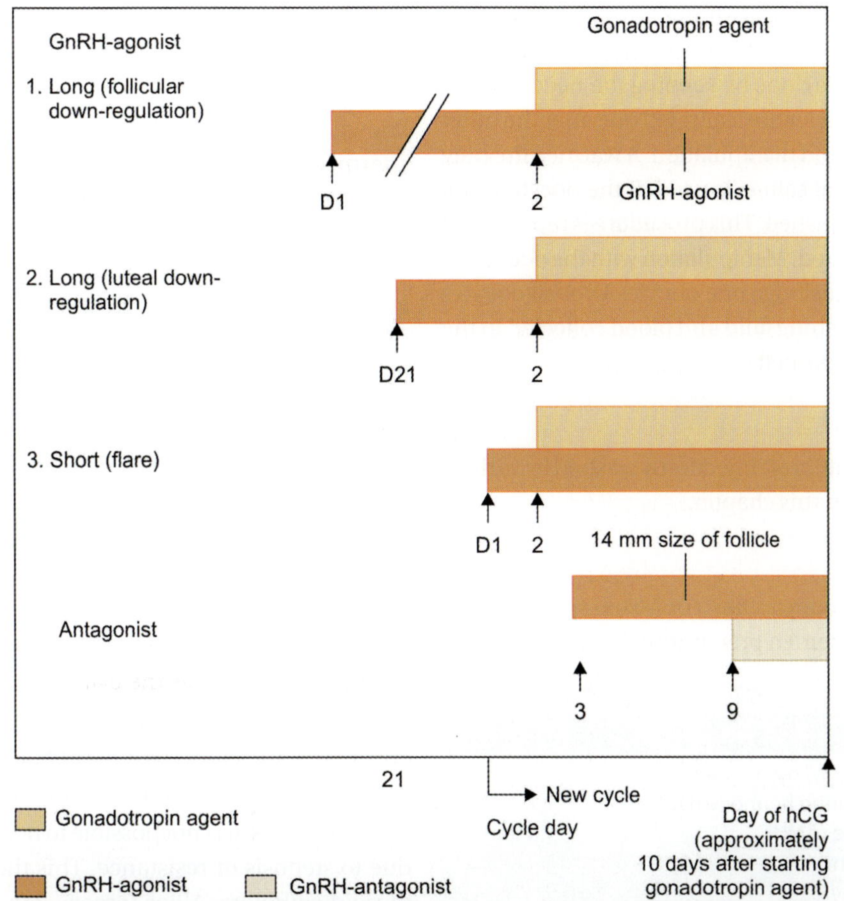

Fig. 2: In vitro fertilization protocols with gonadotropins in controlled ovarian hyperstimulation. (hCG: human chorionic gonadotropin; GnRH: gonadotropin-releasing hormone)

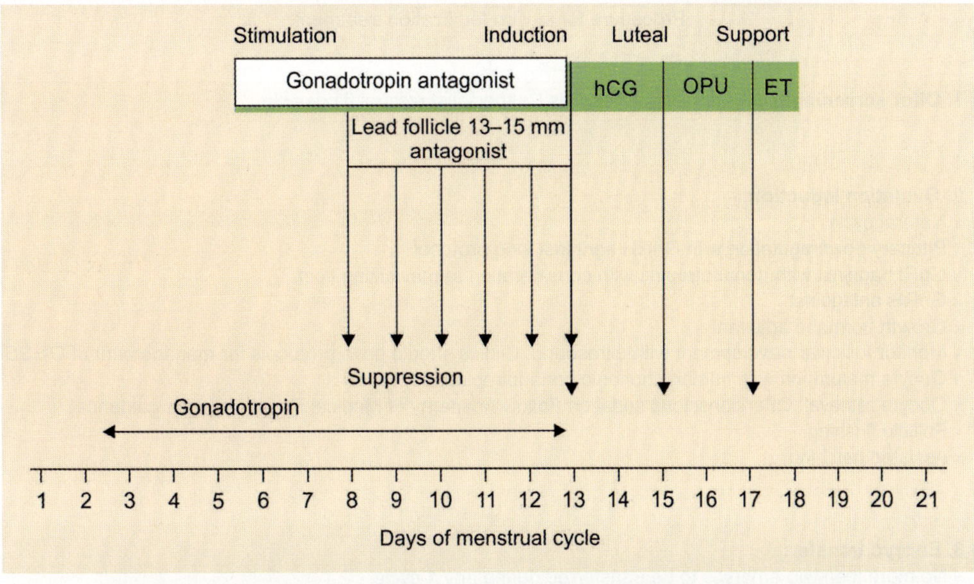

Fig. 3: Gonadotropin-releasing hormone antagonist down-regulation protocol. (hCG: human chorionic gonadotropin; OPU: ovum pick-up; ET: embryo transfer)

It was previously done with laparoscopy and percutaneously. But with the easy availability of TVS, its simplicity and safety, it is now mostly done transvaginally. This is the easiest, most accurate, and patient-friendly method. In rare situations like inaccessible ovary, vaginal infection, a perurethral oocyte pick-up can also be done under guidance of a transabdominal ultrasound probe. To fix the ovaries to prevent the ovary from slipping, sharp beveled, disposable needles are used and gentle suprapubic pressure is applied with one hand by the assistant.

It is generally preferable to make minimum punctures in the vagina and in the ovary. This reduces risk of pelvic infections and bleeding. This can be done by keeping the needle in the ovary so that, several follicles are aspirated one after the other by careful maneuvering and manipulation. A warmed flushing medium, warmed normal saline, is used. If the oocyte is not recovered, the follicle is flushed. This procedure is repeated till all the oocytes are recovered. Manipulation with the needle tip may help to aspirate or dislodge one oocyte. After all oocytes have been recovered, flushing fluid and blood collected in the pouch of Douglas are aspirated.

Semen Preparation

Semen used for insemination or injection is washed by various methods covered later in this chapter.

INSEMINATION

For insemination of the oocytes fresh or frozen sperm can be used. The technique of semen preparation is described later in this chapter. IVF insemination with less than 50,000 sperm/egg decreases the fertilization rate, so ICSI is done.

BOX 2: Predictive factors for assessment of correct stimulation protocol.

- Age
- Baseline follicle-stimulating hormone (D2/3)
- Anti-Müllerian hormone (AMH)
- Basal antral follicle count
- Body mass index

Whereas the risk of fertilization with multiple sperms known as polyspermy, it is increased with more than 500,000 sperm/egg. The sperms and oocytes are incubated under controlled conditions. After 16–18 hours, they are checked for the presence of two pronuclei, which confirms fertilization. The zygotes are further cultured in the incubator to allow growth and cleavage to the 2-4-8 cell stage when they are ready for transfer to the uterus. They can be followed till the blastocyst stage, which usually form on day 5 of sperm insemination **(Flowchart 1)**.

EMBRYO TRANSFER

Embryo transfer is done 48–50 hours after oocyte recovery, i.e., 46–48 hours after insemination.

Embryo transfer catheter is taken and it is flushed with Earle's medium. Two or three embryos suspended in 15–25 μL of fluid are transferred 1–1.5 cm below the fundus or lower, i.e., about 5–6 cm from the external os, and the catheter checked to ensure that the embryos have not been expelled. The patient is made to rest for 30 minutes after the procedure.

Sometimes, it is not possible to negotiate the cervical canal due to stenosis or resistance. This then may require the use of rigid catheters. Allies forceps, etc. and rarely the patient

Flowchart 1: Algorithm for management of infertility patient with bilateral tubal occlusion.

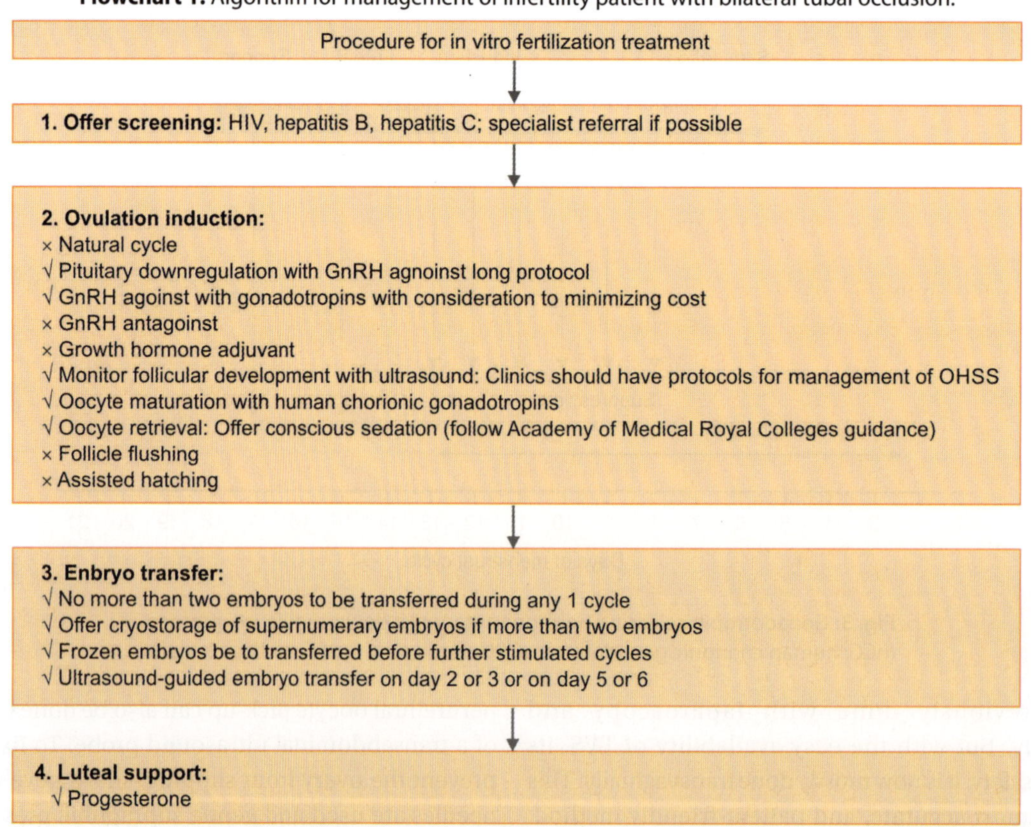

(GnRH: gonadotropin-releasing hormone; HIV: human immunodeficiency virus; OHSS: ovarian hyperstimulation syndrome)

may require to have the ET done under general anesthesia. It can be prevented by proper examination and mock ET before actual ET.

Post-transfer, the patient receives progesterone vaginal suppositories 600–800 mg daily in divided doses, or IM progesterone 25–50 mg daily.

Factors Affecting Embryo Transfer

- *Cervical mucus:* It may plug catheter tip leading to retention of embryos
- Failed negotiation of cervical canal: Acute flexion or version
- Irritation of uterus and initiation of uterine contractions.

To improve success rate of ET:
- Dummy transfer—mock transfer
- Ultrasonography-guided transfer
- Avoiding initiation of contractions
- Using soft malleable catheter to avoid trauma
- Cervix should not be held with any instrument to avoid irritation of uterus
- Cervical infection reduces pregnancy rate
- Loading of embryos into catheter should be done carefully with small volume 30–40 μL.

OUTCOME

The pregnancy through IVF like any natural conception can have abortion, preterm delivery, or live birth. A preclinical abortion is a biochemical pregnancy, which ends within 28 days of fertilization diagnosed by a minimum of two raised beta hCG values. This is reported in 9–16% of pregnancies.

A clinical abortion is the spontaneous termination of pregnancy of at least 28 days after oocyte pick-up and is seen in 18–30% of pregnancies.

In general, women with tubal disease, mild and treated endometriosis or unexplained infertility have a better outcome. Increasing female age, antisperm antibodies, and sperm dysfunction affect success rates adversely.

A better outcome is seen in those women who undergo a repeat attempt after having a live birth following an IVF cycle; and in women who have had an unsuccessful pregnancy in the previous cycle, whether a miscarriage, an ectopic or a biochemical pregnancy, as compared to a woman who did not conceive at all in the first cycle. The average clinical pregnancy rate is about 26% per retrieval. The live-birth rate varies from 9 to 26% per cycle, the overall rate is 21%. Of these, 66–72% are singleton, 22–24% twins, 3–11% triplets, and less than 1% are higher order multiple pregnancies.

Pregnancy rates increases as number of embryos transferred increase. With 1, 2, 3, and 4 embryos transferred pregnancy rate is 9.6%, 15.9%, 24.2%, and 30.6% per cycle, respectively, but the con is multiple pregnancy rate is also correspondingly increased.

The cumulative conception rate (CCR) below 35 years of age is similar too of the normally cohabiting fertile population. After 6 cycles of IVF, CCR varies from 56 to 72%, whereas in the normal fertile population, it is about 55%. 18% show vanishing fetus 4–6% have ectopic pregnancy. Risk of ectopic pregnancy in these patients is because of the following reasons:
- *Preexisting tubal pathology:* It was common practice earlier to occlude the tubes at the time of laparoscopy to prevent future ectopic pregnancy but with ultrasound-guided oocyte retrieval, laparoscopy is no longer necessary.
- Multiple embryo transfer
- *Technique of transfer:* using increased volume of transfer fluid. Use of excessive force in the transfer, placing the ET catheter too far above in mid cavity or extending into the tube itself.
- Retrograde migration of embryos to the tubes.
- Bilateral tubal pregnancy is the rarest form of binovular twins. More commonly the twin sacs are seen in the same tube or there may be simultaneous intrauterine and extrauterine gestation (heterotopic pregnancy). In women with an IVF pregnancy, the presence of an intrauterine gestation sac on TVS, one has to be careful to rule out an extrauterine pregnancy, which may be located in the cervix or the ovary.

Maternal complications can be associated with: (1) ovarian stimulation; (2) oocyte retrieval; and (3) embryo transfer.

In stimulation, it is the OHSS, which is seen in 1% of women undergoing superovulation, and ovarian cyst formation, which is seen during down-regulation with GnRHa or as a result of previous gonadotropin therapy. It usually settles with continued administration of GnRHa.

With oocyte retrieval, it is mainly the risks of intravenous sedation and regional anesthesia, and pelvic infection. There is also the risk of needle damage to adjacent organs—bowel, bladder, uterus, and vascular structures, and of pelvic infection.

Obstetric complications seen with IVF-ET are mainly multiple births, low birth weight and ectopic pregnancy. Selective fetal reduction is recommended, if there are more than three or four fetuses. In some countries, the law prohibits the transfer of more than three embryos.

Delivery by cesarean section is common. Low birth-weight babies comprise 32% of births, mainly because of multiple pregnancies. Risk of major congenital abnormalities is present in 2–3% of the children, which is similar to the general population. The use of vitrified or frozen gametes or embryos does not increase congenital abnormalities and developmental milestones are similar in all groups.

CRYOPRESERVATION

Freezing of semen is a time tested technique and has been in use for over a century. Multiple follicle stimulation techniques yield oocytes or embryos in excess of the number required for fresh transfer. Embryo cryopreservation is an accepted method for these excess embryos as survival of frozen embryos is more than 90%. With frozen ET pregnancy rates are improved by up to 10%. No adverse effects have been seen in babies born by this technique. The technique involves cooling of embryos in the pronucleate or early cleavage state to very low temperatures with the help of cryoprotectants, e.g., 12-propanediol, dimethyl sulfoxide (DMSO) or glycerol with sucrose, which minimizes damage to the embryos. They are then preserved in liquid nitrogen till required. Over 95% of the embryos survive the thawing process. Since the past decade with advancement of techniques Oocyte preservation has also been very successful and popular method of fertility preservation.

OOCYTE DONATION (FIG. 4)

Oocyte donation is also a treatment option in cases of women with premature ovarian failure or resistant ovary syndrome, surgical castration, following chemotherapy or radiotherapy, ovarian dysgenesis, in women with hereditary genetic disease or poor quality of oocyte in IVF treatments. It is also useful for women with diminished ovarian reserve due to common diseases like endometriosis, PID, iatrogenic or idiopathic causes.

Oocytes may be obtained from unrelated or known donors, oocytes sharing from IVF programs are allowed in certain countries with consent of the couple. In some countries, the practice of obtaining oocytes from patients undergoing sterilization prior to operation or from professional donors has been noted. In the future, cadaveric oocyte donation or oocyte recovery from fetuses may also become possible.

Pregnancy rates are improved in oocyte donation cycles (50–60% per cycle). However, there is also a higher risk of first trimester bleeding, preeclampsia and intrauterine growth restriction **(Boxes 3 and 4)**.

EMBRYO DONATION

Embryo donation may be indicated in some menopausal or perimenopausal women with a subfertile partner, in cases of recurrent implantation failure or in couples with genetic disease or chromosomal abnormality.

SURROGACY

Surrogacy is an option for women without a uterus as in cases with congenital absence of the uterus or those who have undergone hysterectomy for severe hemorrhage or ruptured uterus and also for those with very much diseased uterus such as Asherman's syndrome that is unlikely to implant the embryos. Some patients with recurrent miscarriages or those with medical conditions, which may make pregnancy life-threatening even though long-term health prospects are otherwise good, may also prefer to opt for surrogacy. They may have one or both ovaries functioning.

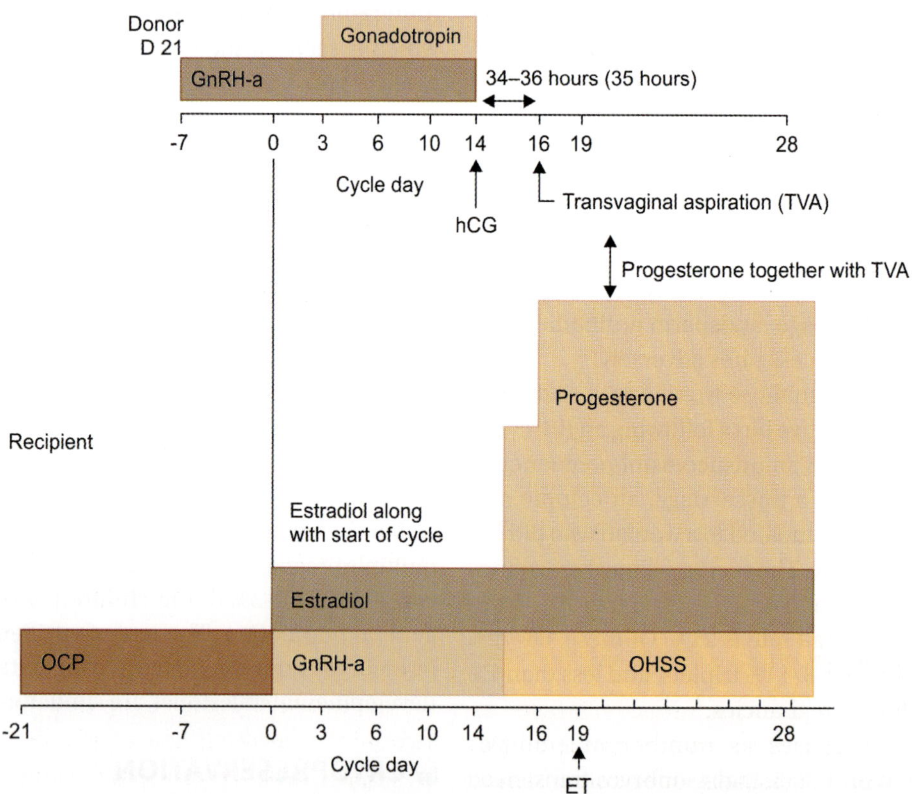

Fig. 4: Regimens of ovarian stimulation and hormone replacement used to synchronize the development of ovarian follicles in the oocyte donor and the endometrial cycle in the recipient. (ET: embryo transfer; hCG: human chorionic gonadotropin; OHSS: ovarian hyperstimulation syndrome; GnRH: gonadotropin-releasing hormone; OCP: oral contraceptive pill)

BOX 3: Indications for oocyte donation.

- Premature ovarian failure
- Ovarian agenesis
- Surgical removal of bilateral ovaries
- Radiotherapy or chemotherapy for ovarian cancer
- Postmenopausal patient
- Risk of inheritable genetic disease in children
- Failed in vitro fertilization due to poor oocyte quality
- Inaccessible ovaries

BOX 4: Evaluation of oocyte recipient.

- Complete medical and reproductive history
- Blood group, RH, VDRL, HIV, HbsAg, HBC, blood sugar
- Pelvic sonography to assess endometrium
- Hysteroscopy

(HbsAg: hepatitis B surface antigen; HBC: hepatitis B core; HIV: human immunodeficiency virus; RH: rhesus; VDRL: venereal disease research laboratory)

The host mother should be normal, healthy, not more than 38 years of age, with at least one child. Her husband or partner should be fully aware of the implications. Investigations of the host mother are kept to a minimum. Because of the risk of human immunodeficiency virus (HIV) infection, it is recommended that frozen sperm be used after waiting to cross the stipulated window period of 6 months. The procedure is relatively simple, cheap, with fewer complications than IVF and permits better bonding with the child although it is not genetically related. However, very few such cases are possible.

As was expected, the success of IVF has posed many ethical, social, and legal problems, which are being debated extensively in those countries where these procedures are carried out. Some of these issues were posed by Professor Jeffcoate in the fourth edition, well before the success of Edwards and Steptoe. The answers to some of these issues are known, but many are still not fully resolved, particularly those related to the freezing and storage of donor ova or embryos, to the use of stored embryos, and to the disposal of those embryos not directly required in the management of infertility. At present, developments in this field are ahead of legal decisions. Public opinion is also changing; what was not acceptable a decade ago is now regarded as a normal event. It seems probable that fairly strict legislation will ultimately apply to certain infertility procedures and their performance in recognized institutions or centers.

INTRAUTERINE INSEMINATION (BOXES 5 TO 7; TABLE 1)

Intrauterine insemination is a procedure, which involves collection of semen by ejaculation or masturbation), and its transfer into the uterus by processing by one or other semen preparation techniques.

Intrauterine insemination is indicated when there is an ejaculatory disorders, which may be anatomical, e.g., hypospadias, neurological problems, secondary to spinal cord injury, retrograde ejaculation, which may occur in multiple sclerosis and in impotence. Male subfertility as reflected in abnormal semen analysis findings with oligospermia or hypospermia, asthenozoospermia or teratozoospermia [though some of these patients may require ICSI (see later)]. Immunological factors like antisperm antibodies in the male or female partner; hostile or poor cervical mucus; disease or deformity of the cervix making it difficult for sperm to enter. In recent times, the processed semen of an HIV-positive partner has been used to inseminate an HIV-negative woman. Advancement in techniques of cryopreservation of semen now make it possible for men with cancer undergoing surgery,

BOX 5: Indications of intrauterine insemination.

- Unexplained infertility
- Cervical factor
- Mild male factor
- Ejaculatory failure
- Immunological causes
- Mild-to-moderate endometriosis

BOX 6: Pre-requisites for intrauterine insemination.

- Age less than 40 years
- At least one patent fallopian tube
- Occurrence of spontaneous or induced ovulation
- Post wash sperm count >5 million motile sperm

BOX 7: Steps of intrauterine insemination.

- Patient selection and workup
- Ovarian stimulation
- Semen wash
- Insemination
- Luteal support

TABLE 1: Patient workup.

Wife	*Husband*
CBC, ESR, VDRL, HIV, HbsAg, HCV	CBC, VDRL, blood sugar, HIV, HbsAg, HCV
D2/3- FSH, LH, E2, Prolactin, TSH, Hormonal evaluation	Semen analysis
Rule out tuberculosis	Optional: Semen culture, Kruger sperm morphology, sperm antibodies, FSH, testosterone, prolactin, scrotal Doppler
Hysterosalpingography or diagnostic laparoscopy, hysteroscopy, dilation and curettage	
Ovulation study: Serial vaginal ultrasound for follicular study (Others: BBT, serum progesterone D21, endometrial biopsy)	

(BBT: basal body temperature; CBC: complete blood count; E2: estradiol; ESR: erythrocyte sedimentation rate; FSH: follicle-stimulating hormone; HCV: hepatitis C virus; HIV: human immunodeficiency virus; HbsAg: hepatitis B surface antigen; HBC: hepatitis B core; LH: luteinizing hormone; TSH: thyroid-stimulating hormone; USG: ultrasound; VDRL: venereal disease research laboratory)

chemotherapy, radiotherapy, or orchidectomy to store their semen to be used for IUI after cure of the disease.

Intrauterine insemination can be done in natural or stimulated cycles but results are better with the latter. Standard protocols of oral ovulogens such as clomiphene or letrozole, or combined with gonadotropins such as SH or HMG may be used. With the development of up to four mature follicles, there are better chances of implantation. Human chorionic gonadotropin is administered when the lead follicle is 18–20 mm in size. Follicle monitoring is done by ultrasound and hormonal profile.

Semen Preparation

Semen consists of seminal fluid with sperm and other cellular debris from the urogenital tract. Prostaglandins, enzymes, and protease inhibitors present in the seminal fluid are detrimental to the fertilization process in the Fallopian tube or in vitro, as they provoke strong uterine contractions and impair sperm capacitation. The object of sperm preparation is to separate the sperm from the seminal fluid and provide a concentrated number of motile, capacitated sperm resuspended in a small volume of protein-supplemented medium **(Boxes 8 and 9)**.

The swim-up technique is commonly used and is suitable for samples with normal sperm count and motility. The semen is divided into 0.5 mL aliquots per centrifuge tube and diluted 2:1 with protein-supplemented medium to decrease viscosity and improve pellet formation. The tubes are centrifuged for 10 minutes at a speed not greater than 400 g to avoid damage to the sperm. The supernatant is removed and the pellets are overlaid with 0.5 mL of medium. They are incubated at 37°C for 1 hour. Motile sperms swim up into the supernatant, which is collected from all the tubes and centrifuged at 300 g for 5 minutes **(Box 10)**. The final pellet is resuspended in 0.5 mL of medium.

Techniques using a density gradient are better for samples with a low-sperm count and/or motility as they also significantly decrease bacterial contamination. Each milliliter of semen is placed on a column of silica particles or bovine albumin in centrifuge tubes and centrifuged for 20 minutes at 400 g. The sperm pellets are washed off the gradient matrix with media, combined and resuspended in 0.5 mL medium **(Box 11)**.

Sperm wash is used for severely low sperm counts and motility.

In these cases the technique described earlier cannot provide adequate sperms. The undiluted semen is divided into 1 mL aliquots, centrifuged at 300 g for 5 minutes, the supernatant removed and the pellet resuspended in 0.5 mL of fresh medium.

Insemination is done using a flexible sterile IUI catheter made of nonsperm toxic latex materials. The washed sperms are reconstituted in 0.5 mL of HTF medium and gently injected into the uterus to avoid endometrial trauma, which can cause cramping and bleeding resulting in poorer sperm survival. For a good chance of pregnancy in IUI cycles minimum inseminated motile count (IMC) should be at least 1 million /mL, better results are seen with IMC more than 5 million/mL. Undiluted or raw semen is never used because of the need of high volumes and risk of infection. The technique has the advantage of being relatively simple, cheap, effective, and noninvasive. It can also be performed in low cost non-IVF units. However, IVF units have the advantage that rarely if hyperstimulation occurs, they may convert the cycle to an IVF cycle and freeze surplus embryos.

When IUI is used for retrograde ejaculation it necessitates alkalinizing the male urine, collecting a specimen after coitus, centrifuging that sample for spermatozoa and then using these for insemination after washing. Sperm retrieved from this technique can be used in ICSI.

BOX 8: Essential requirements for semen preparation.

- Motile sperm count
- Volume
- Viscosity
- Presence of leucocytes, cells and debris
- Whether it is for IUI, IVF or ICSI

(IUI: intrauterine insemination; IVF: in vitro fertilization; ICSI: intracytoplasmic sperm injection)

BOX 9: Different methods for semen preparation.

- Direct swim up (used for semen with normal parameters)
- Pellet and swim up method
- Density gradient

BOX 10: Swim-up method for semen preparation.

- Take two test tubes, label them, put 1 mL of semen sample in each
- Add 2 mL of flushing medium in each tube and mix
- Centrifuge for 10 minutes at 1,500 rpm
- Aspirate supernatant
- Layer pellet with 1 mL flushing or culture media
- After 30–40 minutes, remove 0.5 mi of supernatant from each tube and use for intrauterine insemination, in vitro fertilization, intracytoplasmic sperm injection

BOX 11: Density gradient for semen preparation.

- Take two conical tubes, label them and put 1 mL of 90% sperm gradient
- Layer 1 mL of 40% sperm gradient over it
- Layer 1–2 mL of sperm on top of the two layers
- Centrifuge at 1,500 rpm for 20 minutes
- Pipette out supernatant and transfer pellet to new tube with 5 mL of flushing medium
- Centrifuge at 1,500 rpm for 10 minutes
- Pipette out supernatant
- Pellet is resuspended in 0.8 mL of culture media and sample used for intrauterine insemination, in vitro fertilization, intracytoplasmic sperm injection

The success rate of IUI is about 18–20% per cycle. After failing to achieve pregnancy after 4–6 cycles IVF can be considered.

Those couples with male factor infertility who fail treatment with artificial insemination, and those who have semen parameters that make insemination an inferior approach, in these couples, use of ART, especially ICSI, may be better treatment choice. ICSI allows even patients with severe male factor infertility patients to father their own biological child. Therefore, ICSI should be considered if the total motile sperm count is less than 0.5×10^6 because the IUI success rates are extremely low with such sperm counts. Finally, ICSI should be recommended after three to four failed IUI cycles in a couple with male factor infertility.

DONOR INSEMINATION

Donor insemination (DI) is indicated when the woman is normal but the man is infertile, when there are genetic diseases or there is severe rhesus incompatibility (to produce a rhesus-negative fetus) for the woman who has had previous repeated losses of babies due to isoimmunization despite advances in perinatal medicine.

With the advances of microsurgical epididymal sperm aspiration (MESA), percutaneous epididymal sperm aspiration (PESA) and testicular sperm extraction (TESE) for ICSI (see later) in male infertility, with the availability of preimplantation genetic diagnosis (see below) in conditions such as hemophilia and cystic fibrosis (which allows transfer of normal embryos only) and with the decreasing incidence of rhesus isoimmunization in developed countries, the demand for DI is decreasing except in developing countries, as the costs of these alternative procedures is much higher **(Box 12)**.

It is essential that adequate counseling of the couple concerned is done so that it can be ascertained that this method is acceptable and that they are likely to be suitable parents. The criteria are similar to those used for adoption but the upper age limit for the wife is usually 37 years. The couple should understand all the implications of DI and the risks of the pregnancy itself. Because of anonymity of the donor, genetic abnormalities cannot be looked for.

There is debate about the number of successful pregnancies which should be allowed per donor. Although at one time 20 seemed acceptable, the increasing use of DI suggests that 5 or 10 would be more appropriate. An exception could be considered when a second child by DI is requested by a couple.

BOX 12: Donor insemination.

Donor insemination for couple with:
- Azoospermia
- Generic/infectious disease in male partner
- Severe rhesus isoimmunization
- Severe semen defects

The risk of transmission of acquired immunodeficiency syndrome (AIDS) by DI suggests that fresh semen would rarely be used. Tests for freedom from infection must be repeated after 6 months, before stored specimens can be used.

The general practice is to inseminate the woman for up to six or nine confirmed ovulatory cycles. The majority of successful inseminations occur within three ovular cycles and the success rate is certainly less in women with infertility problems which required treatment.

Overall, the success of DI varies considerably from 10 to 35%.

OTHER ART METHODS

Though ICSI is most reliable and effective ART method many other have been developed over the years, such as gamete intrafallopian transfer (GIFT); zygote intrafallopian transfer (ZIFT), fallopian tube sperm perfusion (FSP) or intrafallopian insemination (IFI); direct intraperitoneal transfer (DIPI) peritoneal oocyte sperm transfer (POST); pronuclear stage tubal transfer (PROST); tubal embryo stage transfer (TEST); tubal embryo transfer (TET); embryo intrafallopian transfer (EIFT); surgical embryo transfer (SET); transmyometrial embryo transfer (TM-ET); direct oocyte transfer (DOT); and intravaginal culture (IVC). Many of them have been discarded in favor of IUI, IVF, or ICSI (see later).

Many of the terms are self-explanatory. DIPI and IUI give similar results; the IUI is a simpler technique unless there is severe cervical stenosis when DIPI can be performed. FSP has been replaced by IUI or IVF. POST is a good rescue procedure for IUI or FSP if hyperstimulation develops requiring cancellation of the cycle. ZIFT, PROST, TEST, TET, and EIFT have been replaced by IVF since these procedures need general anesthesia and laparoscopy. SET or TM-ET has a place in cases of severe cervical stenosis. In some patient profiles higher pregnancy rates is reported with ZIFT, TET, GIFT, as compared to uterine ET. Intravaginal culture (IVC) or intravaginal culture of oocytes (INVO) involves incubating the tubes containing the gametes in the vagina, Though this reduces costs and steps of laboratory set up, but this is not acceptable to many women. With the development of transport IVF and portable incubators this is not required. In transport IVF, the complete clinical phase, i.e., initial oocyte recovery as well as subsequent follow-up after ET, is done at a facility near the patient's home. The oocyte is transported by the husband to the central IVF unit which takes care of the laboratory phase and ET. Thus, the wife has to come to the central IVF unit only for ET.

Intracytoplasmic Sperm Injection (Flowchart 2)

Patients with severe male factor infertility with defects in sperm motility or morphology, various techniques can be used to aid sperm penetration. Partial zona dissection (PZD) and subzonal insemination (SUZI) have been used to improve

Flowchart 2: Indications of intracytoplasmic sperm injection.

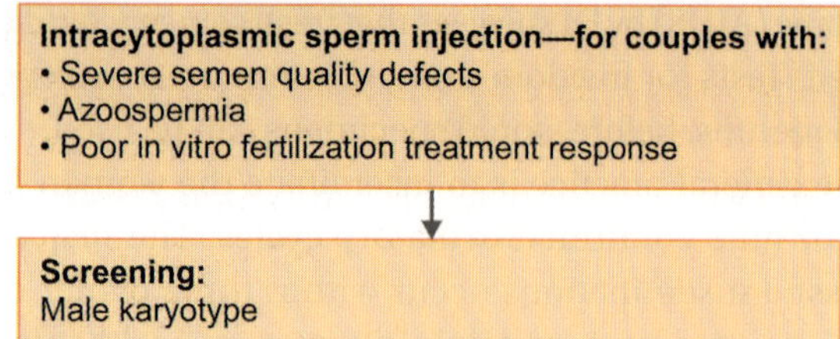

sperm penetration, but with limited success. In ICSI, special needles known as pipettes are used to stabilize oocyte and inject sperm respectively under an inverted microscope.

The technique is useful in cases of oligozoospermia, where conventional IVF has failed, or in azoospermia and aspermia. Various surgical sperm recovery techniques are available for these patients. These include rete testis aspiration (RETA), PESA, TESA, spermatocele aspiration (SPAS), microsurgical epididymal sperm extraction (MESA), and testicular sperm extraction (TESE). The choice of method depends on the diagnosis and that the procedure is diagnostic or therapeutic, and whether sperm will be used immediately for oocyte injection or it will be cryopreserved.

Percutaneous testicular sperm fine-needle aspiration (TESA, also called fine-needle aspiration, or FNA) is most commonly used technique. This may be used to in cases of post-testicular azoospermia or obstructive azoospermia (in which spermatogenesis is expected to be normal), with a successful sperm recovery in 96% of patients. TESA is simple procedure and well tolerated. It is usually done using a 21-gauge needle with local anesthesia. Alternatively, if the nature of the obstruction needs to be investigated by a full scrotal exploration, or if attempted surgical correction of the obstruction will be performed at the time of sperm recovery, MESA may be the preferred procedure. On the other hand, MESA is a useful surgical treatment in obstruction, if planned at the same time of sperm extraction. It is performed with general or regional anesthesia using a microsurgical approach. Advantage of MESA is that a large number of spermatozoa are usually retrieved, so that cryopreservation can be done and repeated procedures avoided. Fresh or frozen-thawed epididymal or testicular spermatozoa have similar fertilization and ongoing pregnancy rates when used for ICSI. PESA is done using a 19-gauge needle with local or regional anesthesia. Sperm recovery rate is greater than 80% with 55% fertilization and 33% ongoing pregnancy rates after ICSI. Although, this procedure is less invasive than others but it is blind. Bleeding and epididymal injury are possible, and postsurgical fibrosis may result. In contrast, men with testicular azoospermia or gonadal failure require TESE, and possibly multiple biopsies, to retrieve sperm. However, the sperm recovery rate with TESE is only about 50%, and clinical outcomes also variable.

Lower fertilization rates but comparable ongoing pregnancy rates have been reported for ICSI using testicular spermatozoa recovered from testicular azoospermia, compared with epididymal spermatozoa, post-testicular azoospermia. Sperm at all stages have been used to establish successful pregnancies using ICSI. However, the fertilization and pregnancy rates associated with maturation-arrested spermatid are very low, and proper counseling should be done about prognosis and alternative options.

Both fresh and frozen sperm can be used for further ICSI cycles. With a combination of different methods a 90–94% success in sperm retrieval can be reached. Regardless of sperm recovery method fertilization rates of 55% per oocyte, and pregnancy rates of 21–39% per ET have been achieved. Pregnancy outcome is similar to that with other ART pregnancies.

In addition, ICSI should be considered for those couples in whom a previous IVF cycle has resulted in failed or poor fertilization.

Laser-assisted Hatching

- Indium-Gallium-Arsenic phosphorus laser is used
- 1.48 μm wavelength.

Indications

- Thick zona pellucida
- Elderly patient
- Elevated basal FSH
- Failed implantation cycles
- Poor responders
- Unexplained infertility
- Few embryos
- IVF cycles
- Laser can also be used in ICSI where it prevents excessive cell deformation during injection. Zona thinning is advantageous with no loss of blastomeres. Generally, assisted hatching is done on Day 3 at 6–8 cell stage. A laser mounted micromanipulation is used. Multiple small holes are drilled.

Preimplantation Genetic Diagnosis

Medicine is evolving in the field of genetic analysis. When IVF cycles are considered, preimplantation genetic testing (PGT) is significant. Preimplantation genetic testing refers to genetic testing of oocyte or embryo done specially for those couples in whom one or both genetic parents have a known genetic abnormality and testing is performed on resultant embryo to determine, if it also carries same or different genetic abnormality. Preimplantation genetic screening (PGS) is another technique where embryos from presumed chromosomally normal genetic parents are checked for aneuploidy. Both techniques involve extraction of cell(s) from a developing embryo and subjected to genetic analysis and the results obtained are used as a guide to make a decision for an ET. An increase awareness and application of the technology has grown in the recent years.

There are three types of PGT, formerly known as PGD or preimplantation genetic diagnosis

1. *Preimplantation genetic testing for monogenic (single-gene) disorders (PGT-M):* PGT-M is a targeted genetic testing done on embryo when we are already aware of any known genetic abnormality in one or both parents. It can also be used to select embryos for transfer that has specific characteristics, gender, or compatible human leukocyte antigen complex type.
2. *Preimplantation genetic testing for structural rearrangements (PGT-SR):* This is done to detect any structural chromosomal abnormality (translocation) in the embryo in a couple with known balanced translocation or deletion/duplication. With technological advancement, it can be distinguished between normal noncarrier embryos from balanced carriers.
3. *Preimplantation genetic testing for aneuploidy (PGT-A) (formerly called PGS):* The goal of PGT-A is to identify in couples who are presumed to be normal any de novo aneuploidy, including subchromosomal deletions and additions (duplications). This can reduce the risk of miscarriage and improve the chance of conceiving a viable pregnancy.

These technologies are offered to older women, couples who have had a family history of chromosome anomalies, or who have undergone several miscarriages and failed IVF-attempts.

Benefits of PGT:

- Improved IVF success or pregnancy rates
- Decreases the risk for miscarriage and failed transfers.
- Increases the chance of a healthy pregnancy across all age groups
- Fewer cycles of IVF treatment needed (cost and time reduction)
- Allows for single-embryo transfer by identifying the embryo that has the best chances of implanting and leading to a healthy child.
- It can reduce the amount of time in between IVF cycles. IVF is required as part of this process even though many of these couples have no known difficulties conceiving a pregnancy. The inconvenience, risks, and expense of PGT limit the utilization of this technology.

OUTCOMES OF INFERTILITY TREATMENT

In women awaiting a successful pregnancy by IVF or other infertility treatment, 3–4% may conceive by chance naturally in the process of waiting for their turn.

On the other hand having an IVF baby does not mean that an IVF would be required for subsequent pregnancy. There have been incidences of second natural pregnancy in women with previous IVF birth especially in couple with unexplained infertility, pregnancy in an infertile woman, carry special risks. The chance of tubal pregnancy in those with tubal disease is fivefold greater than normal and that of abortion is double. The overall chance of obstetric complications such as prematurity, PIH, GDM is increased by one-third to a half. This increased incidence of complications is also due to increased age of infertile mother and associated medical problems. When, therefore, a pregnancy after prolonged infertility demands rigorous attention.

COMPLICATIONS OF ART

Twins and Higher-order Multiple Gestation

Multiple pregnancies especially higher-order multiple pregnancies is a serious complication of infertility treatment and has significant medical, psychological, social, and financial implications. 80% of higher order gestations are attributable to reproductive interventions, ART or non-ART infertility treatment.

Ovarian Hyperstimulation Syndrome

Ovarian hyperstimulation syndrome is a medical complication that is completely iatrogenic and unique to the treatment of infertility. The pathophysiology of OHSS is multifactorial but most can be attributed to local and systemic increase in capillary permeability. These changes, in turn, result in the depletion of intravascular volume, hemoconcentration, at the expense of third-space fluid accumulation.

Ovarian hyperstimulation syndrome has a varied spectrum of presentation. A staging system for OHSS is developed that would reflect symptom severity. This classification categorizes patient into mild, moderate, and severe disease. In mild OHSS, patients often complain of mild abdominal distension and soreness, nausea, and vomiting. Ovarian enlargement can be 5–12 cm. Moderate disease is marked by the presence of abdominal ascites on ultrasound examination. Severe disease is diagnosed when there are clinical signs of tense ascites, hydrothorax, shortness of breath, hemoconcentration, hypercoagulability, or any complications of OHSS such as renal failure, thromboembolism, or acute respiratory distress syndrome (ARDS) **(Table 2)**.

Golari's Classification of Ovarian Hyperstimulation Syndrome

Mild

- *Grade I:* Abdominal distension pain
- *Grade II:*
  - Grade I + nausea, vomiting, diarrhea
  - Ovary enlarge (<5 cm)
  - Weight gain (<3 kg)

Moderate

- *Grade III:*
  - Mild + Ultrasound evidence of ascites + hyponatremia, hypokalemia, hypoproteinemia

TABLE 2: Differences between early and late ovarian hyperstimulation syndrome.

Early ovarian hyperstimulation syndrome	*Late ovarian hyperstimulation syndrome*
Within 9 days of oocyte retrieval	After 9 days
Higher serum estradiol	Lower serum estradiol
Increased follicle number	Less follicle number
Increased follicular response	Multiple gestation
By exogenous human chorionic gonadotropin	By endogenous human chorionic gonadotropin of pregnancy

- Ovary less than or equal to 10 cm in size
- Weight gain 10 lbs
- Decreased urine output

Severe

- *Grade IV:*
  - Moderate + clinical ascites/hydrothorax, ARDS, ovary (>12 cm)
  - Weight gain (>5 kg)
- *Grade V:*
  - Grade IV + hypovolemia, hyponatremia, hyperkalemia
  - Increased blood viscosity, hypercoagulability
  - Decreased renal perfusion, oliguria, hypertension, hypoproteinemia, thrombosis, coagulation failure, electrolyte imbalance
  - Leucocytes more than 15,000/mm^3
  - Liver and kidney failure.
  - Severe OHSS mandates hospitalization.

Principles of Management

- *Monitor:* Fluid intake/urine output, hematocrit, electrolytes, AG/liver function, coagulation profile
- *Replace:* Crystalloids, fresh frozen plasma (FFP), human
- Serum albumin
- *Aspirate:* Ascitic tapping is therapeutic
- *Operate:* Only if hematoperitoneum or torsion or life-threatening OHSS
- *Conservative in mild to moderate:*
  - Bed rest
  - Intravenous fluids
  - Anti-inflammatory, antiemetics.

Age and Decreased Ovarian Reserve

An association between the age of the woman and reduced fertility has been well documented, with the decline in fecundability beginning in the early 30s but accelerating during the late 30s and early 40s. Chronologic age is the strongest determinant of reproductive success in spontaneous and ART cycles because it is a predictor of ovarian reserve.

The fecundability of women undergoing DI whose husbands are azoospermic provides insight into the effects of age on the fertility of the female alone. A French group that studied women enrolled in artificial insemination programs found that fertility rates begin to drop after 30 years of age. The pregnancy rate after 1 year of inseminations was 74% in women aged 30 years and younger, 62% in women aged 30–35 years, and 54% in women older than 35 years of age.

The physiology of declining fertility in older women is better understood in the light of data from oocyte donation programs. When embryos produced from oocytes retrieved from younger women are transferred into older women, the pregnancy rates among the older women approximate those of the younger women, and variations in pregnancy rates are directly dependent on the age of the donors, not that of the recipients. Several observations strongly support that it is the age of the oocyte, rather than the age of the endometrium, that accounts for the age-related decline in female fertility.

This oocyte-related decline in fertility is also known as decreased ovarian reserve. Absolute evidence of decreased ovarian reserve often can be ascertained only after ART treatment shows decreased ovarian responsiveness to COH. In ART, decreased ovarian reserve is reflected by an increased requirement for gonadotropins (FSH ± LH), small numbers of ovarian follicles and oocytes, and low serum estradiol levels during exogenous stimulation of folliculogenesis. These clinical outcomes probably reflect a decreased number of ovarian antral follicles as well as poor quality of granulosa cells and oocytes. Although age is the best predictor of ovarian reserve as reflected by ovarian responsiveness to COH, there is a subset of women who demonstrate an ovarian reserve that is prematurely diminished based on their chronologic age. Appropriate ovarian reserve test should be done that can be used to diagnose and then counsel patients in their management. But on the other hand there are women who respond well to COH and achieve pregnancies despite their advanced age. So, clinical response and laboratory finding can be varied in different patients.

Ovarian reserve tests (ORT) include serum day 3 FSH, clomiphene citrate challenge test (CCCT), serum inhibin B, and TVS to assess antral follicle number or ovarian size. Measurement of day 3 FSH is based on evidence that small increase in basal serum FSH levels correlates with the decreased fecundability seen among women in their late 30s. Antra follicle count is a good guide for a woman has less than four antral follicles, they usually are poor responders in IVF.

Serum inhibin B is produced by ovarian granulosa cells during the follicular phase of the menstrual cycle. It suppresses the production of FSH by the pituitary gland. Women with low ovarian reserve have a lower rise in the day 10 serum inhibin B levels in response to the CCCT. In addition, women with diminished ovarian reserve and normal day 3 FSH have been found to have low day 3 inhibin B levels. This finding suggests that a decrease in day 3 serum inhibin B levels may precede detectable changes in day 3 FSH levels. But does not predict pregnancy outcomes after AR, as inhibin B reflect granulosa cell function and thereby only predict ovarian response in ART.

ADOPTION

The adoption of a child is an individual choice, or on which individual outlooks vary. As in case of DI, adoption should be suggested as a possible option to consider. They should be guided and supported in this decision and made aware of the long waiting lists and limited availability of children.

If the husband and wife decide to opt for adoption, they should do so by the legal machinery operating in their area. The doctor cannot be a mediator or take responsibility in this they can only facilitate the process.

CONCLUSION

Infertility is rarely absolute. It may be seen in couples with congenital or acquired permanent loss of gametes in either partner or the absence of a uterus in the female. These couples should be counseled regarding their options of adoption, the use of donor gametes, or surrogacy. Most couples who have difficulty conceiving have subfertility. These couples could conceive spontaneously in time sometimes due to prolonged problem and impatience seeks medical intervention. Another reason to seek medical attention, is falling ovarian reserve and fecundity as woman ages.

Assisted reproductive techniques should be used to assist and decrease physical and mental pain of subfertility and infertility wherever possible. This is the aim and success of medical science ART has changed the methodology of treatment and seems to be an effective method of infertility treatment.

KEY MESSAGES

- *Assisted reproduction technology:* Topics covered.
- Indication of ART, COH, IUI, oocyte retrieval, semen preparation, IVF, ICSI, ET, cryopreservation, oocyte donation, sperm donation, male factor infertility, perimplantation genetic diagnosis, complications of ART, surrogacy, and adoption.

FURTHER READING

1. Brezina PR, Kutteh WH. Clinical applications of preimplantation genetic testing. BMJ. 2015.
2. Joshi N, Dmitry K, Anderson J. Trends and correlates of good perinatal outcomes in assisted reproductive technology. Obstet Gynecol. 2012;120(4):843-51.
3. Kushnir VA, Barad DH, Albertini DF. Systematic review of worldwide trends in assisted reproductive technology 2004-2013. Reprod Biol Endocrinol. 2017;15(1):6.
4. Luke B. Pregnancy and birth outcomes in couples with infertility with and without assisted reproductive technology: with an emphasis on US population-based studies. Am J Obstet Gynecol. 2017;217(3):270-81.

LONG QUESTIONS

1. Describe OHSS prevention and management.
2. Explain semen preparation techniques.
3. Explain third party reproduction.
4. Enumerate factors affecting embryo transfer.
5. Discuss controlled ovarian hyperstimulation.

SHORT QUESTIONS

Write short notes on:

1. Enumerate ART techniques
2. Indications of IUI
3. Semen analysis normal parameters
4. PGD
5. Laser-assisted hatching.

MULTIPLE CHOICE QUESTIONS

1. Full form of ART is:
   a. Artificial reproduction technology
   b. Artificial regenerative techniques
   c. Assisted reproduction technology
   d. Assisted reproduction techniques
2. Sperm retrieval techniques are all, except:
   a. TESA b. TESE
   c. MESA d. PZD
3. Sperm injection techniques are all, except:
   a. ICSI b. IMSI
   c. PICSI d. ZIFT
4. Embryo transfer, volume of fluid transferred is:
   a. 2 mL b. 0.2 mL
   c. 0.02 mL d. 0.05 mL
5. GnRH agonist are all, except:
   a. Leuprolide b. Buserelin
   c. Ganirelix d. Nafarelin
   e. Goserelin
6. OPU is performed how many hours after ovulation trigger?
   a. 32 hours b. 40 hours
   c. After ovulation d. 36 hours
7. Best protocol for OHSS prevention is:
   a. Long agonist b. Flare protocol
   c. Ultra long protocol d. Antagonist protocol
   e. Short protocol
8. Complication unique to ART:
   a. Multiple pregnancy b. Ectopic pregnancy
   c. Ovarian torsion d. OHSS
9. Cryoprotectants are all, except:
   a. 12-propanediol b. Glycerol
   c. Pentoxifylline d. DMSO
10. Surrogate mother in ART is a:
    a. Genetic mother b. Biological mother
    c. Gestational carrier d. Oocyte donor

Answers

1. c 2. d 3. d 4. c 5. c 6. d
7. d 8. d 9. c 10. c

12.12 ASSISTED REPRODUCTIVE TECHNOLOGIES: NEW TECHNIQUES AND RESEARCH

Hrishikesh Pai, Sunita Arora, Nandan Roongta, Rishma Dhillon Pai, Nandita Palshetkar

Be not the first by whom the new are tried;
nor yet the last to lay the old aside.

—Alexander Pope

INTRODUCTION

Since their inception, assisted reproduction technologies (ART) have followed the simplest of human physics; the fertilization of an oocyte by a sperm to create an embryo, to create life. The difference today lies in the path taken to achieve this same aim. Over the years that ART has been practiced, there has been a constant endeavor to improve the technology and overcome any obvious or presumed drawbacks. This endeavor has led to tremendous research in the field and a constant inflow of newer techniques. Some of these improvised techniques have led to better and safer results, while some have been cast away after an unsatisfactory trial.

There have been concerns regarding the iatrogenic propagation of certain genetic conditions, since ART also involves "forced" fertilization and the bypassing of certain natural filters to abnormal genes. These concerns have led research analysts to once again turn toward the basics and encourage the achievement of results by the least intervention possible.

All this then makes ART one of the most active research fields with ongoing improvisations aiming toward perfection. In this chapter we outline the main aspects of some of the newer technologies and research in ART.

FERTILITY ANALYSIS

Male Infertility Tests[1]

- *Sperm meiotic studies:*[2] Since the early 1990s male infertility has correctly been dealt with via way of means of intracytoplasmic sperm injection (ICSI), though concerns were raised concerning the genetic risk of ICSI. Chromosome aneuploidy (the presence of more or lacking chromosomes) is the leading cause of pregnancy loss and intellectual retardation in humans. While the bulk of chromosome aneuploidies are maternal in origin, the paternal contribution to aneuploidy is clinically relevant particularly for the sex chromosomes. Given that it is hard to contemplate female gametes examinations are overwhelmingly led in male meiotic recombination and sperm aneuploidy. Research suggests that infertile men have increased levels of sperm aneuploidy and that this is likely due to increased errors in meiotic recombination and chromosome synapses within these individuals.
- *Sperm-fluorescent in situ hybridization (FISH):*[3] Since the development of human sperm karyotyping, problems such as teratozoospermia, oligozoospermia, and translocations, have been identified. The current technique is an application of FISH which is used at interphase stage with careful enumeration of the labeled chromosomes to determine sperm ploidy. Typically, five to seven chromosomes are evaluated in ejaculated samples to determine the percent of aneuploid sperm present. This protocol will detail the procedures for: preparation of specimens, exposure of the sperm nuclei to the FISH probes, hybridization, detaining, and scoring criteria.
- *DNA fragmentation test:*[4] DNA integrity of sperm is of paramount importance for a healthy embryo. Increased DNA fragmentation index is associated with morphologically and genetically poor-quality embryos. Therefore, it is prudent to look for DNA integrity of sperms more so if unexpected poor quality embryos or apparent male factor. Smokers are seen to have higher levels of DNA fragmentation index. Semen samples with severe ologoasthenozoospermia are seen to have high index too. DNA fragmentation index 35% or more need to be addressed. As per some reports in literature, TESA samples may be better than ejaculated samples and may stand a better option.

Mutation Carrier and Genetic Studies[5]

Diminished fertility in either partner can potentially be due to chromosomal irregularity in one or both partners. Chromosomal aberrations comprise of numerical abnormality such as Klinefelter syndrome, XYY karyotype or Turner syndrome and its variants, sex reversion, such as XX males or XY females and structural abnormalities such as Robertsonian or reciprocal translocations and inversions. Other disorders such as cystic fibrosis, Fragile X syndrome, factor V Leiden, *prothrombin* gene, and *MHTFR* gene mutations should be ruled out. Infertility caused due to chromosomal aberrations if diagnosed in time has a prognostic value as it improves the management of pregnancies obtained after IVF ICSI and may also so we suggest prenatal or preimplantation genetic testing.

FERTILITY PRESERVATION

Mature Oocyte Cryopreservation

Substantial evidence now suggest that fertilization and pregnancy rates are similar when IVF ICSI is done that is fresh oocytes versus cryopreserved oocytes. There is no increase in incidence of chromosomal abnormalities, birth defects and developmental deficits in offspring born from cryopreserved oocytes versus conventional IVF ICSI in the general population. Evidence, though limited, indicates that oocyte vitrification and thawing should no longer be considered experimental.[6]

Success of oocyte cryopreservation was limited by the fragility of metaphase II (MII) oocytes related to its large size, water content and chromosomal arrangement mature oocytes (MII) retrieved after superovulation have the metaphase chromosomes lined up by the meiotic spindle along the equatorial plate. Studies demonstrate that the spindle apparatus may be damaged by intracellular ice formation during freezing or thawing technique. This damage may also be dependent on patient age, technique used and time Interval after thawing.

Alterations in methodology of slow freeze cryopreservation technique might be responsible for elevated survival of slow freezed-cryopreserved mature oocytes.

- *Modifications in technique include:*
  - Initial temperature of cryoprotectant
  - Seeding temperature
  - Timing after oocyte retrieval
- *Modifications in composition of cryoprotectant:* Recent studies suggest that vitrification for oocyte cryopreservation significantly improves oocyte survival and pregnancy rate.
- As stated in most studies that survival rates of oocytes which are vitrified are superior than those which have underground slow freeze technique.
- Also, the recovery rate of meiotic spindle was faster in vitrified oocytes as compared oocytes which were cryopreserved using slow freezing protocols.

Some existing concerns:

- To minimize ice crystal formation by maximized ultra-rapid cooling the US size are directly exposed to liquid nitrogen in an "open" system this is used in most vitrification techniques.

  A theoretical concern regarding this "open" system is a risk of exposure of sides to any infectious organisms which might be present in contaminated liquid nitrogen. Methods to sterilize liquid nitrogen are being developed like microfiltration technique and ultraviolet radiation (UV) though infectious transmission has never been observed as such in reproductive tissue. Vitrification can also be done in a "closed" system but currently data does not exist if it is as successful as open system.
- Cumulus cells are removed from oocytes to assess the maturity before cryopreservation. ICSI is generally used for fertilizing previously cryopreserved thawed oocytes as removing the cumulus cells has shown to decrease fertilization after standard insemination, also zona hardening has been elicited after thawing cryopreserved oocytes. While some studies may suggest that ICSI may improve fertilization by overcoming changes in zona pellucida caused by freezing, it is still not documented if ICSI is actually necessary for fertilization of frozen thawed oocytes.

Embryo Cryopreservation[7-9]

Vitrification has many advantages over slow freezing for cryopreservation of cleavage stage embryos such as higher post thaw survival, minimal ill effects on morphology and better clinical outcome. Vitrification and slow freezing technique when used for blastocyst give the same percentage of implantation and clinical pregnancy rate. For slow growing blastocysts cryopreservation can be done on day 6 which has yielded a better survival, implantation, and pregnancy rate.

Ovarian Tissue Cryopreservation[10,11]

First ovarian tissue cryopreservation (OTC) was done in 1997 which resulted in first successful birth in September 2004 by Professor Donnez of Louvain in Belgium.

Indications

- When prophylactic oophorectomy is indicated in case of any benign ovarian disease requiring ablative surgery (surgical menopause)
- Before exposure to gonadotoxic drugs and radiation (cancer, autoimmune disease, hematologic disorders requiring a bone marrow transplant)
- Women at increased risk of premature ovarian failure (Turner's, Trisomy, Fragile X syndrome, autoimmune disease)
- Fertility preservation for social reasons.

Advantages

- Large number of primordial follicles are preserved and these being small and undifferentiated are less likely to be damaged by freezing technique
- Ovarian tissue can be preserved at any stage of menstrual cycle thereby minimizing delay in cancer treatment or radiation therapy
- Once reimplanted patient will have restored endocrine and fertility function
- No requirement of spermatozoa
- No dilemma of embryo storage and disposal (ethical reasons).

Disadvantages

- It is a surgical procedure
- Loss of 60% of all follicles
- Graft has a shorter lifespan
- Cancers which metastasize to ovary result in harboring malignant cells in ovary
- Low rate of survival of follicles
- Experimental study.

Major advances in ovarian tissue cryopreservation have occurred and are still under research.

Follicle Culture In Vitro

Metastatic spread of certain cancers can occur if the ovarian tissue grafted has any evidence of malignancy at the time of preservation. Additional precautionary methods need to be utilized to minimize risk of cancer potentiation. In vitro follicle culture technique would allow follicles to be isolated from frozen thawed tissue and grow to maturity in-vitro. Inception of this technique is recent. Overcoming the growth arrest observed in current in vitro culture systems requires better understanding of physical environment of follicle, growth factors, metabolic needs of preantral follicles and physiology of follicle growth initiation.

Once outside the natural environment, follicles have to cope with changes in oxygen tension, temperature, and uptake of nutrients thereby compelling ovarian follicle culturist to take assistance of tissue engineers.

In Vitro Maturation of Oocytes

Cha et al. reported first in vitro maturation (IVM) birth from immature oocytes derived from oocyte donors. The first IVM baby from mothers own immature oocytes was in 1994. Worldwide over 5,000 IVM babies have still been born.

Oocyte retrieval is performed according to a simple protocol with decreased or no hormonal stimulation. After retrieval oocytes are matured in vitro with LH supplemented media and ICSI is then performed. By minimizing or eliminating ovarian stimulation, this protocol is less expensive and time consuming. In addition it completely avoids the risk of OHSS. IVM can be particularly useful in cancer patients undergoing fertility preservation as it can avoid potentially toxic exposure to high doses of estradiol and may expedite the introduction of appropriate oncological treatment.

In vitro maturation of oocytes has been suggested to avoid ovarian stimulation and time requirement in patients with cancer and can be combined with ovarian tissue cryobanking.[12]

IMPROVING THE IN VITRO FERTILIZATION RESULTS

The "raw material" decides the quality of the "final product", so also in assisted reproduction. Hence it is very important to have good "quality" of oocytes, sperm, and hence embryos **(Fig. 1)**.

Assessment of the Oocyte

Polar Body Biopsy

Biopsy for implantation genetic profiling can be done at three stages by testing the first polar body, second polar body, and trophectoderm (D5/D6) biopsy.

Opening the zona pellucida is done mechanically (partial zona dissection) or chemically (acidic Tyrode's solution), now with introduction of noncontact laser, this method has become indispensable.

It is well acknowledged that biopsy is an invasive technique.

It is believed that removal of polar bodies from MII oocytes and fertilized zygotes, may have the least detrimental effects on subsequent embryo thereby increasing its application.

Polarization Microscopy (PolarAIDE)[13-15] (Fig. 2)

Main features:

- Quantification of the bifringement of zona pellucida
- Automatic scoring of the developmental potential of oocytes in seconds
- Orientation independent live imaging of meiotic spindle
- Simultaneous view of oocyte morphology and spindle
- Spindle imaging under normal light intensity (bright field).

Structures within the oocyte (like the meiotic spindle and the zona pellucida) possess natural by fringes which have been identified by introduction of polarizing light microscopy systems.[16] This imaging is a novel approach in assessment of oocyte and embryo viability. Studies on the use of polarization microscopy on sperm are still under research.

Automatic assessment and scoring of oocyte quality and developmental potential: Transfer of embryos fertilized by

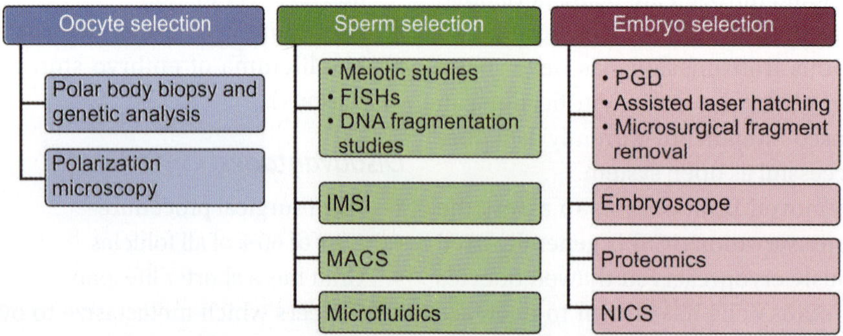

Fig. 1: Techniques to improve the in vitro fertilization results.
(IMSI: intracytoplasmic morphologically selected sperm injection; FISH: fluorescent in situ hybridization; PGD: preimplantation genetic diagnosis; MACS: magnetic-activated cell sorting; NICS: noninvasive chromosome screening)

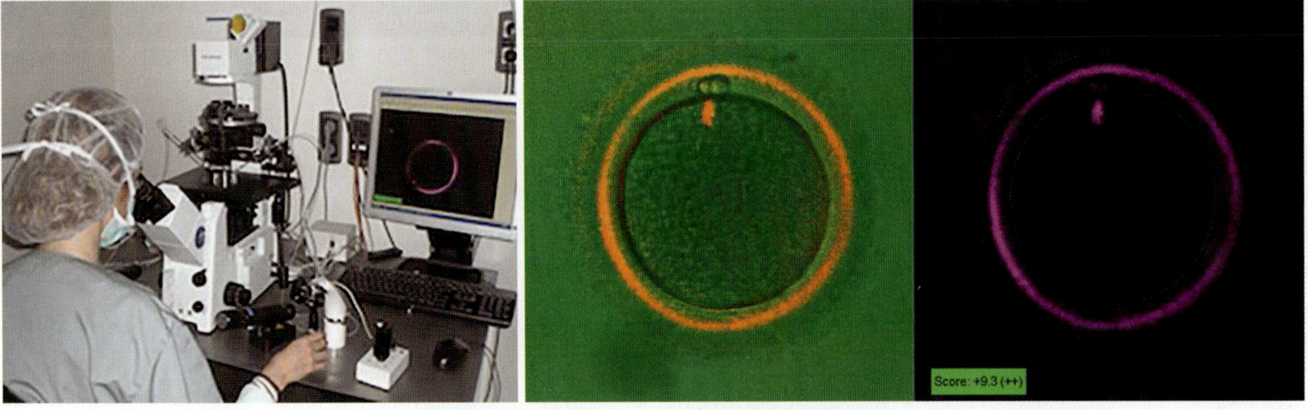

Fig. 2: Polarization microscopy (PolarAIDE).[13-15]

oocytes with high birefringence of zona pellucida resulted in significantly elevated pregnancy rates as compared to the conventional pronuclear scoring. Inspecting the zona birefringence to recognize the best zygotes resulted in significantly higher pregnancy rates.

Oocyte maturity evaluation: Different meiotic stages can be identified distinctly. Oocyte maturity is evaluated after in vitro maturation (IVM) in cases of low responders or before polar body biopsy and to optimize the timing of ICSI or polar body biopsy.

Quality control: The spindle is delicate and highly sensitive to suboptimal pH and temperature. Increased number of oocytes displaying spindles indicate suitable temperature and pH environment in dish placed under the microscope.

Assessment of the Sperm

IMSI[15-17] (Fig. 3)

Intracytoplasmic sperm injection is a potent tool in male factor infertility. Intracytoplasmic morphologically selected sperm injection (IMSI) is a progressive technique where prior to ICSI the sperm morphology is evaluated under high magnification.

Intracytoplasmic morphologically selected sperm injection is an automated software solution for live sperm morphology analysis, based on the motile sperm organelle morphology examination (MSOME) in magnifications in excess of 6000X to select sperm with morphologically normal nuclei **(Table 1)**.

Parameters studied are the head shape, size, the middle piece, and number of vacuoles. Many authors have suggested a market rise in ICSI outcomes following IMSI especially in male factor infertility.[18,19] Study conducted by Schachter et al. in 2019 suggested that IMSI can Improve IVF results in severe cases of male infertility.[20]

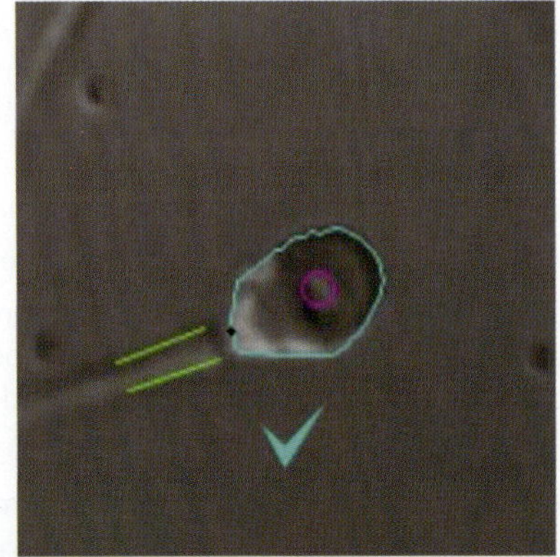

Parameter:	Value:
Object type:	Cell
Head length:	5.4 μm
Head width:	3.8 μm
Head area:	19.3 μm²
No. of vacuoles:	1

Cell classification:	
Head size:	Normal
Shape:	Slight
Vacuoles:	Acceptable
Mid-piece:	Normal
OUTCOME:	Sub-normal

Fig. 3: Live sperm morphology analysis using IMSI, an automated software solution based on the Motile Sperm Organelle Morphology Examination (MSOME).[15-17]

ASSESSMENT AND SELECTION OF THE EMBRYO

Improving outcomes in IVF pregnancies in terms of pregnancy rates and Implantation rates involves selecting the morphologically best embryos for transfer. With great advances in embryo assessment and selection procedures the morphology of each embryo can be assessed in a better way thus providing substantial success in IVF procedures.

ANNEXIN V MAGNETIC ACTIVATED CELL SORTING[17]

Annexin V magnetic activated cell sorting (MACS) is an efficient method of sperm selection used for separating nonapoptotic spermatozoa. It was first reported by Grunewald et al. in 2001.[21] The negatively charged phospholipid phosphatidylserine is present in the cytosolic leaflet of plasma membrane lipid bilayer and its redistribution is an early event in apoptosis. Annexin V has a high affinity for phosphatidylserine and sperms magnetically labeled with Annexin V microbeads are passed through MACs column placed in magnetic field.

TABLE 1: Live sperm morphology analysis using IMSI based on the Motile Sperm Organelle Morphology Examination (MSOME).[15-17]

IMSI	*Classification parameters*	
Normal	To be classified as *normal, all* sperm parameters must match normal criteria	
Size	Normal	Within the range of: 4.0 µm > Length > 6.0 µm 2.5 µm > Width> 4.0 µm
Shape	Normal	Perfect oval shape
Vacuoles	Normal	No vacuoles
Mid-piece	Normal	Straight and thin without cytoplasmic droplets
Subnormal	To be classified as *subnormal*, at least *one* sperm parameter must match subnormal criteria, but none should match abnormal criteria	
Size	Marginal	The marginal classification is used to allow for slight tolerances in image pixel resolution (magnification changed slightly after initial slide calibration). Marginal size classification using 15% tolerance will accept sperm cell heads of: Length is in range of: *Low:* 3.4 µm < Length < 4.0 µm *High:* 6.0 µm < Length < 6.9 µm Width is in range of: *Low:* 2.1 µm < Width < 2.5 µm *High:* 4.0 µm < Wldlh < 4.6 µm
Shape	Slight	Slightly amorphous shape that is almost normal, but has a minor deviation
Vacuoles	Acceptable	1 or 2 vacuoles detected
Mid-piece	Unknown	Mid-piece classification of "unknown" means that the software was not able to characterize the mid-piece, either because of complexities in the background image (other objects near-by) or because the mid-piece is not very clear
Abnormal	To be classified as *abnormal*, at least *one* sperm parameter must match abnormal criteria	
Size	Abnormal	Abnormal size applies to any cell head dimension outside the marginal tolerances. For 15% tolerance, the abnormal classifications are: • *Long:* Length is more than 6.9 µm • *Short:* Length is less than 3.4 µm • *Wide:* Width is more than 4.6 µm • *Narrow:* Width is less than 2.1 µm
Shape	Amorphous	Amorphous indicates any shape that does not satisfy normal or subnormal criteria
Vacuoles	Abnormal	More than two vacuoles detected
Mid-piece	Abnormal	The following mid-piece abnormalities are detected: • Thick mid-piece • Skew mid-piece junction into cell head • Conical shape either due to wide attachment to cell head or presence of debris at junction

The magnetically labeled phosphatidylserine exposing cells are retained in the column allowing recovery of non-apoptotic spermatozoa.[22] However this technique is not applicable in asthenozoospermic samples. Studies have shown that when AV-MACS is combined with double density gradient before ICSI there is a higher implantation rate.[23]

Sperm Selection Based on Sperm Motility (Microfluidics)[24]

Microfluidics is a technique where small amounts of microfluids are passed through traversal devices. Microfluidics allows sperm selection not only in a very gentle but fast way without leading to procedure associated loss of DNA.[25] Microfluidic chip method may be recommended in patients with recurrent IVF/ICSI failure.[26]

Preimplantation Genetic Testing: Monogenetic Disorders/Preimplantation Genetic Testing for Aneuploidy[27,28]

Preimplantation genetic testing identifies genetic aberrations in the embryos in preimplantation stage by biopsying the embryos obtained by IVF/ICSI. It can be used for screening single gene disorders (PGT-M) and aneuploidy (PGT-A). It was first described in 1990 by Handyside et al. after their team was able to transfer only female embryos in two women known to be carriers of X-linked disease.

Genetic testing can be done from different stages of embryo development like polar body biopsy, Blastomere biopsy from Day 3 cleavage stage embryo or trophectoderm biopsy from blastocyst stage embryo and either fluorescence in situ hybridization or polymerase chain reaction is used to identify specific genetic or chromosomal traits. Till now out of different stages, trophectoderm biopsy at blastocyst stage is supposed to be the best. PGT-M and PGT-SR are more encouraging and more accepted as compared to PGT-A worldwide. Though theoretically it seems to improve the implantation rates and decrease the miscarriage rates.[29]

Noninvasive Chromosomal Screening[30]

Invasiveness and complexity of PGS may limit its clinical applicability. Unlike PGS, noninvasive chromosomal screening/testing (NICS) avoids need for embryo biopsy and is based on MALBAC (multiple annealing and looping based amplification cycle) technique for WGA (whole genome amplification). The technique is based on sequencing of genomic DNA secreted into the culture medium from the developing blastocyst. Study by Juan et al.[30] indicates positive predictive value and negative predictive value respectively 78.9 % and 91.3%

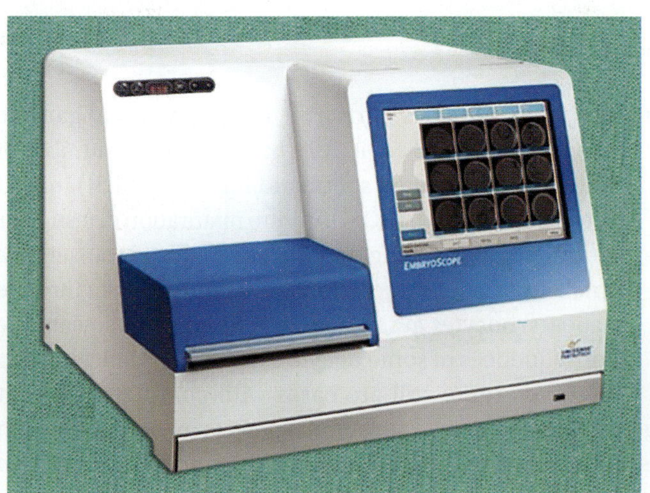

Fig. 4: Embryoscope.[31]

- *Embryoscope* **(*Fig. 4*)**:[31] The embryoscope is a highly sophisticated instrument containing an incubator, microscope and computer. This time-lapse video **(Fig. 5)** observation of the embryo may be used to gain a broader understanding of embryo viability. The principal advantages of the embryoscope are less manipulation of embryos reduces risk of harm, instant and continuous monitoring of all embryos, accurate regulation of CO_2 and unique temperature control, and complete and accurate documentation of all embryos.
- *Proteomics:*[32,33] Proteomics and metabolomics the Omics technologies) are useful[1] tools for assessing the development potential of an embryo. There are different Omics sciences such as *genomics, transcriptomics, metabolomics,* ***(Fig. 6)*** *and proteomics.* Now it is possible to test the culture environment of a developing embryo to check its viability. The oxygen consumption of the embryos can be tested by using these techniques and one can also test the soluble HLA-G present in the human embryo secretome in[1] the environment as it is associated with higher implantation rates. Amino acid turnover (*asparagine, glycine and leucine*) are an indicator of embryo viability as they are correlated to the development of the blastocyst. Predicting embryo viability by analyzing the metabolome of different stage embryos and embryo selection using the metabolomics

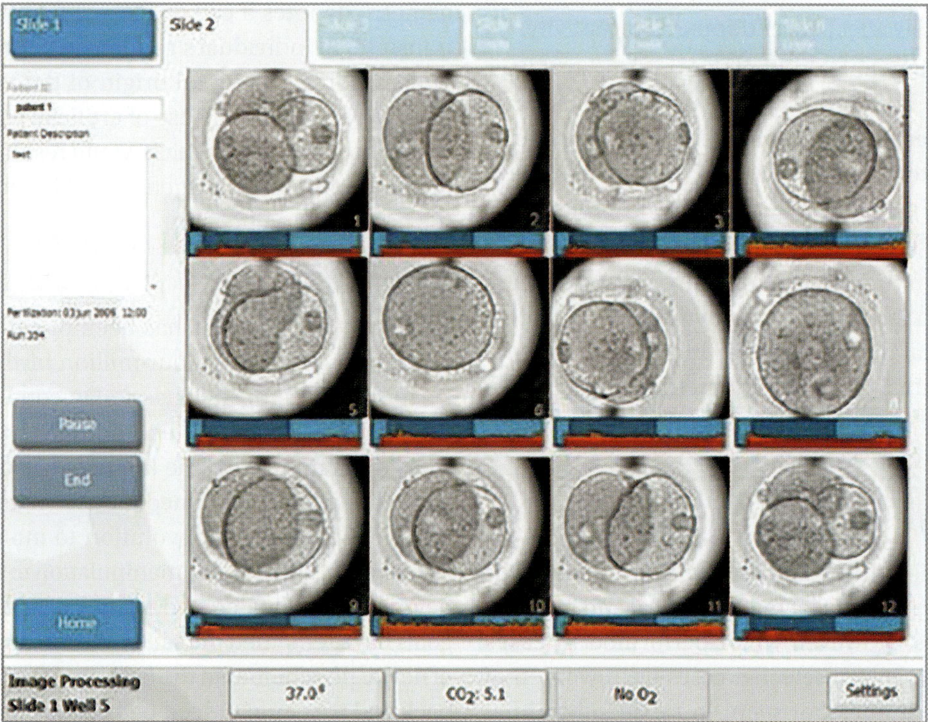

Fig. 5: Time-lapse video observation of the embryo.[31]

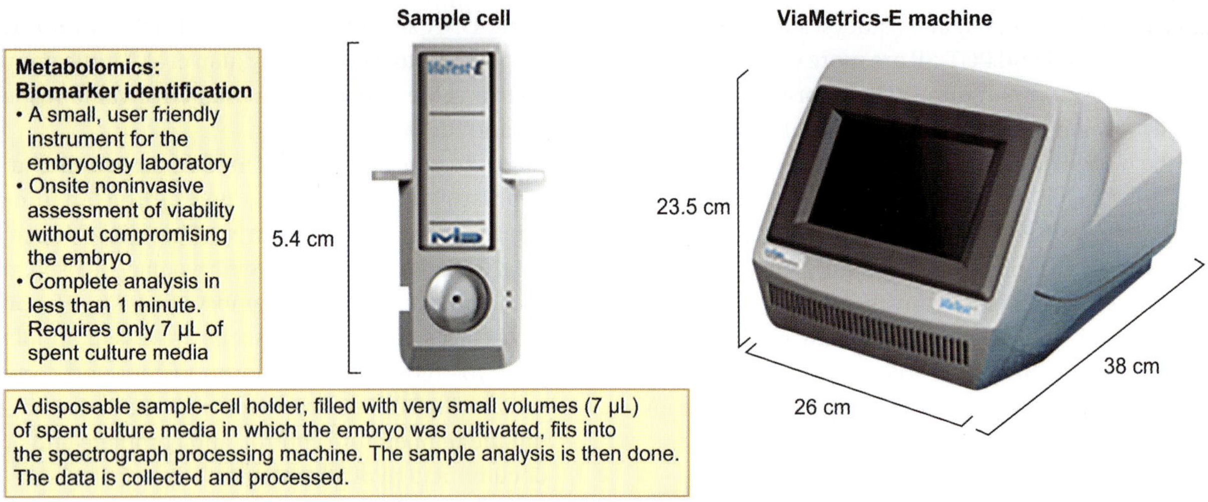

Sample cell

ViaMetrics-E machine

Metabolomics: Biomarker identification
- A small, user friendly instrument for the embryology laboratory
- Onsite noninvasive assessment of viability without compromising the embryo
- Complete analysis in less than 1 minute. Requires only 7 µL of spent culture media

5.4 cm

23.5 cm

26 cm

38 cm

A disposable sample-cell holder, filled with very small volumes (7 µL) of spent culture media in which the embryo was cultivated, fits into the spectrograph processing machine. The sample analysis is then done. The data is collected and processed.

Fig. 6: Metabolomics.[32,33]

profile helps improve implantation and pregnancy rates. From a clinical perspective, the morphologic assessment of embryo and invasive analysis of human embryo secretome will improve IVF success rates and pave the way for higher possibility of single embryo transfers. This research will have a major social impact as well as great commercial application.

Improving the Implantation Chances

Proteomic analysis of the endometrium:[34] Abnormal endometrial receptivity is a major cause of Implantation failures. During the window of implantation the endometrium has a different proteomic repertoire. Various gynecological disorders such as endometriosis, polycystic ovarian syndrome or tubal diseases can adversely affect the endometrial receptivity.

With the advancing Omics technologies investigators have been able to define both molecular signatures and specific biomarkers of a receptive endometrium. New research involving transcriptomic and proteomic technologies have been able to analyze gene- or protein-expression-profile shifts between the pre-receptive and receptive secretory stages.

Secretomics is another useful alternative to assess endometrial maturation and receptivity without need of an invasive endometrial biopsy by collecting the endometrial cell secretions poured into the endometrial cavity. It can give additional useful information regarding endometrial physiology and day of cycle.

Assisted Hatching

- In repeated IVF failures and frozen-thawed embryos assisted hatching leads to increased clinical and multiple pregnancy rates. However, when performed in cases of fresh transfers in nonselected cases or in women of advanced age[35] it does not seem to cause substantial increase in clinical pregnancy rates.
- *Artificial gametes:* For the couple with a gamete abnormality or lack of it, ART has helped in a number of ways: ICSI, elongated spermatid injection (ELSI), round spermatid injection (ROSI), in vitro maturation of testicular germ cells, genetic engineering that involved transfer of a small amount of cytoplasm from a donor oocyte into the patients' oocytes at the time of ICSI helped alleviate the consequences of some oocyte cytoplasmic deficiencies.

However, there still are cases with completely absent germline or gametes with serious defects incompatible with embryo creation. Though gamete donation is an efficient therapeutic tool in these situations, it is not always accepted by the infertile couple. It is for them that ART has been researching the "artificial gametes".[36,37] The term "artificial gamete" denotes a cell or cell component which is able to transmit the individual's genome to a biparentally gendered embryo. This biparental origin of the embryos makes the difference between the use of artificial gametes for ART, and reproductive cloning, which would result in mono parentally derived embryos whose genome will be identical with that of the parent of origin.

CONCLUSION

Reproductive medicine has been practiced since 1978 and has resulted in almost four million births worldwide. With a rapid evolution, ART has today come a long way and a number of IVF-related techniques have been introduced since then, more so in the last two decades. There has been a rapid transition from medicine to surgery and now we are experiencing a further evolution to molecular and genetic approaches. Today micromanipulation in the laboratory is the new operative theater. And to think of it, all along the way, the goals have remained the same. With an ever increasing range of newer possibilities in the field, there seems to be no looking back and we could indeed be heading towards a new world, a "Brave New World"![38]

REFERENCES

1. The Male Infertility Best Practice Policy Committee of the American Urological Association and the Practice Committee of the American Society for Reproductive Medicine. Report on optimal evaluation of the infertile male. Fertil Steril. 2006;86(Suppl 4):2-9.
2. Tempest HG. Meiotic recombination errors, the origin of sperm aneuploidy and clinical recommendations. Syst Biol Reprod Med. 2011;57(1-2):93-101.
3. Emery BR. Sperm aneuploidy testing using fluorescence in situ hybridization. Methods Mol Biol. 2013;927:167-73.
4. Sakkas D, Alvarez JG. Sperm DNA fragmentation: mechanisms of origin, impact on reproductive outcome, and analysis. Fertil Steril. 2010;93(4):14-9.
5. Chantot-Bastaraud S, Ravel C, Siffroi JP. Underlying karyotype abnormalities in IVF/ICSI patients. Reprod Biomed Online. 2008;16(4):514-22.
6. The Practice Committees of the American Society for Reproductive Medicine and the Society for Assisted Reproductive Technology. Mature oocyte cryopreservation: a guideline. Fertil Steril. 2012:S0015-0282(12)02247-9.
7. Liebermann J, Tucker MJ. Comparison of vitrification and conventional cryopreservation of day 5 and day 6 blastocysts during clinical application. Fertil Steril. 2006;86(1):20-6.
8. Sifer C, Sermondade N, Dupont C, Poncelet C, Cédrin-Durnerin I, Hugues JN, et al. [Outcome of embryo vitrification compared to slow freezing process at early cleavage stages. Report of the first French birth]. Gynecol Obstet Fertil. 2012;40(3):158-61.
9. Li Y, Chen ZJ, Yang HJ, Zhong WX, Ma SY, Li M. Comparison of vitrification and slow-freezing of human day 3 cleavage stage embryos: post-vitrification development and pregnancy outcomes. Zhonghua Fu Chan Ke Za Zhi. 2007;42(11):753-5.
10. Smitz J, Dolmans MM, Donnez J, Fortune JE. Current achievements and future research directions in ovarian tissue culture, in vitro follicle development and transplantation: implications for fertility preservation. Hum Reprod Update. 2010;16(4):395-414.
11. Grynberg M, Poulain M, Sebag-Peyrelevade S, LeParco S, Fanchin R, Frydman N. Ovarian tissue and follicle transplantation as an option for fertility preservation. Fertil Steril. 2012;97(6):1260-8.
12. Grynberg M, Hesters L, Bénard J, Trèves R, Fanchin R, Frydman R, et al. In vitro maturation of oocytes: an option for fertility preservation in women. J Gynecol Obstet Biol Reprod (Paris). 2011;40(2):103-8.
13. Montag M, van der Ven H. Symposium: innovative techniques in human embryo viability assessment. Oocyte assessment and embryo viability prediction: birefringence imaging. Reprod Biomed Online. 2008;17(4):454-60.
14. Montag M, Köster M, van der Ven K, van der Ven H. Gamete competence assessment by polarizing optics in assisted reproduction. Hum Reprod Update. 2011;17(5):654-66.
15. Simon L, Wilcox A, Carrell DT. Intracytoplasmic morphology-selected sperm injection. Methods Mol Biol. 2013;927:247-56.
16. Berkovitz A, Eltes F, Lederman H, Peer S, Ellenbogen A, Feldberg B, et al. How to improve IVF-ICSI outcome by sperm selection. Reprod Biomed Online. 2006;12(5):634-8.
17. Oseguera-López I, Ruiz-Díaz S, Ramos-Ibeas P, Pérez-Cerezales S. Novel techniques of sperm selection for improving IVF and ICSI outcomes. Front Cell Development Biol. 2019;7:2.
18. Knez K, Zorn B, Tomazevic T, Vrtacnik-Bokal E, Virant-Klun I. The IMSI procedure improves poor embryo development in the same infertile couples with poor semen quality: a comparative prospective randomized study. Reproduct Biol Endocrinol. 2011;9(1):123.
19. Dalal RY, Pai HD, Palshetkar NP, Mishra AP. Intracytoplasmic Morphologically selected Sperm Injection vs Intracytoplasmic Sperm Injection: a Retrospective Analysis. Int J Infertil Fetal Med. 2011;3:101-5.
20. Schachter-Safrai N, Karavani G, Reuveni-Salzman A, Gil M, Ben-Meir A. Which semen analysis correlates with favorable Intracytoplasmic morphologically selected sperm injection (IMSI) outcomes? Eur J Obstet Gynecol Reprod Biol. 2019;234:85-8.
21. Grunewald S, Paasch U, Glander HJ. Enrichment of non-apoptotic human spermatozoa after cryopreservation by immunomagnetic cell sorting. Cell Tissue Bank. 2001;2(3):127-33.
22. Gil M, Sar-Shalom V, Sivira YM, Carreras R, Checa MA. Sperm selection using magnetic activated cell sorting (MACS) in assisted reproduction: a systematic review and meta-analysis. J Assist Reprod Genet. 2013;30(4):479-85.
23. García-Ferreyra J, Villegas L, Romero R, Zavala P, Hilario R, Dueñas-Chacón J. High pregnancy and implantation rates can be obtained using Magnetic-Activated Cell Sorting (MACS) to selection Spermatozoa in patients with high levels of spermatic DNA fragmentation. JFIV Reprod Med Genet. 2014;2(133):17-9.
24. Samuel R, Feng H, Jafek A, Despain D, Jenkins T, Gale B. Microfluidic—based sperm sorting & analysis for treatment of male infertility. Translat Androl Urol. 2018;7(Suppl 3):S336.
25. Nosrati R, Gong MM, San Gabriel MC, Pedraza CE, Zini A, Sinton D. Microfluidics based quantification of male fertility potential. Clin Chem. 2016;62(3):458-65.
26. Yildiz K, Yuksel S. Use of microfluidic sperm extraction chips as an alternative method in patients with recurrent in vitro fertilisation failure. J Assist Reprod Genet. 2019;36(7):1423-9.
27. Levin I, Almog B, Shwartz T, Gold V, Ben-Yosef D, Shaubi M, et al. Effects of laser polar-body biopsy on embryo quality. Fertil Steril. 2012;97(5):1085-8.
28. Xu K, Montag M. New perspectives on embryo biopsy: not how, but when and why? Semin Reprod Med. 2012;30(4):259-66.
29. Munné S. Preimplantation genetic diagnosis for aneuploidy and translocations using array comparative genomic hybridization. Curr Genomics. 2012;13(6):463-70.
30. Xu J, Fang R, Chen L, Chen D, Xiao JP, Yang W, et al. Noninvasive chromosome screening of human embryos by genome sequencing of embryo culture medium for in vitro fertilization. Proceed Nat Acad Sci. 2016;113(42):11907-12.
31. Kovacs P. Embryo selection: the role of time-lapse monitoring. Reprod Biol Endocrinol. 2014;12(1):124.
32. Katz-Jaffe MG, McReynolds S, Gardner DK, Schoolcraft WB. The role of proteomics in defining the human embryonic secretome. Mol Hum Reprod. 2009;15(5):271-7.
33. Nel-Themaat L, Nagy ZP. A review of the promises and pitfalls of oocyte and embryo metabolomics. Placenta. 2011;32(Suppl 3):S257-63.
34. Berlanga O, Bradshaw HB, Vilella-Mitjana F, Garrido-Gómez T, Simón C. How endometrial secretomics can help in predicting implantation. Placenta. 2011;32(Suppl 3):S271-5.

35. Martins WP, Rocha IA, Ferriani RA, Nastri CO. Assisted hatching of human embryos: a systematic review and meta-analysis of randomized controlled trials. Hum Reprod Update. 2011;17(4): 438-53.
36. Gardner DK, Rizk BR, Falcone T. Human Assisted Reproductive Technology: Future Trends in Laboratory and Clinical Practice. Cambridg: Cambridge University Press; 2011.
37. Kashir J, Jones C, Child T, Williams SA, Coward K. Viability assessment for artificial gametes: the need for biomarkers of functional competency. Biol Reprod. 2012;87(5):114.
38. Huxley A. Brave New World. Albatross Library. 1934.

LONG QUESTIONS

1. Enumerate and explain the available and experimental technologies for oocyte, sperm, and embryo selection in the IVF laboratory.
2. Explain the fertility preservation technologies available today.

SHORT QUESTIONS

1. Explain preimplantation genetic diagnosis (PGD) and preimplantation genetic screening (PGS).
2. What are the main features of polarization microscopy?
3. What are the main features of embryoscopy?
4. What are the fertility preservation options for a woman affected by cancer prior to the treatment of the cancer?
5. What are the advantages of the IMSI technology?
6. Explain the application of the proteomics technology in embryo selection.

MULTIPLE CHOICE QUESTIONS

1. Oocyte selection techniques include:
   a. 1st polar body biopsy and genetic studies
   b. Polarization microscopy
   c. Follicular fluid assessment
   d. Ultrasonographic assessment of the oocyte
2. Sperm selection techniques include:
   a. Sperm meiotics
   b. Sperm FISH studies
   c. Sperm DNA fragmentation test
   d. Sperm microscopy IMSI
3. Embryo selection techniques include:
   a. Embryo PGD b. Embryoscopy
   c. Embryo "Omics" d. Embryo size
4. The Embryoscope consists of:
   a. Incubator b. Microscope
   c. Computer d. Embryo biopsy devices
5. Preimplantation genetic diagnosis (PGD) can be done at the following stages:
   a. 1st polar body from oocyte
   b. 2nd polar body from fertilized zygote
   c. Blastomere(s) from Day-3 embryos
   d. Trophectoderms from day 5/6 Blastocysts
6. Polarization microscopy uses the principle of:
   a. Oocyte polar body microscopy
   b. Detection of structures within oocytes that possess a natural birefringence
   c. Magnification of the oocyte by more than 6000X
   d. Detecting the axis of the opposite poles of the oocyte
7. In IMSI the sperm are examined under a magnification of:
   a. More than 6000X
   b. More than 2000X
   c. Approximately 16 times more than for ICSI
   d. Approximately 60 times more than for ICSI
8. Metabolomics assessment of embryo culture environment includes study of:
   a. Oxygen consumption
   b. Soluble HLA-G on the human embryo secretome
   c. Amino acid turnover
   d. Color of the spent media
9. In vitro maturation (IVM) can be used in:
   a. PCOS cases to avoid OHSS
   b. IVM of immature cryopreserved oocytes for fertility preservation
   c. For research purposes
   d. Low cost setups to reduce treatment costs
10. Fertility preservation technology does not include:
    a. Oocyte and sperm cryopreservation
    b. Ovarian tissue preservation
    c. Ovarian transposition procedure
    d. Embryo cryopreservation

Answers

1. a, b	2. a, b, c, d	3. a, b, c	4.	a, b, c
5. a, b, c, d	6. b	7. a, c	8.	a, b, c
9. a, b, c, d	10. c			

12.13 RECURRENT PREGNANCY LOSS

Mala Arora

INTRODUCTION

Recurrent pregnancy loss (RPL) was earlier defined as three or more consecutive pregnancy losses at 20 weeks or less or with fetal weight of less than 500 g.[1,2] The ACOG changed it to two or more spontaneous miscarriages for clinical purposes.[3] American Society of Reproductive Medicine (ASRM) defines *recurrent pregnancy loss* as two or more failed clinical pregnancies, which should be documented by either ultrasound or histopathological examination. None of the definitions include biochemical pregnancies, ectopic pregnancies or pregnancy of uncertain location.

CAUSES OF RECURRENT MISCARRIAGES

The causes of recurrent miscarriages are:

- *Immunological: Autoimmune*
  - Primary antiphospholipid syndrome (PAPS)
  - Secondary antiphospholipid syndrome (SAPS): SLE, autoimmune conditions
  - Any systemic autoimmune disorder, e.g., rheumatoid arthritis, may lead to abnormal immunological response to pregnancy.
- *Immunological: Alloimmune (currently classified as unexplained)*
  - Normally the maternal immune system tolerates the fetal allograft which is foreign. Lack of this immunotolerance leads to miscarriage. This may be manifest in the endometrium as:
    - Abnormalities of cytokine production—lack of shift of Th 1 to Th 2 response
    - Lack of alpha V beta 3 integrin
    - Increased levels of tumor necrosis factor alpha (TNF) in the endometrium
    - Increased uterine natural killer cells
    - Low concentration of macrophage inhibitory cytokines (MIC)
  - Asynchronous timing of ovulation and implantation window as seen in polycytic ovarian disease (PCOD) also leads to poor implantation and miscarriage
- *Genetic*
  - *Fetal aneuploidy:* Trisomy/monosomy and polyploidies
  - Parental balanced translocations, inversions, deletions, duplications
  - Skewed inactivation of X chromosome, Fragile X syndrome
  - Single gene defects, e.g., alpha thalassemia major, Rett syndrome, etc.
- *Hormonal*
  - Polycystic ovarian syndrome
  - Progesterone receptor gene polymorphism and luteal phase defects
  - Hyperandrogenism
  - Hypothyroidism/hyperthyroidism
  - Hyperprolactinemia
  - Low anti-Müllerian hormone (AMH)/poor ovarian reserve
  - Adrenal hyperplasia/Addison's disease
  - Deficiency of Vitamin D
  - Uncontrolled diabetes mellitus
- *Anatomical*
  - Müllerian abnormalities, septate uterus
  - Myomas—submucous, intramural
  - Uterine synechiae and polyps
  - T-shaped uterus
  - Cervical incompetence
- *Inherited thrombophilia*
  - Antithrombin III deficiency
  - Deficiency of protein C and protein S
  - Activated protein C resistance
  - Factor V Leiden mutation
  - *Methyltetrahydrofolate* gene homozygosity and hyperhomocysteinemia
  - *Prothrombin* gene mutation
  - Plaminogen activator inhibitor
- *Semen factors*
  - High sperm DNA fragmentation index
  - Male urogenital infections
- *Infections*
  - Genital bacterial vaginosis, chlamydia, latent tuberculosis
  - Subclinical chronic endometritis diagnosed by increased plasma cells in the endometrium.
  - Abnormal Uterine microbiome: Non-lactobacilli dominated microbiome
  - Systemic syphilis, Lyme's disease, toxoplasmosis, brucellosis
- *Systemic conditions*
  - Hypertension
  - Chronic renal disease
  - Chronic pulmonary disease
  - Heart disease
  - Severe rhesus sensitization

- Other diseases associated with RPL are Sickle cell anemia, Myotonic dystrophy, Marfan's syndrome, homocystinuria, factor VIII deficiency, dysfibrinogenemia and Ehlers-Danlos syndrome.

- *Lifestyle factors*
  - Maternal age > 35 years
  - Maternal obesity BMI > 30
  - Paternal age
- *Environmental*
- Endocrine disrupters
- Smoking, alcohol, drugs
- Exposure to irradiation
- Exposure to environmental toxins, pesticides, DDT, dry-cleaning chemicals
- Exposure to anesthetic gases.

Chemicals which have been associated with RPL include nitrous oxide, arsenic, aniline dyes, benzene, ethylene oxide, lead, pesticides, mercury, and cadmium.

Although an exhaustive list of causes exists, we still have 40–50% patients that fall in the unexplained category. In many patients more than one factor may lead to miscarriage and in some each miscarriage may have a different etiology. This poses a diagnostic difficulty to the physician.

Lifestyle and Environmental Factors

Maternal age has a very positive correlation with recurrent pregnancy loss.[4] Over the age of 40 years majority of pregnancies are lost with autologous oocytes. Hence reproduction should be encouraged before the age of 35 years.

Parental obesity should be addressed positively[5] and parental smoking, alcohol and drug exposure should be strongly discouraged. Exposure to environmental toxins such as pesticides, anesthetic gases, dry cleaning chemicals, and endocrine disruptors released from plastic should be avoided.

Systemic Conditions

Maternal comorbidities such as chronic kidney, liver, cardiac or respiratory illness can result in pregnancy loss. Such mothers need to be counseled regarding surrogacy to safe guard their health and fulfill their reproductive desires. Women with true rhesus sensitization are managed with intrauterine blood transfusions and early delivery.

Infections

Genital tract infections often result in Infertility. However milder forms may result in recurrent pregnancy loss, e.g., bacterial vaginosis,[6] latent genital tuberculosis[7] and nonspecific bacterial endometritis post intrauterine procedures such as dilatation and curettage. There is growing evidence that alteration of the microbiome of the vagina and endometrial cavity will lead to implantation failure and miscarriages.[8] Although microbiome testing is still a research tool and not available in the clinical setting, probiotics like lactobacilli may play a role in correcting the uterine microbiome.

Certain systemic infections such as brucellosis, Lyme's disease and toxoplasmosis are also associated with sporadic miscarriages.[9] These are rare and may be diagnosed by positive serology if suspected.

Semen Factors

An unhealthy paternal lifestyle, exposure to alcohol and smoking are associated with increased sperm DNA fragmentation, which in turn, can lead to poor embryo quality and RPL.[10] These patients need lifestyle modification and long-term (i.e., 3 months or longer) treatment with antioxidants to reverse the damage.

Male accessory gland infections (MAGI), e.g., seminal vesiculitis and prostatitis will coat the sperm with bacteria prior to ejaculation. This in turn may cause chronic endometritis, and RPL.

Inherited Thrombophilia

These are most commonly associated with second & third trimester pregnancy loss. However some disorders such as *prothrombin* gene and factor V Leiden mutation may be associated with recurrent pregnancy loss.[11]

Anatomical

An estimated 15% of couples (one in six) with recurrent miscarriage have an anatomic abnormality of the uterus as the primary cause.[12] These abnormalities include the following:

- Defects of Müllerian fusion include septate uterus, unicornuate uterus and bicornuate uterus with unequal uterine horns **(Fig. 1)**.
- Acquired anatomical defects, such as, submucous or intramural myomas, endometrial polyps and uterine synechiae.

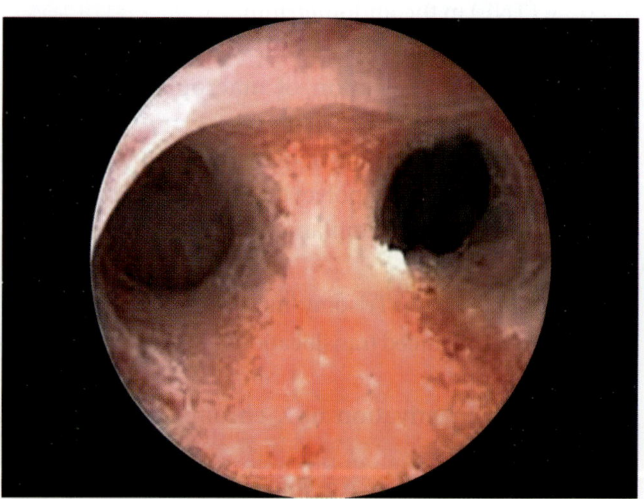

Fig. 1: Hysteroscopy showing a uterine septum.

- Small tubular uterine cavity: This may be congenital, secondary to diethylstilbestrol exposure *in utero* or genital tuberculosis.
- Cervical incompetence, which is diagnosed by visualizing the cervix with an empty bladder on transvaginal ultrasound scan and assessing the width at the internal os as well as the cervical length from internal to external os.[13] It may be a congenital weakness or secondary to repeated cervical dilatation. It is also associated with unicornuate or bicornuate uteri.

Hormonal

A multitude of endocrinal disorders can cause recurrent miscarriage.

Polycystic ovarian syndrome is one of the most common endocrinal abnormalities affecting female reproductive performance. Besides infertility, it presents higher risks of first and second-trimester miscarriages.[14]

Factors associated with a high miscarriage rate are *hyperandrogenism, hyperinsulinemia* and/or *ovulatory dysfunction* that accompanies high levels of luteinizing hormone and low levels of progesterone.

Women with poorly controlled *type 1 (insulin-dependent) diabetes mellitus* with glycated hemoglobin (HbA1C) levels greater than four standard deviations above the mean had a higher pregnancy loss rate. Well-controlled diabetes had pregnancy loss rates similar to those of non-diabetics. Apart from frank diabetes, syndrome X,[15] which comprises of impaired glucose tolerance test (GTT), hypertension, hypertriglyceridemia and a procoagulant state with increased coronary heart disease, could also potentially cause recurrent pregnancy loss.

Abnormal maternal thyroid functions have been implicated as a cause of recurrent miscarriage.[16] However, mild or subclinical thyroid dysfunction is not associated with recurrent miscarriage, as it more often leads to infertility, but increased levels of thyroid peroxidase and/or microsomal antibodies have been associated with recurrent miscarriage.[17] In autoimmune thyroid disease (AITD), the risk of miscarriage was the same whether the status was hypothyroid or euthyroid, indicating that AITD negatively affects fetal implantation. Hence, all women with positive thyroid antibodies should be treated with a low dose of thyroxin replacement to suppress thyroid autoimmunity and achieve a favorable maternal and perinatal outcome.[17]

Hyperprolactinemia usually causes infertility due to luteolysis; however, in partially treated cases, the picture may change to early pregnancy loss due to corpus luteum deficiency.

Although rare, the patient with an untreated late onset *congenital adrenal hyperplasia* may have an increased chance of recurrent miscarriage owing to hyperandrogenism. On the other hand, incipient *Addison's disease* will also cause recurrent miscarriages; the patient often has low blood pressure and hyperpigmentation.

Poor ovarian reserve, diagnosed by low levels of AMH and a poor antral follicle count, remains an important factor responsible for recurrent miscarriage, owing to increased rate of aneuploidy in oocytes. Women with AMH levels below 1 ng/mL not only experience difficulty in conceiving but also have a higher rate of pregnancy loss due to a higher rate of aneuploidy in the embryo.[18] Therapy with dehydroepiandrostenedione sulfate (DHEAS) and Coenzyme Q 10 (CoQ 10) has been tried but there is no robust evidence to support it.

Genetic

Genetic Abnormalities in Karyotypically Normal Parents

Various studies demonstrate that at least 50% of clinically recognized pregnancy loss results from a cytogenetic abnormality,[19] of which 51% show autosomal trisomies, 22% show polyploidy, 19% show monosomy, 4% show translocations, and the rest are unclassified genetic defects. The autosomal trisomies commonly encountered are those of chromosomes 3, 4, 9, 13–16, 19, 21 and 22.[12]

Products of conception should be routinely submitted for genetic testing preferably with array complete genomic hybridization (CGH) and couples with abnormal genetic testing should have parental karyotyping[20] and if normal should be counseled regarding an optimistic outcome in future pregnancies.

Genetic Abnormalities in Karyotypically Abnormal Parents

Women may have structural chromosomal abnormality in the following forms:

- Deletions and duplications produce large chromosomal defects, which may cause severe phenotypic anomalies, thus individuals with these anomalies rarely reproduce.
- Dicentric and ring chromosomes are mitotically unstable, so the chances of offspring acquiring these anomalies are very small.
- In balanced translocations in men, the reproductive fitness is only slightly diminished. In spite of their good reproductive performance, these individuals show a significant decrease in live births, and a significant increase in both fetal death and interval infertility; hence, they will present with recurrent miscarriage.
- In unbalanced translocations in men, not only is there productive fitness greatly decreased but the risk of abnormal offspring is also increased.
- In single gene defects, diagnosis can only be made by a detailed family history coupled with array CGH testing.

Alternatively if the gene locus is well identified PCR testing or SNP will help in diagnosis.

Immunological Causes

Antiphospholipid antibody syndrome is the most common immunological cause of recurrent miscarriage. It is the most rewarding as far as the treatment is concerned. Antibodies are directed against negatively charged phospholipids, which are the major constituents of trophoblast. These antibodies can cause impaired trophoblastic function, abnormal placentation, and placental thrombosis/infarction. This may lead to pregnancy-induced hypertension, intrauterine growth retardation (IUGR), intrauterine fetal death, and recurrent miscarriage. Both early first-trimester losses and late third-trimester losses can occur. There is usually an ultrasound confirmation of a viable pregnancy prior to the pregnancy loss in most first trimester losses.

The diagnosis of APS is made by the presence of *one clinical criterion and one-laboratory criterion, which must be positive on two occasions 3 months (12 weeks) apart.*

Clinical criteria include the following:[21,22]

- One or more unexplained deaths of a morphologically normal fetus of more than 10 weeks' gestation documented by ultrasonography or direct examination.
- One or more preterm births at or before 34 weeks' gestation due to severe preeclampsia or placental insufficiency with evidence of IUGR.
- Three or more consecutive miscarriages before 10 weeks' gestation with no maternal hormonal, anatomic abnormalities, normal fetal genetic testing, and other causes of recurrent losses being ruled out.

Laboratory criteria include detection of any of the following:

- Lupus anticoagulant by DRVVT, APTT or PTT
- Anticardiolipin antibodies
- Antiphospholipid antibodies
- Anti-beta-2-glycoprotein antibodies
- Antiphosphatidylserine antibodies.

Autoimmune disorders, such as systemic lupus erythematosus, systemic sclerosis, and autoimmune thrombocytopenia are associated with recurrent miscarriage, and are often classified as SAPS. The mechanism of loss and the treatment are the same as those for primary APS.

Treatment with steroids is not recommended based on current evidence. A combination of low dose aspirin and unfractionated/low molecular weight heparin currently gives the best pregnancy outcome. Heparin is not only an anticoagulant, it has a potent complement inhibitory action which is beneficial in preventing complement mediated damage in APS syndrome. Aspirin should be started preconceptually and heparin after a positive pregnancy test and continued until the time of delivery. Postpartum thromboprophylaxis is recommended for 2 weeks to prevent deep vein thrombosis.

In cases of SAPS due to systemic lupus erythematosus, hydroxychloroquine (HCQ) has been used with good success rates during pregnancy. It is started in the preconception period and continued throughout pregnancy in a dose of 400 mg once or twice daily after meals. It is a pregnancy category C drug and it controls both disease activity and flares during pregnancy. It also prevents heart block in the fetus.[23]

Intravenous immunoglobulins (IVIG) therapy is indicated in women with secondary recurrent miscarriages, very high titers of antibodies where treatment with aspirin and low molecular weight heparin fails to prevent a pregnancy loss.[24]

CONCLUSION

All women presenting with two or more miscarriages need to be worked up to identify the cause of miscarriages. All women should have the following:

- Uterine cavity evaluation by 3D ultrasound scan/ sonohysterogram for cavity lesions such as polyps/myoma. Alternatively a hysterosalpingogram may be done and in positive cases hysteroscopy is both a confirmatory and therapeutic option.
- *Hormonal profile:* Thyroid function test and antithyroid antibodies. HbA1C and in women with galactorrhea serum prolactin levels. In women over 35 years serum AMH.
- Autoimmune screening for APLA syndrome. Antinuclear antibodies (ANA) testing could be considered.[25]
- Infection screening—for bacterial vaginosis, cervicitis and endometritis.
- Semen analysis and culture and sperm DNA fragmentation index if indicated.

If all above investigations are normal, a diagnosis of unexplained RPL should be made. Any subsequent pregnancy losses should have genetic screening of products of conception by array CGH for genetic abnormalities. In women with recurrent aneuploidy miscarriages, IVF with PGD or oocyte donation have been suggested.

Treatment of specific causes has been discussed in each section, however treatment in unexplained RPL is largely empirical. Evidence for use of empirical therapy with the following is lacking:

- Heparin or low dose aspirin
- Vaginal progesterone supplementation[26]
- IVIG
- Glucocorticoids
- Intralipid therapy

Vitamin D3 deficiency should be corrected and these patients should be offered tender loving care with reassurance scans in early pregnancy.

Progesterone therapy is widely prescribed, although there is evidence that use of vaginal progesterone does not improve pregnancy rates. Immune modulation with dydrogesterone may show some benefit.

Flowchart 1: A clinician's approach to a patient with recurrent pregnancy loss.

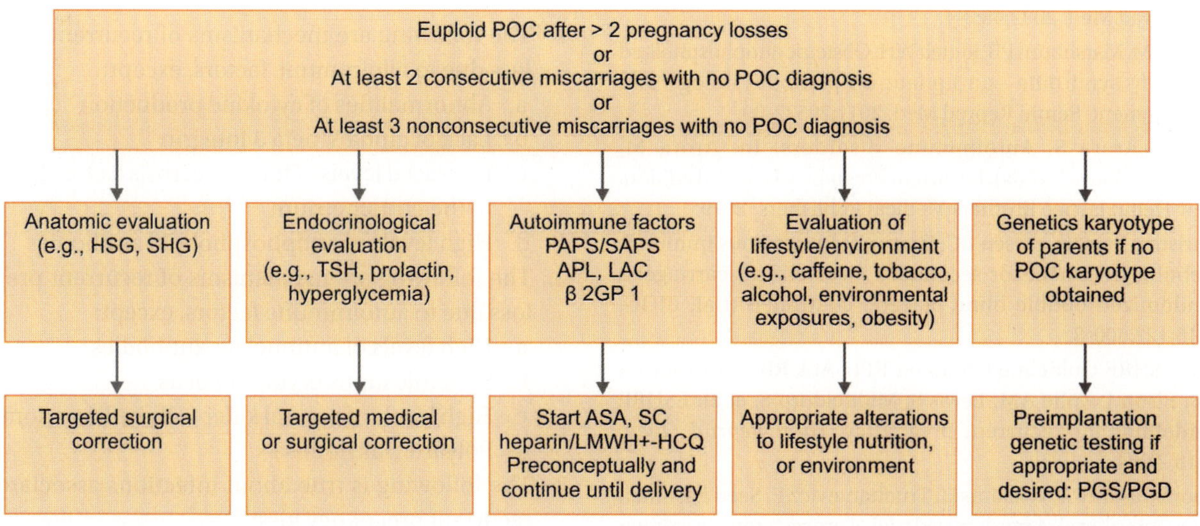

(HCQ: hydroxychloroquine; POC: products of conception; PGD: preimplantation genetic diagnosis; PGS: preimplantation genetic screening; HSG: hysterosalpingogram; SHG: sonohysterogram; PAPS: primary antiphospholipid syndrome; SAPS: secondary antiphospholipid syndrome; ASA: acetye salicylic acid (aspirin); APL: antiphosholipid; LAC: lupus anti-coagulant; LMWH: low molecular weight heparin; SC: subcutaneous; TSH: thyroid stimulating hormone)

Complementary therapies: Acupuncture, reflexology and other stress relieving therapies can also be tried.

There is an 80% chance that these women will achieve a live birth, however they may have an increased incidence of pregnancy complications such as gestational diabetes, preterm deliveries and hepatic cholestasis.[27]

The **Flowchart 1** summarizes the clinician's approach to a patient with RPL. For a full workup all the possible causes have to be looked into.[28]

REFERENCES

1. Royal College of Obstetricians and Gynecologists. The investigation and treatment of couples with recurrent first-trimester and second-trimester miscarriage. Green-top Guideline No.17. London: RCOG; 2011.
2. Bhattacharya S. Recurrent miscarriage: should the definition be revised? World Clin Obstet Gynecol. 2011:1:1.
3. Practice Committee of the American Society for Reproductive Medicine. Definitions of infertility and recurrent pregnancy loss. Fertil Steril. 2008;89:1603.
4. Practice Committee of the American Society for Reproductive Medicine. Aging and infertility in women. Fertil Steril. 2006;86(5 Suppl):S248-52.
5. Pandey S, Bhattacharya S. Obesity and miscarriage. World Clin Obstet Gynecol. 2011:1:1-8.
6. Kuppusamy R, Visvanathan D, Hollingworth T. Pregnancy loss and bacterial vaginosis. World Clin Obstet Gynecol. 2011;1:9.
7. Jaiswar SP, Gautam S. Latent genital infections and subclinical endometritis. In: Arora M, Mukhopadhaya N (Eds). Recurrent Pregnancy Loss, 3rd edition. New Delhi: Jaypee Brothers Medical Publishers; 2019.
8. Moreno I, Codoner FM, Vilella F. Evidence that the endometrial microbiota has an effect on implantation success or failure Am J Obstet Gynecol. 2016;215(6) 684-703.
9. Pal N. Thyroid and medical disorders. In: Arora M, Konje N (Eds). Recurrent Pregnancy Loss, 2nd edition. New Delhi: Jaypee Brothers Medical Publishers; 2007.
10. Opuwari CS, Henkel RR, Agarwal A. Sperm DNA fragmentation Index. In: Arora M, Mukhopadhaya N (Eds). Recurrent Pregnancy Loss, 3rd edition. New Delhi: Jaypee Brothers Medical Publishers; 2019.
11. Mishra S. Inherited Thrombophilia. In: Recurrent Pregnancy Loss, 3rd edition. New Delhi: Jaypee Brothers Medical Publishers; 2019.
12. Basiri A, Kabessa M, Gvenetadze A. Anatomical factors. In: Arora M, Mukhopadhaya N (Eds). Recurrent Pregnancy Loss, 3rd edition. New Delhi: Jaypee Brothers Medical Publishers; 2019.
13. O'Brien J. Cervical causes of Preterm labor. World Clin Obstet Gynecol. 2012;2:1.
14. Venkataraman M, Thanawala U. Pregnancy complication in Polycystic ovaries. World Clin Obstet Gynecol. 2017;6:1.
15. Zaveroni I, Bonini L, Fantuzzi M. Hyperinsulinemia, obesity and AQ Syndrome X. J Intern Med. 1994;235: 51-6.
16. Alexander EK, Pearce EN, Brent GA, Brown RS, Chen H, Dosiou C, et al. American Thyroid association guidelines for thyroid disease in pregnancy. 2017;27(3):315-89.
17. Lata K, Dutta P, Sridhar S. Thyroid autoimmunity and obstetric outcomes in women with recurrent miscarriage: a case control study. Endocrine connect 2013;2(2):118-24.
18. Atasever M, Soyman Z, Demirel E, Gencdal S, Kelekci S. Diminished ovarian reserve: is it a neglected cause in the assessment of recurrent miscarriage? A cohort study. Fertil Steril. 2016;105(5):1236-40.
19. Boui J, Boui A, Lazar P. Retrospective and prospective epidemiological studies of 1500 karyotyped spontaneous human abortions. Teratology. 1975;12:11.
20. Kasak L, Rull K, Laan M. Overview of Genetic Causes. In: Recurrent Pregnancy Loss, 3rd edition. In: Arora M, Mukhopadhaya N (Eds). New Delhi: Jaypee Brothers Medical Publishers; 2019.

21. Rai RS. Antiphospholipid syndrome and recurrent miscarriages. J Post grad Med. 2002;48:3-4.
22. Ernest JM, Marshburn PB, Kutteh WH. Obstetric antiphospholipid antibody syndrome—an update on pathophysiology and management. Semin Reprod Med. 2011;29522-39.
23. Pal N, Arora S. Autoimmune disorders. In: Arora M, Mukhopadhaya N (Eds). Recurrent Pregnancy Loss, 3rd edition. New Delhi: Jaypee Brothers Medical Publishers; 2019.
24. Christiansen OB, Larsen EC, Egerup P. Intravenous immunoglobulin treatment for secondary recurrent miscarriage: a randomized double blind placebo controlled trial. BJOG. 2015;122:500-8.
25. The ESHRE Guideline Group on RPL, Atik RB, Christiansen OB, Elson J, Kolte AM, Lewis S, Middeldorp S, et al. ESHRE guidelines for recurrent pregnancy. *Hum Reprod Open.* 2018;2:004.
26. Coomarasamy A, Williams H, Truchanowicz E, Seed PT, Small R, Quenby S, et al. A randomized trial of progesterone in women with recurrent miscarriages. Promise study. N Engl J Med. 2015;373:2141-8.
27. Cozzolino M, Rizzello F, Riviello C, Romanelli C, Coccia Elisabetta M. Ongoing pregnancies in patients with unexplained recurrent pregnancy loss: adverse obstetric outcomes. Hum Fertil (Camb). 2019;22(3):219-25.
28. Brezina PR, Ke RW, Kutteh WH. Preimplantation genetic screening: a practical guide. Clin Med Insight Reprod Health. 2013:197-208.

LONG QUESTIONS

1. What are the possible, probable and unlikely causes of recurrent pregnancy loss in the first trimester?
2. Discuss the etiopathogenesis, diagnostic approach and therapeutic interventions for anatomical factors in recurrent pregnancy loss.
3. How do immunological factors contribute to recurrent pregnancy loss? Discuss laboratory testing, criteria for diagnosis and therapeutic approach to these conditions.

SHORT QUESTIONS

1. What is the currently accepted definition of recurrent pregnancy loss?
2. What is the contribution of lifestyle and stress to the occurrence of recurrent pregnancy loss?
3. Which infections may have a role in the etiology of recurrent pregnancy loss?
4. What are the common genetic and chromosomal errors leading to recurrent pregnancy loss?
5. What is the immune rejection hypothesis in recurrent pregnancy loss?

MULTIPLE CHOICE QUESTIONS

1. The following are mechanisms of recurrent pregnancy loss due to alloimmune factors, except:
   a. Abnormalities of cytokine production
   b. Lack of alpha V beta 3 integrin
   c. Increased levels of tumor necrosis factor alpha (TNF) in the endometrium
   d. High levels of antiphospholipid antibodies
2. The following are mechanisms of recurrent pregnancy loss due to autoimmune factors, except:
   a. High levels of antinuclear antibodies
   b. Systemic lupus erythematosus
   c. High levels of natural killer cells in the endometrium
   d. Polyarteritis nodosa
3. The following is true about infections associated with recurrent pregnancy loss:
   a. The most common etiology of recurrent pregnancy loss is TORCH infections
   b. Bacterial vaginosis is associated with recurrent pregnancy loss in the second trimester
   c. Tuberculosis resulting in blocked tubes can cause recurrent pregnancy loss
   d. Lyme disease is a common cause of recurrent pregnancy loss in medical professionals
4. The following is true about laboratory testing for autoimmune etiology of recurrent pregnancy loss:
   a. False positive results may be seen due to cross reactivity of infections
   b. Tests should be done only once
   c. Tests should be repeated after 4 weeks
   d. Four fold rise in titer is necessary to confirm the etiology
5. A small tubular uterine cavity leading to recurrent miscarriage may be due to all the following, except:
   a. Tuberculosis
   b. Asherman syndrome
   c. Exposure to diethylstilbesterol in utero
   d. Cervical insufficiency
6. The following are acceptable regimens to treat primary autoimmune etiology of recurrent pregnancy loss, except:
   a. Aspirin
   b. Aspirin + unfractionated heparin
   c. Aspirin + fractionated heparin
   d. Aspirin + steroids

Answers

1. d 2. c 3. b 4. a 5. d 6. d

12.14 THIRD PARTY REPRODUCTION

Nayana Patel, Molina Patel, Niket Patel, Yuvraj Jadeja, Harmi Thakkar

INTRODUCTION

Third party reproduction refers to a process where another person provides sperm or eggs or where another woman provides her uterus so that a woman can have a child. However, the third party's involvement is limited to the reproductive process and does not extend into the raising of the child.

There are four different types of third-party reproduction arrangements:[1]

1. *Egg donation:* An egg donor provides ova for fertilization in the in vitro fertilization (IVF) process. The embryo is placed into the uterus/womb for the future mother.
2. *Sperm donation:* A third party provides sperm that can be used for insemination of the future mother or to fertilize an ovum for reinsertion of the resulting embryo into the mother, or by embryo transfer into a Surrogate mother.
3. *Embryo donation:* With the Unused embryos after the woman for whom they were originally created has successfully carried one or more pregnancies to term or where embryos are specifically created for donation using donor eggs and sperms.
4. Surrogacy.

STAGES OF THIRD PARTY IN VITRO FERTILIZATION[2]

- Identify couples/individual that need egg donation and/or surrogacy
- Psychological counseling of the receipt
- Sources of egg donors/surrogates
- Screening of egg donors/surrogates
- Agreement and/or contract
- Preparation of the recipient.

Egg Donation

The use of donor oocytes has become an option for family building since the 1980s, with the first egg donor pregnancy occurring in 1984. Though initially used for women with primary ovarian insufficiency (POI), egg donation is now used successfully to treat a wide range of conditions including women who have survived cancer, experienced multiple pregnancy losses, carry genetic diseases and have poor egg quality due to advanced maternal age.[3]

Indications for Donor Oocyte

The indications are as follows:

Ovarian dysfunction:

- Premenopausal
  - Poor ovarian responders
  - Diminished ovarian reserve
  - Premature ovarian failure (includes genetic autoimmune, iatrogenic causes, surgical oophorectomy, etc.)
  - Previous ART failure
  - Unexplained
- Postmenopausal
  - Oncology related chemoradiotherapy
  - Genetic
  - Unexplained
- Normal ovarian function
  - Genetic transmittable disorder
    - Autosomal/sex chromosomal related
  - Recurrent pregnancy loss
    - With/without recurrent aneuploidy
  - Same sex couples
  - Research
  - Older women with reduced ovarian reserve/diminished oocyte quality
  - Female survivors of cancer in childhood and adolescence treated with bone marrow transplant including total body irradiation (Tbi). X-ray therapy or chemotherapy
  - Ovarian resistance syndrome.

Cause of premature ovarian failure:

- *Gonadal dysgenesis:*
  - Turner Syndrome
  - Perrault Syndrome
  - 46, XX gonadal dysgenesis/46, XY gonadal dysgenesis
  - Genetic associations
  - Familial ovarian failure
  - Galactosemia
  - Enzyme defects - P450c17
  - FRA-XA premutation
  - Blepharophimosis, ptosis, and epicanthus inversus syndrome
  - Small X chromosome Defects
  - FSH receptor mutations/LH receptor mutations
- *Autoimmune:*
  - Autoimmune polyendocrinpathy syndrome 1
  - APECED/autoimmune polyendocrinopathy syndrome 2
  - Association with various autoimmune diseases
  - Isolated autoimmune ovarian failure
  - Iatrogenic autoimmune ovarian failure
  - Iatrogenic chemotherapy
  - Radiotherapy
  - Pelvic Surgery
  - Environmental toxins
  - Idiopathic.

Counseling of Donors and Recipients

Counseling is the integral part as all the patients and their partners require a detailed explanation of the procedures involved in egg donation and the moral, ethical, and legal implications.

Egg donation can be anonymous, known or by directed donors or by IVF programs.

In IVF programs donation, women undergoing IVF cycles may agree to donate their excess eggs to infertile patients.[1]

There are many alternative sources of donor oocytes by using the emerging technologies such as:

- In vitro maturation of eggs
- Ovarian rejuvenation techniques
- Oocyte vitrification and cryopreservation
- Egg banks
- Use of preimplantation genetic screening
- Optimizing treatment of male infertility to counterbalance the egg subfertility.

Selection and Screening of Oocyte Donors According to the Indian Council of Medical Research[3]

- Donors should be healthy, well screened, and in the age-group of 21–35 years.
- Relevant information regarding the donor, such as age, height, weight, blood group, educational qualifications, profession, color of the skin and the eyes must be recorded.
- Detailed history to rule out hereditary disease and to exclude individuals who might be at high risk for HIV, sexually transmitted infections, or other infections that might be transmissible via gamete donation.
- Basic investigations should include endocrine profile (FSH, LH, estradiol levels, serum TSH, prolactin and serum progesterone), blood profile, screening for sexually transmitted diseases (STDs such as HIV, Hepatitis B/C, HCV, syphilis, gonorrhea, chlamydia) detailed pelvic ultrasound examination, genetic karyotyping and hemoglobin electrophoresis to rule out conditions such as thalassemia.
- Psychological evaluation and counseling for the oocyte donor and her partner. In circumstances involving known donors, this counseling should be offered to the donor and her partner, as well as the recipient and her partner.
- The donor must be informed that the offspring will not know her identity.
- A Written and Informed consent according to Indian Council of Medical Research (ICMR) guidelines.
- It is advisable that a single person donates not more than six times with a gap of 3 months between subsequent egg retrievals.
- Additional testing can be performed based on the ethnicity of the donors.

Selection and Screening of Egg Recipient

- Hormonal profile
- HbsAg, HIV, blood group and Rh factor, Pap smear
- Tansvaginal sonography (TVS)—to see for pelvic pathology and assess mock cycle
- Hysterosalpingogram (HSG)/hysteroscopy
- Medical conditions—heart disease, hypertension, DM
- Counseling
- Male partner assessment.

Evaluation of the Partner of the Oocyte Recipient

- Semen analysis for male partners
- Blood type and Rh factor
- Serologic test for syphilis
- Hepatitis B surface antigen
- Hepatitis B core antibody (IgG and IgM)
- Hepatitis C antibody and NAT
- HIV-1 (AB and NAT), HIV-2 AB testing
- Appropriate genetic screening and testing based on history counseling.

Test/consultation:

- Hysterosalpingogram, saline hysterosonography or hysteroscopy: Within 2 years
- *Pap Smear:* Within 1 year
- *Mammogram:* Within 5 year if recipient is between ages 35 and 40, within 2 years if she is 51 years or older
- *Fasting glucose level:* Within 3 years if anyone in recipient's immediate family or two or more people among her relatives have diabetes, if she is obese, or if she has had diabetes while pregnant
- *Electrocardiogram:* Within the year if recipient is aged 40 years or more
- *Total cholesterol level:* Within the year if a parent or sibling of the recipient has/had a total >240 mg/dL, if members of her family developed premature (<55 years) cardiovascular disease, if she has diabetes, or if she smokes
- *Preconceptual counseling:* If recipient is age 35 years or more, with an obstetrician, to review risks of pregnancy
- *General medical screening:* If recipient is age 45 years or more, or gets short of breath, has a heart murmur, or has an abnormal electrocardiogram, a high total cholesterol, or blood in her stools
- *Psychological counseling:* Recommended for all.

CYCLE MANAGEMENT

Preparation of the Donor

The donor is treated with a period of long downregulation with the GnRH analog, leuprolide or buserelin for up to 2 weeks, after which the serum levels of estradiol, LH and progesterone are measured **(Figs. 1 and 2)**. A baseline pelvic scan is conducted and then follicular stimulation can begin with recombinant FSH/HMG, etc., (150 IU or 225 IU daily,

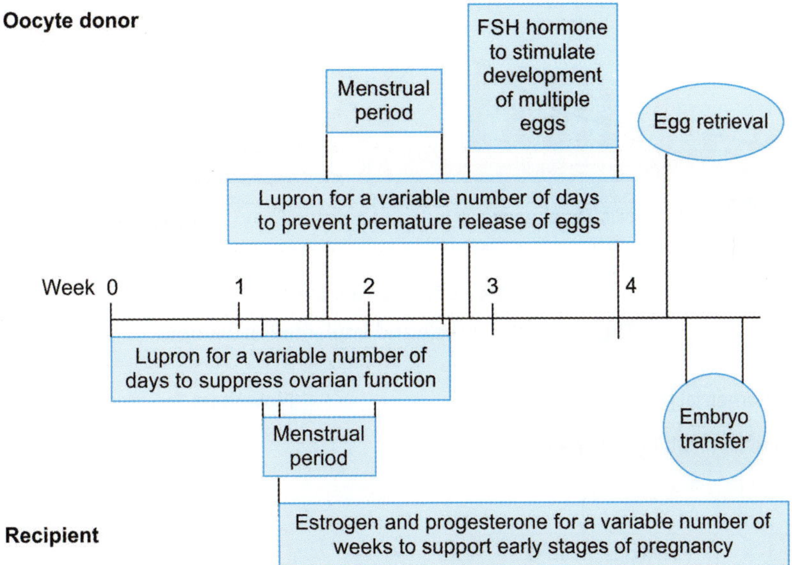

Fig. 1: Agonist protocol.

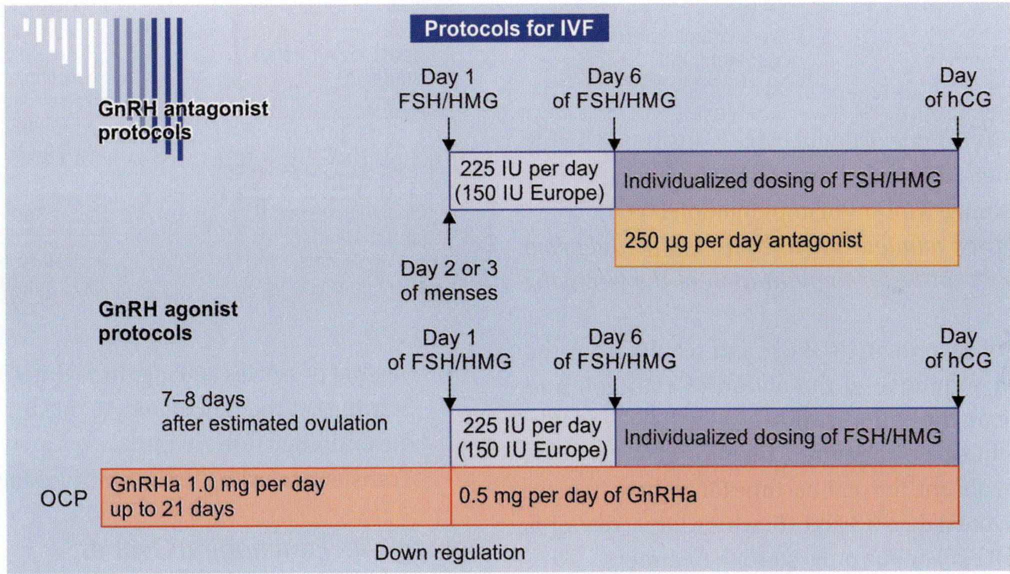

Fig. 2: Antagonist protocol.
(FSH: follicle stimulating hormone; hCG: human chorionic gonadotropin; HMG: human menopausal gonadotropin; OCP: oral contraceptive pill)

depending on various clinical parameters and hormone profile).

Monitoring of the follicles is done using TVS and blood hormone profile and dose adjustments are made accordingly. When we can see at least three follicles of 17 mm with normally rising estradiol levels, a suitable trigger such as hCG 10,000 IU is given 34–36 hours before the intended time of oocyte retrieval.

Note: The aim being optimal stimulation with prevention of the ovarian hyperstimulation syndrome (OHSS), tailored protocols for every individual donor should be the norm. In donors at risk of OHSS, the use of the antagonist protocol, and with replacement of the hCG trigger with recombinant LH or GnRH agonists (only in an antagonist protocol cycle) helps in prevention of OHSS.

Key points to remember while stimulating a donor:

- Preferably antagonist cycle
- OHSS prevention
- Optimal oocyte number around 10–15 (minimum 7)
- Safety and well-being of donor
- Complication free stimulation and oocyte retrieval procedure.

Preparation of the Recipient for Embryo Transfer (Fig. 3 and Flowchart 1)

- Endometrial preparation is the most optimal step in third party cycles
- Endometrial preparation of the recipient is modeled on the natural menstrual cycle

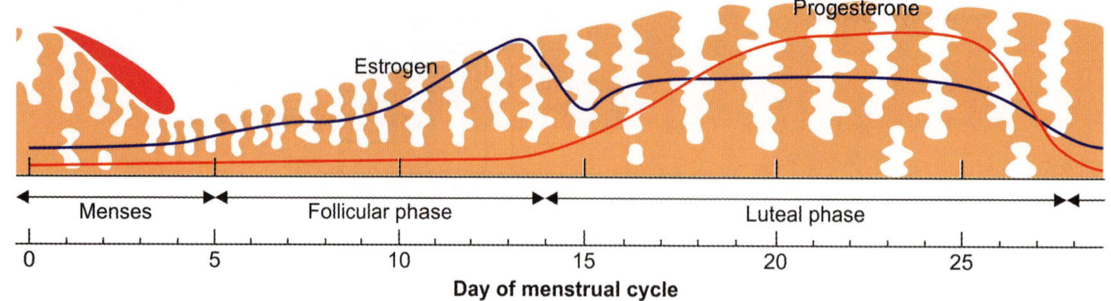

Fig. 3: Menstrual cycle and implantation window.

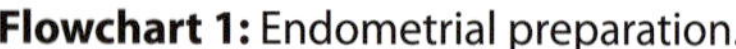

Flowchart 1: Endometrial preparation.

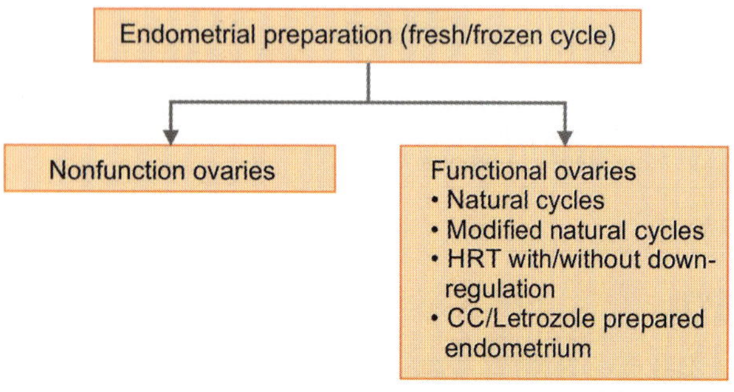

- The higher success rate of donor cycle is attributed highly to the endometrial preparation techniques
- Trying to optimize window of implantation (WOI)
- *The implantation window is defined as that period when the uterus is receptive for implantation of the free-lying blastocyst*
- This period of receptivity is short and results from the programmed sequence of the action of estrogen and progesterone on the endometrium
- In cycles where endogenous hormonal activity is suppressed or absent, the optimal time for embryo transfer lies between luteal days +3 and +5, where luteal day +1 is the first day of exogenous progesterone treatment
- In the human, blastocyst apposition begins about LH day +6 and is complete by LH +10.

Aim is to get recipient's menstruation 2 days (1-2 days) before the donor or simultaneously to synchronization.

- Synchronize the donor and recipient cycle by BCP or GnRH agonist or progesterone
- When both donor and recipient are downregulated, recipient starts estrogen and donor starts ovarian stimulation 2–3 days later.

Women with Nonfunctioning Ovaries (Flowchart 2)

- HRT-estradiol valerate
  - 6–8 mg daily, fixed or variable dose regimen
  - Starting 2–3 days before stimulation of the donor
  - Transdermal estrogen 0.2–04 mg
  - Ideally, 12–14 days of estrogen
- Progesterone replacement
  - Injectable 100 mg daily or

Flowchart 2: Complications with oocyte donation.

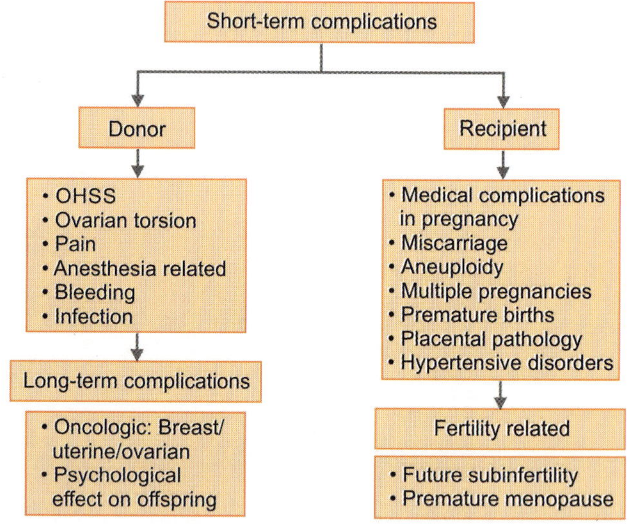

  - Vaginal pessaries 200 mg three times a day
  - Starting on the day of oocyte pickup (OPU) or when the endometrium ≥ 8 mm
  - Transfer according to the embryo staging.

Women with Functioning Ovaries

- Natural cycle
- HRT cycle
- Semi-HRT cycle
- GnRHa + HRT cycle
- CC/aromatase inhibitors.

Natural cycle:
No HRT supplementation to be given.

To decide follow up based on cycle length

- ET to be evaluated along with follicular growth strictly from Day 8/Day 10 of cycle
- Ovulation cannot be missed (LH kit can be used in mid cycle or daily ultrasound)

Transfer is planned on LH surge + 7 days or ovulation + 5 days.

Modified natural cycle: No HRT treatment is given. To decide the follow-up based on cycle length

- Endometrium and follicular growth meticulously evaluated

- With ET ≥8 mm and follicle ≥18 mm, hCG trigger (5,000 IU/ 10,000 IU) is given
- Ovulation is checked
- Transfer is planned hCG + D7.

CC/Letrozole induced endometrium: Oral ovulogens are sometimes used to stimulate development of follicle which would cause natural development of endometrium. hCG can be given at follicle ≥18 mm and adequate ET can be planned accordingly.

Endometrial Receptivity

Endometrial receptivity is the window of time when the uterine environment is conductive to embryo acceptance and subsequent implantation

- Endometrial receptivity can be accessed by
- Parameters for assessing endometrial receptivity:
  - Transvaginal USG
  - Color Doppler
  - Recently using 3D/4D USG
  - Hormonal evaluation
  - Endometrial thickness (>7 to <14 mm)
  - Endometrial pattern (triple-line pattern)
  - Endometrial and subendometrial blood flow (within zone 3)
  - Uterine artery RI/PI.

SPERM DONATION

The use of artificial insemination by donor (AID) has expanded since the late 1960s and has become a therapeutic option for male infertility in many countries. But since the 1980s, with the emergence of HIV, donor insemination has been performed only with frozen and quarantined sperm to allow for time to test the donors. Sperm should be quarantined for at least 6 months before being used.[4]

Indications for Sperm Donation

- Nonobstructive azoospermia with failure to retrieve testicular sperms
- Obstructive and nonobstructive azoospermia, which may be congenital or acquired
- Severe azoospermia (CBAVD or vasectomy)
- Severe oligospermia
- Ejaculatory dysfunction
- Failed fertilization on ICSI
- Hereditary genetic defect in male partner not willing for PGD
- The couple has Rh incompatibility
- Absence of a male partner (Single women/lesbian couples).

Psychological consultation for recipients:

- The decision to proceed with donor insemination is complex, may benefit from psychological counseling
- The clinician should strongly recommend psychological counseling by a qualified mental health professional
- Directed donations, not allowed in India.

Selection of sperm donors:

- The main qualities to seek in selecting a donor for TDI are an assurance of good health status and the absence of known genetic abnormalities.
- The assisted reproductive technology banks shall obtain semen from males between 21 and 45 years of age, both inclusive and cannot donate semen more than 25 times (ART Bill, 2015).
- Selection of donors with established fertility is desirable but not required.
- Psychological evaluation and counseling.
- No owner, operator, laboratory director, patient's physician or employee of a facility performing TDI may serve as a donor in that practice.

Screening and Testing of Sperm Donors

1. *Semen testing:*
   - More than one sample be examined (each after a 2- to 5-day abstinence interval)
   - The sample should be examined within 1–2 hours
   - The minimum criteria for normal semen quality can be applied
2. *Genetic evaluation:*
   - Genetic screening for heritable diseases should be performed
   - Testing for cystic fibrosis carrier status
3. *Medical history:*
   - Donors should be healthy and give no history to suggest hereditary disease
   - Complete personal and sexual history to exclude high risk for HIV, STIs, or other infections
4. *Physical examination:* Before acceptance, and every 6 months while remaining an active donor, donors should undergo a complete physical examination.

EMBRYO DONATION

Technologies have approved their efficacy in treating infertile couples. One such technique is embryo donation. It is relatively simple, safe and cost effective procedure compared to oocyte or IVF procedure.

Embryo donation is one of the most important achievements in the present century. This method is used when one or both spouses suffer from infertility lacking the ability to participate in the biological embryo formation. In this therapeutic method, the embryo formed from the sperm and ovum of a legal couple is transferred to the woman's uterus after fertilization to facilitate pregnancy and childbirth in the recipient.[5] The embryo donation method has been used for more than 25 years in many countries; such as gamete donation method, it has led to the birth of many children.[6,7]

Embryo donation is a unique therapy among the IVF techniques since the offspring born in this way has no genetic relation to its parents.

Indications for Embryo Donation Program

- Menopausal and perimenopausal women with subfertile partner
- Recurrent IVF failures
- Carriers of genetic or chromosomal abnormalities such as germ cell disease, etc.
- Financial constraints
- Untreatable infertility in one/both partners.

Pregnancy following embryo donation depends on the quality of the embryos that were frozen, the age of the woman who provided the eggs, and the number of embryos transferred.

SURROGACY

Surrogacy, also known as surrogate motherhood, is a fertility treatment in which a woman other than the intended mother carries the pregnancy to term and delivers the baby for the intended parents. This technique is the one involving a greater degree of complexity from the ethical, psychological, moral and technical points of view.

Surrogacy is of two types: Traditional and gestational

1. Traditional (genetic/partial/straight) surrogacy is the result of artificial insemination of the surrogate mother with the intended father's sperm, making her a genetic parent along with the intended father.

   The ICMR does not allow traditional surrogacy in India.
2. Gestational surrogacy (host/full surrogacy) is defined as arrangement in which an embryo from the intended parents or from a donated oocyte or sperm is transferred to the surrogate uterus. In gestational surrogacy, the woman who carries the child has no genetic connection to the child.

Surrogacy may be commercial or altruistic, depending upon whether the surrogate receives financial reward for her pregnancy.

If surrogate receives money for the surrogacy arrangement, it is considered commercial, and if she receives no compensation beyond reimbursement of her medical and other pregnancy-related expenses along with the insurance coverage for her, it is referred to as altruistic.[8,9]

Current Status of Surrogacy in India

On August 5th 2019, the bill states certain changes from the Surrogacy (Regulation) Bill, 2016.

- The Bill Prohibits Commercial Surrogacy and Allows Altruistic Surrogacy
- Use of Brokers/Intermediaries to Arrange Surrogate
- Ban on Advertisement of Commercial Surrogacy
- Abandoning or Exploitation of Children Born through Surrogacy
- Exploitation of Surrogate
- Selling of Human Embryos/Gametes
- Import or Aiding in Import of Human Embryos
- Sex Selection in any Form.

Indications in Surrogacy

- Absolute indication for surrogacy is the absence of uterus.
- Causes for it can be Mayer-Rokitansky-Kuster-Hauser syndrome (MRKHS) or history of obstetrics hysterectomy or hysterectomy for gynecological indications such as cervical cancer or endometrial cancer.
- Apart from this, significant structural abnormalities such as small unicornuate uterus, T-shaped uterus, or multiple fibroids with failed fertility treatment attempts also constitute indications.
- Women with severe medical conditions (heart or renal diseases) which are contraindication of pregnancy are the other indications for surrogacy.
- Surrogacy can also be considered as a last resort for the treatment of patient with repeated miscarriage and recurrent implantation failure where all possible tools for self-pregnancy have been exhausted.
- Biological impossibility to conceive or bear a child which applies to same-sex couples or single men also may necessitate surrogacy.

Steps in Surrogacy[10]

- Proper patient selection
- Source of surrogate (ART bank)
- Proper selection and screening of the surrogate
- Intensive counseling – the key factor
- Proper controlled ovarian stimulation and IVF technique
- Preparing the surrogate
- Synchronizing the cycles of the surrogate and the genetic mother
- Window period for embryo transfer
- Taking care of the legalities and financial contracts
- Transparency of the whole arrangement.

Screening of the Surrogate

According to Indian Council of Medical Research:

- The surrogate should be in the age group of 21–35 years.
- Tested for Blood group, HIV, HBsAg, HCV and VDRL.
- A thorough medical history and extensive medical testing and physical examination.
- A complete personal and sexual history to exclude individuals who might be at high risk for sexually transmitted infections.
- Psychological evaluation and counseling by a qualified professional is recommended for the surrogacy and her partner, and immediate family.

- The surrogate should be well informed about the procedure and the possible complications.
- The surrogate should be free from any medical conditions, hereditary disorders, hemoglobinopathies, infectious diseases, and personal addictions like smoking or alcohol consumption.

Before starting the cycle, a physical examination and PAP smear, infectious disease screening, hysteroscopy, a mock cycle must be done.

COUNSELING

The role of counseling is of utmost importance in surrogacy arrangement. This is to prepare all parties contemplating in this last resort treatment regarding the psychological, social, legal, emotional aspects. Counseling ensures that they should be confident and comfortable with their various decisions, and have trust in each other.

Couples should also be informed realistically, about the failures of the treatment. Legal considerations and financial obligations are to be discussed carefully. An attorney knowledgeable in reproductive law may also be consulted, whenever the need arises.

Counseling for the Couple

- The medical and psychological risks of surrogacy
- Potential psychological risk to the child
- The chances of having a multiple pregnancy
- The importance of obtaining legal advice.

Counseling for the Surrogate

- The full implications of undergoing treatment by IVF surrogacy
- The possibility of multiple pregnancy
- The possibility of her family and friends being against her having treatment
- The medical risks associated with pregnancy and delivery
- The implications of guilt on both sides if the host should spontaneously abort a pregnancy
- The possible effect on her own children of acting as a surrogate
- The possibility that the host may fell a sense of bereavement when she gives the baby to the commissioning couple.

ICMR Code of practice, and ethical considerations in gestational surrogacy (salient points):

- A child born through surrogacy must be adopted by the genetic (biological) parents, unless they can establish by genetic (DNA) fingerprinting that the child is theirs.
- Advertisements regarding surrogacy should not be made by the ART clinic. The responsibility of finding a surrogate mother, through advertisement or otherwise, should rest with the couple, or a registered agency.
- Legal papers regarding the contract agreement should be made by a lawyer, and as per the rules of the court.
- Payments to surrogate mothers should cover all genuine expenses associated with the pregnancy. Documentary evidence of the financial arrangement for surrogacy must be available. The ART center should not be involved in this monetary aspect.
- A relative, a known person, as well as a person unknown to the couple may act as a surrogate mother for the couple. In the case of a relative acting as a surrogate, the relative should belong to the same generation as the woman desiring the surrogate. The consent of the surrogate's spouse is essential in all cases.
- A surrogate mother should not be over 45 years of age.
- No woman may act as a surrogate more than thrice in her lifetime.
- Sex selection at any stage after fertilization, or abortion of the fetus of any particular sex should not be permitted, except to avoid the risk of transmission of a genetic abnormality assessed through genetic testing of biological parents or through preimplantation genetic diagnosis (PGD).
- A surrogate mother carrying a child biologically unrelated to her must register as a patient in her own name. The birth certificate shall be in the name of the genetic parents.
- The surrogate mother must relinquish in writing all parental rights concerning the offspring and vice versa.

REPRODUCTIVE TOURISM[11]

Regulations governing oocyte/sperm donation and surrogacy greatly vary from country to country. As a result, there exists a huge disparity in not only the spectrum of services, but the cost at which they are available to the infertile couple.

Due to these differences, we have witnessed the birth of fertility tourism, also known as *reproductive tourism*. This concept is defined as the process of traveling abroad to undergo a fertility treatment.

Singles and couples who opt for this option are usually forced to do so because of the restrictions they find in their own country, or because the process or part of it does not accommodate their needs.

Disclosure to Children

There exist many opinions regarding this issue, but the truth is that it depends on each family. Nonetheless, the ASRM considers that disclosure might be beneficial for the child for various reasons, including:

- Knowing your biological origins reinforces your autonomy
- Understanding your identity improves your decision-making skills
- Parents are able to build a relationship with the child based on openness and honesty
- Knowing your genetic heritage allows you to deal more accurately with severe health problems
- It helps protect the child against later inadvertent consanguinity.

On the other hand, those who are against disclosure argue that it would subject the child to a psychological turmoil, thereby affecting his long-term capacity of developing social skills. Nevertheless, researchers have found a greater interaction and skills between child and mothers who opted for third party reproduction than naturally conceived. More studies in this respect are needed to draw a conclusive evidence.

Different Consent Forms

- *Form D:* IVF/ICSI
- *Form I:* Consent form for oocyte retrieval
- *Form J:* Agreement for surrogate
- *Form K:* Consent form of donors
- *Form M(1):* Information on egg donor
- *Form M(2):* Information on surrogate mother
- *Form N:* Results of screening of semen donors/oocyte donors/surrogate mothers
- *Form O:* Record of use of donor gametes and surrogates
- *Form R(1):* Contract between the semen bank and the oocyte donor
- *Form R(2):* Contract between the semen bank and the surrogate
- *Form S:* Contract between the semen bank and the patient
- *Form T:* Contract between the semen bank and the ART clinic.

CONCLUSION

- Third party reproduction refers to the use of oocytes, sperm, embryos, or uterus that has been provided by a third person (donor) to enable an infertile individual or couple (intended parent) to become parents.
- Indications for treatment using donor oocytes include advanced maternal age, premature ovarian failure or poor ovarian reserve, recurrent IVF failure, genetic or chromosomal disorder in the female partner.
- Indications of donor sperm include severe male infertility (azoospermia), genetic or chromosomal disorders in the male partner, same sex couples or in single women.
- Indications for surrogacy include the absence of uterus (women with congenital absence of uterus or previous hysterectomy), unexplained recurrent miscarriage, repeated implantation failure, previous radiotherapy to pelvic structures or any medical condition due to which pregnancy is harmful for the recipient.
- Management options should include thorough counseling of the donor as well as the recipient.
- All donors should have a detailed medical and family history with emphasis on inherited disorders and STDs. The donors should be thoroughly screened for karyotype, CGT, CMV and any type of STD.
- Synchronization of donor's and recipient's cycle in a donor oocyte program is required.
- Endometrial preparation for recipients should be simplified and should be ideally customized.
- The ultimate goal of physicians and attorneys specializing in reproductive law is to enable this process to move forward as smoothly as possible and bring joy and satisfaction to all parties involved in ensuring conception and delivery of healthy child.
- Third party reproduction has got legal, moral, and ethical prescriptions along with the medical prescription.

KEY MESSAGES

Natural conception occurs in the presence of ovulation, normal sperm count and motility and patent pair of fallopian tubes. In the absence or dysfunction of any of the mentioned parameters pregnancy can still be achieved using donated gametes. Third party reproduction is mode of using the donor gametes or Surrogates in order to attain pregnancy. This chapter aims to provide the latest modes available, the complete screening and guidance and the medical and psychological impact on the donors as well as recipients by choosing this way of reproduction.

REFERENCES

1. American Society for Reproductive Medicine. Guidelines for oocyte donation. Fertil Steril. 2002;77:S6-S8.
2. Lutjen P, Trouson A, Leeton J. The establishment and maintenance of pregnancy using in vitro fertilization and embryo donation in a patient with primary ovarian failure. Nature 1984;307:174-5.
3. ICMR. The Assisted Reproductive Technologies (Regulation) Bill 2010. [online] Available from: http://icmr.nic.in/guide/ART%20REGULATIO%20Draft%20Bill1.pdf.[Last accessed December, 2021].
4. Meirow D, Schenker JG. The current status of sperm donation in assisted reproductive technology: ethical and legal considerations. J Assist Reprod Genet. 1997;14:133-8.
5. Zenke U, Chetkowski RJ. Transfer and uterine factors are the major recipient-related determinants of success with donor eggs. Fertil Steril. 2004;82(4):850-6.
6. Abbasi-Shavazi MJ, Nasrabad HBR, Ardekani ZB, Akhondi MM. Attitudes of infertile women towards gamete donation: a case study in Tehran. J Reprod Fertil. 2006;7(2):9.
7. Hershberger P. Recipients of oocyte donation: an integrative review. J Obstet Gynecol Neonatal Nurs. 2004;33(5):610-21.
8. Government of Bill. (2016). Surrogacy (Regulation Bill). Available from: http://164.100.47.4/BillsTexts/LSBillTexts/Asintroduced/257_LS_2016_Eng.pdf. [Last accessed December, 2021].
9. Lindenman E, Shepard MK, Pescovitz OH. Müllerian agenesis: an update. Obstet Gynecol. 1997;90:307-12.
10. Patel NH, Jadeja YD, Bhadarka HK, Patel MN, Patel NH, Sodagar NR. Insights into different aspects of surrogacy practices. J Hum Reprod Sci. 2018;11(3):212-8.
11. Deonandan R, Green S, van Bienum A. Ethical concerns for maternal surrogacy and reproductive tourism. J Med Ethics. 2012;38:742-5.

LONG QUESTIONS

1. Explain endometrial preparation procedure.
2. Enumerate the steps in third party reproduction.
3. Discuss the concept of counseling in third party reproduction.
4. Discuss the screening of surrogates in third party reproduction.
5. Discuss the screening of gametes in donor cycles.

SHORT QUESTIONS

1. What is the third party reproduction?
2. What are the indications for donor eggs?
3. What are the indications for sperm donor?
4. What are the indications for embryo donation?
5. What are the indications for surrogacy?

MULTIPLE CHOICE QUESTIONS

1. The ideal age group for donor egg cycle is:
   a. 20–30 years b. 21–35 years
   c. 25–40 years d. 30–50 years
2. The important factor to consider while screening egg donors is:
   a. STIs
   b. Caste
   c. Hormonal profile
3. _______ should be prevented while stimulating in donors.
   a. OHSS b. Bleeding
   c. Infection d. Ovarian torsion
4. _______ is the most optimal step in third party cycles.
   a. Endometrial preparation
   b. Blood profiling
   c. Patience
   d. Embryo transfer
5. Endometrial thickness should be:
   a. >7 to <14 mm b. >3 to <6 mm
   c. >10 to <14 mm d. >7 mm
6. Donor sperm should be quarantined for ___ time period.
   a. 6 months b. 15 days
   c. 1 week d. 1 year
7. The ideal age group for sperm donation is—
   a. 15–25 years b. 21–45 years
   c. 21–35 years d. 30–50 years
8. __________ of surrogacy where the surrogate is not compensated.
   a. Commercial b. Altruistic
   c. Compensated d. Traditional
9. _______ is an indication for surrogacy.
   a. MRKH b. Advanced age
   c. Male factor infertility
10. A mock cycle is done in _______
    a. Surrogacy b. Donor cycle
    c. Embryo donation d. Sperm donation

Answers

1.	b	2.	a	3.	a	4.	a	5.	a	6.	a
7.	b	8.	b	9.	a	10.	a				

12.15 ADOPTION

T Ramani Devi, D Gayathri

INTRODUCTION

Children are essential part of life for people in almost all culture whereas not having children is a personal tragedy causing impact on the entire family and the surrounding community which imposes a negative psychological consequence upon the family.[1]

Infertile people face problems ranging from overt ostracism or divorce leading to mental distress or isolation. Approximately 70 million couples are infertile worldwide. Recent advances in diagnosis and treatment have revolutionized the management of infertility. However, adequate health care facilities and high cost of ART remains a limiting factor to most couples. As a result of which 2–7% of people remain infertile in their reproductive period.[2]

Adoption has been considered by many as a privileged and unique lifestyle. Existence of an extensive adoption community encompassing a wide range of interesting aspects is noteworthy. In fact, adoption is not just procuring guardianship of a child by law but has factors way beyond.

The numerous facts and figures associated with adoption are of a wide range. Legally, adoption includes transferring birth parents rights and responsibility to the adoptive parents.[3] Regulation of adoption procedure and granting of adoption orders are done by the adoption board authority.

Adoption board authorities provide all required information and guide the couple through the entire process involved thereby helping them to decide whether adoption would be the best choice.

Adoption is a process which legally facilitates placement of a child with a married couple (to adopt a child) or a single female/male (to adopt only a male child) who agrees to raise the child as their own and assume all responsibilities for the child.

LAWS GOVERNING ADOPTION

- Hindu Adoption and Maintenance Act of 1956 (Hindus, Jain, Sikhs or Buddhists)
- Guardian and Wards Act of 1890 [Foreign citizens, nonresident Indians (NRIs) and Indian nationals who are Muslims, Christians or Jews]
- Juvenile Justice Act of 2000 (a part of which deals with Adoption of children by non-Hindu parents).

Requirements for a Valid Adoption

An adoption is valid only if it fulfills the following:

- The adopter is capable of taking in adoption legally.
- The person giving in adoption is capable of doing so by law.
- The child so adopted is capable of being taken in adoption legally.
- The adoption is completed by an actual giving and taking and after the ceremony called *Datta Homam* (oblation to the fire) has been performed. However this may not be essential in all cases as to the validity of adoption.

Who may Adopt a Child?

An Indian, NRI, a foreign citizen, a single female (unmarried, widowed or divorced) or single male (only male child) or a married couple can adopt a child.

Criteria for Children to be Considered for Adoption

- The child should be legally free for adoption.
- Two unrelated children cannot be adopted at the same time.
- A child may be placed in adoption before 12 years of age.
- Consent has to be obtained from children who are around 7 years of age.
- Siblings/twins/triplets cannot be separated.
- In case inter country adoption clearance from State Adoption Resource Authority-Adoption Coordinating Agency (SARA-ACA) is mandatory for all children. After adopting a child the birth certificate bears the name of adoptive parents mentioning the birth place (city or village) instead of the orphanage name. The child's name is liable to change by the adoptive parents if desired.

Capacity to Give the Child for Adoption

- Father or mother or guardian of the child.
- The father alone if mother has completely and finally renounced the world or has ceased to be a Hindu, or has been declared by a court of competent jurisdiction to be of unsound mind.
- The mother may give the child in adoption if the father is dead or has completely and finally renounced the world or has ceased to be a Hindu, or has been declared by a court of competent jurisdiction to be of unsound mind.
- Where both the father and mother are dead or have completely and finally renounced the world or have abandoned the child or have been declared by a court of competent jurisdiction to be of unsound mind or where the parentage of the child is unknown. The guardian of the child may give the child in adoption with the previous permission of the court.

CONDITIONS TO BE FULFILLED BY AN ADOPTIVE PARENT

- Fitness in medical and financial grounds to take care of a child.
- Should be 21 years old or above.
- Upper age limit legally not applicable for parents.
- Criteria on age limit of the parents may be relaxed if the adoption is of older children.
- Criteria on age limit of parents may be relaxed if the adoption is of a child with special needs.
- If the child to be taken in by adoption is a son, the adoptive father or mother must not have a son living at that time.
- If the child to be taken in by adoption is a daughter, the adoptive father or mother must not have a daughter living at that time.

Eligibility Criteria for Prospective Adoptive Parents

- Financial, physical, and emotional stability is essential among prospective adoptive parents.[4]
- Prospective parents irrespective of their marital status and even if they have a biological daughter or son they can adopt a child with following necessities.
- In case of a married couple consent of both spouses for adoption is mandatory. A single female can adopt child of any gender.
- A single male cannot adopt a girl child.
- 2 years of marital stability is essential among a couple prior to adoption.
- The age of prospective parent as per registration date shall be considered for deciding eligibility for adoption.
- If adoption is carried out by a couple, their composite age shall be considered.
- The age difference between the child and the adopter shall not be less than 25 years. This, however, may not be applicable in cases where the adopter is a relative or a step parent.
- As per subregulation (21) of regulation 2, couples with three or more biological children (except in case of special children) shall not be considered for adoption **(Table 1)**.

Hindu Adoption and Maintenance Act 1956

- An adopter has rights to ask for a child based on his/her preferences (age, gender, skin color, religion, specific features, and health condition) in adoption.

TABLE 1: Eligibility criteria for prospective adoptive parents.

Age of the child	Maximum composite age of prospective adoptive parents (couple)	Maximum age of single prospective adoptive parent
Up to 4 years	90 years	45 years
Above 4 and up to 8 years	100 years	50 years
Above 8 and up to 18 years	110 years	55 years

- Adoption of more than one child of the same sex by a single parent or a married couple is not permissible.

PROCESS OF ADOPTION STEPS

Step 1: Registration

- Register in a genuine adoption coordinating agency
- Never register with multiple agencies
- Adoption agencies in most of the states have been recognized by the Central and State Governments
- Preparation of the documentation and submission in a recognized agency is for registration.

Step 2: Home Study and Counseling

- Home study at the couple's residence
- Evaluate the adopter's parenting capabilities, applicant's motivations, their preparations, strengths, and weaknesses on the process of adoption
- This step is drafted into a report for submission to the honorable court.

Step 3: Referral of the Child

- The agency should show health records and other such reports pertaining to the child who is to be taken in adoption.
- Once this meets the adopter's preferences and they show willingness, the agency will arrange for a physical meet with the child.
- The couple then interacts with the child.
- Once comfortable, future formalities are to be carried out.

Step 4: Acceptance of the Child

Once the couple identifies the child, they can sign the documents pertaining to the acceptance of the child.

Step 5: Filing of Petition

- Documentations from the adopters along with those of the child are sent across to the lawyer for petition preparation.
- When the petition is ready, the adopter will be called and asked to sign the same at court in the presence of the court officer.

Step 6: Court Hearing

- Adopters, with the adopted child, should attend the court hearing.
- The Judge may pose a few simple questions. On receiving satisfactory answers, he will pass the order and mention the details regarding the investment to be made on the child's name.

Step 7: Court Order

- On making the investment and producing the receipt for the same to the Judge, the order will finally be issued.
- If the adoption is under *Hindu Adoption and Maintenance Act of 1956,* then a Deed of Adoption is prepared and the same needs to be registered with the local registrar's office.
- There is no such requirement in adoptions done under *Guardian and Wards Act of 1890 and Juvenile Justice Act of 2000 Acts.*

Step 8: Follow-up

- Following final adoption, the agency is required to submit follow-up reports regarding the child's wellbeing spanning over a period of 1–2 years to the court.
- Reports to the court about the child's wellbeing (For 1–2 years).

GUARDIAN AND WARDS ACT OF 1890

- Under this Act a foreign national is eligible to adopt an Indian child.
- The adopter is guardian of the adopted child until he/she becomes 18 years old.
- An adopter is permitted to ask for a child in adoption based on his/her preferences (age, gender, skin color, religion, etc.).
- Adoption by foreign citizens and NRIs are to be done based on the procedures pertaining to the adoption laws in the country of their residence.
- Registration of adoption in a Social/Child Welfare Agency recognized by the government of the residential country of the foreign adopter is necessary.
- Home study report will be compiled by a professional social worker for the agency.
- It is mandatory for the foreign adopter to submit the application and declaration of willingness along with the supporting documents.
- Filling of the application will be duly performed by the Indian welfare agency or any other person authorized by them.
- The court of the District Judge within whose jurisdiction the Social and Welfare Child Agency in India that handles the application of the foreign adopter will handle the application for guardianship as well.
- The initial step consists of hearing of concerned parties by the court followed by examination of all the documents.

- The foreign adopter should give the court assurance that he/she will be a suitable adoptive parent and the court should be satisfied that the child will be provided tender loving care in a secure home.
- On satisfaction of the above mentioned points, the court will then pass an order.
- *LK Pandey vs. Union of India:* The Supreme Court of India has laid down certain guidelines for foreign adoption in an attempt to safeguard the interests of the children.
- Applications made under the Guardians and Wards Act, 1890 has to be disposed of within 2 months.
- Requirement for personal presence of the foreign national.

JUVENILE JUSTICE ACT OF 2000

Children who have been abused and not those children who have voluntarily put up for adoption.

Placement of Child shall be Treated Illegal

- If adoption of an orphan, abandoned or surrendered child is a private arrangement.
- A child is placed without involvement of recognized agencies or authorities.
- A child is adopted without ensuring safety in the family which he or she is adopted.
- If prospective adoptive parents are of the same sex adoption shall be declared illegal.
- Any payment made to mothers or parents to place their babies.
- Direct placement by advocates or intermediaries or by biological parents without following guideline procedures.

PSYCHOLOGICAL ASPECTS OF ADOPTION ON THE CHILD

Adoption causes unique psychological impact on adopted children, birth parents and adoptive parents. Coping with these feelings is a difficult task and a challenge that must be met. In addition to the normal development issues, every child goes through a cycle of adjustment and development issues as he or she grows. These issues are correlated with anxiety, grief, self-esteem, and identity. Adopted children over-presents with mental, emotional and behavioral problems than nonadopted children because it will take time for them to adopt with a family.

When older children are adopted from faster care they may have to overcome with loss of siblings, grandparents who were or might have been are part of their life.

Many studies have shown that adopted persons have less self-esteem and self-confidence than non-adopted counterparts. Hence, psychiatrist advices to explain the child about adoption in a way that they can understand, because knowledge on adoption intentionally or accidentally from someone other than parents causes anger or mistrust toward parents.[5]

Effects on Adoptive Parents

Although the excitement of actual adoption anticipated by couples persists. Sometimes they may unknowingly enter into a phase called post adoption depression syndrome (PADS).[6] This phase may arise self-doubt in the adopters on their parenting capabilities due to the difficulties they encounter in getting attached to the new child. As time passes, slowly depression vanishes out as the parents adjust to the new life. Sometimes, a therapist is needed when depression persists over weeks or hinders the adopters' individual ability.

CONCLUSION

Adoption is the establishment of an emotional bond and a new relationship of unconditional love between the adopter and the adopted. After which, there is no legal difference perceived between an adopted child and a child by birth. Open communication acceptance and supporting family environment defines a successful adoption. Let us make families out of couples.

KEY MESSAGES

Adoption is creating parent child relationship between persons who are not biologically related. It is a sociolegal process that confers mutual rights and obligations. As a result of adoption the child gets identity of his/her adoptive parents in the society. We believe that "every child has a right to a family" and adoption is a better option for homeless children. In India two main acts which are involved with adoption includes the Hindu Adoption and Maintenance Act (HAMA) 1956 and the Guardians and Ward Act (GAWA) 1890. Legally adopted children can enforce his/her rights in the court of law. On the contrary, informal adoptions are considered as gross violation.

REFERENCES

1. Dyer SJ. The value of children in African countries–insights from studies on infertility. J Psychosom Obstet Gynecol. 2007;28(2):69-77.
2. Aina OF. An overview of sociocultural and psychiatric aspects of women's reproductive health in West Africa. Niger Postgrad Med J. 2007;14:231-7.
3. Draft Guidelines on Adoption of Indian children without parental care. New Delhi: Ministry of Women and Child development of India; 2008.
4. Brand AE, Brinich PM. Behavior problems and mental health contacts in adopted, foster, and nonadopted children. J Child Psychol Psychiatr Allied Disc. 1999;40(8):1221-9.
5. AACAP. Facts for families. Washington DC: American Academy of child and Adolescent Psychiatry; 2011.
6. Eldridge S. 20 things adoptive parents need to succeed. New York: Random House; 2009.

LONG QUESTIONS

1. Define adoption. Discuss the requirements for valid and legal adoption in India.
2. Describe the laws governing adoption of a baby in India.

SHORT QUESTIONS

1. What are the conditions to be fulfilled by adoptive parents?
2. What are the possible psychological aspects of adoption on the child and parents?

MULTIPLE CHOICE QUESTIONS

1. Which of the following is not a law governing adoption?
   a. Hindu Adoption and Maintenance Act of 1956
   b. Guardian and Wards Act of 1890
   c. Juveline Justice Act of 2000
   d. Surrogacy Act 2020
2. Which of the following is considered illegal?
   a. Child is placed without involvement of recognized agencies or authorities
   b. Child is adopted without ensuring safety in family
   c. Any payment to mother and parents to place their babies
   d. All of the above
3. Conditions to be fulfilled by an adoptive parent does not include one of the below:
   a. > 21 years old
   b. Upper age limit of 50 years
   c. Adoption of older children, age of parent may be relaxed
   d. Adopted child with special needs the age limit may be relaxed
4. Who has the capacity to give the child for adoption?
   a. Father/mother or guardian of the child
   b. Father alone if mother has completely and finally renounced the world or has ceased to be a Hindu
   c. Mother may give the child in adoption if father is dead or has been declared by a court of competent jurisdiction to be of unsound mind
   d. All of the above

Answers

1. d 2. d 3. b 4. d

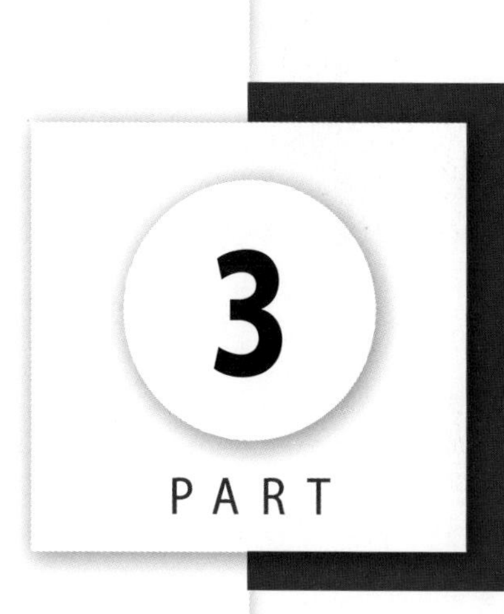

Urogynaecology and Gynaecological Oncology

Urogynaecology

13.1 ASSESSMENT OF LOWER URINARY TRACT COMPLAINTS AND FUNCTION

Achla Batra, Karishma Thariani

INTRODUCTION

The lower urinary tract (LUT) is composed of the bladder and urethra, and the two defining functions of the LUT are urinary storage (continence) and emptying (micturition) **(Fig. 1)**. The proper conduction of these two functions depends on an integrated system, comprising of the central nervous system, the peripheral nervous system, bladder smooth muscles, urethra and the pelvic floor. Any disturbances in the smooth functioning of this integrated system can lead to lower urinary tract dysfunction (LUTD) which manifests in the form of lower urinary tract symptoms (LUTS).

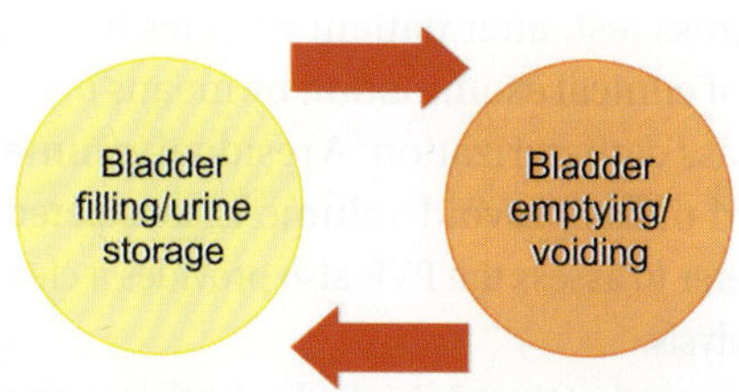

Fig. 1: The two main functions of the lower urinary tract.

Lower urinary tract symptoms are the subjective indicator of a disease or change in condition as perceived by the patient, carer, or partner and may lead him/her to seek help from health care professionals.[1] Symptoms may either be volunteered by or elicited from the patient at the time of history taking. They are usually qualitative and cannot be used alone to make a definitive diagnosis and hence require further evaluation to understand the lower urinary tract dysfunction.

CLASSIFICATION OF THE LOWER URINARY TRACT SYMPTOMS

The lower urinary tract symptoms are divided into three groups: (1) storage, (2) voiding and (3) postmicturition symptoms **(Table 1)**.

ASSESSMENT OF LOWER URINARY TRACT SYMPTOMS

A thorough assessment of LUTS is extremely essential as it helps in coming to a definitive diagnosis. It involves multiple steps, comprising of a detailed history, examination, urinalysis,

TABLE 1: Classification of lower urinary tract symptoms (LUTS).

Storage symptoms	***Voiding symptoms***	***Postmicturition symptoms***
Increased day time frequency	Hesitancy	Feeling of incomplete emptying
Urgency	Intermittency	Postmicturition dribble
Nocturia	Slow stream	Position-dependent micturition
Urinary incontinence: • Stress urinary incontinence • Urgency urinary incontinence • Mixed urinary incontinence • Continuous urinary incontinence	Splitting or spraying of stream	Dysuria
	Straining to void	Urinary retention
	Terminal dribble	

bladder diary, imaging, and other tests depending on the need. We shall be discussing each of these points in detail.

History Taking

- *History of LUTS:* A detail and well taken history helps in understanding the severity, frequency and duration of the LUTS volunteered by the patient and also helps in eliciting certain other complaints which the patient may be suffering from, but does not consider them to be significant. Early in the history, one should elicit a description of the patient's main complaint, including duration and frequency. A clear understanding of the severity of the problem or disability and its effect on quality of life should be sought. Assessment of mobility and living environment is especially important in certain patients. Questions should be asked about access to toilets or toilet substitutes and about social factors such as living arrangements, social contacts, and caregiver involvement. **Box 1** enumerates questions that help in evaluation of a woman presenting with incontinence.[2]
- *Menstrual history:* It is of importance as menopause may lead to worsening of certain LUTS. Also, women with vesicovaginal fistulas may be amenorrhic due to hypothalamic suppression or present with menouria as in uterovesical fistula.
- *Obstetric history:* The obstetric history should include gravidity, parity, number of vaginal deliveries, any instrumental delivery and or cesarean section. Any history of difficult delivery, vaginal lacerations or cervical tears, birth of a large baby, and the time interval between deliveries should be recorded. Pregnancies and deliveries per se predispose to SUI. In case patient complains of continuous incontinence after childbirth then the interval between the delivery and onset of symptoms should be noted.
- *Medical history:* The clinical assessment should seek to identify relevant coexistent predisposing and precipitating factors. The medical history should identify contributing factors such as diabetes mellitus, chronic lung disease, stroke, lumbar disk disease, fecal impaction, cognitive impairment, congestive heart failure, obesity, connective tissue disorders, chronic urinary tract infection, urinary tract stones, and cancer of pelvic organs. History of all the drugs that the patient is taking should be obtained as certain medications cause incontinence and some may cause difficulty in passing urine **(Table 2)**.
- *Personal history:* The effect of UI on the quality of life of the woman should be assessed. Lifestyle issues such as smoking, alcohol or caffeine abuse, and occupational and recreational factors causing repeated increase in intra-abdominal pressure should be inquired.

BOX 1: Evaluation of a woman with lower urinary tract symptoms (LUTS).

- Do you leak urine when you cough, sneeze or laugh?
- Do you ever have such an uncomfortably strong need to urinate that if you do not reach the toilet you will leak?
- If "Yes" to question 2, do you ever leak before you reach the toilet?
- How many times during the day do you urinate?
- How many times do you void during the night after going to bed?
- Do you have to use a pad to stay dry?
- Do you have recurrent urinary tract infections?
- Do you have pain on passing urine?
- Do you find it difficult to start urinating?
- Do you suffer from thin urinary stream, intermittent stream, interrupted flow or feeling of incomplete bladder emptying?
- Do you dribble urine as you stand or walk after passing urine?

Physical Examination

Physical examination is extremely essential in the evaluation of all patients with LUTD. It should include general physical examination including calculation of BMI, abdominal, pelvic, perineal, and a focused neurological examination.

- *Abdominal examination:* Abdomen should be inspected and palpated for any surgical scars, masses, etc. Bladder may be felt suprapubically in patients with urinary retention.
- *Local perineal/genital examination:* This should include description of the skin such as presence of atrophy, excoriation, scar marks, ulcerations or any other anatomic abnormality. It also allows for demonstration of incontinence by means of cough stress Test. The patient in full bladder is made to perform Valsalva or cough. Any escape of urine per urethra is observed and is suggestive of stress urinary incontinence. Extra urethral leakage may be observed in patients of vesicovaginal fistulas.
- *Measurement of postvoid urine:* This may be done after the cough stress test, after patient empties her bladder, or in the end of clinical examination by means of ultrasound or single-pass catheterization. A residual volume of less than one-third of the prevoid volume is considered normal. Use of a catheter to assess the PVR also provides a clean sample for urine analysis.
- *Vaginal examination:* It includes both per speculum and bimanual examination. It helps in observing changes of

TABLE 2: Effect of drugs on lower urinary tract symptoms (LUTS).

Medication	*Effect on lower urinary tract function*
Diuretics	Urgency, frequency
Antidepressants	Sedation, retention
Caffeine	Frequency, urgency
Narcotics	Retention, constipation
Anticholinergic	Retention, difficulty in voiding
Calcium channel blockers	Retention
Alpha adrenergic blockers	Urinary leakage

vaginal atrophy, presence of pelvic organ prolapse and its quantification or presence of any cyst or diverticulum. A thorough bimanual examination helps in ruling out any other co existent pelvic pathology, lump or any focus of tenderness **(Fig. 2)**.

- *Pelvic floor muscle function:* Pelvic floor muscle function can be qualitatively defined by the tone at rest and the strength of a voluntary or reflex contraction as strong, weak or absent or by a validated grading system (e.g., Oxford 1–5).
- *Neurological examination:* A screening neurological examination should always be performed. It includes evaluation of mental status, sensory and motor function of both lower extremities, and also a screening lumbosacral neurologic examination. The screening lumbosacral examination should include assessments of: (1) pelvic floor muscle strength, (2) anal sphincter resting tone, (3) voluntary anal contraction, and (4) perineal sensation. This simple screening examination can be performed quickly and easily as part of the gynecologic examination.
- *Rectal examination:* Perrectalexaminationis done to evaluate the tone of anal sphincter, any fecaliths, any rectal growth or rectovaginalfistula.

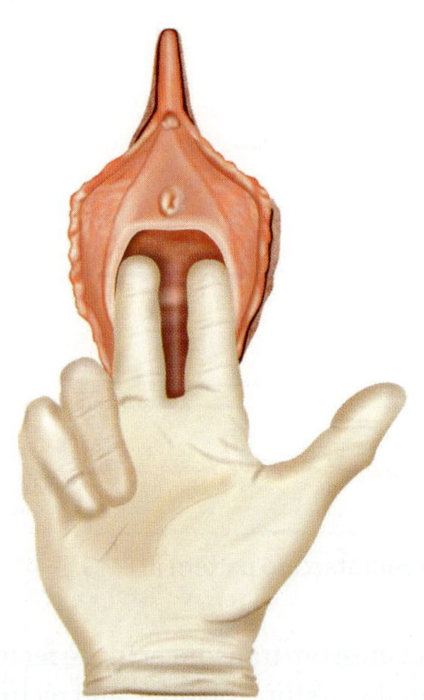

Fig. 2: Bonney's test for stress incontinence.

Bladder Diary

It records the times of micturition and voided volumes, incontinence episodes, pad usage, and other information such as fluid intake, the degree of urgency, and the degree of incontinence. A 3-day diary is generally sufficient. This is not only helpful for pretreatment assessment but also help in objective assessment ofpost-therapy outcomes **(Table 3)**.

Investigations

- *Urine analysis:* Urine routine, microscopy and culture sensitivity are common methods of urine analysis. Urine routine and microscopy should be undertaken in all women presenting with LUTS.
- *Ultrasonography:* Ultrasonography offers a noninvasive method of assessing postvoid residual urine in patients. Any abdominal or adnexal mass can also be detected on ultrasound. Transperineal USG and endovaginal USG may

TABLE 3: Picture of a bladder diary of a patient with mixed urinary incontinence.

Date	***Drink***		***Urine***		***Leakage***		
Time	Type	How much (mL)	Volume of urine (mL)	How urgent 0–3 3 = most urgent	Leakage with urgency	Leakage with activities	Pad change
0200			150 mL		Y		
0700	Mug coffee	250 mL	250 mL				
0800			60 mL			Cough	P
0900	Cup orange juice	200 mL				Sneeze	
1000			100 mL				
1200	2 mugs coffee	500 mL					
1400			300 mL		Y		
1530	Cup of tea	200 mL				Jogging	P
1600			100 mL				
1800	Cup of tea	200 mL					
1900			100 mL		Y		
2000	Glass of beer	200 mL	20 mL				
2030	Glass of wine	50 mL				Cough	
2200							P
2300			150 mL				

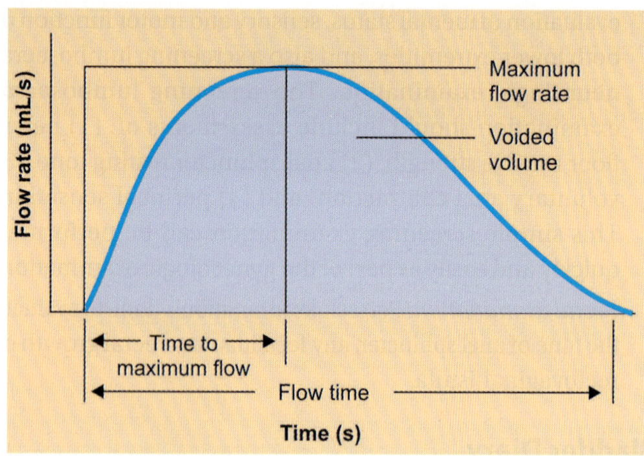

Fig. 3: A normal uroflow pattern.

TABLE 4: Validated questionnaires.

Questionnaire	*Symptom evaluated*	*Goal*
UDI-6 (Urogenital Distress Inventory)	Urinary incontinence	Symptom distress
IIQ (Incontinence Impact Questionnaire)	Urinary incontinence	Life impact
PFIQ (Pelvic Floor Impact Questionnaire)	UI, POP, colorectal dysfunction	Life impact
OABS	Overactive bladder	Symptom distress

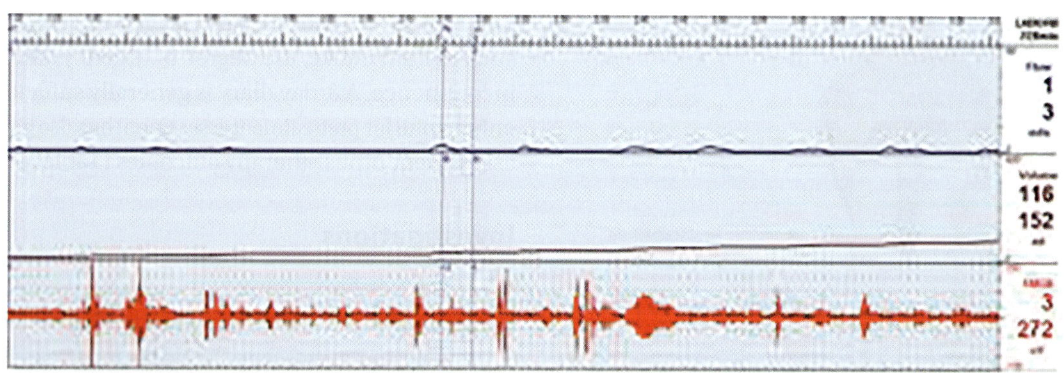

Fig. 4: Uroflowmetry with surface EMG showing interrupted flow with staccato pattern in EMG.

be used to document urethral hypermobility and other pelvic floor defects.

- *Uroflowmetry:* Uroflowmetry is noninvasive, inexpensive and is best used as a screening test in patients who may have LUTS. It should ideally be done before the other urodynamic studies. It measures the urine flow rate and its pattern. Normally, the maximum flow rate of urine is 15 mL/s and the pattern is bell-shaped with an early peak flow rate **(Fig. 3)**. In women with obstruction the flow rate is slow. Uroflowmetry combined with postvoid residual urine can use for diagnosing voiding dysfunction. Since small voided volumes may affect the curve shape only voided volumes >150 mL are interpretable. A normal uroflowmetry and residual volume of less than 100 mL, may be useful in ruling out voiding dysfunction. In cases where pelvic floor dyssynergia is suspected, a uroflowmetry with surface EMG may be preferred **(Fig. 4)**.
- *Multichannel urodynamics*: This may be reserved for cases where a clear diagnosis is not possible only by means of history and clinical examination alone, in cases where symptoms persists despite treatment, cases of neurogenic bladder, patients planned for incontinence surgery, cases of urinary incontinence with prolapse or in patients with outflow obstruction.[2] The aim of urodynamics is to replicate symptoms and record the pressure and flow changes in the bladder and recognize the basic cause for the symptoms. It is an invasive investigation, involving catheterization of the bladder and pressure transducer in the rectum to measure pressures in the urethra, bladder, and rectum.
- *Use of validated questionnaires*: The severity of symptoms and their effect on the patient's quality of life are vital parameters which should be recorded by means of standard validated questionnaires. Few important questionnaires are listed in **Table 4**.[3]
- *Cystoscopy*: Cystourethroscopy may help in identifying bladder and urethral lesions such as urethral diverticulum, stricture, fistulas, features of bladder wall inflammation and foreign bodies. Bladder mucosal biopsy may be coupled with this investigation to diagnose interstitial cystitis. It is also used for the evaluation of incontinence suspected to be due to surgical trauma.

REFERENCES

1. Abrams P, Cardozo L, Fall M, Griffiths D, Rozier P, Ulmsten U, et al. The standardization of terminology of lower urinary tract function: report from the Standardisation Sub-committee of the International Continence Society. Neurobiol Urodynam. 2002;21:167-78.
2. Kobashi KC, Albo ME, Dmochowski RR. Surgical treatment of female stress urinary incontinence (SUI): AUA/SUFU guideline 2017. J Urol. 2017;198:875.
3. Capobianco G, Madonia M, Morelli, Desole F. Management of female stress urinary incontinence; a care and update pathway. Maturitas. 2018;109:32-8.

LONG QUESTIONS

1. Mention the important points in history for evaluation of LUTS.
2. What are the different diagnostic tests which may help in evaluation of LUTS?

SHORT QUESTIONS

1. Describe the indications of urodynamic evaluation in women.
2. Enumerate the various lower urinary tract symptoms in women and their etiological causes.
3. What is the significance of post void urine?

MULTIPLE CHOICE QUESTIONS

1. LUTS are classified as:
   a. Storage symptoms
   b. Voiding symptoms
   c. Postmicturition symptoms
   d. All
2. Alpha blockers can cause:
   a. Urine retention b. Burning
   c. Urine leak d. None
3. What is abnormal PVR:
   a. >50 mL b. >100 mL
   c. >1/3rd of prevoid d. None
4. Cough stress test is used to demonstrate:
   a. Urgency urinary incontinence
   b. Stress urinary incontinence
   c. Both a and b
   d. None
5. Oxford score measures:
   a. Pelvic floor muscle strength
   b. Urethral sphincter strength
   c. Anal tone
   d. None
6. Bladder diary is:
   a. Measure of no. of voids only
   b. Measure of volume of voids only
   c. Frequency–volume chart
   d. None
7. Minimum voided volume for interpretation of UFM is:
   a. >100 mL b. >200 mL
   c. >250 mL d. >150 mL
8. Voiding dysfunction is best diagnosed by:
   a. UFM b. UFM with surface EMG
   c. Both d. None
9. Multichannel UDS should be done in:
   a. All cases of incontinence
   b. In all cases of SUI
   c. Pelvic organ Prolapse
   d. POP with SUI
10. Choose the correct statement:
    a. UFM is invasive
    b. UDS is mandatory for diagnosis of incontinence
    c. Cystoscopy helps in diagnosis of type of incontinence
    d. None

Answers

1.	d	2.	c	3.	c	4.	b	5.	a	6.	c
7.	d	8.	b	9.	d	10.	d				

13.2 NONSURGICAL AND SURGICAL TREATMENT OF STRESS URINARY INCONTINENCE

N Rajamaheswari, Vaishnavy

INTRODUCTION

Stress urinary incontinence (SUI) is common in women. Though not a life-endangering problem, it does significantly compromise the quality of life of the sufferers.

The International Continence Society describes *stress urinary incontinence* as involuntary leakage of urine with an increase in intra-abdominal pressure such as coughing and sneezing.

Stress urinary incontinence usually results from weak or damaged muscles and connective tissues of the pelvic floor, or due to weakness of the urethral sphincter itself.

Among young adults and middle-aged, SUI is reported approximately in 25% of women and its prevalence increases further with the increase in age.

Apart from increasing age, pregnancy, vaginal delivery, instrumental delivery, menopause, obesity, intra-abdominal mass, extensive pelvic surgery, chronic cough and constipation are the other risk factors implicated.

MANAGEMENT OF STRESS URINARY INCONTINENCE

Assessment of a Patient with SUI

All patients presenting with SUI should have a detailed assessment, which includes a general, abdominal, vaginal and rectal examination **(Box 1)**. This is primarily to look for contributing factors such as abdominal/pelvic mass, prolapse, neurological problems, etc.

Patients should have a routine urine examination to rule out infections and stone disease. A urine culture is necessary if an infection is suspected. Besides an ultrasound scan and basic blood tests provide information about other causes.

Preoperative Urodynamic Evaluation

The role of preoperative urodynamics for patients who have SUI has long been a matter of debate.

A urodynamic evaluation helps to avoid unnecessary intervention and enables a better understanding of the lower urinary tract symptoms (LUTS) **(Box 2)**. It is a must at least before surgical management.

Preoperative urodynamic study:

- Confirms the occurrence of leakage with physical exertion in the absence of detrusor contraction.
- Detects coexisting detrusor overactivity and voiding problems.
- Recognition of preexisting voiding problems with pressure-flow study demands discreet use of surgical interventions.
- *Low urethral mucosal closure pressure*: Low leak point pressure points out to intrinsic sphincter deficiency (ISD) and alerts the surgeon to select retropubic slings [pubovaginal slings (PVS)/retropubic-midurethral sling (RP-MUS)].

Urodynamic evaluation thereby ensures effective treatment and is instrumental in reducing treatment failures.[1]

History of mixed incontinence or atypical urinary leakage, previous surgical failures (persistent and recurrent SUI) and features suggestive of neurogenic bladder demand a full urodynamic evaluation.

Treatment of SUI can be conservative, pharmacological, or surgical. Mostly less severe and infrequent episodes of SUI are managed by nonsurgical treatment options.

Behavioral and Lifestyle Modifications

Weight Reduction

Maintaining an ideal body weight helps with the management of SUI.[2] Avoiding excess caffeine and smoking helps indirectly too.

Regular exercises and in particular exercises that engage the core muscles to make a significant difference.

Pelvic Floor Exercises

Supervised pelvic floor exercises done diligently and regularly are helpful in the management of SUI. They have to be done for at least 3–6 months to make a significant impact. Biofeedback and electrical stimulation can be used to augment the effectiveness of pelvic floor exercises.[3]

Kegel's exercises have been in practice since the 1940s **(Box 3)**. However, the biggest problem is the awareness of the right group of muscles in this population.

In the past, vaginal cones and short-term electrical stimulation have been used to assist the patients to identify and exercise the appropriate group of pelvic floor muscles. Biofeedback using a probe in the vagina that is connected to a monitor provides visual feedback is extremely helpful.[4]

Containment and Support Devices

The indications for using support devices are given in **Box 4**.

Pessaries with urethral support are available, though of limited use. It can be particularly helpful if urinary incontinence is associated with a prolapse.

Pessary: The Pessaries help by restoring the urethrovesical angle. The pessaries are of two types—(1) supportive (ring pessary) and (2) obstructive (Gellhorn or donut pessary).[5,6] The type and size of the pessary depend on the severity of the prolapse, the patient's age, sexual function, and presence of a uterus. In the majority, the doctor inserts the pessary

BOX 1: Patient assessment.

- History
- Examination
- Pelvic organ prolapse-quantification (POP-Q) grading
- Q-tip test
- Urine-routine examination, culture and sensitivity and cytology
- Blood tests to rule out diabetes and renal diseases

BOX 2: Urodynamics in stress urinary incontinence.

- Flow rates and postvoid residual volume
- Detrusor contractions and detrusor over activity
- Bladder capacity and compliance
- Valsalva leak point pressure
- Mean urethral closure pressure
- Voiding detrusor pressure and flow

BOX 3: Kegel's exercises.

- The patient is asked to empty her bladder
- The exercises can be done either in a lying down or sitting posture
- The patient will be advised to contract their pelvic floor and hold for 10 seconds and relax for 10 seconds
- They should do 10 slow contractions and 10 quick contractions or "the Knack" at a time and repeat this 5–10 times a day
- These exercises are not done when a woman is passing urine

BOX 4: Indications for using support devices.

- In patients who are keen to avoid surgery
- For patients not fit for surgery
- Occasionally as primary management of prolapse
- During pregnancy

and regular follow-up at least every 3 months is advised. The common complications are infection, vaginal erosion, and ulceration. Fistula formation is rare in current-day practice unless the pessary is forgotten.

Urethral insert: It is a device that is inserted into the urethra. It is particularly helpful for short-term use, for example for women who leak during a gym session or high-impact sports only. They are designed for single use only. Patients need proper training to insert this device and remove it. The most common side effects are infection, pain and hematuria. They cannot be used if the patient has an infection, neoplasia or significant overactivity of the bladder.

Medical Treatment

Duloxetine

Duloxetine is a noradrenergic serotonin reuptake inhibitor. It was originally used for the management of depression and was found to have a significant beneficial effect on stress urinary incontinence in the elderly population.[7] However, this medication's efficacy is only 40–50% and therefore used when all alternatives are exhausted **(Box 5)**.

Sudden withdrawal of this medication is associated with nightmares and suicidal thoughts and patients need to be warned regarding this. The most common side effects of this medication are nausea and fatigue. These medications are not FDA approved for the management of incontinence. The maximum permissible dose is 40 mg twice a day but is typically started at a small dose and titrated against the effect.

Estrogen

Local vaginal creams or oral estrogen have been used for the management of urogenital atrophy and incontinence.[8]

Indications: Urogenital atrophy with incontinence.

The Cochrane review of the matter in 2009 found that vaginal estrogen is better than oral estrogen and found that oral estrogen either alone or in combination with progesterone caused a worsening of urinary incontinence. The estrogen cream when applied vaginally is thought to increase vascularity of the vaginal and periurethral region and increases the thickness of the urethral mucosa and thereby facilitates coaptation of the urethra. Estrogen is also thought to increase the alpha-adrenergic receptors in the bladder and urethra and improve continence.

Estrogen cream is usually prescribed once a day for 6–8 weeks, followed by a maintenance regime of once or twice a week.

BOX 5: Indications for using duloxetine.

- Not willing for surgery
- Unfit for surgical procedures
- As a temporary measure prior to surgery

Surgical Treatment

When conservative measures fail, surgical treatment becomes the main treatment for SUI.

The objective of continence surgery is to restore continence without creating outlet obstruction. The procedures used in the treatment of SUI, either aim to reposition the bladder neck or enhance the urethral sphincter function. Though hundreds of surgical procedures have been improvised, no surgical technique has been identified to suit all incontinent patients. Therefore, the surgeon should individualize each case and select the technique best suited to the patient.

The choice of surgery is decided based on the patient's expectations, day-to-day activities of the patient, comorbid pelvic pathology, physical fitness, surgeon's expertise, etc.

Most importantly, the pathogenesis of sphincter incompetence, whether urethral hypermobility or ISD is the predominant factor that determines the site or route of the sling.

Women who have significant SUI with minimal physical exertion or leakage with an empty bladder are more likely to have ISD. On the contrary, SUI predominately due to urethral hypermobility tends to present with less severe symptoms.

The other signs of ISD include:

- Patulous external urethral meatus with well-supported urethra on clinical examination
- Failure of closure of bladder neck during cystourethroscopy
- Low urethral mucosal closure pressure (<20 cm of water)
- Low leak point pressure (<60 cm of water).

Often urethral hypermobility and ISD coexist. Treatment is planned based upon the predominant factor.

Women with SUI due to ISD will greatly benefit from retropubic sling (MUS or PVS) or urethral bulking agents.

Stress urinary incontinence due to hypermobility-related sphincter incompetence can be successfully managed by colposuspension or transobturator MUS.

Pubovaginal slings and retropubic MUS can effectively take care of both ISD and urethral hypermobility-related sphincter incompetency.

Retropubic MUS provides a classical obstructive sling effect compared to the hammock effect provided by transobturator MUS **(Fig. 1)**.

Sling Procedures

Sling procedures are well established in the surgical management of SUI. The technique relies on a strip of material autologous or synthetic placed under the proximal or mid urethra to provide support.

Natural slings are commonly autologous fascia either from the thigh, such as fascia lata or rectus fascia, or allogeneic from cadaveric fascia or porcine dermis. If synthetic slings are used, macroporous, monofilament polypropylene mesh slings are preferred over others.

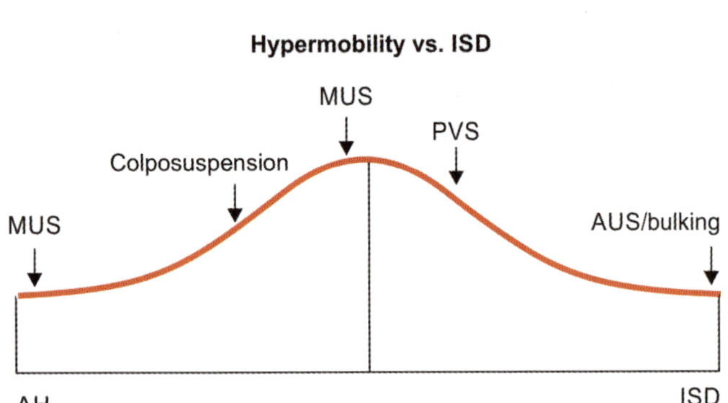

Fig. 1: Retropubic MUS provides a classical obstructive sling effect. (AUS: artificial urinary sphincter; ISD: intrinsic sphincter deficiency; MUS: midurethral sling; PVS: pubovaginal slings; SUI: stress urinary incontinence)

Proximal Urethral Slings (or) Pubovaginal Sling

Pubovaginal sling is an autologous sling, placed under the proximal urethra through the retro pubic route. The sling procedure is done by a combined abdominal-vaginal approach using rectus fascia or fascia lata.[9] While the cure rates range from 85 to 90%, the complications reported include pain, voiding dysfunction (10%), urinary tract infections and de novo urgency (16.6%) **(Box 6)**.

Pubovaginal slings were initially reserved for women with previous failed surgery with restricted vaginal mobility. It used to be a long, complicated procedure involving extensive dissection and blood loss. The high occurrence of voiding problems and other complications prevented its use as a primary procedure.

Overtime PVS technique was subjected to several modifications. Small incision, minimal dissection and placement of the retropubic PVS by a minimally invasive needle technique were introduced. These modifications shortened the duration of the operation. Most importantly, these suburethral slings are placed under the proximal urethra, in a tension-free manner, which minimized postoperative voiding problems. Eventually, newer PVS sling procedures were performed quickly, with minimal complications and have been found to be equally effective.

Thus "sling on a string type of PVS" using autologous fascia lata or rectus sheath (harvested through a lower abdominal incision) has gained momentum and popularity as it avoids mesh-related complications completely.

Pubovaginal sling is intentionally placed tension-free to minimize postoperative voiding complications.

Pubovaginal sling surgically augments intraurethral pressure, thereby resulting in urethral compression and improves the transmission of intra-abdominal pressure to the proximal urethra. Coaptation is accomplished without causing the obstruction.

BOX 6: Indications for using PVS.

- In patients with stress urinary incontinence (SUI) with intrinsic sphincter deficiency (ISD)
- In patients who are reluctant to have the mesh procedure
- In patients who have had mesh complications and removal
- In patients with significant pelvic pain issues

BOX 7: Indications for using retropubic midurethral slings.

- Urodynamic stress incontinence significantly affecting quality of life
- Sphincter incompetency due to ISD
- Failed transobturator tape/colposuspension
- Failed urethral bulking agents

The efficacy of this procedure is found to be superior or comparable to the mid-urethral sling procedure. Based on the evidence, PVS is now recommended as a primary procedure for women with SUI.

Sandy Kim et al.[10] reported a success rate of 53% after nearly a decade and a half following PVS surgery and opined that the autologous fascia PVS remains an effective and lasting treatment option for both simple and complex SUI.

Midurethral Slings

The tension-free vaginal tape (TVT) initially described by Ulmsten differs from the conventional PVS. With TVT, the polypropylene mesh tape is placed under the midurethra via the vaginal approach exiting abdominally through the retropubic space. TVT is deliberately placed tension-free and support is achieved by causing a tissue reaction with a subsequent collagen formation.

The standard slings are made of monofilament, macroporous polypropylene mesh. They have been the gold standard for the management of SUI since the late 1990s.

Retropubic Midurethral Slings

These are slings inserted through a small 1 cm incision in the vagina, in the region of the midurethra. They course through the retropubic space and exit through small wounds in the suprapubic area **(Box 7)**. Peroperative cystoscopy is mandatory to recognize inadvertent entry into the bladder or urethra.

Retropubic MUS are effective and most studies report 85–95% efficacy. It is a minimally invasive procedure and is usually done as a day case procedure under anesthesia.

The complications reported with this procedure are bladder injuries, infections, voiding dysfunction, mesh extrusion, and pelvic pain.[11]

Early case series with TVT, quoted objective cure rates of 84–100% for up to 2 years. Higher success rates have persisted in the long-term studies with a 95% cure rate at 5 years and an 82% cure rate at 7 years.[12]

The risk of voiding disorders is around 2% and that of de novo detrusor overactivity is around 5%. The largest randomized trial comparing TVT and colposuspension has shown similar objective cure rates for both the procedures (66% with TVT and 57% with colposuspension).

The largest RCT compares TVT with colposuspension. Apart from providing the cure rates this study also brought to light various complications encountered with TVT. Vascular, bladder and bowel injuries have been reported with TVT procedure. These were thought to be related to the blind entry of the needle into the retropubic space and modified devices were introduced attempting to reduce it.

The suprapubic-arc sling (SPARC) procedure advocates the passage of the device from above downward in an attempt to minimize vascular damage (i.e., antegrade versus retrograde).

Transobturator Midurethral Sling

The risk of bladder injury associated with the retropubic slings led to the innovation of MUS through the obturator foramen.

Placing MUS by the transobturator route was introduced by Delorme.[13] De Leval[14] modified the surgical technique bypassing the MUS from inside out through the obturator foramen. The results of a multicenter trial with short-term follow-up have shown cure rates of 80.5% with no vascular, bowel or nerve injury **(Figs. 2 and 3)**.

Transobturator tape (TOT) is beneficial in obese patients and in women who have had previous retropubic operations **(Box 8)**.

Concerns regarding bladder, vascular, and bowel injuries with the TVT have been somewhat alleviated by the TOT procedure. The incidence of bladder injury was minimal compared to the retropubic MUS.[15] However, the long-term efficacy and safety of the TOT are unknown.

The learning curve was less steep compared to the retropubic MUS. Peroperative cystoscopy is performed at the discretion of the surgeon. Hence a larger group of gynecologists were able to perform TOT. Postprocedure voiding problems and de novo detrusor overactivity were less frequently reported. The complications frequently reported were meshing exposure, dyspareunia, and groin pain.

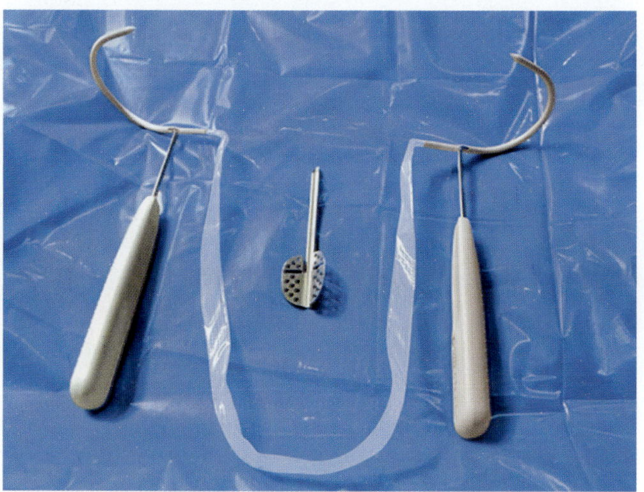

Fig. 2: Transobturator tape (TOT).

Gradually, MUS procedures have been widely accepted as the primary surgical treatment of SUI.

Single-incision Slings

These are mid-urethral slings inserted through a single incision in the vagina.

The failure rates were higher compared to the traditional slings through postoperative pain and urinary tract infections were less common.[16]

Adjustable retropubic slings are available, which enables the alteration of sling tension postoperatively depending upon the requirement of the patient.

Burch Colposuspension

Burch colposuspension has been the standard operation for SUI for many decades before the advent of mid-urethral slings.[17] It involved anchoring the paravaginal tissue, lateral to the bladder neck to the Cooper's ligament with a non-absorbable suture. The surgery was mostly done through a lower abdominal transverse incision and elevated the bladder neck and proximal urethra to a retropubic position **(Fig. 4)**.

Indications:

- Stress urinary incontinence due to urethral hypermobility
- Concomitant pelvic pathology.

The reported complications include voiding dysfunction, de novo detrusor overactivity, venous bleeding, and injury to the bladder, urethra and ureter. Infection and prolonged hospital stays were a big problem. Posterior wall defects and enteroceles were reported in patients undergoing this operation.

The above complications and the technical difficulties in performing the surgery, along with the invention of the MUS procedure led to this operation becoming obsolete. However, with the controversy around tape and meshes, there has been a resurgence of this operation.

Laparoscopic Colposuspension

Laparoscopic colposuspension became popular in the 1990s in keeping with the trend toward less invasive procedures to provide shorter hospital stay and recovery. The laparoscopic approach has enabled better precision, less bleeding and less pain.

The success rate at 1 year was 84% with laparoscopic approach compared to 95.6% with open procedures. There was a precipitous decline in the success rates with long-term

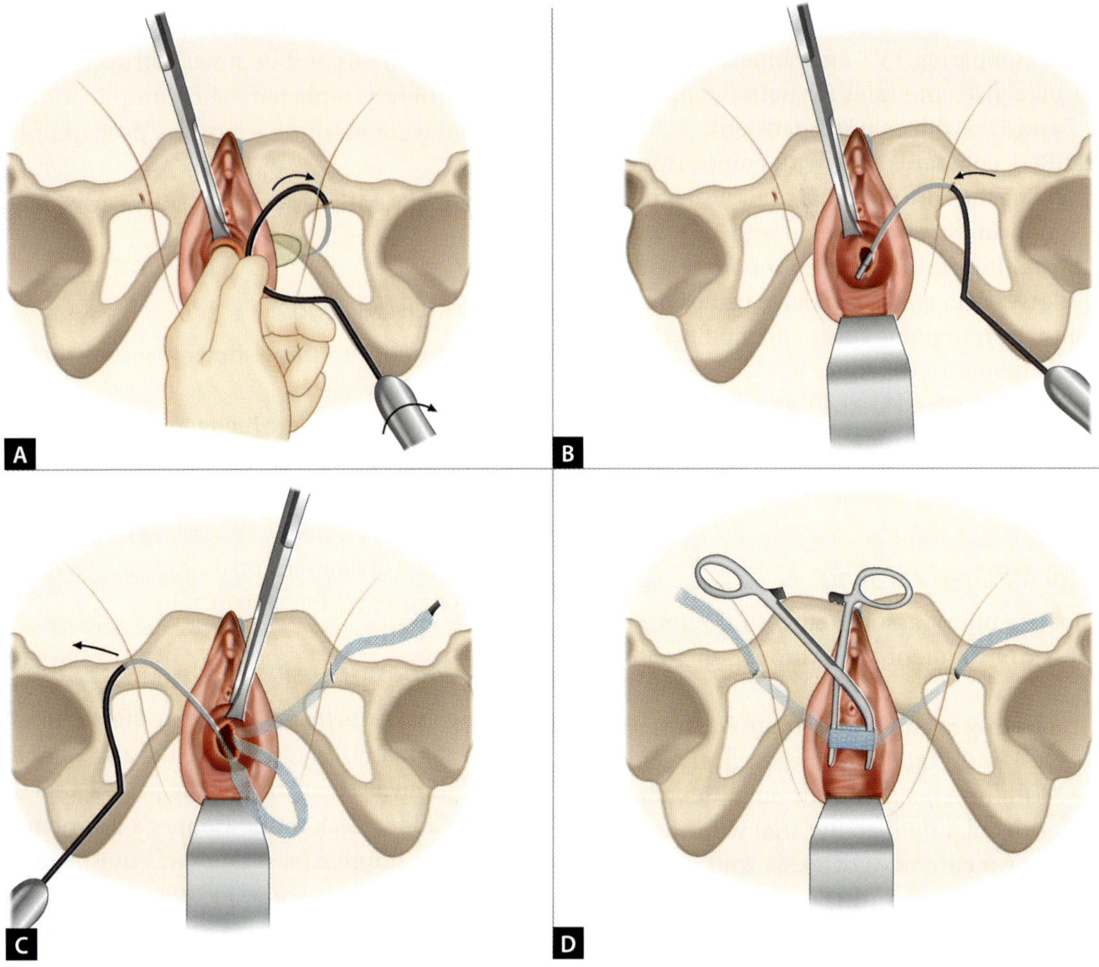

Figs. 3A to D: Transobturator tape (TOT) surgical steps.

BOX 8: Indications for using transobturator tape (TOT).

- Urodynamic stress incontinence affecting quality of life significantly
- Previous pelvic surgery causing extensive scarring in the retropubic area
- Lack of expertise to perform cystoscopy

follow-up. With the laparoscopic approach, the incidence of urinary tract injury was also higher at 10%.

In comparison with the open procedure, no significant differences were observed in postoperative urgency, voiding dysfunction or de novo detrusor overactivity. Several studies showed a trend toward a higher complication rate, longer operating time, less intraoperative blood loss, less postoperative pain, shorter hospital stay, quicker return to normal activities, and shorter duration of voiding problems for laparoscopic, compared with open colposuspension.

One of the early problems with the laparoscopic approach was the long learning curve and the difficulty of intracorporeal suture tying. Ankardal et al.[18,19] prospectively randomized patients into open Burch with sutures versus laparoscopic Burch with staples and mesh. With 1-year follow-up, the

Name of surgical procedure	*Supporting structure in the anterior pelvis*
Paravaginal procedure	Arcus tendineus
Modified Marshall-Marchetti-Krantz procedure	Back of pubic symphysis
Burch colposuspension	Iliopectineal ligament (Cooper's ligament)
Turner-Warwick vaginal obturator shelf procedure	Fascia over obturator internus

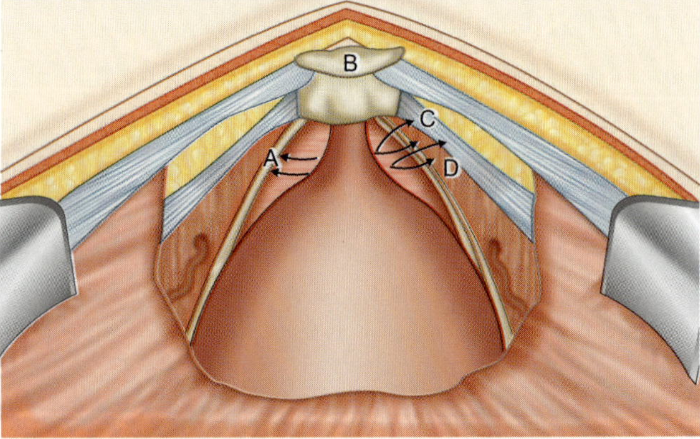

Fig. 4: Bladder neck suspension operations.

subjective cure (89 vs. 62%), objective cure (92 vs. 74%), subjective improvement, quality of life, and satisfaction rate were all significantly higher in the open group. However, the laparoscopic group had less blood loss and significantly shorter hospital stay. Despite the low morbidity with laparoscopy, based on the poor long-term results and the increased risk of urinary tract injuries, a Cochrane review concluded that the performance of the laparoscopic approach was poor compared to the open approach.

Urethral Bulking Agents

This is a short, minimally invasive procedure done under anesthesia with cystoscopic guidance **(Box 9)**. Repeat sessions can be done under local anesthesia. The urethral bulking agents commonly used are polydimethylsiloxane elastomer or polyacrylamide hydrogel.

The bulking agent is injected submucosally in the proximal urethra through sharp needles at multiple points, using a preloaded syringe, taking care to avoid the urethral sphincters. They act as cushions underneath the mucosa and occlude the lumen, thereby helping in coaptation **(Fig. 5)**.

The effectiveness of urethral bulking agents is between 40 and 75%. The main problems are urinary tract infection, voiding dysfunction demanding catheterization and loss of effectiveness with time. Most patients need a repeat injection after 9–12 months.

Their use has significantly increased with the current controversy around the use of midurethral slings.

Artificial Urinary Sphincter

Use of artificial sphincters is rarely employed in the treatment of SUI. The sphincter is usually placed by a combined abdominal/vaginal approach. Though successful, it is associated with high complication rates. The main problems are the failure of the device and erosion of the cuff.

BOX 9: The indications for use of urethral bulking agents (UBA).

- Patients physically unfit for surgery
- Patients not willing for a mesh procedure
- Persistent stress urinary incontinence (SUI) (sling failures)
- Recurrent SUI after slings

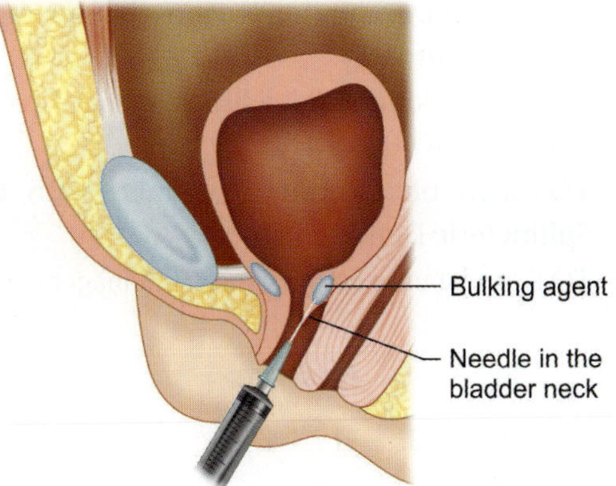

Fig. 5: Paraurethral bulking injections.

INNOVATIONS

Novel molecular techniques such as gene therapy and tissue engineering are promising new advances in the field of incontinence treatment. The goal is to provide tissue repair and to enhance the biological function of damaged tissue, which is the basic pathophysiology of incontinence. This may truly revolutionize the treatment of incontinence therapy in the future.

A new minimally invasive technique using radiofrequency micro remodeling, that relies on the focal denaturation of submucosal collagen is noteworthy. The efficacy of these interesting modalities remains to be tested.

CONCLUSION

Stress urinary incontinence when mild and infrequent is managed with nonsurgical modalities. If day-to-day activities are disturbed to the extent of requiring pads to contain leakage, surgical intervention is justified. Though pubovaginal and mid-urethral slings are effective, the autologous pubovaginal sling scores higher as it is devoid of mesh-related complications. Irrespective of the kind of sling material used and site of sling placement, the sling should be tension-free to minimize the post-operative voiding problems. Women with ISD will benefit from PVS, retropubic MUS or urethral bulking agents. Colposuspension or transobturator MUS will correct urethral hypermobility-related sphincter incompetence. The selection of appropriate surgery to suit the patient is the key to the success.

KEY MESSAGES

- Conservative treatment should be the first line of treatment for SUI.
- Preoperative urodynamic evaluation is essential to rule out detrusor over activity and voiding problems.
- All surgical procedures should be done tension free and should be performed after appropriate training.

REFERENCES

1. Abrams P. Urodynamics, 2nd edition. London: Springer;1997.
2. Single-blind randomized controlled trial of pelvic floor exercises, electrical stimulation, vaginal cones, and no treatment in the management of genuine stress incontinence in women. BMJ. 1999;318:487.
3. Bø K, Talseth T, Bump R, Sugerman H, Fantl J. Obesity and lower urinary tract function in women: effect of surgically induced weight loss. Am J Obstet Gynecol. 1992;166:392.
4. Hagen S, Stark D. Conservative prevention and management of pelvic organ prolapse in women. Cochrane Database Syst Rev. 2011;CD003882.
5. Lipp A, Shaw C, Glavind K. Mechanical devices for urinary incontinence in women. Cochrane Database Syst Rev. 2011;7:CD001756.

6. Abu-Sitta MI, Kapur G, Enhorning G. Stress incontinence alleviated by an intravaginal device. Int Urogyn J. 1995;6:95.
7. Mariappan P, Alhasso AA, Grant A, N'Dow JMO. Serotonin and noradrenaline reuptake inhibitors (SNRI) for stress urinary incontinence in adults. Cochrane Database Syst Rev. 2005;3:CD004742.
8. Cody JD, Richardson K, Moehrer B, Hextall A, Glazener CMA. Oestrogen therapy for urinary incontinence in post-menopausal women. Cochrane Database Syst Rev. 2009;7:CD001405.
9. McGuire EJ, Lytton B. Pubovaginal sling procedure for stress incontinence. J Urol. 1978;119(1):82-4.
10. Kim S, Wong DG, Lee D, Christie AL, Zimmern PE. Very long-term follow-up of autologous pubovaginal fascia slings in women with stress urinary incontinence. Int Urogynecol J. 2021.
11. Abouassaly R, Steinberg JR, Lemieux M. Complications of tension-free vaginal tape surgery: multi-institutional review. BJU Int. 2004;94:110.
12. Nilsson CG, Kuuva N, Falconer C, Rezapour M, Ulmsten U. Long-term results of the tension-free vaginal tape (TVT) procedure for surgical treatment of female urinary stress incontinence. Int Urogynecol J. 2001;12:S5-8.
13. Delorme E. Transobturator urethral suspension: a noninvasive procedure in the treatment of stress urinary incontinence in women. Prog Urol. 2001;11:1306-13.
14. De Leval J. Novel surgical technique for the treatment of female stress urinary incontinence: transobturator vaginal tape inside-out. EUR Urol. 2003;44:724-30.
15. Abdel-Fattah M, Mostafa A, Young D, Ramsay I. Evaluation of transobturator tension-free vaginal tapes in the management of women with mixed urinary incontinence: one-year outcomes. Am J Obstet Gynecol. 2011;205:150.e1.
16. Abdel-Fattah M, Ford JA, Lim CP, Madhuvrata P. Single-incision mini-slings versus standard midurethral slings in the surgical management of female stress urinary incontinence: a meta-analysis of effectiveness and complications. EUR Urol. 2011;60:468.
17. Burch JC. Urethrovaginal fixation to Cooper's ligament for correction of stress incontinence, cystocele, and prolapse. Am J Obstet Gynecol. 1961;81:281.
18. Ankardal M, Ekerydh A, Crafoord K. A randomized trial comparing open Burch colposuspension using sutures with laparoscopic colposuspension using mesh and staples in women with stress urinary incontinence. BJOG. 2004;111:974.
19. Ankardal M, Milsom I, Stjerndahl JH, Engh ME. A three-armed randomized trial comparing open Burch colposuspension using sutures with laparoscopic colposuspension using sutures and laparoscopic colposuspension using mesh and staples in women with stress urinary incontinence. Acta Obstet Gynecol Scand. 2005;84:773-9.

LONG QUESTIONS

1. Discuss recent treatment options for managing SUI.
2. A patient attends your clinic and is undecided between having a retropubic sling and a Burch colposuspension. What would your discussion be? Set out salient points.

SHORT QUESTIONS

1. What are conservative methods of SUI treatment?
2. What are different surgical procedures adopted for SUI?
3. Explain the role of urodynamic evaluation in managing women with SUI.
4. Write about pelvic floor physiotherapy in the management of SUI.
5. Differentiate between midurethral slings versus pubovaginal slings.
6. Compare and contrast the TVT and TOT sling operations.

MULTIPLE CHOICE QUESTIONS

1. Which statement is incorrect about pubovaginal sling (PVS)?
   a. Is an autologous sling
   b. Ideal for extrinsic sphincter deficiency
   c. Is a proximal urethral sling
   d. Has long term efficacy
2. Which statement is correct about colposuspension?
   a. Involves anchoring the paraurethral tissue at the bladder neck and proximal urethra to the Coopers ligament
   b. Is not preferred if there is an associated pelvic pathology
   c. Uses a tape or mesh
   d. Is obsolete now a days
3. Which statement is correct about transobturator tape (TOT)?
   a. TOT will not be beneficial for obese women with SUI
   b. TOT is ideal for SUI due to intrinsic sphincter deficiency
   c. TOT is ideal for women who have recurrent SUI
   d. None of the above
4. Which answer is correct about tension-free vaginal tape (TVT)?
   a. TVT is placed through the trans obturator route
   b. TVT is not beneficial for women who have an intrinsic sphincter deficiency
   c. TVT is a mid- urethral sling
   d. TVT is not suitable for recurrent SUI
5. Which of the following statement is false within management of SUI
   a. Urodynamic evaluation is a must before reoperation for recurrent SUI
   b. Urethral bulking agents will be beneficial in persistent or recurrent SUI
   c. TOT can be offered to women with Intrinsic Sphincteric Defieciency
   d. TOT can be used as first-line for management of SUI

Answers

1. b 2. a 3. d 4. c 5. c

13.3 OVERACTIVE BLADDER

Subhash Ch Biswas, Ramprasad Dey

INTRODUCTION

Overactive bladder (OAB) is defined as urgency, usually with frequency and nocturia with or without urgency incontinence in the absence of pathologic or metabolic conditions that might explain these symptoms.[1,2] Urgency is the key symptom of OAB.[3]

When it occurs with incontinence it is known as "wet OAB", when it occurs without incontinence it is known as "dry OAB". These combinations of symptoms suggest detrusor muscle overactivity, but can result from other forms of urethrovesical dysfunction.[4]

This definition focuses on the symptoms of OAB rather than on urodynamic parameters and is much more clinically useful for physicians, because most do not conduct urodynamic studies on patients with OAB.

IMPORTANT COMPONENTS OF OVERACTIVE BLADDER

Urgency is a sudden compelling desire to urinate that is difficult to defer. Urge urinary incontinence is involuntary leakage that is associated with urgency. Normal urge sensation is normal, but urgency is pathologic. Frequency is defined as eight or more visits to the toilet per 24-hour period, two or more of which may be during the night. Nocturia is waking up to urinate at night; usually more than two times per night is abnormal.

Urge incontinence is defined as the sudden, involuntary loss of urine. Urge urinary incontinence is caused by uncontrollable contractions of the detrusor muscle; there may be very little warning time, and the volume of leakage is usually large.

In contrast, stress incontinence occurs at the time of coughing or sneezing when the pressure on the bladder is greater than the urethral pressure, resulting in a sudden loss of urine (usually a small volume). Stress incontinence is typically due to weakened or damaged pelvic floor muscles.

Mixed incontinence occurs when the symptoms of OAB and stress incontinence are present in the same person. Individuals with mixed incontinence may experience leakage of urine due to a sudden uncontrollable urge to urinate and also with coughing or sneezing.

INCIDENCE AND EPIDEMIOLOGY

Overactive bladder incidence underreported, the data of OAB is like "Tip of Iceberg". In majority of the cases, OAB remains as a hidden condition since many patients with OAB attempt to self-manage their problem by voiding frequently, reducing fluid intake, and wearing pads. Nearly two-thirds of patients experience symptoms for 2 years before seeking treatment.

Worldwide prevalence of OAB is 12.8% for women and 10.8% for men. The data from various epidemiologic studies describes that the prevalence of all incontinence increases with age.[5,6] It is not an untreatable disorder and appropriate management can decrease morbidity.[7]

Prevalence of OAB in USA is more common than many other chronic conditions such as asthma, osteoporosis, diabetes, or Alzheimer's disease. 63% of cases of OAB are classified as dry and other 37% as wet in the United States.[8] There is paucity of Indian data.

Overactive bladder has a significant impact on quality of life (QoL) and thereby lessen work productivity.

It does impact on daily activities in different ways. Physically, they are less productive due to lack of concentration, sleep disturbances, and tiredness. Psychologically, it do affects self-esteem and hinders there social and sexual life. Finally, it carries negative impact on their occupational productivity.

PATHOPHYSIOLOGY

Many neurological and anatomical components are actively involved to maintain urinary continence as well as urination. These are CNS, spinal cord, peripheral autonomic, somatic, sensory afferent innervations as well as pelvic floor muscle. Disorders of this structure may contribute urinary incontinence.[9] The symptoms of OAB are due to involuntary contraction of the detrusor muscle during filling phase of the micturition cycle. These involuntary contractions are termed detrusor over activity and are mediated by acetylcholine induced stimulation of bladder muscarine receptors. Under normal circumstances, as the bladder volume increases, the detrusor muscles fills like a balloon and maintain a low bladder pressure. At the time of urination, generally in and around volume of 300–400 mL, phasic detrusor muscle contraction empties the bladder.[9] In detrusor instability, the symptoms are usually associated with involuntary contractions of detrusor muscles. Overactivity of bladder may be of neurogenic or idiopathic in origin can result in urgency or urge incontinence depending upon the urethral sphincter mechanisim.[10] Etiology of overactive bladder may be due to decreased inhibitory control, increased afferent activity or increased sensitivity to efferent activity.[11] However symptoms of OAB may also present without any demonstrable detrusor over activity. OAB is not synonymous with detrusor overactivity as the former is symptom based diagnosed and the latter is an urodynamic diagnosis. 64% of patients with OAB have urodynamic proven detrusor overactivity and 83% of patients of detrusor overactivity have symptoms suggestive of OAB.

CLINICAL PRESENTATION AND DIAGNOSIS OF OVERACTIVE BLADDER

A presumptive diagnosis of OAB can be based on

- Patient history, symptom assessment
- Physical examination
- Urinalysis.

Initiation of noninvasive treatment may not require an extensive further workup:[12.]

1. The clinician should engage in a diagnostic process to document symptoms and signs that characterize OAB and exclude other disorders that could be the cause of the patient's symptoms. Minimum requirements for this process are a careful history, physical examination, and urinalysis.
2. In some patients, additional procedures and measures may be necessary to validate an OAB diagnosis, to exclude other disorders and to formulate the treatment plan. At the clinician's discretion, a urine culture and/or postvoid residual assessment may be performed and information from bladder diaries and/or symptom questionnaires may be obtained.
3. Urodynamic study, cystoscopy and diagnostic renal and bladder ultrasound should not be used in the initial workup of the uncomplicated patient.
4. OAB is not a disease; it is a symptom complex that generally is not a life-threatening condition. After evaluation, counseling should be done to guide proper acceptable mode of treatment by the care givers.
5. Clinicians should provide education to patients regarding normal lower urinary tract function, what is known about OAB, the benefits versus risks/burdens of the available treatment alternatives and the fact that acceptable symptom control may require trials of multiple therapeutic options before it is achieved.

Healthcare professionals should routinely ask patients whether they have bladder problems that are troublesome or whether they ever leak urine. If the answer is yes, the clinician should proceed with an assessment of the patient's history and symptoms, as well as tests such as urinalysis, to determine whether a diagnosis of OAB can be established.

Overactive bladder screening can help diagnose other causes of bladder symptoms. Bladder symptoms may be caused by a wide variety of factors other than OAB. Screening for OAB can help uncover these disorders. Bladder symptoms may be due to local pathology, metabolic factors, the use of certain medications, or other medical or psychological factors. A simple symptom assessment can differentiate between OAB, stress incontinence, and mixed incontinence.

INVESTIGATIONS

1. *Initial investigations*
   - Urinalysis to exclude infection, hematuria and glycosuria
   - Urinary tract ultrasound and measurement of postresidual volume
   - Frequency/volume chart for at least 3 days
   - Bladder diary for a minimum of 3 days
2. *Secondary investigations*[13]
   - Urine cytology and culture
   - Urodynamic study
   - Cystoscopy
   - Imaging of upper urinary tract or spine.
3. *Indications for urodynamic study:*[14]
   - Suspicion of occult diagnosis that may alter management
     - Bladder outlet obstruction
     - Detrusor hyperactivity with impaired contractility
     - Impaired bladder compliance
     - Dysfunctional voiding
     - Mixed incontinence
   - Risk of upper urinary tract deterioration
     - History of pelvic irradiation
     - Radical pelvic surgery (abdominoperineal resection, radical hysterectomy)
     - Spina bifida
     - Neurogenic voiding dysfunction (e.g., multiple sclerosis, spinal cord injury)
   - Other
     - Failed or unsatisfactory response to empiric medical therapy
     - Uncertain diagnosis
     - Unaware incontinence
     - Prior lower urinary tract surgery (e.g., transurethral resection of prostate, anti-incontinence surgery).

MANAGEMENT OF OVERACTIVE BLADDER

Barriers to treatment: There are several barriers to the treatment of OAB. Among the most important are patients' misconceptions and fears. Individuals with OAB are often under the wrong impression that bladder dysfunction is a normal part of aging or everyday life. Some may feel that their symptoms are not severe enough or frequent enough to warrant treatment. Embarrassment comes into play, as many individuals feel ashamed of their problem and are reluctant to discuss it with a health care professional. Another common misperception is that there is no effective treatment available for OAB.

OAB treatment goals: Eliminate or reduction in urinary urge incontinence. The treatment goals are just basically to eliminate the symptoms or improve urinary incontinence. To get the patients 100% dry would be difficult but it should reduce the urgency/frequency, i.e., reduce the amount of times they have to go to the bathroom. Ensure treatment compliance as well as improve quality of life.

Treatment options: Behavioral therapy, medication, combined therapy—behavioral and pharmacologic therapy, minimally invasive therapies—botulinum A-toxin, neuromodulation surgery.

Patients with UUI/overactive bladder can be managed by urologists, gynecologists, geriatricians, general practitioners (GPs), nurses/continence advisors, others, e.g., pediatricians, neurologists, physiotherapists, and psychologists.

Behavioral Therapy: First-line Treatment

- Simple advice regarding fluid intake
- Weight loss in morbidly obese
- Avoidance of smoking, tea, caffeine
- Bladder retraining-prompted and timed voiding, habit retraining and bladder drill
- Pelvic floor muscle training (PFMT).

Behavioral therapies may be combined with pharmacologic management.

Medication: Drug therapy is becoming increasingly important and is currently the mainstay in the treatment for overactive bladder. Medications used to treat overactive bladder can be highly effective in providing relief of symptoms.

Pharmacologic Management: Second-line Treatments (Table 1)

Clinicians should offer oral antimuscarinics or oral β-adrenoceptor agonists as second-line therapy. If an immediate release (IR) and an extended release (ER) formulation are available, then ER formulations should preferentially be prescribed over IR formulations because of lower rates of dry mouth. Transdermal (TDS) oxybutynin (patch or gel) may be offered.

If a patient experiences inadequate symptom control and/or unacceptable adverse drug events with one antimuscarinic medication, then a dose modification or a different antimuscarinic medication or a β-adrenoceptor agonist may be tried.

Clinicians may consider combination therapy with an antimuscarinic and β-adrenoceptor agonist for patients' refractory to monotherapy with either anti-muscarinics or β-adrenoceptor agonists.

Clinicians should not use antimuscarinics in patients with narrow-angle glaucoma unless approved by the treating ophthalmologist and should use antimuscarinics with extreme caution in patients with impaired gastric emptying or a history of urinary retention.

Clinicians should manage constipation and dry mouth before abandoning effective antimuscarinic therapy. Management may include bowel management, fluid management, dose modification or alternative antimuscarinics.[15]

Clinicians must use caution in prescribing antimuscarinics in patients who are using other medications with anticholinergic properties. Clinicians should use caution in

TABLE 1: Drugs available for treatment of OAB.

Drug	*Adverse effects*	*Remarks*
Oxybutynin ER 5–15 mg/day	• Dry mouth (68%) • Constipation (10%)	Dose response observed
Oxybutynin transdermal 3.9 mg twice weekly	• Itching at site (14%) • Erythema at site (8%) • Dry mouth (7%) • Constipation (2.1%)	Transdermal delivery reduces the typical anticholinergic side effects of dry mouth and constipation
• Trospium chloride • 20 mg BID dose	Theoretically harder to pass through blood/brain barrier with less side effects	• Not metabolized by liver • 60% excreted in the urine unchanged
Tolterodine 2 mg twice per day	• Dry mouth (23%) • Constipation (6%) • Dry eyes (4%)	• Dose dependent effect with immediate release • Safe in men with bladder outlet obstruction
Solifenacin 5–10 mg/day	• Dry mouth (26%) • Constipation (12%) • Blurred vision (5%)	Steady state at 10 days due to long half-life
Darifenacin 7.5–15 mg/day	• Dry mouth (35%) • Constipation (21%)	• Steady state 4–5 hours • Dose response, safety, efficacy and tolerability maintained with long-term use
Mirabegron, *The first USFDA approved B_3 agonist*. Dose is 25–50 mg once dailya	• Mirabegron is not recommended for use in patients with severe uncontrolled hypertension • Angioedema of the face, lips, tongue, and/or larynx has been reported with mirabegron. Caution should be used if mirabegron is co-administered with metoprolol and desipramine and especially NTI drugs such as thioridazine, flecainide and propafenone	• Proven long-term efficacy and safety in treatment of OAB. Comparable efficacy with solifenacin • Proven efficacy in patients who have discontinued antimuscarinic therapy
Vaginal estrogen (topical) 0.5 g cream every night for 2 weeks then twice per week	• Increased risk of breast cancer • Breast discomfort and pain • Local reactions	• For postmenopausal women with vaginal atrophy • *Contraindications*: Past history of breast cancer

prescribing antimuscarinics or β-adrenoceptor agonists in the frail OAB patient.

Patients who are refractory to behavioral and pharmacologic therapy should be evaluated by an appropriate specialist if they desire additional therapy.

Contraindication for antimuscarine agents: Closed angle glaucoma—anticholinergic medications substantially increase intraocular pressure which may impair vision. A history of impaired gastric emptying or urinary retention.

Elderly patients: Antimuscarinic agents will be used in caution.

- Central adverse effects include sedation, confusion, delirium, cognitive impairment, and psychotic symptoms
- Signs of toxicity include urinary retention, agitation, hallucinations, seizures, cardiac arrhythmias, and heart block
- Close monitoring is required.

Third-line Treatments

1. Clinicians may offer intradetrusor botulinum toxin A (100 U) as third-line treatment in the carefully-selected and thoroughly-counseled patient who has been refractory to first- and second-line OAB treatments.[16,17] The patient must be able and willing to return for frequent postvoid residual evaluation and also willing to perform self-catheterization if necessary.
2. Clinicians may offer peripheral tibial nerve stimulation (PTNS) as third-line treatment in a carefully selected patient population. The success of PTNS are variable (54–79%) in different trial.[18,19]
3. Clinicians may offer sacral neuromodulation (SNS) as third-line treatment in a carefully selected patient population characterized by severe refractory OAB symptoms or patients who are not candidates for second-line therapy and are willing to undergo a surgical procedure. Different study showed success of SNS as 50% decrease of incontinence episodes.[20]

Practitioners and patients should persist with new treatments for an adequate trial in order to determine whether the therapy is efficacious and tolerable. Combination therapeutic approaches should be assembled methodically, with the addition of new therapies occurring only when the relative efficacy of the preceding therapy is known.

Fourth-line Treatments: Augmentation Cystoplasty and Urinary Diversion

In rare cases, augmentation cystoplasty or urinary diversion for severe, refractory, complicated OAB patients may be considered.

Refractory OAB: Patients with refractory OAB have failed first-line treatment modalities such as conservative measures and bladder retraining with, or without antimuscarinic therapy. Insufficient duration of prescription or poor patient compliance is the main cause of treatment failure. Some patients do have therapeutic improvement in symptoms but tolerate adverse effects poorly. Management of refractory OAB includes the following.

Medical therapy:

- Shift from one antimuscarinic to another
- Combination of antimuscarinics.

Neuromodulation:

- Percutaneous tibial nerve stimulation
- Sacral nerve modulation.

Intravesical therapy: Botulinum toxin type A (BTX A).

Reconstructive surgery: Small number of patients who have failed to respond to alternative options may benefit from reconstructive surgery. It includes:

- Ileovesicostomy
- Bladder augmentation
- Cystectomy.

With neuromodulation and BTX therapy, it is hopeful that these surgical procedures will be used in a small number of patients.

CONCLUSION

Overactive bladder is a disturbing problem. It is not due to aging. It can be treated and improved. For the treatment of OAB to be successful, patient should be willing and engaged in the treatment process. Behavioral therapies may be combined with drug therapies to optimize patient symptom control and quality of life. All antimuscarinics have similar efficacy profile and they differ in their safety profile. Hence, selection of a particular antimuscarinic agent depends on its safety profile. Persistence to antimuscarinic therapy is a major challenge. Balance between efficacy and safety of an antimuscarinic agent is a critical predictor of continuation of treatment. Patients with refractory OAB, and who have failed medical therapy, may benefit from intravesical botulinum toxin or neuromodulation. Good understanding of pathophysiology, better understanding of receptor action and interaction and future research may allow the patients to choose optimal treatment regimen.

KEY MESSAGES

- Overactive bladder is a syndrome affecting millions of women worldwide and prevalence increases as the population ages.
- OAB has significant impact on quality of life which can lead to depression and also affect relationships.
- OAB is a symptomatic diagnosis but detrusor over activity is diagnosed on the basis of urodynamic study.
- All women require through assessment to exclude urinary tract infection and voiding dysfunction. Pathology such as urinary infection, diabetes, bladder stones, malignancy

or an underlying neurological cause should be excluded. Urodynamic study is useful in persistent symptoms and mixed incontinence.

- Pelvic floor exercise and muscle retraining is the first therapy. Initial treatment consists of a combination of lifestyle interventions, pelvic floor exercises, bladder training, and antimuscarinic medications.
- Antimuscurine drugs are presently the mainstay of therapy but side effects is a matter of concern for discontinuation. Care should be taken when prescribing antimuscarinic therapy in the elderly.
- Newer therapy such as intradetrusor injection of botulinum toxin, neuromodulation is beneficial for refractory OAB.
- Reconstructive surgery should be reserved for those women who are nonresponsive to all other treatment modalities.
- Further research is needed for the best treatment option for OAB.

REFERENCES

1. Haylen BT, de Ridder D, Freeman RM. An International Urogynecological Association (IUGA)/International Continence Society (ICA) joint report on the terminology for female pelvic floor dysfunction. Int Urogynecol J. 2010;21:5-26.
2. Chapple C, Gormley EA. Developments in pharmacological therapy for the overactive bladder. BJU Int. 2006;98(1 Suppl):78-87.
3. Hashim H, Abrams P. Overactive bladder: an update. Curr Opin Urol. 2007;17:231-6.
4. NICE. Urinary incontinence in women. [online] Available from: www.nice.org.uk/guidance/qs77. [Last accessed November, 2021].
5. Botlero R, Davis SR, Urquhart DM, Bell RJ. Incidence and resolution rates of different types of urinary incontinence in women: findings from a cohort study. J Urol. 2011;185: 1331-7.
6. Irwin DE, Milsom I, Hunskaar S. Population-based survey of urinary incontinence, overactive bladder, and other lower urinary tract symptoms in five countries: results of the EPIC study. Eur Urol. 2006;50:1306-14.
7. Andersson KE. Antimuscarinics for treatment of overactive bladder. Lancet Neurol. 2004;3:46-53.
8. Hu TW, Wagner TH, Bentkover JD, Leblanc K, Zhou SZ, Hunt T. Costs of urinary incontinence and overactive bladder in the United States: a comparative study. Urology. 2004;63(3): 461-5.
9. Ouslander JG. Management of overactive bladder. N Engl J Med. 2004;350:786-99.
10. Flisser AJ, Walmsley K, Blaivas JG. Urodynamic classification of patients with symptoms of overactive bladder. J Urol. 2003;169(2):529-33.
11. Brading AF. A myogenic basis for the overactive bladder. Urology. 1997;50(6A Suppl):57-67.
12. Diagnosis and Treatment of Non-Neurogenic Overactive Bladder (OAB) in Adults: an AUA/SUFU Guideline (2019). AUA/SUFU Guideline (2012); Amended 2014, 2019. Silver Spring, Maryland: American Urogynecologic Society (AUGS); 2019.
13. Nitti V. Clinical testing for overactive bladder. Can Urol Assoc J. 2011;5(5 Suppl 2):S137-8.
14. Rovner ES, Goudelocke CM. Urodynamics in the evaluation of overactive bladder. Curr Urol Rep. 2010;11:343-7.
15. American Urological Association. Overactive Bladder (OAB) Guideline. [online] Available from: https://www. auanet.org/guidelines/overactive-bladder-(oab)-guideline 3/70. [Last Accessed November, 2021].
16. Dmochowski R, Chapple C, Nitti VW, Chancellor M, Everaert K, Thompson C, et al. Efficacy and safety of onabotulinumtoxinA for idiopathic overactive bladder: a double-blind, placebo controlled, randomized, dose ranging trial. J Urol. 2010;184(6): 2416-22 .
17. Tincello DG, Kenyon S, Abrams KR, Mayne C, Toozs-Hobson P, Taylor D, et al. Botulinum toxin a versus placebo for refractory detrusor overactivity in women: a randomised blinded placebo-controlled trial of 240 women (the RELAX study. Eur Urol. 2012;62(3):507-14..
18. Gaziev G, Topazio L, Iacovelli V, Asimakopoulos A, Di Santo A, De Nunzio C, et al. Percutaneous Tibial Nerve Stimulation (PTNS) efficacy in the treatment of lower urinary tract dysfunctions: a systematic review. BMC Urol. 2013;13:61.
19. Burton C, Sajja A, Latthe PM. Effectiveness of percutaneous posterior tibial nerve stimulation for overactive bladder: a systematic review and meta-analysis. Neurourol Urodyn. 2012;31(8):1206-16.
20. Groen J, Blok BF, Bosch JL. Sacral neuromodulation as treatment for refractory idiopathic urge urinary incontinence: 5-year results of a longitudinal study in 60 women. J Urol. 2011;186(3):954-9.

LONG QUESTIONS

1. Define urinary incontinence. What are the types of urinary incontinence? How to evaluate a case of urinary incontinence to clinch the diagnosis of OAB?
2. Discuss the etiopathology of OAB.
3. Discuss the pharmacotherapy of OAB.

SHORT QUESTIONS

Write short notes on:

1. Non-pharmacotherapy of OAB.
2. Efficacy and indication of use of mirabegron on OAB.

MULTIPLE CHOICE QUESTIONS

1. All of the following are the components of overactive bladder (OAB), except:
   a. Urgency b. Frequency
   c. Nocturia d. Polyuria
2. Which is the key symptom of OAB?
   a. Urgency b. Frequency
   c. Nocturia d. Incontinence
3. Worldwide prevalence of OAB in women is:
   a. 5% b. 12%
   c. 20% d. 25%

4. Initial investigations of overactive bladder include all, except:
   a. Urinalysis to exclude infection, hematuria and glycosuria
   b. Urinary tract ultrasound and measurement of postresidual volume
   c. Urodynamic testing
   d. Frequency/volume chart for at least 3 days
   e. Bladder diary for a minimum of 3 days
5. All of the following are Indications for urodynamic study, except:
   a. SUI
   b. Mixed incontinence
   c. Detrusor hyperactivity with impaired contractility
   d. Neurogenic voiding dysfunction
6. First-line treatment for OAB include all, except:
   a. Pharmacologic drug therapy
   b. PFMT (pelvic floor muscle training)
   c. Bladder retraining-prompted and timed voiding, habit retraining and bladder drill
   d. Simple advice regarding fluid intake
   e. Weight reduction
7. All of the following drugs used for treatment for OAB are anticholinergic agents, except:
   a. Oxybutynin b. Tolterodine
   c. Solifenacin d. Darifenacin
   e. Mirabegron
8. Bladder specific muscarinic receptor are:
   a. M2 and M3 b. M1 and M2
   c. M1 and M3 d. M2 and M4
9. All of the following are side effects of anticholinergic therapy, except:
   a. Pain abdomen b. Constipation
   c. Dry mouth d. Loose motion
10. Mirabegron is the first USFDA approved:
   a. B_3 agonist b. B_1 agonist
   c. B_2 agonist d. B_4 agonist

Answers

1.	d	2.	a	3.	b	4.	c	5.	a	6.	a
7.	e	8.	a	9.	d	10.	a				

13.4 URINARY TRACT INFECTIONS

Susheela Rani BS

INTRODUCTION

Infections of the urinary tract are one of the most common bacterial infections. The infections can range from asymptomatic bacteriuria (AUB) to acute pyelonephritis and to gram-negative septicemia. Urinary tract infection (UTI) is 14 times more common in women than men. This is because

- Women have shorter urethra as compared to men
- The urethra, particularly the lower third, is continuously exposed to pathogens from the vagina and the rectum
- Women generally do not empty their bladders as completely as men do
- Proximity of the urethra to the vagina makes it more vulnerable to exposure to bacteria during intercourse.

Pregnant women are even more susceptible to urinary tract infections as compared to their nonpregnant counter parts. The mechanical and hormonal changes of pregnancy cause increased urinary stasis and vesicoureteric reflux. Along with the difficulty with hygiene due to distended abdomen, the changes of pregnancy make UTI the most common bacterial infection in pregnancy (**Box 1**).[1] The prevalence of asymptomatic bacteriuria in pregnant women is 2.5–11%, as opposed to 3–8% in nonpregnant women. 40% of women with asymptomatic bacteriuria in pregnancy may progress to symptomatic upper UTI or pyelonephritis.

BOX 1: Urinary tract infection.
- 14 times more common in women
- Most common bacterial infection in women
- Most common medical complication

CLASSIFICATION

Urinary tract infection can be classified depending upon the anatomical part that is infected. Upper UTI when the kidneys and ureters are infected, and lower UTI when the bladder and urethra are infected. Based on the presence of symptoms, UTI can be classified as symptomatic and asymptomatic. However, the most common classification of UTI is *uncomplicated UTI and complicated UTI.*

Uncomplicated UTI is defined as "acute, sporadic or recurrent UTI, limited to nonpregnant, premenopausal women with no known relevant anatomical and functional abnormalities within the urinary tract or comorbidities."

The rest belong to the complicated UTI category.[2]

ETIOLOGY

Most of the organisms responsible for UTI are considered part of the normal fecal and/or vaginal flora. *E. coli* is the most common organism and is seen in 80–90% of infections. Other gram-negative bacteria such as *Klebsiella, Proteus,*

Enterobacter, group B streptococci, enterococci are responsible for the remainder.

EPIDEMIOLOGY

The incidence of UTI varies with age. The prevalence of UTI in the neonatal period is very low and when it does occur, it is usually associated with bacteremia. Quite often, there is functional or anatomic abnormality of the urinary tract. Between one-third and one half of UTI in the age group of 1–5 years are associated with vesicoureteral reflux. There is a striking increase in the incidence of UTI during adolescence with almost 80% having had at least one episode of UTI by the age of 25. This increase is attributed to exposure to sexual intercourse at this time.[3]

In the elderly postmenopausal woman, asymptomatic bacteriuria though not uncommon, is transient and does not need treatment. Symptomatic UTI are seen in women who have functional disability, diabetes, recent gynecological surgery, urinary incontinence or incomplete emptying of the bladder. Though symptoms of frequency, urgency, nocturia and incontinence may have multiple causes in this age group, an evaluation for UTI with urine culture is important.

PATHOGENESIS

The region around the urethra gets contaminated by organisms which normally reside in the gut. These organisms then ascend the urethra and into the bladder with help of appendages such as flagella and pili. They multiply in the bladder and subsequent course depends upon the ability of the bladder to mount an immune response. Adequate immune response will eliminate the organism and if the organism overpowers the bladder's immune response it establishes infection **(Fig. 1)**.[4]

Environmental Factors

Vaginal Ecology

Colonization of the vaginal introitus with enteric organisms is the most important factor in UTI. Sexual intercourse, use of vaginal spermicide/diaphragm increases the risk of colonization. Change in vaginal flora due to decreased lactobacilli that occurs in postmenopausal women promotes infection.

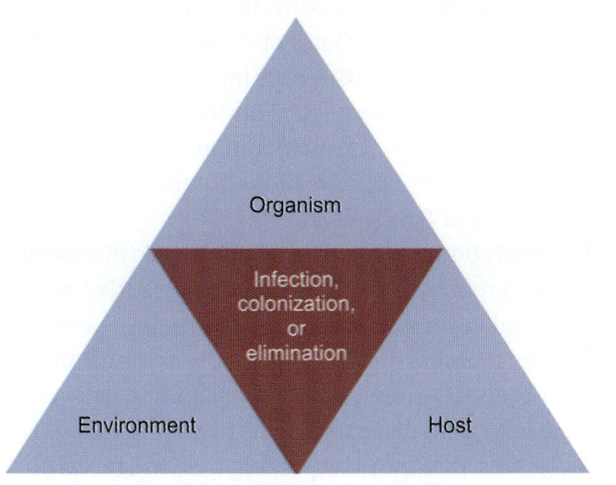

Fig. 1: The disease triangle in UTI.

Anatomic and Functional Abnormalities

Anatomic features such as short urethra, proximity to vagina and anus predispose a woman to UTI. Stasis or obstruction to the flow of urine that can occur in functional abnormalities such as vesicoureteral reflux, ureteral obstruction, neurogenic bladder can provide an optimum environment for UTI. Additionally, any foreign body in the urinary tract like a catheter or stone provides a nidus for bacterial colonization. In pregnancy, hormonal changes can cause inhibition of ureteral peristalsis, decreased ureteral tone, both of which can lead to functional vesicoureteral reflux.

Organism

The uropathogens, such as *E. coli*, have appendages called filaments or pili. These help the bacteria to adhere to the uroepithelium of the bladder wall. They invade the epithelium, produce toxins and proteases and synthesize siderophores to obtain iron. They then ascend to the kidneys where they adhere to the renal epithelium and produce toxins. Subsequently they cross the tubular epithelial barrier and gain access to the blood stream where they can lead to bacteremia.

Meanwhile the host epithelium mounts an immune response which is overcome by the uropathogens by forming biofilms and undergoing morphological changes. Morphological changes like filamentation help in resisting phagocytosis by macrophages and neutrophils. Extracellular DNA (eDNA), extracellular polymeric substances, pili, flagella and other adhesive fibers create a scaffold within which the bacteria remain protected from the host's immune response and antimicrobial agents. These changes allow the uropathogens to persist and cause recurrent infections.[5]

Host Factors

Urinary bladder is usually resistant to bacterial colonization. The forward flow of urine acts like a flushing mechanism. Other defense mechanisms include urine inhibitors (PH, osmolality, urea), uroepithelial defenses such as cytokines, PMNs, and Tamm-Horsfall protein or uromodulin. Genetic predilection is often found in women with recurrent UTI. A maternal history of UTI is more likely to be present in women who have recurrent UTI. Diseases that cause immunosuppression can promote UTI. Diabetes is an important comorbid condition that is associated with UTI. Women with diabetes are twice likely to have asymptomatic bacteriuria as compared to nondiabetic women. Longer the duration of diabetes, greater is the risk of developing UTI. Similarly, women on insulin are more likely to have UTI than women who are on oral antidiabetic agents.

INVESTIGATIONS

Microscopic Examination of Urine

- *Bacteriuria*: Presence of bacilli in a centrifuged sediment indicates significant bacteriuria since only approximately 10% of patients with less than 10^5 CFU/mL show bacteria.
- *Pyuria*: Presence of 10 neutrophils per high power field in an uncentrifuged midstream specimen is considered pyuria. Pyuria is indicative of UTI. Sterile pyuria is urine which contains white blood cells while appearing sterile by standard culturing techniques. Causes of sterile pyuria are listed in **Box 2**.

Urine Culture

The diagnosis of UTI from simple cystitis to complicated pyelonephritis with sepsis can be established with absolute certainty only by cultures of urine. However, simple, uncomplicated UTI does not warrant urine culture. The major indications for urine cultures are listed in **Box 3** and the method of collection is listed in **Box 4**.

Organisms grown on culture specimens depend largely on the clinical setting. About 80–90% of acute uncomplicated cystitis, acute pyelonephritis grow *E. coli* on culture. Proteus is grown in those with staghorn calculi. *Klebsiella, Pseudomonas* and *Enterobacter* are usually seen in culture of hospital acquired infections. *Staphylococcus aureus* grown in urine culture is often due to UTI acquired by hematogenous spread.

BOX 2: Causes of aseptic pyuria.

- Self-medication before urine culture
- Sample contamination by cleansing solution
- Vaginal discharge
- Urinary stone
- Urinary tract tumor
- Chronic interstitial nephritis (especially due to analgesics)
- Fastidious microorganisms requiring special culture medium *(Ureaplasma urealyticum, Chlamydia, Candida)*

BOX 3: Indications for urine culture.

- Suspicion of complicated urinary tract infection (UTI)
- Symptoms not characteristic of UTI
- UTI symptoms persisting after antibiotic treatment and new antibiotic needs to be started
- Symptoms recur within 1 month of antibiotic treatment and a culture was not done in the previous episode

BOX 4: Collection of urine specimen for culture.

- The specimen should be mid-stream. Cleansing with water and holding the labia apart are not essential
- Cleansing with antiseptic leads to false negatives
- Catheter specimen—the distal end of the catheter, or preferably the sampling port if present, should be cleansed with a disinfectant, and urine then aspirated with a sterile needle and syringe
- Suprapubic needle aspiration

Imaging Studies[6]

Diagnosis of UTI is made on clinical grounds. However, imaging is useful when there is no response to appropriate treatment, when an obstruction or an anatomical abnormality is suspected and in complicated urinary tract infections.

Plain X-ray of abdomen: KUB radiography (plain X-ray of the kidney, ureter, bladder region) is useful in evaluating in patients with known calculi to assess the passage or movement of the stones. However, it is not useful when there is acute pain.

Intravenous urography (IVU): It is also called intravenous pyelography (IVP) or excretory urography (EU), is used to evaluate the kidneys, ureters and the urinary bladder. CT urography gives better results and is therefore used instead of IVU.

Computed tomography: Among all the imaging methods, CT with and without contrast helps best in identifying calculi and evaluating them. CT is also useful in the evaluation of the pelvicalyceal system, the diagnosis of renal abscess, perinephric collections, etc. However, CT is more expensive and its use is associated with the hazards of exposure to radiation and the risks of contrast media. It is therefore preferred only as a second line in the investigation of recurrent or complicated UTI.

Ultrasound: Ultrasound is noninvasive and does not have the ill effect of radiation. Hence, it is the chosen imaging method in patients with recurrent UTI or when obstruction or structural abnormality is suspected. It is a useful in evaluating the bladder wall thickness, urine residue, dilatation of the ureter, dilatation of pelvicalyceal system, kidney stones, scars, and abscesses.

ACUTE UNCOMPLICATED CYSTITIS

Uncomplicated cystitis is defined as acute, sporadic or recurrent cystitis limited to nonpregnant, premenopausal women with no known relevant anatomical and functional abnormalities within the urinary tract or comorbidities.

Acute uncomplicated cystitis is so common that half the women will experience at least one episode of cystitis during their lifetime. Common risk factors include sexual intercourse, use of spermicides, history of UTI during childhood, history of UTI during pregnancy. The most common causative organism is *E. coli*, followed by *Staphylococcus saprophyticus, Klebsiella pneumoniae* and *P. mirabilis*.

It is most commonly seen in young women of reproductive age, who can present with acute onset dysuria, frequency, urgency and lower abdominal or pelvic pain. The urine may be cloudy, malodorous or bloody. Dysuria and frequency are also seen in women with vulvovaginitis. However, the absence of vaginal discharge helps to differentiate UTI from vulvovaginitis. Routine urine examination will reveal pus cells >8/HPF. RBC may be seen in one-third of the cases. Bacteriuria is demonstrable on Gram stain 60–70% of cases. With this clinical picture in a healthy young woman, antimicrobial treatment can be given and a urine culture and sensitivity need not be done. Urine culture is required in women with atypical symptoms or in those whose symptoms have not resolved with antimicrobial therapy. In patients presenting with symptoms of uncomplicated cystitis a colony count of 10^3 CFU/mL of uropathogens confirms the diagnosis.[7]

Treatment: Fosfomycin 3 g, single dose or nitrofurantoin monohydrate macrocrystals 100 mg BID for 5 days are preferred. However, in resistant cases, trimethoprim/sulfamethoxazole 160/800 mg BID for 3 days or cephalosporins 500 mg BID for 3 days are preferred.

For symptoms persisting even after a course of antimicrobial therapy, urine culture is done and sensitive antibiotic is sought. If culture is negative, other infections like chlamydial, gonococcal or herpes must be considered.

It is often difficult to differentiate between cystitis, urethritis, and vaginitis. **Table 1** enlists the common causes of acute dysuria.

ACUTE PYELONEPHRITIS (TABLE 2)

In acute pyelonephritis the infection can be mild with fever and loin pain or severe with septicemia. Symptoms include low back, flank or abdominal pain and systemic symptoms such as fever, rigors, malaise, sweating nausea, vomiting, and prostration. Acute pyelonephritis may or may not be associated with acute cystitis. Presence of fever distinguishes acute pyelonephritis from cystitis. Fever is typically, high, spiking, and resolves over 72 hours of therapy. Tachycardia may accompany fever. Urine microscopy may show pyuria and gram stain of urine may demonstrate bacteriuria. The course of illness can be complicated by the presence of bacteremia. Bacteremia could progress to septic shock and disseminated intravascular coagulation. A majority of the patients with acute pyelonephritis have upper urinary tract calculi causing obstruction necessitating emergency drainage by a ureteral stent or percutaneous nephrostomy.

Acute papillary necrosis is seen in some cases of acute pyelonephritis complicated by obstruction, sickle cell disease or analgesic nephropathy. This condition is often seen in diabetic women and in women in whom bacteremia persists after antimicrobial treatment. In acute papillary necrosis, the ureters may be obstructed by the sloughed papillae. One of the serious forms of pyelonephritis seen only in diabetic patients is emphysematous pyelonephritis. There is necrotizing infection of the renal parenchyma which extends beyond the renal capsule into the perinephric tissues with the production of gas. Acute pyelonephritis may also result in necrotizing intrarenal or perinephric abscesses.[9] A perinephric abscess results when an intrarenal abscess opens into the space between the Gerota's fascia and renal capsule.

In severe cases treatment consists of hospitalization, IV fluids to replenish volume loss due to recurrent vomiting, antipyretics and appropriate antibiotics. Once clinical improvement is achieved, antibiotics can be switched from parenteral to oral which can be continued for 10 days.

RENAL AND PERIRENAL ABSCESSES

These are macroscopic abscesses in the renal and perirenal region. The causative organisms are usually *S. aureus* when the infection occurs by the hematogenous route and Enterobacteriaceae when infection occurs by ascending infection of the urinary tract. An ascending infection can get complicated by the presence of urinary calculi or any obstruction to the flow of urine leading to abscess formation.

TABLE 1: Common causes of acute dysuria.[8]

Condition	*Pathogen*	*Lab findings*			*Symptoms, onset and factors*
		Pyuria	*Hematuria*	*Urine culture*	
Cystitis	*Escherichia coli* (most common), *Staphylococcus saprophyticus*, *Proteus* species, *Klebsiella* species	Usual	Often	10^2 to 10^5 (CFU/mL)	Abrupt onset, multiple symptoms (dysuria, increased frequency, and urgency), suprapubic or low back pain, suprapubic tenderness on examination
Urethritis	*Chlamydia trachomatis*, *Neisseria gonorrhoeae*	Usual	Rare	$<10^2$ (CFU/mL)	Gradual onset, mild symptoms, vaginal discharge or bleeding (caused by herpes simplex virus concomitant cervicitis), lower abdominal pain, new sexual partner, cervicitis or vulvovaginal herpetic lesions on examination
Vaginitis	*Candida* species, *Trichomonas vaginalis*	Rare	Rare	$<10^2$ (CFU/mL)	Vaginal discharge or odor, pruritus, dyspareunia, external dysuria, no increased frequency or urgency

TABLE 2: Suggested regimens for empirical oral antimicrobial therapy in uncomplicated pyelonephritis.[10]

Antimicrobial	*Daily dose*	*Duration of therapy*
Ciprofloxacin	500–750 mg BID	7 days
Levofloxacin	750 mg OD	5 days
Trimethoprim sulfamethoxazole	160/800 mg BID	14 days
Cefpodoxime	200 mg BID	10 days

Renal cysts can get infected and form an abscess. Clinical presentation could be chronic fever, night sweats, anorexia, weight loss, flank pain. However, abscesses could present with acute symptoms of severe pain in back or flank, high grade fever with or without symptoms of UTI such as dysuria or hematuria. Costovertebral angle tenderness and a tender mass may be present on clinical examination. An ultrasound, CT or MRI may clinch the diagnosis. Treatment consists of drainage of the abscess and antibiotics.

COMPLICATED URINARY TRACT INFECTIONS

Complicated UTIs occur in situations where there are structural, functional or metabolic abnormalities. Complicated UTIs are associated with significantly increased incidence of treatment failures. They are generally seen among premenarchal girls and post-menopausal women. The clinical manifestations of complicated UTI are more often atypical and nonspecific. Antimicrobial resistance is more common and even when treated with sensitive antimicrobials response to therapy may be delayed or absent. Complications of UTI are more frequently encountered and recurrences are common.

Asymptomatic Bacteriuria

Asymptomatic bacteriuria is defined by a mid-stream sample of urine showing bacterial growth 10^5 CFU/mL in two consecutive samples in a woman who is asymptomatic. Asymptomatic bacteriuria occurs in an estimated 1–5% of healthy premenopausal females, increasing to 4–19% in otherwise healthy elderly females, 0.7–27% in patients with diabetes, 2–10% in pregnant women, and 15–50% in institutionalized elderly women.[1] ABU may protect against superinfecting symptomatic UTI. Asymptomatic bacteriuria should be treated only in cases of proven benefit for the patient in order to avoid the risk of developing antimicrobial resistance and eradicating a potentially protective ABU strain. Therefore, ABU treatment with antimicrobials is warranted only in pregnant women and in those undergoing urological procedures which are likely to breach mucosa. Women without risk factors, well-regulated diabetics, post-menopausal women, elderly institutionalized women and in women with renal transplants, ABU need not be treated.[11] Treatment of ABU in pregnancy with a short course (2–7 days) of antimicrobials is associated with lower rates of symptomatic UTI, FGR and preterm delivery.

Recurrent Urinary Tract Infections

Recurrent UTI is defined as three episodes of urinary tract infection with 3 positive urine cultures in the previous 12 months or two episodes in the last 6 months. A "relapse" is a recurrent UTI after therapy resulting from persistence of the pretherapy isolate in the urinary tract. "Reinfection" is urinary tract infection which recurs due to infection with an organism originating from outside of the urinary tract, either a new bacterial strain or a strain previously isolated that has persisted in the colonizing flora of the gut or vagina.[12] Despite having anatomically and physiologically normal urinary tracts it is not uncommon for young, healthy women to have recurrent urinary tract infections.

Behavioral risk factors such as lack of postcoital urination, vaginal douches, use of hot tubs, restrictive underwear, hygiene, and circumcision status of male partners, earlier linked with recurrent UTI have not found evidence. In the post-menopausal woman, vulvovaginal atrophy due to lack of estrogen, anterior vaginal wall prolapse, post void residue due to incomplete emptying of bladder are risk factors for recurrent UTI. Treatment is with appropriate antimicrobials but the possibility of antibiotic resistance is higher.

The prevention of UTI in women with recurrent infection can be classified into two categories:

1. Nonantimicrobial
2. Antimicrobial.

Nonantimicrobial Strategy

- Cranberries and other berries containing proanthocyanidins have not shown any benefit in preventing UTI.[13,14]
- Evidence for the use of lactobacillus for the prevention of UTI remains inconclusive and controversial.[15]
- Intravaginal estriol cream is effective in preventing recurrent UTI in postmenopausal women.[16]
- Vaccines are being developed for prevention of recurrent UTI but have not been licensed for use as yet.

Antimicrobial Strategies[17]

- Low-dose continuous antimicrobial prophylaxis nitrofurantoin (100 mg daily), cephalexin daily, and TMP-SMX (daily or 3 times a week)
- Postcoital prophylaxis for women who develop UTI after intercourse with a single dose of antibiotic following intercourse
- Self-start therapy where the woman diagnoses UTI herself with a urine dipstick or by recognizing incipient UTI symptoms and starts a 3-day course of antibiotics immediately.

Catheter-associated Urinary Tract Infections

Catheter-associated UTI refers to UTIs occurring in a person whose urinary tract is currently catheterized or has been catheterized within the past 48 hours

Catheter-associated UTI constitutes 35–40% of all hospital-acquired infections. The significance of these infections lies in the fact that catheter AUB is the most common cause of gram negative bacteremia in hospitalized patients and is associated with a threefold increase in mortality, prolonged hospital stay and increased hospital costs.[18]

Introduction of Bacteria into the Urinary Tract

Bacteria may enter along the external surface of the catheter in the urethral mucus sheath (periurethral route). Alternatively, they may enter by contamination of the collecting bag urine. Bacteria can also enter the catheter during disconnection of the junction between the catheter and the collecting tube of the urobag (intraluminal route). However, introduction of the closed sterile drainage systems has remarkably reduced the incidence of CA-UTI. Currently, the periurethral route appears to be the most frequent route of bacterial entry in women. Antecedent rectal and periurethral colonization plays an important role in the subsequent development of catheter AUB. The overall risk of infection increases with the length of time the catheter is in place. About 50% of women with catheter in place for 2 weeks become bacteriuric and all women with permanent indwelling catheter eventually become infected. Risk of catheter-associated UTI is greater in women, in patients in whom sterile closed drainage system is disconnected, patients not receiving antibiotics.

Clinical diagnosis: Fever—new onset or worsening of existing fever, rigors, malaise, lethargy, hematuria, pelvic discomfort, pain in the flanks, in a catheterized woman along with costovertebral tenderness, altered mental status suggest CA-UTI. Dysuria, urgency, frequency and suprapubic pain are symptoms in woman whose catheter has been recently removed.

Laboratory diagnosis: Urine culture showing a microbial growth of 10^3 CFU/mL of one or more bacterial species in a single catheter specimen (or a mid-stream voided urine specimen in a person in whom the catheter has been removed in the previous 48 hours) is diagnostic of CA-UTI. Pyuria is not diagnostic of CA-UTI.

Treatment: Antimicrobial therapy is started only after removing or replacing the urinary catheter. A urine specimen for culture should be obtained before starting antimicrobial therapy. Antimicrobial therapy is given for 7 days in those whose symptoms resolve promptly and 14 days in whom there is a delayed response to treatment.

Prevention: Bacteriuria can be prevented in majority of the patients for up to 10 days with modern sterile closed collecting systems and catheters. A variety of additional preventive approaches to further reduce the occurrence of bacteriuria have been evaluated but not found to be useful. For example, application of antibiotic ointment to the urethral meatus has not been protective. Systemic antibiotics may be useful in the prevention of infection in short term catheterization in high risk patients but is probably unwise for long-period catheterizations because of the development of resistant bacterial strains. Catheter associated bacteriuria should be treated only in symptomatic patients. Concretions on the inner surface of catheter serve as reservoirs of infection. These concretions often grow resistant bacteria and fungi like candida. Thus, symptomatic CA-UTI should be treated with sensitive antibiotics for 7 days. Fungi in urine clear with change in catheter and do not usually need treatment.

KEY MESSAGES

- UTI are the most common bacterial infection in women.
- Acute uncomplicated cystitis does not need urine culture for diagnosis and can be treated with a short course of antimicrobials for 3 days.
- Acute pyelonephritis is characterized by fever, chills, flank pain and vomiting and may need admission for administration of IV fluids and IV antibiotics.
- Preventing growth of resistant organisms while preventing recurrent UTI is a formidable challenge.
- Asymptomatic bacteriuria needs to be treated only in pregnant women and in women likely to undergo traumatic urological interventions.
- Catheter-associated infections can be largely avoided by following guidelines for catheter care.

REFERENCES

1. Mazor-Dray E, Levy A, Schlaeffer F, Sheiner E. Maternal urinary tract infection: is it independently associated with adverse pregnancy outcome? J Matern Fetal Neonatal Med. 2009;22(2):124-8.
2. Sweet RL, Gibbs RS. Infectious Diseases of the Female Genital Tract, 5th edition. Philadelphia: Lippincott Williams and Wilkins; 2009. pp. 254-8.
3. Foxman B. Epidemiology of urinary tract infections: incidence, morbidity, and economic costs. Am J Med. 2002;113:5S.
4. Flores-Mireles AL, Jennifer N. Walker Urinary tract infections: epidemiology, mechanisms of infection and treatment options. Nat Rev Microbiol. 2015;13(5):269-84.
5. Horvath DJ Jr. Morphological plasticity promotes resistance to phagocyte killing of uropathogenic Escherichia coli. Microbes Infect. 2011;13:426-37.
6. Najar MS, Saldanha CL, Banday KA. Approach to urinary tract infections. Indian J Nephrol. 2009;19:129-39.
7. Fihn SD. Clinical practice. Acute uncomplicated urinary tract infection in women. N Engl J Med. 2003;349:259.
8. Hooton TM, Stamm WE. Diagnosis and treatment of Uncomplicated UTI. Infect Dis Clin North Am. 1997;11:551.

9. Root RK. Clinical Infectious Diseases: A Practical Approach. New York: Oxford University Press; 1099. p. 654-56.
10. Bonkat G, Bartoletti RR, Bruyère F, Cai T, Geerlings SE, Köves B, et al. EAU guidelines on Urological infections. Arnhem, Netherlands: European Association of Urology; 2019.
11. Nicolle LE. Infectious diseases society of America guidelines for the diagnosis and treatment of asymptomatic bacteriuria in adults. Clin Infect Dis. 2005;40:643.
12. Mohsin R, Siddiqui KM. Recurrent urinary tract infections in females. J Pak Med Assoc. 2010;60(1):55.
13. Kontiokari T, Sundqvist K, Nuutinen, M. Randomized trial of cranberrylingonberry juice and Lactobacillus GG drink for the prevention of UTI in women. BMJ. 2001;322(7302):1571.
14. Barbosa-Cesnik C, Brown MB, Buxton M, Zhang L, DeBusscher J, Foxman B. Cranberry juice fails to prevent recurrent uti: results from a randomized placebo-controlled trial. Clin Infect Dis. 2011;52(1):23-30.
15. Barrons R, Tassone D. Use of Lactobacillus probiotics for bacterial genitourinary: a review. Clin Ther. 2008;30(3):453-68.
16. Society of Obstetricians and Gynaecologists. Recurrent UTI. Clinical Practice Guidelines. Ottawa: SOGC; 2010.
17. Dielubanza EJ, Schaeffer AJ. Urinary Tract Infections in Women. Med Clin North Am. 2011;95:27-41.
18. Stamm WE. Catheter associated UTI: epidemiology, pathogenesis and prevention. Am J Med. 1991;91:65S-71S.

LONG QUESTIONS

1. Describe the pathogenesis of urinary tract infections.
2. How would you manage a 35-year-old woman with acute uncomplicated cystitis?
3. What are the complications of acute pyelonephritis and describe briefly how you would manage each?
4. How can catheter associated infection be prevented?
5. How would you manage a woman with recurrent UTI?

SHORT QUESTIONS

1. Why are women more susceptible to develop urinary tract infections?
2. What are the factors responsible for UTI in a woman of reproductive age?
3. What are the changes in the urinary tract during pregnancy and how does it predispose a woman to UTI?
4. Which are the organisms commonly associated with UTI?
5. How does a woman with uncomplicated cystitis present?
6. How do you manage acute cystitis? How does the management differ in pregnancy?
7. What is aseptic pyuria?
8. What caution would you exercise to prevent contamination while collecting a specimen of urine for culture?
9. What are the indications for culture of urine?
10. What is the role of ultrasound and CT in the management of UTI?
11. What is asymptomatic bacteriuria?
12. What are the guidelines to treat asymptomatic bacteriuria?
13. How would you diagnose a woman with perinephric abscess?
14. What are the non-antimicrobial methods to prevent recurrent UTI?
15. What is the significance of catheter associated UTI?

MULTIPLE CHOICE QUESTIONS

1. UTI is more common among women than men because:
   a. Women are genetically predisposed to UTI
   b. The urethra is shorter in women
   c. Women are more temperamental than men
   d. Women tend not to completely empty their urinary bladder
2. Which of these statements is not true with regard to UTI in pregnancy?
   a. Hormonal and mechanical changes increase the risk of urinary stasis
   b. The risk of vesicoureteral reflux is increased
   c. UTI is less common in pregnancy than non-pregnant
   d. Poor vulval hygiene due to distended abdomen predisposes to UTI
3. Treatment for asymptomatic bacteriuria is indicated in:
   a. Long standing diabetes
   b. Pregnancy
   c. Postmenopausal women
   d. Children below 5 years
4. Which is the most common uropathogen?
   a. *Escherichia coli (E. coli)*
   b. *Staphylococcus aureus (S. aureus)*
   c. *Chlamydia*
   d. *Mycoplasma*
5. On average, what percentage of pregnant women develops UTIs?
   a. 50% b. 25%
   c. 10–15% d. 2–4%
6. Which antibiotics are used in the treatment of uncomplicated UTIs?
   a. Trimethoprim/sulfamethoxazole
   b. Amoxicillin
   c. Norflox, Ciproflox, Levoflox
   d. All of the above
7. A pregnant woman who develops a UTI needs prompt treatment to avoid:
   a. Premature delivery of her baby
   b. High blood pressure
   c. (A) and (B)
   d. None of the above
8. What percentage of women who have a UTI will have another?
   a. 5% b. 50%
   c. 20% d. None of the above
9. The following are indications for urine culture, except:
   a. Suspicion of complicated UTI
   b. Symptoms not characteristic of UTI

c. UTI symptoms persisting after antibiotic treatment and new antibiotic needs to be started
d. Uncomplicated acute cystitis

10. Common cause of dysuria includes all, except:
a. Urethritis b. Vaginitis
c. Cystitis d. Appendicitis

11. The symptoms which distinguishes pyelonephritis from cystitis is:
a. Fever and flank pain b. Frequency and urgency
c. Hematuria d. None of the above

12. The only non-antimicrobial therapy approved by Cochrane for prevention of UTI:
a. Cranberry juice
b. Lactobacillus
c. Vaccine
d. Topical estrogen cream

13. Which of the following statement is not true?
a. Acute uncomplicated cystitis does not need urine culture for treatment
b. Significant Asymptomatic bacteriuria is >105 CFU
c. Recurrent UTI can be treated with postcoital antimicrobials
d. Catheter associated UTI is not associated with the duration of the catheter in situ

14. Complications of acute pyelonephritis include all, except:
a. Septicemia b. Shock
c. Perinephric abscesses d. Liver failure

15. Which of these statements about recurrent UTI is not true?
a. History of UTI before 15 years age
b. Maternal history of UTI
c. Affects women of low BMI
d. Resistance to commonly used drugs
e. Women with recurrent UTI

Answers

1.	c	2.	c	3.	b	4.	a	5.	d	6.	d
7.	c	8.	c	9.	d	10.	d	11.	a	12.	d
13.	d	14.	d	15.	c						

13.5 UROGENITAL PROLAPSE: ASSESSMENT AND TREATMENT APPROACHES

RM Saraogi, Chirag Patel

DEFINITION

- Descent of pelvic organs into the vagina, often accompanied by urinary, bowel, sexual or local pelvic symptoms.

or

- Leading edge of any vaginal segment > -1 cm above the hymenal remnant.
- Most women take genital prolapse as a part of aging process.

INCIDENCE

- 50% of parous women have prolapse
- Maximum prevalence is seen in India in worlds.

PATHOPHYSIOLOGY

Basic defect lies in weakness of one or more supports of the uterus.

Supports of the Uterus

- *Level 1*: Maintain vaginal length and axis. Uterosacral and cardinal ligaments.
- *Level 2*: Paravaginal attachment of lateral vaginal and endopelvic fascia to the arcus tendineus to maintain the midline position of the vagina (Levator ani).
- *Level 3*: Supports distal vagina-made up of muscles and supportive tissue surrounding the distal vagina and perineum.
- If the level 2 muscles are relaxed and level 3 ligaments are strong then prolapse will not occur.
- If level 2 support is intact-descent will not occur beyond second degree.
- Intact perineal body can present as 3rd degree prolapse.
- Coordinated action of the levator ani muscles (active support), in the presence of intact fascia (passive support) and neural component maintains pelvic organ support intact.
- Anal and urethral sphincter control fecal and urinary incontinence respectively.
- During insult of child birth, muscles and ligaments are still able to prevent prolapse until further insults of repeated child birth and/or atrophy of pelvic floor due to menopause-results in prolapse.
- Prolapse gets precipitated due to chronic factors such as chronic cough, constipation, etc.

ETIOLOGY/RISK FACTORS

- Pregnancy and repeated vaginal childbirth
- Aging and menopause
- Chronically increased intra-abdominal pressure
- Hypoestrogenism
- Trauma
- Genetic factors
- Race

- Musculoskeletal diseases
- Chronic diseases
- Smoking
- Prior surgery.

Hence, the etiology of pelvic organ prolapse (POP) is multifactorial.

A recent case-controlled study of young women operated on for POP reported a 30% family history of genital prolapse. The study group also had a significantly higher rate of operations for abdominal hernias than did the control group (6 vs. 1%). Several prior studies have documented a decrease in total collagen content in women with genital prolapse. These patients have lower amounts of type I collagen (the native collagen), and higher amounts of type III collagen, which is more elastic. Norton et al. showed an increased prevalence of joint hypermobility among women with genital prolapse. This may be a result of connective tissue changes, which can allow ligaments and tendons to stretch abnormally, and can also allow for POP.

Women with connective tissue disorders such as Marfan's (33%) or Ehlers–Danlos (75%) syndromes have higher rates of POP.

POP is more common in older women. A decrease in the ratio of collagen to matrix substance with aging has been noted in certain studies.

As we all know following angioplasty for coronary heart disease, recurrence of blockage will occur may be after 10 years due to the factors which were responsible to cause the disease earlier. Hence, correction of those factors will prevent further recurrence of coronary heart disease. Similarly correction of prolapse without correcting the chronic factors may cause recurrence.

VARIOUS CLASSIFICATIONS OF PROLAPSE

Shaw's Classification

- *Primary*: Descent of uterus and cervix within introitus
- *Secondary*: Descent of uterus cervix projects up to introitus
- *Tertiary*: Projects out through vulva
- *Quaternary*: Complete procedentia [Procedentia (Latin): Procedure to fall].

Baden Walker's Classification

- *Grade 1*: Prolapsed tissue halfway to hymen
- *Grade 2*: Tissue extends to level of hymen
- *Grade 3*: Prolapsed tissue extends outside the hymen with straining
- *Grade 4*: Prolapsed tissue extends outside the hymen without straining.

Jeffcoate's Classification

- Uterine prolapse
- Vaginal prolapse.

Uterine Prolapse

- *1st degree:* Descent of the uterus but cervix is within the introitus
- *2nd degree:* Cervix projects through the vulva when woman is standing or straining
- *3rd degree:* Entire uterus prolapses outside the vulva.

Vaginal Prolapse (Figs. 1A to C)

- *Anterior*: Vaginal wall prolapse. It comprises of cystocele, urethrocele, and Stress urinary incontinence (SUI)
- *Middle*: Vault prolapse and enterocele
- *Posterior vaginal wall prolapse*: It involves rectocele and lax perineum.

Malpas' Classification

Type 1

- It is uterovaginal prolapse occurring due to congenital weakness or damaged Mackenrodt's/uterosacral ligaments.
- In this cervix prolapses up to the introitus.

Type 2

It is uterovaginal prolapse in which paravaginal fascia are maximally damaged resulting in cystocele, rectocele, enterocele and later uterocervical descent.

Type 3

It is bladder neck descent due to damage of bladder neck supports resulting in urethral descent and SUI.

Type 4

Total prolapse where all supports are damaged resulting in procidentia.

International Continence Society

Pelvic organ prolapse-quantification (POP-Q) staging **(Fig. 2)**:

- *Stage 0*: No prolapse is demonstrated.
- *Stage I*: Most distal portion of the prolapse is more than 1 cm above the level of the hymen.
- *Stage II*: The most distal portion of the prolapse is situated between 1 cm above the hymen and 1 cm below the hymen.
- *Stage III*: The most distal portion of the prolapse is more than 1 cm beyond the plane of the hymen but everted at least 2 cm less than the total vaginal length.
- *Stage IV*: Complete eversion or eversion at least within 2 cm of the total length of the lower genital tract is demonstrated.

The POP-Q classification involves the identification of nine locations in vagina and vulva and estimating their distance in centimeters in relation to hymen, which is used to quantify the stage of prolapse at its most advanced site **(Figs. 3 and 4)**:

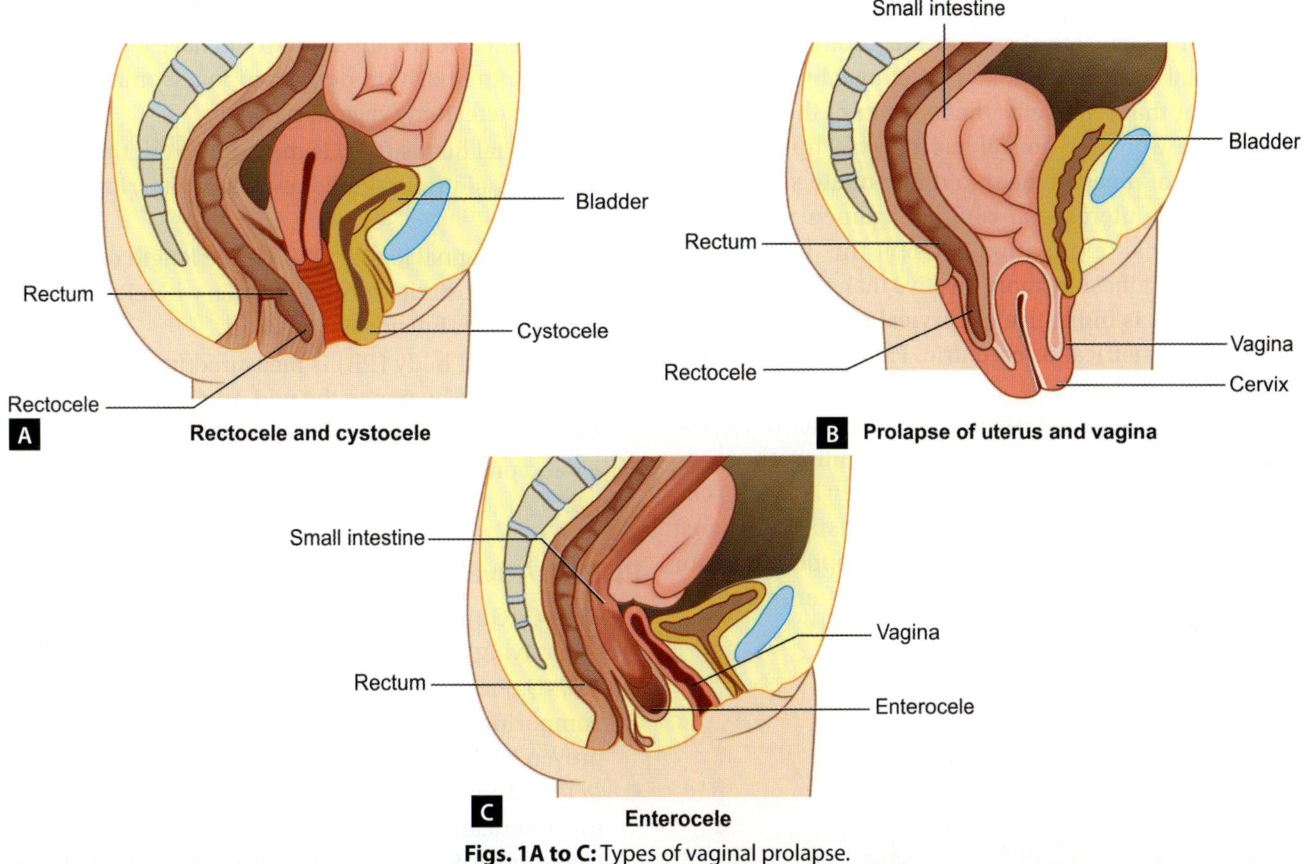

Figs. 1A to C: Types of vaginal prolapse.

Fig. 2: Staging of prolapse using the leading edge of cervix.

- *Aa:* A point located in the midline of the anterior vaginal wall 3 cm proximal to the external urethral meatus. By definition, the range of position of Point Aa relative to the hymen is –3 to + 3 cm.
- *Ba:* A point that represents the most distal (i.e., most dependent) position of any part of the upper anterior vaginal wall. From the vaginal cuff or anterior vaginal fornix to Point Aa. By definition, Point Ba is at 3 cm in the absence of prolapse and would have a positive value equal to the position of the cuff (Point C) in women with total uterine prolapse or posthysterectomy vaginal eversion.

- *C:* A point that represents either the most distal (i.e., most dependent) edge of the cervix or the leading edge of the vaginal cuff (hysterectomy scar) after total hysterectomy.
- *D:* A point that represents the location of the posterior fornix in a woman who still has a cervix. It is included as a point of measurement to differentiate suspensory failure of the uterosacral-cardinal ligament "complex" from cervical elongation. When the location of Point C is significantly more positive than the location of Point D, this is indicative of cervical elongation which may be symmetrical or eccentric. Point D is omitted in the absence of the cervix.
- *Ap:* A point located in the midline of the posterior vaginal wall 3 cm proximal to the hymen. By definition, the range of position of Point Ap relative to the hymen is –3 to +3 cm.
- *Bp:* A point that represents the most distal (i.e., most dependent) position of any part of the upper posterior vaginal wall from the vaginal cuff or posterior vaginal fornix to Point Ap. By definition, Point Bp is at - 3 cm in the absence of prolapse and would have a positive value equal to the position of the cuff in a woman with total post-hysterectomy vaginal eversion.
- The genital hiatus (GH) is measured from the middle of the external urethral meatus to the posterior margin of the hymen.
- The total vaginal length (TVL) is the length of the vagina (cm) from posterior fornix to hymen when Point C or D is reduced to its full normal position.
- The perineal body (PB) is measured from the posterior margin of the hymen to the mid-anal opening.

Measurements distal to hymen are marked as positive values and proximal or above hymen are marked as negative values.

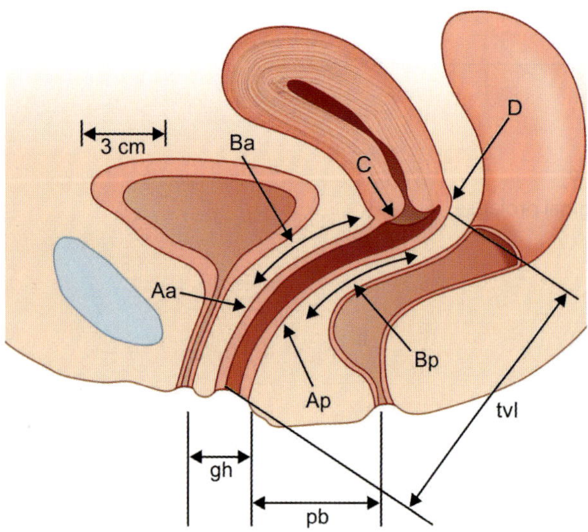

Fig. 3: The nine reference points in POP-Q Classification.

POP-Q: Advantages

- *POP-Q*: Objective, site-specific system for describing, quantifying, and staging pelvic support in women
- *POP-Q*: Provides standardized means for documenting, comparing, and communicating clinical findings with proven inter observer and intraobserver reliability
- *POP Q*: Approved by the International Continence Society, the American Urogynecologic Society, and the Society of Gynecologic Surgeons for the description of female pelvic organ prolapse.

POP-Q: Disadvantages

- *POP-Q*: Too many variations to allow grouping patients into comparable populations for study purposes
- *POP-Q*: Too complex for simple clinical communication, such as describing a patient briefly to a colleague.

Results: Staging system created to make comparative analyses and clinical communications more practical.

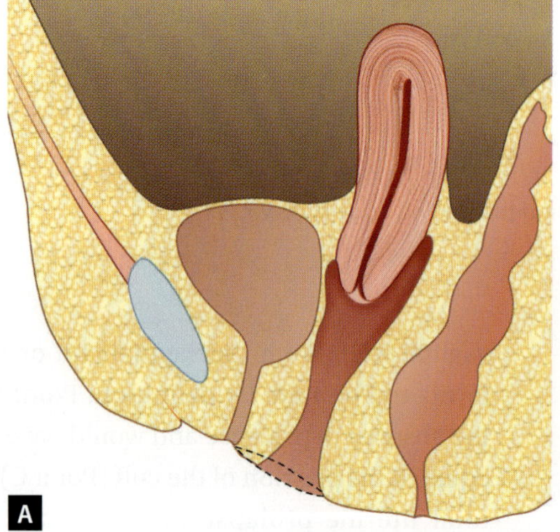

Anterior wall Aa	Anterior wall Ba	Cervix or cuff C
Genital hiatus gH	Perineal body pB	Total vaginal length TVL
Posterior wall Ap	Posterior wall Bp	Posterior fornix D

B

Figs. 4A and B: (A) Simplified POP-Q; (B) Grid presentation of POP-Q.

SYMPTOMS

Symptoms Related to Urination

- Incontinence of urine
- Urinary urgency
- Urinary frequency
- Weak or prolonged urinary stream
- Hesitancy while urination
- Feeling of incomplete emptying
- Manual reduction of prolapse to start or complete voiding
- Position change to start or complete voiding
- Urinary dribbling on coughing or sneezing.

Bowel Symptoms

- Incontinence of flatus or liquid/solid stool
- Feeling of incomplete emptying
- Hard straining to defecate
- Urgency to defecate
- Digital evacuation to complete defecation
- Splinting vagina or perineum to start or complete defecation
- Feeling of blockage or obstruction during defecation.

Symptoms of Bulge

- Seeing or feeling a vaginal or perineal bulge
- Feeling of something coming out per vaginum
- Feeling pelvic or vaginal pressure
- Feeling of heaviness in pelvis or vagina.

Sexual Symptoms

- Dyspareunia
- Decreased lubrication
- Decreased sensation
- Decreased arousal or orgasm
- Inability to retain semen.

Pain

- Pain in vagina, bladder or rectum
- Pelvic pain
- Low back pain.

Abnormal Bleeding, Discharge Per Vaginum or Infection of Vagina

Splinting/Digitation: Complaint of the need to digitally replace the prolapse or to otherwise apply manual pressure, e.g., to the vagina, perineum or perianal area (splinting), or rectally (digitation) to assist voiding or defecation.

CLINICAL EXAMINATION/ ASSESSMENT/SIGNS

Position: Standing—ideal but awkward and impractical; dorsal lithotomy position—more practical.

The bladder of the patient should be empty.

What to Look while doing Examination?

- Look for gapping of introitus and size, take measurements
- Integrity of perineal body
- Measurement of all prolapsed parts preferably in centimeters
- *After replacement of prolapsed parts*: Ask patient to cough and note order of descent
- *Cervix first*: Cervix comes first in nulliparous followed by cystocele or rectocele
- *Cervix last*: Cervix comes last in multiparous. First comes the cystocele, then rectocele
- Look for keratinization, ulceration (decubitus ulcer) and fibrosis at dependent part of prolapsed part
- Take UCL
- With the help of tenaculum or vulsellum- give traction to prolapsed part-will give idea about degree and type of prolapsed and difficulty in subsequent vaginal hysterectomy or any other operative procedure
- Once patient's bladder is full, look for SUI
- Bimanual examination to be done to rule out any associated adnexal pathology and to see size of uterus
- *A composite examination*: Inspection and palpation—vaginal, rectal, rectovaginal or even under anesthesia may be required to arrive at a correct diagnosis
- Etiological aspect of prolapse should be evaluated.

Cystocele (Fig. 5)

- Bulge of the anterior vaginal wall which increases on straining.
- It can be demonstrated by separating the labia or depressing the posterior vaginal wall using a speculum.
- Essentially a hernia in the anterior vaginal wall is due to weakness or defect in pubovesicovaginal fascia
    - Midline weakness allows bladder to descend causing central cystocele
    - Tearing of endopelvic fascial connections from lateral sulci to arcus tendineus causes lateral or displacement cystocele
    - Detachment of pubocervical fascia from pericervical ring causes a transverse or apical cystocele.

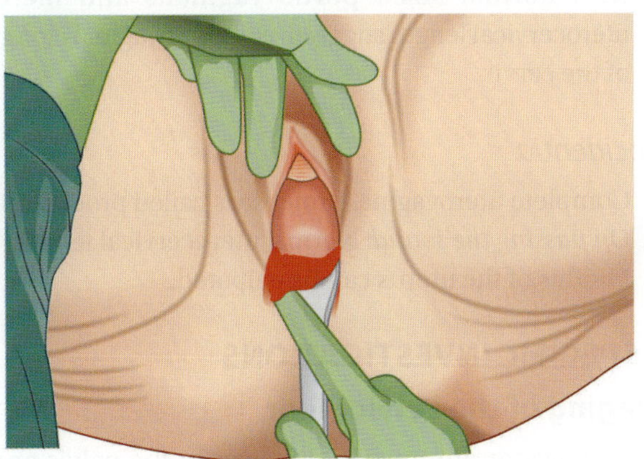

Fig. 5: Cystocele.

Rectocele

After retracting the anterior vaginal wall the bulge of the posterior middle third vaginal wall on valsalva, with diffuse margins and being reducible.

Perineal Deficiency

Gaping introitus with or without straining due to retraction of heads of bulbocavernosus and superficial transverse muscles.

Perineal Descent

- Sagging and funneling of the levator ani around the perineum such that anus becomes most dependent
- Difficulty during defecation
- Sexual dissatisfaction.

Enterocele

- The bulge on the posterior vaginal wall which is close to the cervix in upper third of the posterior vaginal wall
- A true hernia of the rectouterine or cul-de-sac pouch (pouch of Douglas)
- Descent of bowel in a peritoneum-lined sac between posterior vaginal apex and anterior rectum
- Pulsion enterocele is filled with bowel and distended by abdominal pressure bowel peristalsis confirms diagnosis
- It can occur anteriorly as well
- Generally after a surgical change in vaginal axis following vaginal/abdominal hysterectomy in previously missed enterocele
- The differentiation between the two is by rectal and rectovaginal examination.

Uterine Prolapse

- For first degree descent speculum examination with the cervical descent below the level of ischial spines confirms diagnosis
- In second to third degree prolapse inspection can reveal the external os coming out through the introitus
- Bimanual examination reveals shallow vaginal fornices with normal sized portio vaginalis and increases uterocervical length suggestive of supravaginal elongation of the cervix.

Procidentia

- Complete uterovaginal prolapse is called procidentia
- *On passing the sound*: Normal uterocervical length
- Fundus of the uterus can be palpated.

SPECIFIC INVESTIGATIONS

Imaging of the Pelvic Floor

- The levator ani muscles lie deep in the pelvis and are difficult to assess clinically.
- It is seen that patients with stage III and stage IV prolapse all have abnormal levator ani morphological features.
- *Two-dimensional translabial scanning is now a standard technique*: Reported for assessing position and mobility of the bladder neck and proximal urethra, stress incontinence, bladder wall thickness, levator ani activity (with perineal scanning), and prolapse quantification.
- Three-dimensional ultrasound has been used to image the urethra, levator-ani complex, paravaginal supports, prolapse, and synthetic implant materials.
- Intravenous pyelography (IVP) particularly in cases of procidentia for evaluating the course of the ureters.
- Cystoscopy and urodynamic studies may be required in the evaluation of incontinence.
- MRI allows noninvasive in vivo measurement of the structure and function of the pelvic floor muscles.

DIFFERENTIAL DIAGNOSIS

- Cyst of anterior vaginal wall
- Urethral caruncle
- Cervical polyp
- Hypertrophy and elongation of infravaginal cervix
- Inversion of uterus
- Rectal prolapsed.

COMPLICATIONS OF PROLAPSE

- Hypertrophy, hyperplasia and supravaginal elongation of cervix
- Congestion and edema of prolapsed parts
- Decubitus ulcer
- Infection of urinary system
- Obstructive lesions of urinary tract.

MANAGEMENT

Conservative

- Pessary
- Kegel's exercise
- Weight loss
- Treatment of underlying chronic disease
- Cessation of smoking
- Physical therapy
- Estrogen supplement
- Vaginal splinting.

Use of Pessary (Fig. 6)

- The pessary is most commonly used in the management of pelvic support defects such as cystocele and rectocele. Pessaries can also be used in the treatment of stress urinary incontinence.
- The type of pessary that is appropriate for each patient depends on the condition being treated.

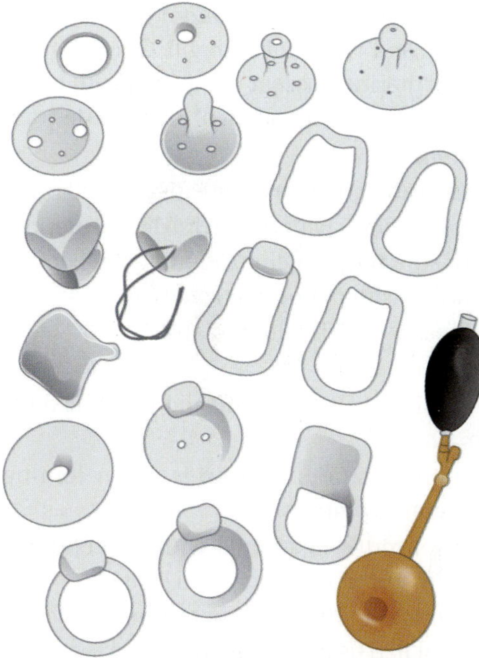

Fig. 6: Types of pessaries used in urogenital prolapse.

- It remains a useful temporary device for nonsurgical management of a number of gynecologic conditions.
- Selection of an appropriate pessary depends primarily on the condition for which the patient is being treated. Gellhorn pessary can offer excellent support for uterine prolapse as long as the perineal body is intact. If the perineal body is weak, a cube or Donut pessary will be more effective.
- An incontinence ring pessary usually helps with SUI, but if the patient has some degree of cystocele, a Hodge with support or a Gehrung pessary may be more effective.
  "In women with POP of stage 2 or higher undergoing surgery, prolapse symptoms were less severe than in those who were treated with a pessary, but 72% of women who were treated with a pessary did not opt for surgery."
- Most common side effects of pessary are vaginal discharge and vaginal pain.
- The reasons for discontinuation are mostly spontaneous expulsion, urinary incontinence, vaginal pain, discharge, no reduction in prolapse symptoms.
- "Likelihood of preferring pessary treatment over surgery increases with increasing patient age—surgery is preferred over pessary as POP stage increases and if POP symptoms are more bothersome and affect general well-being and that patients who are sexually active tend to prefer surgery over conservative treatment.
- A strategy of pessary treatment followed by surgery if needed, or strategy with immediate surgery both seem to be effective options for the treatment of POP in women.
- Two prospective cohort studies comparing pessary treatment and surgery have shown similar improvements in urinary and bowel symptoms, sexual function, and quality of life at 12 months.

Kegel's Exercise

- A pelvic floor exercise, more commonly called a Kegel exercise (named after Dr Arnold Kegel), consists of repeatedly contracting and relaxing the muscles that form part of the pelvic floor, now sometimes colloquially referred to as the "Kegel muscles".
- The aim of Kegel's exercises is to improve muscle tone by strengthening the pubococcygeus muscles of the pelvic floor.
- A meta-analysis of randomized controlled trials by the Cochrane Collaboration concluded that "there is now some evidence available indicating a positive effect of pelvic floor muscle exercises for prolapse symptoms and severity."
- Guided pelvic floor muscle training is more beneficial than self-taught Kegel's exercise, though may not be effective for high stage or apical prolapse.
- Pelvic floor physical therapy (PFPT) with a physical therapist is the best approach to conservative management of apical prolapse.

Surgical Approach

The basic idea is to concentrate on restoring anatomy, i.e., structure and physiology, i.e., function.

It is classified as:

- Restorative
- Compensatory
- Obliterative

Surgeries done are for prophylaxis, therapeutic and preventing recurrence of prolapse. *Hysterectomy per se is not the treatment for prolapse.*

Ideally the patient should have completed her child bearing before undergoing any surgery for prolapse.

Restorative Surgeries

- *Principle*: Use of patient's endogenous tissues for repair provided they are strong enough to support the descending organ.
- It is based on the principle that due to pregnancy or birth trauma the involution of only some part of the support is poor and incomplete, while rests of the tissues are normal.
- When patient has 2nd to 3rd degree uterine descent with supravaginal elongation of cervix, the muscular support (levator ani) of the uterus is invariably weak/torn, as a result there is compensatory hypertrophy and hyperplasia of ligamentous supports like uterosacrals and Mackenrodt's ligaments.
- In such cases, if the ligaments are detached and shortened; and fixed back on anterior surface of the cervix, the prolapse gets corrected.

The surgeries are site specific repair—defect-specific, or site-specific defect repair, was introduced by Richardson in 1972. It attempts to identify and repair specific areas of deficiency in the endopelvic fascia.

Vaginal **(Figs. 7A to E)**:

1. *Anterior colporrhaphy*:
   - *Indications*:
     - Cystocele
     - Urethrocele
   - *Principle*: Mobilize bladder, push it upwards plicate endopelvic and pubocervical fascia under bladder neck in midline (excise a portion of relaxed anterior vaginal wall)

   Complications
   - Injury to bladder/urethra
   - *Intraoperative hemorrhage*: Injury to vesical venous plexus
   - Hematoma between vagina and bladder infected necrosis of adjacent walls
   - UTI
   - SUI due to overcorrection
   - Difficult micturition—overtightening of bladder neck
2. *Posterior colpoperineorrhaphy—for rectocele and lax perineum*:
   - The common sites of injury to the rectovaginal septum are transverse apical defect due to detachment of rectovaginal septum from pericervical ring, midvaginal defects may be central or lateral due to injury to levator fascia and inferior defect due to detachment from perineal body.

   Technique: A transverse incision was made at the vaginal introitus, and the posterior vaginal wall was incised in the midline to a point cephalad to the rectocele. The rectovaginal septum was identified, and the vaginal epithelium and smooth muscle were dissected away from it by means of sharp and blunt dissections. This was extended laterally to the arcus tendineus levator ani muscles and inferiorly to the perineal body. An effort was made to leave as much endopelvic connective tissue on the rectum as possible in an avascular plane. A rectal examination was performed to identify location of site-specific defects in the Denonvilliers' fascia.
3. *Shirodkar's uterosacral advancement* ***(Table 1)***:

   Indications:
   - Young patients with completed child bearing function.
   - Patients in whom menstrual function is desired.
   - This surgery is useful in patients with enterocele and those requiring tubal ligation.
   - Patients with 2nd or 3rd degree uterine prolapse without much uterocervical elongation and with healthy cervix.
   - Uterosacral ligaments are advanced anteriorly on cervix after detaching them from posterior surface of the cervix (after opening the pouch of Douglas).
4. *Fothergill's/Manchester's operation* **(Table 1)**: It was devised by Donald and William Fothergill. Operation is designed to correct uterine descent associated with cystocele and rectocele, when preservation of uterus is desirable.

   Indications:
   - Preservation of menstrual functions
   - Young patients with 2nd or 3rd degree uterine prolapse with supravaginal elongation of cervix of more than 4 inches with cystocele/rectocele
   - Unhealthy cervix with prolapse.

   Principles of surgery:
   - Preliminary D&C is done and cervix is dilated up to no. 12.
   - Racquet shaped incision is taken joining all the Fothergill's points.
   - Mackenrodt's ligaments with descending cervical arteries are clamped, cut and ligated.
   - Cervix is amputated and posterior lip is covered by the vaginal flap using Sturmdorf suture.
   - Plication of Mackenrodt's in front of cervix using Fothergill's stitch.
   - Correct the uterus from retroversion to anterversion manually.

Fothergill's 4 points:

1. Immediately above the urethral meatus.
2. Slightly posterolateral to cervix on one side-depends on extent of prolapsed.
3. Similarly on other side.
4. Midline of the posterior fornix at the point where vaginal skin can be picked up freely from the cervix.

Fothergill's stitch **(Fig. 8)**:

- The needle is inserted at Fothergill's lateral point on the patient's left side, through the vaginal skin, through the Mackenrodt's divided ligament and through the midpoint of the anterior lip of the amputated cervix, from without inwards into the canal
- Needle is then passed in a reverse direction from within outwards and the process exactly repeated on patient's right side
- When the suture is tied-effect is elevation of the cervix and anteversion of the uterus.

Enterocele:

a. Abdominal
   - Halban's operation
   - Moskowitz operation

   These surgeries are performed for prevention or correction of entereocele.
b. Vaginal
   - Iliococcygeus fascia suspension
   - *McCall culdoplasty*: For enterocele and prevention of vault prolapsed.

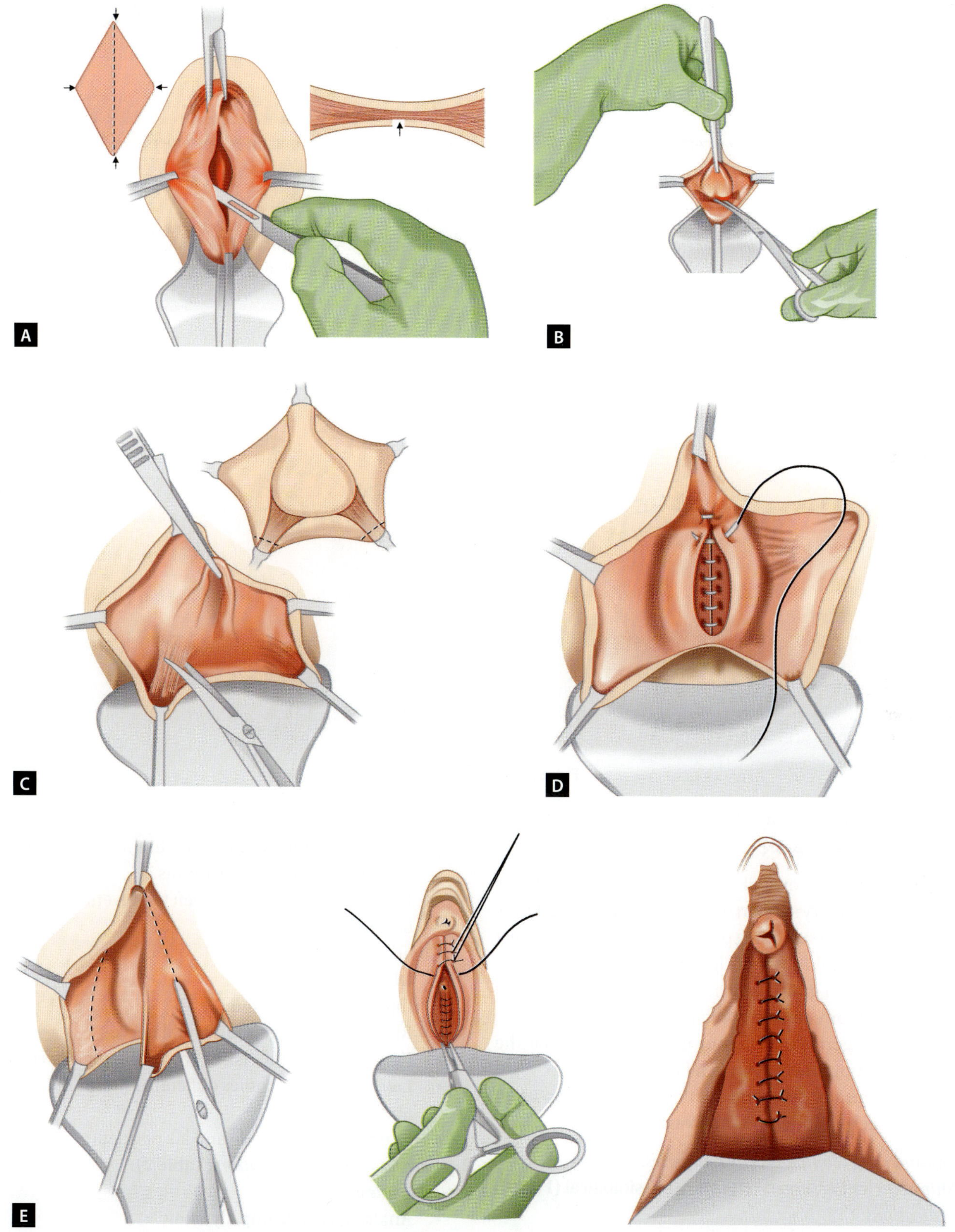

Figs. 7A to E: (A) Inverted T incision on anterior vaginal wall; (B) Raised triangular flaps and dissection of endopelvic fascia; (C) Bladder with covering endopelvic fascia; (D) Pubocervical fascia plicated with interrupted sutures and hernial sac reduced; (E) Redundant portion of vaginal mucosa cut on either sides and cut margins apposed with interrupted sutures.

TABLE 1: Comparison of Fothergill's repair and Shirodkar's repair.

Fothergill's repair	***Shirodkar's repair***
Prior dilatation of cervix is done	Not done
POD not opened	POD opened
Cardinal ligaments are used for advancement	Uterosacral ligaments are used for advancement
Cervical dystocia can occur	No cervical dystocia
Cervical amputation done	Cervical amputation not done
Risk of abortion and preterm labor increased	Risk not increased
No necrosis of cervix	Sloughing and autoamputation of cervix can occur and cervicovaginal fistula can occur

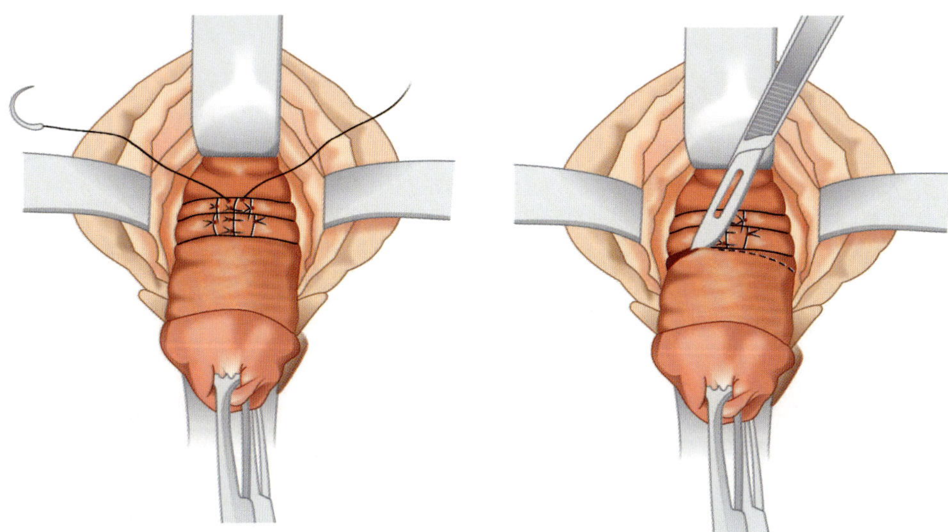

Fig. 8: Fothergill's stitches.

Compensatory Surgeries

- Whenever there is overall weakness of the muscular as well as ligamentary support of the uterus due to weakness of the collagen tissue; using patients own tissue to correct the prolapse would not result in cure. Hence these patients require artificial grafts; which will act as supports of the uterus, thus correcting the prolapse.
- In these surgeries an attempt is made to replace the weakened supports with artificial grafts.
- The compensatory surgeries can be divided based upon the approach as abdominal and vaginal.

Abdominal sling (compensatory) surgeries:

1. *Shirodkar's sling surgery*: It is more physiological **(Fig. 9)**.
   Indications:
   - Nulliparous prolapse
   - Following child birth without cystocele/rectocele
   - Procidentia in a young patient
   - Vault prolapse

   Principles:
   - Posterior, closed loop, static
   - A mersilene tape is anchored to the L-5 vertebra and the posterior aspect of isthmus.
   - Psoas loop is made on the left to prevent compression of sigmoid colon.

   Complications:
   - Difficult to perform
   - Injury to sigmoid colon
   - Risk of injury to genitofemoral nerve
   - If it becomes tight, risk of bowel obstruction is there.
   - Later on D&C becomes difficult as uterus becomes an abdominal organ
   - Cannot cure rectocele and lax perineum
2. *Purandare's pexy operation* **(Table 2)**:
   Principles:
   - Anterior, closed loop, dynamic
   - This involves anchoring the anterior aspect of uterine isthmus to the anterior abdominal wall with the help of mersilene tape
   - Plication of round ligaments done to antevert the uterus
   - Moskowitz stitch taken to prevent enterocele.

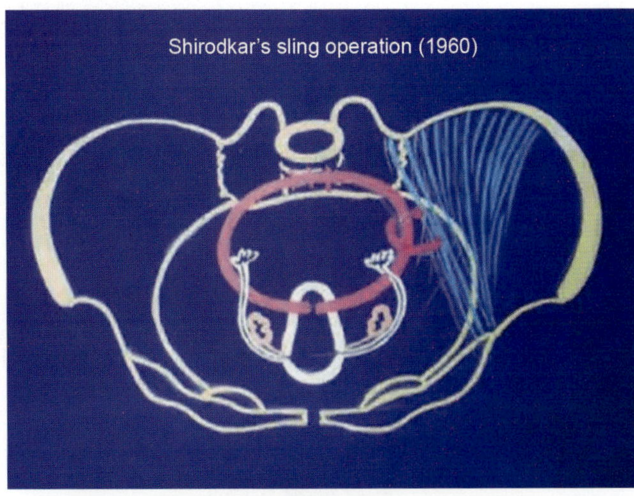

Fig. 9: Shirodkar's sling surgery.

TABLE 2: Comparison of Shirodkar's sling and Purandare's pexy.

Shirodkar's sling	***Purandare's pexy***
Pulls the cervix upwards and backwards so the uterus remains anteverted	Pulls the cervix upwards and forwards so the uterus becomes retroverted
Does not increase the chance of enterocele	Increases the chances of enterocele
Static sling	Dynamic sling
Technically more difficult	Technically easier

3. *Khanna's sling operation*
   Principles:
   - Static and neutral
   - Mersilene tape is anchored to the anterior aspect of isthmus and anterior superior iliac spine
   - Static, neutral

   Complications:
   - Tape is superficial and can be easily felt by the patient
   - Infection results in periostitis
4. *Sonavala's sling operation*
   Principle: Shirodkar's sling is more difficult to perform on left side due to presence of sigmoid colon so Sonawala thought of doing it only on right side.
5. *Virkud's composite sling*
   Principle: Tape is anchored to sacral promontory on right side such as Shirodkar's sling and to anterior rectus sheath on left side like Purandare's cervicopexy. However, it causes twist of uterus hence plication of uterosacral ligament is required.
6. *Congenital prolapse*
   - Complete prolapse of uterus at birth is rare anomaly
   - Associated with breech presentation
   - *Associated with an anomalous baby*: Hydrocephalus, spina bifida with meningocele, cervical prolapsed
   - Spina bifida is the most important etiological factor
7. Nulliparous prolapse.

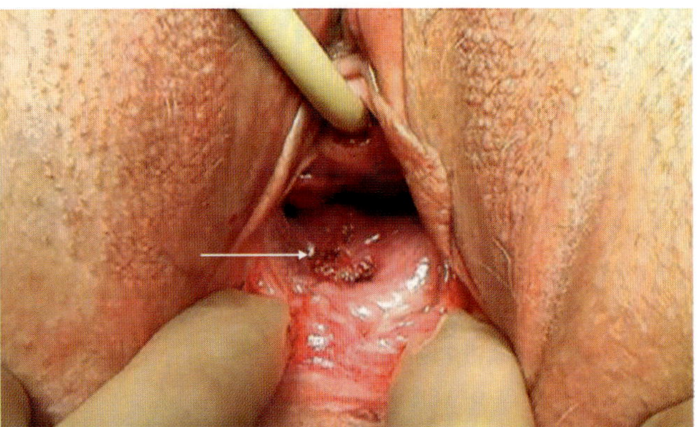

Fig. 10: Mesh extrusion (arrow).

Vaginal compensatory surgeries:

Role of mesh

Principles:
- Used for patients with endogenous weak tissues
- Fibrous reaction around the tape/mesh acts to strengthen and replace weakened tissues

Complications:
- Mesh extrusion (5–15%), most common **(Fig. 10)**
- Incidence decreasing due to recent lighter softer mesh and improved surgical techniques
- Deeply placed mesh have lower extrusion rates
  - Surgisis
    - Surgisis is a new biomaterial for pelvic floor repairs using SIS (small intestine submucosa of pig)
    - Tissue graft for surgical reinforcement and strengthening of pelvic floor tissues
    - Takes on the natural form of the area it is surgically inserted into, known as tissue remodeling
  - *APOGEE*: New minimal invasive procedure for posterior vaginal wall defects using mesh.
  - *PERIGEE*: For surgery of anterior vaginal wall defect mesh.
  - Posterior intravaginal slingplasty (infracoccygeal sacropexy)
    - First reported by PE Papa Petros in 1997
    - To create neouterosacral ligaments, using polypropylene tape
    - Helping to relocate vaginal apex (Level 1 support) to its original level above the levator plate and restore vaginal axis.

Obliterative Surgeries

Principles:
- To close the vagina partially or completely with the prolapse reduced above.
- These surgeries are generally carried out in very old postmenopausal high risk patients where anesthesia is contraindicated.
- It should be done in patients who do not desire sexual function.
- There should not be any uterine or pelvic pathology.

Types of obliterative surgeries:

1. *Partial colpocleisis:* LeFort colpocleisis

   Indications:
   - Old postmenopausal patient with 3rd degree uterine prolapse with healthy cervix
   - Sexual function is not desired
   - Medically unfit for surgery

   Principles:
   - Denudation of rectangular vaginal flap from anterior and posterior vaginal walls
   - Apposition of the denuded anterior and posterior vaginal walls

   Complications:
   - Pyometra
   - Stress urinary incontinence
2. *Goodall Power's Modification:* Total colpocleisis
   - Dani's stitch (introital tightening)
   - Though we have so many surgeries every surgery has its own indications, contraindications, advantages, and disadvantages.
   - The operative techniques should be combined with appropriate clinical evaluation to obtain maximum benefit for the patients.
   - Some patients have concomitant prolapse of anterior vagina, posterior vagina, cul de sac and even rectum. Such patients may require correction of all pathologies in one sitting.

SURGERIES FOR VAULT PROLAPSE (FIGS. 11 AND 12)

1. *Sacrospinous ligament fixation*

   Principles: Delayed absorbable suture is passed through sacrospinous ligament on both sides or preferably the right side 2 cm medial to ischial spine and then fixed to the vaginal vault.

   Complications:
   - Injury to bowel, ureter, pudendal vessels
   - High failure rates

   Anterior sacrospinous vaginal vault suspension: Sacrospinous ligament is accessed through the paravesical space. This maintains the anterior orientation of vagina and does not cause apical narrowing as seen with the traditional posterior sacrospinous vaginal vault suspension.

   Anterior placement of vagina minimizes tension on the anterior vaginal wall. Fewer recurrent cystoceles were noted with anterior sacrospinous suspension than with posterior sacrospinous suspension.

   A recent analysis of Medicare claims data found that, at 10 years follow-up, women who had undergone a combined apical prolapse procedure and cystocele repair had significantly lower prolapse reoperation rate than those who had undergone an isolated anterior repair (11.6 vs. 20.2%, $p<0.01$), demonstrating the importance of correcting the apical component.

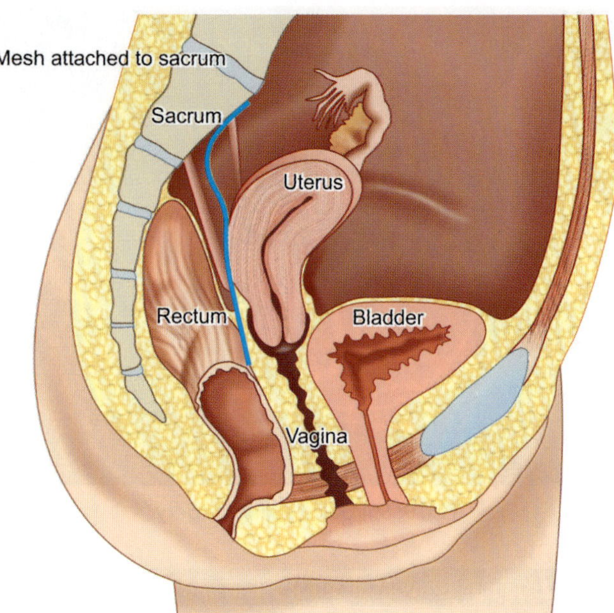

Fig. 11: Sacrohysteropexy procedure.

2. *Aldrich procedure*: Fixation of vault using mersilene tape.
3. *Sacrohysteropexy* **(Fig. 11)**: First described by Falk who attached the vaginal vault directly to the sacrum
   - Subsequently, Lane used mersilene vascular graft to bridge the gap between the vault and the sacral promontory
   - Performed to cure vaginal vault prolapse (sacrocolpopexy) or prolapse of the uterus (sacrohysteropexy).
   - Lifts the vagina or uterus back into its normal position by attaching a piece of synthetic mesh between the top of the vagina and the sacrum
4. *Laparoscopic sacrohysteropexy*
   - Involves the use of a permanent polypropylene mesh, which is attached to the cervix and the sacral promontory (the first and second vertebra of the sacrum).
   - The uterus and cervix are suspended, restoring a normal anatomy, enhancing sexual function, and preserving childbearing capability.
   - If there is posthysterectomy vaginal vault prolapse, then same procedure is called a laparoscopic sacral colpopexy.
   - Two randomized control trials have demonstrated equal efficacy between robotic and laparoscopic sacrocolpopexy.

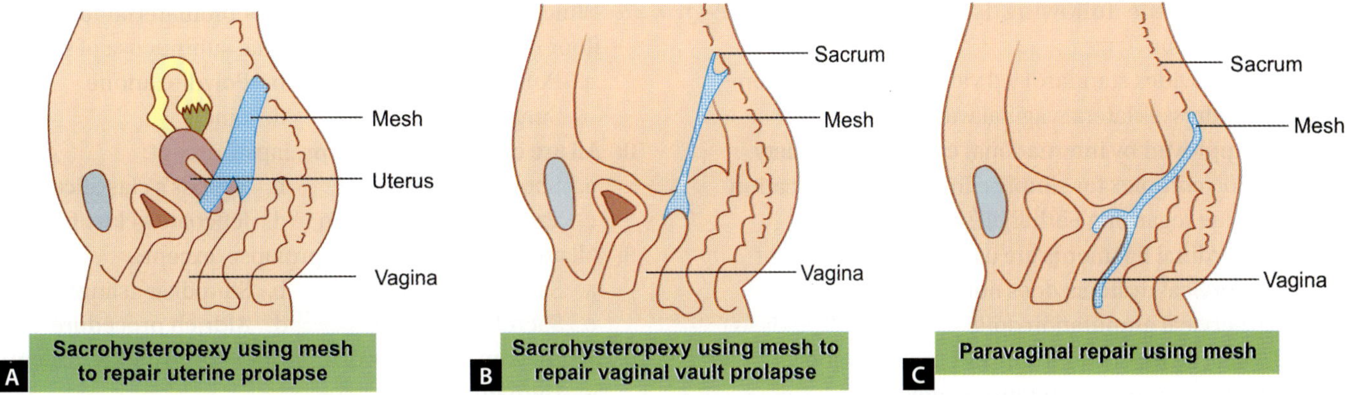

Figs. 12A to C: Sacrocolpopexy and paravaginal repair for total pelvic floor prolapse.

FURTHER READING

1. Abdool Z, Thakar R, Sultan AH, Oliver RS. Prospective evaluation of outcome of vaginal pessaries versus surgery in women with symptomatic pelvic organ prolapse. Int Urogynecol J. 2011;22:273-8.
2. Abrams P, Cardozo L, Fall M. The standardisation of terminology of lower urinary tract function. Report from the standardisation subcommittee of the International Continence Society. Neurourol Urodyn. 2002;21:167-78.
3. Ajit Virkud. Modern Gynaecology, 2017; 2nd Edition. APC Publications.
4. Bump RC, Mattiasson A, Bo K. The standardization of female pelvic organ prolapse and pelvic floor dysfunction. Am J Obstet Gynecol. 1996;175:10-1.
5. Bump RC, Mattiasson A, Bo K. The standardization of terminology female pelvic organ prolapsed and pelvic floor dysfunction. Am J Obstet Gynecol. 1996;175:10.
6. Carley ME, Schaffer J. Urinary incontinence and pelvic organ prolapse in women with Marfan or Ehlers-Danlos syndrome. Am J Obstet Gynecol. 2000;182:1021-3.
7. Coolen AWM, Troost S, Mol BWJ, Roovers JPWR, Bongers MY. Primary treatment of pelvic organ prolapse: pessary use versus prolapse surgery. Int J Urogynaecol. 2018;29(1):99-107.
8. Eilber KS, Alperin M, Khan A. Outcomes of vaginal prolapse surgery among female medicare beneficiaries: the role of apical support. Obstet Gynecol. 2013;122(5):981-7.
9. Hagen S, Stark D, Glazener C. Individualised pelvic floor muscle training in women with pelvic organ prolapse (POPPY): a multicentre randomised controlled trial. Lancet. 2014;383(9919):796-806.
10. Haylen BT, Freeman RM, de Ridder D. An International Urogynecological Association (IUGA)—International Continence Society (ICS) Joint Report into the Terminology for Female Pelvic Floor Dysfunction. Neurourology and Urodynamics. Int Urogynecol J. 2010;21:5-26.
11. Jackson S, Avery N, Eckford S. Connective tissue analysis in genitourinary prolapse. Neurourol Urodyn. 1995;14:412-4.
12. Lamers BH, Broekman BM, Milani AL. Pessary treatment for pelvic organ prolapse and health-related quality of life: a review. Int Urogynecol J. 2011;22:637-64.
13. Norton PA, Baker JE, Sharp HC, Warenski JC. Genitourinary prolapse and joint hypermobility in women. Obstet Gynecol. 1995;85:225-8.
14. Norton PA. Pelvic floor disorders: the role of fascia and ligaments. Clin Obstet Gynecol. 1993;36:929-38.
15. Parekh M, Swift S, Lemos N. Multicentre inter-examiner trial of the validation of simplified POPQ system. Int Urogynecol J. 2011;22:645-50.
16. Rinne KM, Kirkinen PP. What predisposes young women to genital prolapse? Eur J Obstet Gynecol Reprod Biol. 1999; 84:23-5.
17. Swift S, Morris S, McKinnie V. Validation of a simplified technique for using the POPQ pelvic organ classification system. Int Urogynecol J. 2006;17:615-20.
18. Thakar R, Stanton S. Management of genital prolapse. BMJ. 2002;324(7348):1258-62.
19. Winkler HA, Tomeszko JE, Sand PK. Anterior sacrospinous vaginal vault suspension for prolapse. Obstet Gynecol. 2000;95:612-5.

LONG QUESTIONS

1. Describe various classifications of pelvic organ prolapse.
2. Write principles of Fothergill's repair and difference between Fothergill's repair and Shirodkar's repair.
3. Describe abdominal compensatory surgical approaches.
4. Describe anterior colporrhaphy.

SHORT QUESTIONS

1. Describe POP-Q classification.
2. Write principles of anterior colporrhaphy.
3. What are presenting symptoms and signs of prolapse?
4. Write short note on "pessary".
5. Write short note on Kegel's exercise.

MULTIPLE CHOICE QUESTIONS

1. All are included in supports of uterus, except:
   a. Uterosacral and cardinal ligaments
   b. Infundibulopelvic ligaments
   c. Levator ani
   d. Lateral pelvic fascia
2. Which of the following is a risk factor for prolapse of uterus?
   a. Chronic diarrhea b. Hemorrhoids
   c. Repeated vaginal birth d. Pelvic endometriosis

3. Which of the following is not correct for POP-Q classification?
   a. It provides standardized values for comparison
   b. Addresses lateral vaginal wall defect
   c. Approved by international continence society
   d. Too complex for simple clinical communication
4. Not true regarding Fothergill's repair:
   a. Cardinal ligaments are used for advancement
   b. Cervical dystocia does not occur
   c. Cervical amputation done
   d. Risk factors of abortion and preterm labor
5. Which one is not obliterative surgery?
   a. LeFort's colpocleisis
   b. Goodall power modification
   c. Shirodkar sling surgery
   d. Dani's stitch
6. Which of the following surgery is dynamic sling surgery?
   a. Shirodkar's sling b. Khanna's sling
   c. Sonawala's sling d. Purandare's pexy
7. Which of the following is a new biomaterial for pelvic floor repair using small intestinal submucosa of sheep?
   a. Polyglecaprone b. Polydioxanone
   c. Surgisis d. Linen
8. All are classifications for prolapse, except:
   a. Show's classification b. Malpas's classification
   c. Tanner's classification d. Jeffcoate's classification
9. All are surgeries for vault prolapse, except:
   a. Sacrospinous fixation b. Shirodkar's sling surgery
   c. Sacrohysteropexy d. Aldrich procedure
10. All are complications of anterior colporrhaphy, except:
   a. Hematoma
   b. Injury to vesical venous plexus
   c. Fecal incontinence
   d. Difficulty in micturition

Answers

1.	b	2.	a	3.	b	4.	b	5.	c	6.	d
7.	c	8.	c	9.	b	10.	c				

13.6 POSTHYSTERECTOMY VAGINAL VAULT PROLAPSE

L Krishna, N Shailaja

INTRODUCTION AND BACKGROUND EPIDEMIOLOGY

There is no precise definition of posthysterectomy vaginal vault prolapse (PHVP); however, the International Urogynecological Association (IUGA)/International Continence Society (ICS) joint report on female pelvic floor dysfunction defines it as "descent of...the apex of the vagina (vaginal vault or cuff scar after hysterectomy)". The vaginal cuff scar corresponds to point C on the Pelvic Organ Prolapse Quantification (POP-Q) grid. Prolapse of the vaginal vault after hysterectomy may occur when the structures that support the top of the vagina and uterus are not reattached at the time of the initial procedure or due to weakening of these supports over time **(Fig. 1)**.[1]

Case series dating back to 1960 have identified the incidence of PHVP as ranging from 0.2 to 43%. More recently, PHVP has been reported to follow 11.6% of hysterectomies performed for prolapse and 1.8% for other benign diseases. A large study from Austria estimated the frequency of PHVP requiring surgical repair to be between 6 and 8%.

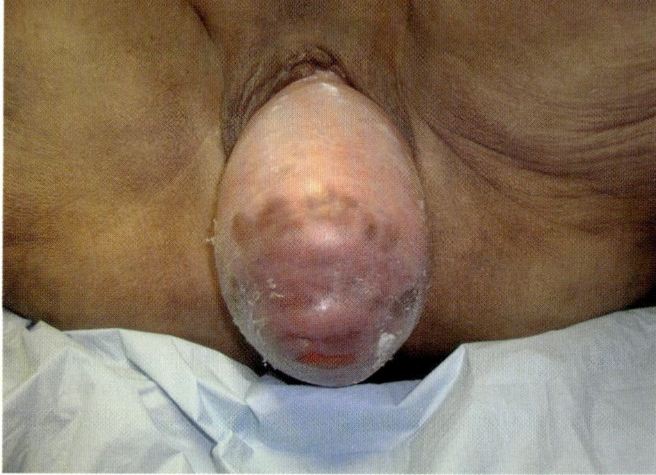

Fig. 1: Vault prolapse—clinical presentation. Keratanization and ulceration of the vault are seen.

DIAGNOSIS AND INVESTIGATION

A number of classification systems for POP are used in both research and clinical settings. Standardized classification systems should be used for the assessment and documentation of pelvic organ prolapse (POP), including vault prolapse as it enables assessment of outcomes for individual woman and facilitates the comparison of results for audit and research purposes.

The ICS POP-Q system is the most comprehensive and widely used.

Routine urodynamic assessment is not recommended in women with PHVP. Performing preoperative urodynamic testing with and without prolapse reduction in continent women undergoing POP surgery does not always predict postoperative stress incontinence. Prophylactic treatment for women thought to have occult stress urinary incontinence (SUI) will result in unnecessary treatment for some women. Clinical assessment remains the most important assessment tool.

In the Colpopexy and Urinary Reduction Efforts (CARE) trial, patients undergoing sacrocolpopexy, who were asymptomatic for SUI, were randomized to undergo either a concomitant Burch colposuspension or no Burch colposuspension (control group). The group demonstrated that the preoperative incidence of urodynamic stress incontinence (USI) increased from 3.7 to 19% following manual prolapse reduction, while using pessaries or speculum reduction for prolapse was associated with detection rates of 6% and 30% respectively. Women who demonstrated preoperative USI were at higher risk of postoperative SUI, even if they underwent a concomitant Burch colposuspension. Preoperative urodynamic testing did not, however, accurately predict USI in all cases, with 38% of women with negative testing in the control group and 21% in the Burch group still developing symptomatic postoperative SUI.

Clinicians should work as part of a pelvic floor multidisciplinary team (MDT). Clinicians involved in the management of patients with PHVP should demonstrate an appropriate level of training and clinical practice. Involvement of other specialties (e.g., coloproctology or urology) or allied health professionals may be useful in the management of PHVP in patients with concomitant bladder/bowel symptoms.

Patient assessment should address quality of life (QoL) issues using standardized tools.

PREVENTION

McCall culdoplasty at the time of vaginal hysterectomy is effective in preventing subsequent PHVP. Suturing the cardinal and uterosacral ligaments to the vaginal cuff at the time of hysterectomy is effective in preventing PHVP following both abdominal and vaginal hysterectomies. Sacrospinous fixation (SSF) at the time of vaginal hysterectomy should be considered when the vault descends to the introitus during closure.

A small RCT compared vaginal Moschcowitz-type operation, McCall culdoplasty and peritoneal closure of the cul-de-sac as preventive measures against the development of enterocele. It showed that McCall culdoplasty was more effective than vaginal Moschcowitz or simple closure of the peritoneum in preventing enterocele at 3 years' follow-up.

McCall culdoplasty involves approximating the uterosacral ligaments using continuous sutures, so as to obliterate the peritoneum of the posterior cul-de-sac as high as possible. A similar approach has been described for abdominal hysterectomy. No comparative studies are available to assess the value of such a step at the time of abdominal hysterectomy, which is often carried out for indications other than prolapse.

Attaching the uterosacral and cardinal ligaments to the vaginal cuff and high circumferential obliteration of the pouch of Douglas have been shown to prevent PHVP and subsequent enterocele formation. Incorporation of the cardinal-uterosacral ligaments into the vaginal cuff margins at the time of total abdominal hysterectomy may help to minimize subsequent apical vault prolapse.

Subtotal hysterectomy is not recommended for the prevention of PHVP. There is no evidence to support the role of subtotal hysterectomy in preventing PHVP.

There is inadequate and conflicting evidence over the use of permanent sutures in the short term and no evidence of benefit in the long term; they can be associated with high suture exposure rates.

CONSERVATIVE MANAGEMENT

Pelvic floor muscle training (PFMT) is an effective treatment option for women with stage I–II vaginal prolapse, including PHVP. No trials looking specifically at the role of PFMT in women with PHVP were identified. A large multicenter RCT [the Pelvic Organ Prolapse Physiotherapy (POPPY) trial] showed that one-to-one PFMT for prolapse is effective for the improvement of prolapse symptoms. This study included, but did not exclusively address, women with PHVP. There is growing evidence, including a small number of RCTs, to indicate that PFMT has a positive effect on prolapse symptoms and severity in women with POP-Q stage I–II vaginal prolapse compared with no treatment. These trials included, but were not specific to, PHVP. Both the National Institute for Health and Care Excellence and the American College of Obstetricians and Gynecologists list PFMT as a treatment option in women with all types of vaginal prolapse.

Vaginal pessaries are an alternative treatment option for women with stage II–IV PHVP. A randomized crossover trial (the PESSRI study) compared two different vaginal pessaries (Gellhorn versus ring) in women with stage II–IV prolapse and showed clinically significant improvements in prolapse symptoms with both types of pessaries, but no significant differences between pessary groups. Pessaries should be considered in all women with POP, including PHVP. Consideration needs to be given to sexual function, regular pessary changes and possible complications such as ulceration, vaginal bleeding and a small risk of fistula formation.

SURGICAL MANAGEMENT

Surgical treatment should be offered to women with symptomatic PHVP after appropriate counseling. The decision to offer surgical treatment for PHVP should primarily be determined by the woman's symptoms, her response to conservative treatment, the impact of PHVP on her QoL and daily activities, and also on her fitness for surgery. The planned procedure should be fully discussed, including success rates, recurrence, potential complications, and the impact of treatment and potential complications on women's QoL and sexual function.

Posthysterectomy vaginal vault prolapse surgery should be performed by a subspecialist urogynecologist, or gynecologists who can demonstrate an equivalent level of training or experience. No studies were identified that evaluated the level of training and/or experience that a surgeon is required to achieve prior to undertaking PHVP surgery, nor the workload per year that is required to maintain skills. A clear referral pathway should be in place to refer the patient to the appropriate surgeon to undertake the required procedure.

Patient-reported outcomes, including patient-reported success rates and relief of presenting symptoms, should be the primary assessment outcomes. Objective cure is important as it correlates to symptoms of vaginal bulge; a POP-Q stage of I or O in the apical compartment seems to be acceptable and widely used as the optimum postoperative result. The primary aims of surgical treatment are the restoration of normal vaginal anatomy, improvement in vaginal bulge symptoms and the restoration/maintenance of normal bladder, bowel and sexual function. Most of the studies in the literature, however, have used the anatomical outcome as the primary outcome, with POP-Q stages I or 0 defined as the anatomical cure. A recent qualitative study based on patient interviews showed that women are most affected by the actual physical symptoms of prolapse (bulge, pain and bowel problems) as well as by the impact that prolapse has on their sexual function. The prevalence of pelvic floor dysfunction symptoms was found to be quite high 6 years after primary POP surgery: urinary leakage (once or more/week, 41%), vaginal bulge (18%), fecal incontinence (15%), and refraining from sexual intercourse (15%). Surgical failure is point C greater than (two-thirds × total vaginal length), i.e., the vaginal apex descending below the upper third of the vagina, or one of points Ba or Bp being greater than 0 cm, i.e., the anterior (Ba) or posterior (Bp) vaginal wall prolapsing beyond the hymen. The outcome reporting scheme proposed by IUGA/ICS is recommended.

The type of operation performed should be tailored to the individual patient's circumstances.

A variety of procedures exist for surgical treatment of PHVP in women who are deemed fit for surgery. There is no robust evidence to guide the clinician as to the best surgical technique for a particular patient. The type of operation performed should be tailored to the individual patient's circumstances, such as concomitant prolapse in other compartment(s), sexual activity, previous abdominal surgery, previous prolapse surgery, the total vaginal length, and associated comorbidities. Women with multiple compartment prolapse and/or a history of extensive abdominal surgery can be quite challenging with the abdominal/laparoscopic approach and a vaginal approach may be appropriate. An abdominal approach would be more appropriate in women with short vaginal length and those undergoing concomitant abdominal surgery. An elderly, sexually inactive woman or a woman unfit for a long surgical operation would be a candidate for colpocleisis.

Women should be aware that both open abdominal sacrocolpopexy (ASC) and vaginal sacrospinous fixation (SSF). Surgical management are effective treatments for primary PHVP. ASC is associated with significantly lower rates of recurrent vault prolapse, dyspareunia, and postoperative stress urinary incontinence (SUI) when compared with SSF. However, this is not reflected in significantly lower reoperation rates or higher patient satisfaction. SSF is associated with earlier recovery compared with ASC. SSF may not be appropriate in women with short vaginal length and should be carefully considered in women with preexisting dyspareunia.

Sacrospinous fixation involves unilateral anchoring of the vaginal vault to the sacrospinous ligament (usually the right side) using either absorbable or non-absorbable sutures and can be done bilaterally **(Figs. 2 and 3)**. Several systematic reviews have shown that SSF is a highly effective therapy for vault prolapse, with low recurrence and complication rates and good patient satisfaction. One concern is the high incidence (8–30%) of postoperative anterior compartment prolapse and SUI, presumably due to posterior fixation of the

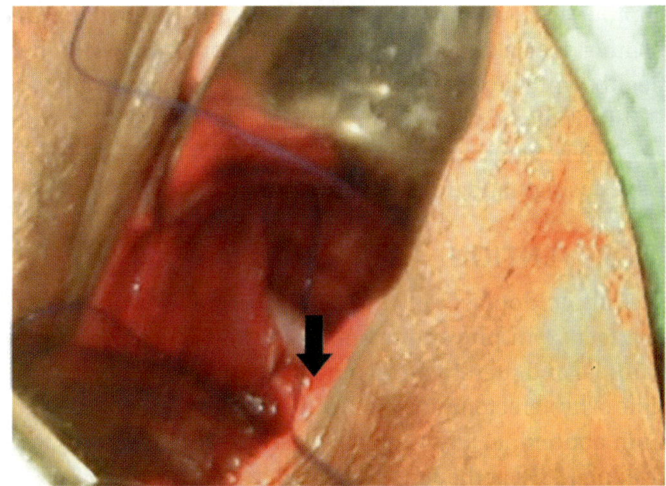

Fig. 2: Sacrospinous fixation. Suture has been passed through the sacrospinous ligament on the right side (black block arrow).

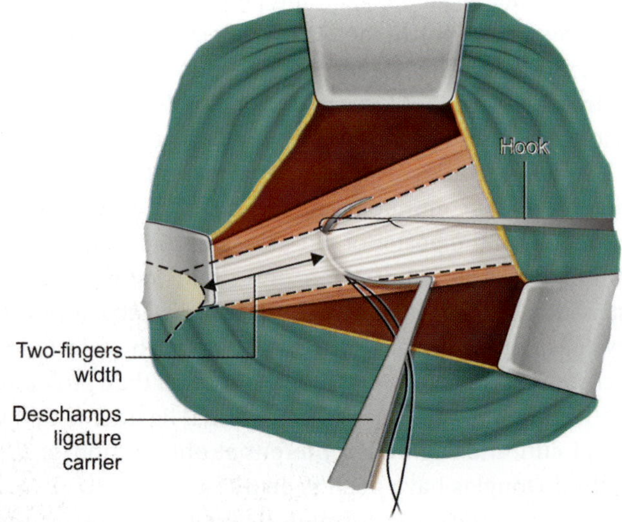

Fig. 3: Sacrospinous fixation—suture placement.

upper vagina which predisposes the anterior compartment to excess intra-abdominal pressure. Postoperative buttock pain has an estimated incidence of 18%, although this usually resolves within 2–3 months and rarely requires any additional treatment apart from analgesics and anti-inflammatory agents. There are case reports of pudendal nerve injury with SSF, primarily owing to the anatomical variations in the course of the pudendal nerve on crossing the ischial spine. However, placing the SSF sutures 1.5–2 cm medial to the ischial spines is recommended. One large study showed temporary irritation of the sciatic nerve in 7.5% and temporary partial ureteral obstruction in 5.5% of 200 women who underwent SSF. There is no evidence that bilateral SSF or using permanent suture material is associated with better success rates. Long-term follow-up studies showed patient-reported prolapse symptoms in 16% of women at 2–15 years' follow-up.

Laparoscopic sacrocolpopexy (LLCS) can be equally effective as ASC in selected women with primary PHVP **(Fig. 4)**. LSC can include mesh extension or be combined with other vaginal procedures to correct other compartment prolapse. There is limited evidence on the effectiveness of robotic sacrocolpopexy (RSC); therefore, it should only be performed in the context of research or prospective audit following local governance procedures.

One prospective single-blinded RCT75 compared the outcomes of LSC (n = 33) versus RSC (n = 35) in patients with stages II–IV PHVP. The primary outcome measure was operative time from incision to closure. Results showed that LSC had a shorter operating time (199 ± 46 minutes versus 265 ± 50 minutes) and less use of postoperative analgesia and that it was significantly less expensive compared with RSC. At 1 year, both groups reported significant and similar improvements in objective assessment and functional outcomes; however, the study was not powered to show significant differences in cure rates.

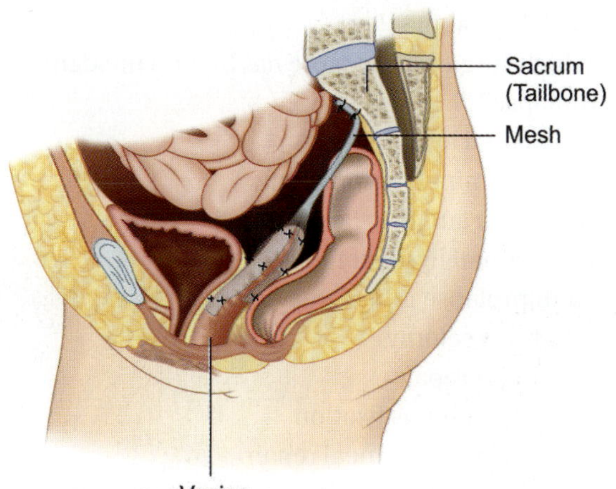

Fig. 4: Abdominal sacrocolpopexy—surgical principle and mesh placement.

High uterosacral ligament suspension (HUSLS) should only be offered as first-line management in women with PHVP within the context of research or prospective audit following local governance procedures. Clinicians should be aware of the risk of ureteric injury, especially in the laparoscopic approach.

High uterosacral ligament suspension can be done vaginally, abdominally or laparoscopically and involves bilateral suspension of the vaginal vault, using sutures, to the uterosacral ligaments near the level of the ischial spine. The evidence regarding the value of HUSLS as first-line management in women with vault prolapse is limited and contradictory.

The limited evidence on transvaginal mesh (TVM) kits does not support their use as first-line treatment of PHVP. If TVM is considered, women should be fully informed of the permanent nature of the mesh and potential mesh complications, some of which are serious and have long-term effects that can be difficult to treat. If TVM is considered, women should be fully informed of alternative surgical and nonsurgical options and referral to other surgeons/units arranged as appropriate. TVM should only be performed by an appropriately trained urogynecologist, after discussion of each individual case in an MDT meeting. The results of all surgical procedures involving mesh should be prospectively audited and submitted to a national surgical database.

Transvaginal mesh has mesh arms that bilaterally anchor the vaginal vault to both sacrospinous ligaments, achieving level I support. These were originally delivered with trocars through anatomical landmarks via the obturator membrane/ischiorectal fossa; however, more recently they have been anchored through single vaginal incisions.

Colpocleisis is a safe and effective procedure that can be considered for frail women and/or women who do not wish to retain sexual function.

Colpocleisis entails closure of the vagina. Different techniques have been described, including vaginectomy, purse-string closure, colpocleisis after performing standard anterior and posterior vaginal wall repair, purse-string closure of enterocele followed by approximation of perivesical and rectovaginal fascia and high levator plication and LeFort colpocleisis, where a bridge of tissue is created between the anterior and posterior vaginal wall to stop the vault prolapse from protruding. Colpocleisis has a short operating time and a low incidence of complications. The procedure can also be performed under local anesthesia, which suits frail women who may be difficult to anesthetize **(Figs. 5A to C)**.

There are no trials that evaluated performing prophylactic mid-urethral sling surgery at the time of SSF or ASC/LSC for occult SUI.

Colposuspension at the time of ASC does not appear to be effective treatment for SUI. Concomitant midurethral sling surgery may be considered when vaginal surgical approaches are used for the treatment of PHVP.

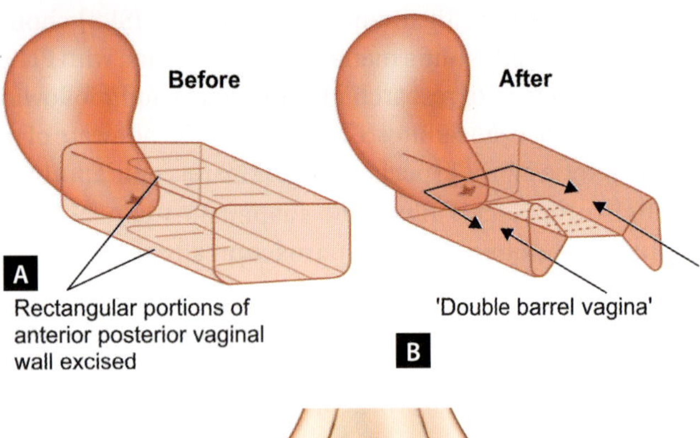

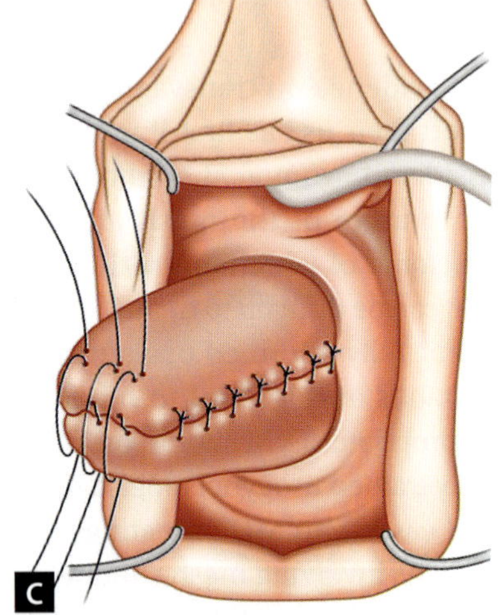

Figs. 5A to C: Colpocleisis—surgical principles.

The management of recurrent vault prolapse should be through a specialist MDT with experience and training in this field.

A number of case series have reported good outcomes after vaginal HUSLS and LSC for recurrent vault prolapse. Evidence in relation to other management options, including PFMT and the use of pessaries, is very limited. Patients should be counseled about the likely benefits and potential risks of each management option. These patients should be assessed by those with expertise in the management of recurrent vaginal vault prolapse, ideally a subspecialist urogynecologist (or those with equivalent experience) working within MDTs.

CLINICAL GOVERNANCE

National databases should be used to document surgical outcomes and complications. Reporting of the complications of surgery for PHVP should describe the nature of the complication in terms of category, time, and site. It should also describe any involvement of adjacent structures, such as the urinary tract or bowel, as well as any systemic effect. The use of a standard method to report the outcome of surgery, including complications, for POP enables comparison for audit and research. Utilizing the schemes proposed by IUGA/ICS facilitates the standardization of terminology and the comparison of results for audit and research purposes.

RECOMMENDATIONS FOR FUTURE RESEARCH

- The role of concomitant continence surgery in patients with PHVP
- The correlation of surgical workload and outcome
- Robotic versus other abdominal and vaginal procedures for the treatment of PHVP
- The use of mesh in the treatment of PHVP.

REFERENCE

1. Royal College of Obstetricians and Gynaecologists. Post-Hysterectomy Vaginal Vault Prolapse Green-top Guideline No. 46 RCOG/BSUG Joint Guideline. London: RCOG; 2015.

LONG QUESTIONS

1. Discuss the surgical anatomy and conservative management of vault prolapsed.
2. What are the curative surgical therapies for vault prolapse? Discuss the possible complications after such repairs.

SHORT QUESTIONS

1. Enumerate the risk factors for posthysterectomy vault prolapsed.
2. What are the anatomical protective features against a vault prolapse?
3. What is colpocleisis? Enumerate its advantages and disadvantages.

MULTIPLE CHOICE QUESTIONS

1. What are risk factors for prolapse?
   a. Chronic cough
   b. Increased abdominal pressure
   c. Obstructive airway disease
   d. All the above
2. Which surgical procedure has highest incidence of vault prolapse?
   a. Vaginal hysterectomy
   b. Abdominal hysterectomy
   c. Both a and b
   d. Subtotal hysterectomy
3. Vault prolapse is best treated with:
   a. Hysterectomy
   b. LeFort repair
   c. Sacrospinous fixation
   d. Abdominoperineal repair
4. Damage to level-1 Delancey support causes:
   a. Cystocele b. Rectocele
   c. Enterocele d. Urethrocele

5. What percentage of women develop vault prolapse after sling operations?
   a. 15% b. 20%
   c. 40% d. 50%
6. Conservative management of vault prolapsed includes:
   a. Pelvic floor exercises b. Pessaries
   c. Both a and b d. None
7. All are vaginal procedures, except:
   a. Sacrospinous fixation
   b. McCall Culdoplasty
   c. Abdominal sacrocolpopexy
   d. None
8. Obliterative vaginal procedures include:
   a. LeFort's partial colpocleisis
   b. Colpectomy
   c. Both a and b
   d. Abdominal sacrocolpopexy
9. Sacrospinous fixation is done at:
   a. Right side b. Left side
   c. Both sides d. None
10. What are the early complications of prolapse surgeries?
    a. Hemorrhage
    b. Injury to adjacent structures
    c. Both a and b
    d. Narrowing of vagina causing dyspareunia

Answers

1.	d	2.	b	3.	c	4.	c	5.	a	6.	c
7.	c	8.	b	9.	c	10.	c				

13.7 ANAL INCONTINENCE

Pranav Mandovra, Roy Patankar

"If one can laugh, sneeze, cough, fart and poop all at the same time, it is not multitasking; it is rather due to anal incontinence."

INTRODUCTION

Anal incontinence is the inability to control bowel movements causing recurrent involuntary unexpected leakage of stools, mucous and flatus from the anus. Anal incontinence encompasses all the types of bowel incontinence, i.e., fecal, mucous and flatus incontinence. Anal incontinence can be either passive or urge or functional. Leakage of stool without being aware of the passage of feces is the passive fecal incontinence (FI). Urge fecal incontinence is the leakage of feces related with defecation urgency. Functional incontinence is the leakage of stools owing to linked problems of cognition or inadequate mobility.[1] Prevalence of FI is estimated to be 8.39%.[2] FI is a distressing condition associated with social stigma and being embarrassing. FI is also a risk factor for skin irritation and inflammation of perianal skin. There is significant negative effect of FI on quality of life of patients.

ETIOPATHOLOGY

To maintain a normal continence is a complex mechanism. It involves collaboration of the sensory function, rectal compliance, anal sphincter function, coordination of the pelvic floor muscles, and consistency of feces. Failure of any of these can cause incontinence. Anatomical structures with their role in defecation and continence are summarized in **Table 1**.[3]

TABLE 1: Anatomical structures and reflexes for maintaining continence.

Structure, reflex, or function	*Contribution toward continence*
Anal canal	Stores feces until an acceptable place for defecation is found
Longitudinal anal muscle	Occludes the anal canal
Internal anal sphincter	Accounts for 50–85% of the resting sphincter pressure
External anal sphincter	Accounts for 25–30% of the resting anal sphincter pressure
Anal vascular cushions	Accounts for 15% of resting anal pressure
Rectoanal inhibitory reflex	Sampling mechanism that allows flatus to be expelled without feces
Rectal distension	Signals the central nervous system that defecation is needed and accommodates accumulation of feces until defecation
Postural reflex	Contraction of the puborectalis when sampling reflex occurs and when finishes defecation
Continence-preserving reflex	Contraction of the levator ani when a sudden urgency to evacuate occurs

Source: Bliss DZ. Management of Fecal Incontinence for the Advanced Practice Nurse. London: Springer; 2018.

Any disturbance one or more mechanisms that maintain continence can lead to FI if the other mechanisms fail to compensate.[4]

The most common factor of FI in a female is prior obstetric trauma. About 10% of normal vaginal deliveries have clinically significant sphincter injury due to the obstetric trauma and around 21–35% of normal deliveries may have occult sphincter damage. Other probable causes pudendal nerve injury during child birth causing pelvic floor denervation, sphincter disruption due to previous anorectal procedure (fistulectomy, fissurectomy with internal sphincterotomy), prolapse of the rectum, neurological conditions (myelomeningocele, Alzheimer's, stroke), personality disorders or a noncompliant rectum (due to prior irradiation causing radiation proctitis or inflammatory bowel disease).[5] Encopresis is condition in which a child avoids to defecate thereby leading to collection of impacted stools in the colon and rectum and lead to leakage.

PATIENT ASSESSMENT

A detailed clinical history helps to find out the cause of FI. Physical examination must include per vaginal examination and abdominal examination with focused physical examination of the perineum. Perineum should be carefully examined to see for any signs of previous perineal injury. Per rectal examination must be carried out to rule out any other condition (such as tumor, fistula, polyp, prolapsed rectum) and the assessment of sphincter anatomy and function, resting muscle tone and squeeze augmentation should be noted during per rectal examination. Patient should be examined in left lateral, lithotomy and squatting position. Proctoscopy can be helpful to note proctitis. Neurological examination of the patient should also be performed to rule out neural cause for FI.

There are several assessment scores to determine the severity of fecal incontinence and quality of life of patients such as Cleveland Clinic Florida Incontinence Score, FI severity index, Fecal incontinence QOL score, etc. Another scoring tool was suggested by Pescatori et al., which included both frequency and degree of symptoms. Incontinence to flatus or mucous was denoted by A, incontinence to liquid stools was denoted by B, and C indicated incontinence solid stool. Indicating the frequency of FI, 1, 2, and 3 was used to determine occasional, weekly, and daily FI. Most severe was C3 that meant daily incontinence for solid stools.[5] But all these scoring systems are cumbersome to use and are rarely used in clinical practice.[6]

Diagnostic Investigations

Laboratory tests for diabetes, thyroid function tests, celiac disease, and colorectal cancer screening test should be done to rule out secondary causes which can attribute to FI. Sigmoidoscopy should be performed to visualize the mucosa and to look for any underlying condition. Anorectal physiology testing is useful in the evaluation of patients with FI. Anorectal manometry is an important aid which helps in the assessment of FI. It measures the sphincter length, distal rectal and anal canal pressures including the resting and maximal (squeeze) anal pressures, rectal compliance and rectoanal inhibitory reflex.[7] Reduced squeeze pressures can be due to injury to external anal sphincter or poor compliance of the patient. Compliance and rectal sensitivity are measured by inflating a balloon with air or saline in the distal rectum. Feedback of the patient regarding the first sensation, first desire to defecate, and the maximum volume tolerated is noted. Rectal hypersensitivity is a can cause urge FI, whereas hyposensitivity may lead to passive or overflow FI.[1] Literature suggests that there are chances of pudendal nerve injury during vaginal child birth. Pudendal neuropathy can also cause FI. Pudendal nerve conduction study can also be done to measure the velocity of nerve conduction.[8]

Magnetic resonance imaging (MRI) of the perineum and/or 3-dimensional endoanal ultrasound assesses the perineal anatomy with precision and gives sufficient details regarding sphincter muscle thickness and site and size of the defect in the sphincter if any due to previous surgery. Endoanal ultrasound is an accurate and useful method for preoperative sphincter mapping.[9] Defecography has limited diagnostic usefulness for the assessment of FI.

MANAGEMENT

Conservative management in the form of medication and lifestyle modification along with biofeedback/physiotherapy should be considered as first-line management before subjecting patients to more aggressive treatment options. Local skin care should be taken and zinc based ointments should be applied to the perianal skin to prevent excoriation.

Diet tolerance may differ as per individual preference. Food containing lactose, caffeine, artificial sweeteners are thought to aggravate the symptoms and should be discontinued.

A Cochrane review for medical management in FI was done which included 16 trials but most of the trials observed FI in the background of diarrhea and had a limited follow-up. They examined the effect of antimotility drugs on FI concluded that the studies focused on treating diarrhea rather than FI.[10]

FIRM trial compared loperamide and psyllium fiber for the treatment of FI and concluded that both improved FI but loperamide was associated with more adverse effects especially constipation.[11] Loperamide is a derivative of opioid. It increases the time taken by food bolus for its transit through the small bowel and proximal large bowel, thereby it promotes water reabsorption. It also reduces secretion in the bowel and henceforth improves the consistency of stools. It also acts by impairing the rectoanal inhibitory reflex and also increases resting pressure inside the anal canal.[12] Codeine acts alike loperamide but has more adverse effects like drowsiness. In addition to oral medications few patients choose to take care of rectal evacuation through transanal irrigation suppositories at a more socially appropriate time.[13] For the management of patients with intractable FI due to neurogenic bowel transanal irrigation is an effective and safe option. Tube cecostomy can be created and antegrade enemas can be administered through it. Antegrade Continence Enema can also be administered using appendix as a conduit as described by Malone et al. For the purpose of colonic irrigation via the abdominal wall, a one way valve mechanism is formed through which catheterization of the appendix can be done for the purpose of administration of antegrade enema.[14]

Use of anal plugs has been mentioned to reduce FI. "Peristeen® Anal Plug" has been designed by Coloplast. It has of a small polyurethane foam plug which is cup-shaped and has a string at one end for easy removal. Upon insertion, the plug fits the contour of the lower rectum and the anal canal thereby plugging it and preventing leakage. Although anal plug is temporary solution it definitely helps in preventing socially awkward situations.[15]

Behavioral Therapies

Pelvic floor physiotherapy and biofeedback may be used along with medical management. The biofeedback equipment provides info on how the pelvic floor muscles are being contracted during the act of defecation. Patients can utilize this data towards learning on how to do the pelvic floor exercises more efficiently. Studies indicate atleast some improvement in 64–89% of patients.[16] There is no standard protocol in the literature regarding the regimen of biofeedback treatment and they vary from 6 to 12 weekly or twice a week sessions.

Another treatment modality in the management of FI is electrical stimulation, although it has lower success rate.[1] To the pelvic floor and sphincters, electrical stimulation can be delivered either by surface electrodes or intrarectal probes. Electrical stimulation aims to improve the strength of sphincter muscle contraction. In case of FI the goal is to strengthen the external sphincter.

When the conservative treatment fails other treatment modalities should be considered. Evaluation should be done to find out the cause of FI and it should be treated. Patients having FI with rectal prolapse should undergo surgery for their prolapse. A step wise algorithm suggested by American Society of Colon and Rectal Surgeons (ASCRS) is mentioned in **Flowchart 1**.[6]

Overlapping Sphincteroplasty

It is the treatment of choice for FI in young females with obstetric sphincter injury. It can also be performed when patient has FI following previous anorectal surgery the defect in external sphincter is less than 120°. Approximately 80% of patients have reasonable function following this surgery in short term,[17] but the efficacy of the repair decreases with time.[18] Patient should be counseled regarding this beforehand. American College of Obstetricians and Gynecologists state that both kinds of repairs, i.e., end to end repair or the overlap repair, are acceptable.[19]

It should be done under anesthesia. Mechanical bowel preparation is preferred and a broad spectrum antibiotic

Flowchart 1: Management of fecal incontinence (FI).

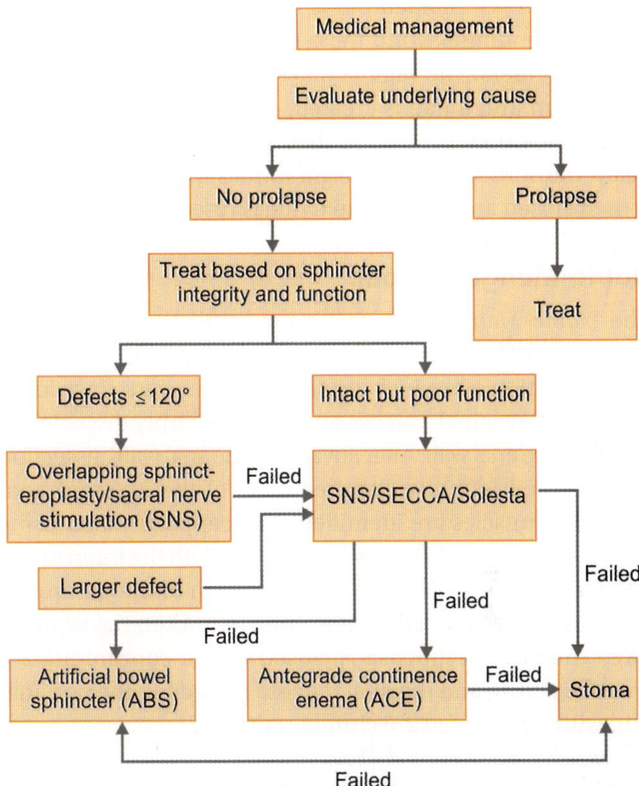

Source: Steele SR, Hull TL, Read TE, Saclarides TJ, Senagore AJ, Whitlow CB. The ASCRS Textbook of Colon and Rectal Surgery. London: Springer; 2016.

coverage is given. Surgery can be done either in jack-knife position or lithotomy position according to surgeons preference and a preoperative perurethral catheterization is advised. Local anesthetic with 1:200,000 adrenaline is infiltrated which helps in better hemostasis.

To separate the vagina from the anus, an incision is made in a curvilinear fashion parallel to the outer edge of the external sphincter. The damaged external anal sphincter and the perineal body scar are meticulously detached from the skin, vagina and anoderm without buttonholing the anoderm or the vagina. The scarred sphincter should be mobilized adequately with the objective of eventually overlapping it anteriorly. Dissection should not be done beyond 180° to prevent injury to pudendal nerves. Sphincter anatomy is clearly defined by separating the external and internal sphincters and subsequently separate repair should be done for them. Following the dissection anterior levatorplasty is performed using absorbable suture. Following this mobilized sphincter is overlapped anteriorly and sutured with strong delayed absorbable suture material using horizontal mattress technique. Wound irrigation is done and skin is loosely approximated with interrupted sutures.

Warren Flap

It is a relatively simple dissection of the thinned septum between the rectum and vagina, to provide additional length and depth while minimizing the risk of infectious sequelae.[20] An inverted "U" shaped cut is made in the mucosa of the vagina extending beyond the retracted ends of the external sphincter fibers. The vaginal mucosa is sharply dissected off the rectum and a flap is created. After identification of the external sphincter muscles, they are reapproximated with delayed absorbable figure of eight sutures. The vaginal mucosa is then closed and excess flap tissue is resected.

Noble-Mengert Repair

The *Noble-Mengert repair* (or anal pull-through repair) provides increased rectovaginal septal length while avoiding contamination of the incision site.[21,22] A transverse incision is made in the vaginal mucosa and then is sharply dissected to mobilize the anal wall. After advancing the anal wall, dissection is continued laterally and free ends of the external anal sphincter muscles are identified and reapproximated using interrupted delayed absorbable sutures. With the interrupted 2-0 delayed-absorbable stitches placation of the pararectal fascia and subvaginal tissues is done to thicken the septum. Then the vaginal mucosa is closed with a continuous 2-0 chromic suture and the anal mucosa sutured to the perianal skin with interrupted 2-0 chromic stitches.

Sphincter Augmentation: Muscle Transposition Repair

Muscle transposition repairs can be used whenever there is a substantial loss of the tissues preventing sphincteroplasty or earlier futile repair. It can be a stimulated or non-stimulated transposition. Graciloplasty is the most common nonstimulated choice. It can also be augmented by implanting an electrical stimulator which augments the contraction of the transferred muscle (dynamic graciloplasty). Whenever there is an extensive sphincter tissue loss or in cases of anorectal congenital malformations, this procedure may be helpful. Owing to variable results and associated high morbidity, dynamic graciloplasty has not gained much acceptance.[23]

Sacral Nerve Stimulation

It can be offered to patients who have structurally normal sphincter but poor function or in patients with failed sphincteroplasty. S3 nerve root nerve impulse is modulated. It is hypothesized that sacral nerve stimulation (SNS) may modify colorectal motility and transport by helping antegrade neuromodulation of the brain.[24] Sacral neuromodulation is performed in two stages. The first phase is a temporary external neurostimulator which is used to modulate S3 nerve root. For around next 1–2 weeks patient is asked to keep a record of bowel movements and episodes of FI and a diary is maintained. If the results of SNS are promising then the second stage of the procedure is done which comprises of placement of the whole system in one setting. Other forms of neromodulation like percutaneous tibila nerve stimulation may also be effective in the treatment of FI,[25] but now only SNS is permitted by FDA for the management of FI. SNS has shown decrease in the incidence and severity of FI in the patients.[26] The downside of this modality is the need for replacement of the neurotransmitter in long term due to loss of battery or lead migration. Also the device is contraindicated for MRIs.

Sphincter Augmentation Procedure

Several augmentation procedures with differing success have emerged as a substitute to sphincter repair. These treatments include radiofrequency energy delivery and injection of some biomaterial. Delivery of radiofrequency energy is contraindicated in patients who had previous biomaterial injection.

Radiofrequency Energy Delivery

Secca® is a special patented anoscope used to deliver the radiofrequency energy.[27] It permits putting of four curved needles made of titanium-nickel containing electrodes at 5 mm distance inside the anal canal. After deploying the electrodes, radiofrequency energy is dispensed to the internal anal sphincter. This treatment leads to hypertrophy of the internal anal sphincter. Increase in the bulk of the muscularis propria layer leads to the thickening of the internal anal sphincter.[28] Literature suggests that this method has uncertain improvements in continence scores both in long term as well as in short term. Although few patients have reported very good response with complete resolution of FI.[27,29] Side effects include pain, infection and rectovaginal fistula.

Biomaterial Injection

Injection of a biomaterial is done between the internal anal sphincter and the mucosa. A non-degrading dextranomer stabilized in hyaluronic acid gel is used. Studies suggest that it reduces the severity of FI. They are more successful in mild FI and in the case of sphincter defect its role still needs to be determined.[30] It is contraindicated in inflammatory bowel diseases, pelvic radiation and rectal prolapse. Other substances such assilicon and collagen have also been tried.

Vaginal Bowel Control System: Eclipse™ System

Eclipse™ system is a unique vaginal bowel control system **(Figs. 1A and B)**. It was made with an aim to give an effective and patient-managed method to prevent inadvertent stool leakage.[31] It comprises of a pressure-regulated user controlled pump and a vaginal insert. The balloon of the insert is inflated and then it is pushed posteriorly which helps to occlude the rectum. By mechanically occluding the rectum, it helps to prevent leakage and patient immediately regains the control.

Sphincter Replacement Methods

Patients with persistent FI despite treatment, having well maintained tissue around their anal canal and without any major medical comorbidity can be offered artificial bowel sphincter system. Patients of inflammatory bowel disease, immunosuppression, prior pelvic irradiation should

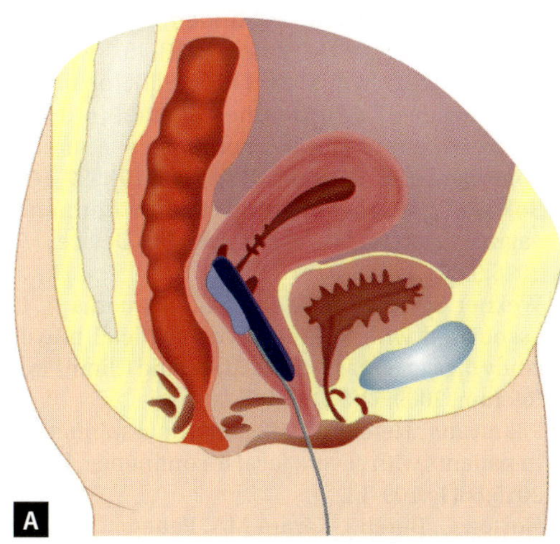

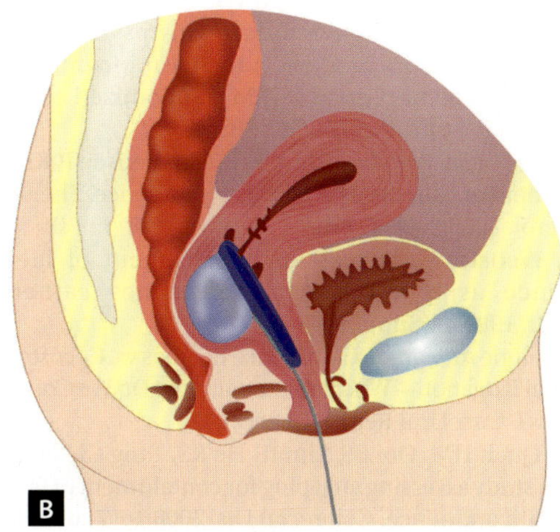

Figs. 1A and B: Eclipse™ system: (A) Insert deflated; (B) Inflated.
Source: Sokol ER. Management of fecal incontinence–focus on a vaginal insert for bowel control. Medical devices (Auckland, NZ). 2016;9:85.

be excluded. Presently there are two artificial bowel sphincter devices, magnetic anal sphincter reinforcement (MAS) and artificial bowel sphincter (ABS). The artificial bowel sphincter comprises of tubing, pump and a silicone cuff. The tubing is fixed along the perineum which is coupled to a pump in the labium or scrotum and an inflatable silicone cuff which is positioned around the upper anal canal. The pump has a button that controls the active deflation and passive reinflation of the silicone cuff. Infection and cuff perforation are the main indications for explanation, with rates of up to 72%.[32]

Magnetic anal sphincter has tiny magnets on a flexible string. It is positioned surrounding the anal sphincter, just below puborectalis. In the usual position of MAS, the magnets direct to the closing of the anal canal thereby preventing stool leakage. During defecation the stool bolus pushes apart the magnets during expulsion. It has reported promising results in continence with reduction in the Wexner Fecal Incontinence Severity Score.[33] Around 15% required device explantation.

Stomas

Creation of a stoma is considered as a last choice for patients with FI who failed all other options. A well created colostomy significantly improves the quality of life for the patient.[34]

KEY MESSAGES

- Anal incontinence is the inability to control bowel movements causing recurrent involuntary unexpected leakage of stools, mucus and flatus from the anus.
- Anal incontinence encompasses all the types of bowel incontinence, i.e., fecal, mucus and flatus incontinence.
- Anal incontinence can be either passive or urge or functional.
- Leakage of stool without being aware of the passage of feces is passive fecal incontinence.
- Urge fecal incontinence is the leakage of feces related with defecation urgency.
- Functional incontinence is the leakage of stools owing to linked problems of cognition or inadequate mobility.
- Fecal incontinence is a distressing condition associated with social stigma.
- Fecal incontinence is also a risk factor for irritation and inflammation of perianal skin.
- There is significant negative effect of fecal incontinence on quality of life of patients.

REFERENCES

1. Bliss DZ, Mimura T, Berghmans B, Bharucha A, Chiarioni G, Emmanuel A, et al. Assessment and conservative management of faecal incontinence and quality of life in adults. In: Abrams P, Cardozo L, Wagg A, Wein A (Eds). Incontinence, 6th edition. Bristol: International Continence Society; 2017. pp. 1993-2085.
2. Ditah I, Devaki P, Luma HN, Ditah C, Njei B, Jaiyeoba C, et al. Prevalence, Trends, and Risk Factors for Fecal Incontinence in United States Adults, 2005-2010. Clin Gastroenterol Hepatol. 2014;12(4):636-43.e2.
3. Bliss DZ. Management of Fecal Incontinence for the Advanced Practice Nurse. London: Springer; 2018.
4. Rao SSC. Diagnosis and management of fecal incontinence. Am J Gastroenterol. 2004;99(8):1585-604.
5. Pescatori M, Anastasio G, Bottini C, Mentasti A. New grading and scoring for anal incontinence. Dis Colon Rectum. 1992;35(5):482-7.
6. Steele SR, Hull TL, Read TE, Saclarides TJ, Senagore AJ, Whitlow CB. The ASCRS Textbook of Colon and Rectal Surgery. London: Springer; 2016.
7. Yamada T, Inadomi J, Bhattacharya R, Dominitz J, Hwang J. Yamada's handbook of gastroenterology, 3rd edition. Hoboken, New Jersey: Wiley; 2013.
8. Brouwer R, Duthie G. Sacral nerve neuromodulation is effective treatment for fecal incontinence in the presence of a sphincter defect, pudendal neuropathy, or previous sphincter repair. Dis Colon Rectum. 2010;53(3):273-8.
9. Meyenberger C, Bertschinger P, Zala GF, Buchmann P. Anal sphincter defects in fecal incontinence: correlation between endosonography and surgery. Endoscopy. 1996;28(02):217-24.
10. Omar MI, Alexander CE. Drug treatment for faecal incontinence in adults. Cochrane Database Syst Rev. 2013;6:CD002116.

11. Markland AD, Burgio KL, Whitehead WE, Richter HE, Wilcox CM, Redden DT, et al. Loperamide versus psyllium fiber for treatment of fecal incontinence: the fecal incontinence prescription (Rx) management (FIRM) randomized clinical trial. Dis Colon Rectum. 2015;58(10):983-93.
12. Duelund-Jakobsen J, Worsoe J, Lundby L, Christensen P, Krogh K. Management of patients with faecal incontinence. Ther Adv Gastroenterol. 2016;9(1):86-97.
13. Walker J, Webster P. Successful management of faecal incontinence using the enema continence catheter. Z Kinderchir. 1989;44(Suppl 1):44-5.
14. Kelly MS. Malone Antegrade Continence Enemas vs. Cecostomy vs. Transanal Irrigation—What Is New and How Do We Counsel Our Patients?. Curr Urol Rep. 2019;20(8):41.
15. Chew MH, Quah HM, Ooi BS, Lim JF, Ho KS, Tang CL, et al. A prospective study assessing anal plug for containment of faecal soilage and incontinence. Colorectal Dis. 2008;10(7):677-80.
16. Lacima G, Pera M, Amador A, Escaramis G, Pique JM. Long-term results of biofeedback treatment for faecal incontinence: a comparative study with untreated controls. Colorectal Dis. 2010;12(8):742-9.
17. Glasgow SC, Lowry AC. Long-term outcomes of anal sphincter repair for fecal incontinence: a systematic review. Dis Colon Rectum. 2012;55(4):482-90.
18. Lamblin G, Bouvier P, Damon H. Long-term outcome after overlapping anterior anal sphincter repair for fecal incontinence. Int J Colorectal Dis. 2014;29(11):1377-83.
19. American College of Obstetricians and Gynecologists Committee on Practice Bulletins. Practice Bulletin No. 165: prevention and management of obstetric lacerations at vaginal delivery. Obstet Gynecol. 2016;128(1):e1-e15.
20. Warren JC. A new method of operation for the relief of rupture of the perineum through the sphincter and rectum. Trans Am Gynecol Soc. 1882;7:324.
21. Noble GH. A new operation for complete laceration of the perineum designed for the purpose of eliminating danger of infection from the rectum. Trans Am Gynecol Soc. 1902;27(357):63.
22. Mengert WF, Fish SA. Anterior Rectal Wall Advancement Technic for repair of complete perineal laceration and rectovaginal fistula. Obstet Gynecol. 1955;5(3):262-7.
23. Chapman AE, Geerdes B, Hewett P, Young J, Eyers T, Kiroff G, et al. Systematic review of dynamic graciloplasty in the treatment of faecal incontinence. Br J Surg. 2002;89(2):138-53.
24. Lundby L, Moller A, Buntzen S. Relief of fecal incontinence by sacral nerve stimulation linked to focal brain activation. Dis Colon Rectum. 2011;54(3):318-23.
25. Shafik A, Ahmed I, El-Sibai O, Mostafa RM. Percutaneous peripheral neuromodulation in the treatment of fecal incontinence. Eur Surg Res. 2003;35(2):103-7.
26. Hull T, Giese C, Wexner SD, Mellgren A, Devroede G, Madoff RD, et al. Long-term durability of sacral nerve stimulation therapy for chronic fecal incontinence. Dis Colon Rectum. 2013;56(2):234-45.
27. Lam TJ, Visscher AP, Meurs-Szojda MM, Felt-Bersma RJ. Clinical response and sustainability of treatment with temperature-controlled radiofrequency energy (Secca) in patients with faecal incontinence: 3 years follow-up. Int J Colorectal Dis. 2014;29(6):755-61.
28. Frascio M, Mandolfino F, Imperatore M, Stabilini C, Fornaro R, Gianetta E, et al. The SECCA procedure for faecal incontinence: a review. Colorectal Dis. 2014;16(3):167-72.
29. Herman RM, Berho M, Murawski M, Nowakowski M, Rys J, Schwarz T, et al. Defining the histopathological changes induced by non-ablative radiofrequency (RF) treatment of faecal incontinence—a blinded assessment in an animal model. Colorectal Dis. 2015;17:433-40.
30. Graf W, Mellgren A, Matzel KE, Hull T, Johansson C, Bernstein M. Efficacy of dextranomer in stabilised hyaluronic acid for treatment of faecal incontinence: a randomised, sham-controlled trial. Lancet. 2011;377(9770):997-1003.
31. Sokol ER. Management of fecal incontinence-focus on a vaginal insert for bowel control. Med Devices (Auckland, NZ). 2016;9:85.
32. Wexner SD, Jin HY, Weiss EG, Nogueras JJ, Li VK. Factors associated with failure of the artificial bowel sphincter: a study of over 50 cases from Cleveland Clinic Florida. Dis Colon Rectum. 2009;52(9):1550-7.
33. Pakravan F, Helmes C. Magnetic anal sphincter augmentation in patients with severe fecal incontinence. Dis Colon Rectum. 2015;58(1):109-14.
34. Norton C, Burch J, Kamm MA. Patients' views of a colostomy for fecal incontinence. Dis Colon Rectum. 2005;48(5):1062-9.

LONG QUESTIONS

1. Explain the management of anal incontinence.
2. Explain the various surgical options available for treatment of anal incontinence?

SHORT QUESTIONS

1. State the causes of anal incontinence?
2. State different investigation for anal incontinence?
3. What are anatomical structures and reflexes for maintaining continence?

MULTIPLE CHOICE QUESTIONS

1. Muscle which is primarily responsible for rectal continence:
   a. External sphincter
   b. Internal sphincter
   c. Puborectalis
   d. Sacrococcygeus
2. Internal sphincter of rectum is formed by:
   a. Levator ani
   b. Puborectalis
   c. Longitudinal muscle fibers condensation
   d. Circular muscle fibers condensation
3. External anal sphincter is innervated by:
   a. S2,S3,S4
   b. S2,S3
   c. L5,S1
   d. L2,L3
4. The following are important in maintainance of normal fecal continence, except:
   a. Anorectal angulation
   b. Rectal inervation
   c. Internal sphincter
   d. Haustral valve
5. Which of the following is not a component of anorectal ring?
   a. External anal sphincter
   b. Puborectalis
   c. Anococcygeal raphe
   d. Internal anal sphincter
6. Not true about the anal canal is:
   a. Completely lined by stratified squamous epithelium
   b. Supplied by pudendal nerve
   c. Drained by veins forming portosystemic anastomosis
   d. Part below pectineal line is supplied by inferior rectal artery

Answers

1. c 2. d 3. a 4. d 5. c 6. a

13.8 FISTULAS IN OBSTETRICS AND GYNAECOLOGY

Manu Sobti

GENITOURINARY FISTULAS

INTRODUCTION

Genitourinary fistulas are severely morbid conditions caused by leakage of urine through the vagina. Occasionally ureterovaginal fistulas can impair renal function as they are often associated with ureteral obstruction. Genitourinary fistulas include vesicovaginal, ureterovaginal, urethrovaginal and uterovesical.

ETIOLOGY

Genitourinary fistulas may be classified into obstetric and surgically induced. Obstetric fistulas are the result of pressure necrosis of the anterior vaginal wall, bladder neck and proximal urethra.[1] Poor perinatal obstetric care and immature motherhood are principal causes in developing countries. Gynecological or surgically induced fistulas are caused by inadvertent suture placement through both vagina and bladder or through the ureter, thermal necrosis due to inappropriate use of cautery, especially during laparoscopic hysterectomy and devascularization of the bladder wall by rough attempts at blunt dissection. Significantly the advent of laparoscopic hysterectomy has been attended by a rise in the incidence of ureterovaginal fistulas, most probably due to the learning curve.

Radiation for pelvic malignancies can result in urinary fistulas several months or even years later. The median interval from the completion of radiation therapy to presentation of the vesicovaginal fistulas is about 8.7 months.

MANAGEMENT

Principles

- Thoroughly evaluate the fistula and the patients' general health.
- Individualize treatment for each patient, planning the timing, approach, and method of surgical repair.

Evaluation

Detailed evaluation of a genitourinary fistula commences with a focused clinical examination and is followed by imaging studies and finally by cystoscopy.

Clinical Examination

A logical sequence would proceed as follows:

- A good pelvic examination with visualization of the vagina. Leakage of methylene blue instilled into the bladder readily confirms the presence of a vesicovaginal fistula.
- Should there be no such leakage, it becomes necessary to ascertain whether the leaking fluid is urine (and not peritoneal fluid, lymphomas or inflammatory exudates), and also whether the leak is from a ureterovaginal fistula. This involves the intravenous injection of indigo carmine or methylene blue or oral administration of phenazopyridine (Pyridium) (the three vaginal swab test).
- An essential part of the clinical examination is to assess the state of the local tissues (slough, foreign body, inflammatory process, infection and residual tumor).
- Accessibility of the fistula from the vaginal route should also be assessed.

Imaging Studies

Every genitourinary fistula needs radiological imaging to determine the following:

- Whether there is ureteric involvement.
- Whether there is abscess formation or unresolved urinoma in the surrounding tissue planes.
- Whether residual malignancy is present in postradiation fistulas.

A spiral CT scan with 3-D reconstruction is now the standard of care. In addition to renal and ureteric anatomy, it can reveal fluid collections, abscesses, and residual tumor. It also offers detailed perspectives of the fistulous track in any desired plane. If CT scan is not available, an intravenous urogram or even only an ultrasonogram may be used to assess the pathology.

Cystoscopy

Cystoscopy is vital. It helps to document the following **(Fig. 1)**:

- The number and size of the vesicovaginal fistulas with their exact location in relation to the ureter and bladder neck.
- The state of the margins of the fistula (slough, suture material, residual tumor, inflammation). A biopsy is

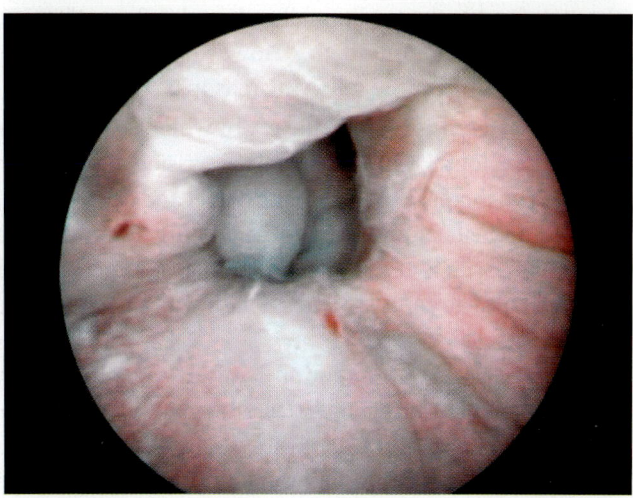

Fig. 1: Vesicovaginal fistula (VVF)—endoscopic view.

mandatory in a post radiation fistula. If ureteric involvement has been revealed on radiological imaging, a retrograde ureterogram and a double J stenting can be attempted. For this reason, imaging studies should precede cystoscopy.

THE PLAN FOR TREATMENT

The approach for repair of genitourinary fistulas has turned progressively in favor of early intervention, moving away from earlier dictum of a compulsory waiting period or allowing the inflammation to subside.

Indications for Conservative Management

- In a recently developed small vesicovaginal fistula, urinary drainage by indwelling catheter, anticholinergics and antibiotics may be tried for up to 3 weeks. The patients' general condition and ability to withstand another surgery also plays a role influencing this discussion in favor of conservative treatment. In general one may expect conservative treatment to succeed no more than (7–12.5%) of the time.
- Established vesicovaginal fistulas with epithelized tracks of a diameter of less than 3 mm may be cured by ablating the epithelial lining (by a metal screw or cautery) and draining the bladder for 2–3 weeks. Fibrin sealant can also be used.
- Ureterovaginal fistulas often heal if a double J stent can be maneuvered across the injured ureteral segment and left indwelling for 8 weeks. An aggressive attempt should be made to pass a double J-stent across the defect, employing ureteroscopy if called for.

Surgical Treatment

Timing of surgical treatment is crucial, and a distinctly different approach is used to schedule surgical repair for vesicovaginal fistulas as compared to ureterovaginal fistulas.

Vesicovaginal Fistulas

Successful repair of vesicovaginal fistulas at an early stage without enforcing the traditionally advised 3–6 months wait is increasingly recommended.[6,7] However, this enthusiasm must be tempered for the following reasons:

- Ischemic necrosis is often the way by which vesicovaginal fistula develops. Early repair involves excision of the slough which can increase the size of the defect and cause further insult to the local tissue microvasculature. Identification of viable tissue is easier and surer when slough has been allowed time to separate and a healthy margin allowed to declare itself.[8]
- A urinary fistula at inception is often complicated by local infection. An infective bacterial load is detrimental to the wound environment directly by bacterial toxins and indirectly by stimulating macrophages to produce collagenase.

A balance must then be struck between the disease for early relief and the need to await optimization of local tissue condition before attempting surgical repair of the fistula. Repeated examination to determine the absence of infection and inflammatory phlegmon will help to optimize the timing of repair.

Patients with multiple failed repairs, associated enteric fistulas or those with pelvic irradiation should wait at least 6–8 months before undergoing repair.[5]

Ureterovaginal Fistulas

Generally are taken up for immediate repair for the following reasons:

- Ureterovaginal fistulas are often associated with ureteral obstruction.
- Almost always it is the distal ureter which is involved and repair involves re implantation of the ureter into a healthy bladder. Procedures like the psoas hitch or Boari flap allow a tension free anastomosis to be made between the bladder and the healthy part of the ureter proximal to the site of the ureterovaginal fistula.

When an extensive or infected urinoma is present or generalized sepsis and anemia would compromise repair, temporizing measures to divert urine from the affected kidney, viz. percutaneous nephrostomy are needed.

Principles of successful fistula surgery:

- Adequate preoperative correction of anemia, nutritional state and infection. Local urinomas and abscesses should have been fully resolved.
- Appropriate surgical approach, vaginal, abdominal or laparoscopic.
- Adherence to certain surgical principles during handling of tissues.

Surgical Approach

Vaginal repair is less traumatic (no cystoscopy and no repeat laparotomy) less expensive (shorter hospital stay) and significantly easier on the patient (less postoperative discomfort).

Clear indications for abdominal repair are:

- Recurrent fistulas and post radiation fistulas which necessarily require the interposition of omentum.
- Vesicovaginal fistula repair where a ureter needs to be re implanted
- Complex uroenteric fistulas
- Severe scarring makes vaginal access difficult
- Shrunken bladders which require augmentation cytoplasty.

Laparoscopic approach offers the advantage of reduced morbidity. Omental interposition and even ureteral reimplantation are well within the reach of a skilled laparoscopic surgeon.[11]

Principles of Tissue Handling Technique

The cardinal principle in surgical repair of any fistula which involves a hollow viscus, is to concentrate on the repair of the viscus. It is the bladder which will bear the brunt of dehisive forces on the line of repair due to its storage function. Hence, a secure double layered closure of the bladder defect is vital. The vaginal defect may even be left open or loosely sutured **(Figs. 2A to E)**.

Some points of basic tissue handling techniques are as follows:

- Wide separation of the plane between bladder and vagina to permit a multilayered and tension free closure of the bladder defect. This will also allow interposition of a viable tissue buttress (omentum or Martius flap).
- Avoid excision of the fistulous track as this will enlarge the tissue defect and may even compromise local vascularity when cautery is used for homeostasis.[3]
  In addition in chronic fistulas, a strong fistulous ring forms outside the epithelized track that maintains some strength through the repair if this layer is incorporated into the closure.[3]
- Use of adjuvant flaps and grafts to allow for the interposition of healthy tissue.
- Uninterrupted and secure postoperative urinary drainage.

PREVENTION OF GENITOURINARY FISTULAS

- Ensure an empty bladder during all gynecological operations by constant catheter drainage.
- Perform sharp dissection along anatomical tissue planes; dissect and develop extra peritoneal spaces.
- Clamp, cut, suture under direct vision while avoiding large tissue pedicles.
- Avoid frantic blind attempts to clamp and ligate bleeding vessels. Sustained application of pressure will almost always control the bleeding to allow accurate identification and control of the bleeding vessel.
- Avoid excessive use of monopolar cautery during laparoscopic surgery.
- When planning to operate difficult cases take care of the following:
  - Position, prepare and drape the patient so as to allow both abdominal and vaginal access.
  - Identify the course of each ureter and safeguard from injury. Preoperative placement of ureteral catheters is neither practical nor desirable as the catheters themselves can cause injury to the ureteral mucosa or impart stiffness to a ureter that may predispose it to a devascularization or a laceration.[10]
  - Intraoperative testing of the integrity of the urinary track should be ready resorted to, so that primary repair may be immediately undertaken. This can easily be done by the instillation of methylene blue into the bladder or into the ureter.[10] Intraoperative cystoscopy or cystotomy should be practised without hesitation.

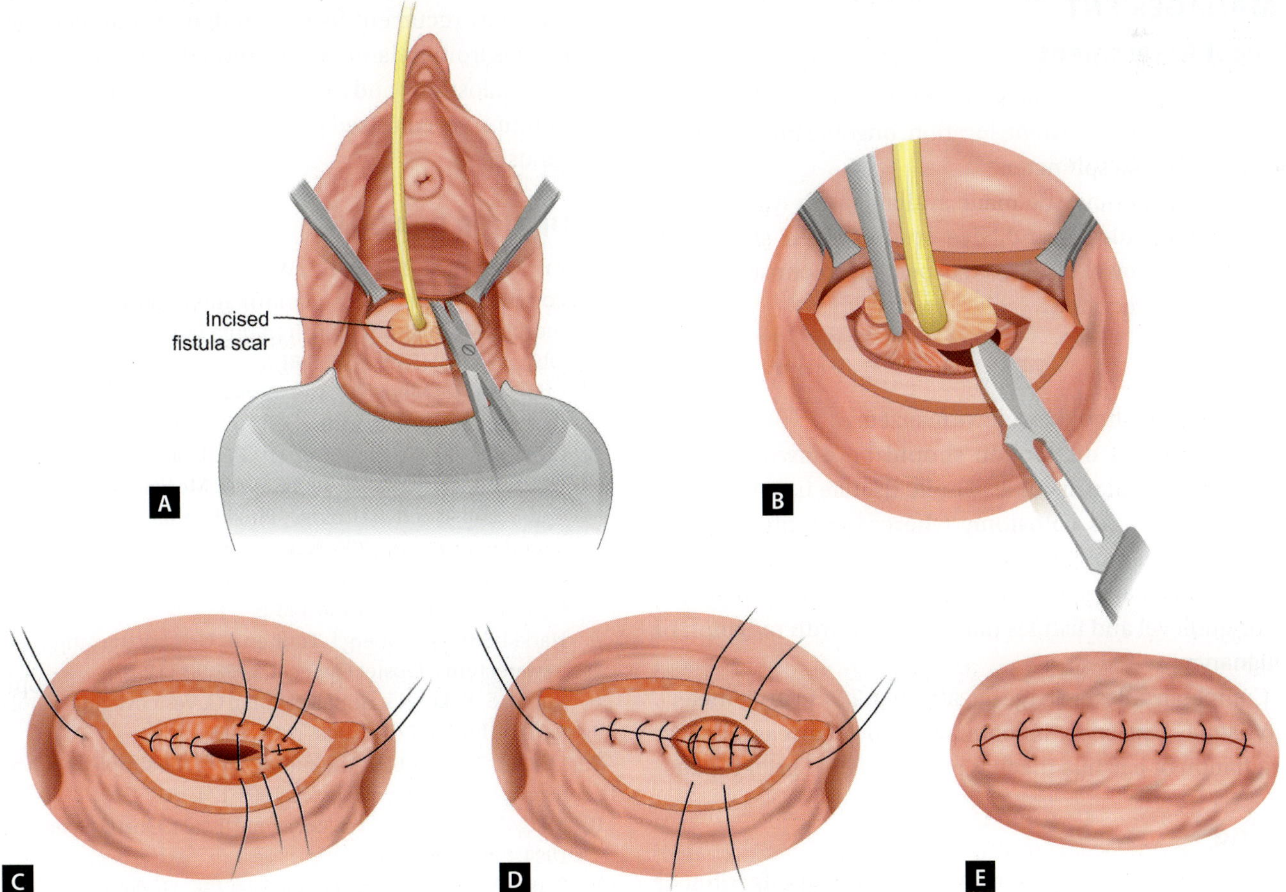

Figs. 2A to E: Vesicovaginal fistula repair—surgical principles.

RECTOVAGINAL FISTULAS

INTRODUCTION

A rectovaginal fistula is an epithelium lined track between the vagina and the rectum.

ETIOLOGY

Trauma (obstetric, operative, trauma), infection, inflammatory bowel disease, carcinoma, and radiation.

The most common cause remains obstetric trauma; usually associated with a laceration or episiotomy during delivery which has developed an infection or has been inadequately repaired.

Surgical trauma during anorectal or vaginal operations.

Perianal infections such as perianal abscess or Bartholin gland abscess, diverticulitis, tuberculosis can lead to rectovaginal fistulae. Ulcerative colitis and more commonly Crohn's disease can both result in rectovaginal fistula.

Carcinoma (commonly rectal, cervical and vaginal)—tissue and vascular damage resulting from radiation therapy is another common cause (0.5–0.6%). The incidence of these fistulas is dose related and usually occurs within 2 years of treatment. Biopsy of the fistula is imperative to look for recurrence of the original malignancy.

MANAGEMENT

Clinical Assessment

Thorough history and physical examination to determine causative factors and extent, location, ongoing inflammation and state of rectal sphincter.

Further detail may be made available with transvaginal or endorectal ultrasound, dye studies, MRI studies. If inflammatory bowel disease is suspected, colonoscopy with biopsy may be required.

Repair

Treatment plan should be individualized.

An important distinction should be drawn between simple and complex fistulae. Simple fistulae usually do not require a proximal colostomy whereas complex fistulae require diversion of fecal stream by a proximal colostomy. Simple fistulas are small (less than 2.5 cm in diameter), a low or midlevel and fistulas not associated with radiation or malignancy.

Complex fistulas are large (greater than 2.5 cm in diameter), high fistulas caused by inflammatory bowel disease, cancer or radiation or a fistula that has multiple failed prior repairs.

Timing

It is essential to wait for resolution of any infection or inflammation of the surrounding tissue before attempting a repair. Usually 12–14 weeks may be needed. An added advantage is spontaneous closure of anal fistulae during this period.

If the patient is planning more children, one need not wait till completion of child bearing, as C-section may be electively performed.

Principles of surgical repair:
- Full bowel preparation to reduce fecal load and bacterial content.
- Excision of the epithelium lined fistulous communication.
- Interposition of well vascularized tissue between the rectum and vagina.

The basic principle of repair on the high pressure side namely the rectum should be adhered to. The vaginal side may be left open for drainage.

There are four major approaches for repairing a simple rectovaginal fistula:
1. Transvaginal
2. Conversion of the fistula into a complete perineal laceration with subsequent repair
3. Transperineal
4. Transanal

In small fistulas, closure may be attempted by fibrin glue.

Complex Fistulas

High fistulas, recurrent fistulas, radiation induced fistulas and fistulas from inflammatory bowel disease may require a proximal colostomy and interposition of vascular grafts such as omentum, vascularized patch of sigmoid colon, gracilis or other muscles.

FURTHER READING

1. Arrowsmith S, Hamlin EC, Wall LL. Obstructed labour injury complex: Obstetric Fistula formation and the multifaceted morbidity of maternal birth trauma in the developing world. Obstet Gynecol Surv. 1996;51:568-74.
2. Cooke SA, De Moor NG. The surgical treatment of the radiation damaged rectum. Br J Surg. 1981;68:488-92.
3. Ganabathi K, Sirls L, Zimmern PE, Leach GE. Vesicovaginal fistulas. Reconstructive Techniques. McAninch JW. Traumatic and Reconstructive Urology. Philadelphia, Pennsylvania: WB Saunders; 1996. pp. 295-325.
4. Greenwald JC, Hoexter B. Repair of rectovaginal fistulas. Surg Gynecol Obstet. 1978;146:443-5.
5. Harkki-Siren P, Sjoberg I, Tutinen A. Urinary tract injuries after hysterectomy. Obstet Gynecol. 1998;92:112-8.
6. Kumar S, Kekre NS, Gopalkrishnan G. Vesicovaginal fistula. An update. Indian J Urol. 2007;23:187-91.
7. Lescher TC, Pratt JH. Vaginal repair of the simple rectovaginal fistula. Surg Gynecol Obstet. 1967;124:1317-21.
8. Margolis T, Mercer I. Vesicovaginal fistula. Obstet Gynecol Surv. 1994;49:840-7.
9. Persky I, Heman Ackah CV, Gelister JSK. Ureteroscopic Salvage of a Ureterovaginal fistula. Br J Urol. 1997;13:273.

10. Radcliffe AC, Ritchie JK, Jawley PR, Lennard-Jones JE, Northover JM. Anovaginal and Rectovaginal fistulas in Crohn's disease. Dis Colon Rectum. 1988;31:94-9.
11. Ramalingam K, Senthil V, Vekatesh V. Laparoscopic repair of Ureterovaginal fistula. Successful outcome by laparoscopic ureteral implantation. J Endourol. 2005;19(10):1174-6.
12. Reddy CJ, Heman Ackah CV, Gelister JSK. Ureteroscopic salvage of a Ureterovagial fistula. Br J Urol.1997;80:817-8.
13. Rovner ES. Urinary Tract fistula. In: Wein AJ, Kavoussi LR, Novick AC, Partin AW, Peters CA (Eds). Campbell Walsh Urology, 9th edition. Philadelphia: WB Saunders; 2007. pp. 2322-60.
14. Vasavda S, Rayman Rackley E. Urinary incontinence. Medicine specialities. Updated: Jul 12, 2021. https://emedicine.medscape.com/article/452289-overview.
15. Venkatesh KS, Ramanujam P. Fibrin glue application in the treatment of recurrent anorectal fistulas. Dis Colon Rectum. 1999;42(9):1136-44.
16. Wang Y, Hadley G, Gurrier K. Nondelay in Vesicovaginal Fistula Repair of high lying vesicovaginal fistula. J Urol. 1990;144:34.

LONG QUESTIONS

Genitourinary Fistulas

1. Discuss the etiology and pathophysiology of genitourinary fistulae.
2. Enumerate and discuss principles for successful repair of vesicovaginal fistula.
3. How will you evaluate a patient with persistent watery vaginal discharge after abdominal hysterectomy?
4. Discuss the advantages and disadvantages of various operative approaches for the repair of vesicovaginal fistula.
5. Discuss the management of a case in which trauma to a ureter is suspected 2 days after hysterectomy.

Rectovaginal Fistulas

6. Discuss etiology of rectovaginal fistulas associated with practice of obstetrics and gynecology.
7. Discuss the planning, surgical technique, and post-operative care for a woman who has a rectovaginal fistula after a difficult forceps delivery.

SHORT QUESTIONS

Geniturenary Fistulas

1. What are the surgical steps that can lead to genitourinary fistulae?
2. What is the role of imaging and cystoscopy in evaluating genitourinary fistulae?

Rectovaginal Fistulas

3. Describe preoperative evaluation of a patient with rectovaginal fistula.
4. Describe the surgical management of rectovaginal fistula.
5. Classify rectovaginal fistulae and discuss principles of their management.

MULTIPLE CHOICE QUESTIONS

Genitourinary Fistulas

1. Early repair of vesicovaginal fistula should be avoided in:
   a. Obstetric fistulas b. Large fistulas
   c. Ureterovaginal fistulas d. Postradiation fistulas
2. The following tissues can be used for interposition in repair of vesicovaginal fistulas:
   a. Omentum
   b. Peritoneum
   c. Pad of fat from Labium Majus
   d. All of the above
3. Conservative management of vesicovaginal fistulas does not include:
   a. Suprapubic cystostomy b. Anticholinergics
   c. Steroids d. Diapers
4. Recommended measures for prevention of genitourinary fistulae are all, except:
   a. Indwelling catheter drainage during surgery
   b. Abdominoperineal access for difficult cases
   c. Sharp dissection of tissue planes
   d. Preoperative placement of ureteric catheters.
5. Laparoscopic repair of vesicovaginal fistulas is not recommended when:
   a. Fistula is large
   b. Ureteral re-implantation is needed
   c. Omental interposition is needed
   d. Bowel involvement has occurred

Rectovaginal Fistulas

6. A complex rectovaginal fistula is classified as such by:
   a. Obstetric trauma
   b. Operative trauma
   c. Involvement of rectal sphincter
   d. Presence of inflammatory bowel disease
7. Proximal diversion of fecal stream by a colostomy is usually not indicated when cause of fistula is:
   a. Radiation induced
   b. Associated with inflammatory bowel disease
   c. Associated with malignancy
   d. Obstetric trauma
8. In the surgical repair of rectovaginal fistulae the nonessential procedure is:
   a. Thorough mobilization of rectum from vagina
   b. Secure closure of rectum in two layers
   c. Stretching of anal sphincter
   d. Secure closure of vagina

Answers

1. d 2. d 3. b 4. d 5. d 6. d
7. d 8. d

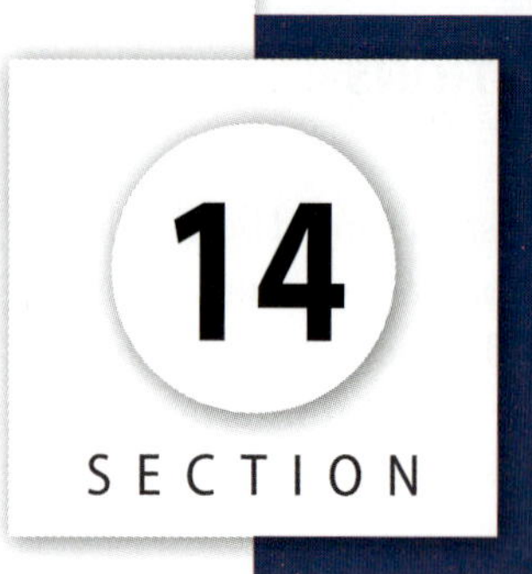

SECTION 14: Gynaecological Oncology

14.1 NEOPLASTIC DISEASES OF VULVA

Niranjan Chavan, Dinesh Wade, Prathamesh Kane, Richa Deshmukh

VULVAR ATYPIA: INTRAEPITHELIAL NEOPLASIA

Lichen Sclerosus

Characteristics

- A change in the vulvar skin that often appears whitish **(Fig. 1)**.
- Microscopically the epithelium becomes markedly thinned with a loss or blunting of the rete ridges.
- There is also a thickening or hyperkeratosis of the surface layers.
- Inflammation is usually present.
- Irritation or itching is common symptom.
- Whitish discoloration is due to a thickened keratin layer.
- Vulvar skin often appears thin, and there may be scarring and contracture. Fissuring of the skin is often present, accompanied by excoriation secondary to itching.

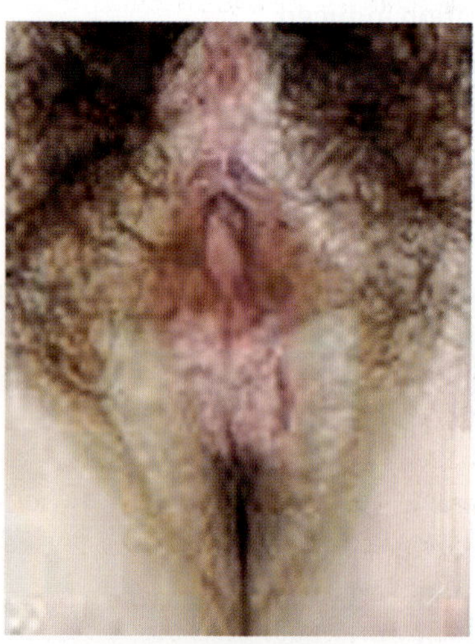

Fig. 1: Lichen sclerosus.

Management of Lichen Sclerosus

- Relief of itching is often the main concern of the patient.
- Representative vulval biopsy is recommended prior to starting treatment as it is important to rule out any underlying invasive or preinvasive malignancy.
- Topical potent steroid is usually given as first line treatment. Clobetasol or halobetasol propionate 0.05% is used for topical application. It is advised to apply it carefully only on the affected areas and the patient is also taught to do the same using mirrors. The duration of treatment may be over weeks depending on response. Patients may also require maintenance therapy to prevent relapses.
- Topical testosterone was used in the past. However, due to androgenic side effects (clitoral hypertrophy, increased hair growth), it is not a preferred treatment now. Effective preparation is 2% testosterone propionate in petrolatum, which is used twice daily for 6–8 weeks followed by twice weekly maintenance.
- Although lichen sclerosus can be associated with the development of squamous cell carcinoma in less than 5% of cases, some believe that use of a potent steroid cream has a protective effect from malignant transformation. It is advisable to keep these patients under close surveillance so that any malignant change should be identified at the earliest.
- Local measures to diminish irritation such as use of cotton underclothes, avoidance of strong soap/detergents, and avoidance of synthetic undergarments are advised.

Carcinoma In Situ (Vulvar Intraepithelial Neoplasia)

- Diagnosed if a part of thickness of vulvar epithelium has dysplasia.

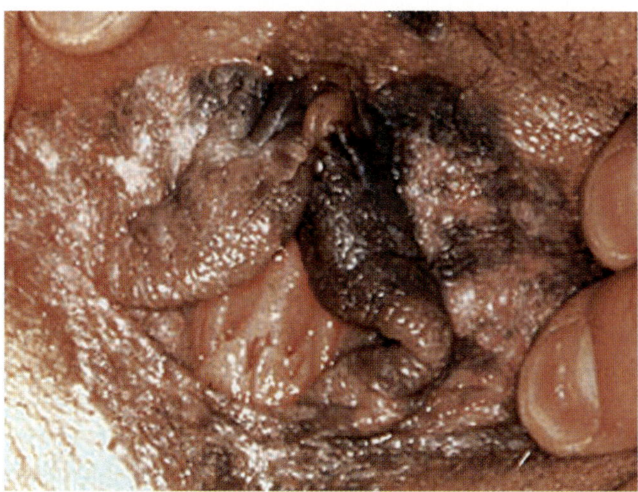

Fig. 2: High grade vulvar intraepithelial neoplasia (VIN).

- Occasionally, the process may histologically resemble carcinoma in situ of the cervix, and in many lesions, there are multinucleated cells, abnormal mitoses, an increased density in cells, and an increase in the nuclear-to-cytoplasmic ratio.

Earlier vulvar intraepithelial neoplasia (VIN) was classified as follows based on the degree of histological abnormality:

- *VIN1:* Abnormal cellular changes confined to lower one-third of epithelium
- *VIN2:* Lower one-third to two-thirds epithelium involved
- *VIN3:* Full thickness of the epithelium involved

The current classification of VIN was given by ISSVD in 2015. This terminology is similar to the lower anogenital squamous terminology (LAST) classification and it incorporates the pathogenesis of VIN:

- *Low-grade vulvar lesions,* referred to as vulvar low-grade squamous intraepithelial lesions (vL-SIL).

  These are benign lesions (flat condyloma or HPV effect) associated with low-risk HPV infection.
- *High-grade vulvar lesions,* further classified into:
  - *High-grade squamous intraepithelial lesion of the vulva* ***(Fig. 2)***: VIN usual type (uVIN), are associated with high-risk HPV infection, and can progress to invasive vulvar cancer.
  - Differentiated VIN lesions (dVIN), develop in chronic skin lesions (like lichen sclerosus), and have a potential for malignant transformation.

Management of Vulvar Intraepithelial Neoplasia (Box 1)

Although VIN is often diagnosed in younger women, the risk of progression to invasive cancer is higher in older women and in those who are immunosuppressed, such as transplant recipients or HIV positive patients. HPV types 6 and 11 are most frequently found in benign vulvar warts, whereas high risk HPV types 16, 18, 31, 33, and 35 are more frequently associated with intraepithelial neoplasia or invasive carcinoma. Surgical removal has been effectively used, but the type of procedure has changed in recent years.

BOX 1: Management of vulvar intraepithelial neoplasia (VIN).

- *Excisional:*
  - Wide Local Excision
  - Simple vulvectomy
  - Skinning vulvectomy
  - Laser excision
- *Ablative:*
  - CO_2 laser ablation
  - Cavitational ultrasonic surgical ablation
- *Topical application:*
  - 5-Flurouracil cream
  - Imiquimod cream

- *Wide local excision* is the preferred initial management for localized unifocal lesion.
- *Skinning vulvectomy* is mainly useful in confluent multifocal lesions. This removes the superficial vulvar skin, preserving the clitoris, and replaces the removed skin with a split-thickness vulvar graft.
- *Simple vulvectomy* was widely practiced to treat carcinoma in situ of the vulva, but this disfiguring operation is now infrequently used, particularly because the disease is occurring in younger women.
- *Carbon dioxide laser* can be used for excisional treatment or ablative treatment. The ablative therapy has been used to treat VIN, usually to a depth of 1–3 mm, with deeper depth being used for areas that contain hair. This results in eradication of the abnormal vulvar tissue and healing without scarring. It is particularly useful for younger patients. The advantage of excisional therapy includes the retrieval of specimen for histological examination. Hence, it is essential to be certain that the patient does not have invasive disease before using laser for ablative procedure.
- *Cavitational ultrasonic surgical aspiration (CUSA)* is the newer modality of the treatment available for these lesions.
- *5-Fluorouracil (5-FU)* cream has been tried to treat VIN, but it causes severe burning and irritation of skin and is generally not used. Median time to response is 7–8 weeks.
- *Imiquimod,* an immune response modulator, is an effective new therapy for management of VIN. 5% imiquimod is used three times a week over the affected area for 12–20 weeks. Erythema and vulval pain are common side effects of this treatment.

Paget's Disease

A rare intraepithelial disorder that occurs in the vulvar skin and histologically resembles Paget's disease in the breast. Generally seen in postmenopausal women and typically appears grossly as a diffuse erythematous eczematoid lesion **(Fig. 3)** that has usually been present for a long time. Itching is common presenting symptom.

- Paget cells are large pale cells. The cells often occur in nests and infiltrate upward through the epithelium. Frequently

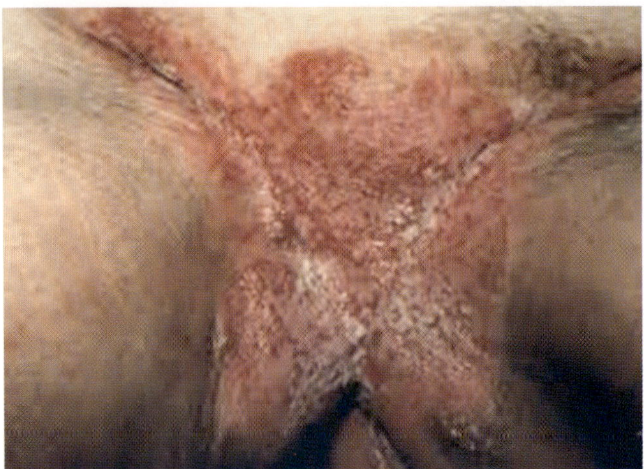

Fig. 3: Paget's disease of vulva.

histologic abnormalities of the apocrine glands of the skin may be noted in these lesions.

- Paget's disease often has a reddish, eczematoid appearance. It should be reemphasized that this condition cannot be accurately diagnosed from clinical appearance, and biopsy is needed.
- There is an increased association of Paget's disease of the vulva with underlying invasive adenocarcinoma of the vulva, vagina, and anus as well as distant sites including the bladder, cervix, colon, stomach, and breast.
- Paget's disease of the vulva tends to spread, often in an occult fashion, and recurrences are frequent after treatment. The disease is primarily seen in whites, and the average age of the patient is approximately 65 years.
- Paget's disease of the vulva can be classified as follows (Wilkinson and Brown classification):
    - Type I Paget's disease of primary cutaneous origin which is further divided into:
        - Type Ia: intraepithelial Paget's disease
        - Intraepithelial Paget's disease with stromal invasion
        - As a manifestation of underlying adenocarcinoma of skin appendage or subcutaneous vulvar gland.
    - Type II Paget's disease includes lesions of non-cutaneous origin such as adenocarcinoma of rectum, bladder or upper genital tract.

Management of Paget's Disease of the Vulva

- Once a diagnosis of Paget's disease of the vulva is made, it is important to rule out the presence of primary Paget's disease of breast and gastrointestinal or genitourinary.
- If no local or distant primary malignancy is uncovered, a wide excision of the affected area can be performed.
- It is important to remove the full thickness of the skin to the subcutaneous fat to be certain that all the skin adnexal structures are excised, as they may have a subclinical malignancy.
- Even if resection margins are free of Paget's disease at the time of surgical excision, local recurrence remains a risk.
- Women who have been diagnosed with Paget's disease of the vulva should have as part of their routine workup, mammography of the breast, cytological evaluation of the cervix and vulva, and screening for genitourinary disease and gastrointestinal disease.

CONCLUSION

Various types of vulval lesions may encountered in various age groups of women. These could range from premalignant conditions like lichen sclerosus to VIN, i.e., high grade and low grade intraepithelial lesions (HSIL and LSIL) which are HPV associated. These lesions are managed depending upon the histopathological diagnosis and nature and extent of the disease with appropriate topical and surgical treatment options and each case has to be individaulized.

KEY MESSAGES

- Lichen sclerosus is a premalignant condition. The lesions tend to be clitoral in location and are seen in patients older than age 40 years.
- Ultrapotent corticosteroid cream is the most commonly used treatment for lichen sclerosus. Although, indiscriminate and unsupervised usage can lead to complications such as dermal thinning.
- Topical testosterone is often beneficial to treat lichen sclerosus but can lead to masculinizing side effects, hence not commonly used now.
- VIN is classified into high grade and low grade intraepithelial lesions (HSIL and LSIL) which are HPV associated and dVIN which is not associated with HPV.
- HPV-positive tumors tend to occur in younger patients, and these tumors have a better prognosis than HPV-negative tumors.
- Intraepithelial neoplasia of the vulva is usually treated by local excision. Laser therapy of the atypical area may be used in younger patients.
- Paget's disease generally occurs in postmenopausal women and is usually treated by wide excision. Invasive carcinomas at other sites should be ruled out.

REFERENCES

1. Iyengar S, Acheson N. Premalignant vulval conditions. Obstet Gynaecol Reprod Med. 2008;18(3):60-3.
2. Olsson A, Selva-Nayagam P, Oehler MK. Postmenopausal vulval disease. Menopause Int. 2008;14(4):169-72.
3. Bowen AR, Vester A, Marsden L, Florell SR, Sharp H, Summers P. The role of vulvar skin biopsy in the evaluation of chronic vulvar pain. Am J Obstet Gynecol. 2008;199:467.
4. Kelekci KH, Adamhasan F, Gencdal S, Sayar H, Kelekci S. The impact of the late classification system of benign vulvar diseases on the management of women with chronic vulvar pruritus. Indian J Dermatol Venereol Leprol. 2011;77:294-9.
5. Tyring SK. Vulvar squamous cell carcinoma: guidelines for early diagnosis and treatment. Am J Obstet Gynecol. 2003;189:S17-S23.

LONG QUESTIONS

1. Explain types of neoplastic diseases of vulva, clinical features, diagnosis and management of Paget's disease.
2. Classify VIN, describe clinical features, diagnosis and management of VIN.

SHORT QUESTIONS

1. What is VIN?
2. Write in brief about Lichen sclerosis of vulva.
3. Describe Paget's diseases of vulva.
4. Describe the diagnostic method for neoplastic diseases of vulva.
5. Describe the newer treatment modalities for VIN.

MULTIPLE CHOICE QUESTIONS

1. Lichen sclerosus of vulva is:
   a. A type of skin reaction b. Premalignant condition
   c. Metastasis d. None of the above
2. Paget's disease of vulva is seen in age group of:
   a. 25–35 years b. 35–45 years
   d. 45–55 years d. >65 years
3. All are treatment modalities for VIN, except:
   a. Radiotherapy b. Simple vulvectomy
   d. Skinning vulvectomy d. CO_2 laser
4. Most common HPV associated with VIN is:
   a. HPV 16 b. HPV 18 c. HPV 31 d. HPV 45
5. All of following are neoplastic diseases of vulva, except:
   a. Lichen sclerosis b. Intraepithelial neoplasia
   c. Paget's disease d. Lichen planus
6. There is increased association of Paget's disease of vulva with:
   a. Adenocarcinoma of vulva
   b. Adenocarcinoma of cervix
   d. Adenocarcinoma of anus
   d. All of these
7. CO_2 laser ablation has been used to treat lesions up to the depth of:
   a. 7–8 mm b. 5–6 mm
   c. 2–3 mm d. 1.0 cm
8. Which of the following is not a diagnostic modality of neoplastic diseases of vulva?
   a. Cytological smear
   b. FNAC
   c. Biopsy of vulva using keys dermal punch
   d. Colposcopy
9. Blunting of rete ridges and hyperkeratosis of surface layer is seen in:
   a. Paget's disease b. Lichen sclerosis
   c. Lichen planus d. VIN
10. Neoplastic disease of vulva can present as all of the following, except:
    a. Vulval itching
    b. Whitish change in the vulval skin
    d. Fissuring and excoriation of vulva
    d. Vaginal discharge

Answers

1.	b	2.	d	3.	a	4.	a	5.	d	6.	d
7.	c	8.	b	9.	b	10.	d				

14.2 VULVAL CARCINOMA

SP Somashekhar

INTRODUCTION

Vulvar cancer is the fourth most common gynecologic cancer accounting for 5% of all gynecological cancers.[1] Approximately, 27,000 cases have been reported annually and 58% of cases are from developed countries. The incidence of vulvar cancer is highest in North America, South America, and Europe. The incidence rates are between 1 and 1.5 per 100,000. Vulvar cancer is rare in developing countries, including Asia.[2] In India vulvar cancer accounts for 1–3% of gynecological cancers.[3] The incidence as per cancer registry in India is given in **Table 1**.

Vulvar carcinoma is encountered most frequently in postmenopausal women. Vulvar carcinoma encompasses any malignancy that arises in the skin, glands, or underlying stroma of the perineum, including the mons, labia minora, labia majora, Bartholin glands, or clitoris. Metastatic tumors have also been described but occur relatively infrequently. The mean age at diagnosis is 65 years. Cigarette smoking, vulvar dystrophy, vulvar or cervical intraepithelial neoplasia, human papillomavirus (HPV) infection, immunodeficiency syndromes, a prior history of cervical cancer, and northern European ancestry are some of the risk factors for vulvar cancer.[4]

- 4th most common gynecological cancer
- 5% of malignancies of female genital tract in India
- Disease of 6–7th decade
- Incidence of VIN increasing

Epidemiology
- Cigarette smoking
- Vulvar dystrophy
- VIN or CIN
- HPV infection subtypes 16, 18, 31, 33
- Immunodeficiency syndromes
- Prior history of cervical cancer
- Northern European ancestory

TABLE 1: Incidence of vulvar cancer by cancer registry in India.

Cancer registry	*Period*	*N cases**	*Crude rate†*	*ASR†*
Chennai	1998–2002	53	0.5	0.6
Karunagappally	1998–2002	1	0.1	0.1
Mumbai	1998–2002	65	0.2	0.3
Nagpur	1998–2002	28	0.6	0.7
New Delhi	1998–2002	82	0.3	0.5
Poona	1998–2002	80	0.1	0.1
Trivandrum	1998–2002	10	0.3	0.3

Standardized rates have been estimated using the direct method and the World population as the reference.
*Accumulated number of cases during the period.
†Rates per 100,000 women per year.
Data sources: IARC, Cancer Incidence in 5 Continents, Vol IX.
(ASR: age-standardized rate)

At present two pathways of vulvar carcinogenesis exist. The first is related to mucosal HPV infection and the second to chronic inflammatory (vulvar dystrophy) or autoimmune processes.[5] HPV has been shown to be responsible for 60% of vulvar cancers (predominantly HPV 16 and 33).[6] The fall in the mean age at diagnosis may be due to increasing incidence of HPV-related vulvar intraepithelial neoplasia (VIN). HPV DNA is found more commonly in vulvar cancers of young women who smoke as compared to older nonsmokers.[6] Early detection and treatment of VIN prevents development of cancer.

CLINICAL FEATURES AND DIAGNOSIS

Pruritus is the most common symptom especially if associated with vulvar dystrophy. Most patients present with unifocal vulvar plaque, ulcer, or mass on the labia majora (**Figs. 1 and 2**). The involvement of labia minora, perineum, clitoris, and mons is considerably less.

Presentation
- Unifocal vulvar plaque, ulcer or mass on labia majora
- Multifocal in 5%
- Clitoris involved 5–15%
- Posterior fourchette 15%
- Synchronous second malignancy 22%

Multifocality is seen in 5% of cases requiring evaluation of perianal skin along with vagina and cervix. Approximately, 20% will have a synchronous malignancy, commonly in cervix.[7] Less frequently vulvar bleeding or discharge, dysuria or enlarged lymph nodes in the groin suggestive of advanced disease may be present.

- Diagnosis is based upon of biopsy.
- Biopsy is taken from the center of the lesion to reflect the most severe histology of the lesion.
- If multiple abnormal areas are present, then multiple biopsies should be taken to "map" all potential sites of vulvar pathology.
- No gross lesion, colposcopic examination using 5% acetic acid soln

Vulvar cancer is a histological diagnosis based upon a vulvar biopsy. Visual inspection is done during pelvic examination to look for any suspicious lesion, which might be raised or fungating or showing pigmentation. Colposcopy with application of 5% acetic acid is done, if no lesion is grossly evident. Simultaneous examination of cervix can also be performed. All acetowhite areas with abnormal vascular pattern are biopsied. Differential diagnosis includes epidermal inclusion cysts, lentigos, disorders of Bartholin

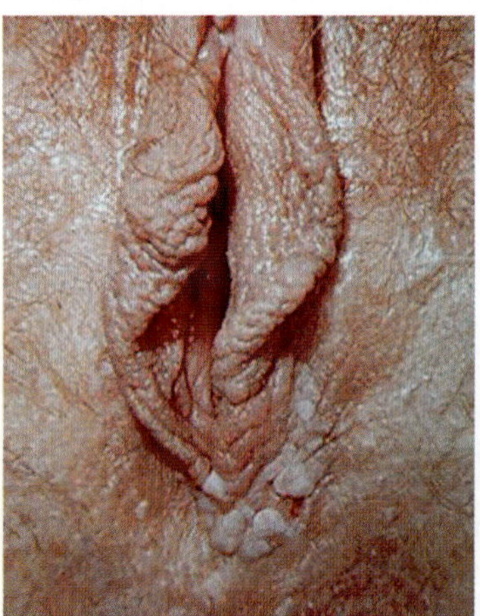

Fig. 1: Vulvar intraepithelial neoplasia (Raised white plaques).

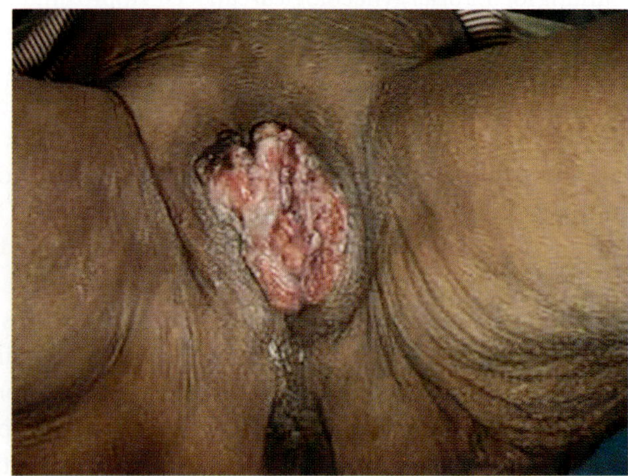

Fig. 2: Locally advanced vulvar carcinoma.

gland, acrochordons, seborrheic keratoses, hidradenomas, lichen sclerosus and other dermatoses, and condyloma acuminata.

HISTOLOGICAL TYPES

Most vulvar cancers are squamous cell carcinomas; other histologies include melanoma, Bartholin gland adenocarcinoma, sarcoma, Paget disease, or basal cell carcinoma.

> ***Histological types***
> - Squamous cell carcinoma > 90%
> - Melanoma 5%
> - Basal cell carcinoma 2%
> - Soft tissue sarcoma 1–2%
> - Extramammary pagets < 1%
> - Bartholin gland adenocarcinoma

Squamous Cell Carcinoma

Over 90% of vulvar malignancies are squamous cell carcinomas. There are two subtypes, both of which usually occur on the labia or vestibule:

1. The keratinizing differentiated or simplex type is more common, occurs in older women, is not related to HPV infection, but is associated with vulvar dystrophies and chronic venereal granulomatous disease.
2. The classic, warty, or Bowenoid type is predominantly associated with HPV 16, 18, and 33, and found in younger women.[8] Early age at first intercourse, multiple sexual partners, human immunodeficiency virus (HIV) infection, and cigarette smoking are risk factors with HPV infection.[9]

Typical SCC	*Basaloid carcinoma*	*Warty carcinoma*
65% >65 years HPV uncommon Well differentiated Keratinizing Sq cell Keratin pearls	28% < 60 years HPV 16,18 VIN III associated Basal cell type No keratin pearls	7% Young patients HPV + Bowenoid epithelium

Verrucous Carcinoma

Verrucous carcinoma is a variant of squamous cell cancer with cauliflower-like in appearance. Biopsy shows papillary fronds without the central connective tissue core typical of condylomata acuminata. The lesion grows slowly and may be locally destructive, but rarely metastasizes to lymph nodes.

Melanoma

Melanoma is the second most common vulvar cancer histology, accounting for approximately 5–10% of primary vulvar neoplasms.[10] It occurs predominantly in postmenopausal white non-Hispanic women and is usually a pigmented lesion, but amelanotic lesions also occur.[10]

Basal Cell Carcinoma

A 2% of vulvar cancers are basal cell cancers and 2% of basal cell cancers occur on the vulva.[11] The typical appearance is that of a "rodent" ulcer with rolled edges and central ulceration. Basal cell carcinomas are associated with a high incidence of concomitant malignancy elsewhere in the body.

Sarcoma

Soft tissue sarcomas (including leiomyosarcomas, rhabdomyosarcomas, liposarcomas, angiosarcomas, neurofibrosarcomas, fibrous histiocytomas, and epithelioid sarcomas) constitute 1–2% of vulvar malignancies. Their prognosis is generally poor.

Extramammary Paget Disease

Extramammary Paget disease, an intraepithelial adenocarcinoma, accounts for less than 1% of all vulvar malignancies. Invasive adenocarcinomas may be present within or beneath the surface lesion (4–17%) and 20–30% of these patients have a noncontiguous carcinoma.[12]

Bartholin Gland Adenocarcinoma

Cancers arising in Bartholin gland are most often adenocarcinomas or squamous cell carcinomas, but transitional cell carcinomas, adeno-squamous, and adenoid cystic carcinoma may also develop. Enlargement of the Bartholin gland in a postmenopausal woman should evoke suspicion of malignancy. Metastases are common in cancers of Bartholin gland because of the rich vascular and lymphatic network in this area.

> ***Mode of spread***
> - Direct extention – contiguous
>   – continuous
> - Lymphatic
> - Hematogenous dissemination

MODE OF SPREAD

Vulvar carcinoma metastasizes by direct extension to adjacent structures (e.g., vagina, urethra, clitoris, and anus) or by lymphatic spread to regional lymph nodes.

Lymph node involvement can occur early in the course of disease, even in patients with small lesions. The risk of lymph node metastasis based on the depth of invasion ranges from 0% in lesions with invasion to less than or equal to 1 mm to 43% in lesions with invasion deeper than 5 mm. The pathway for lymphatic drainage of the vulva begins at the superficial inguinal nodes, followed by drainage to the deep inguinal and femoral lymph nodes below the cribriform fascia, and then to the pelvic lymphatics. Lateral lesions spread to the ipsilateral nodal group; central lesions may metastasize to ipsilateral, contralateral, or both groups of nodes **(Fig. 3)**.

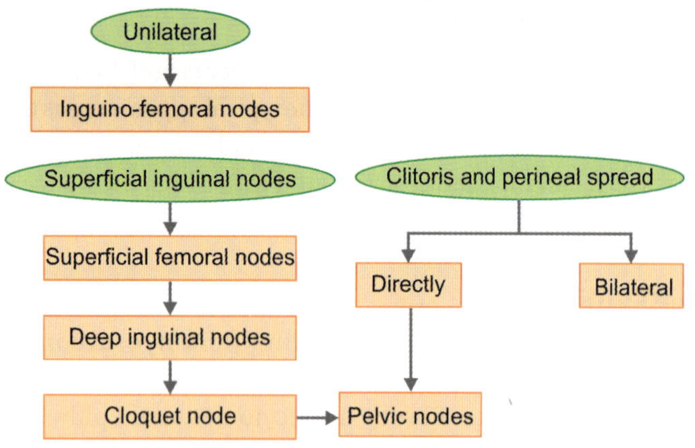

Fig. 3: Lymphatic drainage of vulva and perineum.

Hematogenous dissemination is rare without inguino-femoral lymph node involvement and occurs late in the course of the disease. Common sites involved by hematogenous spread are, lung, bone, and liver.

EVALUATION

Vulvar cancer is surgically staged based on the International Federation of Gynecology and Obstetrics (FIGO) recommendations. A thorough clinical evaluation helps in planning the choice of treatment modality to be used. Particular attention is paid to measurement of the diameter of the primary tumor and palpation for inguinal, axillary, or supraclavicular lymphadenopathy along with cervical cytology and colposcopy of the cervix, vagina, and vulva. For women with large tumors (≥2 cm) or suspected metastases, an abdominal/pelvic computed tomography may be performed to detect lymphadenopathy or other metastases.

The FIGO staging uses a surgical-pathologic staging system for vulvar cancer based upon findings from the biopsy of the vulvar lesion(s) and the inguino-femoral lymph nodes rather than a clinical staging system, which was in use prior to 1988.[13] Surgical staging is preferable as inguino-femoral lymph node status is the most important predictor of overall prognosis. In patients with clinically normal lymph nodes, 16–24% have metastases, while 24–41% of those with clinically enlarged nodes are negative at histological examination, making palpation of groin inadequate for lymph node assessment.[14] FIGO 2009 staging is given in **Table 2**.

TABLE 2: FIGO staging of cancer of vulva.

Stage	*Clinical and pathological findings*
IA	Tumor confined to the vulva or perineum, ≤2 cm in size with stromal invasion ≤1 mm, negative nodes
IB	Tumor confined to the vulva or perineum, >2 cm in size or with stromal invasion > 1 mm, negative nodes
II	Tumor of any size with adjacent spread (1/3 lower urethra, 1/3 lower vagina, anus), negative nodes
IIIA	Tumor of any size with positive inguino-femoral lymph nodes; 1 lymph node metastasis greater than or equal to 5 mm; 1–2 lymph node metastasis(es) of less than 5 mm
IIIB	Two or more lymph nodes metastases greater than or equal to 5 mm; three or more lymph nodes metastases less than 5 mm
IIIC	Positive node(s) with extracapsular spread
IVA	Tumor invades other regional structures (2/3 upper urethra, 2/3 upper vagina), bladder mucosa, rectal mucosa, or fixed to pelvic bone; fixed or ulcerated inguino-femoral lymph nodes
IVB	Any distant metastasis including pelvic lymph nodes

SURGICAL APPROACH

In the early part of the 20th century, patients with vulvar cancer usually died of disease. The overall survival rate for vulvar cancer after simple surgical excision was less than 25%. Basset in 1912 described a more radical procedure to improve outcomes for patients with vulvar cancer. An improved survival rate using an en bloc dissection radical vulvectomy with an inguinal and pelvic lymphadenectomy was demonstrated by Way. The Bassett-Way operation resulted in a 5-year survival rate of 74%.[15] Fred Taussig collected a large series of vulvar cancer cases from 1911–40.[16] He initially started his series with a radical excision of the primary tumor with an en bloc dissection of the inguinal lymph nodes.

Later, he modified his technique for patients with small lesions in an attempt to decrease operative morbidity. He used separate incisions for the groin dissection and the vulvar excision. This less radical operation for small lesions was not routinely used until Hacker reported his experience with 100 patients in 1981. He reported using three separate incisions, as described by Taussig, for patients with clinical stage I disease. The 5-year survival rate was 97%[17] **(Fig. 4)**.

Way's radial excision—Butterfly incision-1960
- Mortality 33%
- High morbidity
- Secondary healing usually

Taussig-1940
- Three separate incisions
- Wound problems <15–30%
- Primary healing
- Early mobilization
- Pre-op antibiotics
- Subcutaneous heparin
- Suction drains in the groin-prevents lymphocysts and facilitates healing
- Trim margins of skin before closure

- Spread is by embolization rather than by contiguous permeation
- Keeping intervening bridge of skin b/w vulva and groin nodes is safe in early disease
- Spread follows a predictable course to nodes so very good model for sentinel node study

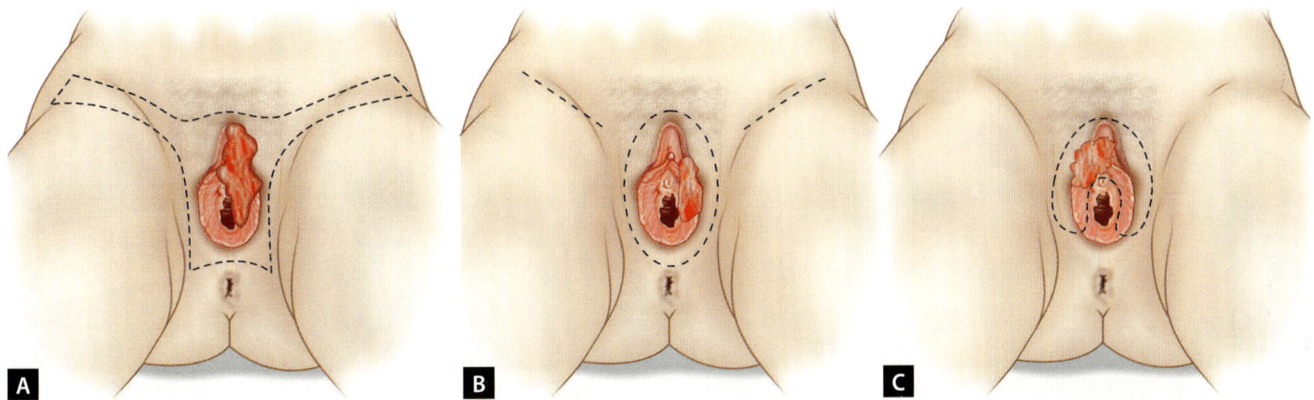

Figs. 4A to C: Incisions for radical vulvectomy. (A) Modified butterfly incision; (B) Triple incision technique—a skin bridge is left between the radical vulvectomy and the groin incisions; (C) Anterior horseshoe incision.

MANAGEMENT OF PRIMARY TUMOR

Current approach is to utilize most conservative procedure thereby optimizing survival while minimizing perioperative morbidity and maximizing long-term psychosexual and physical well being.[18] Standard radical vulvectomy consists of removal of the entire vulva down to the level of the deep fascia of the thigh, the periosteum of the pubis, and the inferior fascia of the urogenital diaphragm. This is performed through a single incision that circumscribes the labia majora and extends to the groins bilaterally to include en bloc inguino-femoral lymph node dissection. There is considerable morbidity associated with this procedure in form of wound breakdown, psychosexual effects from distortion of the vulva, and lymphedema.[19]

Alternative approaches where the depth of the dissection is the same as in standard radical vulvectomy but less of the vulvar and surrounding skin is removed are most commonly performed. A tumor-free margin of at least a 1 cm decreases the risk of local recurrence.[20] An alternative to radical vulvectomy in women with stage III or IV disease is the three-incision technique. Radical excision of the primary lesion and bilateral groin node evaluation is performed while retaining skin over the groin thereby lowering the risk of postoperative wound breakdown and lower extremity lymphedema and improves cosmesis **(Figs. 5 to 7)**.

MANAGEMENT OF LYMPH NODES

In all stages of disease except stage IA inguino-femoral lymph node dissection (removal of the superficial inguinal and deep femoral lymph nodes) is performed **(Figs. 8 and 9)**. Pelvic lymph node dissection is not required. Morbidity rates are high including wound infection and breakdown (20–40%) and lower extremity lymphedema (30–70%) leading some to propose nodal debulking followed by groin irradiation to minimize morbidity.[21]

Unilateral lymph node dissection (LND) is associated with a <1% risk of contralateral groin node in Stage IB disease which is unifocal lateral (>1 cm from the vulvar midline), not located in the anterior portion of the labia minora (defined anatomically as the area just posterior to the clitoris), with no palpable lymphadenopathy in either groin or metastases found at time of unilateral lymph node dissection.[22] Bilateral lymph node dissection is performed for stage II or greater disease as the rate of bilateral groin metastases in women with unilateral lesions with stromal invasion ≥3 mm is more than 2.8%.[23] The reported rate of groin recurrence after inguino-femoral lymph node dissection ranges from 1 to 10%. Inclusion of deep lymph nodes is generally preferred to reduce groin recurrence. Incision for groin dissection is shown in **Figure 10** and inguino-femoral LND is shown in **Figure 11**.

SENTINEL LYMPH NODE BIOPSY

Sentinel lymph node biopsy (SLNB) for vulvar cancer is under investigation as an alternative to inguino-femoral LND.[24] This procedure has less morbidity without compromising detection of lymph node metastases or increasing the risk of a groin recurrence.

Sentinel lymph node is the first echelon draining node in the lymph node basin from the primary tumor; accordingly tumor cells metastasizing via lymphatics enter the sentinel node (SN) before spreading to other lymph nodes along the lymphatic chain. This sentinel node is the most likely lymph node to contain tumor cells if regional nodal metastasis has occurred **(Fig. 12)**. The first area to receive lymphatic drainage from a lateral vulvar lesion is usually the ipsilateral superficial inguinal nodes. If the SLN shows no evidence of metastatic involvement, then all other nodes should be negative, rendering complete nodal dissection unnecessary.

The best candidates for intraoperative lymphatic mapping are women with uninfected tumors limited to the lateral vulva, with no palpable enlarged groin nodes and no history of vulvar surgery that could disrupt lymphatic drainage.

Intraoperative lymphatic mapping of SLN is performed using either of two general methods: Peritumoral injection

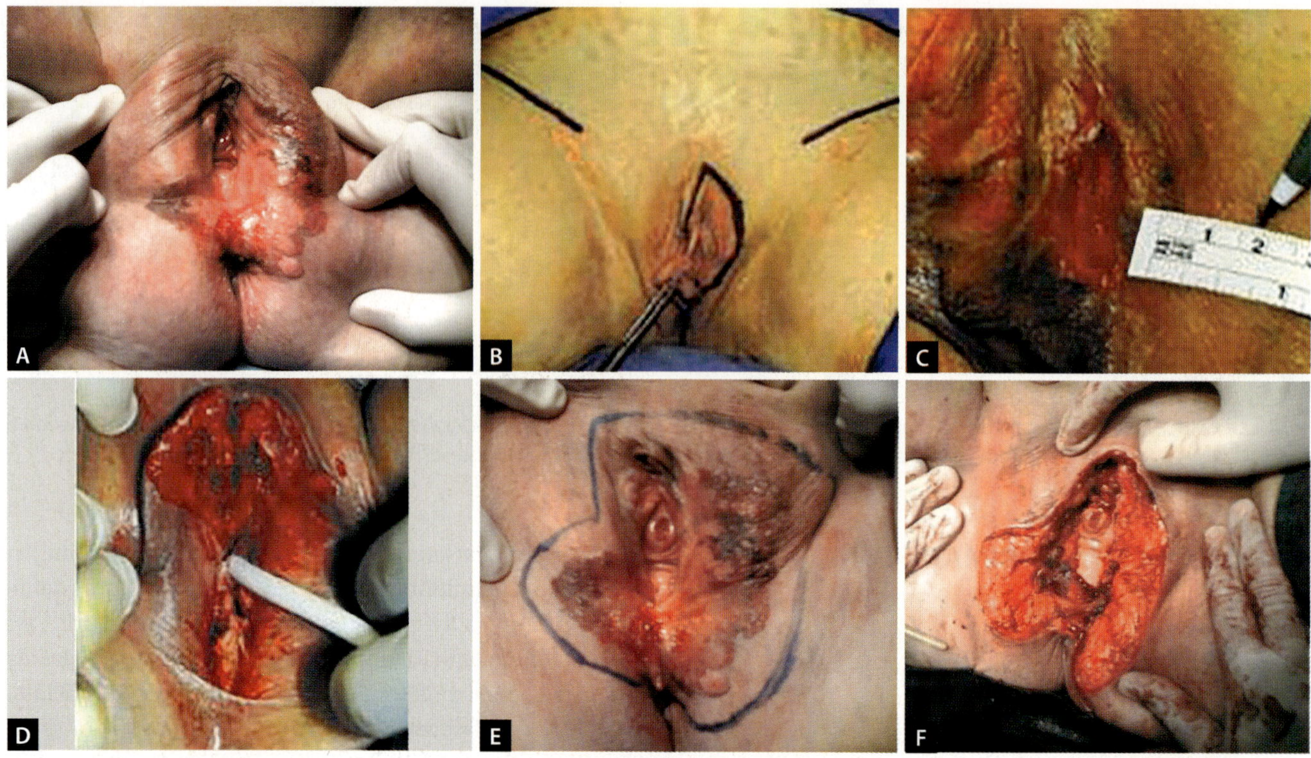

Figs. 5A to F: Radical vulvectomy.

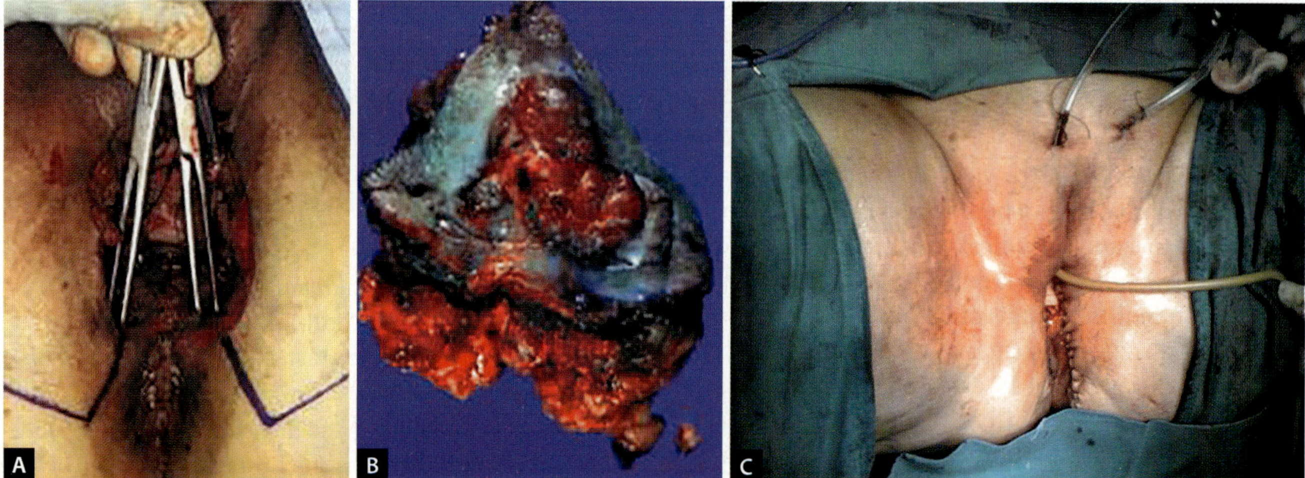

Figs. 6A to C: Bilateral rhomboid flap.

of isosulfanblue or methylene blue dye (sensitivity 95%) or preoperative lymphoscintigraphy using radiolabeled colloid followed by node detection with an intraoperative gamma-detecting probe (sensitivity 97%) **(Figs. 13A and B)**. Use of a combination of blue dye and radiolabeled colloid is preferred so as to yield more accurate results than either test alone. The groin recurrence rate in women with a negative SLNB in all study participants was 2.9%.[25]

- Vulvar cancer is staged using surgical-pathologic staging system based upon findings from the biopsy of the vulvar lesion(s) and the inguino-femoral lymph nodes.
- Clinical staging is inadequate

- Women with stage IA disease with no clinically palpable groin nodes do not require inguino-femoral LND
- Sentinel lymph node biopsy (SLNB) appears to be a promising approach

TREATMENT OF SQUAMOUS CELL CARCINOMA

Stage IA: Radical local excision without lymph node dissection is the treatment of choice in patients with less than 1 mm of stromal invasion (lymph node involvement < 1%).[26]

Stage IB disease should undergo radical local excision with inguino-femoral lymph node dissection. (>8% lymph node

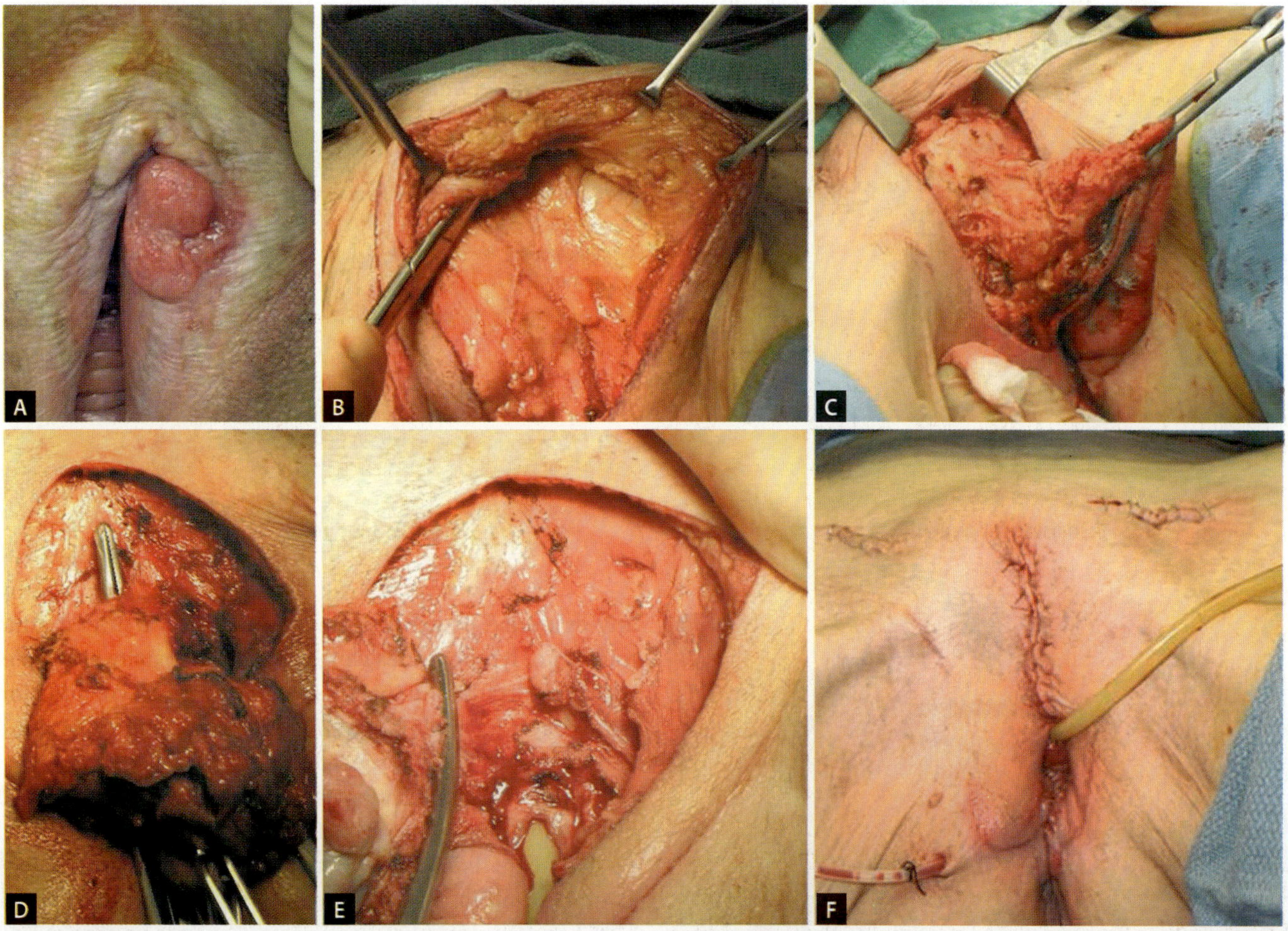

Figs. 7A to F: Anterior horse-shoe incision.

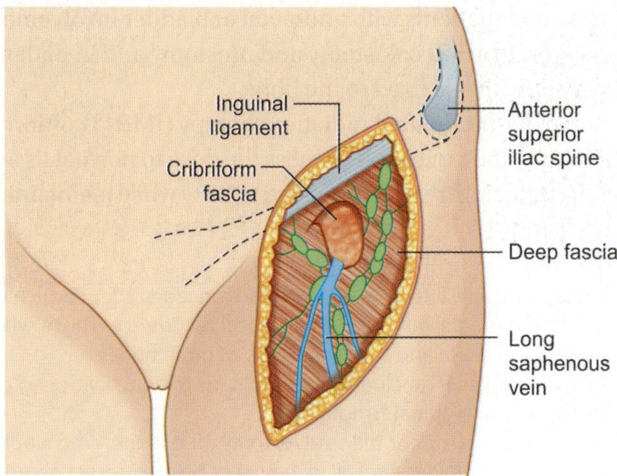

Fig. 8: Superficial inguinal nodes.

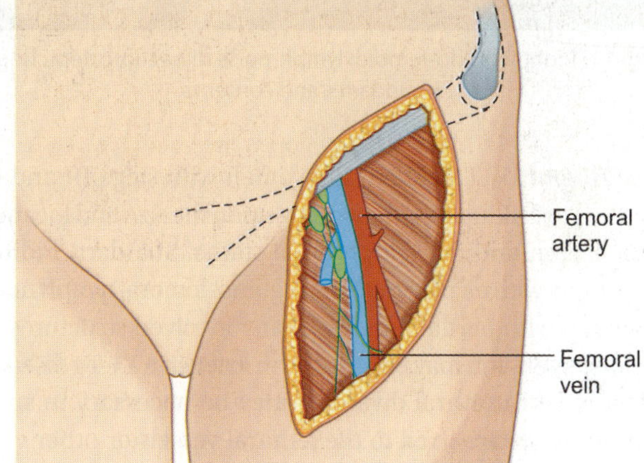

Fig. 9: Deep inguinal nodes.

involvement). Depending upon the location of the lesion decision made regarding unilateral or bilateral lymph node dissection.[27]

Stage II disease: The most conservative excision technique resulting in a ≥1 cm tumor-free margin is performed (Radical local excision, partial radical vulvectomy, or the three-incision technique).[26]

Due to associated morbidity, primary radiation therapy (RT) is generally avoided for management of early stage vulvar cancers. In patients not fit enough to tolerate surgery, RT results in more groin recurrences than surgery. There is benefit with RT in patients with positive or close (<8 mm) margins but re-excision is preferred to avoid the toxicity associated with RT.[14]

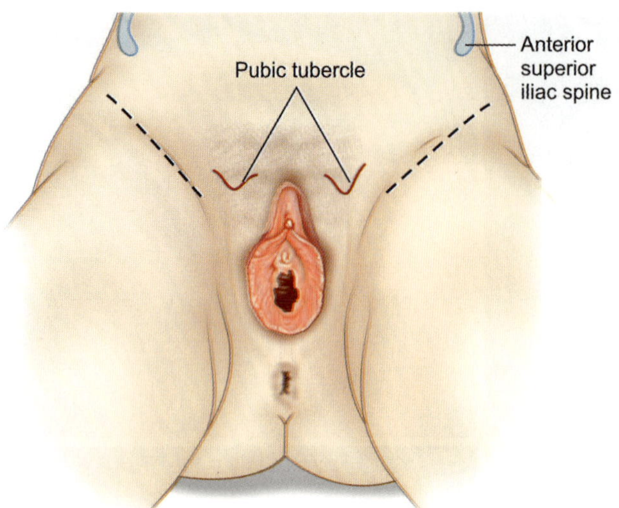

Fig. 10: Incision for groin dissection.

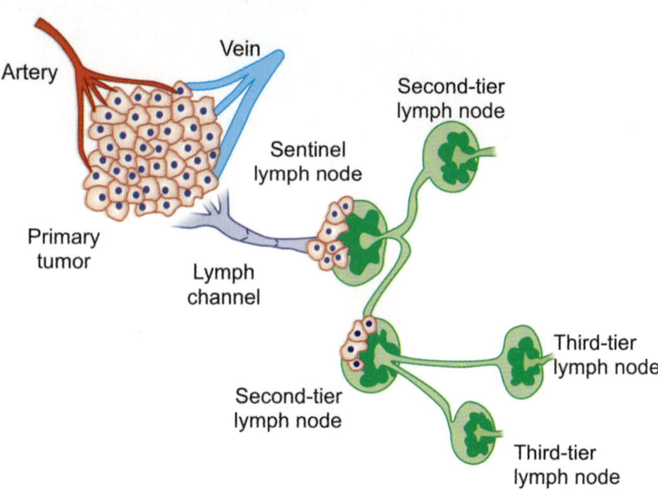

Fig. 12: Sentinel node concept.

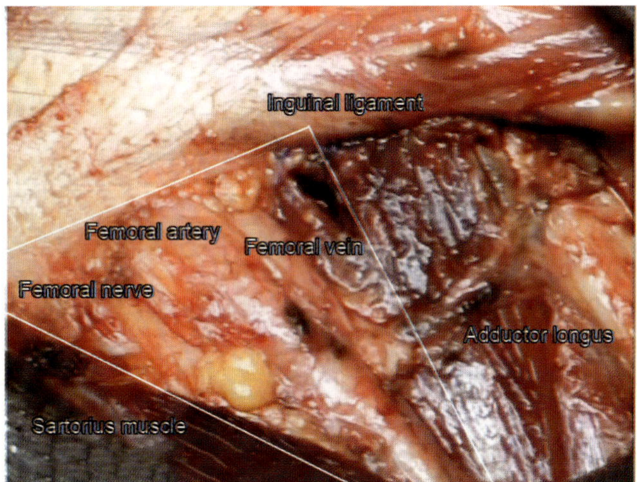

Fig. 11: Right inguino-femoral lymph-node dissection, depicting the boundaries and contents.

Stage III and IV: Treatment for women with stage III and IV disease is individualized depending upon the size and location of the lesion and the lymph node status. Standard radical vulvectomy with en bloc bilateral inguino-femoral lymph node dissection with partial removal of any involved structures or pelvic exenteration may be required in extensive T3–T4 disease. Colostomy or urethral diversion may be necessary in such cases. If nodes are fixed to the femoral vessels or other vital structures lymphadenectomy may not be feasible.

- Traditional radical vulvectomy with en bloc inguino-femoral LND results in significant morbidity
- Tumor-free margin ≥1 cm minimizes the risk of local recurrence
- Stage I or II disease with margins <1 cm after excision, we suggest re-excision rather than radiation therapy (RT)

Ipsilateral groin and pelvic irradiation are recommended when there are two or more microscopically positive groin nodes, one or more macroscopically involved lymph nodes, any evidence of extracapsular spread, or if only a small number of lymph nodes were sampled.[28] Toxicity associated with groin irradiation includes wound breakdown, infection, lymphocyst formation, lymphedema, and long-term risk of femoral fracture or hip replacement.[21]

Primary chemoradiation has been used to treat women with locally advanced (stage III to IVA) or inoperable disease with no significant difference in death rates compared to surgery.[29] Chemoradiation is associated with high rates of pathologic (70%) and clinical (48%) complete response rates with 55% recurrence free survival at 50 months. Radical resection is preferred to chemoradiation.[29] However; chemoradiation is an option for patients with anorectal or bladder involvement in an effort to avoid colostomy and urostomy and in patients with disease that is fixed to the bone.

Intensity-modulated radiation therapy (IMRT) conforms radiation to the target and reduces the dose to normal tissue, thereby reducing treatment-related toxicity while maintaining tumor control.

- Postoperative RT to the vulva for advanced stage, surgically resected patients with high-risk of local recurrence: Those with stage IV A disease and a large number of groin nodes.
- Adjuvant pelvic RT including the groin for patients with two or more positive inguinal lymph nodes.
- Chemoradiation rather than vulvectomy for patients who would require an ostomy as a result of bowel or bladder resection and for patients with disease that is fixed to the bone.
- Chemotherapy, radiation therapy, and surgery are options for management of regional recurrences and metastatic disease.
- Local perineal recurrences can be treated successfully by reexcision.
- Follow patients at least twice yearly for five years with a gynecologic examination.

Palliative chemotherapy: In stage IVB metastatic disease or for frail, inoperable patients. Response rates are poor and

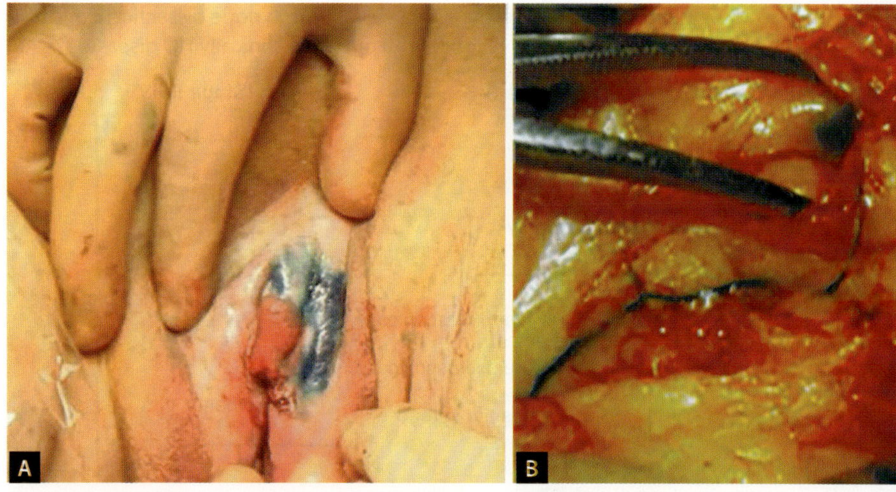

Figs. 13A and B: (A) Blue dye injected around tumor; (B) Blue streaked lymphatics leading to the SN.

of short duration. Cisplatin and 5 FU are traditionally used chemotherapeutic agents with some improvement seen with use of taxanes. Novel agents such as anti-EGFR tyrosine kinase inhibitors, erlotinib, have shown promising results in small series.[30]

- Radical wide excision and selective inguinal lymphadenectomy is the main approach to patients with early stage disease.
- Chemoradiation is an alternative to radical vulvectomy with en bloc inguino-femoral LND for advanced disease.

Prognosis: The presence of inguino-femoral node metastases is the most important prognostic factor for survival in patients with vulvar cancer. Five-year survival ranges from 70 to 93% for patients with negative nodes to 25–41% for those with positive nodes.[31] Other prognostic factors include capillary lymphatic space invasion, and older age.

5-year survival	***Prognostic factors***
Node +ve 60%	• Grade
Node -ve 96%	• Lymphnode metastasis
One node + 94%	• Depth of lesion/invasion
2 node s + 80%	• Lympho-vascular invasion
≥ 3 nodes + 12%	
Stage I 98%	
Stage II 90%	
Stage III 60%	

The majority of relapses of vulvar cancer occur in the first year, but recurrences are known to seen ≥5 years after diagnosis.[32] For low-risk disease (early stage, treated with surgery alone, no adjuvant therapy) follow up with clinical examination for the first 2 years, every 6 months; and then annually. For high-risk disease (advanced stage, treated with primary chemotherapy/radiation therapy or surgery plus adjuvant therapy)—for the first 2 years, every 3 months; for year 3 through 5, every 6 months, and then annually. Vulvar colposcopy and biopsy are indicated, if abnormalities are noted on physical examination. Cervical cytology (or vaginal cytology if the cervix has been removed) is done annually. Routine use of imaging studies was not recommended. If recurrence is suspected computed tomography and/or positron emission tomography should be performed.

RECURRENT DISEASE

Recurrences following primary surgery are most commonly seen in perineum (53%) followed by groin (19%), pelvis (6%), distant recurrence (8%), and multiple sites (14%). Local perineal recurrences can often be treated successfully by re-excision whereas inguinal recurrences are associated with a much worse prognosis.[33] RT may be added to surgery or chemotherapy, or used as a sole modality in patients with recurrent vulvar cancer. For patients with distant metastases salvage chemotherapy can be considered **(Flowchart 1)**.

Follow-up
- Every 3 monthly for 2 years
  - 6 monthly for up to 5 years
  - After 5 years—annually
- Gynecologic examination with visual inspection and palpation of the vulva, skin bridge, and inguinal nodes.
- Vulvar colposcopy and biopsy are indicated, if abnormalities are noted.

TREATMENT OF OTHER HISTOLOGIES

Melanoma

Mostly located on labia minora and clitoris. Prognosis depends on size of the lesion and depth of invasion. Staging is similar to that of skin melanoma. Radical vulvectomy with inguinal and pelvic lymphadenectomy, taking 2 cm margins for thin (up to 7 mm) and 3–4 cm margin for thicker lesions.

Basal Cell

As basal cell carcinomas are locally aggressive but rarely metastasize radical local excision without lymphadenectomy is adequate.

Flowchart 1: Treatment algorithm for stage-wise management of carcinoma vulva. Lymph node dissection done for lesions > 2 cm in size or with >1 mm invasion in Stage IB. SN biopsy is an option in clinically NO disease.

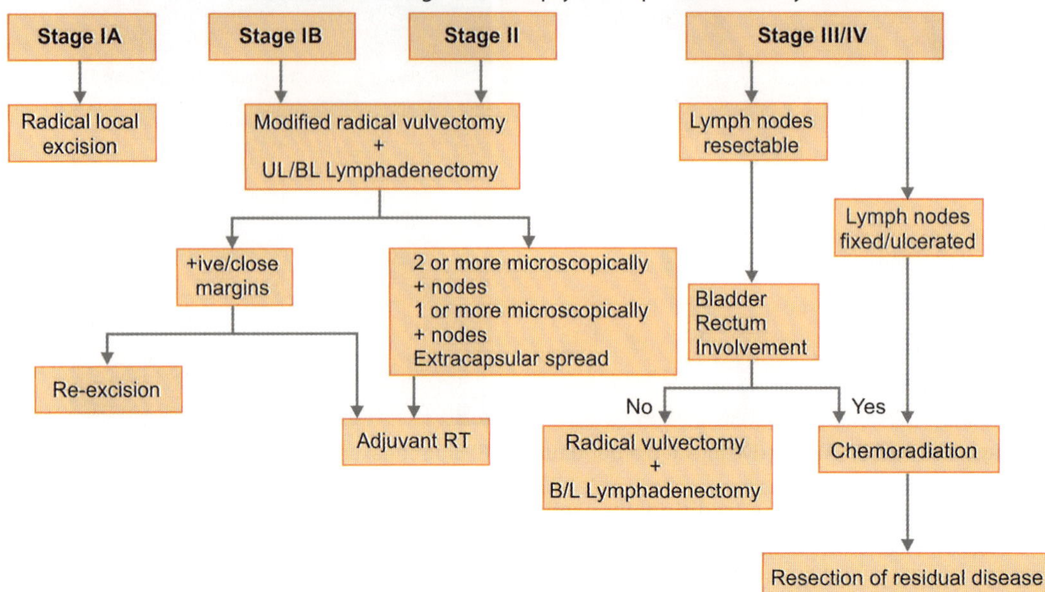

Sarcomas

Wide local excision is the standard approach to treatment of most vulvar sarcomas. Lymphatic metastases are uncommon.

Paget Disease of the Vulva

The vulva is one of the most common sites for extramammary Paget disease. Treatment consists of wide local excision or vulvectomy, depending upon the extent of disease. Radical excision in not required, but a 2 cm margin is preferred. Greater depth of invasion and lymphovascular involvements are poor prognostic markers.[34] Inguinal lymphadenectomy be performed in cases with invasive disease or an underlying adenocarcinoma. Due to multicentricity and microscopic extension of disease beyond the clinically visible margins 12–58% of women experience a local recurrence despite negative surgical margins. Treatment with Moh's micrographic surgery (i.e., microscopically controlled systematic excision of cancerous tissue) may be associated with a lower recurrence rate, particularly for recurrent tumors.[35] The roles of definitive RT, cytotoxic chemotherapy, and topical imiquimod in the treatment of Paget disease of the vulva are also not well-defined, but may be an option for some patients who are not suitable surgical candidates. Overexpression of HER2 suggests a possible role for trastuzumab therapy.

Bartholin Gland Adenocarcinoma

Traditionally treated with radical vulvectomy with bilateral groin and pelvic lymphadenectomy. The lesions are typically deep within the vulva so extensive deep dissection is generally required.

Surgical margins are frequently microscopically positive and require postoperative RT to reduce the incidence of local recurrence. If ipsilateral groin nodes are involved, pelvic and bilateral groin radiation may decrease the frequency of regional recurrence.

Verrucous Carcinoma

Radical local excision is usually adequate. Suspicious lymph nodes should be biopsied and if positive, then inguino-femoral lymphadenectomy should be performed. RT is contraindicated because it can induce anaplastic transformation and increase the likelihood of metastases.

- Radical vulvectomy is a procedure usually performed for the treatment of vulvar carcinoma.
- The treatment of nonsquamous cell vulvar malignancies depends upon the histologic type, but in general, surgery is the primary therapy.
- Ancillary procedures performed with radical vulvectomy include distal urethrectomy, vaginectomy, pubic symphysectomy, anovulvectomy, posterior exenteration, sigmoid colostomy and superficial and deep groin lymph node dissection.
- Modifications limit the extent of tissue removal and morbidity of the procedure-less radical resection, the introduction of sentinel node sampling.
- Treatment of carcinoma of the vulva should be tailored to each patient.
- Bladder and anal sphincter function may be able to be preserved by limiting the extent of surgery and treating patients with chemotherapy or radiation.
- Musculocutaneous transposition flaps may be necessary to close large defects on the vulva and perineum.

REFERENCES

1. Siegel R, Ward E, Brawley O, Jemal A. Cancer statistics, 2011: The impact of eliminating socioeconomic and racial disparities on premature cancer deaths. CA Cancer J Clin. 2011;61:212.
2. Ferlay J, Shin HR, Bray F, Forman D, Mathers C, Parkin DM. GLOBOCAN 2008 v1.2, Cancer Incidence and Mortality

Worldwide: IARC Cancer Base No. 10 Lyon, France: International Agency for Research on Cancer; 2010.
3. Devi UK. Current status of gynecological cancer care in India. J Gynecol Oncol. 2009;20(2):77-80.
4. Madsen BS, Jensen HL, van den Brule AJ, Wohlfahrt J, Frisch M. Risk factors for invasive squamous cell carcinoma of the vulva and vagina—population-based case-control study in Denmark. Int J Cancer. 2008;122:2827-34.
5. de Koning MN, Quint WG, Pirog EC. Prevalence of mucosal and cutaneous human papillomaviruses in different histologic subtypes of vulvar carcinoma. Mod Pathol. 2008;21:334.
6. Monk BJ, Burger RA, Lin F, Parham G, Vasilev SA, Wilczynski SP. Prognostic significance of human papillomavirus DNA in vulvar carcinoma. Obstet Gynecol. 1995; 85:709.
7. Collins CG, Lee FY, Roman-Lopez JJ. Invasive carcinoma of the vulva with lymph node metastasis. Am J Obstet Gynecol. 1971;109:446.
8. Iwasawa A, Nieminen P, Lehtinen M, Paavonen J. Human papillomavirus in squamous cell carcinoma of the vulva by polymerase chain reaction. Obstet Gynecol. 1997;89:81.
9. Elit L, Voruganti S, Simunovic M. Invasive vulvar cancer in a woman with human immunodeficiency virus: case report and review of the literature. Gynecol Oncol. 2005;98:151.
10. Sugiyama VE, Chan JK, Shin JY, Berek JS, Osann K, Kapp DS. Vulvar melanoma: a multivariable analysis of 644 patients. Obstet Gynecol. 2007;110:296.
11. de Giorgi V, Salvini C, Massi D, Raspollini MR, Carli P. Vulvar basal cell carcinoma: retrospective study and review of literature. Gynecol Oncol. 2005;97:192.
12. Parker LP, Parker JR, Bodurka-Bevers D, Deavers M, Bevers MW, Shen-Gunther J, et al. Paget's disease of the vulva: pathology, pattern of involvement, and prognosis. Gynecol Oncol. 2000;77:183.
13. Benedet JL, Bender H, Jones H 3rd, Ngan HY, Pecorelli S. FIGO staging classifications and clinical practice guidelines in the management of gynecologic cancers. FIGO Committee on Gynecologic Oncology. Int J Gynaecol Obstet. 2000;70:209.
14. Gonzalez Bosquet J, Kinney WK, Russell AH, Gaffey TA, Magrina JF, Podratz KC. Risk of occult inguinofemoral lymph node metastasis from squamous carcinoma of the vulva. Int J Radiat Oncol Biol Phys. 2003;57:419.
15. Morley GW. Infiltrative carcinoma of the vulva: results of surgical treatment. Am J Obstet Gynecol. 1976;124:874-8.
16. Taussig FJ. Cancer of the Vulva. Am J Obstet Gynecol. 1940;40:764.
17. Hacker NF, Leuchter RS, Berek JS, Castaldo TW, Lagasse LD. Radical vulvectomy and bilateral inguinal lymphadenectomy through separate groin incisions. Obstet Gynecol. 1981;58(5): 574-9.
18. Barton DP. The prevention and management of treatment related morbidity in vulval cancer. Best Pract Res Clin Obstet Gynaecol. 2003;17:683.
19. DiSaia PJ, Creasman WT, Rich WM. An alternate approach to early cancer of the vulva. Am J Obstet Gynecol. 1979;133:825.
20. Heaps JM, Fu YS, Montz FJ, Hacker NF, Berek JS. Surgical-pathologic variables predictive of local recurrence in squamous cell carcinoma of the vulva. Gynecol Oncol. 1990;38:309-14.
21. Rouzier R, Haddad B, Dubernard G, Dubois P, Paniel BJ. Inguinofemoral dissection for carcinoma of the vulva: effect of modifications of extent and technique on morbidity and survival. J Am Coll Surg. 2003;196:442.
22. Hacker NF. Vulvar cancer. In: Practical Gynecologic Oncology, 4th edition. Philadelphia: Lippincott Williams & Wilkins; 2005. p. 543.
23. Homesley HD, Bundy BN, Sedlis A, Yordan E, Berek JS, Jahshan A, et al. Prognostic factors for groin node metastasis in squamous cell carcinoma of the vulva (a Gynecologic Oncology Group study). Gynecol Oncol. 1993;49:279-83.
24. Selman TJ, Luesley DM, Acheson N, Khan KS, Mann CH. A systematic review of the accuracy of diagnostic tests for inguinal lymph node status in vulvar cancer. Gynecol Oncol. 2005;99:206-14.
25. Van der Zee AG, Oonk MH, De Hullu JA, Ansink AC, Vergote I, Verheijen RH, et al. Sentinel node dissection is safe in the treatment of early-stage vulvar cancer. J Clin Oncol. 2008; 26:884-9.
26. Farias-Eisner R, Cirisano FD, Grouse D, Leuchter RS, Karlan BY, Lagasse LD, et al. Conservative and individualized surgery for early squamous carcinoma of the vulva: the treatment of choice for stage I and II (T1-2N0-1M0) disease. Gynecol Oncol. 1994;53:55-8.
27. Hacker NF, Berek JS, Lagasse LD, Nieberg RK, Leuchter RS. Individualization of treatment for stage I squamous cell vulvar carcinoma. Obstet Gynecol. 1984;63:155-62.
28. Fons G, Groenen SM, Oonk MH, Ansink AC, van der Ze AGJ, Burger MPM, et al. Adjuvant radiotherapy in patients with vulvar cancer and one intra capsular lymph node metastasis is not beneficial. Gynecol Oncol. 2009;114:343-5.
29. Montana GS, Thomas GM, Moore DH, Saxer A, Mangan CE, Lentz SS, et al. Preoperative chemo-radiation for carcinoma of the vulva with N2/N3 nodes: a gynecologic oncology group study. Int J Radiat Oncol Biol Phys. 2000;48:1007-13.
30. Olawaiye A, Lee LM, Krasner C, Horowitz N. Treatment of squamous cell vulvar cancer with the anti-EGFR tyrosine kinase inhibitor Tarceva. Gynecol Oncol. 2007;106:628.
31. Gadducci A, Cionini L, Romanini A, Fanucchi A, Genazzani AR. Old and new perspectives in the management of high-risk, locally advanced or recurrent, and metastatic vulvar cancer. Crit Rev Oncol Hematol. 2006;60:227-41.
32. Gonzalez Bosquet J, Magrina JF, Gaffey TA, Hernandez JL, Webb MJ, Cliby WA, et al. Long-term survival and disease recurrence in patients with primary squamous cell carcinoma of the vulva. Gynecol Oncol. 2005;97:828-33.
33. Maggino T, Landoni F, Sartori E, Zola P, Gadducci A, Alessi C, et al. Patterns of recurrence in patients with squamous cell carcinoma of the vulva. A multicenter CTF Study. Cancer. 2000;89:116-22.
34. Shepherd V, Davidson FJ, Davies-Humphreys J. Extramammary Paget's disease. BJOG. 2005;112:273.
35. Tebes S, Cardosi R, Hoffman M. Paget's disease of the vulva. Am J Obstet Gynecol. 2002;187:281.

LONG QUESTIONS

1. Discuss etiopathogenesis and prognostic factors of carcinoma vulva.
2. Discuss the current FIGO staging and management of carcinoma vulva.

SHORT QUESTIONS

Write short notes on:

1. Indications for adjuvant RT in carcinoma vulva.

2. SLNB—sentinel node in carcinoma vulva.
3. Mode of spread of carcinoma vulva and its implication on treatment.
4. Lymphadenectomy in carcinoma vulva.
5. FIGO staging for carcinoma vulva.
6. Risk factors for carcinoma vulva and discuss briefly role of HPV.

MULTIPLE CHOICE QUESTIONS

1. Vulvar cancer accounts for what percentage of gynecological cancers:
   a. 7% b. 10%
   c. 5% d. 15%
2. Mean age of diagnosis is:
   a. 5th decade b. 6th decade
   c. 7th decade d. 8th decade
3. Carcinoma vulva is multifocal in:
   a. 3% b. 5%
   c. 7% d. 9%
4. Involvement of clitoris in carcinoma vulva is seen in:
   a. 5–15% b. 18–20%
   c. 20–25% d. 30%
5. Most common site of synchronous malignancy in carcinoma vulva is:
   a. Vagina b. Endometrium
   c. Ovary d. Cervix
6. Most common histopathology seen in carcinoma vulva is:
   a. Squamous cell carcinoma
   b. Basal cell carcinoma
   c. Adenocarcinoma
   d. Melanoma
7. Involvement of lower urethra is which stage as per FIGO?
   a. Stage I b. Stage II
   c. Stage III d. Stage IV
8. In Stage I disease, lymphadenectomy can be avoided, if invasion is:
   a. <1 mm b. <2 mm
   c. < 3 mm d. <4 mm
9. First node to receive lymphatics from a lateral vulvar lesion is usually is:
   a. Ipsilateral superficial inguinal node
   b. Contralateral superficial inguinal node
   c. Ipsilateral deep inguinal node
   d. Contralateral deep inguinal node
10. All are indications for adjuvant RT to groin and pelvis, except:
    a. ≥2 microscopically positive groin nodes
    b. ≥1 macroscopically involved lymph nodes
    c. Evidence of extracapsular spread
    d. ≥1 microscopically positive groin nodes
11. All are prognostic factors, except:
    a. Grade
    b. Lymphnode metastasis
    c. Depth of lesion/invasion
    d. Site

Answers

1.	c	2.	c	3.	b	4.	a	5.	d	6.	a
7.	b	8.	a	9.	a	10.	d	11.	d		

14.3 INTRAEPITHELIAL DISEASE OF THE CERVIX

Nikhil Parwate, Sabina Hasan Ali Moman

INTRODUCTION

Cervical cancer is a major public health problem in India with an incidence of 122,844 cases and mortality of 67,477 cases every year. Carcinoma cervix is the second most common gynecological malignancy among Indian women aged 25–44 years with an incidence of 3.5% after carcinoma breast (28.6%).

Almost all cervical cancer cases (99%) are linked to infection with high-risk human papillomaviruses (HPV), an extremely common virus transmitted through sexual contact. Although most infections with HPV resolve spontaneously and cause no symptoms, persistent infection can cause cervical cancer in women.

Cervical cancer is the fourth most common cancer in women. In 2018, an estimated 570,000 women were diagnosed with cervical cancer worldwide and about 311,000 women died from the disease.

Effective primary (HPV vaccination) and secondary prevention approaches (screening for, and treating precancerous lesions) will prevent most cervical cancer cases.

When diagnosed, cervical cancer is one of the most successfully treatable forms of cancer, as long as it is detected early and managed effectively. Cancers diagnosed in late stages can also be controlled with appropriate treatment and palliative care.

With a comprehensive approach to prevent, screen, and treat, cervical cancer can be eliminated as a public health problem within a generation.

HISTORY

The concept of cervical cancer precursors dates back to the late 19th century, when areas of noninvasive atypical epithelial changes were recognized in tissue specimens adjacent to invasive cancers. The term carcinoma in situ (CIS) was introduced in 1932 to denote those lesions in which the undifferentiated carcinomatous cells involved the full thickness of the epithelium, without disruption of the basement membrane.

The association between CIS and invasive cervical cancer was subsequently reported.

The term dysplasia was introduced in the late 1950s to designate the cervical epithelial atypia that is intermediate between the normal epithelium and CIS.

Dysplasia was further categorized into three groups—mild, moderate, and severe—depending on the degree of involvement of the epithelial thickness by the atypical cells.

Subsequently, for many years, cervical precancerous lesions were reported using the categories of dysplasia and CIS, and are still widely used in many developing countries.

A system of classification with separate classes for dysplasia and CIS was increasingly perceived as an arbitrary configuration, based upon the findings from a number of follow-up studies involving women with such lesions. It was observed that some cases of dysplasia regressed, some persisted and others progressed to CIS. A direct correlation with progression and histological grade was observed.

These observations led to the concept of a single, continuous disease process by which normal epithelium evolves into epithelial precursor lesions and on to invasive cancer.

On the basis of the above observations, the term cervical intraepithelial neoplasia (CIN) was introduced in 1968 to denote the whole range of cellular atypia confined to the epithelium. CIN was divided into grades 1, 2, and 3.

CIN 1 corresponded to mild dysplasia, CIN 2 to moderate dysplasia, and CIN 3 corresponded to both severe dysplasia and CIS.

ETIOPATHOGENESIS

Epidemiological studies have identified a number of risk factors that contribute to the development of cervical cancer precursors and cervical cancer.

These include infection with certain oncogenic types of HPV, sexual intercourse at an early age, multiple sexual partners, multiparity, long-term oral contraceptive use, tobacco smoking, low-socioeconomic status, infection with *Chlamydia trachomatis*, micronutrient deficiency, and a diet deficient in vegetables and fruits. HPV types 16, 18, 31, 33, 35, 39, 45, 51, 52, 56, 58, 59, and 68 are strongly associated with CIN and invasive cancer.

Persistent infection with one or more of the above oncogenic types is considered to be a necessary cause for cervical neoplasia.

HPV DNA was detected in 99.7% of 1,000 evaluable cervical cancer biopsy specimens obtained from 22 countries. HPV 16 and 18 are the main viral genotypes found in cervical cancers worldwide. Several cohort (follow-up) studies have reported a strong association between persistent oncogenic HPV infection and high risk of developing CIN.

Human papillomaviruses infection is transmitted through sexual contact and the risk factors, therefore are closely related to sexual behavior (e.g., lifetime number of sexual partners, sexual intercourse at an early age). In most women, HPV infections are transient.

- The natural history of HPV infection has been extensively reviewed. Although the prevalence of HPV infection varies in different regions of the world, it generally reaches a peak of about 20–30% among women aged 20–24 years, with a subsequent decline to approximately 3–10% among women aged over 30 years. About 80% of young women who become infected with HPV have transient infections that clear up within 12–18 months.
- HPV infection is believed to start in the basal cells or parabasal cells of the metaplastic epithelium. If the infection persists, integration of viral genome into the host cellular genome may occur.
- The normal differentiation and maturation of the immature squamous metaplastic into the mature squamous metaplastic epithelium may be disrupted as a result of expression of E6/E7 oncoproteins and the loss of normal growth control.
- This may then lead to development of abnormal dysplastic epithelium.
- If the neoplastic process continues uninterrupted, the early low-grade lesions may eventually involve the full thickness of the epithelium.
- Subsequently the disease may traverse the basement membrane and become invasive cancer, extending to surrounding tissues and organs.
- The invasion may then affect blood and lymphatic vessels and the disease may spread to the lymph nodes and distant organs.

CERVICAL ANATOMY

The cervix is composed of columnar epithelium, which lines the endocervical canal, and squamous epithelium, which covers the exocervix. The point at which they meet is called the squamocolumnar junction (SCJ).

The Squamocolumnar Junction

- The SCJ appears as a sharp line with a step, due to the difference in the height of the squamous and columnar epithelium. The location of the SCJ in relation to the external os is variable over a woman's lifetime and depends upon factors such as age, hormonal status, birth trauma, oral contraceptive use, and certain physiological conditions such as pregnancy. The SCJ visible during childhood, perimenarche, after puberty, and early reproductive period is referred to as the original SCJ, as this represents the junction between the columnar epithelium and the "original" squamous epithelium laid down during embryogenesis and intrauterine life.

- During childhood and perimenarche, the original SCJ is located at, or very close to, the external os.
- After puberty and during the reproductive period, the female genital organs grow under the influence of estrogen. Thus, the cervix swells and enlarges and the endocervical canal elongates. This leads to the eversion of the columnar epithelium of the lower part of the endocervical canal on to the ectocervix. This condition is called ectropion or ectopy, which is visible as a strikingly reddish-looking ectocervix on visual inspection.
- It is sometimes called "erosion" or "ulcer", which are misnomers and should not be used to denote this condition. Thus, the original SCJ is located on the ectocervix, far away from the external os. Ectropion becomes much more pronounced during pregnancy.

  The buffer action of the mucus covering the columnar cells is interfered with when the everted columnar epithelium in ectropion is exposed to the acidic vaginal environment.
- This leads to the destruction and eventual replacement of the columnar epithelium by the newly formed metaplastic squamous epithelium.
- Metaplasia refers to the change or replacement of one type of epithelium by another. The metaplastic process mostly starts at the original SCJ and proceeds centripetally toward the external os through the reproductive period to perimenopause. Thus, a new SCJ is formed between the newly formed metaplastic squamous epithelium and the columnar epithelium remaining everted onto the ectocervix.
- As the woman passes from the reproductive to the perimenopausal age group, the location of the new SCJ progressively moves on the ectocervix toward the external os.

Hence, it is located at variable distances from the external os, as a result of the progressive formation of the new metaplastic squamous epithelium in the exposed areas of the columnar epithelium in the ectocervix. From the perimenopausal period and after the onset of menopause, the cervix shrinks due the lack of estrogen, and consequently, the movement of the new SCJ toward the external os and into the endocervical canal is accelerated. In postmenopausal women, the new SCJ is often invisible on visual examination.

The new SCJ is hereafter simply referred to as SCJ in this manual. Reference to the original SCJ will be explicitly made as the original SCJ.

Transformation Zone

- The region of cervix where the columnar epithelium has been replaced and/or is being
- Replaced by the new metaplastic squamous epithelium is referred to as the Transformation zone (TZ) **(Fig. 1)**.
- It corresponds to the area of cervix bound by the original SCJ at the distal end and proximally by the furthest extent that squamous metaplasia has occurred as defined by the new SCJ.
- Histologically, it is the zone of metaplasia or transitional epithelium.
- In premenopausal women, the TZ is fully located on the ectocervix.

After menopause, the cervix shrinks with the decreasing levels of estrogen and hence TZ may move partially and later completely into the cervical canal.

It is the most important cytologic and colposcopic landmark, as this is where 90% of cervical neoplasia occurs.

Types of Transformation Zone

- *Type 1:* When the TZ is completely visible on cervix.
- *Type 2:* TZ is partially visible on ectocervix and partially in endocervical canal.
- *Type 3:* Complete TZ is not visible even with colposcope and manipulation.
- *Type 4:* TZ extends caudally to upper vagina called the congenital TZ, fine mosaic may be present, may partially stain with Lugol's iodine.

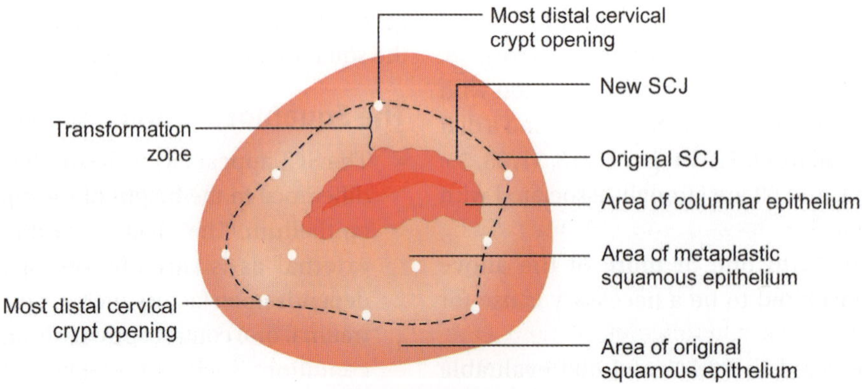

Fig. 1: Transformation zone.
(SCJ: squamocolumnar junction)

Transformation zone will show following landmarks on colposcopy: Nabothian cyts, island of columnar epithelium, glandular openings with secretions, mature squamous epithelium, and squamous metaplasia.

Human Papillomavirus

Persistent infection with oncogenic types of HPV has been shown to be the necessary cause of cervical cancer.

About 6.6% of Indian women in the general population have HPV infection at any given time. Most of the time, HPV infection does not cause any manifestations and is self-limited. It has been observed that approximately 70% of all newly acquired HPV infections are cleared within 1 year, and approximately another 20% in the next 1 year. In some women infection persists and may cause cervical cancer and other manifestations including oropharyngeal cancers, anogenital cancers, and genital warts.

Human papillomavirus is a nonenveloped, small, double stranded DNA of the family papilloma viridae. The viral genome consists of 7,200–8,000 base pairs and the early fragments of the genome regulates DNA replication (e1, e2), transcription (e2) and cell transformation (e5, e6, e7) and late fragments (l1 and l2) encode structural proteins of the virion. Purified l1 protein form empty shells resembling a virus, called Virus-like Particles (VlPs).

Human papillomaviruses are largely nonlytic and restricted to the epithelium. Antibodies will be formed in serum against many different viral proteins. The most characterized antibodies formed are those directed against conformational epitopes of the l1 capsid and detectable antibodies are not found in all infected persons. In a study by Carter et al., 54–69% of women who were found to be infected with HPV 6, 16, or 18 infections had type-specific antibody.

More than 100 types of HPV have been recognized on the basis of DNA sequence showing genomic differences. infection with HPV types 1 and 2 cause warts in some individuals while HPV-5 may cause lifelong infection without any clinical manifestation. Infection with HPV types 6 and 11 can cause laryngeal papillomatosis and genital warts. HPV types 16, 18, 31, 33, 35, 39, 45, 51, 52, 56, 58, 59, 68, 73, and 82 are considered to be carcinogenic. HPV 16 and 18 are high-risk types and account for over 75% of invasive cervical cancers in South Asia.

In India approximately 80% of cervical cancer and 63% of high-grade cervical lesions are linked with infection due to HPV 16 and 18. age and sexual activity are the major influencing factors for HPV transmission. About 75% of sexually active individuals harbor at least one HPV type. Risk of HPV infection can be reduced by an HPV type-specific targeted vaccine. Abstinence or lifetime mutual monogamy is helpful in preventing genital HPV infection. There is limited evidence to suggest the protective role of condoms and male circumcision against HPV infection.

DIAGNOSIS AND GRADING OF CIN BY HISTOPATHOLOGY

Cervical intraepithelial neoplasia may be suspected through cytological examination using the Papanicolaou technique or through colposcopic examination. Final diagnosis of CIN is established by the histopathological examination of a cervical punch biopsy or excision specimen. A judgment of whether or not a cervical tissue specimen reveals CIN, and to what degree, is dependent on the histological features concerned with differentiation, maturation and stratification of cells and nuclear abnormalities. The proportion of the thickness of the epithelium showing mature and differentiated cells is used for grading CIN. More severe degrees of CIN are likely to have a greater proportion of the thickness of epithelium composed of undifferentiated cells, with only a narrow layer of mature, differentiated cells on the surface.

Nuclear abnormalities such as enlarged nuclei, increased nuclear-cytoplasmic ratio, increased intensity of nuclear staining (hyperchromasia), nuclear polymorphism, and variation in nuclear size (anisokaryosis) are assessed when a diagnosis is being made. There is often a strong correlation between the proportion of epithelium revealing maturation and the degree of nuclear abnormality. Mitotic figures are seen in cells that are in cell division; they are infrequent in normal epithelium and, if present, they are seen only in the parabasal layer. As the severity of CIN increases, the number of mitotic figures also increases; these may be seen in the superficial layers of the epithelium. The less is the differentiation in an epithelium, the higher is the level at which mitotic figures are likely to be seen. Abnormal configurations of mitotic figures also are taken into account in arriving at final diagnosis.

In CIN 1, there is good maturation with minimal nuclear abnormalities and few mitotic figures. Undifferentiated cells are confined to the deeper layers (lower third) of the epithelium. Mitotic figures are present, but not very numerous. Cytopathic changes due to HPV infection may be observed in the full thickness of the epithelium.

CIN 2 is characterized by dysplastic cellular changes mostly restricted to the lower half or the lower two- thirds of the epithelium, with more marked nuclear abnormalities than in CIN 1. Mitotic figures may be seen throughout the lower half of the epithelium.

In CIN 3, differentiation and stratification may be totally absent or present only in the superficial quarter of the epithelium with numerous mitotic figures. Nuclear abnormalities extend throughout the thickness of the epithelium. Many mitotic figures have abnormal forms.

A close interaction between cytologists, histopathologists, and colposcopists improves reporting in all three disciplines. This particularly helps in differentiating milder degrees of CIN from other conditions with which there can be confusion **(Table 1)**.

TABLE 1: Comparison of cytology and histological classification systems.

Cytological classification (used for screening)		*Histological classification (used for diagnosis)*	
Pap	Bethesda system	CIN	WHO descriptive classifications
Class I	Normal	Normal	Normal
Class II	ASC-US ASC-H	Atypia	Atypia
Class II	LSIL	CIN 1 including flat condyloma	Koilocytosis
Class III	HSIL	CIN 2	Moderate dysplasia
Class III	HSIL	CIN 3	Severe dysplasia
Class IV	HSIL	CIN 3	Carcinoma in situ
Class V	Invasive carcinoma	Invasive carcinoma	Invasive carcinoma

(ASC-US: atypical squamous cells—undetermined significance; ASC-H: atypical squamous cells—cannot rule out high grade squamous intraepithelial lesion; CIN: cervical intraepithelial neoplasia; HSIL: high grade squamous intraepithelial lesion; LSIL: low grade squamous intraepithelial lesion)

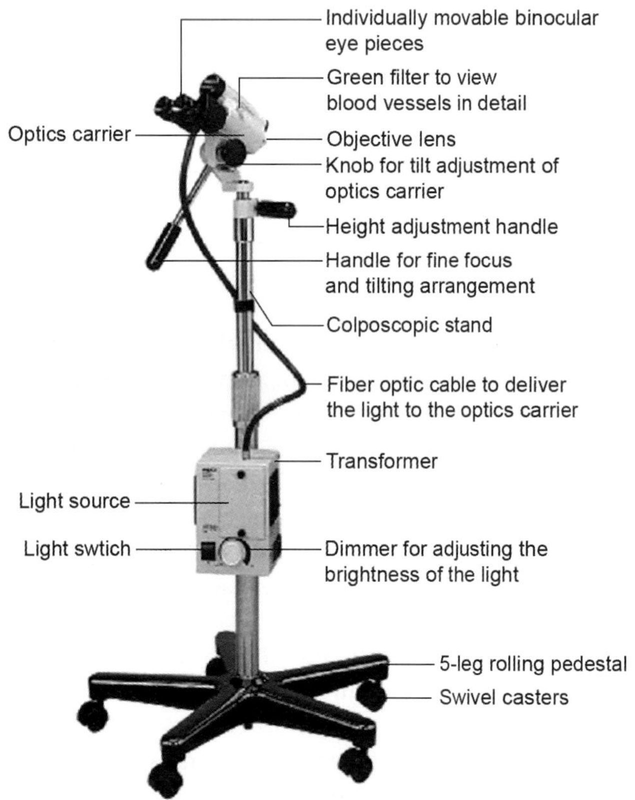

Fig. 2: Colposcope.

COLPOSCOPY

- A colposcope **(Fig. 2)** is a low-power, stereoscopic, binocular field microscope with a powerful light source used for magnified visual examination of the uterine cervix to help in the diagnosis of cervical neoplasia.
- The most common indication of referral for colposcopy is positive screening tests [e.g., positive cytology, positive on visual inspection with acetic acid (VIA), etc.]. The management protocol for VIA positive lesions is outlined in **Flowchart 1**.
- The key ingredients of colposcopic examination are the observation of features of the cervical epithelium after application of normal saline, 3–5% dilute acetic acid, and Lugol's iodine solution in successive steps.
- The characteristics of acetowhite changes, if any, on the cervix following the application of dilute acetic acid are useful in colposcopic interpretation and in directing biopsies.
- The color changes in the cervix following the application of Lugol's iodine solution, depends on the presence or absence of glycogen in the epithelial cells. Areas containing glycogen turn brown or black; areas lacking glycogen remain colorless or pale or turn mustard or saffron yellow.

Instruments in Colposcopy

Colposcopy is an outpatient procedure requiring basic instrumentation. The detailed list is given in **Table 2**. The instruments are illustrated in **Figures 3 to 8** and the arrangement is shown in **Figure 9**.

Indications for Colposcopy

- Suspicious-looking cervix invasive carcinoma on cytology
- *CIN 2 or CIN 3 on cytology:* Persisting (for more than 12–18 months) low-grade (CIN 1) abnormalities on cytology CIN 1 on cytology
- Persistently unsatisfactory quality on cytology
- Infection with oncogenic HPV
- Acetopositivity on visual inspection with acetic acid (VIA)
- Acetopositivity on VIA using magnification (VIAM)
- Positive on visual inspection with Lugol's iodine (VILI).

Principles of Acetic Acid Test

The other key ingredient in colposcopic practice, 3–5% acetic acid, is usually applied with a cotton applicator (cotton balls held by sponge forceps, or large rectal or small swabs) or with a small sprayer. It helps in coagulating and clearing the mucus. Acetic acid is thought to cause swelling of the epithelial tissue, columnar and any abnormal squamous epithelial areas in particular. It causes a reversible coagulation or precipitation of the nuclear proteins and cytokeratins. Thus, the effect of acetic acid depends upon the amount of nuclear proteins and cytokeratins present in the epithelium. When acetic acid

Flowchart 1: Screening by VIA.

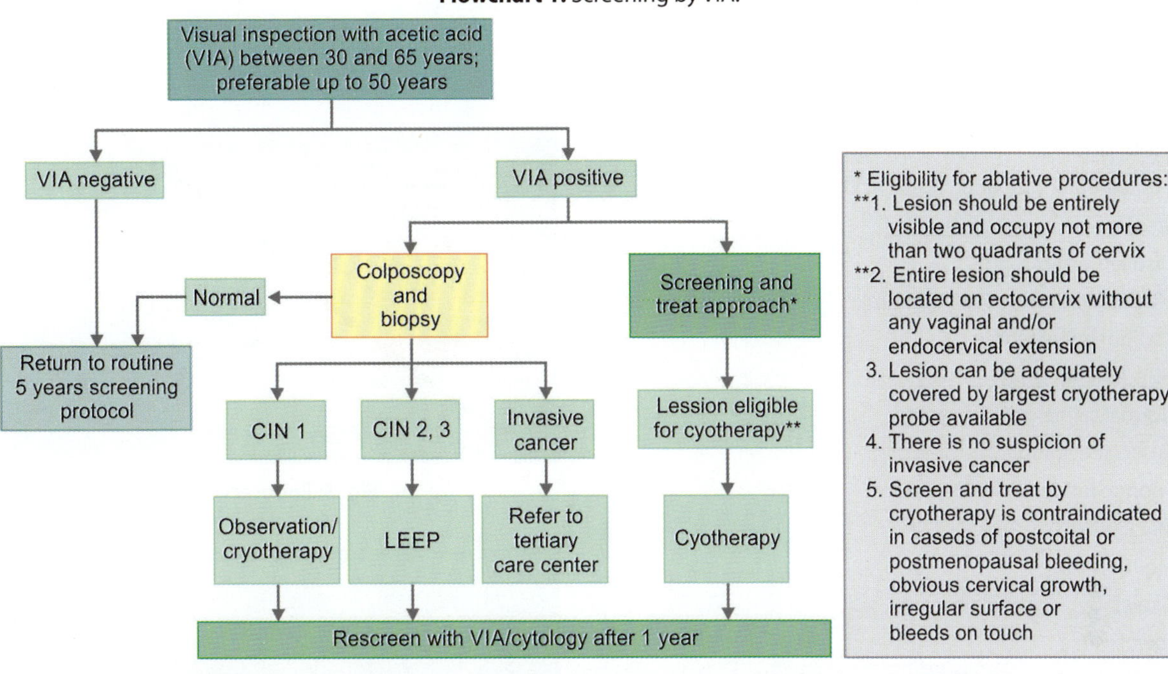

(CIN: cervical intraepithelial neoplasia; LEEP: loop electrosurgical excision procedure)

is applied to normal squamous epithelium, little coagulation occurs in the superficial cell layer, as this is sparsely nucleated. Though the deeper cells contain more nuclear protein, the acetic acid may not penetrate sufficiently and, hence, the resulting precipitation is not sufficient to obliterate the color of the underlying stroma. Areas of CIN undergo maximal coagulation due to their higher content of nuclear protein and prevent light from passing through the epithelium. As a result, the subepithelial vessel pattern is obliterated and less easy to see and the epithelium appears white. This reaction is termed acetowhitening, and produces a noticeable effect compared with the normal pinkish color of the surrounding normal squamous epithelium of the cervix, an effect that is commonly visible to the naked eye.

With low-grade CIN, the acetic acid must penetrate into the lower one-third of the epithelium (where most of the abnormal cells with high nuclear density are located). Hence, the appearance of the whiteness is delayed and less intense due to the smaller amount of nuclear protein compared to areas with high-grade CIN or preclinical invasive cancer. Areas of high-grade CIN and invasive cancer turn densely white and opaque immediately after application of acetic acid, due to their higher concentration of abnormal nuclear protein and the presence of large numbers of dysplastic cells in the superficial layers of the epithelium.

The acetowhite appearance is not unique to CIN and early cancer. It is also seen in other situations when increased nuclear protein is present, e.g., in immature squamous metaplasia, congenital transformation zone, in healing and regenerating epithelium (associated with inflammation), leukoplakia (hyperkeratosis), and condyloma. While the acetowhite epithelium associated with CIN and preclinical early invasive cancer is more dense, thick and opaque with well-demarcated margins from the surrounding normal epithelium, the acetowhitening associated with immature squamous metaplasia and regenerating epithelium is less pale, thin, often translucent, and patchily distributed without well-defined margins. Acetowhitening due to inflammation and healing is usually distributed widely in the cervix, not restricted to the transformation zone. The acetowhite changes associated with immature metaplasia and inflammatory changes quickly disappear, usually within 30–60 seconds.

Acetowhitening associated with CIN and invasive cancer quickly appears and persists for more than 1 minute. The acetic acid effect reverses much more slowly in high-grade CIN lesions and in early pre-clinical invasive cancer than in low-grade lesions, immature metaplasia and sub-clinical HPV changes. It may last for 2–4 minutes in the case of high-grade lesions and invasive cancer.

Acetowhitening also occurs in the vagina, external anogenital skin, and anal mucosa. The acetowhite reaction varies in intensity, within and between patients. The reaction is often associated with other visual signs in the same area, and is not specific for intraepithelial preneoplasia. Invasive cancer may or may not be acetowhite; it usually has other distinguishing features that will alert the colposcopist. For these reasons, practical training is necessary to develop knowledge, skills and experience in colposcopy. Learning colposcopy requires more supervised practice than most other endoscopic procedures, because of the microscopic interpretation that must occur *in vivo*, in addition to the technical aspects of the endoscopic procedure.

As previously stated, the main goal of colposcopy is to detect the presence of high-grade CIN and invasive cancer.

TABLE 2: Instruments required for colposcopy.

1.	Drum-autoclaved (with speculum, sponge-holding forceps, steel bowl, green towel)
2.	Drum-autoclaved containing sterile cotton balls
3.	Acetic acid
4.	Container for preparing acetic acid solution
5.	Steel bowl
6.	Distilled water
7.	Measuring cylinder, syringe: 5 mL
8.	Sodium hypochlorite
9.	70% ethanol spray
10.	Normal saline
11.	Cusco speculum
12.	Sponge holder
13.	Mackintosh
14.	Mouth mask
15.	Gloves
16.	Towel
17.	Dustbins 3
18.	Disposable bags
19.	Gloves boxes 3, plastic gloves (if required)
20.	Boiler with plug
21.	Writing pad/board with clip for holding the forms
22.	Address cards, prescription pad
23.	Table/trolley
24.	Table fan
25.	Trolley, green towel
26.	Cryo machine with probe and filled N2O cylinder (optional)
27.	Extension board (for boiling instruments)
28.	Torch-2, extra cells (LED torch preferably with four batteries)
29.	Register for keeping log
30.	Gynec examination table, stool, writing table, chairs, hand sanitizer/soap, etc.
31.	Consent forms to be signed by the beneficiaries
32.	Client record sheet

(LED: light-emitting diode; VIA: visual inspection with acetic acid)

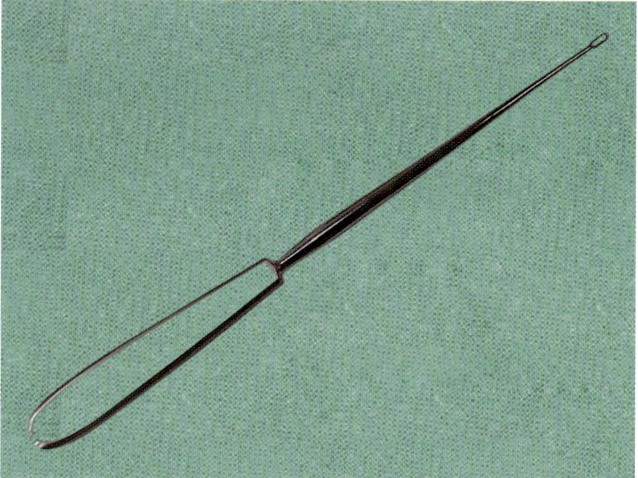

Fig. 3: Endocervical curette.

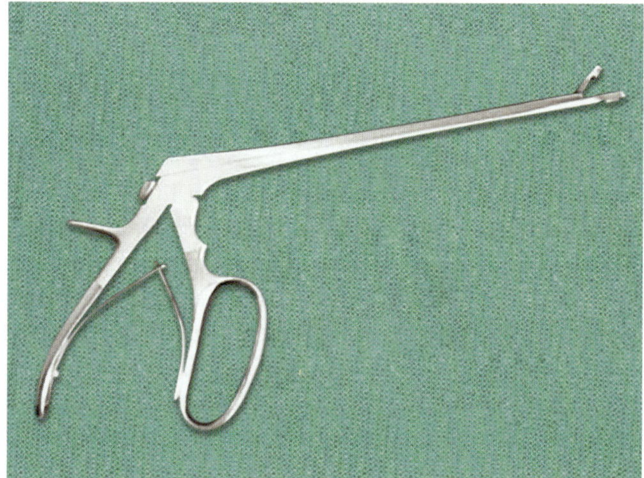

Fig. 4: Cervical punch biopsy forcep with sharp cutting edges.

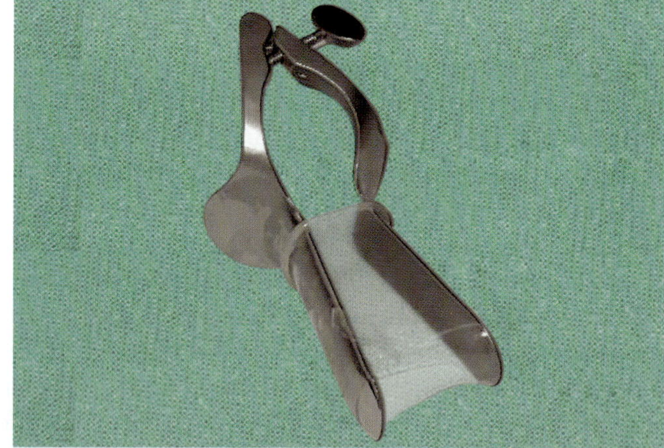

Fig. 5: Vaginal speculum covered with a latex condom.

To effectively achieve this, the entire epithelium at risk should be well visualized, abnormalities should be identified accurately and assessed for their degree of abnormality, and appropriate biopsies must be taken. The colposcopic documentation and the biopsies taken by a colposcopist are important indicators for quality management in colposcopy clinics.

Principles of Schiller's (Lugol's) Iodine Test

The principle behind the iodine test is that original and newly formed mature squamous metaplastic epithelium is glycogenated, whereas CIN and invasive cancer contain little or no glycogen. Columnar epithelium does not contain glycogen. Immature squamous metaplastic epithelium usually lacks glycogen or, occasionally, may be partially glycogenated. Iodine is glycophilic and hence the application of iodine solution results in uptake of iodine in glycogen-containing epithelium. Therefore, the normal glycogen-containing

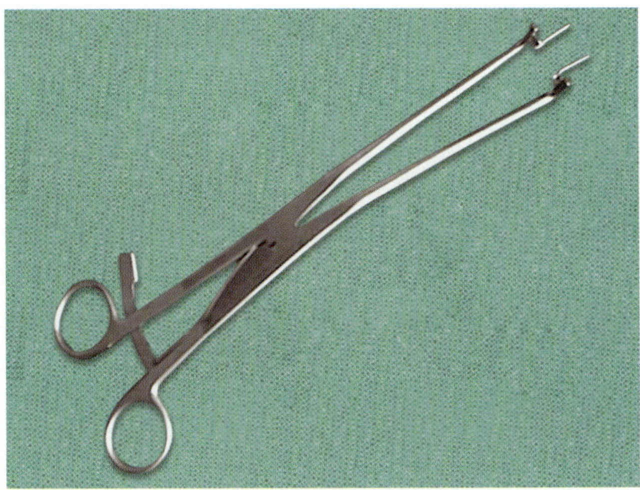
Fig. 6: Endocervical speculum.

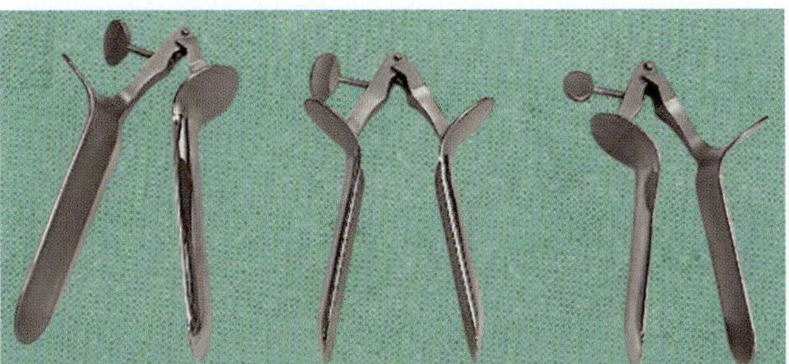
Fig. 7: Collins bivalve speculum of different sizes.

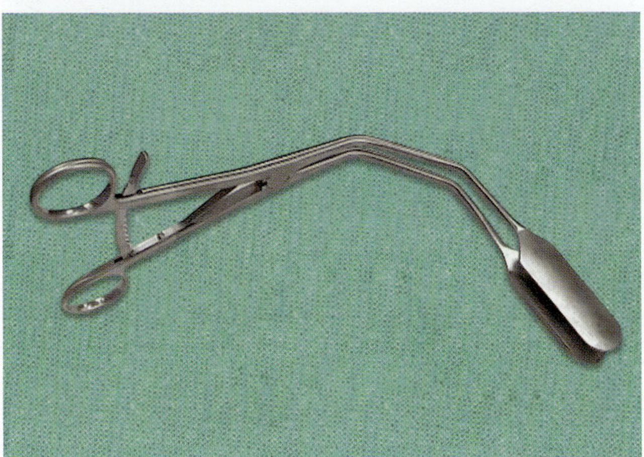
Fig. 8: Vaginal side wall retractor.

squamous epithelium stains mahogany brown or black after application of iodine. Columnar epithelium does not take up iodine and remains unstained, but may look slightly discolored due to a thin film of iodine solution; areas of immature squamous metaplastic epithelium may remain unstained with iodine or may be only partially stained. If there is shedding (or erosion) of superficial and intermediate cell layers associated with inflammatory conditions of the squamous epithelium, these areas do not stain with iodine and remain distinctly colorless in a surrounding black or brown background. Areas of CIN and invasive cancer do

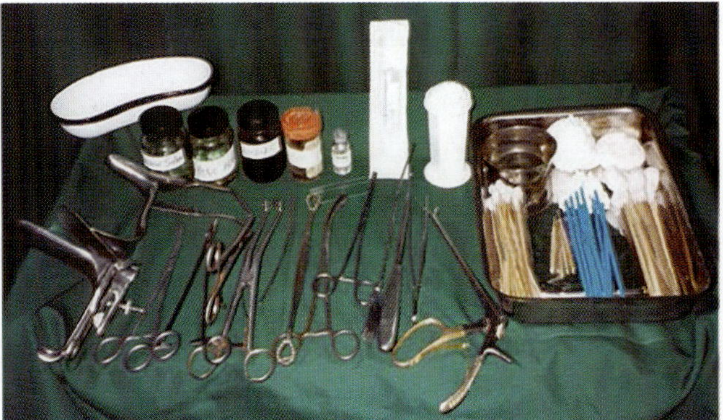
Fig. 9: Colposcopy trolley.

not take up iodine (as they lack glycogen) and appear as thick mustard yellow or saffron-colored areas. Areas with leukoplakia (hyperkeratosis) do not stain with iodine. Condyloma may not, or occasionally may only partially, stain with iodine. We recommend the routine use of iodine application in colposcopic practice as this may help in identifying lesions overlooked during examination with saline and acetic acid and will help in delineating the anatomical extent of abnormal areas much more clearly, thereby facilitating treatment.

Documentation of Colposcopic Findings

The record of colposcopic findings for each visit should be documented carefully by the colposcopists themselves, immediately after the examination. This record, which can be stored on paper or electronically, forms the backbone of any medical record system that can be used for continuing patient care and performance. An example of a colposcopy record containing the important attributes of a colposcopic assessment is shown in **Table 3**. Colposcopists or clinics can adapt this form to suit their needs; the structured format is intended to prompt the colposcopist to use quantitative data, whenever possible, and to capture qualitative data in a drawing. Colposcopists, even in the same clinic, generally record their findings in a wide variety of ways. Various experts have recommended standardized representations of colposcopic findings in a drawing; the symbolic representations suggested by René Cartier are a good example of what may be useful in this context.

Since an examination of the entire lower genital tract should be performed whenever a woman is referred for colposcopy, the colposcopist must be able to record the clinical findings in the vaginal, vulvar, perianal and anal epithelium. These findings can be combined with the cervical record on one page or kept on a separate page.

Examination Points

- It is important to explain the examination procedure and reassure the woman before colposcopy. This will ensure that the woman relaxes during the procedure.

TABLE 3: 2011 IFCPC Nomenclature.[1]

Accepted in Rio World Congress, July 5, 2011 Nomenclature Committee Chairman: Jacob Bornstein MD			
2011 IFCPC colposcopic terminology of the cervix[1]			
General assessment		• Adequate/inadequate for the reason... (i.e., cervix obscured by inflammation, bleeding, scar) • Squamo-columnar junction visibility: completely visible, partially visible, not visible • Transformation zone types 1, 2, 3	
Normal colposcopic findings		*Original squamous epithelium:* • Mature • Atrophic *Columnar epithelium:* Ectopy *Metaplastic squamous epithelium:* • Nabothian cysts • Crypt (gland) openings Deciduosis in pregnancy	
Abnormal colposcopic findings	General principles	*Location of the lesion*: Inside or outside the T-zone Location of the lesion by clock position *Size of the lesion:* Number of cervical quadrants the lesion covers Size of the lesion in percentage of cervix	
	Grade 1 (Minor)	Thin aceto white epithelium Irregular, geographic border	Fine mosaic Fine punctation
	Grade 2 (Major)	Dense aceto white epithelium Rapid appearance of acetowhitening Cuffed crypt (gland) openings	Coarse mosaic Coarse punctation Sharp border Inner border sign Ridge sign
	Nonspecific	Leukoplakia (keratos is, hyperkeratosis), Erosion Lugol's staining (Schiller's test): Stained/ non-stained	
Suspicious for invasion		Atypical vessels *Additional sign:* Fragile vessels, irregular surface, exophytic lesion, necrosis, ulceration (necrotic), tumor/gross neoplasm	
Miscellaneous finding		Congenital transformation zone Condyloma Polyp (Ectocervical/endocervical) Inflammation	Stenosis Congenital anomaly Post-treatment consequence Endometriosis

- Written informed consent should be obtained from the woman before the colposcopic examination.
- Relevant medical and reproductive history should be obtained before the procedure.
- A strict adherence to the essential steps involved in colposcopic examination ensures that common errors are avoided.
- It is important to visualize the SCJ in its entire circumference, otherwise, the colposcopic procedure is termed "unsatisfactory".
- One should identify the transformation zone (TZ) during the colposcopic procedure. The proximal limit of the TZ is defined by the SCJ, while the distal limit of the transformation zone is identified by finding the most distal crypt openings or nabothian follicles in the lips of the cervix and by drawing an imaginary line connecting these landmarks.
- It is essential to obtain directed biopsies, under colposcopic control, from abnormal/-suspicious areas identified.
- Colposcopy during pregnancy requires considerable experience. As pregnancy progresses, cervical biopsy is associated with increased probability and severity of bleeding, which is often difficult to control. The risk of biopsy should always be weighed against the risk of missing an early invasive cancer. Noninvasive lesions may be evaluated postpartum.

Explain the Procedure to the Woman

Women referred to a colposcopy clinic may not have had the procedure explained to them in detail before their arrival. For literate women, pamphlets on what an abnormal cervical cytology or other screening test means and an explanation of the colposcopic examination may be helpful. It is important for all women to have a prior explanation of the procedure and reassurance by the clinic nurse or the colposcopist. Colposcopic examination may prove difficult and yield suboptimal results if the woman does not relax during the procedure. Privacy during the consultation and examination is of utmost importance.

Obtain Informed Consent

After the procedure has been explained to the woman, written informed consent should be obtained, before colposcopy. The written consent form should include information about the colposcopic examination and the usual procedures that may accompany it, such as biopsy, endocervical curettage and photography, and summarize the usual complications (less serious and more frequent ones, as well as more serious but less frequent ones) that may occur. It may be preferable to obtain informed consent each time, if a woman requires subsequent colposcopic examinations.

Obtain a Relevant Medical History

The woman's medical history is usually taken after her written informed consent has been obtained. Most women are referred after a screening examination and it is ideal to have the result of the screening test available at the time of colposcopic examination. If the woman has been referred because of abnormal cytology results, it is ideal to have a written copy of the previous smear(s) on hand at the time of the colposcopy appointment. Relevant obstetric and gynecological history and history of any relevant exposures (e.g., number of pregnancies, last menstrual period, history of oral contraceptive use, hormonal supplements, sexually transmitted infections, etc.) should be obtained and recorded with the aid of a form designed for this purpose. It is important to enquire about the last menstrual period in order to assess the possibility of pregnancy or menopause.

Insert the Vaginal Speculum and Inspect the Cervix

The woman should be in a modified lithotomy position on an examining table with heel rests, or stirrups or knee crutches. It is preferable to place the buttocks slightly over the end of the table. It is important to ask the woman to relax. Positioning the buttocks in this way makes it much easier to insert the speculum and to manipulate it in different axes, if needs be. An instrument tray with essential instruments for colposcopy is placed beside the couch. A medium-size bivalve speculum (Cusco, Grave, Collin's or Pedersen's) is usually adequate. Warm, clean water on the speculum is the preferred lubricant, as it warms the metal, but does not interfere with the interpretation of cervical specimens, such as a cytology smear. If the woman has extremely lax vaginal walls, a lateral vaginal side-wall retractor or a latex condom on the speculum (with the tip of the condom cut 1 cm from the nipple) is helpful. Particular care should be taken to align the blades of the vaginal side-wall retractor perpendicular to the vaginal speculum to prevent vaginal pinching. The skills for this maneuver come with practice. In very obese women, it may be preferable to use two Sim's specula to retract the anterior and posterior vaginal walls.

Once the speculum is inserted and the blades are widely separated, a good view of the cervix and the vaginal fornices is obtained. This may also result in some eversion of the lips of the multiparous cervix, allowing the lower portion of the endocervical canal to come into view. After exposing the cervix, one should assess the nature of the cervico-vaginal secretions and note any obvious findings such as ectropion, polyp, nabothian follicles, congenital transformation zone, atrophy, inflammation and infection, leukoplakia (hyperkeratosis), condylomata, ulcer, growth and any obvious lesions in the vaginal fornices. Following this, excess mucus should be removed gently rom the cervix with saline-soaked cotton swabs. Swabbing with dry cotton balls is discouraged, as these may induce traumatic bleeding and subepithelial petechiae. Loss of epithelium and bleeding due to rough and traumatic manipulation of the speculum and swabs should be avoided.

Apply Normal Saline Solution

Normal saline is applied to the cervix with a sprayer or cotton balls and excess liquid is removed afterward. This is not only the ideal way to conduct a preliminary inspection for surface abnormalities (e.g., leukoplakia, condylomata), but also the best way to examine the detail of cervical capillaries and surface blood vessels. The examination of the blood vessels is further aided by using the green (or blue) filter on the colposcope to enhance the contrast of the vessels, and by using higher levels of magnification (about 15 ×). Although some experienced colposcopists do not routinely perform an examination after saline has been applied (instead going directly to the application of acetic acid), it has been argued that an examination should be done in all cases, since the information obtained on the location of abnormal vessels can be noted and integrated with the findings from later steps, which will determine the appropriate biopsy site(s), if any. The application of acetic acid, and even Lugol's iodine solution, to the cervix can result in tissue swelling and consequent opacity. This swelling and opacity tend to obscure some of the details of the vessels in the subepithelial tissue, so it is always best to assess the capillaries and vessels with saline before the application of any other solution.

The other important task at this step is to identify the distal and proximal borders of the TZ. The inner border is defined by the entire 360-degree circumference of the SCJ. If the junction is proximal to the external os, in the canal, it requires additional effort to visualize the entire junction. Opening the blades of the vaginal speculum and using a cotton-tipped applicator to pry the anterior lip up or the posterior lip down will often allow visualization if the junction is close enough to the os.

Apply Acetic Acid

This step may be carried out using 3–5% dilute glacial acetic acid. We prefer to use 5% dilute acetic acid as the acetowhite changes may occur faster and be more obvious than with a 3–4% solution. If white table vinegar is used, it is usually 5% acetic acid, but it is preferable to confirm the strength of the solution. The two main purposes of applying acetic acid are, first, to conduct another inspection of the entire new SCJ and second, to detect and evaluate any areas of abnormal or atypical transformation zone (ATZ). Acetic acid should be liberally applied to the cervix with a cotton-tipped swab or cotton balls or using a 2 × 2 inches gauze or with a sprayer so that it covers the entire cervical surface, including the external os.

Wiping the cervix a few times with a cotton ball or other large applicator assists in the coagulation and removal of mucus, which in turn helps the acetic acid to penetrate to the epithelium in full strength. The mucus in the canal may be difficult to extract, but it can be easily and temporarily pushed into the os with an acetic acid–soaked cotton swab, particularly if it is obscuring the assessment of an important feature, such as the SCJ. In the latter case, the swab also helps to apply the acid to the area of the SCJ, which may be just inside the os, and can also be used to manipulate the cervix to view otherwise hidden areas of interest. Patience is required during this step because the acetowhitening effect of acetic acid develops gradually over the course of 60 seconds and the effect may fade afterward. Hence, acetic acid may be reapplied every 2–3 minutes during the examination. A swab may be used to reapply, using the acetic acid pooled in the posterior aspect of the vagina.

Apply Lugol's Iodine Solution

Normal squamous (both original and mature metaplastic) epithelial cells contain stores of glycogen that give a mahogany brown or nearly black stain when an iodine-containing solution, such as Lugol's, is applied. In contrast, normal columnar epithelium does not contain glycogen and does not take up the iodine stain. Similarly, immature squamous metaplasia, inflammatory and regenerating epithelium and congenital TZ contain very little or no glycogen and either do not or only partially stain with iodine. Condylomata also either do not or only partially stain with iodine. Abnormal TZ, such as those with CIN or invasive cancer, contain very little or no glycogen. The degree of differentiation of the cells in a preneoplastic squamous lesion determines the amount of intracellular glycogen and thus the degree of staining observed. Therefore, one would expect to see a range of staining from partially brown to mustard yellow across the spectrum from low- to high-grade CIN. Usually, high-grade CIN takes up less of the stain, appearing as mustard or saffron yellow areas. In the case of high-grade CIN, vigorous or repeated application of iodine may occasionally peel off the abnormal epithelium and the underlying tissue stroma may appear pale, as it lacks glycogen.

It is important always to integrate the findings of the saline, acetic acid, and iodine tests to make a colposcopic assessment. The iodine test is also very helpful for determining whether vaginal lesions are present. Application of iodine will clearly delineate the borders of a lesion before a biopsy, or treatment of the lesion, is attempted.

Perform Cervical Biopsies, if Necessary

Once an abnormal TZ is detected, the area is evaluated and compared with other areas of the cervix. If any other abnormal zones are present, the colposcopist should then decide from where a biopsy or biopsies should be taken. It is essential to obtain one or more directed punch biopsies from areas colposcopically identified as abnormal and/or doubtful. Biopsy should be obtained from the area of the lesion with worst features and closest to the SCJ. Biopsy always should be done under colposcopic control by firmly applying the biopsy instrument, with the jaws wide open, to the cervical surface to be sampled. The cervix may move back somewhat with this maneuver, but that is normal.

To obtain a tissue sample, the biopsy forceps is guided under colposcopic visualization to the area from which the tissue specimen is to be obtained. The cervix may tend to slip away on pressure, but it is usually easy to grasp and remove tissue, if the forceps used for biopsy has wide and sharp cutting edges, with one or two teeth to anchor the forceps while taking the biopsy. A tenaculum may be also used to fix the cervix before taking the biopsy. The jaws are then closed completely, and the specimen is removed and immediately placed in formalin. The biopsy performed should be deep enough to obtain adequate stroma, in order to exclude invasion. Cutting the specimen should be carried out by quick and firm closure of the jaws. Repeated cutting and rotation of the forceps should be avoided, as they can crush the tissue sample. The procedure is usually painless if carried out efficiently using a sharp and toothed biopsy forceps. A skin hook is sometimes useful to anchor a potential biopsy site if it is difficult to grasp with the biopsy instrument. After the biopsy has been obtained, it is advisable to indicate the site of the target area which has been biopsied, on the diagram of cervix in the reporting form. It is important to place the freshly obtained biopsy specimen in a labeled bottle containing 10% formalin. The biopsy site(s) may be cauterized with Monsel's paste or with a silver nitrate stick immediately after the procedure to control any bleeding.

Apply Monsel's Paste after Biopsy

It is usual practice to ensure hemostasis by applying Monsel's (ferric subsulfate) paste to the biopsy site. This is done by gently applying pressure with a cotton-tipped applicator, the tip of which has been coated with Monsel's paste. Monsel's solution is the most common hemostatic agent used after cervical biopsy or excision, and it performs well when it has a thick, toothpaste-like consistency. The paste-like consistency may be produced by exposing the stock solution to the air in a small container, which results in evaporation and thickening of the agent, or using a microwave oven. The paste-like consistency may be preserved by keeping the paste in a closed container and by adding small amount of Monsel's solution whenever it becomes dry and excessively thick.

A silver nitrate stick can also be used to cauterize a biopsy site. The hemostatic action of these chemicals is much better if the chemical is applied promptly, before bleeding begins, allowing direct contact of the chemical with the tissue rather than with blood.

Perform Endocervical Curettage, if Necessary

There are three commonly encountered circumstances, in which an endocervical curettage (ECC) should be performed using an endocervical curette. First, if the colposcopic examination of the ectocervix has not revealed any abnormality, yet the woman has been referred because of a cytological abnormality, an ECC should be performed to properly evaluate the endocervical canal, which may contain a hidden invasive cancer or other lesion. Second, if the referral cytology indicated that a glandular lesion may be present, an ECC should be performed (regardless of the findings of the colposcopic examination). Third, an ECC should be performed if the colposcopic examination has been unsatisfactory.

COLPOSCOPIC ASSESSMENT OF CERVICAL INTRAEPITHELIAL NEOPLASIA

- The colposcopic diagnosis of cervical neoplasia depends on the recognition of four main features: (1) intensity (color tone) of acetowhitening, (2) margins and surface contour of acetowhite areas, (3) vascular features, and (4) color changes after iodine application.
- The occurrence of abnormal features in a localized area in the transformation zone increases the probability of diagnosis of a neoplastic lesion.
- Considerable skill may be required to differentiate between low-grade CIN, immature squamous metaplasia and inflammatory lesions.
- Biopsy should be directed whenever in doubt.
- The observation of well-demarcated, dense, opaque, acetowhite area(s) in the transformation zone close to or abutting the SCJ is the hallmark of colposcopic diagnosis of CIN.
- Low-grade CIN is often seen as thin, smooth acetowhite lesions with well-demarcated, but irregular, feathery or digitating or angular margins.
- High-grade CIN are associated with thick, dense, dull, opaque, or greyish-white acetowhite areas with well-demarcated, regular margins, which sometimes may be raised and rolled out. They may be more extensive and complex lesions extending into the endocervical canal. The surface contour of the acetowhite areas associated with high-grade CIN lesions tend to be less smooth, or irregular and nodular. Visualization of one or more borders within an acetowhite lesion or an acetowhite lesion with varying color intensity is associated with high-grade lesions.
- Abnormal vascular features such as punctation and mosaics are significant only if these are seen confined to acetowhite areas.
- Vascular features, such as fine punctation and/or fine mosaics in acetowhite areas, may be associated with low-grade CIN.
- Coarse punctation and/or coarse mosaics in acetowhite areas tend to occur in high-grade lesions.
- CIN lesions do not contain glycogen and thus do not stain with iodine and remain mustard or saffron-yellow areas.
- Using a scoring system such as Reid's colposcopic index may guide colposcopic interpretation and diagnosis.

The colposcopic diagnosis of cervical neoplasia requires an understanding and recognition of four main features: color tone and intensity of acetowhitening, margins and surface contour of acetowhite areas, vascular pattern and iodine staining. Colposcopy with directed biopsy is described as the reference investigation or "gold standard" for the diagnosis of cervical precancer. Colposcopy has a reported sensitivity ranging from 87 to 99% to diagnose cervical neoplasia, but its specificity is lower, between 23 and 87%.

The colposcopic features of CIN are described in this chapter to equip the student with the skills to distinguish the colposcopic findings associated with high-grade CIN (CIN 2–3) from those of low-grade lesions (CIN 1). Although the appearance of a single abnormal features alone is not a strong indicator that a lesion is present, the occurrence of abnormal features together in a localized area in the transformation zone increases the probability of a lesion. It will become obvious during colposcopic practice that considerable skills are required to differentiate between low-grade lesions, immature squamous metaplasia and certain inflammatory conditions. The student is encouraged to obtain biopsies whenever in doubt, and to review the histopathological findings with the pathologist. Close collaboration with pathologists is obligatory and useful in improving one's diagnostic skills. At the end of this chapter, a system that enables the colposcopist to score abnormalities is presented. This system is useful as a basis for the choice of which area(s) to select for biopsy. It is essential to biopsy the "worst" area(s), i.e., the area(s) with the most severe changes in features.

The colposcopic findings of an abnormal or atypical TZ can involve the whole TZ but more commonly affect only a portion of it and there may be multiple distinct lesions. There is usually a distinct demarcation between normal and abnormal epithelium.

The colposcopic features that differentiate an abnormal TZ from the normal include the following: color tone of acetowhite areas; surface pattern of acetowhite areas; borderline between acetowhite areas and the rest of the epithelium; vascular features and color changes after application of iodine.

After Application of Normal Saline Solution

Following application of saline, abnormal epithelium may appear much darker than the normal epithelium.

Vasculature

Using the green (or blue) filter and higher-power magnification when necessary, the best opportunity to evaluate any abnormal vasculature patterns is before the application of acetic acid, the effect of which may obscure some or all of the changes, especially in an acetowhite area. The abnormalities of interest are punctation, mosaics, and atypical vessels **(Figs. 10 to 12)**.

Capillaries

The afferent and efferent capillaries within the villi **(Fig. 13)** of columnar epithelium become compressed during the normal metaplastic process and are not incorporated within the newly formed squamous epithelium. Instead, they form a fine network below the basement membrane. When CIN develops as a result of HPV infection and atypical metaplasia, the afferent and efferent capillary system may be trapped (incorporated) into the diseased dysplastic epithelium through several elongated stromal papillae **(Figs. 14 and 15)**, and a thin layer of epithelium may remain on top of these vessels. This forms the basis of the punctate and mosaic blood vessel pattern.

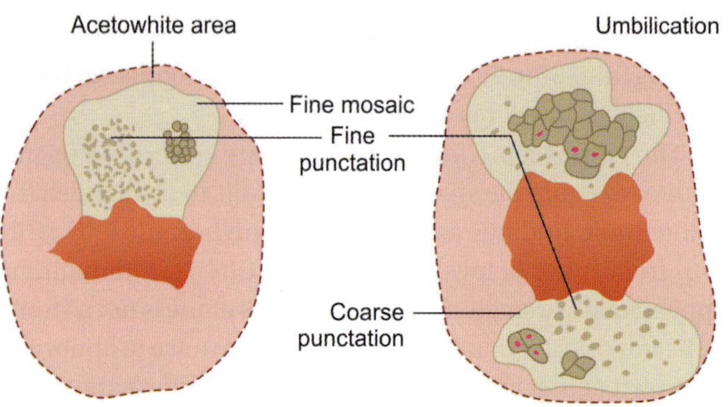

Fig. 10: Mosaics and punctations on colposcopy.

The terminating vessels in the stromal papillae underlying the thin epithelium appear as black points in a stippling pattern in an end-on view under the colposcope, making what are called punctate areas. The inter-connecting blood vessels in the stromal papillae surrounding the rete pegs of the epithelium, running parallel to the surface, are observed colposcopically as cobbled areas of mosaic pattern. In mosaic areas, the epithelium appears as individual small, large, round, polygonal, regular or irregular blocks. Punctation and mosaic areas may be classified as either fine or coarse. Coarse changes tend to be associated with more severe degrees of abnormality. When both punctation and mosaic patterns are found to coexist, the same evaluation criteria for colposcopic prediction of disease are used as when they exist separately.

Vessels exhibiting punctation and mosaics are usually more strikingly obvious than the normal stromal vessels because these vessels penetrate into the epithelium and are thus closer to the surface. When acetic acid is applied, these abnormal vascular patterns seen to be confined to the acetowhite areas.

Fine punctation refers to looped capillaries—viewed end-on—that appears to be of fine caliber and located close to one another, producing a delicate stippling effect. *Fine mosaics* are a network of fine-caliber blood vessels that appear in close proximity to one another, as a mosaic pattern, when

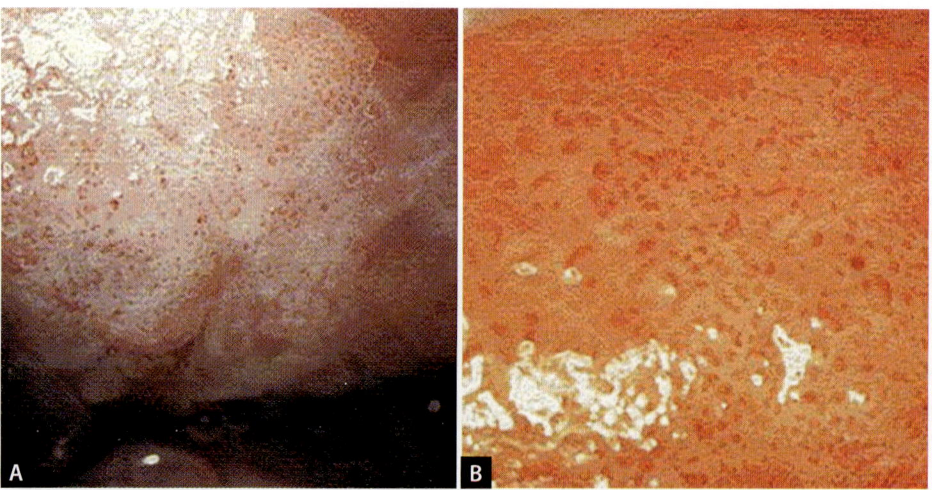

Figs. 11A and B: Coarse punctation before (A) and after (B) application of acetic acid.

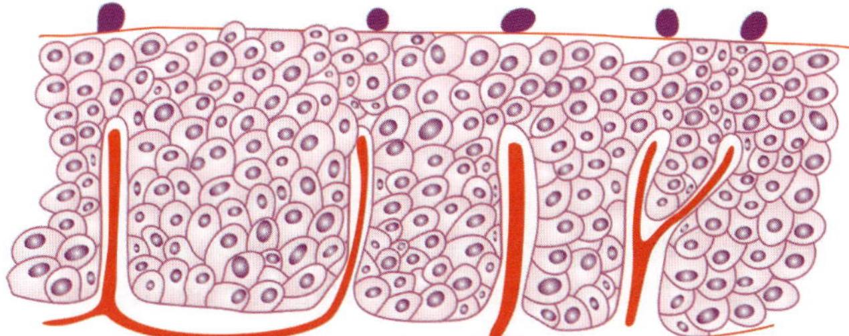

Fig. 12: Rete pegs and stromal capillaries which on end view appears as punctations.

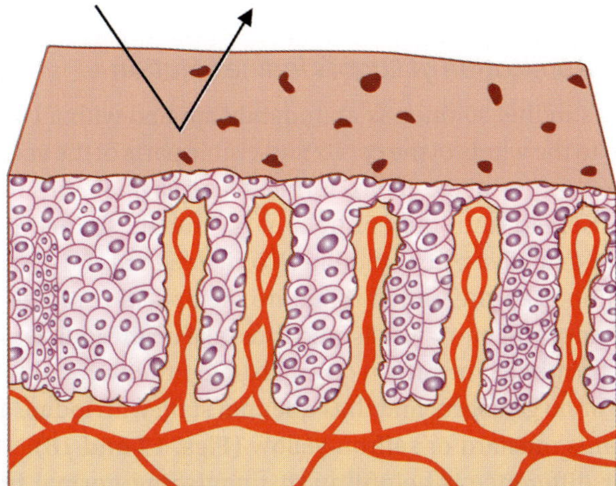

Fig. 13: Afferent and efferent capillaries within villi form a fine network below basement.

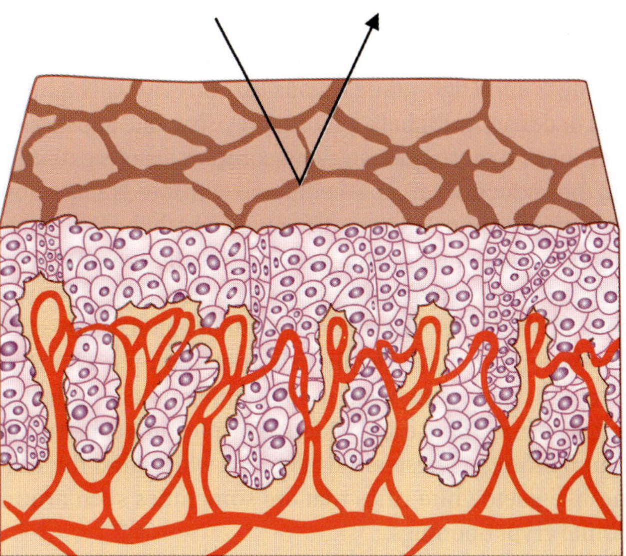

Fig. 14: Trapping of afferent and efferent capillaries into diseased dysplastic.

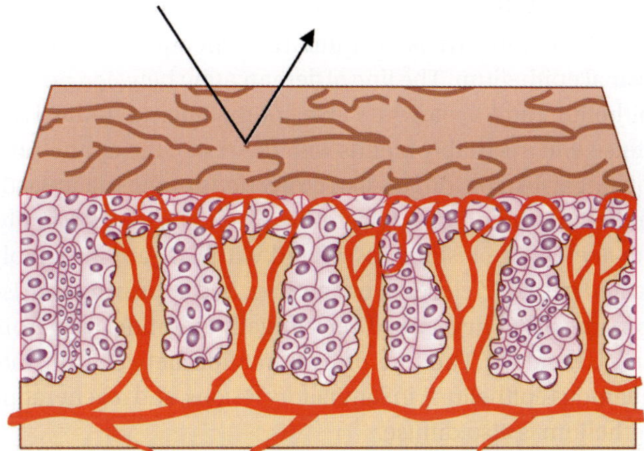

Fig. 15: Afferent and efferent vessels now getting converted into atypical.

viewed with the colposcope. These two vascular appearances may occur together and may be found in low-grade (CIN 1) lesions. The patterns do not necessarily appear throughout the whole lesion.

Coarse punctation and *coarse mosaics* are formed by vessels having larger caliber and larger intercapillary distances, in contrast to the corresponding fine changes. Coarse punctation and mosaicism tend to occur in more severe neoplastic lesions such as CIN 2, CIN 3 lesions and early preclinical invasive cancer. Sometimes, the two patterns are superimposed in an area so that the capillary loops occur in the center of each mosaic "tile". This appearance is called umbilication.

After the Application of 5% Acetic Acid Solution

The observation of a well-demarcated, dense, opaque, acetowhite area closer to or abutting the SCJ in the TZ after application of 5% acetic acid is critical. In fact, it is the most important of all colposcopic signs, and is the hallmark of colposcopic diagnosis of cervical neoplasia. The degree to which the epithelium takes up the acetic acid stain is correlated with the color tone or intensity, the surface shine, and the duration of the effect, and, in turn, with the degree of neoplastic change in the lesion. Higher-grade lesions are more likely to turn dense white rapidly **(Fig. 16)**. Abnormal vascular features such as punctation, mosaicism, and atypical vessels are significant only if these are seen in acetowhite areas.

The acetic acid dehydrates cells and reversibly coagulates the nuclear proteins. Thus, areas of increased nuclear activity and DNA content exhibit the most dramatic color change. The most pronounced effects are observed in high-grade lesions and invasive cancer. A direct correlation exists between the intensity of the dull, white color and the severity of the lesion. Less differentiated areas are associated with an intensely opaque, dull-white appearance of lesions in the transformation zone.

Flat condyloma and low-grade CIN may uncommonly present as thin, satellite acetowhite lesions detached (far away) from the SCJ with geographical patterns (resembling geographical regions) and with irregular, angular, or digitating or feathery margins . Many low-grade CIN lesions reveal less dense, less extensive and less complex acetowhite areas close to or abutting the SCJ with well demarcated, but irregular, feathery, or digitating margins compared with high-grade

CIN lesions. High-grade lesions show well demarcated, regular margins, which may sometimes have raised and rolled out edges and High-grade lesions like CIN 2 or CIN 3 have a thick or dense, dull, chalk-white or greyish-white appearance. They may be more extensive and complex lesions extending into the endocervical canal compared with low-grade lesions. High-grade lesions often tend to involve both the lips. Severe or early malignant lesions may obliterate the external os.

The line of demarcation between normal and abnormal areas in the TZ is sharp and well-delineated. High-grade lesions tend to have regular, sharper borders. The crypt openings that are involved in high-grade precursor lesions may have thick, dense and wide acetowhite rims called cuffed crypt openings. These are whiter and wider than the mild, line-like acetowhite rings that are sometimes seen around normal crypt openings.

The cardinal features that should differentiate between the CIN lesions and immature metaplasia are the less dense and translucent nature of the acetowhitening associated with metaplasia, and the lack of a distinct margin between the acetowhite areas of immature metaplasia and the normal epithelium. The line of demarcation between normal epithelium and acetowhite areas of metaplasia in the TZ is diffuse and invariably blends with the rest of the epithelium. The finger-like or tongue-like projections of the metaplastic epithelium often point toward the external os centripetally. The acetowhite lesions associated with CIN are invariably located in the TZ closer to or abutting, and appearing to arise from, the SCJ. They spread centrifugally, pointing away from the external os. The line of demarcation between normal squamous epithelium, inflammatory lesions, and regenerating epithelium is also diffuse.

To summarize, acetowhite staining is not specific for CIN and may also occur, to some extent, in areas of immature squamous metaplasia, the congenital TZ, inflammation and healing and regenerative epithelium. However, acetowhite changes associated with CIN are found localized in the TZ, abutting the SCJ and well-demarcated from the surrounding epithelium. Low-grade lesions tend to be thin, less dense, less extensive, with irregular, feathery, geographic or angular margins and with fine punctation and/or mosaic; sometimes, low-grade lesions may be detached from the SCJ; and atypical vessels are seldom observed in low-grade lesions. On the other hand, high-grade lesions are associated with dense, opaque, grey white, acetowhite areas with coarse punctation and/or mosaic and with regular and well-demarcated borders; these lesions often involve both lips and may occasionally harbor atypical vessels; CIN 3 lesions tend to be complex, involving the os.

After Application of Lugol's Iodine Solution

Lugol's iodine solution is abundantly applied with a cotton swab to the whole of the cervix and visible parts of the vagina. The periphery of the cervix, fornices, and vaginal walls must be observed until the epithelium is strongly stained dark brown or almost black by iodine. Normal vaginal and cervical squamous epithelium and mature metaplastic epithelium contain glycogen-rich cells, and thus take up the iodine stain and turn black or brown. Dysplastic epithelium contains little or no glycogen, and thus does not stain with iodine and remains mustard or saffron yellow **(Figs. 17 and 18)**. This color difference is helpful in distinguishing normal from abnormal areas in the transformation zone that have shown faint acetowhitening. Columnar epithelium does not stain with iodine and immature metaplasia only partially stains, if at all. Atrophic epithelium also stains partially with iodine and this makes interpretation difficult in postmenopausal women. Condylomatous lesions also do not, or only partially, stain with iodine.

After the findings of colposcopy are documented, the Swede score should be calculated as given in **Table 4**.

Atypical epithelium of CIN may be less firmly attached to the underlying stroma, from which it may easily detach or

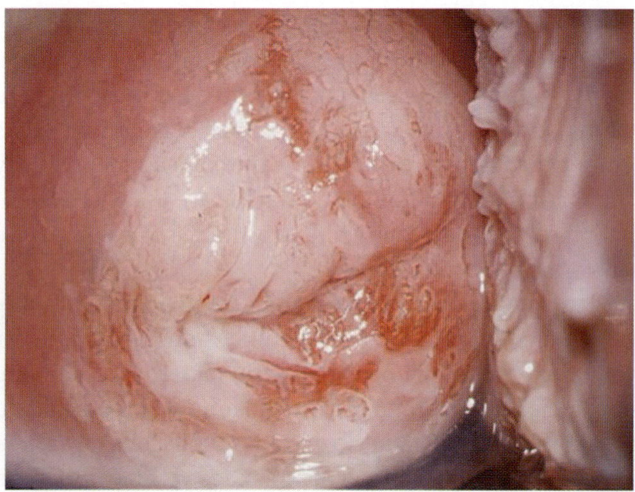

Fig. 16: A dense acetowhite, opaque, complex, circumorificial CIN 3 lesion.

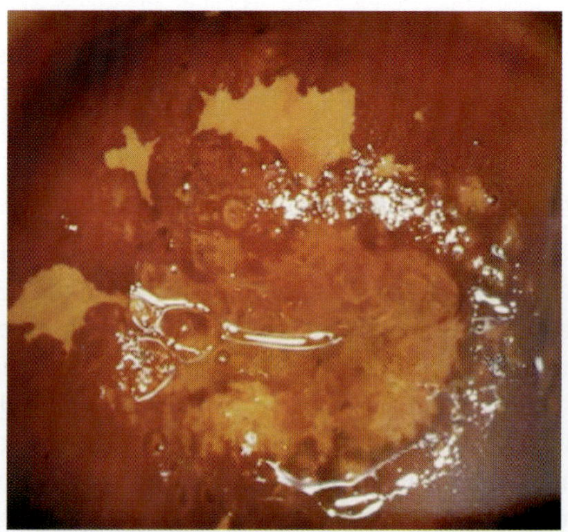

Fig. 17: CIN 1 lesion with a mustard yellow iodine- negative area with irregular margins.

peel off, after repeated application with different solutions, resulting in a true erosion (epithelial defect) exposing the stroma. Such true erosions may easily be observed after iodine application, as the stroma does not stain with iodine.

SALIENT FEATURES

- Invasive squamous cell cervical cancers are preceded by a long phase of preinvasive disease, collectively referred to as CIN.
- CIN may be categorized into grades 1, 2, and 3 depending upon the proportion of the thickness of the epithelium showing mature and differentiated cells.
- More severe grades of CIN (2 and 3) reveal a greater proportion of the thickness of the epithelium composed of undifferentiated cells.
- Persistent infection with one or more of the oncogenic subtypes of HPV is a necessary cause for cervical neoplasia.
- Most cervical abnormalities caused by HPV infection are unlikely to progress to high-grade CIN or cervical cancer.
- Most low-grade CIN regress within relatively short periods or do not progress to high-grade lesions.

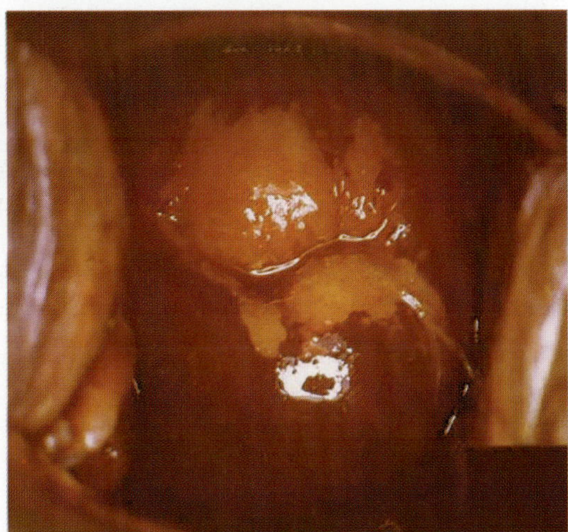

Fig. 18: Satellite lesions do not stain with iodine after the application of Lugol's iodine solution and remain as thin yellow areas.

- High-grade CIN carries a much higher probability of progressing to invasive cancer.

TREATMENT OF CIN

In an era where the indications of hysterectomies done are severely challenged and rightly so, it is very important to understand that entire precancer lesion of cervix do not require hysterectomy as the mode of treatment.

The management depends on the degree of abnormality. The management of CIN 1 is given in **Flowchart 2** and for CIN 2 and 3 in **Flowchart 3**. Pregnancy represents a special situation and the management of CIN in pregnancy is shown in **Flowchart 4**.

Methods of Treatment

- Cryotherapy
- Large loop excision of transformation zone (LLETZ)) also called loop excision
- Cold Knife conization
- Conization
- Therma coagulation.

Of these cryotherapy and LLETZ are most commonly performed short procedures while others are based on individual choice and availability of infrastructure.

Cryotherapy

- *Indication:* Low-grade lesion of cervix, unhealthy cervix with persistent discharge not responding to medical treatment—high-grade lesion being ruled out by colposcopy biopsy.
- Can be performed under local anesthesia, day care hospitalization, if patient not cooperative—short IV sedation.
- *Equipment:* Colposcope, Cryogun with attached air pressure gauze, NO_2/CO_2 gas cylinder, wide-angled cusco speculum.
- *Principle:* Involves 3-3-3 minute freeze-thaw-freeze cycle using available gas (NO_2/CO_2), ensuring ice formation going 5 mm beyond tip of the cryoprobe.

TABLE 4: Swede score.

Swede score	***0***	***1***	***2***
Aceto uptake	Zero or transparent	Shady, milky (not transparent not opaque)	Distinct, opaque white
Margins/surface	Diffuse	Sharp but irregular, jagged, "geographical" satellites	Sharp and even, difference in surface level including "cuffing"
Vessels	Fine, regular	Absent	Coarse or atypial
Lesion size	<5 mm	5–15 mm or 2 quadrants	>15 mm or 3–4 quadrants or endocervically undefined
Iodine staining	Brown	Faintly or patchy yellow	Distinct yellow
			Total score

Swede score (minimum: 0; maximum: 10):
- Total score 0–4: Normal/CIN 1
- Total score 5–6: CIN 2/CIN 3
- Total score 7–10: CIN 3/cancer.

Flowchart 2: Management of CIN 1.

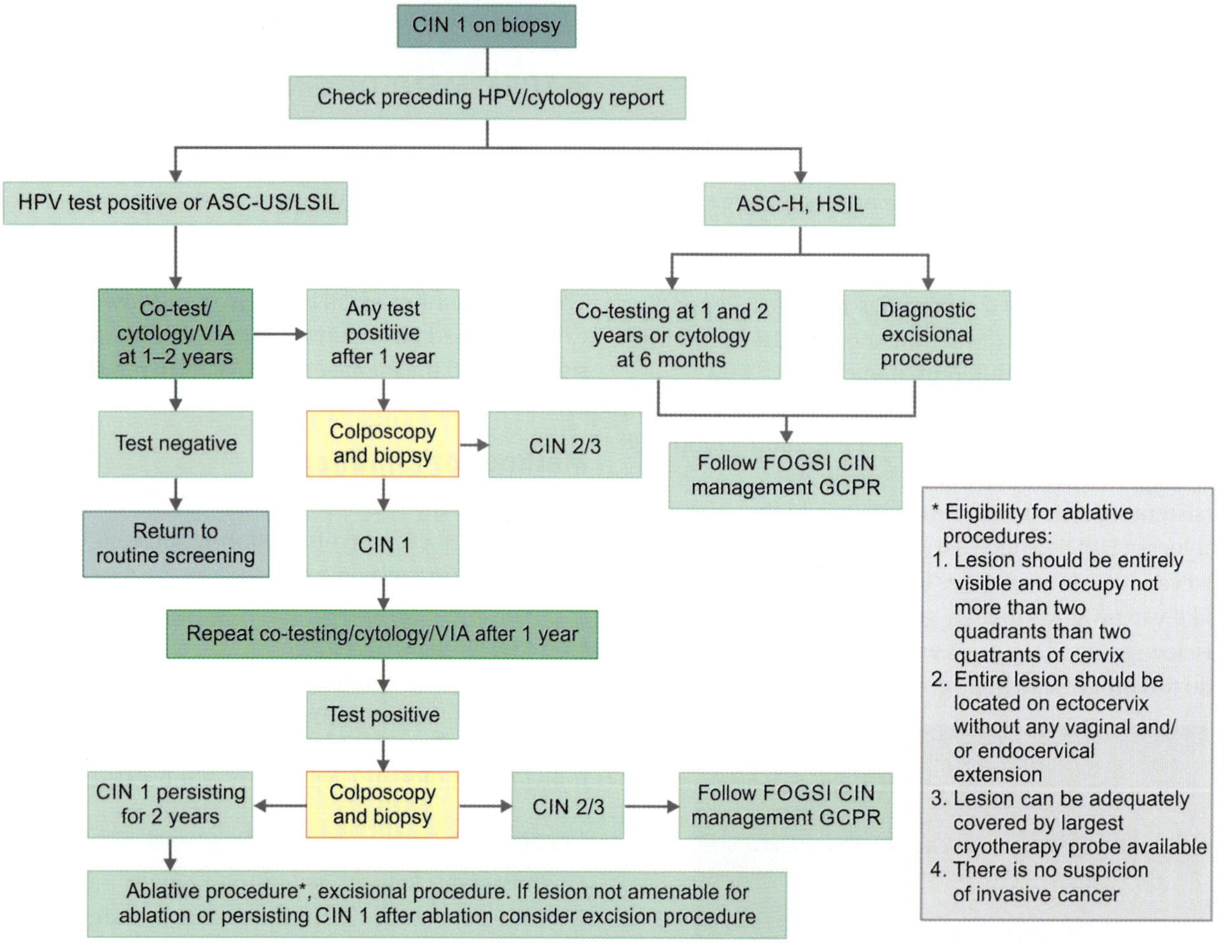

CIN 1 on biopsy
Check preceding HPV/cytology report
HPV test positive or ASC-US/LSIL
ASC-H, HSIL
Co-test/ cytology/VIA at 1–2 years
Any test positiive after 1 year
Co-testing at 1 and 2 years or cytology at 6 months
Diagnostic excisional procedure
Test negative
Colposcopy and biopsy
CIN 2/3
Follow FOGSI CIN management GCPR
Return to routine screening
CIN 1
Repeat co-testing/cytology/VIA after 1 year
Test positive
CIN 1 persisting for 2 years
Colposcopy and biopsy
CIN 2/3
Follow FOGSI CIN management GCPR
Ablative procedure*, excisional procedure. If lesion not amenable for ablation or persisting CIN 1 after ablation consider excision procedure
* Eligibility for ablative procedures:
1. Lesion should be entirely visible and occupy not more than two quadrants than two quatrants of cervix
2. Entire lesion should be located on ectocervix without any vaginal and/ or endocervical extension
3. Lesion can be adequately covered by largest cryotherapy probe available
4. There is no suspicion of invasive cancer

(ASC-US: Atypical squamous cells—undetermined significance; ASC-H: Atypical squamous cells—cannot rule out high grade squamous intraepithelial lesion; CIN: cervical intraepithelial neoplasia; GCPR: good clinical practice recommendations; HPV: human papillomaviruses; HSIL: high grade squamous intraepithelial lesion; LSIL: low grade squamous intraepithelial lesion)

Flowchart 3: Management of CIN 2 and CIN 3.

CIN 2/3 on histology
Review colposcopy report
Adequate
Inadequate/ECC positive/recurrent CIN
Excision of T zone/ablation*
Diagnostic excisional procedure
Repeat HPV and cytology/VIA at 1–2 years
Margin negative
Test negative at 1–2 years
Margin positive
Repeat HPV and cytology/VIA at 3 years
Repeat cone biopsy/ hysterectomy if technically repeat, cone not feasible or patient noncompliant
Repeat cytology and ECC at 6 months
Return to routine screening
Follow FOGSI CIN management GCPR
* Eligibility for ablative procedures:
1. Lesion should be entirely visible and occupy not more than two quadrants of cervix
2. Entire lesion should be located on ectocervix without any vaginal and/or endocervical extension
3. Lesion can be adequately covered by largest cryotherapy probe available
4. There is no suspicion of invasive cancer
5. N.B. In CIN 3, excision is preferred especially for large lesions, lesions not fully accessible for ablation, or recurrent lesion

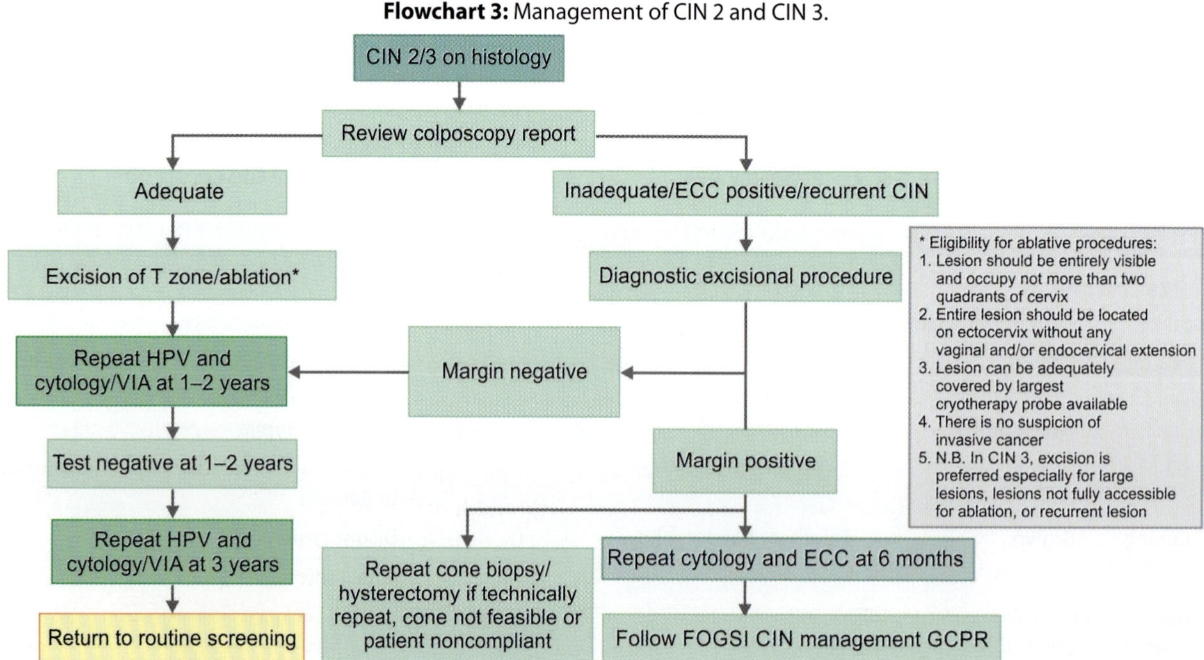

(CIN: cervical intraepithelial neoplasia; ECC: endocervical curettage; GCPR: good clinical practice recommendations; HPV: human papillomaviruses; VIA: visual inspection with acetic acid)

Flowchart 4: CIN in pregnancy.

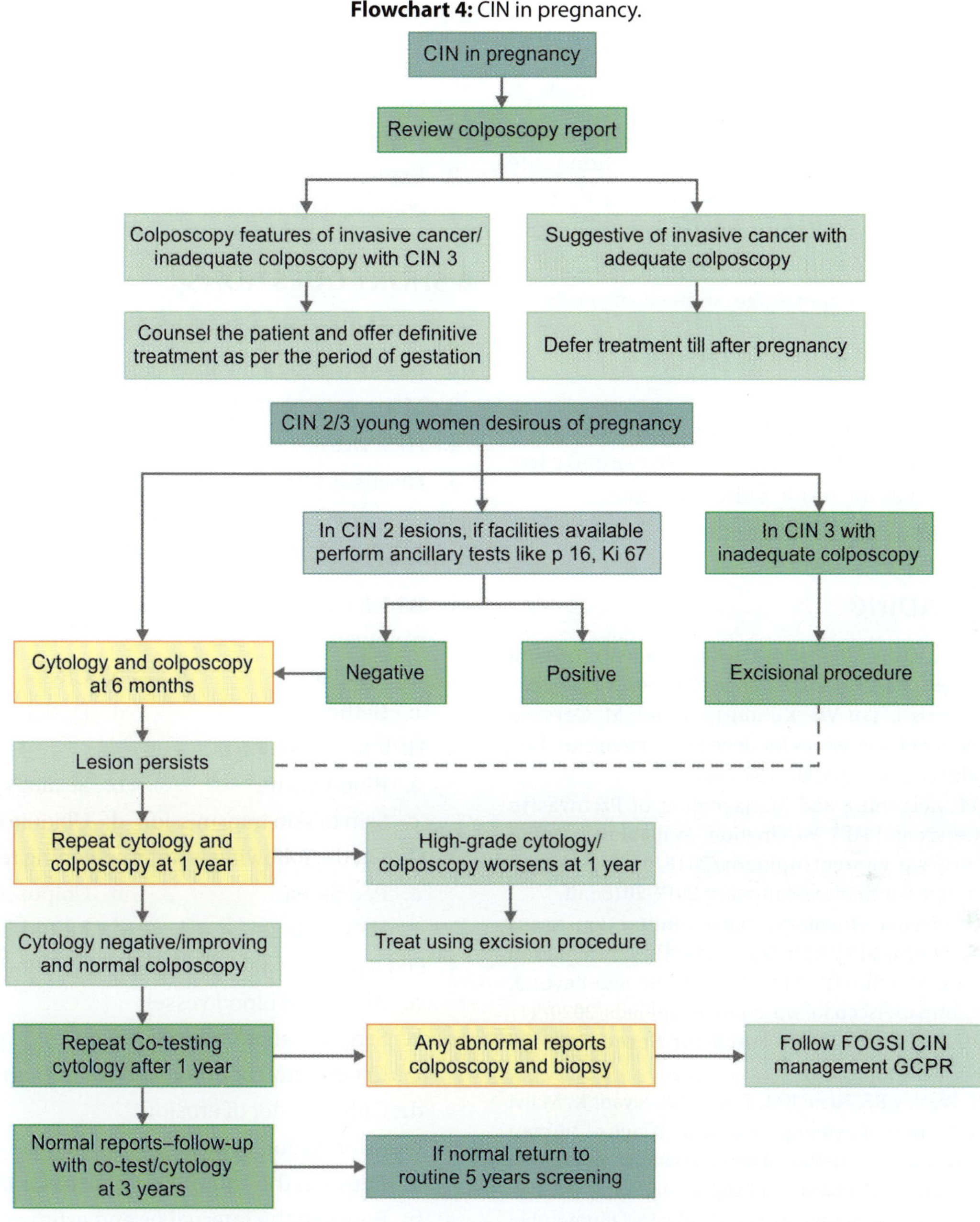

(CIN: cervical intraepithelial neoplasia; GCPR: good clinical practice recommendations)

- *Complication:* Nil, except for copious watery discharge, which the patient may experience for 15 days and make her uncomfortable.
- Best in "see and treat policy" of treatment where patient is not sure to follow up, do colposcopy detect low-grade lesion and there itself do cryotherapy.

Large Loop Excision of Transformation Zone

- *Indications:*
  - High grade CIN lesion—serves both as diagnosis and treatment
  - HSIL cytology with inadequate colposcopy.
  - High suspicion of high grade lesion but TZ type 3
  - Fertility sparing treatment for C.A. CERVIX 1A1/ selected cases of 1A2, squamous variety.
- Can be done under local anesthesia but many a times requires short sedation in a day care set up.
- *Equipment:* Colposcope, Cautery machine, suction machine, wide bore cusco speculum with smoke evacuator, various diameters of loop electrodes, ball point cautery, Monsel's paste, and sutures for hemostasis.
- *Principle:* Based on the type of TZ loop electrode is selected to get adequate depth of the endocervical canal and breadth of the lesion.
- The loop is passed from one side to other IN ONE PASS so that the entire lesion along with the TZ is EXCISED. If the lesion is very big involving both the lips of cervix it is than done in two passes, anterior lip and posterior lip and specimen sent separately.
- *Complications:* Bleeding, stenosis of cervix.

Conization

- Here the indications remain same as that of LLETZ, it is an old traditional method of treating and diagnosing high grade lesion.
- *Principle:* Under GA, cervix is amputed with adequate endocervical depth and excised in such a way that the specimen looks like a cone, sutures are taken to achieve hemostasis, and patient hospitalized for 2/3 days.
- *Complications:* Severe hemorrhage, stenosis of cervix.

Thermacoagulation

- Its like an alternate to the cryotherapy, here there is no need to use gas, it is battery operated easy to use and carry equipment, achieves the result within a minute.
- *Indications:* Same as for cryotherapy.

FURTHER READING

1. Basu P, Taghavi K, Hu SY, Mogri S, Joshi S. Management of cervical premalignant lesions. Curr Probl Cancer. 2018;42(2):129-36.
2. Bishop A, Sherris J, Tsu VD, Kilbourne-Brook M. Cervical dysplasia treatment: key issues for developing countries. Bull Pan Am Health Organ. 1996;30(4):378-86.
3. FOGSI GCPR Screening and Management of Preinvasive Lesions of Cervix and HPV Vaccination. Available at: http://www.fogsi.org/wp-content/uploads/2018/01/fogsi-gcpr-smplc-cervix-hpv-vaccination-summary-2017-2018.pdf
4. ISCCP, FOGSI Gynae Oncology, AOGIN India, Consensus Guidelines for Cervical Cancer Screening, HPV vaccination and Management in the COVID-19 Pandemic and beyond. Available at: https://isccp.in/wp-content/uploads/2020/11/ISCCP-AOGIN-FOGSI-Guidelines-for-Screening-in-COVID_27-10-2020.pdf
5. Muwonge R, Wesley RS, Nene BM, Shastri SS, Jayant K, Malvi SG, et al. Evaluation of cytology and visual triage of human papillomavirus-positive women in cervical cancer prevention in India. Int J Cancer. 2014;134(12):2902-9.
6. Santesso N, Mustafa RA, Schünemann HJ, Arbyn M, Blumenthal PD, Cain J, et al.; Guideline Support Group. World Health Organization Guidelines for treatment of cervical intraepithelial neoplasia 2-3 and screen-and-treat strategies to prevent cervical cancer. Int J Gynaecol Obstet. 2016;132(3):252-8.
7. Santesso N, Mustafa RA, Wiercioch W, Kehar R, Gandhi S, Chen Y, et al. Systematic reviews and meta-analyses of benefits and harms of cryotherapy, LEEP, and cold knife conization to treat cervical intraepithelial neoplasia. Int J Gynaecol Obstet. 2016;132(3):266-71.
8. Santesso N, Schünemann H, Blumenthal P, De Vuyst H, Gage J, Garcia F, et al.; World health Organization Steering Committee for Recommendations on Use of Cryotherapy for Cervical Cancer Prevention. World Health Organization Guidelines: Use of cryotherapy for cervical intraepithelial neoplasia. Int J Gynaecol Obstet. 2012;118(2):97-102.
9. WHO Guidelines for Screening and Treatment of Precancerous Lesions for Cervical Cancer Prevention. Geneva: World Health Organization; 2013.

LONG QUESTIONS

1. Discuss the anatomy of cervix and clarify how HPV brings changes in cervical cells.
2. Discuss the histopathology, diagnosis of CIN lesion.
3. Explain nomenclature, scoring, basic requirements of colposcopy examination.

SHORT QUESTIONS

1. Corelation between dysplasia and Bethesda system.
2. Basis of acetic acid and lugols iodine test.
3. Management of CIN as per guidelines.
4. HPV virus
5. Discuss LLETZ and cryotherapy.

MULTIPLE CHOICE QUESTIONS

1. Which is the current accepted nomenclature for reporting of smears?
   a. Dysplasia b. CIN
   c. Bethesda d. Dyskaryosis
2. HPV transmission is:
   a. Blood borne b. Sexually transmitted
   c. Skin to skin transmission d. Ubiquitous
3. One of the following is not a screening test:
   a. Pap Smear b. Colposcopy
   c. HPV testing d. Liquid-based cytology
4. Old squamo-columnar junction is identified by:
   a. Abnormal blood vessels
   b. Signs of inflammation
   c. Crypt/gland opening and Nabothian cyst
   d. Outer border of erosion
5. Transformation zone is:
   a. Between the anterior and posterior lip of cervix
   b. Between the internal os and external os
   c. Between the old and new squamo-columnar junction
   d. Within the endocervical canal
6. 5% acetic acid is:
   a. Readily available commercially
   b. Prepared by mixing equal amount of acetic acid and normal saline
   c. Always freshly prepared by adding 1 mL of acetic acid to 19 mL normal saline
   d. Prepared by adding 1 mL of normal saline to 19 mL of acetic acid
7. CIN 3 is treated by:
   a. Cryotherapy
   b. Thermacoagulation
   c. Observation
   d. LLETZ or conization

8. Indication of colposcopy is:
   a. Unhealthy cervix
   b. Abnormal cytology
   c. Positive VIA examination
   d. All of the above
9. Colposcopy is done as a:
   a. Outpatient test
   b. Procedure under short GA
   c. Procedure under spinal anesthesia
   d. Procedure under IV sedation
10. Mosaics and punctations are called so if:
   a. They are seen outside the transformation zone
   b. They are seen within an acetowhite area
   c. They are seen at the internal os
   d. They are seen at either the old or new squamo-columnar junctions.

Answers

1.	c	2.	b	3.	b	4.	c	5.	c	6.	c
7.	d	8.	d	9.	a	10.	b				

14.4 MALIGNANT DISEASES OF VAGINA

Shalini Rajaram, Bindiya Gupta

INTRODUCTION

Primary vaginal cancer is tumor confined to vagina and not arising from cervix, uterine body or vulva which can be excluded by clinical examination, imaging, endometrial biopsy, colposcopy, vulvoscopy and hysteroscopy. It is a rare malignancy and accounts for less than 2% of all gynecologic malignancies.[1]

Squamous cell carcinoma is the most common histology (80–90%) followed by adenocarcinoma with a clear cell histology (4–10%). Other rare histological types include malignant melanoma, neuroendocrine carcinomas and papillary squamo-transitional cell carcinomas.[2] Metastatic tumors in the vagina are quite common extending from cervix, vulva, urinary bladder, rectum and urethra. They may also occur following lymphatic and hematogenous spread from endometrial cancer and gestational trophoblastic disease respectively.[3]

Histologically, tumor grading is classified as Gx: grade cannot be assessed; G1, well differentiated; G2, moderately differentiated and G3, poorly differentiated or undifferentiated (G3).[4] Vaginal adenosis is usually the precursor lesion for adenocarcinoma, which may be present in women with intrauterine exposure to diethylstilbestrol.[5] Diethylstilbestrol (DES) associated cancers are rarely seen today and they are associated with good prognosis while non DES associated vaginal adeno cancers (NDAV) occur in older women between 37 and 77 years, are more aggressive and have a high recurrence rate.[6]

RISK FACTORS

The incidence of vaginal cancer increases with advancing age with 50% presenting at 70 years and 20% beyond 80 years, median age being 63 years.[7] According to GLOBCAN 2020 Indian data, annually there were 5,518 new cases and 2,723 deaths due to vaginal cancer. The 5 year prevalence was 12,315 cases.[8] High risk factors for vaginal cancer include black race, five or more lifetime sexual partners, early age at first intercourse (<17 years), smoking, coexistent HIV infection and previous treatment for an anogenital tumor. History of anogenital warts, male partner's lifetime number of other sexual partners and cumulative alcohol consumption may be other probable risk factors. Approximately one third of all cases had history of abnormal cervical cytology and (OR = 3.9; 95% CI = 2.5–6.1).[7] The risk factors are summarized in **Box 1**.

High-risk human papillomaviruses (HPVs) are implicated as causative factor for vaginal cancer; HPV16, HPV33, and HPV45 in VaIN and HPV18, and HPV33 in VaSCC and these tumors show positive p16 expression.[9] It has been calculated that approximately 60% of vaginal carcinomas may be avoided by currently available prophylactic vaccines against HPV 16/18.

CLINICAL PRESENTATION AND PATTERNS OF SPREAD

Women usually present with symptoms similar to cervical cancer and most common clinical presentation is vaginal bleeding. Other symptoms include foul smelling vaginal discharge, urinary and bowel symptoms, post coital bleeding

BOX 1: Risk factors of vaginal cancer.

- Advanced age (>60 years)
- Black women
- Multiple sexual partners of self or of male partner
- Early age at first intercourse
- Current smokers
- Previous treatment for an anogenital tumor
- Cumulative alcohol consumption.
- Human papillomavirus (types 16, 18, 33, 45)
- Human immunodeficiency virus (HIV) infection

and constitutional symptoms. Clinically it appears as an ulcerating or fungating vaginal mass or an annular constricting lesion in the vagina. Squamous cell cancers tend to occur more commonly in the proximal third of vagina in the posterior wall while adenocarcinomas are usually seen in the anterior wall.[10] In a retrospective analysis it was found that tumor involved the upper third of the vagina in 46.2% of the cases, the middle third in 11%, the distal third in 23.1%, and the whole vagina in 19.8%.[11]

Vaginal cancer spreads by direct extension to adjacent structures like cervix, vulva, bladder and rectum, and by lymphatics to locoregional nodes. The lymphatic drainage of upper two-thirds of the vagina is to obturator, hypogastric and external iliac nodes, while lower one-third drains to the groin nodes. Lymphatics from posterior vaginal wall also drain to presacral nodes via pararectal lymphatics. Distant metastases are uncommon, and when present, mainly involve the lungs, liver and bones.[12]

PREOPERATIVE WORKUP

The diagnosis is made once a suspicious vaginal lesion is seen on a speculum examination and is confirmed on biopsy using a punch (Baker's or Keyes) or cervical (Tischler or Kevorkian) biopsy forceps. The lesion may appear as an exophytic mass, a plaque, or an ulcer and it is important to take multiple biopsies from the margin of the growth to avoid necrotic cells. Occasionally, the diagnosis is made on presence of malignant cells on cytology and the lesion is visualized and biopsied during colposcopy. Careful vaginal examination by inspecting all vaginal walls to avoid missing high or lateral lesions, must be carried out and sometimes one may need to carry out an examination under anesthesia especially in postmenopausal women. In cases of palpable lymph nodes, biopsy or fine-needle aspiration may be performed to exclude malignancy.

According to FIGO, other ancillary aids that can be used for staging include intravenous pyelogram to evaluate for hydronephrosis, cystoscopy and/or proctoscopy in patients with urinary or rectal symptoms and Chest X-ray. Advanced imaging modalities such as contrast enhanced magnetic resonance imaging (MRI), positron emission tomography (PET)-computed tomography (CT)/contrast-enhanced computed tomography (CECT)/ultrasound cannot be used to revise staging but to guide therapy.[13]

Magnetic Resonance Imaging

It is useful in delineating tumor size and extent both in primary, recurrent and metastatic cancers specially to delineate local paravaginal and parametrial spread.[14] Primary vaginal tumors are best visualized on T2-weighted images and appear as intermediate or high signal intensity in contrast to the hypointense muscularis and submucosa.[15] On T-1 weighted imaging there is low to intermediate signal intensity. Dynamic contrast enhancement may be also helpful in distinguishing tumor type, distinguishing recurrence from fibrosis and evaluating tumor extension.[15] In order to appreciate the tumor thickness and volume more accurately, a vaginal gel or a dry vaginal tampon can be instilled to distend the vaginal walls. For stage 1 disease the documented accuracy of MRI is 88–97% and the accuracy for detecting bladder and rectal invasion is 96–99%.[16,17]

PET/CT/Ultrasound

Positron emission tomography imaging is very sensitive in detecting nodal metastasis, more than CT or MRI alone.[18] PET-CT is also useful in management of recurrent disease. CT is primarily used for three-dimensional (3D) conformal treatment planning for radiotherapy delivery.[19]

Transvaginal and/or transrectal sonography helps to delineate the precise morphology, location, and topography of the tumor in the vagina and may be used in the initial workup of patient.

Staging

The 2009 International Federation of Gynecology and Obstetrics (FIGO) clinical staging system is summarized in **Table 1**.

Another pathological staging system used, is the TNM staging system which is based FIGO staging with additional information on histopathological confirmation of the resected specimen and nodes. The pT, pN, and pM categories correspond to the T, N, and M categories. "p" stands for pathologic staging while "c" denotes clinical staging. The definitions of the T categories (T1-T4) correspond to the stages accepted by the FIGO. Lymph nodes are assessed as Nx (regional lymph nodes cannot be assessed), N0 (no regional lymph nodes), and N1 (pelvic or inguinal lymph nodes). Staging of metastasis (M) is assessed as Mx (distant metastases cannot be assessed), M0 (no distant metastases), and M1 (distant metastases).

TABLE 1: FIGO 2009 staging of vaginal cancer.

Stage	*Description*
Stage I	Tumor should be confined to the vaginal wall
Stage II	The carcinoma has involved the subvaginal tissue but has not extended to pelvic wall
Stage III	The carcinoma has extended to the pelvic side wall, with involvement of the obturator internus, levator ani, or piriformis, external or internal iliac vessels, or bony structures
Stage IVA	Tumor invades adjacent organs, involving the mucosal layer of the bladder, rectum, or urethra, or extension beyond the true pelvis. Bullous edema of bladder does not permit a case to be allotted to stage IV
Stage IVB	Presence of distant metastases, including disease in the lungs or liver

TREATMENT

The factors deciding the mode of treatment are tumor size and histology, tumor location, stage at presentation, age of the patient and performance status. Various modalities of treatment include surgery, radiotherapy, chemotherapy or its combination.[20]

Surgery

Surgery is limited to early and small lesions confined to the vaginal mucosa (less than 2 cm).[20] It is more important in the management of stage I and II adenocarcinoma (especially clear cell adenocarcinoma) as it is poorly sensitive to radiation.[3] Surgical management is limited by anatomical constraints as vagina is in close proximity to critical pelvic structures such as the bladder, urethra, and rectum.

In tumors of upper vagina, surgery includes radical hysterectomy, or modified radical hysterectomy and pelvic lymphadenectomy, and vaginectomy with sufficient excision margin. The aim is to attain a 1 cm disease-free margin.[21] For disease in lower half of vagina, regional lymph nodes involvement is similar to ones involved in vulval cancer; hence, bilateral groin node dissection in addition to radical wide local excision should be offered. The role of sentinel lymph nodes is still experimental. Pelvic exenteration may be considered in case of isolated central recurrence or even in stage IVa disease. Extensive counseling regarding the risks and morbidity of surgery and impact on quality of life and body image should be discussed in detail with the patient.

Other surgical treatments used include ovarian transposition in women before radiation therapy and laparoscopic resection of bulky nodes in advanced disease for staging. Occasionally, a palliative urinary diversion or colostomy before radiation may be done in recurrent or advanced settings.[20,21]

Adjuvant radiation is recommended in case of positive margins or presence of lymph node metastasis.

Radiation

Radiation therapy (brachytherapy, external beam irradiation, or a combination of the two) remains the main modality of treatment for vaginal cancer especially in advanced stages. Concurrent chemotherapy with a single platinum-based drug or combination with 5-FU has been used. Depending on the tumor stage, radiotherapy alone can achieve high local control rates, ranging from 85–95% for FIGO stage I, to 70–80% for FIGO stage II and around 50–70% for FIGO stages III–IVA.[22]

MRI is also helpful in treatment as it is often used to assess response after external beam radiotherapy, to assess and localize initial tumor volume prior to brachytherapy, guide placement and evaluate response.[14]

Stage 1 vaginal cancer (tumor thickness of ≤5 mm): High dose irradiation (HDR) brachytherapy alone may be considered, although it may have intrapelvic recurrences ranging from 20 to 30%.[23] Interstitial brachytherapy is used especially if there is any doubt of submucosal invasion.[24]

Stage I (tumor thickness >5 mm – Stage IVA): Both external beam irradiation (EBRT) and brachytherapy are given. Maximum dose of EBRT given is 45–50 Gy.[21] Depending on the site of tumor nodal boost is administered. Pelvic nodes are irradiated, in addition groin and rectal lymphatics are included if the tumor is in distal vagina or in the posterior vaginal wall respectively. A higher dose of EBRT (65–70 Gy) may be given if response by decrease in tumor size is inadequate, if brachytherapy cannot be administered appropriately based on physicians discretion or brachytherapy facility is not available.[21,25]

Intensity modulated radiation therapy (IMRT) results in improved dosages and fewer adverse effects; more evidence is required on its use.[26]

PROGNOSIS

The main determinant of prognosis in carcinoma of the vagina is the stage of disease at the time of diagnosis. Squamous cell cancer has better prognosis compared to other histologic variants. Additional factors are tumor volume (>4 cm), location outside of the upper third of the vagina, HPV status, and MIB-1 index for squamous cell cancers.[12,20]

Five-year survival rate for stage I is 90% for surgical therapy and 63% for radiation therapy while in stage II, the survival is 70 and 57%, respectively. The 5-year survival rate in stage III and IV is 47% for surgical therapy alone and 35% for radiation therapy alone and 60% using combined modality.[27]

VAGINAL MELANOMA

Malignant melanoma of vagina is a rare tumor and accounts for less than 3% of all vaginal malignancies, and for 0.3–0.8% of all malignant melanomas.[28] It is usually seen in post-menopausal women and common presentation is vaginal bleeding, vaginal discharge or a palpable mass. On examination the mass can be blue-black or black-brown, with plaques or ulceration or sometimes it may not be pigmented as in case of amelanotic melanoma (<10%). It is usually unifocal but may present as multifocal lesion in 20%. The most common location is the distal third of anterior vaginal wall. Preoperative biopsy is advisable for confirmation of diagnosis. Immunohistochemical markers such as HMB-45 and S-100 can be used to confirm the diagnosis. Due to high propensity of local extension, lymphatic and hematogenous spread a thorough work up includes imaging using CT scan, MRI or PET CT. Due to paramagnetic properties of melanin, specific signal intensity on MRI like high signal intensity on T1-weighted images and low signal intensity on T2-weighted images, not suppressed by fat-saturated sequences helps to distinguish melanoma from other malignancies besides accurately estimating the local extension of disease.[29]

Wide local excision is the mainstay of treatment and the aim is to completely resect the tumor with a 1–2 cm tumor free margin.[30] Radical approach may be used in multifocal disease. In patients presenting with large masses involving the urethra, the bladder, and/or the rectum, total pelvic exenteration may be considered with removal of enlarged groin and/or pelvic nodes.[31] Sentinel lymph node mapping has been used in melanoma instead of complete lymphadenectomy in order to reduce the morbidity, but reports are few.[31,32]

Radiotherapy is used as primary definitive primary treatment in patients with surgically unresectable disease or in patients who refuse surgery. It is also used for adjuvant postoperative treatment in patients with no clear surgical margins, tumor size >3 cm or positive groin or pelvic nodes.[33]

Platinum-based chemotherapy, either alone or in combination with dacarbazine and temozolomide, has not proved to be of much benefit. Immunotherapy using various multikinase inhibitors (including sorafenib), PDL1 inhibitors may be effective. Application of high-dose interferon-α-2b may also be an effective neoadjuvant treatment in melanoma.[34]

Tumor stage, tumor size (3 cm cut off), and nodal status are the strongest predictors of clinical outcome.[31] Vaginal melanomas are associated with high risk of recurrence, distant metastases and 5-year survival of 18–20%.[30,35]

CONCLUSION

Squamous cell cancer is the most common histologic subtype of vaginal cancer. Radiation is the mainstay of treatment while surgery is reserved for stage 1 disease. Tumor stage is the most important prognostic factor. With earlier diagnosis and advances in radiotherapy, survival is improving. Vaginal melanomas carry a bad prognosis.

KEY MESSAGES

- The mainstay of treatment for invasive squamous cell cancer of vagina is usually concurrent chemoradiation.
- Surgery for management of vaginal cancer is limited to stage 1 disease.
- Poor prognosis factors include old age, advanced stage at presentation, tumor size >4 cm and tumor outside the upper third of the vagina.
- Interferon and immunotherapy may be useful in management of melanoma.

REFERENCES

1. Siegel R, Naishadham D, Jemal A. Cancer statistics, 2013. CA Cancer J Clin. 2013;63:11-30.
2. Khurana A, Gupta G, Gupta M, Kaur M. Primary neuroendocrine carcinoma of the vagina with coexistent atypical vaginal adenosis: a rare entity. J Cancer Res Ther. 2013;9(2):328-30.
3. Hacker NF, Eifel PJ, van der Velden J. Cancer of the vagina. Int J Gynaecol Obstet. 2012;119(Suppl 2):S97-S99.
4. Beller U, Benedet JL, Creasman WT, Ngan HY, Quinn MA, Maisonneuve P, et al. Carcinoma of the vagina. FIGO 26th Annual Report on the Results of Treatment in Gynecological Cancer. Int J Gynaecol Obstet. 2006;95(Suppl 1): S29-42.
5. Conlon JL. Diethylstilbestrol: potential health risks for women exposed in utero and their offspring. JAAPA. 2017;30(2):49-52.
6. Frank SJ, Deavers MT, Jhingran A, Bodurka DC, Eifel PJ. Primary adenocarcinoma of the vagina not associated with diethylstilbestrol (DES) exposure. Gynecol Oncol. 2007;105(2):470-4.
7. Madeleine MM, Daling JR. Cancers of the vulva and vagina. In: Schottenfeld D, Fraumeni JF (Eds). Cancer epidemiology and prevention. New York: Oxford University Press; 2006. pp. 1068-74.
8. IARC. Global Cancer Statistics 2020. Available from: https://gco.iarc.fr/today/data/factsheets/populations/356-india-fact-sheets.pdf. [Last accessed November, 2021].
9. Daling JR, Madeleine MM, Schwartz SM, Shera KA, Carter JJ, McKnight B, et al. A population-based study of squamous cell vaginal cancer: HPV and cofactors. Gynecol Oncol. 2002;84(2):263-70.
10. Bertoli HK, Rasmussen CL, Sand FL, Albieri V, Norrild B, Verdoodt F, et al. Human papillomavirus and p16 in squamous cell carcinoma and intraepithelial neoplasia of the vagina. Int J Cancer. 2019;145(1):78-86.
11. Morrow CP, Curtin JP. Tumors of the vagina. In: Synopsis of Gynecological Oncology, 5th edition. Philadelphia, PA: Churchill Livingstone; 1998. pp. 89-105.
12. Slomovitz BM, Coleman RL. Invasive Cancer of the vagina. In: DiSaia PJ, Creasman WT (Eds). Clinical Gynecologic Oncology, 8th edition. Philadelphia: Elsevier Saunders; 2012. pp. 245-59.
13. Gadducci A, Fabrini MG, Lanfredini N, Sergiampietri C. Squamous cell carcinoma of the vagina: natural history, treatment modalities and prognostic factors. Crit Rev Oncol Hematol. 2015;93(3):211-24.
14. Rajaram S, Maheshwari A, Srivastava A. Staging for vaginal cancer. Best Pract Res Clin Obstet Gynaecol. 2015;29(6):822-32.
15. Bipat S, Glas AS, van der Velden J, Zwinderman AH, Bossuyt PM, Stoker J. Computed tomography and magnetic resonance imaging in staging of uterine cervical carcinoma: a systematic review. Gynecol Oncol. 2003;91(1):59-66.
16. Gardner CS, Sunil J, Klopp AH. Primary vaginal cancer: role of MRI in diagnosis, staging and treatment. Br J Radiol. 2015;88(1052):20150033.
17. Donati OF, Lakhman Y, Sala E, Burger IA, Vargas HA, Goldman DA, et al. Role of preoperative MR imaging in the evaluation of patients with persistent or recurrent gynaecological malignancies before pelvic exenteration. Eur Radiol. 2013;23(10):2906-15.
18. Kim WY, Chang SJ, Chang KH, Yoo SC, Lee EJ, Ryu HS. Reliability of magnetic resonance imaging for bladder or rectum invasion in cervical cancer. J Reprod Med. 2011;56(11-12):485-90.
19. Robertson NL, Hricak H, Sonoda Y, Sosa RE, Benz M, Lyons G, et al. The impact of FDG-PET/CT in the management of patients with vulvar and vaginal cancer. Gynecol Oncol. 2016;140(3): 420-4.

20. Lee LJ, Jhingran A, Kidd E, Cardenes HR, Elshaikh MA, Erickson B, et al. Acr appropriateness criteria management of vaginal cancer. Oncology (Williston Park). 2013;27(11):1166-73.
21. Adams TS, Cuello MA. Cancer of the vagina. Int J Gynaecol Obstet. 2018;143(Suppl 2):14-21.
22. Saito T, Tabata T, Ikushima H, Yanai H, Tashiro H, Niikura H, et al. Japan Society of Gynecologic Oncology guidelines 2015 for the treatment of vulvar cancer and vaginal cancer. Int J Clin Oncol. 2018;23(2):201-34.
23. Schnürch HG, Ackermann S, Alt-Radtke CD, Angleitner L, Barinoff J, Beckmann MW, et al. Diagnosis, Therapy and Follow-up of Vaginal Cancer and Its Precursors. Guideline of the DGGG and the DKG (S2k-Level, AWMF Registry No. 032/042, October 2018). Geburtshilfe Frauenheilkd. 2019;79(10):1060-78.
24. Frank SJ, Jhingran A, Levenback C. Definitive radiation therapy for squamous cell carcinoma of the vagina. Int J Radiat Oncol Biol Phys. 2005;62:138-47.
25. Vargo JA, Kim H, Houser CJ, Sukumvanich P, Olawaiye AB, Kelley JL, et al. Image-based multichannel vaginal cylinder brachytherapy for vaginal cancer. Brachytherapy. 2015;14(1):9-15.
26. Moran MS, Castrucci WA, Ahmad M. Clinical utility of the modified segmental boost technique for treatment of the pelvis and inguinal nodes. Int J Radiat Oncol Biol Phys. 2010;76:1026-36.
27. Rajagopalan MS, Xu KM, Lin J. Patterns of care and brachytherapy boost utilization for vaginal cancer in the United States. Pract Radiat Oncol. 2015;5(1):56-61.
28. Creasman WT, Phillips JL, Menck HR. The National Cancer Data Base report on cancer of the vagina. Cancer. 1998;83(5):1033-40.
29. Gökaslan H, Sişmanoğlu A, Pekin T, Kaya H, Ceyhan N. Primary malignant melanoma of the vagina: a case report and review of the current treatment options. Eur J Obstet Gynecol Reprod Biol. 2005;121(2):243-8.
30. Sugiyama VE, Chan JK, Kapp DS. Management of melanomas of the female genital tract. Curr Opin Oncol. 2008;20(5):565-9.
31. Gadducci A, Carinelli S, Guerrieri ME, Aletti GD. Melanoma of the lower genital tract: Prognostic factors and treatment modalities. Gynecol Oncol. 2018;150(1):180-9.
32. Nakagawa S, Koga K, Kugu K, Tsutsumi O, Taketani Y. The evaluation of the sentinel node successfully conducted in a case of malignant melanoma of the vagina. Gynecol Oncol. 2002;86:387-9.
33. Siu SS, Lo KW, Chan AB, Yu MY, Cheung TH. Nodal detection in malignant melanoma of the vagina using laparoscopic ultrasonography. Gynecol Oncol. 2004;92:985-8.
34. Kirschner AN, Kidd EA, Dewees T, Perkins SM. Treatment approach and outcomes of vaginal melanoma. Int J Gynecol Cancer. 2013;23(8):1484-9.
35. Terzakis E, Androutsopoulos G, Adonakis G, Zygouris D, Grigoriadis C, Decavalas G. Vaginal primary malignant melanoma: report of four cases and review of the literature. Eur J Gynaecol Oncol. 2011;32(1):122-4.

LONG QUESTIONS

1. What is the epidemiology and risk factors of vaginal cancer?
2. Outline the various therapeutic modalities and stage wise management of vaginal cancer.

SHORT QUESTIONS

Write short notes on:

1. Staging of vaginal cancer.
2. Vaginal melanoma.
3. Radiation treatment of vaginal cancer.

MULTIPLE CHOICE QUESTIONS

1. What is false about DES associated cancers?
   a. Adenocarcinoma usually develops from vaginal adenosis in women with intrauterine exposure to diethylstilbestrol
   b. DES associated cancers are rare
   c. Associated with good prognosis
   d. Occur in older women
2. What is true about tumor presentation in vaginal cancer?
   a. Squamous cell cancers tend to occur more commonly in the posterior wall
   b. Adenocarcinomas are usually seen in the anterior wall
   c. Most common site of tumor is middle third of the vagina
3. What is true about MRI in vaginal cancer?
   a. It is only useful in primary disease
   b. Primary vaginal tumors are best visualized on T2-weighted images
   c. MRI accuracy is 50–60% for local extension
   d. Best modality for lymph node metastasis
4. Which statement is not true for malignant melanoma?
   a. Always visible as a pigmented lesion in the vagina
   b. Wide local excision is the mainstay of treatment
   c. It is not chemosensitive
   d. Immunotherapy and high-dose interferon-α-2b may also be an effective

Answers

1. d 2. c 3. b 4. a

14.5 MALIGNANT DISEASE OF VAGINA

Saritha Shamsunder

INTRODUCTION

Carcinoma cervix represents a major public health problem accounting for significant morbidity and mortality. This genital cancer of women has the greatest potential for secondary prevention. The incidence of carcinoma cervix is decreasing due to implementation of various screening and prevention strategies, but it is still high in resource limited settings.

Human papillomavirus (HPV) can be detected in 99.7% of cases of cervical cancer and is central to its development.[1] Around 20% patients present in early stage of cervical cancer whereas 80% patients present with advanced disease.[2] It is very important to pick up preinvasive lesions when the treatment is simple with very low treatment related morbidity.

EPIDEMIOLOGY

Globally carcinoma cervix is the fourth most common cancer and fourth leading cause of cancer related mortality in women, and accounts for about 604,000 new cancer cases and 342,000 deaths annually.[3]

As per the National Cancer Registry of India (Cancer Statistics 2020), the crude incidence rate of cervical cancer is 10.9 with cumulative risk of 1 in 75.[4]

RISK FACTORS

Early onset of sexual activity: Risk is 1.5 fold for 18–20 years and two-fold for younger than 18 years.[5]

- Multiple sexual partners[5]
- History of sexually transmitted infections
- Early age at first child birth (younger than 20 years)[5]
- Multiparity (three or more full term births)
- History of cervical, vulvar or vaginal squamous intraepithelial neoplasia
- Immunosuppression
- *Oral contraceptive use:* Risk increases with increasing duration of use (>5 years = RR 1.9) and returns to normal after 10 years of stoppage.[6]
- Low socioeconomic status
- Cigarette smoking-associated with increased risk of squamous cell carcinoma[5]

ETIOPATHOGENESIS

Human papillomavirus is a small double stranded deoxyribonucleic acid (DNA) virus of approximately 7,900 base pairs. It is the most common sexually transmitted infection and is responsible for a substantial proportion of pre malignant and malignant lesions of the cervix, vagina and vulva. The broad separation of HPV genotypes is based on their associated risk of cervical cancer and include 14 high-risk types: 16, 18, 31, 33, 35, 39, 45, 51, 52, 56, 58, 59, 66, and 68 and 12 low-risk genotypes of HPV are 6, 11, 40, 42, 43, 44, 53, 54, 61, 72, 73, and 81.

Types 16 and 18 are the most commonly isolated HPV types in carcinoma cervix, with type 16 being found in approximately 50% of cases.[1]

Carcinogenesis pathway of HPV: The HPV genome encodes DNA sequences for six early (E) proteins that are primarily associated with viral gene regulation and cell transformation, two late (L) proteins that form the shell of the virus, and a region of regulatory DNA sequences known as the long control region or upstream regulatory region.

The two most important HPV proteins in the pathogenesis of malignant disease are E6 and E7 which act in a cooperative manner to immortalize epithelial cells.[7] At the molecular level, the ability of E6 and E7 proteins to transform cells relates in part to their interaction with two intracellular proteins, p53 and retinoblastoma (Rb). Following E6 binding of p53, it is degraded.[8] This allows unchecked cellular cycling, and has an antiapoptotic effect, permitting the accumulation of chromosomal mutations without DNA repair which leads to chromosomal instability in high-risk HPV containing cells.[9] E7 interacts with Rb protein via an E2F/Rb protein complex, E2F is released and allows cyclin A to promote cell cycling. These processes allow unchecked cell growth in the presence of genomic instability that may lead to malignant change.

Histological Types and Subtypes[10]

- *Squamous epithelial tumors:* Mimics of squamous precursor lesions
  - Squamous metaplasia
  - Atrophy of the uterine cervix
- Squamous cell tumors and precursors
  - Condyloma acuminatum
  - Squamous intraepithelial lesions of the uterine cervix
  - Squamous cell carcinoma, HPV associated, of the uterine cervix
  - Squamous cell carcinoma, HPV independent, of the uterine cervix
  - Squamous cell carcinoma, NOS of the uterine cervix
- Glandular tumors and precursors
  - Benign glandular lesions
    - Endocervical polyp
    - Müllerian papilloma of the uterine cervix
    - Nabothian cyst
    - Tunnel clusters
    - Microglandular hyperplasia
    - Lobular endocervical glandular hyperplasia

- Diffuse laminar endocervical hyperplasia
- Mesonephric remnants and hyperplasia
- Arias Stella reaction of the uterine cervix
- Endocervicosis of the uterine cervix
- Tuboendometrioid metaplasia
- Ectopic prostate tissue
- Adenocarcinomas
  - Adenocarcinoma in situ, HPV associated, of the uterine cervix
  - Adenocarcinoma, HPV associated, of the uterine cervix
  - Adenocarcinoma in situ, HPV independent, of the uterine cervix
  - Adenocarcinoma, HPV independent, gastric type, of the uterine cervix
  - Adenocarcinoma, HPV independent, clear cell type, of the uterine cervix
  - Adenocarcinoma, HPV independent, mesonephric type, of the uterine cervix
  - Other adenocarcinomas of the uterine cervix
- Other epithelial tumors
  - Carcinosarcoma of the uterine cervix
  - Adenosquamous and mucoepidermoid carcinomas of the uterine cervix
  - Adenoid basal carcinoma of the uterine cervix
  - Carcinoma of the uterine cervix, unclassifiable
- Mixed epithelial and mesenchymal tumors
- Adenomyoma of the uterine cervix
  - Mesonephric type-adenomyoma
  - Endocervical type adenomyoma
- Adenosarcoma of the uterine cervix
  - Germ cell tumors: Germ cell tumor NOS
  - Mature teratoma NOS
  - Dermoid cyst NOS
  - Endodermal sinus tumor
  - Yolk sac tumor NOS
  - Choriocarcinoma NOS

Squamous cell carcinoma accounts for 70% of cases followed by adenocarcinoma in 25%.[2]

The HPV genotypes leading to SCC of cervix are HPV 16 (59%), 18 (13%), 58 (5%), 33 (5%), 45 (4%).[11] The important subtypes such as large cell keratinizing tumors have better prognosis than small cell variant. Small cell anaplastic carcinoma lesions resemble oat cell carcinoma of the lung. It behaves aggressively and has a poor prognosis. Other rare variants include verrucous carcinoma, which may resemble giant condyloma acuminatum and rarely metastasize and papillary (transitional) carcinoma which histologically resembles transitional cells of the bladder.

Adenocarcinoma commonly affects younger women in their 2nd or 3rd decade of life.[12] The commonly found HPV genotypes are HPV 18 (37%), 16 (36%), 45 (5%),31 (2%), 33 (2%).[11] Important subtypes such as mucin producing endocervical cell variant comprises of nearly 80% of the cases.

Adenoma malignum (minimal deviation adenocarcinoma) is a special variant which may not be identified as malignant in small biopsy specimen, causing delay in diagnosis and may require special immunohistochemistry staining for the same **(Figs. 1 and 2)**. Other subtypes such as Villoglandular papillary adenocarcinoma, has limited risk of spread beyond the uterus and is generally seen in young women.[13]

Neuroendocrine tumors of the cervix though rare, have high propensity to metastasize and have aggressive behavior. These are usually disseminated at the time of diagnosis with bone, brain, liver and bone marrow being the most common sites.[14]

PATTERNS OF SPREAD

Carcinoma of the uterine cervix spreads by direct invasion, by lymphatic dissemination or by hematogenous route.

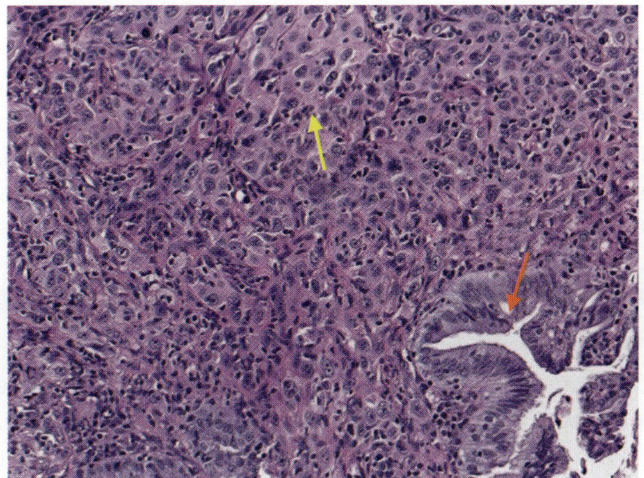

Fig. 1: Squamous cell carcinoma in high power view with yellow arrow indicating atypical squamous cells in stroma and orange arrow indicating normal endocervical gland.

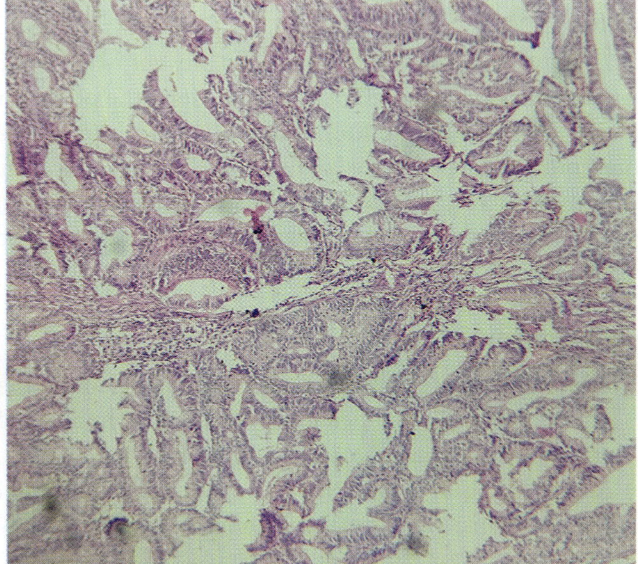

Fig. 2: Adenocarcinoma in low power view with red circle showing atypical glandular epithelium with moderate nuclear atypia.

- *Direct extension* may involve the uterine corpus, vagina, parametria, encasement of ureters, bladder, or rectum. Ovarian involvement is rare and in early-stage may occur in approximately 1.7% of adenocarcinomas and 0.5% of squamous cell carcinomas.[15]
- *Lymphatic spread:* The risk of lymph node involvement increases with increase in stage. The incidence of pelvic lymph node metastasis is 0.5% in Stage IA1, 4.8% in IA2, 15.9% in IB, 24.5% in IIA, 31.4% in IIB, 44.8% in III, 55% in IVA and para-aortic metastasis is 0% in Stage IA1, <1% in IA2, 2.2% in IB, 11% in IIA,19% in IIB, 30% in III, 40% in IVA.[16,17]
- *Hematogenous spread:* Rare, but if it happens, the common sites involved are the lungs, liver, and bone; the bowel, adrenal glands, spleen, and brain are less frequent sites.

Earlier, it was reported that obturator lymph node was the first draining node and was considered the sentinel node, but recently it has been seen that any of the pelvic lymph node groups, or rarely para-aortic lymph nodes, can be the first draining lymph node from cervical cancer.[18] The distribution of sites of nodal metastasis is as follows: external iliac (43%), obturator (26%), parametrial (21%), common iliac (7%), presacral (1%), and para-aortic (1%).[19]

CLINICAL FEATURES

History

The patients are usually parous, sexually active, of low socioeconomic status and are around the age of 48–50 years.

In early cervical cancer, the patients generally present with heavy or irregular vaginal bleeding, post-coital bleeding, or with vaginal discharge that may be watery, mucoid, or purulent and/or malodorous. Rarely carcinoma cervix may be asymptomatic if the growth is small and may be picked up during examination for some other condition or during screening.

In advanced disease, patients may present with pelvic or lower back pain, which may radiate along the posterior side of the lower extremities. Lump abdomen can be the chief complaint if pyometra has developed. Bowel or urinary symptoms, such as pressure-related complaints, hematuria, hematochezia, or vaginal passage of urine or stool can be present in some women.

Examination

- A careful general examination must be done to look for the presence of pallor, leg edema, supra clavicular lymph node enlargement or palpable inguinal lymph nodes.
- Abdominal examination is generally normal except when there is increase in size of uterus due to pyometra or if any other concurrent pathology is present.
- Local vulvar examination, purulent discharge may be seen at fourchette. Concurrent multifocal HPV related changes should be looked for during vulval and vaginal examinations.
- Speculum examination may reveal a superficial ulceration or exophytic tumor on the ectocervix, which can also infiltrate into the endocervix. If the growth is totally endophytic, cervix appears enlarged, smooth, and indurated, often referred to as a "barrel shaped cervix". Among cervical adenocarcinomas, approximately one-half are exophytic, others are diffusely enlarged or ulcerative lesions over the cervix, and approximately 15% have no visible lesion because the carcinoma is within the endocervical canal.
- *Vaginal examination:* Cervix may feel firm to hard which bleeds on touch or obvious growth can be felt involving a part or whole of the cervix. Note should be made of size, character, consistency and mobility of the growth and if there is any extension to vagina. Uterus can be normal or enlarged in size due to pyometra. Vaginal walls may be involved.
- Rectovaginal examination is done to check for involvement of parametrium, involvement of the rectal mucosa, status of uterosacral ligaments and confirmation of the vaginal examination findings.

Differential diagnosis: Cervical lesions leading to irregular vaginal bleeding, postcoital bleeding or cervical growth must be differentiated from:

- *Cervical erosions:* The cervix appears red velvety non-indurating, and does not bleed on light touch, oozing might occur on rubbing.
- *Cervical polyp:* It is nonfriable, smooth pedunculated mass arising from cervix or protruding through os. Diagnosis is confirmed on biopsy.
- *Cervical tuberculosis:* It can present as vegetative or ulcerative or hypertrophic growth mimicking carcinomatous lesion which may even bleed on touch. Diagnosis is confirmed on histopathological examination which may show epithelioid granulomatous lesion with giant cells with or without caseous necrosis and presence of acid fast bacilli.
- *Cervical syphilitic ulcer:* It may present with punched out ulcer with syphilitic base. History of exposure or multiple sexual partners might be present.

Diagnosis: It requires thorough history, examination and investigations. The diagnosis is confirmed by histological evaluation of cervical biopsy.

Cervical biopsy: Punch biopsy is taken from the junction of healthy and unhealthy appearing tissue on the cervix or from obvious growth, avoiding the grossly necrotic areas which are often nondiagnostic. Biopsy in patients with gross lesions may result in significant bleeding, and one should be prepared with hemostatic agents such as Monsel solution and/or packing material to control the bleeding.

Sometimes, women may present with abnormal cervical cytology showing squamous cell carcinoma but cervix has no obvious growth. In these cases colposcopy and directed biopsy is required.

Pretreatment Workup

Pretreatment workup of the patient mandates clinical staging by physical examination including gynecological examination, and imaging modalities to assign proper stage for deciding appropriate management, to determine prognosis and follow up.

Staging: The Federation of Obstetric and Gynaecological Societies of India (FIGO) 2018 **(Table 1)** has revised the staging of the carcinoma of the cervix uteri incorporating imaging and/or pathological findings along with the clinical assessment of the tumor size and disease extent. Size of the tumor and stage are closely related to prognostic parameters. Lymph node involvement is the most significant prognostic parameter in early stages of cervical cancer.

Various imaging modalities used are ultrasound, magnetic resonant imaging (MRI), computed tomography (CT) and positron emission tomography (PET-CT). For primary tumor characterization and parametrial and vaginal spread, MRI or USG are more accurate than CECT scan.

Performance of imaging modalities in terms of parametrial invasion shows sensitivity and specificity of CT scan to be 17–84% and 64% and that of MRI to be 40–57% and 77–80%, respectively.

For assessment of lymph node metastasis, sensitivity and specificity of CT scan is 31% and 86%, MRI is 30–73% and 69–95% and that of PET CT is 78–91% and 94–100%, respectively.[21] For detection of metastasis in para-aortic lymph nodes MRI, CT and PET-CT have equal sensitivity (84%) **(Fig. 3)**.

Pretreatment surgical evaluation of para-aortic lymph nodes: Para-aortic lymph nodes can be enlarged due to infection or metastasis. In the regions where tuberculosis is prevalent one has to make sure that the enlarged para-aortic nodes are sampled to define the pathology. Pathological evaluation can be done by either CT guided fine needle aspiration biopsy or laparoscopic excision biopsy. If metastasis is proved then patient will require extended beam radiotherapy.

Pre-treatment investigations: Patients should have a complete blood count, liver and renal function tests, viral markers and a chest radiograph prior to treatment. Management is done based on stage **(Table 2)**.

TABLE 1: FIGO staging carcinoma of the cervix uteri (2018).[20]

Stage	Description
I	The carcinoma is strictly confined to the cervix (extension to the uterine corpus should be disregarded)
IA	Invasive carcinoma that can be diagnosed only by microscopy with maximum depth of invasion ≤5 mm[a]
IA1	Measured stromal invasion ≤3 mm in depth
IA2	Measured stromal invasion >3 mm and ≤5 mm in depth
IB	Invasive carcinoma with measured deepest invasion >5 mm (greater than stage IA), lesion limited to the cervix uteri[b]
IB1	Invasive carcinoma >5 mm of stromal invasion, and ≤2 cm in greatest dimension
IB2	Invasive carcinoma >2 cm and ≤4 cm in greatest dimension
IB3	Invasive carcinoma >4 cm in greatest dimension
II	The carcinoma invades beyond the uterus but has not extended onto the lower third of the vagina or the pelvic wall
IIA	Involvement limited to the upper two-thirds of the vagina without parametrial involvement
IIA1	Invasive carcinoma ≤4 cm in greatest dimension
IIA2	Invasive carcinoma >4 cm in greatest dimension
IIB	With parametrial involvement but not up to the pelvic wall
III	The carcinoma involves the lower third of the vagina and/or extends to the pelvic wall and/or causes the hydronephrosis or nonfunctioning kidney and/or involves pelvic and/or para-aortic lymph nodes
IIIA	The carcinoma involves the lower third of the vagina, with no extensions to the pelvic wall
IIIB	Extensions to the pelvic wall and/or hydronephrosis or non-functioning kidney (unless known to be due to another cause)
IIIC	Involvement of pelvic and/or para-aortic lymph nodes (including micrometastasis), irrespective of tumor size and extent (with r and p notations)[c]
IIIC1	Pelvic lymph node metastasis only
IIIC2	Para-aortic lymph node metastasis
IV	The carcinoma has extended beyond the true pelvis or has involved (biopsy proven) the mucosa of the bladder or the rectum, (A bullous edema, as such, does not permit a case to be allotted to stage IV)
IVA	Spread to adjacent pelvic organs
IVB	Spread to distant organs

When in doubt the lower staging should be assigned.
[a]Imaging and the pathology can be used where available to supplement the clinical findings with respect to tumor size and extent in all stages.
[b]The involvement of vascular/lymphatic spaces does not change the staging.
[c]Adding notations of r (imaging) and p (pathology) to indicate the findings that are used to allocate the case to stage IIIC. For example: If imaging indicates pelvic lymph node metastasis the stage allocation would be stage IIIC(r), and if confirmed by pathologic findings, it would be stage IIIC1(p).
(FIGO: The Federation of Obstetric and Gynaecological Societies of India)

TREATMENT MODALITIES

Basic Principle

All stages of cervical cancer are amenable to primary treatment with radical radiation with or without chemotherapy. However, surgical modality is preferred for women in early stages with good performance status in view of lower long-term morbidity. Some of these women might require adjuvant treatment as well depending on the final histopathological risk

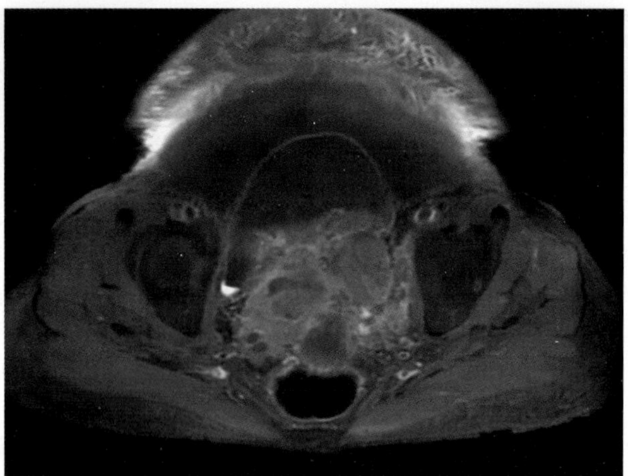

Fig. 3: Preaxial T1 weighted post-contrast MRI pelvis showing cervical growth with red circle and parametrial invasion with blue circle.

TABLE 2: Stage based management of cervical cancer.

IA1	≤3 mm without LVSI ≤3 mm with LVSI	• Conization or extrafascial hysterectomy • Radical trachelectomy or • Modified radical hysterectomy + pelvic lymphadenectomy or SLN
IA2	>3 mm to ≤5 mm	• Radical trachelectomy or • Modified radical hysterectomy + pelvic lymphadenectomy or SLN
IB1	>5 mm to ≤2 cm	Radical trachelectomy or Modified radical/radical hysterectomy + pelvic lymphadenectomy or SLN
IB2	≥2 cm to ≤4 cm	Radical Hysterectomy + pelvic lymphadenectomy
IB3	>4 cm	• Concurrent chemoradiation, (EBRT - pelvic field + brachytherapy) (preferred) • Radical hysterectomy pelvic lymphadenectomy
IIA1	≤4 cm + upper two-thirds vagina	Radical hysterectomy + pelvic lymphadenectomy or chemoradiation
IIA2	>4 cm + upper two-thirds vagina	Chemoradiation, pelvic field
IIB	+ Parametria not to pelvic wall	Chemoradiation, pelvic field
IIIA	+ Lower vagina	Chemoradiation, pelvic field + groin node irradiation
IIIB	+ Pelvic wall or hydronephrosis	Chemoradiation, pelvic ± extended field
IIIC1	+ Pelvic lymph node	Chemoradiation, pelvic ± extended field
IIIC2	+ Para-aortic lymph node	Chemoradiation, pelvic + extended field ± systemic chemotherapy
IVA	+ Adjacent pelvic organs	Chemoradiation, pelvic ± extended field or pelvic exenteration
IVB	+ Distant organs	Systemic therapy (chemotherapy + targeted therapy) ± radiation, pelvic or modified field

(EBRT: external beam radiation therapy; LVSI: lymphovascular space invasion; SLN: sentinel lymph node)

factors. However, the goal is to avoid dual modality treatment in the form of radical surgery and adjuvant treatment in view of increased toxicity without any survival advantage. Therefore, a careful selection of patients for surgical management is essential.

Surgical Management

In young women, where ovarian function preservation is important, surgery has an advantage over radiotherapy in early-stage cervical cancer. In lesions larger than 4 cm in diameter, concurrent chemoradiation is preferred over radical surgery because a substantial number of these women will require adjuvant treatment.

Various Surgical Procedures for Carcinoma Cervix

- Cone biopsy of the cervix
- Hysterectomy
  - Extrafascial hysterectomy with lymph node dissection
  - Modified radical hysterectomy with lymph node dissection
  - Radical hysterectomy with lymph node dissection
  - Nerve sparing radical hysterectomy
  - Exenteration procedures
- Trachelectomy
  - Simple trachelectomy
  - *Radical trachelectomy:* Abdominal or vaginal.

Cone biopsy of cervix: It serves as a diagnostic and therapeutic procedure in microinvasive cervical cancer. Cold knife conization is the resection of a cone shaped portion of the cervix using a surgical knife.

Indications:
- To confirm the diagnosis
- To treat stage IA1 disease when fertility is desired.

For cone biopsy alone to be therapeutic, there should be no evidence of lymphovascular space invasion (LVSI) and both endocervical margins and curettage findings must be negative for carcinoma or dysplasia **(Fig. 4)**.

Side effects: Hemorrhage, cervical incompetence, preterm labor and cervical stenosis.

Hysterectomy: The steps of type A, B and C are described in **Table 3 (Fig. 5)**.

Nerve sparing radical hysterectomy: Oncologically relevant tissues surrounding the cervical lesion are removed while preserving pelvic autonomic nerves. Here, the neural part of the uterosacral and cardinal ligaments which contain autonomic nerves are preserved. The hypogastric nerve plexus as well as the distal part (bladder branch), remains intact. Thus, the bladder's innervation is safe with resultant rapid functional recovery of urinary bladder.

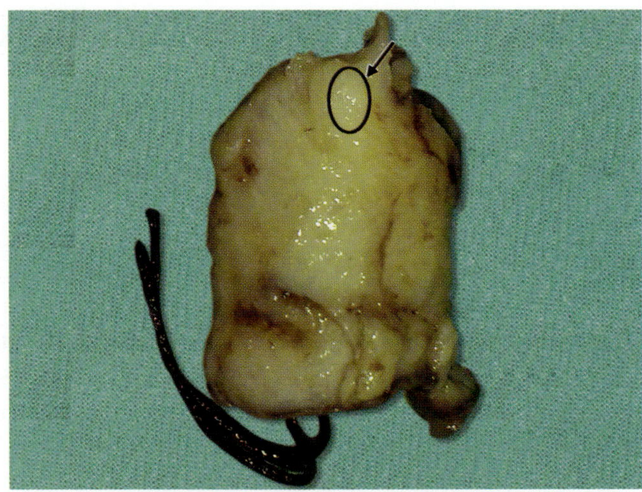

Fig. 4: Cone biopsy specimen of cervix marked at 12 O'clock position.

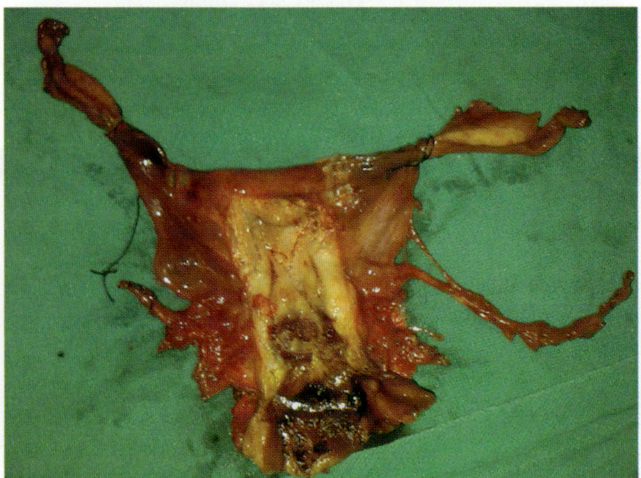

Fig. 5: Radical hysterectomy specimen showing uterus, cervix, vaginal cuff, parametrium, bilateral fallopian tubes and ovaries.

Complications of radical hysterectomy:

Intraoperative:

- Blood loss.
- Injuries to pelvic blood vessels, bladder, rectum or obturator nerves.

Postoperative:

Early complications:

- Fever (25–50%)
  - Urinary tract infections
  - Pulmonary infections
  - Surgical site infections (wound infection/pelvic abscess)
- Urinary complications such as bladder dysfunction, fistula formation (ureterovaginal fistula: 1–2%, vesicovaginal fistula)
- Deep vein thrombosis and pulmonary embolism (1–2%)
- Vesicovaginal fistula (1%)
- Ileus (1%).

Late complications:

- Bladder dysfunction
- Lymphocyst formation, lymphedema.

Trachelectomy

Indications: Fertility preserving surgery done in selected young women with cervical cancer for stage IA2 or stage IB1 lesions of ≤2 cm in diameter. Difference between simple and radical trachelectomy are described in **Table 4**.

Prerequisites for trachelectomy: Young age, desirous of fertility, small tumor size, adequate distance from internal os (at least 1 cm margin after surgery), low risk histology—squamous cell/adenocarcinoma (to be avoided in gastric type of adenocarcinoma, neuroendocrine carcinoma, adenoma malignum), MRI to confirm size and rule out parametrial/LN involvement.

Complications: Postoperative pain, vaginal discharge and bleeding, infertility, incompetence, increased incidence of abortion, second trimester loss, preterm labor.

SENTINEL LYMPH NODE IDENTIFICATION

The sentinel lymph node (SLN) is the first lymph node to receive drainage from the primary tumor (cervical lesion) and is first site for nodal metastasis. SLN identification procedure can replace pelvic lymphadenectomy in early cervical cancer and therefore has the potential to reduce complications associated with lymphadenectomy.

The usual dye includes the use of indocyanine green dye or blue dye and technetium 99 alone or in combination.[23]

Indications for SLN mapping:

- Early stage disease - preferably tumors <2 cm[24]
- No suspicious/enlarged lymph nodes on imaging
- Availability of ultrastaging (i.e., enhanced pathologic review, including additional sectioning and immunohistochemistry for pan cytokeratin of the SLN)

Sentinel lymph node biopsy appears to perform better than imaging studies. The sensitivity and specificity for the detection of lymph node metastasis by various approaches was found to be: SLN biopsy (91% and 100%), PET (75 and 98%), MRI (56 and 93%), and CT (58 and 92%).[25]

PROGNOSTIC FACTORS AND ADJUVANT TREATMENT

Disease stages followed by lymph node status represent the most important prognostic variables. The survival of surgically treated patients of carcinoma cervix depends on the following risk factors.[26]

Intermediate risk factors (any two out of three):

1. Large tumor size > 4 cm
2. Lymphovascular space invasion
3. Cervical stromal invasion to middle or deep one-third.

High risk factors (any one positive):

1. Positive margins
2. Positive lymph nodes
3. Microscopic parametrial involvement.

TABLE 3: Main steps of different types of hysterectomies (Querleu and Morrow Classification).[22]

	Extra facial hysterectomy (Type A)	*Modified radical hysterectomy (Type B)*	*Radical hysterectomy (Type C1/C2)*
Indication	Stage IA1 without LVSI	Stage IA1 with LVSI and IA2	Local disease without obvious metastasis, including: Stage IB1-IIA1
Uterus	Removed	Removed	Removed
Ovaries	Optional removal	Optional removal	Optional removal
Cervix	Completely removed	Completely removed	Completely removed
Vaginal margin	Length of vaginal cuff is adjusted to the extent of tumor; 10 mm of vagina from cervix/tumor		
Ureteral dissection	Not mobilized	Ureters unroofed and dissected from cervix	Ureters are mobilized completely from the ureteric tunnel
Parametrial resection	None	Resection at the level of ureter bed (horizontal resection 1–2 cm)	Divided at medial aspect of internal iliac vessels. The deep margin is the deep uterine vein
Uterosacral ligaments	Divided at cervical border	1–2 cm dorsal from cervix (preserves hypogastric nerve plexus)	Divided at least 2 cm dorsal from cervix (close to the rectum)
Bladder	Mobilized caudal to cervix	Mobilized to upper vagina	Mobilized to middle vagina
Rectum	Not mobilized	Mobilized below cervix	Mobilized till upper vagina

(LVSI: lymphovascular space invasion)

TABLE 4: Difference between simple and radical trachelectomy.

	Simple trachelectomy	*Radical trachelectomy*
Indication	Carcinoma in situ and stage IA1	Stage IA2-IB1 Select IB2
Uterus	Spared	Spared
Ovaries	Spared	Spared
Cervix	Majority removed (approximately 5–10 mm of cranial aspect of the cervix typically left for cerclage)	Majority removed (approximately 5–10 mm of cranial aspect of the cervix typically left for cerclage)
Vaginal margin	Minimal	1–2 cm margin
Ureteral dissection	Not mobilized	Ureters unroofed and dissected from cervix
Parametrium	Resected at cervical border	Resection at the level of ureter bed (horizontal resection 1–2 cm)
Uterosacral ligaments	Divided at cervical border	1–2 cm dorsal from cervix (preserves hypogastric nerve plexus)
Bladder	Mobilized to peritoneal reflection	Mobilized to upper vagina
Rectum	Mobilized to peritoneal reflection	Mobilized below cervix
Approach	Vaginal or laparotomy or minimally invasive	Vaginal or laparotomy or minimally invasive

Patients with intermediate and high risk factors have recurrence risk of 30% and 40%, respectively within 3 years. Therefore, adjuvant radiation therapy (RT) is indicated in women with intermediate risk factors and chemoradiation therapy in women with high risk factors.[27]

- *Lesion size:* patients with lesions <2 cm have survival rate of 90% while >2 cm is 60%.[28]
- *Depth of invasion:* If depth of invasion is <1 cm, a 5-year survival rate of approximately 90% and if more than 1 cm, survival rate of 63–78% is expected.[29]
- *Parametrial involvement:* survival rate is 69% if parametrium is involved and 95% if negative. If involved with positive pelvic lymph nodes, 5-year survival rate drops to 39–42%.[26]
- *Lymphovascular space involvement:* It is the predictor of lymph node metastasis. There is 50–70% 5-year survival rate if LVSI is present and 90% if absent.[30]
- *Lymph node status:* It is an independent predictor of survival. Patients with negative nodes have survival rate of 85–90%, whereas with positive nodes have 20–74% survival rate depending on the number, location of nodes involved and size of metastasis.[31]

FOLLOW-UP

The main aim of follow-up is early detection of the recurrence that might be amenable to potentially curative therapy. A follow-up visit should consist of a detailed history, general

TABLE 5: Survival rate of the patients as per 1999–2001 FIGO statistics.[32]

FIGO stage	*5-year survival rate (%)*
IA1	97.5
IA2	94.8
IB1	89.1
IB2	75.7
IIA	73.4
IIB	65.8
IIIA	39.7
IIIB	41.5
IVA	22.0
IVB	9.3

(FIGO: The Federation of Obstetric and Gynaecological Societies of India)

and pelvic examination. The Society of Gynecologic Oncology, states to avoid routine imaging for cancer surveillance in women with cervical cancer and it should be reserved for patients with symptoms of recurrence **(Table 5)**.[33]

History and physical examination every 3–4 months for 2 years, every 6–12 months for up to 5 years, and then annually as the primary surveillance modality. Symptoms that raise concern for a cervical cancer recurrence include: vaginal bleeding or discharge, abdominopelvic pain, urinary symptoms, and/or change in bowel habits.

Physical examination findings suspicious of recurrence include: Enlarged lymph nodes, in particular groin or supraclavicular nodes; a vaginal lesion that is friable, raised, or nodular; nodularity in the rectovaginal septum; or a palpable mass at any location, most commonly in the pelvis.

For women who have undergone RT, cervicovaginal cytology is not routinely performed as part of surveillance because of high false positive rates. However, in patients who undergo surgery without RT (e.g., those treated with primary hysterectomy for very early disease), annual cervical cytology should be performed.[34]

RECURRENT CERVICAL CANCER

It can present as a local recurrence or as metastatic disease. Locally recurrent cervical cancer usually presents with vaginal symptoms (i.e., discharge, pain, bleeding, dyspareunia).

By comparison, patients with metastatic cervical cancer usually present with either no symptoms or nonspecific complaints (i.e., fatigue, nausea, or weight loss); however, they may have symptoms related to the site of metastases.

The most commonly used imaging modalities to evaluate recurrent cervical cancer include CT and positron emission tomography (PET) with or without CT. It has a sensitivity of 93–96% and specificity of 93–95%.[5]

For women who present with a local relapse confined to the cervix or vagina, treatment is directed according to the site of recurrence. Options include hysterectomy or pelvic exenteration in patients who have received prior RT, or RT in those who have not received RT or are not surgical candidates; the choice depends on the patient's prior treatment.

Patients who have previously been treated with RT and who are not candidates for surgical resection should be offered chemotherapy. The approach to these patients is identical to the treatment of women with metastatic disease.

Candidates for surgical resection: Patients who experience a local recurrence should be offered surgical resection with curative intent. Commonly employed criteria to identify those women most likely to benefit from surgery include:[10]

- A central pelvic recurrence without side wall fixation or associated hydronephrosis
- A long disease-free interval
- Tumor size of the recurrence less than 3 cm in diameter

Surgical Procedure

- Hysterectomy
- *Pelvic exenteration:* It includes anterior exenteration (removal of bladder, uterus, cervix and vagina), posterior exenteration (removal of rectum, vagina, cervix and uterus) and total exenteration.

Contraindication to exenteration:

- Metastatic disease confirmed by imaging
- Extension of the tumor to pelvic sidewall

Clinical triad of: Unilateral leg edema + sciatic pain + ureteral obstruction - pathognomonic of unresectable disease in pelvic sidewall.

Candidates for RT: Radiation therapy is a reasonable option for the following patients:

- Women who have not been previously treated with RT
- Women with operable disease who opt not to proceed with pelvic exenteration. As palliative therapy in patients with localized metastatic lesions that are incurable.

Candidates for chemotherapy: For patients who are not candidates for surgical resection or salvage RT, chemotherapy is the only option.

Carboplatin and paclitaxel ± bevacizumab is the preferred regimen.

Acutely Symptomatic Patients (Palliative Care)

For women with pelvic pain or bleeding from locally advanced disease, and for patients with symptomatic metastatic disease, single-dose or short-course external beam RT may be helpful.

For the treatment of visceral or distant metastases, large fractions of RT administered in a short treatment course may also be used for local treatment of symptoms related to metastatic disease, such as alleviation of pain from skeletal metastases, or symptoms associated with brain lesions.

Locally Advanced Cervical Cancer

Women with locally advanced cervical cancer (stage IB3 to IVA) have a higher rate of recurrence and worse survival than those with early-stage disease (stage IA to IB2).

Bulky stage IB3 to IIA2 disease may be treated either with radical surgery or primary chemoradiation. Primary chemoradiation is the preferred modality of treatment in order to avoid dual modality treatment and ensuing morbidity. If surgical therapy is desired, a type III radical hysterectomy with pelvic lymphadenectomy should be offered. Adjuvant chemoradiation therapy is considered in those who have intermediate or high risk factors post-operatively.

Stage IIB to IIIB cancers are managed primarily by chemoradiation therapy, with cisplatin being the therapeutic agent of choice.

Stage IIIC1 cancer reflects metastatic disease to pelvic lymph nodes where chemoradiation to pelvic lymph nodes is given. While stage IIIC2 includes involvement of para-aortic lymph nodes, where concurrent chemoradiation with extended filed radiotherapy covering the para-aortic lymphnodes is offered.

Stage IVA disease includes involvement of adjacent pelvic organs where patients are either treated with primary chemoradiation therapy or pelvic exenteration surgery which is rarely performed.

In patients with stage IVB disease, the primary concern is control of symptoms with least morbidity. These are candidates of chemotherapy and palliative pelvic radiation therapy.

CONCLUSION

Cancer of uterine cervix is one of the common cancers among women, especially in low and middle-income countries. It is amenable to primary and secondary preventions by HPV vaccination and screening. The revised FIGO2018 cervical cancer staging has incorporated radiological and histopathological findings along with clinical features. Surgery is the standard of care for early-stage cervical cancer, while concurrent chemo-radiation is the treatment of choice for locally advanced stage disease. In recurrent cervical cancer, treatment options are limited and depend on the site of recurrence and previous lines of treatment.

REFERENCES

1. Walboomers JM, Jacobs MV, Manos MM, Bosch FX, Kummer JA, Shah KV, et al. Human papillomavirus is a necessary cause of invasive cervical cancer worldwide. J Pathol. 1999;189:12.
2. Ries LAG, Melbert D, Krapcho M. SEER Cancer Statistics Review, 1975-2004. Bethesda, MD: National Cancer Institute; 2007.
3. Bray F, Ferlay J, Soerjomataram I, Siegel RL, Torre LA, Jemal A. Global cancer statistics 2018: GLOBOCAN estimates of incidence and mortality worldwide for 36 cancers in 185 countries. CA Cancer J Clin. 2018;68:394.
4. Mathur P, Sathishkumar K, Chaturvedi M, Das P, Sudarshan KL, Santhappan S, et al. ICMR-NCDIR-NCRP Investigator Group. Cancer Statistics, 2020: Report From National Cancer Registry Programme, India. JCO Glob Oncol. 2020;6:1063-75.
5. International Collaboration of Epidemiological Studies of Cervical Cancer. Comparison of risk factors for invasive squamous cell carcinoma and adenocarcinoma of the cervix: collaborative reanalysis of individual data on 8,097 women with squamous cell carcinoma and 1,374 women with adenocarcinoma from 12 epidemiological studies. Int J Cancer. 2007;120:885.
6. Castellsagué X, Bosch FX, Muñoz N. Male circumcision, penile human papillomavirus infection, and cervical cancer in female partners. N Engl J Med. 2002;346:1105.
7. Münger K, Phelps WC, Bubb V, Howley PM, Schlegel R. The E6 and E7 genes of the human papillomavirus type 16 together are necessary and sufficient for transformation of primary human keratinocytes. J Virol. 1989;63:4417.
8. Scheffner M, Huibregtse JM, Vierstra RD, Howley PM. The HPV-16 E6 and E6-AP complex functions as a ubiquitin-protein ligase in the ubiquitination of p53. Cell. 1993;75:495.
9. Tommasino M, Adamczewski JP, Carlotti F, Barth CF, Manetti R, Contorni M, et al. HPV16 E7 protein associates with the protein kinase p33CDK2 and cyclin A. Oncogene. 1993;8:195.
10. Kurman RJ, Norris HJ, Wilkinson EJ. Atlas of tumor pathology: Tumors of the cervix, vagina, and vulva, 3rd edition. Washington, DC: Armed Forces Institute of Pathology; 1992.
11. Li N, Franceschi S, Howell-Jones R, Snijders PJ, Clifford GM. Human papillomavirus type distribution in 30,848 invasive cervical cancers worldwide: variation by geographical region, histological type and year of publication. Int J Cancer. 2011;128:927.
12. Kjorstad KE. Adenocarcinoma of the uterine cervix. Gynecol Oncol. 1977;5:219-23.
13. Young RH, Scully RE. Villoglandular papillary adenocarcinoma of the uterine cervix: a clinicopathologic analysis of 13 cases. Cancer. 1989;63:1773-9.
14. Sheets EE, Berman ML, Hrountas CE, Liao SY, DiSaia PJ. Surgically treated, early stage neuroendocrine small-cell cervical carcinoma. Obstet Gynecol. 1988;7:10-4.
15. Sutton GP, Bundy BN, Delgado G, Sevin BU, Creasman WT, Major FJ, et al. Ovarian metastases in stage IB carcinoma of the cervix: a Gynecologic Oncology Group study. Am J Obstet Gynecol. 1992;166:50.
16. Boyce J, Fruchter R, Nicastri A. Prognostic factors in stage I carcinoma of the cervix. Gynecoloncol. 1981;12:154-65.
17. Averette HE, Ford JH Jr, Dudan RC, Girtanner RE, Hoskins WJ, Lutz MH. Staging of cervical cancer. Clin Obstet Gynecol. 1975;18:215-32.
18. Levenback C, Coleman RL, Burke TW, Lin WM, Erdman W, Deavers M, et al. Lymphatic mapping and sentinel node identification in patients with cervix cancer undergoing radical hysterectomy and pelvic lymphadenectomy. J Clin Oncol. 2002;20:688.
19. Bader AA, Winter R, Haas J, Tamussino KF. Where to look for the sentinel lymph node in cervical cancer. Am J Obstet Gynecol. 2007;197:678.e1.
20. Bhatla N, Berek JS, Cuello Frede M, Denny LA, Grenman S, Karunaratne K, et al. FIGO committee report. Revised FIGO staging for carcinoma of the cervix uteri. Int J Gynecol Obstet. 2019:1-7.

21. Siegel CL, Andreotti RF, Cardenes HR, Brown DL, Gaffney DK, Horowitz NS, et al. ACR Appropriateness Criteria pretreatment planning of invasive cancer of the cervix. J Am Coll Radiol. 2012;9(6):395-402.
22. Querleu D, Cibula D, Abu-Rustum NR. 2017 Update on the Querleu-Morrow Classification of Radical Hysterectomy. Ann Surg Oncol. 2017;24(11):3406-12.
23. Zapardiel I, Alvarez J, Barahona M, Barri P, Boldo A, Bresco P, et al. Utility of Intraoperative Fluorescence Imaging in Gynecologic Surgery: Systematic Review and Consensus Statement. Ann Surg Oncol. 2021;28:3266.
24. Abu-Rustum NR, Yashar CM, Bean S, Bradley K, Campos SM, Chon HS, et al. NCCN Guidelines Insights: Cervical Cancer, Version 1.2020. J Natl Compr Canc Netw. 2020;18:660.
25. Selman TJ, Mann C, Zamora J, Appleyard TL, Khan K. Diagnostic accuracy of tests for lymph node status in primary cervical cancer: a systematic review and meta-analysis. CMAJ. 2008;178:855.
26. Inoue T, Okumura M. Prognostic significance of parametrial extension in patients with cervical carcinoma in stage IB, IIA, and IIIB. Cancer. 1984;54:1714-9.
27. Peters WA, Liu PY, Barrett RJ, Everett EN, Bondurant AE, Drescher CW. Concurrent chemotherapy and pelvic radiation therapy alone as adjuvant therapy after radical surgery in high-risk early-stage cancer of the cervix. J Clin Oncol. 2000:18;1606-13.
28. Chung C, Nahhas W, Stryker J. Analysis of factors contributing to treatment failures in stage IB and IIA carcinoma of the cervix. Am J Obstet Gynecol. 1980;138:550-6.
29. Van Nagell J Jr, Greenwell N, Powell D. Microinvasive carcinoma of the cervix. Am J Obstet Gynecol. 1983;145:981-91.
30. Van Nagell J, Donaldson E, Parker J. The prognostic significance of cell type and lesion size in patients with cervical cancer treated by radical surgery. Gynecol Oncol. 1977;5:142-51.
31. Tinga DJ, Timmer PR, Bouma J, Aalders JG. Prognostic significance of single versus multiple lymph node metastasis in cervical carcinoma stage IB. Gynecol Oncol. 1990;39:175-80.
32. Quinn MA, Benedet JL, Odicino F, Maisonneuve P, Beller U, Creasman WT, et al. Carcinoma of the cervix uteri. Int J Gynecol Obstet. 2006;95:S43.
33. Choosing Wisely. An initiative of the ABIM Foundation. [online] Available from: http://www.choosingwisely.org/about-us/. [Last accessed December, 2021].
34. Salani R, Backes FJ, Fung MF, Holschneider CH, Parker LP, Bristow RE, et al. Post-treatment surveillance and diagnosis of recurrence in women with gynecologic malignancies: Society of Gynecologic Oncologists recommendations. Am J Obstet Gynecol. 2011;204:466.

LONG QUESTIONS

1. Classify various types of hysterectomies and their indication in cervical cancer.
2. Mrs X, a 52-year-old, P3L3 postmenopausal lady presents with the chief complain of irregular vaginal bleeding associated with foul smelling discharge for past 3 months. How will you manage this case?
3. Mrs Y, a 55-year-old P2L2 postmenopausal lady presents with the MRI report showing cervical growth of size 2.5 cm × 2.5 cm with no parametrial, vaginal or lymph node involvement. Assign the stage and discuss the stage wise management of this case.
4. Discuss in detail about various prognostic indicators for carcinoma cervix.
5. Enumerate the revised FIGO 2018 staging for carcinoma of the cervix uteri. What changes have been made in FIGO staging of 2018 as compared to 2009?

SHORT QUESTIONS

1. Write a short note on etiopathogenesis of cervical cancer.
2. What are the complications of hysterectomy?
3. Write a note on fertility sparing surgeries for carcinoma cervix.
4. Enumerate various histological types and subtypes of carcinoma cervix.
5. How will you follow-up a woman who has undergone modified radical hysterectomy for carcinoma cervix?

MULTIPLE CHOICE QUESTIONS

1. What constitutes a stage IA cervical cancer?
   a. Depth of stromal invasion less than 5 mm
   b. Lesion not seen by naked eye
   c. horizontal spread less than 7 mm
   d. All of the above
2. Which statement is not correct for FIGO 2018 cervical cancer staging?
   a. Width of lesion is measured in stage IA cancers
   b. Stage IB2 constitutes lesions of size between 2 cm and 4 cm
   c. Pelvic lymph node positivity comes in stage III
   d. All of the above
3. What is true for FIGO 2018 staging?
   a. Staging can be done based on clinical examination
   b. Staging can be done based on radiological findings
   c. Histopathological report can be used to stage the disease
   d. All of the above
4. 65-year-old patient has 4 × 4 cm cervical growth with involvement of upper 2 cm of vagina and B/L parametria. On USG, both kidneys show hydroureteronephrosis with serum creatinine value of 2.5. Cervical biopsy is clear cell carcinoma. What is the stage of the disease?
   a. Stage IB3 b. Stage II A2
   c. Stage III B d. Stage III C
5. Which of these is not a risk factor for development of cervical cancer?
   a. Multiple sexual partners
   b. Early marriage/onset of sexual relationships
   c. HPV vaccination
   d. HIV positive status
6. Which of these is not an indication to receive adjuvant chemoradiation after radical hysterectomy?
   a. Positive vaginal margins
   b. Positive parametrium

c. Deep stromal invasion
d. Positive lymph nodes

7. Which of these is not considered to be an intermediate risk factor to decide adjuvant radiation after radical hysterectomy (Sedlis criteria)?
   a. Deep stromal invasion
   b. Lymph vascular space invasion
   c. Tumor size more than 4 cm
   d. Adenocarcinoma histology
8. What is the preferred treatment for a 45-year-old lady with 3 cm cervical growth without involvement of vagina and parametrium. HPR shows adenocarcinoma and MRI shows no enlarged lymph nodes
   a. Extrafascial type I hysterectomy with BSO
   b. Type III radical abdominal hysterectomy with bilateral pelvic lymph node dissection (BPLND)
   c. Type IIII radical abdominal hysterectomy with BSO with BPLND
   d. Concurrent chemoradiation
9. What's the preferred treatment for a 55-year-old lady with 4 × 5 cm cervical growth with vaginal extension and B/L medial parametrium involvement. HPR shows squamous cell carcinoma.
   a. Concurrent chemoradiation
   b. External beam radiotherapy alone
   c. Chemotherapy followed by surgery
   d. Surgery
10. What constitutes radical chemoradiation for cervical cancer?
   a. External beam radiotherapy (EBRT)
   b. Weekly cisplatin given along with EBRT
   c. Intracavitary brachytherapy
   d. All of the above

Answers

1.	a	2.	a	3.	d	4.	c	5.	c	6.	c
7.	d	8.	c	9.	a	10.	d				

14.6 PREMALIGNANT AND MALIGNANT DISEASES OF THE UTERUS

SK Giri, BL Nayak

INTRODUCTION

This topic is discussed under two major headings:

1. Premalignant diseases of uterus
2. *Malignant diseases of uterus:* divided in to two groups according to tissue of origin:
   a. *Diseases arising from the epithelium of the uterus:* Endometrial carcinoma (EC)
   b. *Diseases arising from the mesenchymal tissue of uterus:* Sarcoma uterus.

PREMALIGNANT DISEASES

The premalignant diseases of endometrium are believed to be the precursors of EC, whereas malignant mesenchymal neoplasm, such as leiomyosarcomas (LMS), endometrial stromal sarcomas, etc., does not have a recognized premalignant phase. So, our discussion on premalignant diseases of uterus will focus on premalignant diseases of endometrium, i.e., endometrial hyperplasia (EH) **(Fig. 1)**.

Endometrial Hyperplasia

Endometrial hyperplasia is described as a nonphysiological, noninvasive proliferation of endometrial glands of irregular size and shape, visibly resulting in an increase in the volume of endometrial glands in relation to endometrial stroma. Both EH and endometrioid adenocarcinoma commonly share many genotypic alterations, including microsatellite instability, *PTEN* and *K-ras* gene mutations.[1]

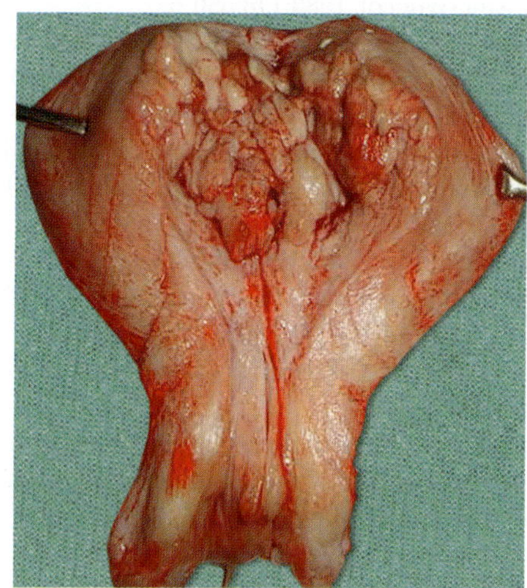

Fig. 1: Hyperplastic endometrium.

Classification of EH

The most followed classification of EH was WHO 1994 classification. This system characterizes the glandular and architectural pattern as simple or complex and describes the presence or absence of nuclear atypia to differentiate between atypical and typical EH.[2]

WHO 1994 classification of EH:[2]

- Simple hyperplasia without atypia
- Complex hyperplasia without atypia
- Simple hyperplasia with atypia
- Complex hyperplasia with atypia.

Atypical EH (AEH) does have increased risk of subsequent development of adenocarcinoma[3] **(Table 1)**. Besides, there is substantial risk of coexisting EC in patients with biopsy report of atypical hyperplasia. A prospective GOG study found concurrent invasive adenocarcinoma in 42.6% of hysterectomy specimen in 306 patients with preoperative biopsies of AEH.[4]

Mutter and the Endometrial Collaborative Group (ECG) simplified the WHO classification by entertaining two, rather than four categories—"endometrial hyperplasia" and "endometrial intraepithelial neoplasia" (EIN). EIN is the immediate precursor of endometrioid adenocarcinoma with 45-fold increased cancer risk. EIN lesion can be diagnosed, if it fulfills the following criteria.[5]

- Monoclonal growth
- Size greater than 1 mm in diameter or more than ten glands
- Closely packed glands with a gland area greater than stromal area
- Cytological change different from that of the adjacent normal endometrium.

WHO in 2014 classified EH accordingly into two groups:[6]

1. Hyperplasia without atypia
2. Atypical EH or endometrioid intraepithelial neoplasia.

Atypical EH or EIN: The two interchangeable terminologies are precursors for development of estrogen dependent Type-I EC, whereas endometrial intraepithelial carcinoma (EIC)[7] (which shows intense p53 protein expression) is the precursor for estrogen independent type-II serous carcinoma.

Risk Factors of EH/EC

- *Estrogen replacement therapy:*[8] Unopposed estrogen use increases the risk of EC, but addition of progestogen reduces the risk.
- *Early menarche before 12 years and late menopause after 52 years:* Prolonged exposure of uterus to progesterone-deficient menstrual cycles.
- *Obesity:* Peripheral conversion of adrenally-derived androstenedione to estrone.
- *Nulliparity:* Infertility and a history of irregular menses as a result of anovulatory cycles (prolonged exposure to estrogen without sufficient progesterone) increase the risk.
- *Diabetes:* Diabetes is association with insulin resistance.
- *Feminizing ovarian tumors:* Due to estrogen secretion.
- *Polycystic ovarian syndrome (PCOS):* The absence of ovulation inhibits the production of progesterone to counteract estrogen.
- *Tamoxifen therapy for breast cancer:* Tamoxifen, a SERM, is an estrogen antagonist in breast cancer tissue but can also cause EH by acting as a partial agonist on the uterus.
- Women with Lynch syndrome/hereditary nonpolyposis colorectal cancer (HNPCC) syndrome, germline mutations in mismatch repair (MMR) genes *MLH1, MSH2,* and *MSH6,* have a 40–60% lifetime risk for endometrial as well as many other cancers including colon cancer.

Protective Factors for EH/EC

- Term pregnancy/multiparity
- Menarche after 15 years
- *OCP:* Protective effect of OCP used for 1 year lasts for even 10 years after cessation.
- Raloxifene
- Smoking
- Soy consumption.

Clinical Features and Diagnosis of Endometrial Hyperplasia/Cancer

The most common clinical presentation of patients with EH and cancer is abnormal uterine bleeding, in the form of heavy menstrual bleeding (HMB), irregular bleeding, abnormal vaginal discharge, or postmenopausal bleeding (PMB). Less than 5% of ECs are asymptomatic. Glandular abnormalities in Pap smear are suspicious of EC.

A detailed history and careful clinical examination guides towards diagnosis. The source of vaginal discharge or bleeding, the size of the uterus and any pelvic masses should be noted. In absence of any lesion in cervix, vulva, and vagina, endometrial abnormality needs to be excluded primarily by transvaginal ultrasound (TVS). In postmenopausal women, TVS has a sensitivity of greater than 96% for ruling out EC by measuring endometrial thickness. In a study on menopausal women with total endometrial thickness ≥ 4 mm, 22% were reported to have EC, and no women with thickness < 4 mm had carcinoma endometrium.[9] In another study, it was observed that in symptomatic postmenopausal woman, the risk of cancer is approximately 7.3% if endometrial thickness is >5 mm and < 0.07%, if thickness is ≤ 5 mm.

TABLE 1: Natural progression of endometrial hyperplasia.[3]

Degree of hyperplasia	*No. of patients N = 170*	*Regressed*	*Persisted*	*Progressed to CA*
Simple	92	74 (80%)	17 (19%)	1 (1%)
Complex	29	23 (80%)	5 (17%)	1 (3%)
Simple atypical	13	9 (69%)	3 (23%)	1 (8%)
Complex atypical	25	20 (57%)	5 (14%)	10 (29%)

Kurman et al. 1985

In asymptomatic postmenopausal women, the risk of cancer is approximately 6.7%, if the thickness is > 11 mm and 0.002%, if the endometrium is thin.[10] In a recent study, it was observed that the probability of endometrial malignancy increased by 1.012, 1.769, and 4.737-fold in the group with endometrial thickness 5–8 mm, 8–11 mm and > 11 mm, respectively compared to the control group with endometrial thickness < 5 mm.[11] In women with thin endometrium, invasive procedures to evaluate endometrium with histopathology can be avoided. But in women with persistent or recurrent bleeding, even if the endometrial echo complex is less than 5 mm, endometrial biopsy is required,[12] and thin endometrium does not exclude type II ECs.[13] There is insufficient evidence of CT scan, MRI, or biomarkers as aids in the management of EH.

Once TVS indicates any abnormality, pathologic evaluation is to be done to exclude AEH/EIN/EC. Various devices such as Gravlee jet wash; Vabra aspirator and Pipelle are used for endometrial aspiration cytopathology. Pipelle (a soft flexible plastic suction canula) biopsy is reliable with 97.5% sensitivity.[14] The diagnostic accuracy of a fractional curettage is high, though there is chance of over staging in 40–50% to stage II. If hyperplasia is diagnosed by office biopsy, one should consider D&C/hysteroscopy to rule out atypia or cancer prior to conservative medical management.

Hysteroscopic-guided biopsy is regarded as a gold standard in diagnostic evaluation of EC. Hysteroscopic-guided biopsy prevents missing of small lesion and polyp, which can be missed by blind curettage alone. Additional information like tumor diameter, tumor extension to cervix can also be obtained. Direct visualization and biopsy of the uterine cavity using hysteroscopy should be undertaken where EH has been diagnosed within a polyp or other discrete focal lesion. Accurate histological diagnosis is the ultimate aim. Pathologist should provide minimum information like type of hyperplasia, and if malignancy, the histologic type and degree of differentiation.

Management

Management of EH depends upon following factors:

- Age of the patient and desire for fertility
- Presence of cytological atypia.

Before planning for conservative treatment, one should be sure about the histological diagnosis and risk of coexistent malignancy.

Management of EH without atypia: The risk of progression to endometrial cancer is less than 5% over 20 years and the majority of cases of EH without atypia usually regress spontaneously over time. However, treatment with progesterone has higher disease regression rate in comparison to observation alone **(Flowchart 1)**.

- *Premenopausal women:* Conservative treatment with progesterone is usually preferred in young and women desirous of fertility.
    - Levonorgestrel-releasing intrauterine system (LNG-IUS) (Mirena) gives encouraging result in the treatment of EH and is recommended as first-line therapy.[15] Histopathological regression usually occurs by 6 months. If fertility is an issue, LNG-IUS can be removed after 6 months once regression is confirmed. Otherwise, it can be retained for 5 years to prevent relapses.[16]
    - Continuous oral medroxyprogesterone acetate (MPA) 10–20 mg/day or norethisterone 10–15 mg/day) for 6 months can be prescribed for women who decline the LNG-IUS.[16] Cyclical progesterone does not offer adequate therapeutic response, hence not recommended.

Flowchart 1: Schematic diagram of management of premalignant disease of uterus.

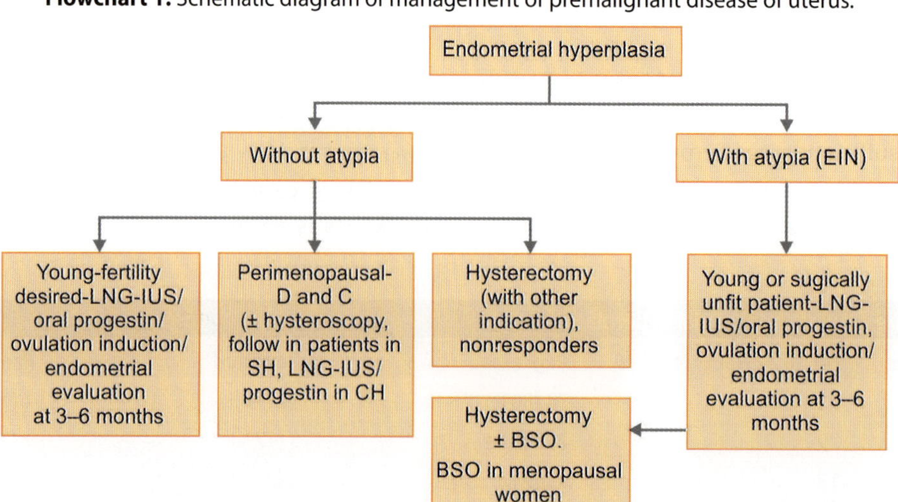

(BSO: bilateral salpingo-oophorectomy; CH: complex hyperplasia; EIN: endometrial intraepithelial neoplasia; LNG-IUS: levonorgestrel-releasing intrauterine system; SH: simple hyperplasia)

- As risk of relapse is high in women with a BMI > 35 longer follow-up is recommended with 6 monthly biopsies for 2 years.
  Endometrium should be sampled at least twice every 6 months to confirm regression and to stop therapy. Patients should be counseled about initial irregular bleeding with progesterone therapy.
- *Perimenopausal women:* Same doses of progesterone may be tried after review of histopathological report. In practice, cases of simple hyperplasia without atypia can be left untreated and kept on follow-up, whereas, complex hyperplasia without atypia warrants treatment with progestin. Hysteroscopic biopsy should be done annually as surveillance measure. Hysterectomy should be considered in refractory lesions.

Hysterectomy is indicated in:[16]

- Women not desirous of fertility preservation
- Progression to atypical hyperplasia during follow-up
- No histological regression despite 12 months of treatment
- There is relapse of hyperplasia after treatment
- Persistent bleeding
- Noncompliance to follow up

Management of atypical endometrial hyperplasia: Hysterectomy is the preferred treatment in woman of any age with AEH, because of high incidence of concurrent subclinical invasive disease and higher probability of progression to cancer. Women desirous of fertility or with high-surgical risk are candidate for progestin therapy. LNG-IUS is preferred as first-line treatment in such situation. Continuous oral progesterone can be used as second-best option. Endometrial biopsy should be done every 3 months until two consecutive reports of complete response, failing which hysterectomy is recommended.

Summary of Premalignant Diseases of Uterus

- Can be prevented by preventing the risk factors.
- Presence of atypia is the most important indicator of risk for cancer.
- Main purpose of treatment is to detect/prevent cancer.
- Medical versus surgical—depending upon age, fertility desire
- Conservative treatment with endometrial monitoring every 3 months
- LNG-IUS offer promise for EH as first-line therapy in EH with or without atypia
- Oral progestins are the second option for EH with or without atypia.
- Perimenopausal women with atypical hyperplasia should, in most instances, be treated with hysterectomy.

MALIGNANT DISEASES OF UTERUS

Endometrial Carcinoma

Endometrial carcinoma is the most common gynecological malignancy in developed countries with an age standardized incidence rate of 8.4 per 100,000 across the world.[17] In developing countries, though cervical cancer still remains the leading cause of gynecological cancers, there is a recent rise in the incidence of endometrial cancer. The rise is mainly attributed to the changing trends in the lifestyle and reproductive profile of women, especially in urban areas. In India, as per GLOBOCAN 2020, the estimated number of new cases of endometrial cancer per year is 16,413 with 6, 385 deaths. The age standardized incidence rate (ASIR) of endometrial cancer in India is 2.3/100,000 women.[17,18] The majority of cases present in 6th and 7th decade of life with the mean age at the time of diagnosis being 60 years.[19] Usually, these women do have concomitant morbidities such as obesity, hypertension, and diabetes. A 85–90% of EC occur in women over 50 years of age, with less than 5% occurring in women less than 40 years of age and this malignancy is increasingly aggressive in advance age.

Endometrial carcinoma is an epithelial malignant lesion arising in the endometrium usually with glandular differentiation, which has the potential to invade the myometrium and spread to lymph nodes and distant sites.

With introduction of molecular classifiers and better understanding of their implications in management of EC, WHO in 2020 has modified their classification of 2014 **(Table 2)**.[20,21]

Carcinosarcoma, previously termed as "malignant mixed Müllerian tumor (MMMT)" comprises of both carcinoma

TABLE 2: WHO classification of endometrial carcinoma.[20,21]

WHO-2014[20]	*WHO-2020*[21]
• Endometrioid adenocarcinoma – Squamous differentiation – Villoglandular – Secretory • Mucinous carcinoma • Serous endometrial intraepithelial carcinoma • Serous carcinoma • Clear cell carcinoma • Neuroendocrine tumors – Low-grade neuroendocrine tumor - Carcinoid tumor – High-grade neuroendocrine carcinoma - Small cell neuroendocrine carcinoma - Large cell neuroendocrine carcinoma • Mixed cell adenocarcinoma • Undifferentiated carcinoma • Dedifferentiated carcinoma	• Endometrioid carcinoma NOS – POLE ultramutated endometrioid carcinoma – Mismatch repair-deficient endometrioid carcinoma – P53-mutant endometrioid carcinoma – No specific molecular profile (NSMP) endometrioid carcinoma • Serous carcinoma NOS • Clear cell carcinoma NOS • Carcinoma, undifferentiated NOS • Mixed cell adenocarcinoma • Mesonephric adenocarcinoma • Squamous cell adenocarcinoma • Mucinous carcinoma intestinal type • Mesonephric–like carcinoma • Carcinosarcoma-NOS

(NOS: not otherwise specified; POLE: polymerase ε)

and sarcoma elements is classified under EC. It appears as a large, soft, polypoid mass involving the endometrium and myometrium. They are regarded as "metaplastic" ECs instead of true sarcoma,[22] and should be dealt like type-II EC. The carcinomatous component is usually high grade and have poor prognosis.

All endometrioid carcinoma are graded as grade-1, 2, and 3 depending on degree of differentiation. Adenosquamous tumors contain malignant elements of both glandular and squamous epithelium. Presence of squamous differentiation does not affect prognosis. Clear cell and papillary serous carcinoma are histologically similar to those noted in ovary and fallopian tubes and have poor prognosis. Mucinous, neuroendocrine tumors and undifferentiated tumors are rare.

Two distinct subtypes of EC were described by Bokhman in 1983,[23] which have different incidence, clinical picture, molecular pattern, and biological behavior.

- Type I (80–90% of all cases), or low-grade endometrioid carcinomas, with favorable prognosis, having > 90% 5-year survival rate
  - Present at low stage in perimenopause
  - Associated with unopposed estrogen stimulation, obesity, and infertility.
  - Prognosis depends on depth of myometrial invasion and stage.
  - Grading is based on both, architectural and nuclear features
  - Molecular changes include microsatellite instability, mutations of p-TEN, k- RAS, and β-catenin
- Type II (10–20%) [Serous carcinoma, clear cell carcinoma (CCC), carcinosarcoma], have worse prognosis
  - Arises in atrophic endometrium, in postmenopausal, multiparous, nonobese, smokers, and tamoxifen users.
  - Estrogen independent
  - High grade and aggressive biological behavior
  - p53 mutations and genetic instability are characteristic

Molecular Classification of Endometrial Carcinoma[24]

In 2013, The Cancer Genome Atlas Research (TCGA) network performed a comprehensive genomic and transcriptomic analysis of endometrioid and serous carcinomas and classified them into four molecular subgroups:

1. POLE ultramutated
2. MSI unstable/hypermutated (Lynch syndrome)
3. Copy-number (CN) low
4. CN high

Pole ultramutated and MSI hypermutated constitute 30% of EC.

The TCGA Genomic classification provides significant prognostic and potential therapeutic information.

- POLE-ultramutated tumors were associated with the best disease-free survival (DFS)
- CN high tumors were associated with the worst DFS
- The other two groups were associated with intermediate DFS

It is interesting to note that FIGO grade 3 endometrioid carcinomas did not segregate into a single molecular cluster, but were represented in all four TCGA subgroups, unlike serous carcinoma which were largely confined to CN high group.

TCGA classification is based on whole genome sequencing, is expensive and time consuming to be employed in any clinical setting. To overcome these issues, a simple, inexpensive, and clinically useable molecular classification system, i.e., **ProMisE** (**Pro**active **M**olecular R**is**k Classifier for **E**ndometrial Cancer) has been developed.[25] This uses immunohistochemical (IHC) stains like MMR proteins for MSI and p53 and POLE exonuclease domain hotspot sequencing.

The resultant molecular subtypes are termed

- POLE exonuclease domain mutant (POLE EDM, surrogate of POLE-ultramutated group)
- MMR deficient (MMR-D, surrogate of MSI-hypermutated group)
- p53 wild type/nonspecific molecular profile (p53wt/NSMP, surrogate of CN low)
- p53 abnormal (p53 abn for staining patterns) surrogate of copy number high

The result of undergoing PORTEC 4a trial is expected to validate prognostic and therapeutic implications of molecular classification.[26]

Management

Preoperative workup: After diagnosis by histology, routine investigations for surgical staging are done. Imaging is done as per resource availability. A good TVS/MRI has proved to be the most accurate modality for assessing the size and extent of tumor, myometrial invasion, extension to cervix and adnexal pathology. Contrast enhanced MRI to exclude myometrial invasion and cervical extension is mandatory when planning fertility preserving treatment.[27] CT and MRI are equivalent in evaluating nodal metastasis, but neither is good enough to replace surgical lymph node assessment. Routine PET-CT is not recommended in early lesions, but can be used in advanced and recurrent disease.

Elevated serum CA-125 correlates with extrauterine spread of disease. Pretreatment CA-125 elevation indicates extrauterine spread in patients with uterine papillary serous carcinoma (UPSC). However, CA-125 elevation is not an independent prognostic factor for recurrence or survival.[28] Cystoscopy, sigmoidoscopy, intravenous urography, etc., are done only when indicated.

Treatment

Endometrial carcinoma cases are staged surgicopathologically. However, clinical staging is useful in advanced stage and surgically unfit cases, who are treated with nonsurgical modalities **(Flowchart 2)**.

Flowchart 2: Treatment algorithm of endometrial carcinoma.

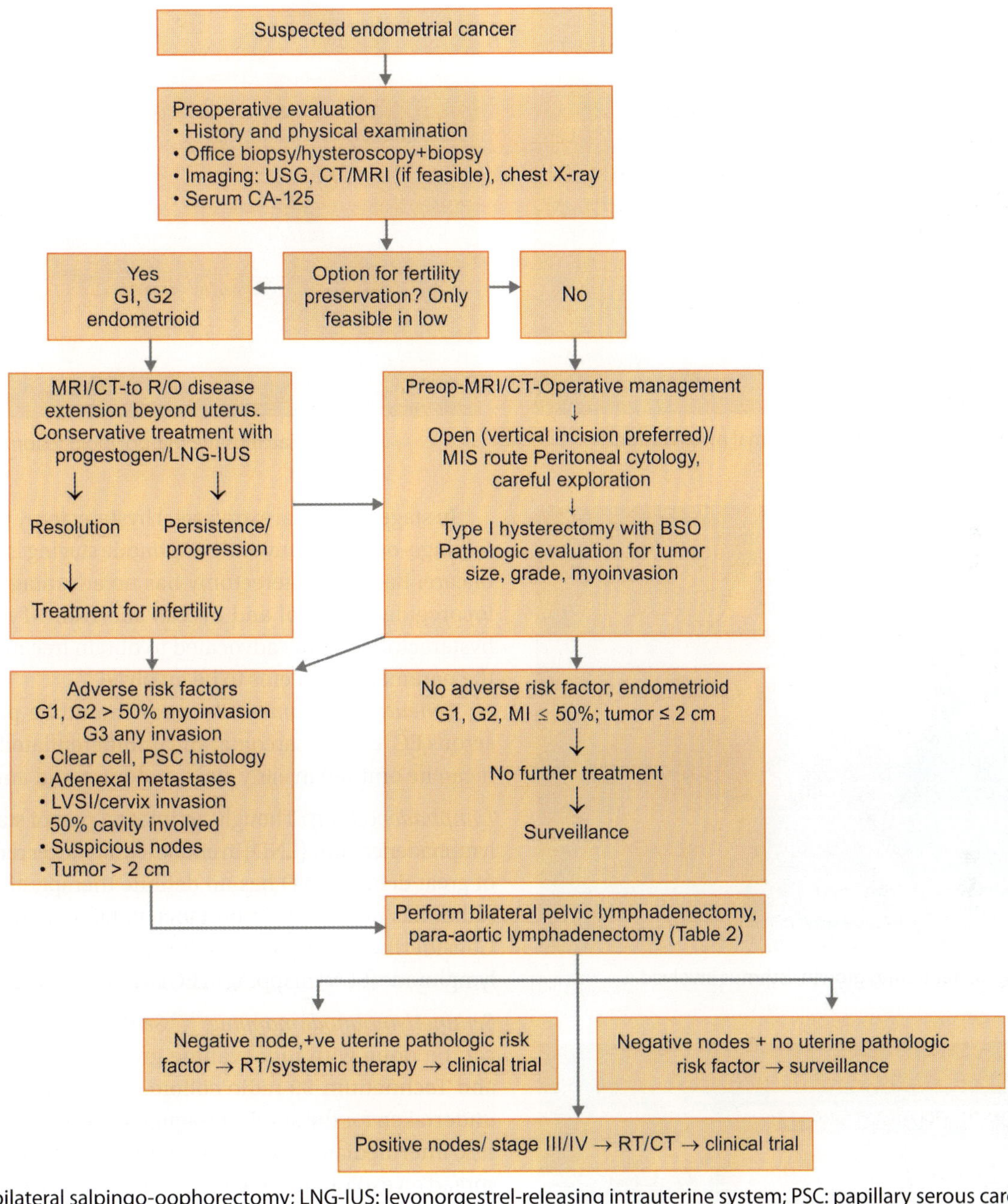

(BSO: bilateral salpingo-oophorectomy; LNG-IUS: levonorgestrel-releasing intrauterine system; PSC: papillary serous carcinoma)

Management of Early-stage Disease

The surgico pathological staging provides precise information about the extent of the disease and identifies risk factors to decide upon adjuvant treatment. Usually, an exploratory laparotomy is done by suprapubic midline vertical incision, which facilitates surgical staging procedures in assessing upper abdomen. However, presently less morbid minimally invasive surgery is preferred over open technique. Peritoneal washings are taken from the pelvis and abdomen with 100–150 mL of saline. This is followed by systematic exploration of intra-abdominal contents like the omentum, liver, peritoneal cul-de-sac, and adenexal surfaces along with palpation of pelvic and para-aortic regions for possible metastases. Extrafascial hysterectomy (type-I radical hysterectomy) with bilateral salpingo-oophorectomy is done (even if both adenexae appear normal, as they may contain micrometastases). Type of hysterectomy (simple vs. type-I vs. type II) has not shown to impact locoregional control and survival.[29] Normal looking ovaries may be preserved in very young women with low-risk disease after counseling. Vaginal cuff removal or parametrial tissue removal has no survival benefit.

The uterus is cut opened and assessed by either visual inspection or on frozen section to determine the size of tumor, depth of myometrial invasion, and cervical extension **(Figs. 2 to 5)**. Both the techniques have a 5–10% inaccuracy rate for depth of myometrial invasion.[30] Hence, this step may

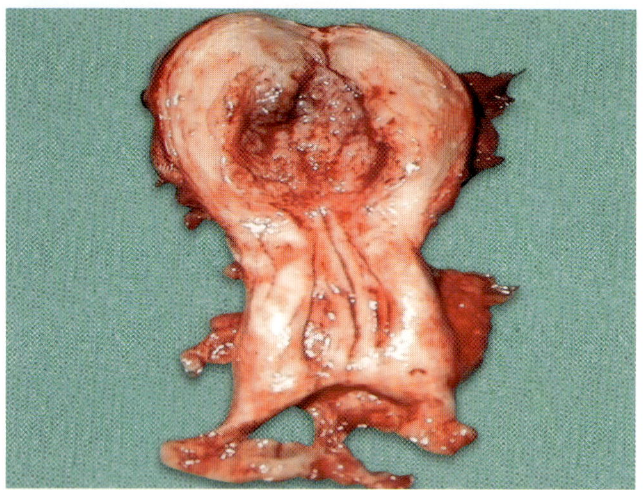

Fig. 2: Fundal growth with minimal myoinvasion.

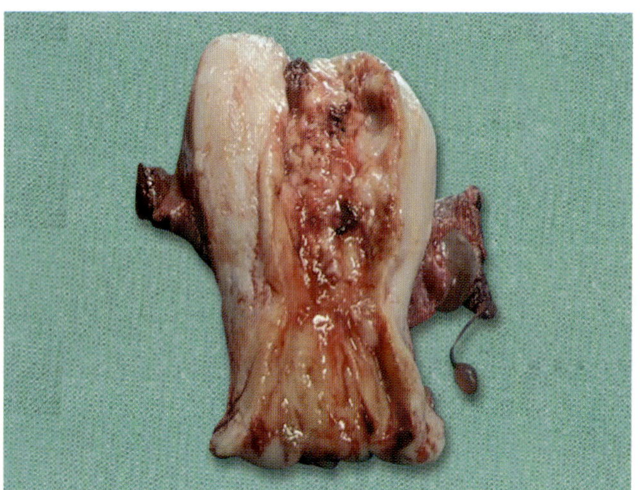

Fig. 3: Infiltrating growth, isthmus involved.

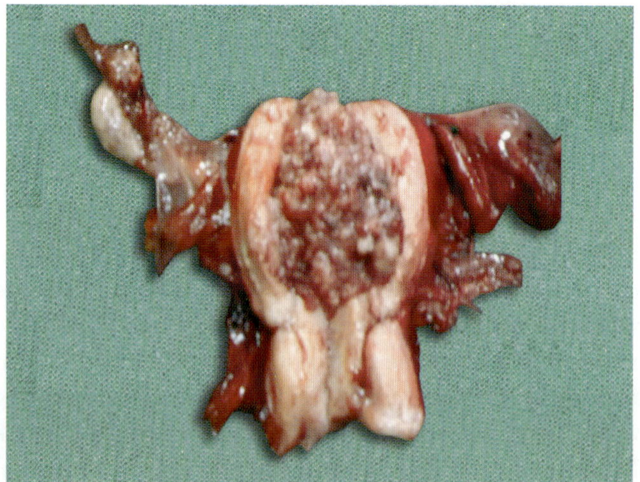

Fig. 4: Large growth filling uterine cavity.

be omitted, if the above information is available preoperatively by a proper imaging (MRI). Moreover, frozen section to detect the depth of myoinvasion has poor accuracy and leads to difficulty in final histopathological diagnosis.[31]

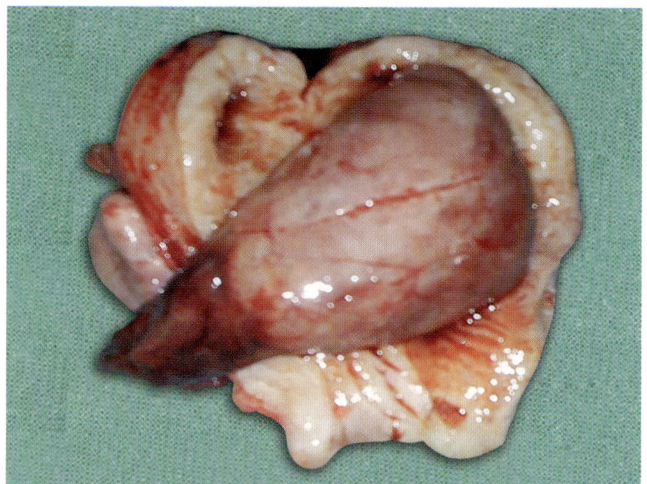

Fig. 5: Carcinosarcoma-polypoid lesion.

In stage II EC total extrafascial hysterectomy with bilateral salpingo-ophorectomy and lymphnode staging is the standard of care. Radical hysterectomy has no advantage in terms of locoregional control and overall survival.[32] Type II radical hysterectomy is only advocated to obtain free margins when the parametrium seems to be involved.[33]

Omentectomy/omental biopsy should be performed in serous EC, carcinosarcoma, and undifferentiated carcinoma. It can be omitted in early stage endometrioid and CCC.[34]

Lymphadenectomy: Though, an integral part of staging, role of lymphadenectomy (LND) in endometrial cancer remains a topic of great debate. LND has no definite therapeutic advantage; rather has prognostic importance to tailor adjuvant therapy. Considering the high morbidity of extensive LND, sentinel lymphnode (SLN) mapping in EC is under extensive evaluation.

Sentinel lymphnode mapping:[31,35] *Sentinel lymphnode mapping* can be done with indocyanine green (ICG) dye, blue dye, and Technetium-99 radio colloid. SLN mapping should be undertaken for the surgical staging of uterine-confined (low-risk/intermediate-risk) disease with no obvious extrauterine spread on exploration and where imaging reveals no evidence of distant metastasis or enlarged nodes. It can be omitted in cases with no myoinvasion. SLN mapping in high-risk types including serous carcinoma, CCC or carcinosarcomas is not routinely recommended and should be done with caution in experienced hands.

The dissected sentinel node is subjected to ultra-staging for any evidence of micrometastasis. All suspicious nodes need to be removed irrespective of mapping. When no SLN is detected, systematic LND is recommended.

Systematic lymphadenectomy: **(Table 3)**[36,37]

- *LND is not indicated* in patients with low-risk endometrioid carcinoma (Low grade—grade 1/2, < 50% myoinvasion).[36]
- *LND is indicated in the following situations.*[37]
    - For patients with intermediate risk (deep myometrial invasion > 50% or grade 3 with < 50% myometrial

TABLE 3: Decision for lymphadenectomy.[36, 37]

Lymphadenectomy omitted	*Pelvic and para-aortic lymphadenectomy*
• Grade I–II • <50% myoinvasion • No evidence of extrauterine disease • Absence of cervical involvement	• FIGO Grade 3 tumor • Stage II • Evidence of extrauterine disease • Nonendometrioid endometrial cancer • Depth of myoinvasion >50% • When pelvic node(s) positive • Previously incompletely staged high risk cases

invasion, and in high-risk patients (grade 3 with > 50% myoinvasion).
- Stage II
- Previously incompletely staged high risk cases to tailor adjuvant therapy.
- Nonendometrioid EC (NEEC)

When systematic LND is indicated, both pelvic and para-aortic LND up to the level of renal veins should be performed.[38] When metastatic pelvic node is detected during surgery, further pelvic dissection is omitted. But all bulky lymph nodes should be removed and para-aortic lymphnode staging should be considered.

However, Hacker et al., advocate only pelvic lymphadenectomy in all of the above high-risk groups and in grade 2 tumors more than 2 cm. They practice para-aortic LND only when pelvic node(s) are positive. With positive pelvic node(s), the risk of para-aortic metastasis is about 50%, compared to only 2% when pelvic nodes are negative.[39]

Laparoscopic/Robotic surgical procedure: Laparoscopic-assisted surgical staging (LASS) and robotic surgery in EC is feasible and safe. It is especially useful in obese and elderly high-risk women. There is level-I evidence on oncological safety of minimally invasive surgery in patients with early-stage EC. Moreover, it has definite role in incompletely staged patients for comprehensive staging to decide adjuvant treatment. The safety and feasibility of the minimally invasive surgery are limited to early-stage endometrial cancers and appear suboptimal for the advanced stages.[40]

Vaginal hysterectomy:[33] In selected patients with marked obesity, poor medical status or uterovaginal prolapse, vaginal hysterectomy with BSO has a place; particularly in low-risk tumor (grade 1 or 2, < 50% myoinvasion, tumor diameter < 2 cm), where lymph node assessment is not warranted. The major limitations of vaginal surgery are inadequate surgical staging procedure including LND and chance of intraperitoneal spillage during the procedure.

Fertility preservation:[31] Fertility preservation option can be offered to women with AEH/EIN or with grade 1 EC without myoinvasion after thorough counseling. Pretreatment hysteroscopic cavity evaluation and endometrial biopsy is recommended. A good quality ultrasound or MRI is prerequisite to exclude myometrial invasion and cervical involvement. Continuous MPA (300–600 mg/day) or megestrol acetate (160–320 mg/day) is commonly recommended for minimum 6 months with hysteroscopic biopsy at 3- and 6-month interval. Levonorgestrel intrauterine device can be used in combination with continuous oral progestins for minimum 6 months. If there is no response after 6 months, standard treatment for EC is recommended.

Adjuvant Treatment: Depends on Risk Stratification

Risk stratification: After surgical staging the patients are classified into low-risk, intermediate-risk, high-intermediate risk, and high-risk depending on risk factors **(Table 4)**.[31] Here, the authors have brought about the novel modification in risk stratification by incorporating the molecular characteristics. Until the molecular markers are universally available, histopathological factors will help in decision making.

The patients are classified into groups at different risk of relapse **(Table 5)**[31] and adjuvant therapy planned accordingly.

Adjuvant therapies are in the form of radiotherapy, chemotherapy, and hormone therapy. While vaginal vault recurrence is common in tumor extending to cervix, upper abdomen failure is typical in papillary serous carcinoma. The anticipated pattern of failure plays an important role in selecting adjuvant therapy. Radiotherapy would take care of the local recurrence at vault, while chemotherapy can exert a systemic effect. Radiotherapy should be initiated within 6–8 weeks of surgery. Though, it is evident that UPSC/CC tumor carries a bad prognosis, only brachytherapy or no adjuvant therapy may be considered in adequately staged IA disease with no myoinvasion.[31,41]

Adjuvant radiotherapy: Most studies indicate that advanced age, grade 3 tumors lymph vascular space invasion (LVSI), deep myometrial invasion, and adverse pathologic types relate to a high risk of disease recurrence. Postoperative radiotherapy in such cases has demonstrated significant reduction in the 5-year vaginal and pelvic recurrence rate, but without any survival benefit and with higher rate of treatment related complications (PORTEC study), and EC-related death rates were 9% in RT group and 6% in control group.[42] Vaginal irradiation (IVRT) is given in intermediate risk group for better local control.[43] Pelvic irradiation—both teletherapy and IVRT are given in high-risk patients.

Extended field radiotherapy used in para-aortic nodal metastasis or in multiple pelvic node metastasis. The place of whole abdomen radiation (WAR) is not established.

Adjuvant chemotherapy: The results from trials are inconsistent regarding any survival benefit of adjuvant chemotherapy. It plays an important role in groups of patients with high-risk features like high grade disease (type II histology), and extrauterine disease (stage III disease), to prevent distant metastasis.[44]

TABLE 4: Risk group and adjuvant treatment with level of evidence and grade of recommendation.[31]

Risk description	*Adjuvant treatment*
Low risk	
Stage IA endometrioid + low-grade (Grade 1–2) LVSI negative or focal Pole mutant-St-I-II- No Res Stage-IA-MMRd /NSMP: Low grade	No adjuvant (I, A)
Intermediate risk	
Stage IB endometrioid + grade-1–2 + LVSI negative or focal Stage IA endometrioid + grade 3 + LVSI negative or focal Stage IA nonendometrioid (serous, clear cell, undifferentiated carcinoma, carcinosarcoma, mixed) without myometrial invasion St-I-MMRd/NSMP-LVSI negative	Adjuvant brachytherapy can be recommended to decrease vaginal recurrence (I, A) Omission of adjuvant brachytherapy can be considered (III, C), especially for patients aged < 60 years (II, A)
High intermediate risk	
Stage I endometrioid + substantial LVSI regardless of grade and depth of invasion Stage IB endometrioid grade-3 regardless of LVSI status Stage II Stage-I-MMRd/NSMP+LVSI Stage-IB-G3,St-II-MMRd/NSMP ±LVSI Stage-II-MMRd/NSMP	*Lymph node staging performed –Node negative*
	Adjuvant brachytherapy can be recommended to decrease vaginal recurrence (II, B). EBRT can be considered for substantial LVSI and for stage II (I, B) Adjuvant chemotherapy can be considered, especially for high grade and/or substantial LVSI (II, C). Omission of any adjuvant treatment is an option (IV, C)
	Lymph node staging not performed
	Adjuvant EBRT is recommended, especially for substantial LVSI and/or for stage II (I, A). Additional adjuvant chemotherapy can be considered, especially for high-grade and/or substantial LVSI (II, B) Adjuvant brachytherapy alone can be considered for high-grade LVSI negative and for stage II grade 1 endometrioid carcinomas (II, B).
High risk	
Stage III–IVA with no residual disease Stage I–IVA non-endometrioid (serous, clear cell, undifferentiated carcinoma, carcinosarcoma, mixed) with myometrial invasion, and with no residual disease) p53 regardless of stage NSMP/MMRd, no residual tumor	EBRT with concurrent and adjuvant chemotherapy (I, A) or alternatively sequential chemotherapy and radiotherapy is recommended (I, B). Chemotherapy alone is an alternative option (I, B). Carcinosarcomas should be treated as high-risk carcinomas (not as sarcomas) (IV, B).

(EBRT: external beam radiation therapy; LVSI: lymphovascular space invasion; MMRd/NSMP: MMR-deficient/no specific molecular profile)

Adjuvant hormone therapy: Meta-analysis of different trials failed to demonstrate any survival benefit of progesterone as an adjuvant maintenance therapy in endometrial cancer. Progestogen therapy (MPA 300–600 mg per day) may prove a viable alternative to surgery in young women desirous of fertility in early-stage disease with well-differentiated adenocarcinoma, as discussed above. Hormonal therapy also has a role in metastatic or recurrent disease.

Management of Advanced Endometrial Carcinoma

Management of Stage III

In operable *Stage IIIa* disease the treatment of choice is surgico-pathological staging with TAH, BSO, pelvic and para-aortic LND and omentectomy. This is followed by radiotherapy and/or chemotherapy as required. With surgery along with adjuvant treatment survival rate at 5 years is around 50%.

In Stage III b and c—(when inoperable)—pelvic radiation or neoadjuvant chemotherapy followed by surgery or external pelvic RT or extended field RT followed by intrauterine and intravaginal brachytherapy (in unresectable or medically unfit patient) is the treatment of choice. Concurrent chemoradiation as adjuvant therapy, showed 11% absolute improvement of failure-free survival only in stage III disease[45] as shown in PORTEC3 trial.

Extended field radiation therapy or systemic therapy with cytotoxic medications or hormones is warranted in the presence of extra-pelvic metastases, depending on patient's conditions.

Management of Stage IV

Patients with extra-pelvic metastases are managed with systemic chemotherapy or hormone therapy. GOG study on WAR versus chemotherapy showed improved progression

TABLE 5: Simplified approach for adjuvant treatment according to the risk stratification with level of evidence and grade of recommendation.[31]

	Adjuvant treatment		
Risk group	***Brachy therapy***	***External beam radiotherapy***	***Chemotherapy CCRT +CT***
Low risk	No (I, A)	No (I, A)	No (I, A)
Intermediate risk	Yes (I, A) Can be omitted in 1. <60 years (II, A) 2. Pole mut, P53 abn 3. NEEC-without MI	No	No
High intermediate risk pN0 (Surgical staging or SLN Neg)	Yes (II, B) Stage IB G3 without LVSI Can be omitted in Pole mut	If substantial LVSI and Stage II (I, B)	No Can be considered only in G3 and substantial LVSI (II, C)
High intermediate risk cN0/pNX (No surgical staging nor SLN)	Yes- G3-LVSI –ve St-II G1 (II, B) Can be omitted in Pole mut	If substantial LVSI and/or St-II (I, A)	Especially for NSMP/G3/Substantial LVSI (II, B) PORTEC 3 protocol
High risk	No	Concurrent chemoradiation + Chemo (PORTEC3 protocol) (I, A) Only chemotherapy is an alternative option In case of contraindication of chemo- EBRT recommended Carcinosarcomas should be treated as high-risk carcinomas (not as sarcomas)	

(CCRT: concurrent chemoradiation; LVSI: lymphovascular space invasion; NEEC: nonendometrioid EC; SLN: sentinel lymphnode)

free and overall survival with chemotherapy compared with WAR.[46] Local radiation may be beneficial, particularly in brain or bone metastases, and occasionally pelvic radiotherapy may help in providing local tumor control and preventing bleeding or complications from local disease. Palliative hysterectomy may have a role in select patients.

Prognostic variables: Prognostic indicators are defined in EC to prognosticate the disease outcome and plan therapy **(Box 1)**.[33]

Post-treatment surveillance: Patient should be seen every 3–4 months in first 2 years, every 6 months in next 3 years and annually thereafter. At each visit, patient should have a complete physical and pelvic examination. The role of routine vault smear is controversial. Ultrasonography and CA-125 measurement, CT scan, MRI may be done as appropriate. Pelvic and distant recurrences, if suspected, should be confirmed by histology.

Hormone replacement therapy: As 80% of recurrences occur within 2 years it is worthwhile to withhold hormone replacement therapy during this period. Short course of conjugated estrogen 0.625 mg along with MPA 2.5 mg daily may be used thereafter in stage IA after counseling the woman about risk of recurrence. Symptomatic women with vaginal dryness, dyspareunia may be treated with short course of topical estrogen alone. MPA injection 150 mg every 3 months or nonhormonal agents may be of use for symptomatic relief of hot flushes.[34]

Endometrial cancer diagnosed after hysterectomy: NCCN guidelines suggest that patients with unstaged endometrial cancer with >50% myoinvasion of any grade should undergo imaging to rule out metastasis before deciding treatment modalities.[47] If high-risk factors (deep myoinvasion,

BOX 1: Prognostic variables of endometrial carcinoma.[33]

- *Age* > 60 years have more chance of recurrence
- *Histological type:* Non-endometrioid subtypes—increased risk
- *Histological grade:* The higher the grade the worse the prognosis
- *Myometrial invasion:* More the invasion, more is extrauterine spread and recurrence
- *LVSI:* An independent risk factor
- *Lymph node metastasis:* Carries a poor prognosis
- *Tumor size:* Tumor size > 2 cm, has 21% incidence of nodal metastasis whereas tumor < 2 cm with < 1/2 myometrial invasion rarely has nodal metastasis
- *Cervical extension:* Increased extrauterine disease, lymph node metastasis, and recurrence
- *Adnexal metastasis:* Correlate with pelvic and PA nodal metastasis and survival
- *Intraperitoneal tumor* is highly correlated with lymph node metastasis and survival
- *Peritoneal cytology:* Positive peritoneal cytology in the absence of other evidence of extrauterine disease or poor prognostic factors has no significant effect
- *Hormonal receptors:* Positive receptors levels have better survival benefit
- *DNA polyploidy/Proliferative indices:* DNA polyploidy tumors are regarded as low- risk category—regardless of stage, grade, and myometrial invasion, they can be treated with simple hysterectomy/HT, whereas aneuploid tumors, (20–30% of all ECs), tend to recur early with poor prognosis
- *Genetics/molecular tumor markers:* Type I cancers frequently have PTEN, KRAS, and PIK3CA mutations, whereas type II cancers are more likely to have TP53 mutations

substantial lymph vascular space invasion, grade 3 histology, type II carcinomas) are identified, complete surgical staging including lymph node assessment and removal of both the adnexae is recommended. Alternately, adjuvant therapy (including EBRT, VBT, and chemotherapy) may be decided based on histopathology report and uterine factors. Patient with grade 1 or 2 lesion with ≤ 50% myometrial invasion and no LVSI generally require no further therapy.[48]

Treatment of recurrence: Most of the recurrences are detected by physical examination and treatment depends on primary therapy. Pelvic recurrence is common in surgery alone group and treated with RT. Pelvic exenteration is also an option in highly selected patients. Recurrences after surgery with adjuvant RT or RT alone are usually extra-pelvic. In these cases, chemotherapy like platinum and taxane are used. Local RT can be tried in isolated recurrences outside the previous RT field. Treatment with tamoxifen, MPA alone or in combination may be used in metastatic disease. However, the response to treatment is not encouraging. Patients can be put on clinical trial.

Targeted therapy: Targeted therapies are under clinical trial in management of EC, mostly in recurrent setting and advanced EC. EGFR, human epidermal growth factor receptor-2 (HER2), mTOR, and VEGFR inhibitors have been tested in phase I and II trials, with modest response rates.[49] Pembrolizumab and Dostarlimab have been approved by FDA as immunotherapeutic agents for patients with unresectable or metastatic MSI-H or MMRd endometrial cancer.

FIGO Staging-2009 (Box 2)[50]

Survival of EC:
- Histologic type and survival (Stage-I, EC) (**Table 6**)[51]
- Stage and survival (**Table 7**).[52]

Summary of Endometrial Carcinoma

- ECs are usually disease of elderly who often have multiple comorbidities.
- Presently, there is definite rise in the incidence of EC in younger population.
- Endometrioid adenocarcinoma is more common sub-type and have good prognosis. UPSC, CCC, carcinosarcoma are uncommon with poor prognosis.
- Surgery is the mainstay of treatment, preoperative evaluation with information about type and grade of lesion is a must.
- Surgical staging defines the extent of disease and predicts outcome.
- Role of LND is controversial, although it is required for staging purpose—it guides adjuvant treatment and is also prognostic but systematic LND failed to have a therapeutic value.
- Adjuvant therapy is tailored according to risk stratification.
- Adjuvant RT does not improve overall survival in most instances but reduces pelvic recurrences.
- Chemotherapy as adjuvant is recommended in advanced nonendometroid cancers or in patients with higher stage (extrauterine) disease.

BOX 2: Surgical staging classification endometrial carcinoma–FIGO-2009.[50]

- *Stage IA:* G123 Tumor limited to endometrium or invades less than half of myometrium
- *Stage I B:* G123 Tumor invades to more than half of myometrium
- *Stage II** G123 Cervical stromal invasion
- *Stage III* G123 Local and/or regional spread of the tumor
  - *Stage IIIA* G123 Tumor invading serosa of the corpus uteri and/or adnexae#
  - *Stage IIIB* G123 Vaginal/Parametrial metastases
  - *Stage IIIC* G123 Metastases to pelvic and/or paraaortic lymphnodes#
    - *Stage III C1* G123 Positive pelvic node
    - *Stage III C2* G123 Positive para-aortic LN ± Positive pelvic node
- *Stage IVA* G123 Tumor invasion of bladder and/or bowel mucosa
- *Stage IVB* G123 Distant metastases, including intra-abdominal metastasis and/or inguinal nodes

FIGO Committee on Gynecologic Oncology. Revised FIGO staging for carcinoma of vulva, cervix, and endometrium. Int J Gynecol Obstet 2009;105:103-4.

*Endocervical glandular involvement only should be considered as Stage I, no longer in Stage II.

#Positive cytology has to be reported separately without changing the stage.

TABLE 6: Histologic type and survival (FIGO stage-I, EC).[51]

Histologic type	*Overall survival in years (%)*				
	1 year	*2 years*	*3 years*	*4 years*	*5 years*
Endometroid	98.4	96.3	94.00	91.8	90.1
Adenosquamous	98.9	95.6	95.0	93.1	93.1
Mucinous	100.0	100.0	100.0	100.0	93.3
Papillary	97.7	89.0	82.3	81.4	79.9
Clear cell	96.1	93.4	89.1	87.5	85.1
Squamous	89.5	78.3	78.3	78.3	78.3
Others	95.5	89.1	84.0	82.0	77.3

TABLE 7: Stage and survival of EC.[52]

Stage	*Survival*
IA	88%
IB	75%
II	69%
IIIA	58%
IIIB	50%
IIIC	47%
IVA	17%
IVB	15%

(EC: endometrial carcinoma)

- Concurrent chemoradiation has shown promising results in stage III disease and type II histology.
- Targeted therapies are clinical trials and hold promise.

SARCOMA UTERUS

The malignant tumors arising from stroma of the endometrium or from the mesenchymal elements of the uterus are termed as sarcomas. *GOG has classified uterine sarcoma in to two types according to tissue of origin.*[53]

1. Pure nonepithelial neoplasm
   - *Endodermal stromal tumors:*
     - Stromal nodule
     - Low-grade stromal sarcoma
     - High-grade stromal sarcoma
   - Smooth muscle tumor of uncertain malignant potential (STUMP)
   - Leiomyosarcoma
     - Epitheloid
     - Myxoid
   - Mixed endometrial stromal and smooth muscle tumor
   - Poorly differentiated (undifferentiated) endometrial sarcoma
   - Other soft tissue tumors
     - Homologous
     - Heterologous
2. Mixed epithelial and nonepithelial tumor
   - Adenosarcoma
     - Homologous
     - Heterologous
   - Carcinosarcoma
     - Homologous
     - Heterologous.

It is to note that carcinosarcoma is now classified under EC.[21] According to the 2003 WHO classification,[54] uterine sarcoma is classified into mesenchymal tumors and mixed epithelial and mesenchymal tumors. Mesenchymal tumors are further classified into LMS, endometrial stromal sarcoma, and undifferentiated uterine sarcoma. Mixed tumors include carcinosarcoma (now included under EC) and adenosarcoma **(Table 8)**.[54] The incidence of different histological subtypes, after exclusion of carcinosarcoma, is as follows; LMS (63%), endometrial stromal sarcoma (21%), adenosarcoma (6%), undifferentiated uterine sarcoma (6%) **(Table 9)**.[55]

- *Leiomyosarcoma* accounts for 1.3% of all uterine malignancies and most of them are intramural. Median age of occurrence is somewhat lower than other uterine sarcomas (45–50 years) and has a poor prognosis; postmenopausal patients have a better chance of survival. Diagnosis of LMSs is made with the histologic evidence of:
  - Coagulative tumor necrosis, cytologic atypia, and any number of mitotic activity, or
  - More than 10 mitotic figures/10 HPF and coagulative tumor necrosis even in absence of cytologic atypia.[56]

TABLE 8: Classification of uterine sarcoma.[54]

- *Pure:* Non-epithelial sarcoma in which only malignant mesodermal elements are present:
  - *Homologous:* Native uterine elements present (e.g., leiomyosarcomas and endometrial stromal sarcomas, stromal nodule)
  - *Heterologous:* Made up of elements which are not native to uterus (e.g., rhabdomyosarcoma, chondrosarcoma, osteosarcoma, liposarcoma)
- Mixed-epithelial and non-epithelial elements—homologous and heterologous:
  - *Malignant mixed Mullerian tumor* in which malignant mesodermal and malignant epithelial elements are present (MMMT)—(e.g., carcinosarcoma)
  - *Adenosarcoma* in which malignant mesodermal and benign epithelial elements are present

TABLE 9: Distribution of uterine sarcoma.[55]

Type	*% of uterine sarcoma*
LMS	63
ESS	21
Adenosarcoma	06
Undifferentiated uterine sarcoma	06
Others	05

(ESS: endometrial stromal sarcoma; LMS: leiomyosarcoma)

Though LMS may be sometimes graded is graded as low-grade (Grade-1) and high- grade (Grade 2 and 3), majority are high grade. Morphologically, they are classified into (a) spindloid, (b) epitheloid, and (c) myxoid types. But usually, tumor has more than one component. LMSs spread by local extension, peritoneal implantation, and more commonly through hematogenous route.

- *Endometrial stromal sarcoma (ESS)* is a rare tumor. It occurs primarily in women between ages 45 and 50 years; about one-third occurs in postmenopausal women. It is typically subdivided into low-grade (fewer than 5–10 mitosis per 10 HPF and minimal cellular atypia) and high-grade stromal sarcoma. It is now suggested that low-grade stromal sarcoma be designated as *"endometrial stromal sarcoma"*[57] and high grade tumors without recognizable evidence of a definite endometrial stromal phenotype be termed as *"Endometrial sarcoma or undifferentiated uterine sarcoma".*[58] *Recently, WHO has classified endometrial sarcomas in the following three* main categories:
  1. Low-grade endometrial stromal sarcoma
  2. High-grade endometrial stromal sarcoma
  3. Undifferentiated sarcoma.[59]
- *Adenosarcoma* is characterized by Müllerian epithelium resembling benign proliferative or hyperplastic endometrium admixed with sarcomatous stroma with two or more mitotic activity per HPF. It arises from the endometrium as a sessile or polypoid growth. It is a low-grade lesion with good prognosis.

Clinical Features of Uterine Sarcoma

The usual presenting symptom is irregular vaginal bleeding or postmenopausal bleeding. Sometimes, pelvic or abdominal pain may be the presenting symptom. Rarely do they present with pelvic mass and fever. Sarcoma should be suspected when there is history of rapidly enlarging uterus, large polypoid friable mass seen extending through a dilated cervix into vagina. Diagnosis is confirmed by imaging and biopsy of polypoid lesion or endometrial curettage.

Management

Surgery is the mainstay of treatment in uterine sarcomas. Intraoperatively, the peritoneal cavity should be thoroughly explored and peritoneal washings obtained for cytology. Total abdominal hysterectomy and bilateral salpingo-oophorectomy is the standard surgical procedure **(Figs. 6 to 9)**. Ovaries may be preserved in early stage LMS in a young patient. Role of systematic LND is controversial in ESS; however, removal of enlarged nodes is recommended. A routine LND is not indicated in LMS; the risk of lymph node metastasis is low and therapeutic and diagnostic value of LND is not established. All extrauterine tumors should be removed. Primary radiotherapy is reserved for patients who are not suitable for surgery for medical or technical reasons. Adjuvant radiotherapy is beneficial in decreasing pelvic recurrence without any survival benefit. Adjuvant chemotherapy has also not shown any survival benefit though it prevents the incidence of distant metastasis. Targeted therapies are under investigation and may open new avenues in future.

FIGO Staging for Uterine Sarcomas-2009[50] (Table 10)

Management of Recurrent Disease

Stage of the disease is the most important prognostic factor. The other factors are age, LVSI, and mitotic count. Recurrences

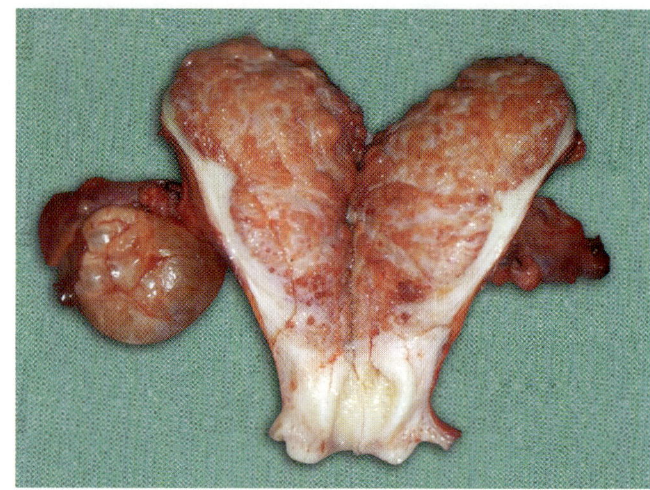

Fig. 7: Endometrial stromal sarcoma.

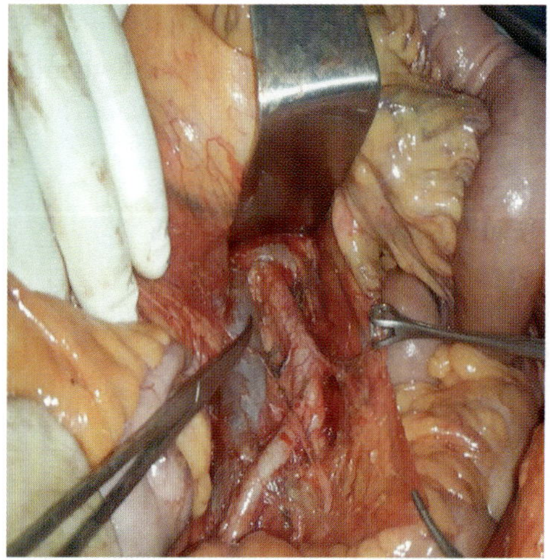

Fig. 8: PALND up to renal vein.

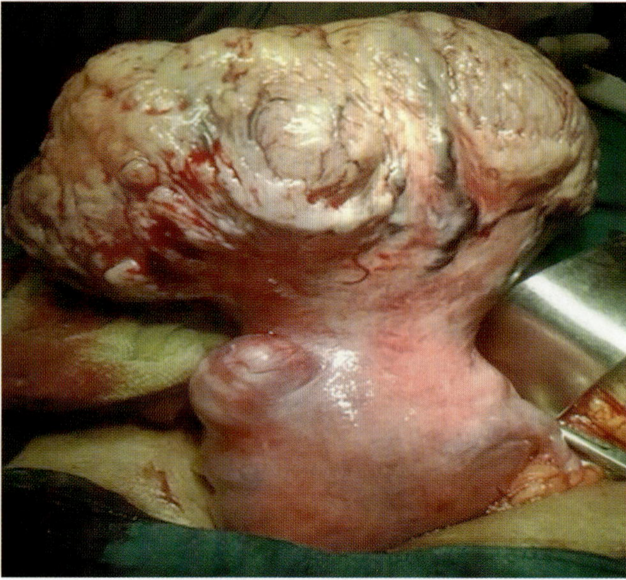

Fig. 6: Leiomyosarcoma.

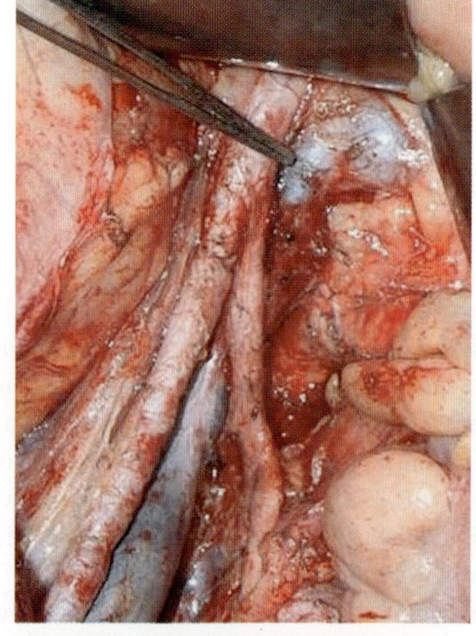

Fig. 9: Pelvic lymphadenectomy.

TABLE 10: FIGO staging for uterine sarcomas-2009.[50]

Leiomyosarcomas and endometrial stromal sarcoma	
Stage	***Definition***
Stage I	Tumor limited to uterus
IA	< 5 cm
IB	> 5 cm
Stage II	Tumor extends beyond the uterus within the pelvis
IIA	Adnexal involvement
IIB	Involvement of other pelvic tissues
Stage III	Tumor invades abdominal tissues (not just protruding into the abdomen)
IIIA	One site
IIIB	> one site
IIIC	Metastasis to pelvic and/or para-aortic lymph node
Stage IV	
IVA	Tumor invades bladder and/or rectum
IVB	Distant metastasis
Adenosarcoma	
Stage	***Definition***
Stage I	Tumor limited to uterus
IA	Tumor limited to endometrium/endocervix with no myometrial invasion
IB	Less than or equal to half myometrial invasion
IC	More than half myometrial invasion
Stage II	Tumor extends to the pelvis
IIA	Adnexal involvement
IIB	Tumor extends to extrauterine pelvic tissue
Stage III	Tumor invades abdominal tissues (not just protruding into the abdomen)
IIIA	One site
IIIB	> one site
IIIC	Metastasis to pelvic and/or para-aortic lymph node
Stage IV	
IVA	Tumor invades bladder and/or rectum
IVB	Distant metastasis
Carcinosarcoma	should be staged as carcinoma of the endometrium

develop in more than 50% of cases, even when the disease is apparently localized at the time of diagnosis. More than 50% recurrences occur outside the pelvis, with isolated pelvic failures accounting for less than 10%. The most common sites of recurrences are live and lungs. Treatment of recurrent disease is individualized.

Summary of Uterine Sarcoma

- Uterine sarcomas are derived from Müllerian mesoderm and arise in the connective tissues of either the endometrium or myometrium.
- They are rare but highly malignant group of tumors with poor prognosis.
- Surgery is the mainstay of treatment of uterine sarcoma.
- A total abdominal hysterectomy with bilateral salpingo-oophorectomy is the surgical procedure of choice. Oophorectomy may be avoided in young women with early-stage LMS. A routine systematic LND is controversial in sarcomas.
- Adjuvant radiation therapy and chemotherapy are given as per indication.
- Adjuvant treatment reduces recurrence but does not improve overall survival.
- Advanced, recurrent low grade ESS patients benefit from progestin and aromatase inhibitor.

REFERENCES

1. Orbo A, Nilsen MN, Arnes MS, Pettersen I, Larsen K. Loss of expression of MLH1, MSH2, MSH6, and PTEN related to endometrial cancer in 68 patients with endometrial hyperplasia. Int J Gynecol Pathol. 2003;22:141-8.
2. Scully RE, Bonfiglio TA, Kurman RJ, Silverberg SG, Wilkinson EJ. Uterine corpus. In Histological Typing of Female Genital Tract Tumour. New York: Springer-Verlag; 1994. pp. 13-31.
3. Kurman RJ, Kaminski PF, Norris HJ. The behavior of endometrial hyperplasia. A long-term study of "untreated" hyperplasia in 170 patients. Cancer. 1985;56(2):403-12.
4. Trimble CL, Kauderer J, Zaino R, Silverberg S, Lim PC, Burke 2nd JJ, et al. Concurrent endometrial carcinoma in women with a biopsy diagnosis of atypical endometrial hyperplasia: a Gynecologic Oncology Group study. Cancer. 2006;106(4):812-9.
5. Mutter GL. Endometrial intraepithelial neoplasia (EIN): will it bring order to chaos? The Endometrial Collaborative Group. Gynecol Oncol. 2000;76:287-90.
6. Emons G, Beckmann MW, Schmidt D, Mallmann P. New WHO classification of endometrial hyperplasias. Geburtsh Frauenheilk. 2015;75:135-6.
7. Roelofsen T, van Kempen LT, van der L Jeroen AWM, van Ham MA, Johan B, Massuger Leon FAG. Concurrent Endometrial Intraepithelial Carcinoma (EIC) and Serous Ovarian Cancer: Can EIC Be Seen as the Precursor Lesion? Int J Gynecol Cancer. 2012;22:457-64.
8. Beral V, Bull D, Reeves G. Endometrial cancer and hormone-replacement therapy in million women study. Lancet. 2005; 365:1543-51.
9. Osmers R, Volksen M, Schauer A. Vaginosonography for early detection of endometrial carcinoma? Lancet. 1990; 335:1569-71.
10. Bindman RS, Weiss E, Feldstein V. How thick is too thick? When endometrial thickness should prompt biopsy in postmenopausal women without vaginal bleeding. Ultrasound Obstet Gynecol. 2004;24:558-65.
11. Tofiloska V, Stefanovska VV, Dimitrov LG. The connection between the endometrial thickness and the risk of endometrial malignancy in postmenopausal women. Open Access Maced J Med Sci. 2019;7(14):2263-6.

12. American College of Obstetricians and Gynecologists. Practice Bulletin No. 149: Endometrial cancer. Obstet Gynecol. 2015;125:1006-26.
13. Wang J, Wieslander C, Hansen G, Cass I, Vasilev S, Holschneider CH. Thin endometrial echo complex on ultrasound does not reliably exclude type 2 endometrial cancers. Gynecol Oncol. 2006;101(1):120-5.
14. Strovall TG, Photopulos GJ, Poston WM, Ling FW, Sandles LG. Pipelle endometrial sampling in patients with known endometrial carcinoma. Obstet Gynaecol. 1991;77:954-56.
15. Gallos ID, Shehmar M, Thangaratinam S, Papapostolou TK, Coomarasamy A, Gupta JK. Oral progestogens vs. levonorgestrel-releasing intrauterine system for endometrial hyperplasia: a systematic review and meta-analysis. Am J Obstet Gynecol. 2010; 203(6):547.e1-10.
16. Royal College of Obstetrician and Gynecology. Management of Endometrial Hyperplasia RCOG/BSGE Joint Guideline. London: RCOG; 2016.
17. Cancer Today (2018). Global cancer observatory [online]. Available from: https://gco.iarc.fr/today/home. [Last accessed December, 2021].
18. Balasubramaniam G, Sushama S, Rasika B, Mahantshetty U. Hospital-based study of endometrial cancer survival in Mumbai, India. Asian Pac J Cancer Prev. 2013;14:977-80.
19. McMeekin DS, Yashar C, Campos SM, Zaino RJ. Corpus: epithelial tumors. In: Barakat RR, Berchuk A, Markman M, Randall M (Eds). Principles and Practice of Gynecologic Oncology, 6th edition. Philadelphia: Lippincott Williams & Wilkins; 2013. pp. 661-714.
20. Kurman RJ, Carcangiu ML, Herrington CS, Young RH. WHO Classification of Tumours of the Female Reproductive Organs, 4th edition. Lyon: IARC; 2014.
21. WHO Classification of Tumours Editorial Board. WHO Classification of Tumours, Female Genital Tumours, 5th edition. Lyon: IARC; 2020. p. 6.
22. McCluggage WG. Uterine carcinosarcoma (Malignant mixed Mullerian tumours) are metaplastic carcinomas. Int J Gynecol Cancer. 2002;12:687-90.
23. Bokhman JV. Two pathogenetic types of endometrial carcinoma. Gynecol Oncol. 1983;15(1):10-7.
24. Stelloo E, Nout RA, Osse EM, Jürgenliemk-Schulz IJ, Jobsen JJ, Lutgens LC, et al. Improved risk assessment by integrating molecular and clinicopathological factors in early-stage endometrial cancer-combined analysis of PORTEC cohort. Clin Cancer Res. 2016;22:4215-24.
25. Talhouk A, McConechy MK, Leung S, Yang W, Lum A, Senz J, et al. Confirmation of ProMisE: A simple, genomics-based clinical classifier for endometrial cancer. Cancer. 2017;123:802-13.
26. van den Heerik ASVM, Horeweg N, Nout RA, Lutgens LCHW, van der Steen-Banasik EM, Westerveld GH, et al. PORTEC-4a: International randomized trial of molecular profile-based adjuvant treatment for women with high-intermediate risk endometrial cancer. Int J Gynecol Cancer. 2020;30(12): 2002-7.
27. Sala E, Rockall A, Kubik-Huch RA. Advances in magnetic resonance imaging of endometrial cancer. Eur Radiol. 2011;21:468-73.
28. Gupta D, Marc JG, Kathleen Y, Stephen L, Lisa Z, Chen LM, et al. Performance of serum CA125 as a prognostic biomarker in patients with uterine papillary serous carcinoma. Int J Gynecol Cancer. 2011;21:529-34.
29. Signorelli M, Lissoni AA, Cormio G, Katsaros D, Pellegrino A, Selvaggi L, et al. Modified radical hysterectomy versus extra fascial hysterectomy in the treatment of stage I endometrial cancer: results from the ILIADE randomized study. Ann Surg Oncol. 2009;16:3431-41.
30. Shim JU, Rose PG, Reale FR, Soto H, Tak WK, Hunter RE. Accuracy of frozen- section diagnosis at surgery in clinical stage I and II endometrial carcinoma. Am J Obstet Gynecol. 1992; 166:1335-8.
31. Concin N, Matias-Guiu X, Vergote I, Cibula D, Mirza MR, Marnitz S, et al. ESGO/ESTRO/ESP guidelines for the management of patients with endometrial carcinoma. Int J Gynecol Cancer. 2020;31(1):12-39.
32. Liu T, Tu H, Li Y, Liu Z, Liu G, Gu H. Impact of radical hysterectomy versus simple hysterectomy on survival of patients with stage 2 endometrial cancer: a meta-analysis. Ann Surg Oncol. 2019;26:2933-42.
33. Dowdy SC, Mariani A, Lurain JR. Uterine Cancer. In: Berek JS (Ed). Berek and Novak Gynaecology, 5th edition. US: Lippincott William & Wilkins; 2012. pp. 1250-303.
34. Joo WD, Schwartz PE, Rutherford TJ, Seong SJ, Ku J, Park H, et al. Microscopic omental metastasis in clinical stage I endometrial cancer: a meta-analysis. Ann Surg Oncol. 2015;22:3695-700.
35. Abu-Rustum NR. Sentinel lymph node mapping for endometrial cancer: a modern approach to surgical staging. J Natl Compr Canc Netw. 2014;12:288-97.
36. Vargas R, Rauh-Hain JA, Clemmer J, Clark RM, Goodman A, Growdon WB, et al. Tumor size, depth of invasion, and histologic grade as prognostic factors of lymph node involvement in endometrial cancer: a SEER analysis. Gynecol Oncol. 2014; 133:216-20.
37. Benedetti PP, Basile S, Maneschi F, Lissoni AA, Signorelli M, Scambia G, et al. Systematic pelvic lymphadenectomy versus no lymphadenectomy in early-stage endometrial carcinoma: randomized clinical trial. J Natl Cancer Inst. 2008;100:1707-16.
38. Todo Y, Kato H, Kaneuchi M, Watari H, Takeda M, Sakuragi N, et al. Survival effect of paraaortic lymphadenectomy in endometrial cancer (SEPAL study): a retrospective cohort analysis. Lancet. 2010;375:1165-72.
39. Hacker NF, Friedlander ML. Uterine cancer. In: Berek JS, Hackerm NF (Eds). Berek & Hacker's Gynecologic Oncology. 7th edition. US: Wolters Kluwer; 2020. pp. 371-413.
40. Palomba S, Ghezzi F, Falbo A, Mandato VD, Annunziata G, Lucia E, et al. Laparoscopic versus abdominal approach to endometrial cancer: A 10 year retrospective multicentre analysis. Int J Gynecol Cancer. 2012;22(3):425-33.
41. Kwon JS, Abrams J, Sugimoto A, Carey MS. Is adjuvant therapy necessary for stage IA and IB uterine papillary serous carcinoma and clear cell carcinoma after surgical staging? Int J Gynecol Cancer. 2007;18(4):820-4.
42. Creutzberg CL, van Putten WL, Koper PC, Lybeert ML, Jobsen JJ, Wárlám-Rodenhuis CC, et al. Surgery and postoperative radiotherapy versus surgery alone for patients with stage I endometrial carcinoma: multicenteric randomised trial. PORTEC Study Group: PostOperative Radiation therapy in Endometrial Carcinoma. Lancet. 2000;355:1404-11.
43. Rittenberg PV, Lotocki RJ, Heywood MS, Jones KD, Krepart GV. High-risk surgical stage I endometrial cancer: outcome with vault brachytherapy alone. Gynecol Oncol. 2003;89:288-94.
44. Tangjitgamol S, See HT, Kavanagh J. Adjuvant chemotherapy for endometrial cancer. Int J Gynecol Cancer. 2011;21:885-95.

45. De Boer SM, Powel EM, Mileshkin L, Katsaros D, Bessette P, Haie-Meder C, et al. Adjuvant chemotherapy versus radiotherapy alone in women with high-risk endometrial cancer (PORTEC-3): pattern of recurrence and post-hoc survival analysis of a randomized phase 3 trial. Lancet Oncol. 2019;20(9):1273-85.
46. Randall ME, Filiaci VL, Muss H, Spirits NM, Mannel RS, Fowler J, et al. Randomised chemotherapy in advanced endometrial carcinoma: A Gynaecologic Oncology Group Study. J Clin Oncol. 2006;24:36-44.
47. NCCN (2005). NCCN guidelines Uterine Neoplasms Version 2 [online]. Available from: https://www.nccn.org/patients/guidelines/content/PDF/uterine-patient.pdf. [Last accessed December, 2021].
48. Amant F, Mirza MR, Koskas M, Creutzberg CL. Cancer of the corpus uteri. FIGO Cancer Rep. 2018;37-50.
49. Tsoref D, Welch S, Lau S, Biagi J, Katia Tonkin K, Martin LA, et al. Phase II study of oral ridaforolimus in women with recurrent or metastatic endometrial cancer. Gynecol Oncol. 2014;135:184-9.
50. Pecorelli S. Revised FIGO staging for carcinoma of vulva, cervix, and endometrium. Int J Gynecol Obstet. 2009;105:103-4.
51. Creasman WT, Odicino F, Maisonneuve P, Quinn MA, Beller U, Benedet JL, et al. Carcinoma of the corpus uteri. FIGO annual report Vol 26, Int J Gynecol Oncol. 2006;95(1):S105-43.
52. The American Cancer Society medical and editorial content team (2018). Endometrial Cancer Survival Rates [online]. Available from: https://www. cancer.org/cancer/ endometrial-cancer/detection-diagnosis staging/survival-rates.html. [Last accessed December, 2021.
53. McMekin DS. Sarcoma of the uterus. In: Clinical Gynaecologic Oncology, 8th edition. Philadelphia: Elseiver, Saunders; 2012. pp. 175-87.
54. Genest DR, Berkowitz RS, Fisher RA. World Health Organization Classification of Tumours, Pathology and Genetics, Tumours of the Breast and Female Genital Organs. Lyon, France: IARC Press; 2003. pp. 250-4.
55. Benson C, Miah AB. Uterine sarcoma–current perspectives. Int J Women's Health. 2017;9:597.
56. Bell SW, Kemson RL, Hendrickson MR. Problematic uterine smooth muscle neoplasms: A clinicopathological study of 203 cases. Am J Surg Pathol. 1994;18:535.
57. Clement PB, Young RH. Mesenchymal and mixed epithelial-mesenchymal tumors of the uterine corpus and cervix. In: Clement PB, Young RH (Eds). Atlas of Gynaecologic Surgical Pathology. Philadephia: WB Saunders; 2000. pp. 177-210.
58. Evans HL. Endometrial stromal sarcoma and poorly differentiated endometrial sarcoma.Cancer. 1982;50:2170-82.
59. Oliva E. Cellular mesenchymal tumors of the uterus: A review emphasizing recent observations. Int J Gynecol Pathol. 2014;33:374-84.

LONG QUESTIONS

1. Define and classify endometrial hyperplasia. Describe the management of atypical endometrial hyperplasia.
2. How do you evaluate a case of postmenopausal bleeding? Describe the management strategies of early stage endometrial carcinoma.
3. Describe the risk factors of endometrial hyperplasia and cancer; describe the current recommendation for screening in endometrial carcinoma.
4. Can you prevent endometrial cancer? Describe strategies to prevent.
5. Adjuvant treatment of endometrial carcinoma—how do you decide and what is advocated—their result thereof?
6. Describe the molecular characterisation of endometrial cancers and its therapeutic implication?
7. Describe molecular classification of endometrial cancer and how will itimpact treatment of EC?
8. What are the prognostic variables in endometrial cancer? what are their implications in management in EC?
9. Classify the different types of mesenchymal uterine tumors and describe their management strategies.
10. What you mean by HNPCC? How it is related to endometrial cancer?

SHORT QUESTIONS

1. Describe EIN and its implication in terms of diagnosis and management.
2. Conservative management of endometrial hyperplasia and cancer
3. Transvaginal ultrasonography - its role in evaluation of postmenopausal bleeding.
4. Describe surgical staging procedure in endometrial carcinoma.
5. Sentinel nodal sampling in endometrial cancer—its implication in management.
6. Indications and justification of systematic lymphadenectomy in endometrial carcinoma.
7. Diagnosis and management of leiomyosarcoma/ endometrial stromal sarcoma.
8. Carcinosarcoma—how it is different from other sarcomas?
9. Describe role of imaging in endometrial carcinoma.
10. Write in brief about uterine papillary serous carcinoma of endometrium.

MULTIPLE CHOICE QUESTIONS

1. Which of the following endometrial hyperplasias is most prone to develop cancer:
   a. Simple hyperplasia
   b. Complex hyperplasia
   c. Simple hyperplasia with atypia
   d. Complex hyperplasia with atypia
2. All of the following are regarded as risk-factors for development of endometrial carcinoma, except:
   a. Estrogen replacement therapy
   b. Menopause after 52 years and menarche before 12 years
   c. Tamoxifen therapy for breast cancer >2 years
   d. OCP

3. In conservative management of endometrial hyperplasia the followings are true, except:
   a. MPA, OCP, Depo-provera are commonly used
   b. The drugs are used for 3–6 months
   c. Endometrial cavity should be sampled by endometrial biopsy every 3 months
   d. Levonorgestrel-releasing intrauterine system (Mirena) is never used
4. Staging of endometrial carcinoma is:
   a. Clinical b. Histological
   c. Surgicopathological d. Imaging
5. Which histological criteria are correlated to lymph node metastases in endometrial carcinoma?
   a. Histology type
   b. Depth of myometrial invasion
   c. Microscopic grading
   d. All of above
6. Systematic pelvic and para-aortic lymphadenectomy is recommended in all cases of endometrial carcinoma, except:
   a. Grade III tumors
   b. Grade I-II tumor with < 50% myoinvasion
   c. Uterine papillary serous and clear cell carcinoma
   d. Carcinosarcoma
7. Omentectomy/Omental biopsy recommendedin all, except:
   a. Serous, clear cell
   b. MMMT
   c. G3 EC
   d. Grade I-II endometrioid EC with < 50% myoinvasion
8. Which is the least significant prognostic factor in early endometrial carcinoma?
   a. Positive peritoneal fluid
   b. Histological grade
   c. Lymph node metastases
   d. Deep myometrial invasion
9. All the statements are correct, except:
   a. Non-endometrioid cancers account for approximately 10% of endometrial carcinoma
   b. Adenoacanthoma is a variant of endometrioid tumors
   c. Patients with papillary serous carcinoma have a poor prognosis
   d. Adenosquamous carcinoma do have higher rate of recurrence
10. Tumor involvement of the inguinal lymph nodes in endometrial cancer is staged as:
   a. III b b. IV a c. IV b d. III a
11. All are true in positive peritoneal fluid cytology in EC, except:
   a. Has poor prognosis if associated with other risk factors
   b. Should be mentioned separately
   c. Does not affect survival in early EC
   d. The disease is upstaged
12. Follow-up of treated cases of endometrial cancer – the standard of care:
   a. Annually
   b. Every 6 months for first 2 years
   c. Only when they are symptomatic
   d. Every 3–4 months in first 3 years, every 6 months during 4th and 5th year and annually thereafter
13. Which of the following uterine sarcoma should be staged as that of endometrial carcinoma?
   a. Leiomyosarcoma
   b. Endometrial stromal sarcoma
   c. Carcinosarcoma
   d. Adenosarcoma
14. In management of uterine sarcomas all are true, except:
   a. TAH with BSO
   b. Ovaries may be conserved in Leiomyosarcoma
   c. Lymphadenectomy should be performed in all
   d. Omentectomy along with lymphadenectomy is recommended in MMMT
15. Adjuvant radiotherapy in uterine cancers:
   a. Increases survival
   b. Decreases survival
   c. Decreases pelvic recurrences
   d. None of the above
16. If paraaortic lymphnode is positive in EC—it is staged as:
   a. Stage II b. Stage IIIa
   c. Stage IIIc1 d. Stage IIIc2
17. In molecular classification of EC—the worst prognosis is with:
   a. Pole ultramutated b. Pole hypermutated
   c. Copy number low d. Copy number high
18. Carcinosarcoma of uterus all are true, except:
   a. Pure non-epithelial sarcoma
   b. Both epithelial and non-epithelial components
   c. Staged under endometrial carcinoma
   d. Poor prognosis
19. Incidence of complex hyperplasia without atypia developing to carcinoma if untreated is:
   a. 1% b. 3%
   c. 8% d. 29%
20. Ovaries can safely be conserved in perimenopausal women in:
   a. ESS b. MMMT
   c. LMS d. Adenosarcoma

Answers

1.	d	2.	d	3.	d	4.	c	5.	d	6.	b
7.	d	8.	a	9.	d	10.	c	11.	d	12.	d
13.	c	14.	c	15.	c	16.	d	17.	d	18	a
19.	b.	20.	c								

14.7 BENIGN OVARIAN NEOPLASIA

Neerja Bhatla, Anju Singh, Seema Singhal

INTRODUCTION

Ovarian masses can have varied etiology, ranging from non-neoplastic to neoplastic, with an overlapping spectrum of clinical presentation. Establishing the diagnosis of ovarian neoplasms is important to allow appropriate management of each case.

The ovary is made up of tissue derived from coelomic epithelium, germ cells, and stromal (mesenchymal) cells. Tumors can arise from any of these structures, triggered by various genetic, environmental, and other factors. Certain non-neoplastic ovarian masses need to be mentioned as they constitute an important differential diagnosis of benign neoplasms. These are the tumors formed due to physiological variations in the process of ovulation, or during pregnancy, under the influence of various hormones **(Table 1)**.

CLASSIFICATION OF OVARIAN TUMORS

Based on the most probable tissue of origin, the World Health Organization (WHO) has classified ovarian neoplasms into surface epithelial (65%), germ cells (15%), sex-cord stromal

TABLE 1: Non-neoplastic ovarian tumors resulting from physiological variation.

Type of cyst	*Key features*	*Management*
	Related to ovulation	
Follicular cyst	• Most common in reproductive-age women • Results when mature follicles does not rupture at ovulation and continues to grow • Thin-walled simple cyst (usually <10 cm) • Clear fluid-filled cyst lined by an inner layer of granulosa cell and an outer layer of theca-interna cells	• Spontaneous resolution in 3–6 months • Hormonal suppression in the form of oral contraceptive pills (OCPs) can be given • Surgical intervention needed rarely if torsion, hemoperitoneum or persistent larger cysts (>10 cm) • Cystectomy is the surgical treatment of choice
Corpus luteal cyst	• Develop when corpus luteum fails to involute and enlarges abnormally • Cystic lesion with clear or hemorrhagic fluid • Rupture may lead to hemoperitoneum	
Theca lutein cyst	• Resulting from overstimulation of ovary by hCG • Seen in molar pregnancy and choriocarcinoma • Characterized by presence of significant luteinization of stroma surrounding the follicle	• Treatment of molar pregnancy or GTN is required and it usually resolves the cysts • Surgical intervention of these cysts is usually not needed
Polycystic ovaries	• Endocrine disorder characterized by oligomenorrhea, hyperandrogenism, and polycystic ovaries • Bilateral ovarian enlargement (2–5 times) consisting of multiple 2–9 mm follicles arranged peripherally • "String of pearls" appearance on ultrasonography	• Hormonal treatment (OCPs)
Ovarian hyperstimulation syndrome	• Iatrogenic form of hyper-reaction luteinalis (HL) seen in women undergoing ovulation induction • Characterized by marked enlargement of ovaries, high concentration of sex steroids and extravascular fluid accumulation due to increased vascular permeability	• Adequate hydration, strict vital monitoring • Use of dopamine agonist (cabergoline) • Might need drainage of ascites • Surgical intervention is needed rarely only in cases of torsion or rupture
	Related to pregnancy	
Hyper-reactioluteinalis	• Formation of multiple luteinized follicular cysts due to hCG stimulation • Grossly, bilateral enlargement of ovaries (up to 30–35 cm) with thin-walled cyst and intervening stroma • "Spoke-wheel" appearance on USG • Microscopically, follicular cysts are seen with prominent luteinization of theca-interna cells	• Spontaneous resolution in 6–8 months postpartum • Surgical removal may be needed in case of infarction, hemorrhage or to reduce ovarian size to decrease androgen production in virilized patients
Luteoma of pregnancy	• hCG–induced proliferation of luteinized ovarian stromal cells • Bilateral ovarian enlargement • Multiple, solid-cystic, fleshy, reddish-brown nodules of varying size (microscopic to 15–20 cm), which replace the normal parenchyma of ovaries	• A benign, self-limiting condition, which resolves spontaneously after pregnancy

TABLE 2: Common benign tumors of ovary.

Benign epithelial tumors	*Benign germ cell tumors*	*Benign sex-cord stromal tumors*
• Serous tumors – Cystadenoma – Adenofibroma – Surface papilloma • Mucinous tumors Cystadenoma • Endometrioid tumors – Endometriotic cyst – Endometrioid cystadenoma – Endometrioid cystadenofibroma • Clear cell tumors – Cystadenoma – Adenofibroma • Brenner tumor • Seromucinous tumors – Seromucinous cystadenoma – Seromucinous adenofibroma	Benign cystic teratoma (dermoid cyst)	• Fibroma • Thecoma • Sertoli-Leydig cell tumor

(10%), metastatic (5%), and miscellaneous tumors. Epithelial neoplasms are further subclassified based on the cell type (serous, mucinous, endometrioid type, etc.) and the degree of atypia (benign, borderline, or malignant) **(Table 2)**.

Benign Epithelial Ovarian Tumors

Epithelial neoplasms account for approximately 40% of all benign ovarian tumors. These are derived from surface epithelial cells of the ovary. WHO (2020) has subclassified epithelial tumors into six subtypes, which include serous, mucinous, endometrioid, clear cell, seromucinous, Brenner, and mixed tumors.[1,2] Benign tumors can be differentiated from malignant ones based on history, clinical examination, imaging findings and tumor markers **(Table 3)**. In the following sections of this chapter, our discussion will focus on benign tumors of the ovary.

Benign Serous Tumors

These are tumors composed of epithelium resembling fallopian tube or in some cases the surface epithelium of the ovary, constituting 20% of all benign ovarian tumors. These affect women in reproductive age at 30–50 years but cases in premenarchal, adolescents, and postmenopausal females, have been reported. Small tumors can be asymptomatic and diagnosed incidentally on routine pelvic examination or ultrasound. Large tumors present as a unilateral, large abdominopelvic mass associated with nonspecific pain, heaviness in the lower abdomen and pressure symptoms. Subtypes include cystadenoma, adenofibroma, and surface papilloma. Among serous tumors, 10–15% are bilateral and are usually smaller than mucinous tumors.

On ultrasonography, they appear as well-defined unilocular or bilocular cyst with homogenous echogenicity with thin septa and no vegetation. Different subtypes can be identified based on the histological findings.

Serous cystadenoma: Grossly, these appear as a simple cyst with a smooth glistening surface filled with serous (clear, watery) fluid, which may be blood-tinged **(Fig. 1A)**. On cut section, these have a smooth cyst wall. Presence of a large papillary growth, any solid nodule or area of necrosis should raise the suspicion of malignancy. On microscopy, the cysts are lined by a single layer of ciliated pseudostratified cuboidal or columnar epithelium **(Fig. 1B)**. These do not contain basophilic cytoplasmic vacuoles or granules characteristic of mucinous neoplasms. Psammoma bodies are a characteristic feature of serous neoplasm present in approximately 30% of benign serous cystadenoma. Focal papillary excrescences are present and formed by focal epithelial proliferation without cellular or nuclear atypia. Presence of these papillary projections in <10% of tumors differentiates benign tumors from borderline serous tumors.[3,4]

Serous cystadenoma composed of scattered glands with a prominent cellular and fibrous stroma are subclassified as serous adenofibroma and cystadenofibroma, if cystic.

Benign Mucinous Tumors

Mucinous tumors represent 15–20% of all ovarian tumors. They may be benign (85%), borderline (10%), or malignant (5%). They account for 10–15% of all benign ovarian tumors and are subclassified as mucinous cystadenoma and adenofibroma. The clinical presentation resembles that of serous tumors. KRAS is the most common genetic alteration present in approximately 50–60% cases.[4,5]

Mucinous cystadenoma: On gray-scale ultrasound, these appear as thin-walled, large, uni- or multiloculated cysts filled with fluid of low-level echogenicity. The multiple thin-walled locules may contain fluid of different echogenicity due to differences in the consistency of mucin. On gross examination, these appear as a large cystic mass of variable size (ranging from a few cm up to 30 cm) with smooth outer surface. On cut section, the multilocular cyst with a smooth cyst wall is filled with mucin-like gelatinous material. Papillary projections may be present in the cyst wall **(Fig. 2A)**.

Histologically, mucinous cystadenomas are composed of multiple cysts and glands lined by simple nonstratified tall columnar epithelium with basal nuclei-secreting mucin. The epithelium resembles gastric mucosa or intestinal epithelium with goblet cells. Focal papillae may be present which show no features of atypia **(Fig. 2B)**.

TABLE 3: Features to differentiate between benign and malignant ovarian neoplasm.

Key features	*Benign neoplasm*	*Malignant neoplasm*
	Clinical evaluation	
History	Abdominal pain, abdominal fullness, pressure symptoms	Abdominal fullness, pressure, pain, pressure symptoms, weight loss, anorexia
Examination	Palpable adnexal mass, no ascites, no lymphadenopathy	Cachexic look, palpable adnexal mass, ascites ±, lymphadenopathy ±, palpable omental caking ±
Ultrasound features (IOTA classification)	B-rules • Unilocular cyst • Presence of solid components where the largest solid component is <7 mm • Presence of acoustic shadows • Smooth multilocular tumor with largest diameter <100 mm • No blood flow	M-rules • Irregular solid tumor • Presence of ascites • At least four papillary structures • Irregular multilocular solid tumor > 100 mm • Strong blood flow
Tumor markers	Within normal range or mildly deranged	Elevated depending upon the type of malignancy
	Intraoperative findings	
Gross examination	Cystic or solid	Solid-cystic mass, ascites ±, usually bilateral, capsular breach, surface excrescences, large or multiple papillary projections +, necrosis and area of hemorrhages,
Cut section	Smooth cyst wall, Thin septa if present	Irregular cyst wall, thick septa, solid nodules +
Omental caking	–	+
Peritoneal deposit	–	+
E/O distant metastasis	–	+

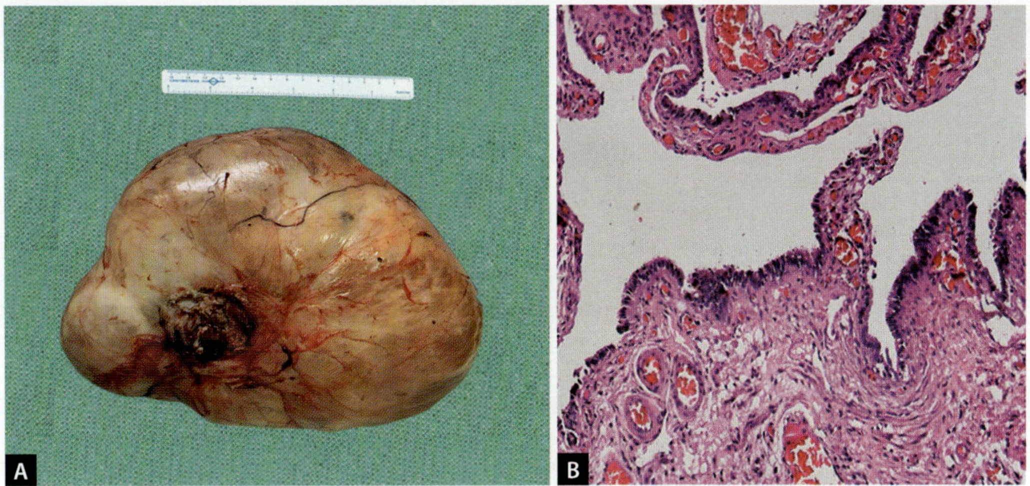

Figs. 1A and B: Gross and histopathological images of serous cystadenoma.
Courtesy: Professor Sandeep Mathur, Department of Pathology, AIIMS, Delhi

Adenofibroma: Adenofibromas are smaller in size and have a solid appearance as compared to mucinous cystadenoma. On histology, these have dense and fibrous stroma.

Differences between benign serous and mucinous tumors are enumerated in **Table 4**.

Brenner Tumor

It is a rare type of epithelial tumor, accounting for 5% of all benign ovarian tumors, derived from surface epithelial cells that have undergone transitional cell metaplasia. These clusters of metaplastic transitional cells are also known as "Walthard cell nests" when they invaginate into paratubal or ovarian tissue. These are seen in women at 50–60 years of age, are usually smaller in size (<2 cm), therefore they may remain asymptomatic and are often diagnosed incidentally. Occasionally, they may be larger and present as an adnexal mass.

On gross examination, a well-circumscribed, firm, and rubbery mass with a smooth or bosselated outer surface

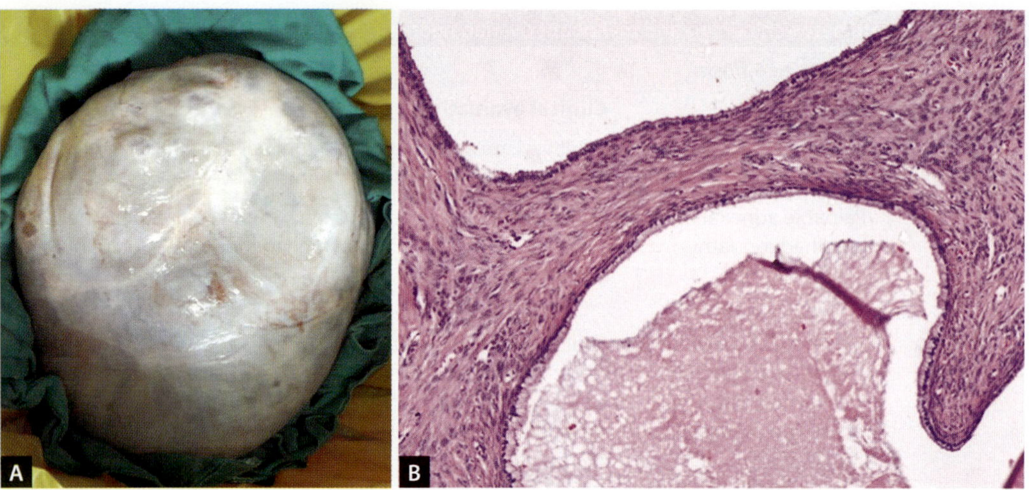

Figs. 2A and B: Gross and histopathological images of benign mucinous cystadenoma.
Courtesy: Professor Sandeep Mathur, Department of Pathology, AIIMS, Delhi

TABLE 4: Differences between mucinous and serous tumors.

Characteristic feature	*Benign mucinous tumor*	*Benign serous tumor*
Incidence	10–15% of all benign ovarian tumors	20% of all benign ovarian tumors
Clinical Features	20–40 years of age Mostly unilateral	30–50 years of age 10–15% can be bilateral
• Ultrasonography – Size – Locule – Opacity – Papillaryprojection	 • Mostly large • Uniloculated / multiloculated • Low-level echogenicity (variable) • Rare	 • Smaller than mucinous • Unilocular or bilocular cyst • Homogeneous echogenicity • Often seen
Gross examination	• Large cystic mass, smooth outer surface • Multiseptated • Size: few cm up to 30 cm • Filled with mucin	• Simple cyst with smooth glistening surface • Serous (clear, watery) fluid, may be blood-tinged
Cut section	Smooth cyst wall, filled with mucin-like gelatinous material	Smooth cyst wall, filled with serous material
• Microscopy – Epithelial lining – Papillary excrescences – Psammoma bodies	 • Simple non-stratified tall columnar epithelium with basal nuclei secreting mucin • Focal papillae may be rarely present which shows no features of atypia • Absent	 • Ciliated pseudostratified cuboidal or columnar epithelium • Focal papillary excrescences often seen with no feature of cellular or nuclear atypia in <10% of tumor • Present
Treatment	Ovarian cystectomy or oophorectomy, either laparoscopically or via laparotomy Take all precautions to prevent cyst rupture	Ovarian cystectomy or oophorectomy, either laparoscopically or via laparotomy Take all precautions to prevent cyst rupture

is palpated. It appears solid, gray-white, or yellow surface on the cut section with whorled or lobulated appearance. On histopathology, sharply demarcated epithelial cell nests resembling urothelium are seen in a background of dense, fibrous stroma.

Epithelial cells are uniform in size with sharp borders, ovoid nuclei, and a longitudinal groove giving "coffee-bean appearance". These are strongly positive for immunohistochemical markers like keratin, EMA, GATA3, and CK7; they are stain negative for calretinin, inhibin, WT1, CK20, PAX8, PAX2, ER, and PR. Rarely, a borderline and malignant form of Brenner tumor may be seen.[4,6]

Endometroid Tumors

The ovary is the most common site of endometriosis and it has also been implicated as a precursor lesion for epithelial ovarian neoplasms, which can be benign, borderline, or malignant. Benign tumors associated with endometriosis and presenting as adnexal mass are endometriotic cyst, endometriotic cystadenoma, or cystadenofibroma.

This condition commonly affects women of reproductive age group with a peak incidence at 35–45 years and more common in nulliparous women. In a patient with adnexal mass, dysmenorrhea, dyspareunia, and infertility are the specific symptoms, which favor the diagnosis of endometriosis. On examination, these tend to be tender with restricted mobility due to surrounding adhesions and nodularity of uterosacral ligaments can be felt. Serum CA-125 levels are often increased in patients with endometriosis (usually within 10 X of normal), above-mentioned features on history and examination may help in differentiating benign endometriotic lesions from other benign and malignant ovarian tumors preoperatively.

Endometriotic cyst: Ovarian endometriosis most commonly presents as a cyst-containing old blood of dark-brown color called an endometriotic cyst or chocolate cyst. It is seen in 17–44% of women with endometriosis, tends to involve both ovaries and adhesions to surrounding structures is frequently seen. These cysts show homogeneous echogenic ground-glass appearance on ultrasound. On magnetic resonance imaging (MRI), it shows high intensity in both T1-weighted and T2-weighted images, reflecting the blood element in the cyst. Lack of fat suppression helps to distinguish an endometriotic cyst from a dermoid cyst. These cysts are easily identifiable on histopathology by their characteristic lining of endometrial epithelium and stroma and pigmented histiocytes within their walls **(Fig. 3)**.

Endometriotic cystadenoma and adenofibroma: Cystic tumors with endometriotic features.

Benign Clear Cell Tumor

Clear cell tumors are a rare variety of epithelial ovarian tumors that are mostly malignant but can rarely be benign or borderline. Benign types include clear cell cystadenoma and adenofibroma. These show a close association with endometriosis, similar to endometrioid tumors. These usually present in women of reproductive age-group as adnexal mass, pelvic pain/dysmenorrhea and pressure symptoms. They have a lobulated external surface with honey-comb appearance due to closely packed minute cysts embedded in the firm-rubbery stroma (parvilocular) on cut section. Clear cell cystadenoma is cystic in appearance containing clear fluid while adenofibroma is solid. Histopathologically, tubular glands lined by 1–2 layers of hobnail cells or large polyhedral cells are seen in a background of compact and fibrocollagenous stroma. The cytoplasm is often scanty in hobnail cells while abundant, eosinophilic, and granular in large polyhedral cells. Benign tumors are distinguished from malignant ones by no cytological atypia and the presence of relatively uniform nuclei with minimal nuclear atypia with <1 mitotic figure (MFs)/10 high-power fields (HPF).

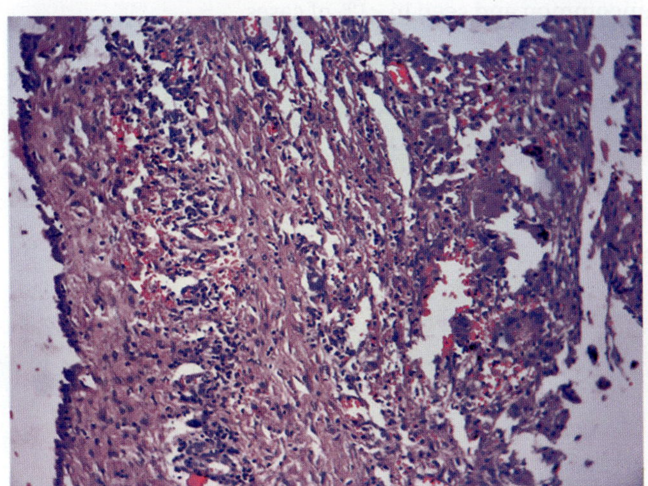

Fig. 3: Histopathological image of endometriotic cyst.
Courtesy: Professor Sandeep Mathur, Department of Pathology, AIIMS, Delhi

Seromucinous Tumor

This distinctive group of tumors is the addition to the epithelial group of ovarian tumors in the WHO (2014) classification. These constitute approximately 1% of all benign epithelial neoplasms and include seromucinous cystadenoma or adenofibroma. The term seromucinous is a misnomer as they are not composed of serous and mucinous epithelium only, but are characterized by two or more Müllerian cell types including endocervical-type mucinous, endometrioid, and squamous type epithelium. These tumors show a close resemblance to endometriosis and not to serous tumors.[7]

The characteristic features of these tumors are bilaterally (20–40%), frequent association with endometriosis (30–70%), and absence of gastrointestinal differentiation, as evidenced by admixtures of goblet cells and/or Paneth cells.[8]

On gross examination, these are thin-walled unilocular or paucilocular cysts with smooth outer and inner surfaces filled with thin mucinous /serous fluid. The cyst wall is lined by endocervical-type columnar cells with abundant intracytoplasmic mucin admixed with scattered ciliated cells, endometrioid cells, and less often, transitional or squamous cells. Seromucinous adenofibromas are mostly solid lesions with few cystic spaces **(Fig. 4)**.

Benign Germ Cell Tumors (GCT): Teratoma

Teratomas are a group of ovarian tumors derived from pluripotent germ cell tumors. Three histological subtypes include:

- *Immature teratoma*: Malignant teratomas. Composed of tissues derived from all three germ cell layers, histologically these tissues are immature/embryonic.
- *Mature cystic teratoma (dermoid cyst):* Benign teratomas containing well-differentiated tissue from all three germ cell lines.

- *Monodermal teratomas:* Predominantly composed of one particular cell line. Main types are struma ovarii, ovarian carcinoid tumors, and tumors with neural differentiation, etc.

Mature Cystic Teratomas (Dermoid Cyst)

Dermoid cyst is the most common type of GCT among adults and the most common type of teratoma. These benign tumors are diploid (46XX) in nature and are believed to arise from germ cells after the first meiotic division. These tumors can affect women of all age groups and clinically present as an adnexal mass and are bilateral in 10–20% of cases.[9]

Characteristic features on USG include:

- Cystic lesion with a densely echogenic tubercle (Rokitansky nodule) projecting into the cyst lumen
- Diffusely or partially echogenic mass with the echogenic area usually demonstrating sound attenuation owing to sebaceous material and hair within the cyst cavity

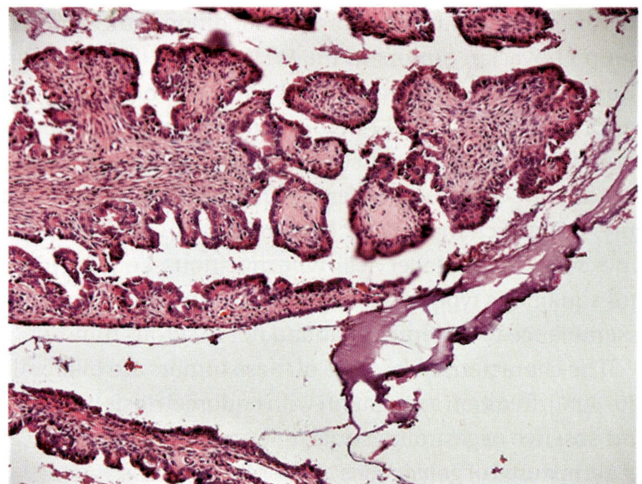

Fig. 4: Histopathological image of benign seromucinous tumor.
Courtesy: Professor Sandeep Mathur, Department of Pathology, AIIMS, Delhi

- Fluid-fluid levels result from sebum floating above aqueous fluid, which appears more echogenic than the sebum layer.

Computed tomography (CT) and MRI are helpful to differentiate teratoma from hemorrhagic cyst. On CT scan, fat attenuation within a cyst, with or without calcification in the wall, is diagnostic for mature cystic teratoma. On MRI, the sebaceous component of dermoid cysts has very high-signal intensity on T1-weighted images, similar to retroperitoneal fat. The signal intensity of the sebaceous component on T2-weighted images is variable, approximating that of fat.

Grossly, these are of variable size, cystic to firm appearance containing yellow, sebaceous material. The cyst is lined by skin composed of keratinized squamous epithelium with abundant sebaceous and eccrine glands. Cyst lining may be of mature respiratory or gastrointestinal epithelium type **(Figs. 5A and B)**. These are easily identified due to the distinguished presence of ectodermal tissue (hair follicle, nails, neural tissue), mesodermal tissue (fat, bone, muscle, cartilage), and endodermal tissue (bronchial epithelium, thyroid tissue) inside. Rokitansky nodule is a raised protuberance projecting into the cyst cavity from which most of the hair, bone, teeth, etc., typically arise. This site should always be carefully sampled during histopathological examination.

These cysts may undergo a malignant transformation in 1–2% of cases, most common being squamous cell carcinoma (SCC). Other malignant transformations can be mucinous carcinoma, basal cell carcinoma, malignant melanoma, carcinoid tumor, etc. Advanced age (>50 years), large-sized cysts (>10 cm), elevated CA-125, and SCC antigen are some of the features which raise the possibility of malignancy.

Treatment of choice is cystectomy and all precautions must be taken to prevent spillage of contents as it may result in chemical peritonitis. Complete cyst excision with removal of the cyst wall should be the desired aim of cystectomy to prevent recurrence. Local recurrence after cyst excision is uncommon and seen in <1% of cases.

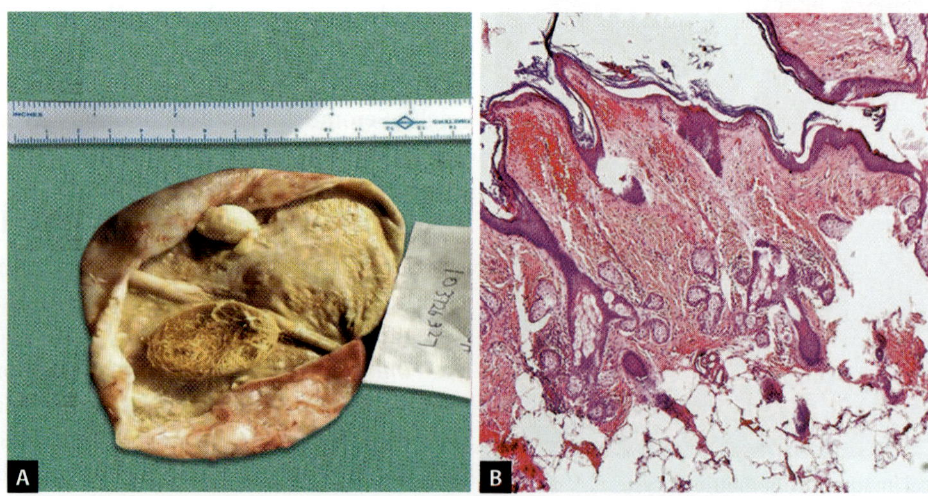

Figs. 5A and B: Gross and histopathological images of mature cystic teratom.
Courtesy: Professor Sandeep Mathur, Department of Pathology, AIIMS, Delhi

Struma Ovarii

It is a monodermal type of teratoma composed predominantly of thyroid tissue and constitutes approximately 3% of ovarian teratomas. Clinical presentation is similar to a dermoid cyst except it may be associated with enlargement of the thyroid gland.

It is usually unilateral, of varying size (<10 cm) with a smooth surface. On cut section, it appears light-tan with glistening thyroid tissue. Microscopically, it is composed of thyroid follicles lined by a single layer of columnar epithelium filled with eosinophilic, PAS-positive colloid. Treatment involves cystectomy or unilateral oophorectomy. Uncommon complications associated with struma ovarii include malignant transformation (malignant struma ovarii resembling papillary thyroid carcinoma), pseudo-Meigs syndrome (presence of ascites and pleural effusion), and extra-ovarian spread.

Sex-cord Stromal Tumors

Sex-cord stromal tumors (SCSTs) are a heterogeneous group of benign and malignant neoplasm arising from either gonadal sex cord cells (granulosa and Sertoli cells), gonadal stromal cells (Leydig cells, theca cells, or fibroblasts) or a combination of these (Sertoli-Leydig cells). They account for 5–8% of all primary ovarian tumors. These tumors can be differentiated with the help of immunohistochemical markers which include the presence of ?-inhibin, calretinin and steroidogenic factor-1 (SF-1), FOXL2 and absence of epithelial and germ cell tumor markers.[10] Based on the clinical behavior, these may be classified as enumerated in **Table 5**.

Fibroma

Fibroma is a rare benign ovarian tumor comprising approximately 1–4% of all ovarian tumors.[4,10] It is the most common benign tumor among SCSTs, which arise from stromal cells of the ovary. These can occur at all age groups but most commonly seen in reproductive-age women and present as an adnexal mass. Knowledge about these tumors is essential to differentiate these from uterine fibroids, which also present as a solid mass. If these solid tumors are associated with ascites/pleural effusion or elevated CA-125 levels then they can be misdiagnosed as ovarian malignancy.

TABLE 5: Classification of sex-cord stromal tumors according to clinical behavior.

Malignant SCSTs	*Benign SCSTs*	*Benign/ malignant SCSTs*
• Adult granulosa cell tumor • Juvenile granulosa cell tumor • Sertoli cell tumor	• Fibroma • Cellular fibroma • Thecoma • Luteinized thecoma associated with sclerosing peritonitis	Sertoli–Leydig tumors

- *Imaging findings:* On USG, these tumors appear as a solid hypoechoic adnexal mass with ultrasound beam attenuation and cast striped shadows due to the cellular bundles and intersecting strips of hyaline-like collagen and fibrous tissue. Additional imaging modalities like Doppler ultrasound, CT, or MRI can be helpful to distinguish these tumors from uterine fibroid. On Doppler ultrasound, a subserosal myoma appears as a well-vascularized solid pelvic mass with the high-speed flow whereas a less vascularized tumor with the low-speed flow will mostly indicate an ovarian tumor. On CT scan, these appear as a solid mass with delayed/poor contrast enhancement. On MRI, these tumors appear as a homogenous mass with low signal intensity on both T1 and T2-weighted images. Sometimes in the case of large tumors, it may show scattered hyperintense areas on T2 images due to various degenerative changes such as cystic and myxomatous changes as well as hemorrhagic infarction thus mimicking solid ovarian malignancies.
- *Histopathological findings:* Fibromas are composed of spindle-shaped fibroblasts with abundant cytoplasm that produce collagen. Presence of lipid-laden theca cells along with fibroblasts points towards a diagnosis of fibrothecoma. Cellular fibromas are a variant with dense cellular proliferation of fibroblasts with mild-to-moderate nuclear atypia, a mitotic count of ≤3 MFs/10 HPF, and low malignant potential **(Figs. 6A and B)**.

Management

After a thorough preoperative evaluation, surgery is the treatment of choice. If the diagnosis is confirmed preoperatively, then less extensive surgery in the form of excision of the tumor or unilateral oophorectomy can be performed, thus fertility is preserved. Intraoperative frozen section may be considered if facilities are available.

Sertoli-Leydig Cell Tumor (SLCTs)

These rare tumors constitute < 0.5% of all ovarian neoplasm and are derived from both sex-cord (Sertoli cells) and stromal cells (Leydig cells) of the ovary. They are more commonly seen in the second and third decades of life and rarely can be seen in postmenopausal women. These also present clinically as adnexal mass associated with pain and pressure symptoms. Some of the symptoms are due to hormone production (mostly androgen and rarely estrogen) by these tumors include virilism, hirsutism, and hoarseness of voice, clitoromegaly, oligomenorrhea, and amenorrhoea.

These tumors may occur sporadically or due to germ line mutation in DICER1 (DICER 1 syndrome or pleuropulmonary blastoma familial tumor susceptibility syndrome), a gene encoding the RNAase III enzyme in the microRNA maturation pathway. Their clinical behavior (benign/ malignant) varies depending upon histological subtype

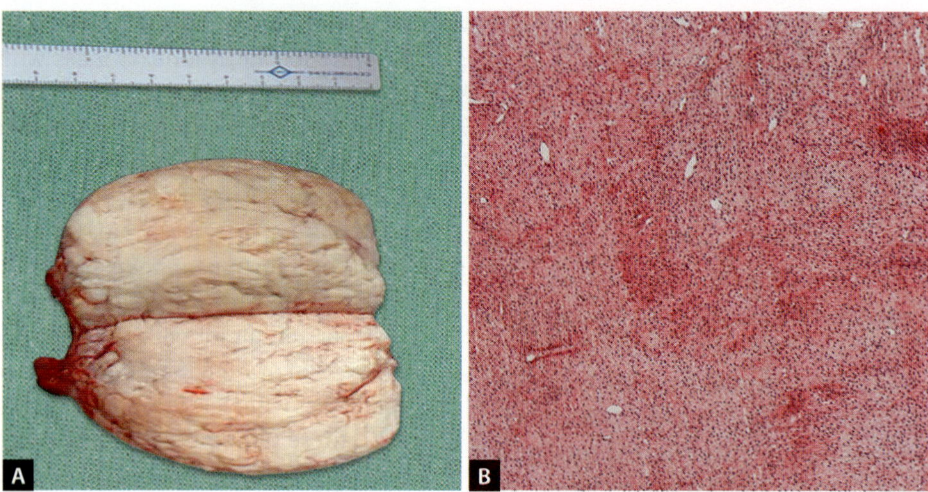

Figs. 6A and B: Gross and histopathological images of fibroma.
Courtesy: Professor Sandeep Mathur, Department of Pathology, AIIMS, Delhi

and tumor grade. Various histological subtypes of these tumors include:

- Sertoli-Leydig cell tumor
  - Well-differentiated (11%)
  - Moderately differentiated/intermediate grade (54%)
  - Poorly differentiated (13%)
- SLCTs with heterologous elements (22%) which include carcinoid, mesenchymal, and mucinous epithelial tissues with the most common being gastrointestinal-types
- SLCTs, retiform variant.

Well-differentiated subtype is essentially benign and presents as a unilateral, solid adnexal mass with a yellow, lobulated appearance on cut section. These tumors have varied appearances on gross examination and are not easily identifiable. Microscopically, these are made up of tubules lined by Sertoli cells and intervening nests of Leydig cells. Sertoli cells form tubular structures lined by single or multiple layers of cuboidal-columnar cells with well demarcated margins, oval dark nuclei, inconspicuous nucleoli, and eosinophilic or vacuolated cytoplasm. Leydig cells are typically found in clusters in the interstitial stroma and exhibit polygonal cells with well-defined margins, centric nuclei, prominent nucleoli, and eosinophilic cytoplasm.

Fertility-sparing surgery (unilateral salpingo-oophorectomy) can be considered as the treatment of choice in all patients with well-differentiated ovarian SLCTs. Long-term follow-up is advised in all the patients.

CLINICAL FEATURES OF BENIGN OVARIAN TUMORS

Benign ovarian tumors are most commonly seen in women of the reproductive age group. However, cases in premenarchal and postmenopausal women have also been reported. These can also be detected for the first time during pregnancy. Dermoid is the most common benign ovarian neoplasm detected during pregnancy.

Symptoms

All benign ovarian neoplasms may share common clinical presentation, which may be:

- *Asymptomatic*: These may remain asymptomatic for years and detected incidentally on routine pelvic examination or ultrasonography. Usually occurs with serous cystadenoma or teratoma.
- *Acute presentation:* Patients may present to emergency with acute onset pain with or without features of shock in case of torsion, rupture, or hemorrhage.
- *Chronic presentation*: The clinical presentation may be in the form of chronic symptoms from months or years. The most common clinical presentation is chronic abdominal pain, which is dull-aching and may be associated with abdominal fullness or gradually increasing abdominal mass/distension. Large tumors may have pressure symptoms of bladder and bowel, which include frequency of micturition, hesitancy or feeling of incomplete evacuation of bladder or constipation. Certain hormone-producing tumors like Sertoli-Leydig cell tumors may be associated with menstrual irregularities, feminizing or virilizing symptoms depending upon the hormones produced.

EXAMINATION FINDINGS

General Physical Examination

In the acute presentation, the patient may have sick look, tachycardia and hypotension. In the chronic presentation, vitals are essentially stable.

Per Abdomen Examination

A palpable abdominopelvic mass with well-defined or ill-defined borders is the most common presentation. The lower border is usually not reachable suggesting a pelvic origin. This mass may have a cystic to firm consistency, mostly non-tender and with restricted mobility. These are not associated with ascites and lymphadenopathy, unlike their malignant counterparts. However, a fluid thrill may be noted in some very large tumors with thin cyst wall and watery contents. Coexisting ascites and right side hydrothorax may be associated with fibroma or benign Brenner tumor and is known as Meig's syndrome.

Per Vaginal Examination

On bimanual examination, adnexal mass can be palpated in one or both of the lateral fornices. Approximate size, consistency, mobility, and any tenderness, if present to be noted. The uterus is mostly of normal size if no associated uterine pathology and usually deviated to one side due to adnexal mass. In the case of very big tumors, fullness is appreciated in all the fornices with difficulty in making out the uterus separately. Dermoid cysts are usually felt anterior to the uterus and with good mobility.

Since, almost all of the tumors have a similar clinical presentation, can be differentiated with the help of imaging findings and tumor markers, which are discussed above with specific tumor type.

Different multimodalities scoring systems for triaging of ovarian masses are Risk of Malignancy Index (RMI), Risk of Ovarian Malignancy Algorithm (ROMA), and Risk of Ovarian Cancer Algorithm (ROCA) score **(Table 6 and Box 1)**.

TABLE 6: Risk of malignancy index (RMI)-1 scoring system for evaluation of adnexal mass.

U= Ultrasound characteristics	*M is menopausal status*	*Serum CA -125 levels*
Multilocular cysts Bilateral lesions Presence of ascites Evidence of solid areas Evidence of metastasis *Score:* U = 0: None of above features U = 1: One of these U = 3: Two or more features	M=1: Premenopausal, M=3: Postmenopausal,	Value in Unit per mL
RMI = USG score × Menopausal status score × CA 125 value RMI <200: Low risk RMI >200 indicates high probability of ovarian malignancy		

BOX 1: Risk of Malignancy Algorithm (ROMA) score.

Premenopausal predictive index (PI): -12.0 + 2.38 × HE4 + 0.0626 × CA-125

Postmenopausal predictive index (PI): -8.09 + 1.04 × HE4 + 0.732 × CA-125

ROMA = exp (PI)/[1 + exp (PI)] × 10
Premenopausal: <1.14 (low-risk)
Postmenopausal: < 2.99 (low-risk)

MANAGEMENT

Observation

Asymptomatic patients with ultrasound features suggestive of benign etiology and normal serum CA-125 levels are the best candidates who can be managed conservatively by observation. With rare exceptions, most are simple, asymptomatic and uniloculated cysts up to 10 cm in premenopausal and < 5 cm in postmenopausal women with normal CA-125 levels, which tend to be benign and do not need surgical intervention. During the period of observation, the patient should be monitored by serial ultrasound monitoring 3–6 monthly.[11-13]

Medical Management

Benign ovarian endometriotic cysts can be managed medically tailored according to patient's age, symptomatology and need for future fertility. Medical therapy is best suited for young patients with mild to moderate symptoms and small (< 4 cm) endometriomas. It includes the use of oral contraceptive pills, progestogens, gonadotropin-hormone releasing (GnRH) agonists or aromatase inhibitors.

Surgical Intervention

Cystectomy is the surgical treatment of choice for benign tumors in premenopausal women, which can be done via laparotomy or preferably by laparoscopic route. In the presence of large tumors where no healthy ovarian tissue can be appreciated, oophorectomy may be done. In peri- and postmenopausal women, hysterectomy and bilateral salpingo-oophorectomy may be considered. Some practical points, which can be adopted while performing surgery, are as follows:

- A longitudinal incision for laparotomy may be preferred, if in doubt. It will also ease the process of abdominal exploration and scope for extending the incision, if the tumor inadvertently turns out to be malignant intraoperatively.
- Careful inspection and palpation of the uterus, contralateral ovary, abdominal viscera and lymph nodes should be done.
- Peritoneal fluid or washings should be sent for cytological examination.
- All efforts to be made to deliver the tumor intact and prevent spillage of contents.
- If in any doubt due to gross appearance and cut section features, frozen section can aid in diagnosis, if available. This is especially useful in younger women for considering fertility preserving surgery.

In a minimally invasive approach (laparoscopy), techniques for safe removal without spillage of content should be practiced. The detached cyst/mass should be placed into an intraperitoneal specimen bag, and the edges of the bag drawn up through one of the abdominal incisions. This skin incision is then enlarged and the cyst can be drained in-bag with a large bore needle attached to a syringe or with a suction device without risking peritoneal contamination. However, if at any point of time spillage is deemed likely, prompt conversion to laparotomy should be considered.

COMPLICATIONS OF BENIGN OVARIAN NEOPLASMS

Torsion

Torsion is the most common complication seen with non-neoplastic and neoplastic tumors of the ovary especially large, mobile, pedunculated cysts. It is more commonly seen with benign cystic teratoma and serous cystadenoma. Patients present with an acute abdomen with severe pain and vomiting, and a tender adnexal mass may occasionally be palpated depending on the size. Treatment includes emergency surgery with reduction of torsion and concomitant ovarian cystectomy, if fertility is to be preserved. Ovarian function is preserved in up to 90% of cases 3 months after intervention, despite the presence of ischemia and necrosis at time of exploration. Ovarian fixation, though controversial, can be considered in cases of recurrent torsion.

Rupture or Hemorrhage

Ovarian cyst may undergo intracystic hemorrhage or may rupture into the peritoneal cavity. It is seen more commonly with physiological cysts like corpus luteal cyst and less commonly may be seen with pathological cysts like a dermoid cyst, cystadenoma, etc. Rupture may lead to hemoperitoneum or irritation of the peritoneal cavity by cyst contents. It may present with features of acute abdomen with or without shock or peritonitis. This condition can be managed conservatively if the patient is hemodynamically stable. Surgical intervention is needed in the presence of hemodynamic instability or rupture of pathological cysts like dermoids.

Infection

Infection of an ovarian mass may lead to the formation of ovarian abscess and present clinically with fever, chills, abdominal pain and tenderness, and foul-smelling discharge. It can be managed conservatively with broad-spectrum antibiotics or may need surgical exploration if it does not respond to medical treatment or if features of sepsis are present.

Meig's Syndrome

Meig's syndrome is characterized by the presence of ascites and right-sided pleural effusion in association with a benign ovarian fibrous tumor. It is most commonly seen in fibromas and the underlying pathophysiology is believed to be seepage of fluid from the serosal surface of the tumor into the peritoneal cavity and subsequent passage to the pleural cavity via lymphatics. This condition usually resolves after removal of the primary tumor.

Malignant Transformation

Rarely, benign tumors may undergo malignant transformation such as serous adenocarcinoma from serous cystadenoma, SCC from dermoid cyst, or clear cell carcinoma from endometriosis.

KEY MESSAGES

- Benign ovarian tumors can be differentiated from malignant by history, clinical examination, imaging, and tumor markers.
- Fibromas are benign solid tumors, associated with ascites/ pleural effusion or elevated CA-125 levels and can be misdiagnosed as ovarian malignancy.
- Sex-cord stromal tumors can secrete hormones (mostly androgen, rarely estrogen) and present with menstrual irregularities, virilizing, or masculinizing symptoms.
- Simple cysts up to 10 cm in premenopausal women are usually functional. If surgery is needed, ovarian cystectomy is preferred, via laparotomy or preferably laparoscopically. Techniques for safe removal without spillage are essential.
- In peri- and postmenopausal women, hysterectomy and bilateral salpingo-oophorectomy may be considered for benign tumors.

REFERENCES

1. Kurman RJ, Carcangiu ML, Herrington S, Young RH. World Health Organization Classification of tumors of the female reproductive organs. 4th edition. Lyon, France: IARC; 2014.
2. Cree AI, White AV, Indave IB, Lokuhetty D. Revising the WHO classification : female genital tract tumors . Histopathology. 2020;76(1):151-6.
3. Berek JS, Hacker NF. Berek & Hacker's Gynecologic Oncology. 7th edition. Philadelphia: Wolters Kluwer Health; 2020.
4. Kurman JR, Ellenson HL, Ronnett MB. Blaustein's Pathology of female genital tract. 7th edition. Berlin/Heidelberg: Springer; 2019.
5. Mills MA, Shanes ED. Mucinous ovarian tumors. Surg Pathol. 2019;12(2):565-8.
6. Kuhn E, Ayhan A, Shih I, Seidman JD, Kurman RJ. Ovarian Brenner tumor: a morphologic and immunohistochemical analysis suggesting an origin from fallopian tube epithelium. Eur J Cancer. 2013;49:3839-49.
7. Kurman JR, Shih I. Seromucinous tumors of the ovary. What's in a name? Int J Gynecol Pathol. 2016;35(1):78-81.
8. Nagamine M, Mikami Y. Ovarian seromucinous tumors: Pathogenesis, morphologic spectrum, and clinical issues. Diagnostics. 2020;10:77.
9. Nogales F, Dulcey I, Preda O. Germ cell tumors of the ovary: An update. Arch Pathol Lab Med. 2014;138:351-62.
10. Lim D, Olivia E. Ovarian sex cord-stromal tumors: an update in recent molecular advances. Pathology. 2017;1-12.

11. Royal College of Obstetricians and Gynaecologists (RCOG). Ovarian cysts in premenopausal women. London, UK: Royal College of Obstetricians and Gynaecologists; 2011.
12. Royal College of Obstetricians and Gynaecologists (RCOG). Ovarian cysts in postmenopausal women. London, UK: Royal College of Obstetricians and Gynaecologists; 2016.
13. The American College of Obstetricians and Gynecologists (ACOG). Evaluation and management of adnexal masses. Practice Bulletin No 174. Washington, D.C.: ACOG; 2016.

LONG QUESTIONS

1. Mention the WHO classification of benign epithelial ovarian tumors. How will you differentiate between benign mucinous and serous tumors.
2. Describe in brief about the benign ovarian tumors which show association with endometriosis.
3. A 28-year-old, pregnant female presents at 16 weeks period of gestation with pain lower abdomen and 6 cm adnexal mass . What are the common differential diagnosis. Describe the gross, histopathological features and management of mature cystic teratoma.
4. Mention in brief about complications of benign ovarian neoplasms.
5. A 25-year-old female presents to the outpatient department with complaints of oligomenorrhea, lump in the lower abdomen and hoarseness of voice. Describe the benign ovarian tumor with similar presentation.

SHORT QUESTIONS

1. How will you differentiate between benign and malignant ovarian neoplasm?
2. Write a short note on:
   a. Luteoma of pregnancy
   b. IOTA classification
   c. Sertoli-Leydig cell tumors
   d. Multimodal scoring system for triaging of ovarian masses
   e. Benign seromucinous tumor.

MULTIPLE CHOICE QUESTIONS

1. Which of the following benign ovarian tumors is most prone to undergo torsion during pregnancy?
   a. Theca lutein cyst
   b. Serous cystadenoma
   c. Mucinous cystadenoma
   d. Dermoid cyst
2. All of the following are features of Meig's syndrome, except:
   a. Ascites
   b. Mucinous tumor
   c. Fibroma
   d. Pleural Effusion
3. All of the following are characteristic features of benign seromucinous tumor, except:
   a. Frequent association with endometriosis
   b. Composed of serous and mucinous epithelium only
   c. Bilaterality in 20–40% cases
   d. Absence of gastrointestinal differentiation
4. Epithelial cells with "Coffee-bean appearance" are characteristic of:
   a. Clear cell tumor
   b. Brenner tumor
   c. Seromucinous tumor
   d. Sertoli-Leydig cell tumor
5. All are correctly matched, except:
   a. Dermoid cyst: Bone
   b. Mucinous tumor: Psammoma bodies
   c. Brenner tumor: Walthard cell nests
   d. Clear cell tumor: Hobnail cells
6. Most common benign ovarian tumor is:
   a. Serous cystadenoma
   b. Mucinous cystadenoma
   c. Mature cystic teratoma
   d. Endometriotic cyst
7. What will be the RMI of post-menopausal women with serum CA-125 of 15 U/mL, ultrasound showing 6 cm bilateral multi-loculated cyst with no ascites?
   a. 90
   b. 135
   c. 95
   d. 130
8. Endometriosis has close association with all of the following, except:
   a. Endometriotic cyst
   b. Seromucinous tumor
   c. Brenner tumor
   d. Clear cell tumor
9. Which of the following gene mutation is seen in Sertoli-Leydig cell tumor?
   a. KRAS mutation
   b. PTEN gene mutation
   c. DICERI mutation
   d. P 53 gene
10. Most common malignant transformation seen in mature cystic teratoma is:
   a. Mucinous carcinoma
   b. Basal cell carcinoma
   c. Malignant melanoma
   d. Squamous cell carcinoma

Answers

1. d 2. b 3. b 4. b 5. b 6. c
7. b 8. c 9. c 10. d

14.8 MALIGNANT OVARIAN NEOPLASIA

Harshad Parasnis, Suchita Dabhadkar

INTRODUCTION

In India, ovarian cancer accounts for 6.7% of all cancers in women and 4.8% mortality due to cancer in women. According to Globocan 2020 data, the age standardized incidence rates of cancers in females in India are: breast (26.3%), cervix uteri (18.3%), ovary (6.7%), oral cavity (4.6%), and colorectal (3.7%).[1]

According to the cell of origin, there are three broad categories of malignant ovarian tumors: epithelial ovarian cancers, ovarian germ cell tumors, and sex cord stromal tumors. Epithelial ovarian cancers constitute 90% of all ovarian malignancies.[2] More than 70% of patients present with advanced disease. Epithelial ovarian cancer carries the highest mortality rate among all gynecological cancers **(Fig. 1)**.

EPIDEMIOLOGY AND RISK FACTORS FOR EPITHELIAL OVARIAN CANCER

Age: 50% of ovarian cancers are seen above 65 years of age.[3]

Genetic factors: 18–24% of invasive epithelial cancers have an autosomal dominant germ line mutation and have a strong family history of breast and ovarian cancer. BRCA1/2 is the most commonly identified genetic mutation, followed by Hereditary Nonpolyposis Colon cancer (Lynch syndrome), showing MLH1, MSH2, MSH6, PMS2 mutations.[4-6] Lynch syndrome associated cancers occur at various sites like colorectum, ovary, uterus (endometrial), stomach, liver, kidney, brain, and certain types of skin cancers.

Hormonal and reproductive factors: Early menarche, late menopause, endometriosis, nulliparity increase the chance of ovarian cancer.[7] High parity, breastfeeding, and oral contraceptive (OC) pill use are protective against ovarian cancer.[8] The common mechanism involved in these reproductive factors is the increase or decrease in the number of ovulations that a woman experiences in her lifetime. Suppression of ovulation prevents injury to surface epithelial cells of the ovary. A 5-year use of OC pills reduces the chance of developing ovarian cancer by 50%.

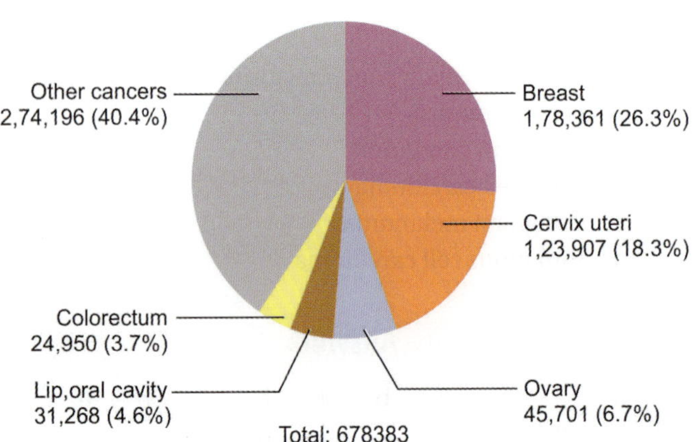

Fig. 1: Estimated number of new cases (age standardized incidence rates) in females in India in the year 2020.

History of tubal ligation and hysterectomy are protective against ovarian cancer.[8]

Pelvic inflammatory disease (PID) and endometriosis are found to be associated with ovarian cancer.[9] The intensive release of cytokines and inflammatory infiltrates are responsible for increased risk of cancer in these patients.

Lifestyle factors like diet, smoking, and physical exercise have not directly implicated in ovarian carcinogenesis.[10] But long-term interventions like low-fat high vegetarian diet and cessation of smoking have shown to reduce incidence of ovarian cancer and improve survival rate.[11,12]

PATHOLOGY

The World Health Organization histological classification for ovarian tumors separates ovarian neoplasms according to the most probable tissue of origin: surface epithelial (65%), germ cell (15%), sex cord-stromal (10%), metastases (5%), and miscellaneous.

Surface epithelial tumors are further classified by cell type (serous, mucinous, endometrioid, etc.) and atypia [benign, borderline (atypical proliferation, low malignant potential) or malignant]

Most malignant tumors are surface epithelial (90%).

The classification of ovarian tumors (2020) is summarized in **Box 1**.[13]

Serous Epithelial Tumors

Borderline (Low Malignant Potential) Tumors

About 10–20% of the common epithelial tumors are histologically and clinically intermediate between the innocuous benign tumors and invasive malignant carcinomas. By definition (WHO, 1973), a borderline tumor is one that has some, but not all, of the morphological features of malignancy, with obvious lack of stromal invasion. These tumors have a high cure rate when confined to the ovaries and an indolent behavior when disseminated. The diagnosis of borderline tumor is made by histologic examination of the primary neoplasm without consideration of whether it has spread beyond the ovary.

- *Serous borderline tumors:* They comprise 9–15% of all serous tumors of ovary. About 14–40% are bilateral, with up to 46% extraovarian involvement. The histological features include multilayering and budding of the epithelium,

BOX 1: Classification of ovarian tumors.

- Surface epithelial—stromal tumors
  - *Serous tumors:*
    - Benign (cystadenoma)
    - Borderline tumors (serous borderline tumor)
    - Malignant (serous adenocarcinoma)
  - *Mucinous tumors, endocervical-like and intestinal type:*
    - Benign (cystadenoma)
    - Borderline tumors (mucinous borderline tumor)
    - Malignant (mucinous adenocarcinoma)
  - *Endometrioid tumors:*
    - Benign (cystadenoma)
    - Borderline tumors (endometrioid borderline tumor)
    - Malignant (endometrioid adenocarcinoma)
  - *Clear cell tumors:*
    - Benign
    - Borderline tumors
    - Malignant (clear cell adenocarcinoma)
  - *Transitional cell tumors:*
    - Brenner tumor
    - Brenner tumor of borderline malignancy
    - Malignant Brenner tumor
    - Transitional cell carcinoma (non-Brenner type)
  - *Epithelial-stromal:*
    - Adenosarcoma
    - Carcinosarcoma (formerly mixed Müllerian tumors)
    - Seroumucinous tumors
    - Mesenchymal tumors
    - Mixed epithelial mesenchymal
    - others
- Sex cord—stromal tumors
- Pure stromal
- Pure sex cord stromal tumor
- Mixed sex cord stromal tumors
  - *Granulosa tumors:*
    - Fibromas
    - Fibrothecomas
    - Thecomas
  - *Sertoli cell tumors:*
    - Leydig cell tumors
    - Sex cord tumor with annular tubules
    - Gynandroblastoma
    - Steroid (lipid) cell tumors
- Germ cell tumors
- *Teratoma:*
  - Immature
  - Mature
    - Solid
    - Cystic (dermoid cyst)
- Monodermal (e.g., struma ovarii, carcinoid)
- Dysgerminoma
- Yolk sac tumor (endodermal sinus tumor)
- Mixed germ cell tumors
- Non-gestational choriocarcinoma
- Embryonal carcinoma
- *Miscellaneous tumors:*
  - Malignant, not otherwise specified
  - Metastatic cancer from nonovarian primary:
    - Colonic, appendicle
    - Gastric
    - Breast

apparent detachment of cell clusters in the lumen, cellular atypia, increased mitotic activity, and absence of stromal invasion. Invasive peritoneal implants have a worse prognosis than noninvasive ones. Actuarial 5-year survival rates for all stages range from 92 to 100% and 10 year rates from 75 to 95%.[14] Recurrence may develop after a long period of 20–50 years.

- *Mucinous borderline tumors:* They are less common than their serous counterparts. Due to marked morphological variation, it is common to find benign, borderline, and sometimes malignant changes in the same section. The presence of stromal invasion is more difficult to determine in mucinous than serous tumors because the glandular structures lying in the stroma may be the result of budding from a larger gland rather than true invasion. Only 10% of these tumors are bilateral, and 15% may have extraovarian spread at diagnosis.[15]

The borderline mucinous tumors have a better prognosis than serous borderline tumors. The 5- and 10-year actuarial survival rates for stage I tumors are 98% and 96%, respectively.[15]

Serous Epithelial Cystadenocarcinoma

- 35–55% of serous tumors are bilateral with size of around 10 cm.
- Malignant tumors are typically multilocular, cystic, and solid.
- The external surfaces often display papillae.
- On the cut section, solid areas are pink to gray. Hemorrhage and necrosis are often present.
- Cystic cavities are soft with friable papillae. The cysts contain serous, turbid, or bloody fluid.
- At least two sections per cm are needed to confidently exclude invasion.

Microscopically, characteristic stratification and budding is seen. Cells show coarse nuclei with pleomorphism, prominent nucleoli and atypia, and psammoma bodies are seen in the majority of cases. Low-grade serous ovarian cancer (LGSOC) have less than 12 mitotic figures per 10 HPF while high-grade serous ovarian cancer (HGSOC) which have more than 12 mitotic figures per 10 HPF.[16]

High grade serous carcinoma is epithelial carcinoma of serous cell lineage with papillary, glandular and solid growth patterns and high grade cytologic atypia. Often present as bilateral, solid and cystic ovarian masses. The most important prognostic factor is stage. In advanced stage disease, the amount of residual tumor present after staging and debulking is the most important factor.

Endometrioid carcinomas: It is the second most common histology in epithelial cancers. These can be low grade or high grade. These are usually diagnosed at early stages. They are associated with endometriosis/endometriotic cyst (15%), endometrioid adenofibroma, synchronous endometrial endometrioid adenocarcinoma, or endometrial hyperplasia (15–30%).[17] These have better prognosis due to earlier presentations. Stage is the most important prognostic factor. The survival rates are >95% for stage IA and IB and 51% for stage III and IV.[18] High-grade endometrioid adenocarcinomas behave like high-grade serous cancers and have poorer prognosis.

Mucinous cystadenocarcinoma: They constitute less than 3% 5–10% of all epithelial ovarian cancers. Benign and borderline tumors have good prognosis. About 77% of all ovarian mucinous carcinomas are metastases, 23% are ovarian primaries.[19] Ovarian primary invasive tumors are typically large (>10 cm), unilateral, multicystic, and contain mucin and most arise in a benign or borderline tumor. The metastatic mucinous tumors from GIT and are usually bilateral with exophytic growths on surface of ovary. Stromal invasion > 10 mm^2 distinguishes these tumors from borderline tumors. Distant metastases are rare. Survival is usually 95% for stage I disease while stages II or greater have 32% survival.

Clear cell carcinoma: These are malignant epithelial tumor composed of clear, eosinophilic, or hobnail cells with tubulocystic, papillary, and solid growth patterns with uniform nuclear atypia without brisk mitotic figures. Usually, positive for CK7, PAX8, napsin A, and HNF1β, and negative for ER, PR, and WT1, with aberrant p53 expression in up to 24% of cases. They may be associated with endometriosis. Stage is the most important prognostic factor. Beyond stage 1, prognosis is poor. Clear cell tumors have been found to be resistant to conventional chemotherapy using platinum and taxane.

Pseudomyxoma peritonei describes the collection of abundant mucinous material in pelvis and abdominal cavity surrounded by thin fibrous capsule. The appendix has to be evaluated for primary tumor in all these cases.

Pathogenesis of Epithelial Ovarian Cancer

The cell of origin of ovarian cancer and the mechanisms by which cancer develops have been long debated. The traditional view of ovarian carcinogenesis has been that the various types of tumors are all derived from the ovarian surface epithelium (mesothelium). The metaplasia of mesothelium leads to the development of the different cell types [serous, endometrioid, clear cell, mucinous and transitional cell (Brenner)], which morphologically resemble the epithelia of the Fallopian tube, endometrium, gastrointestinal tract or endocervix and urinary bladder, respectively.

Dualistic model of ovarian carcinogenesis postulates that serous tumors develop from the fimbriated portion of the fallopian tube, endometrioid and clear cell tumors from endometrial tissue passing through the fallopian tube resulting in endometriosis and mucinous and Brenner tumors from transitional-type epithelium located at the tubal-mesothelial junction where the fimbria makes contact with the peritoneum.[20]

Dualistic model highlights the heterogeneity of ovarian carcinoma.

Epithelial ovarian tumors are divided into two groups based on clinical, pathological, and molecular characteristics—type 1 and type 2.

Type I tumors (low-grade serous, low-grade endometrioid, clear cell, and mucinous) are slow growing and attain a large size while still confined to the ovary. They are easily detected by pelvic examination and/or transvaginal ultrasound. They constitute, however, only 25% of ovarian cancers and account for approximately 10% of ovarian cancer deaths. These tumors are characterized by specific mutations including KRAS, BRAF, ERBB2, CTNNB1, PTEN and PIK3CA but rarely TP53. They are relatively genetically stable.

The majority of type II tumors, rather than developing de novo from the ovary as previously proposed, appear to arise from a STIC (serous tubal intraepithelial carcinoma) in the fimbriated end of the Fallopian tube that spreads to the ovary.[21] Another possible mechanism for the development of "ovarian" carcinoma is dislodgement of normal tubal epithelium from the fimbria, which implants on the site of rupture where ovulation occurred resulting in the formation of an inclusion cyst that may then undergo malignant transformation.

The type II tumors include high-grade serous, carcinosarcomas and undifferentiated tumors, represent approximately 75% of all ovarian carcinomas and are responsible for 90% of ovarian cancer deaths. They have a very high frequency of TP53 mutations but rarely harbor the mutations detected in type I tumors. They are genetically highly unstable.

It is the type II tumors that should be targeted for screening as they have high mortality but unfortunately these tumors are rarely confined to the ovary, even at their inception.

Natural History of Disease and Patterns of Spread

Serous Ovarian Cancer

Clinically it is impossible to differentiate between the cancers arising from ovary, fallopian tube or peritoneum.

All of these three tumors grow quickly, disseminate by exfoliating cells in the peritoneal cavity. These exfoliated cells follow the current of peritoneal fluid and spread in pouch of Douglas, right paracolic gutter, undersurface of diaphragm and virtually can spread to all peritoneal and pleural surfaces. This causes development of ascites and pleural effusion. Locoregional spread occurs to the opposite ovary, recto sigmoid, and pelvic peritoneum. Most common distant metastasis occurs in infracolic omentum. In extensive disease, lesser omentum is also involved.

Lymph Node Metastasis

It is the second common mode of spread. Common lymphatic pathway is via infundibulo-pelvic ligaments through lymphatics draining in the para-aortic group up to the level of renal vessels, may spread upwards till mediastinal and supraclavicular groups. Second common lymphatic spread is through the parametrial channels to internal iliac, external iliac, common iliac, and obturator groups.

CLINICAL PRESENTATION

Variable clinical presentation is seen depending upon the size and extent of spread of the tumor. Most of the time ovarian cancer remains asymptomatic till it becomes huge in size. Once it is big enough to compress the surrounding structures, it presents with various symptoms.

- Pressure symptoms like chronic pelvic pain, backache
- Urinary symptoms like urgency, dysuria, and frequency
- Recto sigmoid pressure symptoms like constipation
- Sometimes complications in tumors like torsion, rupture, hemorrhage presents like acute abdomen
- Nonspecific symptoms like anorexia, fatigue, and early satiety are common in advanced malignant tumors
- Bloating, diffuse abdominal pain is observed due to peritoneal infiltration
- Large volume ascites presents as abdominal distention, dyspnea, and electrolyte imbalance
- DVT and hypercoagulopathy features could also be seen.

As symptoms often develop late, ovarian cancer is called a "silent killer". Initial symptoms are quite vague and often presented to general practitioners. Combination of four most common symptoms among these are: increased abdominal size/bloating, early satiety, pelvic/abdominal pain, urinary urge/incontinence. There is a symptom index called the "Goff index" based on frequency, intensity of these symptoms.[21] These patients are suggested to be screened with USG abdomen/ pelvis and serum cancer antigen 125 (CA 125). Though routine screening of asymptomatic women for ovarian cancer is not found to be effective in large trials.[22]

DIFFERENTIAL DIAGNOSIS

The nonspecific early symptoms mimic conditions like irritable bowel syndrome, dyspepsia and menopause.

Most important point to consider in adnexal mass is the patient's age.

- *Premenarchal girls:* germ cell tumors, mature teratomas, rhabdomyosarcomas.
- Adnexal mass in reproductive age group could be: ectopic pregnancy, functional ovarian cyst, benign ovarian tumors like serous and mucinous cystadenomas, germ cell tumors (both benign and malignant), peritoneal inclusion cysts, fibroids, and endometriosis, ovarian tumors like juvenile granulosa tumor, endodermal sinus tumor or mature teratomas.
- Acute complications like torsion can mimic other acute abdomen conditions like PID, appendicitis, and diverticulitis, etc.
- *Advanced reproductive age group (35–45 years):* Pedunculated fibroids, peritoneal cysts, stromal cell tumors like fibroma, adult granulosa cell tumors, cystadenomas, and borderline tumors.
- *Perimenopausal age group:* Functional cysts, fibroids, ovarian cancer, and endometrial cancer.
- *Postmenopausal age group:* Benign/borderline serous/ mucinous cystadenoma, fibroid, ovarian cancer, and colon cancer. Though malignant ovarian cancers are more prevalent in postmenopausal age group, most common cause of an adnexal mass in a postmenopausal patient is still a benign cyst.

DIAGNOSIS OF OVARIAN CANCER

Consider following important factors: age, history/ symptomatology, menopausal status, clinical examination, family history, imaging USG/CT scan, tumor markers CA-125, HE-4, CEA, and CA 19.9.

Clinical Examination

Apart from routine, general examination findings following points to be stressed in general examination: palpate supraclavicular lymph nodes, breast examination, and inguinal lymph nodes.

Per abdominal examination: Look for distension, scars, and distended veins on abdominal wall. Because of reduced central venous return due to large mass "caput medusa" may be seen. Size and mobility of mass should be assessed. Demonstrate ascites, costo-vertebral angle tenderness due to hydronephrosis.

On gynecological examination, a prominent cystocele may indicate ascites. The bimanual examination should assess adnexal mass with respect to size, location, bilaterality, borders, mobility, and surface. Invasive malignant ovarian tumors often have irregular borders, nodular surface and restricted mobility. Uterus may not be palpable separately performing rectovaginal examination throws a better light on findings.

The clinical features arousing suspicion of malignancy preoperatively are as follows.

- Postmenopausal age of presentation.
- Rapid growth of mass.
- Pyrexia.
- Postmenopausal bleeding.
- Cachexia.
- Pressure symptoms.
- Metastasis - palpable supraclavicular lymph nodes.
- Tumor characteristics
    - Bilateral
    - Solid
    - Fixed
    - Irregular, nodular
    - Large
    - Ascites.

Laboratory Tests

Blood tests are done to assess general health of patients and specific tests done for diagnostic purposes. Blood investigations may show hemoconcentration, thrombocytosis, and low albumin level. Hypoalbumenia occurs due to tumor cachexia and malnutrition. Liver function tests, kidney function tests to be done for functional assessment.

Serum CA 125 is the most studied tumor marker in cases of epithelial ovarian cancer with a cut off value of 35 U/mL. It is useful for differentiating between benign and malignant neoplasms. Also helps in judging response to chemotherapy, prognosis, and recurrence after therapy. Apart from CA ovary, CA 125 can be raised in other carcinomas as well (both gynec and non gynec). It is also elevated in physiological and benign conditions like menstruation, pregnancy, PID; endometriosis. CA 125 is elevated in nongynecological conditions like cirrhosis of liver, inflammatory bowel disease, SLE.

Human epididymis (HE) 4 is a secreted glycoprotein by human ovarian cancer cells. Combined results with CA 125 are better for prediction of ovarian cancer.

ROMA score (risk of ovarian malignancy algorithm) **(Table 1)**[23]: CA125, HE4, and menopausal status are used, to predict the risk of malignancy in ovarian tumors.

The serum level of HE4 protein can be combined with the serum level of CA 125 to produce a predictive ROMA.

In patients with early stages of ovarian cancer, use of ROMA correctly detected 85% of women with ovarian cancer, compared with 65% detected using the "Risk of Malignancy" Index **(Table 2)**.[24]

OVA 1 is a combination of five different serum proteins CA125, beta 2 micro globulin, prealbumin, apo lipoprotein A1 and transferrin. Presently, OVA1 is approved by US FDA for clinical use.

Imaging: Most widely used imaging for establishing a diagnosis of ovarian cancer is USG.

TABLE 1: Reference cut offs of tumor markers used in ovarian CA.

Test	*Normal range*
CA 125	< 35 u/ML
HE4 (Premenopausal)	<70 pmol/L
HE4 (Postmenopausal)	<140 pmol/L

TABLE 2: Comparison of multiple markers for the prediction of ovarian cancer.

Tumor marker	*Sensitivity*	*Specificity*
CA 125	50–74%	69–87%
HE4	74%	87%
Combined CA125 and HE4	90%	85%

USG: Features suggestive of malignancy on ultrasonography are:
- Bilaterality.
- Ascites.
- Omental, nodal or hepatic metastases.
- Adherent tumor.
- *Tumor characteristics:* Presence of septation, solid and cystic tissue, papillary excrescences, and large mass with scattered internal echoes.

Risk of Malignancy (RMI) score (RMI 3) considers various USG features (U), menopausal status (M) and CA 125 value **(Figs. 2A to C and Table 3)**[25]

RMI score = U × M × CA 125 value

- Score of > 200 cut off
- M - 1 pre-menopausal
  M - 3 post-menopausal
- U - 0 No features of malignancy
  1 - multilocular with thick septa, solid area, bilateral, ascites, metastases
  U =1 (score 0–1) U = 3 (score 2–5)

IOTA model: The model was developed by clinicians and statisticians from the International Ovarian Tumor Analysis (IOTA) group, and is based on clinical and ultrasound data from almost 6,000 women recruited at 24 centers in 10 countries.[26]
- *IOTA risk calculation:*[27] Simple rules risk
- *Low risk:* More B features and no M
- *Intermediate risk:* B feature except B1, no M features
- *Elevated risk:* Equal number of M and B features
- *Very high risk:* More M than B features

CT and MRI: May be complementary to USG to diagnose and assess the spread and extent of disease.

Staging: The most important factor in prognosis of ovarian cancer is FIGO stage and amount of disease remaining after debulking surgery. The current staging system used for malignant ovarian cancers is 2014 FIGO Staging **(Table 4)**.[28]

Both the old and new FIGO staging systems require that surgery be performed to confirm the histological diagnosis and to determine the true extent of the disease.

The following discussion regarding treatment is on epithelial ovarian carcinomas, which are the most common ovarian cancers.

Surgery: surgical staging is the key stone in management. It is recommended that all patients should undergo surgery by an experienced gynecologic oncologist.[29]

Signs suggestive of malignancy intraoperatively are as follows.
- Blood stained ascitic fluid.
- Solidity.
- Fixity.

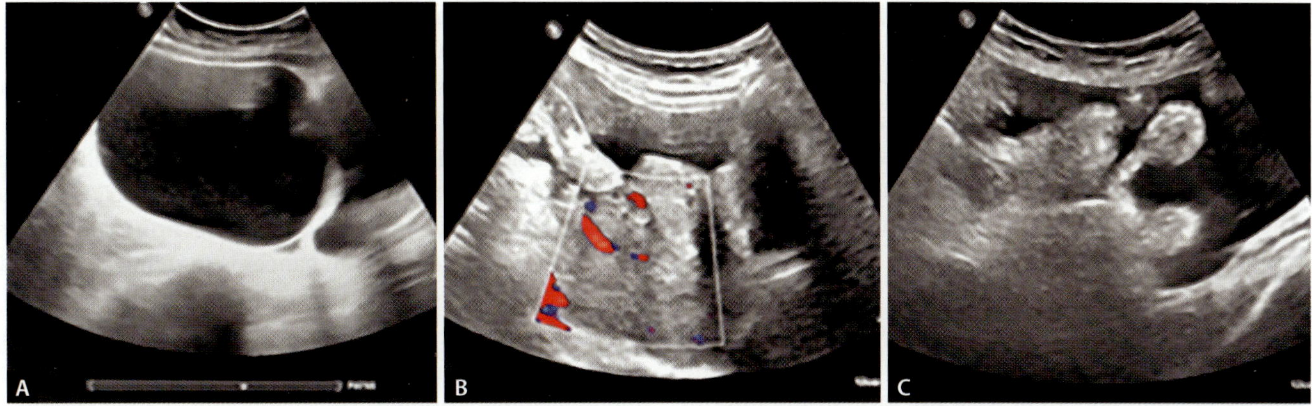

Figs. 2A to C: Ultrasonographic images: (A) Benign cyst; (B and C) Malignant cysts.
Courtesy: Dr. Mangal Mahajan, Department of Radiology, BVDUMC, Pune.

TABLE 3: Benign vs malignant features of an ovarian tumor.

Benign features	***Malignant features***
B1 Unilocular	M1 Irregular solid tumor
B2 Presence of solid component <7 mm	M2 Presence of ascites
B3 Presence of acoustic shadows	M3 At least four papillary structures
B4 Smooth multilocular tumor with largest diameter <100 mm	M4 Irregular multilocular solid tumor with largest diameter >100 mm
B5 No blood flow (color score 1)	M5 Very strong blood flow (color score 4)

- Bilaterality.
- Peritoneal deposits.
- Omental deposits.
- Tumor characteristics.
  - Tumor excrescences on the surface.
  - Large blood vessels over the tumor surface.
  - Hemorrhagic areas in the wall of the tumor.
  - Solid - cystic areas.
  - Cut surface shows soft pultaceous areas with interspersed hemorrhage and necrosis.

In Early-stage ovarian cancer, surgery is performed with following two aims:

1. To establish the correct FIGO stage in order to determine choice of therapy (chemotherapy vs. observation) and prognosis.
2. To perform effective surgical removal of tumor.

Principles of Surgery in Early Stage Disease[30-32]

- Liberal midline vertical incision.
- Collect peritoneal fluid for cytology.
- Systematic inspection, palpation, and scrapings/biopsies of suspicious areas or peritoneal surfaces clockwise from right paracolic gutters, liver, diaphragm, omentum. Pelvic exploration including palpation of opposite ovary, bladder,

TABLE 4: FIGO (2014) Staging of ovarian cancer.

Stage I: Tumor confined to ovaries or fallopian tube(s)
IA: Tumor limited to 1 ovary (capsule intact) or fallopian tube; no tumor on ovarian or fallopian tube surface; no malignant cells in the ascites or peritoneal washings IB: Tumor limited to both ovaries (capsules intact) or fallopian tubes; no tumor on ovarian or fallopian tube surface; no malignant cells in the ascites or peritoneal washings IC: Tumor limited to 1 or both ovaries or fallopian tubes, with any of the following: IC1: Surgical spill IC2: Capsule ruptured before surgery or tumor on ovarian or fallopian tube surface IC3: Malignant cells in the ascites or peritoneal washings
Stage II: Tumor involves 1 or both ovaries or fallopian tubes with pelvic extension (below pelvic brim) or peritoneal cancer
IIA: Extension and/or implants on uterus and/or fallopian tubes and/or ovaries IIB: Extension to other pelvic intraperitoneal tissues
Stage III: Tumor involves 1 or both ovaries or fallopian tubes, or peritoneal cancer, with cytologically or histologically confirmed spread to the peritoneum outside the pelvis and/or metastasis to the retroperitoneal lymph nodes
IIIA1: Positive retroperitoneal lymph nodes only (cytologically or histologically proven): IIIA1(i) Metastasis up to 10 mm in greatest dimension IIIA1(ii) Metastasis more than 10 mm in greatest dimension IIIA2: Microscopic extrapelvic (above the pelvic brim) peritoneal involvement with or without positive retroperitoneal lymph nodes IIIB: Macroscopic peritoneal metastasis beyond the pelvis up to 2 cm in greatest dimension, with or without metastasis to the retroperitoneal lymph nodes IIIC: Macroscopic peritoneal metastasis beyond the pelvis more than 2 cm in greatest dimension, with or without metastasis to the retroperitoneal lymph nodes (includes extension of tumor to capsule of liver and spleen without parenchymal involvement of either organ)
Stage IV: Distant metastasis excluding peritoneal metastases
Stage IVA: Pleural effusion with positive cytology
Stage IVB: Parenchymal metastases and metastases to extra-abdominal organs (including inguinal lymph nodes and lymph nodes outside of the abdominal cavity)

and cul-de-sac peritoneum, pelvic and para-aortic lymph nodes, etc.

- BSO and hysterectomy should be performed with every effort to keep an encapsulated mass intact during removal. For selected patients desiring to preserve fertility, USO or BSO with uterine preservation may be considered. Uterine preservation allows for potential future assisted reproductive approaches.
- Omentectomy should be performed.
- Para-aortic lymph node dissection should be performed by stripping the nodal tissue from the vena cava and the aorta bilaterally to at least the level of the inferior mesenteric artery and preferably to the level of the renal vessels. The preferred method of dissecting pelvic lymph nodes is bilateral removal of lymph nodes overlying and anterolateral to the common iliac vessel, overlying and medial to the external iliac vessel, overlying and medial to the hypogastric vessels, and from the obturator fossa at a minimum anterior to the obturator nerve.

Both the pelvic and infrarenal para-aortic lymph nodes provide an important prognostic and staging information for patients and highlight the need for adjuvant chemotherapy.

About 33% of previously thought stage I or II tumors will be found to have advanced-stage disease on staging laparotomy.

ADVANCED EPITHELIAL OVARIAN CANCER

In advanced disease, cytoreductive surgery reduces tumor bulk to a point where subsequent chemotherapy will exert a maximal effect. Every effort should be made during a primary cytoreduction procedure to achieve maximum cytoreduction of all abdominal, pelvic, and retroperitoneal disease. Residual disease <1 cm defines optimal cytoreduction; however, maximal effort should be made to remove all gross disease since this offers superior survival outcomes.

Aspiration of ascites (if present) should be performed for peritoneal cytologic examinations.

It is helpful to stratify patients with advanced cancer as having either low- and high-volume disease preoperatively/intraoperatively because different approach to management (surgical strategies) are associated with each classification.

Patients with advanced ovarian cancer but low-volume disease should have debulking surgery, including a total abdominal hysterectomy, bilateral salpingo-oophrectomy, and infragastric omentectomy between the hepatic flexure and the splenic hilum. If the patient can be rendered macroscopically disease free, a pelvic and high para-aortic lymph node dissection is reasonable (debulking of enlarged nodes to achieve optimal cytoreduction) .

Patients with advanced ovarian cancer and high-volume disease usually have extensive tumor burden in the pelvis with encasement of the reproductive organs and sigmoid colon. This requires a modified posterior exenteration, an en bloc resection of the tumor-studded bladder, peritoneum, uterus, sigmoid colon, and proximal rectum, as well as ovarian/fallopian tube masses, cul-de-sac tumors, and possibly the appendix.

A low colorectal anastomosis should follow; a colostomy is rarely required in patients with serous cancers because serous cancers grow above the peritoneal reflection. The current practice in advanced ovarian cancer is to remove enlarged/suspicious lymph nodes as part of tumor debulking.

Procedures that may be considered for optimal surgical cytoreduction (in all stages) include bowel resection and/or appendectomy, stripping of the diaphragm or other peritoneal surfaces, splenectomy with or without distal pancreatectomy, partial cystectomy, and/or ureteroneocystostomy, partial hepatectomy, partial gastrectomy, cholecystectomy.

NEOADJUVANT CHEMOTHERAPY

Neoadjuvant platinum-containing chemotherapy followed by interval debulking surgery is a reasonable choice in cases of advanced ovarian cancer cases, where optimal cytoreduction is not feasible or in patients with poor performance status. This reduces the complicated extensive surgeries resulting into less blood loss, less complications and reduced perioperative morbidity. Usually, 3–4 cycles of chemotherapy are given before surgery and remaining three cycles (total 6–8 cycles) are given after the surgery. Before initiation of neoadjuvant chemotherapy, histologic confirmation of ovarian cancer should be obtained (by FNA, biopsy, or paracentesis) in this group of patients.

Interval Debulking Surgery (IDS) after Neoadjuvant Chemotherapy

The principles of IDS are similar to primary cytoreductive surgery.

As with a primary debulking procedure, every effort should be made to achieve maximum cytoreduction during an interval debulking procedure. Maximal effort should be made to remove all gross disease in the abdomen, pelvis, and retro-peritoneum. IDS should be performed after 3–4 cycles of neoadjuvant chemotherapy for women with a response to chemotherapy or stable disease.

Hyperthermic intraperitoneal chemotherapy (HIPEC) with cisplatin (100 mg/m^2) can be considered at the time of IDS for stage III disease and optimally cytoreduced patients.[33] All peritoneal surfaces should be visualized, and any peritoneal surface or adhesion suspicious for harboring metastasis should be selectively excised or biopsied.

An omentectomy should be performed.

Suspicious and/or enlarged nodes should be resected, if possible. Removal of lymph nodes noted to have potential metastasis at the time of initial diagnosis should be considered, even if not currently suspicious or enlarged.

Palliative Surgery

A malignant bowel obstruction is the most common reason for a hospital admission for patients with ovarian cancer during the last year of her life. Management options are percutaneous endoscopic gastrostomy (PEG) tube, parenteral nutrition, palliative chemotherapy, stents for gastric outlet obstruction or single-site colonic obstruction, and as last resort, palliative surgery. Initial treatment for a malignant bowel obstruction should be conservative and may include bowel rest and hydration to correct metabolic abnormalities. Because the purpose of palliative surgery is to improve the quality of life, the procedure must be short and limited, with the lowest possible complication rate.

ADJUVANT CHEMOTHERAPY

Patients comprehensively staged as stage IA or IB low-grade epithelial ovarian cancer should receive no postoperative chemotherapy.

Patients with early-stage disease and unfavorable prognostic markers (stage IA or IB grade 3, clear cell, stage IC, and completely resected stage II) should receive 3–6 cycles of intravenous chemotherapy.

The recommended intravenous chemotherapy regimens include:

- Paclitaxel, 175 mg/m^2 over 3-hour intravenous infusion, followed by carboplatin, dosed at an area under the curve (AUC) of 5–6 intravenous over 1 hour on day 1, given every 3 weeks for 6 cycles (category 1)
- Dose-dense paclitaxel, 80 mg/m^2 intravenous over 1 hour on days 1, 8, and 15 plus carboplatin AUC 5–6 intravenous over 1 hour on day 1, every 3 weeks for 6 cycles (category 1)
- Paclitaxel 60 mg/m^2 over 1 hour followed by carboplatin AUC 2 intravenous over 30 minutes, weekly for 18 weeks (category 1)
- Docetaxel, 60–75 mg/m^2 over 1-hour intravenous infusion followed by carboplatin, dosed at AUC of 5–6 intravenous over 1 hour on day 1, every 3 weeks for 6 cycles (category 1)
- Carboplatin AUC 5 plus pegylated liposomal doxorubicin 30 mg/m^2 every 4 weeks for 6 cycles (category 2A).

Fertility-Sparing Surgery

Fertility-sparing surgery with USO (preserving the uterus and contralateral ovary) or BSO (preserving the uterus) can be considered for patients with apparent early-stage disease and/or low-risk tumors (early-stage invasive epithelial tumors, low malignant potential tumors, malignant germ cell tumors, mucinous, or malignant sex cord-stromal tumors) who wish to preserve fertility. High-grade cancers like high-grade serous, high-grade endometrioid, clear cell cancers are not suitable for fertility preservation even in early stage.

Evaluation by reproductive endocrinologist should be done if clinically indicated. Comprehensive surgical staging should still be performed to rule out occult higher stage disease but may be omitted in pediatric/adolescent patients with clinically apparent early-stage malignant germ cell tumors based on the pediatric surgical literature.[34]

POST-THERAPY FOLLOW-UP

Patients should be monitored by physical examination, USG/CT/MRI/PET CT (as clinically indicated) and tumor markers (CA125) to diagnose recurrence. Follow-up should be done 3 monthly for initial 2 years, 6 monthly for next 3 years and annually thereafter lifelong.

Recurrence

After pathologic complete response to initial chemotherapy, about 40–60% patients of ovarian cancer relapse, thereby requiring second line treatment. The suboptimal sensitivities of tumor markers and lack of precision in predicting the presence or absence of disease by noninvasive imaging methods for determining the disease status after completion of therapy, reflect their limitations in detecting recurrence. The Gynecologic Oncology Group (GOG) have identified the following characteristics associated with increased likelihood of recurrence.[35]

- Higher stage.
- Histologic type (mucinous or clear cell).
- Nonplatinum based therapy.
- Poor performance status.
- Older age.
- Clinically measurable disease.
- Larger residual tumor volume
- Ascites.

Patients who relapse 6 months or more after initial chemotherapy are termed to have *platinum-sensitive disease*. Those who relapse within 6 months after initial treatment are termed to have *platinum-resistant disease*. When the disease progresses, while on platinum-based chemotherapy, it is termed platinum refractory disease.

Platinum-based combination chemotherapy is preferred in patients with platinum-sensitive disease, especially for first recurrence.

For platinum-resistant disease, non-platinum-based agents or regimens are preferred like gemcitabine, liposomal doxorubicin, topotecan, docetaxel, cyclophosphamide, etoposide. These can be given in combination with bevacizumab.

Targeted single agent therapy using bevacizumab, niraparib, olaparib, and rucaparib can be used for maintenance therapy.

Immunotherapy using pembrolizumab can be used in patients with MSI-H or dMMR solid tumors or TMB-H tumor >10 mutations and no satisfactory alternative treatment options.

Flowchart 1: The treatment of ovarian cancer integrating the role of targeted therapy.

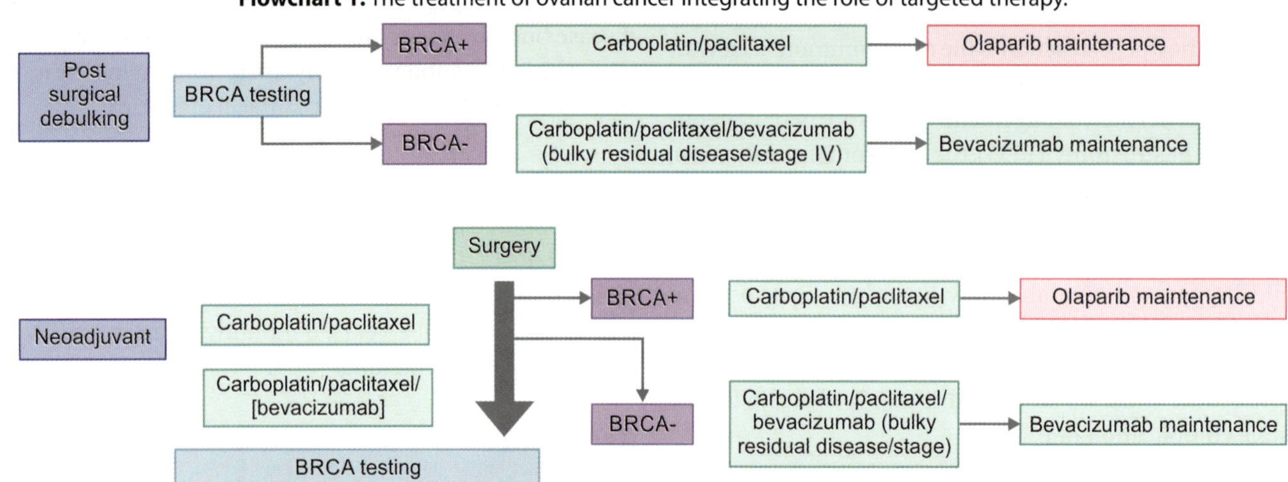

Current guidelines recommend germline testing for BRCA mutation all high grade non-mucinous ovarian cancers. This is especially important for young patients and those with significant family history. This has therapeutic implications as well, as PARP inhibitors have shown excellent disease control in women with BRCA mutation. The **Flowchart 1** outlines the treatment of ovarian cancer integrating the role of targeted therapy based on BRCA mutation status (germline or somatic).

GERM CELL TUMORS

Ovarian malignant germ cell tumors (OMGCTs) are heterogeneous tumors that are derived from the primitive germ cells of the embryonic gonad. OMGCTs are rare, accounting for about 2.6% of all ovarian malignancies, and typically manifest in adolescence, usually with abdominal pain, a palpable mass, and elevated serum tumor marker levels, which may serve as an adjunct in the initial diagnosis, monitoring during therapy, and post-treatment surveillance.[36]

Dysgerminoma, the most common malignant germ cell tumor, usually manifests as a solid mass. Immature teratomas manifest as a solid mass with scattered foci of fat and calcifications. Yolk sac tumors usually manifest as a mixed solid and cystic mass. Capsular rupture or the bright dot sign, a result of increased vascularity and the formation of small vascular aneurysms, may be present. Embryonal carcinomas and polyembryomas rarely manifest in a pure form and are more commonly part of a mixed germ cell tumor.

Some OMGCTs have characteristic features that allow a diagnosis to be confidently made, whereas others have nonspecific features, which make them difficult to diagnose. However, imaging features, the patient's age at presentation, and tumor markers (AFP, β-hCG, LDH) may help establish a reasonable differential diagnosis. Malignant ovarian germ cell tumors spread in the same manner as epithelial ovarian neoplasms but are more likely to involve regional lymph nodes.

Preoperative imaging may depict local extension, peritoneal disease, and distant metastases. Suspicious areas may be sampled during surgery. Because OMGCTs are almost always unilateral and are chemosensitive, fertility-sparing surgery is the standard of care. Surgery, when appropriate, should be unilateral oophorectomy, peritoneal washing, omental biopsy and selective removal of enlarged lymph nodes. Ultraradical surgeries like those advised in epithelial ovarian cancers are not advised in OMGCTs in upfront setting as these tumors are very chemosensitive. Biopsy of a normal contralateral ovary is not indicated. Surgery should be by an open procedure to enable removal of the affected ovary with its tumor intact rather than broken or ruptured.[37]

The combined BEP regimen is the international standard of care, usually administered for three cycles in completely resected disease and four cycles for macroscopic residual disease.[38,39]

Though OMGCT are rare, but early diagnosis and multiagent chemotherapy are associated with high cure rates of 85.6% (range 81.2–90.0%).[40]

5-YEAR SURVIVAL RATES

The 5-year survival rates for all histologies in stage I, II, III, and IV are 90%, 70%, 39%, and 17%, respectively.[41]

REFERENCES

1. Sung H, Ferlay J, Siegel RL, Laversanne M, Soerjomataram I, Jemal A, et al. Global cancer statistics 2020: GLOBOCAN estimates of incidence and mortality worldwide for 36 cancers in 185 countries. CA Cancer J Clin. 2021;71:209-49.
2. Carcangiu ML, Kurman RJ, Carcangiu ML, Herrington CS. WHO Classification of Tumours of Female Reproductive Organs. Lyon: IARC; 2014.
3. Chan JK, Cheung MK, Husain A, Teng NN, West D, Whittemore AS, et al. Patterns and progress in ovarian cancer over 14 years. Obstet Gynecol. 2006;108(3):521-8.
4. Rebbeck TR, Mitra N, Wan F, Sinilnikova OM, Healey S, McGuffog L, et al. Association of type and location of BRCA1

and BRCA2 mutations with risk of breast and ovarian cancer. JAMA. 2015;313(13):1347-61.
5. Lancaster JM, Powell CB, Kauff ND, Cass I, Chen LM, Lu KH, et al. Society of Gynecologic Oncologists Education Committee statement on risk assessment for inherited gynecologic cancer predispositions. Gynecol Oncol. 2007;107(2):159-62.
6. Liu G, Yang D, Sun Y, Shmulevich I, Xue F, Sood AK, et al. Differing clinical impact of BRCA1 and BRCA2 mutations in serous ovarian cancer. Pharmacogenomics. 2012;13(13): 1523-35.
7. Torre LA, Trabert B, DeSantis CE, Miller KD, Samimi G, Runowicz CD, et al. Ovarian cancer statistics, 2018. CA Cancer J Clin. 2018;68(4):284-96.
8. Hankinson SE, Hunter DJ, Colditz GA, Willett WC, Stampfer MJ, Rosner B, et al. Tubal ligation, hysterectomy, and risk of ovarian cancer: a prospective study. JAMA. 1993;270(23):2813-8.
9. Lin HW, Tu YY, Lin SY, Su WJ, Lin WL, Lin WZ, et al. Risk of ovarian cancer in women with pelvic inflammatory disease: a population-based study. Lancet Oncol. 2011;12(9):900-4.
10. Barakat RR, Markman M, Randall M. Principles and Practice of Gynecologic oncology. Philadelphia: Lippincott Williams & Wilkins; 2009.
11. Mørch LS, Løkkegaard E, Andreasen AH, Krüger-Kjær S, Lidegaard Ø. Hormone therapy and ovarian cancer. JAMA. 2009;302(3):298-305.
12. Olsen CM, Nagle CM, Whiteman DC, Ness R, Pearce CL, Pike MC, et al.et al. Obesity and risk of ovarian cancer subtypes: evidence from the Ovarian Cancer Association Consortium. Endocrine Relat Cancer. 2013;20(2):251-62.
13. De Leo A; Santini D, Ceccarelli C, Santandrea G, Palicelli A, Acquaviva G, et al. What is new on ovarian carcinoma: integrated morphologic and molecular analysis following the new 2020 World Health Organization Classification of female genital tumors. Diagnostics. 2021;11:697.
14. Katzenstein AA, Mazur MT, Morgan TE, Kao MS. Proliferative serous tumors of the ovary: histologic features and prognosis. Am J Surg Pathol 1978; 2:339.
15. Hart WR, Norris HJ. Borderline and malignant mucinous tumors of the ovary: histologic criteria and clinical behaviour. Cancer. 1973; 31:1031.
16. Vang R, Shih IM, Kurman RJ. Fallopian tube precursors of ovarian low-and high-grade serous neoplasms. Histopathology. 2013;62(1):44-58.
17. Machado-Linde F, Sánchez-Ferrer ML, Cascales P, Torroba A, Orozco R, Silva-Sánchez Y, et al. Prevalence of endometriosis in epithelial ovarian cancer. Analysis of the associated clinical features and study on molecular mechanisms involved in the possible causality. Eur J Gynaecol Oncol. 2015;36:21.
18. Peres LC, Cushing-Haugen KL, Köbel M, Harris HR, Berchuck A, Rossing MA, et al. Invasive epithelial ovarian cancer survival by histotype and disease stage. JNCI. 2019;111(1):60-8.
19. Seidman JD, Kurman RJ, Ronnett BM. Primary and metastatic mucinous adenocarcinomas in the ovaries. Am J Surg Pathol. 2003;27(7):985-93.
20. Kurman RJ, Shih IeM. The dualistic model of ovarian carcinogenesis: revisited, revised, and expanded. Am J Pathol. 2016;186(4):733-47.
21. National Academies of Sciences, Engineering, and Medicine. Ovarian cancers: evolving paradigms in research and care. Washington (DC): National Academies Press; 2016.
22. Menon U, Gentry-Maharaj A, Hallett R, Ryan A, Burnell M, Sharma A,et al. Sensitivity and specificity of multimodal and ultrasound screening for ovarian cancer, and stage distribution of detected cancers: results of the prevalence screen of the UK Collaborative Trial of Ovarian Cancer Screening (UKCTOCS). Lancet Oncol. 2009;10(4):327-40.
23. Romagnolo C, Leon AE, Fabricio AS, Taborelli M, Polesel J, Del Pup L, et al. HE4, CA125 and risk of ovarian malignancy algorithm (ROMA) as diagnostic tools for ovarian cancer in patients with a pelvic mass: an Italian multicenter study. Gynecol Oncol. 2016;141(2):303-11.
24. Moore RG, Jabre-Raughley M, Brown AK, Robison KM, Miller MC, Allard WJ, et al. Comparison of a novel multiple marker assay vs the Risk of Malignancy Index for the prediction of epithelial ovarian cancer in patients with a pelvic mass. Am J Obstet Gynecol. 2010;203(3):228.e1-6.
25. Javdekar R, Maitra N. Risk of Malignancy Index (RMI) in evaluation of adnexal mass. J Obstet Gynaecol India. 2015;65(2):117-21.
26. Timmerman D, Calster DV, Testa A, Savelli L, Fischerova D, Froyman W, et al. Predicting the risk of malignancy in adnexal mases based on Simple ultrasound rules from International Ovarian Tumor Analysis group. Am J Obstet Gynecol. 2016; 214(4):424-37.
27. Kaijser J, Sayasneh A, Van Hoorde K, Ghaem-Maghami S, Bourne T, Timmerman D, et al. Presurgical diagnosis of adnexal tumours using mathematical models and scoring systems: a systematic review and meta-analysis. Human Reprod Update. 2014;20(3):449-62.
28. Prat J; FIGO Committee on Gynecologic Oncology. Staging classification for cancer of the ovary, fallopian tube, and peritoneum. Int J Gynaecol Obstet. 2014;124(1):1-5.
29. Eisenkop SM, Spirtos NM, Montag TW, Nalick RH, Wang HJ. The impact of subspecialty training on the management of advanced ovarian cancer. Gynecol Oncol. 1992;47(2):203-9.
30. Fleming GF, Seidman J, Yemelyanova A, Lengyl E. Epithelial ovarian cancer. In: Chi DS, Berchuck A, Dizon D, Yashar CM (Eds). Principles and Practice of Gynecologic Oncology, 7th edition. Philadelphia: Lippincott Williams & Wilkins; 2017. pp. 611-705.
31. Whitney CW, Spirtos N. Gynecologic Oncology Group Surgical Procedures Manual. Philadelphia: Gynecologic Oncology Group; 2010.
32. Chi DS, Eisenhauer EL, Zivanovic O, Sonoda Y, Abu-Rustum NR, Levine DA, et al. Improved progression-free and overall survival in advanced ovarian cancer as a result of a change in surgical paradigm. Gynecol Oncol. 2009;114:26-31.
33. van Driel WJ, Koole SN, Sikorska K, van Leeuwen JHS, Schreuder HWR, Hermans RHM, et al. Hyperthermic intraperitoneal chemotherapy in ovarian cancer. N Engl J Med. 2018;378:230-40.
34. Billmire D, Vinocur C, Rescorla F, Cushing B, London W, Schlatter M, et al. Outcome and staging evaluation in malignant germ cell tumors of the ovary in children and adolescents: an intergroup study. J Pediatr Surg. 2004;39:424-9.
35. Ozols RF. Gynecologic Oncology Group (GOG-USA) trials in ovarian cancer.Adv Exp Med Biol. 2008;622:131-43
36. Shaaban AM, Rezvani M, Elsayes KM, Baskin Jr H, Mourad A, Foster BR, et al. Ovarian malignant germ cell tumors: cellular classification and clinical and imaging features. Radiographics. 2014;34(3):777-801.

37. Mahdi H, Swensen RE, Hanna R, Kumar S, Ali-Fehmi R, Semaan A, et al. Prognostic impact of lymphadenectomy in clinically early stage malignant germ cell tumour of the ovary.Br J Cancer. 2011;105:493-7.
38. Satoh T, Aoki Y, Kasamatsu T, Ochiai K, Takano M, Watanabe Y, et al. Administration of standard-dose BEP regimen (bleomycin+etoposide+cisplatin) is essential for treatment of ovarian yolk sac tumour. Eur J Cancer. 2015;51:340-51.
39. Dimopoulos MA, Papadimitriou C, Hamilos G, Efstathiou E, Vlahos G, Rodolakis A, et al.Treatment of ovarian germ cell tumors with a 3-day bleomycin, etoposide and cisplatin regimen: a prospective multicenter study. Gynecol Oncol. 2004;95:695-700.
40. Oberaigner W, Minicozzi P, Bielska-Lasota M, Allemani C, de Angelis R, Mangone L, et al.; Eurocare Working Group. Survival for ovarian cancer in Europe:The across-country variation did not shrink in the past decade. Acta Oncol. 2012;51:441-53.
41. Elattar A, Bryant A, Winter-Roach BA, Hatem M, Naik R. Optimal primary surgical treatment for advanced epithelial ovarian cancer. Cochrane database of systematic reviews. 2011; 2011(8): CD007565.

LONG QUESTIONS

1. A 58-years-old P2L2, postmenopausal lady, came for routine gynecological checkup. Her transabdominal USG finding is showing of 9 cm complex mass, possibly arising from right ovary. Discuss the differential diagnosis, investigations and management plan for this patient.
2. Describe the 2014 FIGO staging of carcinoma Ovary. Discuss management of stage 1C serous ovarian cystadeno-carcinoma in a 64 years old postmenopausal lady.
3. Discuss principles of surgery for malignant ovarian tumor.
4. A 65-years-old postmenopausal lady comes abdominal distension. On USG a large ovarian mass of 12 x 11 cm with gross ascites is noted. Discuss treatment of advanced stage ovarian cancer
5. Discuss various theories for pathogenesis of ovarian cancer.

SHORT QUESTIONS

Write short notes on:

1. CA 125
2. Tumor markers in epithelial ovarian cancers
3. Hereditary ovarian cancers
4. USG risk scoring in adnexal masses
5. Fertility sparing surgery in ovarian tumors
6. Borderline ovarian tumors

MULTIPLE CHOICE QUESTIONS

1. Which of the following decrease a woman's risk of developing epithelial ovarian cancer?
   a. Smoking
   b. Endometriosis
   c. Use of menopausal hormone therapy
   d. Tubal ligation
2. Which one of the following symptoms is an uncommon presentation of ovarian cancer?
   a. Abdominal pain
   b. chest pain
   c. Weight loss
   d. abdominal distension
3. Which of the following is true of staging of ovarian cancer?
   a. Stage 1 tumors are common
   b. Stage 2 describes tumor spread beyond true pelvis
   c. Stage 2 describes tumor spread in retroperitoneal lymph nodes.
   d. Stage 3 describes tumor spread beyond true pelvis
4. In women who develop relapsed EOC more than 6 months since their last platinum-based chemotherapy:
   a. Re-treatment with platinum and taxane is the treatment of choice for most women.
   b. Treatment should commence when relapsed disease is confirmed on the basis of a rising CA125 tumor marker.
   c. Platinum hypersensitivity reactions are common.
   d. Carboplatin hypersensitivity precludes the use of cisplatin.
5. Which of the following statements relating to surgical staging of early ovarian cancer is/are true?
   a. The main purpose of staging is to detect subclinical residual tumor spread.
   b. Without complete surgical staging early ovarian carcinoma cannot be established.
   c. The upstaging potential of a proper surgical staging procedure is around 16%.
   d. The staging procedure in itself does not change the survival of patients.
   e. Apparent early stage disease can harbor subclinical or microscopic tumor seeding in the upper abdomen or retroperitoneal area.
6. Risk factors for ovarian cancer include which of the following?
   a. Young age
   b. Nulliparity
   c. Multiple pregnancies
   d. Prolonged use of oral contraceptive pills
7. Which of the following statements is true of first line chemotherapy for epithelial ovarian cancer?
   a. Following platinum/taxane chemotherapy 5 year survival is >40%
   b. Response rates to platinum/taxane chemotherapy are approximately 50%
   c. Median survival following platinum/taxane chemotherapy is 2–3 years
   d. The most commonly used chemotherapy is a combination of docetaxel and oxaliplatin
8. Which among the following is not a feature of borderline ovarian tumor?
   a. Mitotic figures are 3/10 high-power field
   b. Stromal invasion

c. 90% survival rate
d. occurs in young age

9. Bilateral ovarian tumor with involvement of pelvic lymph node and liver capsule is stage ______.
   a. Stage 2A b. Stage 2B
   c. Stage 3 d. Stage 4
10. Pseudomyxoma peritonei is associated with:
   a. Serous cystadenoma b. Mucinous cystadenoma
   c. Brenner tumor d. Dermoid
11. Signet ring cells are seen in:
   a. Mucinous cystadenoma
   b. Krukenberg's tumor
   c. Endodermal sinus tumor
   d. Dysgerminoma
12. Which of the following conditions have raised CA 125 levels?
   a. Epithelial ovarian tumor
   b. Endometriosis
   c. Acute peritonitis
   d. All of the above

Answers

1.	d	2.	b	3.	d	4.	a	5.	e	6.	b
7.	c	8.	b	9.	c	10.	b	11.	b	12.	d

14.9 NEOPLASTIC DISEASES OF FALLOPIAN TUBE

Uma Singh, Manjulata Verma

INTRODUCTION

Neoplastic growths arising exclusively from fallopian tube are thought to be uncommon. Clinical importance of this entity is increasing as emerging evidence suggests that the origin of many pelvic serous tumors may be in fallopian tubes. A primary fallopian tube neoplasm is an entity in which the tumor exclusively involves the fallopian tube or predominantly involves the fallopian tube with minimal involvement of the ovary or the uterus or in presence of significant tumors in other organs, differs in histology from those. WHO has classified fallopian tube tumors on the basis of their origin and behavior as given in **Box 1**.

BOX 1: WHO classification of fallopian tube tumors.

Epithelial tumors
- 9014/0 Serous adenofibroma NOS
- 8442/1 Serous borderline tumour NOS
- 8461/3 High-grade serous carcinoma
- 8380/3 Endometrioid adenocarcinoma NOS
- 8980/3 Carcinosarcoma NOS

Mixed epithelial and mesenchymal tumors
- 8933/3 Adenosarcoma

Germ cell tumors
- 9080/0 Mature teratoma NOS
- 9080/3 Immature teratoma NOS

Tumor-like lesions
- Paratubal cysts
- Tubal hyperplasia
- Tubo-ovarian abscess
- Salpingitis isthmica nodosa
- Metaplastic papillary lesion
- Placental site nodule
- Mucinous metaplasia
- Endosalpingiosis

Source: WHO. Female Genital Tumors. In: WHO Classification of Tumors, 5th edition. Geneva: WHO; 2020.

BENIGN TUMORS OF FALLOPIAN TUBE

Epithelial benign Tumors

These are solid tumors and clearly limited to fallopian tube. They arise from intramural or serosal surface of the fallopian tube. Papillomas are defined as lesions which may obstruct fallopian tube and have fibrovascular stacks with epithelial linings. Adenofibroma and cystadenofibroma are incidentally found during other surgeries and vary in size between 0.5 and 3 cm. They can be located intramurally, on serosal surface or at fimbrial end of fallopian tube and have both stromal and papillary structures. Bundle like leiomyoma cells and endometrial remnants are seen in adenomyomas. Endometrial polyps are found at interstitial end and may result in infertility.

Metaplastic papillary tumor of fallopian tube is rare, usually detected incidentally during pregnancy or in the postpartum period. They originate from the mucosa, project into the tubal lumen and have papillary projections with fine connective tissue cores lined by a single or double layer of large columnar cells. In association with ovarian or cervical tumors, tubal endocervical type of mucinous metaplasia can be seen especially in women with Peutz-Jeghers syndrome. Epithelial papillomas may arise in the tubal mucosa but are very rare.

Mesothelial Tumor: Adenomatoid Tumor

Adenomatoid tumor is the most common benign tumor of fallopian tube. It originates from the serosal and subserosal surface of fallopian tube and round ligament and can later involve full thickness of the tubal wall. It is usually limited to a particular area and does not infiltrate into adjacent structures. These may be found incidentally as yellow to white nodules of up to 2 cm in diameter. These are similar to adenomatoid tumor of other sites histologically, including uterus.

Soft Tissue Tumor: Leiomyoma

It originates from muscular layer of fallopian tube or from blood vessel walls and is benign smooth muscle tumor. Tubal musculature does not show marked morphological or functional changes such as uterine myometrium under hormonal influence during the menstrual cycle, hence tubal leiomyoma is less common than uterine leiomyoma. Histologically it is similar to uterine leiomyoma. Smooth muscle cells are elongated and are arranged in interweaving, intersecting bundles and fascicles which stain positive for α smooth muscle actin on immunohistochemistry. They are usually unilateral and more common on left side.

Tumor-like Lesions

Serosal Mesothelial Inclusion Cyst

These are found incidentally and have no clinical significance. Usually these cysts are small, clear or light tan cysts on the serosal or subserosal aspects of the tubes. When transitional type metaplasia occurs in the mesothelial epithelium of the inclusions, the cell rests are seen as Walthard's cell rest.

Hyperplasia of Tubal Epithelium

Acute and chronic salpingitis, unopposed estrogen exposure, tamoxifen and carcinoma of reproductive tract leads to hyperplasia of tubal epithelium.[1]

On rare occasions, it occurs independently. Although hyperplasia of tubal epithelium is a benign condition. Sometimes this may have associated tubular epithelial atypia. When this atypia is associated with BRCA positivity, it may be precursor of adnexal serous carcinomas.

It has been seen from recent studies that women with BRCA mutation having tubular epithelial atypia suggest that these atypical lesions are precursor to all adnexal serous carcinomas, especially if atypical cells are positive for both p 53 and MIB-1. Presence of these lesions is associated with increased risk of development of serous carcinoma of ovaries, uterus, peritoneal surface and opposite fallopian tube.

Isolated Necrotizing Arteritis

This self-limiting arteritis is seen in tubes and is similar to poly-arteritis nodosa (PAN). Although it is self-limiting and localized, a search for systemic disease should be done. Giant cell arteritis may involve the uterus, cervix, fallopian tubes and ovaries. It may also be associated with adenomyoma, cystadenofibroma, adenofibroma, tubal hemangioma, lipoma, angiomyolipoma and angiomyofibroblastoma.

Salpingitis isthmica nodosa: It is a benign condition. It is also known as diverticulosis of tubes. It is usually seen in young women with mean age of 26 years. It is associated with infertility in 50% of cases. The diagnostic signs are presence of isthmic diverticula and outpouching of tubal epithelium. Nodularity is present in this condition which is because of diverticulae that communicate with central tubal lumen invading the surrounding muscularis layer, which provoke secondary smooth muscle hypertrophy.

Endosalpingiosis: Ectopic presence of cystic glands of tubular epithelium of columnar type cells is known as endosalpingiosis. Chronic tubal inflammation and genetic composition are proposed as etiological factors for the development of endosalpingiosis. Endosalpingiosis is usually present in the visceral pelvic peritoneum covering the uterus, fallopian tubes, ovaries and cul-de-sac. Sometimes it may be seen in the pelvic parietal peritoneum, omentum, bladder/bowel serosa, periaortic area and within the skin.[2]

Clinical presentation is chronic pelvic pain. Sometimes it may be associated with ovarian and cervical neoplasm. It may also undergo malignant change. Laparoscopic excision is considered better treatment than ablation for endosalpingiosis.

DIAGNOSIS AND TREATMENT OF BENIGN TUMORS

These are mainly incidental findings and are usually asymptomatic. Sometimes patient may present with symptoms such as vague pelvic discomfort, heaviness, palpable mass or abdominal pain secondary to obstructed tubal lumen. On examination, these lesions are palpable separate from the uterus as an ovoid, pedunculated, smooth, and soft to firm mass. Torsion, degeneration of leiomyoma, and acute abdomen are some complications associated with these lesions. They are generally not associated with malignant transformation.

Diagnosis is established by transvaginal ultrasonography on which they are seen as hypoechoic mass distinct from the ovary and uterus. Some of these lesions are homogenously hyperechoic but mixed echogenic lesions are also noted. Malignant neoplasms can be ruled out with the help of MRI. Surgery, such as salpingectomy or tumor excision, is the mainstay of treatment of benign neoplasms of fallopian tubes, taking care to conserve the ovaries in young patients.

Borderline Fallopian Tube Tumors

These are rare tumors showing serous, mucinous and endometrioid differentiation and are histologically similar to borderline ovarian tumors. Overall prognosis is good.

Malignant Tumors of Fallopian Tube

Renaud described the first case of fallopian tube malignancy in 1847 and an authentic case report on the same was submitted by Orthmann in 1888.

Although malignant primary fallopian tube lesions are uncommon, accounting only for 0.3–1.1% of female genital tract malignancies, the incidence of these lesions is increasing.

Annual incidence of 3.3 per 1,000,000 women has been reported from USA.[3] A four- fold increase in the incidence has been observed in Finland from 1.2 to 5.4 per 100,000 women from 1950s to 1990s. This increase in incidence may be due to improved diagnostic facilities, increased longevity, decreased parity, higher socioeconomic status and increase in pelvic inflammatory disease. The true incidence of fallopian tube cancers may also be actually higher because in situations of an advanced stage disease, when anatomy is not clear, it is presumed to be of ovarian origin.

Serous tubal intraepithelial carcinoma (STIC): There is growing evidence suggesting that the origin of certain high-grade serous adenocarcinomas of ovary is from the fimbrial end of fallopian tube. To investigate this, salpingectomy specimens of asymptomatic BRCA mutation carriers' were examined by SEE-FIM (sectioning and extensively examining fimbriated ends) protocol. It was found that 5–6% of the specimens of these women had serous tubal intraepithelial carcinoma (STIC) of fallopian tube. STIC lesion has been deemed to be the precursor of ovarian malignancy. STIC lesions are focal and microscopic, hence extensive examination of fallopian tube has to be done. For achieving this, SEE FIM protocol was developed with an aim to carefully examine the full tube in toto with emphasis on maximizing the cross section of visible fimbria, which is the most likely site of STIC lesions.[4-6] In SEE FIM protocol tube is amputated and longitudinal sectioning is done at infundibular and fimbrial end (distal 2 cm) and isthmus and ampulla is cut transversely at 2–3 mm intervals.

STIC is characterized by loss of nuclear polarity with stratification, nuclear pleomorphism, increased nuclear cytoplasmic ratio, mitotic activity and apoptotic bodies. Genetic identity between STIC and high grade epithelial ovarian cancer has also been proven by molecular sequencing studies of *p53 gene* and others by shared genetic lineage.[7,8] Most patients with STIC have uneventful course without disease recurrence. However, 4–11% of patients develop primary peritoneal cancer even after salpingectomy. Etiology may be that the tubal lesion has already seeded into the peritoneal cavity before salpingectomy.

Management of STIC in risk reducing salpingo-oophorectomy (RRSO) samples: High-risk population for developing ovarian cancer include women with BRCA 1 and 2 mutation and literature supports role of RRSO in these patients for reduction of risk of ovarian and fallopian tube cancer. However, there is no definitive guideline for further management if STIC lesions incidentally detected in salpingectomy specimens. But since STIC carries a possibility of development of peritoneal cancers, these patients need to be strictly followed up frequently with CA 125 and imaging by ultrasonography or CT scan for long periods. Role of postoperative chemotherapy is also not well established.

ETIOLOGY AND RISK FACTORS

Most commonly fallopian tube cancer is seen after menopause with the mean age of 56 year. High-risk factors for development of these cancers are nulliparity or low parity, infertility, genetic abnormalities such as gene mutations, alteration in gene copy number, loss of heterozygosity and protein level changes. An increased association of BRCA mutation with fallopian tube cancer is reported by recent studies accounting to be as high as 3% in this subgroup of women, which is 120 times higher than in general population.

The hypothesis that serous carcinoma in the ovary or other pelvic sites originates from the fallopian tubes is justified by detection of STIC in fallopian tubes of BRCA mutation carriers. From the protocol it was found that approximately 50% of patients with HGSC were found to have coexisting STIC. Somatic mutations in TP53[9] and certain molecular markers like elevated stathmin 1[10] shortened telomeres,[11] and cyclin E[12] amplification are also associated with STIC mutation in ovarian neoplasm.

PATHOLOGY

Fallopian tube cancers can be primary and secondary. Most common types include serous papillary adenocarcinoma (80%) followed by endometrioid and transitional cell type (5-10% each), Rarely, they can be of mixed cell type, clear cell or adenosquamous histologically. A study by Alvarado-Cabrero and colleagues on 105 patients[13] showed a histological distribution as follow: 50% serous cancers, 25% endometrioid, 20% transitional cell or undifferentiated carcinoma and 5% others. Serous adenocarcinomas mostly have poor prognosis. Sometimes, histologically immune cell invasion can be confused as salpingitis and this delays the diagnosis.[14] Strict criteria are required to differentiate tubal cancers from ovarian cancers due to the close similarity. PFTC usually distends the tubal lumen or may protrude through the fimbrial end. Most common site is the distal portion, followed by middle portion for the development of carcinoma. Considering the difficulty in differentiating between epithelial ovarian carcinoma and primary fallopian tube carcinoma, the following criteria have been laid out for making a diagnosis of PFTC:[15]

- Primary tumor is in tube arising from endosalpinx
- Growth pattern is of papillary type involving mucosa
- The transition between benign and malignant epithelium should be demonstrable if wall involvement occurs
- Ovaries and endometrium are spared or minimally involved.

Differentiation between primary ovarian and primary tubal carcinoma becomes difficult if ovarian involvement is also present. In primary ovarian cancer, pattern of tubal involvement is serosal with spared endosalpinx in contrast to primary fallopian tube cancer which mostly originate in the mucosa of endosalpinx.

PFTC has an extremely unstable genotype, with highly scattered DNA ploidy patterns and frequent genetic alterations as shown by molecular biology studies. Prophylactic salpingo-oophorectomy performed in BRCA mutation carriers reported carcinoma in-situ or atypical hyperplasia in 18% of fallopian tubes removed.[16]

Women on tamoxifen therapy have been observed to have diffused atypical hyperplasia. Patients undergoing tubal ligation and those with Peutz-Jeghars syndrome have been reported to have mucinous metaplasia and neoplasia. In 20% cases, it may be bilateral.[17]

CLINICAL PRESENTATION AND DIAGNOSIS

Fallopian tube cancers commonly seen in postmenopausal women show a classical Latzko's triad which includes intermittent profuse serosanguinous vaginal discharge, colicky lower abdominal pain relieved by discharge, and abdominopelvic or pelvic mass (although found only in 15% of patients). Most common presenting feature is postmenopausal bleeding seen in 50% of patients. Bleeding comes from fallopian tube to endometrial cavity and exits from vagina. Sometimes colicky pain is associated with passage of accumulated blood or watery discharge.

An important clue to fallopian tube cancers in post-menopausal women is profuse watery discharge, referred as hydrops tubae profluens. In contrast to epithelial ovarian cancers, primary fallopian tube cancers are usually symptomatic in early stages of disease. Ascites is seen in 5–10% of patients in advanced disease.

Tumor Markers

Tumor markers play an important role in diagnosis, monitoring response to treatment and in follow-up for detecting recurrences. Most commonly used tumor marker is serum CA 125. A study by Hefler[18] found elevated levels of serum CA125 in 80% patients with median value of 183 U/mL. In this study the sensitivity, specificity, positive predictive, and negative predictive values of serum CA 125 levels in the follow-up of patients with PFTC were 92%, 90%, 67%, and 98%, respectively. In addition, pretreatment serum CA125 level has independent correlation with disease free and overall survival of patients with PFTC and response to chemotherapy. Increased levels precede the clinical and radiologic diagnosis of disease recurrence in 90% of patients with median lead time of 3 months.

Imaging

Imaging is an important investigation in the diagnostic workup of patients with gynecological neoplasms including PFTC. PFTC usually presents as a pelvic mass with anechoic or low level echoes with papillary projections or intraluminal masses on ultrasound studies. As most of the echographic appearances of fallopian tube are nonspecific, differential diagnosis with other pelvic masses such as tubo-ovarian abscess, ovarian tumor and ectopic pregnancy should be kept in mind.

On imaging, the dominant component in the tumor dictates echogenicity and appearance. On ultrasonography, predominantly a solid component appears like a sausage shaped adnexal mass. In contrast, a hydrosalpinx will have the appearance of a fluid filled tubular adnexal structure, containing papillary, solid or nodular components, or a multilocular cystic mass with a cog wheel appearance. On contrast enhanced CT imaging, the mass lesion has attenuation similar to other pelvic soft tissue, but less enhancing than myometrium. A solid papillary intratubal mass allows easy prediction of PFTC. MRI findings suggesting PFTC are hydrosalpinx with mural papillary nodules or sausage shaped mass with mild-to-moderate enhancement of solid components, intrauterine fluid accumulation, and rim enhancement.

Staging

Fallopian tube carcinomas are staged according to the 2014 FIGO staging classification for cancer of the ovary, fallopian tube, and peritoneum **(Table 1)**.

PROGNOSTIC FACTORS

As compared to ovarian cancers, this disease is diagnosed at an earlier stage, probably due to presenting symptoms of postmenopausal vaginal discharge and bleeding.

Stage at diagnosis	*% patients*
Stage I:	20%
Stage II:	20%
Stage III:	50%
Stage IV:	10%

Age, stage at diagnosis, grade of cancer, lymph vascular space invasion, and residual disease at surgery are important prognostic factors. Disease originating from fimbrial end has poorer prognosis. Stage wise prognosis is better than ovarian cancers.

Stage wise prognosis

Heintz (2003)[19] reported 5-year survival as follows:

- Stage I: 82%
- Stage II: 79%
- Stage III: 60%
- Stage IV:29%
- Overall: 69%

MANAGEMENT

Exploratory laparotomy and comprehensive staging is usually undertaken in suspected early stage cancers. Steps of staging surgery include collecting peritoneal fluid for cytological examination and total abdominal hysterectomy, with bilateral

TABLE 1: FIGO staging classification for cancer of the ovary, fallopian tube, and peritoneum.

Stage I: Tumor confined to ovaries or fallopian tube(s)
IA: Tumor limited to 1 ovary (capsule intact) or fallopian tube; no tumor on ovarian or fallopian tube surface; no malignant cells in the ascites or peritoneal washings IB: Tumor limited to both ovaries (capsules intact) or fallopian tubes; no tumor on ovarian or fallopian tube surface; no malignant cells in the ascites or peritoneal washings IC: Tumor limited to 1 or both ovaries or fallopian tubes, with any of the following: IC1: Surgical spill IC2: Capsule ruptured before surgery or tumor on ovarian or fallopian tube surface IC3: Malignant cells in the ascites or peritoneal washings
Stage II: Tumor involves 1 or both ovaries or fallopian tubes with pelvic extension (below pelvic brim) or peritoneal cancer
IIA: Extension and/or implants on uterus and/or fallopian tubes and/or ovaries IIB: Extension to other pelvic intraperitoneal tissues
Stage III: Tumor involves 1 or both ovaries or fallopian tubes, or peritoneal cancer, with cytologically or histologically confirmed spread to the peritoneum outside the pelvis and/or metastasis to the retroperitoneal lymph nodes
IIIA1: Positive retroperitoneal lymph nodes only (cytologically or histologically proven): IIIA1(i) Metastasis up to 10 mm in greatest dimension IIIA1(ii) Metastasis more than 10 mm in greatest dimension IIIA2: Microscopic extrapelvic (above the pelvic brim) peritoneal involvement with or without positive retroperitoneal lymph nodes IIIB: Macroscopic peritoneal metastasis beyond the pelvis up to 2 cm in greatest dimension, with or without metastasis to the retroperitoneal lymph nodes IIIC: Macroscopic peritoneal metastasis beyond the pelvis more than 2 cm in greatest dimension, with or without metastasis to the retroperitoneal lymph nodes (includes extension of tumor to capsule of liver and spleen without parenchymal involvement of either organ)
Stage IV: Distant metastasis excluding peritoneal metastases
Stage IVA: Pleural effusion with positive cytology
Stage IVB: Parenchymal metastases and metastases to extra-abdominal organs (including inguinal lymph nodes and lymph nodes outside of the abdominal cavity)

salpingo-oophorectomy, infracolic omentectomy, pelvic and para-aortic lymphadenectomy and peritoneal biopsies. For cancers presenting in advanced stages, debulking should be done. For staging in clinically early stage disease, systematic lymphadenectomy is required. Except for stage IA, grade 1 and 2 all patients require adjuvant chemotherapy. Alvarado-Cabrera et al.[13] have suggested that patients of stage IA with spread to muscularis layer should be given adjuvant chemotherapy. Current recommendations include combination chemotherapy in the form of platinum and paclitaxel for 4–6 cycles. Several studies have shown use of carboplatin based combination chemotherapy for patients with advanced stage PFTC, with overall response rates of 53–92%.[20,21] Follow-up requires thorough clinical evaluation, CA125 estimation and imaging if clinically indicated. For refractory and recurrent disease, second line combination chemotherapy consisting of docetaxel, etoposide, topotecan, gemcitabine or doxorubicin may be considered.

Fallopian Tube Sarcomas and Other Rare Malignancies

These are rare tumors and mainly seen in elderly age group but can also occur in adolescents. They are usually diagnosed at advanced stage and clinical presentation is similar to tubal carcinoma.

Surgery followed by doxorubicin, ifosfamide, and DTIC (dacarbazine)[22] chemotherapy is the mainstay of treatment but overall prognosis is poor. Carcinosarcomas are treated along the same lines as epithelial carcinomas. Neuroendocrine carcinoma, para fallopian tube transitional cell carcinoma, mixed malignant germ cell tumors, T-cell lymphoma and marginal zone B-cell lymphoma, trophoblastic lesions including placental site nodule or tumor or choriocarcinoma are some rare types of malignant fallopian tube tumors.

Tumors Metastatic to Fallopian Tube

Fallopian tube tumors may be metastases from other sites such as endometrium, ovary, appendix, stomach, colon, and breast. Any part of the fallopian tube including fimbria, serosa, muscularis mucosa, lymphovascular spaces, and tube lumen can be involved. Metastatic lesions may mimic histological pattern of STIC and also p53 staining. Mucosal metastasis and STIC can be differentiated by IHC staining. Although metastasis from HPV positive endocervical primaries have same IHC staining with p16 as STIC but they lack p 53 staining and have apical mitotic figures. In difficult cases human papillomavirus tissue testing can be used. If metastasis is suspected, immunohistochemistry for CK7, CK20, CDX2 or SATB2 (colonic), GATA-3 (breast), and SMAD4 (lost in half of metastatic pancreatic adenocarcinomas) can be performed. Müllerian origin primaries are confirmed using PAX 8 IHC. Most important feature to raise the possibility of a mucosal metastasis is history of malignancy. A thorough search for the primary site of cancer should be made in order to guide appropriate therapy.

REFERENCES

1. Chene GN, Radosevic-Robin AS, Cayre TA, Raoelfils I, Dechelotte P, Dauplat J, et al. Morphological and immunohistochemical study of ovarian and tubal dysplasia associated with tamoxifen. Eur J Histochem. 2014;58(2):2251.
2. Ong NC, Maher PJ, Pyman JM, Readman E, Gordon S. Endosalpingiosis, an unrecognized condition: report and literature review. Gynecol Surg. 2004;1:11-4.
3. Stewart SL, Wike JM, Foster SL, Michaud F. The incidence if primary fallopian tube cancer in the United States. Gyecol Oncol. 2007;107:392.

4. Salvador S, Scott S, Francis JA, Agrawal A, Giede C. No. 344-Opportunistic Salpingectomy and Other Methods of Risk Reduction for Ovarian/Fallopian Tube/Peritoneal Cancer in the General Population. J Obstet Gynaecol Can. 2017;39:480-93.
5. Kindelberger DW, Lee Y, Miron A, Hirsch MS, Feltmate C, Medeiros F, et al. Intraepithelial carcinoma of the fimbria and pelvic serous carcinoma: evidence for a causal relationship. Am J Surg Pathol. 2007;31:161-9.
6. Labidi-Galy SI, Papp E, Hallberg D, Niknafs N, Adleff V, Noe M, et al. High grade serous ovarian carcinomas originate in the fallopian tube. Nat Commun. 2017;8:1093.
7. Patrono MG, Iniesta MD, Malpica A. Clinical outcomes in patients with isolated serous tubal intraepithelial carcinoma (STIC): a comprehensive review. Gynecol Oncol. 2015;139(3):568-72.
8. Chay WY, McCluggage WG, Lee CH. Outcomes of incidental fallopian tube high-grade serous carcinoma and serous tubal intraepithelial carcinoma in women at low risk of hereditary breast and ovarian cancer. Int J Gynecol Cancer. 2016;26(3):431-6.
9. Kuhn E, Kurman RJ, Vang R. TP53 mutations in serous tubal intraepithelial carcinoma and concurrent pelvic high-grade serous carcinoma–evidence supporting the clonal relationship of the two lesions. J Pathol. 2012;226:421-6.
10. Novak M, Lester J, Karst AM. Stathmin 1 and p16(INK4A) are sensitive adjunct biomarkers for serous tubal intraepithelial carcinoma. Gynecol Oncol. 2015;139:104- 11.
11. Kuhn E, Meeker A, Wang TL, Sehdev AS, Kurman RJ, Shih IEM. Shortened telomeres in serous tubal intraepithelial carcinoma: an early event in ovarian high-grade serous carcinogenesis. Am J Surg Pathol. 2010;34:829-36.
12. Sehdev AS, Kurman RJ, Kuhn E, Shih IEM. Serous tubal intraepithelial carcinoma upregulates markers associated with high grade serous carcinomas including Rsf-1 (HBXAP), cyclin E and fatty acid synthase. Mod Pathol. 2010;23:844-55.
13. Alvarado-Cabrero I, Young RH, Vamvakas EC, Scully RE. Carcinoma of the fallopian tube: a clinicopathological study of 105 cases with observations on staging and prognostic factors. Gyecol Oncol. 1999:72:367.
14. Cheung AN, Young RH, Scully RE. Pseudocarcinoamtous hyperplasia of the fallopian tube associated with salpingitis: a report of 14 cases. Am J Surg Pathol. 1994;18(11):1125-30.
15. Hu CY, Taymor ML, Hertig AT. Primary carcinoma of the fallopian tube. Am J ObstetGynecol. 1950;59:58-67.
16. Carcangiu ML, Radice P, Manoukian S, Spatti G, Gobbo M, Pensotti V, et al. Atypical epithelial proliferation in fallopian tubes in prophylactic salpingo-oophorectomy specimens from BRCA1 and BRCA2 germline mutation carriers. Int J Gynecol Pathol. 2004;23(1):35-40.
17. Markman M, Zaino RJ, Fleming PA, Barakat RR. Carcinoma of the fallopian tube. In: Hoskins WJ, Perez CA, Young RC (Eds). Principles and Practice of Gynecologic Oncology. Philadelphia: Lippincott Williams and Wilkins; 2000. pp. 1099-112.
18. Hefler LA, Rosen AC, Graf AH, Lahousen M, Klein M, Leodolter S, et al. The clinical value of serum concentrations of cancer antigen 125 in patients with primary fallopian tube carcinoma: a multicenter study. Cancer. 2000;89:1555-60.
19. Heintz AP, Odicino F, Maisonneuve P. Carcinoma of the fallopian tube. FIGO 26th Annual Report on the Results of Treatment in Gynaecological Cancer. Int J Gynaecol Obstet. 2006;95(Suppl 1): S145.
20. Kurjak A, Kupesic S, Ilijas M. Preoperative diagnosis of primary fallopian tube carcinoma. Gyecol Oncol. 1998:68:29.
21. Pectasides D, Pectasides E, Economopoulos T. Fallopian tube carcinoma: a review. Oncologist. 2006;11:902e12.
22. You D, Wang Q, Jiang W, Lin L, Yi T, Zhao L, et al. Primary leiomyosarcoma of the fallopian tube: a case report and literature review. Med Baltimore. 2018;97(17):e0536.

LONG QUESTION

1. How will you diagnose and manage a case of primary fallopian tube malignancy?

SHORT QUESTIONS

1. Write short note on STIC.
2. What is clinical presentation of fallopian tube tumors?
3. Enumerate criteria for differentiation between primary fallopian tube neoplasm and epithelial ovarian malignancy.
4. What are the treatment modalities for fallopian tube malignancy?

MULTIPLE CHOICE QUESTIONS

1. High risk factors for development of fallopian tube cancer are all, except:
   a. Multiparity
   b. Infertility
   c. History of breast cancer
   d. Menopausal age
2. Which benign tumor of fallopian tube is commonly present in pregnancy?
   a. Papilloma
   b. Adenofibroma
   c. Endometrial polyp
   d. Metaplastic papillary tumor
3. Latzko's triad includes all, except:
   a. Intermittent profuse serosanguinous vaginal discharge
   b. Colicky pain relieved by discharge
   c. Abdominal or pelvic mass
   d. Heavy menstrual bleeding
4. What is correct statement about fallopian tube sarcomas?
   a. They are usually present in younger patients
   b. Usually present in early stage
   c. Have bad prognosis
   d. Radiation is mainstay of treatment
5. What is correct about primary fallopian tube cancer?
   a. Usually diagnosed in early stage
   b. Ascites is present in 50% of patients
   c. Adnexal mass is rarely present
   d. Fallopian tube cancer is asymptomatic in most of patients
6. Most common benign fallopian tube tumor is:
   a. Papilloma
   b. Adenomatoid tumor

c. Leiomyoma
d. Metaplastic papillary tumor

7. What is correct about isolated necrotizing arteritis of fallopian tube?
   a. It is progressive disease
   b. It may be associated with adenomyoma
   c. It is generalized in nature
   d. It has very poor prognosis
8. Increased association of BRCA mutation with fallopian tube cancer is as high as:
   a. 3% b. 10%
   c. 25% d. 38%
9. Tubal endocervical type of mucinous metaplasia of fallopian tube is associated with:
   a. HNPCC b. Peutz–Jegher'ssyndrome
   c. Lynch syndrome d. Li-Fraumeni Syndrome
10. Most common malignant tumor of fallopian tube is:
   a. Serous papillary adenocarcinoma
   b. Endometrioid tumor
   c. Transitional cell carcinoma
   d. Clear cell carcinoma

Answers

1.	a	2.	d	3.	c	4.	a	5.	b	6.	b
7.	b	8.	a	9.	a	10.	a				

14.10 PRINCIPLES OF RADIATION THERAPY

Umesh Mahantshetty, Gargee Mulye, Lavanya Gurram

INTRODUCTION

Cancer management principles include a comprehensive multidisciplinary and multimodality approach after thorough evaluation and staging. Major treatment modalities for gynecological cancers include surgery, radiation therapy, and chemotherapy. The aim of this chapter is to introduce the basic principles, rationale, indications, radiation therapy details, relevant clinical evidence, radiation-related side effects, and its management in gynecological cancers.

Radiation oncology is a discipline of human medicine concerned with the generation, conservation, and dissemination of knowledge concerning the causes, prevention, and treatment of cancer and other diseases involving special expertise in the therapeutic applications of ionizing radiation. Radiation therapy is use of ionizing radiation for the treatment of malignant and rarely, benign diseases. Radiation therapy has been utilized as curative/definitive, adjuvant postsurgery, consolidation after chemotherapy, and for palliation of moderate-to-severe symptoms due to cancer.

HOW DOES RADIATION WORK?

This needs some understanding of basic physics and biological effects on living cells/tissues/organs.

Basic Physics of Radiation

Ionizing radiation is of two types; electromagnetic waves comprising of packets of energy (photons) or charged particles like electrons, protons, neutrons, and heavy ions. Photons are the most commonly used ionizing radiation in clinical practice, and may be in the form of X-rays or gamma rays. The physical or biological effects are comparable and the difference is in origin or the source. X-rays are produced by machines called linear accelerators that accelerate electrons across large potential difference and are made to strike a high atomic number target to produce X-rays of desired energy, while gamma rays are produced as a consequence of decay of unstable nuclei (radioisotope). The X-rays used in radiology are of low energy, i.e., in kilovoltage (KV) while it is in megavoltage (MV) in radiotherapy. The therapeutic effect of photons is caused by a phenomenon called Compton scattering, where a photon on interaction with a free electron transfers some of its energy to the electron resulting in production of a recoil electron and scattering of the photon from its original path. The scattered photon produces further secondary electrons, albeit with lower energy. The effects of radiation are produced by these secondary electrons, which cause excitation or ionization in the target tissue. The dose in therapeutic radiation is measured as absorbed dose with SI unit Gray (Gy) where 1 Gy is equal to 1 joule of energy absorbed per kg of material. 1 Gy = 100 cGy = 100 Rads.[1]

Biological Effect of Radiation

The interaction of radiation with matter causes physical, chemical, and biological events in that order to produce a meaningful cellular event. Physical event consists of interaction between radiation and atoms, resulting in excitation or ionization. Useful interactions are ionizations comprising of ejection of the electron from its orbit due to absorption of energy from the photon. These high-energy electrons then trigger chemical reactions. Chemical event is a rapid process of further interaction of high-energy electron with molecules of biological significance. Most of the body tissue is composed of water with which electrons react in presence of oxygen to form free radicals (hydroxyl, hydrogen peroxide, and perhydroxyl radicals). These free radicals form the basis for biological damage, by entering the nucleus and causing base damage, single-strand breaks, double-strand breaks, and sugar damage, as well as DNA-DNA, and DNA-protein cross links. Of these biological events, double-stranded breaks in DNA induce inactivation and cell death. This implies that radiation therapy would result in cell death for both normal and cancer tissues. However, intact inherent DNA repair mechanism in normal tissues allows recovery, resulting in relatively increased cell killing of cancer tissues.[2]

Cellular injury triggers various processes depending on the local environmental conditions. From radiation perspective, the mechanisms relevant are 5R's—repair, reassortment, repopulation, reoxygenation, and radiosensitivity. Repair of normal as well as tumor tissue occurs between radiation fractions, hence dividing radiation dose into smaller fractions reduce toxicities. Repopulation is the increase in surviving fraction of a tissue during the course of fractionated radiotherapy. Reassortment is the movement of cells into more radiosensitive phase of the cell cycle between fractions. Reoxygenation is a process where a hypoxic tumor becomes well oxygenated between fractions due to tumor shrinkage and opening up of blood vessels. Radiosensitivity is the relative susceptibility of cells and tissues to radiation, which varies for various normal and cancer tissues. The normal cells/tissues have inherent mechanisms favoring normal tissue sparing while some processes such as increased radiosensitivity, reoxygenation, and reassortment result in more damage of cancer tissues. This ratio of increased cancer cell kill and recovery of normal tissues and inherent radiosensitivity forms the basis of radiation treatment for cancers.[2]

HOW DO WE DELIVER RADIATION THERAPY?

Based on delivery systems, radiation therapy is known as external radiation or teletherapy and internal radiation or brachytherapy (BT).[3] The radiotherapy machines are usually placed in specialized rooms with adequate shielding in the walls commonly labelled as bunkers with specific radiation protection principles.

Teletherapy

Teletherapy uses radiation source (X-rays/gamma rays) placed far away from the body. The external beam is delivered through cobalt 60 unit (gamma rays) or a linear accelerator (X-rays). External beam radiotherapy (EBRT) is the most common form of radiation treatment practiced.

Teletherapy over past few decades has evolved with the incorporation of advances in technology. Based on the delivery technology, it is labelled as

- Two-dimensional (2D) conventional radiation therapy (RT)
- Three-dimensional conformal radiation therapy (3D-CRT)
- Intensity-modulated RT (IMRT)
- Image-guided RT (IGRT).

Conventional 2D radiation is based on defining the radiation fields using bony landmarks either by fluoroscopy or by X-rays to target the disease. For example, **Figure 1** shows a 2D-based radiation plan for cervical cancer. 3DCRT, IMRT, and IGRT are based on defining the targets and planning the radiation fields using multiplanar images generated from computed tomography (CT) scans. CT imaging is performed with the patient aligned in treatment position (e.g., supine), following which images are transferred to treatment planning system. The tumor tissues including organ, potential areas of cancer spread (e.g., cervix, uterus, parametrium, and pelvic nodes for cervical cancer), and neighboring normal structures (e.g., bladder, rectum, small bowel, and femoral heads for cervical cancer) are delineated by the radiation oncologist. These are assigned certain nomenclature for uniform reporting and recording. Target volumes [gross tumor target volume (GTV), clinical target volume (CTV), and planning target volume (PTV)] are related to cancer and organs at risk related to normal tissues. The clinical or radiological tumor is called gross tumor volume, the microscopic subclinical disease extent is labeled as clinical target volume. Planning target volume is formed by applying a geometric margin to

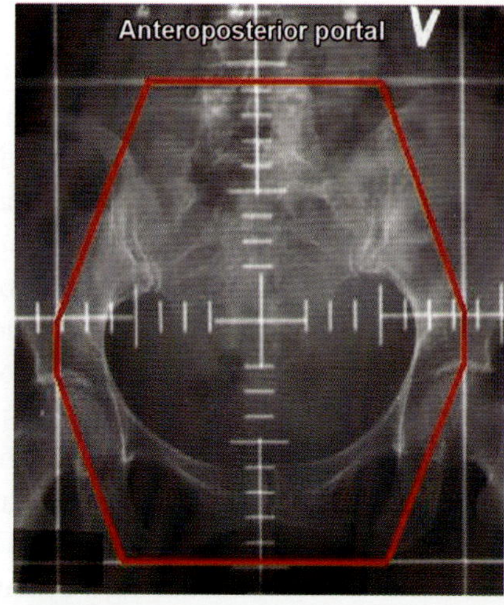

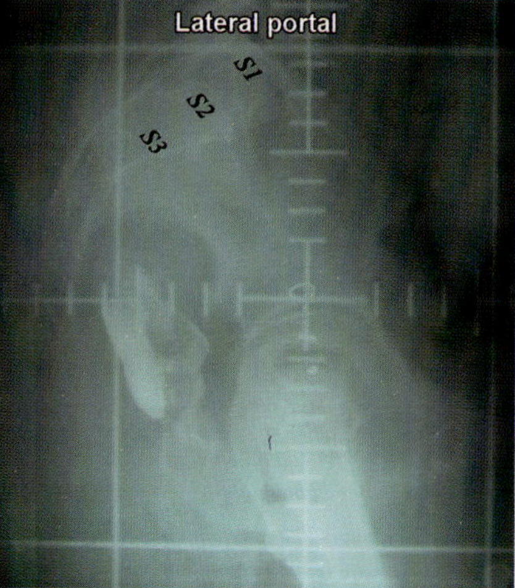

Fig. 1: X-ray field borders on two-dimensional planning for external beam radiotherapy (EBRT) in cervical cancer.

the CTV to account for daily organ motion (internal motion due to rectal or bladder filling) and patient set up errors on the treatment machine. The organs at risk include any adjacent normal tissue which needs to be spared from radiation and has no disease involvement, e.g., bladder, rectum, sigmoid, small bowel, pelvic bone marrow, femur, etc. The aim of teletherapy is to deliver homogenous dose to this PTV with minimal doses to surrounding normal tissues. The medical physicist derives an appropriate plan depending on the technique as explained here.

In case of 2D or 3D treatments, the field directions are prefixed and after setting the field borders, the total dose is calculated. In IMRT the field directions, therapeutic doses to target volumes along with constraints to the normal tissues are predetermined and this information is passed to the planning system, which uses optimization algorithms to obtain desired dose distribution. Imaging (planning CT scan called as CT simulation) used for treatment planning in 3D conformal radiotherapy ensures that target volume is well encompassed in the treating fields, as X ray-based planning using bony landmarks may lead to miss of critical target tissue owning to patient-to-patient anatomical variations. In 3DCRT, the RT beams are shaped according to the target and to spare surrounding normal tissues. IMRT has greater capacity for sparing of normal tissue due to its ability to produce nonuniform dose across the treatment beam and extremely sharp dose falls at the edge of the treated volume.[4-6] Thus, IMRT also poses the risk of missing the tumor, especially in moving targets such as cervix and uterus, whose position depends on daily rectal and bladder filling. To mitigate the movement issues during daily radiation treatment, IGRT was developed and established. The principles of IGRT include image guidance usually using a cone beam or megavoltage CT scan of the region of interest (related to radiation treatment, e.g., pelvic region for radiation treatment of cervical cancer) taken on the treatment machine just prior to treatment, review, and adjust couch parameters to match to patient anatomy so that all target structures are covered in the radiation beam. This ensures radiation treatment efficiency and maybe utilized on twice/thrice weekly or daily basis.

Volumetric arc therapy (VMAT) is a more advanced form of IMRT, where the gantry rotates continuously around the patient while the radiation beam is on. It has the potential to better spare normal tissue and shorten treatment delivery. This sophisticated treatment delivery needs image guidance as a quality check. **Figure 2** shows the isodose color wash difference between 3D-CRT and IMRT techniques for treatment of cervical cancer.

Internal Radiation or Brachytherapy

Brachytherapy uses radiation source (radioactive isotopes like iridium, Co60) near/within the tissues/body cavities. It is called intracavitary/endoluminal (within body cavities) or interstitial (within the tissues) or surface mold (body surfaces) BT depending on the placement of radioactive sources. It has the advantage of sharp dose fall off, delivering high radiation doses to the tumor with minimal doses to the surrounding tissues but has limitation of applicability in small tumors at accessible sites only. BT alone is given in relatively small tumors or as boost after external radiation to improve the local

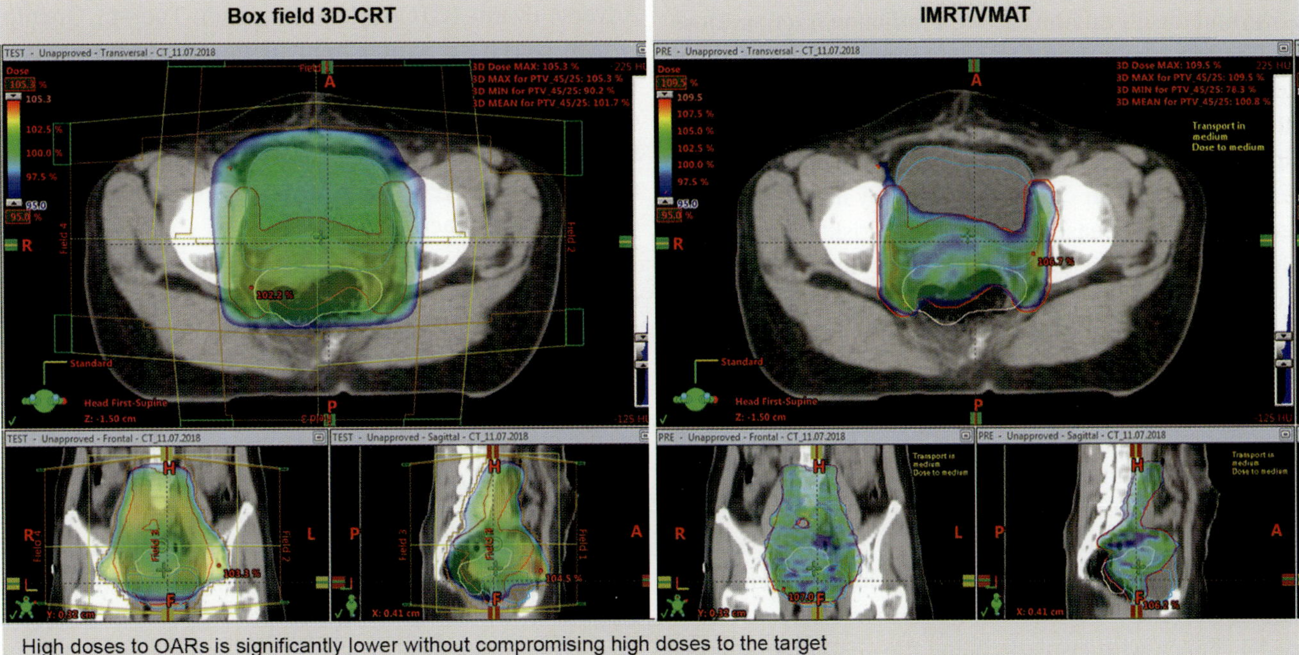

Fig. 2: Newer radiation techniques and isodose color wash and comparison between 3D-CRT and IMRT for EBRT in cervical cancer. (3D-CRT: three-dimensional conformal radiation therapy; EBRT: external beam radiotherapy; IMRT: intensity-modulated radiation therapy; OAR: organs at risk; RT: radiation therapy; VMAT: volumetric arc therapy)

control rates. BT plays a very important role in management of gynecological cancers except ovarian cancers. For example, BT treatment is indispensable for radiotherapeutic management of cervical cancers.[3]

Based on the treatment time, BT treatment is labelled as low dose rate (LDR), medium dose rate (MDR), high dose rate (HDR), and pulse dose rate (PDR). This is simply based on dose delivered per minute. For example, LDR is <200 cGy per minute, MDR is 2–12 Gy per minute, HDR is >12 Gy per minute, and PDR is HDR delivered in pulses of small doses for 10–30 minutes at a time, every hour to give a cumulative dose equivalent to that given in LDR BT.

In modern era, BT is mainly delivered using HDR. The classical example to understand the basic principles of radiation therapy is radiotherapeutic management of cervical cancer patients who receive a combination of both teletherapy (EBRT) and HDR BT.

CONCURRENT CHEMORADIATION

The rationale of using concurrent chemotherapy with radiation is to increase the local tumor control by enhancing radiation action using radiosensitizing effects of various chemotherapeutic drugs, which would translate into better survival. Cisplatin is the most effective chemotherapeutic drug in treating cervical cancer. It acts synergistically with radiation by binding to DNA; and causing inter- and intrastrand cross-links, it prevents repair of DNA damage caused by radiation. Cisplatin in nephrotoxic, ototoxic, and myelosuppressive. It must be administered with adequate hydration and periodic monitoring of blood counts, renal function, and audiometry. For cervical cancer, cisplatin is administered weekly, at 40 mg/m^2, and ideally an hour before a radiation fraction. Dose modification is required in patients with impaired renal function. Multiple randomized phase III trials comparing concurrent chemotherapy with radiation to RT alone, and their meta-analysis have shown an absolute benefit in disease-free and overall, with chemoradiotherapy in patients with stage IB2 to IVA disease as well as high-risk patients after hysterectomy.[7-10] A recent trial from our country exclusively included patients with III B cervical cancer, demonstrated an absolute benefit in disease-free survival (DFS) of 8.5% and overall survival (OS) of 6% at 5 years with addition of chemotherapy **(Table 1)**.[11] This reiterates the benefit of chemotherapy in our patient population, a larger number of who present with more advanced disease and were earlier thought to be poor candidates for concurrent chemotherapy due to poor nutritional/performance parameters as a result of poor socioeconomic status. Thus, concomitant chemoradiotherapy is the standard of care for locally advanced cervical cancer, with cisplatin being the chemotherapeutic agent of choice. Carboplatin can be used as an alternative in patients who cannot tolerate cisplatin, however the outcomes have generally been inferior.

TABLE 1: Stagewise 5-year overall survival in gynecological cancers.

	Stage I	*Stage II*	*Stage III*	*Stage IV*
Cervix	80–90%	70%	40%	10–15%
Endometrium	95%	80–85%	70%	20%
Ovary	80–90%	70%	30–50%	20%
Vagina	85%	75%	30–40%	5%
Vulva	90%	70–80%	50%	20%

RADIATION-RELATED TOXICITIES: BASIC UNDERSTANDING AND CLINICAL IMPLICATIONS

Broadly, reactions may be divided into acute, subacute, and late. Acute reactions are those, which manifest while on treatment or within 3 months, subacute reactions arise between 3 and 6 months and late reactions become apparent after 6 months of treatment. Early reactions manifest clinically during the course of radiotherapy, and are generally due to mitotic-linked cell death in rapidly dividing tissues and secondary impaired tissue function. In general, with conventionally fractionated radiotherapy, the acute normal tissue reactions are within tolerable limits. Use of concurrent chemotherapy with radiation increases rates of severe acute radiation toxicity. Most common acute toxicities with concurrent chemoradiation are nausea, vomiting, increased frequencies of bowel and bladder emptying, neutropenia, and electrolyte imbalance. There are validated criteria to grade the toxicities [Common Terminology Criteria for Adverse Events (CTCAE) and Radiation Therapy Oncology Group (RTOG)], which help in monitoring and timely intervention. Treatment interruptions are not advised for optimal oncological outcomes and hence, assessment of early toxicities is crucial. Acute toxicities if not addressed may lead to impaired/delayed healing of normal tissues which leads to consequential reactions.

Variables impacting normal tissue tolerance may be classified into host, organ, tumor, and treatment-related factors. *Host-related factors* include age, individual response to radiation, and comorbid conditions such as collagen vascular disease and diabetes mellitus. *Organ-related variables* include preradiation organ function compromise or loss, volume of organ irradiated, geographical variation in the radiosensitivity within the organ, and the functional organization of the organ (i.e., whether it is a serial or parallel type and if damage to one part affects only that portion or has more widespread effect). *Treatment-related variables* include total dose, fraction size, overall treatment time, beam energy, and volume irradiated. For example, in a classic pelvic radiation field, the small and large bowel mainly rectosigmoid, and urinary bladder are at an increased risk of treatment-related complications.

BOX 1: The International Federation of Gynecology and Obstetrics (FIGO) 2018 staging for cervical cancer.[12]

Stage I: The carcinoma is strictly confined to the cervix uteri (extension to the corpus should be disregarded)
- *IA* Invasive carcinoma that can be diagnosed only by microscopy, with maximum depth of invasion <5 mm
  - *IA1* Measured stromal invasion <3 mm in depth
  - *IA2* Measured stromal invasion ≥3 mm and <5 mm in depth
- *IB* Invasive carcinoma with measured deepest invasion ≥5 mm (greater than stage IA), lesion limited to the cervix uteri
  - *IB1* Invasive aircinoma ≥5 mm depth of stromal invasion and <2 cm in greatest dimension
  - *IB2* Invasive aircinoma ≥2 cm and <4 cm in greatest dimension
  - *IB3* Invasive aircinoma ≥4 cm in greatest dimension

Stage II: The carcinoma invades beyond the uterus, but has not extended onto the lower third of the vagina or to the pelvic wall
- *IIA* Involvement limited to the upper two-thirds of the vagina without parametrial involvement
  - *IIA1* Invasive carcinoma <4 cm in greatest dimension
  - *IIA2* Invasive carcinoma ≥4 cm in greatest dimension
- *IIB* With parametrial involvement but not up to the pelvic wall

Stage III: The carcinoma involves the lower third of the vagina and/or extends to the pelvic wall and/or causes hydronephrosis or non-functioning kidney and/or involves pelvic and/or para-aortic lymph nodes
- *IIIA* Carcinoma involves the lower third of the vagina, with no extension to the pelvic wall
- *IIIB* Extension to the pelvic wall and/or hydronephrosis or non-functioning kidney (unless known to be due to another cause)
- *IIIC* Involvement of pelvic and/or para-aortic lymph nodes, irrespective of tumor size and extent (with r and p notations)
  - *IIIC1* Pelvic lymph node metastasis only
  - *IIIC2* Paraaortic lymph node metastasis

Stage IV: The carcinoma has extended beyond the true pelvis or has involved (biopsy proven) the mucosa of the bladder or rectum. A bullous edema, as such, does not permit a case to be allotted to stage IV
- *IVA* Spread of the growth to adjacent organs
- *IVS* Spread to distant organs

RADIATION TREATMENT FOR GYNECOLOGICAL CANCERS

Cervical Cancer

In 2018, the International Federation of Gynecology and Obstetrics (FIGO) revised the staging of cervical cancer **(Box 1)**,[12] to include pelvic and para-aortic nodal involvement as a part of staging. In early invasive cervical cancer (FIGO Stage IB1 and IIA1) the standard of care is either surgery (radical/modified radical hysterectomy) or radiotherapy with equivalent outcomes. However, combination of surgery and radiation in early stages does not improve outcomes in terms of local control rates or survival but definitely increases the treatment related toxicities due to both modalities. Hence, proper patient selection and single radical treatment is associated with excellent outcome. This is possible in current era with the use of newer imaging modalities like MRI to identify adverse features such as early parametrial involvement, depth of stromal invasion, significant uterine segment invasion, and better selection for single modality treatment. Patients in whom need of postoperative adjuvant radiation is anticipated, radiotherapy should be preferred over surgery, as surgery followed by adjuvant radiotherapy is associated with significantly higher morbidity such as hydroureteronephrosis, intestinal obstruction and lower limb edema, compared to radical radiotherapy (28% vs. 12%).[9]

Nevertheless, in patients undergoing surgery, the decision regarding adjuvant therapy is a risk adapted approach based on final histopathology report and adverse features including tumor size, vaginal cuff, parametrial dissection and number of nodes dissected on gross pathology while histopathological type, grade, vaginal and parametrial cut margins, depth of stromal infiltration, presence or absence of lymphovascular space invasion (LVSI) and nodal involvement. Assessment of these risk factors prior to surgery may help to prevent multimodality treatments. Patients planned for radical surgery, lymph node assessment intraoperatively and frozen section evaluation if feasible and abandoning the primary surgery to offer chemoradiation may be useful.[13]

Patients are deemed high risk in the presence of any one of the following features: presence of lymph node metastases, or positive surgical margins or positive parametrial extension and adjuvant chemoradiation with external pelvic radiation therapy with concurrent weekly cisplatin chemotherapy is recommended. Intermediate risk as defined by the Sedlis criteria, in the absence of above high-risk features and presence of any two factors on final histopathology—deep cervical stromal invasion, presence of LVSI or tumor size >4 cm, and adjuvant pelvic radiation alone is recommended. Low-risk patients are defined as absence of both high and intermediate risk features and requires no further adjuvant.[10]

Adjuvant radiation is delivered as EBRT (preferably with IMRT to reduce small bowel and hematological toxicity) to the pelvis to a dose of 45–50 Gy.[14,15] A BT boost to the vaginal cuff may be added in patients at a high risk of local recurrence—close/positive surgical margins, simple hysterectomy with inadequate vaginal cut margins, parametrial or vaginal involvement, extensive LVSI, and large tumor size.

Patient with locally advanced disease (FIGO IB3–IIIC2 and IVA with good general condition) radical radio(chemo) therapy with concomitant platin based radiosensitizing chemotherapy is recommended. Definitive radiation therapy should include EBRT and BT. The aim is to deliver 40–50 Gy using EBRT and BT with a dose of 35–40 Gy equivalent to achieve a total tumoricidal dose of 80–85 Gy.

If toxicity and comorbidities preclude chemoradiation, radiation alone should be tried. In the paucity of radiation facilities, use of neoadjuvant chemotherapy for down-staging the tumor followed by surgery has been tried as an alternative approach. However, a recently published randomized trial from our country has shown this to provide inferior disease outcomes compared to radical (chemo) radiotherapy.[16] Overall treatment time (OTT) is a crucial factor affecting outcomes in cervical cancer, and each day of increase in OTT over 7 weeks is associated with worsening local control and OS.[17]

Principles of External Beam Radiotherapy for Cervical Cancer

The main principle of EBRT for cervical cancer is to treat the target and the surrounding tissues with potential areas of spread (cervix uterus, parametria, vagina, and ovaries in case of adenocarcinoma histology) including the regional lymphatics to a dose of 45–50 gray in 25 fractions, 5 days through the week to reduce the primary tumor burden to make it amenable for BT and to eradicate the microscopic disease.

It is delivered with the patient lying in the supine position. Arms are placed overhead/over the chest to keep them away from the radiation beam. A knee rest is placed below the knees to straighten the spine and fix the pelvis. Patients are treated with a comfortably full bladder, with a fixed bladder protocol, to push the small bowel out of the radiation portal and to ensure reproducibility during the entire treatment. In 2D planning, the field borders are fixed corresponding to the bony landmarks of the patients, as seen on the simulator X-ray. A box field technique is usually used for the pelvis (*see* **Fig. 1**), where four radiation beams—anteroposterior (AP), posteroanterior (PA), and two lateral beams are used for treatment delivery. The superior border of the AP-PA fields is placed at the L4-L5 interspace to adequately cover the common iliac nodes, inferior border is placed 2 cm below the gross tumor in the vagina, which is marked with a radio-opaque marker during simulation. The lateral borders are placed 1.5–2 cm beyond the widest part of the pelvic brim. The superoinferior borders of the lateral fields are same as those of the AP-PA fields, the anterior border is placed at the anterior edge of the pubic symphysis, and the posterior border at the junction of S2-S3 vertebrae. 3D-CRT involves the use of multileaf collimators (MLCs) for shaping the radiation fields to the target volume. The advantage of CT images is the identification of the metastatic lymph nodes and adaptation of the target volumes accordingly. In addition, many patients have the aortic bifurcation at L3-L4 level and the coverage of common iliac lymph nodes may be suboptimal if planned on 2D technique. IMRT in the treatment of cervical cancer is particularly useful in the postoperative setting as the small bowel falls into the pelvis and is within the radiation portal in hysterectomized patients. In summary, conformal RT for locally advanced with newer EBRT techniques have potential to reduce toxicities, especially in postoperative settings. The use of IMRT in definitive settings (intact cervix) is challenging due to organ motion (cervix, uterus, and bladder/rectal volume reproducibility). This introduces uncertainty in daily treatment and hence image guidance before treatment is mandatory. **Figure 2** shows the isodose color wash comparison of 3D-CRT versus IMRT for cervical cancer.

Principles of Brachytherapy for Cervical Cancer

With EBRT and concomitant chemotherapy, adequate shrinkage of primary tumor and sterilization of draining lymph nodes is achieved. BT boost is delivered to treat the primary tumor to high doses for complete eradication of the primary tumor. The main advantage of BT is the principle on which it stands. There is rapid dose fall off from the center to the periphery and hence the doses to the surrounding normal tissues are minimal.

The principles of BT include, BT application, imaging, planning, and treatment. The BT application is done under anesthesia/sedation—bidigital pelvic examination is mandatory to assess residual disease, identification and sounding of uterine canal (assisted by ultrasonography, if available), insertion of BT applicator assembly which consists of a straight tube in uterine canal called tandem, and a vaginal component placed in the lateral fornices, either in the form of a ring or two ovoids which are usually perpendicular to axis of tandem, followed by vaginal packing to stabilize the applicator assembly. Imaging (orthogonal X-rays or CT/MRI) of the pelvic region is done. **Figure 3** illustrates different types of BT applicators currently available for cervical cancer BT. Treatment planning is performed by medical physicist. The principles of planning include identification and reconstruction of applicator channels, source loading, defining patient/applicator related points, dosimetry, plan evaluation, and finalization as shown in **Figure 4**. BT treatment delivery is done using BT machine (commonly HDR-BT). The radioactive source (Ir192/Co60) is introduced into the applicator via a remote afterloading machine, thus causing minimal exposure to the radiation personnel.

Point "A", Point "B", and ICRU

Point "A" is a point in the paracervical triangle identified as 2 cm superior and lateral to the upper most part of lateral fornices **(Fig. 4)**. This is defined in relation to the applicator channels and uterine canal axis on orthogonal X-rays/CT/MR as shown in the **Figure 4**. The BT dose prescription is done to point "A" for uniform prescription, reporting, and comparison with clinical outcome in the community. Apart from point "A", point "B" is defined in the transverse plane of point "A" and is 5 cm lateral to the midline of the body axis. This represents the pelvic node point and serves as a surrogate for lateral pelvic wall lymph nodes and dose estimation. Apart from point "A" and "B", bladder and rectal reference points are also defined mainly on X-rays, which act as surrogate for doses to rectum and bladder. All these details have been described in detail in International Commission for Radiation Units and Measurements (ICRU) reports No. 38 and 89.[18] The prescription and recording of doses delivered to point "A" and

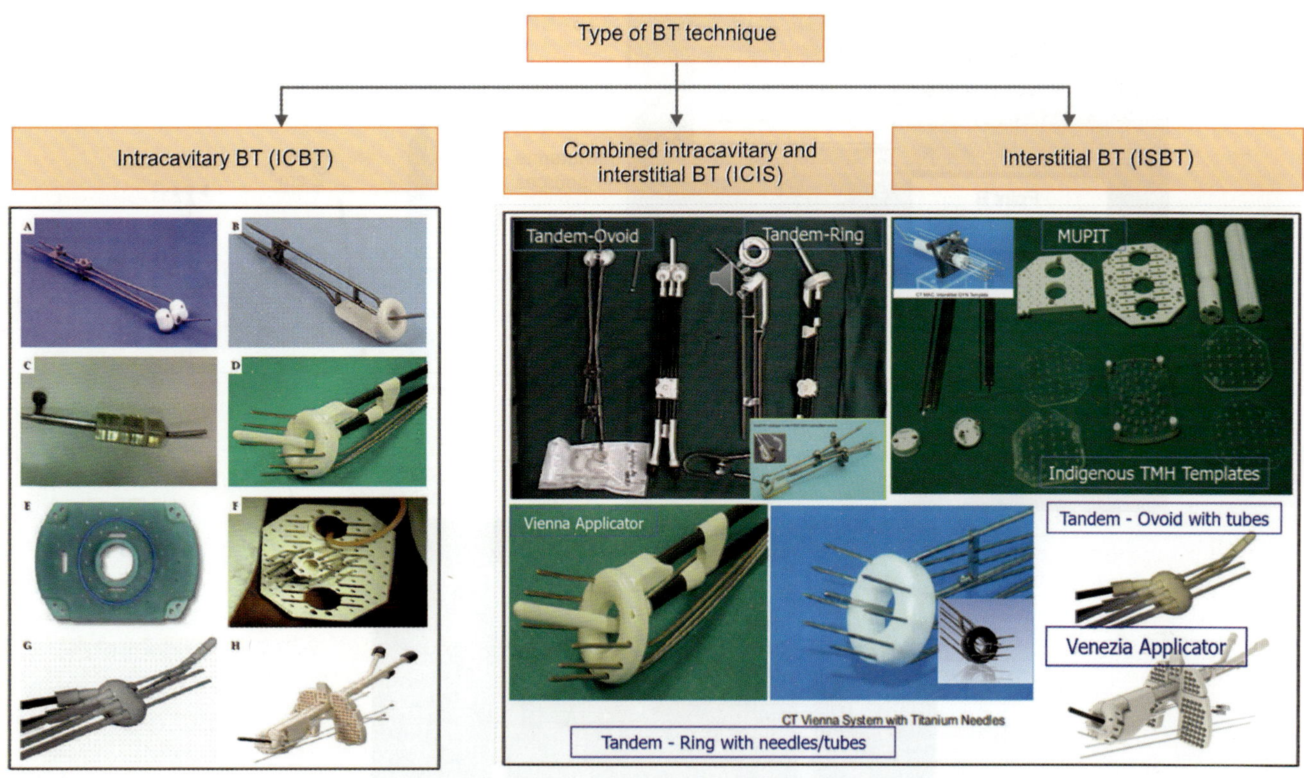

Fig. 3: Brachytherapy (BT) applicators for cervical cancer.

reference points have shown excellent correlation with control rates and acceptable late toxicity.

Recent Advances in Cervical Cancer Brachytherapy

Three-dimensional imaging with CT/MRI has been incorporated in BT treatment planning and is described as *image-guided adaptive brachytherapy (IGABT)*. Instead of conventional orthogonal X-rays, 3D CT/MR imaging of primary tumor is obtained to identify the tumor details better at diagnosis and BT, target the BT doses to the residual disease at cervix and optimal sparing of doses to rectum, bladder, sigmoid, and bowel rather than various surrogate points defined. The detailed process of IGABT is described in ICRU 89 report and is out of the scope of this chapter. Promising results are being reported with IGABT approach with local control rates > 90% even for advanced stages, even including developing countries.[19] The use of MRI for IGABT, especially in developing countries, seems beneficial in terms of economic models.[20-23]

An example of the workflow of MR IGABT for cervical cancer is as shown in **Figures 5A to D**. An MRI at diagnosis and at BT forms the basis of IGABT. The high-risk target volume (HRCTV) is contoured on the MRI at the time of BT after the insertion of applicator, and dose is prescribed to this volume, in place of prescription to point A. The aim is to the deliver 85–90 Gy to the HRCTV while restricting dose to the bladder to 90–95 Gy and that to the rectum and sigmoid to 75 Gy. IGABT allows tailoring of the BT dose according to the response of the tumor to EBRT, leading to better local control and decreased toxicities. In case of unfavorable responses after EBRT, advanced MRI compatible applicators (with provisions for insertion of tubes into the parametrium as shown in **Figure 5)** should be used. On similar lines CT IGABT for cervical cancer is adopted, especially in resource constraint settings where MRI may not be available and is also current area of research.

Summary: Radiation therapy with/without concomitant chemotherapy is mainstay of treatment for cervical cancers, especially locally advanced disease (FIGO IB2–IVA) with radical surgery restricted to very early disease—preinvasive and early invasive (up to FIGO stage IB1). All patients should receive a combination of EBRT and BT mandatorily with an overall treatment time not exceeding 7–8 weeks for optimum clinical outcomes, both survivals and toxicities.

Endometrial Cancer

Endometrial cancers have shown a rising incidence in India, with the number new cases each year being approximately 13,000 according to The Global Cancer Observatory (GLOBOCAN) 2018. Endometrial cancers are broadly divided into two types. Type I (endometrioid type) that is associated with prolonged estrogen exposure, obesity, earlier age at presentation, and has better prognosis. Type II (nonendometrioid) endometrial cancers present at a later age, are not associated with estrogen excess, and have

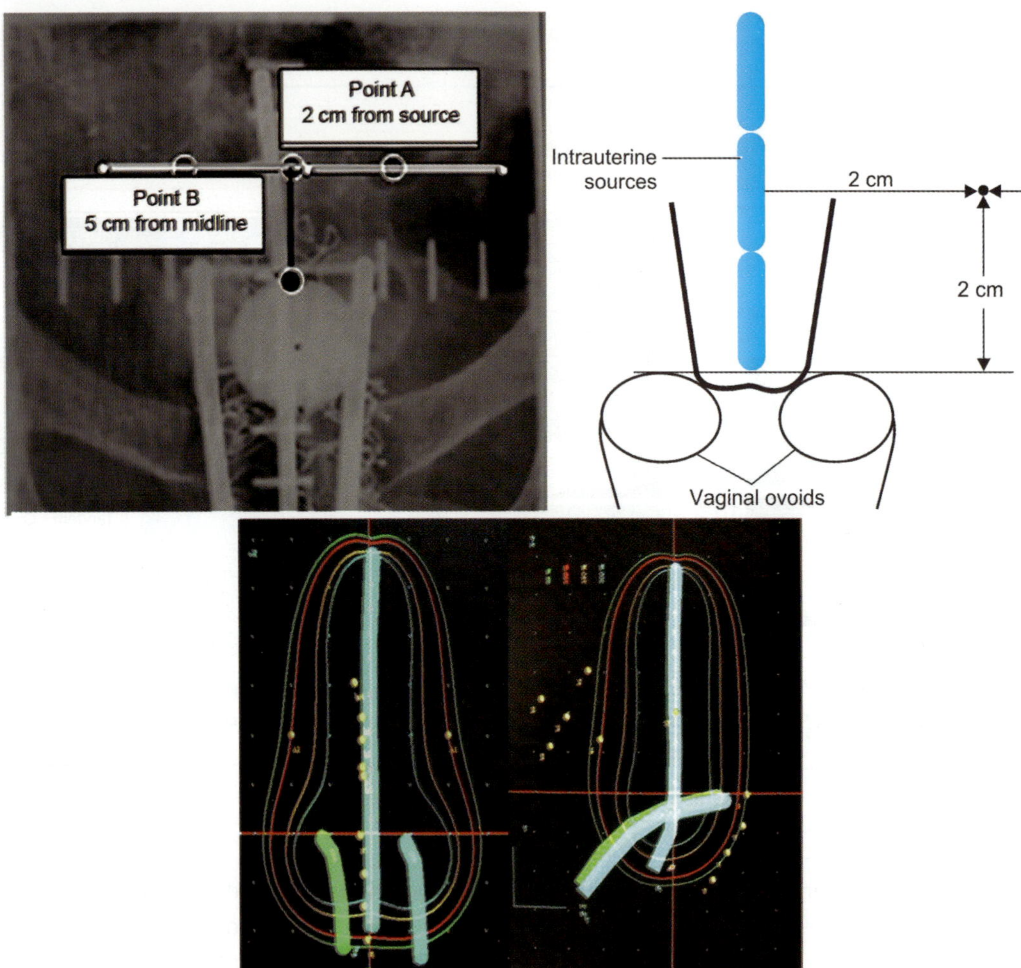

Fig. 4: Definition of point A and point B on X-ray/schematic and isodose lines on planning by two-dimensional (2D) X-ray-based brachytherapy.

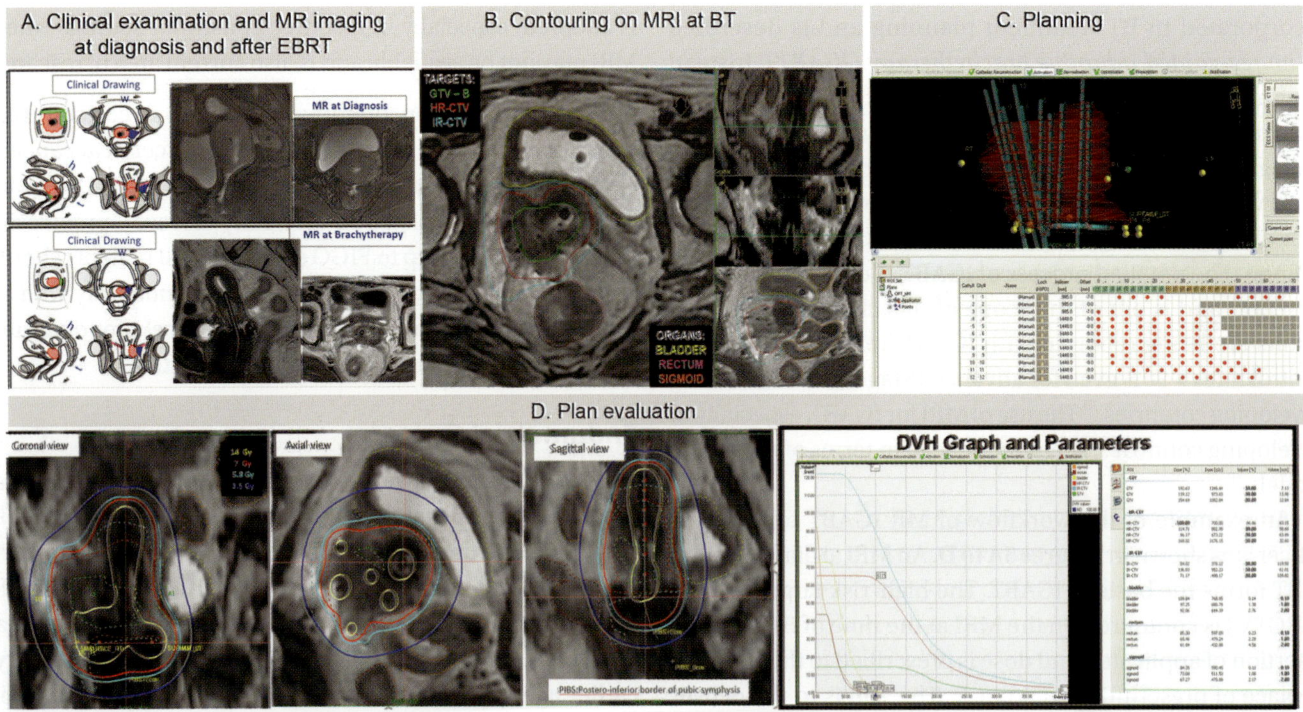

Figs. 5A to D: Schematic presentation of the workflow for MRI-guided adaptive brachytherapy (BT) for cervical cancer. (DVH: dose-volume histogram; EBRT: external beam radiotherapy)

TABLE 2: ESMO-ESGO-ESTRO consensus risk stratification for endometrial cancers.[24]

Risk group	***Description***
Low risk	Stage I endometrioid, grade 1–2, <50% myometrial invasion, lymphovascular space invasion (LVSI) negative
Intermediate risk	Stage I endometrioid, grade 1–2, >50% myometrial invasion, LVSI negative
High-intermediate risk	Stage I endometrioid, grade 3, <50% myometrial invasion, regardless of LVSI status Stage I endometrioid, grade 1–2, LVSI unequivocally positive, regardless of depth of invasion
High risk	Stage I endometrioid, grade 3, >50% myometrial invasion, regardless of LVSI status Stage II Stage III endometrioid, no residual disease, non-endometrioid (serous or clear cell or undifferentiated carcinoma, or carcinosarcoma)
Advanced	Stage III residual disease and stage IVA
Metastatic	Stage IVB

poor prognosis. The initial treatment for endometrial cancer is comprehensive surgical staging—extrafascial hysterectomy with bilateral salpingo-oophorectomy, with cytological examination of peritoneal washings, with or without pelvic lymphadenectomy with omentectomy for type II histology only. Lymphadenectomy may be avoided in patients with low-risk features such as grade 1 or 2 tumors and with less than half of myometrial invasion. Surgicopathological staging is vital and mandatory after patients undergo initial surgery.

The adjuvant therapy in endometrial cancer is also based on the risk adapted approach and many risk classifications have been utilized based on surgical details and final histopathological features. Various histopathological features include histology type, depth of endomyometrial invasion, grade, LVSI (absent/present)—if present focal or extensive, involvement of cervix/adnexa/vagina, lymph node involvement, and final histopathological staging. The most recent one is the ESMO-ESGO-ESTRO risk stratification **(Table 2)**.[24] Patients with low risk may be observed. For intermediate or high-intermediate risk patients, vaginal cuff BT or rarely pelvic radiation (mini-pelvis), while in high-risk patients, adjuvant pelvic irradiation (EBRT) is recommended.

Patients who are high risk on account of having stage I, high grade, deep myometrial invasion will benefit from adjuvant pelvic EBRT, while stage II patients will benefit with addition of vaginal BT along with EBRT. In patients with high-risk disease and more advanced stage, i.e., stage IIIC disease and nonendometrioid histology, adjuvant chemotherapy may also be beneficial.[25]

Radiation Therapy Details

Vaginal cuff BT alone patients undergo BT application consisting of intravaginal cylinder-shaped applicators inserted into whole length of vagina up to the apex. The upper 3–4 cm of the vaginal cuff is treated to a dose prescribed at a depth of 5 mm from the mucosa, in order to adequately treat the submucosal lymphatic channels with high-dose rate BT. If BT alone, the commonly dose-fraction schedule utilized is 5–7 Gy × 1# once or twice weekly for 3–5 fractions. Patients who are candidates to receive pelvic EBRT are on similar principles as mentioned in the postoperative radiation and cervical cancer. The EBRT protocol consist of radiation dose delivery of 45–50 Gy/25# over 5 weeks, preferably with IMRT to reduce toxicity. In patients receiving vaginal cuff BT after EBRT, a dose of 5–7 Gy per fraction × 2–3 fractions once/twice weekly is delivered.

Recently, the TCGA (The Cancer Genome Atlas) used gene sequencing to characterize endometrial cancers into four molecular subtypes: (1) POLE ultramutated, (2) microsatellite instability hypermutated, (3) copy-number low, (4) and copy-number high. POLE ultramutated tumors are seen in younger women and associated with good prognosis, while copy-number high tumors are associated with inferior outcomes. Its use has been limited due to high cost, however surrogate immunohistochemical (IHC) markers have now been developed to make molecular classification more feasible. IHC for p-53 staining is used to identify copy-number high subtypes, IHC for mismatch repair proteins is used as surrogate for microsatellite instability (MSI) hypermutated tumors, POLE mutations are identified using sequencing, while tumors lacking any of the above molecular features are identified as copy-number low.[26] Tailoring of adjuvant treatment based on the molecular classification is still under investigation. The PORTEC 4a trial aims to de-escalate therapy in patients with a favorable molecular profile in high intermediate risk factors.

Vaginal Cancer

Primary vaginal cancer is a rare malignancy, accounting for 1–2% of all gynecological malignancies and occurs in the 6th and 7th decade more commonly. FIGO stage I comprises of cancer limited to the vaginal wall, stage II is cancer that has involved the subvaginal tissue, but not extended to the pelvic wall, stage III is cancer extending to the pelvic wall, while stage IV consists of cancer that has extended beyond the true pelvis, or has involved the mucosa of the bladder or rectum. The diagnostic workup, as with all cancers, should include history and physical examination. Particular attention must be paid to the inguinal nodes; 5–20% cases have inguinal nodal involvement depending on the stage of involvement. Cross-sectional imaging (CT/MRI) is used to ascertain local extent as well as lymph nodal involvement. Insertion of ultrasound jelly in the vagina during MRI helps in better characterization of tumor. An fluorodeoxyglucose-positron emission tomography (FDG-PET) scan may be used when available, as it has higher sensitivity for detecting involved nodes and distant metastases in locally advanced cases. Cystoscopy and proctosigmoidoscopy is indicated in patients with symptoms suggestive of bladder and rectal infiltration.

Radical surgery is very uncommon since it amounts to exenteration and associated with severe morbidity. Radiation therapy is the primary treatment modality in majority of patients with vaginal cancer. On similar lines as cervical cancer, these patients usually receive a combination of EBRT with/without concomitant platin based chemotherapy and BT boost whenever feasible. Upper and middle vagina has higher chances of spread to pelvic nodes than lower vagina, which spreads to inguinal nodes, and treatment volumes are modified accordingly.

During EBRT, along with treatment of the pelvis, as in cervical cancer, inguinal nodes are to be treated in case of distal one-third vaginal involvement. When inguinal nodes are to be treated, the patient is placed with thighs externally rotated to reduce skin folds in the groin, to decrease skin toxicity. EBRT with IMRT may be particularly beneficial in such cases to reduce toxicities. After pelvic EBRT to a dose of 50 Gy, BT is in the form of vaginal BT or advanced BT intracavitary/combined intracavitary and interstitial treatments using different perineal templates. Patients treated with intracavitary BT alone receive a dose equivalent of 25–30 Gy, while those treated with perineal templates receive a dose equivalent to 15–20 Gy via BT.[27]

Vaginal stenosis is a common toxicity postradiotherapy for vaginal cancer. All patients should be prescribed and counseled regarding use of vaginal dilators after healing of acute mucositis has taken place.

Vulvar Cancer

Vulvar cancers account for <5% of all gynecological cancers. Similar to cervical and vaginal cancers, vulvar cancers too are associated with persistent human papillomavirus (HPV) infection or lichen chronic sclerosis and squamous cell carcinomas are the most common histology. In preinvasive cancers, management is essentially surgical or topical application of various agents. FIGO stage I consists of cancer confined to the vulva/perineum, stage II involved adjacent spread to distal one-third of urethra and/or vagina or anus. Involvement of inguinal lymph nodes comprises of stage III, stage IVA involves extension to proximal one-third of urethra and or vagina, bladder/rectal mucosa, or fixation to pelvic bone. Fixed or ulcerated inguinal nodes are also a part of stage IVA. Stage IVB consists of distant metastases (including involvement of pelvic nodes). Imaging may be omitted in small, early lesions with little chance of lymph nodal involvement. The treatment depends on clinical findings, appropriate staging, and availability of expertise.

In patients with early stage, wide local excision with inguinofemoral nodal evaluation is preferred. Alternatively, if patient is not suitable for surgery due to severe obesity or comorbidities, radiation therapy is an effective alternative. After radical surgery, adjuvant radiation is offered in patients with close/positive surgical margins and nodal metastasis (>1 node positive) or perinodal extension (PNE).

In patients with locally advanced vulvar cancer; not amenable to upfront radical vulvectomy; preoperative radiation with or without concurrent chemotherapy, or neoadjuvant chemotherapy followed by assessment for locoregional therapy by surgery or definitive (chemo) radiation has been attempted. All attempts should be made to avoid mutilating surgeries and compromise in quality of life. Preoperative multimodality therapy (radiation therapy of neoadjuvant chemotherapy or chemoradiotherapy) followed by conservative surgery to achieve clear margins, organ-function sparing and better QOL should be discussed and offered through a multidisciplinary joint clinic discussion. Alternatively, radio(chemo) therapy with either EBRT alone or combination of EBRT and BT boost with curative intent can also be offered. EBRT is usually delivered using AP fields with field borders as follows: Superior border is placed at middle of sacroiliac joints to adequately cover external and internal iliac nodes, inferior border should cover the entire vulva, and superficial, inferior inguinal nodes. The lateral border is kept 1.5–2 cm beyond the widest part of the pelvic brim. Advanced techniques like IMRT/VMAT may be used with adequate knowledge of target volume approach and image guidance. BT is an important option to be considered for patients after completion of 45–50 Gy. In select group of patients, it may be considered and performed using free-hand needles or a perineal template depending on the location of the tumor. However, expertise is needed to perform the procedure and should be attempted in high-volume centers. The total radiation dose required for curative treatment is 60–70 Gy depending upon the response to primary phase of RT. IMRT should be the technique of choice for vulvar cancers, however with the knowledge of the present uncertainties during implementation of treatment.[28] Radical BT using interstitial implant is an option for organ preservation for suitable cases **(Figs. 6A to H)**. Adjuvant radiation involves treatment of bilateral pelvic and inguinal nodes to 45–50 Gy.

Ovarian Cancer

Ovarian cancer is the second most common gynecological malignancy in the developed world. Advanced age, early menarche, late menopause, and low parity are risk factors for developing ovarian cancer. Staging (FIGO) of ovarian

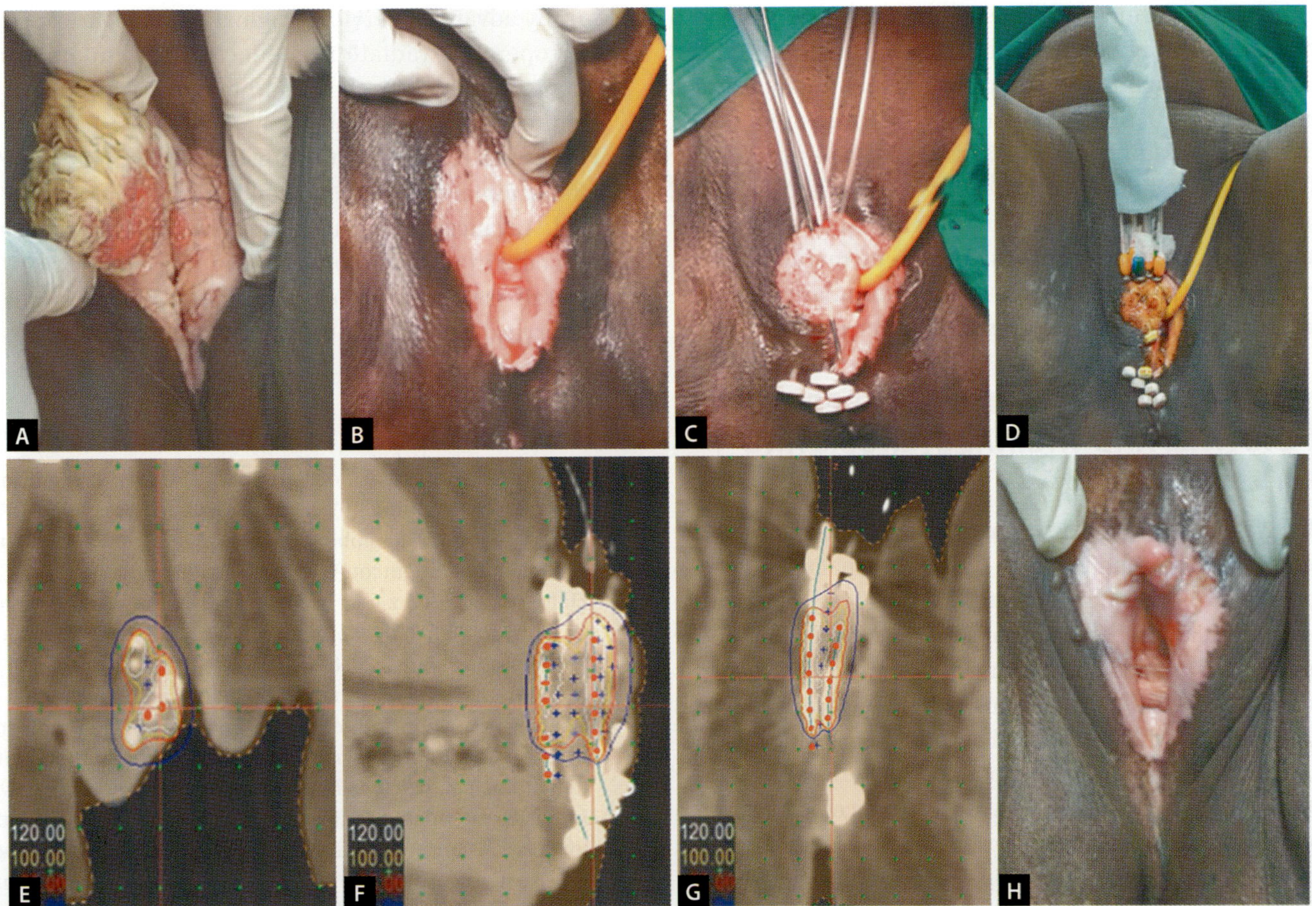

Figs. 6A to H: An example of a vulval cancer treated with radical radiation therapy including brachytherapy. (A) Cancer at presentation; (B) Post EBRT; (C and D) Catheter placements; (E to G) Representative coronal, sagittal and axial CT images with isodose distributions; (H) Post treatment 3 months showing complete response.
(EBRT: external beam radiotherapy)

cancer is surgical. Stage I comprises of tumor limited to the ovaries or fallopian tube and stage II comprises of tumor involving one or both ovaries with pelvic extension or primary peritoneal cancer. Involvement of retroperitoneal lymph nodes/pathologically confirmed peritoneal implants outside the pelvis is stage III disease, while stage IV consists of distant metastases outside the peritoneal cavity.

The patient usually presents with a pelvic mass, and an ultrasonography (USG) is the initial investigation of choice to differentiate between a benign and malignant mass. 3D imaging (CT/MRI) is used next to assess disease extent and plan the surgery. CA-125 is mainly used as a screening tool, while levels of β-human chorionic gonadotropin (β-hCG), alpha-fetoprotein (AFP), lactate dehydrogenase (LDH) are elevated in nonepithelial germ cell tumors.

The mainstay of treatment is surgery. The detailed treatment algorithms are out of scope of this chapter. Radiation therapy has been explored historically in epithelial ovarian cancers. In 1980s, adjuvant radiation to pelvis and/or whole abdominal radiation was extensively evaluated in prospective studies. With the introduction of platinum-based chemotherapy in late 1980s landmark studies showed superior outcome and less toxicities in favor of platin chemotherapy replacing radiation in adjuvant settings.[29] In the recent past, with advent of newer radiation techniques for whole abdomen radiation treatment with IMRT/IGRT phase I/II studies have shown promising results and is being tested further in ongoing phase II clinical studies. Nevertheless, radiation therapy is used for palliation of pelvic mass, vaginal recurrences, tumor mass causing severe symptoms like pain, bone/brain metastasis.

RADIATION-RELATED TOXICITIES OF RADIATION FOR GYNAECOLOGICAL CANCERS

Acute Toxicities

During the course of radiation, RT toxicities are seen primarily in rapidly dividing tissue. Radiation dermatitis consists of dry followed by moist desquamation, along with epilation and loss of xerosis. Acute gastrointestinal (GI) toxicity presents as diarrhea and acute genitourinary (GU) toxicity presents as dysuria and frequency. EBRT to the pelvis, especially along with concurrent chemotherapy causes myelosuppression as about 40% of active marrow in present in the pelvic bones.

Incidence of dermatitis is reduced by asking the patient to wear loose fitting cotton clothes. Steroid creams are used for moist desquamation and placental membrane extracts for moist desquamation. GI and GU toxicities are reduced in conformal radiation, urine alkalizing agents are used for GU toxicities while antidiarrheal drugs may be used for GI toxicities. Hematological toxicities are also reduced with conformal radiation, and management includes blood transfusion, hematinics, and colony-stimulating factors. Severe toxicity may warrant treatment interruption.

LATE RADIATION TOXICITIES: RT PROCTITIS, CYSTITIS, AND VAGINAL STENOSIS AND ITS MANAGEMENT

The two most common problems in clinics for late toxicity are radiation cystitis and proctitis. Cystitis is usually seen at 3–5 years post-treatment, while proctitis generally presents within 2 years. Radiation cystitis usually presents as blood in urine or acute obstruction due to clots and is seen in 3–7% patients postradiation. In both conditions, patients are to be managed conservatively with catheterization and clot evacuation. Three-way catheter is inserted with continuous saline lavage.[30] Biopsy is strictly avoided to rule out disease recurrence if clinically it is not suspected on per vaginum examination. It is a self-limiting condition which heals with time. Hyperbaric oxygen therapy (HBOT) can be tried in resistant cases.[31] Similarly, in proctitis, seen in 5–20% patients, and presents with loose stools with blood and is to be manage conservatively with sucralfate/steroid enema, argon plasma coagulation, and if required HBOT.[32,33] Other late toxicities that may be seen are vaginal stenosis, small bowel obstruction secondary to adhesions, or malabsorption. Intestinal obstruction is usually managed conservatively, with surgery limited to cases not responding to conservative management. Malabsorption is managed with dietary modification.

KEY MESSAGES

- Radiation therapy is an established treatment modality for gynecological cancers.
- Radiation therapy forms an integral part of treatment for cancers of uterine cervix, endometrium, vagina, and vulva.
- Radiation therapy is utilized in the form of definitive, postoperative, and palliative settings.
- Radiation therapy can be delivered by external source (teletherapy) or by placing radioactive sources in and around tumor (brachytherapy).
- Biological effect of radiation is by double-stranded deoxyribonucleic acid (DNA) breaks.
- Radiation therapy with concurrent platinum-based radio sensitizing chemotherapy (if feasible) is as effective alternate to surgery in early stage cervical and vulvar cancers while it is the treatment of choice in locally advanced cervical, vaginal, and vulvar cancers. Postoperative radiation is effective for endometrial, cervical and vulvar cancers in patients with high-risk features on post-surgical histopathology.
- For cervical cancer radiotherapy, brachytherapy treatment after external radiation and concurrent chemotherapy is vital. Advances in brachytherapy have shown promising outcome in terms of local control rates and toxicities. Overall treatment time significantly affects survival in cervical cancer, and every attempt must be made to complete treatment within 7 weeks.

REFERENCES

1. Khan FM. The Physics of Radiation Therapy, 3rd edition. Philadelphia: Lippincott Williams & Wilkins; 2003.
2. Hall EJ, Giaccia AJ. Radiobiology for the Radiologist, 6th edition. Philadelphia: Lippincott Williams & Williams; 2006.
3. Halperin EC, Perez CA, Brady LW. Principles and Practice of Radiation Oncology, 5th edition. Philadelphia: Lippincott Williams & Williams; 2008.
4. Mahantshetty U, Krishnatry R, Chaudhari S, Kanaujia A, Engineer R, Chopra S, et al. Comparison of 2 contouring methods of bone marrow on CT and correlation with hematological toxicities in non-bone marrow-sparing pelvic intensity-modulated radiotherapy with concurrent cisplatin for cervical cancer. Int J Gynecol Cancer. 2012;22(8):1427-34.
5. Roeske JC. Incorporation of SPECT bone marrow imaging into intensity modulated whole-pelvic radiation therapy treatment planning for gynecologic malignancies. Radiother Oncol. 2005;77:11-7.
6. Portelance L, Chao KS, Grigsby PW, Bennet H, Low D. Intensity modulated radiation therapy (IMRT) reduces small bowel, rectum, bladder doses in patients with cervical cancer receiving pelvic and para-aortic irradiation. Int J Radiat Oncol Biol Phys. 2001;51(1):261-6.
7. Chemoradiotherapy for Cervical Cancer Meta-Analysis Collaboration (CCCMAC). Reducing uncertainties about the effects of chemoradiotherapy for cervical cancer: individual patient data meta-analysis. Cochrane Database Syst Rev. 2010;2010(1):CD008285.
8. Kirwan JM, Symonds P, Green JA, Tierney J, Collingwood M, Williams CJ. A systematic review of acute and late toxicity of concomitant chemoradiation for cervical cancer. Radiother Oncol. 2003;68:217-26.
9. Landoni F, Maneo A, Colombo A, Placa F, Milani R, Perego P, et al. Randomized study of radical surgery versus radiotherapy for stage Ib-lla cervical cancer. Lancet. 1997;350:535-40.
10. Sedlis A, Bundy BN, Rotman MZ, Lentz SS, Muderspach LI, Zaino RJ. A randomized trial of pelvic radiation therapy versus no further therapy in selected patients with stage IB carcinoma of the cervix after radical hysterectomy and pelvic lymphadenectomy: a Gynecologic Oncology Group Study. Gynecol Oncol. 1999;73(2):177-83.
11. Shrivastava S, Mahantshetty U, Engineer R, Chopra S, Hawaldar R, Hande V, et al. Cisplatin Chemoradiotherapy vs Radiotherapy in FIGO Stage IIIB Squamous Cell Carcinoma of the Uterine Cervix: a Randomized Clinical Trial. JAMA Oncol. 2018;4(4):506-13.

12. Bhatla N, Berek JS, Cuello Fredes M, Denny LA, Grenman S, Karunaratne K, et al. Revised FIGO staging for carcinoma of the cervix uteri. Int J Gynaecol Obstet. 2019;145(1):129-35.
13. Chopra SJ, Mathew A, Maheshwari A, Bhatla N, Singh S, Rai B, et al. National Cancer Grid of India Consensus Guidelines on the Management of Cervical Cancer. J Glob Oncol. 2018;(4):1-15.
14. Lewis S, Chopra S, Naga P, Pant S, Dandpani E, Bharadwaj N, et al. Acute hematological toxicity during post-operative bowel sparing image-guided intensity modulated radiation with concurrent cisplatin. Br J Radiol. 2018;91(1092):20180005.
15. Klopp AH, Moughan J, Portelance L, Miller BE, Salehpour MR, Hildebrandt E, et al. Hematologic toxicity in RTOG 0418: a phase 2 study of postoperative IMRT for gynecologic cancer. Int J Radiat Oncol Biol Phys. 2013;86(1):83-90.
16. Gupta S, Maheshwari A, Parab P, Mahantshetty U, Hawaldar R, Sastri Chopra S, et al. Neoadjuvant Chemotherapy Followed by Radical Surgery Versus Concomitant Chemotherapy and Radiotherapy in Patients with Stage IB2, IIA, or IIB Squamous Cervical Cancer: a Randomized Controlled Trial. J Clin Oncol. 2018;36(16):1548-55.
17. Perez CA, Grigsby PW, Castro-Vita H, Lockett MA. Carcinoma of the uterine cervix. I. Impact of prolongation of overall treatment time and timing of brachytherapy on outcome of radiation therapy. Int J Radiat Oncol Biol Phys. 1995;32(5):1275-88.
18. Prescribing, Recording, and Reporting Brachytherapy for Cancer of the Cervix. J ICRU. 2016;13(1-2):NP.
19. Mahantshetty U, Krishnatry R, Hande V, Jamema S, Ghadi Y, Engineer R, et al. Magnetic Resonance Image Guided Adaptive Brachytherapy in Locally Advanced Cervical Cancer: An Experience From a Tertiary Cancer Center in a Low and Middle Income Countries Setting. Int J Radiat Oncol Biol Phys. 2017;99(3):608-17.
20. Pötter R, Georg P, Dimopoulos JC, Grimm M, Berger D, Nesvacil N, et al. Clinical outcome of protocol-based image (MRI) guided adaptive brachytherapy combined with 3D conformal radiotherapy with or without chemotherapy in patients with locally advanced cervical cancer. C Radiother Oncol. 2011;100:116-23.
21. Mahantshetty U, Swamidas J, Khanna N, Engineer R, Merchant NH, Deshpande DD, et al. Reporting and validation of gynaecological Groupe Euopeen de Curietherapie European Society for Therapeutic Radiology and Oncology (ESTRO) brachytherapy recommendations for MR image-based dose volume parameters and clinical outcome with high dose-rate brachytherapy in cervical cancers: a single-institution initial experience. Int J Gynecol Cancer. 2011;21(6):1110-6.
22. Mahantshetty U, Khanna N, Swamidas J, Engineer R, Thakur MH, Merchant NH, et al. Transabdominal ultrasound (US) and magnetic resonance imaging (MRI) correlation for conformal intracavitary brachytherapy in carcinoma of the uterine cervix. Radiother Oncol. 2012;102:130-4.
23. Krishnatry R, Patel FD, Singh P, Sharma SC, Oinam AS, Shukla AK. CT or MRI for image-based brachytherapy in cervical cancer. Jpn J Clin Oncol. 2012;42(4):309-13.
24. Colombo N, Creutzberg C, Amant F, Bosse T, González-Martín A, Ledermann J, et al. ESMO-ESGO-ESTRO Consensus Conference on Endometrial Cancer: diagnosis, treatment and follow-up. Ann Oncol. 2016;27(1):16-41.
25. Gurram L, Mahantshetty U, Chopra S, Gupta S, Ghosh J, Gulia S, et al. Adjuvant therapy in endometrial cancer with special emphasis and reference to indian setting. Indian J Gynecol Oncol. 2019;17(4):95.
26. Kandoth C, Schultz N, Cherniack AD, Akbani R, Liu Y, Shen H, et al. Integrated genomic characterization of endometrial carcinoma. Nature. 2013;497(7447):67-73.
27. Pingley S, Shrivastava SK, Sarin R, Agarwal JP, Laskar S, Deshpande DD, et al. Primary carcinoma of the vagina: Tata Memorial Hospital experience. Int J Radiat Oncol Biol Phys. 2000;46(1):101-8.
28. Sciacero P, Cante D, Piva C, Casanova Borca V, Petrucci E, Gastaldi L, et al. The role of radiation therapy in vulvar cancer: review of the current literature. Tumori. 2017;103(5):422-9.
29. Fields EC, McGuire WP, Lin L, Temkin SM. Radiation treatment in women with ovarian cancer: past, present, and future. Front Oncol. 2017;7:177.
30. Eifel PJ, Levenback C, Wharton JT. Time course and incidence of late complications in patients treated with radiation therapy for FIGO stage IB carcinoma of the uterine cervix. Int J Radiat Oncol Biol Phys. 1995;32(5):1289-300.
31. Feldmeier J, Hampson N. A systematic review of the literature reporting the application of hyperbaric oxygen prevention and treatment of delayed radiation injuries: an evidence-based approach. Undersea Hyperb Med. 2002;29:4-30.
32. Andreyev J. Gastrointestinal symptoms after pelvic radiotherapy: a new understanding to improve management of symptomatic patients. Lancet Oncol. 2007;8(11):1007-17.
33. Denton A, Forbes A, Andreyev HJN, Maher EJ. Non-surgical interventions for late radiation proctitis in patients who have received radical radiotherapy to the pelvis. Cochrane Database Syst Rev. 2002;1:CD003455.

LONG QUESTIONS

1. Describe role of radiation treatment in cervical cancer with special emphasis on brachytherapy.
2. Describe rationale and role of adjuvant radiation in cervical and endometrial cancers.

SHORT QUESTIONS

1. Describe mechanism of radiation action.
2. Describe the role radiation in uterine cancer.
3. Describe role of chemoradiation in cervical cancer.
4. Describe in short about modern radiation techniques.
5. Describe role of brachytherapy in cervical cancer.
6. Describe role of radiotherapy in vaginal and vulvar cancer.

MULTIPLE CHOICE QUESTIONS

1. The following are types of ionizing radiation, except:
   a. X-rays b. Gamma rays
   c. UV rays d. Protons
2. The principal target for radiation induced cell kill is:
   a. Mitochondria b. Cell membrane
   c. Ribosomes d. DNA
3. Following are true in the treatment of locally advanced cervical cancer, except:
   a. Chemotherapy increases radiation effect
   b. Dose of radiation can be compromised for toxicity of chemotherapy
   c. Cisplatin is used as chemotherapy
   d. Total treatment time should not exceed 6–8 weeks

4. The following is true regarding the use of IMRT:
   a. Decreases toxicity
   b. Requires the use of image guidance (IGRT) for safe delivery
   c. Is more beneficial in postoperative cases
   d. All of the above
5. The new FIGO 2018 staging incorporates the following changes, except:
   a. Stage IB divided three components—IB1, IB2, and IB3
   b. Involvement of pelvic and para-aortic nodes causes upstaging of disease
   c. Stage IVA involves spread to lower third of the vagina
   d. Horizontal spread of 7 mm removed as a part of stage IA1
6. Indications of adjuvant chemoradiotherapy in cervical cancer are all, except:
   a. Positive surgical margins
   b. Involvement of uterine fundus
   c. Parametrial involvement
   d. Involvement of pelvic lymph nodes
7. The following are true regarding endometrial cancer, except:
   a. The initial treatment consists of comprehensive surgical staging
   b. Adjuvant chemotherapy is indicated only in high-risk cases
   c. Adjuvant radiation may be in the form of pelvic EBRT, vaginal brachytherapy, or both
   d. Surgery is in the form of radical hysterectomy in all cases
8. The following is an indication for adjuvant radiation in vulvar cancer:
   a. Positive surgical margins
   b. Multiple nodal involvement
   c. Extracapsular spread
   d. All of the above
9. The following is true regarding late radiation cystitis and proctitis, except:
   a. Generally occurs as a consequence of high dose received during brachytherapy
   b. Always manifests within 1 year of treatment
   c. Treatment includes use of HBOT
   d. Surgical management may be required in severe cases
10. Acute radiation reactions occur:
    a. within 3 months of treatment
    b. 3–6 months
    c. After 6 months
    d. Any of the above

Answers

1.	c	2.	d	3.	b	4.	d	5.	c	6.	b
7.	d	8.	d	9.	b	10.	a				

14.11 PRINCIPLES OF CHEMOTHERAPY

Anant Ramaswamy, Sudeep Gupta

INTRODUCTION AND BRIEF HISTORY

The word chemotherapy was coined by Nobel Prize winner and German scientist, Dr Paul Ehrlich, while expounding on his concept of "Corpora non agunt nisi fixate" or "agents only work when bound" in the treatment of infections such as syphilis and malaria.[1] Although the action of estrogen in breast cancer, and estrogens and androgens in metastatic prostate cancers was known in the early 1900s, major interest in the activity of chemotherapy emerged post World War II.[2,3] The effect of an accidental spill of mustard gas resulting in marked depletion of bone marrow and lymph nodes in the exposed army personnel set the ball rolling in terms of active and sustained research into chemotherapeutic agents.[4]

PRETREATMENT VARIABLES MODULATING THE USE OF CHEMOTHERAPY

Before evaluating the requirement for chemotherapy, certain disease related and patient related characteristics require determination. These include:

- *Histological diagnosis:* Current treatment paradigms for a majority of cancers have gone beyond pathological identification of site and histology. The use of immunohistochemical staining for accurate identifications of primary tumors coupled with subtyping of various tumors [e.g., hormone positive or hormone negative breast cancers, epithelial growth factor receptor (EGFR) positivity or negativity, etc.] has helped individualize treatment to great extents in the current era.[5,6]
- *Staging:* Management strategies are crucially based on an accurate staging of tumors, based on a combination of clinical assessment, pathology radiology, evaluation of surgical specimens and operative findings. The American Joint Committee on Cancer (AJCC) regularly releases updated versions of the staging of various tumors and is the most widely followed classification. The AJCC 8th edition is the current version in use.[7]
- *Patient related factors:* A key aspect of the management of cancer patients involves an in-depth assessment of patient related factors including physiological age, comorbidities, Eastern Cooperative Oncology Group score, and pharmacogenomic differences in terms of potential for drug susceptibility.[8,9]

PRINCIPLES OF MAXIMUM TOLERATED DOSE CHEMOTHERAPY

Chemotherapy is the backbone of systemic therapy of cancers and in this context refers to cytotoxic maximum tolerated dose (MTD) chemotherapy. Maximum drug doses are evaluated in dose escalating phase I clinical trials until a balance is achieved between efficacy and intolerable side effects.[10] Advances in oncology means that there are now systemic anti-cancers agents such as targeted therapy, hormonal therapy, and immunotherapy that do not necessarily follow the same mechanisms of action as MTD chemotherapy. The principles described here largely pertain to MTD chemotherapy alone:

- *Skipper's laws:* These were the first set of biological principles that were postulated to govern the action of chemotherapy and their efficacy.[11] They were based on laboratory experiments conducted in mouse leukemia models. The first law states that the doubling time of tumor volume is constant over the life of the tumor, i.e., if a graph was plotted for tumor growth, it would form a straight line on a semi-log plot **(Fig. 1)**. Thus, the corollary is that survival of the patient is directly proportional to the burden of tumor at the time of diagnosis.

  Skipper's 2nd law states that the percentage of cells killed by a given drug dose is constant, implying that a linear increase in drug dose causes a log increase in cell kill. This is also known as the kill law. The law also suggests that repeated subsequent further dosing will ensure lesser cell kill, with the remaining cells being the toughest to kill.[12]

  It is important to understand these laws pertain predominantly to proliferative cells, which are present in the majority of cancers like leukemias. The majority of non-hematological malignancies only have a small minority of rapidly proliferative cells.
- *Gompertzian growth:* The Gompertzian growth curve is a concept that taken into consideration the ideas of tumor heterogeneity as well as tumor growth. It proposes a growth curve based on different types of cells in a tumor, processes such as blood supply (or limitations of blood supply), oxygen availability and diffusion, interaction between stroma and tumor and pharmacologic action.[13,14] This kind of "S-shaped" growth curve is the one approximated by human solid tumors and is a consequence of the increasing population of cells due to the birth of cells and decreasing population due to cell death.

  The growth curve is composed of different phases of growth and stabilization: An initial rate of slow growth as the number of dividing cells is small, then an increased rate of growth because of an increased number of dividing cells with a maximum. This means that growth rate of a tumor is always changing, a concept further explained by the Norton Simon hypothesis.
- *Norton-Simon model:* The Norton-Simon model is based on the Gompertzian growth curve. For purpose of explanation, we assume that a tumor has "x" size and is growing at the rate of "y". By the Gompertzian concept, the growth rate of a tumor is always changing. Norton-Simon conceptualized that if tumor with size "'x" grew at rate "y", then the rate of regression of the tumor in response to chemotherapy would be "y"/"x" at size "x" and less than "y"/"x" at size 2"x". This explains an important aspect of the action of chemotherapy - log kill of tumor cells would be much greater in a smaller tumor than a larger tumor. This model forms the rationale for the successful use of adjuvant chemotherapy in patients where the primary solid tumor has been resected.[15]

  Both the Gompertzian and Simon-Norton models also contribute partly to the rationale of sequential and multidrug chemotherapy.
- *Goldie-Coldman hypothesis (Somatic mutation therapy):* The Goldie-Coldman hypothesis states that somatic mutations arise spontaneously within a tumor, thereby leading to drug resistance.[16] The hypothesis further states that mutations will occur inevitably with cell proliferation at the rate of 1 in 10^5 cells. Hence, larger the tumor size, greater the chances of finding cells with resistance to chemotherapy. The corollary of this hypothesis was that debulking of the tumor would reduce the number of resistant clones. An additional application of this theory was to use combination chemotherapy, as opposed to monotherapy, to reduce the chances of resistant clones emerging during treatment.[17]

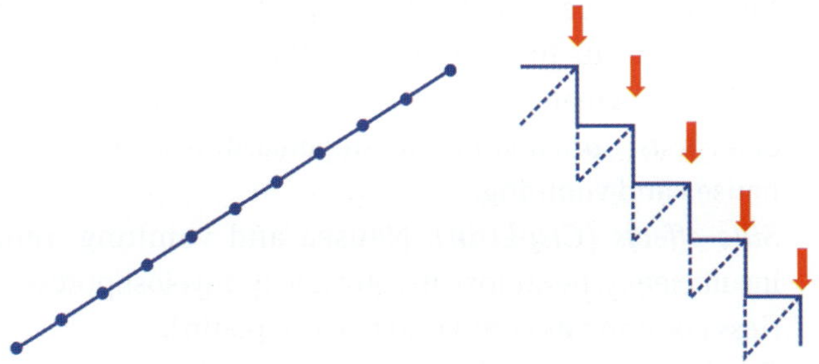

Fig. 1: The Skipper-Schable-Wilcox "log-kill model. Tumor growth appears exponential when plotted on a logarithmic scale (left). With each dose of chemotheraphy, a constant fraction of cells are killed (right).

PRINCIPLES OF METRONOMIC CHEMOTHERAPY

While chemotherapy usually refers to MTD chemotherapy and the advantages of this form of systemic therapy are well known, there are a number of factors that limit the efficacy of MTD chemotherapy. Predominantly amongst these limitations are the side effects of chemotherapy with increasing doses as well as the development of resistance. In as early as 1972, Judah Folkman proposed a different method of treatment that targeted the angiogenesis seen in tumors with continuous low dose chemotherapy.[18] This continuous low dose anti-angiogenic chemotherapy showed potential efficacy with minimal side effects in well conducted cell line and animal studies.[19,20] A number of retrospective and phase II studies in recent years have increased interest in this form of systemic therapy, but conclusive phase III studies in a majority of tumors are lacking.[21]

PRINCIPLES OF IMMUNOTHERAPY: CHECKPOINT INHIBITORS

The immune system has always been a focus of anti-cancer therapy, be it in the form of vaccines, immunomodulators or passive transfer of antitumor antibodies in lymphomas (e.g., Rituximab in B-cell lymphomas). Allogeneic stem cell transfer (ASCT, commonly known as bone marrow transplants) also exploits the action of donor derived lymphocytes recognizing and rejecting host tumor cells, thereby partially coming under the ambit of immunotherapy.[22]

However, immunotherapy as a wide-spread and successful option against cancers got a major push with successful development of checkpoint inhibitors.[22,23] Checkpoint inhibition uses the regulatory mechanisms in the body which normally maintain immune responses within a desired physiologic range and protect the host from autoimmune responses. This autoregulation is mediated by a host of mechanisms, with a predominant role for T cells and its various subtypes. Based on complex interplays between a tumor and the body's immune system, tumors coopt immune suppressive and tolerance mechanisms to avoid recognition and destruction by the body's immune system. These pathways involve positive and negative feedback stimulation (i.e., stimulation and suppression) via T-cells and their associated checkpoints.[24]

Checkpoint inhibitors inhibit T-cell mediated negative co-stimulation, i.e., remove the block in the body's immune system recognizing tumor antigens, thereby allowing the body's immune system to actively cause regression of the tumor. During normal physiological maintenance of activation and tolerance, T cell activation and inhibitory receptors such as CTLA-4 (cytotoxic T lymphocyte associated protein 4) and PD-1 (programmed cell death ligand 1), are simultaneously induced to limit overstimulation of the immune system after antigen encounter. This scenario continues to persist in the presence of an active tumor, with T-cells failing to actively recognize tumors. Checkpoint inhibitors, in the form of antibodies, reverse inhibitory signals transmitted to T-cells and allow reactivation and reprogramming of T-cells. The reprogrammed T-cells will be able to recognize and cause regression of active tumors. The most commonly used checkpoint inhibitors act against CTLA-4 (e.g., ipilimumab) and PD-1 (e.g., Nivolumab).[25,26] Other checkpoint targets under evaluation include VISTA. Lag3 and Tim-3.

Checkpoint inhibitors are now recommended in many advanced tumors with deficient mismatch repair protein status (dMMR) or high microsatellite instability (MSI–H) tumors; trials are ongoing in the adjuvant and neoadjuvant settings to evaluate their use.

COMMONLY USED CHEMOTHERAPEUTIC AGENTS IN GYNAECOLOGICAL MALIGNANCIES

Some of the commonly used drugs, their mechanism(s) of action and side-effect profile in gynecological malignancies are described in brief here.

- *Paclitaxel:* Paclitaxel was initially isolated from the Pacific yew tree *Taxus brevifolia* Nutt. It is one of the key drugs in the management of ovarian, endometrial, and cervical malignancies.
  Mechanism of action: It acts by targeting microtubules, which are a key component of cell division. Microtubules are required for formation of mitotic spindle during cell division, besides maintenance of cell structure and motility. Paclitaxel prevents cell division by promoting the assembly of stable microtubules and inhibiting their depolymerization. By this arrest of depolymerization, cells cannot progress from the G2 to M phase of the cell cycle, thus inhibiting cell division and replication.[27] Besides targeting microtubules, other mechanisms of action have also been postulated.
  Common side-effects: Neutropenia, thrombocytopenia, peripheral neuropathy, hypersensitivity reactions, nausea and vomiting, myalgias, arthralgias, alopecia.
- *Carboplatin and Cisplatin:* Both drugs are members of the platinum group of compounds, which is one of the oldest and most widely used group of chemotherapeutic agents. Both drugs are commonly used in ovarian, endometrial, and cervical malignancies, with some overlap in use. Cisplatin is also the most common radio sensitizing agent used concurrently with radiotherapy in cervical cancers.
  Mechanism of action: The platinum group of drugs act predominantly by forming DNA adducts, i.e., covalently binding to purine DNA bases, thereby disrupting the functions of cellular DNA. These DNA adducts maybe intrastrand or interstrand, but therapeutic efficacy is related to a greater extent to the formation of intrastands.[28]
  Side effects (Carboplatin): Neutropenia, thrombocytopenia, nausea and vomiting.
  Side effects (Cisplatin): Nausea and vomiting, renal insufficiency, neurotoxicity, ototoxicity, myelosuppression (less common as compared to carboplatin).
- *Pegylated liposomal doxorubicin (PLD):* PLD, is a modified form of doxorubicin, which is a member of the group of drugs known as anthracyclines. It is used in recurrent ovarian cancer.

Mechanism of action: Doxorubicin acts by forming protein associated DNA breaks through formation of a complex consisting of doxorubicin, DNA and an enzyme, DNA topoisomerase II. This complex inhibits the action of topoisomerase II, and prevents resealing of DNA strand breaks. Though is likely the major mechanism of action of doxorubicin, other methods of activity include stimulation of apoptosis and generation of reactive oxygen intermediates.

Pegylated liposomal doxorubicin is a liposomal formulation of doxorubicin, which has the same action as doxorubicin, but has an extended circulation time and reduced volume of distribution. This ensures greater tumor uptake and potentially greater action as compared to doxorubicin (which is a weak drug against ovarian cancers).[29]

Side effects: Hand-foot-syndrome, infusion reactions, myelosuppression.

- *Gemcitabine:* Gemcitabine belongs to a group of drugs called fluoropyrimidine analogs. It is primarily used in relapsed refractory ovarian cancers.
  Mechanism of action: Gemcitabine is a potent inhibitor of DNA synthesis. A phosphorylated form of gemcitabine post cellular uptake, gets incorporated into DNA, thereby terminating DNA elongation. Gemcitabine also inhibits ribonucleotide reductase and inhibiting DNA repair.[30]
  Side effects: Neutropenia, thrombocytopenia, transient flu-like reactions, fatigue.
- *Irinotecan:* Irinotecan belongs to a group of drugs called camptothecins and is indicated in refractory ovarian cancers.
  Mechanism of action: Irinotecan is a prodrug that requires conversion to an intermediate called SN-38. SN-38 inhibits an enzyme called DNA topoisomerase I, which is involved in multiple aspects of DNA and RNA activity, including DNA metabolism, RNA transcription, DNA replication, recombination, chromatin remodeling, and repair. SN-38 forms a complex with topoisomerase I, and this results in an irreversible arrest of DNA replication and formation of a double-strand break when DNA replication is attempted at the replication fork.[31]
  Side-effects: Diarrhea (early and delayed), neutropenia, thrombocytopenia.
- *Actinomycin-D:* It is an antibiotic that has a limited spectrum of activity. It is an important drug in the management of gestational trophoblastic neoplasia (GTN).
  Mechanism of action: Actinomycin-D binds strongly to DNA by intercalation and inhibits topoisomerase I and topoisomerase II. It also inhibits RNA and protein synthesis.
  Side effects: Neutropenia, thrombocytopenia, nausea and vomiting, erythema, veno-occlusive disease of liver, radiation recall, tissue necrosis with extravasation.
- *Methotrexate:* Methotrexate is one of the oldest chemotherapeutic agents discovered and is primarily used to treat GTNs in the context of gynecological malignancies.
  Mechanism of action: Methotrexate is a modified folate, with the modification allowing the drug to bind to and inhibit dihydrofolate reductase (DHFR), an enzyme critical for intracellular folate metabolism. Additionally, polyglutamate derivatives of methotrexate and dihydrofolate inhibit purine and thymidylate biosynthesis, which are essential in DNA and RNA synthesis.
  Side effects: Mucositis, diarrhea, myelosuppression, acute renal insufficiency, pneumonitis, transient derangements in liver function tests.

MONOCLONAL ANTIBODIES AND TARGETED THERAPY IN GYNAECOLOGICAL MALIGNANCIES

"Monoclonal antibodies" and "targeted therapy" are anticancer agents that act specifically against certain cell targets or molecules involved in promoting oncogenesis. These terms are often used interchangeably, though they are not mutually inclusive. Some of the commonly used drugs in this category are:

- *Bevacizumab:* Bevacizumab is a recombinant humanized monoclonal antibody (IgG type). It is commonly used in advanced ovarian, uterine and cervical malignancies in combination with chemotherapy.
  Mechanism of action: Bevacizumab acts by binding and inactivating all active forms of vascular endothelial growth factor (VEGF). VEGF and its pathway are important in homeostatic as well as pathogenic angiogenesis. By binding to VEGF, Bevacizumab inhibits the binding of VEGF to their receptors on endothelial cells.[32]
  Side effects: Hypertension, proteinuria, bleeding, impaired surgical wound healing, arterial and venous thromboembolism, gastrointestinal perforation.
- *Olaparib (O), Rucaparib (R), Neliparib (N):* These drugs belong to a group called poly (ADP-ribose) (PARP) inhibitors. They are selectively used in patients with ovarian cancer who have germline (or germline like phenotype) mutations in the BReast CAncer (BRCA) *BRCA1 or BRCA2* genes.
  Side effects: Anemia, neutropenia (N>R>O), thrombocytopenia (N>R>O), nausea and vomiting, fatigue, diarrhea, renal insufficiency (predominantly rucaparib), hypercholesterolemia.
  Mechanism of action: PARP inhibitors act on the basis of synthetic lethality, i.e., a mutation in either of two genes by itself has no negative effect, but combining the two mutations leads to cell death. PARP is an enzyme that is involved in repair of single strand breaks (SSB) in DNA and

its inhibition leads to failure of SSB repair. Persistent SSBs cause collapse of the replication fork resulting in double strand breaks (DSB). In the background of BRCA (which are involved in repair of DSBs) deficiency, DSB repair is also impaired causing chromosomal instability, and cell death.[33]

INDICATIONS FOR CHEMOTHERAPY IN GYNAECOLOGICAL MALIGNANCIES

Common terminologies that are applicable when chemotherapy is planned in the context of solid tumors are as follows:

- *Adjuvant chemotherapy:* Chemotherapy that is administered post resection of the primary tumor to reduce the risk of recurrence as well as treat micrometastatic disease.
- *Neoadjuvant chemotherapy:* Chemotherapy that is administered prior to resection of the primary tumor in order to assess disease biology, debulk the tumor, ensure potentially lesser extent of resection as well as treat micrometastatic disease.
- *Perioperative chemotherapy:* This approach refers to initial neoadjuvant chemotherapy, followed by resection and further chemotherapy (adjuvant chemotherapy). This approach combines the concepts of adjuvant and neoadjuvant chemotherapy with resection (or rarely concurrent chemoradiation) sandwiched between.
- *Palliative chemotherapy:* This is a term used in the management of stage IV cancers where the intent is to reduce symptoms, decrease disease burden and improve survival. It usually does not result in long term cures.
- *Concurrent chemotherapy (chemoradiation):* It refers to the simultaneous use of radiotherapy and chemotherapy. In the context of gynecological malignancies, the best example would be external beam radiotherapy (EBRT) with "concurrent" cisplatin, which acts as a radiosensitizing agent.
- *Maintenance therapy:* The term does not have a fixed definition, but usually refers to continuation of a "less intensive" treatment regimen after an initially more intensive treatment approach. The idea behind such treatment would be to keep the malignancy in remission; a remission which would have been achieved by an initially aggressive cytotoxic chemotherapy. An apt example is the use of PARP inhibitors in advanced ovarian malignancies after achievement of remission with platinum-based chemotherapy.

It should also be noted there is a fair degree of overlap in the way these terms are used as well as the fact that a percentage of stage IV cancers survive for long periods of time, based on biological nature of tumors, as well as response to therapy.

Table 1 provides a short summary of the recommendations for the use of chemotherapy in common gynecological malignancies. This is not an exhaustive list of all available treatment options for these tumors.

TABLE 1: Indications and chemotherapeutic agents in gynecological malignancies.

Type of malignancy	*Stage of disease*	*Type of therapy*	*Commonly used regimens*
Epithelial ovarian tumors	Resected, Ib – IV	Adjuvant	• Paclitaxel plus Carboplatin (IV) • Docetaxel plus Carboplatin (IV) • Paclitaxel plus Carboplatin also combined with intraperitoneal (IP) chemotherapy • Paclitaxel plus Carboplatin plus Bevacizumab (R+ resections)
	IIIC–IV	Perioperative	Paclitaxel plus Carboplatin (IV)
	IV, recurrent/metastatic	Palliative	• Paclitaxel plus Carboplatin (IV) • Paclitaxel plus Carboplatin plus Bevacizumab • PLD plus Carboplatin (IV) • Irinotecan (IV) • Pazopanib (PO)
	IV, BRCA positive	Palliative, targeted, maintenance	• Olaparib (PO) • Rucaparib (PO) • Neliparib (PO) • Veliparib (PO) • Talazoparib (PO)
Germ cell ovarian tumors	All patients except stage IA dysgerminoma and grade 1 immature teratoma	Adjuvant	Bleomycin plus Etoposide plus Cisplatin (IV)
Cervical cancers	IB3–IIIB (treated with radiotherapy)	Concurrent chemoradiation	Weekly Cisplatin (IV) with radiotherapy

Contd...

Contd...

Type of malignancy	*Stage of disease*	*Type of therapy*	*Commonly used regimens*
GTN	Low risk		• Single agent Methotrexate (IV/IM) • Single agent Actinomycin-D (IV)
	High risk		• EMA-CO (IV) • EMA-EP (IV)
Uterine cancers	II–III (select stage II patients)	Adjuvant	Paclitaxel plus Carboplatin ± EBRT ± brachytherapy
	IV	Palliative	• Paclitaxel plus Carboplatin (IV) • Paclitaxel plus Carboplatin plus Bevacizumab (IV) • Docetaxel plus Carboplatin (IV) • Irinotecan (IV) • PLD (IV) • Hormonal therapy (PO)

(IV: intravenous; PO: per oral; EMA-EP: etoposide, methotrexate, actinomycin D, and cisplatin; EMA-CO: etoposide, methotrexate, and dactinomycin alternating with cyclophosphamide and vincristine; EBRT: external beam radiotherapy; GTN; gestational trophoblastic neoplasia; PLD: pegylated liposomal doxorubicin)

KEY MESSAGES

The principles and roles of chemotherapy have evolved from the 1940s till today, wherein chemotherapy is an integral component of the treatment of the majority of gynecological malignancies. Biological concepts such as the Gompertzian curve, Norton–Simon hypothesis and Goldie–Coldman hypothesis still form the basis of the development of chemotherapy protocols.

Research has expanded the number of options of systemic treatment that we possess beyond chemotherapy, though chemotherapy still forms the backbone of the systemic management of gynecological malignancies. Newer treatment modalities in the treatment of malignancies include targeted therapy, immunotherapy, and biological agents.

REFERENCES

1. Nature Reviews. (2020). Paul Ehrlich: founder of chemotherapy. [online] Available from: https://www.nature.com/articles/nrd2582#Abs1. [Last accessed December, 2021].
2. Huggins C, Hodges CV. Studies on prostatic cancer. I. The effect of castration, of estrogen and androgen injection on serum phosphatases in metastatic carcinoma of the prostate. CA Cancer J Clin. 1972;22(4):232-40.
3. Beatson GT. On the Treatment of Inoperable Cases of Carcinoma of the Mamma: Suggestions for a New Method of Treatment, with Illustrative Cases (Meeting IX—May 20, 1896). Trans Med Chir Soc Edinb. 1896;15:153-79.
4. AACR. A History of Cancer Chemotherapy. [online]. Available from: https://cancerres.aacrjournals.org/content/68/21/8643. [Last accessed December, 2021].
5. Curtis C, Shah SP, Chin SF, Turashvili G, Rueda OM, Dunning MJ, et al. The genomic and transcriptomic architecture of 2,000 breast tumours reveals novel subgroups. Nature. 2012;486(7403):346-52.
6. Bethune G, Bethune D, Ridgway N, Xu Z. Epidermal growth factor receptor (EGFR) in lung cancer: an overview and update. J Thorac Dis. 2010;2(1):48.
7. AJCC. AJCC 8th Edition Cancer Staging Form, Histology and Topography Supplements. [online]. Available from: https://cancerstaging.org/About/news/Pages/AJCC-8th-Edition-Cancer-Staging-Form-and-Histology-and-Topography-Supplements-Available-Now.aspx. [Last accessed December, 2021].
8. Sarfati D, Koczwara B, Jackson C. The impact of comorbidity on cancer and its treatment. CA Cancer J Clin. 2016;66(4):337-50.
9. Moen EL, Godley LA, Zhang W, Dolan ME. Pharmacogenomics of chemotherapeutic susceptibility and toxicity. Genome Med. 2012;4(11):90.
10. Frei E, Canellos GP. Dose: a critical factor in cancer chemotherapy. Am J Med. 1980;69(4):585-94.
11. Skipper HE, Schabel FM Jr, Wilcox WS. Experimental evaluation of potential anticancer agents. XIII. On the criteria and kinetics associated with "curability" of experimental leukemia. Cancer Chemother Rep. 1964;35:1-111.
12. West J, Newton PK. Chemotherapeutic dose scheduling based on tumor growth rates provide a case for low-dose metronomic high entropy therapies. Cancer Res. 2017;77(23):6717.
13. Lloyd HH. Estimation of tumor cell kill from Gompertz growth curves. Cancer Chemother Rep. 1975;59(2 Pt 1):267-77.
14. Kendal WS. Gompertzian growth as a consequence of tumor heterogeneity. Math Biosci. 1985;73(1):103-7.
15. López ÁG, Iarosz KC, Batista AM, Seoane JM, Viana RL, Sanjuán MAF. Nonlinear cancer chemotherapy: modelling the Norton-Simon hypothesis. Commun Nonlinear Sci Numer Simul. 2019;70:307-17.
16. Woodhouse JR, Ferry DR. The Genetic Basis of Resistance to Cancer Chemotherapy. Ann Med. 1995;27(2):157-67.
17. Goldie JH, Coldman AJ. The Genetic Origin of Drug Resistance in Neoplasms: Implications for Systemic Therapy. Cancer Res. 1984;44(9):3643-53.
18. Folkman J. Anti-angiogenesis: new concept for therapy of solid tumors. Ann Surg. 1972;175(3):409-16.
19. Klement G, Baruchel S, Rak J, Man S, Clark K, Hicklin DJ, et al. Continuous low-dose therapy with vinblastine and VEGF receptor-2 antibody induces sustained tumor regression without overt toxicity. J Clin Invest. 2000;105(8):R15-24.

20. Browder T, Butterfield CE, Kräling BM, Shi B, Marshall B, O'Reilly MS, et al. Antiangiogenic Scheduling of Chemotherapy Improves Efficacy against Experimental Drug-resistant Cancer. Cancer Res. 2000;60(7):1878-86.
21. Simsek C, Esin E, Yalcin S. Metronomic Chemotherapy: A Systematic Review of the Literature and Clinical Experience. J Oncol. 2019:e5483791.
22. Dougan M, Dranoff G, Dougan SK. Cancer immunotherapy: beyond checkpoint blockade. Annu Rev Cancer Biol. 2019; 3(1):55-75.
23. Kruger S, Ilmer M, Kobold S, Cadilha BL, Endres S, Ormanns S, et al. Advances in cancer immunotherapy 2019 – latest trends. J Exp Clin Cancer Res. 2019;38(1):268.
24. Granier C, Guillebon ED, Blanc C, Roussel H, Badoual C, Colin E, et al. Mechanisms of action and rationale for the use of checkpoint inhibitors in cancer. ESMO Open. 2017;2(2):e000213.
25. Tarhini A, Lo E, Minor DR. Releasing the Brake on the Immune System: Ipilimumab in Melanoma and Other Tumors. Cancer Biother Radiopharm. 2010;25(6):601-13.
26. Guo L, Zhang H, Chen B. Nivolumab as Programmed Death-1 (PD-1) Inhibitor for Targeted Immunotherapy in Tumor. J Cancer. 2017;8(3):410-6.
27. Kampan NC, Madondo MT, McNally OM, Quinn M, Plebanski M. Paclitaxel and Its Evolving Role in the Management of Ovarian Cancer. Bio Med Res Int. 2015:e413076.
28. Makovec T. Cisplatin and beyond: molecular mechanisms of action and drug resistance development in cancer chemotherapy. Radiol Oncol. 2019;53(2):148-58.
29. Gabizon A, Shmeeda H, Barenholz Y. Pharmacokinetics of Pegylated Liposomal Doxorubicin. Clin Pharmacokinet. 2003;42(5):419-36.
30. Plunkett W, Huang P, Xu YZ, Heinemann V, Grunewald R, Gandhi V. Gemcitabine: metabolism, mechanisms of action, and self-potentiation. Semin Oncol. 1995;22(4 Suppl 11): 3-10.
31. Liu LF, Desai SD, Li TK, Mao Y, Sun M, Sim SP. Mechanism of Action of Camptothecin. Ann N Y Acad Sci. 2000;922(1):1-10.
32. Keating GM. Bevacizumab: a review of its use in advanced cancer. Drugs. 2014;74(16):1891-925.
33. Cancer Treatment Reviews. PARP inhibitors in ovarian cancer. [online]. Available from: https://www.cancertreatmentreviews.com/article/S0305-7372(18)30200-7/fulltext. [Last accessed December, 2021].

LONG QUESTIONS

1. Explain the rational for the use of neoadjuvant chemotherapy in ovarian cancers.
2. Explain the principles of chemotherapy based on the Gompertzian curve and Norton–Simon hypothesis.

SHORT QUESTIONS

1. Write a short note on "synthetic lethality" and PARP inhibitors.
2. Write a short note on Goldie–Coldman hypothesis.
3. Write a short note on mechanism of action of immune checkpoint inhibitors.

MULTIPLE CHOICE QUESTIONS

1. Systemic chemotherapy most commonly used in the initial management of gynecological malignancies is based on:
   a. Metronomic dosing
   b. Maximum tolerated dosing (MTD)
   c. Area under curve in all drugs
   d. None of the above
2. Skipper's laws of chemotherapy are mainly applicable to:
   a. Quiescent cells
   b. Rapidly proliferating cells
   c. Both of the above
   d. None of the above
3. The Gompertzian curve is shaped as:
   a. Parabolic
   b. Straight line
   c. Quadratic
   d. Sigmoid (S shaped)
4. The Gompertzian curve implies the following about growth in a tumor cell population:
   a. The doubling time of tumor volume is constant over the life of the tumor
   b. The growth rate of a tumor cell population is always changing over the life span of a tumor
   c. The log kill of tumor cells would be much lesser in a smaller tumor than a larger tumor
   d. The Gompertzian curve is not relevant to growth of tumor cell populations
5. Implications of the somatic mutation theory include:
   a. Somatic mutations arise spontaneously within a tumor, causing drug resistance
   b. Larger tumors have lesser chances of harboring cells with intrinsic resistance to chemotherapy as compared to smaller tumors.
   c. Combination chemotherapy is preferable to monotherapy to reduce the chances of resistant clones emerging during treatment
   d. Both A and C
6. The most commonly recommended chemotherapeutic regimen in adequately resected stage III epithelial ovarian cancer is:
   a. Single agent pegylated liposomal doxorubicin
   b. Paclitaxel plus carboplatin
   c. Nivolumab
   d. Irinotecan
7. The appropriate chemotherapeutic regimen in high risk GTN is:
   a. Single agent methotrexate
   b. Single agent dactinomycin
   c. Methotrexate plus dactinomycin
   d. EMACO regimen

8. Concurrent chemoradiation with EBRT and cisplatin is not indicated in which of the following patients with cervical cancer?
   a. Stage 1B, but not fit for surgery
   b. Stage IIIA
   c. Stage IIA
   d. Stage IV with metastases to lung
9. Which of the following side-effects in not commonly seen with bevacizumab?
   a. Neutropenia
   b. Hypertension
   c. Proteinuria
   d. Bleeding
10. PARP inhibitors are not currently indicated in the management of which of the following malignancies?
   a. Pancreatic cancer
   b. Cervical cancer
   c. Breast cancer
   d. Ovarian cancer

Answers

1.	b	2.	b	3.	d	4.	b	5.	d	6.	b
7.	d	8.	d	9.	a	10.	b				

14.12 PALLIATIVE CARE IN GYNAECOLOGIC ONCOLOGY

Jayaraman Nambiar M, Thiencherry Rema

INTRODUCTION

World Health Organization (WHO) has defined palliative care as an approach that improves the physical, psychosocial, and spiritual wellbeing of patients and their family through early assessment and treatment of pain and other problems.[1] Palliative care is an integral part of cancer care, just like medical and surgical treatments. Palliative care must be incorporated early in the course of the treatment. The aim of palliative care is neither hastening nor delaying death but giving good palliation of symptoms. American Society of Clinical Oncology (ASCO) recommends that "patients with advanced cancer, whether inpatient or outpatient, should receive dedicated palliative care services, early in the disease course, concurrent with active treatment. Referring patients to interdisciplinary palliative care teams is optimal, and services may complement existing programs. Providers may refer caregivers of patients with early or advanced cancer to palliative care services."[2] Palliative care provides support to the patient and their families. It reduces the cost of treatment.[3] Palliative care mainly involves compassion and does not include costly equipment, and therefore, can be offered in low resource settings.[3] When giving palliative care, we must ensure we do not cause harm, and consideration must be given to relieving symptoms. All treatment must be directed in conjunction with the patient's wishes. Everyone involved in the care of gynecological malignancies must undergo basic training in palliative care. Gynecologic oncologists can provide palliative care and if needed, seek assistance by specialists in palliative care. An interdisciplinary approach is always preferred for managing patients with advanced cancers for handling various problems associated with terminal cancer.

OBSTACLES IN PALLIATIVE CARE

There are many obstacles to palliative care. Many people are not willing to undergo palliative care early in the course of treatment, as they equate it with death. The public generally is not aware of importance of palliative care. Most physicians are not adequately trained in palliative care. Many doctors consider referring patients to palliative care as a failure of treatment. Drugs like morphine are restricted in many countries.

PRINCIPLES OF PALLIATIVE CARE

When giving palliative care, we must adhere to the following principles:

- Give care with compassion and respect
- Good communication about the treatment options and prognosis
- Alleviate pain and other distressing symptoms
- Take help from other disciplines if needed. Palliative care often requires multidisciplinary actions. Involvement of palliative care physicians and pain management specialists is of paramount importance.
- Respect the patient's decision to refuse treatment
- Explain complications of treatment
- Understand and support the end of life care
- Maintain continuity of care till death

WHEN TO START PALLIATIVE CARE?

Palliative care should be available for patients at the time of diagnosis of cancer. It should be instituted early in the course of the disease. A recent Cochrane review has suggested that the early introduction of palliative care improves survival in cancer patients.[4,5] Many patients die without ever receiving any palliative care.[6] Palliative care may be given in hospitals or as home-based care. Palliative care can be basic or complex. Basic care includes basic management of pain, depression, anxiety, and general discussion about treatment and prognosis. Complex palliative care includes managing refractory pain, complex depression and anxiety, and conflict resolution regarding treatment. National Compressive Cancer Care Network (NCCCN) has defined trigger points for palliative care.[7]

The trigger points for palliative care:
- Uncontrolled symptoms
- Moderate or severe symptoms related to cancer
- Serious comorbid conditions
- Potentially life-limiting disease
- Advanced cancer with poor prognosis
- Request from patient or family caregiver
- Evidence of worsening prognosis as evidenced by malignant effusions, poor performance status, malignant bowel obstruction, CNS metastasis with delirium, etc.

Psychological Support

Palliative care involves counseling and treatment of symptoms that are distressing to the patient. Cancer patients need psychosocial support apart from the treatment of symptoms. Psychological counseling can help a long way in end-stage cancer patients.[8] When the patient's family requests to do "everything possible", a realistic option about disease status and prognosis should be provided. Often aggressive treatments are not beneficial in end-stage disease. We cannot reliably predict the time a patient is going to survive. A study showed that physicians were inaccurate most times regarding the time left till death.[9] Anxiety and depression are common among patients with malignancy. This may necessitate the use of serotonin-norepinephrine reuptake inhibitors (SNRIs). Studies have shown that ketamine infusion could be beneficial for patients with severe depression.[10,11]

Pain

One of the most important symptoms that needs treatment is pain. Pain is experienced by almost 80% of patients during the course of disease.[12] The patient should be given adequate analgesia so to allow her to perform daily activities. Pain may be due to direct involvement of nerves by cancer, related to therapy, or other causes unrelated to cancer. Pain associated with cancer can be nociceptive or neuropathic. Nociceptive pain occurs due to direct invasion by cancer, and neuropathic pain occurs due to alteration in neuronal pathways. Nociceptive pain may be somatic or visceral. Somatic pain is more localized and sharp in quality, whereas visceral pain is poorly localized and ill-defined. Visceral pain occurs due to the involvement of the viscera. Nociceptive pain associated with cancer usually needs opioids for relief.[13]

Initially pain treatment is started with nonsteroidal anti-inflammatory drugs (NSAIDs) followed by milder opioids like codeine and finally more potent opioids like morphine. Continuous round the clock pain relief should be provided. Opioids are used when NSAIDs do not control pain or if the pain is of moderate to severe degree. Side effects such as constipation, vomiting, and dry mouth are not uncommon with the use of morphine. Neuropathic pain tends to be resistant to opioids and may require drugs such as tricyclic antidepressants (TCAs), serotonin-norepinephrine reuptake inhibitors (SNRIs), GABA agonists.[14] Ketamine is another drug that helps manage cancer-related pain.[10,11] When given in subanesthetic doses, it can reduce the need for opioids. There is a risk of addiction with ketamine, and caution must be used with its use. Corticosteroids are also used in the treatment of neuropathic pain. While giving analgesics, the least invasive mode is preferred, i.e., oral or sublingual is preferred over the parenteral route. Opioids, when given for a long time, can cause addiction, and this should be born in mind.

Bony metastasis may be treated by local radiotherapy to alleviate pain. It may take about 7–14 days for the pain to subside after radiotherapy. A nerve block helps in reducing pain from local lesions.[15] Brain metastasis may be treated with steroids and brain irradiation. If a brain lesion is amenable to resection, stereotactic resection may be considered. Lumbar epidural can also be considered when all methods fail to provide pain relief.[16] A summary of common drugs used for management of pain is summarized in **Table 1**.

Nonpharmacological Methods for Relief of Pain

Physical methods such as heat, massage, and positioning may also help relieve cancer associated pain.[17]

Anorexia

Loss of appetite and fatigue are expected at the end of life. Eating gives a patient psychological satisfaction, and loss of appetite can be worrying. Steroids given can often increase appetite and instill a sense of wellbeing. The use of cannabinoids may increase appetite.

Other Gastrointestinal Symptoms

Constipation is a common symptom in patients using opioids for pain relief. Constipation may occur due to bowel obstruction or infiltration of nerves in the pelvis. Immobility, dehydration and electrolyte imbalances can also add to constipation. Opioid-induced constipation is also a possibility. Ambulation and correction of dehydration may help remove constipation. Sennoside is the usual drug that is used in the treatment of opioid-related constipation. Osmotic laxatives

TABLE 1: Drugs used in the management of pain.

Drug	*Indication*	*Dose*	*Side effect*
Nonsteroidal anti-inflammatory drugs (NSAIDs)	Mild pain	• Acetaminophen 650 mg every four hourly or 1 g every s6 hourly (maximum 4 g/day) • Ibuprofen 400 mg 4 times a day • Celecoxib 200 mg twice a day • Topical Diclofenac gel	Bleeding in the presence of a gastric ulcer, caution in elderly patients with compromised renal function
Opioids	Moderate-to-severe pain	• The noninvasive route is preferred over the parenteral route • Morphine 30 mg orally every 4-hourly • Morphine IV 10 mg every 4-hourly • Codeine 200 mg orally 4-hourly	Constipation, delirium, respiratory depression, motor and cognitive impairment
Tricyclic antidepressants	Neuropathic pain	Nortriptyline 10–25 mg at night increase the dose to 50–100 mg if needed	• Drowsiness • Blurred vision • Constipation • Dry mouth hypotension
Serotonin norepinephrine reuptake inhibitors	Neuropathic pain	Duloxetine 10–20 mg per day	• Dry mouth • Dizziness • Headache • Excessive sweating
Anticonvulsants	Neuropathic pain	Gabapentin 100–300 mg at night	Drowsiness, dizziness, tiredness, loss of coordination
Corticosteroids	Neuropathic pain	Methylprednisolone 16–32 mg orally	Side effect related to steroids osteopenia, impaired glucose tolerance

also may be used. However, it is essential to rule out bowel obstruction before the administration of laxatives.

Vomiting may be due to mechanical obstruction, renal failure or cerebral metastasis. Nausea and vomiting can also occur as a result of chemotherapy or opioids used for pain. Nausea and vomiting are commonly treated with serotonin antagonists. Dopamine antagonists may be added if serotonin antagonists do not work. Severe, intractable vomiting may necessitate the use of steroids and benzodiazepines. Olanzapine may be of benefit in severe, uncontrollable vomiting. Apart from this, it also improves anxiety associated with malignancy. Opioid-induced vomiting may need drug-like haloperidol.

Breathlessness

Many cases of end-stage malignant diseases have dyspnea either due to pleural effusion or metastasis in the lungs. A trial of oxygen therapy and drainage of pleural fluid may give symptomatic relief. Cognitive behavioral therapy and breathing exercises may be helpful in subjective improvement of the symptom of dyspnea. Passing air using a fan over the face may be beneficial in relieving dyspnea.[17] Opioids and benzodiazepines can be used in symptomatic relief of dyspnea.

Malignant Bowel Obstruction

Malignant bowel obstruction is usually a terminal event in patients with ovarian cancer and generally not amenable to definitive treatment. The diagnostic criteria of malignant bowel obstruction are: (1) clinical evidence of bowel obstruction, (2) obstruction distal to the Treitz ligament, (3) the presence of intra-abdominal or extra-abdominal cancer with peritoneal involvement. The idea of not eating anything is not well accepted by patients. Median survival is only months to 1 year after malignant obstruction happens in terminal ovarian cancer. In the presence of ascites, carcinomatosis, palpable intra-abdominal mass, multiple bowel obstructions, prior radiation, advanced disease, or poor overall status, surgical treatment to relieve obstruction should not be undertaken. If the expected life span is good, surgery to relieve obstruction may be undertaken after a detailed CT evaluation in carefully selected patients.

The obstruction in ovarian cancer is often at multiple sites and is not amenable to definitive surgical correction. Pharmacological treatment depends on whether maintaining bowel function is essential and feasible. If bowel function can be supported, then opioids, antiemetics and anticholinergics are given. If bowel function cannot be maintained, then somatostatin analogs such as octreotide and anticholinergics are used. Dexamethasone and octreotide, which decreases bowel secretions, may be tried.[18] Total parental nutrition is rarely indicated in a patient whose bowel obstruction is amenable to surgical resection.[19] In general, patients with advanced malignancies do not do well when malignant obstruction. Venting procedures such as gastrostomy or placement of an endoscopic stent are an option in some patients. A colostomy may be done in cases of pelvic disease. Malignant obstruction may also occur due to peristaltic failure. This can be treated with metoclopramide if there is no evidence of mechanical obstruction.

Fistulae

Bowel or urinary fistulas which occur in terminal malignancies are not amenable to surgical treatment. A fistula may be due to recurrent disease or late toxicity of radiotherapy. Fistula can be very distressing to the patient. They are usually treated with skincare and local hygienic measures. Urinary tract catheterization may be helpful. Sometimes even per cutaneous nephrostomy may be done. For rectal fistulas, a diverting colostomy is an option.

Ascites

Malignant ascites often appears in late stage of disease in endometrial and ovarian cancers and can cause pain and discomfort. It may be due to secondary deposits on peritoneal surfaces or due to lymphatic obstruction. It can lead to shortness of breath and considerable discomfort. Intravenous chemotherapy remains first line therapy for reducing abdominal disease burden and thereby ascites. There are no accepted protocols for the treatment of malignant ascites in presence of a chemoresistant disease. It can be treated by serial paracentesis. Repeated paracentesis carries a risk of infection and even visceral perforation. Bevacizumab has shown to decrease ascites in some patients.[20] There is no place for diuretics in the management of ascites.

Limb Edema

Limb edema could be due to low albumin or lymphatic obstruction. Massage and elevation of limbs may help in relieving it. The use of stockings, physiotherapy can also help to reduce limb edema.

Bleeding

Bleeding may be a terminal event in patients with advanced malignancies such as cervical, vaginal or vulval cancer. Bleeding is usually due to the invasion of the tumor to the surrounding structures, including blood vessels. Bleeding may also be due to chemotherapy induced thrombocytopenia. Excessive bleeding can be the cause of death in patients with terminal cancer. It may be treated with palliative blood transfusion. Vaginal packing may be useful. Topical application of adrenaline or uterine artery embolization can be used to control bleeding. A heavy dose of radiation (hemostatic radiotherapy) can also be given to control bleeding in cases of advanced pelvic cancers.

Ureteric Obstruction

Ureteric obstruction may be seen in patients with advanced gynecological cancer. It occurs due to the invasion of ureters or bladder trigone by the tumor. Treatment mainly aimed at relieving the obstruction by retrograde stenting. If retrograde stenting is not possible per cutaneous nephrostomy may be an option. Performance status of patient, tumor histology and disease extent should be evaluated properly prior to planning intervention.

Deep Vein Thrombosis

Patients with terminal malignancies are prone to develop deep vein thrombosis (DVT). Active or passive leg movements and anticoagulation should be considered to prevent deep vein thrombosis. Anticoagulation should be considered based on patient's prognosis, quality of life and balanced against the risk of bleeding. Thromboprophylaxis is indicated if there is a high risk of thrombosis such as acute illness with previous history of venous thromboembolism, hypercoagulable state, stroke, acute MI, acute respiratory failure, or acute cardiac failure.[21] Low molecular weight heparin like enoxaparin 40 mg SC once daily is the preferred method of thromboprophylaxis in patients with normal renal function. The presence of bleeding or platelet count less than 50,000 is a contraindication for thromboprophylaxis.

CONCLUSION

- Palliative care should be instituted early in the course of disease.
- The patient and the family should be involved in palliative care.
- Palliative care is mainly about treating distressing symptoms.
- Pain usually treated with NSAIDs followed by opioids.
- Other distressing symptoms that need attention include bleeding, dyspnea, refractory ascites, and bowel obstruction.
- A realistic approach should be used, and care should be tailored depending on the situation.

REFERENCES

1. World Health Organization. Definition of Palliative Care. Available from: http://www.who.int/cancer/palliative/definition/en. [Last accessed November, 2021].
2. Ferrell BR, Temel JS, Temin S, Alesi ER, Balboni TA, Basch EM, et al. Integration of palliative care into standard oncology care: ASCO clinical practice guideline update summary. J Oncol Pract. 2017;13(2):119-21.
3. Merriman A. Compassion: the basis of our care. Plenary Session: Hospice Palliative Care Association of South Africa Conference. 2014.
4. Haun MW, Estel S, Rücker G, Friederich HC, Villalobos M, Thomas M, et al. Early palliative care for adults with advanced Cancer. Cochrane Database Syst Rev. 2017;6:CD011129.
5. Wright AA, Zhang B, Ray A, Mack JW, Trice E, Balboni T, et al. Associations between end-of-life discussions, patient mental health, medical care near death, and caregiver bereavement adjustment. JAMA. 2008;300:1665-73.

6. Taylor JS, Brown AJ, Prescott LS, Sun CC, Ramondetta LM, Bodurka DC. Dying well: how equal is end of life care among gynecologic oncology patients? Gynecol Oncol. 2016;140:295-300.
7. Case AA, Dalal S, Edwards H, Thomas Fitch PR, Kapo J, Kutner JS, et al. NCCN Guidelines Version 2. Fort Washington, PA: National Comprehensive Cancer Network; 2017.
8. Irwin SA, Ferris FD. The opportunity for psychiatry in palliative care. Can J Psychiatry. 2008;53:713-24.
9. Cheon S, Agarwal A, Popovic M. The accuracy of clinicians' predictions of survival in advanced Cancer: a review. Ann Palliat Med. 2016;5:22-9.
10. Serafini G, Howland RH, Rovedi F, Girardi P, Amore M. The role of Ketamine in treatment-resistant depression: a systematic review. Curr Neuropharmacol. 2014;12(5):444-61.
11. Caddy C, Amit BH, McCloud TL. Ketamine and other glutamate receptor modulators for depression in adults. In: Cipriani A (Ed). Cochrane Database of Systematic Reviews. Chichester, UK: John Wiley and Sons Ltd.; 2015. pp. CD011612.
12. Vainio A, Auvinen A. Prevalence of symptoms among patients with advanced cancer: an international collaborative study. Symptom Prevalence Group. J Pain Symptom Manage. 1996; 12:3-10.
13. Wiffen PJ, Wee B, Derry S. Opioids for cancer pain – an overview of Cochrane reviews. In: Wiffen PJ (Ed). Cochrane Database of Systematic Reviews. Chichester, UK: John Wiley and Sons, Ltd.; 2017. pp. CD012592.
14. Lohman D, Schleifer R, Amon JJ. Access to pain treatment as a human right. BMC Med. 2010;8:8.
15. Plancarte R, de Leon-Casasola OA, El-Helaly M. Neurolytic superior hypogastric plexus block for chronic pelvic pain associated with Cancer. Reg Anesth. 1997;22:562-8.
16. Platt M. Pain Challenges at the End of Life - Pain and Palliative Care Collaboration. Rev Pain. 2010;4(2):18-23.
17. Bausewein C, Booth S, Gysels M, Higginson IJ. Non-pharmacological interventions for breathlessness in advanced stages of malignant and nonmalignant diseases. In: Bausewein C (Ed). Cochrane Database of Systematic Reviews. Chichester, UK: John Wiley and Sons, Ltd.; 2008.
18. Feuer DJ, Broadley KE. Corticosteroids for the resolution of malignant bowel obstruction in advanced gynaecological and gastrointestinal Cancer. In: Feuer DJ (Ed). Cochrane Database of Systematic Reviews. Chichester, UK: John Wiley and Sons Ltd.; 2000.
19. Brard L, Weitzen S, Strubel-Lagan SL. The effect of total parenteral nutrition on the survival of terminally ill ovarian cancer patients. Gynecol Oncol. 2006;103:176-80.
20. Zhao H, Li X, Chen D. Intraperitoneal administration of cisplatin plus bevacizumab for the management of malignant ascites in ovarian epithelial cancer: results of a phase III clinical trial. Med Oncol. 2015;32:37.
21. Palliativedrugs.com. Recommendations for Primary Thromboprophylaxis In Palliative Care. [online] Available from: https://www.palliativedrugs.com/download/081126_Network_Primary_Thromboprophylaxis_Guidance%20_Version%202c.pdf. [Last accessed November, 2021].

LONG QUESTIONS

1. A 65-year-old woman has recurrence following ovarian cancer treatment. She has undergone surgery and chemotherapy. Now she presents with features of widespread metastasis in abdomen and intestinal obstruction. How will manage the case?
2. Mention the pathways of pain management in advanced gynecological malignancy.

SHORT QUESTIONS

Write short notes on:

1. Principles of palliative care in gynecological oncology.
2. Management of bleeding in terminal cases of carcinoma cervix.

MULTIPLE CHOICE QUESTIONS

1. Palliative care should be instituted:
   a. Early in the course of disease
   b. Late in the disease
   c. Only if there is pain
   d. When life expectancy is poor
2. Palliative care in oncology ideally should be given by:
   a. Gynecologist b. Oncologist
   c. Anesthetist d. Multidisciplinary team
3. Palliative care is associated with:
   a. Poor survival b. Better survival
   c. Early Death d. More pain
4. First drug that is to be used in cancer related pain is:
   a. NSAIDs b. Morphine
   c. Ketamine d. Diazepam
5. Which of the following statement about malignant bowel obstruction is *true*?
   a. Always is treatable
   b. TPN should always be given
   c. Associated with poor prognosis
   d. Is commonly associated with cervical cancer
6. Ascites associated with terminal malignancy is best treated with:
   a. Serial paracentesis b. Diuretics
   c. Oxygen d. Morphine

Answers

1. a 2. d 3. b 4. a 5. c 6. a

14.13 SCREENING FOR OVARIAN CANCER CURRENT PERSPECTIVE

Usha B Saraiya, Nidhi Shah Gandhi

INTRODUCTION

Ovarian cancer is the 5th leading cause of cancer related deaths among women in developed countries.[1] The global projections of ovarian cancer incidence and mortality for 2020 was 313,959 and 207,252, respectively. In USA, the reported number of new cases per year is 26,630 and 16,451 deaths. In India, with its large population the reported number per year is 45,701 with a mortality of 32,077. Hence, we can conclude that mortality is uniformly high all over. The life time risk of ovarian cancer is 1–2% in the low risk group and about 10–40% in the high risk group.[2]

Ovaries are deep seated organs and the symptoms are noted in late stages of the disease. Hence, diagnosis of ovarian cancer is often delayed, more than 70% patients present with advanced disease and have poor prognosis. With liberal availability of sonography and tumor markers such as CA-125, an attempt at early detection by screening has been made.

Since treatment with a combination of surgery and chemotherapy in early stages gives good survival rates, it has become imperative to make an early diagnosis. 5-year survival rate in stage 1 disease is as high as 90%.[3] This has prompted an interest in ovarian cancer screening to detect disease in early stage. Unfortunately, there is no well-defined precancerous lesion as is the case in cervical or endometrial cancers. Research is going on to unravel the mystery of this disease.

It is also encouraging to know that many screening tests are currently available. Important ones are enumerated in **Box 1**.

ULTRASOUND

This test has revolutionized the detection and evaluation of adnexal masses. It is easily available and affordable. It is important to know whether the tumor is cystic or solid or both, whether it is bilateral and whether extraovarian disease is present in the abdomen. Intra-abdominal spread can also be evaluated. Ascites, if present is an ominous sign.[4]

BOX 1: Screening tests available in current picture.

- Ultrasonography of pelvis
- Tumor markers
  - CA-125
  - Human epididymis protein 4 (HE4)
  - Multiplex immunoassay
  - Multivariate index assay (OVA1)
- Multimodal screening
  - Risk of malignancy index (RMI)
  - Risk of malignancy algorithm (ROMA)
  - Risk of ovarian cancer algorithm (ROCA)

There are many benign asymptomatic lesions which are detected on sonography. It is difficult to make a diagnosis of malignancy only on morphological characteristics. The addition of color Doppler to detect increased vascularity may aid in differentiating between benign and malignant masses.[5] If sonography is used along with estimation of a tumor marker, the diagnostic accuracy is further increased. At times ovaries are not visible. Shrinkage due to age, obesity and a previous pelvic surgery can also affect the findings.[6] Transvaginal scan gives a much better resolution and more reliable information and hence should be recommended. Women may find transvaginal scan painful, but are ready to accept it when the advantages are explained. The experience and knowledge of the sonologist will make a difference as it is a subjective assessment.

International Ovarian Tumor Analysis: ADNEX Model

The International Ovarian Tumor Analysis (IOTA) group has introduced the Assessment of Different Neoplasias in the adnexa (ADNEX) model in 2014. IOTA - ADNEX model is based on data was collected from 24 centers and 10 countries and included 6,000 women. This model is very useful to distinguish between benign and malignant adnexal masses.

The ADNEX model uses nine predictors (three clinical predictors and six ultrasound predictors):

1. Patients age (years)
2. Serum CA-125
3. Type of center (oncology referral center versus other)
4. Maximal diameter of lesion (in mm)
5. Maximum diameter of the largest solid tissue (in mm)
6. Presence of more than 10 cyst locules (yes/no)
7. Number of papillary projections (0, 1, 2, 3, >3)
8. Presence of acoustic shadows (yes/no)
9. Presence of ascites (yes/no)

This model aids in categorizing an adnexal tumor as benign, borderline, stage I cancer, stage II–IV cancer, or secondary metastatic cancer, thereby helping the clinician in making decisions on management.

Other imaging techniques are also of great value if cancer is suspected: A contrast enhanced computed tomography (CT) scan is very important to assess metastatic disease. A magnetic resonance imaging (MRI) pelvis helps in characterization of the adnexal mass and will indicate local spread into adjacent organs and help detect adhesions. It will also estimate the volume of the disease. Positron emission tomography (PET) scan will indicate distant metastasis. Thus, a thorough assessment of extent of disease is possible prior to planning treatment.

TUMOR MARKERS

They are recent introduction in our armamentarium.

- *Cancer antigen-125 (CA-125):* Of all the tumor markers available, CA-125 is most widely used and may be elevated in epithelial ovarian cancers. Cancer antigen-125 is a protein derived from cancerous epithelial cells which is secreted in the blood. It is also known as MUCIN 16. It is made up of 22,000 amino acids. It was discovered by Robert Bast, Knapp and their team in the year 1981,[7] and has received FDA approval as a diagnostic test. The normal value is 0–35 units/mL. It can be used for screening asymptomatic women in the high risk group. It is useful to monitor the treatment response and is also used in the follow up of treated cases. It also has a prognostic value. However, it is not specific to ovarian cancer and may be raised in other cancers and benign conditions like endometriosis, tuberculosis and some inflammatory conditions.

  Serum CA-125 levels may be elevated many years before the diagnosis of ovarian cancer. The trend of CA-125 is more important for screening purposes. Hence if a repeat test indicates a rise in the level, it may be significant and warrants a further evaluation by a pelvic ultrasound.[8]

  A multimodal approach for screening that involves sequential measurements of CA-125 level as a first line test and an ultrasound as a second line test, if there is a rising trend in CA-125 level. This approach has shown to improve sensitivity and specificity.[9]
- *Human epididymis protein 4 (HE4):* It is a new marker which has received US Food and Drug Administration (FDA) approval in 2008 for its use in the diagnosis of recurrent and progressive ovarian cancer and monitoring.[10] It is used in the evaluation of an adnexal mass. It rises as a result of an over expression of *W7DC2* gene in patients with serous and endometrioid ovarian carcinoma. A value of ≤150 picomol/L (pM) is the upper 95th percentile for both pre- and postmenopausal women. Range is different for premenopausal and postmenopausal women.

  Risk of malignancy index (RMI) is a multimodality approach. It includes serum CA-125 level, pelvic ultrasound and menopausal status. For RMI 1, score ≥ 200 is considered significant and referral to an oncologist is recommended.

  Risk of ovarian malignancy algorithm (ROMA) is another multimodal evaluation. It got US-FDA approval in 2011. It includes serum CA-125, HE4 and menopausal status.

  Risk of ovarian cancer algorithm (ROCA) includes the age of the woman and serial CA-125 levels and there by gives us a risk estimation of the patient and classifies them into three categories: (1) elevated, (2) intermediate and (3) normal based on statistically derived change point.[11]

  All these algorithms are calculated by a statistical software program.

ADVANTAGES AND DRAWBACKS OF OVARIAN CANCER SCREENING

Screening can detect cases early and in curable stage of the disease. They do solve some clinical dilemmas and reduce mortality as a result of early diagnosis. On the other hand, there are many disadvantages of routine screening. Screening tests may be falsely positive and patients suffer physical, psychological, and financial losses. False positive test also results in increased surgical interventions and associated complications. Results from large population based studies have shown that screening for ovarian cancer in general population does not cause reduction in mortality and may lead to unnecessary surgery and anxiety. Therefore, United States Preventive Services Task Forces categorically stated in 2018 that only women with high risk factors need screening.[12]

PROTECTIVE AND HIGH RISK FACTORS FOR OVARIAN CANCER

Protective Factors

- *Oral contraceptive pills:* A significant factor which lowers the risk of ovarian cancer is the long-term use of oral contraceptives for more than 5 years, shown to be effective in both general population and in *BRCA* gene mutation carriers. Absence of ovulation seems to protect the surface epithelium of the ovary from potential carcinogens.

  The risk is 50% lower for women who have history of OCP use as compared to never users. However, breast cancer risk may be increased marginally and regular monitoring is recommended. Protection is for epithelial ovarian cancer and not for germ cell and stromal tumors.[12]
- *Lactation* lowers the risk.
- *Multiparity* also reduces the risk of developing ovarian cancer.
- Maintaining a normal body weight and physical activity are also considered protective.

High-risk Factors

- *Age:* The risk of developing ovarian cancer increases with increasing age. The lifetime risk of developing ovarian cancer is about 1% for general population. Although it can occur at any age, peri- and postmenopausal women are at a higher risk of development of epithelial ovarian malignancy. In fact, menopausal status is taken into account for multimodal screening.
- *Race:* Caucasians have the highest risk, followed by Hispanics and Africans. Asians reportedly have the lowest risk.[12]
- *Use of talcum powder:* Application of talcum powder on vulva and perineum has been associated with an increase in ovarian cancer.[13]

- *Use of hormones:* Women who have been on hormone replacement therapy are likely to be at increased risk of ovarian cancer. A study of Danish women aged 50–79 years observed over a period of 10 years showed a slightly increased risk of ovarian cancer, irrespective of the formulation of estrogen, progesterone or the combination. Hormone replacement therapy (HRT) users should be monitored carefully.[14]

  A study by Jacob and Menon et al. indicated that HRT with estrogen only as well as combined estrogen and progesterone increases the risk of ovarian cancer. This risk remains even 10 years after stopping the therapy.[15]
- *Genetic predisposition:* Currently this has received a lot of interest. Every woman should be asked if there is a family history of breast and/or ovarian cancer and to elicit this history in the last three generations. A first degree relative, i.e., mother or sister or daughter having these cancers is very significant.

There are many genes which are involved in ovarian carcinogenesis. The most important are *BRCA1* and *BRCA2*, and mismatch repair genes (MMR) - *MLH1, MSH2, MSH6* and *PMS2*.[16] Currently, genetic testing is too complicated to be universally available in clinical practice. If it gets simplified and freely available, it would be of great help in the early detection of ovarian cancer. However, it is to be considered in high risk groups, like in women having significant family history of related cancers.

Evidence suggests that:
- Every woman should be asked if there is any family history of cancer on maternal and paternal side. History of any cancer breast, ovarian and colon cancer has to be elicited in the last three generations.
- The life time risk of developing ovarian cancer in women with *BRCA1* gene mutation is 40% while those with *BRCA2* gene mutation is 20%.
- Women with Lynch syndrome especially those with *MSH2* gene have a life time risk of 10–15% for ovarian cancer and 40–60% risk for endometrial cancer.[16]

Therefore, in these women a more aggressive preventive strategy may be considered. This was possible only by introduction of risk reducing salpingo-oophorectomy (RRSO). Prophylactic risk reducing surgery (RRSO) has shown to significantly reduce lifetime risk of developing ovarian cancer in susceptible women with pathogenic germ-line mutations. In BRCA mutated women, the risk of developing ovarian cancer reduces to less than 5% after RRSO.[17]

Therefore, the National Comprehensive Cancer Network (NCCN) recommendation is as follows: to perform a RRSO in women with pathogenic BRCA mutation after the completion of child bearing or between the ages of 35 and 40 years. For those not willing/suitable for surgery an alternative is a regular screening at 4–6 monthly interval with serum CA-125 and a transvaginal scan is recommended.[9]

ROLE OF FIMBRIAL END OF THE FALLOPIAN TUBE IN THE DEVELOPMENT OF OVARIAN CANCER (A HYPOTHESIS)

The histopathological examination of the ovary and the fallopian tube, in *BRCA* gene mutants who had undergone prophylactic salpingo-oophorectomy, revealed an interesting finding **(Figs. 1 to 3)**. The fimbrial end of fallopian tube showed precursor lesion called serous tubal intra-epithelial cancer (STIC).[2,17] However, no such lesion was found in the ovary. Further, these STIC lesions had the same *p53* gene mutation that was found in high grade ovarian cancer. This led to the hypothesis that ovarian cancer could be originating

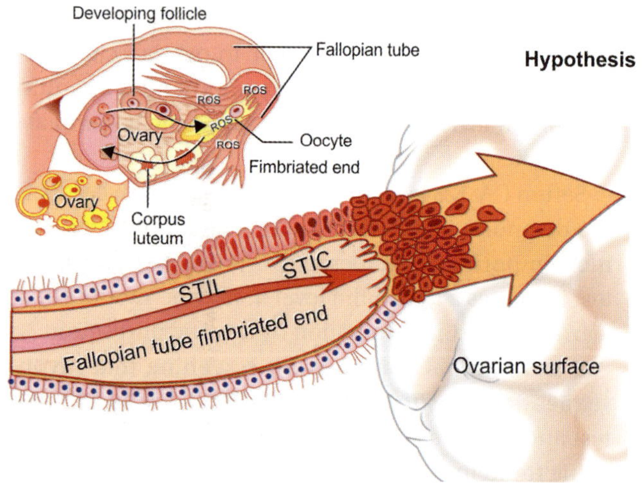

Fig. 1: Proposed development of ovarian HGSC by direct shedding and implantation of STIC cells from the fimbria onto the ovarian surface. [CIN: cervical intraepithelial neoplasia; ROS: reactive oxygen species (free radicals; HSGC: high-grade serous ovarian carcinoma; STIC: serous tubal intra-epithelial cancer; STIL: serous tubal intraepithelial lesions)]
Source: Vang R, Kurman RJ, Visvanathan K, Shaw P, Soslow R, Parkash V, et al. Ovarian Cancer Prevention, Detection and Treatment. Johns Hopkins Medicines; 2011.

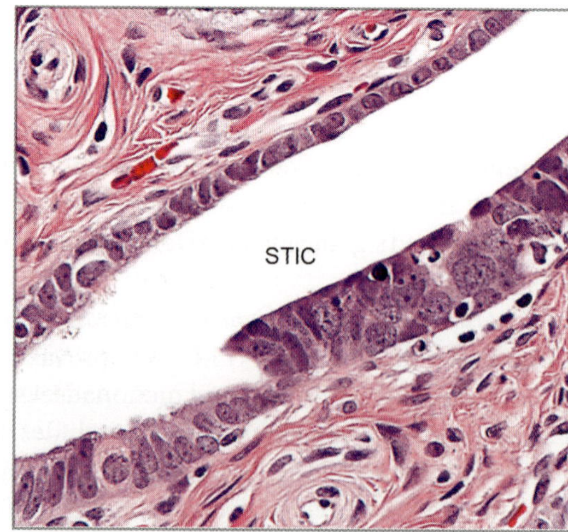

Fig. 2: Serous tubal intraepithelial carcinoma.
Source: Vang R, Kurman RJ, Visvanathan K, Shaw P, Soslow R, Parkash V, et al. Ovarian Cancer Prevention, Detection and Treatment. Johns Hopkins Medicines; 2011.

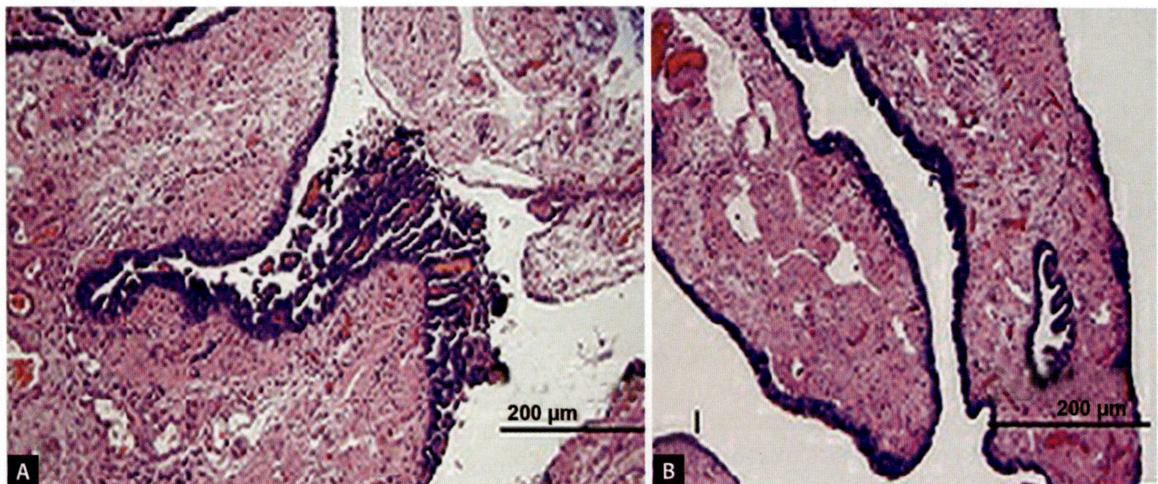

Figs. 3A and B: Serous tubal intraepithelial carcinoma and p53 signature pattern.
Source: Vang R, Kurman RJ, Visvanathan K, Shaw P, Soslow R, Parkash V, et al. Ovarian Cancer Prevention, Detection and Treatment. Johns Hopkins Medicines; 2011.

in the fimbrial end of the fallopian tube and those malignant cells then get implanted on the surface of the ovary by direct spread.[18] It has been reported that 33–59% of high grade serous ovarian and primary peritoneal cancers coexist with STIC lesions.[19]

This information is of great value in women undergoing hysterectomy for benign lesions. It is a standard recommendation that ovaries need to be preserved in women till the age of 65 years as they safeguard against cardiovascular and bone diseases. However, to reduce the risk of developing ovarian cancer, risk reducing surgery in the form of either fimbriectomy or total salpingectomy, should be done. Care should be taken to preserve the vascularity of retained ovaries.

Current research indicates that although the final diagnosis may be primary invasive epithelial ovarian cancer (ICD-10), it is a part of a group of malignancies which include fallopian tube cancer (ICD-10 C 57.0) and primary peritoneal cancer (ICD-10 C 48). These cancers are Müllerian in origin and are staged and treated along similar lines, as their pathogenesis is similar and may perhaps be a single entity.

Many genetic alterations have been found in epithelial ovarian cancers and based on these, tumors are divided in to type I and type II. Type 1 or low grade ovarian cancers show alterations of K-ras/B-raf pathway and generally have a better prognosis. However, Type II or high grade cancers show p53 mutations and have a poor prognosis. Therefore, further molecular profiling and immunohistochemistry would be of considerable value in planning the suitable treatment.

REVIEW OF LITERATURE

- US Preventive Services Task Force published in July 2017, an update evidence review on screening for ovarian cancer. The objective was to update previous systematic review and suggest screening guidance. Four RCTs (n = 293,587) were included. Two trials were conducted in USA and two in UK, in postmenopausal women with average risk. The analysis concluded that ovarian cancer mortality did not differ between control and screening groups.
- United Kingdom Collaboration Trial of Ovarian Cancer Screening (UKCTOCS): One of the largest studies reported is from UK consisting of 202,638 cases observed over 11½ years. The pilot study was reported in 1999 and the complete study in 2016.

  The study comprised of random allocation of cases from general population into a control arm and an intervention (screening) arm. The intervention group was further divided into two groups: (1) one multimodal screening group (transvaginal ultrasonography following an annual CA-125 screening) and (2) the other TVS alone group. Screen abnormalities were retested and women with persistent abnormality were clinically evaluated and underwent surgical intervention when indicated. Complications of surgery occurred in 15% of the cases. Initial analysis showed no reduction in ovarian cancer mortality in intervention group. However, once the prevalent cases were excluded there was a 20% reduction in mortality in the multimodal screening (MMS) group.[15]

  Flowchart 1 explains the number of women included in the study, number of cancers detected, and number of women died in each group.

  Some degree of psychological trauma was also noted in the subjects undergoing investigation especially those post-menopausal women between 50 and 74 years with no known risk of ovarian cancer. Hence the UKCTOCS suggested that screening may be restricted to women with high risk which includes women with family history or confirmed mutations.
- United Kingdom Familial Ovarian Cancer Study (UKFOCSS) was carried out in women with estimated

Flowchart 1: The United Kingdom Collaborative Trial of Ovarian Cancer Screening (UKCTOCS).

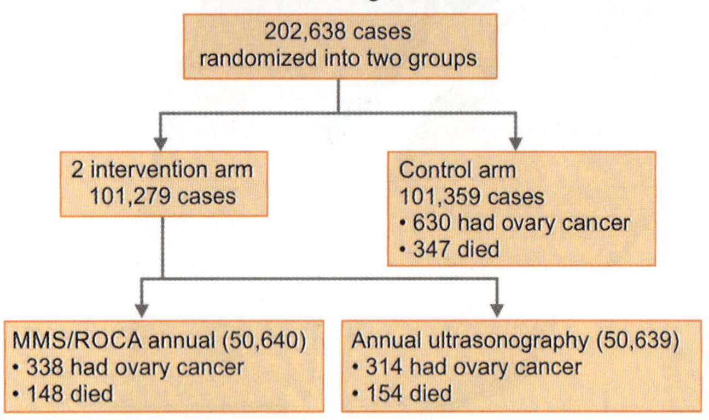

(MMS: multimodal screening; ROCA: risk of ovarian cancer algorithm)

lifetime risk of developing ovarian/fallopian tube cancer of ≥10%. This trial was carried out in two phases. It comprised of 3,563 high risk women with mutation in high penetrance genes such as *BRCA1 and 2*. The conclusion after phase 2 was that ROCA based screening could be an option for high risk women who declined risk reducing surgery. The authors reported that there was evidence of stage shift in phase 2 thereby reducing mortality. However, further studies are needed.[20]

- American College of Obstetricians and Gynecologists (ACOG) and American Cancer Society (ACS) recommend screening of high risk women with a physical gynecological examination, transvaginal sonography and a CA-125 test.[12] Frequency can be determined by the attending clinicians.
- Memorial Sloan Kettering Cancer Center (MSK, New York) has given clear guidelines for screening women with germline genetic mutations. For women at high risk other than genetic mutation it is advised that a thorough counseling be done, followed by screening undertaken within the framework of research studies.
- National Comprehensive Cancer Network (NCCN) has also given similar guidelines including RRSO or RR salpingectomy for women with *BRCA1 and BRCA2* mutation. Women with specific *MMR* gene mutations (Lynch syndrome) require hysterectomy along with salpingo-oophorectomy as risk reducing surgery. They further state that screening cannot be a recommendation in this group and risk reducing surgery remains definitive preventive strategy.

ROLE OF CANCER DETECTION CLINICS

In general, there is a demand for cancer detection package for women after all the awareness has been created. The demand is for safe, affordable, reliable, and comprehensive screening for common cancers. The current recommendations are for cervical and breast cancer screening.

- *Cervical cancer:* Pap smear, HPV test, and visual inspection of cervix with acetic acid are standard detection tests in use. Screening should start at the age of 25–30 years and should continue till the age of 65 years. Acceptable frequency of screening is every 3–5 years. Cotesting may be considered.
- *Endometrial cancer:* Routine screening in low risk women (general population) is not recommended. Pelvic sonography (transvaginal) and endometrial aspiration cytology if the endometrial thickness is out of range for age in symptomatic women can be considered.
- *Ovarian cancer:* As discussed earlier, screening with sonography and CA-125 is considered in high risk women. Universal screening of general population is not recommended.
- *Breast cancer:* Clinical breast examination is suggested and mammography to be considered if required. Self-breast examination is to be taught to women. Screening is advocated after 45 years of age along with creating awareness, about regular check-ups.

An integral part of cancer detection clinics is counseling, advise about healthy lifestyle, follow-up and data analysis. If such a facility is made widely available at all medical colleges and hospitals, both in private and public sectors, there is hope for reduction in incidence and mortality of gynecological and breast cancers.

ON-GOING RESEARCH, FUTURE TRENDS, AND CONCLUSION

Ovarian cancer screening has come a long way in the first two decades of the 21st century. Currently CA-125 and HE4 protein are approved tumor markers for ovarian cancer screening. Research is going on for better screening tests which will be more valuable in clinical practice. What is in the realm of research today will come into clinical practice tomorrow.

There are many other serum markers and other screening approaches under research. Angiogenesis or neovascularization occurs early in the development of a cancer. Real time imaging with contrast showing micro bubbles which are small enough to go through the capillaries has been found to be useful. It is the microvascular pattern rather than macrovascular pattern which is important. The kinetics of blood flow has to be measured.

Angiogenesis occurs due to the release of a chemical called angiogenic factor which helps in the development of new capillaries. It was first described by Judah Folkman in 1971.[21] Subsequent research done by Folkman and Cao helped develop an angiogenesis blocking factor called angiostatin and endostatin in 1998. This opened up a new chapter in the therapy of cancer with possibility of reversal of progression of a malignant tumor. Angiostatin is now commercially available.[22] It has been recommended for delaying progression in cases of metastatic breast, colon and ovarian cancers. Therefore, early detection of neovascularization would help in early detection and therapy and thus reduce the mortality. *At present, it does not have a role in screening.*

The closest we have come to detection of a precancerous phase in ovarian cancer is the identification of STIC. Future developments may show that imaging or cytology of the peritoneal or fallopian tube wash, to predict ovarian cancer in early stages and assist us in making an early diagnosis.

The Report of the 11th Biennial Ovarian Cancer Research Symposium was published in November 2019. The Researchers from all over the world concluded that although progress is being made in areas of prevention, screening and early detection, these advances have not yet translated into tangible clinical benefits for patients. However, research work presented offers a glimmer of hope for improved outcome for patients in future.[23]

Perhaps a new era for ovarian cancer screening is about to come giving more hope and success in controlling and bringing down mortality from ovarian cancer.

To conclude, preventive gyneco-oncology has a bright future to prevent death and disability caused by cancer. For this to happen everyone has to follow the dictum:

"Be Forewarned
Be Aware and
Take Care"

REFERENCES

1. IARC/WHO. GLOBOCAN 2020: Estimated cancer incidence, mortality and prevalence worldwide in 2020. Ovarian cancer Fact Sheet. [online] Available from: http://gco.iarc.fr/today/data/factsheets/cancers/25-Ovary-factsheet.pdf. [Last accessed December, 2021].
2. Jani P, Iyer R. Screening for Ovarian Cancer. New York: Intech Open; 2017. pp. 215-26.
3. Howlader N, Noone AM, Krapcho M, Miller D, Bishop K, Kosarv CL, et al. SEER Cancer Statistics. Review. 1975-2014.
4. Timmerman D, Valentin L, Bourne TH, Collins WP, Verrelst H, Vergote I. Terms, definitions and measurements to describe the sonographic features of adnexal tumors: A consensus opinion from the International Ovarian Tumor Analysis (IOTA) group. Ultrasound Obstet Gynaecol. 2000;16(5):500-5.
5. Van Calster B, Van Hoorde K, Valentin L, Testa AC, Fischerova D, Van Holsbeke C, et al. Evaluating the risk of ovarian cancer before surgery using the ADNEX model to differentiate between benign, borderline, early and advanced stage invasive, and secondary metastatic tumours: prospective multicentre diagnostic study. BMJ. 2014;349:g5920.
6. Sharma A, Burnell M, Gentry-Maharaj A, Campbell S, Amso NN, Seif MW, et al. Factors affecting visualization of postmenopausal ovaries: Descriptive study from the multicenter United Kingdom Collaborative Trial of Ovarian Cancer Screening (UKCTOCS). Ultrasound Obstet Gynecol. 2013;42(4):472-7.
7. Bast RCJ, Klug TL, John ES, Jenison E, Niloff JM, Lazarus H, et al. A radioimmunoassay using a monoclonal antibody to monitor the course of epithelial ovarian cancer. N Engl J Med. 1983;309(15):883-7.
8. Jacobs I, Davies AP, Bridges J, Stabile I, Fay T, Lower A, et al. Prevalence screening for ovarian cancer in postmenopausal women by CA 125 measurement and ultrasonography. Br Med J. 1993;306(6884):1030-4.
9. Menon U, Griffin M, Gentry-Maharaj A. Ovarian cancer screening—current status, future directions. Gynec Onco. 2014;132:490-5.
10. Moore RG, McMeekin DS, Brown AK, DiSilvestro P, Miller MC, Allard WJ, et al. A novel multiple marker bioassay utilizing HE4 and CA125 for the prediction of ovarian cancer in patients with a pelvic mass. Gynecol Oncol. 2009;112(1):40-6.
11. Skates SJ, Menon U, Macdonald N, Rosenthal AN, Oram DH, Knapp RC, et al. calculation of the risk of ovarian cancer from serial CA-125 values for preclinical detection postmenopausal women. Journal of Clinical Oncology. 2003;21(10 Suppl):206-10.
12. Henderson JT, Webber EM, Sawaya GF. Screening for Ovarian Cancer: An Evidence Review for the US Preventive Services Task Force: Evidence Synthesis No. 157. Rockville, MD: Agency for Healthcare Research and Quality; 2018.
13. Cramer DW, Vitonis AF, Terry KL, Welch WR, Titus LJ. The association between talc use and ovarian cancer. A retrospective case-control study in the two US states. Epidemiology. 2016;27:334-46.
14. Mørch LS, Løkkegaard E, Andreasen AH, Krüger-Kjær S, Lidegaard Ø. Hormone therapy and ovarian cancer. JAMA. 2009;302(3):298-305.
15. Jacobs IJ, Menon U, Ryan A, Gentry-Maharaj A, Burnell M, Kalsi JK, et al. Ovarian cancer screening and mortality in the UK Collaborative Trial of Ovarian Cancer Screening (UKCTOCS): a randomised controlled trial. Lancet. 2016;387(10022):945-56.
16. Bonadona VBB, Olschwang S, Grandjouan S, Huiart L, Longy M, Guimbaud R, et al. Cancer risks associated with germline mutations in mlh1, msh2, and msh6 genes in lynch syndrome. J Am Med Assoc. 2011;305(22):2304-10.
17. Patni R. Screening for ovarian cancer: An update. J Midlife Health. 2019;10:3-5.
18. Gilks CB, Irving J, Kobel M, Lee C, Singh N, Wilkinson N, et al. Incidental nonuterine high-grade serous carcinomas arise in the fallopian tube in most cases: Further evidence for the tubal origin of high-grade serous carcinomas. The American J Surg Pathol. 2015;39(3):357-64.
19. Vang R, Kurman RJ, Visvanathan K, Shaw P, Soslow R, Parkash V, et al. Ovarian Cancer Prevention, Detection and Treatment. John Hopkins Medicines; 2011.
20. Rosenthal AN, Fraser LSM, Philpott S, Manchanda R, Burnell M, Badman P, et al. Evidence of stage shift in women diagnosed with ovarian cancer during phase II of the United Kingdom Familial Ovarian Cancer Screening Study. J Clin Oncol. 2017;35(13):1411-20.
21. Folkman J. Tumour angiogenesis: therapeutic indications. N Engl J Med. 1971;285:1182-6.
22. Saraiya U, Miniello G. Cytology and Colposcopy in Gynaecological Practic. New Delhi: Jaypee Brothers Medical Publishers; 2009. pp. 179-80.
23. Chein J, Poole E. Ovarian Cancer Prevention, Screening abd early Detection: report from the 11th Biennial Ovarian Cancer research Symposium. Int J Gynecol Cancer. 2017;27(9): S20-22.

LONG QUESTIONS

1. What are the features on ultrasound examination suggesting that the ovarian tumor could be malignant?

2. What is the current recommendation for management of a patient with BRCA gene mutation?
3. Role of fimbriectomy in ovarian cancer prevention.
4. Your views on the harms of screening for ovarian cancer.

SHORT QUESTIONS

1. Explain Risk of Malignancy Index (RMI).
2. How does CA-125 estimation help in the management of a case of cancer of the ovary, other than screening.
3. Explain tumor angiogenesis.
4. Briefly describe ovarian cancer screening guidelines by the United States Preventive Services Task Forces (USPSTF).
5. Enumerate risk factors of ovarian cancer.

MULTIPLE CHOICE QUESTIONS

1. Characteristics of ideal screening test are:
   a. It is reasonable and safe
   b. High sensitivity and specificity
   c. Widely available
   d. Demonstrates improved health outcomes
   e. All of the above
2. All of the following are high risk factors for ovarian, cancer, except:
   a. Hormone therapy
   b. LYNCH syndrome
   c. Women with history of good lactation
   d. Liberal use of talcum powder on vulva and perineum
   e. Obesity, infertility and menopause
3. Prophylactic salpingo-oophorectomy is recommended in case of:
   a. BRCA1 and BRCA2 mutation carriers
   b. Polycystic ovarian syndrome
   c. Endometriosis
   d. Multiple fibroids
4. All of the following are characteristic features of ovarian malignancy on ultrasonograpghy, except:
   a. High impedance flow on color Doppler
   b. Irregular walls with/without thick septations
   c. Cystic and solid areas
   d. Papillary excrescences
   e. Ascites
5. The following statements of cancer antigen-125 are true/false:
   a. Also known as Mucin 16, it is made up of 22,000 amino acids (True/False)
   b. Was 1st isolated by Robert Bast, Robert Knapp and his research team in 1981 (True/False)
   c. Originates from the epithelial lining of the pleura, peritoneum, pericardium and mullerian tissues (True/False)
   d. Is raised exclusively in epithelial ovarian malignancy (True/False)
6. Match the following molecular markers for ovarian cancer with the grade of tumor:
   a. Grade I (better prognosis)
   b. Grade II (worse prognosis)
   c. p53 mutations
   d. Alterations in K-ras/B-raf pathways
7. Disadvantages of implementing ovarian cancer screening in asymptomatic women:
   a. Unnecessary surgical interference
   b. Anxiety
   c. Not cost effective
   d. Requires repetitive periodic screening
   e. All of the above

Answers

1. e 2. c 3. a 4. a
5. a True, b True, c True; d False
6. a & d, b & c 7. e

Index

Page numbers followed by *b* refer to box, *f* refer to figure, *fc* refer to flowchart, and *t* refer to table.

B

D

E

F

N

Q

R

V